Mosby's
Dictionary of Medicine, Nursing and Health Professions
UK Edition

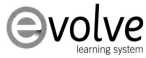
learning system

Evolve Learning Resources for Students and Lecturers:

See the instructions panel on the inside cover for access to the web site.

Think outside the book...evolve

For Elsevier

Commissioning Editor: *Mairi McCubbin*
Development Editor: *Helen Leng*
Project Manager: *Alan Nicholson*
Designer: *Stewart Larking*
Illustration Manager: *Bruce Hogarth*

Mosby's
Dictionary of Medicine, Nursing and Health Professions
UK Edition

Edited by

Chris Brooker BSc MSc RGN SCM RNT

Author and Editor, Norfolk, UK

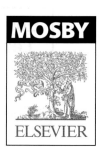

Edinburgh London New York Oxford Philadelphia St Louis Sydney Toronto 2010

MOSBY
ELSEVIER

First published 2010, © Elsevier Limited. All rights reserved.

ISBN 978-0-7234-3504-4

British Library Cataloguing in Publication Data
A catalogue record for this book is available from the British Library

Library of Congress Cataloging in Publication Data
A catalog record for this book is available from the Library of Congress

Notice
Neither the publisher nor the editor assumes any responsibility for any loss or injury and/or damage to persons or property arising out of or related to any use of the material contained in this book. It is the responsibility of the treating practitioner, relying on independent expertise and knowledge of the patient, to determine the best treatment and method of application for the patient.

The Publisher

ELSEVIER your source for books, journals and multimedia in the health sciences
www.elsevierhealth.com

Working together to grow libraries in developing countries
www.elsevier.com | www.bookaid.org | www.sabre.org

ELSEVIER   BOOK AID International   Sabre Foundation

The Publisher's policy is to use paper manufactured from sustainable forests

Printed in China

Contents

Preface

Medicine, nursing and the health professions continue to change at a breathtaking pace and all those concerned need easy access to information from a range of medical specialties, nursing roles and other healthcare disciplines. This first fully UK version of the hugely successful *Mosby's Dictionary of Medicine, Nursing & Health Professions* aims to meet the needs of a broad group of students and practitioners in medicine, nursing and health professions that include midwifery, dentistry, physiotherapy, occupational therapy, speech and language therapy, nutritional science, optometry, radiography, sport and exercise science and medicine, podiatry, etc. It will also be relevant to others working in the medical/health fields, such as medical secretaries and receptionists, and members of the public.

The dictionary has over 20 000 main entries, many of which cover topics in some depth. Many less common conditions are covered, allowing readers to obtain basic information from a single source. The A-Z entries are supported by 200 two-colour illustrations and photographs. A full colour section provides a selection of colour photographs of conditions that includes skin disorders, infectious diseases, eye conditions, etc. and many full-colour line drawings that illustrate anatomical structures, physiological processes and various abnormal conditions. Cross references in the dictionary entry alert readers to a relevant colour illustration.

Many subject areas are included: anatomy, critical care, complementary medicine, cytology, epidemiology, ethics, management, medicine, nursing, nutrition, occupational medicine, oncology, pathology, physiology, podiatry, public health and health promotion, quality issues, research, sports and exercise science and medicine, surgery, etc. The entries reflect the increasingly multiprofessional and interprofessional approaches to healthcare. The pharmacological entries are mainly general and most relate to drug groups rather than specific drug names. However, further drug information is provided in Appendix 5.

The book is supported by a related website on Evolve with a spellchecker, 'Word of the Day', useful websites and the full image bank for the dictionary.

Fourteen appendices provide information about a range of topics.

I hope that the UK version of the dictionary will prove to be a valuable resource for students, registered practitioners and all those with an interest in health and healthcare.

Norfolk, 2010   *Chris Brooker*

Acknowledgements

The editor would like to thank Mairi McCubbin, Helen Leng and Alan Nicholson at Elsevier; Jennifer Creek, who updated the entries for occupational therapy; and the European Network of Occupational Therapy in Higher Education (ENOTHE) Terminology Project, 2008.

The editor would like to thank the authors, editors and contributors of the following works and books, all of which have been used as a source of text or artwork, or photographs for *Mosby's Dictionary of Medicine, Nursing and Health Professions UK Edition*.

Alexander MF, Fawcett JN, Runciman PJ 2006 Nursing Practice Hospital and Home 3rd edn. Churchill Livingstone, Edinburgh.

Bale S, Jones V 1997 Wound Care Nursing A patient-centred approach. Baillière Tindall, London.

Boon NA, Colledge NR, Walker BR 2006 Davidson's Principles & Practice of Medicine 20th edn. Churchill Livingstone, Edinburgh.

Brooker C 1998 Human Structure and Function 2nd edn. Mosby, Edinburgh.

Brooker C 2002 Churchill Livingstone Dictionary of Nursing 18th edn. Churchill Livingstone, Edinburgh.

Brooker C, Nicol M 2003 Nursing Adults The Practice of Caring. Mosby, Edinburgh.

Brooker C 2005 Churchill Livingstone's Mini Encyclopaedia of Nursing. Churchill Livingstone, Edinburgh.

Brooker C 2006A Mosby Nurse's Pocket Dictionary 33rd edn. Mosby, Edinburgh.

Brooker C 2006B Churchill Livingstone Dictionary of Nursing 19th edn. Churchill Livingstone, Edinburgh.

Brooker C, Waugh A 2007 Foundations of Nursing Practice Fundamentals of Holistic Care. Mosby, Edinburgh.

Brooker C 2008 Churchill Livingstone Medical Dictionary 16th edn. Churchill Livingstone, Edinburgh.

Downie G, Mackenzie J, Williams A 2003 Pharmacology and Medicines Management for Nurses 3rd edn. Churchill Livingstone, Edinburgh.

European Network of Occupational Therapy in Higher Education (ENOTHE), Terminology Project. 2008.

Fraser DM, Cooper MA 2003 Myles Textbook for Midwives 14th edn. Churchill Livingstone, Edinburgh.

Gangar E (ed) 2001 Gynaecological Nursing A Practical Guide. Churchill Livingstone, Edinburgh.

Gates B 2002 Learning disabilities Towards inclusion 4th edn. Churchill Livingstone, Edinburgh.

Graham DT 1996 Principles of Radiological Physics 3rd edn. Churchill Livingstone, Edinburgh.

Greenstein C, Gould D 2004 Trounce's Clinical Pharmacology for Nurses 17th edn. Churchill Livingstone, Edinburgh.

Gunn C 2008 Churchill Livingstone Pocket Radiology and Medical Imaging Dictionary. Churchill Livingstone, Edinburgh.

Hagedorn R 2000 Tools for Practice in Occupational Therapy A Structured Approach to Core Skills and Processes. Churchill Livingstone, Edinburgh.

Heasman P, McCracken G 2007 Harty's Dental Dictionary 3rd edn. Churchill Livingstone, Edinburgh.

Hinchliffe SM, Montague SE, Watson R 1996 Physiology for Nursing Practice 2nd edn. Bailliere Tindall, London.

Huband S, Trigg E (eds) 2000 Practices in Children's Nursing Guidelines for Hospital and Community. Churchill Livingstone, Edinburgh.

Jamieson E, McCall J, Whyte L 2002 Clinical Nursing Practices 4th edn. Churchill Livingstone, Edinburgh.

Jennett S 2008 Churchill Livingstone Dictionary of Sport and Exercise Science and Medicine. Churchill Livingstone, Edinburgh.

Kanski JJ 1999 Clinical Ophthalmology A Systematic Approach 4th edn. Butterworth Heinemann, Oxford.

Mallik M, Hall C, Howard D 1998 Nursing Knowledge and Practice A Decision-making Approach. Baillière Tindall, London.

Maclean H 2002 The Eye in Primary Care. Butterworth Heinemann, Oxford.

McMillan A, Scott GR 2000 Sexually Transmitted Infections: A Colour Guide. Churchill Livingstone, Edinburgh.

Millodot M 2004 Dictionary of Optometry and Visual Science 6th edn. Butterworth Heinemann, Edinburgh.

Montague SE, Watson R, Herbert R 2005 Physiology for Nursing Practice 3rd edn. Bailliere Tindall, Edinburgh.

Mosby's Dictionary of Medicine, Nursing and Health Professions 7th edn. 2006, Mosby, St Louis.

Nicol M, Bavin C, Bedford-Turner S, Cronin P, Rawlings-Anderson K 2004 Essential Nursing Skills 2nd edn. Mosby, Edinburgh.

Parsons M, Johnson M 2001 Diagnosis in Colour: Neurology. Mosby, Edinburgh.

Peattie P, Walker S 1995 Understanding Nursing Care 4th edn. Churchill Livingstone, Edinburgh.

Porter S 2005 Dictionary of Physiotherapy. Butterworth Heinemann, Edinburgh.

Pudner R 2000 Nursing the Surgical Patient. Baillière Tindall, Edinburgh.

Rodeck C, Whittle M 1999 Fetal Medicine Basic Science and Clinical Practice. Churchill Livingstone, Edinburgh.

Tiran D 2008 Baillière's Midwives' Dictionary 11th edn. Baillière Tindall, Edinburgh.

Walsh M 2002 Watson's Clinical Nursing and Related Sciences, 6th edn. Baillière Tindall, Edinburgh.

Watson R 2000 Anatomy and Physiology for Nurses, 11th edn. Baillière Tindall, Edinburgh.

Waugh A, Grant A 2006 Ross and Wilson Anatomy and Physiology In Health and Illness 10th edn. Churchill Livingstone, Edinburgh.

Westwood O 1999 The Scientific Basis for Health Care. Mosby, London.

Wilson J 1995 Infection Control in Clinical Practice. Baillière Tindall, London.

Wilkinson J, Shaw S, Orton D 2005 Dermatology in Focus. Churchill Livingstone, Edinburgh.

Winson N, McDonald RS 2005 Illustrated Dictionary of Midwifery. Butterworth Heinemann, Edinburgh.

Zhu H 2005 Running a Safe and Successful Acupuncture Clinic. Churchill Livingstone, Edinburgh.

How to use this dictionary

Main entries

These are listed in alphabetical order and appear in **bold** type. Derivative forms of the main entry also appear in **bold** type and are to be found at the end of the definition, along with their parts of speech. For example:

ketonaemia *n* ketone bodies in the blood—**ketonaemic** *adj.*

Separate meanings of main entry

Different meanings of the same word are separated by means of an Arabic numeral before each meaning. For example:

kinanaesthesia **1**. loss of the ability to sense movement. **2**. decreased awareness of the position or movement of part of the body.

Subentries

Subentries relating to the defined main entry are listed in alphabetical order and appear in *italic* type, following the main definition. For example:

ligation *n* tying off; usually reserved for *ligation of the uterine (fallopian) tubes*, a method of sterilization.

Parts of speech and other abbreviations

The parts of speech follows single word main entries and derivative forms of the main entry, and appear in *italic* type. The parts of speech and other abbreviations used in the dictionary are:

abbr	**abbreviation**
acron	**acronym**
adj	**adjective**
adv	**adverb**
Am	**American**
e.g.	**for example**
i.e.	**that is**
n	**noun**
npl	**noun, plural**
opp	**opposite**
pl	**plural**
sing	**singular**
syn	**synonym**
v	**verb**
vi	**intransitive verb**
vt	**transitive verb**

Cross-references

Cross-references alert you to related words and additional information elsewhere in the dictionary. A single symbol has been used for this purpose—an arrow ⊃. Either within or at the end of the definition, the arrow indicates the word(s) you can then look up for related subject matter. For example:

overgrowth an overall increase in the size of a tissue either by an increase in the size of its cells, or in their number. ⊃ hyperplasia, hypertrophy.

Most drug entries relate to drug groups rather than specific drug names and the cross-reference will be to Appendix 5 for more information. For example:

penicillins *npl* a large group of β-lactam antibiotics. Many have activity against a broad range of bacteria (known as broad spectrum antibiotics) but they produce hypersensitivity reactions and many micro-organisms have developed resistance. Some penicillins are β-lactamase resistant. ⊃Appendix 5.

Many anatomical structures or terms are cross-referenced to the appropriate figure(s) in the Colour Section - Illustrations to show the structures/term's position in the body. For example:

vena cava one of two large veins emptying into the right atrium of the heart. The superior vena cava drains venous blood from the head, neck and upper limbs, and the inferior vena cava drains venous blood from structures below the diaphragm—**venae cavae** *pl*, **vena caval** *adj.* ⊃ Colour Section Figures 8, 10.

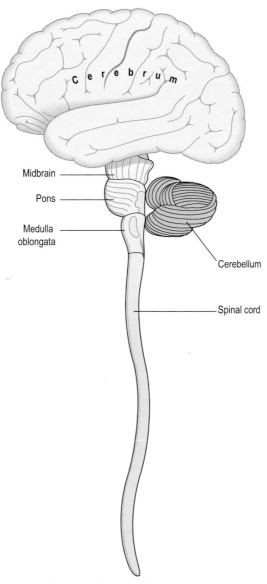

Figure 1 The parts of the central nervous system (brain and spinal cord)

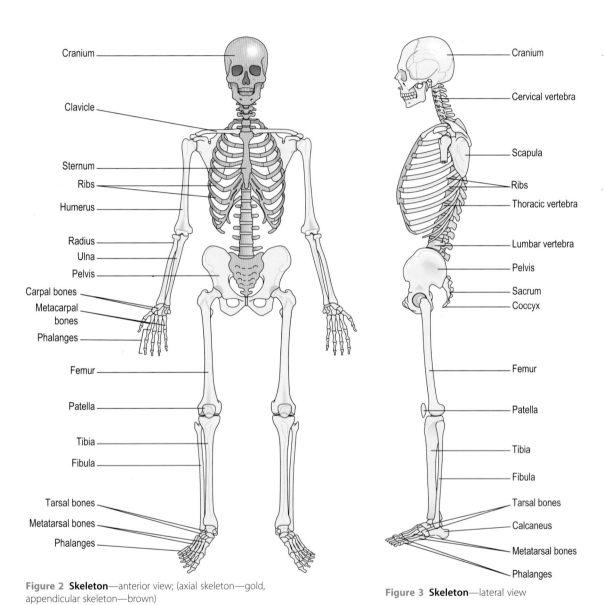

Cranium

Clavicle

Sternum

Ribs

Humerus

Radius

Ulna

Pelvis

Carpal bones

Metacarpal bones

Phalanges

Femur

Patella

Tibia

Fibula

Tarsal bones

Metatarsal bones

Phalanges

Cranium

Cervical vertebra

Scapula

Ribs

Thoracic vertebra

Lumbar vertebra

Pelvis

Sacrum

Coccyx

Femur

Patella

Tibia

Fibula

Tarsal bones

Calcaneus

Metatarsal bones

Phalanges

Figure 2 Skeleton—anterior view; (axial skeleton—gold, appendicular skeleton—brown)

Figure 3 Skeleton—lateral view

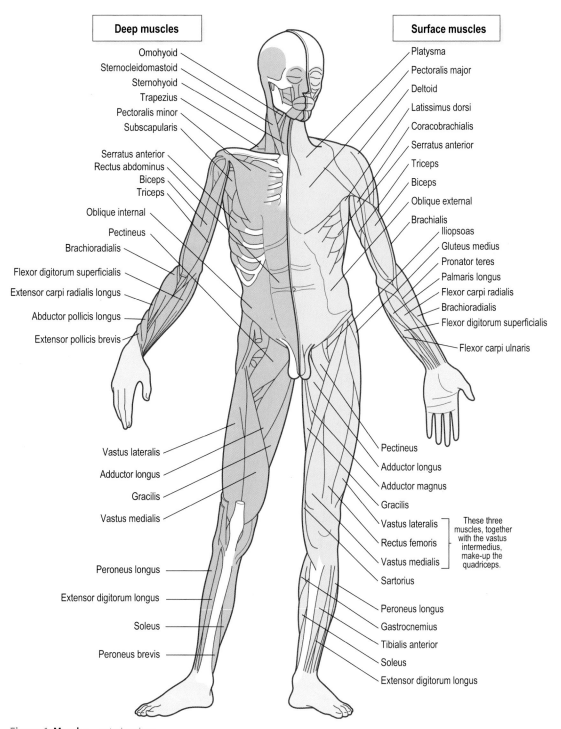

Deep muscles

Omohyoid
Sternocleidomastoid
Sternohyoid
Trapezius
Pectoralis minor
Subscapularis

Serratus anterior
Rectus abdominus
Biceps
Triceps

Oblique internal

Pectineus

Brachioradialis

Flexor digitorum superficialis

Extensor carpi radialis longus

Abductor pollicis longus

Extensor pollicis brevis

Vastus lateralis

Adductor longus

Gracilis

Vastus medialis

Peroneus longus

Extensor digitorum longus

Soleus

Peroneus brevis

Surface muscles

Platysma
Pectoralis major
Deltoid
Latissimus dorsi
Coracobrachialis
Serratus anterior
Triceps
Biceps
Oblique external
Brachialis
Iliopsoas
Gluteus medius
Pronator teres
Palmaris longus
Flexor carpi radialis
Brachioradialis
Flexor digitorum superficialis

Flexor carpi ulnaris

Pectineus
Adductor longus
Adductor magnus
Gracilis
Vastus lateralis
Rectus femoris
Vastus medialis

These three muscles, together with the vastus intermedius, make-up the quadriceps.

Sartorius
Peroneus longus
Gastrocnemius
Tibialis anterior
Soleus
Extensor digitorum longus

Figure 4 **Muscles**—anterior view

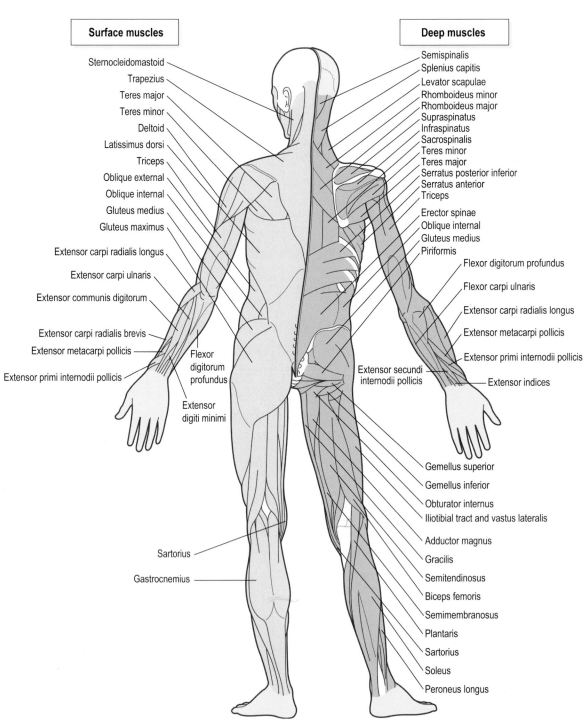

Surface muscles

- Sternocleidomastoid
- Trapezius
- Teres major
- Teres minor
- Deltoid
- Latissimus dorsi
- Triceps
- Oblique external
- Oblique internal
- Gluteus medius
- Gluteus maximus
- Extensor carpi radialis longus
- Extensor carpi ulnaris
- Extensor communis digitorum
- Extensor carpi radialis brevis
- Extensor metacarpi pollicis
- Extensor primi internodii pollicis
- Flexor digitorum profundus
- Extensor digiti minimi
- Sartorius
- Gastrocnemius

Deep muscles

- Semispinalis
- Splenius capitis
- Levator scapulae
- Rhomboideus minor
- Rhomboideus major
- Supraspinatus
- Infraspinatus
- Sacrospinalis
- Teres minor
- Teres major
- Serratus posterior inferior
- Serratus anterior
- Triceps
- Erector spinae
- Oblique internal
- Gluteus medius
- Piriformis
- Flexor digitorum profundus
- Flexor carpi ulnaris
- Extensor carpi radialis longus
- Extensor metacarpi pollicis
- Extensor primi internodii pollicis
- Extensor indices
- Extensor secundi internodii pollicis
- Gemellus superior
- Gemellus inferior
- Obturator internus
- Iliotibial tract and vastus lateralis
- Adductor magnus
- Gracilis
- Semitendinosus
- Biceps femoris
- Semimembranosus
- Plantaris
- Sartorius
- Soleus
- Peroneus longus

Figure 5 Muscles—posterior view

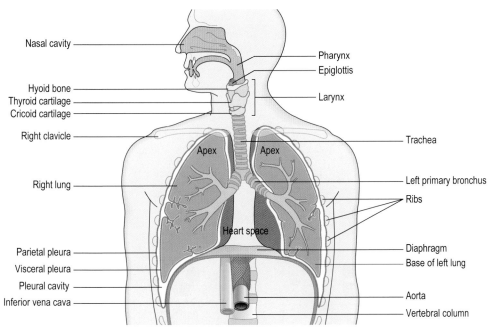

Nasal cavity

Pharynx
Epiglottis

Hyoid bone
Thyroid cartilage
Cricoid cartilage

Larynx

Right clavicle

Trachea

Apex   Apex

Right lung

Left primary bronchus

Ribs

Heart space

Parietal pleura
Visceral pleura
Pleural cavity
Inferior vena cava

Diaphragm
Base of left lung

Aorta
Vertebral column

Figure 6 Respiratory system and related structures

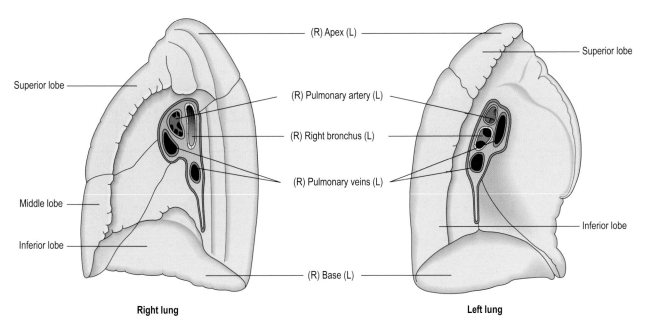

(R) Apex (L)

Superior lobe

Superior lobe

(R) Pulmonary artery (L)

(R) Right bronchus (L)

Middle lobe

(R) Pulmonary veins (L)

Inferior lobe

Inferior lobe

Inferior lobe

(R) Base (L)

Right lung

Left lung

Figure 7 Respiratory system—lungs showing lobes and vessels and airways of each hilum (medial views)

A5

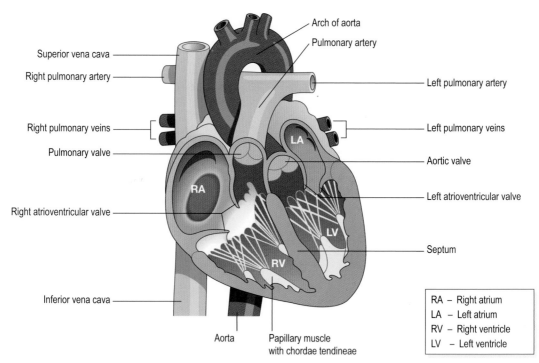

Superior vena cava

Right pulmonary artery

Right pulmonary veins

Pulmonary valve

Right atrioventricular valve

Inferior vena cava

Arch of aorta

Pulmonary artery

Left pulmonary artery

Left pulmonary veins

Aortic valve

Left atrioventricular valve

Septum

Aorta

Papillary muscle
with chordae tendineae

RA – Right atrium
LA – Left atrium
RV – Right ventricle
LV – Left ventricle

Figure 8 Circulatory system—interior of the heart

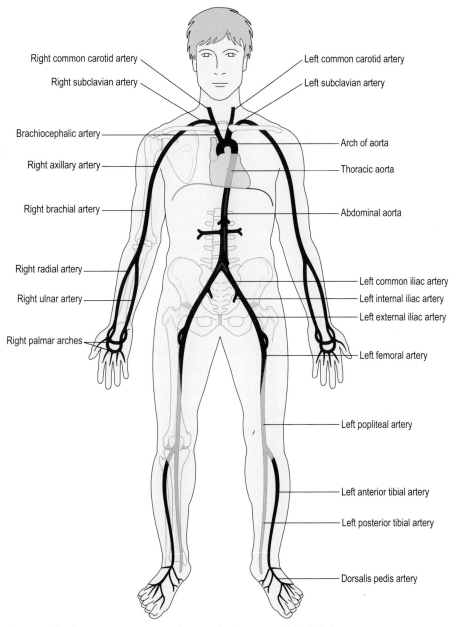

Right common carotid artery

Right subclavian artery

Brachiocephalic artery —

Right axillary artery —

Right brachial artery —

Right radial artery —

Right ulnar artery —

Right palmar arches —

Left common carotid artery

Left subclavian artery

Arch of aorta

Thoracic aorta

Abdominal aorta

Left common iliac artery

Left internal iliac artery

Left external iliac artery

Left femoral artery

Left popliteal artery

Left anterior tibial artery

Left posterior tibial artery

Dorsalis pedis artery

Figure 9 Circulatory system—arteries (aorta and main arteries of the limbs)

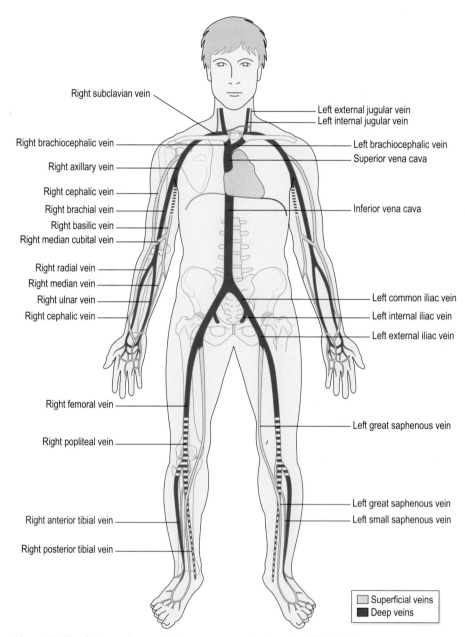

Right subclavian vein

Left external jugular vein
Left internal jugular vein

Right brachiocephalic vein

Left brachiocephalic vein
Superior vena cava

Right axillary vein

Right cephalic vein

Right brachial vein

Inferior vena cava

Right basilic vein

Right median cubital vein

Right radial vein

Right median vein

Right ulnar vein

Left common iliac vein

Right cephalic vein

Left internal iliac vein

Left external iliac vein

Right femoral vein

Left great saphenous vein

Right popliteal vein

Left great saphenous vein
Left small saphenous vein

Right anterior tibial vein

Right posterior tibial vein

Superficial veins
Deep veins

Figure 10 Circulatory system—veins (venae cavae and main veins of the limbs)

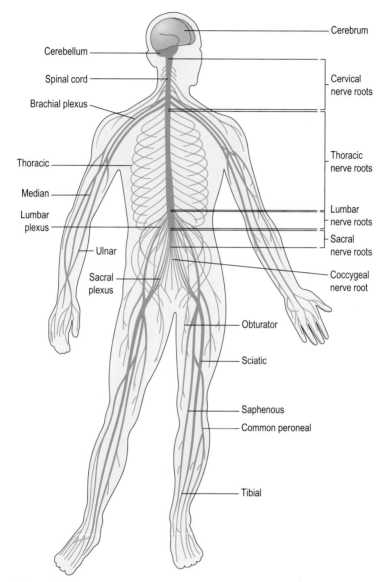

Cerebrum

Cerebellum

Spinal cord

Brachial plexus

Cervical
nerve roots

Thoracic

Thoracic
nerve roots

Median

Lumbar
plexus

Lumbar
nerve roots

Sacral
nerve roots

Ulnar

Sacral
plexus

Coccygeal
nerve root

Obturator

Sciatic

Saphenous

Common peroneal

Tibial

Figure 11 **Nervous system**

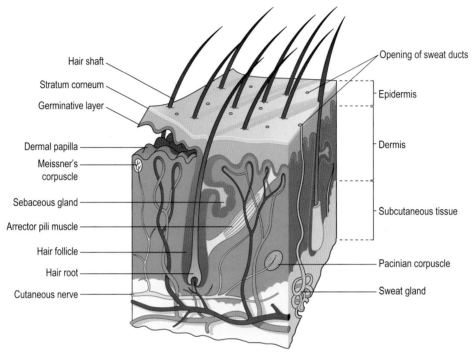

Figure 12 **Skin**

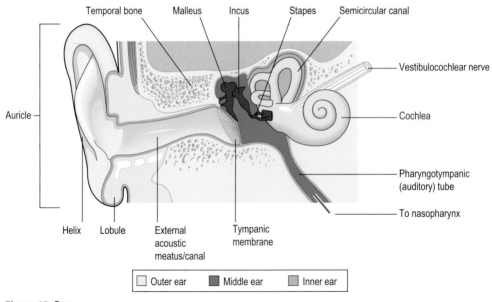

Figure 13 **Ear**

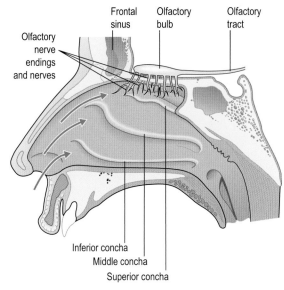

Olfactory nerve endings and nerves

Frontal sinus

Olfactory bulb

Olfactory tract

Inferior concha

Middle concha

Superior concha

Figure 14 **Nose**—olfactory structures

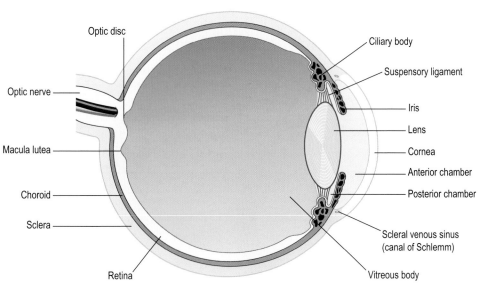

Optic disc

Optic nerve

Macula lutea

Choroid

Sclera

Retina

Ciliary body

Suspensory ligament

Iris

Lens

Cornea

Anterior chamber

Posterior chamber

Scleral venous sinus (canal of Schlemm)

Vitreous body

Figure 15 **Eye**

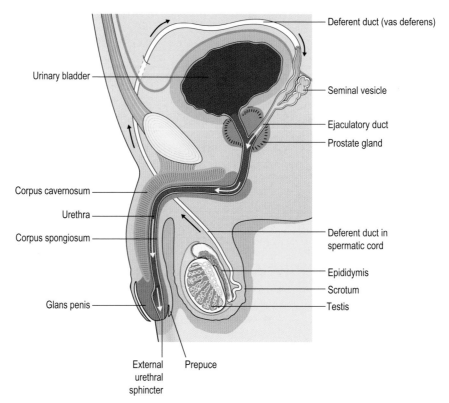

Figure 16 Male reproductive system (showing route taken by spermatozoa during ejaculation)

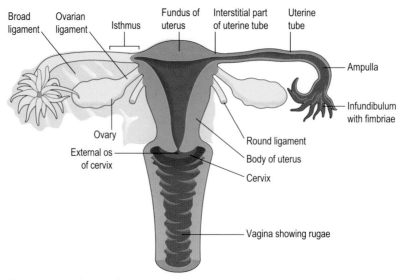

Figure 17 Female reproductive system

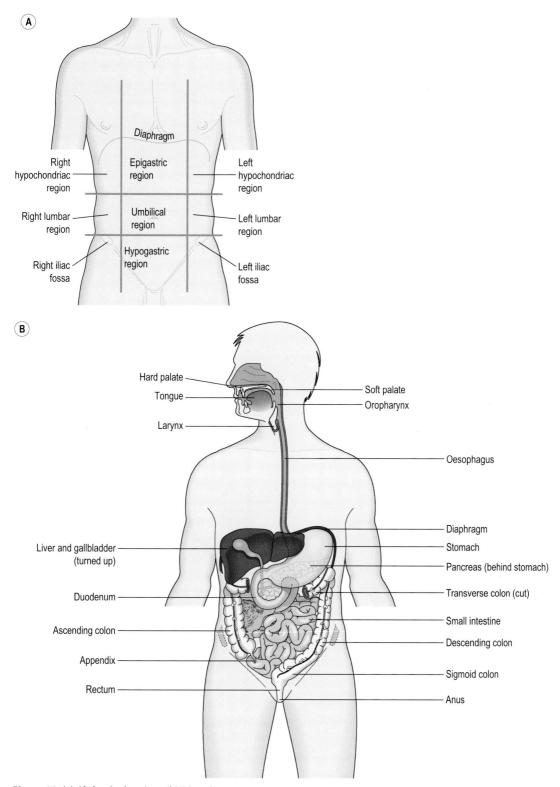

Figure 18 (a) Abdominal regions (b) Digestive system

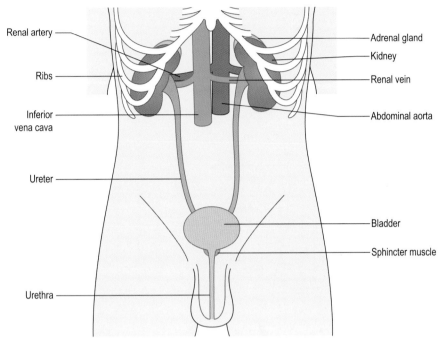

Figure 19 Urinary system

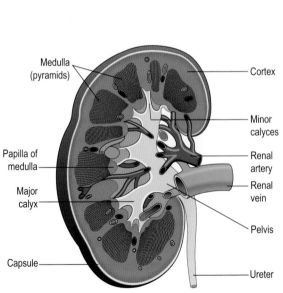

Figure 20 **Urinary system**—the kidney (longitudinal section)

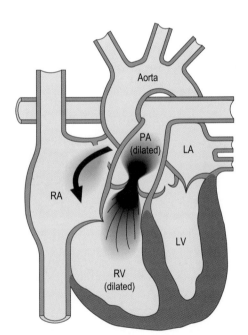

Figure 21 **Atrial septal defect.** Blood flows across the atrial septum (arrow) from left to right. The murmur is produced by increased flow velocicty across the pulmonary valve, as a result of left-to-right shunting and a large stroke volume. The density of the shading is proportional to velocity of blood flow.

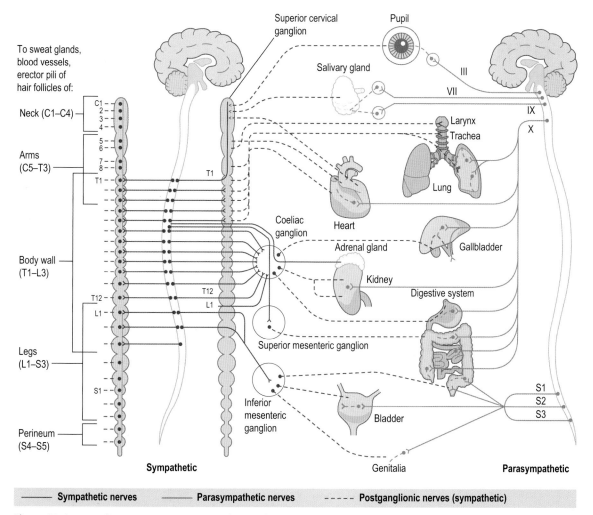

To sweat glands, blood vessels, erector pili of hair follicles of:

Neck (C1–C4)

Arms (C5–T3)

Body wall (T1–L3)

Legs (L1–S3)

Perineum (S4–S5)

C1
2
3
4
5
6
7
8
T1

T12
L1

S1

Superior cervical ganglion

Pupil

Salivary gland

III

VII

IX

X

Larynx

Trachea

Lung

Coeliac ganglion

Heart

Adrenal gland

Gallbladder

Kidney

Digestive system

Superior mesenteric ganglion

Inferior mesenteric ganglion

Bladder

Genitalia

S1
S2
S3

T1

T12
L1

Sympathetic

Parasympathetic

——— **Sympathetic nerves**   ——— **Parasympathetic nerves**   - - - - **Postganglionic nerves (sympathetic)**

Figure 22 Autonomic nervous system – sympathetic and parasympathetic systems. For clarity peripheral and visceral nerves of the sympathetic system are shown on separate sides of the cord.

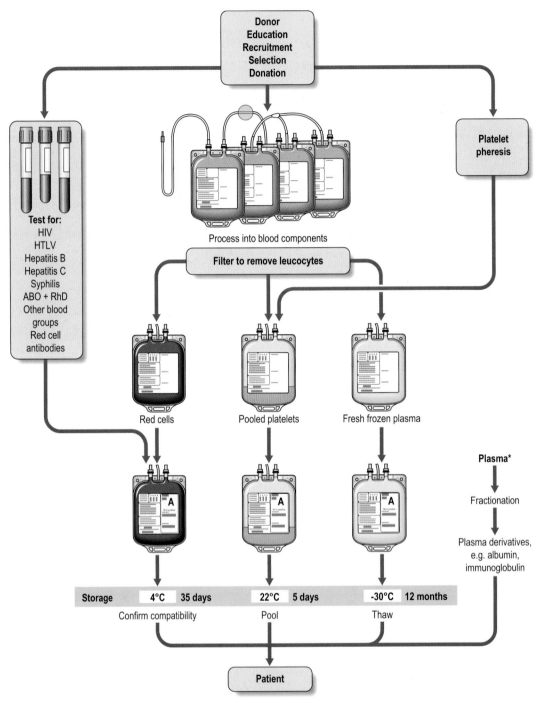

Figure 23 Blood donation, processing and storage. *In the UK, plasma for fractionation is imported as a precautionary measure against vCJD

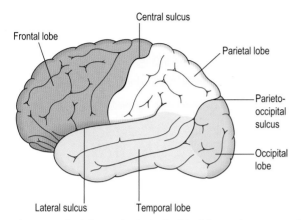

Figure 24 **The lobes and principal sulci of the cerebrum.** Viewed from the left side

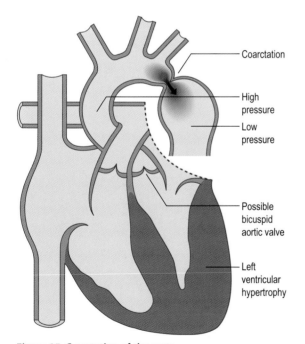

Figure 25 **Coarctation of the aorta**

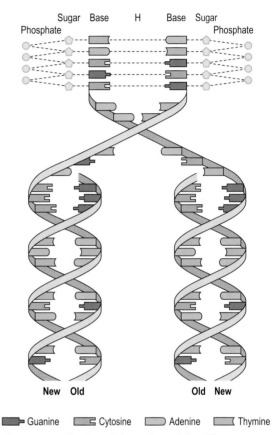

Figure 26 **Replication of deoxyribonucleic acid**

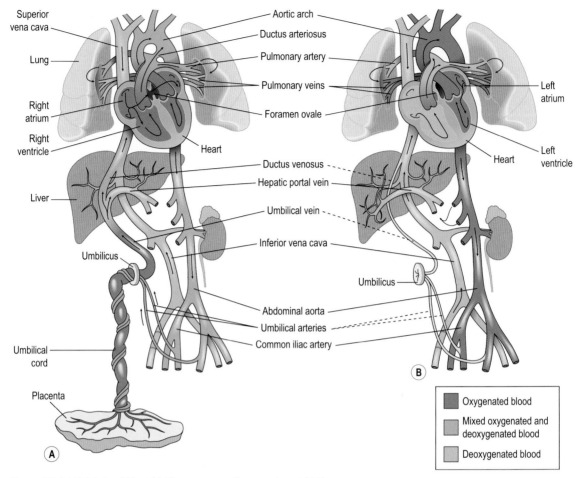

Figure 27 (a) Fetal circulation (b) Changes normally occurring at birth

■	Oxygenated blood
■	Mixed oxygenated and deoxygenated blood
■	Deoxygenated blood

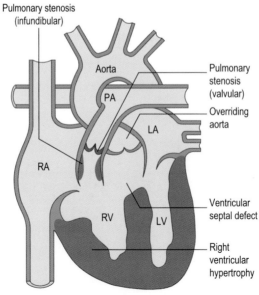

Figure 28 Fallot's tetralogy

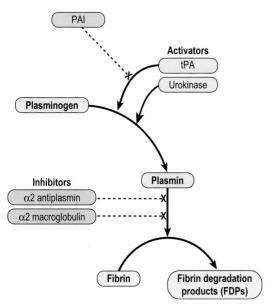

Figure 29 **Fibrinolysis** (t-PA = tissue plasminogen activator; PAI = plasminogen activator inhibitor)

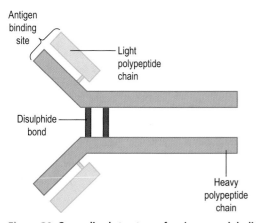

Figure 30 **Generalized structure of an immunoglobulin molecule**

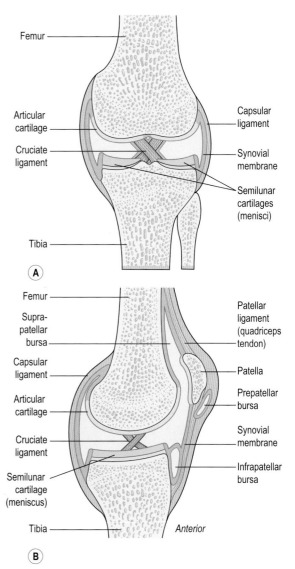

Figure 31 **Knee joint** (a) Section viewed from the front (b) Section viewed from the side.

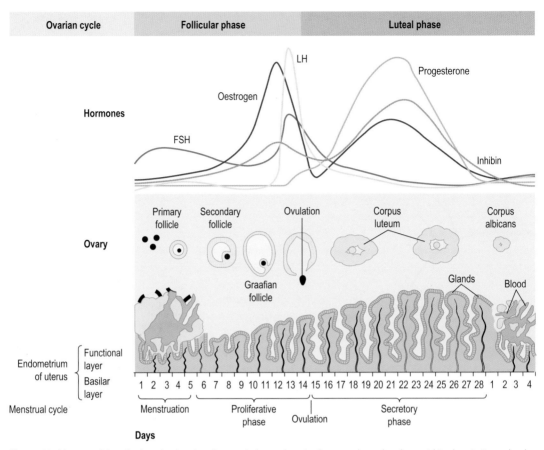

Figure 32 Menstrual (uterine) cycle showing the precisely synchronized events that take place within the pituitary gland, ovary and the endometrium lining of the uterus

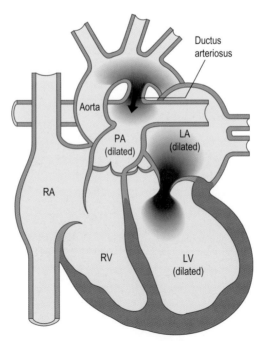

Figure 33 Persistent ductus arteriosus. There is a connection between the aorta and the pulmonary artery with left-to-right shunting and dilatation of the pulmonary artery, left atrium and left ventricle

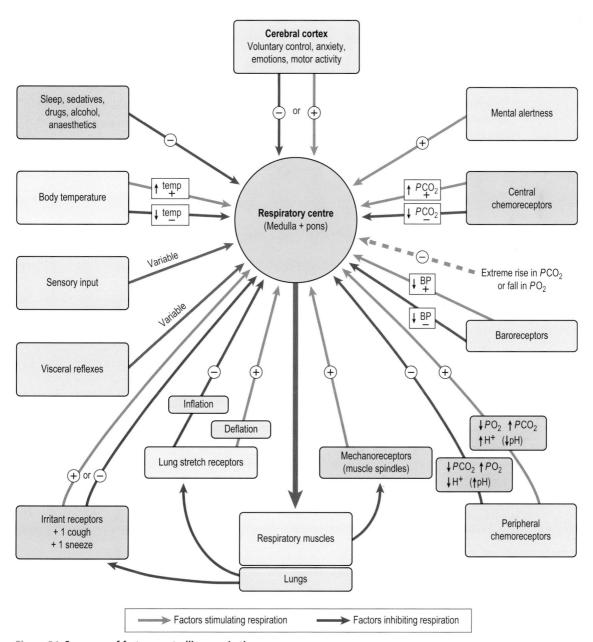

Figure 34 **Summary of factors controlling respiration**

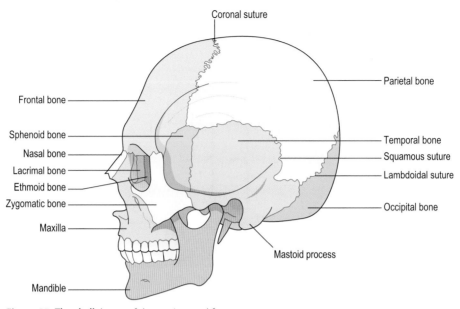

Figure 35 **The skull:** bones of the cranium and face

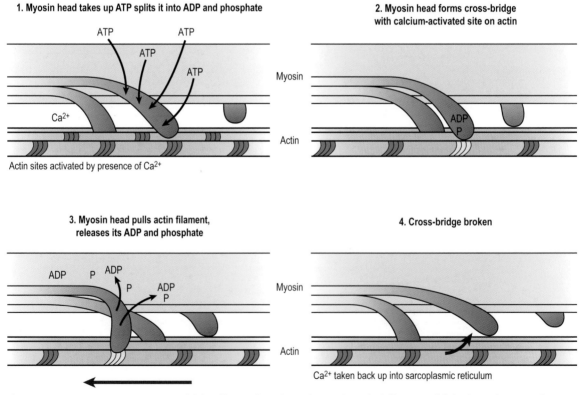

1. Myosin head takes up ATP splits it into ADP and phosphate

ATP ATP

ATP

ATP

Ca²⁺

Myosin

Actin

Actin sites activated by presence of Ca²⁺

2. Myosin head forms cross-bridge with calcium-activated site on actin

Myosin

ADP
P

Actin

3. Myosin head pulls actin filament, releases its ADP and phosphate

ADP   P   ADP

P   ADP
            P

Myosin

Actin

4. Cross-bridge broken

Myosin

Actin

Ca²⁺ taken back up into sarcoplasmic reticulum

Figure 36 Diagrammatic representation of sliding filament hypothesis showing how thick filaments of skeletal muscle move relative to one another as cross-bridges are formed and broken

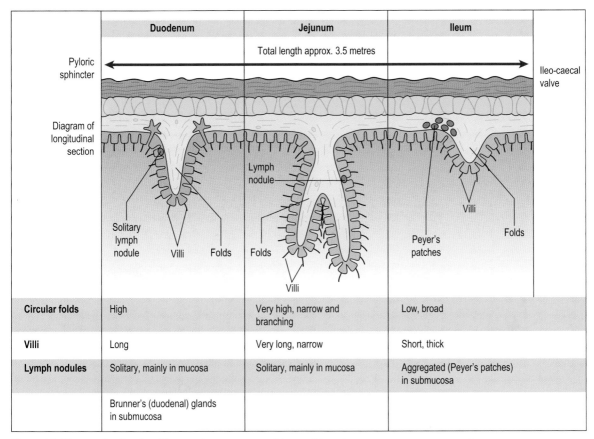

	Duodenum	Jejunum	Ileum
		Total length approx. 3.5 metres	
Circular folds	High	Very high, narrow and branching	Low, broad
Villi	Long	Very long, narrow	Short, thick
Lymph nodules	Solitary, mainly in mucosa	Solitary, mainly in mucosa	Aggregated (Peyer's patches) in submucosa
	Brunner's (duodenal) glands in submucosa		

Figure 37 Diagram showing the differences between areas of the small intestine

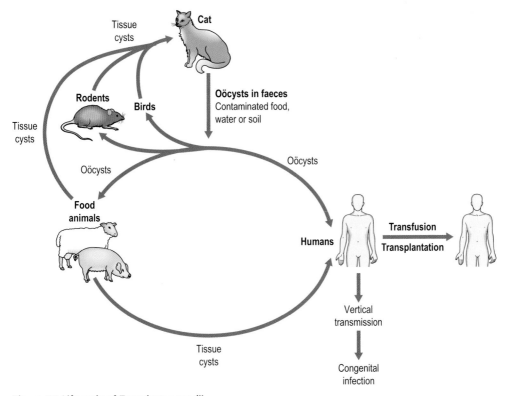

Figure 38 Life cycle of *Toxoplasma gondii*

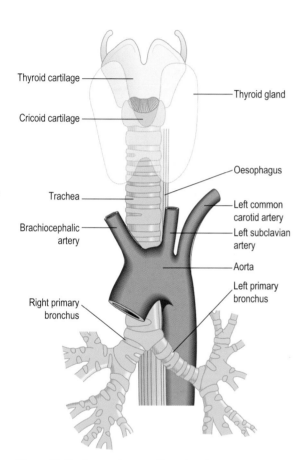

Thyroid cartilage

Cricoid cartilage

Trachea

Brachiocephalic artery

Right primary bronchus

Thyroid gland

Oesophagus

Left common carotid artery

Left subclavian artery

Aorta

Left primary bronchus

Figure 39 Trachea and some of its related structures

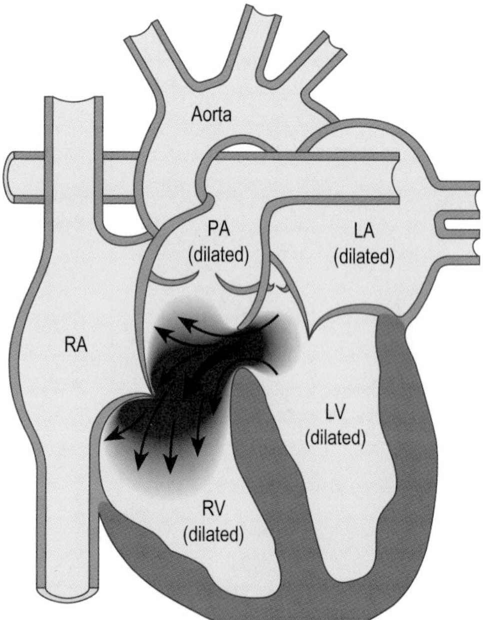

Aorta

PA (dilated)

LA (dilated)

RA

LV (dilated)

RV (dilated)

Figure 40 Ventricular septal defect. In this example a large left-to-right shunt (arrows) has resulted in chamber enlargement

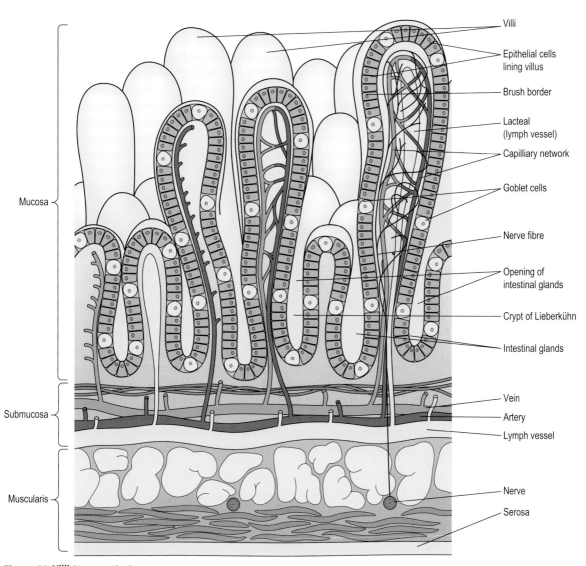

Mucosa

Submucosa

Muscularis

Villi

Epithelial cells
lining villus

Brush border

Lacteal
(lymph vessel)

Capilliary network

Goblet cells

Nerve fibre

Opening of
intestinal glands

Crypt of Lieberkühn

Intestinal glands

Vein

Artery

Lymph vessel

Nerve

Serosa

Figure 41 Villi (cross section)

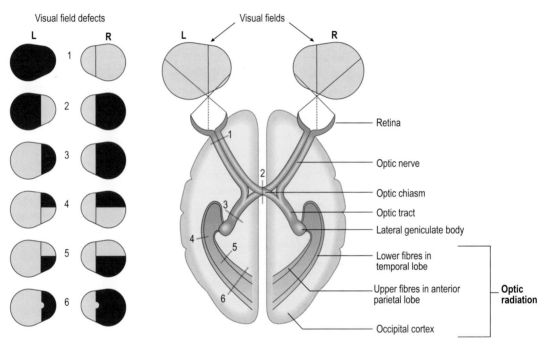

Figure 42 Visual pathways and visual field defects. Schematic representation of the eyes and brain in transverse section

Clinical photographs

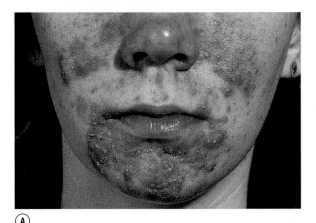

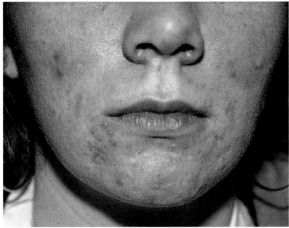

Figure 43 Acne in a teenager (a) Before treatment (b) After prolonged systemic antibiotic treatment.

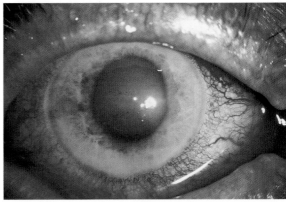

Figure 44 Acute angle-closure glaucoma

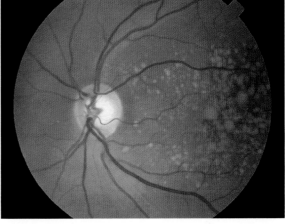

Figure 45 Macular drusen. These appear as yellow lumps and represent areas of worn out retina

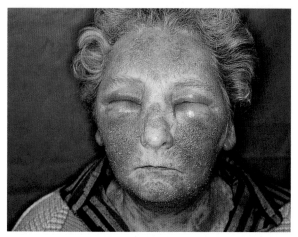

Figure 46 Allergic contact eczema

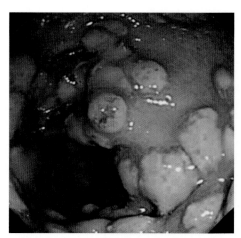

Figure 49 Colonoscopic view showing numerous adherant 'pseudomembranes' on the intestinal mucosa. Caused by *Clostridium difficile* superinfection (antibiotic-associated colitis, pseudomembranous colitis)

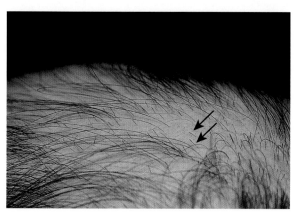

Figure 47 Alopecia areata

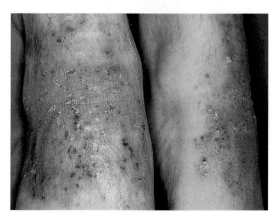

Figure 50 Atopic subacute eczema

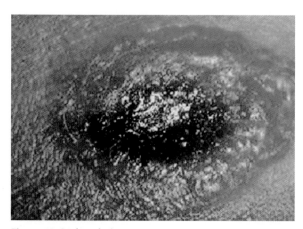

Figure 48 Anthrax lesion

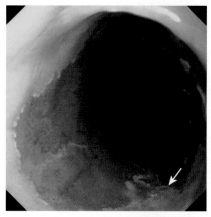

Figure 51 Barrett's oesophagus. Pink columnar mucosa extends up the oesophagus. Small islands of squamous mucosa remain (arrow)

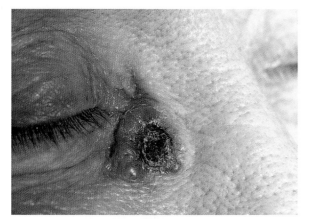

Figure 52 Basal cell carcinoma (BCC)

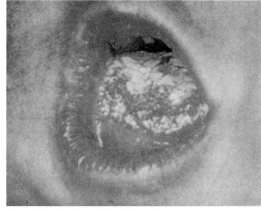

Figure 55 Oral candidiasis (thrush)

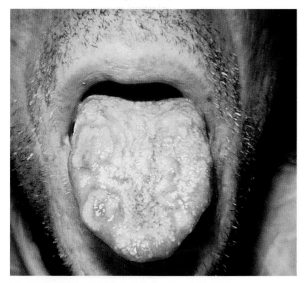

Figure 53 Oral ulceration in Behçet's syndrome

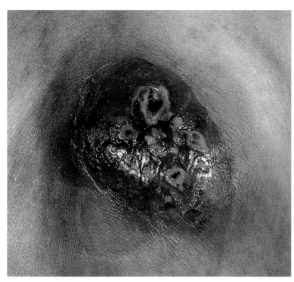

Figure 56 Carbuncle (staphylococcal)

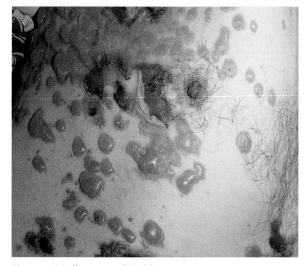

Figure 54 Bullous pemphigoid

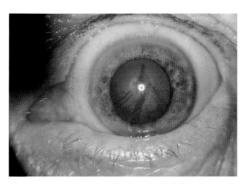

Figure 57 Cataract in the lens is highlighted against the red reflex.

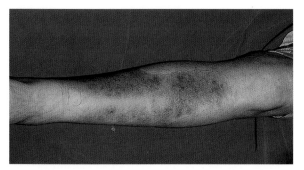

Figure 58 **Acute cellulitis**

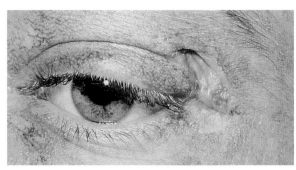

Figure 62 **Typical eyelid appearance in dermatomyositis**

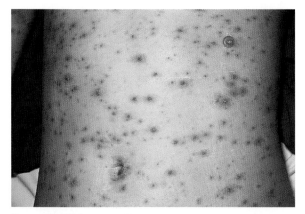

Figure 59 **Chickenpox rash**

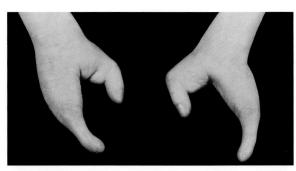

Figure 63 **Ectrodactyly**

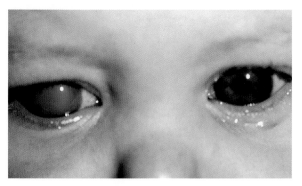

Figure 60 **Congenital glaucoma**

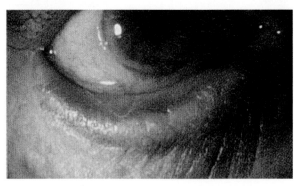

Figure 64 **Ectropion.** Secondary conjunctivitis is not uncommon

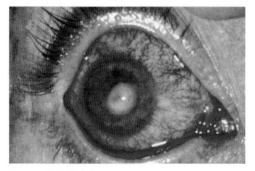

Figure 61 **Bacterial corneal ulcer**

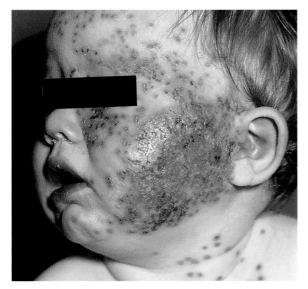

Figure 65 **Eczema herpeticum**

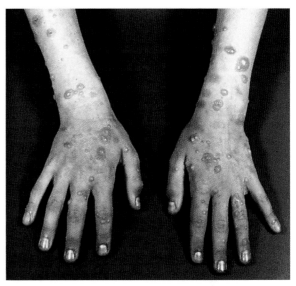

Figure 68 **Erythema multiforme.** With blistering lesions

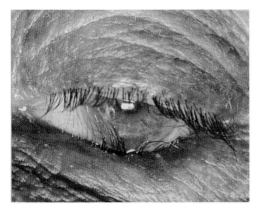

Figure 66 **Entropion**

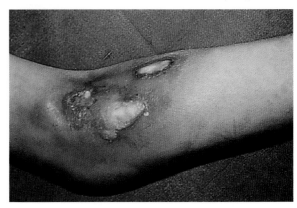

Figure 69 **Extravasation.** Skin necrosis due to extravasation of anthracycline chemotherapy (e.g. doxorubicin, daunrubicin)

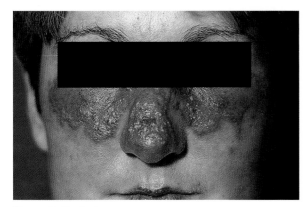

Figure 67 **Erysipelas**

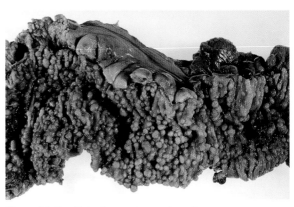

Figure 70 **Familial adenomatous polyposis**

A31

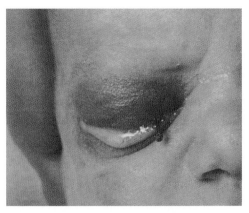

Figure 71 **Gonococcal ophthalmia neonatorum**

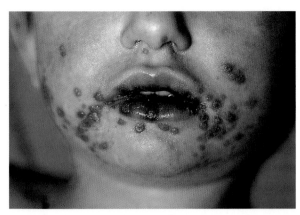

Figure 74 **Acute herpes simplex (HSV-1).** There are also vesicles in the mouth

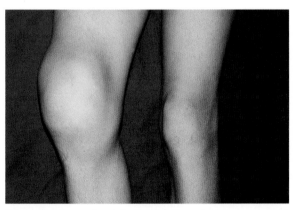

Figure 72 **Haemarthrosis in the right knee** (with haemophilia A)

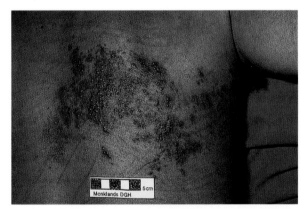

Figure 75 **Typical herpes zoster (shingles)** reactivation in a thoracic dermatome

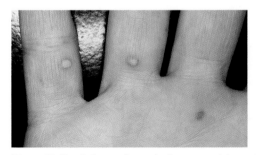

Figure 73 **Hand, foot and mouth disease**—vesicles on hand

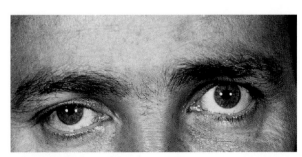

Figure 76 **Horner's syndrome** (right side). Due to paravertebral metastasis at T1 with ipsilateral ptosis, and a small pupil

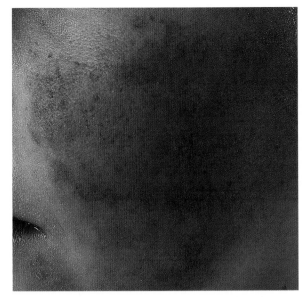

Figure 77 **Human erythrovirus 19**—'slapped cheek' syndrome

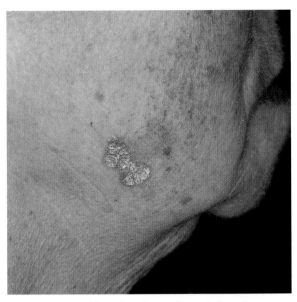

Figure 79 **Intraepidermal carcinoma** (Bowen's disease)

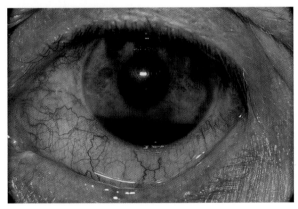

Figure 78 **Hyphaema.** Blood in the anterior chamber will precipitate, and form a fluid level inferiorly. Movement will stir up blood cells and reduce visual acuity

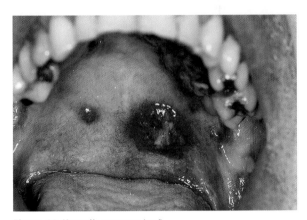

Figure 80 **Kaposi's sarcoma** (oral)

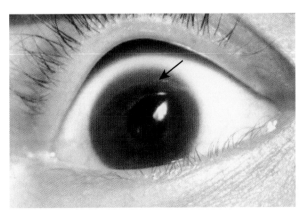

Figure 81 **Kayser–Fleischer ring**

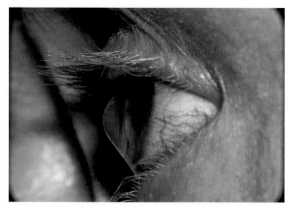

Figure 82 Keratoconus. The shape of the cornea causes irregular astigmatism, blurring the person's vision

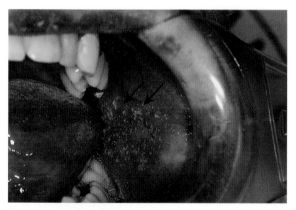

Figure 83 **Koplik's spots**

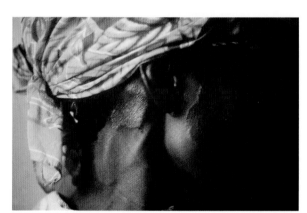

Figure 85 **Tuberculoid leprosy**

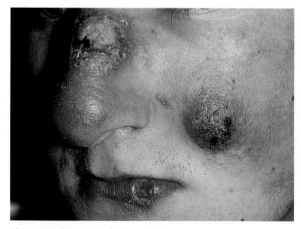

Figure 84 **Cutaneous leishmaniasis**

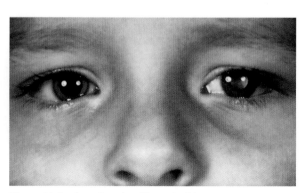

Figure 86 **Leukocoria caused by retinoblastoma**

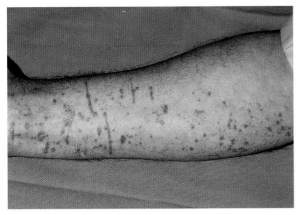

Figure 87 Lichen planus

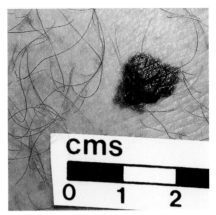

Figure 89 Malignant melanoma

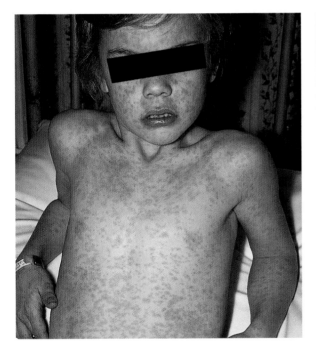

Figure 88 Measles rash

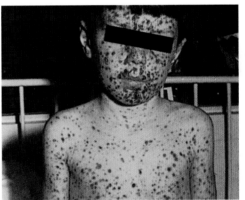

Figure 90 Petechial rash in meningococcal septicaemia

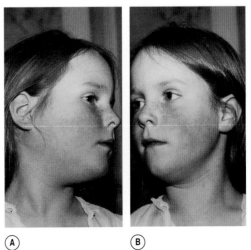

(A)　　　　　(B)

Figure 91 Typical unilateral mumps. (a) Note the loss of angle of the jaw on the affected (right) side. (b) Comparison showing normal (left) side

A35

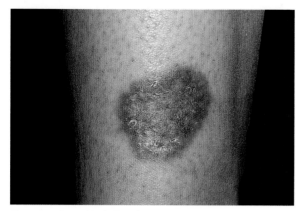

Figure 92 Necrobiosis lipoidica

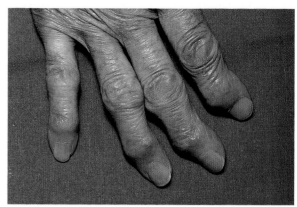

Figure 95 **Nodal osteoarthritis.** Heberden's nodes, lateral deviation of distal interphalangeal joints, with mild Bouchard's nodes at the proximal interphalangeal joints

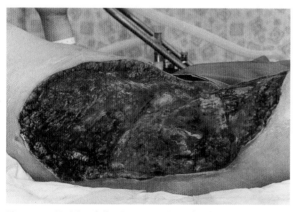

Figure 93 **Excision following necrotizing fasciitis in an intravenous drug-user**

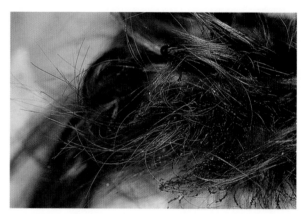

Figure 96 **Head lice.** 'Nits' (empty egg cases) adhere strongly to the hair shafts.

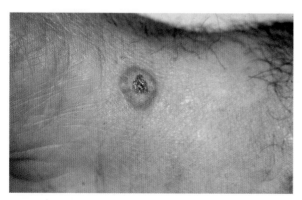

Figure 94 **Orf**—lesions on forearm and hand

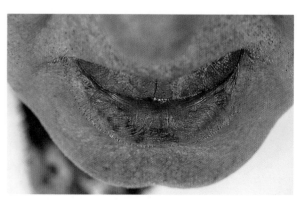

Figure 97 **Peutz–Jeghers syndrome**

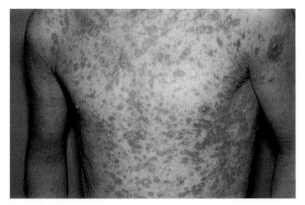

Figure 98 **Pityriasis rosea**—rash

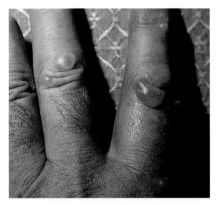

Figure 100 **Skin blistering in porphyria**

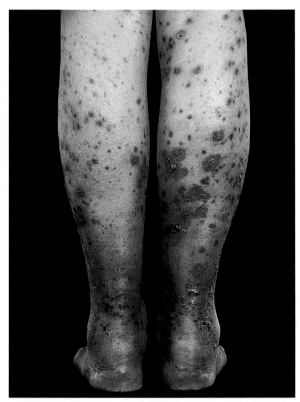

Figure 99 **Rash of systemic vasculitis** (palpable purpura)

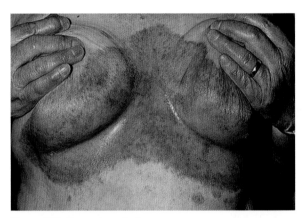

Figure 101 **Flexural psoriasis**

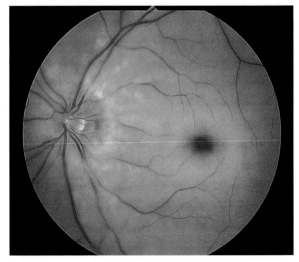

Figure 102 **Central retinal artery occlusion.** The whole retina is infarcted and oedematous, like a giant cotton-wool spot. The thin retina at the fovea allows a red glow from the unaffected choroidal circulation to show through

A37

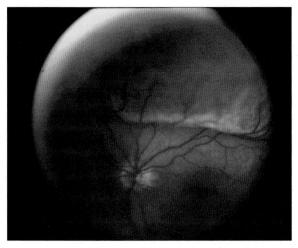

Figure 103 Retinal detachment. The advancing front of detached retina is approaching the optic disc and macula

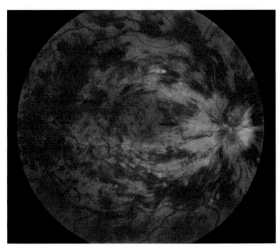

Figure 104 Central retinal vein occlusion

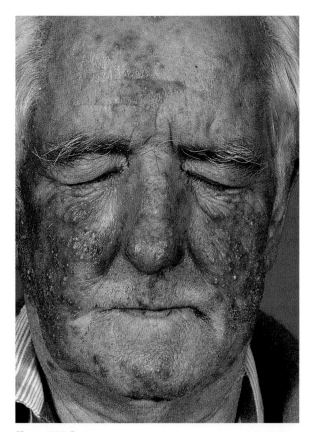

Figure 105 Rosacea

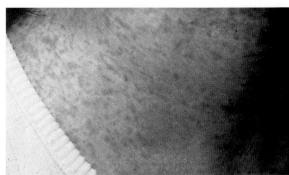

Figure 106 Rubella rash

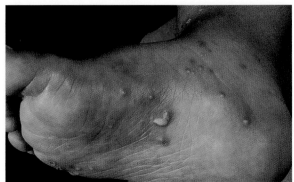

Figure 107 Scabies

A38

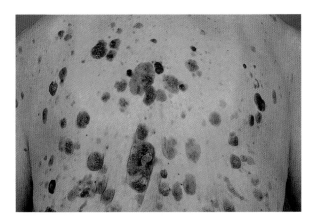

Figure 108 Seborrhoeic warts

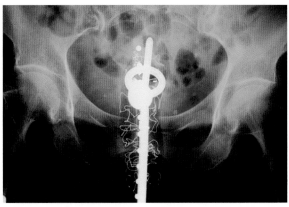

Figure 109 Selectron treatment of cervical cancer

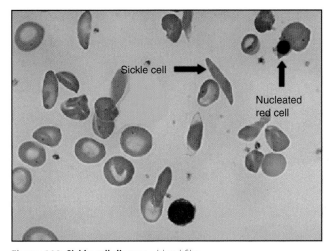

Sickle cell →

Nucleated
red cell

Figure 110 Sickle cell disease—blood film

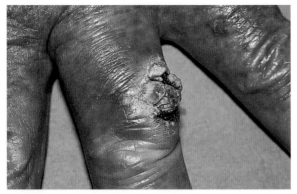

Figure 111 Squamous cell carcinoma (SCC)

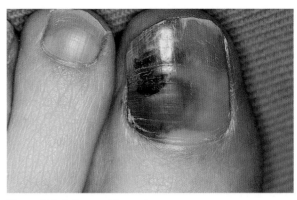

Figure 114 Subungual haematoma

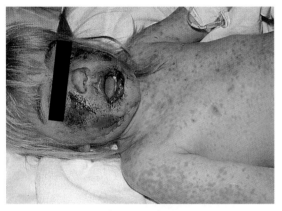

Figure 112 Stevens-Johnson syndrome

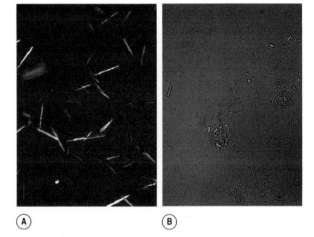

(A)　　　　　(B)

Figure 115 Compensated polarized light microscopy of synovial fluids (x 400) (a) Monosodium urate crystals showing bright birefringence (negative sign) and needle-shaped morphology. (b) Calcium pyrophosphate crystals showing weak birefringence (positive sign), scant numbers and a predominantly rhomboid morphology. These are clearly more difficult to detect than urate crystals.

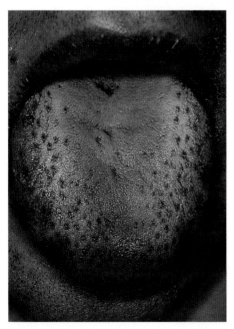

Figure 113 'Strawberry tongue' of acute streptococcal disease

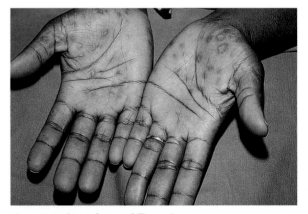

Figure 116 Secondary syphilis—rash

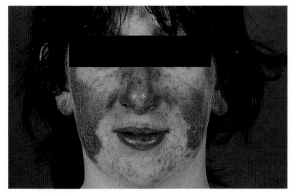

Figure 117 **Butterfly** (malar) rash of systemic lupus erythematosus

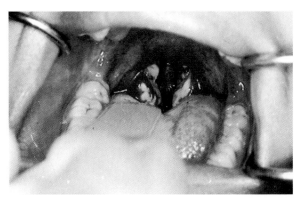

Figure 120 **Tonsillitis**

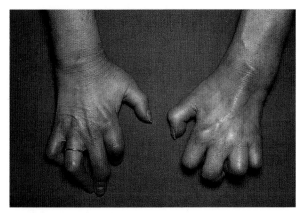

Figure 118 **Systemic sclerosis.** Hands showing tight shiny skin, sclerodactyly, flexion contractures of the fingers and thickening of the left middle finger extensor tendon sheath

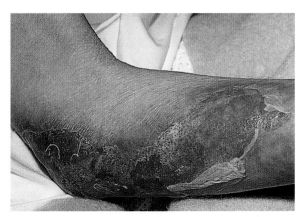

Figure 121 **Toxic epidermal/epidermolytic necrolysis (TEN)**

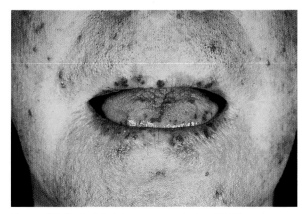

Figure 119 **Typical facial appearance in the CREST syndrome**

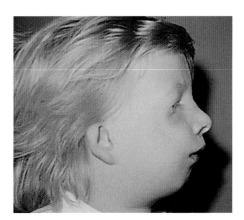

Figure 122 **Treacher Collins syndrome**

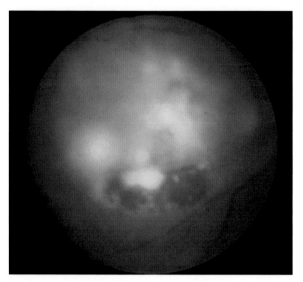

Figure 123 Retinochoroiditis due to toxoplasmosis

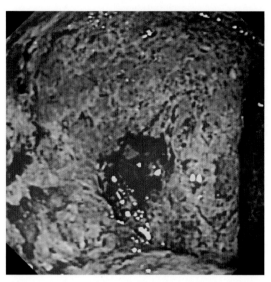

Figure 125 Sigmoidoscopic view of moderately active ulcerative colitis. Mucosa is erythematous and friable with contact bleeding. Submucosal blood vessels are no longer visible.

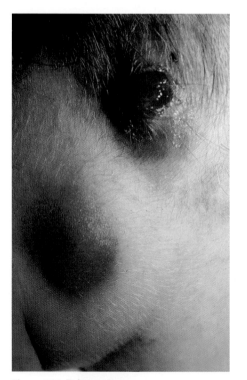

Figure 124 Tularaemia

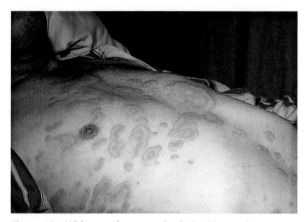

Figure 126 Widespread acute urticaria (in this case due to penicillin allergy)

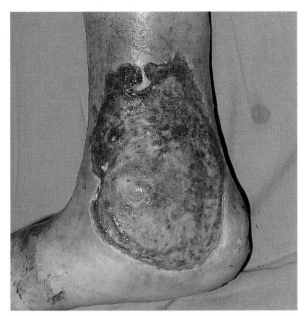

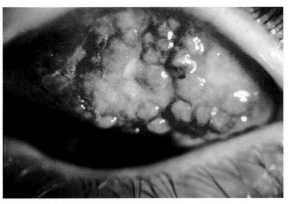

Figure 128 Vernal conjunctivitis/keratoconjunctivitis. Giant 'cobblestone' papillae are seen on everting the upper lid

Figure 127 Venous ulcer. Overlying the medial malleolus

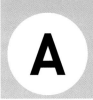

A *abbr* ampere.

a- a prefix that means 'lack of, without, not', e.g. *apyrexia*.

AA *abbr* Alcoholics Anonymous.

AAA *abbr* abdominal aortic aneurysm.

AACG *abbr* acute angle-closure glaucoma.

AAMI *abbr* age-associated memory impairment.

AAT *abbr* alpha₁ (α)-antitrypsin deficiency.

ab-, abs- a prefix that means 'away from', 'from' or 'off', e.g. *abduct, abstract*.

A–B ratio used in pregnancy ultrasound scans to assess the amount of blood through the umbilical cord; a low ratio is normal, a high ratio may indicate intrauterine growth retardation.

abacterial *adj* without bacteria. A condition, such as inflammation that is not caused by bacteria.

A band the dark constrictions formed in muscle myofibrils when the actin and myosin filaments overlap. They are visible on electron microscopy.

abatement reduction in the severity of pain or symptoms.

Abbé Estlander's operation transfer of a full-thickness flap from one lip to repair a defect in the other lip, using an arterial pedicle to ensure survival of the graft.

Abbé's condition ⊃ sine condition.

Abbé's number ⊃ constringence.

Abbé's refractometer ⊃ refractometer.

Abbreviated Injury Scale (AIS) a scoring system (1 to 6) used to provide a ranking of the severity of injuries and the threat to life. ⊃ Advanced trauma life-support.

ABCs of proprioception agility, balance and coordination. ⊃ proprioception.

abdo- a prefix that means 'abdomen', e.g. *abdominal*.

abdomen *n* the largest body cavity. The portion of the body between the thorax and the pelvis. It is separated from the thorax by the diaphragm. This cavity contains the abdominal viscera and is enclosed by the abdominal wall (comprising the abdominal muscles, fascia, fat and skin), the vertebral column and the iliac bones.

abdominal *adj* pertaining to the abdomen.

abdominal aorta *n* that part of the aorta within the abdomen. Smaller arteries branch from it to supply oxygenated blood to abdominal structures, such as the renal arteries which supply the kidneys. ⊃ Colour Section Figures 9, 19.

abdominal aortic aneurysm (AAA) a swelling in the abdominal aorta. AAAs are present in 5% of men aged over 60 years and 80% are confined to the infrarenal segment. Men are affected three times more commonly than women. About two-thirds of AAAs are sufficiently calcified to show up on a plain abdominal X-ray. Ultrasound is used for establishing the diagnosis; an approximate size may be obtained, and the technique can be used to follow up patients with asymptomatic aneurysms that are not yet large enough to warrant surgical repair. Computed tomography (CT) provides much more accurate information about the size and extent of the aneurysm, the surrounding structures and whether there is any other intra-abdominal pathology, and is the standard pre-operative investigation; however, it is not suitable for surveillance. Arteriography is usually only indicated if there are concerns about associated lower limb, renal and/or visceral occlusive disease. Until an asymptomatic AAA has reached a maximum of 5.5 cm in diameter, the risks of surgery generally outweigh the risks of rupture. All symptomatic AAAs should be considered for repair, not only to rid the patient of symptoms but also because pain often predates rupture. Distal embolization is a strong indication for repair, regardless of size, because otherwise limb loss is common. Most patients with a ruptured AAA do not survive to reach hospital, but if they do and surgery is appropriate, there must be no delay in getting them to the operating theatre. Open repair is the established treatment of choice in both the elective and the emergency setting, and entails replacing the aneurysmal segment with a prosthetic (usually Dacron) graft. The 30-day mortality for this procedure is approximately 5–8% for elective asymptomatic AAA, 10–20% for emergency symptomatic AAA, and 50% for ruptured AAA. However, patients who survive operation to leave hospital have a long-term survival which approaches that of the normal population. Some AAAs may be treated with a covered stent placed via a femoral arteriotomy under radiological guidance. ⊃ aneurysm, aortic dissection.

abdominal breathing more than usual use of the diaphragm and abdominal muscles to increase the input of air to and output from the lungs. May occur voluntarily. It can occur in disease as a compensatory mechanism for inadequate oxygenation.

abdominal cavity that below the diaphragm; the abdomen. The largest cavity in the body; it is oval in shape. It is situated in the main part of the trunk and its boundaries are: superiorly—the diaphragm, which separates it from the thoracic cavity; anteriorly—the muscles forming the anterior abdominal wall; posteriorly—the lumbar vertebrae and muscles forming the posterior abdominal wall; laterally—the lower ribs and parts of the muscles of the abdominal wall; and inferiorly—the pelvic cavity with which it is continuous. Most of the space in the abdominal cavity is occupied by the organs and glands involved in the digestion and absorption of food. These are: the stomach, small intestine and most of the large intestine, the liver, gall-bladder, bile ducts and pancreas. Other structures include: the spleen, 2 kidneys and the upper part of the ureters, 2 adrenal (suprarenal) glands, numerous blood vessels, lymph vessels, nerves and lymph nodes. By convention the the the surface anatomy is divided into nine regions. ⊃ abdomen, abdominal regions.

abdominal delivery birth of an infant through an incision into the abdominal wall and uterus; this includes caesarean section.

abdominal enlargement during pregnancy the abdomen becomes progressively larger as the uterus increases in size; it is visible externally from about 16 weeks' gestation. Excess enlargement may be due to multiple pregnancy, polyhydramnios, uterine fibroids, or abnormal ovum development (molar pregnancy).

abdominal examination during pregnancy and puerperium systematic examination of the woman's abdomen by visual inspection for shape, scars, striae gravidarum, skin tension and contour; symphysis–fundal distance measurement, gentle palpation and auscultation. The uterus is palpable above the symphysis pubis from 12 weeks' gestation, increasing steadily in size until term. Fetal growth is estimated by measuring the symphysis–fundal distance in centimetres and plotting this on a growth chart to detect deviations in growth rate. Presentation is assessed by palpation after 36 weeks and may need to be confirmed by an ultrasound assessment. The fetal heart is auscultated with a Pinard's stethoscope or electric monitor for rate, rhythm and regularity and should be differentiated from the uterine souffle. Postnatally the abdomen is palpated to monitor uterine involution, to assess that the uterus is regaining its non-pregnant size and position and to elicit deviations from normal such as constipation or urinary retention.

abdominal excision of the rectum an operation sometimes performed for rectal cancer. The rectum is mobilized via an abdominal approach. The bowel is divided well proximal to the cancer. The proximal end is brought out as a permanent colostomy. Excision of the distal bowel, containing the cancer and the anal canal, is completed through a perineal incision.

abdominal girth measurement of the abdominal circumference, taken at the umbilicus. It may be carried out to detect abdominal distension, due for instance to ascites with ovarian cancer. During pregnancy it may be used to detect rapid increase that may be diagnostic of polyhydramnios.

abdominal hernia a hernia protruding through a defect or weakness in the abdominal wall, e.g. an umbilical hernia is a type of abdominal hernia.

abdominal injury damage to the abdomen and/or its contents, such may occur in a road traffic accident or violence. Can occur in sport, especially contact sports. Injury may be superficial, to the abdominal wall only, but significant trauma can damage the internal organs and lead to significant blood loss. Accumulation of blood in the abdominal cavity may be undetected, with potential fatality.

abdominal muscles the five pairs of muscles that form the abdominal wall. From the surface inwards they are the: rectus abdominis, external and internal obliques, transversus abdominis and the quadratus lumborum. The anterior abdominal wall is divided longitudinally by a very strong midline tendinous cord, the linea alba (meaning 'white cord') which extends from the xiphoid process of the sternum to the symphysis pubis. The structure of the abdominal wall on each side of the linea alba is identical. *rectus abdominis* is the most superficial muscle. It is broad and flat, originating from the transverse part of the pubic bone then passing upwards to be inserted into the lower ribs and the xiphoid process of the sternum. Medially the two muscles are attached to the linea alba. *external oblique* extends from the lower ribs downwards and forward to be inserted into the iliac crest and, by an aponeurosis, to the linea alba. *internal oblique* lies deep to the external oblique. Its fibres arise from the iliac crest and by a broad band of fascia from the spinous processes of the lumbar vertebrae. The fibres pass upwards towards the midline to be inserted into the lower ribs and, by an aponeurosis, into the linea alba. The fibres are at right angles to those of the external oblique. *transversus abdominis* is the deepest muscle of the abdominal wall. The fibres arise from the iliac crest and the lumbar vertebrae and pass across the abdominal wall to be inserted into the linea alba by an aponeurosis. The fibres are at right angles to those of the rectus abdominis. These paired muscles form the strong muscular anterior wall of the abdominal cavity. When the muscles contract together they compress the abdominal organs and flex the vertebral column in the lumbar region. Contraction of the muscles on one side only bends the trunk towards that side. Contraction of the oblique muscles on one side rotates the trunk. *quadratus lumborum* is a muscle of the back and forms the posterior wall. It originates from the iliac crest, then it passes upwards, parallel and close to the vertebral column and it is inserted into the 12th rib. Together the two muscles fix the lower rib during respiration and cause extension of the vertebral column (bending backwards). If one muscle contract is causes lateral flexion of the lumbar region of the vertebral column.

abdominal reflex a superficial reflex where the abdominal muscles contract when the skin is lightly stroked.

abdominal regions where the surface anatomy is divided into nine regions used to describe the location of organs or symptoms, such as pain. ⊃ Colour Section Figure 18a.

abdominal thrust a first aid measure for choking. The manoeuvre is never practised on volunteers. ⊃ Heimlich's manoeuvre, Appendix 10.

abdominal striae ⊃ striae.

abdominal wall defects neonatal defects which develop in utero, usually requiring immediate surgical intervention, e.g. exomphalos and gastroschisis.

abdomin/o- a prefix that means 'abdomen', e.g. *abdominopelvic*.

abdominocentesis *n* paracentesis (aspiration) of the peritoneal cavity. ⊃ amniocentesis, colpocentesis, thoracentesis.

abdominopelvic *adj* pertaining to the abdomen and pelvis or pelvic cavity.

abdominoperineal *adj* pertaining to the abdomen and perineum.

abdominoplasty *n* plastic surgical procedure used to tighten the abdominal muscles and remove surplus skin. It may be performed following a large reduction in weight that has resulted in a pendulous abdomen with the anterior abdominal wall hanging down over the pubis. It is also undertaken for cosmetic reasons. Known colloquially as a 'tummy tuck'.

abducens muscle an extraocular muscle. ⊃ lateral rectus muscle.

abducens nerve (abducent) the sixth pair of cranial nerves. They control the lateral rectus muscle of the eyeball, which turns the eyeball outwards.

abduct *vt* to draw away from the median line of the body ⊃ adduct *opp*.

abduction *n* the act of moving (or abducting) away from the midline. Such as moving the arm away from the body, or the outward rotation of the eyeball. ⊃ adduction *opp*.

abductor *n* a muscle which, on contraction, draws a part away from the median line of the body. ⊃ adductor *opp*. abductor digiti minimi, abductor hallucis, abductor pollicis brevis, abductor pollicis longus.

abductor digiti minimi small muscles in the feet and hands. In the foot its origin is on the calcaneus and it inserts onto the lateral side of the proximal phalanx of the fifth toe; it contracts to abduct the little toe. In the hand its origin is on the pisiform bone and the flexor retinaculum, and it inserts into the ulnar side of the base of the proximal phalanx; it contracts to abduct the little finger to the ulnar side.

abductor hallucis a muscle in the foot. Its origin is on the calcaneous and it inserts into the medial side of the proximal phalanx of the great toe; it contracts to abduct the great toe (especially in bare-footed people).

abductor pollicis brevis one of the thenar muscles in the hand. Its origin is on the scaphoid and flexor retinaculum, and it inserts into the radial side of the base of the first phalanx; it contracts to abduct the thumb and to abduct and rotate the first phalanx, thus aiding opposition of the thumb.

abductor pollicis longus one of the muscles of the extensor compartment of the forearm. Its origin is on both the ulna and radius and the interosseous membrane, and it inserts into the base of the first metacarpal; when it contracts alone the movement produced is between abduction and extension of the thumb. It can aid abduction and flexion of the wrist. ⊃ Colour Section Figure 4.

aberrant *adj* deviating from the normal; usually applied to a blood vessel or nerve which does not follow the normal course.

aberration *n* a deviation from normal—**aberrant** *adj*. ⊃ chromosomal aberration, optical aberration.

aberration prism additional effects of a prism on light, in addition to the expected change in direction of light. These effects include different magnifications, curvature of field and chromatic aberration.

aberrometry ⊃ wavefront aberration.

aberroscope an instrument for observing optical aberration. Such an instrument was designed by Tscherning to measure his own spherical aberration. It consists of a planoconvex lens with a grid made up of squares ruled on its plane surface.

ABGs *abbr* arterial blood gases.

ability *n* **1.** in sport, the physical and/or cognitive capability to perform a task without further training. ⊃ perceived ability, performance, skill. **2.** in occupational therapy practice, a personal characteristic that supports occupational performance. (Reproduced with permission from the European Network of Occupational Therapy in Higher Education (ENOTHE) Terminology Project, 2008.)

ablation *n* removal. In surgery, the word means excision or eradication (destruction). Various means of ablation exist, e.g. radiation, photocoagulation, etc.—**ablative** *adj*.

ablatio retinae ⊃ retinal detachment.

-able, -ible a suffix that means 'able to, capable of', e.g. *permeable*.

ablepharia *n* absence or partial absence of the eyelids.

ablepsia ⊃ visual impairment.

abnormal moulding ⊃ moulding.

abnormal retinal correspondence (ARC) (*syn*. anomalous retinal correspondence, retinal incongruity) a type of retinal correspondence in which the fovea of one eye is associated with an extrafoveal area of the other eye to give rise to a perception of a single object. This phenomenon is common in strabismus, but may also occur as a result of a macular lesion. ARC is often classified in three types: *harmonious* in which the angle of anomaly is equal to the objective angle of deviation—indicates that the ARC fully corresponds to the strabismus; *unharmonious* in which the angle of anomaly is less than the objective angle of deviation; *paradoxical*, when the angle of anomaly is greater than the objective angle of deviation. ARC can be detected by examination with a major amblyoscope, with the after-image test, or by comparison between the objective and the subjective angles of deviation measured with the alternate cover test and either a Maddox rod or the von Graefe's test, respectively (a difference between the objective and the subjective angles indicates ARC). ⊃ after-image test, angle of anomaly, Bagolini's glass, incongruous diplopia, phi movement, physiological diplopia.

ABO blood group system comprises four main blood groups – A, B, AB and O discovered in 1901 by Nobel laureate Karl Landsteiner (1868–1943). ⊃ anti-D, blood groups, Rhesus incompatibility.

ABO incompatibility in pregnancy occurs in about 1 in 200 pregnancies where the maternal blood group is O, the plasma containing anti-A and anti-B antibodies. If the fetus is group A, B or AB, an antibody differing immunologically from normal anti-A and anti-B may cross the placenta and cause haemolysis in the neonate, even in a first baby.

A
B

Jaundice appears within 24 hours of birth but is usually mild. The bilirubin level rises very rapidly but anaemia is less obvious. The Coombs' test is usually negative, unlike in Rhesus incompatibility. The jaundice is treated with phototherapy or, in severe cases, by exchange transfusion. ➲ blood groups, isoimmunization, Rhesus incompatibility isoimmunization.

abort *vt, vi* to terminate before full development.

abortifacient *adj* causing abortion, such as the drug mifepristone.

abortion *n* **1**. abrupt termination of a process. **2**. the induced expulsion from the uterus of the product of conception before viability by medical or surgical means. NB. The preferred term for unintentional loss of the product of conception prior to 24 weeks' gestation is miscarriage. *criminal abortion* intentional evacuation of the uterus by other than trained licensed personnel, or where abortion is prohibited by a country's law.

ABPA *abbr* allergic bronchopulmonary aspergillosis.

ABPI *abbr* ankle-brachial pressure index.

abrachia congenital absence of arms.

abrasion *n* **1**. superficial injury to skin or mucous membrane from scraping or rubbing; excoriation. **2**. abnormal wearing away of a substance or structure by a mechanical process. ➲ dental abrasion. **3**. a therapeutic procedure sometimes used for removal of scar tissue (dermabrasion).

abrasive in dentistry, a substance which wears away, scours or grinds down a surface, sometimes in preparation for polishing, e.g. diamonds, carborundum, sand, emery, garnet, pumice, cuttle. ➲ abrasive disc, abrasive paste, abrasive strip, abrasive wheel.

abrasive disc metal, plastic or cardboard disc having one surface carrying an abrasive, glued or bonded to it. Mounted on a mandrel, it may be used to abrade or polish restoration surfaces or to sharpen instruments. ➲ mandrel.

abrasive paste paste used for polishing or cleaning, e.g. prophylactic paste.

abrasive strip metal, linen or plastic strip coated with an abrasive on one or both sides and used to modify and polish the surface of a tooth or restoration.

abrasive wheel wheel-shaped rotary instrument containing an abrasive in a rubber base and used to shape and polish metal restorations and prostheses.

abruptio tearing asunder. *abruptio placentae* or *placental abruption* partial or complete separation of the placenta from its site, usually in the upper uterine segment, after 24 weeks of pregnancy, causing pain and haemorrhage. ➲ antepartum haemorrhage, Couvelaire uterus, placenta, placenta praevia.

abscess *n* localized collection of pus produced by pyogenic organisms. May be acute or chronic. An acute abscess is a relatively short-lived abscess accompanied by painful local inflammation. A chronic abscess is slow to develop and is accompanied by mild inflammation, it is slow to heal and generally draining through a sinus. ➲ blind abscess, Brodie's abscess, cold abscess, dentoalveolar abscess, periapical abscess, periodontal abscess, psoas abscess, pulp (or pupal) abscess.

absences (petit mal) ➲ epilepsy.

Absidia *n* a genus of fungus. Some species cause lung and ear infections in humans.

absolute detector efficiency the ability of a detector to measure the total events emitted by a source of ionizing radiation.

absolute glaucoma the final stage of the disease which has been either untreated or unsuccessfully treated. The eye is blind and hard, the optic disc is white and the pupil dilated.

absolute poverty ➲ poverty.

absolute refractive index ➲ refractive index.

absolute refractory period ➲ refractory period.

absolute risk reduction in a comparative study the difference in the event rate between the control group the group having the treatment.

absolute poverty ➲ poverty.

absolute threshold in psychophysics, the smallest magnitude of a sensory input that can be detected, typically defined as the magnitude that can be detected over a proportion of presentations (e.g. 75%). Also known as absolute limen. ➲ difference threshold.

absorbance spectrum ➲ absorption spectrum.

absorbed in radiology, describes when a photon interacts with an object and as a result loses all its energy.

absorbed dose in radiology, is the measure of the amount of radiation absorbed by an object. The SI unit is the gray (Gy).

absorbed fraction the quantity of radiation absorbed by the tissues in radionuclide imaging.

absorbent substance which attracts and takes up gases or liquids.

absorbent point ➲ paper points.

absorption **1**. the transformation of radiant energy into a different form of energy, usually heat, as it passes through a medium. Light that is absorbed is neither transmitted nor reflected. It may, however, be re-emitted as light of another wavelength as, for example, ultraviolet radiation is converted into visible radiation on absorption by a luminescent material. A substance that absorbs all radiations is called a black body. ➲ absorption factor, black body, fluorescence, optical density, transmission. **2**. in electrotherapy – absorption varies with the type, intensity and properties of the energy as well as the types and distribution of tissues through which it passes. Absorption is the inverse of penetration, therefore, higher frequency ultrasound (e.g. 3 MHz) with its shorter wavelength is absorbed more readily than lower frequency ultrasound (e.g. 1 MHz or less). **3**. a radiological term – in intensifying screens the incident photons are absorbed by the phosphor, 95% as a result of the photoelectric effect and 5% by the Compton scattering (effect). ➲ Compton scattering (effect), photoelectric absorption.

4. the incorporation of a fluid, gas or other substance into the body of a material or tissue.

absorption factor the ratio of the absorbed luminous flux to the incident flux.

absorption rate constant a value describing the amount of a drug absorbed in a unit of time.

absorption spectrum (*syn* absorbance spectrum) the curve representing the relative absorption of a pigment or chemical substance as a function of the wavelength of light. For example, the absorption spectrum of rhodopsin. ⊃ rhodopsin, visual pigment.

absorptive able to absorb, absorbent.

absorptive lens a lens which absorbs a proportion of the incident radiation. Some lenses absorb mostly in the infrared region of the spectrum, others absorb mostly in the ultraviolet region and others absorb more or less equally throughout the visible spectrum. ⊃ coated lens, infrared radiations/rays (IRR), light, pterygium, ultraviolet (UV) rays.

absorptive state the metabolic state immediately after a meal and continuing for about four hours. Absorbed nutrients are used as energy or to build up other substances through anabolic processes, such as glycogenesis. ⊃ postabsorptive state.

abstract a clear and concise summary of a research paper. It details the study design, results and implications for practice.

abulia (aboulia) *n* inability or reduced capacity to make decisions or to show initiative.

abuse *n* **1.** deliberate injury to another person. It may be either physical, sexual, psychological or through neglect, such as failure to feed or keep clean. The term can apply to any group of individuals, especially those most vulnerable, such as children, older people, and those with mental health problems or learning disabilities. ⊃ child abuse, elder abuse. **2.** misuse of equipment, drugs and other substances, power and position.

abut to have a common boundary. To touch or border upon.

abutment support to receive lateral and horizontal thrust. In dentistry, a tooth, crown or part of an implant used to provide support, stabilization, anchorage or retention for a fixed or removable prosthesis. *abutment replica* a prefabricated laboratory copy of an implant fixture or abutment that is combined with an impression coping prior to casting of an impression. The replica will then be cast within the stone model. *customizable abutment* an implant abutment that may be modified (trimmed) intra- or extraorally to allow placement of a definitive restoration. *custom made abutment* an implant abutment that has been made to order to fit an underlying implant fixture. *healing abutment* (*temporary abutment*) an abutment designed to be connected to an underlying implant fixture which sits transmucosally to allow healing of the soft tissues prior to the placement of a definitive abutment and restoration. *implant abutment* that part of an implant that supports a prosthesis.

AC *abbr* **1.** alternating current. **2.** approved clinician.

AC/A ratio ratio of the accommodative convergence AC (in prism dioptres) to the stimulus to accommodation A (in dioptres). The most common method of determining this ratio is by the gradient method (or gradient test) in which the phoria at near is measured after changing the accommodation with a spherical lens (usually $+1.00$ D or -1.00 D) placed in front of the two eyes. ⊃ accommodative convergence, prism dioptre, proximal convergence.

academic title the title of an academic member of staff, e.g. from most junior upwards—lecturer, senior (principal) lecturer, professor, dean, pro vice chancellor, provost, vice chancellor, chancellor.

academic unit the term used to describe a distinct academic part of a university, e.g. in progressive order of size—section, department, division, school, faculty, college.

acalculia *n* inability to do simple arithmetic.

Acanthamoeba *n* a genus of amoebae typically present in water and soil. May cause local infections or infections of the respiratory system, nervous system or genitourinary system.

acanthamoebiasis meningoencephalitis caused by *Acanthamoeba*. Cleaning contact lenses in water containing *Acanthamoeba* can cause keratitis and serious corneal ulceration.

acanth/o- a prefix that means 'spiny', e.g. *acanthosis*.

acanthosis thickening of the epidermis. There is diffuse proliferation of the cells in the prickle layer of the epidermis, associated with skin conditions, such as eczema.

acanthosis nigricans a velvety thickening and pigmentation of the major flexures, particularly the axillae and groin. There are several types of acanthosis nigricans: (a) the most common form is a weight-dependent mild acanthosis nigricans (obesity-associated). When the person loses weight the cutaneous features regress; (b) secondly, acanthosis nigricans can be associated with various syndromes, some of which have insulin resistance as a feature; (c) finally, acanthosis nigricans can be associated with malignancy, particularly gastric (60%). Pruritus is a feature of malignancy-associated acanthosis and regression occurs after the tumour is excised. Acanthosis nigricans sometimes recurs with metastatic disease. ⊃ insulin resistance, metabolic syndrome.

acapnia *n* ⊃hypocapnia.

acardia *n* absence of the heart. A rare congenital abnormality, except in conjoined twins where one twin has the heart which circulates blood to both twins. It can be detected by ultrasound scan and termination of pregnancy offered.

acardiac twin twin which develops without a viable cardiac structure; life is maintained in utero via the placental circulation of the other, viable twin.

acardius acephalus absence of heart, head and upper parts of the body.

acariasis *n* a condition caused by an acarid (mite), e.g. scrub typhus which is transmitted by mites.

acarid *n* a mite belonging to the order Acarina.

acatalasia (Takahara's disease) *n* a rare genetic condition caused by the lack of catalase activity. It is usually asymptomatic but can cause mouth ulceration.

ACBT *abbr* active cycle of breathing technique.

accelerated fractionation in radiotherapy it is the method of delivering small doses of radiation several times a day, over a reduced number of days compared with a standard course of treatment.

accelerating voltage the kilovoltage peak (kV_p) determining the minimum wavelength in the spectrum, in a constant potential unit it will be present throughout the exposure.

acceleration change in motion of a body or object: the rate of change of velocity with respect to time. ⊃ angular acceleration, gravitational acceleration, instantaneous acceleration, linear acceleration, tangential acceleration.

acceleration of labour ⊃ augmentation of labour.

acceleration phase period of labour during which the greatest cervical dilation is achieved, between 3 and 10 cm.

accelerator in radiology, a chemical that controls activity by assuring the correct pH values are maintained; in developer sodium or potassium hydroxide is used.

accelerator (promotor) in dentistry, substance used in small quantities to increase the rate of a chemical reaction. ⊃ catalyst.

acceptable daily intake (ADI) the quantity of a food additive that could be ingested daily for the entire lifespan without appreciable risk.

acceptance tests tests done on newly installed radiotherapy equipment and include checking that the agreed specification has been met with regard to the radiotherapy beam, movement of the tube stand, electrical aspects, radiation safety requirements and accessories.

access cavity in dentistry, coronal opening into a pulp cavity required for effective shaping, cleaning and filling of the pulp space during root canal treatment.

accessory bone the os trigonum in the ankle joint—a bone present in only <10% of the population. In practice, rarely injured in sport but can be confused on X-ray with an avulsed fragment of bone or loose body.

accessory lacrimal glands they are the glands of Krause and Wolfring. These glands are histologically identical to the main lacrimal gland, but are located within the eyelids. These glands are responsible for basal (not reflex) tear secretion and appear to be under sympathetic neural control. ⊃ tear secretion.

accessory motion sliding, gliding or rolling motion that occurs within and between joint surfaces during active or passive joint movement.

accessory nerve *n* sometimes referred to as the spinal accessory nerve. The eleventh pair of cranial nerves. They supply the muscles of the larynx and pharynx, and the muscles of the neck and shoulder, sternocleidomastoid and the trapezius muscles, to control movement of the head and shoulders.

accessory oculomotor nucleus ⊃ Edinger–Westphal nucleus.

accessory parasympathetic nucleus ⊃ Edinger–Westphal nucleus.

accessory placenta placental tissue supplementary to the main organ and connected to it by blood vessels.

Access to Health Records Act (1990) the Act allows access to both manual and computerized health records made after 1991, with certain exceptions. Patients must apply to gain access to their records. The Data Protection (Subject Access Modification) (Health) Order 1987 restricted access to health information which might cause serious physical or mental harm to an individual or reveal the identity of another person. ⊃ data protection legislation.

accident rates (in sport) accidents are common in sport, particularly in contact sports, and result in a significant workload for hospital emergency departments. Currently there are 20 million sports injuries in the UK each year, 50% of them football related, at an estimated cost in treatment and lost productivity of £1 billion.

acclimation *n* the chronic adaptation caused by artificially imposed stress, which mimics the natural environmental stress. In sport, the artificial approximation to natural acclimatization, to either heat or altitude, achieved by exposure in a thermal or hypobaric chamber for several hours a day, typically for 2–3 weeks before going to the challenging new environment.

acclimatization *n* the body's ability to adapt physiological processes in response to a change from the accustomed environment: to heat or cold, or to high altitude. For example, repeated exercise in the heat leads to an increase in maximal sweating rate, but with reduced sodium concentration in the sweat; low oxygen content in the blood at high altitude leads among other adjustments to increased breathing and cardiac output, assisting oxygen supply. ⊃ altitude acclimatization, heat acclimatization.

accommodating resistance muscle activity during which the resistance provided changes as the muscle moves through its range of motion. Also known as isokinetic activity.

accommodation *n* **1.** the adjustment of the dioptric power of the eye. It is generally involuntary and made to see clearly objects at any distance. In humans, this adjustment is brought about by a change in the shape of the crystalline lens. The normal or positive accommodation that occurs when looking from a distant to a near object. ⊃ accommodation reflex, ciliary muscle, Fincham's theory, Helmholtz's theory of accommodation, mechanism of accommodation, objective accommodation, subjective accommodation. **2.** decreased sensitivity to stimuli demonstrated by neurons that have been exposed to subthreshold stimuli for long periods of time.

accommodation lag 1. (*syn* lazy lag of accommodation) the amount by which the accommodative response of the eye is less than the dioptric stimulus to accommodation. **2.** the condition occurring in dynamic retinoscopy in which the neutral point is situated further from the eyes than is the retinoscopic target. ⊃ accommodation lead, ciliary muscle, dynamic retinoscopy.

accommodation lead the amount by which the accommodative response of the eye is greater than the dioptric stimulus to accommodation. ⊃ accommodation lag.

accommodative convergence (*syn* accommodative vergence, associative convergence) that component of convergence which occurs reflexly in response to a change in accommodation. It is easily demonstrated by having one eye fixate from a far point to a near point along its line of sight, while the other eye is occluded. The occluded eye will be seen to make a convergence movement in response to the accommodation. Alternatively, one eye fixates while the other is occluded. If a minus lens is placed in front of the fixating eye, the occluded eye will be seen to converge. ➲ fusional convergence, initial convergence, motor fusion, proximal convergence, tonic vergence.

accommodative facility (*syn* accommodative rock) the ability of the eye(s) to focus on stimuli at various distances and in different sequences in a given period of time. Clinically, this is measured either monocularly or binocularly usually by having the subject fixate a small target alternately through plus and minus lenses which are interchanged as soon as the target appears clear. The operation is repeated many times and the results are commonly presented in cycles per minute (one cycle indicates that both plus and minus lenses have been cleared). ➲ accommodative insufficiency, lens flippers.

accommodative insufficiency (*syn* premature presbyopia) an insufficient amplitude of accommodation which is unequivocally below the appropriate level for the age. It may be due to extreme fatigue, influenza, high stress, systemic medication, ocular inflammation, head trauma, thyroid disease or type 1 diabetes mellitus. The condition is often associated with convergence insufficiency, general fatigue, measles, multiple sclerosis, myotonic dystrophy, etc. It is the most common accommodative dysfunction. Patients complain of blurred vision, or difficulty in sustaining clear vision at near; this is often accompanied by a frontal headache and even sometimes by pain in the eye. A mild form of convergence insufficiency is often referred to as ill-sustained accommodation in which the response may be initially normal but cannot be maintained. It is easily discovered with accommodative facility exercises. Ill-sustained accommodation may be a precursor of accommodative insufficiency. Treatment is aimed at the primary cause, but plus lens correction, and in some cases exercises such as accommodative facility training are prescribed. ➲ accommodative facility, convergence insufficiency, ocular headache, presbyopia, thyroid ophthalmopathy.

accommodative reflex (*syn.* near reflex; near-triad reflex; synkinetic near reflex) the reflex evoked by a blurred retinal image, as when fixating from far to near. It consists of three responses: increased convexity of the crystalline lens; constriction of the pupils; and convergence of the eyes. This reflex is not a pure reflex since each of the three components can act independently of the other two; convergence by means of prisms, accommodation by means of lenses and miosis by light stimulation.

accommodative response the response of the accommodative system when the eye changes fixation from one point in space to another. The reaction time for the accommodative response is about 370 ms. Clinically it can be estimated by measuring the accommodative lag or accommodative lead. ➲ accommodation lag, accommodation lead, accommodative reflex, Mandelbaum effect, mechanism of accommodation.

accommodative rock ➲ accommodative facility.

accommodative vergence ➲ accommodative convergence.

accouchement *n* delivery in childbirth. Confinement.

accoucheur a professionally trained person who attends women in childbirth; midwife or obstetrician.

accountability *n* health professionals have a duty to care according to law. In some countries the statutory body, and/or the professional organization, develop a code of conduct via which each practitioner can accept responsibility and accountability for the professional service delivered to each patient/client. ➲ duty of care, malpractice, negligence.

accreditation process of evaluation of an institution or individual in order to obtain official recognition of standards set against agreed criteria, e.g. education.

accreditation of prior experiential learning (APEL) credit is awarded towards a current programme of study for previously acquired professional experience which has not been formally assessed; this may entail completing a professional development portfolio.

accreditation of prior learning (APL) system in which credit is awarded towards a current programme of study for courses or modules which have been previously completed.

accretion *n* an increase of substance or deposit round a central object, e.g. plaque and calculus on teeth—**accrete** *adj*, *vt*, *vi*, **accretive** *adj*.

accuracy in radiology, the ability of a detector to correctly indicate dose.

ACD *abbr* anaemia of chronic disease.

ACE inhibitor *acron* Angiotensin-Converting-Enzyme inhibitor.

acellular 1. free from cells. In medicine a vaccine may be described as acellular if it contains no cells. 2. not characterized by a cellular structure. An organism which is not divided into cells, often referred to as unicellular or single-celled.

acentric 1. in genetics, describes a chromosome fragment without a centromere. 2 without a centre.

acephalous *adj* without a head.

acesulfame-potassium intense sweetener with approximately 130 times the sweetness of sucrose (beet or cane sugar). Commonly used in low calorie soft drinks. ➲ sweeteners.

acetabular labrum a fibrocartilaginous ring attached around the margin of the acetabulum in the pelvis, it serves to deepen the socket and aids joint stability. The glenoid of the shoulder also possesses a labrum.

acetabul/o- a prefix that means 'acetabulum', e.g. *acetabular.*

acetabuloplasty *n* an operation to improve the depth and shape of the hip socket (acetabulum); necessary in such conditions as developmental dysplasia of the hip and osteo-arthritis of the hip.

acetabulum *n* a cup-like socket on the external lateral surface of the pelvis into which the head of the femur fits and articulates to form the hip joint—**acetabula** *pl*.

acetate *n* a salt of acetic acid.

acetic acid an organic acid present in vinegar. Used in radiology as the acid in fixing solutions and is used in combination with aluminium chloride as the hardener.

acetoacetate *n* an acidic ketone produced during an intermediate stage of fat oxidation in the body. Some can be utilized as a fuel by tissues, such as the kidney. In situations where carbohydrate molecules are not available for metabolism, such as in diabetes mellitus or starvation, excess is produced and the high levels in the blood result in ketoacidosis with severe disturbances of pH, fluid and electrolytes.

acetonaemia *n* ⊃ ketonaemia.

acetone *n* inflammable liquid with odour of 'pear drops'; used as a solvent. *acetone bodies* ⊃ ketones.

acetonuria *n* acetone and other ketones in the urine. ⊃ ketonuria—**acetonuric** *adj*.

acetylcholine (ACh) *n* a chemical neurotransmitter released from nerve endings to allow the transmission of a nerve impulse at the neuromuscular junction in voluntary (skeletal) muscle, in preganglionic sympathetic neurons and across all synapses in parasympathetic neurons. The nerve fibres releasing this chemical are described as 'cholinergic'. Cholinergic receptors occur in two different pharmacological groups: nicotinic, e.g. at skeletal muscle motor endplates, and muscarinic, e.g. in cardiac and smooth muscles. Acetylcholine is broken down into choline and acetate by the enzyme acetylcholinesterase. ⊃ myasthenia gravis, neurotransmitters.

acetylcholinesterase *n* enzyme that inactivates acetylcholine following the transmission of a nerve impulse across the synapse.

acetyl coenzyme A (*syn* acetyl-CoA) a molecule formed from coenzyme A linked with an acetyl group. An important metabolic intermediate, involved in various metabolic pathways, including glycolysis, fatty acid oxidation and degradation of some amino acids. It also represents a key intermediate in lipid biosynthesis. ⊃ Krebs' cycle.

acetylsalicylic acid better known as aspirin. Developed by the pharmaceutical group Bayer in Germany in 1899. Used at lower doses (2–3 g per day) as an analgesic and antipyretic. At higher doses (>4 g per day) it is a very powerful anti-inflammatory agent and therefore effective in soft tissue injury, but its use is limited by side effects, especially those affecting the gastrointestinal tract. ⊃ acetylsalicylic acid burn, non-steroidal anti-inflammatory drugs.

acetylsalicylic acid burn an opaque, wrinkled, sloughing burn produced within 30 minutes if aspirin tablet remains on the mucous membrane of the mouth.

ACG *abbr* angle-closure glaucoma.

ACh *abbr* acetylcholine.

ACH index arm, chest, hip index.

achalasia *n* loss of oesophageal peristalsis and failure of lower oesophageal sphincter relaxation. ⊃ cardiomyotomy.

achievement goal a goal focused on demonstrating high ability to oneself or others, or to avoid demonstrating low ability.

achievement goal orientation a person's general tendency to act in an ego-involved or task-involved manner.

achievement motivation form of motivation characterized by a competitive drive to meet high standards of performance, also known as need for achievement.

Achilles tendon also known as tendo calcaneus. The tendinous termination of the soleus and gastrocnemius muscles inserted into the heel bone (os calcis, calcaneus or calcaneum) (Figure A.1). The tendon is commonly injured in sport either by direct trauma (resulting in partial or complete rupture) or by repeated micro-trauma or overuse resulting in inflammation. The test that diagnoses a ruptured Achilles tendon is the Thompson test. ⊃ Achilles tendonitis (tendinitis), Thompson test.

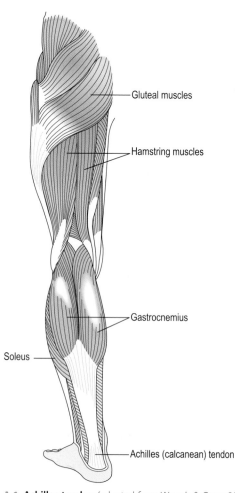

A.1 Achilles tendon (adapted from Waugh & Grant 2006 with permission).

Achilles tendonitis (tendinitis) inflammation of the Achilles tendon. It is most commonly the result of poor technique, poor footwear, hard running surface, high-intensity or long-distance running. Treatment is with RICE, anti-inflammatory medication, a heel raise and correction of causes. Surgery may be required in severe cases.

achlorhydria *n* the absence of gastric acid (hydrochloric). Found in pernicious anaemia and gastric cancer—**achlorhydric** *adj*.

acholia *n* the absence of bile—**acholic** *adj*.

acholuria *n* the absence of bile pigments from the urine. ⊃ jaundice—**acholuric** *adj*.

achondroplasia *n* an inherited condition characterized by arrested growth of the long bones resulting in short-limbed dwarfism with a large head. The intellect is not impaired. Inheritance is dominant—**achondroplastic** *adj*.

achromasia ⊃ achromatopsia.

achromat ⊃ achromatic lens.

achromatic *adj* the condition of being totally colour blind. ⊃ achromatic lens, achromatopsia, equal energy spectrum, white light.

achromatic axis a line in the eye along which light passes through all the optical elements and emerges without chromatic dispersion. Although it may lie close to the optical axis it does not necessarily coincide with it. ⊃ chromatic chromostereopsis, chromatic parallax, dispersion.

achromatic lens (*syn* achromat) a compound lens designed to reduce or eliminate chromatic aberrations. The most common type is called a doublet. ⊃ apochromatic lens, doublet, hyperchromatic lens.

achromatic prism a prism that deviates light without dispersion. It consists of two prisms, usually one of crown glass and the other of flint, of equal angular dispersions and mounted so that the apex of one is against the base of the other. ⊃ dispersion.

achromatic vision ⊃ achromatopsia.

achromatism ⊃ achromatopsia.

achromatizing lens a lens aimed at reducing or eliminating the chromatic aberration of the eye. It consists of either a doublet or a triplet which possesses longitudinal chromatic aberration opposite to that of the eye and thereby neutralizes it. Thus the lens system has negative power for short wavelengths and positive power for long wavelengths of an amount similar to that of the eye for those wavelengths. ⊃ doublet, longitudinal chromatic aberration, triplet.

achromatopsia *n* (*syn.* achromasia, achromatic vision, achromatism, acritochromacy, monochromatism) the inability to see colours. Total colour blindness. ⊃ defective colour vision, monochromat.

acid *n* **1**. any substance that has an excess of hydrogen ions over hydroxyl ions, e.g. hydrochloric acid. They have a pH below 7 and turn blue litmus red. They react with alkalis to form salts plus water. **2**. in radiography, the chemical in the fixer solution that neutralizes the alkaline developer as soon as the film reaches the fixing tank and therefore prevents further development, the acid used is either acetic acid or sulphuric acid and depends on the hardener used.

acidaemia *n* a high level of acid (hydrogen ions) in the blood resulting in a below normal blood pH <7.35 (hydrogen ion concentration >44 mmol/L) —**acidaemic** *adj*. acid–base balance, acidosis, arterial blood gases, metabolic acidosis, respiratory acidosis.

acid-alcohol-fast *adj* in microbiology, describes a micro-organism which, when stained, is resistant to decolorization by alcohol as well as acid, e.g. *Mycobacterium tuberculosis*. ⊃ Ziehl–Neelsen technique.

acid–base balance refers to the mechanisms that keep body fluids close to their normal pH (i.e. neither too alkaline nor too acidic), vital for normal cellular function. The equilibrium between the acid and base elements of the blood and body fluids. The net rate at which acids or bases are produced in the body is equal to the net rate at which acids and bases are excreted. Four primary acid–base disturbances disrupting the balance, with changes to pH, $PaCO_2$ and PaO_2, are recognized. They are respiratory acidosis, respiratory alkalosis, metabolic acidosis and metabolic alkalosis. ⊃ acidosis, alkalosis, arterial blood gases, metabolic acidosis, metabolic alkalosis, respiratory acidosis, respiratory alkalosis.

acid bath in dentistry, acid solution, generally 50% hydrochloric or sulphuric acid, used to cleanse the surface of a metal casting of its oxide coating. The process is known as *pickling*. The casting is placed in the acid in a test tube and heated. Boiling should be avoided because of the acid fumes evolved.

acid etchant liquid or gel form, typically 37% phosphoric acid, used in bonding resins to tooth structure. Modifies and roughens dentine and enamel surfaces.

acid etching in dentistry, the partial demineralization of a selected area of tooth substance by the use of dilute acid, usually phosphoric acid, in order to provide a clean and mechanically retentive surface for the retention of selected types of restorative materials such as composite, glass ionomer cements or orthodontic brackets and sealant.

acid-fast *adj* in microbiology, describes a micro-organism which, when stained, does not become decolorized when washed with dilute acids.

acid-fast bacilli (AFB) a type of bacteria identified using acid-fast techniques, for example *Mycobacterium tuberculosis*.

acid foods, basic (alkaline) foods describes the residue of the metabolism of different foods. Foods containing phosphorus, sulphur and chlorine are acid-forming while those containing sodium, potassium, calcium and magnesium are base-forming. The predominate foods in the diet determines the nature of the residue; meat, cheese, eggs and cereals produce an acidic residue, whereas milk, vegetables and some fruits leave a basic (alkaline) residue.

acidity *n* the state of being acid or sour. The degree of acidity can be measured on the pH scale where a pH below 7 is acid and pH 6 denotes a weak acid and pH 1 a strong acid.

acidogenic theory most commonly accepted theory on the aetiology of dental caries, postulated by W Miller in 1890. According to Miller, plaque bacteria metabolize refined carbohydrates to produce acid which demineralizes enamel.

acidosis *n* process leading to the accumulation of excess acid in the body (acidaemia). It may have a metabolic or respiratory cause—**acidotic** *adj*. ⊃ acid–base balance, acidaemia, ketoacidosis, ketosis, metabolic acidosis, respiratory acidosis.

acid phosphatase *n* an enzyme which synthesizes phosphate esters of carbohydrates in an acid medium. An increase of this enzyme in the blood may be indicative of cancer of the prostate gland.

acid–pumice microabrasion a technique using a strong acid (hydrochloric or phosphoric) and pumice for controlled removal of surface enamel to improve the aesthetics of teeth with dental opacities and hypoplasia. Often used to treat dental fluorosis.

acidulated rendered acidic in reaction.

acidulated phosphate fluoride (APF) sol, gel or foam preparation professionally applied to cleaned teeth, usually for 4 minutes in a tray, to reduce dental caries incidence.

aciduria *n* excretion of an acid urine. It can be caused by the intake of acid-forming foods, inborn errors of metabolism and certain medications.

acinar secretion the saliva formed in the acinus that has a similar ionic composition to that of blood plasma and tissue fluid. ⊃ serous secretion.

Acinetobacter *n* a genus of aerobic bacteria of the family Neisseriaceae. They cause infections that include wound infection, pneumonia and meningitis. The micro-organism has developed antibiotic resistance and is a particular danger to critically ill patients who require intensive or high dependency care.

acini *npl* minute saccules or alveoli, lined or filled with secreting cells. Several acini combine to form a lobule—**acinus** *sing*, **acinous, acinar** *adj*.

ACJ *abbr* acromioclavicular joint.

ACL *abbr* anterior cruciate ligament.

acme *n* **1**. the highest point. **2**. crisis or critical point of a disease.

acne, acne vulgaris *n* a condition in which the pilosebaceous units are overstimulated by circulating androgens and the excessive sebum is trapped by a plug of keratin, one of the protein constituents of human skin. Skin bacteria then colonize the glands and convert the trapped sebum into irritant fatty acids responsible for the swelling and inflammation (pustules) which follow. Treatment options include topical benzoyl peroxide, topical or oral antibiotics, topical azelaic acid, topical or oral retinoids, or anti-androgen hormone therapy (for young women). ⊃ Colour Section Figure 43.

acne rosacea a skin disorder that results from chronic inflammation of the cheeks, nose, chin, forehead and or eyelids. It is treated with antibiotics.

acneiform *adj* resembling acne.

acorea the absence of the pupil of the eye.

acoustic *adj* pertaining to sound or the sense of hearing.

acoustic cavitation a potential biological effect of ultrasound imaging, marked by large amplitude oscillations of microscopic gas bubbles.

acoustic enhancement an artefact that occurs in ultrasound imaging when an object with a low level of absorption causes objects which are further away from the probe to be brighter than they should be.

acoustic impedance (Z) the term describing the resistance of tissues to the passage of ultrasound. A value given to a substance and is calculated by multiplying the density of the medium by the velocity of the ultrasound travelling through the medium and is independent of frequency.

acoustic neuroma a benign tumour (schwannoma) affecting the eighth cranial nerve (vestibulocochlear nerve) as it passes through the skull into the brainstem, causing problems in hearing and balance. It usually presents with hearing loss in the side affected. Other symptoms can occur especially as it grows and presses on the trigeminal nerve, including dizziness, poor balance, facial pain and tinnitus. It is usually successfully removed by surgery, but in many cases the hearing loss is permanent. The main complication of surgery is damage to the facial nerve for which the patient may be referred to physiotherapy.

acoustic shadow in ultrasound imaging, the absence of echoes produced by a dense structure such as a calculus (stone) which prevents the transmission of ultrasound waves by reflection.

acoustic shadowing tissues and structures which reflect or absorb ultrasound, for example gallstones, will cast a shadow on the image. The tissue interface has to be similar to or larger than the ultrasound beam to cause shadowing.

acoustic streaming the unidirectional movement of fluid in an ultrasound field. It is thought to stimulate cell activity if it occurs at boundaries, such as between the cell membrane and surrounding tissue fluid. It may alter cell membrane permeability resulting in: increased protein synthesis; increased secretion from mast cells; increased mobility of fibroblasts; and release of growth factors by macrophages.

acoustic window an area of the body used to allow imaging of underlying structures, for example, the intercostal spaces between the ribs, the liver.

ACPSM *abbr* Association of Chartered Physiotherapists in Sports Medicine.

acquired aplastic anaemia (secondary aplasia) the causes of this condition include: (a) drugs—cytotoxic drugs (idiosyncratic), antibiotics (e.g. chloramphenicol, sulphonamides), antirheumatic agents (e.g. penicillamine, gold, phenylbutazone, indometacin), antithyroid drugs, anticonvulsants, immunosuppressives (e.g. azathioprine); (b) chemicals—benzene toluene solvent misuse, insecticides (e.g. chlorinated hydrocarbons [DDT], organophosphates and carbamates); (c) radiation; (d) viral hepatitis; (e) pregnancy; (f) paroxysmal nocturnal haemoglobinuria. It is not practical to list all the drugs which have been suspected of causing aplasia. It is important to check the reported side-effects of all drugs taken over the preceding months. In some instances the cytopenia is more selective and affects only one cell line, most often the neutrophils. Frequently, this is an incidental finding with no ill health. It probably has an immune basis but this is difficult to prove. The clinical features and methods of diagnosis are the same as for primary idiopathic aplastic anaemia. An underlying cause should be treated or removed but otherwise management is as for the idiopathic form.

acquired haemolytic anaemia ⊃ autoimmune haemolytic anaemia, non-immune haemolytic anaemia.

acquired immune deficiency syndrome (AIDS) a term used to denote a particular stage of infection with human immunodeficiency virus (HIV). The Centers for Disease Control and Prevention (CDC) define AIDS as the development of an AIDS-defining illness in a patient with HIV infection. A low CD4+ T cell count of less than 200 per μL (or less than 14% of lymphocytes) in an HIV-positive person is also regarded as AIDS-defining, regardless of symptoms or opportunistic infections.

acquired megacolon ⊃ megacolon.

acquired myopathies muscle weakness caused by a range of metabolic, endocrine and inflammatory disorders, and a wide range of toxins and drugs. Causes include: (a) inflammatory—polymyositis, dermatomyositis; (b) endocrine and metabolic—hypothyroidism, hyperthyroidism, acromegaly, Cushing's syndrome (including iatrogenic), Addison's disease, Conn's syndrome, osteomalacia, hypokalaemia (liquorice, diuretic and purgative misuse), hypercalcaemia (disseminated body metastases); (c) toxic—alcohol (both chronic and acute syndromes), vitamin E toxicity, organophosphates, snake venom; (d) drugs—ε-aminocaproic acid, amiodarone, β-blockers, chloroquine, ciclosporin, clofibrate, corticosteroids (especially fluorinated), opiates, statins, vincristine, zidovudine; (e) paraneoplastic—carcinomatous neuromyopathy, dermatomyositis. Disorders affecting the muscles' structural integrity can be distinguished by electromyogram (EMG) from those caused by metabolic derangement. In metabolic disorders, weakness is often acute and generalized, while a proximal myopathy predominantly affecting the pelvic girdle is a feature of some endocrine disorders. This may develop without other manifestations of hormonal disturbance.

acritochromacy ⊃ achromatopsia.

acro- a prefix that means 'extremity', e.g. *acrodynia.*

acrocentric *adj* describes a chromosome that has the centromere at or close to one end.

acrocephalia; acrocephaly *n* a congenital malformation whereby the top of the head is pointed and the eyes protrude, due to premature closure of sagittal and coronal skull sutures—**acrocephalic, acrocephalous** *adj.*

acrocephalosyndactyly *n* a congenital malformation consisting of a pointed top of head, with fusion of fingers and/or toes. ⊃ Apert's syndrome.

acrocyanosis *n* coldness and blueness of the extremities due to circulatory disorder—**acrocyanotic** *adj.*

acrodermatitis enteropathica *n* an inherited disorder of zinc malabsorption. The zinc deficiency leads to vesicles and bullae affecting the skin and mucosae, poor growth, chronic diarrhoea and alopecia. Treatment is with zinc supplements.

acrodynia *n* acute, painful reddening of the extremities, such as occurs in erythroedema polyneuropathy.

acromegaly *n* enlargement of the hands, face and feet, occurring due to excess growth hormone in an adult, almost always from a pituitary adenoma. Treatment may be with drugs, radiation or surgery—**acromegalic** *adj.*

acromicria *n* smallness of the hands, face and feet.

acromioclavicular *adj* pertaining to the acromion process (of scapula) and the clavicle.

acromioclavicular joint (ACJ) the small synovial joint between the acromion process of the scapula and the end of the clavicle, linking them to form the shoulder girdle. Parts of the trapezius and deltoid muscles are attached to the joint capsule. Commonly injured in contact sports especially rugby football.

acromion *n* the point or summit of the shoulder: the triangular process at the extreme outer end of the spine of the scapula—**acromial** *adj.*

acropachy clubbing and enlargement of the extremities. A rare sign associated with hyperthyroidism.

acrophobia *n* morbid fear of being at a height.

acrosome *n* structure surrounding the nucleus of a spermatozoon. It contains lytic enzymes, which when released by many spermatozoa (during the acrosome reaction) facilitate the penetration of an oocyte by a single spermatozoon.

acrylamide *n* chemical formed when starchy foods, such as crisps and chips, are cooked at high temperatures.

acrylic referring to synthetic resins derived from acrylic acid and used in the manufacture of medical and dental prostheses.

acrylic denture denture made from acrylic resin.

acrylic resin ⊃ resin.

acrylic trimmer in dentistry, a rotary instrument used to remove and shape acrylic resin. Manufactured in various shapes and may be of steel or an abrasive material having a wide pore structure (pumice-like).

ACTH *abbr* adrenocorticotrophic hormone.

actin *n* a globular contractile protein which readily links with other proteins (with consumption of energy in the form of adenosine triphosphate [ATP]) to form long, double-helical strands. Such actin filaments are found in a wide variety of animal and plant cells, as well as forming the structural core and main (but not only) component of the thin filaments in the myofibrils of all animal muscles. Actin is thus a protein of great evolutionary antiquity and vertebrate striated muscles are unusual only in having a very high content of it (80% of total protein), and in its highly ordered locations within the cells, where thin filaments alternate with thick filaments containing the protein myosin, to form the cross-striated pattern. ⊃ myosin, tropomyosin, troponin.

acting out reducing distress by the release of disturbed or violent behaviour, which is unconsciously determined and reflects previous unresolved conflicts and attitudes.

actinic pertaining to the chemical activity of radiant energy (especially ultraviolet) on absorption by certain substances. In the eye, the cornea, in particular, but also the lens and retina are most susceptible. ⊃ actinic keratoconjunctivitis.

actinic dermatoses skin conditions in which the integument is abnormally sensitive to ultraviolet radiation.

actinic keratoconjunctivitis inflammation of the cornea and conjunctiva caused by exposure to ultraviolet light as, for example, from sun lamps, welder's arc or reflection from the snow. Both cornea and conjunctiva are usually involved although one tissue may be more affected than the other, hence the terms 'actinic conjunctivitis' or 'actinic keratitis'. Some time after exposure (4–8 hours) to the ultraviolet radiations, the patient experiences a marked sandy feeling in the eye, lacrimation, photophobia, blepharospasm, with congestion of the conjunctiva and swelling of the eyelids. The condition is usually self-limited and heals within 48 hours. Symptoms are relieved with cold compresses, firm patching and an analgesic. A local anaesthetic may sometimes be used but this delays the regeneration of the corneal epithelium and is not usually recommended. A topical antibiotic may also be used to prevent secondary infection. Sunglasses or suitable protection may prevent the condition. Also known as: arc eye, flash blindness, photokeratitis, photokeratoconjunctivitis, photophthalmia, snow blindness (although this is not a strictly correct synonym it is often used as such), sun lamp conjunctivitis, ultraviolet keratitis. ⊃ actinic, blepharospasm, ultraviolet radiation (UVR).

actinism *n* the chemical action of radiant energy, especially in the ultraviolet spectrum—**actinic** *adj*.

actinobiology *n* study of the effects of radiation on living organisms.

Actinomyces *n* a genus of branching micro-organisms. *Actinomyces israeli* causes disease in humans. ⊃ actinomycosis.

actinomycosis *n* a disease caused by *Actinomyces israeli*, the sites most affected being the face, neck, lung and abdomen. When it affects the jaw it is also known as '*wooden*' or '*lumpy*' jaw. There is pus containing yellow 'sulphur granules', abscess formation with sinuses and necrosis—**actinomycotic** *adj*.

actinotherapy *n* electrotherapy term. An alternative name for ultraviolet radiations (UVR) used therapeutically in certain skin disorders.

action *n* the activity or function of any part of the body. ⊃ specific action.

action potential change in electrical potential and charge that occurs across excitable cell membranes during the transmission of an electrical impulse along an axon, i.e. nerve impulse conduction or when muscles contract (Figure A.2). Initiated by a receptor (e.g. pain receptors in the skin, afferent nerve) or centrally (e.g. at spinal level if motor nerve, efferent nerve). The impulse is an electrochemical change, an action potential, that can travel proximally or distally

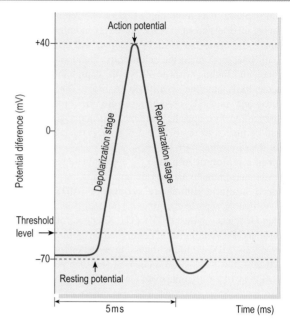

A.2 **Action potential** (reproduced from Brooker & Nicol 2003 with permission).

along the axon. The action potential has five distinct phases: normal state (potential difference inside the axon with respect to outside); depolarization (if increasing level of sodium ions inside axon membrane and proportionately fewer potassium ions is sufficient, nerve reaches 'threshold' and action potential is inevitable – 'All or none law'); peak (overshoot of charge – to same level irrespective of strength of stimulus); absolute refractory period (stimulation not possible as ion balance starts to revert to normal state); relative refractory period (stimulation possible but requires high intensity stimulus); normal state (stable ion balance level). ⊃ nerve impulse.

action research a type of social research involving a systematic and planned implementation of a cycle of social interventions and an evaluation of the change within the environment/situation being researched. The aims are to solve practical problems within the environment/situation and augment knowledge.

activated partial thromboplastin time (APTT) a test of blood coagulation ability.

activator *n* **1.** a substance which renders something else active, e.g. the hormone secretin, the enzyme enterokinase—**activate** *v*. **2.** in radiology, impurities which stimulate the phosphor of an intensifying screen to emit light.

activator (orthodontics) myofunctional removable orthodontic appliance constructed to lie in contact with all or part of the teeth in both dental arches. It does not fit firmly to the teeth and provides its activation by displacing muscles in and around the mouth from their natural resting position, e.g. Fraenkel, monobloc and Andresen appliances. ⊃ orthodontic appliance.

active *adj* energetic. ➲ passive *opp*.

active hyperaemia ➲ hyperaemia.

active immunity immunity which is acquired, naturally during an infection or artificially by immunization. It involves the production of antibodies and specific T cells in response to exposure to an antigenic stimulus. The primary response to exposure is followed by a 2–3 week lag phase before enough antibodies are produced, but the secondary response following a subsequent exposure is more intense and has a much reduced lag phase because the memory cells are able to produce antibodies very quickly. This type of immunity tends to be of long duration. ➲ immunity.

active assisted movement exercise that involves the person's own efforts combined with assistance from the therapist or the use of equipment. ➲ active movement, movement classification, passive movement, resisted movement.

active cycle of breathing technique (ACBT) techniques used to clear excessive pulmonary secretions in people with dyspnoea. The techniques include control of breathing, chest expansion exercises and 'huffing' out through the mouth. Great care is needed in patients prone to bronchospasm because strenuous huffing and insufficient relaxation between techniques can lead to bronchospasm. Care should also be taken post-operatively as patients tire easily. ➲ forced expiration technique.

active eruption normal movement of an erupting tooth into the oral cavity.

active insufficiency affects muscles that span two joints, it occurs when the muscle cannot contract maximally across both joints at the same time. An example would be the finger flexors. When you make a strong fist, you may notice that the wrist is in a neutral or an extended position. Now, if you attempt to actively flex your wrist joint whilst keeping your fingers flexed, you will find that the strength of the grip is greatly diminished. This is because the wrist and finger flexors are unable to shorten any further and, therefore, the fingers begin to extend or lose grip strength. ➲ passive insufficiency.

active management of labour obstetric intervention to prevent prolonged labour and its complications. First stage delay may be diagnosed from the partogram and may be accelerated by amniotomy (artificial rupture of membranes) and/or oxytocic infusion. ➲ augmentation of labour. The midwife's responsibilities include monitoring progress and carrying out medical instructions for the care of these women.

active management of third stage of labour involves administration of an oxytocic injection (e.g. Syntometrine®) to facilitate placental separation, either with crowning of the head or delivery of anterior shoulder; placental separation occurs within 2 ½ minutes, then the midwife can manually deliver placenta and membranes. ➲ controlled cord traction.

active movement movement performed by a person unaided by any external factor or influence. ➲ active assisted movement, active range of motion, movement classification, passive movement, resisted movement.

active principle an ingredient which gives a complex drug its chief therapeutic value, e.g. atropine is the active principle in belladonna.

active range of motion (AROM) the movement of a joint without assistance through a range of motion. Those produced by patients using their own neuromuscular mechanisms.

active transport movement of substances across cell membranes that requires the use of energy, usually adenosine triphosphate (ATP). For example moving substances against a concentration gradient. Substances transported by active transport include nutrients and ions, e.g. the sodium-potassium pump in cell membranes. ➲ diffusion, filtration, osmosis.

activins glycoproteins secreted by the pituitary gland, the ovaries, testes and other structures. They act locally to stimulate the production of follicle stimulating hormone, and have wider effects on cell differentiation and the development of the embryo. ➲ inhibins.

activities of daily living (ADLs) the things that a person does every day that are necessary to maintain personal health and wellbeing, such as cooking, eating and washing. ➲ DADL, IADL, PADL.

activities of daily living (ADLs) assessment and training the formal and informal evaluation of a person's ability to perform activities of daily living followed by a therapy/treatment programme designed to maintain or improve function.

Activities of Living (ALs) those activities that meet the holistic needs of an individual, e.g. breathing, working and playing, etc. They form the basis of some commonly used behavioural models of nursing. For example, the Roper, Logan and Tierney model which has twelve ALs; breathing, communication, controlling body temperature, dying, eating and drinking, elimination, expressing sexuality, maintaining a safe environment, mobilizing, personal cleansing and dressing, sleeping and working and playing.

activity a structured series of actions or tasks that contribute to occupations. (Reproduced with permission from the European Network of Occupational Therapy in Higher Education (ENOTHE) Terminology Project, 2008.)

activity adaptation modifying the components or task sequence of an activity to meet the needs, skills, interests and values of the client.

activity analysis the process of identifying the inherent properties and task sequence of an activity for the purposes of ascertaining the skills required for its performance and its potential as a therapeutic medium.

activity components the building blocks of activity that include skills, movements, task sequence, techniques, tools, materials, people and physical environment.

activity grading adapting an activity to make it progressively more difficult as the client's performance improves or easier as her/his function deteriorates.

activity limitation inability to perform an activity to a satisfactory level.

activity performance choosing, organizing and carrying out activities in interaction with the environment.

A
B

(Reproduced with permission from the European Network of Occupational Therapy in Higher Education (ENOTHE) Terminology Project, 2008.)

activity programme a number of pre-planned activities that are carried out over a period of time for therapeutic purposes. The programme may be designed for a specific client or group of clients, or it may be designed so that clients do not attend the whole programme but are assigned to the most appropriate activities.

activity sequencing providing a series of different but related activities that incrementally increase or decrease the demands made on the individual in particular aspects of performance. For example, the sequence might be designed to incorporate progressively longer periods of standing as the client's standing tolerance improves.

activity synthesis combining activity components into new activities designed to enable the assessment of particular aspects of performance or the achievement of therapeutic goals.

activity theory a psychosocial theory of ageing that supports the view that older people who develop different roles and are socially active into old age gain benefit and satisfaction. It describes a process whereby, while people do disengage from certain activities as they become older, they replace these with others as they are able physically and economically to do. For example, there are those who retire from work who take up new hobbies and interests and, indeed, become more active in old age than they were in their younger years. ➲ continuity theory, disengagement theory.

actomyosin *n* the protein complex of actin and myosin formed during muscle fibre contraction.

actomyosin ATPase (amATPase) an enzyme present in skeletal muscle. It is associated with the contractile mechanism. It is located in the myosin head groups. Catalyses the hydrolysis (magnesium-dependent [Mg^{2+}] and triggered by a rise in calcium [Ca^{2+}]) of the terminal phosphate group of adenosine triphosphate (ATP) when head-group is in interaction with actin, releasing the energy that powers force generation. ➲ muscle enzymes.

Act of Parliament most English law is in the form of Acts of Parliament (statutes). An Act of Parliament is primary legislation, e.g. Disability Discrimination Act 2005, Health and Social Care Act 2008. Statutory instruments (subordinate or secondary legislation) made under delegated powers provide the regulations needed to implement a particular Act. An Act results from a Bill (a draft proposal). Proposals for legislative changes may be contained in Government White Papers. Consultation papers, sometimes called Green Papers, which set out Government proposals and seek comments from interested parties including the public, may precede these. The draft proposal or Bill is introduced into either the House of Commons (the elected Lower House) or the House of Lords or Upper House (currently an unelected body). The procedure of passing a Bill is similar in both Houses, and has seven stages (Figure A.3). If both Houses vote for the proposal then

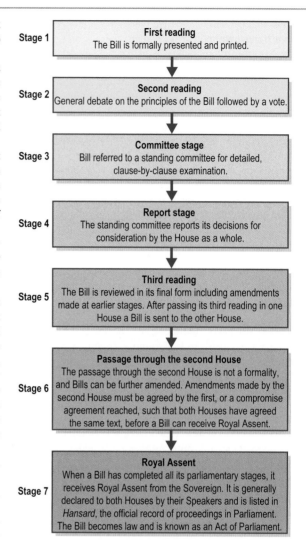

Stage 1	**First reading** The Bill is formally presented and printed.
Stage 2	**Second reading** General debate on the principles of the Bill followed by a vote.
Stage 3	**Committee stage** Bill referred to a standing committee for detailed, clause-by-clause examination.
Stage 4	**Report stage** The standing committee reports its decisions for consideration by the House as a whole.
Stage 5	**Third reading** The Bill is reviewed in its final form including amendments made at earlier stages. After passing its third reading in one House a Bill is sent to the other House.
Stage 6	**Passage through the second House** The passage through the second House is not a formality, and Bills can be further amended. Amendments made by the second House must be agreed by the first, or a compromise agreement reached, such that both Houses have agreed the same text, before a Bill can receive Royal Assent.
Stage 7	**Royal Assent** When a Bill has completed all its parliamentary stages, it receives Royal Assent from the Sovereign. It is generally declared to both Houses by their Speakers and is listed in *Hansard*, the official record of proceedings in Parliament. The Bill becomes law and is known as an Act of Parliament.

A.3 How a Bill becomes law (reproduced from Brooker & Waugh 2007 with permission).

the Bill is ready to become an Act, however it only becomes law after receiving Royal Assent. The law undergoes constant reform in the courts as established principles are interpreted, clarified or reapplied to meet new circumstances; laws become outdated, new policies require new laws, or new laws are needed to ensure that the UK complies with international or European Law, for example, The Human Rights Act 1998.

actual scores each score has a real value.

acuity *n* clearness, sharpness, keenness. ➲ auditory acuity, visual acuity.

acupressure component of Chinese medicine in which pressure is applied to various points on the body to stimulate or sedate internal energies. A more contemporary form is the Japanese technique of shiatsu. Acupressure has been used successfully to treat nausea and vomiting in pregnancy and relieve pain in labour.

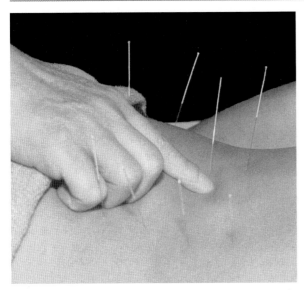

A.4 **Acupuncture (photograph)** (reproduced from Zhu 2005 with permission).

acupuncture *n* a technique that involves the insertion of fine needles into specific parts of the body (Figure A.4). There are approximately 365 points along meridians (channels through which energy known as *Qi* flows) at which needles can be inserted into the body to stimulate or depress the energy flow. Sometimes the herb moxa is also used to warm and stimulate certain points. This is known as moxibustion. Used for the treatment of many diseases, relief of pain or production of anaesthesia.

acute 1. describes a condition of severe rapid onset and short duration. Opposite to chronic. **2.** describes intense symptoms such as sharp and severe pain.

acute abdomen a pathological condition within the abdomen requiring immediate surgical intervention. Causes include a perforated viscera, acute appendicitis, diverticulitis or intestinal obstruction.

acute angle-closure glaucoma (AACG) (*syn*. acute glaucoma, congestive glaucoma) a form of raised intraocular pressure in which the pressure within the eye increases rapidly due to blockage of the trabecular meshwork. Symptoms include: intense pain, redness, blurred vision, haloes around lights, as well as nausea. Findings on examination include: reduced visual acuity, greatly elevated intraocular pressure (in the range of 40–50 mmHg), corneal epithelial oedema, semi-dilated and fixed pupil, shallow anterior chamber and mild aqueous cell and flare. Elevated intraocular pressure often causes glaucomatous optic nerve damage, as well as iris atrophy and damage to the anterior epithelial cells of the lens (glaukomflecken). Immediate treatment is initiated and is directed at lowering the intraocular pressure. Therapeutic agents include: topical beta-adrenergic agents, oral or topical carbonic anhydrase inhibitors, and oral hyperosmotic agents. Surgery is often necessary, e.g. laser

iridotomy to provide a pathway for the drainage of aqueous humour. ➲ Colour Section Figure 44.

acute bronchitis ➲ bronchitis.

acute confusional state sudden onset confusion with loss of awareness and disorientation due to a physical or metabolic disturbance affecting brain function. It may be misdiagnosed as dementia when it occurs in older people. Often there is an acute medical cause, such as stroke, urinary tract or chest infection, but may be caused by medications or recent loss or bereavement.

acute conjunctivitis conjunctivitis characterized by an onset of hyperaemia (most intense near the fornices), purulent or mucopurulent discharge and symptoms of irritation, grittiness and sticking together of the eyelids on waking. In severe cases there will be chemosis, eyelid oedema, subconjunctival haemorrhages and photophobia. The bacterial type is caused by *Staphylococcus epidermidis*, *S. aureus*, *Haemophilus influenzae*, *Streptococcus pneumoniae* (pneumococcus). A rare form of acute conjunctivitis is caused by the *Neisseria* spp. (gonococcus, meningococcus, e.g. gonococcal conjunctivitis) which produce a more severe form of the disease referred to as hyperacute bacterial conjunctivitis or acute purulent conjunctivitis. These require immediate treatment with systemic and topical antibiotics. Acute conjunctivitis is also caused by viruses, such as herpes simplex or adenoviruses. All forms of acute conjunctivitis occasionally spread to the cornea. Bacterial conjunctivitis often resolves without treatment within two weeks. Treatment consists of topical antibiotic therapy (e.g. chloramphenicol, erythromycin) and warm wet compresses. Acute allergic conjunctivitis most typically resolves spontaneously, otherwise treatment includes sodium cromoglicate. Acute follicular conjunctivitis is treated by antiviral agents (e.g. aciclovir), although in many cases the condition is self-limiting.

acute constipation ➲ constipation.

acute coronary syndromes describes the spectrum of events ranging from chest pain, the partial occlusion of a coronary artery resulting in unstable angina, a minor heart attack and a major heart attack. ➲ myocardial infarction.

acute defibrination syndrome ➲ hypofibrinogenaemia.

acute dilatation of the stomach sudden enlargement of this organ due to paralysis of the muscular wall. ➲ gastrectasia, paralytic ileus.

acute fatty liver of pregnancy (AFLP) acute yellow atrophy. A rare complication of pregnancy of unknown aetiology, characterized by rapid progressive atrophy of the liver with massive fatty necrosis and a mortality rate of over 80%. Typically, an obese woman presents with third trimester vomiting, headache, malaise, drowsiness, tender, but not enlarged, liver and jaundice. Concomitant hypertension and symptoms of fulminating pre-eclampsia can mask the diagnosis. The liver enzymes are slightly raised, hypoglycaemia and renal failure follow quickly. Fatty infiltration of the liver is seen on ultrasound or computed tomography, but liver biopsy is contraindicated due to risk of coagulopathy. Management involves correction of any coagulopathy and immediate delivery of the infant, preferably vaginally, although Caesarean section may be safer for the infant.

acute glaucoma ⊃ acute angle-closure glaucoma (AACG).

acute haemorrhagic conjunctivitis a highly contagious viral infection of the anterior segment resulting in haemorrhage of the bulbar conjunctiva. The infection is caused by a picornavirus, often associated with pre-auricular adenopathy and a follicular conjunctivitis. The infection is self-limited and lasts 7–10 days. No specific treatment is presently available.

acute heart failure cessation or impairment of heart action, in previously undiagnosed heart disease, or in the course of another disease.

acute injury an injury that presents with a rapid onset and has a short duration, due to a traumatic episode. Term used to describe the first 24–48 hours after onset of an injury, such as that sustained during a sporting activity.

acute interstitial pneumonia (AIP) one of the idiopathic interstitial pneumonias (IIPs). Onset is often preceded by a viral upper respiratory tract infection. There is severe exertional dyspnoea, widespread pneumonic consolidation and diffuse alveolar damage (DAD) on biopsy. The prognosis is often poor.

acute inversion of the uterus turning inside out of the uterus, a rare, serious complication of labour. It is caused by mismanagement of the third stage of labour, such as by attempting Credé's expression, or by applying umbilical cord traction when the uterus is relaxed and placenta incompletely separated, or occasionally it occurs spontaneously. Sudden profound maternal shock is accompanied by severe abdominal pain, bleeding if the placenta is wholly or partially separated, palpation of a concave-shaped fundus in the abdomen, or no uterus felt at all if inversion is complete, presence of the uterus in cervix or vagina, felt on examination or visible at the vulva. The foot of the bed/table should be raised to relieve tension and alleviate shock and the midwife should urgently call for the doctor who will attempt to replace the uterus by applying pressure to the lower segment near the cervix and working upwards to the fundus. If replacement of a totally inverted uterus is not possible it should be gently placed inside the vagina to reduce traction on the uterine (fallopian) tubes and ovaries. Severe shock is treated by replacing fluids and blood, narcotic analgesic and general anaesthetic to enable manual replacement of the uterus, or the hydrostatic method may be used. If all attempts fail a hysterectomy will be required.

acute leukaemia ⊃ leukaemia.

acute mountain sickness (AMS) ⊃ altitude sickness/illness (acute mountain sickness, AMS).

acute necrotizing ulcerative gingivitis (ANUG) now known as necrotizing ulcerative gingivitis (NUG). A recurrent periodontal condition characterized by ulceration and necrosis affecting the interdental tissues. ⊃ necrotizing ulcerative gingivitis (NUG)

acute otitis media (AOM) acute inflammation of the middle ear, common during childhood. AOM often follows an upper respiratory tract infection (URTI). Mucopurulent fluid collects in the middle ear and increased pressure causes the ear drum (tympanic membrane) to bulge and in some cases perforate, thus allowing the fluid to discharge. The child has a fever, pain, otorrhoea and will be irritable and miserable. Antibiotics are not routinely recommended, but they may be used for very young children and in cases where no improvement occurs.

acute pain pain of brief duration usually associated with tissue injury (nociceptive pain) which reduces as healing occurs. ⊃ chronic pain, nociceptive pain.

acute pancreatitis ⊃ pancreatitis.

acute phase proteins a class of proteins produced by the liver. They include C-reactive protein, etc., and are produced in response to inflammation, trauma and with malignancy.

acute/adult respiratory distress syndrome (ARDS) characterized by difficulty breathing, poor oxygenation, stiff lungs and typical changes on a chest X-ray, following a recognized cause of acute lung injury. Analysis of arterial blood gases reveals a fall in PaO_2 and eventually an increased $PaCO_2$ and a fall in pH.

acute suppurative otitis media (ASOM) an acute infection of the middle ear, often due to bacterial infection.

acute tubular necrosis (ATN) rapid onset necrosis of the renal tubules. It is usually caused by renal ischaemia due to shock, but may be due to the nephrotoxic effects of bacterial toxins or chemical toxins. ⊃ renal failure.

acute ulcerative gingivitis (AUG) now known as necrotizing ulcerative gingivitis (NUG). ⊃ necrotizing ulcerative gingivitis (NUG).

acute ulcerative necrotizing gingivitis (AUNG) now known as necrotizing ulcerative gingivitis (NUG). ⊃ necrotizing ulcerative gingivitis (NUG).

acute wound usually describes a surgical incision or uncomplicated trauma. The wound usually heals quickly. ⊃ chronic wound, wound healing.

acute yellow atrophy acute diffuse necrosis of the liver; icterus gravis; malignant jaundice. ⊃ acute fatty liver of pregnancy.

acyanosis *n* without cyanosis.

acyanotic *adj* without cyanosis; a word used to differentiate congenital cardiovascular defects.

acyesis *n* absence of pregnancy—**acyetic** *adj*.

acystia *n* congenital absence of the bladder—**acystic** *adj*.

ad- a prefix that means 'towards' , e.g. *adduct*.

adamantinoma ⊃ ameloblastoma.

Adam's apple the laryngeal prominence in the anterior part of the neck, especially in the adult male, formed by the junction of the two wings of the thyroid cartilage.

Adams' arrowhead clasp clasp of stainless steel wire used to retain removable orthodontic appliances and consisting of a buccal wire connecting two arrowhead formations to fit into the mesio- and disto-buccal undercuts. The wire is continuous over the occlusal surfaces, to be held in place in the base-plate by several bends.

adaptability *n* the ability to adjust mentally and physically to circumstances in a flexible way.

adaptation *n* **1**. the changes that an individual makes to her/his performance and patterns of occupation in order to meet environmental demands and/or compensate for loss of function. **2**. in sports medicine describes the long term physical changes that occur from the training effects produced as a result of overload. ⊃ aerobic adaptations, anaerobic adaptations.

adaptive behaviour advantageous or appropriate behaviour that follows a change.

adaptive thermogenesis the thermic effect of factors such as cold, heat, fear, stress and various drugs that can increase the rate of energy expenditure above normal baseline levels.

addiction *n* craving for chemical substances, such as a drug, alcohol and tobacco, which the addicted person finds difficult to control. Also more recently applied in exercise settings to a dependency on regular exercise. ⊃ exercise dependence.

Addison's disease (T Addison, British physician, 1793–1860) deficient secretion of cortisol and aldosterone due to primary failure of the adrenal cortex, causing electrolyte imbalance, diminished blood volume, hypotension, weight loss, hypoglycaemia, muscular weakness, gastrointestinal upsets and pigmentation of skin.

addisonian crisis ⊃ adrenal crisis

addisonian pernicious anaemia ⊃ pernicious anaemia.

additive a substance not usually considered to be or used as a food which is added to foods to assist processing/manufacture, or to enhance flavour, texture, colour, keeping properties, appearance, or stability of the food, or as a convenience to the consumer. Nutrients, such as vitamins and minerals, added to enhance the nutritional value of food are not included as additives. Other substances that include spices, salt, herbs, yeast, air and water are also usually excluded.

address a number which designates a particular storage area in the memory of the computer.

adduct *vt* to draw towards the midline of the body. ⊃ abduct *opp*.

adduction *n* the act of adducting, drawing towards the midline of the body. ⊃ abduction *opp*.

adductor *n* any muscle which moves a part toward the median axis of the body. ⊃ abductor *opp*, adductor brevis, adductor hallucis, adductor longus, adductor magnus, adductor pollicis.

adductor brevis one of the adductor muscles in the medial compartment of the thigh. Its origin is on the body and inferior ramus of the pubic bone and it inserts into the upper part of the linea aspera close to the insertions of the pectineus and adductor longus muscles; it contracts to adduct and laterally rotate the thigh.

adductor hallucis one of the muscles in the foot. It has two heads and its large oblique head arises from the long plantar ligament and the bases of the second, third and fourth metatarsals and the muscle inserts into the lateral side of the plantar surface of the proximal phalanx of the great toe; it functions to move the great toe towards the metatarsal axis and helps in maintaining the transverse arch of the foot.

adductor longus one of the adductor muscles in the medial compartment of the thigh. Its origin is on a circular area between the symphysis pubis and the pubic crest (the tendon may become ossified 'rider's bone') and it inserts into the middle third of the femoral shaft (lower part of the linea aspera); it contracts to adduct and flex the thigh. ⊃ Colour Section Figure 4.

adductor magnus one of the adductor muscles in the medial compartment of the thigh. It is a composite muscle formed by adductor muscle and a hamstring muscle (there is no septum between the medial and posterior compartments of the thigh). The adductor part is innervated by the obturator nerve and the hamstring part by the sciatic nerve. Its origin is on the ischiopubic ramus and ischial tuberosity, and it inserts into the adductor tubercle and linea aspera of the femur; the adductor part adducts, flexes and laterally rotates the thigh, whereas the hamstring part functions as a synergist of the hamstring muscles. ⊃ Colour Section Figures 4, 5.

adductors of the thigh the muscles of the medial compartment of the thigh; the adductor brevis, adductor longus and the adductor magnus that move the thighs together. ⊃ gracilis muscle, pectineus.

adductor pollicis one of the muscles in the hand. It has two heads. The transverse head arises from the palmar border of the third metacarpal and the oblique head arises from the bases of the second and third metacarpals and the trapezoid and capitate bones (carpals). The fibres from the two heads converge on the ulnar sesamoid; it contracts to approximate the thumb to the index finger.

ADE *abbr* acute demyelinating encephalitis.

aden/o- a prefix that means 'gland, glandular', e.g. *adenoma*.

adenectomy *n* surgical removal of a gland.

adenine *n* a nitrogenous base derived from purine. With other bases, one or more phosphate groups and a sugar it is part of the nucleic acids DNA and RNA. ⊃ deoxyribonucleic acid, ribonucleic acid.

adenitis *n* inflammation of a gland, or lymph node. ⊃ dacr(y)oadenitis, hilar adenitis, lymphadenitis, sialoadenitis.

adenoacanthoma a tumour of glandular tissue which may be benign or malignant and is identified by changes in the squamous epithelial cells.

adenocarcinoma *n* a malignant, epithelial cell tumour of glandular tissue—**adenocarcinomata** *pl*, **adenocarcinomatous** *adj*.

adenofibroma *n* ⊃ fibroadenoma.

adenohypophysis the glandular anterior lobe of the pituitary gland. It develops from the ectoderm of the mouth/pharynx in the embryo. ⊃ pituitary gland.

adenoid *adj* resembling a gland. ⊃ adenoids.

adenoidectomy *n* surgical removal from the nasopharynx of enlarged pharyngeal tonsil (adenoid tissue).

A
B

adenoid facies open mouthed, vacant expression due to deafness from enlarged pharyngeal tonsils (adenoids).

adenoids *npl* abnormally enlarged pharyngeal tonsils. Lymphoid tissue situated in the nasopharynx which can obstruct breathing and impede hearing.

adenoma *n* a benign tumour of glandular epithelial tissue—**adenomata** *pl*, **adenomatous** *adj*.

adenomatous polyp a benign tumour of the large intestine which may develop into a malignant tumour.

adenomyoma *n* a benign tumour composed of muscle and glandular elements, usually applied to benign growths of the uterus—**adenomyomata** *pl*, **adenomyomatous** *adj*.

adenopathy *n* any disease of a gland—**adenopathic** *adj*.

adenosine a nucleoside formed from the sugar ribose and adenine. With the addition of one, two or three phosphate groups forms the three nucleotides: *adenosine monophosphate, adenosine diphosphate* and *adenosine triphosphate*.

adenosine deaminase the enzyme that facilitates the conversion of adenosine to the nucleoside inosine. ⊃ adenosine deaminase deficiency.

adenosine deaminase deficiency a genetic condition that affects lymphocyte function and can lead to severe combined immunodeficiency syndrome.

adenosine diphosphate (ADP) an important cellular metabolite involved in energy exchange within the cell. Chemical energy is conserved in the cell, by the phosphorylation of ADP to ATP primarily in the mitochondrion, as a high energy phosphate bond.

adenosine monophosphate (AMP) an important cellular metabolite involved in energy release for cell use. ⊃ cyclic adenosine monophosphate (cAMP).

adenosine triphosphate (ATP) an intermediate high energy compound which on hydrolysis to ADP releases chemically useful energy. ATP is generated during catabolism and utilized during anabolism.

adenosis a disease or enlargement of a gland or glandular tissue.

adenotonsillectomy *n* surgical removal of the pharyngeal tonsil (adenoid tissue) and palatine tonsils.

adenovirus *n* a group of DNA-containing viruses. They cause upper respiratory and gastrointestinal infections, cystitis and conjunctivitis.

adequate intake in situations where there is insufficient scientific evidence to confirm needs and reference intakes for a particular nutrient for which deficiency is rarely, if ever, seen, the observed intake levels are assumed to be greater than requirements, and thus give an approximation of intakes that are greater than adequate to meet needs.

ADH *abbr* antidiuretic hormone ⊃ antidiuretic hormone, vasopressin (or arginine vasopression [AVP].)

ADHD *abbr* attention deficit hyperactivity disorder.

adherence extent to which a person maintains a behavioural regimen, such as regular exercise. ⊃ compliance, concordance.

adherent placenta an abnormally adherent placenta which is firmly attached to the uterine wall, and which fails to separate during the third stage of labour. It may be due to a placenta accreta, placenta increta or a placenta percreta. ⊃ placenta accreta, placenta increta, placenta percreta, retained placenta.

adhesion *n* 1. action of sticking to, by molecular attraction of certain dissimilar molecules, by viscosity of surface or by grasping. 2. abnormal union of two parts, occurring after inflammation; a band of fibrous tissue which joins such parts. In the abdomen such a band may cause intestinal obstruction; in joints it restricts movement; between two surfaces of pleura it prevents complete pneumothorax. 3. in dentistry, the force which retains an upper denture in place without the use of adhesive gums or mechanical aids such as 'suction' cups—**adherent** *adj*, **adherence** *n*, **adhere** *vi*.

adhesion molecules *npl* specific cell-surface molecules that bind cells to each other within tissues.

adhesive substance causing surface attachment. ⊃ dentine adhesive, denture adhesive, orthodontic adhesive, tray adhesive.

adhesive bridge generic term for a dental bridge dependent upon adhesive technology to allow metal wing(s) to be bonded to a minimally prepared retainer(s). ⊃ bridge, Maryland bridge, Rochette bridge.

adhesive capsulitis ⊃ frozen shoulder.

ADI *abbr* acceptable daily intake.

Adie's pupil (W Adie, British physician, 1886–1935) (*syn* myotonic pupil, pupillotonia, tonic pupil; some authors use this last term when the cause is known and Adie's pupil when the cause is unidentified) a pupil in which the reactions to light, direct or consensual, are almost abolished, with a reaction occurring only after prolonged exposure to light or dark. The reaction of the pupil to a near target is also delayed and slow. The condition is usually unilateral with the affected pupil being the larger of the two. It may be due to a disease of, or injury to, the ciliary ganglion or to the short ciliary nerves. Other causes include temporal arteritis in older people, syphilis or diabetes. ⊃ Adie's syndrome, pupillary light reflex.

Adie's syndrome (W Adie) (*syn* Holmes–Adie syndrome) a condition characterized by one pupil reacting more slowly to light, convergence and accommodation than the other pupil. There is also a reduction in, or absent tendon reflexes, such as the ankle relexes. It typically affects adult women. ⊃ Adie's pupil, aniscoria, pupillary light reflex.

adipocyte a fat (adipose) cell (Figure A.5). Able to store fat as triglycerides (triacylglycerol).

adiponectin a hormone produced by adipose tissue, which may be concerned with energy balance. Its effects include increased insulin sensitivity and glucose tolerance, and oxidation of fatty acids in muscle tissue.

adipose *n, adj* fat; of a fatty nature. A specilized connective tissue; there is white and brown adipose tissue. White adipose tissue (or fat) is stored by the body, under the skin, within body cavities, e.g. in the abdominal cavity, and around organs. It contains cells, the adipocytes, that are able to synthesize and store fat in the form of triacylglycerols

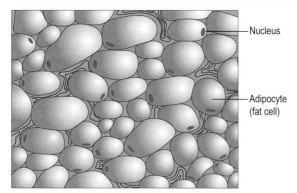

— Nucleus

— Adipocyte
(fat cell)

A.5 Adipocyte (reproduced from Waugh & Grant 2006 with permission).

(triglycerides), releasing it into blood as fatty acids to be used as an energy source in the fasted state or during endurance exercise. It also provides a protective and insulating layer. Brown adipose tissue is metabolically more active and is important for the production of heat needed for maintaining body temperature within the normal range. ➲ body composition, body fat, brown adipose tissue.

adiposity *n* excessive accumulation of fat in the body.

adiposogenital dystrophy Fröhlich's syndrome. Affects males, it is characterized by obesity with female fat distribution, underdevelopment of the genitalia and female secondary sexual characteristics, somnolence, disturbance of temperature regulation and diabetes insipidus due to damage of the pituitary and hypothalamus.

adipsia absence of thirst.

aditus *n* in anatomy, an entrance or opening.

ADJ amelo-dentinal junction.

adjective checklist in psychometrics, a list of adjectives that can be endorsed as applying or not applying to oneself or others.

adjustable articulator an articulator used by the dental technician, which can be adjusted to accommodate the many positions and movements of the mandible relative to the maxilla as recorded in the mouth.

adjustable axis face-bow face-bow with adjustable arms, used in conjunction with an adjustable articulator, to record the retruded hinge axis. Also known as hinge axis locating face-bow or hinge bow, kinematic face-bow. ➲ face-bow.

adjustable template used in radiology. A large number of parallel rods or pins which can be adjusted to the patient shape and clamped into position to show the patient contour.

adjustment *n* **1.** process of modifying a state. In dentistry, an alteration made to a denture. ➲ occlusal adjustment, correction or equilibration. **2.** stability within an individual and an acceptable relationship between the individual and his or her environment. **3.** the mechanism used in focusing a microscope.

adjuvant *n* a substance included in a prescription to assist the action of other drugs, e.g. a preservative.

adjuvant therapy additional treatment, such as a drug, that acts synergistically to assist or increase the action of other drugs or therapies. Especially used to describe the use of drugs, such as antidepressants, e.g. amitriptyline, given with an analgesic for pain relief. It is also applied to the treatment of cancer where cytotoxic drugs are used after removal of the tumour by surgery or radiotherapy. The purpose of treatment being to enhance the chance of cure and prevent recurrence. ➲ neoadjuvant therapy.

ad lib (Latin, *ad libitum*) give freely, to the desired amount.

ADLs *abbr* activities of daily living.

admixed amalgam alloy alloy containing particles of different composition. ➲ alloy.

adnexa *npl* structures that are in close proximity to a part—**adnexal** *adj.*

adnexa oculi structures close to the eyeball, the lacrimal apparatus.

adnexa uteri structures close to the uterus, the ovaries and uterine (fallopian) tubes.

adolescence *n* the period between the onset of puberty and full maturity; youth—**adolescent** *adj, n.*

adolescent athlete an athlete in the period between the onset of puberty and full maturity. This is the period of final bone growth and skeletal maturation, which increases the risk from contact injuries to the epiphyses (the ends of the long bones, not yet fused with the main shaft). The psychological changes that accompany the physical changes may result in problems with self-esteem, compliance and motivation.

adoption *n* the acquisition of legal responsibility for a child who is not a natural offspring of the adopter.

ADP *abbr* adenosine diphosphate.

adrenal *adj* near the kidney. ➲ adrenal glands.

adrenal cortex the outer part of the adrenal gland secretes three groups of steroid hormones derived from cholesterol. They are known collectively as the adrenocorticocoids (corticosteroids, corticoids). They are the glucocorticoids, mineralocorticoids and sex hormones which control metabolism, the chemical constitution of body fluids and secondary sexual characteristics. The hormones in each group have different characteristic actions but due to their structural similarity their actions may overlap. Secretion is under the control of the pituitary gland via the secretion of adrenocorticotrophic hormone (ACTH). ➲ glucocorticoids, mineralocorticoids, sex hormones, zona fasciculata, zona glomerulosa, zona reticularis.

adrenal crisis (addisonian crisis) acute life-threatening situation occurring in patients with adrenal cortex (adrenocortical) insufficiency. It may present as shock in previously undiagnosed Addison's disease, or in a patient who is having insufficient corticosteroid replacement therapy during a concurrent illness. There is low blood pressure with weakness and commonly fever and abdominal tenderness.

adrenal function tests tests to identify adrenocortical hypofunction or hyperfunction; random cortisol may identify gross abnormalities in function, but for the vast majority dynamic testing of the hypothalamo-pituitary-adrenal axis is needed. ⊃ dexamethasone suppression tests, glucagon stimulation test, insulin tolerance test, tetracosactide (Synacthen) test.

adrenal glands (*syn* suprarenal glands) two endocrine glands, one situated on the upper pole of each kidney enclosed within the renal fascia. They are about 4 cm long and 3 cm thick. The arterial blood supply to the glands is by branches from the abdominal aorta and renal arteries. The venous return is by suprarenal veins. The right gland drains into the inferior vena cava and the left into the left renal vein. The glands are composed of two parts which have different structures and functions. The outer part is the cortex and the inner part the medulla. The adrenal cortex is essential to life but the medulla is not. ⊃ adrenal cortex, adrenal medulla, Colour Section Figure 19.

adrenal medulla the medulla or middle part of the adrenal gland is completely surrounded by the cortex. It develops from nervous tissue in the embryo and is part of the sympathetic division of the autonomic nervous system. It is stimulated by its extensive sympathetic nerve supply to produce the catecholamine hormones adrenaline (epinephrine) and noradrenaline (norepinephrine). Noradrenaline is the postganglionic neurotransmitter of the sympathetic division of the autonomic nervous system. Adrenaline and some noradrenaline are released into the blood from the adrenal medulla during stimulation of the sympathetic nervous system. They are structurally very similar and this explains their similar effects. Adrenaline has a greater effect on the heart and metabolic processes whereas noradrenaline has more influence on blood vessels. Together they potentiate the 'fight or flight' response after initial sympathetic stimulation by: increasing heart rate, increasing blood pressure, diverting blood to critical organs such as the brain, heart and the skeletal muscles by dilating their blood vessels and constricting those of less essential organs, such as the skin or digestive tract, increasing metabolic rate, increasing blood glucose, dilating the bronchioles, dilating the pupils. ⊃ adrenaline (epinephrine), noradrenaline (norepinephrine).

adrenalectomy *n* removal of an adrenal gland, usually for tumour. If both adrenal glands are removed, replacement administration of cortical hormones is required.

adrenaline (epinephrine) *n* a catecholamine hormone, produced by the adrenal medulla. It enhances the effects of the sympathetic nervous system during times of physiological stress by preparing the body for 'fight or flight' responses. These include increased heart rate, bronchodilation and increased respiratory rate and glucose release. Also acts as a neurotransmitter but, in mammals, only within the central nervous system. Adrenaline (epinephrine) is used therapeutically as a sympathomimetic in situations that include: acute allergic reactions, and in local anaesthetic to prolong the anaesthetic effects. Used topically, in dentistry, to reduce haemorrhage, and in gingival retraction cords. ⊃ adrenal medulla, alpha (α)-adrenoceptor agonist, alpha (α)-adrenoceptor antagonist, beta (β)-adrenoceptor agonist,

beta (β)-adrenoceptor antagonist, monoamine, noradrenaline (norepinephrine)

adrenarche increased adrenal cortex activity occurring at around 6–8 years of age. Hormone secretion is increased, especially androgens.

adrenergic *adj* describes nerves which liberate the catecholamine noradrenaline (norepinephrine) from the terminations. Most postganglionic sympathetic neurons release noradrenaline as the neurotransmitter at the tissue or organ supplied. The exceptions to this are the postganglionic sympathetic neurons that supply the skin, sweat glands and the blood vessels in skeletal voluntary muscle (structures having no parasympathetic supply); these generally use acetylcholine ⊃ cholinergic *opp*.

adrenoceptor *n* (*syn* adrenergic receptor) receptor sites on the effector structures innervated by sympathetic nerves. The adrenoceptors are transmembrane proteins on cells that are activated by noradrenaline (norepinephrine) released at sympathetic nerve endings or by circulating catecholamines. There are three main types: alpha$_1$ (α$_1$), alpha$_2$ (α$_2$) and beta (β) which mediate responses by different cellular mechanisms and are activated preferentially by different agonists. Each type has three subtypes. All subtypes respond strongly to noradrenaline (norepinephrine), beta (β) most strongly to adrenaline (epinephrine), and certain synthetic dugs can distinguish between alpha$_1$ and alpha$_2$ receptors. Such differences account, for example, for smooth muscle relaxation in some tissues (beta-mediated vasodilatation in skeletal muscle; bronchodilation in the lungs) and vasoconstriction in others (alpha-mediated, in gut and skin) during heightened sympathetic activity. International agreement is for 'adrenoceptor' but the use of 'adrenergic receptors' is still common in the USA.

adrenocorticotrophic hormone (ACTH) (*syn* corticotrophin) secreted by the anterior lobe of the pituitary gland it stimulates the production of hormones by the adrenal cortex.

adrenogenital syndrome an endocrine disorder, usually congenital, resulting from abnormal activity of the adrenal cortex. A female child will show enlarged clitoris and possibly labial fusion, perhaps being confused with a male. The male child may show pubic hair and enlarged penis. In both male and female there is rapid growth, muscularity and advanced bone age.

adrenoleucodystrophy (ALD) a group of neurodegenerative disorders associated with adrenocortical insufficiency. X-linked inheritance. ⊃ Schilder's disease.

adrenolytic *adj* describes a substance that inhibits the function of adrenergic nerves.

ADRs *abbr* adverse drug reactions.

Adson–Caffey syndrome (A Adson, American neurosurgeon, 1887–1951; I Caffey, American physician) ⊃ thoracic outlet syndrome.

Adson's sign (A Adson) the radial pulse cannot be felt when the arm is abducted and externally rotated. A sign that may be indicative of thoracic outlet syndrome.

adsorbents *npl* solids that bind dissolved substances or gases on their surfaces. Charcoal can be used to adsorb gases to act as a deodorant, such as in certain wound dressing products. Bacterial and other toxins are adsorbed by kaolin, which may be used in the treatment of food poisoning.

adsorption *n* the property of a substance to attract and to hold to its surface a gas, liquid or solid in solution or suspension—**adsorptive** *adj*, **adsorb** *vt*.

adult basic life support the basic resuscitation measures used in people who have reached puberty. ⊃ Appendix 10.

adult congenital heart disease there are increasing numbers of children who have had surgical correction of congenital defects and who may have further cardiological problems as adults. For example, those who have undergone correction of coarctation of the aorta may develop hypertension in adult life. Those with transposition of the great arteries who have had a 'Mustard' repair, where blood is re-directed at atrial level leaving the right ventricle connected to the aorta, may develop right ventricular failure in adult life. The right ventricle is unsuited for function at systemic pressures and may begin to dilate and fail when patients are in their twenties or thirties. Those who have had surgery involving the atria may develop atrial arrhythmias, and those who have ventricular scars may develop ventricular arrhythmias. Such patients require careful follow-up from the teenage years through adult life so that problems can be identified early and appropriate medical or surgical treatment instituted. The management of these adult or 'grown-up' congenital heart disease patients has developed as a cardiological subspecialty. ⊃ congenital heart disease (CHD).

adult inclusion conjunctivitis (*syn* trachoma inclusion conjunctivitis [TRIC]) an acute conjunctivitis caused by infection with the serotypes D to K of *Chlamydia trachomatis* and typically occurring in sexually active adults in whom the genitourinary tract is infected. Signs in the eye usually appear 1 week following sexual exposure. It may also be caused by the unhygienic use of personal articles, using contaminated eye cosmetics or soon after having been in a public swimming pool. Infants born to infected women may be infected by contact during birth with vaginal secretions. The infant develops signs of disease (also called neonatal inclusion conjunctivitis or neonatal chlamydial conjunctivitis) some 5 to 14 days after birth. The conjunctivitis is mucopurulent with follicles in the fornices which often spread to the limbal region. The condition is commonly associated with punctate epithelial keratitis, preauricular lymphadenopathy, marginal infiltrates and, in long-standing infection, micropannus in the superior corneal region may also appear. Differentiation from viral follicular conjunctivitis is made through culture, serological and cytological studies. Treatment consists of using both systemic and topical tetracyclines, although in pregnant or lactating women, or for children, other antibiotics are prescribed. ⊃ conjunctival follicle, follicular conjunctivitis, ophthalmia neonatorum, punctate epithelial keratitis, trachoma.

adulteration *n* the addition of cheaper substances to foods etc. in order to increase the bulk and reduce the cost, with intent to mislead and defraud the customer.

adult polycystic kidney diseases (APKD) ⊃ polycystic kidney disease.

adumbration poor edge definition of an image on a radiographic film due to cross-over X-rays. ⊃ penumbra.

advance directive referred to as an advance decision to refuse treatment in the Mental Capacity Act 2005 but also known colloquially as a 'living will'. It is a written declaration made by a mentally competent adult before they lose the capacity to make decisions about medical treatment. An advance directive is legally binding if it is in the form of an advanced refusal and the adult is competent at the time of making it. An advance directive allows a competent adult to specify which medical interventions they wish to refuse and the situations/circumstances where the refusal would apply. There must be a clear refusal to have a specified treatment and if there is any doubt about the validity a declaration may be sought or treatment is given that is in the best interests of the person.

advanced life support (ALS) the use of drugs, artificial aids and advanced skills to save or preserve life during resuscitation procedures. Including tracheal intubation, intravenous drugs, etc. ⊃ Broselow™ paediatric resuscitation system, cardiopulmonary resuscitation, paediatric advanced life.

Advanced Trauma Life Support (ATLS) a simple systematic method of managing patients with major trauma, such as following a road traffic accident, explosions, gunshot, etc., and dealing with the most life-threatening injury. Specialist courses prepare doctors, nurses and paramedics to use the approach.

advancement *n* surgical detachment of a tendon or muscle followed by reattachment at an advanced point.

adventitia *n* the external coat, especially of an artery or vein—**adventitious** *adj*.

adventitious *adj* **1.** occurring outside the usual location, in an inappropriate place. **2.** relating to an accidental condition. **3.** acquired not hereditary.

adverse neural tension (ANT) the term that refers to restricted movement of the nervous system, such as is seen with a case of nerve root tethering following a prolapsed intervertebral disc.

adverse drug reactions (ADRs) *npl* a term describing any unwanted effects of a drug. They range from very minor through to extremely unpleasant or life-threatening. They are usually classified into five types: A–E. Type A or augmented effects are adverse effects that occur as a result of the drug's pharmacology, i.e. they are pharmacologically predictable. They are sometimes referred to as side-effects, for example the dry mouth and constipation caused by morphine; Type B or bizarre effects are unpredictable adverse effects that are not dose-related, for example hypersensitivity reactions to penicillin. Although the occurrence of type B ADRs is relatively uncommon, they do have a high morbidity and mortality rate; Type C or chronic effects occur after prolonged drug usage, for example tardive dyskinesia, that occurs with typical antipsychotic drugs (neuroleptics) the phenothiazines used to manage symptoms in serious mental health problems; Type D or delayed effects occur years after the original drug therapy, for example cancers caused by the use of cytotoxic drugs for childhood leukaemia. In some cases, the adverse effect may affect the offspring of the original recipient, as in the case of a rare vaginal cancer occurring in the daughters of women who took diethylstilbestrol (a sex hormone) during pregnancy; Type E or ending-of use effects are adverse effects that occur when the drug is stopped suddenly, i.e. withdrawal effects, illustrated by delirium tremors which occurs when a person stops misusing alcohol. ➲ Commission on Human Medicines, drug eruptions, side-effects, yellow card reporting.

advocacy *n* process by which a person supports or argues for the needs of another. Healthcare professionals may act as advocate for their patients or clients, or assist individuals to develop the skills needed for self-advocacy by, for instance, providing sufficient information for the person to make an informed decision. ➲ self-advocacy.

AE *abbr* air entry.

AED *abbr* automated external defibrillator.

Aedes *n* a genus of mosquitoes which includes *Aedes aegypti*, an important vector of dengue and yellow fever.

-aemia a suffix that means 'blood', e.g. *leukaemia*.

aer/o- a prefix/combining for that means 'air, gas', e.g. *aerosol* .

aerobe *n* a micro-organism that requires oxygen to maintain life—**aerobic** *adj*. ➲ anaerobe, aerobic micro-organisms.

aerobic *adj* requiring free oxygen or air to support life or a specific process.

aerobic adaptations long term physical changes that result from aerobic exercise. They increase the body's ability to deal with endurance exercise. ➲ anaerobic adaptations.

aerobic capacity the maximum rate at which an animal or human subject can take up oxygen from the air; also known as maximal oxygen consumption/uptake ($\dot{V}O_{2max}$). Aerobic capacity of individual muscles is the maximum rate at which they can utilize oxygen. ➲ aerobic power.

aerobic endurance period for which aerobic work can be maintained by an individual; may vary from a few tens of seconds in a sedentary person and a few minutes in a sprint or power athlete, to more than 24 h in an ultra-marathoner.

aerobic energy the production of adenosine triphosphate (ATP) by oxidative phosphorylation. ➲ anaerobic energy.

aerobic exercise physical activity that requires the heart and lungs to work harder in order to obtain and supply increased oxygen to strenuously contracting skeletal muscles. It is furnished with energy by aerobic metabolism; regular repetition enhances the capacity of the cardio-respiratory system to deliver oxygen to muscles. Compare anaerobic exercise.

aerobic fitness the capacity to deliver oxygen to the strenuously contracting muscles and to use it to produce energy during exercise.

aerobic metabolism ➲ glycolysis, oxidative phosphorylation.

aerobic micro-organisms (aerobes) *npl* micro-organisms that require oxygen for growth. Micro-organisms may be facultative aerobes or obligate aerobes. ➲ facultative aerobes, microaerophiles, obligate aerobes.

aerobic power a term that is widely, but loosely, used as interchangeable with aerobic capacity, or maximal oxygen consumption/uptake ($\dot{V}O_{2max}$) though the units for this are those of oxygen uptake rate, not power.

aerobic threshold work rate considered to be minimum for achievement of aerobic training effects (not that at which aerobic metabolism starts, which is of course zero). ➲ metabolic and related thresholds.

aerobic training training aimed at enhancement of aerobic power or endurance; consists of intensive (for power) or sustained (for endurance) exercise below $\dot{V}O_{2max}$. ➲ target heart rate.

aerodontalgia ➲ barodontalgia.

aerogenous *adj* gas producing.

aerophagia, aerophagy *n* excessive air swallowing.

aerosol *n* small particles finely dispersed in a gas phase. May be used: to deliver inhalation drug therapy, such as bronchodilators, in insect control and for skin application. Aerosols produced during sneezing and coughing can be responsible for the spread of infection.

aerotolerant describes anaerobic micro-organisms that can grow in the presence of air (oxygen).

aesthesia the capacity of feeling, sensing or perceiving.

-aesthesia a suffix that means 'sensibility, sense-perception', e.g. *paraesthesia*.

aesthetic dentistry term used to describe the treatment techniques used to improve the position and symmetry of the teeth, jaws and face in order to improve the appearance, as well as the function of the teeth, mouth and face.

aetiology *n* (etiology) the science of the causation of disease—**aetiological** *adj*, **aetiologically** *adv*.

AF *abbr* atrial fibrillation.

AFB *abbr* acid-fast bacillus.

AfC *abbr* Agenda for Change.

AFD *abbr* anode to film distance. ➲ focus to film distance.

afebrile *adj* without fever.

affect *n* in psychology, a general term for subjectively experienced feelings encompassing emotion and mood. *affective response* is subjectively experienced feeling in response to an environmental event. May be negative or positive—**affective** *adj*. ➲ circumplex model, negative affect, positive affect.

affection *n* the feeling or emotional aspects of mind; one of the three aspects. ➲ cognition, conation.

affective *adj* pertaining to emotions or moods.

affective psychosis a mental health problem characterized by mood disturbance together with psychotic symptoms. ➲ mood, psychosis.

afferent *adj* conducting inward to a part or organ; used to describe nerves, blood and lymphatic vessels Describes nerves that carry impulses towards the central nervous system, or to relay stations outside it, from neural receptors (e.g. sensory nerves from the skin, those conveying proprioceptive information from muscles and joints or visceral afferents from internal organs). Also describes blood or lymph vessels in which flow is towards some point of reference, e.g. afferent arterioles to the glomeruli of the kidney. ⊃ efferent *opp*.

afferent degeneration that which spreads up sensory nerves.

afferent fibre a nerve fibre conducting impulses to a nerve centre or spinal cord.

affiliation *n* settling of the paternity of an illegitimate child on the putative father.

affiliation order court order by which an absent father is required to make regular payments towards his child's maintenance.

affinity *n* describes the chemical attraction between two substances, e.g. oxygen and haemoglobin.

affirmative action policies or practices that favourably support disadvantaged groups (including women, ethnic minorities and people with disabilities) who have experienced institutionalized discrimination. It is also referred to as positive discrimination. The concept is complex and the practice of affirmative action can, in some circumstances, be illegal.

affordance a property of an object or a feature of the environment that offers an organism the opportunity to act in a particular way.

AFI *abbr* amniotic fluid index.

afibrinogenaemia *n* a lack of fibrinogen resulting in a serious disorder of blood coagulation—**afibrinogenaemic** *adj*.

aflatoxin *n* carcinogenic metabolites of certain strains of *Aspergillus flavus* that can affect peanuts and carbohydrate foods stored in warm humid climates. Hepatic enzymes produce the metabolites of aflatoxins which predispose to liver cancer.

AFLP *abbr* acute fatty liver of pregnancy.

AFO *abbr* ankle foot orthosis.

AFP *abbr* alphafetoprotein.

afterbirth *n* the placenta, cord and membranes which are expelled from the uterus after childbirth.

aftercare *n* a word denoting the care given during convalescence and rehabilitation. It may be within the remit of health professionals including therapists or nurses, or may be provided by social care staff or family members.

aftercoming head fetal head (coming after the trunk) in a breech delivery. ⊃ breech presentation.

aftereffect *n* a response occurring after the initial effect of a stimulus.

after-glow the production of light from a crystal after the irradiation of the crystal stops. ⊃ phosphorescence.

after-image *n* a visual impression of an object persisting after the object has been removed. May be 'positive' when the image is seen in its natural bright colours or 'negative' if the dark parts are light and the bright parts become dark.

after-image test (*syn* Hering's after-image test) a subjective test used to determine the presence or absence of abnormal retinal correspondence (ARC). The subject is instructed to fixate the centre of a vertical light filament for some 15 s with one eye and then the centre of a horizontal light filament for some 15 s with the other eye. Looking at the after-images of the two filaments on a uniform surface (e.g. a wall), the subject sees either a cross, which indicates normal retinal correspondence or two separated filaments, indicating ARC. ⊃ abnormal retinal correspondence, after-image.

after-image transfer test (*syn* Brock's after-image test) a test aimed at detecting and measuring the angle of eccentric fixation in an amblyopic eye in a patient with normal retinal correspondence. The normal eye fixates an illuminated vertical line and is then occluded, while the amblyopic eye fixates a dot. If the after-image and the fixation point coincide the amblyopic eye has no eccentric fixation, otherwise the relative position of one to the other indicates the angle of eccentric fixation. ⊃ eccentric fixation, retinal corresponding points.

afterload the pressure of blood in aorta and vessel constriction that forms the resistance or load that left ventricular contraction must overcome to pump blood into the circulation. ⊃ preload.

afterloading the method of inserting a number of guides into a body cavity and then mechanically inserting a radioactive source over the guides. This technique reduces the radiation dose to the hands of the operator.

afterpains *n* the pains felt after childbirth, due to contraction and retraction of the uterine muscle fibres. Occurs in the early puerperium, common in multiparous women, and frequently felt during breastfeeding. Severe and persistent afterpains may indicate a blood clot, membrane or fragment of placenta may have been retained in the uterus. ⊃ 'let down' reflex.

AGA *abbr* appropriate for gestational age.

agalactia *n* non-secretion or imperfect secretion of milk after childbirth—**agalactic** *adj*.

agammaglobulinaemia *n* absence of gammaglobulin in the blood, with consequent inability to produce immunity to infection—**agammaglobulinaemic** *adj*. ⊃ Bruton's agammaglobulinaemia, ⊃ dysgammaglobulinaemia.

aganglionosis *n* absence of ganglia. For example the parasympathetic ganglion cells of the distal bowel ⊃ Hirschsprung's disease, megacolon.

agar *n* a gelatinous substance obtained from certain seaweeds. It is used as a bulk-increasing laxative and for solidifying bacterial culture media.

agate very hard gemstone. Used to make spatula blades which are resistant to abrasion.

age *n* ⊃ mental age.

ageing and exercise certain risks, especially involving the cardiovascular system, increase with age. Ageing is associated with degenerative conditions; there is a reduction in bone density and deterioration of lung function, aerobic fitness and muscle strength. The benefits of activity in advancing years include a reduced incidence of heart disease, maintenance of bone mineral content (reducing fracture risk), muscle strength and balance (reducing falls) and an increased life expectancy. ⊃ osteoporosis.

age-associated memory impairment (AAMI) an abnormal decline in memory (greater than one standard deviation from the normal) with age where there is no premorbid problem with IQ or the presence of dementia.

age-related macular degeneration (AMD/ARMD) (*syn* age-related maculopathy) degenerative changes of the retina in the macular region which may lead to loss of central vision. There are problems with reading and distinguishing fine features. AMD is found in a large percentage of older people (and sometimes middle-aged people), in which there is a degeneration of the photoreceptors of the macular area of the retina. It is a leading cause of blindness in people aged over 50. Two types of AMD are described, it may be 'dry' or atrophic when Bruch's membrane accumulates debris known as drusen, or 'wet' which involves the growth of a new, abnormal blood vessels in Bruch's membrane: (a) the 'dry' type is characterized by the presence of fine pigment stippling with the later appearance of gross pigment clumps and yellowish clumps/spots (drusen) in the macular region while the surrounding retinal area remains usually relatively healthy. ⊃ Colour Section Figure 45. Visual acuity becomes markedly reduced and the condition usually becomes bilateral developing over several years. Management of this condition is essentially by the use of low vision aids; (b) a less common form which is known as neovascular or exudative 'wet' age-related macular degeneration in which the clinical picture is the same initially but is followed by the formation of new blood vessels (choroidal neovascularization - CNV) and fibrous tissue in the macular region resulting in total loss of central vision. Drug therapy is available for 'wet' AMD. A monoclonal antibody that inhibits vascular endothelial growth factor, such as ranibizumab or pegaptanib is administered as a course of intravitreal injections. If detected early (usually with an Amsler chart), treatment with laser photocoagulation will reduce the risk of further visual loss. Photodynamic therapy (PDT) is another method of reducing the risk of visual loss. It allows selective destruction of the choroidal neovascularization with minimal damage to the overlying retinal tissue. It consists of injecting a photosensitizing agent (e.g. verteporfin) that is taken up by the abnormal vessels and when activated by a laser light of a given wavelength (e.g. 689 nm) it damages and shrivels up the vessels. ⊃ Amsler chart, drusen, fluorescein angiography, low vision, photocoagulation, photodynamic therapy, photostress test.

age-related maculopathy (ARM) ⊃ age-related macular degeneration (AMD/ARMD).

ageism *n* stereotyping people according to chronological age: overemphasizing negative aspects to the disadvantage of more positive points. Discriminatory attitudes in society disadvantage older people on the basis of age alone. Ageism is also interpreted to be stigmatizing and to separate the older person from others who are younger. Ageist behaviours are often demonstrated in the choice of terms or labels used. For example, 'elderly', 'seniors', 'senile' and 'geriatric'. The media often reinforce this negative stereotyping. Furthermore, ageist views can impact on people of any age. For example, a group of teenagers chatting on a street corner may be perceived, by others, as a potential threat.

agenesis *n* incomplete and imperfect development—**agenetic** *adj*.

agenitalism a body without recognizable sex organs.

ageusia loss or impairment of the sensation of taste.

agglutination *n* the clumping of bacteria, red blood cells or antigen-coated particles by antibodies called 'agglutinins', developed in the blood serum of a previously infected or sensitized person or animal. Agglutination forms the basis of many laboratory tests—**agglutinable, agglutinative,** *adj*, **agglutinate** *vt, vi*.

agglutinins *npl* antibodies that agglutinate or clump organisms or particles.

aggressive periodonitis ⊃ periodontis.

agility *n* the ability to control the direction of the body or body part during rapid movement.

aglossia *n* absence of the tongue—**aglossic** *adj*.

aglutition *n* dysphagia.

agnathia *n* absence or incomplete development of the jaw.

agnathocephaly a congenital abnormality in which there is a small chin, displaced mouth and approximate fusion of the eyes, which are low set.

agnosia *n* inability to perceive the nature of sensory impressions. People and things are not recognized; usually classified by the sense or senses affected—**agnosic** *adj*. *spatial agnosia* loss of spatial appreciation.

agonal *adj* relating to the events occurring just before death. ⊃ agonal rhythm, Cheyne–Stokes respiration.

agonal rhythm the terminal arrhythmia recorded just prior to death. Usually there is broad-based bradycardia without a cardiac output.

agonist *n* **1.** a prime mover muscle that shortens to perform a movement. For example, when raising a glass to the mouth, the biceps brachii and brachialis muscles are agonists, triceps would be the antagonist in this example. **2.** also describes a drug or other chemical that imitates the response of the ligand (natural chemical such as a neurotransmitter or hormone) at a receptor site. ⊃ antagonist *opp*.

agoraphobia *n* morbid fear of being alone in large open places—**agoraphobic** *adj*.

agranulocyte *n* a non-granular leucocyte.

agranulocytosis *n* marked reduction in or complete absence of granulocytes (the polymorphonuclear leucocytes neutrophils, eosinophils and basophils). Usually results from bone marrow depression caused by: (a) hypersensitivity to drugs; (b) cytotoxic drugs; (c) or irradiation. Symptoms include fever, ulceration of the mouth and throat. There is an inability to fight infection and this can lead to overwhelming infection and ultimately to death. ⊃ neutropenia—**agranulocytic** *adj.*

agraphia *n* loss of language facility—**agraphic** *adj.* ⊃ motor agraphia, sensory agraphia.

agreeableness one of the big five personality factors characterized by a tendency to be kind, generous, sympathetic and unselfish.

AGREE instrument a tool developed by the AGREE Collaboration that facilitates systematic evaluation of the quality of a clinical guideline. The AGREE Collaboration is an international group of researchers and policy makers whose aim is to improve the quality and effectiveness of clinical practice guidelines.

AHF/G *abbr* antihaemophilic factor/globulin.

AHI *abbr* apnoea hypopnoea index.

AHP *abbr* allied health profession.

AICD *abbr* automatic implantable cardioverter defibrillator.

Aicardi syndrome (J Aicardi, French paediatrician/neurologist, b. 1926) a rare genetic defect affecting females. There is abnormal brain development with the partial or total absence of the corpus callosum which normally connects the two hemispheres of the brain. Affected children have seizures, a learning disability and retinal abnormalities.

AID *abbr* artificial insemination of a female with donor semen.

aid a piece of equipment designed to assist a person to carry out a task or activity independently.

AIDS *abbr* acquired immune deficiency syndrome.

AIDS-defining illness the US Centers for Disease Control and Prevention (CDC) criteria for AIDS in a patient infected with HIV disease. Examples include candidiasis of bronchus, trachea, lungs or oesophagus, invasive cervical cancer, Kaposi's sarcoma, pulmonary tuberculosis or other mycobacterial infection, and *Pneumocystis jirovecii* (former name *Pneumocystis carinii*) pneumonia.

aids to independence any articles that enable a person to retain or regain independence. They include those used for eating and drinking; those used for personal hygiene, dressing and undressing; those for walking and so on; and those used for transit. ⊃ walking aids.

AIH *abbr* artificial insemination of a female with her husband's (partner's) semen.

ainhum *n* the spontaneous amputation of the fifth toe. It may be due to the formation of a constricting fibrous band. It may occur in Africa, in people who habitually walk barefoot.

AIP *abbr* acute interstitial pneumonia.

air *n* the gaseous mixture which makes up the atmosphere surrounding the earth. It consists of approximately 78% nitrogen, 20% oxygen, 0.04% carbon dioxide, 1% argon, and traces of ozone, neon, helium, etc., and a variable amount of water vapour.

air embolism obstruction to the flow of blood resulting from an air bubble entering the circulation. This may occur during surgery, during intravenous fluid infusion or injection, cardiac catheterization or trauma.

air hunger a deep indrawing of breath which characterizes the late stages of uncontrolled haemorrhage.

air knives are used in the drier section of automatic film processors to increase the velocity of the air as it strikes the film surface.

air motor in dentistry. A drill motor, driven at medium speeds by compressed air and coupled directly to a conventional handpiece having no driving cable.

air rotor in dentistry, a handpiece incorporating an air-driven high-speed rotor.

air swallowing (aerophagia) swallowing of excessive air particularly when eating: it may result in belching or the passage of flatus from the anus.

air syringe ⊃ syringe.

air turbine ⊃ air rotor.

airway *n* used to describe the entry to the larynx from the pharynx. *Brook airway* oropharyngeal airway used in expired air resuscitation. *nasopharyngeal airway* a curved airway introduced into the pharynx via the nostril. It is located behind the tongue and so prevents a flaccid tongue from obstructing the airway in an unconscious patient. *oropharyngeal airway* a flexible oval tube, such as a Guedel airway (Figure A.6), which can be placed along the upper surface of the tongue to prevent a flaccid tongue from resting against the posterior pharyngeal wall, thereby obstructing the airway, and is commonly used during general anaesthesia. Also used during cardiopulmonary resuscitation.

airway conductance the ease in which air/gas flows through the airways. It is the reciprocal of airways resistance.

airways the passages to the lungs consisting of upper and lower respiratory tracts. The upper respiratory tract consists of the nose, pharynx and larynx and warms, filters and moistens the inhaled air prior to its passage down the lower

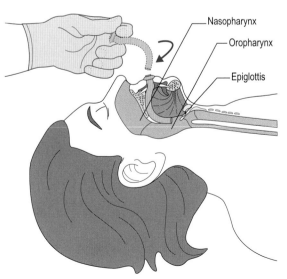

Nasopharynx

Oropharynx

Epiglottis

A.6 Airway (reproduced from Nicol et al 2004 with permission).

respiratory tract. The upper respiratory tract is also important for the functions of speech, taste and smell. The lower respiratory tract comprises the conducting system and begins at the trachea, which bifurcates, to the point of the terminal bronchioles before the formation of the gas exchange unit of the lung (alveolar sacs). ⇨ bronchial tree.

airways resistance (R$_{aw}$) the pressure required to elicit airflow between the mouth and the alveolus. Airway resistance increases as the calibre of the airway is reduced, e.g. through inflammation, bronchial smooth muscle contraction or thickening of the airway walls through remodelling in various disease processes. R$_{aw}$ is calculated by the change in pressure along a tube, divided by the flow.

AIS *abbr* abbreviated injury scale.

AJC *abbr* acrylic jacket crown.

A-K amputation *abbr* above-the-knee amputation.

akathisia *n* a subjective state of persistent motor restlessness: it can occur as a side-effect of antipsychotic (neuroleptic) drugs.

akinesia *n* impairment in initiation of movement or delay in reaction time, such as with parkinsonism—**akinetic** *adj.*

ALA *abbr* alpha (α)-linolenic acid.

ala a wing-like process, e.g. the ala of the nose—**alae** *pl.*
ala nasi the cartilagenous wing of the nostril.

alacrima the absence of secretion from the lacrimal gland. However, the typical picture is one of reduced tear secretion more correctly termed hypolacrima. It may occur as a result of occlusion of the orifices of the lacrimal gland due to trauma, cicatrization, diseases (e.g. trachoma); it may be congenital (e.g. Riley-Day syndrome) or it may be due to a neurogenic cause (secondary to brain damage) or to a systemic disease (e.g. Sjögren's syndrome). Treatment includes artificial tears, bland ointments, sealed scleral contact lenses and in very severe cases tarsorrhaphy. ⇨ artificial tears, lacrimal gland, keratitis sicca, Riley-Day syndrome, Sjögren's syndrome, tarsorrhaphy, tears.

alactacid (alactic) anaerobic system a series of chemical reactions occurring within the cells whereby adenosine triphosphate (ATP) for energy use is produced, without oxygen, from adenosine diphosphate (ADP) and creatine phosphate (CP) (phosphocreatine).

alactacid oxygen debt component the amount of oxygen required to replace the adenosine triphosphate (ATP) and creatine phosphate (phosphocreatine) stores in cells during the process of recovery from exercise.

alactasia the deficiency (partial or total) of the intestinal enzyme lactase. The affected person is unable to digest lactose (sugar) in milk. ⇨ lactase deficiency.

Alagille sydrome a dominantly inherited autosomal condition. There is jaundice due to faulty development of the intrahepatic bile ducts. It may be associated with pulmonary stenosis and other heart defects, and abnormalities affecting the eyes and nervous system.

-al, ale a suffix that means 'characterized by, pertaining to', e.g. *meningeal.*

alanine *n* a non-essential (dispensable) amino acid.

alanine aminotransferase (ALT) an enzyme that facilitates the reversible transfer of amino groups during amino acid metabolism. ⇨ aminotransferases.

ALARA an overarching principle which states that the radiation dosage to patients and staff should be kept **as low as reasonably achievable.**

alar ligaments a ligament in the upper cervical spine that extends from the side of the dens of the axis to the medial occipital condyle, may be ruptured following certain disorders, such as rheumatoid arthritis.

alba, albicans white. ⇨ corpus albicantes, linea.

ala-tragal line also known as Camper's line. An imaginary line running from the inferior border of the ala of the nose to the superior border of the tragus of the ear. Used as a reference plane in orthodontics, radiography and prosthetics, when determining the occlusal plane.

alb- a prefix that means 'white', e.g. *albinism.*

Albers-Schönberg disease (H Albers-Schönberg, German surgeon/radiologist, 1865–1921) ⇨ osteopetrosis.

albinism *n* a congenital hypopigmentation of the hair, skin and eyes. It is caused by a deficiency of melanin pigment in skin and/or the eye. Other associated eye and neurological defects can contribute to poor vision.

albino *n* a person affected with albinism—**albinotic** *adj.*

Albright's syndrome (F Albright, American physician, 1900–1969) a condition that includes fibrous dysplasia of bone, endocrine problems, such as precocious puberty in female, and brown macular areas on the skin. ⇨ fibrous dysplasia.

albumin *n* a protein found in animal and vegetable material. It is soluble in water and coagulates on heating. *serum albumin* the main protein of blood plasma. ⇨ lactalbumin—**albuminous, albuminoid** *adj.*

albuminuria *n* the presence of albumin in the urine. The condition may be temporary and clear up completely, as in many febrile states. May be indicative of serious kidney disease—**albuminuric** *adj.* ⇨ microalbuminuria, orthostatic albuminuria, proteinuria.

albumose *n* an intermediate substance formed during protein digestion.

alcohol *n* a group of organic compounds. Absolute alcohol is occasionally used by injection for the relief of trigeminal neuralgia and other intractable pain. In dentistry, used as a solvent, surgical antiseptic and during cavity toilet. Ethyl alcohol (ethanol) is the intoxicating constituent of alcoholic drinks: wine, beer, cider and spirits. It potentiates the effects of hypnotics and tranquillizers. ⇨ alcohol dependence/misuse, Korsakoff's syndrome, Wernicke's encephalopathy.

alcohol and sport the anxiety-reducing effects of alcohol can improve confidence and performance, particularly in sports where fine motor control is required, e.g. by snooker players or marksmen. In many sports, particularly team sports, alcohol intake is a part of the culture. Because of the well-known diuretic properties, athletes should be advised against alcohol consumption when fluid replacement is a priority, and alcohol can impair both performance and recovery after exercise. It is banned in some sports (e.g. motor racing, skiing).

alcohol dependence/misuse the morbid state of dependence upon an excessive intake of alcohol. A syndrome of physical, psychological and behavioural responses related to alcohol misuse. Characteristically there are withdrawal symptoms and drinking to relieve the same, tolerance to the effects of alcohol, compulsion to drink alcohol, narrowing of repertoire of drinking, etc. Poisoning resulting from alcoholic dependence may be acute or chronic. Chronic poisoning causes severe damage to most body systems, e.g. the liver, digestive organs with malnutrition, the heart and nervous system. Long term alcohol misuse is associated with hepatitis, cirrhosis, hepatic portal hypertension, oesophageal varices and gastrointestinal haemorrhage, gastritis, iron overload, primary liver cancer, other cancers, e.g. head and neck, pancreatitis, arterial hypertension, coronary heart disease and neurological problems caused by alcohol toxicity or B vitamin deficiency. Misuse of alcohol by a woman during pregnancy can lead to the birth of an infant with fetal alcohol syndrome (FAS). Additionally, the chronic misuse of alcohol causes social, emotional and psychological problems, such as the breakdown of relationships, financial difficulties and debt, the loss of employment, criminality and homelessness.

alcohol-fast *adj* in bacteriology, describes a microorganism which, when stained, is resistant to decolorization by alcohol.

alcohol units a useful way of estimating how much alcohol has been consumed, and in promoting safe intake. One unit of alcohol is defined as 10 mL of absolute alcohol

Alcoholics Anonymous (AA) a fellowship of people who have had problems with alcohol dependence. Their aim is helping others with similar difficulties.

ALD *abbr* adrenoleucodystrophy.

aldehydes *npl* a group of organic compounds. Formed by the oxidation of an alcohol (e.g. acetaldehyde from ethyl alcohol).

aldolase *n* an enzyme present in muscle tissue.

aldolase test increased levels of aldolase and other enzymes in the blood are indicative of some muscle diseases, e.g. severe muscular dystrophy.

aldosterone *n* mineralocorticoid hormone secreted by the adrenal cortex. Secretion is regulated by the action of renin and angiotensin. It enhances the reabsorption of sodium accompanied by water and the excretion of potassium by the renal tubules.

aldosterone antagonist a drug that acts as an aldosterone antagonist. ➲ potassium sparing diuretics, Appendix 5.

aldosteronism *n* ➲ hyperaldosteronism.

Aleppo boil ➲ leishmaniasis.

Alexander technique (F Alexander, Australian actor, 1869–1955) a series of techniques used to improve the functioning of mind and body in movement known as 'psychophysical' re-education. It is based on the belief that poor posture can lead to ill health, injury and chronic pain. The technique aims to promote postural improvement through self-awareness and control, aiming either to remove the cause of, or simply prevent, many forms of ill health, chronic pain, poor posture and inadequate performance. Developed in the late 1890s by an Australian actor who studied and improved his own vocal problems, the technique is now widely recognized as a fundamental tool for establishing good co-ordination, balance and poise. It is valued by athletes as a way to improve performance and prevent or resolve injuries. It is taught on a one-to-one basis and teachers will usually have attended a three-year training course or its equivalent.

alexia *n* word blindness; an inability to interpret the significance of the printed or written word, but without loss of visual power. Can be due to a brain lesion or insufficient/inappropriate sensory experience during an *ab initio* stage of learning—**alexic** *adj*.

alexithymia a personality trait characterized by difficulty in recognizing or describing one's emotions.

ALG *abbr* antilymphocyte globulin.

algesia *n* excessive sensitivity to pain.

-algesic a suffix that means 'sensitivity to pain', e.g. analgesic.

algesimeter *n* an instrument that registers the degree of sensitivity to pain.

-algia a suffix that means 'pain', e.g. *neuralgia*.

alginates *npl* salt of alginic acid. Obtained from seaweed derivatives and used in some wound dressings. These dressings have high absorbency, haemostatic properties and can be removed without damaging delicate tissues. They can be used for wounds with moderate to high exudate, for wet wound débridement and on infected wounds. In dentistry, alginates are mixed with water in the recommended proportions to form an irreversible hydrocolloid gel used for dental impressions.

alginate impression material ➲ impression material, irreversible hydrocolloid.

algodystrophy ➲ complex regional pain syndrome.

algorithm **1**. a step-by-step protocol or guide for the management of particular situation or health problem. **2**. a step-by-step procedure for the solution of a problem with computer software that uses specific mathematical or logical operations. For example, in computed tomography (CT) scanning the mathematical process is used in image reconstruction, different algorithms may be used to produce differing images to better demonstrate particular structures.

aliasing **1**. in ultrasound when high velocities in one direction appear as high velocities in the opposite direction. It occurs when an analogue signal is sampled at a frequency which is lower than half its maximum frequency. All the frequency above half of the sampling frequency is projected below the base line (backfolded) in the low frequency region causing artefacts on the image. **2**. An artefact that occurs in magnetic resonance imaging (MRI) due to the image encoding process, it occurs when the field of view is smaller than the area being imaged.

alienation *n* in psychology and sociology, estrangement from people.

A
B

align 1. to bring into line. **2.** in orthodontics and prosthetics, to move teeth into their correct position so as to conform to the correct occlusal plane and arch form.

aligning power ⊃ vernier visual acuity.

aligning prism ⊃ associated heterophoria.

alignment refers to the postural inter-relationship of body segments, in different planes. Physiotherapists assess alignment in different positions, e.g. standing, sitting, as normal alignment is integral to efficient movement. There is considerable variability of alignment.

alimentary *adj* pertaining to food.

alimentary tract *n* comprises the mouth, oesophagus, stomach, small intestine, ascending colon, transverse colon, descending colon, sigmoid colon, rectum and anal canal. ⊃ Colour Section Figure 18b.

alimentation *n* the act of nourishing with food; feeding.

alkalaemia *n* low level of acid (hydrogen ions) in the blood resulting in an above normal pH >7.45 (hydrogen ion concentration <36 mmol/L)—**alkalaemic** *adj.* ⊃ acid–base balance, alkalosis, arterial blood gases, metabolic alkalosis, respiratory alkalosis.

alkali *n* also called a base. Substances that have an excess of hydroxyl ions over hydrogen ions, e.g. sodium bicarbonate, sodium hydroxide. They have a pH greater than 7 and turn red litmus blue. Alkalis react with acids to produce salts plus water, and with fats to form soaps.

alkaline *adj* **1.** relating to or possessing the properties of an alkali. **2.** containing an excess of hydroxyl over hydrogen ions.

alkaline phosphatase an enzyme present in several tissues, e.g. bone, liver and kidney. An increase of this enzyme in the blood is indicative of obstructive jaundice and increased osteoblast activity associated with some bone diseases.

alkaline reserve the amount of buffered alkali (normally bicarbonate) available in the blood for buffering acids (normally dissolved CO_2) formed in or introduced into the body and limiting pH changes in the blood.

alkaline tide describes the movement of basic bicarbonate (hydrogen carbonate) (HCO_3^-) ions from the parietal (oxyntic) cells of the stomach into the venous blood. The hydrogen carbonate ions are formed during the secretion of hydrochloric acid (HCl) by the oxyntic cells. This results in a small rise in blood pH.

alkalinuria *n* alkalinity of urine—**alkalinuric** *adj.*

alkaloid *n* similar to an alkali. Also describes a large group of organic bases present in plants and which have important pharmacological actions, e.g. morphine, atropine, quinine and caffeine. Also result from fungal action on cereal crops, such as ergot. May be present in animal foods, e.g. puffer fish contains tetrodotoxin—**alkaloidal** *adj.*

alkalosis *n* process leading to low levels of acid (excess of alkali) in the body. It may have a metabolic or respiratory cause. ⊃ acid–base balance, alkalaemia, metabolic alkalosis, respiratory alkalosis.

alkaptonuria *n* the presence of alkaptone (homogentisic acid) in the urine, resulting from only partial oxidation of the amino acids phenylalanine and tyrosine. Condition usually noticed because urine turns black in the nappies, or when left to stand. Apart from this, and a tendency to arthritis in later life, there are no ill-effects from alkaptonuria.

alkylating agents organic molecules that disrupt cell division by binding to the DNA in the nucleus, e.g. busulfan. ⊃ cytotoxic. ⊃ Appendix 5.

ALL *abbr* acute lymphoblastic leukaemia.

all fours position position which the women may assume in the second stage of labour. It has been shown to increase the pelvic outlet, facilitating normal delivery.

allantois a membranous sac projecting from ventral surface of the embryo, which eventually helps to form the placenta.

allele *n* allelomorph. Describes the alternative forms of a gene at the same chromosomal location (locus). Previously used to denote inherited characteristics that are alternative and contrasting, such as normal colour vision contrasting with colour blindness, or the different ABO blood groups.

allelomorph ⊃ allele.

allergen *n* an antigen which produces an allergic, or immediate-type hypersensitivity response—**allergenic** *adj*, **allergenicity** *n.*

allergic conjunctivitis conjunctivitis caused by an allergy. Common allergens are pollens associated with hay fever, grass (seasonal allergic conjunctivitis) and air pollutants, house dust mites, smoke (perennial allergic conjunctivitis). It is characterized by hyperaemia, itching, burning, swelling, tearing, discharge and photophobia. Conjunctival scrapings contain a large number of eosinophils and serum IgE is elevated. The condition is often associated with rhinitis (allergic rhinoconjunctivitis). Treatment commonly includes decongestants, oral antihistamines, drugs such as lodoxamide or sodium cromoglicate and if severe, topical corticosteroid eyedrops. ⊃ antihistamines, decongestants, vernal conjunctivitis.

allergic contact eczema caused by a delayed hypersensitivity reaction following contact with antigens or haptens. Previous exposure to the allergen is required for sensitization and the reaction is specific to the allergen or closely related chemicals. Common allergens and their origin include: (a) nickel—jewellery, jean studs, bra clips; (b) dichromate—cement, leather, matches; (c) rubber chemicals—clothing, shoes, latex gloves, latex-containing medical equipment, tyres; (d) colophony—sticking plaster, colloidion; (e) paraphenylenediamine—hair dye, clothing; (f) balsam of Peru—perfumes, citrus fruits; (g) neomycin, benzocaine—topical applications; (h) parabens—preservatives in cosmetics and creams; (i) wool alcohols—lanolin, cosmetics, creams; (j) epoxy resin—resin adhesives.The eczema reaction occurs wherever the allergen is in contact with the skin and sensitization persists indefinitely. It is important to determine the original site of the rash before secondary spread obscures the picture, as this often provides the best clue to the contactant. There are many easily recognizable patterns, e.g. eczema of the earlobes, wrists and back due to contact with nickel in costume jewellery, watches and bra clips; or eczema of the hands and wrists due to latex gloves. Oedema of the lax skin of the eyelids and genitalia is a frequent concomitant of allergic contact eczema. ⊃ Colour Section Figure 46.

allergy *n* an immune response induced by exposure to an allergen causing a harmful hypersensitivity reaction on subsequent exposure—**allergic** *adj.* ⊃ anaphylaxis, sensitization.

Allied and Complementary Medicine Database (AMED) computerized database of literature relevant to a variety of professions allied to medicine, such as physiotherapy, etc., palliative care and complementary medicine.

allied health profession (AHP) a large and varied group of registered health profession practitioners distinct from medicine, dentistry and nursing. They work autonomously in multiprofessional and interagency teams. Professionals included as allied health vary from country to country but may include: art therapists, biomedical scientists, chiropodists/podiatrists, dental hygienists, dietitians, occupational therapists, operating department practitioners, paramedics, physiotherapists (physical therapists), radiographers (diagnostic and therapeutic), prosthetists/orthotists, speech and language therapists.

Allitt Inquiry (Clothier Report, 1994) the report of an independent inquiry team into the events surrounding deaths and injuries to children in the care of one particular nurse in an English hospital. It includes recommendations designed to strengthen procedures that safeguard children in hospital and prevent any repetition.

allocation concealment a research term, The process used to prevent advance knowledge of group assignment in a randomized controlled trial.

allograft *n* grafting or transplanting an organ or tissue from one person to another who does not share exactly the same transplantation antigens. Also known as a homograft.

alloimmunization immune response to donated blood, bone marrow or a transplanted organ. Rhesus negative pregnant women can become alloimmunized following a sensitizing event with a rhesus positive fetus, e.g. antepartum haemorrhage, miscarriage, through development of antibodies which target the foreign material, causing haemolytic disease of the newborn. ⊃ haemolytic disease of the newborn.

allopathy *n* describes conventional medicine and health care—**allopathic** *adj.* ⊃ homoeopathy.

alloplastic implant ⊃ implant.

all-or-none law/phenomenon *n* relates to the conduction of action potentials in nerve or muscle fibres (excitable tissue). The action potential in a particular fibre is always the same size regardless of the intensity of the stimulus. The nerve or muscle fibre either responds in full or does not respond at all. There is no partial response to a reduced intensity stimulus.

allotriophagy desire for extraordinary or abnormal foods. Also known as cissa, cittosis and pica.

alloy 1. product formed by the fusion of two or more metals that are mutually soluble in the liquid state. 2. product of the fusion of several metals, usually supplied as shavings and mixed with mercury. Amalgam alloy may be lathe cut or spherical forms. The mercury is generally triple distilled for the sake of purity and it is important that the proportion of mercury to alloy is correct in order to obtain the best amalgam properties. A proportioner may be used to obtain the correct amounts of each, and may be adjusted to suit the operator but now generally supplied preproportioned in encapsulated form. Mercury should not be handled nor left exposed because of the highly toxic properties of its vapour. ⊃ admixed amalgam alloy, amalgam, encapsulated alloy, high copper amalgam alloy, lathe cut amalgam alloy, silver tin alloy, spherical amalgam alloy, zinc free amalgam alloy.

alloy blocks shielding blocks of an alloy of lead, bismuth or cadmium placed on a tray on the radiotherapy accessory mount to shape the radiation beam so that it accurately covers the treatment area. Blocks can be individually made for each patient, accounting for beam divergence and pre-mounted on a tray.

alopecia *n* baldness, which can be congenital, premature or part of the aging process (senile). ⊃ alopecia areata, cicatricial alopecia, folliculitis decalvans.

alopecia areata a patchy baldness, usually of a temporary nature. Cause unknown, probably autoimmune, but stress is a common precipitating factor. Exclamation mark hairs are diagnostic. The broken stump found at the periphery of spreading bald patches in alopecia areata is called an exclamation mark hair, from the characteristic shape caused by atrophic thinning of the hair shaft. ⊃ Colour Section Figure 47.

alpha (α)-adrenoceptor agonists (*syn* α stimulants) naturally occurring substances or drugs that act specifically on cellular alpha-adrenoceptors. Also applied to a specific group of drugs that stimulate α-adrenoceptors, e.g. adrenaline (epinephrine). ⊃ adrenoceptors, Appendix 5.

alpha (α)-adrenoceptor antagonists (*syn* α blockers) a substance or group of drugs that block the stimulation of α-adrenoceptors, e.g. doxazosin. The antagonists can be selective for alpha$_1$ (α$_1$) adrenoceptors, alpha$_2$ (α$_2$) adrenoceptors or their further subtypes⊃ adrenoceptors, Appendix 5.

alpha (α) decay the spontaneous emission of an alpha particle from the nucleus of an atom, resulting in the atomic number of the element decreasing by two and the mass number decreasing by four.

alpha (α)-glucosidase (acid maltase) enzyme deficiency ⊃ inherited metabolic myopathies, Pompe's disease.

alpha (α)-glucosidase inhibitor an oral hypoglycaemic drug that slows the digestion and absorption of complex carbohydrates and sucrose from the intestine, e.g. acarbose. ⊃ Appendix 5.

alpha (α)-ketoglutarate an intermediate in the Krebs' cycle; may be depleted in the late stages of endurance exercise, suggesting potential utility as an anticatabolic agent.

alpha (α)-linolenic acid (ALA) a polyunsaturated fatty acid. ⊃ linolenic acids.

alpha(α) motor neuron the type of neuron that innervates the extrafusal fibres of the skeletal muscle. The alpha (α) motor neurons have larger diameter axons and bigger cell bodies than the gamma (γ) motor neurons. ⟳ extrafusal fibres, gamma (γ) motor neurons.

alpha (α) particle the nucleus of a helium-4 atom consisting of two protons and two neutrons.

alpha (α) redistribution phase the point after an intravenous injection when the blood concentration of the drug begins to fall below the peak levels achieved.

alpha thalassaemia ⟳ thalassaemia.

alpha (α)-tocopherols the most biologically active forms of vitamin E, which is the most important antioxidant in cell membranes. Its principal function is to stabilize the structural integrity of membranes by breaking the chain reaction of lipid peroxidation. Vitamin E is also essential for normal function of the immune system. ⟳ reactive oxygen species.

alpha$_1$ (α)-antitrypsin a liver protein that normally opposes the proteolytic enzyme trypsin. Reduced blood levels are linked with a genetic predisposition to emphysema and liver disease.

alpha$_1$ (α)-antitrypsin deficiency (AAT) an inherited form of destructive emphysema resulting from the absence or inadequate levels of the chemical alpha$_1$ antitrypsin that inhibits trypsin (a proteolytic enzyme). Neutrophil elastase may go unchecked in this deficiency resulting in the destruction of elastin and subsequent dissolution of the alveolar walls. This should be suspected in patients around the age of 40 years or less, who present with a chronic obstructive pulmonary disease, a disease usually associated with later years.

alphafetoprotein (AFP) *n* a protein produced by the yolk sac, fetal gut and liver cells and by adult liver cancer cells. Raised levels are found in maternal serum and amniotic fluid in fetal abnormalities including open neural tube defects and abdominal wall defects. Low levels are associated with chromosomal anomalies, e.g. Edwards' syndrome (trisomy 18) and Down's syndrome (trisomy 21). AFP levels for Down's syndrome are assessed in the second trimester of pregnancy in conjunction with human chorionic gonadotrophin (hCG) and unconjugated oestriols (UE$_3$); levels are also dependent on gestation, number of fetuses, maternal weight and diabetes mellitus. Also used as a tumour marker for cancers including those of the liver and the testes affecting children and adults. Also present in the serum in liver cirrhosis. ⟳ oncofetal antigens.

alphaviruses a group of very small togaviruses. They are transmitted by mosquito bites and cause diseases that include Ross River virus disease/fever. ⟳ arboviruses.

Alport's syndrome (A Alport, South African physician, 1880–1959) an inherited disorder characterized by glomerulonephritis and haematuria which, in males, usually progresses to end-stage renal failure. A kidney transplant and some form of dialysis may be successful. Affected females may be asymptomatic. Other problems include progressive sensorineural deafness and eye disorders, such as cataracts and lenticonus.

ALS *abbr* **1.** advanced life support. **2.** amyotrophic lateral sclerosis.

ALT *abbr* alanine aminotransferase. ⟳ aminotransferases.

alternate (alternating) cover test ⟳ cover test.

alternating current (AC) an electrotherapy term. One of three recognized categories of therapeutic currents (pulsed, direct and alternating currents). The electrons flow through a circuit in one direction and then the other. A continuous series (train) of biphasic pulses. Continuous pulses can be interrupted (bursts). ⟳ direct current.

alternative medicine ⟳ complementary and alternative medicine.

altitude the height above sea level. As atmospheric (barometric) pressure decreases progressively with increasing altitude, from the standard 1 atmosphere at sea level, the partial pressure of oxygen (PO_2) decreases proportionately; the air still contains the same ~21% of oxygen but there are fewer molecules of oxygen per unit volume. There is also a drop in temperature and humidity, but the essential problem for human life and activity is shortage of oxygen (hypoxia).

altitude acclimatization physiological adjustments that help to compensate mainly for the shortage of oxygen. When blood is inadequately oxygenated in the lungs, the hypoxic condition (low PO_2) of blood and tissues stimulates changes in: (a) ventilation—increase in rate and depth of breathing brings the partial pressure of oxygen in the lungs (and therefore in the arterial blood) closer to that in the air, whilst decreasing the partial pressure of carbon dioxide (PCO_2); the resulting alkalosis is gradually corrected and the hyperventilation later diminishes; (b) cardiac output (CO)—initial increase at rest, and at any level of activity, provides greater blood flow to the tissues in compensation for the lowered oxygen content of the blood. Over a few days CO decreases again for any given $\dot{V}O_2$ until it has returned to sea-level values, with tissues extracting more oxygen per litre of blood (i.e. the arteriovenous difference increases); (c) oxygen transport and delivery—after an initial increase in packed cell volume (haematocrit) due to reduction in plasma volume, stimulation of erthropoietin secretion enhances red blood cell production in the bone marrow, raising the red cell count and haemoglobin (Hb) concentration in the blood; this increases the amount of oxygen that can be carried per litre of blood at the lowered saturation (but the resulting polycythaemia increases blood viscosity). The affinity of Hb for oxygen is modified by an increase in the enzyme 2,3-diphosphoglycerate (2,3-DPG), causing a rightward shift in the oxygen dissociation curve; this assists offloading in the tissues at a any given local PO_2, but can be offset by a leftward shift of the curve due to low arterial PCO_2. There are also changes in cellular metabolism. The timing and effectiveness of these adjustments vary among individuals, as does tolerance of the negative effects (Figure A.7). ⟳ acclimation, altitude sickness, altitude training, chemoreceptors, erythropoiesis, hypoxia, partial pressure.

altitude sickness/illness (acute mountain sickness, AMS) may occur at altitudes higher than about 8000 ft (~2500 metres) above sea level, although it has been

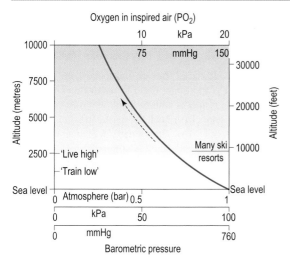

A.7 Altitude: relation between decreasing barometric pressure and PO_2 and levels for athletic training. Broken arrow: altitude sickness in the unacclimatized (reproduced from Jennett 2008 with permission).

reported between 1500 and 2500 metres. It can be encountered during mountaineering or flights in unpressurized aircraft. Incidence is related to the height attained and the rapidity of ascent, as well as to individual susceptibility. Problems range from mild nausea, headache, dizziness, breathlessness, mood changes and disordered sleep (acute mountain sickness) to pulmonary oedema (with cough and frothy sputum) and cerebral oedema (with neurological symptoms and mental confusion) which can be fatal. All are direct or indirect results of low partial pressure of oxygen (PO_2) in the atmosphere. Prevention may include premedication and staging the ascent; those who develop symptoms should go no higher whilst they persist, and descent as a medical emergency may be necessary if symptoms are severe.

altitude training a programme of exercise that aims to produce reversible physiological adaptations that increase a person's tolerance to the reduced PO_2 at altitude. Training at real or simulated altitude sufficient to reduce oxygen partial pressure (PO_2) significantly below that at sea-level, undertaken with a view to increasing packed cell volume (haematocrit) and so oxygen-carrying capacity of the blood, and thus enhancing sea-level aerobic performance. Individual responses vary widely and other effects can be deleterious (e.g. muscle mass is reduced and blood viscosity is increased). A *'live high (e.g. 2500 metres), train lower (e.g. 1250 metre)'* strategy is currently more favoured, as the training itself can then be close to sea-level intensity, while haematocrit increase is still achieved during the less active periods. Some research has suggested that altitude training may also improve sea-level endurance performance by enhancing the running economy (oxygen consumption at a given speed) of the athletes. ⊃ altitude acclimatization.

altitudinal *adj* when describing a visual field defect implies loss of vision in superior or inferior half of field.

altitudinal hemianopsia hemianopsia in either the upper or lower half of the visual field.

alum ⊃ potassium aluminium sulphate.

alumina substance added to porcelain to produce increased strength.

alumina (aluminous) porcelain dental porcelain to which is added a significant amount of recrystallized alumina, in order to increase the strength of the final restoration.

aluminium (Al) a metallic element. It is the third most abundant element. Its physical properties of durability and lightness make it a suitable material for various prostheses and dental appliances. Aluminium salts are used therapeutically as antacids, astringents and antiseptics. They are also used in radiography.

aluminium acetate used in very specific cases as an astringent.

aluminium chloride (AlCl₃) in radiography, used as a hardener in fixing solutions which contain acetic acid as the acid.

aluminium hydroxide (Al(OH)₃) used as an antacid for dyspepsia.

aluminium oxide (Al₂O₃) abrasive sometimes used as a polishing agent and now also added to dental porcelain and cement powders to increase the strength of the final restoration.

aluminium sulphate (Al₂(SO₄)₃) in radiography, used as a hardener in fixing solutions which contain sulphuric acid as the acid.

alveolar *adj* relating to an alveolus.

alveolar abscess ⊃ dentoalveolar abscess.

alveolar–arterial difference for oxygen (P_AO_2–PaO_2 gradient) a measure of lung efficiency for gaseous exchange. Ideally, the two values would be the same but in the normal lung, the alveolar–arterial oxygen difference equates to 0.5–2 kPa. In hypoventilation states, the difference will be small since both are reduced. However, where ventilation perfusion ratio V/Q mismatch is present or diffusion problems experienced, the PaO_2 will be relatively normal, but the P_AO_2 will be reduced, so resulting in a greater A-a PO_2 difference. ⊃ ventilation perfusion ratio.

alveolar bone the bone of the alveolar process that supports and surrounds the teeth. Forms the alveolar process. Develops with the eruption of the teeth and is resorbed when the teeth are lost. ⊃ basal bone, bundle bone.

alveolar crest most coronal portion of the alveolar bone.

alveolar margin coronal aspect of the bone which forms the tooth sockets

alveolar mucosa mucosa covering the base of the alveolar process and the floor of the mouth. It is loosely attached to the periosteum of the bone and is movable.

alveolar process portion of the maxilla or mandible which contains the sockets of erupted teeth and the crypts of the developing teeth.

alveolar resorption the reduction in size of the residual ridges of the mandible and maxillae following the extraction of teeth.

alveolar ridge the residual ridge in which alveolar bone remains after the loss of teeth. ⊃ ridge.

alveolar septum partition of the bone separating individual alveoli of multirooted teeth.

alveolar ventilation ($\dot{V}_A$) alveolar ventilation, refers to the amount of inspired air which reaches the regions of the lungs where gas exchange occurs. It is equal to the total ventilation minus dead space ventilation ($\dot{V}_D$). Normally, at rest, $\dot{V}_A{:}\dot{V}_D = 2{:}1$ or typically, $\dot{V}_E - \dot{V}_D = \dot{V}_A$, $6-2 = 4$ L.min^{-1}.

alveolectomy partial or complete excision of the alveolar process of the maxilla or mandible.

alveolitis *n* inflammation of alveoli. When caused by inhalation of an allergen, such as microbial spores or animal proteins, it is termed *extrinsic allergic alveolitis*.

alveolotomy trimming and moulding of the outer plate of the alveolar process following septal alveolectomy in order to achieve the more aesthetic placing of a denture.

alveolus *n* **1.** an air sac of the lung (pulmonary alveolus). The gas exchange unit of the lung. It is particularly suited to its function of exchanging gases since it has a large cross sectional area, an abundant blood supply and is only a single cell thick, thus facilitating diffusion across the alveolar capillary membrane. **2.** one of the sockets in the alveolar process of the maxilla or mandible which retains teeth by means of the periodontal ligament fibres. Term sometimes incorrectly used to describe the alveolar process. **3.** a gland follicle or acinus—**alveoli** *pl*, **alveolar** *adj*.

alveoplasty a general term used to describe the surgical reshaping of the alveolar ridges.

Alzheimer's disease (A Alzheimer, German neurologist, 1864–1915), a neurodegenerative disorder of the brain with distinct pathology causing a progressive loss of cognitive function (dementia). It is primarily a disease that occurs in older people for no obvious reason but can affect younger patients (i.e.<65 years of age), when it may be familial. Alzheimer's disease is the most common cause of dementia in people under 65 years of age and may be linked to the inheritance of a gene that codes for apolipoprotein E (a transport protein). The brains of people with Alzheimer's disease exhibit specific abnormalities including: plaques containing amyloid (abnormal protein) in the cortex, loss of neurons, brain atrophy with shrinkage and the presence of neurofibrillary tangles. The onset is insidious and some changes may be put down to growing older, and is characterized by progressive memory loss (particularly short term or recent), failing intellectual ability, confusion, restlessness, speech problems, motor retardation, depression and personality changes. As the disease progresses the person becomes bed-bound and completely reliant upon family or carers for every need. ⊃ dementia.

AMA *abbr* antimitochondrial antibody.

amacrine cell a retinal cell located in the inner nuclear layer connecting ganglion cells with bipolar cells. Some have an ascending axon synapsing with receptors.

amalgam *n* dental amalgam. Mercury-containing alloy which becomes a soft silvery paste on mixing and later hardens. ⊃ alloy, amalgam carrier, amalgam condenser, amalgam core, amalgam plugger, amalgam tattoo.

amalgamation mixing together of alloy and mercury to form amalgam. ⊃ trituration.

amalgamator electrically driven mechanical device, often with a built-in proportioner, used to amalgamate alloy and mercury in a capsule. A timing clock controls the mixing time. Should stand in a shallow plastic tray to trap any mercury spillage. Now superseded by the introduction of pre-encapsulated amalgam. Commonly relates to the mechanical device that mixes encapsulated dental amalgam (materials).

amalgam carrier metal or plastic instrument used to convey amalgam, in its plastic state, to the mouth and deposit it into a prepared tooth cavity. Sometimes called an amalgam gun. After use excess amalgam should be expelled immediately from the nozzle to prevent blockage when it has set hard.

amalgam condenser either a hand instrument used to condense amalgam in a cavity preparation, or an engine-driven device which mechanically condenses amalgam.

amalgam core amalgam restoration, usually retained by pins, post or adhesives, designed to support another restoration.

amalgam plugger double-ended hand instrument having round- or oval-shaped ends which may be serrated or plain. Used to plug and condense amalgam into a cavity preparation.

amalgam tattoo brown or black area of pigmentation caused by the accidental implantation of amalgam in the oral tissues.

Amanita a genus of fungi some of which are highly toxic. They include the death cap (*A. phalloides*) mushroom. After some hours following ingestion the toxins cause vomiting, diarrhoea, abdominal pain and acute liver necrosis and failure. Intensive care and support for specific organ failure is required. The mortality rate is high in the absence of treatment.

amastia *n* congenital absence of the breasts.

amATPase *abbr* actomyosin ATPase.

amaurosis *n* partial or total blindness due to a lesion somewhere in the visual pathway, but not in the eye itself.

amaurosis fugax temporary unilateral loss of vision. The visual loss varies from partial to total blindness and rarely lasts longer than 10 minutes. It is usually caused by a temporary occlusion in the internal carotid artery, which produces an insufficient blood flow to the ophthalmic artery and may lead to closure of the central retinal artery. ⊃ fluorescein angiography, retinal arterial occlusion, temporal arteritis.

amb-/ambi- a prefix that means 'both, on both sides', e.g. *ambidextrous*.

ambidextrous *adj* able to use both hands equally well—**ambidexter** *adj*, **ambidexterity** *n*.

ambient light in radiography, describes the light in the room where a film is being viewed.

ambient temperature and pressure the temperature and pressure (atmospheric, barometric) of the body's surroundings. Used when correcting a volume of saturated gas (at ATPS) to standard temperature and pressure dry (STPD), e.g. when measuring the volume of expired gas for assessment of oxygen uptake.

ambivalence *n* **1.** uncertainty that results from an inability to choose between opposites. **2.** the situation where opposite conflicting feelings, drives, desires or attitudes towards the same object, person, or place coexist in a person. For example love and hate or pain and pleasure.

amblyopia *n* defective vision. A condition characterized by reduced visual acuity due to a lesion in the eye or in the visual pathway, which hinders the normal development of vision, and which is not correctable by spectacles or contact lenses. The usual clinical criterion is 6/9 (or 20/30) or less in one eye, or a two-line difference or more, on the acuity chart between the two eyes. Amblyopia may occur as a result of: suppression in the deviated eye in strabismus (strabismic amblyopia which amounts to about 20% of all cases); a blurred image in the more ametropic eye in uncorrected anisometropia (anisometropic amblyopia which amounts to about 50% of all cases); bilateral blurred images in uncorrected refractive errors (isoametropic amblyopia); a blurred image in one of the meridians of high uncorrected astigmatism (meridional amblyopia); any of the above three is also called refractive amblyopia; opacities in the ocular media (e.g. congenital cataract, severe ptosis) in infants (stimulus deprivation amblyopia or visual deprivation amblyopia or image degradation amblyopia) after the lesion has been removed; continuous occlusion of an eye as may occur in occlusion treatment (occlusion amblyopia); arsenic, lead or quinine poisoning (toxic amblyopia) or the more specific types of toxic amblyopia such as those caused by excessive use of alcohol (alcohol amblyopia), methanol (methanol amblyopia), quinine (quinine amblyopia) or tobacco (tobacco amblyopia), although the latter three may actually be due to nutritional deficiencies (nutritional amblyopia); psychological origin or of unknown origin (idiopathic amblyopia). Many of these amblyopias are functional, i.e. in which no organic lesion exists as in psychological, refractive, isoametropic, strabismic or stimulus deprivation amblyopia. Others are organic, i.e. they are due to some pathological (e.g. congenital cataract) or anatomical (e.g. malorientation of retinal receptors) anomalies, as in nutritional, toxic or visual deprivation amblyopia. Amblyopia occurs in 2–4% of the population. There is usually a reduction in the amplitude of accommodation in amblyopic eyes. Treatment of amblyopia depends on the type. However, the younger the patient, the more likely that the treatment will be successful. Typically, the principal treatment is occlusion of the fixating eye (or the eye with the best acuity) by patching or blurring with atropine sulphate to force the other eye to take up fixation, after full refractive correction. Other procedures (alternatives or supplemental to patching) include penalization, kicking a ball towards a specific target, playing catch a ball, bar reading, pleoptics (when there is eccentric fixation as well), and any other procedures which require fixation like drawing, duplicating letter sequences on a keyboard, cutting out patterns, etc.— **amblyopic** *adj.* ◖ amblyopic eye, critical period, eccentric fixation, nystagmus, occlusion treatment, penalization, pleoptics, strabismus, suppression.

amblyopic eye known colloquially as a lazy eye. An eye which has amblyopia. ◖ amblyopia.

amblyoscope an instrument used to assess the angle of strabismus (squint) and the manner in which both eyes are used together.

ambulant *adj* able to walk, i.e. not confined to bed or chair.

ambulatory *adj* mobile, walking about.

ambulatory electrocardiogram (Holter monitoring) recording heart rhythm and rate over a 24-hour period to detect transient ischaemia or arrhythmias. The person continues with their normal activities and keeps a record of times and activities. Continuous recordings of one or more electrocardiograph (ECG) leads may be obtained by attaching them to a small portable solid state or tape recorder for 24 hours or more. This technique is useful for detecting transient episodes of arrhythmia or ischaemia, which seldom occur fortuitously during the short time taken for routine 12-lead ECG recordings. A variety of hand-held or implantable patient-activated devices can be used to record the ECG during symptomatic episodes and are particularly suitable for investigating patients with infrequent but potentially serious symptoms. Many of these devices have the facility to transmit ECG recordings to a cardiac centre through the telephone.

ambulatory surgery (day surgery) surgery carried out on the day of admission and, in the absence of problems, the person is discharged the same day to the care of the primary care team. Examples include hernia surgery, cataract removal, endoscopic examinations and procedures, and minor orthopaedic and gynaecological procedures.

ambulatory treatment interventions, such as blood product transfusion or chemotherapy, provided for patients as day care. ◖ continuous ambulatory peritoneal dialysis.

aMCI *abbr* amnestic mild cognitive impairment.

AMD *abbr* age-related macular degeneration.

AMED *abbr* Allied and Complementary Medicine Database.

amelia *n* a congenital absence of a limb or limbs. ◖ complete amelia.

amelioration *n* a reduction in the severity of symptoms.

ameloblast *n* an ectodermally derived cell primarily responsible for the formation of tooth enamel during the period that the teeth are being formed. ◖ amelogenesis.

ameloblastoma also called adamantinoma. A new growth of tissues of the type characteristic of the tooth enamel organ, but which does not advance to become formed enamel.

amelo-dentinal junction (ADJ) also known as the dentino-enamel junction. The junction between tooth enamel and dentine.

amelogenesis *n* the formation of the tooth enamel, it is finished before the teeth erupt.

amelogenesis imperfecta hereditary condition (autosomal dominant) resulting in the formation of imperfect enamel characterized by either hypoplasia of the tooth enamel (the teeth becoming worn down to the level of the gingivae and stained dark brown) or hypocalcification of the enamel, which becomes pitted, chalky and stained, sometimes having areas in which the enamel is absent.

amenorrhoea *n* absence of the menses. Amenorrhoea is normal before the menarche (the commencement of menstruation) occurring during puberty, during pregnancy and for varying periods during lactation and following the menopause (cessation of menstruation) occurring during the climacteric. When menstruation has not been established at the time when it should have been, it is termed *primary amenorrhoea*. Causes include eating disorders, Turner's syndrome, absence of the uterus or faulty hormone secretion; absence of the menses after they have once commenced is referred to as *secondary amenorrhoea*. Causes include hypothalamic disorders, hormonal disturbances, certain medication, emotional crisis, change in circumstances, eating disorders or some mental health problems—**amenorrhoeal** *adj*.

American Standard Code for Information Interchange (ASCII) defines the decimal and binary code of all the characters stored in a computer.

Ames test a method of in vitro testing for the ability of chemicals, such as potential food additives, to cause mutation in a strain of *Salmonella* bacteria (the mutagenic potential). Frequently used as a preliminary screening test to identify substances likely to be carcinogenic. Also known as the mutagenicity test.

ametria *n* congenital absence of the uterus.

ametropia *n* defective sight due to imperfect refractive power of the eye—**ametropic** *adj*, **ametrope** *n*. ⊃ astigmatism, hypermetropia, myopia.

AMF *abbr* amplitude modulated frequency.

AMHP *abbr* approved mental health professional.

amines *npl* group of organic compounds containing the functional group $-NH_2$. Many are important biochemical molecules, e.g. catecholamines, histamine, dopamine, etc. There are three potentially important amines present in protein foods containing amino acids; phenylethylamine (from the amino acid phenylalanine), tyramine (from the amino acid tyrosine) and tryptamine (from the amino acid tryptophan). These amines can stimulate the activity of the sympathetic nervous system and can cause an increase in blood pressure. In some people they are a possible dietary cause of migraine. The intake of foods high in these amines (e.g. mature cheese, fermented soya bean foods and yeast extract, etc.) is contraindicated for people taking monoamine oxidase inhibitor (MAOI) antidepressant drugs, as a dangerous increase in blood pressure can occur. ⊃ monoamine oxidase inhibitor (MAOI) antidepressant drugs.

amin/o a prefix that means 'containing a NH_2 group', e.g. *amino acid*.

aminoacidopathy *n* disease caused by imbalance of amino acids.

amino acids organic acids in which one or more of the hydrogen atoms are replaced by a basic amino group

$(-NH_2)$, they also contain one or more acidic carboxyl groups $(-COOH)$. They are the end product of protein hydrolysis and from them the body synthesizes its own proteins. In this process individual amino acids are linked together by peptide bonds, in a dehydration reaction, to form new polypeptides or proteins. There are 20 common amino acids which are classified as either essential (indispensable) or non-essential (dispensable). Ten (eight in adults and a further two during childhood) cannot be synthesized in sufficient quantities in the body and are therefore essential (indispensable) in the diet—isoleucine, leucine, lysine, methionine, phenylalanine, threonine, tryptophan and valine. Arginine and histidine are the two amino acids that are essential during childhood. The remainder, which can be synthesized in the body if the diet contains sufficient amounts of the precursor amino acids, are designated non-essential (dispensable) amino acids. They are alanine, asparagine, aspartic acid (aspartate), cysteine, glutamic acid (glutamate), glutamine, glycine, proline, serine and tyrosine. However, some of these are conditionally essential and depend upon adequate amounts of their precursor being present in the diet. ⊃ essential amino acids.

aminoaciduria *n* the abnormal presence of amino acids in the urine; it usually indicates an inborn error of metabolism as in cystinosis, tyrosinaemia and Fanconi syndrome—**aminoaciduric** *adj*.

aminoglycosides *npl* a group of bactericidal antibiotic drugs, e.g. gentamicin, with a wide range of activity. They have toxic effects on the kidney (nephrotoxicity) and on the ear (ototoxicity) and so are only prescribed if, other, safer drugs would be ineffective. ⊃ Appendix 5.

aminopeptidases *npl* intestinal enzymes present in the outer membrane of the enterocytes (intestinal cells) that act upon the amine end $(-NH_2)$ of the peptide chain during the digestion of protein. They break the peptide bond and release the terminal amino acid.

aminotransferases *npl* transaminases. A group of enzymes that catalyse the transfer of an α-amino group from an α-amino acid to an α-keto acid. The major site for these is the liver. *alanine aminotransferase (ALT)* formerly known as serum glutamic pyruvic transaminase (SGPT). *aspartate aminotransferase (AST)* formerly known as serum glutamic oxalacetic transaminase (SGOT). Aminotransferases are released by certain damaged cells and when blood levels are measured may be useful, along with other biochemical tests, in the diagnosis of liver disease (ALT, AST) and myocardial infarction (AST).

amitosis *n* division of a cell by direct fission—**amitotic** *adj*.

AML *abbr* acute myeloblastic/myeloid leukaemia.

ammonia *n* (NH_3) a pungent gaseous compound of nitrogen and hydrogen.

ammonium bicarbonate sometimes used in expectorant cough mixtures but of doubtful value.

ammonium ion (NH_4^+) an ion formed from a reaction between ammonia and hydrogen. Ammonium ions are formed in the liver during amino acid metabolism. Several inherited errors of ammonia/ammonium metabolism can cause a learning disability, seizures and other neurological manifestations. ⊃ urea cycle.

ammonium thiosulphate in radiography, used as a fixing agent in fixer solutions.

amnesia *n* complete loss of memory; can be divided into organic (true) amnesia (e.g. delirium, dementia, post electroconvulsive therapy [ECT]), and psychogenic amnesia (e.g. dissociative states, Ganser's syndrome). The term *anterograde amnesia* is used when there is impaired continuous recall for events following an accident or brain insult, and *retrograde amnesia* when the impairment is of events prior to the insult. *transient global amnesia* is a short period of both of the above usually only lasting hours or days—**amnesic** *adj.*

amnesic syndrome chronic profound impairment of recent memory with preserved immediate recall. Often accompanied by disorientation for time and confabulation (the creation of false memory to fill the gaps in memory). Commonly caused by thiamin(e) deficiency, which can be secondary to chronic alcohol use, dietary deficiency, gastric cancer, etc. ⊃ Korsakoff's (Korsakov's) syndrome.

amniocentesis *n* a diagnostic procedure for detecting chromosomal, metabolic and haematological abnormalities of the fetus. It involves inserting a wide-bore needle under ultrasound guidance through the abdominal wall into the amniotic sac to obtain a sample of amniotic fluid (Figure A.8). Many single gene and chromosome abnormalities can be diagnosed from testing amniotic fluid and fetal cells shed into the amniotic fluid surrounding the fetus. The

cells obtained from the fluid are grown and examined for chromosomal abnormalities, such as Down's syndrome. The amniotic fluid may contain chemical markers for a particular abnormality, e.g. presence of alphafetoprotein (AFP) may indicate neural tube defects. Amniocentesis is usually performed after 15 weeks' gestation. Testing for genetic defects takes time and final results are usually available in about 10–14 days. There are, however, risks associated with amniocentesis, for example spontaneous miscarriage occurs in around 1% of women. ⊃ chorionic villus sampling.

amniocytes desquamated fetal cells in amniotic fluid from fetal skin, respiratory and urinary tracts. They can be isolated and cultured or multiplied with molecular techniques such as fluorescence in situ hybridization (FISH) or polymerase chain reaction (PCR) to determine the fetal karyotype, and for genetic analysis.

amniohook, amnihook *n* an instrument for rupturing the fetal membranes. Also called an amniotome. ⊃ amniotomy.

amnioinfusion procedure to replace fluid which has drained off when membranes have ruptured prematurely and there is a risk of cord compression. Physiologically normal saline at body temperature is introduced into the amniotic cavity. Not currently routine practice in the UK.

amnion *n* membrane of embryonic origin lining the cavity of the uterus during pregnancy containing amniotic fluid and the fetus—**amnionic, amniotic** *adj.* ⊃ chorion.

amnion nodosum nodular condition of the fetal surface of the amnion, as in oligohydramnios. It may be associated with the absence of fetal kidneys.

amnionicity presence/absence of amnion for each fetus in a multiple pregnancy. Diamniotic twins each have an amnion and amniotic cavity, whereas the amnion and amniotic cavity are shared by monoamniotic twins and the risk of entangled umbilical cords increases fetal morbidity and mortality.

amnionitis *n* inflammation of the amnion. May result from infection caused by premature rupture of the fetal membranes.

amnioscope endoscope allowing observation of the fetus and amniotic fluid.

amnioscopy *n* an amnioscope passed through an incision in the abdominal wall and into the amniotic cavity enables direct viewing of the fetus and amniotic fluid. Clear, colourless fluid is normal; yellow or green staining is due to meconium and occurs in cases of fetal hypoxia—**amnioscopic** *adj*, **amnioscopically** *adv*. *cervical amnioscopy* can be performed late in pregnancy. A different instrument is inserted via the vagina and uterine cervix for the same purposes.

amniotic band syndrome neonatal condition in which the infant is born with limb reduction abnormalities, due to possible rupture of the amnion during pregnancy, which then wraps around a developing limb and causes necrosis, strangulation and/or amputation.

amniotic cavity the fluid-filled cavity between the fetus and the amnion.

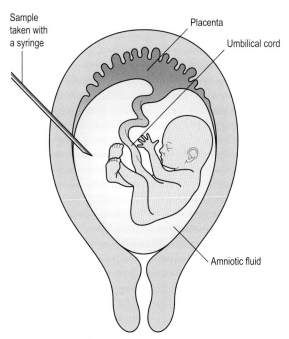

A.8 Amniocentesis (reproduced from Brooker 2006A with permission).

amniotic fluid also called liquor amnii. The fluid produced by the inner fetal membrane (amnion) and the fetus, which surrounds the fetus throughout pregnancy. It is about 99% water and contains proteins, fats and carbohydrates, sodium and potassium in solution; debris consisting of desquamated fetal epithelial cells, vernix caseosa, lanugo; and various enzymes and pigment. Amniotic fluid protects the fetus from temperature variations, and physical trauma by acting as a shock absorber; it allows unhindered fetal growth; distributes pressure evenly around the whole fetus; permits free movement necessary for muscle function; and prevents diminution of the placental site. It is secreted and reabsorbed by cells lining the amniotic cavity and is swallowed by the fetus and excreted as urine. The volume is approximately 1 L at 37–38 weeks' gestation, reduced by half by term. ⮩ amniocentesis, amnioscopy, oligohydramnios, polyhydramnios.

amniotic fluid embolism an embolus caused by amniotic fluid entering the maternal circulation. An extremely rare but very serious complication of pregnancy. ⮩ disseminated intravascular coagulation.

amniotic fluid index (AFI) measurement of amniotic fluid volume. Fluid depth is measured in the four uterine quadrants and added together to estimate the total. A measurement below 5 cm indicates oligohydramnios and above 25 cm indicates polyhydramnios.

amniotic sac bag of amnion or fetal membrane which contains the fetus, suspended in amniotic fluid.

amniotome *n* ⮩ amniohook.

A-mode used in early ultrasound machines, the voltage was produced across the transducer as a vertical deflection on the face of the oscilloscope. The horizontal sweep was calibrated to indicate the distance from the transducer to the reflecting surface. Demonstrates only the position and length of a reflecting structure.

amniotomy *n* artificial rupture of the fetal membranes to induce or expedite labour.

amoeba *n* a unicellular (single cell) protozoon. Strains that are human parasites include *Entamoeba histolytica*, which causes amoebic dysentery (intestinal amoebiasis). ⮩ protozoon—**amoebae** *pl*, **amoebic** *adj*.

amoebiasis *n* infestation of large intestine by the protozoon *Entamoeba histolytica*, where it causes mucosal ulceration leading to pain, diarrhoea alternating with constipation and blood and mucus passed rectally, hence the term 'amoebic dysentery'. Metronidazole or tinidazole is used to treat amoebic dysentery. If the amoebae enter the hepatic portal circulation they may cause a liver abscess. Hepatic involvement is treated with metronidazole or tinidazole followed by a course of diloxanide to destroy any amoebae in the intestine. Diagnosis is by isolating the amoeba in the stools. Cutaneous amoebiasis may cause perianal or genital ulceration in homosexual men.

amoebicide *n* an agent that kills amoebae, such as metronidazole—**amoebicidal** *adj*.

amoeboid *adj* resembling an amoeba in shape or in mode of movement, such as some leucocytes.

amoeboma *n* a tumour (swelling) in the caecum or rectum caused by *Entamoeba histolytica*. Fibrosis may occur and obstruct the bowel.

amorph *n* a gene that is inactive, i.e. does not express a trait.

amorphous *adj* not having a regular shape.

amortization phase the term to describe the time period between eccentric and concentric muscle contractions.

amotivation a state of lacking any motivation to engage in an activity, characterized by a lack of perceived competence and/or a failure to value the activity or its outcomes. ⮩ learned helplessness.

AMP *abbr* adenosine monophosphate.

ampere (A) *n* (A M Ampère, French physicist, 1775–1836), one of the seven base units of the Système International d'Unités (SI) (International System of Units). A measurement of electrical current. The ampere is that constant current which, if maintained in two straight parallel conductors of infinite length, of negligible circular cross-section, and placed one metre apart in vacuum, would produce between these conductors a force equal to 2×10^{-7} newton per metre of length. ⮩ Appendix 2.

amphetamines *npl* a group of sympathomimetic agents. A potent central nervous system (CNS) stimulant. In the UK the amphetamine derivative methylenedioxymethamphetamine (MDMA), 'ecstasy', is classified as a Class A drug, oral amphetamines such as dexamfetamine are Class B drugs and related drugs (e.g. benzfetamine) are Class C drugs. The stimulant effect has led to the increased misuse of and dependence on individual drugs, such as amfetamine. Although clinical use is extremely limited, the amphetamines and related drugs are prescribed by specialists for attention deficit hyperactivity disorder (ADHD); they are also used for daytime sleeping, narcolepsy and sleepiness caused by obstructive sleep apnoea syndrome. ⮩ amphetamine poisoning.

amphetamines and sport potentially harmful group of stimulant drugs currently banned in sport. Scientific evidence as to their beneficial effect is lacking. These drugs primarily affect the central nervous system resulting in euphoria, increased alertness and aggression. Side-effects are common and include drug dependence, depression, impaired co-ordination and judgement, reduced perception of fatigue, cardiovascular effects (increased blood pressure and cardiac output) and an increase in metabolic rate. Also known as 'speed,' 'uppers' and 'pep pills', they were previously prescribed (and are still used illegally) to assist weight loss.

amphetamine poisoning amphetamine poisoning is indicated by signs and symptoms that include hallucinations, delerium, agitation, wakefulness, excessive activity, paranoia, tachycardia, hypertension, exhaustion, seizures, hyperthermia and altered consciousness. Management involves the use of benzodiazepines such as diazepam, anticovulsive drugs, supportive measures including cooling and respiratory support.

amphi-/amph- a prefix that means 'on both sides', e.g. *amphipathic*.

amphiarthrosis *n* a cartilaginous, slightly movable joint. There are two types synchondrosis and symphysis.

amphipathic *adj* describes a molecule that has parts with very different chemical properties. For example, possessing a non-polar (hydrophobic) end and a polar (hydrophilic) end.

amplification gain in radiography, the measure of the extent to which developer increases the initial effect of exposure on the silver halide grains.

amplitude the maximum value of either positive or negative current or voltage that occurs on an alternating current waveform. In ultrasound, the magnitude (height) of the ultrasound beam, the ultrasound pulse is very brief so the power values arranged over a period of time will be low compared to peak intensity. ⊃ peak value.

amplitude of accommodation the maximum amount of accommodation A which the eye can exert. It is expressed in dioptres, as the difference between the far point and the near point measured with respect either to the spectacle plane or the corneal apex or some other reference point. Thus, $A = K - B$, where B is the near point vergence and K is the far point vergence. A is always positive. In the emmetropic eye, $A = -B$, because the far point is at infinity and $K = 0$. So, if the near point of an emmetrope is at 25 cm from the spectacle plane, the amplitude of accommodation is equal to $-[-1/(25 \times 10^{-2})] = 4\,\text{D}$. The amplitude of accommodation declines from about 14 D at age 10 to about 0.5 D at age 60 (although the measured value is usually higher due to the depth of focus of the eye). ⊃ depth of focus, dioptre, minus lens method, push-up method, presbyopia, vergence.

amplitude modulated frequency (AMF) also known as beat frequency. This occurs when using interferential therapy, two medium frequency currents 'interfere' or cancel each other out in a predictable fashion to produce a desired frequency.

ampoule *n* a hermetically sealed glass or plastic phial containing a single sterile dose of a drug.

ampulla *n* any flask-like dilatation, such as that in the uterine (fallopian) tube—**ampullae** *pl*, **ampullar, ampullary, ampullate** *adj*.

ampulla (uterine tube) the wider part of the uterine (fallopian) tube where fertilization usually occurs. It is 5 cm long. ⊃ Colour Section Figure 17.

ampulla of Vater (A Vater, German anatomist, 1684–1751) ⊃ hepatopancreatic ampulla.

ampullary tubal pregnancy a conceptus which implants in the distal end of the uterine (fallopian) tube rather than the uterus.

amputation *n* removal of an appending part of the body, e.g. breast, or a limb or part of a limb. A limb may be amputated following severe trauma, to remove a cancer and in the case of gangrene in peripheral vascular disease. A limb may also be lost by traumatic amputation in an industrial accident, an explosion or a road traffic accident.

amputee *n* a person who has had amputation of one or more limbs.

AMS *abbr* acute mountain sickness.

Amsler chart/grid a series of charts comprising black lines on a white background arranged horizontally and vertically to produce a checkerboard effect with a black or white dot in the centre. It is used to identify central visual field defects that are so slight that they are undetected by the usual methods of perimetry, such as that which occurs with age-related macular degeneration. The person is asked to look at the grid wearing their normal reading spectacles at normal reading distance, to cover one eye and stare at the central spot. This is repeated with the other eye. In order to detect the presence of a potential problem the person is asked to report if any of the lines are blurred, wavy, missing or a different colour, or crooked or bent and whether any of the boxes are distorted in terms of shape or size. ⊃ age-related macular degeneration.

amygdala an almond-shaped nucleus (mass of grey matter) sited deep within the temporal lobe of the cerebrum. It is part of the limbic system and associated with emotional behaviour and the olfactory system, and may have a role in memory processing. It is closely connected to the caudate nucleus, one of the basal nuclei (also known as basal ganglia). ⊃ limbic system.

amyl/o- a prefix that means 'starch', e.g. *amylopectin*.

amylase *n* any enzyme that converts starches into sugars. Found in saliva and pancreatic juice; it converts starchy foods to maltose and disaccharide. The amount of amylase in the blood is increased in disorders of the pancreas, such as pancreatitis, and in some gastrointestinal conditions, e.g. perforation of a peptic ulcer.

amylin *n* also called islet amyloid polypeptide. A polypeptide hormone produced by the beta (β) cells of the islets of the pancreas with insulin. It has a role in glycaemic control in conjunction with insulin and glucagon.

amylodyspepsia a condition characterized by an inability to digest starchy foods.

amyloid *adj*, *n* **1**. resembling starch. **2**. describes the abnormal proteins associated with amyloidosis. It was previously thought to be a starch-like glycoprotein (a protein–carbohydrate complex). ⊃ amyloidosis.

amyloidosis *n* a group of diseases in which amyloid, an abnormal protein, is deposited in one or more organ systems, notably the liver, kidney, heart, gastrointestinal system and nervous system leading to impaired organ function. Amyloidosis can be primary, secondary or familial. There are also other types that include the abnormal protein (β-amyloid protein) associated with Alzheimer's disease. *primary amyloidosis* affects the plasma cells (formed from B-cells) and may be associated with multiple myeloma. *secondary amyloidosis* can occur in conditions where there is chronic inflammation or infection. These include rheumatoid arthritis, tuberculosis, osteomyelitis, bronchiectasis and leprosy. It also occurs in the genetic disease familial Mediterranean fever. *familial amyloidosis* occurs rarely and is caused by the production of an abnormal protein in the liver.

amylolysis *n* starch digestion—**amylolytic** *adj*.

A
B

amylopectin a type of starch that forms a branched chain structure. It forms about 75–80% of most starches.

amylose a type of starch that forms a straight chain structure. It forms about 20–25% of most starches.

amyotrophic lateral sclerosis (ALS) the most common form of motor neuron disease in which there is a loss of the upper motor neurons from the cortex to the brainstem and spinal cord, as well as the loss of the lower motor neurons from the brainstem and spinal cord to the muscles. It is characterized by wasting fasiculated muscles especially in the thenar eminences and brisk reflexes are present indicating involvement of corticospinal tract. This is a deteriorating disease with no proven treatment and so provision of care and management of symptoms by a multidisciplinary team is important.

amyxorrhoea deficiency or lack of mucous secretion.

AN *acron* anorexia nervosa.

an- a prefix that means 'not, without', e.g. *anoxia*.

-an, ian a suffix that means 'belonging to, pertaining to', e.g. *avian*.

ANA *abbr* antinuclear antibody.

anabolic agents substances which have an anabolic effect (tissue building and energy storing). ⊃ anabolic steroids.

anabolic hormones natural or synthetic hormones that stimulate growth and the development of muscle tissue. They include insulin, insulin-like growth factors, growth hormone and the sex hormones oestrogen and testosterone. Compare with catabolic hormones.

anabolic steroids a group of androgens (e.g. nandrolone), that stimulate anabolic effects, such as the synthesis of body protein. They are used therapeutically for aplastic anaemia and are sometimes used to support patients who are very debilitated. In a sports context usually refers to a group of synthetic drugs based on the male sex hormone testosterone, and having similar anabolic and other androgenic actions to this and other androgens from the adrenal cortex in both sexes. These drugs are misused in sports, especially where enhanced power and strength are beneficial such as weight lifting and cycling. Used in conjunction with a training programme, they lead to an increase in muscle size and power. They may also lessen fatigue and improve tissue repair. Use in children can lead to premature fusion of the epiphyses, stunting skeletal growth. Side-effects are common and potentially serious. They include psychological changes (notably aggression), disordered liver function and liver cancer with long term use, cardiovascular (raised blood pressure), acne, oedema and endocrine effects—masculinization in females (voice changes, facial hair and amenorrhoea and testicular atrophy and reduced sperm count in males. ⊃ androgens. ⊃ Appendix 5.

anabolism *n* the series of chemical reactions in the living body requiring energy to change simple substances into complex ones. For example the use of amino acids to form functional proteins such as protein hormones, enzymes, antibodies and plasma proteins—**anabolic** *adj*. ⊃ adenosine triphosphate, catabolism, metabolism.

anachoresis a condition in which micro-organisms or other agents are attracted towards certain local lesions while the rest of the body appears to remain unaffected.

anacidity *n* lack of normal acidity, especially in the gastric juice. ⊃ achlorhydria.

anacrotic *adj* a wave in the ascending curve of an arterial tracing, indicating the opening of the aortic valve (that between the left ventricle and the aorta). An abnormality of this occurs in aortic stenosis. ⊃ dicrotic.

anadidymus conjoined twins joined at the pelvis or lower.

anaemia *n* diminished oxygen carrying capacity of the blood, due to a reduction in the haemoglobin content of the blood. This may be due to reduced amounts of haemoglobin in the red blood cells and/or a reduction in the number of red blood cells. Produces clinical manifestations arising from hypoxaemia, such as lassitude and breathlessness on exertion. There are very many possible causes. ⊃ anaemia of chronic disease, anaemia of pregnancy, aplastic anaemia, haemolytic anaemia, haemolytic disease of the newborn, macrocyte, megaloblastic anaemia, microcyte, pernicious anaemia, sickle cell disease, thalassaemia—**anaemic** *adj*.

anaemia of chronic disease (ACD) a common type of anaemia, particularly in hospital populations. It occurs in the setting of chronic infections, chronic inflammation such as rheumatoid arthritis, or cancer. The anaemia is not related to bleeding, haemolysis or marrow infiltration, is mild, in the range of 85–115 g/L, and is usually associated with a normal mean cell volume (MCV) (normocytic, normochromic), though this may be reduced in long-standing inflammation. The serum iron is low but iron stores are normal or increased, as indicated by the ferritin or stainable marrow iron. The pathogenesis of this type of anaemia is thought to involve abnormalities of iron metabolism, including reduced release of iron to transferrin, and erythropoiesis. Recent interest has been centred on the role of erythropoietin and the inhibitory effect of various cytokines, e.g. interleukin 1 (IL-1) and tumour necrosis factor alpha (TNF-α) on erythropoiesis. Erythropoietin levels appear to be lower than would be expected for the degree of anaemia, and administration of erythropoietin to patients with rheumatoid arthritis has a beneficial effect on the anaemia. It is often difficult to distinguish the anaemia of chronic disease (ACD) associated with a low MCV from iron deficiency. Examination of the marrow may ultimately be required to assess iron stores directly. A trial of oral iron can be given in difficult situations. A positive response occurs in true iron deficiency but not in ACD. Measures which reduce the severity of the underlying disorder generally help to improve the ACD.

anaemia of pregnancy an anaemia caused by a lower concentration of haemoglobin in the blood. It may be physiological because, during pregnancy, the blood is diluted. The plasma volume increases without a corresponding increase in red cell numbers. However, there are pathological causes that include insufficient intake of nutrients required for haemoglobin production, e.g. iron, loss of red cells through bleeding or damage.

anaemic hypoxia due to inadequate amounts of haemoglobin available to carry oxygen. ◒ hypoxia.

anaerobe *n* a micro-organism that is unable to grow in the presence of molecular oxygen. When this is strictly so, it is called an *obligatory anaerobe*. These include *Clostridium tetani, C. perfringens* and *C. botulinum*. Most pathogens are indifferent to atmospheric conditions and will grow whether oxygen is present or not and are therefore called *facultative anaerobes*. Some, however, will grow more vigorously if anaerobic conditions prevail—**anaerobic** *adj*.

anaerobic *adj* relating to the absence of oxygen. Describes processes that occur without oxygen, and certain micro-organisms that survive without free oxygen or air.

anaerobic adaptations long term physical changes that result from anaerobic exercise. They increase the body's ability to deal with powerful dynamic exercise.

anaerobic capacity the total amount of energy that can be obtained from anaerobic sources (creatine phosphate breakdown and anaerobic glycolysis) in a single bout of continuous exercise. Strictly a theoretical concept, since some contribution from aerobic metabolism cannot be prevented in any real-time measurement. Estimated by total work output in 30 s (Wingate test) or 90 s cycle ergometer tests, or by treadmill running up a steep gradient; the longer test periods more closely extract all possible energy from the anaerobic systems, but cannot avoid a small yet significant aerobic contribution.

anaerobic endurance (*syn* short-term endurance) the ability to sustain whole-body work at 'supramaximal' intensity (i.e. above $\dot{V}O_{2max}$), measured in terms of tens of seconds. ◒ endurance.

anaerobic endurance training also known as lactate tolerance training. Anaerobic endurance training aims to place maximum stress on the systems that produce energy when oxygen is in short supply, i.e. anaerobically (ATP-CP pathway, anaerobic glycolysis). The high intensity of training results in fatigue so the repetition of periods of maximal intensity exercise are interspersed with rest periods with a varible exercise:rest ratio, such as 1:1 or 1:4. *long-duration anaerobic endurance training* is a regimen with an exercise:rest ratio of around 1:4. It makes increased demands on the anaerobic glycolysis energy system. *short-duration anaerobic endurance training* involves very short bursts of maximal intensity exercise bouts with an exercise:rest ratio of around 1:10. Short-duration endurance training improves the ATP-CP energy pathway and increases muscular power. ◒ alactacid (alactic) anaerobic system, lactacid (lactic) anaerobic system.

anaerobic energy energy that is produced without using oxygen via two energy systems: alactacid and lactacid.

anaerobic exercise exercise at an intensity exceeding aerobic capacity, which therefore draws a significant fraction of its energy from anaerobic sources. Sprints of any form, jumps and forceful throws are examples. In sustained anaerobic exercise, metabolic products accumulate rapidly; this is indicated by the continual increase of blood lactate concentration $[Lac]_b$ throughout the period of effort, but other products such as phosphate ions, adenosine diphosphate (ADP), adenosine monophosphate (AMP) and adenosine contribute much more to the fatigue which forces termination of the effort after some 10–120 s, depending on its intensity. Also known as supramaximal exercise. Compare aerobic exercise.

anaerobic fitness the ability to perform maximal anaerobic exercise.

anaerobic glycolysis the anaerobic process comprising a series of enzyme catalysed chemical reactions that breakdown stored muscle glycogen or glucose to provide energy for adenosine triphosphate (ATP) resynthesis.

anaerobic metabolism ◒ glycolysis, lactate.

anaerobic power maximum rate of power production, typically measured by Margaria stair test or first 5 s of a Wingate test. ◒ Margaria stair test, Wingate test.

anaerobic threshold (AT, T_{AN}) the work rate at which it has been considered that shortfall in oxygen supply to working muscles causes them to begin drawing on anaerobic pathways. Previously taken as equating to lactate threshold (LT) but there is now good evidence that fully aerobic muscles release lactate. ◒ metabolic and related thresholds.

anaerobic training training at exercise intensities which cannot be maintained by oxygen intake, and are therefore sustainable for not more than a few tens of seconds without a rest interval.

anaesthesia *n* loss of sensation. ◒ caudal anaesthesia, epidural anaesthesia or block, general anaesthesia, local anaesthesia, nerve block anaesthesia, spinal anaesthesia.

anaesthetic practitioner (AP) a non-medically qualified role in anaesthesia care in the UK. Specially trained and qualified individuals will undertake certain parts of anaesthesia care without the direct supervision of an anaesthetist. The diploma course is open to existing healthcare staff and to science graduates.

anaesthesiology *n* the science dealing with anaesthetics, their administration and effect.

anaesthetic *n* 1. *n* a drug that induces general or local anaesthesia. ◒ general anaesthetic, local anaestheic, spinal anaesthetic. 2. *adj* causing anaesthesia. 3. *adj* insensible to stimuli—**anaesthetize** *vt*.

anaesthetic assistant a qualified healthcare professional who provides support for the anaesthetist. A role undertaken by anaesthetic nurses, operating department practitioners (ODP) or operating department assistants (ODA). ◒ anaesthetic practitioner

anaesthetist *n* a doctor with specialist training to administer general anaesthesia.

anaesthetize *vt* to administer drugs or gases to produce general anaesthesia.

anagen the active growth phase (lasting two to three years) in the hair development cycle. Most scalp hairs are in the anagen phase at any given time. ◒ catagen, telogen.

anagen effluvium loss of hair during the active growth phase due to a variety of causes that include chemotherapy drugs used to treat cancer, toxins and alopecia areata.

anaglyph a stereogram consisting of two superimposed and laterally displaced drawings or photographs of the same scene but taken from two directions and in complementary colours (usually red and green). If the anaglyphs are viewed through filters of the same colour, one to each eye, and induce retinal disparity (of a fixed amount) they give rise to the perception of depth or stereopsis. A set of cards, or targets on the same card, to induce various amounts of retinal disparity can be used to detect and train fusion and stereopsis (e.g. Tranaglyphs). ⊃ complementary colour, depth perception, random-dot stereogram, retinal disparity, sensory fusion, stereopsis.

anakinra one of the cytokine inhibitors, it acts to prevent the activity of interleukin 1. A biologic therapy for use in cases of rheumatoid arthritis where methotrexate has not been successful.

anal *adj* pertaining to the anus.

anal canal *n* the last portion of the large intestine. It is about 4cm long in an adult and leads from the rectum to the exterior at the anus. It has the internal and external muscular sphincters, which are involved in the process of defecation. The anal canal is lined with stratified squamous epithelium that is continuous with the rectal mucosa above and merges with the skin (perianal) outside the external sphincter.

analeptic *adj, n* restorative.

anal fissure painful split or break in the anal mucosa or skin, associated with constipation. Also known as a fissure-in-ano.

anal fistula an abnormal opening on the cutaneous surface close to the anus. Also known as a fistula-in-ano. It is usually associated with local abscess formation and often occurs in Crohn's disease.

analgesia *n* loss of sensation of pain without loss of touch— **analgesic** *adj*. ⊃ patient controlled analgesia.

analgesic *n* a drug used to produce analgesia, i.e. relieves pain. For example, paracetamol, codeine or morphine. ⊃ Appendix 5.

analogous *adj* similar in function but not in evolutionary origin.

analogue 1. a chemical, such as a drug, which is similar in structure or composition to other drugs but its action produces different effects. For example an analogue drug may have enhanced potency or cause fewer adverse drug reactions. 2. represents a quantity changing in steps which are continuous, as opposed to digital which is in discrete steps. ⊃ digital.

analogue signal a continuous electrical signal used to transmit images to a computer, television.

analogue to digital converter a device which converts analogue signals into digital signals which can be understood and manipulated by a computer.

anal reflex a superficial reflex. Normally there is reflex contraction of the external anal sphincter when the perianal skin or mucosa is stroked. The reflex is absent if there is disease or damage affecting the relevant segments of the spinal cord.

anal verge the margins or edges of the anal sphincter which closes the rectum. Can be damaged in childbirth.

analysis *n* in chemistry the determination of the component parts of a compound substance. ⊃ psychoanalysis— **analyses** *pl*, **analytic** *adj*, **analytically** *adv*.

analysis by intention-to-treat also known as intention-to-treat analysis. A research term. A method of analysis used in randomized controlled trials (RCT). The analysis is based on all participants who were randomly assigned to the groups, regardless of whether or not they withdrew from the study or received the treatment. After randomization, patients who have been assigned conservative therapy may decide to have surgery instead; conversely, patients assigned to the surgical treatment may decide not to undergo surgery. In an analysis by intention-to-treat, patients would be analysed according to the groups for which they were originally assigned. Using 'intention to treat' rather than 'on treatment' analysis avoids biases.

analysis of variance (ANOVA) a statistical method of comparing sample means.

analytical epidemiology the study of the relationship between different risk factors and the development of disease.

anaphase the third stage of mitosis (Figure M.7, p. 488) and in both divisions of meiosis (Figure M.3, p. 472). During anaphase in mitosis and the second division of meiosis the double chromosomes split at the centromeres with each chromatid arranged in the equatorial region of the mitotic spindle. The fibres of the spindle contract and the chromatids move to opposite poles of the cell where they become complete chromosomes. During anaphase in the first division of meiosis, the 23 pairs (i.e. 46) of homologous chromosomes in humans separate from each other and 23 move intact to one pole and 23 to the other pole of the cell. ⊃ metaphase, prophase, telophase.

anaphylactoid *adj* a systemic reaction, resembling anaphylaxis but not immunoglobulin (Ig) E-mediated.

anaphylactoid syndrome of pregnancy rare but potentially fatal condition associated with amniotic fluid embolism in which the presence of amniotic fluid in the maternal circulation triggers an anaphylactoid response, characterized initally by pulmonary vasospasm causing hypoxia, hypotension, pulmonary oedema and cardiovascular collapse, and then the development of left ventricular failure, uncontrollable haemorrhage and coagulation disorder, with a high risk of maternal morbidity and mortality. ⊃ amiotic fluid embolism.

anaphylaxis *n* an exaggerated systemic reaction due to a type I, or immediate-type, hypersensitivity reaction caused by immunoglobulin E (IgE)-mediated release of inflammatory mediators, e.g. histamine, from mast cells on exposure to an allergen. The allergen that triggers the reaction may be a certain food, such as nuts, eggs or shellfish, drugs that include penicillin, foreign proteins including vaccines, or insect stings especially bees and wasps. Characterized by urticaria, pruritus, angioedema, airway obstruction, bronchospasm, respiratory distress, vascular collapse, hypotension and shock ➲ allergy, sensitization—**anaphylactic** *adj*.

anaplasia *n* loss of the distinctive characteristics of a cell, associated with abnormal proliferative cellular activity as in cancer—**anaplastic** *adj*.

anaplastic carcinoma a malignant tumour of the thyroid gland which grows rapidly and is more common in older people. It is relatively resistant to radiotherapy.

anarthria *n* a severe form of dysarthria. The affected person is unable to produce the motor movements required for speech. The muscle weakness is apparent in the phonatory, articulatory, respiratory and resonatory speech systems. ➲ dysarthria.

anasarca severe generalized oedema. It is associated with renal disease.

anastigmatic lens (*syn* stigmatic lens) **1**. a lens which has a single focal point. **2**. a lens which is corrected for oblique astigmatism and minimum curvature of field. ➲ astigmatic lens, Petzval surface.

anastomosis *n* **1**. the anatomical intercommunication of the branches of two or more tubular structures, e.g. arteries or veins. **2**. in surgery, the establishment of an intercommunication between two hollow organs, ducts, vessels or nerves, such as the anastomosis between two segments of bowel following the resection of a diseased length of bowel. The types of anastomosis are end-to-end or side-to-side—**anastomoses** *pl*, **anastomotic** *adj*, **anastomose** *vt*.

anatomic articulation the rigid or movable function of two or more bones.

anatomical articulator an articulator which attempts to reproduce the normal movements of the jaw during mastication.

anatomical crown that part of a tooth normally covered by, and including, the enamel.

anatomical dead space the area of the conducting airways containing the inspired air that takes no part in gaseous exchange. It has a volume of around 150 mL in an adult and comprises the nasal cavity, pharynx, larynx, trachea and bronchi.

anatomical impression tray ➲ impression tray.

anatomical position for the purpose of accurate description of body parts and their relationship to each other the following position is used. The anterior (front) view is of the upright body facing forward, hands by the sides with palms facing forwards and with feet together. The posterior (back) view is of the back of the upright body in that position.

anatomical position of rest (of the eyes) the position of the eyes when they are completely devoid of tonus, as in death.

anatomical/radiographic apex the external tip of a dental root.

anatomical root that part of a tooth normally covered by, and including, the cementum.

anatomical tooth artificial tooth whose crown simulates the morphology of a natural tooth.

anatomy *n* the science which deals with the structure of the body—**anatomical** *adj*, **anatomically** *adv*.

ANB angle the angle between the points A, N and B in cephalometrics. Used to define the skeletal pattern of the individual. The average ANB angle is 3 degrees (Class I) plus or minus 2 degrees. Angles less than this are described as skeletal Class III and angles greater as skeletal Class II. ➲ cephalometrics.

ANCA *abbr* antineutrophil cytoplasmic antibody.

anchorage in dentistry, the collective term for those areas resisting any forces applied to move certain teeth. Such areas may include other teeth, when the anchorage is intra-oral, or they may be extraoral such as orthodontic headgear. ➲ extra-oral anchorage, orthodontic anchorage, reciprocal anchorage.

anconeus a triangular superficial muscle of the arm. Its origin is on the lateral epicondyle of the humerus and it inserts on the olecranon process of the ulna. Contraction of the muscle extends the forearm and abducts the ulna during forearm pronation.

Ancylostoma *n* a genus of parasitic nematode hookworms that includes *Ancylostoma duodenale* that is mostly found in southern Europe and the Middle and Far East. It is usually only significant when infestation is moderate or heavy. The worm lives in the duodenum and upper jejunum, eggs are passed in faeces, hatch in moist soil and produce larvae that can penetrate bare feet and reinfest individuals. Infestation is prevented by wearing shoes and using latrines. ➲ *Necator*.

ancylostomiasis *n* (*syn* hookworm disease, miners' anaemia) infestation of the human intestine with *Ancylostoma duodenale*, giving rise to malnutrition and severe anaemia.

Andersen's disease (D Andersen, American pathologist, 1901–1963) type IV glycogen storage disease in which there is a deficiency of brancher enzyme. It presents during infancy and is characterized by cirrhosis and severe muscle weakness, which may affect the myocardium.

Andrews' 6 keys to occlusion a definition of optimal occlusion as defined by Andrews. The 6 keys are: **1**. molar relationship: the distal surface of the distobuccal cusp of the upper first permanent molar occludes with the mesial surface of the mesial-buccal cusp of the lower second permanent molar; **2**. crown angulation (mesial-distal tip): the gingival portion of each crown is distal to the incisor portion and varied with each arch tooth type; **3**. crown inclination (labial-lingual, buccal-lingual): anterior teeth (incisors) are at sufficient angulation to prevent overeruption. Upper posterior teeth—lingual tip is constant and similar from canine to second premolar and increased in the molars. Lower posterior teeth—lingual tip increases progressively from the canines to the molars: **4**. no rotations; **5**. no spaces; **6**. flat occlusal planes.

Andrews' straight wire a particular prescription of a pre-adjusted edgewise appliance designed to use a straight arch wire. The brackets incorporate the tip, torque and 'in-out' that is normally bent into the arch wire so simplifying fixed orthodontic appliances.

andro- a prefix that means 'male', e.g. *andrology*.

androblastoma *n* (*syn* arrhenoblastoma) a tumour of the ovary; can produce male or female hormones and can cause masculinization in women or precocious puberty in girls.

androgen insensitivity syndrome a disorder where body tissues are unresponsive to androgen hormones. The affected individual has a male genotype (XY) but has a female phenotype (physical appearance). The relevant gene is inherited on the X chromosome; the disorder is therefore X-linked. The presentation is primary amenorrhoea and although the person has breast development they have no uterus.

androgens *npl* steroid hormones secreted by the testes (testosterone) and adrenal cortex in both sexes. They have widespread anabolic effects, produce the male secondary sex characteristics, e.g. male hair distribution and stimulate spermatogenesis. Applies also to synthetic hormones with similar action—**androgenic, androgenous** *adj.* ⊃ anabolic steroids.

andrology the medical/surgical specialties that deal with men's health. The focus is urological and reproductive problems. It covers diverse areas that include specific, targeted health promotion; diseases that include cancer or infections affecting the penis, testes and epididymis, prostate gland; family planning; infertility; and erectile dysfunction and rapid ejaculation.

android *adj* relating to something that is masculine.

android pelvis a pelvis with masculine characteristics, including a roughly triangular or heart-shaped brim and a narrow funnel shape, with an outlet which is narrower than in the gynaecoid pelvis.

anechoic without echoes.

anembryonic pregnancy 'blighted ovum'. A pregnancy with no visible embryo in the gestation sac, occurs with early embryonic death, although the trophoblast continues to develop. It is a common cause of miscarriage. Diagnosis can only be made when the gestation sac mean diameter is larger than 20 mm and must be differentiated from a viable pregnancy which is too small to visualize the fetal pole.

anencephaly *n* absence of the cranial skull, which begins to ossify at 10 weeks' gestation, and the brain. The condition is incompatible with life. It can be detected by raised levels of alphafetoprotein (AFP) in the amniotic fluid obtained by amniocentesis—**anencephalous, anencephalic** *adj.*

aneuploidy *n* a chromosome number that is not a multiple of the normal haploid number (23). Includes; trisomy, e.g. Down's syndrome, Edward's syndrome, Patau's syndrome, etc. where the individual has 47 chromosomes, and monosomy where there are 45 chromosomes, e.g. Turner's syndrome. ⊃ monosomy, polyploidy, trisomy.

aneurysm *n* a sac formed by localized dilation of a blood vessel, usually an artery, due to a local fault in the wall through defect, disease or injury, producing a swelling, often pulsating, over which a murmur may be heard. They are common in the aorta but also occur elsewhere, e.g. in the popliteal artery, carotid artery and in the cerebral arteries (berry aneurysm). True aneurysms may be saccular, fusiform, or dissecting where the blood flows between the layers

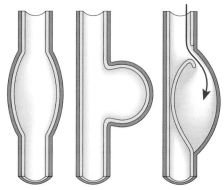

A.9 Aneurysms: fusiform, saccular and dissecting (reproduced from Brooker 2002 with permission).

of the arterial wall (Figure A.9). An aneurysm can predispose to the formation of a thrombus which may enter the circulation as emboli to block a smaller distal vessel, or rupture causing catastrophic haemorrhage—**aneurysmal** *adj.* ⊃ abdominal aortic aneurysm, aortic aneurysm, aortic dissection.

aneurysmal bone cyst lesion of bone that appears radiolucent radiographically and is composed of giant cells and sinusoidal vascular tissue.

Angelman syndrome an inherited condition that arises from mutations in the maternal chromosome 15 during formation of the gamete. Features include: a jerky 'puppet-like' gait and movements, a learning disability, brachycephaly (short, broad skull), hooked nose, tongue protrusion, inappropriate emotional outbursts and seizures. ⊃ Prader–Willi syndrome.

anger management a structured programme used to teach effective skills for recognizing strong emotions, such as rage and aggression, controlling the impulses that these emotions arouse and expressing feelings appropriately.

angi/o- a prefix that means 'vessel (blood)', e.g. *angiogenesis.*

angiectasis *n* abnormal dilatation of blood vessels. ⊃ telangiectasis—**angiectatic** *adj.*

angiitis *n* inflammation of a blood or lymph vessel. ⊃ vasculitis—**angiitic** *adj.*

angina *n* sense of constriction—**anginal** *adj.*

angina pectoris a common condition in developed countries. It is caused by narrowing of the coronary arteries, usually by atherosclerosis, but it may be due to coronary artery spasm. The narrowing of the coronary arteries reduces the blood supply and hence the amount of oxygen reaching the myocardium (myocardial ischaemia), which usually results in severe but transient chest pain that may radiate to the inner aspect of both arms but especially the left, throat, lower jaw, upper abdomen, or the back. There may also be breathlessness. Often the attack is induced by exercise (angina of effort), emotional upsets, cold and windy weather and sometimes after eating a large meal. The pain is promptly relieved by rest and the use of coronary vasodilators, such as glyceryl trinitrate. ⊃ acute coronary syndrome, coronary heart disease, myocardial infarction.

angiocardiography *n* radiographic demonstration of the chambers of the heart and great vessels after injecting a contrast agent via a catheter inserted into the brachial or femoral arteries—**angiocardiographic** *adj*, **angiocardiogram** *n*, **angiocardiograph** *n*, **angiocardiographically** *adv*.

angiodysplasia *n* vascular malformation comprising a collection of small blood vessels initially involving the large bowel, which may cause lower gastrointestinal bleeding.

angiogenesis *n* the formation of new blood vessels (vascularization). Angiogenesis is a feature of wound healing, new blood vessels are formed during stage 2 (inflammation) and stage 3 (proliferation) in response to growth factors released by white blood cells (leucocytes). New blood vessels also develop, in response to growth factors, to supply the blood that supports the growth of cancers. Recent advances in cancer treatment includes drugs that suppress angiogenesis thus reducing the tumour's blood supply. One such drug is the monoclonal antibody bevacizumab, which inhibits vascular endothelial growth factor. It is used with cytotoxic drugs in the management of metastatic colorectal cancer.

angiography *n* demonstration of the blood vessels of the arterial system after injection of a contrast agent into an artery—**angiographic** *adj*, **angiogram** *n*, **angiograph** *n*, **angiographically** *adv*. ⊃ computed tomography angiography, digital subtraction angiography, fluorescein angiography, indocyanine green angiography, magnetic resonance angiography.

angioid streaks degeneration of Bruch's membrane of the choroid characterized by brown or reddish lines or streaks in the fundus of the eye. The condition is bilateral, although one eye may be affected more than the other. Patients may occasionally be aware of some visual impairment in the visual field depending on the location of the streaks. The membrane is very fragile and liable to rupture in the case of ocular trauma, which may lead to macular haemorrhage and visual loss. Angioid streaks are often found in association with pseudoxanthoma elasticum (an eruption of small, superficial, solid elevation of the skin of the neck and other areas), Paget's disease or sickle-cell disease. ⊃ choroid, Bruch's membrane, Ehlers-Danlos syndrome, Paget's disease.

angiokeratoma corporis diffusum also known as Fabry's disease or Anderson–Fabry disease. A rare X-linked recessive familial disease in which the absence of an enzyme leads to the accumulation of a glycolipid in blood vessels, other tissues and organs including the liver and kidneys.

angiology *n* the science dealing with blood and lymphatic vessels—**angiological** *adj*, **angiologically** *adv*.

angioma a benign tumour affecting blood vessels, a haemangioma. Many angiomas are congenital. ⊃ haemangioma, lymphangioma.

angio-oedema *n* (*syn* angioneurotic oedema) a severe form of urticaria which may involve the skin of the face, hands or genitalia and the mucous membrane of the mouth and throat: oedema of the glottis may be fatal. Immediately there is an abrupt local increase in vascular permeability, as a result of which fluid escapes from blood vessels into surrounding tissues. Swelling may be due to an allergic hypersensitivity reaction to drugs, pollens or other known allergens, but in many cases no cause can be found.

angioplasty *n* surgical reconstruction of blood vessels—**angioplastic** *adj*. ⊃ percutaneous transluminal angioplasty.

angiosarcoma *n* a malignant tumour arising from blood vessels—**angiosarcomata** *pl*, **angiosarcomatous** *adj*.

angioscotoma (*syn* Purkinje figures, Purkinje shadows, Purkinje tree) a scotoma produced by the shadow cast by the retinal blood vessels. It looks like the branches of a tree which extend from the blind spot. It is seen only in special conditions of illumination as when illuminating the fundus of the eye by gently moving a penlight over the closed eyelid, or when illuminating the fundus through the sclera, or when plotting the visual field. This phenomenon is sometimes used as a test to predict gross macular function in a patient with dense cataract where visualization of the fundus is impossible, although better results are obtained with the blue field entoptoscope. ⊃ blue field entoptoscope, entoptic image/phenomena.

angiospasm *n* spasm of blood vessels—**angiospastic** *adj*.

angiotensin *n* a polypeptide formed by the action of renin on the precursor protein angiotensinogen in the blood plasma. Renin is mainly released by the juxtaglomerular cells in the kidney. In the lungs angiotensin I is converted in an enzyme catalyzed reaction into angiotensin II, a highly active substance which constricts blood vessels and causes release of aldosterone from the adrenal cortex in the *renin-angiotensin-aldosterone response (*also called *angiotensin-aldosterone response)*. This renin-angiotensin-aldosterone system is important in the normal regulation of blood volume and arterial blood pressure. ⊃ renin, renin-angiotensin-aldosterone response.

angiotensin-converting enzyme (ACE) an enzyme, principally in the kidney and lung endothelia, which catalyses conversion of the inactive form angiotensin I in the blood to angiotensin II; this in turn stimulates release of aldosterone from the adrenal glands and hence sodium reabsorption in kidneys. There are recent indications that either ACE itself, or perhaps some other molecule(s) whose biosynthesis is enhanced in parallel by the ACE gene, favour(s) various aspects of physical performance.

angiotensin-converting enzyme (ACE) inhibitors a group of drugs that inhibit the conversion of angiotensin I to angiotensin II and thereby reduce the angiotensin-aldosterone response, e.g. enalapril maleate. ⊃ Appendix 5.

angiotensin II receptor antagonists a group of drugs that have similar actions to angiotensin-converting enzyme (ACE) inhibitors. They do not, however, prevent the breakdown of kinins such as bradykinin, which may prevent a dry cough. Examples include eprosartan. ⊃ Appendix 5.

angle in anatomy, a corner. ⊃ angle of the eye, angle of the mandible, angle of the mouth, cavosurface angle, line angle.

angle board apparatus for positioning the patient's head during oblique or temporomandibular joint radiography.

angle-closure glaucoma (ACG) (*syn* closed-angle glaucoma, narrow-angle glaucoma) glaucoma in which the angle of the anterior chamber is blocked by the root of the iris which is in apposition to the trabecular meshwork and thus the aqueous humour cannot reach the drainage apparatus to leave the eye. (As the blockage persists, anterior synechia may result.) This condition occurs usually in anatomically shallow anterior chambers, as is often the case in hypermetropes. *Angle-closure* glaucoma can either be *primary* (PACG) or *secondary* following iritis, iridocyclitis, postoperative complications, traumatic cataract, tumours, etc. Moreover, angle-closure glaucoma is divided into *acute* and *chronic*. In *chronic angle-closure glaucoma* (CACG) there may never be an attack but intermittent periods of increased intraocular pressure caused by progressively extensive peripheral anterior synechia. Symptoms may be absent or there may be periodic episodes of mild congestion and blurred vision. Gonioscopy is essential to differentiate this condition from open-angle glaucoma. Treatment of angle-closure glaucoma is essentially surgical. However, initially therapeutic agents are used. They include: miotics (e.g. pilocarpine, carbachol, dapiprazole), the hyperosmotic agents which cause a rapid reduction of the intraocular pressure (e.g. glycerin, isosorbide), beta (β)-adrenoceptor antagonists (e.g. timolol) and carbonic anhydrase inhibitors (e.g. acetazolamide). ➲ anisocoria, gonioscope, iridectomy, iridoschisis, iris bombé, iritis, plateau iris, provocative test, pupillary block, shadow test, synechia, trabeculectomy, van Herick, Shaffer and Schwartz method.

angle of anomaly the angle between the line of visual direction of the fovea and the line of visual direction of the abnormal corresponding point of the same deviated eye. It is usually represented by the difference between the objective and subjective angles of deviation in abnormal retinal correspondence. ➲ abnormal retinal correspondence, angle of deviation, line of direction.

angle of convergence (*syn* angle of triangulation) the angle between the lines of sight of the two eyes which are in a state of convergence. The angle is positive when the lines of sight intersect in front of the eyes, and negative when they intersect behind the eyes. *Note*: some authors regard the angle of convergence as the rotation of one eye only towards the fixation point, and refer to the angle of convergence of both eyes, defined above, as the *total angle of convergence* or the *total convergence*. ➲ base line, interpupillary distance, line of sight, metre angle, prism dioptre.

angle of deviation (angle of squint, angle of strabismus) **1**. an angle through which a ray of light is deviated on reflection by a mirror, or refraction by a lens or prism. **2**. an angle between the visual axis (or line of sight) of the deviated eye in strabismus and the straight ahead position while the other eye fixates straight ahead. It can be assessed subjectively by having the patient report simultaneous perception (e.g. the lion in the cage seen in the amblyoscope) or objectively as

measured by the practitioner either with the amblyoscope or using prisms and cover test, or by the Hirschberg test. ➲ angle of anomaly, prism, visual axis, Worth's amblyoscope.

angle of filtration ➲ angle of the anterior chamber.

angle of incidence **1**. the angle between the incident ray and the normal to the surface at the point of incidence in either reflection or refraction at a surface separating two media. **2**. the angle at which a body, object or vector is moving relative to another (e.g. a stationary surface or environmental factor such as wind), often prior to a collision. For example, when playing a snooker ball at a cushion, the angle between the ball's direction of travel and the cushion.

angle of insonation this is important in pulsed Doppler ultrasound examinations to obtain an accurate representation of blood flow and should be 60° or less.

angle of pull the angle at which a muscle pulls relative to the long axis of the bone on which it pulls. For example, the angle between the biceps brachii tendon and the radius in the forearm.

angle of reflection after a collision, the angle at which one object is moving relative to another (usually a stationary surface or environmental factor such as wind). For example, after a snooker ball has hit a cushion, the angle between the ball's direction of travel and the cushion. It is not necessarily the same size as the angle of incidence. Also known as angle of rebound.

angle of release the angle made between the velocity vector of a body or object (usually the centre of mass) and the ground or other fixed reference frame. Also known as angle of projection or angle of take-off.

angle of stereopsis the difference between the angles subtended at the centres of the entrance pupils of the two eyes by two points located in space at different distances from the eyes. ➲ Howard–Dolman test, stereopsis, stereoscopic visual acuity, three-needle test.

angle of the anterior chamber (*syn* angle of filtration, drainage angle, iridocorneal angle) the angle at the periphery of the anterior chamber formed by the root of the iris, the front surface of the ciliary body and the trabecular meshwork. ➲ anterior chamber of the eye, glaucoma, gonioscope, trabecular meshwork, shadow test, van Herick, Shaffer and Schwartz method.

angle of the eye the outer or inner corner of the eye.

angle of the mandible that part of the mandible formed by the junction of the ramus and the body.

angle of the mouth the point where the upper and lower lips join.

angle of triangulation ➲ angle of convergence.

angle osteotomy excision of a segment of mandible from the region of the angle, either unilaterally or bilaterally, for the correction of prognathism.

angle recession a tear between the longitudinal and circular muscles of the ciliary body. It is most often noted following blunt trauma to the anterior segment. It is typically followed by hyphaemia. This form of injury predisposes the individual to elevated intraocular pressure (i.e. increased risk of glaucoma) in the future. With a gonioscope, angle recession appears with an abnormally wide ciliary body band with a prominent scleral spur and some torn iris processes. There are also marked variations in the width and depth of the angle in different quadrants of the eye. ➲ angle of the anterior chamber, ciliary body, ciliary muscle, cyclodialysis, hyphaema, iridodialysis.

Angle's classification of malocclusion (modified) (E Angle, American orthodontist, 1855–1930) a classification of various forms of malocclusion between the upper and lower teeth. It is based on the mesial position of the lower first molars relative to the upper first molars. The upper first molar's mesiobuccal cusp occludes with the mesiobuccal fossa of the lower first molar.Three classes are described—I, II and III, each with further subdivisions or types. The orthodontic classification is now more related to the position of the upper and lower incisor teeth. ➲ malocclusion.

angstrom (Å) *n* (A J Angström, Swedish physicist, 1814–1874) a unit of measurement equal to 0.1 nanometre or 10^{-10} metre. It is not a SI unit but is sometimes used for wavelength.

angular acceleration the rate of change in angular velocity with respect to time. Measured in degrees per second squared $(°/s^2)$ or radians per second squared (rad/s^2); related to moment by Newton's second angular law of motion (moment = moment of inertia × angular acceleration). ➲ acceleration, gravitational acceleration, instantaneous acceleration, linear acceleration, tangential acceleration.

angular aperture half of the maximum plane subtended by a lens at the axial point of an object or image. (Sometimes the full plane angle is taken as the angular aperture but this is not convenient in optical calculations.). ➲ sine condition.

angular cheilitis condition characterized by dryness, burning, chapping or ulceration of the angle of the mouth. Attributable to candidal and/or bacterial infection in association with haematinic deficiency, vitamin B complex deficiency, loss of vertical dimension and saliva drooling.

angular displacement the angle between the start and finish positions in a rotational movement, including a direction (e.g. clockwise or anticlockwise). Measured in degrees or radians. ➲ displacement, linear displacement.

angular frequency in magnetic resonance, the frequency of oscillation or rotation.

angular impulse moment applied to a rotating body or object multiplied by the duration of the application (newtons × metres × seconds, N. m. s).

angular kinematics the study of rotational motion. ➲ kinematics, linear kinematics.

angular kinetics the study of torques or moments but not linear forces.➲ kinetics, linear kinetics.

angular momentum the product of moment of inertia and angular velocity. Conservation of angular momentum in the absence of an external moment (torque), the angular momentum of a rotating body will remain constant. Often applied to low-velocity flight (e.g. gymnastics) to explain how a body can increase or decrease angular velocity by manipulating moment of inertia (e.g. by 'tucking'). Trading of angular momentum if, in the absence of an external moment (torque), an object or body is rotating about one axis (e.g. somersaulting) and rotation about another axis is introduced (e.g. tilt), the result will be a rotation about a third axis (e.g. twist) due to the vector nature of angular momentum. Transfer of angular momentum can occur from one part of a body to another in the absence of an external moment (torque) (e.g. if one part of a body increases angular velocity, another part must decrease to conserve angular momentum). ➲ linear momentum, momentum.

angular pregnancy implantation of the fertilized ovum in the angle where the uterine (fallopian) tube enters the uterus.

angular speed in degrees per second (°/s) or radians per second (rad/s). ➲ linear speed, speed, velocity.

angular stomatitis ➲ stomatitis.

angular velocity the angular displacement per unit time, i.e. speed of rotation in a particular direction (e.g. clockwise or anticlockwise). ➲ instantaneous velocity, linear velocity, tangential velocity, velocity.

angulation in radiography, the direction in which central X-rays and the cone of the X-ray machine are directed towards the teeth and the radiographic film.

anhedonia *n* a total inability to take pleasure in life. The person is unable to feel happiness in response to events that are ordinarily enjoyable. Associated with severe depressive disorders and schizophrenia.

anhidrosis *n* deficient sweat secretion—**anhidrotic** *adj*.

anhidrotic *n* an agent that reduces perspiration.

anhydraemia *n* deficient fluid content of blood—**anhydraemic** *adj*.

anhydramnios absence of amniotic fluid.

anhydrase *n* an enzyme that catalyses the removal of water molecules. For example carbonic andydrase, which catalyses the removal of water from carbonic acid in the reversible reactions that transport waste carbon dioxide from the cells, maintain normal blood pH and regulate the amount of carbon dioxide excreted by the lungs.

anhydrous *adj* entirely without water, dry.

anicteric *adj* without jaundice.

anion *n* a negatively charged ion, e.g. chloride (Cl^-). They move towards the positive electrode (anode) during electrolysis. ➲ cation.

anion-exchange resin one of several high molecular weight organic substances that exchange anions with other ions. ➲ ion-exchange resins.

anion gap the difference between the amount of anions and cations in the plasma. It is calculated by measuring the concentration of sodium and potassium ions and subtracting the concentration of bicarbonate (hydrogen carbonate) and chloride ions: $(Na^+ + K^+) - (HCO_3^- + Cl^-)$. It may also be determined by subtracting the concentration of bicarbonate and chloride from that of sodium: $(Na^+) - (HCO_3^- + Cl^-)$, normally the gap is between 8 and 14 mmol/L plasma. It is useful in the diagnosis of metabolic acidosis. ➲ metabolic acidosis.

aniridia *n* complete, or almost complete, absence of the iris of the eye. It may be congenitally inherited as an autosomal dominant trait, or can be acquired, due to trauma. The person is photophobic and where the condition is congenital is usually amblyopia and sometimes has nystagmus. Contact lenses incorporating an artificial iris, or tinted spectacle lenses, help in this condition. ➔ cosmetic contact lens, irideremia.

aniseikonia *n* an abnormal condition where each eye perceives the image of an object as being strikingly different (in size and/or shape). This may be due either to unequal axial lengths of the two eyes, to an unequal distribution of the retinal elements or an inequality of the cortical representation of the two ocular images (*basic or intrinsic aniseikonia*). It is most frequently induced by lenses of different power used in the correction of anisometropia (*refractive aniseikonia*). Symptoms include visual discomfort, visual distortion of space and sometimes difficulty in achieving binocular vision, as for example in spectacle corrected unilateral aphakia.

aniso- a prefix that means 'unequal' e.g. *aniscoria*.

anisoaccommodation unequal accommodative response in the two eyes when fixating an object binocularly. It may result from a disease (e.g. glaucoma, ophthalmoplegia, paralysis of the third nerve, unilateral cataract), uncorrected anisometropia, viewing a near object to the side, toxins affecting one eye more than the other, or trauma.

anisochromatic not of uniform colour.

anisochromatopsia a deficiency of colour vision in one eye only, or of unequal severity in the two eyes.

anisochromia ➔ heterochromia.

anisocoria *n* inequality in diameter of the pupils. Typically one pupil is abnormal and cannot either dilate or constrict. It may be physiological (e.g. in antimetropia) or it may be part of a syndrome, the most common being those of Adie's and Horner's. Physiological anisocoria remains constant irrespective of the level of illumination. Anisocoria can occur as a result of injury (e.g. to the iris sphincter muscle), inflammation (e.g. iridocyclitis), diseases of the iris, paralysis of the third nerve, angle-closure glaucoma, systemic diseases (e.g. diabetes, syphilis) or accidental drug instillation into the eye (if the drug or substance has anticholinergic properties the condition is then referred to as anticholinergic mydriasis or 'atropine' mydriasis). The search for the cause of anisocoria is facilitated by testing the pupillary light reflexes and responses to locally instilled drugs. ➔ pupil, pupillary light reflex, pupillometer.

anisocytosis *n* inequality in size of red blood cells. ➔ macrocytosis, microcytosis, poikilocytosis.

anisomelia *n* unequal length of limbs—**anisomelous** *adj.*

anisometropia *n* a difference in the refractive power of the two eyes—**anisometropic** *adj.*

ankle joint *n* the synovial hinge joint between the lower ends of the tibia and fibula, and the talus, where its saddle-shaped upper surface lies in the socket flanked at the sides by the medial and lateral malleoli. Strengthened by four ligaments (anterior, posterior, medial and lateral) between these three bones, and also between them and the calcaneous (calcaneum, os calcis), the heel bone. The two movements occurring at the ankle joint are dorsiflexion (faciltated by the tibialis anterior and toe extensor muscles) and plantar flexion (facilitated by the gastrocnemius, soleus and toe flexor muscles). Note that the movements inversion and eversion occur between the tarsal bones. ➔ anterior talofibular ligament.

ankle-brachial pressure index (ABPI) also known as ankle-arm index. The ratio of ankle systolic blood pressure to systolic blood pressure in the arm. It is calculated by dividing ankle blood pressure by arm blood pressure, this is calculated for both the right and left legs. Doppler ultrasound is used to assess the arterial blood flow to the lower limb (Figure A.10). An ABPI of 1 indicates that 100% of blood is reaching the lower leg, whereas an ABPI of

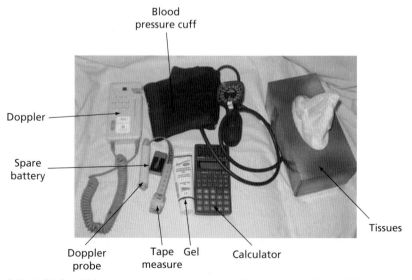

A.10 **Ankle-brachial pressure equipment** (reproduced from Brooker & Waugh 2007 with permission).

0.85 means that only 85% of blood reaches the lower leg and is indicative of arterial disease.

ankle clonus a tendon reflex characterized by a series of rapid muscular contractions of the calf muscle when the foot is dorsiflexed by pressure upon the sole.

ankle equinus a congenital or acquired condition or deformity, which is characterized by deficient dorsiflexion at the ankle joint. During the stance phase of normal gait a minimum 10° of ankle joint dorsiflexion is needed for normal walking. ⊃ talipes.

ankle foot orthosis (AFO) a splint for the ankle foot complex, usually designed to enable function. They are useful in patients with insufficient dorsiflexion to clear the floor on swing through when walking or with unstable ankle and subtalar joints. The orthosis usually allows for some dorsiflexion, but prevents plantarflexion beyond plantargrade. This means that the patient can walk without tripping up. The stability provided by the orthosis can often enable patents to walk more safely and quicker and have greater confidence when walking outside. They are usually made of plastic material. As with all external devices care needs to be taken to ensure correct fitting to prevent skin damage.

ankle sprain overstretch of the ligaments of the ankle joint, most commonly from an inversion injury, resulting in injury to the anterior talofibular ligament.

ankyloblepharon *n* adhesion of the eyelid margins, usually lateral, often secondary to chronic inflammation.

ankyloglossia 'tongue tie', a congenital abnormality. The complete or partial binding of the tongue to the floor of the mouth or alveolar ridge due to an abnormally short lingual frenulum or frenum (fraenum) that limits tongue movement.

ankylosed stiffened: bound by adhesions or fused.

ankylosing spondylitis a seronegative polyarthritis affecting mainly the spine. It is characterized by inflammation involving ligament and tendon attachments to bone (enthesopathy). This results in painful stiffness of ligaments and joints, which in severe cases leads to a forward flexion of the spine ('bamboo' or 'poker' spine). It occurs more commonly in males, M:F ratio is 3:1 and generally affects young men under 30 years of age. It is closely associated with HLA B27, 90% of sufferers are HLA B27 positive, however, a proportion of the population are B27 positive and do not have ankylosing spondylitis. ⊃ human leucocyte antigen (HLA), major histocompatibility complex (MHC), spondylitis.

ankylosis *n* stiffness or fixation of a joint. Fusion of a joint caused by disease, trauma or surgery. ⊃ dental ankylosis, false ankylosis, spondylitis—**ankylosed** *adj*, **ankylose** *vt, vi*.

ankyrins a group of proteins which function to fix the cell cytoskeleton. They are present in the red blood cell membrane where they attach the spectrins to the cell membrane. Ankyrins also exist in other sites including the brain. ⊃ hereditary elliptocytosis, hereditary spherocytosis, spectrins.

annealing low temperature heat treatment of metals to relieve internal stresses.

annular *adj* ring-shaped.

annular array in ultrasound, using crystals of the same frequency which are arranged in a circle and are electronically focussed at several depths.

annular ligaments hold in proximity two long bones, as in the wrist and ankle joints.

annular synechia adhesion of the entire pupillary margin of the iris to the capsule of the crystalline lens. ⊃ iris bombé; pupillary block.

annulus any ring-shaped structure or circular aperture.

annulus fibrosis the ring-shaped outer part of the intervertebral disc. It is formed from sheets of collagen fibres arranged in marginally different orientations. The posterior part is the thinnest part of the annulus fibrosis, which makes it more likely to rupture.

anococcygeal referring to the anus and coccyx, and the muscles between them.

anococcygeal body a mass of muscular and fibrous tissue situated between the anal canal and the coccyx.

anode a conductor with a positive charge, attracting negatively charged atoms or groups of atoms (anions). Usually has a red lead and is used as the indifferent electrode for motor stimulation with a monophasic or an unbalanced pulse. If used distally, the anode may block (anodal block) an action potential as it moves distally down an axon (i.e. positively charged ions at the anode may be sufficient to block the ionic changes that comprise the action potential by creating a local hyperpolarization). **2.** part of an X-ray tube that is made of either copper with a tungsten target embedded in it, or molybdenum with a tungsten/rhenium target; the positive anode can be either stationary or rotating. The target is at an angle to produce a larger effective focal spot.

anode heel effect an effect due to the angle of the target on the anode of an X-ray tube, some of the radiation produced is absorbed by the target and therefore the intensity of the emergent X-ray beam is greater at the cathode end of the tube than at the anode end.

anodontia the failure of the teeth to develop. It may be partial where some teeth develop, or total when all teeth are absent. ⊃ oligodontia.

anodyne a drug, other substance, or treatment that eases or relieves pain.

anogenital *adj* pertaining to the anus and the genital region.

anomaloscope (*syn* Nagel anomaloscope) an instrument for testing colour vision in which the observer is required to match one-half of a circular field which is illuminated with yellow with a mixture of green and red in the other half. The yellow half can be varied in brightness, while the other may be varied continuously from red to green. A certain combination of the red and green mixture is considered normal and variations from that mixture indicate anomalous colour vision. With this instrument one can distinguish between a protanope and a protanomal and between a deuteranope and a deuteranomal. Some anomaloscopes also test for blue-yellow colour vision deficiencies, e.g. Pickford–Nicholson anomaloscope. ⊃ defective colour vision, Rayleigh equation.

anomalous fixation ⟳ eccentric fixation.

anomalous retinal correspondence ⟳ abnormal retinal correspondence (ARC).

anomalous trichromatism ⟳ trichromatism.

anomaly *n* that which is unusual or differs from the normal—**anomalous** *adj*.

anomaly scan an ultrasound scan to detect fetal structural anomalies, and abnormal placental position usually performed between 18 and 21 weeks' gestation although may be undertaken in the first trimester. It involves examination of the skull, vertebral (spinal) column and central nervous system (brain, spinal cord), thorax, heart, abdomen, urogenital tract, skeleton, extremities and face.

anomia *n* a difficulty in word finding that affects many people with aphasia. Most frequently demonstrated when the person is required to perform a naming task but may also be recognized by the use of circumlocutions in spontaneous speech samples.

anomie *n* sociological term that describes a circumstance where the 'norms' that guide behaviour are absent. The 'normless' state that results from weak social controls and moral obligations leads to derangement in social behaviour.

anonychia *n* absence of nails.

anoperineal *adj* pertaining to the anus and perineum.

Anopheles *n* a genus of mosquito. The females of some species are the host of the malarial parasite, and their bite is the means of transmitting malaria to humans.

anophthalmia *n* (*syn* anophthalmos, anophthalmus) the congenital absence of all the tissues of the eyes. It is due to a failure of the outgrowth of the optic vescicle to form the optic cup. However, in many cases some development occurs and there is a rudimentary presence of one or both eyes, such as extreme microphthalmia. ⟳ microphthalmia, optic cup, optic vesicle.

anophthalmos ⟳ anophthalmia.

anophthalmus ⟳ anophthalmia.

anoplasty *n* surgical repair or reconstruction of the anus. Such as may be required after a fourth degree tear during childbirth—**anoplastic** *adj*.

anorchism *n* congenital absence of one or both testes—**anorchic** *adj*.

anorectal *adj* pertaining to the anus and rectum, e.g. a fissure. ⟳ anal fissure.

anorectic *adj* **1**. relating to anorexia. **2**. leading to loss or reduction in appetite, such as drugs that suppress appetite. **3**. lacking appetite.

anorexia *n* lack of appetite for food.

anorexia nervosa (AN) an eating disorder. There is marked weight loss and emaciation, arising from food avoidance, often in combination with bingeing, purging, excessive exercise, or the use of diuretics and laxatives. Occasionally more extreme measures such as blood-letting are encountered. There is profound body image disturbance so that, despite their emaciation, patients still feel overweight and are terrified of weight gain. These preoccupations are intense and pervasive, and the false beliefs at times held with a conviction approaching the delusional. Anxiety and depressive symptoms are common accompaniments. Downy hair (lanugo) may develop on the back, forearms and cheeks. Extreme starvation is associated with a wide range of physiological and pathological bodily changes. All organ systems may be affected, although the most serious problems are cardiac and skeletal. The aetiology is unknown but probably includes genetic and environmental factors, including poor self-esteem, fear of obesity, distorted body image and the social pressure on women to be thin. The condition usually emerges in adolescence, with a marked female preponderance but also affects males and adults. The diagnostic criteria are: (a) weight loss of at least 15% of total body weight (or body mass index ≤17.5); (b) avoidance of high-calorie foods; (c) distortion of body image so that patients regard themselves as fat even when grossly underweight; (d) amenorrhoea for at least 3 months. Differential diagnosis includes other causes of weight loss including psychiatric disorders such as depression, and medical conditions such as inflammatory bowel disease, malabsorption, hypopituitarism and cancer. The diagnosis is made on the presence of a pronounced fear of fatness despite being thin, and on the absence of alternative causes of weight loss. The aims of management are to ensure the patient's physical well-being, whilst helping them to increase their weight to the normal range by addressing abnormal beliefs and behaviour. This requires a good therapeutic relationship. Treatment is usually given on an outpatient basis, inpatient treatment being indicated only if weight loss is intractable and severe (for example, less than 65% of normal), or if there is a risk of death from medical complications or from suicide. There is a limited evidence base for treatment, although individual psychological treatments, particularly cognitive behaviour therapy (CBT) and family therapy, are used. Psychotropic drugs are of little benefit except in those with clear-cut comorbid depressive disorder. Weight gain is best managed in a collaborative fashion. Compulsory admission and re-feeding (including tube feeding) are very occasionally resorted to when patients are at risk of death and other measures have failed. Whilst this may produce a short-term improvement in weight, it probably does not change long-term prognosis. About 20% of patients with anorexia nervosa have a good outcome, a further 20% develop a chronic intractable disorder and the rest have an intermediate outcome. There is a long-term mortality rate of 10–20%, either due to the complications of starvation or from suicide. Anorexia nervosa may also be a feature of certain sports. The sports most often associated with anorexia nervosa include 'aesthetic sports' (e.g. diving, figure skating, gymnastics, synchronized swimming), those in which low body mass and low body fat appear to be a physical and biomechanical advantage (distance running, road cycling, triathlon) and those with weight categories for competition (lightweight rowing, weight lifting, wrestling). A condition described as anorexia athletica is illustrated by similarly disordered eating plus compulsive exercising—**anorexic, anorectic** *adj*. ⟳ eating disorders.

anorgasmy, anorgasmia failure to experience orgasm.

anosmia *n* absence of the sense of smell—**anosmic** *adj*.

ANOVA *abbr* analysis of varience.

anovular *adj* relating to absence of ovulation.

anovular bleeding occurs in dysfunctional uterine bleeding associated with hormone disturbance.

anovular menstruation menstruation not associated with the prior release of an oocyte. Such as that resulting from the use of combined oral contraceptive pills.

anoxaemia *n* literally, no oxygen in the blood. Usually used to indicate hypoxaemia—**anoxaemic** *adj*.

anoxia *n* literally, no oxygen in the tissues. Usually used to signify hypoxia—**anoxic** *adj*.

ANP *abbr* atrial natriuretic peptide.

ANS *abbr* **1**. anterior nasal spine. **2**. autonomic nervous system.

ANT *acron* adverse neural tension.

ant- a prefix that means 'against, counteracting', e.g. *antagonist*.

antacid *n* a substance that neutralizes acidity. Often used in alkaline indigestion medicines, e.g. magnesium trisilicate. ⊃ Appendix 5.

antagonist *n* **1**. a muscle that reverses or opposes the action of an agonist muscle, e.g. the triceps may 'antagonize' flexion of the elbow by the biceps brachii. Antagonistic pairs of muscles allow coordinated control. **2**. also describes a drug or other chemical that blocks the action of a ligand (natural chemical such as a neurotransmitter or hormone) by competing at the receptor sites, e.g. the narcotic antagonist naloxone reverses the action of opioid drugs. **3**. in dentistry, a tooth in one jaw which occludes with a tooth in the other jaw. ⊃ agonist *opp*—**antagonism** *n*, **antagonistic** *adj*.

antagonistic action action performed by those muscles that limit the movement of an opposing group.

antalgia literally away from pain, such as the adoption of a particular posture or gait in order to reduce pain. For example, an antalgic gait is the gait adopted by a person in an attempt to produce the minimum amount of pain when walking.

ante- a prefix that means 'before, in front', e.g. *antenatal*.

anteflexion *n* the bending forward of an organ, commonly applied to the position of the uterus. ⊃ retroflexion *opp*.

antegrade pyelography the radiographic examination of the renal tract following the infusion of contrast agent directly into the renal pelvis.

antemortem *adj* before death. ⊃ postmortem *opp*.

antenatal *adj* prenatal, before birth. ⊃ postnatal *opp*—**antenatally** *adj*.

antenatal care care provided by midwives and obstetricians during pregnancy to ensure that fetal and maternal health are satisfactory to enable early detection and treatment of any deviations from normal. Psycho-emotional preparation of the parents for labour and parenthood and health education are also included.

antepartum *adj* before birth. From 24 weeks' gestation to full term.

antepartum haemorrhage (APH) any bleeding from the genital tract after the 24th week of gestation and before the commencement of labour. Causes include placenta praevia, placental abruption, trauma, cervicitis, genital cancers, etc. ⊃ postpartum *opp*.

anterior *adj* in front of; the front surface of; ventral. ⊃ posterior *opp*—**anteriorly** *adv*.

anterior bite plane platform of acrylic resin in the anterior region of a removable appliance on which the lower teeth occlude, thus preventing posterior tooth contact.

anterior chamber cleavage syndrome ⊃ Peters' anomaly.

anterior chamber of the eye the space between the posterior surface of the cornea and the anterior surface of the iris. Contains aqueous fluid. ⊃ aqueous.

anterior ciliary vein one of many veins which drains the ciliary body, the deep and superficial plexuses, the anterior conjunctival veins and the episcleral veins to empty into the vortex veins. ⊃ vortex vein.

anterior compartment syndrome pain on the front of the lower leg, down the outer side of the tibia, when (mainly) the ankle dorsiflexor (tibialis anterior) and toe extensors are affected. ⊃ chronic exertional compartment syndrome, compartment syndrome, lateral compartment syndrome, posterior compartment syndrome, tibialis syndrome.

anterior cruciate ligament (ACL) a major ligament within the knee joint (Figure A.11). It is important in stabilizing the knee by limiting the chance of hyperextending the tibia beyond the femur, and is also concerned with proprioception. A common sports injury where there is violent twisting combined with rapid deceleration, such as in soccer, rugby football, skiing or basketball. ⊃ anterior (PA) drawer test, cruciate ligaments, cruciate ligament injury.

anterior limiting lamina ⊃ Bowman's membrane.

anterior limiting layer ⊃ Bowman's membrane.

anterior limiting ring of Schwalbe *syn* line of Schwalbe. A bundle of connective tissue and elastic fibres forming

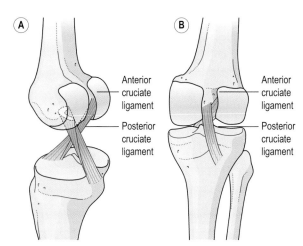

A.11 Cruciate ligaments: (A) oblique view showing twisting of fibres; (B) posterior view showing them crossing in space (reproduced from Porter 2005 with permission).

the junction between the anterior termination of the trabecular meshwork and Descemet's membrane of the cornea. If it is unusually thickened or prominent, it is called posterior embryotoxon. ⊃ Axenfeld's syndrome, gonioscopy, Rieger's syndrome, trabecular meshwork.

anterior membrane dystrophy ⊃ Cogan's microcystic epithelial dystrophy.

anterior oral seal ⊃ seal.

anterior (PA) drawer test a test to detect rupture of the anterior cruciate ligament. The patient lies supine. The therapist sits on the patient's foot to stabilize the leg and grasps around the proximal tibia and tibial tuberosity and pulls the tibia forwards (Figure A.12). A positive sign is elicited by excessive translation of the tibia anteriorly. ⊃ Lachman's test (modified anterior drawer test).

anterior protected articulation a protected arrangement of the teeth in which the vertical and horizontal overlap of the anterior teeth disengages the posterior teeth in all mandibular excursive movements.

anterior superior dental nerve an afferent nerve from the upper central and lateral incisor and canine teeth, passing upwards to join the maxillary division of the trigeminal nerve in the infraorbital canal.

anterior guidance ⊃ guidance.

anterior nares the pair of openings from the exterior into the nasal cavities.

anterior nasal spine (ANS) the top of the anterior nasal spine as seen in a lateral skull radiograph.

anterior occlusal projection ⊃ standard occlusal projection.

anterior open bite occlusion in which the lower teeth are neither overlapped in the vertical plane nor occlude with the upper incisors when the posterior teeth are in occlusion.

anterior pituitary endocrine gland, part of the pituitary gland at the base of the brain. Secretes growth hormone (with widespread actions on growth and metabolism), prolactin (promoting lactation) and 'trophic' hormones that regulate in turn the endocrine secretions of the adrenal cortex, of the thyroid gland, and those from the gonads involved in reproductive function. All these secretory functions are themselves controlled by 'releasing' and in some instances also 'inhibitory' hormones from the hypothalamus via local blood vessels. ⊃ pituitary gland.

anterior protected articulation ⊃ articulation.

anterior talofibular ligament (ATF) the most anterior of the three lateral collateral ankle ligaments and the most commonly injured following inversion injuries. The three ligaments in the complex are: posterior talofibular ligament, calcaneofibular ligament and the anterior talofibular ligament.

anterior tibial syndrome severe pain and inflammation over anterior tibial muscle group, with inability to dorsiflex the foot.

anterior tooth one of the incisor or canine teeth.

antero- a prefix that means 'front', e.g. *anterograde*.

anterograde *adj* proceeding forward. ⊃ retrograde *opp*.

anterograde amnesia ⊃ amnesia.

anteroposterior axis of the eye (*syn* sagittal axis, y-axis) a line passing through the anterior and posterior poles and the centre of rotation of the eye. It is perpendicular to the transverse (or x-axis) and the vertical (or z-axis). ⊃ centre of rotation of the eye, poles of the eyeball.

anteroposterior radiograph a radiograph taken from the front to the back of the body.

anteversion *n* the normal forward tilting, or displacement forward, of an organ or part. ⊃ retroversion *opp*— **anteverted** *adj*, **antevert** *vt*.

anthelmintic *adj* describes a drug for the destruction or elimination of parasitic worms, e.g. mebendazole. ⊃ Appendix 5.

anthracosis *n* coal miners/worker's pneumoconiosis. Accumulation of carbon in the lungs due to inhalation of coal dust; may cause a fibrotic reaction. A form of pneumoconiosis— **anthracotic** *adj*.

anthrax *n* a contagious disease of domestic animals such as cattle, it is caused by the spore-forming bacterium *Bacillus anthracis* (Gram-positive); the extremely resistant spores can survive for decades. Anthrax may be transmitted to humans by cutaneous inoculation (malignant pustule), ingestion (severe gastroenteritis, toxaemia) and inhalation (woolsorter's disease, haemorrhagic bronchopneumonia), the most lethal form, anthrax may also cause meningitis. *cutaneous anthrax* the skin lesion is associated with occupational exposure to anthrax spores, for example during processing of hides and bone products, or with bioterrorism. It accounts for the vast majority of clinical cases. Animal infection is a serious problem in Africa, India, Pakistan and the Middle East. Spores are inoculated into exposed skin. A single lesion develops as an irritable papule on an oedematous haemorrhagic base. This progresses to a depressed black eschar. Despite extensive oedema, pain is

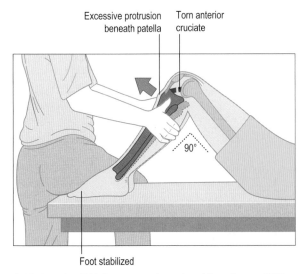

Excessive protrusion beneath patella Torn anterior cruciate

90°

Foot stabilized

A.12 Anterior (PA) drawer test (reproduced from Jennett 2008 with permission).

infrequent. ⊃ Colour Section Figure 48. *B. anthracis* can be cultured from lesional skin swabs. *gastrointestinal anthrax* is associated with the ingestion of meat products that have been contaminated or incompletely cooked. The caecum is the seat of the infection, which produces nausea, vomiting, anorexia and fever, followed in 2–3 days by severe abdominal pain and bloody diarrhoea. Toxaemia and death can develop rapidly thereafter. *inhalational anthrax* is extremely rare unless associated with bioterrorism. Without rapid and aggressive therapy at the onset of symptoms, the mortality is greater than 90%. Fever, dyspnoea, cough, headache and symptoms of septicaemia develop 3–14 days following exposure. Typically, there is little on the chest X-ray other than widening of the mediastinum and pleural effusions. The management depends on the site infected and the severity of the disease. Skin lesions are readily curable with early antibiotic therapy. Treatment is with ciprofloxacin 500 mg daily until penicillin susceptibility is confirmed; the regimen can then be changed to benzylpenicillin 600 000 units i.m. 6-hourly or phenoxymethylpenicillin 500 mg 6-hourly. Aggressive fluid resuscitation and the addition of an aminoglycoside antibiotic may improve the outlook. Respiratory support with mechanical ventilation will be required in inhalational disease. Preventive measures include immunization of humans and animals, post-exposure prophylaxis with antibiotics, e.g. ciprofloxacin, and proper disposal of infected animals. Occupations at high risk include veterinary surgeons, livestock farmers, butchers, and those handling hides and wool. The ease of production of *B. anthracis* spores makes this infection a candidate for biological warfare or bioterrorism. Prophylaxis with ciprofloxacin (500 mg 12-hourly) is recommended for anyone at high risk of exposure to biological warfare. Due to its use in recent years as a bioterrorist weapon, anthrax has assumed considerable significance. ⊃ bioterrorism.

anthropoid *adj* ape-like, resembling man.

anthropoid pelvis a form of contracted pelvis. The brim is long anteroposteriorly and narrow transversely.

anthropological baseline a line joining the infraorbital margin to the superior border of the external auditory meatus.

anthropology *n* the study of humankind. Subdivided into several specialties. ⊃ ethnology.

anthropometry *n* measurement of the human body and its parts for the purposes of comparison and establishing norms for gender, age, weight, race and so on. Used to assess development, nutritional status and as a non-invasive way of assessing body composition. Anthropometric measurements include weight for age; weight for height; height for age; skinfold thickness to assess subcutaneous fat; and mid-upper arm circumference to assess muscle wastage—**anthropometric** *adj*.

anti- a prefix that means 'against', e.g. *antibacterial*.

antianabolic *adj* preventing the synthesis of body protein.

antiandrogens *npl* a group of drugs that block the activity of testosterone, e.g. finasteride. ⊃ Appendix 5.

antiarrhythmic *adj* describes drugs and treatments used to treat a variety of cardiac arrhythmias, e.g. verapamil. ⊃ Appendix 5.

antibacterial *adj* describes an agent that destroys bacteria or inhibits their growth. ⊃ antibiotics, antiseptics, bactericidal, bacteriostatic, disinfectants.

antiberi-beri *adj* against beri-beri, e.g. the thiamin(e) portion of vitamin B complex.

antibilharzial *adj* against *Bilharzia*. ⊃ *Schistosoma*.

antibiosis *n* an association between organisms that is harmful to one of them. ⊃ symbiosis *opp*—**antibiotic** *adj*.

antibiotic-associated colitis also known as antibiotic-associated diarrhoea, or pseudomembranous colitis. A potentially life-threatening condition associated with a superinfection caused by *Clostridium difficile*. Older adults, especially women are affected following surgery. It is linked to the administration of broad-spectrum antibiotics such as clindamycin or the cephalosporins, but it can be associated with any antibiotic drug.These drugs suppress the normal flora of the intestinal tract, thus allowing the colonization and unimpeded growth of micro-organisms such as *C. difficile*. It is characterized by copious watery diarrhoea; if this occurs antibiotic treatment should be stopped. There is necrosis of the epithelium lining the intestine with ulceration; the great danger being perforation of the intestine leading to peritonitis. ⊃ Colour Section Figure 49.

antibiotics *npl* antibacterial substances derived from fungi and bacteria, exemplified by penicillin. However, the term is generally used for all drugs that act against bacteria. Some have a narrow spectrum of activity whereas others act against a wide range of bacteria (broad spectrum). ⊃ aminoglycosides, antituberculosis drugs, bactericidal, bacteriostatic, β-lactam antibiotics, cephalosporins, glycylcyclines, glycopeptide antibiotics, macrolides, penicillins, fluoroquinolones, sulphonamides, tetracyclines. ⊃ Appendix 5.

antibodies *npl* (*syn* immunoglobulins) often used to indicate immunoglobulins with specific antigen-binding activity.

anticardiolipin antibodies (ACAs) antiphospholipid antibodies. They can cause hypercoagulation, are strongly associated with venous and arterial thrombosis, thrombocytopenia and recurrent fetal loss. Often occur with other autoimmune disorders (e.g. systemic lupus erythematosus), in pregnancy. They may react against the trophoblast, causing subplacental clots which interfere with placentation, leading to placental thrombosis and cause fetal loss or growth restriction. ⊃ antiphospholipid antibodies, antiphospholipid antibody syndrome.

anticholinergic *adj* inhibitory to the action of a cholinergic nerve by interfering with the action of the neurotransmitter acetylcholine at synapses. Anticholinergic drugs, therefore, reduce spasm in smooth muscle most notably the bladder, bronchi (causing bronchodilation) and intestines. They also decrease gastric, bronchial and salivary secretions. Certain types of these drugs are used in the treatment of such conditions as Parkinson's disease and dystonia. ⊃ muscarinic antagonists (antimuscarinic).

anticholinesterase *n* any agent that inactivates cholinesterase.

anticipatory postural adjustments small postural adjustments made by postural muscles (e.g. those in the trunk), in anticipation of movement or movement of a body part such as an arm. They form part of the many mechanisms that operate to maintain balance.

anticoagulant *n* an agent that reduces the propensity of blood to clot. Uses: (a) to obtain specimens suitable for pathological examination and chemical analyses where whole blood or plasma is required instead of serum; (b) during the collection of blood for transfusion, the anticoagulant usually being sodium citrate; (c) as therapy in the prophylaxis and treatment of thromboembolic conditions. ➲ Appendix 5, coumarins, heparin.

anticoagulation *n* the process of suppressing or reducing blood coagulation.

anticodon *n* in genetics, the three bases (triplet) in transfer ribonucleic acid (tRNA) concerned with the synthesis of proteins (translation stage). ➲ codon.

anticonvulsant *n* ➲ antiepileptics—**anticonvulsive** *adj*.

anti-curl backing in radiography, used for single emulsion films and coat the opposite side of the base from the emulsion to prevent the film from curling.

anti-D *n* an antibody directed against the rhesus D blood group antigen. It is formed when rhesus negative individuals are exposed to rhesus positive blood, such as being transfused with rhesus positive blood, or a rhesus negative woman who is pregnant with a rhesus positive fetus. ➲ABO blood group system, anti-D (Rh_0) immunoglobulin, blood groups, Rhesus incompatibility.

anti-D (Rh_0) immunoglobulin an immunoglobulin given to prevent the the formation of anti-D antibody by rhesus negative women after the birth of the baby, or following an ectopic pregnancy, threatened miscarriage, spontaneous miscarriage or termination of pregnancy. It is also given after amniocentesis and other invasive procedures, abdominal trauma, antepartum haemorrhage and in cases of intrauterine death or stillbirth. Anti-D (Rh_0) immunoglobulin reduces the risk of isoimmunization and problems with subsequent pregnancies, that include stillbirth or haemolytic disease of the newborn.

antidepressants *npl* drugs used to manage depression. There are three main groups: monoamine oxidase inhibitors (MAOIs) (e.g. phenelzine), selective serotonin reuptake inhibitors (SSRIs) (e.g. fluoxetine), and tricyclic antidepressants (TCA) (e.g. amitriptyline). ➲ Appendix 5.

antidiabetic *adj* literally 'against diabetes'. Used to describe therapeutic measures used for people with diabetes mellitus to control blood glucose. ➲ insulin, hypoglycaemic drugs.

antidiarrhoeals *npl* agents such as drugs used to reduce diarrhoea, e.g. loperamide. ➲ Appendix 5.

anti-discriminatory practice professional codes of practice and policies of healthcare providers that seek to eliminate discrimination experienced by patients/clients, employees and groups, particularly on the basis of their age, gender, sexual orientation, social class, health behaviours, religion, race, disability, political views, or their illness. Specific legislation, such as the UK Sex Discrimination Act (1975), exists to safeguard the interests of people and can be used to challenge discrimatory practices.

antidiuretic *adj* reducing the volume of urine.

antidiuretic hormone (ADH) also called vasopressin, or arginine vasopression (AVP). A hormone formed in the hypothalamus and stored in the posterior lobe of the pituitary gland. ADH increases the permeability of the renal tubule, thereby increasing water reabsorption into the blood stream. ADH is released in response to a reduction in blood volume or increased level of sodium in the blood. When the levels of ADH in the plasma are low, a large volume of dilute urine is excreted (diuresis) by the kidneys. Whereas when plasma levels are high, a small volume of concentrated urine is excreted (antidiuresis). ➲ vasopressin.

antidote *n* a remedy that opposes, counteracts or neutralizes the action of a poison. For example, protamine sulphate is used to counteract the effects of an overdose of heparin.

antiembolic *adj* against embolism.

antiembolism hoisery/stockings elastic hoisery (knee or full length) that exerts linear graduated compression on the superficial veins of the legs. This increases venous return to the heart, thus preventing venous stasis, which predisposes to deep vein thrombosis (DVT) following surgery and in other situations where patients are immobile. Also knows as thromboembolic deterrents (TEDs) stockings.

antiemetic *adj* against emesis. Any agent such as a drug that prevents or treats nausea and vomiting. ➲ cannabinoids, D_2-receptor antagonists, H_1-receptor antagonists, 5-HT_3-receptor antagonists, muscarinic antagonists (antimuscarinic), neurokinin receptor antagonist. ➲ Appendix 5.

antienzyme *n* a substance that exerts a specific inhibiting action on an enzyme. Found in the digestive tract to prevent autodigestion of the mucosa, and in blood where they act as immunoglobulins.

antiepileptic *adj* (*syn* anticonvulsant) describes drugs which reduce the frequency of seizures, e.g. sodium valproate. ➲ Appendix 5.

antifebrile *adj* describes any agent which reduces or allays fever.

antifibrinolytic *adj* describes any agent which prevents fibrinolysis.

anti-frothant in radiography, a chemical added to the developer to reduce foaming due to agitation of the developer by the rollers.

antifungal *adj* describes any agent which destroys fungi, e.g. fluconazole. ➲ Appendix 5.

antigalactic a drug which suppresses the formation of milk in the mammary glands.

anti-GBM disease (*syn* Goodpasture's disease) a disease caused by specific antibodies (linear IgG) that target the glomerular basement membranes. There is autoimmunity to the α3 chain of type IV collagen. The disease is associated with the presence of the human leucocyte antigen HLA-DR15. It is characterized by rapidly progressive glomerulonephritis and pulmonary haemorrhage but either may occur alone. Management includes the administration of corticosteroids, cyclophosphamide and plasma exchange to remove circulating antibodies. ⊃ pulmonary-renal disease/syndrome.

antigen *n* substance inducing a specific immune response which interacts with the product of that immune response. This may be a specific immunoglobulin or T cells bearing T cell receptors specific for that antigen—**antigenic** *adj*.

antigenetic determinant the site on an antigen molecule that binds with the corresponding site on the specific antibody or T-lymphocyte receptor. Also known as an epitope. ⊃ epitope, paratope.

antigenic drift the mutations occurring in a micro-organism over time that alter their antigenic characteristics. This leads to difficulties in the provision of effective vaccines and antimicrobial drugs. For example the changes that occur in the influenza virus, which creates problems for vaccine production, as a new influenza vaccine is required each year.

antigenicity the ability or power of micro-organisms and their products to stimulate the production of antibodies by immune cells, as in a vaccine.

antigen-presenting cells (APC) *npl* part of the immune response. They are cells of the monocyte-macrophage (reticuloendothelial) system that include macrophages, and dendritic cells that are present in the skin (called Langerhans' cells) and in the gastrointestinal tract and respiratory tract. They process antigens so they can be presented to T-lymphocyte receptors. ⊃ macrophages.

antigonococcal *adj* describes any measures used against infections caused by *Neisseria gonorrhoeae*.

antihaemophilic factor (AHF) also called antihaemophilic globulin (AHG). Factor VIII in the blood coagulation cascade, present in plasma. It has two portions, a low molecular weight part and a high molecular weight part, they are involved at different stages of coagulation. A deficiency causes haemophilia A (classical).

antihaemophilic factor B ⊃ Christmas factor.

antihaemorrhagic *adj* describes any agent which prevents haemorrhage.

anti-halation layer in radiography, a coloured dye in the anti-curl backing of a film to absorb any reflected light and therefore prevent unsharpness on the film.

antihelix a curved ridge in the auricle (pina) of the outer/external ear.

antihistamines *npl* drugs which suppress some of the effects of histamine released in the body, e.g. chlorphenamine. ⊃ Appendix 5.

antihypertensive *adj* describes any agent that reduces high blood pressure. ⊃ (α)-adrenoceptor antagonists, angiotensin-converting enzyme inhibitors, (β)-adrenoceptor antagonists, calcium antagonists, diuretics. ⊃ Appendix 5.

anti-infective *adj* describes any agent which prevents infection.

anti-inflammatory *adj* tending to prevent or relieve inflammation. ⊃ non-steroidal anti-inflammatory drugs (NSAIDs). ⊃ Appendix 5.

antileprotic *adj* describing any agent which prevents or cures leprosy, e.g. rifampicin. ⊃ Appendix 5.

antilipidaemic dietary modification, drug, or other treatment used to manage hyperlipidaemia by lowering the level of blood lipids.

antilymphocyte globulin (ALG) an immunoglobulin which binds to antigens on T cells and inhibits T cell-dependent immune responses; occasionally used in preventing graft rejection during organ transplantation.

antimalarial *adj* against malaria, e.g. mefloquine. ⊃ Appendix 5.

antimetabolites *npl* molecules that prevent cell division. They are sufficiently similar to essential cell metabolites to be incorporated into the metabolic pathways, thereby preventing their use by the cell, e.g. methotrexate. ⊃ cytotoxic. ⊃ Appendix 5.

antimicrobial *adj* against microbes.

antimitochondrial antibody (AMA) autoantibodies against mitochondrial components. Certain types are a marker for primary biliary cirrhosis.

antimitotic *adj* preventing cell replication by mitosis. ⊃ cytotoxic.

anti-Monson curve ⊃ reverse curve

antimutagen *n* a substance that cancels out the action of a mutagen—**antimutagenic** *adj*.

antimycotic *adj* ⊃ antifungal.

antineoplastic *adj* describes any substance or procedure that kills or slows the growth of cancerous/neoplastic cells, such as cytotoxic chemotherapy, radiotherapy, or hormonal or biological response modification therapy.

antineuritic *adj* describes any agent which prevents neuritis. Specially applied to vitamin B complex.

antineutrophil cytoplasmic antibodies (ANCA) a group of autoantibodies directed against cytoplasmic components of neutrophils and associated with a range of pathological conditions such as polyarteritis.

antineutrophil cytoplasmic antibodies-associated vasculitis microscopic polyangiitis (MPA), Wegener's granulomatosis (WG) and Churg–Strauss syndrome (CSS) can be grouped together as ANCA-associated vasculitis, although not all patients are ANCA-positive at diagnosis. All patients may present similarly with arthralgia, myalgia and evidence of multisystem disease, the precise 'subtype' being determined by other specific clinical features. Treatment for these conditions should be instituted as early as possible to prevent irreversible damage, even in advance of biopsy confirmation if there is life-threatening or critical organ involvement. Remission can be induced either with oral high-dose prednisolone daily and continuous oral cyclophosphamide or with bolus intravenous methylprednisolone and cyclophosphamide. Doses of cyclophosphamide should be reduced in older adults and those with renal impairment. Once remission has been induced (3–6 months) the dose of oral prednisolone is rapidly reduced and cyclophosphamide is usually replaced with azathioprine. Co-trimoxazole is usually given at a prophylactic dose (thrice weekly) in conjunction with cyclophosphamide to prevent *Pneumocystis* pneumonia (PCP), unless there is a history of drug allergy. Mesna is used with bolus cyclophosphamide to reduce the risks of haemorrhagic cystitis. Occasionally, cyclophosphamide fails to induce a remission, in which case the diagnosis should be reconsidered. Patients who have ANCA-positive vasculitis with acute renal failure (creatinine > 500 μmol/L or 5.66 mg/dL) have a better outcome when also treated with adjunctive plasma exchange.

antinuclear antibody (ANA) a family of many types of autoantibody directed against cell nuclei that are found in connective tissue diseases, particularly in systemic lupus erythematosus (SLE) and Sjögren syndrome. The many types recognized can be used to categorize rheumatological disorders.

antioestrogens *npl* antagonist drugs that block cell surface oestrogen receptors in various body sites, e.g. tamoxifen. ➲ oestrogen receptors, selective (o)estrogen receptor modulators (SERMS). ➲ Appendix 5.

antioppressive practice a term often used interchangeably with antidiscriminatory practice. Antioppressive practice emphasizes the need to change power relations by minimizing power differences in society. This demands fundamental challenges and changes to social values and within relationships and institutions.

antioxidant *n* **1.** molecules that defend body cells against oxidative stress. **2.** a substance that delays the process of oxidation of fats in stored food. Many fats, and especially vegetable oils, contain natural antioxidants, such as vitamin E, which guard against rancidity for some time. ➲ antioxidant enzymes, antioxidant nutrients.

antioxidant enzymes the endogenous antioxidant enzymes include superoxide dismutase, catalase, glutathione peroxidase and glutathione S-transferase and so on; ageing is known to reduce, and exercise training to elevate, their activities. The hormone melatonin, secreted by the pineal gland, has antioxidant properties and there is evidence that it promotes the action of antioxidant enzymes.

antioxidants nutrients a number of nutrients, notably some vitamins and other molecules, contained in a balanced diet, that protect body cells against oxidative stress/damage. Increased cellular concentrations of antioxidants have been claimed to diminish exercise-induced muscle damage, thus reducing the risk of cellular injury. Extremely reactive oxygen radicals are produced normally during metabolism and in response to other insults, such as some chemicals and infection. The reactive oxygen species, some of which are free radicals, disrupt the fatty acids in cell membranes, which eventually leads to damage to cell proteins and DNA. The antioxidant nutrients are vitamins A, C and E, and lipoic acid; in sport the supplementation with these has been demonstrated to protect against exercise-induced oxidative stress/damage and sometimes from delayed onset of

muscle damage, but most studies show no effect on physical performance. Some antioxidants, for example, vitamins E and A, ubiquinone (coenzyme Q10), carotenoids, are fat soluble and located within cell membranes; others such as vitamin C are water soluble, located in the cytosol, mitochondrial matrix or extracellular fluids. ➲ free radical, oxidative stress/damage, reactive oxygen species.

antiparasitic *adj* describes agents that prevent or destroy parasites.

antiparkinson(ism) drugs drugs used in the management of parkinsonism, e.g. orphenadrine. ➲ Appendix 5.

antipellagra *adj* against pellagra; a function of the nicotinic acid portion of vitamin B complex.

antiperistalsis *n* reversal of the normal peristaltic action— **antiperistaltic** *adj*.

antiphospholipid antibodies autoimmune antibodies, e.g. anticardiolipin, lupus anticoagulant. ➲ antiphospholipid antibody syndrome.

antiphospholipid antibody syndrome *n* in this syndrome an antibody in the patient's plasma has activity against enzymic reactions in the coagulation cascade that are dependent on platelet membranes (or in vitro by phospholipid). The antibody in vitro has the effect of prolonging the activated partial thromboplastin time (APTT) because it interacts with phospholipid in the reaction tube and inhibits the binding or enzymic interactions of the coagulation components. It is most sensitively diagnosed by prolongation of the dilute Russell viper venom time (DRVVT) of plasma, an effect that can be neutralized by adding platelet membranes. When the antibody inhibits coagulation in these ways, it is known as the *lupus anticoagulant*. In some individuals the plasma protein β$_2$-glycoprotein-1 undergoes a conformational change after it has bound to anionic phospholipids, and is then recognized by the antibody. In vitro this is usually detected by its ability to bind to the β-glycoprotein-1 in an assay with cardiolipin, when it is known as an *anticardiolipin antibody*. The term antiphospholipid antibody encompasses both a lupus anticoagulant and an anticardiolipin antibody; some individuals are only positive for one of these activities, whereas in others both are present. The antiphospholipid antibody is associated with a constellation of clinical conditions found in association with a history of thromboembolism. The antibody has now been found in some individuals with a history of arterial or venous thromboembolism in one or several organs, often at a young age but without features of systemic lupus erythematosus (SLE); in this case it is known as the primary antiphospholipid antibody syndrome. In those with other conditions associated (e.g. SLE, rheumatoid arthritis, systemic sclerosis, temporal arteritis, Sjögren's syndrome, etc.) with thrombosis it is known as a secondary antiphospholipid antibody syndrome . The antibody is also associated with poor placentation and pregnany loss through miscarriage, fetal death and preterm labour, and with pregnancy-induced hypertension, eclampsia or intrauterine growth restriction. Antenatal care should be provided in a specialist obstetric-haematology centre, as ineffective treatment increases the risk of fetal and maternal mortality. Treatment with low-dose aspirin and low-molecular weight heparin increases the chance of a successful pregnancy and reduces the risk of a thromboembolic condition. The mechanism by which the antibody predisposes to thrombosis is unclear but it may be related either to maintaining platelets in an activated state within the circulation, or to inhibiting the fibrinolytic activity of endothelial cells.

antiplatelet drugs a group of drugs that reduce platelet aggregation, e.g. dipyridamole. ⊃ Appendix 5.

antiprothrombin *n* stops blood coagulation by preventing conversion of prothrombin into thrombin. Anticoagulant.

antiprotozoal *n* a drug used to prevent or cure a protozoal disease, e.g. metronidazole. ⊃ Appendix 5.

antipruritic *adj* describes any agent which relieves or prevents itching.

antipsychotic drugs *adj* also known as neuroleptics. Against psychosis, such as drugs used to treat psychotic episodes. Most are antagonists of dopamine receptors and other receptors. They can be divided into typical and atypical neuroleptics. ⊃ dibenzodiazepines, extrapyramidal, neuroleptic malignant syndrome, phenothiazines, tardive dyskinesia, Appendix 5.

antipyretic *adj* describes any agent which prevents or reduces fever, e.g. aspirin. ⊃ Appendix 5.

antirachitic *adj* describes any agent which prevents or cures rickets, a function of vitamin D.

antireflection (AR) coating (*syn* antireflection film) A thin film of transparent material, usually a metallic fluoride (e.g. magnesium fluoride), deposited on the surface of a lens which increases transmission and reduces surface reflection. ⊃ coated lens, coating, Fresnel's formula, ghost image.

antireflection coated lens ⊃ coated lens.

antireflection film ⊃ antireflection (AR) coating.

antiretroviral *adj* describes a drug (e.g. efavirenz) that acts against retroviruses. ⊃ human immunodeficiency virus, retroviruses, Appendix 5.

antiretroviral therapy during pregnancy (ART) drug therapy that attacks a retrovirus, particularly valuable in treating those with human immunodeficiency virus and acquired immunodeficiency syndrome. Therapy in pregnancy reduces the risk of vertical transmission to the fetus. ⊃ highly active antiretroviral therapy (HAART).

anti-Rhesus ⊃ anti-D.

antischistosomal *adj* describes any agent which destroys *Schistosoma*.

antiscorbutic *adj* describes any agent which prevents or cures scurvy, a function of vitamin C.

antisecretory drug a drug that reduces the secretion of a specific body substance, such as proton-pump inhibitors, (e.g. esomeprazole), reduces the amount of hydrochloric acid secreted by the gastric parietal (oxyntic) cells.

antisepsis *n* prevention of sepsis (tissue infection); introduced into surgical procedures in 1880 by Lord Lister—**antiseptic** *adj*.

antiseptic *n* chemical substances that destroy or inhibit the growth of micro-organisms. They can be applied to living tissues, e.g. chlorhexidine, used for skin preparation before invasive procedures and for routine hand decontamination.

antiserum *n* serum prepared from the blood of an animal or human immunized by the requisite antigen, containing a high concentration of polyclonal antibodies against that antigen.

antisialogogue substance that arrests or reduces salivation.

antisocial *adj* against society. Used to describe a person who does not accept the responsibilities and constraints placed on a community by its members—**antisocialism** *n*.

antispasmodic *adj* (*syn* spasmolytic) describes any measure or drugs used to relieve spasm in muscle, e.g. mebeverine hydrochloride. ⊃ Appendix 5.

antistatic *adj* describes measures to prevent the accumulation of static electricity.

antistreptolysin *adj* against streptolysins. A raised antistreptolysin titre in the blood is indicative of recent streptococcal infection.

antisyphilitic *adj* describes any measures taken to combat syphilis.

antithrombin *n* a substance that inhibits blood coagulation. It is synthesized in the liver and is normally present in the blood, where it restricts coagulation to areas where it is needed. Deficiency is uncommon but is associated with an increased risk of thrombosis. ⊃ antithrombin deficiency, thrombin, thrombophilia.

antithrombin deficiency antithrombin is a protease inhibitor which inactivates coagulation/clotting factors IIa, IXa, Xa and XIa, especially in the presence of heparin (which greatly potentiates its activity). Familial deficiency of antithrombin is a dominantly inherited disorder and is associated with a marked predisposition to venous thromboembolism. ⊃ venous thromboembolism.

antithrombotic *adj* describes any measures that prevent or cure thrombosis.

antithyroid *n* any agent used to decrease the activity of the thyroid gland, e.g. carbimazole. ⊃ Appendix 5.

antitoxin *n* an antibody which neutralizes a given toxin. Made in response to the invasion by toxin-producing bacteria, or the injection of toxoids—**antitoxic** *adj*.

antitreponemal *adj* describes any measures used against infections caused by *Treponema*.

antituberculosis drugs drugs used in the treatment of tuberculosis, e.g. ethambutol—**antitubercular** *adj*. ⊃ Appendix 5.

antitumour antibiotics cytotoxic antibiotics that act against tumour cells by disrupting cell membranes and DNA, e.g. doxorubicin. ⊃ cytotoxic, Appendix 5.

antitussive *adj* describes any measures which suppress cough.

antivenom *n* a serum prepared from animals injected with the venom of snakes; used as an antidote in cases of poisoning by snakebite.

antiviral *adj* acting against viruses. *antiviral drugs*, e.g. aciclovir. ⊃ Appendix 5.

antivitamin *n* a substance interfering with the absorption or utilization of a vitamin, e.g. a large intake of avidin in raw egg white is associated with deficiency of biotin.

antral *adj* pertaining to an antrum.

antral fistula ➲ oro-antral fistula.

antral packing placing of a pack, usually consisting of materials such as ribbon gauze soaked in Whitehead's varnish or paraffin/flavin emulsion, to support the floor of a fractured orbit or part of the zygoma and to reduce haemorrhage.

antrectomy *n* surgical excision of the antrum of the stomach.

antr/o- a prefix that means 'antrum', e.g. *antrostomy*.

antro-oral *adj* pertaining to the maxillary antrum and the mouth.

antroscopy an endoscopic examination of the maxillary air sinus.

antrostomy *n* antral puncture. Surgical opening from nasal cavity to antrum of Highmore (maxillary sinus).

antrum *n* **1.** a cavity, especially in bone. ➲ antrum of Highmore—**antral** *adj*. **2.** the pyloric antrum, the lowest part of the stomach, continuous with the pylorus.

antrum of Highmore (N Highmore, English physician, 1613–1685) an air sinus in the superior maxillary bone.

ANTT® *abbr* Aseptic Non Touch Technique.

ANUG *abbr* acute necrotizing ulcerative gingivitis.

anuria *n* complete absence of urine output by the kidneys. ➲ suppression—**anuric** *adj*.

anus *n* the end of the alimentary canal, at the extreme termination of the rectum and anal canal. The internal and external sphincter muscles relax to allow faecal matter to pass through the anus to the exterior—**anal** *adj*. ➲ anal canal, imperforate anus.

anxiety *n* a subjective experience of fear, apprehension and dread. ➲ anxiety disorder, cognitive anxiety, competetive sport anxiety, somatic anxiety, state anxiety, trait anxiety.

anxiety disorder a mental health problem characterized by recurrent acute anxiety attacks (panic) or by chronic anxiety. The attacks consist of both physical and psychological anxiety signs and symptoms.

anxiolytics *npl* agents that reduce anxiety, e.g. diazepam. ➲ Appendix 5.

AOM *abbr* acute otitis media.

aorta *n* the main artery arising out of the left ventricle of the heart. It comprises four parts: ascending aorta, aortic arch, thoracic descending part and the abdominal descending part. It carries oxygen-rich blood which it supplies to all organs, tissues and cells. Its first branch, the coronary arteries supply oxygen and nutrients to the heart muscle (myocardium). ➲ Colour Section Figures 8, 9.

aortic *adj* pertaining to the aorta.

aortic aneurysm an abnormal dilatation of the aortic wall. The aetiology and types include: (a) 'non-specific' aneurysmal disease, which is associated with smoking and hypertension. It also tends to run in families, and genetic factors are undoubtedly important. The most common site for non-specific aneurysm formation is the infrarenal abdominal aorta. The suprarenal abdominal aorta and a variable length of the descending thoracic aorta may be affected in 10–20% of patients but the ascending aorta is usually spared; (b) associated with the inherited connective tissue disease Marfan's syndrome. Along with effects on other systems, the cardiovascular system is affected by aortic disease and mitral regurgitation. Weakening of the aortic media leads to progressive dilatation of the ascending aorta that may be complicated by aortic regurgitation and aortic dissection. Treatment with β-blockers reduces the rate of aortic dilatation and the risk of rupture. Elective replacement of the ascending aorta may be considered in patients with evidence of progressive aortic dilatation but carries a mortality of 5–10%. ➲ Marfan's syndrome; (c) aortitis is associated with aneurysm formation. Aortitis may be caused by syphilis (a rare cause) that characteristically produces saccular aneurysms of the ascending aorta containing calcification. Other conditions that can cause aortitis and aneurysm formation include Takayasu's disease, Reiter's syndrome, giant cell arteritis and ankylosing spondylitis; (d) abdominal aortic aneurysms (AAA) ➲ abdominal aortic aneurysm; (e) thoracic aortic aneurysms may produce chest pain similar to cardiac pain, associated with expansion of the aneurysm. If they extend proximally they may cause aortic valve regurgitation. They can also cause symptoms by compressing the trachea, main bronchus or superior vena cava. Occasionally, they may erode into the adjacent structures, causing haemorrhage, tamponade and death.

aortic arch a continuation of the ascending aorta that arches over the heart to become the thoracic part of the descending aorta. The left common carotid artery, left subclavian artery and the brachiocephalic artery branch from the aortic arch to supply oxygen-rich blood to the head, neck and upper limbs. ➲ Colour Section Figure 8, 9.

aortic dissection a breach in the integrity of the aortic wall that allows arterial blood to burst into the media of the aorta which is then split into two layers, creating a 'false lumen' alongside the existing or 'true lumen'. Typically, the false lumen eventually re-enters the true lumen, creating a double-barrelled or biluminal aorta, but it may also rupture into the left pleural space or pericardium with fatal consequences. The primary event is often a spontaneous or iatrogenic tear in the intima of the aorta, but many dissections appear to be triggered by a haemorrhage in the media of the aorta which then ruptures through the intima into the true lumen. Aortic disease and hypertension are the most important aetiological factors but a variety of other conditions may be implicated, e.g. non-specific aortic aneurysm, iatrogenic causes, Marfan's syndrome, trauma, etc. The peak incidence is in the sixth and seventh decades of life but dissection can occur in younger patients, most commonly in association with Marfan's syndrome, pregnancy or trauma; men are twice as frequently affected as women. Aortic dissection is classified anatomically and for management purposes into type A and type B, involving or sparing the ascending aorta respectively. Type A dissections account for two-thirds of cases and frequently also extend into the descending aorta. The pain tends to follow the path of the dissection; involvement of the ascending aorta typically gives rise to anterior chest pain, and the descending aorta intrascapular pain. Patients usually present with severe 'tearing' chest pain. The onset of pain is typically very abrupt and collapse is common. Unless there is frank rupture, the patient is invariably hypertensive. There may be asymmetry of the brachial, carotid or femoral pulses, and the signs of aortic reflux may be present in type A dissections. Occlusion of aortic branches may cause a variety of complications including myocardial infarction (coronary), paraplegia (spinal), mesenteric infarction with an acute abdomen (coeliac and superior mesenteric), renal failure (renal) and acute limb (usually leg) ischaemia. Investigations will include a chest X-ray which characteristically shows broadening of the upper mediastinum and distortion of the aortic 'knuckle' but these findings are variable. A left-sided pleural effusion is common. The ECG may show left ventricular hypertrophy in patients with hypertension, or rarely, changes of acute myocardial infarction. Doppler echocardiography may show aortic regurgitation, a dilated aortic root and, occasionally, the flap of the dissection. Transoesophageal echocardiography is particularly helpful because transthoracic echocardiography can only image the first 3–4 cm of the ascending aorta. Computed tomography (CT) and magnetic resonance imaging (MRI) are both highly specific, and angiography of the aortic arch is not usually required unless these techniques are not available. Assessment and treatment are urgent because the early mortality of acute dissection is approximately 1% per hour. Initial management comprises pain control and antihypertensive treatment with labetalol, a combined α- and β-blocking drug, to maintain the systolic pressure below 120 mmHg. Type A dissections require emergency surgical repair. Surgery involves replacing the ascending aorta with a Dacron graft. Type B aneurysms can be treated medically unless there is actual or impending external rupture, or vital organ (gut, kidneys) or limb ischaemia. Percutaneous or minimal access endoluminal repair is possible in some cases and involves either 'fenestrating' (perforating) the intimal flap so that blood can return from the false to the true lumen (so decompressing the former), or implanting a stent graft placed from the femoral artery.

aortic murmur abnormal heart sound heard over aortic area; a systolic murmur alone is the murmur of aortic stenosis, a diastolic murmur denotes aortic regurgitation.

aortic regurgitation (incompetence) regurgitation of blood from the aorta back into the left ventricle.

aortic valve semilunar valve between the aorta and the left ventricle.

aortic valve stenosis narrowing of aortic valve. This is usually due to rheumatic heart disease or a congenital fusion of the valve which predisposes to the deposition of calcium. One of the causes of sudden death in sport. ⊃ mid-systolic murmur.

aortitis *n* inflammation of the aorta.

aorto- a prefix that means 'aorta', e.g. *aortopexy*.

aortocaval compression inability of the inferior vena cava to return blood low in oxygen to the heart, and the aorta to pump oxygenated blood to the lower limbs due to restricted lumen caused by the weight of the pregnant uterus. Occurs when the woman is lying on her back in the third trimester of pregnancy.

aortography *n* demonstration of the aorta after introduction of a contrast agent, either via a catheter passed along the femoral or brachial artery or by direct translumbar injection—**aortographic** *adj*, **aortogram** *n*, **aortograph** *n*, **aortographically** *adv*.

aortopexy a surgical technique used for tracheomalacia, in which the aorta is sutured to the sternum. This moves the trachea forward and prevents it closing, thereby ensuring that the airway remains open. ⊃ tracheomalacia

AP *abbr* **1.** anaesthesia practitioner. **2.** anterioposterior.

ap-/apo- a prefix that means 'away, derived from', e.g. *apoptosis*.

apareunia inability to perform sexual intercourse for physiological or psychological reasons.

apathy *n* **1.** abnormal listlessness and deficiency of activity. **2.** attitude of indifference—**apathetic** *adj*.

apatite inorganic mineral substance. A calcium phosphate found in teeth and bone. Soluble in soft drink acids and carbohydrate fermentations, but when treated with certain fluoride solutions the resulting fluoroapatite is not susceptible to acid destruction and caries.

A, pattern ⊃ pattern, A.

APC *abbr* antigen-presenting cell.

APD *abbr* **1.** auditory processing disorder. **2.** automated peritoneal dialysis.

APEL *abbr* accreditation of prior experiential learning.

aperients *npl* ⊃ laxatives.

aperistalsis *n* absence of peristaltic movement in the bowel. Characterizes the condition of paralytic ileus—**aperistaltic** *adj*.

apertognathia open bite. An occlusion where there is vertical separation between the upper (maxillary) and lower (mandibular) anterior teeth.

Apert's syndrome (E Apert, French paediatrician, 1868–1940) congenital craniosynostosis accompanied by deformities of the hands. ⊃ acrocephalosyndactyly, syndactyly.

apex *n* **1.** a general anatomic term for the top or summit of a body, organ or part, or the pointed end of anything which is cone-shaped, e.g. the tip of a lung. ⊃ Colour Section Figure 7—**apices** *pl*, **apical** *adj*. **2.** that part of a tooth root furthermost from the crown. ⊃ anatomical/radiographic apex, physiological apex.

apex beat the systolic impulse. In a heart of normal size it can be seen or felt in the 5th left intercostal space in the mid-clavicular line (Figure A.13). It is the lowest and most lateral point at which an impulse can be detected and provides a rough indication of the size of the heart.

A
B

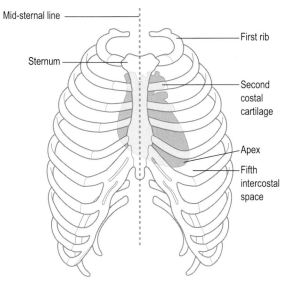

Mid-sternal line

First rib

Sternum

Second costal cartilage

Apex

Fifth intercostal space

A.13 Apex beat (reproduced from Brooker & Nicol 2003 with permission).

apexification more correctly termed *root end closure induction*. Process whereby an immature, open permanent tooth apex is induced to continue root formation, to form a closed apex or to produce a calcific barrier across the root canal. Typically achieved by repeated canal dressing with non-setting calcium hydroxide paste. Increasingly achieved with MTA cement. ⊃ apexogenesis, calcific barrier.

apex locator an electronic device used to measure canal length during root canal treatment.

apexogenesis treatment designed to preserve vital pulp tissue in the apical part of a root canal in order to complete formation of the root apex. ⊃ apexification.

APF *abbr* acidulated phosphate fluoride.

Apgar score (V Apgar, American anaesthetist, 1909–1974) a measure used to evaluate the general condition of a newborn baby. A score of 0, 1 or 2 is given for the criteria of heart rate, respiratory effort, skin colour, muscle tone and response to stimulation (Table A.1). A score between 8 and 10 indicates a baby in good condition.

APH *abbr* antepartum haemorrhage.

aphagia *n* inability to swallow—**aphagic** *adj*.

aphagosis the lack of ability to eat.

aphakia *n* absence of the lens. Describes the eye after removal of a cataract without artificial lens implantation—**aphakic** *adj*.

aphakic eye an eye without the crystalline lens. ⊃ aphakia.

aphakic pupillary block ⊃ pupillary block.

aphasia *n* a language disorder that follows brain damage, due primarily to an impaired linguistic system. The term does not describe language disorders that involve problems with expression or comprehension caused by mental health problems, including psychoses, confusion and dementia, or muscle weakness, or problems with hearing. There are several classifications but generally aphasia is described as being *expressive (motor) aphasia* or *receptive (sensory) aphasia*. However, many people exhibit problems with both language expression and comprehension—**aphasic** *adj*. ⊃ dysarthria, expressive (motor) aphasia, receptive (sensory) aphasia.

apheresis a technique in which blood is transferred from a donor into a cell separator which collects the required components, e.g. red cells, plasma (plasmapheresis), platelets (plateletpheresis), or white cells (leucopheresis) and returns the remainder to the donor. Plasmapheresis may be used in the treatment of some diseases caused by antibodies or immune complexes circulating in the patient's plasma, e.g. myasthenia gravis. ⊃ leucopheresis, plasmapheresis.

aphonia *n* inability to make sound due to neurological, behavioural, psychogenic or organic causes. ⊃ dysarthria—**aphonic** *adj*.

aphrodisiac *n* an agent that stimulates sexual arousal.

aphthae *npl* small ulcers of the gastrointestinal mucosa surrounded by a ring of erythema—**aphtha** *sing*, **aphthous** *adj*.

aphthous stomatitis ⊃ stomatitis.

apical referring to the tip or apex of the tooth root and its immediate surroundings.

apical abscess an abscess involving the apex of a tooth root. ⊃ periapical.

apical clearance the distance between the posterior surface of a contact lens and the apex of the cornea. ⊃ corneal apex.

apical curettage surgical removal of chronic inflammatory tissue surrounding the apex of a tooth.

apical elevator ⊃ elevator (dental).

Table A.1 Apgar score (reproduced from Fraser & Cooper 2003 with permission)

		Score	
Sign	**0**	**1**	**2**
Heart rate	Absent	Less than 100 beats/min	More than 100 beats/min
Respiratory effort	Absent	Slow, irregular	Good or crying
Muscle tone	Limp	Some flexion of limbs	Active
Reflex response	None	Minimal grimace	Cough or sneeze to stimulus
Colour	Blue, pale	Body pink, extremities blue	Completely pink
Reproduced from Fraser & Cooper (2003) with permission.			

apical foramen the opening at or near the apex of a tooth root through which nerve, blood and lymphatics enter and leave.

apical (dental) granuloma a chronic inflammatory lesion at the apical third of a tooth root. It comprises a mass of granulation tissue associated with the apex of a tooth and formed as a sequel to infection of the root canal. ⊃ granuloma.

apical projection a radiographic examination of the lung apices, using an angled beam to project the clavicles away from the lung tissue.

apical (radicular) cyst cyst of inflammatory origin associated with the apical region of a pulpless tooth.

apicectomy (*syn* apicoectomy (USA), root-end resection) more correctly root-end surgery. Surgical procedure to remove the apex of a tooth root together with some of the surrounding tissues. Usually accompanied by root-end cavity preparation and filling. ⊃ retrograde (reverse) root filling.

apicoectomy ⊃ apicectomy.

APKD *abbr* adult polycystic kidney disease.

APL *abbr* accreditation of prior learning.

APL principle anterior pituitary-like hormone of the placenta, chorionic gonadotrophin.

aplanatic lens a lens designed to correct for two monchromatic aberrations; spherical aberration and coma.

aplasia *n* incomplete development of tissue; absence of growth.

aplastic *adj* **1.** without structure or form. **2.** incapable of forming new tissue. ⊃ aplastic anaemia.

aplastic anaemia is the result of complete bone marrow failure. It may be primary or secondary. ⊃ primary idiopathic acquired aplastic anaemia, acquired aplastic anaemia (secondary aplasia).

Apley's test a manoeuvre that tests for a torn meniscus of the knee ('grind test'); or a manoeuvre for testing the range of motion at both shoulders ('scratch test').

apneustic breathing abnormal gasping inspiratory breathing pattern seen after brain injury. It is characterized by a protracted inspiratory phase followed by expiration apnoea.

apneustic centre a respiratory control centre in the pons. Responsible for stimulating the inspiratory centre. It also has a minor role in ensuring a smooth respiratory rhythm. ⊃ pneumotaxic centre.

apnoea *n* a transitory cessation of breathing as seen in Cheyne–Stokes respiration. It is due to lack of the necessary CO_2 tension in the blood for stimulation of the respiratory centre—**apnoeic** *adj*.

apnoea hypopnoea index (AHI) the frequency of periods of apnoea and hypopnoea that occur during sleep. The index is calculated on the number of apnoeic or hypopnoeic periods per hour of sleep. It is used in the diagnosis of various sleep apnoea syndromes and to ascertain its severity. ⊃ obstructive sleep apnoea (hypopnoea) syndrome, sleep apnoea syndrome.

apnoea monitor, apnoea alarm mattress an electronic device that detects changes that indicate that breathing has stopped. The device has an alarm, which is activated when breathing stops for a given time period. Apnoea monitors are used for infants, especially preterm infants and those at risk of sudden infant death syndrome. The alarm may be a pad placed on the cot/bed, a nasal airflow sensor or an abdominal movement sensor.

apnoea of the newborn ⊃ periodic breathing.

Apo-A1 *abbr* apolipoprotein A1.

Apo-B *abbr* apolipoprotein B.

apochromatic lens a compound lens designed to correct chromatic and spherical aberrations. It uses three or more kinds of glass. This lens corrects chromatic aberration more thoroughly than an achromatic lens. ⊃ achromatic lens.

apocrine gland a type of exocrine gland in which the apical portion of the secretory cell buds off and is lost when its secretion is released. ⊃ holocrine gland, merocrine (eccrine) gland.

apocrine sweat glands modified sweat glands, especially in axillae, genital and perineal regions. Responsible after puberty for body odour. ⊃ eccrine.

apodia *n* congenital absence of the feet.

apoenzyme a protein part of an enzyme that needs the specific coenzyme or metal ion to become active.

apogee in medicine, the most severe stage of the climax of a disease.

A point an orthodontic cephalometric landmark defined as the position of the deepest concavity on the anterior profile of the maxilla.

apolipoprotein the protein part of a lipoprotein.

apolipoprotein A1 (Apo-A1) the main protein found in high density lipoproteins (HDL). It is required for the movement of cholesterol to the liver for metabolism and excretion. It activates an enzyme-controlled reaction whereby cholesteryl esters are produced in HDL.

apolipoproteins B (Apo-B) proteins found in low density lipoproteins (LDL), very low density lipoproteins (VLDL) and chylomicrons. Their functions include the binding of LDL to the specific receptor and the production and transport of these lipids. Increased levels in the blood are associated with a higher risk of myocardial infarction.

apolipoproteins B (Apo-B):apolipoprotein A1 (Apo-A1) ratio a blood test that provides an indication of a person's cardiovascular risk.

aponeurosis *n* a broad glistening sheet of tendon-like tissue which serves to invest and attach muscles, e.g. abdominal muscles, to each other, and also to the parts that they move—**aponeuroses** *pl*, **aponeurotic** *adj*.

aponeurositis *n* inflammation of an aponeurosis.

apophyseal joint ⊃ zygapophyseal joint.

apophysis *n* a projection, protuberance or outgrowth. Usually used in connection with bone.

apoplexy *n* historical term for cerebrovascular accident (stroke)—**apoplectic, apoplectiform** *adj*.

apoprotein *n* a protein before it binds to the prosthetic group required for biological activity.

apoptosis *n* programmed cell death.

apparent focal spot the target of an X-ray tube is at an angle to allow a larger area to be struck by electrons while still maintaining the smaller, apparent, focal spot when viewing from the tube port.

appendectomy *n* ➲ appendicectomy.

appendicectomy *n* excision of the appendix vermiformis.

appendicitis *n* inflammation of the appendix vermiformis.

appendicular skeleton the bones of the shoulder girdle, the pelvic girdle and the upper and lower limbs. ➲ axial skeleton, Colour Section Figures 2, 3.

appendix *n* an appendage—**appendices** *pl*, **appendicular** *adj*.

appendix vermiformis a worm-like appendage of the caecum about the thickness of a pencil and usually measuring from 2.5 to 15 cm in length. It contains lymphoid tissue and its position is variable. ➲ Colour Section Figure 18b.

apperception *n* clear perception of a sensory stimulus, in particular where there is identification or recognition—**apperceptive** *adj*.

appetite *n*. the drive to eat. Influenced by the status of energy balance, psychological and behavioural factors and by health status. It may be increased or decreased pharmacologically. The drive to eat can be evaluated by using visual analogue scales (VAS) for self-report ratings of hunger, desire to eat, prospective food consumption (how much food one could eat), satiety and fullness. ➲ anorexia nervosa (AN), bulimia, eating disorders, hypothalamus, obesity.

applanation *n* a way of flattening the cornea during contact tonometry to determine intraocular pressure. ➲ Goldmann applanation tonometer, tonometry.

appliance device used to perform a particular function. ➲ orthodontic appliance.

applicator *n* **1.** in radiotherapy attached to the tube housing to provide an accurate means of setting up the source–skin distance and is a form of secondary collimation. ➲ Fulfield applicator. **2.** also describes an instrument used for local application of remedies, e.g. vaginal medication applicator. **3.** small ball-ended hand instrument used to apply medicaments and cements.

apposition *n* the approximation or bringing together of two surfaces or edges.

appraisal *n* making a valuation. In stress theories, the individual's conscious or subconscious interpretation of the significance of an event; *primary appraisal* the evaluation of the relevance of an event to the person's well-being; *secondary appraisal* the person's evaluation of whether or not they have the resources to cope with an event appraised as a threat to their well-being. ➲ performance appraisal or review.

approach-avoidance conflict a state of behavioural ambivalence with respect to a goal.

approach behaviour behaviour directed toward the attainment of a desired outcome.

apprehension test a test that places a joint in a position that would simulate subluxation or dislocation, visible 'apprehension' on the patient's face is a positive result.

appropriate for gestational age (AGA) a chart which compares the expected and attained growth of a fetus in utero at any stage of pregnancy.

approved clinician (AC) ➲ Mental Health Act 2007.

approved name the generic or non-proprietary name of a drug, such as salbutamol. Should be used in prescribing except in the case of drugs where bioavailability differs between brands. ➲ Recommended International Non-proprietary Name (rINN).

approved mental health professional (AMHP) ➲ Mental Health Act 2007.

approved social worker (ASW) in England and Wales a social worker previously appointed by the local health authority with statutory duties under the Mental Health Act 1983 (England and Wales) including: (a) making applications for compulsory or emergency admission to hospital and conveyance of patients there; (b) applications concerning guardianship, the functions of the nearest relative, or acting as a nearest relative if so appointed; (c) planning and providing aftercare of discharged mentally disordered patients. The Mental Health Act 2007 (England and Wales) makes provision for ASWs to automatically become approved mental health professionals (AMHPs) (Department of Health [DH] 2008 Mental Health Act 2007. online www.dh.gov.uk/). ➲ Mental Health Act 2007.

approximal (proximal) situated close together.

approximal caries (*syn* proximal or interstitial caries) dental caries beginning in the mesial or distal surface of a tooth, usually just below the contact point.

approximal cavity cavity involving a mesial and/or distal surface of a tooth.

approximal surface (*syn* interstitial or interproximal surfaces) adjacent surfaces of teeth in the same dental arch. Usually the mesial surface of one tooth and the distal surface of the next. In the case of the two central incisors the mesial surfaces of each tooth.

approximate power ➲ nominal power.

apraxia *n* inability to perform a motor act or use an object normally, due typically to damage in the parietal lobe of the brain—**apraxic, apractic** *adj*. ➲ constructional apraxia.

apronectomy ➲ abdominoplasty.

apron spring orthodontic fine wire spring, wound on a heavy gauge wire or bow and suspended beneath it to produce a force to move teeth.

aptitude *n* natural ability and facility in performing tasks, either physical or mental.

APTT *abbr* activated partial thromboplastin time.

APUD cells amine precursor uptake and decarboxylation cells. A large group of cells widespread throughout the body, especially in the hypothalamus, pituitary gland, thyroid gland, parathyroid glands, pancreas and the mucosa of gastrointestinal tract. They convert precursor substances to various hormones and physiologically active amines, such as dopamine, 5-hydroxytryptamine (serotonin), etc.

apudoma a hormone or amine-secreting tumour of APUD cells. ➲ argentaffinoma, carcinoid syndrome.

apyrexia *n* absence of fever—**apyrexial** *adj.*

aquanatal exercises antenatal exercises, often in a local swimming pool, run by a trained midwife or other attendant to help women stay fit and develop social networks for post-natal support.

aqueduct *n* a canal. ⊃ cerebral aqueduct, cochlear aqueduct, vestibular aqueduct.

aqueduct of the cochlea ⊃ cochlear aqueduct.

aqueduct of Fallopius a canal in the temporal bone that contains part of the facial nerve (seventh cranial nerve).

aqueduct of the midbrain ⊃ cerebral aqueduct.

aqueduct of the vestibule ⊃ vestibular aqueduct.

aqueduct of Sylvius (F Sylvius, German/Dutch physician, 1614–1672) ⊃ cerebral aqueduct.

aqueous *adj* watery.

aqueous flare the scattering of light seen when a slit-lamp beam is directed, obliquely to the plane of the iris, into the anterior chamber. It occurs as a result of increased protein content, and usually inflammatory cells, in the aqueous humour. Visual impairment depends on the intensity of the flare. It is a sign of intraocular inflammation. ⊃ iritis, Tyndall effect, uveitis.

aqueous humour the fluid contained in the anterior and posterior chambers of the eye. ⊃ Colour Section Figure 15.

aqueous solution a water-based fluid which may carry other substances dissolved in it.

AR *abbr* antireflection coating.

arachidonic acid a polyunsaturated fatty acid with four double bonds. Used in the body for the synthesis of important regulatory lipids that include: prostaglandins, prostacyclins and thromboxanes. A high concentration is found in brain and nervous tissue membranes. Arachidonic acid is important for brain development. The dietary intake of arachidonic acid is associated with birthweight, head circumference and placental weight. It can be synthesized from linoleic acid in the body, but may be considered to be an essential fatty acid (EFA) when linoleic acid is deficient in the diet.

arachis oil oil expressed from peanuts (groundnuts). Used for cooking, in the food industry and for some pharmaceutical products. Contains monounsaturated fatty acids. Should not be used by those with a peanut allergy.

arachn- a prefix that means 'spider', e.g. *arachnoid mater.*

arachnodactyly *n* congenital abnormality resulting in long, slender fingers. Said to resemble spider legs (hence 'spider fingers').

arachnoid *adj* resembling a spider's web—**arachnoidal** *adj.*

arachnoid mater or membrane a delicate membrane enveloping the brain and spinal cord, lying between the pia mater internally and the dura mater externally; the middle membrane of the meninges.

arbor vitae literally, the tree of life. **1.** the tree-like appearance of white matter in the cerebellum. **2.** the appearance of the folds of columnar epithelium lining the cervix uteri.

arborization *n* an arrangement resembling the branching of a tree. Characterizes both ends of a neuron, i.e. the dendrites and the axon as it supplies each muscle fibre.

arboviruses *npl* abbreviation for ARthropod-BOrne viruses. Includes various RNA viruses transmitted by arthropods: mosquitoes, ticks, sandflies, etc. They cause diseases such as yellow fever, dengue, sandfly fever and several types of encephalitis.

ARC *acron* **1.** abnormal retinal correspondence. **2.** AIDS related complex.

arc eye a painful but usually temporary condition of the eyes following exposure to the light from arc welding equipment.

arch structure or structures having a regular curved form. ⊃ arch bar fixation, arches of the foot, archwire, dental arch.

arch aortography the radiographic examination of the aorta and its major branches by injecting a contrast agent via femoral or axillary catheterization.

arch bar fixation ⊃ fixation (dentistry/maxillofacial surgery).

arches of the foot the three arches (two longitudinal and one transverse) are responsible for maintaining the optimum load-bearing position of the foot and thus walking motion (Figure A.14). In the erect position, the arches are maintained primarily by the bones and ligaments, allowing even distribution of body weight. Abnormal foot biomechanics may result in alteration of this balance of load, causing discomfort.

arch of aorta ⊃ aortic arch. ⊃ Colour Section Figures 8, 9.

archwire in orthodontics, a length of fine wire contoured to the dental arch and fitting into brackets or other orthodontic attachments on the buccal or labial aspects of the teeth. ⊃ wiring.

archival permanence the length of time a radiographic film can be stored without significant deterioration of image quality.

arcing spring contraceptive device a diaphragm introduced into the vagina to act as a barrier to sperm penetration.

arcon articulator an articulator which differs from the usual anatomical articulator in that the condylar analogue

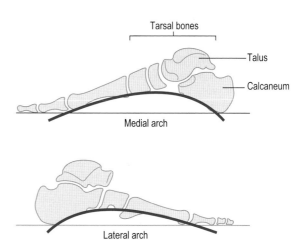

A.14 The longitudinal arches of the foot (reproduced from Jennett 2008 with permission).

is in the mandibular portion of the articulator and the condylar track in the maxillary component.

arc therapy when a source of radiation moves through a prescribed angle during treatment.

arcuate arched, bow-shaped.

arcuate scotoma an arc-shaped blind area in the visual field. Associated with glaucoma. ➲ scotoma.

arcus an arch- or ring-shaped structure.

arcus senilis an opaque ring round the edge of the cornea, seen in older people. ➲ corneal arcus.

arcus tendineus a thickening, generally known as the 'white line' in the pelvic fascia, which gives origin to part of the levator ani.

ARDS *abbr* acute/adult respiratory distress syndrome.

Arenaviridae a family of ribonucleic acid (RNA) viruses. They include the Lassa virus, lymphocytic choriomeningitis virus (LCMV), Machupo virus, etc. They cause serious zoonoses transmitted to human from rodents. ➲ bioterrorism, Bolivian haemorrhagic fever (BHF), Guuanarito virus, Junin virus, Lassa virus, lymphocytic choriomeningitis virus (LCMV), Machupo virus, Sabin virus.

areola *n* the pigmented area round the nipple of the breast. A *secondary areola* surrounds the primary areola in pregnancy—**areolar** *adj.* ➲ Montgomery's glands.

areolar tissue a loose connective tissue comprising cells and fibres in a semisolid matrix.

ARF *abbr* **1.** acute renal failure. ➲ renal failure. **2.** acute respiratory failure. ➲ respiratory failure.

argentaffin cells *npl* cells found, for example, in the mucosa of the gastrointestinal tract. They take up stains containing silver and chromium.

argentaffinoma (carcinoid) *n* tumour affecting argentaffin cells in the gastrointestinal tract, or in those within the bronchi. ➲ carcinoid syndrome.

arginase *n* an enzyme present in the liver, kidney and spleen. It converts arginine into ornithine and urea.

arginine *n* one of the essential amino acids during childhood, it is found in protein foods required for growth and recovery. It is hydrolysed by the enzyme arginase to urea and ornithine. Supplements have been shown to enhance immune function in high risk surgical patients. One of the substances used by some athletes with the intention of stimulating growth hormone release, and so promoting gain in muscle mass and strength, but this action, at least by arginine taken alone, is disputed; there is better evidence for its effectiveness when combined with other amino acids. ➲ ergogenic aids.

argininosuccinuria *n* the presence of arginine and succinic acid in urine. Associated with learning disability and seizures. Also called argininosuccinic aciduria.

argon *n* an insert gas. Forms less than 0.1% of atmospheric air.

argon laser a laser with ionized argon gas as the active medium which emits a blue-green light beam with a wavelength of 514 nm. It may be used to perform iridectomy, iridoplasty, iridotomy, photocoagulation or trabeculoplasty.

Argyll Robertson pupil (D M Argyll Robertson, British ophthalmologist, 1837–1909), small, irregular pupil that responds to accommodation but not to light, associated with neurosyphilis and chronic alcohol misuse.

argyria slate grey discoloration of the skin and conjunctivae resulting from chronic exposure to silver.

ariboflavinosis *n* a deficiency state caused by lack of riboflavin and other members of the vitamin B complex. Characterized by cheilosis, seborrhoea, angular stomatitis, glossitis and photophobia.

arithmetic mean a figure arrived at by dividing the sum of a set of values by the number of items in the set. ➲ central tendency statistic, mean, median, mode.

Arkansas stone especially hard stone used for sharpening metal instruments such as excavators and enamel chisels.

ARM *abbr* **1.** age-related maculopathy. **2.** artificial rupture of the membranes. ➲ amniotomy.

arm, chest, hip index (ACH index) a way of assessing nutritional status using measurements of the arm circumference, chest and hip size.

ARMD *abbr* age-related macular degeneration.

arm prolapse serious complication of uncorrected shoulder presentation in which the fetal arm falls into or through the vagina.

arnica homoeopathic remedy used to prevent and treat bruising, shock and trauma. It is useful postnatally to ease perineal discomfort. Oral arnica is taken within an hour of delivery and thereafter three times daily for three days; arnica cream is useful for bruised buttocks but should not be applied directly over open wounds, e.g. episiotomy suture line.

Arnold–Chiari malformation a group of disorders affecting the base of the brain. Commonly occurs in hydrocephalus associated with meningocele and myelomeningocele. There are degrees of severity but usually there is some 'kinking' or 'buckling' of the brainstem with cerebellar tissue herniating through the foramen magnum at the base of the skull.

AROM *abbr* active range of motion.

aromatase inhibitors *npl* a group of drugs, such as exemestane, used in the treatment of breast cancer in postmenopausal women.

aromatherapy *n* a complementary therapy that involves the use of fragrances derived from essential oils. These may be combined with a base oil, inhaled or massaged into intact skin.

arousal cognitive and physiological activation in response to a situation leading to alertness and reponsiveness to respond. The physiological aspect is also known as physical arousal.

array an arrangement of components. ➲ annular array, curved array, linear array, phased array.

arrectores pilorum *npl* internal, plain, involuntary muscles attached to hair follicles, which, by contraction, erect the hair follicles, causing 'gooseflesh' when the person is cold or aroused, as in fright—**arrector pili** *sing.* ➲ pilomotor reflex, Colour Section Figure 12.

arrested caries dental caries in which progress has become static.

arrhythmia *n* any deviation from the normal rhythm, usually referring to the heart beat. ➲ asystole, extrasystole, fibrillation, heart block, Stokes–Adams syndrome, supraventricular tachycardia, Wolff–Parkinson–White syndrome.

arsenic (As) *n* a poisonous metallic element present in preparations such as herbicides and pesticides. Vegetables, fruit and other foods may contain small amounts. Toxic effects include malaise, gastrointestinal symptoms, pigmentation of the skin, anaemia and nervous symptoms.

ART *acron* **A**nti**R**etroviral **T**herapy during pregnancy.

artefact *n* any artificial product resulting from a physical or chemical agent; an unnatural change in a structure or tissue. In magnetic resonance where an additional image occurs in the reconstructed image which does not match the anatomy or pathology in the patient. In ultrasound an abnormality on an image which is due to data acquisition, processing or the nature of the ultrasound beam.

arteralgia *n* pain in an artery.

arterial blood gases (ABGs) often referred to as blood gases. The measurement of the partial pressure of oxygen (PaO_2) and carbon dioxide ($PaCO_2$), and acid–base (pH or hydrogen ion concentration) content of the arterial blood, following equilibration in the lungs between capillary blood and the gases in the alveoli. Measured as part of the assessment of lung function. There is also a small amount of dissolved nitrogen in equilibrium with alveolar nitrogen. ➲ hypoxia, hypercapnia, oxygen dissociation curve.

arterial haemorrhage bleeding from an artery; the blood is bright red (oxygen-rich – oxygenated) and escapes from the artery/ wound in 'spurts' that correspond to the pumping action of the heart. ➲ haemorrhage.

arterial line a cannula placed in an artery to sample blood for gas analysis and for continuous blood pressure monitoring. Usually only used in specialist units (ITU, HDU and theatre) because of the potential risk of severe blood loss. They should always be attached to a pressure transducer and monitor, and have an alarm that indicates any disconnection. ➲ arterial blood gases, blood pressure.

arterial (systemic) embolism ➲ embolism

arterial ulcer a leg ulcer caused by a defect in arterial blood supply. They are found on the foot, usually between the toes or close to the ankle; the adjacent skin is discoloured, shiny and hairless; and the ulcer is small and deep with some exudate (Figure A.15). They are often associated with a history of cardiovascular disease or diabetes mellitus. ➲ intermittent claudication, peripheral vascular disease.

arteriectomy surgical excision of part of an artery.

arteri/o- a prefix that means 'artery', e.g. *arteriosclerosis*.

arteriography *n* demonstration of the arterial system after injection of a radiographic contrast agent—**arteriographic** *adj*, **arteriogram** *n*, **arteriograph** *n*, **arteriographically** *adv*.

arteriole *n* a small artery, joining an artery to a capillary network. They control the amount of blood entering the

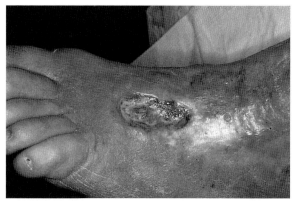

A.15 **Arterial ulcer** (reproduced from Brooker & Nicol 2003 with permission).

capillary network. They are able to constrict and dilate to change peripheral resistance thereby influencing blood pressure.

arteriopathy *n* disease of any artery—**arteriopathic** *adj*.

arterioplasty *n* reconstructive surgery applied to an artery—**arterioplastic** *adj*.

arteriosclerosis *n* degenerative arterial change associated with advancing age. Primarily a thickening of the media (middle) layer and usually associated with some degree of atheroma—**arteriosclerotic** *adj*.

arteriotomy *n* incision or needle puncture of an artery.

arteriovenous *adj* pertaining to an artery and a vein.

arteriovenous (A-V) difference the difference between the arterial and the venous concentration of a substance in the blood, for the whole body (when 'venous' refers to mixed venous blood in the pulmonary artery) or for an organ or region (e.g. for the tissues of the leg if 'venous' refers to blood in the femoral vein). Together with the blood flow, allows calculation of the amount removed in a given time during circulation around the whole body or region. The arteriovenous difference for oxygen is often of interest in exercise physiology. For the whole body, cardiac output (L/min) × arteriovenous difference for oxygen (L/L) = oxygen uptake (L/min) or regional blood flow × arteriovenous difference for oxygen = regional oxygen uptake. ➲ mixed venous blood, oxygen dissociation curve.

arteriovenous extracorporeal membrane carbon dioxide removal (AV ECCO$_2$R) a technique sometimes used in conjunction with extracorporeal membrane oxygenator (ECMO) therapy for critically ill patients, such as those with respiratory failure. Arteriovenous extracorporeal membrane carbon dioxide removal removes excessive carbon dioxide from arterial blood as it passes through a machine with a special filter before returning the blood to the patient's circulation through a tube in a vein. ➲ extracorporeal membrane oxygenator (ECMO), respiratory failure.

arteriovenous fistula the anastomosis of an artery to a vein to promote the enlargement of the latter, to facilitate the removal and replacement of blood during long term haemodialysis.

arteriovenous malformations (AVMs) developmental abnormalities of vasculature. These can be asymptomatic. When they occur in the brain or spinal cord they may cause neurological deficits and if they leak or burst they can lead to subarachnoid haemorrhage.

arteriovenous (A-V) oxygen difference the difference in oxygen content between the arterial and venous blood. It is the arterial oxygen content minus the oxygen content in the central veins.

arteritis *n* an inflammatory disease affecting layers of the arterial wall. It may be due to an infection such as syphilis or it may be part of a systemic vasculitis. The arteries may become swollen and tender and the blood may clot in them. ⇨ endarteritis, giant cell arteritis (GCA), polyarteritis nodosa, Takayasu's disease/arteritis, temporal arteritis—arteritic *adj*.

artery *n* a vessel carrying blood away from the heart to the various tissues. It has three layers. The tunica intima, the internal endothelial lining, provides a smooth surface to prevent intravascular clotting of blood. The tunica media, the middle layer of plain muscle and elastic fibres, allows for distension as blood is pumped from the heart. The outer, tunica adventitia a mainly connective tissue layer prevents overdistension. The lumen is largest nearest to the heart; it gradually decreases in size—**arterial** *adj*.

artery forceps forceps used to achieve haemostasis during surgery. ⇨ forceps.

arthr/o- a prefix that means 'joint', e.g. *arthroplasty*.

arthralgia *n* (*syn* articular neuralgia, arthrodynia) pain in a joint, used especially when there is no inflammation—**arthralgic** *adj*. *intermittent* or *periodic arthralgia* is the term used when there is pain, usually accompanied by swelling of the knee at regular intervals.

arthrectomy surgical excision of a joint.

arthritis *n* inflammation of one or more joints which swell, become warm to touch, and are tender and painful on movement. There are many causes and the treatment varies according to the cause—**arthritic** *adj*. ⇨ arthropathy, gout, juvenile idiopathic arthritis, osteoarthritis, rheumatoid arthritis, Still's disease.

arthrocentesis *n* aspiration of fluid from a synovial joint using a needle and syringe. Synovial fluid samples may be obtained for diagnosis. Therapeutic removal of effusion fluid, pus or blood may be performed. Drugs may also be injected into the synovial cavity.

arthroclasis *n* breaking down of adhesions within the joint cavity to produce a wider range of movement.

arthrodesis *n* the stiffening or fusion of a joint by operative means. Sometimes performed to relieve pain by limiting movement at the joint, or to stabilize an unstable joint.

arthrodynia *n* ⇨ arthralgia—**arthrodynic** *adj*.

arthrography *n* a radiographic examination to determine the internal structure of a joint, outlined by contrast agent—either a gas or a liquid contrast agent or both—

arthrographic *adj*, **arthrogram** *n*, **arthrograph** *n*, **arthrographically** *adv*.

arthrogryposis multiplex congenita *n* a congenital condition characterized by fibrous stiffness of one or more joints. It is often accompanied by poor muscle development of associated muscles and changes to the motor nerves that innervate the muscles.

arthrology *n* the science that studies the structure and function of joints, their diseases and treatment.

arthropathy *n* any joint disease—**arthropathies** *pl*, **arthropathic** *adj*. Arthropathy may be classified as: *enteropathic arthropathies* resulting from chronic diarrhoeal disease; *psoriatic arthropathies* accompanying psoriasis; *seronegative arthropathies* include all other instances of inflammatory arthritis other than rheumatoid arthritis; *seropositive arthropathies* include all instances of rheumatoid arthritis.

arthroplasty *n* surgical remodelling of a joint—**arthroplastic** *adj*. ⇨ cup arthroplasty, excision arthroplasty, Girdlestone arthroplasty, hemiarthroplasty, replacement arthroplasty, total replacement arthroplasty.

arthroscope *n* an endoscopic instrument used for the visualization of the interior of a joint cavity. Used to take tissue biopsies, and also for treatments such as removing loose bodies from the knee joint. ⇨ endoscope—**arthroscopic** *adj*.

arthroscopy *n* the act of visualizing the interior of a joint. Uses an intra-articular endoscopic camera to assess, repair or reconstruct various tissues within and around joints—**arthroscopic** *adj*.

arthrosis *n* degeneration in a joint.

arthrostomy *n* operative procedure to make an opening (temporary) in a joint cavity.

arthrotomy *n* incision into a joint.

articular *adj* pertaining to a joint or articulation. Applied to cartilage, surface, capsule, etc.

articular cartilage the specialized tissue that covers the ends of bones and allows the distribution of compressive loads over the cross section of bones, as well as providing an almost frictionless surface for joint movement.

articular disc an anatomical term used to describe a plate of fibrocartilage attached to the joint capsule and separating the articular surfaces of the bones for a varying distance, it improves joint congruency (fit).

articulate 1. capable of expressing oneself clearly. 2. to join, to unite by joints. 3. in dentistry, to place the teeth in their correct relationship with respect to each other.

articulation 1. the junction of two or more bones; a joint. ⇨ anatomic articulation. 2. enunciation of speech—**articular** *adj*.

articulation (in dentistry) the contact existing between opposing teeth of the maxilla and the mandible while the mandible is moving. ⇨ anterior protected articulation, canine protected articulation, edge-to-edge articulation, free articulation, functional articulation.

articulation of the pelvis the relationship in degrees between the plane of the pelvis with the horizontal plane and the spine.

articulator mechanical device to which models of the upper and lower dental arches are attached and which reproduces recorded positions of the mandible in relation to the maxilla. Assists in the study of occlusion and the construction of prostheses and restorations. ⮑ adjustable articulator, anatomical articulator, arcon articulator, hinge or plane line articulator, plasterless articulator, semi-adjustable articulator.

artificial anus ⮑ colostomy.

artificial blood a fluid able to transport oxygen (O_2).

artificial crown in dentistry, restoration used to cover the part of the tooth that projects above the gum line, usually made of metal, porcelain, or a combination of both. ⮑ crown.

artificial heart ⮑ left ventricular assist device (LVAD).

artificial insemination ⮑ insemination.

artificial kidney ⮑ dialyser.

artificial limb ⮑ orthosis, prosthesis.

artificial lung ⮑ respirator.

artificial menopause ⮑ menopause.

artificial pacemaker ⮑ cardiac pacemaker.

artificial pneumothorax ⮑ pneumothorax.

artificial respiration ⮑ cardiopulmonary resuscitation.

artificial rupture of membranes (ARM) amniotomy. An aseptic procedure in which the amniotic membranes are punctured and amniotic fluid released. It may be carried out to induce labour, speed up labour and to identify if meconium has been passed indicating fetal distress. Problems include increased pain, risk of infection, increased likelihood of further intervention in labour and, occasionally, cord prolapse.

artificial saliva an oral spray useful in saliva deficiency and dry mouth (xerostomia).

artificial stone high-strength model and die material, based on calcium sulphate, used during the construction of crowns and special prostheses.

artificial tears any eye drop solution which can replace tears by approximating its consistency in terms of viscosity and tonicity and may contain many of the substances found in tears. The most common agents found in artificial tears are cellulose derivatives, such as methylcellulose, hydroxymethylcellulose, hydroxypropylcellulose, hydroxypropylmethylcellulose (or hypromellose), hydroxyethylcellulose and carboxymethycellulose, polyvinyl alcohol or polyacrylic acid, as well as a preservative and a substance to produce isotonicity (e.g. sodium chloride). ⮑ alacrima, keratitis sicca, Sjögren's syndrome.

asbestos *n* a fibrous, mineral substance which does not conduct heat and is incombustible. It has many uses, including brake linings, asbestos textiles and asbestos-cement sheeting. Inhalation of asbestos fibres leads to pulmonary fibrous. Long-term contact with asbestos, such as during employment, can cause mesothelioma and lung cancer. ⮑ mesothelioma.

asbestosis *n* a form of pneumoconiosis from inhalation of asbestos dust and fibre. This respiratory disease is a member of the occupational interstitial lung disease group and is one of the three most common (the others being silicosis and pneumoconiosis). Patients with asbestosis will report exposure to asbestos (which may be many years prior to presentation) and demonstrate parenchymal scarring with various symptoms, including dyspnoea on exertion, crackles on auscultation with reduced spirometric values of a restrictive nature, reduced gas diffusing capacity and radiological changes of reticulonodular infiltrates affecting both lung bases, pleural effusion or pleural plaques. ⮑ mesothelioma.

ascariasis *n* infestation by nematodes (roundworms). The ova are ingested and hatch in the duodenum. The larvae pass to the lungs in the blood, from where they ascend to be swallowed and returned to the intestine. They may occasionally obstruct the intestine or the bile ducts.

ascaricide *n* a substance that kills ascarides, e.g. levamisole—**ascaricidal** *adj*.

Ascaris npl a genus of nematode worms of the family Ascaridae, e.g. the roundworm *Ascaris lumbricoides*. ⮑ ascariasis.

ascending colon the part of the colon that passes up the right-hand side of the abdomen from the caecum to the level of the liver where it curves across at the right colonic (hepatic) flexure to continue as the transverse colon. ⮑ colon, Colour Section Figure 18b.

Aschoff's nodules (K A Aschoff, German pathologist, 1866–1942), nodules present in the myocardium in myocarditis caused by rheumatic fever.

ascites *n* (*syn* hydroperitoneum) free fluid in the peritoneal cavity—**ascitic** *adj*.

ASCII *abbr* **A**merican **S**tandard **C**ode for **I**nformation **I**nterchange.

ascorbic acid vitamin C. A water-soluble antioxidant vitamin which is necessary for healthy connective tissue, particularly the collagen fibres and cell membranes. Also enhances absorption of dietary iron and is necessary for functioning of the immune system. Deficiency causes scurvy. Used as nutritional supplement in anaemia and to promote wound healing.

ASD *abbr* atrial septal defect.

-ase a suffix that means 'catalyst, enzyme', e.g. *lipase*.

asepsis *n* the condition of being free from living pathogenic micro-organisms—**aseptic** *adj*.

aseptic technique describes procedures used to exclude pathogenic micro-organisms from an environment. It includes the use of sterile gloves and gowns in theatre, non-touch technique and the use of sterilized equipment. Used where there is a possibility of introducing micro-organisms into the patient's body.

ash the residue of components in a food after all organic matter and water has been burnt off. It is all the non-organic matter in a food, a measure of the total content of minerals in a food.

Ashwell scale (M Ashwell, British scientist and nutritionalist, 20th–21st century) a scale based on waist circumference:height ratio used to calculate the amount of intra-abdominal fat in both women and men ⮑ waist circumference:height ratio, waist circumference:hip ratio.

Ashworth scale a scale to measure muscle tone. It has two versions, a standard and a modified version. It is easy to use in the clinical setting and consists of a five-point graded scale. It has been used extensively in research, although there is considerable debate in the literature as to if it really measures tone or simply the resistance to movement, which could be due to contracture or other factors. It has been modified and more recent research tends to favour the newer Modified Ashworth Scale in which $0 =$ No increase in muscle tone; $1 =$ Slight increase in muscle tone, manifested by a catch and release or by minimal resistance at the end range of motion when the part is moved in flexion or extension/abduction or adduction, etc.; $1+ =$ Slight increase in muscle tone, manifested by a catch, followed by minimal resistance throughout the remainder (less than half) of the range of motion (ROM); $2 =$ More marked increase in muscle tone through most of the ROM, but the affected part is easily moved; $3 =$ Considerable increase in muscle tone, passive movement is difficult; $4 =$ Affected part is rigid in flexion or extension (abduction or adduction, etc.)

asialorrhoea diminished flow or lack of saliva.

ASIS *abbr* anterior superior iliac spine.

Askin tumour highly malignant tumour of the chest wall.

ASO *abbr* antistreptolysin O.

ASOM *abbr* acute suppurative otitis media.

asomatogosia *n* loss of awareness of parts of the body (soma) and their position in space, a perceptual sequela of cerebrovascular accident (stroke) affecting the right parietal lobe of the cerebrum, which may lead to lack of awareness, even denial, of the presence of disability.

asparaginase *n* an enzyme derived from micro-organisms. In the form of crisantaspase, used pharmacologically to treat cancers, e.g. acute lymphoblastic leukaemia. ➲ cytotoxic.

asparagine *n* a non-essential (dispensable) amino acid.

aspartame *n* an intense artificial sweetener. 180 times the sweetness of sucrose (beet or cane sugar). It is converted to phenylalanine in the body and consequently should not be used by people with phenylketonuria. Commonly used in low calorie soft drinks. ➲ sweetener.

aspartate aminotransferase (AST) an enzyme that facilitates the reversible transfer of amino groups during amino acid metabolism. ➲ aminotransferases.

aspartic acid (aspartate) *n* a non-essential (dispensable) amino acid. At physiological pH aspartic acid is negatively charged and is known as aspartate.

Asperger's syndrome (H Asperger, Austrian psychiatrist, 1906–1980), a pervasive developmental syndrome classified as part of the autistic spectrum of disorders. It is diagnosed during childhood and is associated with various problems with social interactions, communication and expressing emotion, but without delay in language or cognitive development. The problems with social interaction frequently continue into adult life. ➲ biographical and health data, evaluation, implementation, planning.

aspergillosis *n* opportunist infection, most frequently of the lungs, caused by any species of *Aspergillus*. ➲ bronchomycosis.

Aspergillus *n* a genus of fungi, found in soil, manure and on various grains. Some species are pathogenic.

aspermia *n* lack of secretion or expulsion of semen—**aspermic** *adj*.

aspheric lens a lens in which one or both surfaces are not spherical, so designed to minimize certain optical aberrations.

asphyxia *n* lack of oxygen reaching the brain leading to unconsciousness and in the absence of effective treatment eventually death.

aspiration *n* (*syn* paracentesis, tapping) **1.** the removal of fluids from a body cavity by means of suction or siphonage such as fluid from the peritoneal cavity, postoperative gastric aspiration, etc. **2.** describes the entry of fluids or food into the airway.

aspiration pneumonia inflammation of lung tissue from inhalation of a foreign body, most often food particles or fluids. ➲ Heimlich's manoeuvre.

aspirator *n* a negative pressure device used for withdrawing fluids or gas from body cavities. In dentistry, apparatus producing a high-volume, low-vacuum suction. When fitted with an *aspirator tip* it may be used to remove fluids, blood, saliva and debris from the mouth, and to assist in keeping the operator's mouth mirror clear.

aspirin ➲ non-steroidal anti-inflammatory drugs. ➲ acetylsalicylic acid, Appendix 5

assault *n* an attempt or offer of unlawful contact in which the person is put in fear of violence or unlawful force. Constitutes a trespass against the person. ➲ battery.

assay *n* a quantitative test used to measure the amount of a substance present or its level of activity, e.g. hormones or drugs.

asseointegrated implant ➲ implant (dental).

assertiveness training **1.** developing self-confidence in personal and professional relationships. It concentrates on the honest expression of feelings, both negative and positive: learning occurs through role playing in a therapeutic setting followed by practice in real-life situations. **2.** a structured programme for teaching effective communication skills through a combination of individual and group exercises, modelling and role play.

assessment the collection of information, including subjective and objective data which are relevant to formulating an individual plan of treatment, a specific therapy or care package.

assessment (nursing) *n* the first stage of the nursing process. Describes the collection by the nurse of relevant data about a patient or client in order to enable individualized nursing. The most detailed information is usually ascertained at the initial interview. Assessment is an ongoing activity, however, and nursing interventions and the goals of patient care should constantly be re-evaluated in the light of this. ➲ biographical and health data, evaluation, implementation, planning.

assessment (occupational therapy) a process of collecting and interpreting information about people's functions and environments, using observation, testing and measurement, in order to inform decision-making and to monitor change. (Reproduced with permission from the European Network of Occupational Therapy in Higher Education (ENOTHE) Terminology Project, 2008.) ⊃ initial assessment, ongoing assessment, screening assessment.

assessment of pelvis in obstetric practice undertaken through observation of the woman's gait, considering previous obstetric history, measuring the pelvic capacity manually or by ultrasound scan or, most accurately, by vaginal examination.

assimilation *n* the process whereby digested foodstuffs are absorbed and used by the cells and tissues—**assimilable** *adj*, **assimilate** *vt, vi*.

assimilation pelvis variation in normal development of the sacrum. *high assimilation pelvis* the last lumbar vertebra is fused into the sacrum, the pelvis is deep, and there may be funnelling and associated difficulty in labour. *low assimilation pelvis* the first sacral vertebra assumes the characteristics of a lumbar vertebra; the pelvis is shallow and the condition does not affect labour.

assisted breech delivery medical approach to delivering the fetus presenting by the breech vaginally; assistance is given by applying forceps to the head to achieve a controlled delivery.

assisted conception techniques used when the normal method of conception has failed. They include in vitro fertilization (IVF) and transcervical embryo transfer or gamete intrafallopian tube transfer (GIFT), zygote intrafallopian transfer (ZIFT), intracytoplasmic sperm injection (ICSI) and microsurgical epididymal sperm aspiration (MESA).

assisted movements movements aided by a therapist, or equipment, another health professional, or carer. May be self-assisted (auto-assisted) when, for instance, a person moves an arm paralysed after a stroke using their unaffected arm.

associated heterophoria (*syn* aligning prism, compensating prism) a term sometimes used to denote the prism power necessary to align the nonius markers of a fixation disparity test. It is not strictly speaking a heterophoria because only part of the visual field is dissociated while the rest of the field is fused (that fused area is often referred to as fusion lock or binocular lock). The dissociation of only part of the field is achieved by using either a method of cross-polarization (e.g. Mallet fixation disparity unit) or a septum (e.g. Turville infinity balance test). ⊃ Disparometer, dissociated heterophoria, Mallett fixation disparity unit, retinal disparity, Turville infinity balance test, uncompensated heterophoria.

associated movements described by some authorities as the normal movements that occur during considerable effort, such as when attempting a new activity. Whilst other authorities use the term to include both normal and abnormal movements.

associated reactions the postural muscle reactions that happen when a muscle is freed from its usual nervous control. They are involuntary stereotyped movements that can occur when a person is having balance problems, or is putting a great deal of effort into a task.

association *n* a term used in psychology. *association of ideas* the principle by which ideas, emotions and movements are connected so that their succession in the mind occurs. *controlled association* ideas called up in consciousness in response to words spoken by the examiner. *free association* ideas arising spontaneously when censorship is removed: an important feature of psychoanalysis.

Association of Radical Midwives an organization originally set up by student midwives who felt that changes were needed in midwifery practice. The term 'radical' relates to a desire to return to the roots of practice rather than indicating a particular political position. Members lobby for political change, woman-centred care and autonomous midwifery practice.

associative convergence ⊃ accommodative convergence.

associative strategy in sport psychology, a strategy used by athletes in which they focus attention on internal sensations in order to identify and reduce muscular tension by relaxation. Also known as association. ⊃ dissociative strategy.

AST *abbr* aspartate aminotransferase. ⊃ aminotransferases.

asteatotic eczema frequently seen in older adults in hospital, care and nursing homes, especially when the skin is dry; low humidity caused by central heating, over-washing and diuretics are contributory factors. It occurs most often on the lower legs as a rippled or 'crazy paving' pattern of fine fissuring on an erythematous background.

astereognosis *n* inability to recognize objects by touch and manipulation, especially inability to perceive the shape, texture and size of objects.

asteroid hyalosis (*syn* Benson's disease) a degenerative condition in which the vitreous body (humour) of the eye contains numerous small opacities. It occurs more commonly in males and mainly in one eye. The opacities consist of numerous small stellate or discoid opacities (called asteroid bodies) suspended in the vitreous body (humour). These opacities appear creamy white when viewed by ophthalmoscopy. They rarely affect vision. ⊃ synchisis scintillans.

asthenia *n* lack of strength; weakness, debility—**asthenic** *adj*.

asthenopia *n* (*syn* eyestrain, near point stress [although this term is restricted to any symptoms arising from near vision]) describes symptoms related to excessive effort of accommodation, e.g. headaches.The causes of asthenopia are numerous: sustained near vision, either when the accommodation amplitude is low or hypermetropia is uncorrected (*accommodative asthenopia*), aniseikonia (*aniseikonic asthenopia*), astigmatism (*astigmatic asthenopia*), pain in the eye (*asthenopia dolens*), heterophoria (*heterophoric asthenopia*), ocular inflammation (*asthenopia irritans*), uncorrected presbyopia (*presbyopic asthenopia*), improper illumination (*photogenous asthenopia*) or retinal disease (*retinal asthenopia*)—**asthenopic** *adj*, **asthenope** *n*. ⊃ ocular headache, visual fatigue.

asthma *n* a condition in which there is chronic airway inflammation and increased airway hyper-responsiveness with bronchospasm leading to symptoms of wheeze, cough, chest tightness and dyspnoea. It is characterized functionally by the presence of airflow obstruction which is variable over short periods of time, or is reversible with treatment. Immunological studies have implicated eosinophils, neutrophils, mast cells, lymphocytes and the release of mediators such as histamine, leukotrienes and many cytokines in an inflammatory cascade leading to bronchial wall hyperactivity and narrowing in response to a stimulus. The prevalence of asthma increased steadily over the latter part of the last century in countries with a Western lifestyle and is also increasing in developing countries. The aetiology of asthma is complex, and multiple environmental and genetic determinants are implicated. Factors include: (a) the exposure to infection in early life—decreased infections bias the immune system towards an allergic phenotype. Some infections, however, such as respiratory syncytial virus (RSV), appear to increase the risk of developing asthma; (b) the association between atopy—a propensity to produce IgE—and asthma suggests that sensitization and exposure to allergens (e.g. house dust mites, animal hair, some food stuffs, such as cow's milk) is an important risk factor; (c) the increase in asthma may also be linked to the rise of obesity in Western society through mechanical mechanisms such as gastro-oesophageal reflux disease (GORD). Shared genetic traits, modification of the immune system by diet, or alteration of airway responsiveness by hormones are, however, alternative explanations. Typical symptoms include recurrent episodes of wheezing, chest tightness, breathlessness and cough. Common precipitants include exercise, particularly in cold weather, exposure to airborne allergens or pollutants, and viral upper respiratory tract infections. In persistent asthma the pattern is one of chronic wheeze and breathlessness. Asthma characteristically displays a diurnal pattern, with symptoms and peak expiratory flow rate (PEFR) being worse in the early morning. Particularly when asthma is poorly controlled, symptoms such as cough and wheeze disturb sleep and have led to the use of the term 'nocturnal asthma'. Cough may be the dominant symptom in some patients and the lack of wheeze or breathlessness may lead to a delay in reaching the diagnosis of so-called 'cough-variant asthma'. In some circumstances the appearance of asthma relates to the use of medications, for example β-adrenoceptor antagonists (β-blockers—even when administered topically as eye drops), aspirin and other non-steroidal anti-inflammatory drugs (NSAIDs) induce bronchospasm. Occupational asthma is now the most common form of occupational respiratory disorder. This should be considered in all adult asthmatics of working age, particularly if symptoms improve during time away from work, e.g. weekends or holidays. Atopic individuals and smokers appear to be at increased risk. In the majority of patients with asthma, the disease can be effectively managed in primary care by the multidisciplinary team of doctors, nurses and physiotherapist and most importantly, patients themselves. Management includes: patient (carer) education and an action plan; avoidance of aggravating factors such as house dust mite, household pets, smoking, etc.; and the use of drugs. A stepwise approach based on disease severity is used in the drug management of asthma. In children aged over 5 years and adults: (a) Step 1—occasional use of inhaled short-acting β_2-adrenoreceptor agonist bronchodilators; (b) Step 2—the introduction of regular preventer therapy. Regular anti-inflammatory therapy (preferably inhaled corticosteroids—ICS) should be started in addition to inhaled β_2-agonists; (c) Step 3—add-on therapy. Short-acting β_2-adrenoreceptor agonist bronchodilator, ICS plus long-acting β_2-agonists (LABAs), such as salmeterol. If contol is not achieved one of the following is started—leukotriene receptor antagonist (e.g. montelukast), an oral theophylline (modified release) or an oral modified release β_2-adrenoreceptor agonist; (d) Step 4—inhaled short-acting β_2-adrenoreceptor agonist bronchodilator, ICS in high doses, an inhaled long-acting β_2-agonist, and in adults one or more of a leukotriene receptor antagonist, an oral theophylline (modified release) or a modified release β_2-adrenoreceptor agonist; (e) Step 5—continuous or frequent use of oral corticosteroids. At this stage prednisolone therapy (usually administered as a single daily dose in the morning). An inhaled short-acting β_2-adrenoreceptor agonist bronchodilator, high dose inhaled ICS and long-acting bronchodilators as needed. (f) Step-down therapy—once asthma control is established, the dose of inhaled (or oral) corticosteroid should be titrated to the lowest dose at which effective control of asthma is maintained. In patients with severe IgE-mediated sensitivity to inhaled allergens who do not respond adequately to other therapies, the monoclonal antibody omalizumab, which binds to immunoglobulin E (IgE), can be used. ⊃ ocupational asthma, severe acute asthma—**asthmatic** *adj*.

astigmatic lens a toric or cylindrical lens which produces two separate focal lines at right angles, instead of a single focal point. Hence it has two principal powers. One of these powers may be zero (cylindrical lens). ⊃ anastigmatic lens, cylinder axis, cylindrical lens, spherocylindrical lens, toric lens.

astigmatism *n* defective vision caused by refractive surfaces, usually corneal, focusing light onto more than one focal plane—**astigmatic, astigmic** *adj*.

astringent *adj* describes an agent which contracts organic tissue, thus lessening secretion. May be used in the management of heavily exuding wounds. In dentistry, agent used to contract gingival tissue away from a crown preparation in order to facilitate impression taking—**astringency, astringent** *n*.

astringency the action of chemicals in foods, such as unripe fruits, on the tongue. They cause contraction of the epithelium of the tongue.

astrocytes *npl* part of the macroglia. Star-shaped neuroglial cells, which are the main supporting tissue in the central nervous system. They are sited close to blood vessel walls where they contribute to the blood–brain barrier.

astrocytoma *n* a slowly growing tumour of astrocytes (neuroglial tissue) of the brain. These can occur in any age group, although most common from 40 to 60 years. They are graded 1–4 depending on the malignancy, with the lowest grade being 1. Management options include neurosurgery, chemotherapy and radiotherapy, with ongoing management of neurological deficits by the multidisciplinary team. Astrocytomas grow more slowly than more malignant tumours such as glioblastomas.

Astrup machine apparatus for the indirect measurement of acid-base parameters of the blood. Uses the measurement of pH and a nomogram to interpolate other parameters, such as PCO_2.

ASW *abbr* approved social worker.

asymmetrical growth restriction fetal growth restriction due to reduced placental nutrition in which head circumference measurements are within normal limits, but abdominal circumference (measured at the level of the liver) is on a lower centile. The growth of vital organs is maintained but subcutaneous fat deposition and glycogen storage in the liver stops. It is sometimes called 'late onset' growth restriction, not to be confused with growth restriction in which the fetal head is small but abdominal growth is conserved.

asymmetric pelvis pelvis with one side distorted due to disease, injury or congenital maldevelopment.

asymmetric tonic neck reflex also called tonic neck reflex. A reflex present in newborns. When an infant is lying on its back with the head turned to one side, the limbs on the side that the head is facing should be straight, while the limbs on the other side should bend. The reflex normally disappears around six months of age.

asymmetry *n* lack of similarity of the organs or parts on each side.

asymptomatic *adj* symptomless.

asymptomatic bacteriuria the presence of $>10^5$/mL bacteria in the urine of individuals who are without symptoms suggestive of infection. Infants and pregnant women with asymptomatic bacteriuria should be treated and the cause investigated. Pregnant women are screened in early pregnancy and treated as necessary as asymptomatic bacteriuria may cause pyelonephritis and be associated with preterm labour.

asynclitism parietal presentation of the fetal head in which the transversely placed sagittal suture lies close to the symphysis pubis or sacrum; a sideways rocking mechanism of fetal descent during labour, in a flat pelvis. In anterior asynclitism the anterior parietal bone moves down behind the symphysis pubis until the parietal eminence enters the brim. The movement is then reversed and the head rocks back until the posterior parietal bone passes the sacral promontory. In posterior asynclitism the movements are reversed, the posterior parietal bone negotiating the sacral promontory before the anterior parietal bone passes behind the symphysis pubis. ⊃ synclitism.

asyndesis a disorder of thought with disruption of the association of ideas. Thought and speech are fragmented because the person cannot assemble related thoughts into a coherent notion.

A syndrome ⊃ pattern, A.

asystole *n* absence of heart beat and output from the heart. One type of cardiac arrest.

AT *abbr* anaerobic threshold.

ataractic *adj* describes drugs that tranquillize and relieve anxiety. ⊃ tranquillizers.

atavism *n* the reappearance of a hereditary characteristic that has missed one or more generations—**atavic, atavistic** *adj*.

ataxia, ataxy *n* ill-timed and incoordinate movements caused by hypotonia, dyssynergia and dysmetria. Failure of muscular co-ordination, varieties include sensory, labyrinthine and cerebellar—**ataxic** *adj*. ⊃ ataxic gait, Friedreich's ataxia, sensory ataxia.

ataxic gait an inco-ordinate or abnormal gait. ⊃ gait.

atelectasis *n* a number of pulmonary alveoli do not contain air due to failure of expansion (congenital atelectasis) or resorption of air from the alveoli (collapse)—**atelectatic** *adj*.

ateliosis a form of dwarfism caused by lack of hormones from the anterior lobe of the pituitary gland. The person appears childlike and sexual development does not occur.

ATF *abbr* anterior talofibular ligament.

atherogenic *adj* capable of producing atheroma—**atherogenesis** *n*.

atheroma *n* plaques of fatty (lipid) material in the intimal (inner) layer of the arteries. Starts as fatty streaks on the intima, deposition of low density lipoprotein and plaque formation (Figure A.16). Eventually the lumen of the artery is reduced and ischaemia results. A thrombus may form if a plaque ruptures, which leads to further occlusion of the

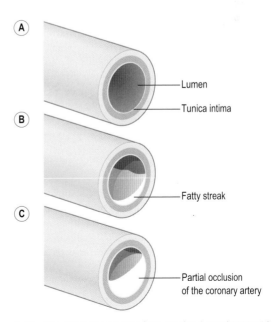

A.16 Atheroma (reproduced from Brooker & Nicol 2003 with permission).

artery. Of great importance in the coronary arteries in predisposing to coronary thrombosis and myocardial infarction—**atheromatous** *adj*.

atherosclerosis *n* coexisting atheroma and arteriosclerosis—**atherosclerotic** *adj*.

athetosis *n* a largely obsolete word used to describe a slow writhing movement disorder typically in the context of cerebral palsy. Made worse by excitement and emotional stress—**athetoid, athetotic** *adj*.

athlete increasingly favoured term for a person involved in any physically demanding sport (not only track and field athletics).

athlete's foot tinea pedis. A fungal infection of the skin of the foot. Symptoms include intense itch, peeling and sometimes painful splits in the skin. Common in sport due to poor hygiene and use of communal changing and showering facilities. Treated by antifungal creams or dusting powders. ⊃ tinea.

athlete's heart the cardiac adaptations associated with physical training. There is hypertrophy of the muscle of the left ventricle as a physiological response to training, especially endurance training. It is not considered to be pathological. The effects include resting bradycardia, changes to the ECG trace, alteration in heart sounds and physical changes to heart muscle.

athletic identity the degree to which a person identifies with an athletic role as part of their self-concept.

athletic trainer a term used in North America for an individual who is trained in the prevention, evaluation, treatment and rehabilitation of athletic injuries.

Atkins' diet (R Atkins, American cardiologist/nutrionalist, 1930–2003) ⊃ low-carbohydrate ketogenic diets.

atlas *n* the first cervical vertebra. An atypical vertebra that consists simply of a ring of bone with two short transverse processes. The anterior part of the large vertebral foramen is occupied by the odontoid process of the axis, which is held in position by a transverse ligament. Thus the odontoid process forms the body of the atlas. The posterior part is the true vertebral foramen and is occupied by the spinal cord. On its superior surface the bone has two articular facets which form joints with the condyles of the occipital bone of the skull. The nodding movement of the head takes place at these joints. ⊃ axis, cervical vertebrae.

ATLS *abbr* advanced trauma life support.

ATN *abbr* acute tubular necrosis.

atom *n* a particle with a nucleus which contains protons which carry a positive charge, surrounded by orbiting electrons which carry a negative charge. The smallest particle of an element capable of existing individually, or in combination with one or more atoms of the same or another element—**atomic** *adj*.

atomic mass number (A) the total number of nucleons in the nucleus of an atom. ⊃ nucleon.

atomic mass unit (amu) or dalton a relative weight used to measure atoms and subatomic particles. Protons and neutrons have both been designated as being 1 amu.

atomic number (Z) the number of protons in the atomic nucleus or the number of electrons, for example hydrogen which, with one of each, has the atomic number 1.

atomic weight (mass) or relative atomic mass. The relative average mass of an atom based on the mass of an atom of carbon-12.

atomizer *n* nebulizer.

atonia *n* total flaccidity or no muscle tone caused by complete loss of motor supply to a muscle—**atonic** *adj*.

atonic bladder a condition marked by overfilling of the urinary bladder and involuntary leakage of small volumes of urine. It arises from some interruption to the nerve pathways to the bladder, such as with diabetes, which leads to loss of the sensation of a full bladder and an inability to empty the bladder normally.

atopic eczema atopy is a genetic predisposition to form excessive immunoglobulin E (IgE) which leads to a generalized and prolonged hypersensitivity to common environmental antigens, including pollen and the house dust mite. Atopic individuals manifest one or more of a group of diseases that includes asthma, hay fever, urticaria, food and other allergies, and this distinctive form of eczema. Although any of these atopic conditions tends to be over-represented in families of persons with any atopic disease, one particular disease type tends to run more strongly in a particular family. A number of operational criteria for the diagnosis of atopic eczema have been proposed for the purpose of research studies, these are itchy skin and at least three of the following: (a) history of itch in skin creases (or cheeks if < 4 years); (b) history of asthma/hay fever (or in a first degree relative if < 4 years); (c) dry skin (xeroderma); (d) visible flexural eczema (cheeks, forehead, outer limbs if < 4 years); (e) onset in first 2 years of life. The aetiology has a clear familial component, a large part of which is due to genetic factors. The disorder is concordant in 86% of monozygotic twins but in only 21% of dizygotes. Atopic diseases show some degree of maternal imprinting—that is, they are inherited more often from the mother than from the father. Atopic dermatitis is therefore genetically complex. More than one genetic locus has been identified that might play a role in the inheritance of atopy and more specifically atopic eczema. The prevalence of atopic eczema is rising and has increased between twofold and fivefold over the last 30 years. It now affects 1 in 10 schoolchildren. Environmental factors, such as exposure to allergens either in utero or during childhood, have been shown to have a role in the aetiology of atopic eczema. Recent evidence suggests that exposure to probiotics in late pregnancy and early infancy reduces the incidence of atopic eczema. The pathogenesis of atopic eczema is still incompletely understood. One unifying view is to consider it as an interplay of genetic susceptibility that causes epidermal barrier dysfunction, a propensity to mount abnormal immune responses, and a positive feedback loop between these two factors. The cardinal feature of atopic eczema is itch ('the itch that rashes'), and scratching may account for many of the signs. Widespread dryness (felt as roughness) of the skin is another feature. The distribution and character of the rash vary with age. In infancy the eczema is often acute and involves the face and trunk; the napkin area is frequently spared. During childhood the rash settles on the backs of the knees, fronts of the elbows, wrists and ankles. ➲ Colour Section Figure 50. In adults the rash involves the face and trunk; lichenification is common. The complications of atopic eczema include: superinfection with bacteria (e.g. *Staphylococcus aureus*) but also importantly with viruses. Herpes simplex virus causes a widespread eruption known as eczema herpeticum. Papillomavirus and molluscum contagiosum superinfections are also more common and are encouraged by the use of local corticosteroids.

atopic syndrome a hereditary predisposition to develop hypersensitivity disorders, such as eczema, asthma, hay fever and allergic rhinitis. Associated with excess immunoglobulin E (IgE) production.

ATP *abbr* adenosine triphosphate.

ATP-CP energy pathway the energy pathway that produces energy from the skeletal muscle stores of the high energy phosphates adenosine triphosphate (ATP) and creatine phosphate (CP). Important during short-duration, high-intensity physical activity.

ATPS *abbr* ambient temperature and pressure dry.

atresia *n* imperforation or closure of a normal body opening, duct or canal such as the oesophagus, bowel, anus or bile duct—**atresic, atretic** *adj*.

atrial fibrillation a cardiac arrhythmia. Chaotic irregularity of atrial rhythm with an irregular ventricular response (Figure A.17). There is a risk of thrombi forming on the atrial wall. When sinus rhythm returns emboli may be dislodged and travel in the circulation to cause, for instance, a stroke. Commonly associated with mitral stenosis, hyperthyroidism (thyrotoxicosis) or heart failure.

atrial flutter a cardiac arrhythmia caused by an irritable focus in atrial muscle and usually associated with coronary heart disease. Speed of atrial beats is between 260 and 340 per minute. The ventricular response is slower and may respond to every four atrial beats.

atrial natriuretic peptides (ANP) peptides produced by cells in the cardiac atria. They are involved in the control of blood pressure by inhibiting the release of antidiuretic hormone and aldosterone when blood pressure rises.

atrial septal defect (ASD) a hole in the atrial septum. Most commonly due to a congenital defect. Types include: ostium secundum defect, which is most common and is situated around the site of the foramen ovale; and ostium primum defects situated lower down on the atrial septum. ➲ Colour Section Figure 21.

atrioventricular (A-V) *adj* pertaining to the atria and the ventricles of the heart. Applied to a node, tract and valves.

atrioventricular bundle also called the bundle of His. Part of the conducting system of the heart. Carries impulses from the atrioventricular node to the ventricles. Divides into right and left bundle branches that transmit the impulses to the apex of each ventricle.

atrioventricular node part of the conducting system of the heart. Situated at the bottom of the right atrium, it transmits impulses from the sinus node (sinoatrial node) to the atrioventricular bundle.

atrioventricular valves valves between the the atria and ventricles in the heart. ➲ mitral (bicuspid), tricuspid.

atrium *n* cavity, entrance or passage. One of the two upper receiving chambers of the heart—**atria** *pl*, **atrial** *adj*. ➲ Colour Section Figure 8.

atrophic rhinitis (*syn* ozaena) chronic infective condition of the nasal mucous membrane with associated crusting and fetor.

atrophy *n* loss of substance of cells, tissues or organs. There is wasting and a decrease in size and function. The process may be physiological such as that occurring as part of normal ageing, or pathological, as in disuse atrophy when a limb is immobilized—**atrophied, atrophic** *adj*. ➲ disuse atrophy.

atropine *n* the principal alkaloid of belladonna. A substance that, by affecting local enzyme actions, leads to destruction (inactivation) of the neurotransmitter acetylcholine at parasympathetic nerve endings. By preventing parasympathetic action where there is dual autonomic innervation, atropine allows the sympathetic influence to predominate, e.g. it increases the heart rate, dilates the pupils, reduces salivary secretion and relaxes intestinal smooth muscle. ➲ muscarinic antagonists.

attached gingiva that part of the gingiva which is attached to the underlying bone and cementum of the teeth.

attachment *n* in psychology a term describing the dependent relationship which one individual forms with another, emanating from the unique bonding between infant and parent figure.

attention *n* ability to select some stimuli for closer examination while discarding others considered less salient.

attention deficit hyperactivity disorder (ADHD) term used to describe children who have short attention spans

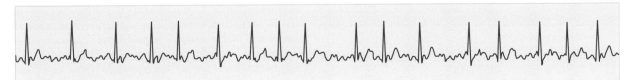

A.17 Atrial fibrillation (reproduced from Brooker & Nicol 2003 with permission).

and are easily distracted. They are frequently overactive, may be aggressive, and often have learning difficulties. ⊃ hyperkinetic disorder/syndrome.

attentional deficits can involve different areas of attention. These include the ability to transfer the focus of attention and to change it between activities; the abililty to avoid being distracted; being able to respond to multiple tasks simultaneously; the ability to sustain concentration; and the ability to be focused and recognize individual pieces of information.

attentional style the way in which an individual tends to focus attention on the environment differentially along two dimensions: width (varying from a broad focus involving attention to a wide range of environmental cues to a narrow focus involving attention to a limited range of cues) and direction (directed internally on one's own thoughts and feelings versus directed externally towards objects and events outside one's body).

attenuation absorption. It is a measure of the absorption of an X-ray beam along a specific path through a substance. Of ultrasound at diagnostic frequencies, attenuation is approximately proportional to frequency, with the higher frequencies being absorbed more than the lower frequencies, the weakening of ultrasound as it goes through tissue due to absorption, reflection and scattering of the sound wave, measured in decibels. ⊃ linear attenuation coefficient.

attenuation coefficient a measure of the attenuation of an X-ray beam along a specific path through a substance. ⊃ linear attenuation coefficient.

attenuation (of micro-organisms) *n* the process whereby pathogenic micro-organisms are induced to develop or show less virulent characteristics. They can then be used in the preparation of vaccines—**attenuant, attenuated** *adj*, **attenuate** *vt, vi*.

atticotomy *n* operation to remove cholesteatoma from the middle ear and mastoid process.

attitude relationship of fetal parts—head, spine and limbs—to each other, normally one of flexion but may be deflexed or extended when the position of the occiput is not anterior.

attitudes *npl* reactions to and evaluations of individuals, situations and objects. They may be positive or negative.

attributable risk ⊃ risk.

attribution *n* in psychology, the theory that deals with the inferences that individuals make regarding the causes of their own and other individuals' behaviour or a behavioural outcome with regard to whether the behaviour or outcome is caused by internal factors (e.g. effort or ability) or external factors (e.g. chance or the influence of other people).

attribution theory a theory designed to explain the types, antecedents and consequences of individuals' attributions.

attrition the loss of tooth substance or of a restoration as a result of mastication or of occlusal or approximal contact between the teeth.

atypical *adj* not typical; unusual, irregular; not conforming to type, e.g. atypical pneumonia.

atypical mole syndrome dysplastic naevus syndrome. A syndrome characterized by the presence of multiple moles.

The moles or naevi are pigmented and irregular in size. Occurs in individuals at risk of familial or non-familial malignant melanoma.

audiogram *n* a graph of the acuity of hearing tested with an audiometer.

audiology *n* the scientific study of hearing—**audiological** *adj*, **audiologically** *adv*.

audiometer *n* apparatus for the clinical testing of hearing. It generates pure tones over a wide range of pitch and intensity—**audiometric** *adj*, **audiometry** *n*.

audiometrist *n* a person qualified to carry out audiometry.

audit *n* investigative methods used to systematically measure outcomes and review performance. ⊃ audit trail, clinical audit, medical audit, quality assurance.

audit trail a way of working and record keeping that allows all processes to be transparent and clear.

Audit Commission within the NHS the main role of the Audit Commission is to promote 'best practice' in terms of economy, effectiveness and efficiency.

auditory *adj* pertaining to the sense of hearing.

auditory acuity ability to hear clearly and distinctly. Tests include the use of tuning fork, whispered voice and audiometer. Hearing can be tested in infants by otoacoustic emission testing (OAE) and automated auditory brainstem response (AABR). ⊃ audiometer, automated auditory brainstem response, neonatal hearing screening, otoacoustic emission testing.

auditory area that portion of the temporal lobe of the cerebral cortex which interprets sound.

auditory canal ⊃ external auditory meatus/canal.

auditory nerves the eighth pair of cranial nerves. More usually called the vestibulocochlear nerve.

auditory ossicles three small bones—malleus, incus and stapes—located within the middle ear.

auditory processing disorder (APD) previously known as central auditory processing disorder. A condition in which the brain does not perceive auditory information despite normal auditory pathways, i.e. there is no sensory impairment. There are several types and it may be genetic or acquired, (e.g. following brain injury). It is characterized by difficulty with the localization of sounds, difficulty remembering spoken instructions, understanding speech in situations with background noise (e.g. television on, parties), etc.

Auerbach's (myenteric) plexus (L Auerbach, German anatomist, 1828–1897) ⊃ myenteric plexus.

AUG *abbr* acute ulcerative gingivitis.

auger electrons electrons ejected during radioactive decay that have discrete energy levels equal to the photon energy minus the binding energy of the electron.

augmentation *n* **1.** enlargement. Commonly applied to plastic surgical procedures using a prosthesis that increases breast size. **2.** the artificial stimulation or acceleration of a normal physiological process.

augmentation of labour intervention to correct slow progress in labour. Correction of ineffective uterine contractions includes amniotomy, administration of oxytocin and amniotomy, or administration of oxytocin in the presence of previously ruptured membranes.

AUNG *abbr* acute ulcerative necrotizing gingivitis.

aura *n* a premonition; a peculiar sensation or warning of an impending attack, such as occurs in epilepsy or migraine. They may include visual disturbances, abnormal sensations such as tingling, or strange tastes.

aural *adj* pertaining to the ear.

auricle *n* **1.** the pinna of the outer/external ear. ⊃ Colour Section Figure 13. **2.** an appendage to the cardiac atrium. **3.** obsolete term for cardiac atrium—**auricular** *adj*.

auricular line a line perpendicular to the anthropological base line through the centre of the external auditory meatus. ⊃ anthropological base line.

auriculotemporal syndrome ⊃ Frey's syndrome.

auriculoventricular *adj* obsolete term ⊃ atrioventricular.

auriscope ⊃ otoscope.

auscultation *n* a method of listening to the body sounds, particularly the heart, lungs and fetal circulation for diagnostic purposes. It may be: (a) immediate, by placing the ear directly against the body, (b) mediate, by the use of a stethoscope—**auscultatory** *adj*, **auscult, auscultate** *v*.

auscultation of the fetal heart sounds is performed during pregnancy and labour, using a Pinard's stethoscope, Doppler ultrasound or cardiotocography.

auscultation of the lungs the art of using a stethoscope to listen to the effects of sound transmission through the lung tissue. These sounds must be taken into consideration with other findings and should not be used in isolation to arrive at a differential or absolute diagnosis. The phase of breathing at which the sound occurs, the loudness and the pitch of the sound, should all be considered. Sounds occur due to the turbulent flow of air through the upper and central airways and constitute high- and low-pitched components. Normally aerated lungs filter out the high-pitched but transmit the low-pitched sounds well. Where disease is present, these sounds may change, e.g. transmission is reduced over areas of pleural effusion, while consolidated lung tissue transmits high-pitched sounds. Semantics are often confusing and the following terminology may be used to describe sounds: bronchial breathing, vesicular breath sounds, creps (crepitations), rhonchi and rhales.

autism *n* a pervasive form of disordered child development characterized by difficulties with social interaction, communication and repetitive stereotyped behaviours. ⊃ Asperger's syndrome.

auto- a prefix that means 'self', e.g. *autoantibody*.

autoagglutination the agglutination of red blood cells (erythrocytes) by the person's own antibodies, such as occurs in autoimmune haemolytic anaemia.

autoantibody *n* an antibody which binds self-antigen expressed in normal tissue.

autoantigen *n* a self-antigen, expressed in normal tissue, which is the target of autoantibodies or self-reactive T cells.

autoclave 1. *n* an apparatus for high-pressure steam sterilization. **2.** *vt* sterilize in an autoclave.

autocrine *adj* describes the action of a hormone or growth factor upon the cells that secrete it. ⊃ endocrine, paracrine.

autodigestion *n* self-digestion of body tissue during life. ⊃ autolysis.

autoeroticism *n* self-gratification of the sex instinct. ⊃ masturbation—**autoerotic** *adj*.

autofluorescence *n* the fluorescence of structures in the eye, for example drusen in the retina. ⊃ fluorescein angiography, indocyanine green angiography.

autogenic *adj* describes a process or condition that originates from within the organism.

autogenic drainage a breathing technique used to clear secretions from the airways. It improves ventilation and ensures optimal chest movements.

autogenic facilitation reflex activation of a muscle through activation of its own sensory receptors; self-generated excitation of muscle, e.g. the stretch reflex.

autogenic inhibition reflex inhibition of a muscle through activation of stretch receptors, the Golgi tendon organs, in its own tendons; self-generated relaxation of muscle that normally prevents build-up of too much, potentially injurious, tension in a muscle.

autogenic therapy a complementary therapy that employs a combination of self-hypnosis and relaxation.

autograft *n* tissue grafted from one part of the body to another.

autohypnosis the ability to induce a trance in oneself, and to become unaware of the world around. Some women use self-hypnosis to enable them to cope with the pain of labour.

autoimmune disease an illness caused by, or associated with, the development of an immune response to normal body tissues.

autoimmune haemolytic anaemia results from increased red cell destruction due to red cell autoantibodies. The antibodies may be IgG or IgM, or more rarely IgE or IgA. If an antibody avidly fixes complement, it will result in intravascular haemolysis, but if complement activation is weak, the haemolysis will be extravascular. Antibody-coated red cells lose membrane to macrophages in the spleen and hence spherocytes are present in the blood. The optimum temperature at which the antibody is active (thermal specificity) is used to classify immune haemolysis: *warm antibodies* bind best at 37°C and account for 80% of cases. The majority are IgG and usually react against Rhesus antigens; *cold antibodies* bind best at 4°C but can bind up to 37°C in some cases. They are usually IgM and bind complement. They account for the other 20% of cases. The incidence of *warm autoimmune haemolysis* is approximately 1/100 000 population per annum; it occurs at all ages but is more common in middle age and there is a female excess. No underlying cause is identified in up to 50% of cases. The remainder are secondary to a wide variety of other conditions that include: (a) lymphoid malignancies—lymphoma, chronic lymphocytic leukaemia, myeloma; (b) solid tumours—lung, colon, kidney, ovary, thymoma; (c) connective tissue disease—systemic lupus erythematosus (SLE), rheumatoid arthritis; (d) drugs—methyldopa, mefenamic acid, penicillin, quinine; (e) miscellaneous—ulcerative colitis, HIV disease. There is evidence of haemolysis and spherocytes on the blood film. The diagnosis is confirmed by the direct Coombs or antiglobulin test. The direct Coombs test can be negative in the presence of brisk haemolysis. The standard Coombs reagent will miss IgA or IgE antibodies. Management includes: (a) treating any underlying cause and any offending drugs stopped; (b) usual treatment is with prednisolone (1 mg/kg orally), there is a response in 70–80% of cases but this may take up to 3 weeks. Once the haemoglobin has reached 100 g/L, the corticosteroid dose can be reduced by 5 mg per week to 10 mg daily, then reduced slowly to nothing over a further 10 weeks. Corticosteroids work by decreasing macrophage destruction of antibody-coated red cells and reducing antibody production; (c) transfusion support may be required for life-threatening problems. The least incompatible blood should be used but may still give rise to transfusion reactions or the development of further alloantibodies; (d) if the haemolysis fails to respond to corticosteroids or can only be stabilized by large doses, then splenectomy should be considered. This removes a main site of red cell destruction and antibody production with a good response in 50–60% of cases. The operation can be performed laparoscopically with reduced morbidity; (e) patients who fail to respond to corticosteroids or for whom splenectomy is not appropriate, alternative immunosuppressive therapy (azathioprine or cyclophosphamide) may be considered. This is least suitable for young patients, for whom long-term therapy may carry a risk of secondary malignancies. *Cold agglutinin disease* is due to antibodies, usually IgM, which bind to the red cells at 4°C and cause them to agglutinate. It may cause intravascular haemolysis if complement fixation occurs. This can be chronic when the antibody is monoclonal, or acute or transient when the antibody is polyclonal. Chronic cold agglutinin disease affects older adults and may be associated with an underlying low-grade B-cell lymphoma. It causes a low-grade intravascular haemolysis with cold, painful and often blue fingers, toes, ears or nose (so-called acrocyanosis). The blood film shows red cell agglutination and the mean cell volume (MCV) may be spuriously raised because the automated analysers count aggregates as single cells. The monoclonal IgM usually has specificity against the I or, more rarely, i antigen and is present in a very high titre. Treatment is directed at any underlying lymphoma but if the disease is idiopathic, then patients must keep extremities warm, especially in winter. Some patients respond to corticosteroid therapy and blood transfusion may be considered, but the cross-match sample must be placed in a transport flask at a temperature of 37°C and blood administered via a blood-warmer. Cold agglutination can occur in association with *Mycoplasma pneumoniae* or with infectious mononucleosis. ➲ non-immune haemolytic anaemia.

autoimmune lymphoproliferative syndrome a primary T-lymphocyte deficiency caused by a failure of apoptosis.

It is characterized by accumulation of lymphocytes and persistence of autoreactive cells, and patients develop lymphadenopathy, splenomegaly and a variety of autoimmune diseases. ➲ primary T-lymphocyte deficiencies.

autoinfection *n* infection resulting from commensals becoming pathogenic, or when commensals or pathogens are transferred from one part of the body to another, for example by the hands. ➲ infection.

autointoxication *n* poisoning from abnormal or excessive metabolic products produced in the body. Some of which may originate from infected or necrotic tissue.

autologous *adj* when a patient acts as the source of cells or a graft.

autologous bone marrow transplant reinfusion of bone marrow cells originating from the recipient. May be performed for patients with leukaemia. Their bone marrow is harvested, stored and replaced after leukaemic cells have been destroyed with cytotoxic chemotherapy or radiotherapy.

autologous implant ➲ implant.

autologous transfusion a patient donates blood or blood products prior to elective surgery to be transfused during surgery or postoperatively. Cross-matching and compatibility problems are avoided, as is the risk of blood-borne infections.

autolysis *n* autodigestion which occurs if digestive enzymes escape into surrounding tissues. Occurs as a physiological process, e.g. of the uterus during the puerperium—**autolytic** *adj.*

automated auditory brainstem response (AABR) a way of testing hearing in newborns. It is performed by exposing the infant (usually when asleep) to clicking sounds via small headphones. Small sensors on the infant's head and neck convey responses to a computer, which analyses the responses to sounds beyond the cochlear of the inner ear. Specific brainstem response testing is being developed for premature infants in order to detect deafness resulting from hypoxia occurring during delivery.

automated external defibrillator (AED) a device that delivers electric shocks to victims of cardiac arrest in order to treat ventricular fibrillation. They are suitable for use by members of the public and health professionals, as they direct the operator with visual and voice prompts. AEDs may be semi-automatic or fully-automatic but all devices analyse the casualty's cardiac rhythm in order to ascertain whether a shock is required and then deliver the shock if needed. ➲ Appendix 10.

automated lamellar keratectomy an operative procedure whereby the cornea is reshaped for the correction of refractive errors.

automated peritoneal dialysis (APD) a type of peritoneal dialysis where the fluid exchanges are performed at night by the use of a mechanical device.

automatic *adj* occurring without the influence of the will; spontaneous; without volition; involuntary acts.

automatic amalgam condenser in dentistry, powered handpiece used on amalgam which has just been packed into a prepared cavity, in order to attain condensation and adaptation. It produces a series of percussions variable in speed.

automatic chemical mixers in radiography, equipment to mix the processing chemicals used to minimize the handling of chemicals by the staff, to promote even mixing and reduce chemical fumes.

automatic implantable cardioverter defibrillator (AICD) used for patients who have recurrent life-threatening arrhythmias, such as ventricular tachycardia and ventricular fibrillation. Also used in the management of patients with some types of sudden adult/arrhythmic death syndrome (SADS). The device detects the arrhythmia and delivers a small electric shock to restore sinus rhythm.

automatic processing information processing that occurs without conscious attention, as in well-learned skills. ➲ controlled processing.

automatic shuttering in digital imaging, the automatic blackening of the film outside the collimated image to increase the subjective contrast of the image. ➲ subjective contrast.

automatism *n* organized behaviour which occurs without subsequent awareness of it. For example somnambulism, hysterical and epileptic states.

autonomic *adj* independent; self-governing.

autonomic dysreflexia a serious condition that can affect people with spinal cord injuries above the level of the 7th thoracic vertebra. It results from a life-threatening sympathetic nervous system response to noxious harmful stimuli, such as bowel distension, constipation, full bladder, etc. It is characterized by tachycardia, hypertension, headache, sweating and flushing above the spinal lesion, seizures, exaggerated reflexes and distension of the bowel or bladder.

autonomic ganglia ➲ ganglion.

autonomic nervous system (ANS) is divided into parasympathetic and sympathetic divisions. They are made up of nerve cells and fibres which cannot be controlled at will. The two divisions are concerned with the control of glandular secretion and involuntary muscle, which regulate body functions which have no direct voluntary control. Consists of motor (efferent) nerves that supply the heart, secretory glands and smooth muscle (e.g. in blood vessels, intestinal tract and airways). In some organs and tissues these have opposing effects, respectively promoting an increase or a decrease in activity, e.g. sympathetic nerves stimulate the heart but quieten the gut, parasympathetic vice versa. Other organs or tissues are supplied by only one of the divisions, e.g. most blood vessels only by sympathetic and digestive secretory glands only by parasympathetic. Preganglionic fibres originate within the central nervous system (CNS) and relay at ganglia outside the CNS; thence postganglionic fibres run to the relevant tissue or organ. Visceral afferents carry information from the various sites which are subject to autonomic reflex control. ➲ Colour Section Figure 22.

autonomy the freedom to make choices based on consideration of internal and external circumstances and to act on those choices. (Reproduced with permission from the European Network of Occupational Therapy in Higher Education (ENOTHE) Terminology Project, 2008)

autopsy *n* the examination of a dead body (cadaver) for diagnostic purposes.

autorefraction 1. a procedure of refraction in which the patient adjusts the controls of the instrument. **2.** refraction carried out with an electronic optometer which is fully objective, generally using infrared light and which can be operated by a non-specialist. ➲ infrared optometer, refractive error.

autorefractor ➲ optometer.

autorefractometer ➲ optometer.

autosome *n* in humans one of 44 (22 pairs) of non-sex chromosomes. The full chromosome complement of 46 (23 pairs) found in somatic cells comprises 44 autosomes and 2 sex chromosomes.

autosomal *adj* relating to autosomes.

autosomal inheritance inheritance determined by the expression or not of genes on the autosomes. It may be dominant or recessive.

autosuggestion *n* self-suggestion; uncritical acceptance of ideas arising in the individual's own mind. Occurs in hysteria.

autotransformer a type of transformer where the primary and secondary coils are wound round a single core; it is used when only low-voltage changes are required.

autotransfusion ➲ autologous transfusion.

auxiliary spring (finger spring) in dentistry, a small gauge wire attached to arches, bows and removable appliances which applies gentle pressure to one or more teeth.

auxotrophe a mutant strain of micro-organisms that needs specific nutrients for growth not needed by the parent micro-organism. Used for microbiological assays of vitamins, etc.

A-V *abbr* **1.** arteriovenous. **2.** atrioventricular.

availability ➲ bioavailability.

avascular *adj* bloodless; not vascular, i.e. without blood supply.

avascular necrosis death of tissue due to complete depletion of its blood supply. Usually applied to that of bone tissue following injury or possibly through disease and other reasons (e.g. hyperbaric exposure [diving], excessive intake of corticosteroids or alcohol). Commonly seen with fractures of the femoral neck, leading to death of the femoral head. Also seen in scaphoid fractures in which the proximal pole may be affected, and head of humerus fractures. Bone receives its blood supply from two sources; from soft tissue structures attached to it or by intraosseous (within the bone) vessels. In certain instances one part of the bone is very dependent on the intraosseous vessels for its blood supply and if this is interrupted because of a fracture, avascular necrosis may occur. This may be a cause of non-union of the fracture and, as the fragment usually includes an articular surface, it can lead to osteoarthritis—**avascularity** *n*, **avascularize** *vt, vi.*

AV ECCO₂R *abbr* arteriovenous extracorporeal membrane carbon dioxide removal.

A
B

average dose in radiotherapy the value of dose calculated by adding together all the individual radiation doses in the area and then dividing the total by the number of doses.

average gradient in radiography, a method of measuring the straight line portion of a characteristic curve to determine the contrast of a film. A right angle triangle is drawn on the characteristic curve with the hypotenuse of the triangle extending from density 0.25 and 2 on the straight line portion of the curve. The angle between the hypotenuse and the horizontal line of the triangle is calculated, therefore the tangent of the angle the slope makes equals the average gradient. ⊃ contrast.

averaging a method of improving the signal-to-noise ratio in magnetic resonance imaging (MRI) scanning. The same magnetic resonance signal is added up and the total is divided by the number of signals.

aversion therapy a method of treatment by deconditioning. Effective in some forms of dependence and abnormal behaviour.

avian *adj* relating to birds.

avian influenza 'bird flu'. An extremely contagious viral disease affecting wild birds and commercially reared and domestic ('back yard') poultry. Some strains are highly pathogenic (H5N1) and cause up to 100% mortality in affected birds. Infection and in some cases death has occurred in humans who had close contact with sick, dead or dying birds, or infected products, such as faeces. In recent years, several epidemics of avian influenza, with subsequent human infection, have been reported, especially from South-east Asian countries and, in 2005, Eastern Europe. Of major concern to health authorities worldwide is the potential for the virus to mutate to a highly infectious form that is passed from person to person to cause an influenza pandemic.

avian tuberculosis is caused by *Mycobacterium avium complex (MAC)* or *M. avium intracellulare (MAI)*, which also cause atypical tuberculosis in humans, especially in immunocompromised individuals.

avidin *n* a high molecular weight protein with an affinity for biotin which can interfere with the absorption of biotin. Found in raw egg white.

avitaminosis *n* any disease resulting from a deficiency of vitamins.

AVM *abbr* arteriovenous malformations.

Avogadro's number ⊃ mole.

avoidance behaviour behaviour directed toward the avoidance of an undesirable outcome.

AVP *abbr* arginine vasopressin.

AVPU scale *n* a simplified tool used to assess level of consciousness. A—alert; V—voice responses present; P—pain response present; U—unresponsive. ⊃ Glasgow coma scale.

avulsion *n* a forcible wrenching away of a structure or part of the body.

avulsion fracture where the insertion of a ligament, muscle or tendon may pull a fragment of bone off when it is damaged.

Axenfeld's syndrome (K Axenfeld, German ophthalmologist, 1867–1930) (*syn* Axenfeld's anomaly) a rare, inherited disease characterized by the adhesion of strands of peripheral iris tissue to a prominent Schwalbe's line. It is occasionally associated with glaucoma. ⊃ anterior limiting ring of Schwalbe, Peters' anomaly, Rieger's syndrome.

axes *npl* the vertical (y axis) and horizontal (x axis) lines on a graph.

axial chromatic aberration ⊃ longitudinal chromatic aberration (LCA).

axial length of the eye the distance between the anterior and posterior poles of the eye. In vivo, it is typically measured by ultrasonography (although strictly speaking, that measurement represents the distance between the anterior pole and the anterior surface of the retina, in most eyes). The axial length of the eye at birth is approximately 17 mm and reaches approximately 24 mm in adulthood. ⊃ poles of the eyeball, ultrasonography in ophthalmology.

axial projection a radiograph taken when either a joint is flexed and/or the beam angled.

axial resolution in ultrasound, the ability to see small structures along the beam; this is dependent on the pulse length which is determined by the wavelength. When the distance between two reflecting surfaces of the object is half the pulse length or less the object will not be demonstrated.

axial skeleton the bones that lie centrally in the body, i.e. the skull, vertebral column, the ribs and sternum, to which the shoulder and pelvic girdles, and the limbs in turn, are linked. ⊃ appendicular skeleton, Colour Section Figures 2, 3.

axilla *n* the armpit.

axillary *adj* applied to nerves, blood and lymphatic vessels, of the axilla.

axillary artery a continuation of the subclavian artery in the axilla. The first part lies deeply; then it runs more superficially to become the brachial artery supplying oxygenated blood to the arm. ⊃ Colour Section Figure 9.

axillary nerve a nerve that arises from the posterior cord of the brachial plexus. It supplies the deltoid and teres minor muscles. ⊃ brachial plexus.

axillary tail of Spence breast tissue normally present in the axillae.

axillary vein part of the system of deep veins of the upper limb, which take the names of the arteries and follow the same route. Sited in the axilla, it is a continuation of the brachial vein and becomes the subclavian vein. ⊃ Colour Section Figure 10.

axis *n* **1.** the second cervical vertebra. An atypical vertebra, the body is small and has the upward projecting odontoid process or dens that articulates with the first cervical vertebra, the atlas. The movement at this joint is turning the head from side to side. ⊃ atlas, cervical vertebrae (spine). **2.** an imaginary line passing through the centre; the median line of the body—**axes** *pl*, **axial** *adj*.

axis (dental) various axes concerning the mandible. ⊃ intercondylar axis (dental), sagittal axis (dental), transverse horizontal axis (dental), vertical axis (dental).

axis of the birth canal/pelvis imaginary line representing the course taken by the fetus in its passage through the pelvic canal, downwards and backwards through the pelvic brim and major part of the cavity; then, at the level of the ischial spines, turning through a right angle to proceed downwards and forwards. ➲ pelvis.

axis traction the process of pulling on the fetal head to aid delivery when progress in the second stage of labour is arrested.

axis traction forceps obstetric forceps designed to allow traction to be applied in the line of the pelvic axis when the head is above the level of the pelvic outlet, rarely used now.

axolemma the membrane of an axon, it covers the cytoplasmic extension of the nerve cell body.

axon *n* the long process of a nerve cell conveying impulses away from the cell body—**axonal** *adj*.

axonotmesis *n* (*syn* neuronotmesis, neurotmesis) peripheral degeneration as a result of damage to the axons of a nerve, through pinching, crushing or prolonged pressure. The internal architecture is preserved and recovery depends upon regeneration of the axons, and may take many months.

axon reflex reflex dilatation of the arterioles occurring when sensory nerves in the skin are stimulated by trauma or massage manipulations. ➲ triple response.

axoplasmic transport the process of transporting materials down an axon.

azoospermia *n* sterility of the male through non-production of spermatozoa.

azotaemia *n* ➲ uraemia.

azygos *adj* occurring singly, not paired. *azygos veins* three unpaired veins of the abdomen and thorax which empty into the inferior vena cava—**azygous** *adj*.

B₀ the symbol used for the static main magnetic field, in magnetic resonance imaging (MRI), which is orientated along the x axis and measured in tesla.

B₁ the symbol used for radiofrequency magnetic field, in a magnetic resonance imaging (MRI) system, and measured in tesla.

Babinski's reflex or sign (J F Babinski, French neurologist, 1857–1932) (*syn* plantar response) movement of the great toe upwards (dorsiflexion) instead of downwards (plantar flexion) on stroking the sole of the foot. It is indicative of disease or injury to upper motor neurons. Babies exhibit dorsiflexion, but after learning to walk they show the normal plantar flexion response.

baby blues a colloquial term for the transient low mood and tearfulness experienced by some women a few days after childbirth.

baby bottle tooth decay dental decay in children aged between 12 months and 3 years. It results from a child being given a bottle just before being put to bed and the consequent prolonged exposure to sugars in the milk or fruit juice.

Baby Friendly Initiative (BFI) the World Health Organization (WHO) and United Nations Children's Fund (UNICEF) campaign to ensure that all mothers are facilitated in order to benefit from the health and social advantages. The WHO/UNICEF initiative, *Ten Steps to Successful Breastfeeding*, offers health professionals an inexpensive, effective means by which to promote breastfeeding and an award incentive: a hospital which implements all 10 steps and achieves a 75% breastfeeding rate is awarded a Global Award; one which implements all 10 steps and achieves a 50–75% breastfeeding rate is awarded the UK Standard; a Certificate of Commitment is given where a hospital is working towards the 10 steps. The ten steps to successful breastfeeding are: breastfeeding policy available and communicated to all staff; all healthcare staff trained to implement the policy; all pregnant mothers informed of the benefits and management of breastfeeding; mothers assisted to commence breastfeeding within half an hour of delivery; education of mothers re breastfeeding and maintening lactation even when separated from their babies; neonates to be given only breast milk unless medically necessary; 24-hour rooming in; on demand breastfeeding; no teats or pacifiers to be given to breastfeeding babies; and establishment of breastfeeding support groups.

Baby Life Support Systems (BLISS) charitable organization which raises money for equipment for babies requiring special and intensive care in neonatal units.

Bach Flower remedies system of complementary medicine, devised by Dr Edward Bach, based partly on homoeopathic principles, in which remedies made from plants are used to treat emotional and psychological disorders. There are 38 flower remedies plus Rescue Remedy. ⊃ homoeopathy.

bacillaemia *n* the presence of bacilli in the blood—**bacillaemic** *adj*.

bacille Calmette–Guérin ⊃ BCG.

bacilluria *n* the presence of bacilli in the urine—**bacilluric** *adj*.

Bacillus *n* (also a colloquial term for any rod-shaped micro-organism). A genus of bacteria consisting of aerobic, Gram-positive, rod-shaped cells that produce endospores. The majority have flagella and are motile. The spores are common in soil and dust. *Bacillus anthracis* causes anthrax in humans and domestic animals. *Bacillus cereus* produces exotoxins and causes food poisoning. It can occur after eating cooked food, e.g. rice, that has been stored prior to reheating.

backache during pregnancy pain located over the lumbar region of the back; occurs frequently in pregnancy due to changes in the centre of gravity as the uterus becomes heavier.

background diabetic retinopathy (*syn* non-proliferative diabetic retinopathy [NPDR]) a progressive microangiopathy of the retinal vessels occurring in the early stage of diabetic retinopathy. It is characterized by microaneurysms, dot-blot haemorrhages, flame-shaped haemorrhages, hard exudates and retinal oedema. Retinal veins may also become dilated and tortuous. If the microvascular occlusion progresses there will be signs of ischaemia and multiple cotton-wool spots will appear, as well as more venous changes and maculopathy, producing the clinical picture of preproliferative diabetic retinopathy. If the macular oedema is not clinically significant the patient remains asymptomatic, although a blue-yellow colour vision defect will usually develop. ⊃ diabetic retinopathy.

backing in dentistry, the metal component of a crown, bridge or denture designed to protect a tooth-coloured facing (usually of porcelain).

back injury injury to the back may affect the bones (vertebral column including the sacrum, also the ilium or the ribs), muscles and ligaments. Sport-related back injuries include fractures and damage from overuse, especially to the soft tissues. Mechanical and postural causes are common and a significant cause of morbidity in the general population. Damage may be prevented by attention to posture, flexibility, muscle strength and fitness. ⊃ ankylosing spondylitis, intervertebral disc, spinal injury/spinal cord injury.

back pointer used in radiotherapy to indicate the central exit point of the radiation. ⊃ front pointer.

back power ⊃ back vertex power (BVP).

back projection mathematical basis for tomographic imaging. In compted tomography (CT) scanning in order to overcome the blurring inherent in this method a filtered back projection is used, resulting in a sharper image.

back scatter radiation that having passed through the object hits a surface, for example the couch, and is reflected onto the original object.

back-slab splint a split specifically produced for the posterior part of a limb, used to immobilize a joint. For example, a lower limb back-slab splint that extends from ankle to hip is designed to prevent movement at the knee. Uses include minimizing the risk of contracture formation.

back toric contact lens a contact lens used to correct corneal astigmatism, in which the surface of the lens facing the cornea is not spherical but toroidal in order to obtain a good physical fit on the cornea. To create better stability of the lens on the eye it usually incorporates a prism ballast.

back up a computer term meaning to store data by copying from the primary data source (hard disk) to a removable device, for example a disk or flash drive.

back vertex power (BVP) (*syn* back power) the symbol is F'_v. It is the reciprocal of the back vertex focal length. It is equal to

$$F'_v = \frac{n'}{SF'}$$

where n' is the refractive index of the second medium, S is the point on the back surface through which passes the optical axis and F' the second principal focus. The back vertex power is the usual measurement made by a focimeter. ⊃ effective power, equivalent power, vergence, vertex focal length.

bacteraemia *n* the presence of bacteria in the blood—**bacteraemic** *adj*.

bacteria *npl* microscopic unicellular organisms widely distributed in the environment. They may be free-living, sacrophytic or parasitic. Bacteria can be pathogenic to humans, other animals and plants, or non-pathogenic. Pathogens may be virulent and always cause infection, whereas others, known as opportunists, usually only cause infection when the host defences are impaired, such as during cancer chemotherapy. Non-pathogenic bacteria may become pathogenic if they move from their normal site, e.g. intestinal bacteria causing a wound infection. Reproduction is generally by simple binary fission when environmental conditions are suitable. Many bacteria have developed adaptations that allow them to exploit environments and survive unfriendly conditions, e.g. flagella, pili, waxy outer capsules, spore formation and enzymes that destroy antibiotics. Bacteria are classified and identified by features that include: shape and staining characteristics with Gram

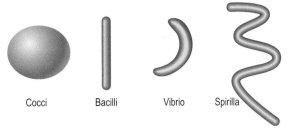

| Cocci | Bacilli | Vibrio | Spirilla |

B.1 Bacterial shapes (reproduced from Brooker 2006A with permission).

stain (positive or negative). Bacteria shapes may be (Figure B.1): (a) round (cocci), paired (diplococci), in bunches (staphylococci) or in chains (streptococci); (b) rod-shaped (bacilli); or (c) curved or spiral (vibrios, spirilla and spirochaetes)—**bacterium** *sing*.

bacterial *adj* pertaining to bacteria.

bacterial vaginosis (BV) vaginal flora overgrowth, e.g. of *Gardnerella vaginalis*, causing vaginal discharge with characteristic fishy odour. It is not sexually transmitted but may be triggered by increased sexual activity, stress, other infections and use of perfumed feminine hygiene products. It occurs in 15–29% of pregnant women and is linked to—pelvic inflammatory disease, preterm labour, recurrent urinary tract infections, postpartum infection, uterine infections following termination, surgery or insertion of intrauterine contraceptive device. Treatment is with antibiotics, e.g. metronidazole.

bactericidal *adj* describes agents that kill bacteria, e.g. some antibiotics—**bactericide** *n*, **bactericidally** *adv*.

bactericidin *n* antibody that kills bacteria.

bacter/io- a prefix that means 'bacteria', e.g. *bacteraemia*.

bacteriologist *n* an expert in bacteriology.

bacteriology *n* the scientific study of bacteria—**bacteriological** *adj*, **bacteriologically** *adv*.

bacteriolysin *n* a specific antibody formed in the blood that causes bacteria to break up.

bacteriolysis *n* the disintegration and dissolution of bacteria—**bacteriolytic** *adj*.

bacteriophage *n* a virus parasitic on bacteria. Some of these are used in phage-typing staphylococci, etc. ⊃ transduction.

bacteriostatic *adj* describes an agent that inhibits bacterial growth, e.g. some antibiotics—**bacteriostasis** *n*.

bacteriuria *n* the presence of bacteria in the urine. Acute cystitis may be preceded by, and active pyelonephritis may be associated with, asymptomatic bacteriuria. ⊃ asymptomatic bacteriuria.

Bacteroides *n* a genus of Gram-negative, anaerobic rod-shaped bacteria, e.g. *Bacteroides fragilis*. They do not form endospores and may be motile or non-motile. They are important commensals in the gastrointestinal flora where they convert complex molecules into simpler substances. The bacteria are also present in the mouth and genital tract.

They can cause appendicitis, peritonitis, pelvic inflammatory disease and infections following gastrointestinal and gynaecological surgery. Some species are opportunistic. They are resistant to many antibiotic drugs.

Badal's optometer (J Badal, French ophthalmologist, 1840–1929) a simple, subjective optometer consisting of a single positive lens and a movable target. The vergence of light from the target, after refraction through the lens, depends upon the position of the target. The person is instructed to move the target towards the lens from a position where it appears blurred until it becomes clear. That point (converted in dioptric value) represents the refraction of the person's eye. This is a crude and inaccurate instrument, in which the measurement is marred by accommodation, variation in retinal image size with target distance, large depth of focus, non-linearity of the scale, etc. Badal's improvement was to place the lens so that its focal point coincides with either the nodal point of the eye or the anterior focal point of the eye or the entrance pupil of the eye, thus overcoming the problems of the non-linear scale and the changing retinal image size. ➲ refractive error.

Bagolini's glass (B Bagolini, Italian opthalmologist, b. 1924) (*syn* Bagolini's lens) a lens on which fine parallel striations have been grooved. It produces a slight reduction in acuity but a light source observed through this lens appears as a streak of light orientated at 90° from the striations. Such a lens is used in the analysis of anomalous correspondence, suppression, etc. For example, in testing suppression the lenses can be placed in a trial frame with the striations at an angle of 135° for one eye and 45° for the other eye. A spotlight stimulus at distance or near is used, and if there is no suppression, the patient will see two diagonal lines crossing at, above or below the light source. If there is suppression, all or part of one line will not be seen. If the two diagonal lines cross at the source when the cover test indicated an ocular deviation, the patient has harmonious, abnormal retinal correspondence. ➲ abnormal retinal correspondence.

Bailey-Lovie chart a visual acuity chart with letter sizes ranging from 6/60 (20/200) to 6/3 (20/10) in 14 rows of 5 letters. Each row has letters which are approximately 4/5 the size of the next larger letters and the letters in each row have approximately the same legibility (within ±10%). It is most useful with low vision patients. This is the most commonly used type of log minimum angle of resolution (MAR) chart (Figure B.2) There is also a Bailey-Lovie Word Reading Chart for near vision. It is composed of words rather than letters. The size progression of each line is logarithmic. The typeface used is the lower case Times Roman customarily used in newspapers and books, and the range of sizes varies between 80-point and 2-point print (or the Snellen equivalent at 40 cm of 6/144 or 20/480 to 6/3.6 or 20/12, respectively). There are 20 such charts, each with a different set of words. ➲ contrast sensitivity chart, low vision.

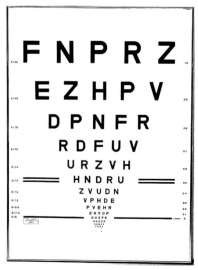

B.2 Bailey-Lovie chart (reproduced from Millodot 2004 with permission).

Bainbridge reflex (F Bainbridge, British physiologist, 1874–1921) stretch receptors in the heart (right atrium) can increase heart rate through sympathetic stimulation when venous return increases.

bake in dentistry, the process by which porcelain restorations are hardened by heating at electrically controlled temperatures generally in a vacuum furnace, the vacuum reducing the possibility of air bubbles. The porcelain is first baked to a biscuit state and then glazed at a higher temperature. ➲ biscuit.

Baker's cyst (W Baker, British surgeon, 1839–1896) an enlargement of the normally small bursa in the popliteal fossa, behind the knee. May cause pain and discomfort if large or inflamed (bursitis). It may occur with rheumatoid arthritis.

baker's itch 1. contact dermatitis resulting from flour or sugar. **2.** itchy papules from the bite of the flour mite *Pyemotes*.

BAL *abbr* **1.** British antilewisite. ➲ dimercaprol **2.** bronchoalveolar lavage.

balance *n* the ability to maintain body equilibrium by controlling the body's centre of gravity over its base of support. Balance reactions are complex responses based on prior experiential learning on a foundation of normal nervous system functioning. The two most commonly described responses are: righting reactions, these are automatic reactions that serve to bring the head and trunk back into midline; equilibrium reactions, these are small often unperceivable reactions that help to maintain posture and position during movement.

balance of probabilities the standard of proof required in civil legal proceedings.

balanced articulation ➲ balanced occlusion.

balanced occlusion a state in which the teeth of complete dentures, or the natural teeth, meet overall without any one tooth causing interference with the occlusion or balance of the prosthesis or dentition.

balanced diet a diet that contains the correct amount of all nutrients (macronutrients and micronutrients) from a wide range of foods. Should also contain the correct proportions of food types, for example, reduced fat, sugar and salt and at least five portions of fruit and vegetables per day. In general, dietary guidelines for the average population are also applicable to athletes, but there are differences for athletes in the recommended intake of macronutrients (carbohydrate, fat and protein), in terms of grams per day, grams per day per kg body mass or percentage of energy intake from each of the main foodstuffs. ⊃ dietary reference values (DRV), Appendix 4.

balancing extraction extraction of a tooth, following the removal of one from the contralateral side or opposite arch, in order to balance space loss, prevent drift from the midline and hopefully preserve symmetry of the dental arch.

balancing test (*syn* equalization test) a test designed to obtain equal focusing or equal accommodative states in the two eyes. This is accomplished either objectively (by retinoscopy) or, more commonly, subjectively using either the duochrome test, or comparing the visual acuity in the two eyes simultaneously or successively, or using prisms to present two images of a chart and ask the patient to compare these images, or using a binocular refraction technique (e.g. Turville infinity balance test). ⊃ duochrome test, Turville infinity balance test, vectogram.

balanitis *n* inflammation of the glans penis.

balanitis xerotica obliterans (BXO) (Csillag's disease) a group of chronic conditions, lichen sclerosis atrophicus is one type. It is characterized by whitish alteration seen on the penis or prepuce. There may be soreness and irritation. If the balanitis affects the glans, it can cause meatal stenosis. It is a common condition and usually benign, but it may occasionally be a premalignant change that could become cancerous.

balanoposthitis *n* inflammation of the glans penis and prepuce.

balantidiasis *n* infestation due to ingesting the cysts of the protozoan *Balantidium coli*. Its presence in the large intestine can cause diarrhoea and possibly ulceration of the intestinal wall with abscesses and ulcers.

Balantidium coli a parasitic protozoan that causes balantidiasis in humans. It is a commensal micro-organism of the gastrointestinal tract of pigs.

balanus *n* the glans of the penis or clitoris.

baldness *n* ⊃ alopecia.

ballast additional weight of material incorporated in a part of a contact lens to maintain it in a given orientation. This is often provided by giving prismatic power to the lens (prism ballast lens).

ballism ⊃ ballismus.

ballismus also known as ballism. A neurological condition chararacterized by uncontrolled ballistic movements. There is jerky, uncoordinated limb movement. It is associated with extrapyramidal conditions. When it affects one side of the body it is termed hemiballismus.

ballistic movement high-intensity movement, such as a long kick, in which a limb or part of a limb is initially accelerated forward by concentric muscle action, then swings pendulum-like through a passive (inertial or 'ballistic') phase of constant velocity, before being eccentrically decelerated.

ballistic stretching the use of a rapid stretch or repetitive bouncing motions at the end of the available range of movement to increase soft tissue flexibility.

ball-and-socket joint enarthrosis. A synovial joint, e.g. the hip or shoulder, where the ball-shaped head of one bone fits into the cuplike depression in another bone. This type of joint allows the greatest range of motion.

ball catcher's projection an anteroposterior oblique projection of both hands.

ballottement literally, bouncing. Tapping a structure in fluid, e.g. the fetus in the amniotic sac, causes it to rebound against the examining fingers. *internal b.* elicited by inserting two fingers *per vaginam* at about 16 to 18 weeks of pregnancy to tap the fetus, causing it to float away and quickly return to the examining fingers. *external b.* elicited during an examination *per abdomen* when the head is not engaged; the fetal head is tapped sharply on one side, floats away and is then felt to return against the examining fingers—**ballottable** *adj.*

balneotherapy *n* the use of therapeutic bathing in a variety of conditions. It can be used, for instance, to improve mobility or reduce pain. ⊃ hydrotherapy.

bamboo spine the term for the X-ray appearance in advanced ankylosing spondylitis, fusion of adjacent vertebrae makes the spine look like a piece of bamboo.

BAN *acron* **B**ritish **A**pproved **N**ame.

band a stainless steel metal ring formed to the circumference of a tooth, most commonly used to retain orthodontic brackets on molar teeth. ⊃ band pusher (or driver), band seater, matrix band, orthodontic band, preformed band.

band pusher (or driver) an instrument used to adapt and place a stainless steel band on a tooth.

band seater a flat-bladed instrument used to push bands onto a tooth by biting force.

bandage *n* material applied to a wound or used to bind an injured part of the body. May be used to: (a) retain a dressing or splint; (b) support, compress, immobilize; (c) prevent or correct deformity. Available in strips or circular form in a range of different materials and applying varying levels of pressure. Compression bandages are widely used in the management of venous leg ulceration.

bandage lens ⊃ therapeutic soft contact lens.

Bandl's ring (L Bandl, German obstetrician, 1842–1892) an abnormally enlarged retraction ring that forms between the upper and lower uterine segments, as the lower segment continues to thin if labour is obstructed. It presents as an oblique ridge seen above the symphysis pubis. Palpable as a transverse ridge across the abdomen; a sign of imminent uterine rupture. ⊃ retraction ring.

bandpass filter a filter which allows the passage of radiations only within a narrow band of wavelengths around a central wavelength. This is done by multilayer coating which produces destructive interference. ⊃ coated lens, coating.

bandwidth the difference between the maximum and minimum frequency in a system. A range of frequencies in magnetic resonance. ⊃ receiver bandwidth, transmitter bandwidth.

Bankart's lesion (A Bankart, British orthopaedic surgeon, 1879–1951) damage to the capsule of the shoulder joint at the rim of the glenoid cavity of the scapula, caused by traumatic anterior dislocation of the shoulder joint and leading to recurrent dislocation with relatively minor injury. The lesion was first described by Bankart in the 1920s. Bankart's operation repairs the defect.

Bankart's operation (A Bankart) for recurrent dislocation of the shoulder joint: the defect of the glenoid cavity is repaired.

banned substance a substance which is on the list of banned doping classes and methods of the World Anti-Doping Agency (WADA). ⊃ doping (in sport), World Anti-Doping Agency (WADA)

Banti's syndrome (G Banti, Italian pathologist, 1852–1925) a syndrome characterized by hepatic portal hypertension, splenomegaly, gastrointestinal bleeding, leucopenia and anaemia. It is associated with liver cirrhosis.

bar in prosthetic dentistry, a metal segment of greater length than width that is used to connect two parts of a removable partial denture. A bar attached to two or more teeth or roots in order to support and retain a complete or partial denture. e.g. *bar attachment* a bar joining two or more roots, teeth or implant superstructures and supporting or retaining a prosthesis. *bar connector* in prosthetics, a bar joining two or more parts of a partial denture. ⊃ connector, Dolder bar, lingual bar.

bar reading test (*syn* Welland's test) a test for determining the presence of binocular vision and also used in the management of amblyopia in which a narrow bar (or a pencil) is held vertically between the reader's eyes and a page of print. The bar occludes a vertical strip of print but the strip is different for the two eyes and if binocular vision is present the subject will experience no difficulty reading the text.

Barbados leg (*syn* elephant leg) ⊃ elephantiasis.

barbiturates *npl* a group of sedative/hypnotic drugs. They are associated with serious problems of dependence and tolerance, and sudden withdrawal may cause a serious withdrawal syndrome that includes anxiety, convulsions and even death. They have been replaced by safer drugs and their use is limited to anaesthesia and sometimes for epilepsy.

barbotage *n* a method of extending the spread of spinal anaesthesia whereby local anaesthetic is directly mixed with aspirated cerebrospinal fluid and reinjected into the subarachnoid space.

bar chart a graph displaying the data in columns, which are separate from each other.

bare lymphocyte syndromes a group of primary T-lymphocyte deficiencies. These are caused by absent expression of human leucoctye antigens (HLA) molecules within the thymus. If HLA class I molecules are affected, CD8+ lymphocytes fail to develop, while absent expression of HLA class II molecules affects CD4+ lymphocyte maturation. In addition to recurrent infections, failure to express HLA class I is associated with systemic vasculitis caused by uncontrolled activation of natural killer cells. ⊃ primary T-lymphocyte deficiencies.

bariatrics a branch of medicine and surgery that deals with obesity, it effects and control.

baritosis a form of pneumoconiosis caused by the inhalation of barium dust.

barium enema a radiographic examination of the large bowel using barium sulphate as the contrast agent. Barium sulphate liquid, followed by a quantity of air, is introduced into the large bowel by means of a rectal tube, during fluoroscopy. It is used for diagnostic purposes, e.g. for colon cancers, in conjunction with endoscopy. ⊃ barium sulphate, colonoscopy.

barium meal, swallow a radiographic examination of the upper gastrointestinal tract (oesophagus and stomach) and the small intestine with follow-through X-rays, using barium sulphate as the contrast agent. The barium sulphate suspension is swallowed and radiographs are taken of the gastrointestinal tract. Pre-examination fasting is required and medicines, e.g. some antacids, that may interfere with the examination should be stopped. Further fasting may be required until follow-through X-rays are completed. ⊃ small bowel enema.

barium sulphate a heavy insoluble powder used, in an aqueous suspension, as a contrast agent in radiographic visualization of the alimentary tract by either being introduced orally, via the rectum or via a colostomy.

Barlow's sign/test a manoeuvre designed to test for congenitally dislocatable hips in the neonate. A modification of Ortolani's test. The baby lies on his back with feet pointing towards the examiner who grasps each leg with knees and hips flexed, places the middle fingers of each hand over the greater trochanter and the thumb of each hand on the inner aspect of the thigh. The thighs are abducted and the middle finger of each hand pushes the greater trochanter forward; if the hip is dislocated the femoral head will 'click' as it enters the acetabulum; the femoral head can be displaced backwards out of the acetabulum by exerting slight pressure when the hips are flexed and adducted (Barlow's sign). ⊃ developmental dysplasia of the hip.

barn a unit of measure used in atomic physics to measure cross sections which equal 10^{-28} m^2. ⊃ scattered cross-section.

barodontalgia *n* also called aerodontalgia. Toothache caused by the reduction in ambient pressure during high-altitude flying and due to the expansion of gas within the pulp chamber of a tooth.

barometric pressure the pressure due to the column of atmosphere above an object or body (measured also in millimetres of mercury or millibars). ⊃ pressure.

baroreceptors *npl* sensory nerve endings which respond to pressure changes. They are present in the cardiac atria, aortic arch, venae cavae, carotid sinus and the inner ear. Those sensory nerve endings in the vascular system respond to changes in pressure within blood vessels, generating afferent nerve impulses which elicit baroreflexes, causing appropriate corrections. The main arterial baroreceptors are in the wall of the carotid sinus on each side of the neck, where the common carotid artery divides into the internal and external carotids, and are responsible for regulation of arterial blood pressure, thereby a rise in pressure elicits reflex reduction in peripheral resistance and/or cardiac output, via control centres in the brain stem.

barotitis also called aerotitis. Inflammation affecting the ear caused by changes in atmospheric pressure.

barotrauma *n* injury due to unequalized changes in atmospheric or water pressure, e.g. ruptured eardrum. Divers can be affected painfully by inequality between high ambient pressure at depth and that in closed internal air-containing spaces such as the the paranasal air sinuses or the middle ear. Aural barotrauma results in an inward bulging or at worst rupture of the tympanic membrane (eardrum), if the pharyngotympanic (eustachian) tube is blocked. During surfacing the danger is pulmonary barotrauma resulting in the rupture of the lung surface by expanding air, with escape into the pleural cavity leading to pneumothorax when surfacing without effective exhalation. ⊃ decompression illness/sickness, diving.

Barr body ⊃ sex chromatin.

barrel chest a term used to describe the shape of the thorax in states of hyperinflation. Most marked is the increased antero-posterior diameter of the chest. A change in the shape of the chest cage that may occur in certain lung diseases.

barrer a unit of oxygen permeability of a contact lens material. The symbol is *Dk*. It is equal to the product of the diffusion coefficient *D* of oxygen through the material (i.e. the speed at which oxygen molecules pass through the material) and the solubility *k* of oxygen in the material (i.e. the number of oxygen molecules that can be absorbed in a given volume of material). ⊃ oxygen permeability, oxygen transmissibility.

Barrett's oesophagus (N R Barrett, British surgeon, 1903–1979). Columnar-lined oesophagus replacing normal squamous mucosa. Related to chronic gastro-oesophageal reflux disease (GORD). Predisposes to oesophageal cancer. ⊃ Colour Section Figure 51.

barrier contraception mechanical barrier to prevent sperm from entering cervical canal, e.g. diaphragm.

barrier nursing a method of preventing the spread of infection from an infectious individual to other people. It is achieved by isolation techniques. ⊃ containment isolation, isolation, protective isolation, source isolation.

Barron's banding apparatus a device used to treat haemorrhoids by elastic band ligation.

Barthel index (D Barthel, American psychiatrist, 20th century) a disability profiles score. It is based on an assessment of a person's ability to selfcare in ten functional areas, which include dressing, hygiene, bladder and bowel control, feeding and walking.

Bartholin's glands (greater vestibular glands) (C Bartholin, Danish anatomist, 1655–1738). Two small glands situated at each side of the external orifice of the vagina. Their ducts open into the vestibule. They produce lubricating mucus that facilitates coitus.

bartholinitis *n* inflammation of Bartholin's (greater vestibular) glands.

Bartonella (A Barton, Peruvian bacteriologist, 1871–1950), a genus of Gram-negative micro-organisms. Various species infect red blood cells, liver, spleen and lymph nodes. *Bartonella bacilliformis* causes bartonellosis, *B. henselae* causes cat-scratch fever. Other species cause trench fever, endocarditis and myocarditis.

bartonellosis *n* an infection caused by *B. bacilliformis*. It is transmitted by the bite of a sandfly and causes anaemia, fever and skin lesions. The infection is endemic in valleys of the Andes across Columbia, Peru and Ecuador. Known as Oroya fever, Carrión's disease or verruga peruana.

Barton's fracture a break in the distal articular surface of the radius which may be associated with dorsal dislocation of the carpus on the radius.

Barts' test a blood test offered at 16–18 weeks' gestation to identify women at high risk of having an abnormal fetus. Now more commonly known as the *double, triple* or *quadruple test*.

Bartter syndrome (F Bartter, American physician, 1914–1983), a rare genetic syndrome, which affects the kidneys resulting in secondary hyperaldosteronism. The blood pressure is usually normal or low even though the levels of renin and angiotensin are raised. There are problems with electrolyte and acid–base balance; hypokalaemia, hypercalciuria and metabolic alkalosis. The infant/child may have excessive thirst (polydipsia) and pass large volumes of urine (polyuria) and life-threatening dehydration can occur if fluids are not replaced. Muscle weakness is a feature and physical growth and mental development may be slowed. Hypercalciuria can lead to kidney stones and possibly end-stage renal failure. Management includes potassium supplements; potassium-sparing drugs, e.g. spironolactone; ACE-inhibitor drugs; and for some types of Bartter syndrome NSAIDs.

BAS *abbr* behavioural activation system.

basal bone that part of the maxilla or mandible which underlies the alveolar process. ⊃ alveolar bone, bundle bone.

basal cell carcinoma (BCC) rodent ulcer. A common type of skin cancer. Often seen on the face which, although locally invasive, does not give rise to metastases. ➲ Colour Section Figure 52.

basal cell papilloma ➲ seborrhoeic warts.

basal dose rate used in brachytherapy and is the average of all dose rates calculated at the minimum dose point in the central transverse plane of a brachytherapy dose distribution. Used in the Paris system of dosimetry.

basal ganglia ➲ basal nuclei.

basal metabolic rate (BMR) some authorities use the term resting metabolic rate. The rate at which energy is consumed at complete rest for essential physiological functions. It is the expression of basal metabolism in terms of kJ per m^2 of body surface per hour. BMR is influenced by nutritional status, age, gender, physiological status, disease, certain drugs and ambient temperature. It is determined by measuring the oxygen consumption when the energy output has been reduced to a basal minimum, that is the person is fasting and is physically and mentally at rest. In clinical practice the resting metabolic rate (RMR) may be measured or BMR is estimated by prediction equations and used to estimate energy requirements. ➲ metabolic equivalent, metabolic rate.

basal narcosis the preanaesthetic administration of narcotic drugs which reduce fear and anxiety and induce sleep.

basal nuclei a collection of interconnected nuclei (masses of grey matter) deep within the cerebral hemispheres concerned with cognition, and modifying and coordinating voluntary muscle movement. Their proper functioning requires the release of the neurotransmitter dopamine. Sometimes erroneously referred to as ganglia, which more properly describes structures in the peripheral nervous system. Site of degeneration in Parkinson's disease. ➲ dopamine.

base *n* **1.** the lowest part, such as the lung. ➲ Colour Section Figure 7. **2.** the major part of a compound. **3.** an alkali. **4.** in radiography, a supporting medium for other layers of either a film or intensifying screens. **5.** in dentistry, that part of a removable prosthesis in contact with the tissues and which supports the artificial teeth—**basal, basic** *adj.* ➲ blue-based films, clear-based films.

base line the line joining the centres of rotation of the two eyes. It is approximately equal to the interpupillary distance

base of support the area between the body part and the surface with which it makes contact. The larger the base of support the less muscle activity is required. For instance, less muscular activity is needed when sitting in a chair than that needed when standing up, or trying to balance on one foot.

baseline fetal heart rate the fetal heart rate as measured in early labour, to which later patterns can be compared and used for diagnosis of possible abnormalities.

baseline measurements 1. the routine recording of vital signs when a person is either admitted to a healthcare facility, or consults a health professional as an outpatient. These might include temperature, pulse, respiration and blood pressure and they provide an initial baseline from which to

compare subsequent recordings. **2.** in sports medicine, the initial physical findings which are usually performed while the athlete is in a healthy state. **3.** in occupational therapy practice, the process of collecting information about the client's current level of functioning in order to provide a point of reference against which change can be measured.

basement membrane *n* the thin layer of tissue that separates the epithelium of mucous surfaces from the underlying structures (see Figure E.7, p. 264).

base metal alloy alloy containing cobalt, chromium and nickel, in varying quantities. Used in conservative and prosthetic dentistry as an inexpensive alternative to the noble metal alloys.

baseplate 1. temporary foundation on which an occlusal rim is built or on which a trial denture is set up. Consists of a combination of waxes and resins or acrylic. **2.** the acrylic resin part of a removable orthodontic appliance, fitting to the necks of standing teeth and the mucosa, and securing in position any springs, wires of clasps.

baseplate wax a hard pink wax used in the laboratory for denture construction.

BASES *abbr* **B**ritish **A**ssociation for **S**port and **E**xercise **S**cience.

BASIC *acron* **B**eginners **A**ll-purpose **S**ymbolic **I**nstruction **C**ode.

basic fog in radiography, the recorded density of a radiographic film base plus the recorded density of chemical blackening on an unexposed part of a film.

basic input/output system (BIOS) describes computer programs which are permanently embedded in a chip (ROM). They are used by the computer operating system to perform fundamental input/output tasks. ➲ chip, read only memory (ROM).

basic life support (BLS) a term that describes the application of artificial respiration, usually by rescue breaths (mouth-to-mouth/nose breathing) and chest compressions (external cardiac massage) to save life without the use of artificial aids or equipment in the case of cardiac or respiratory arrest. Techniques differ between adult BLS, paediatric BLS and newborn life support. ➲ Appendix 10.

basic secretion test measurement of the basal tear secretion independently of reflex tear secretion. A filter paper strip (e.g. Whatman No. 41) is placed in the anaesthetized lower fornix and after 5 minutes the strip is removed and the amount of wetting measured from the folded end. ➲ Schirmer's test, tear secretion test.

basilar artery *n* forms part of the circulus arteriosus (circle of Willis); it supplies blood to the brainstem.

basilar membrane *n* the membrane between the scala media and the scala tympani in the cochlea of the inner ear. It has the specialized cochlear hair cells that contain the auditory receptors. ➲ Reissner's membrane

basilic *adj* prominent.

basilic vein *n* a superficial vein that begins at the back of the hand on the ulnar aspect. It ascends on the medial side of the forearm and upper arm then joins the axillary vein (deep vein). It receives blood from the medial aspect of the hand, forearm and arm. There are many small veins which link the cephalic and basilic veins. ⊃ Colour Section Figure 10.

basket crown cast metal three-quarter crown, with or without a facing, used as a temporary restoration for a fractured or malformed tooth.

basophil *n* **1.** a cell which has an affinity for basic dyes. **2.** a polymorphonuclear granulocyte (white blood cell) which takes up a particular dye: it is phagocytic and has granules containing heparin and histamine.

basophilia *n* **1.** increase in the number of basophils in the blood. **2.** basophilic staining of red blood cells.

Batchelor plaster a type of double abduction plaster, with the legs encased from groins to ankles, in full abduction and medial rotation. The feet are then attached to a wooden pole or 'broomstick'. Alternative to frog plaster, but the hips are free. ⊃ developmental dysplasia of the hip.

bat ears the outer/external ear protrudes away from the head. They can be corrected by surgery if the child/parent, or person is unhappy about their appearance.

bath *n* **1.** the apparatus used for bathing. **2.** the immersion of the body or any part of it in water or any fluid; or the application of spray, jet or vapour of such a fluid to the body. The term is modified according to: (a) temperature, e.g. cold, contrast, hot, tepid; (b) medium used, e.g. mud, water, wax; (c) medicament added, e.g. potassium permanganate; (d) function of medicament, e.g. astringent, antiseptic. ⊃ balneotherapy, hydrotherapy.

Batten's disease (F Batten, British neurologist, 1865–1918) one of a group of genetic diseases that are characterized by disorded metabolism of fatty acids leading to visual impairment, encephalopathy and progressive mental deterioration.

battery *n* legal term. An unlawful touching or contact. Constitutes a trespass against the person. ⊃ assault.

battledore placenta placenta with the umbilical cord attached to the margin instead of the centre. ⊃ placenta.

Battle's sign (W Battle, British surgeon, 1855–1936) ecchymosis or bogginess felt over the mastoid process indicative of a skull fracture.

Bazin's disease (*syn* erythema induratum) (P Bazin, French dermatologist, 1807–1878) a chronic recurrent disorder, involving the skin of the legs of women. There are deep-seated nodules which later ulcerate.

BBA *abbr* born before arrival (at hospital).

BBB *abbr* **1.** blood–brain barrier. **2.** bundle branch block.

BBV *abbr* blood-borne virus.

BCAA *abbr* branched-chain amino acid.

BCC *abbr* basal cell carcinoma.

B cells ⊃ lymphocytes.

BCG *abbr* bacille Calmette–Guérin. An attenuated form of tubercle bacilli: it has lost its power to cause tuberculosis, but retains its antigenic function; it is the base of a vaccine used for immunization against tuberculosis. In the UK it is offered to groups at increased risk, e.g. all newborns and infants who live in a high risk area where TB cases are greater that 40 per 100 000, people in contact with cases of active TB, etc. Also used in urology for the treatment of high risk superficial bladder cancer.

BDD *abbr* body dysmorphic disorder.

bdelygmia an extreme dislike or loathing for food.

BDHA *abbr* British Dental Hygienists' Association.

bead on string ⊃ Brock's string.

beam *n* metal pole attached to a hospital bed to facilitate the use of traction. For example, a Thomas' splint can be slung up, with pulleys and weights attached, to allow movement and provide counterbalance to the weight of the splint and leg.

beam direction device in radiotherapy/radiography, pointers, light sources or laser beams used to indicate the beam direction, the centre of the beam and the source skin distance.

beam direction shell in radiotherapy, a device worn by the patient to enable accurate and reproducible treatment localization, patient positioning, patient contour, beam exit and entry points and a base for additional build-up material. Produced using either clear Perspex or a thermoplastic material.

beam's eye view when an observer looks directly at the planning target volume from the position of the central ray from the X-ray tube, this gives the extent of the beam coverage.

beam guiding instrument position indicating device. Apparatus used in intra-oral radiography to align the X-ray beam onto a film held in a film holder. In the paralleling technique, the apparatus ensures that the central beam strikes the teeth at right angles to their long axis and the film at right angles to its plane.

beam hardening when the total intensity of the X-ray beam is reduced by the addition of filters, as the reduction is much greater at lower energies. An increase in the average energy of an X-ray spectrum caused by greater absorption of the low-energy component by filtration.

beam hardening filters addition of pieces of metal to improve the relative penetration of the X-ray beam, they are not effective at megavoltages. ⊃ compound filters.

beam intensity modulation linear accelerator beam intensity is varied during treatment by altering the collimation leaves to create a better dose distribution over the field.

beam profile the dose of the X-ray beam including any scattered radiation which is added to the primary beam as it passes through the patient. The variation of dose along a line at right angles to the central axis of a radiation beam.

beam quality is the penetrating ability of primary radiation and is influenced by: the accelerating voltage (kVp) across the tube, the voltage waveform, the target material, the inherent filtration and the additional filtration.

beam width the width of an ultrasound beam at a given depth in the patient.

bearing-down 1. describes both the sensation and action of the expulsive contractions experienced during the second stage of labour, where the woman pushes, involuntarily or with added effort, in order to move her baby through the birth canal. **2.** a feeling of weight and descent in the pelvis associated with uterine prolapse or pelvic tumours.

beat *n* pulsation of the blood in the heart and blood vessels. *apex beat* ⊃ apex, dropped beat, premature beat.

Beau's lines (J Beau, French physician, 1806–1865) transverse ridges or grooves which reflect a temporary retardation of the normal nail growth following a debilitating illness (Figure B.3). They first appear towards the proximal nail fold and move towards the free edge as the nail grows. The distance the groove has moved indicates quite accurately the length of time since the illness or trauma (nail growth being about 1 mm per week).

Becker muscular dystrophy (P Becker, German geneticist, 1908–2000) (*syn* benign pseudohypertrophic muscular dystrophy) a type of muscular dystrophy inherited as an X-linked recessive condition; there are deletions in the dystrophin gene. Disease onset occurs during late childhood/early adulthood. The muscles affected are the proximal muscles and limb girdle; there is pseudohypertrophy of the calf muscles and cadiomyopathy. It is less severe than Duchenne muscular dystrophy and has a better prognosis. ⊃ muscular dystrophies.

Beck's triad (C Beck, American surgeon, 1894–1971) hypotension, muffled heart sounds and neck vein distension; the three principal physical signs of cardiac tamponade.

becquerel (Bq) *n* (A H Becquerel, French physicist, 1852–1908) the derived Système International d'Unités (SI) unit (International System of Units) for radioactivity. Equals the amount of a radioactive substance undergoing one nuclear disintegration per second. Has replaced the curie. ⊃ Appendix 2.

BED *acron* biological effective dose.

bedbug *n* a blood-sucking insect belonging to the genus *Cimex*. The commonest species are *Cimex lectularius* in temperate zones and *C. hemipterus* in tropical zones. They live and lay eggs in cracks and crevices of furniture and walls. They are active at night and their bites provide a route for secondary infection.

bedsore *n* obsolete term. ⊃ pressure ulcer.

bedwetting *n* ⊃ enuresis.

Beer Lambert law the greater the distance a ray of light travels in a coloured medium the more it is absorbed.

Beevor's sign movement of the umbilicus as an athlete performs a half sit-up. It indicates an interruption to the nerve supply (innervation) of the abdominal muscles.

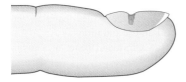

B.3 Beau's lines (reproduced from Boon et al 2006 with permission).

Begg technique a fixed orthodontic technique developed by Dr P Begg and first described in the 1950s. Uses light wires (and hence light forces) in a modified ribbon arch attachment.

Beginners All-purpose Symbolic Instruction Code (BASIC) a high level language for computers.

behaviour *n* the observable behavioural response of a person to an internal or external stimulus.

behavioural activation system (BAS) a neurobehavioural system thought to regulate positive affect and approach behaviour in response to incentives or rewards. Individuals vary in the sensitivity of the system and it is associated with the personality factor of extraversion. ⊃ behavioural inhibition system (BIS).

behavioural analysis applied behaviour analysis application of the principles of operant conditioning to the treatment of behavioural problems. Experimental analysis of behaviour application of the principles of operant conditioning to the study of behaviour. ⊃ conditioning.

behaviour change psychological concept generally applied to lifestyle in relation to health. An approach used in health education, whereby individuals are encouraged to make lifestyle changes by providing information, looking at existing health beliefs and values and increasing self-confidence. The change may be the adoption of health-protective behaviour (e.g. healthy eating, regular exercise) or changing health-threatening behaviour (e.g. excessive alcohol intake, smoking).

behavioural coaching application of the principles of operant conditioning and cognitive behaviour therapy to coaching, especially in sport or the business environment.

behavioural inhibition system (BIS) a neurobehavioural system thought to regulate negative affect and avoidance behaviour in response to threats or punishment. Individuals vary in the sensitivity of the system and it is associated with the personality factor of neuroticism. ⊃ behavioural activation system (BAS).

behavioural intention a person's conscious or deliberate intention to engage in a behaviour.

behaviourism *n* in psychology describes an approach which studies and interprets behaviour by objective observation of that behaviour without regard to any subjective mental processes such as ideas, emotions and will. Behaviour is considered to be a series of conditioned reflexes.

behaviour modification in a general sense, an inevitable part of living, resulting from the consistent rewarding or punishing of response to a stimulus, whether that response is negative or positive. Some education systems deliberately employ a modification approach to maximize learning.

behaviour therapy a type of psychotherapy to modify observable, maladjusted patterns of behaviour by the substitution of a learned response or set of responses to a stimulus. The treatment is designed for a particular patient and not for the particular diagnostic label which has been attached to that patient. Such treatment includes assertiveness training, aversion therapy, conditioning and desensitization.

Behçet's syndrome (H Behçet, Turkish dermatologist, 1889–1948) a form of systemic vasculitis. There is stomatitis, genital ulceration, retinitis and uveitis. There may also be skin nodules, thrombophlebitis and arthritis affecting one or more of the large joints. Gastrointestinal and neurological complications may occur. The syndrome is associated with the presence of a certain human leucocyte antigen (HLA). Treatment is with NSAIDs, corticosteroids and immunosuppressant drugs. ⇨ Colour Section Figure 53.

BEI *abbr* bioelectrical impedance.

bejel *n* a treponemal infection, bejel is the Middle Eastern name for non-venereal syphilis, which has a patchy distribution across sub-Saharan Africa, the Middle East, Central Asia and Australia. It has been eradicated from Eastern Europe. The causative organism is *Treponema pallidum* (ssp. *endemicum*). Transmission is most commonly from the mouth of the mother or child and the primary mucosal lesion is seldom seen. It usually starts in the mouth and affects mucosae, skin and bones. The early and late lesions resemble those of secondary and tertiary syphilis but cardiovascular and neurological disease are rare. It occurs in poor rural populations with low standards of domestic hygiene. It has features in common with pinta, notably that it is transmitted by contact, usually within the family and not sexually, and in the case of bejel, through common eating and drinking utensils. The diagnosis of early stage bejel involves the detection of spirochaetes in exudate of lesions by dark ground microscopy. Both latent and early stage is diagnosed by a positive serological test for syphilis. Treatment of all stages is a single intramuscular injection of 1.2 g of long-acting benzylpenicillin. ⇨ pinta, yaws.

beliefs *npl* a set of ideas and thoughts that a person uses to construct attitudes, views and behaviour. They are formed by culture, family, experiences and many other factors.

belladonna *n* deadly nightshade. The poisonous alkaloid (*Atropa belladonna*) contains atropine and other muscarinic antagonists.

bell and pad a psychological approach to the management of bedwetting in children. A special pad/sheet is placed on the mattress and when the child starts to void urine a buzzer or bell sounds. This wakens the child who completes the voiding of urine in a potty or the lavatory.

'belle indifference' the incongruous lack of appropriate affect in the presence of incapacitating symptoms commonly shown by patients with dissociative disorders.

Bell's palsy (C Bell, British surgeon and anatomist, 1774–1842) usually non-permanent facial hemiparesis due to idiopathic (cause unknown) lesion of the seventh (facial) cranial nerve. Clinical features may include: pain behind or in front of the ear; loss of taste; sensitivity to sound on the affected side; headaches; face feels pulled to one side; problems eating and drinking; facial droop; difficulty with some facial expressions; paralysis of one side of the face; difficulty closing one eye; difficulty with fine facial movements; drooling due to inability to control facial

muscles; and dry eye secondary to being unable to close eye properly because of facial weakness.

Bell's phenomenon a sign present in peripheral facial paralysis. There is upward and outward movement of the eye ball, on the affected side, when the person attempts to close their eye.

Bence Jones protein (H Bence Jones, British physician, 1814–1873) an abnormal protein that is excreted in the urine of some patients with multiple myeloma, composed of fragments of immunoglobulin molecules.

benchmarking *n* part of quality assurance. Involves the identification of examples of best practice from others engaged in similar practice. From this, best practice benchmark scores in agreed areas of care are identified, against which individual units can compare their own performance.

bends *npl* (*syn* caisson disease) ⇨ decompression sickness/illness.

beneficence *n* the principle of doing good that also includes avoiding, removing and preventing harm and promoting good. Ethical dilemmas and problems may arise when the common good is at odds with that for individuals. ⇨ non-maleficence.

benign *adj* 1. non-malignant (of a growth), non-invasive (no capacity to metastasize), non-cancerous (of a growth). 2. describes a condition or illness which is not serious and does not usually have harmful consequences.

benign hypotonia describes infants who are initially floppy but otherwise healthy. Improvement occurs and the infant regains normal tone and motor development.

benign intracranial hypertension (BIH) a condition in which there is raised intracranial pressure with papilloedema and which can lead to the loss of vision, typically in young, obese women. Often associated with thrombosis in the sagittal sinus.

benign monoclonal gammopathy ⇨ monoclonal gammopathy of uncertain significance (MGUS).

benign mucous pemphigoid ⇨ cicatricial pemphigoid.

benign paroxysmal positional vertigo (BPPV) short-lived rotatory vertigo associated with sudden movements of the head. It is a common condition and often occurs after a head injury. It is thought to be caused by chalk-like debris dislodged into the semi-circular canals. The vertigo may last for a few seconds to minutes. Typically it happens when the person lies down or gets up from the bed. Specific manoeuvres, such as the Epley manoeuvre, can improve the condition but may need to be repeated.

benign prostatic enlargement (BPE) also called benign prostatic hyperplasia/hypertrophy. The increase in the size of the prostate gland due either to an increase in cell size or the growth of new cells that generally occurs in older men. It leads to urinary problems that include hesitancy, poor stream, dribbling, frequency and retention. Management may be with drugs, e.g. finasteride, to shrink the gland; minimally invasive techniques that include stent insertion, ultrasound, various laser techniques, vaporization and microwave; or by transurethral resection of the prostate gland (TUR, TURP).

benign prostatic hyperplasia (BPH) ⊃ benign prostatic enlargement (BPE).

benign pseudohypertrophic muscular dystrophy ⊃ Becker muscular dystrophy.

Bennett angle angle formed by the sagittal plane and the path of the advancing condyle during lateral mandibular movement, as viewed in the horizontal plane.

Bennett movement (or shift) lateral shift of the condyles and articular discs during a lateral excursion of the mandible.

Bennett's fracture (E Bennett, Irish surgeon, 1837–1907) fracture of proximal end of first metacarpal involving the articular surface.

Benson's disease ⊃ asteroid hyalosis.

bent lens ⊃ meniscus lens.

benzene *n* a colourless inflammable liquid obtained from coal tar. Extensively used as a solvent. Continued occupational exposure to it results in aplastic anaemia and, rarely, leukaemia.

benzodiazepines *npl* a group of anxiolytic/hypnotic drugs, e.g. diazepam, midazolam. Dependence and withdrawal problems may occur. They may be misused. ⊃ Appendix 5.

benzoic acid an antiseptic and antifungal agent used sometimes in an ointment for ringworm.

benzoin *n* (*syn* Friar's balsam) a resin of balsam used traditionally in inhalations but of doubtful value.

benzotriazole a radiographic developer restrainer.

bereavement *n* a response to a life event involving loss. Includes that which happens to a person after the death of another person who has been important in his or her life. It also occurs in other situations of loss, such as redundancy, loss of home, divorce or loss of a body part, e.g. mastectomy, amputation. ⊃ grieving process.

Berg scale This measures balance during 14 tasks and includes sitting, sit to stand, picking up objects from the floor and turning through 360°. It has good reliability and is easy to undertake in the clinical environment.

Berger's disease/nephropathy (J Berger, French nephrologist, 20th century) also called mesangial IgA nephropathy. A common type of glomerulonephritis characterized by the deposition of immunoglobulin A (IgA) in the glomeruli. There is macroscopic and or microscopic haematuria and proteinuria, which may progress to renal failure.

beri-beri *n* a deficiency disease caused by lack of vitamin B$_1$ (thiamin[e]). It occurs mainly in those countries where the staple diet is polished rice. Beri-beri is usually described as either 'wet' (cardiac) or 'dry' (neurological) depending on the symptoms. The symptoms are pain from neuritis, paralysis, muscular wasting, progressive oedema, mental deterioration and, finally, heart failure.

Bernouille principle the inverse relationship between pressure and velocity in a flowing fluid medium (liquid or gas).

berylliosis *n* an industrial disease: there is impaired lung function because of interstitial fibrosis from inhalation of beryllium. Corticosteroids are used in treatment.

beta (β)-adrenoceptor agonists (*syn* beta stimulants, sympathomimetics) a group of drugs that stimulate β-adrenoceptors, e.g. dobutamine, salbutamol. A subgroup of the β$_2$ agonists used in asthma, usually by inhalation, to dilate the airways by relaxing smooth muscle, acting as a 'reliever' of symptoms of wheeze, cough or breathlessness. In sport, some are allowed under doping regulations (salbutamol and terbutaline) while those with significant anabolic effects (clenbuterol) are prohibited. ⊃ adrenaline (epinephrine), adrenoceptor, Appendix 5.

beta (β)-adrenoceptor antagonists (*syn* beta blockers) a group of drugs that block the stimulation of β$_1$-adrenoceptors in the myocardium and other locations, e.g. atenolol, propranolol. Banned in sport due to the beneficial effect where fine hand movement and avoidance of tremor is important such as in archery, shooting and snooker. ⊃ adrenaline (epinephrine), adrenoceptor, Appendix 5.

beta blockers *npl* ⊃ beta (β)-adrenoceptor antagonists.

beta (β)-carotene precursor of vitamin A, usually ample in a normal diet, which is converted in the body to retinol. This and other carotenoids also function as antioxidants, protecting cells against oxidation stress/damage. Beta-carotene supplements do not appear to have any ergogenic effect. Thus, it is recommended that this pro-vitamin is best obtained through the diet. ⊃ Appendix 4.

beta (β) decay the process of ejecting a beta particle from the nucleus of an atom; if the particle is negative (negatron) the atomic number will increase by one, if the particle is positive (positron) the atomic number will decrease by one.

beta-hydroxy beta-methylbutyrate (HMB) a substance derived from leucine (an amino acid), which is found naturally in small quantities in catfish, various citrus fruits and breast milk. Beta-hydroxy beta-methylbutyrate (HMB) supplementation has been reported to be associated with enhanced gains in muscle mass and strength during resistance training. In addition to affecting protein synthesis, HMB is also claimed to stimulate fat oxidation. According to existing human data HMB is safe and well tolerated. ⊃ ergogenic aids.

beta (β)-lactam antibiotics antibiotics containing a β-lactam ring in their structure (Figure B.4). They include the cephalosporins and penicillins. Many bacteria produce enzymes (β-lactamases) that destroy the β-lactam ring, which renders the antibiotic ineffective.

B.4 Beta lactam ring (reproduced from Wilson 1995 with permission).

beta (β)-lactamases previously known as penicillinases. The enzymes, produced by certain bacteria, e.g. most staphylococci and *Escherichia coli*, that destroy β-lactam antibiotics.

beta (β) oxidation metabolic process whereby fatty acids are converted to acetyl-CoA prior to the production of energy (ATP).

beta (β) particle a mass, equal to that of an electron, which is ejected from the nucleus of an atom and has either a positive or a negative charge.

beta (β) phase the period after the alpha redistribution phase of drug administration. There is a slow decrease in drug blood levels during its metabolism and excretion.

beta thalassaemia ⊃ thalassaemia.

betatron *n* an accelerator device used to produce a stream of high-energy electrons for use during some types of radiotherapy.

bevel the angle that one line makes with another when not at right angles. In dentistry, the inclined edge or surface of a cutting instrument or cavity preparation.

bezoar *n* a compacted mass of hair and or vegetable material found within the stomach. The ingestion of such material can be a feature of some forms of mental distress. The bezoar can eventually obstruct gastric emptying. Strictly speaking, a mass comprising only hair (the person's own hair or that from animals) is called a trichobezoar.

BFI *abbr* Baby Friendly Initiative.

BHF *abbr* Bolivian haemorrhagic fever.

BHL *abbr* bilateral hilar lymphadenopathy.

BHN *abbr* Brinell hardness scale/number.

bi- a prefix that means 'twice, two', e.g. *bicuspid*.

biacromial measure the width of the shoulder.

bibliographical databases details of papers, etc., but sometimes abstracts and full articles, are available electronically via CD-ROM or the Internet, e.g. MEDLINE.

bibliography a list of material used in constructing a piece of written work, but which is not directly cited in the reference list.

bicarbonate (hydrogen carbonate) (HCO_3^-) *n* an anion. Important in pH regulation and the acid–base balance in the body. Also called hydrogen carbonate. The serum (plasma) bicarbonate (that in the blood) represents the alkali reserve. The normal range in arterial blood is 22–28 mmol/L. In sport, bicarbonate supplementation is used to enhance performance in athletic events conducted at near-maximum intensity for 1–7 minutes (400–1500 m running, 100–400 m swimming, kayaking, rowing and canoeing) as they may otherwise be limited by excess hydrogen ion accumulation. ⊃ ergogenic aids. ⊃ Appendix 3.

bicellular *adj* composed of two cells.

biceps *n* two-headed muscle.

biceps brachii the two-headed muscle on the anterior surface of the upper arm. Its origins are on the coracoid process and the glenoid cavity and it inserts on to the radius. It flexes the elbow joint and supinates the forearm and the hand. ⊃ elbow joint, Colour Section Figure 4.

biceps femoris two-headed muscle, the most lateral on the posterior surface of the thigh. Its origins are on the ischial tuberosity and the femur and it inserts in to the fibula and the lateral condyle of the tibia. It extends the thigh and flexes the knee joint. Also rotates the leg laterally when the knee is flexed. It is one of the three hamstring muscles ⊃ semimembranosus, semitedinosus, Colour Section Figure 5.

bichrome test ⊃ duochrome test.

biconcave *adj* concave or hollow on both surfaces, as in the shape of a normal red blood cell, or the shape of a divergent lens used to correct myopia.

bicondylar joint a joint in which two distinct, rounded surfaces of one bone articulate with shallow channels on the corresponding bone. The knee joint is a modified bicondylar joint.

biconvex *adj* convex on both surfaces, as in the shape of a convergent lens used to correct hypermetropia.

bicornuate *adj* having two horns; generally applied to a double uterus or a single uterus possessing two horns.

bicristal measure the width of the hip.

bicuspid *adj* having two cusps or points. *bicuspid teeth* the premolars. *bicuspid valve* the mitral valve between the left atrium and ventricle of the heart.

BID *abbr* brought in (to hospital) dead.

Bielschowsky's head tilt test (A Bielschowsky, German ophthalmologist, 1871–1940) a test used to determine a weakness affecting the superior oblique muscle (extraocular/extrinsic muscle of the eye) caused by damage to the IVth (trochlear) cranial nerve.

bifid *adj* divided into two parts. Cleft or forked.

bifid tongue developmental defect resulting from the incomplete fusion of portions of the tongue along the midline.

bifidus factor a carbohydrate constituent of human milk. It stimulates the growth of the bacterium *Lactobacillus bifidus* in the bowel. The presence of this micro-organism reduces the pH within the bowel contents and inhibits the establishment and growth of pathogenic bacteria.

bifocal lens a lens with two separate parts that have different focal lengths. This facilitates corrected vision for near and distant objects by using a single pair of spectacles or contact lenses.

bifurcation *n* division into two branches, such as the bifurcation of the trachea to form the two main bronchi or the junction of the two roots of the lower molar teeth, or where a blood vessel divides into two—**bifurcate** *adj, vt, vi*.

bigeminal pregnancy a twin pregnancy.

bigeminy *n* a cardiac arrhythmia in which two rapid beats are followed by a longer pause. Every other beat is premature.

big five (personality factors) the widely accepted five fundamental personality factors comprising agreeableness, conscientiousness, extraversion, neuroticism and openness to experience.

bigorexia ⊃ muscle dysmorphic disorder.

biguanides *npl* a group of oral hypoglycaemic drugs, e.g. metformin hydrochloride. ⊃ Appendix 5.

A
B

BIH *abbr* benign intracranial hypertension.

bilateral *adj* pertaining to both sides—**bilaterally** *adv.*

bile *n* a bitter, alkaline, viscid, greenish-yellow fluid secreted by the liver and stored in the gallbladder. 500–1000 mL is produced each day. Bile leaves the gallbladder in response to the secretion of cholecystokinin (CCK) by intestinal cells when fatty foods enter the duodenum. Bile contains water, mineral salts, mucin, lecithin, cholesterol, bile salts (derived from bile acids), the pigments bilirubin and biliverdin and substances (e.g. drug residues) for excretion. Bile emulsifies the fats in food to form smaller particles to allow digestion and absorption, facilitates the absorption of fat-soluble vitamins, stimulates peristalsis and deodorizes faeces.

bile acids *npl* organic acids produced by the liver during the metabolism of cholesterol. They include cholic acid, chenodeoxycholic acid, taurocholic acid and glycocholic acid. The bile acids entering the duodenum in the bile are in the form of bile salts, and most of these are reabsorbed to be reused. ⊃ enterohepatic circulation.

bile ducts *npl* the ducts forming the biliary tract; the right and left hepatic ducts, common hepatic duct and cystic duct, which join to form the common bile duct that empties bile into the duodenum. ⊃ biliary tract.

bile pigments *npl* ⊃ bilirubin, biliverdin.

bile salts *npl* sodium glycocholate and sodium taurocholate present in bile are formed from bile acids. They act as surfactants and reduce surface tension to emulsify fats in the small intestine —**bilious, biliary** *adj.*

Bilharzia *n* ⊃ *Schistosoma.*

bilharziasis *n* ⊃ schistosomiasis.

bili- a prefix that means 'bile', e.g. bilirubin.

biliary *adj* pertaining to bile.

biliary atresia congenital condition characterized by the absence or abnormal development of the bile ducts. Resulting in a failure to drain bile with jaundice and in the absence of effective treatment irreversible damage to the liver and eventually hepatic portal hypertension. Surgical correction is only possible in a few cases but increasingly a liver transplant is a treatment option.

biliary colic pain in the right upper quadrant of abdomen, due to obstruction of the gallbladder or common bile duct, usually by a gallstone (calculus); it may last several hours and is usually steady, which differentiates it from other forms of colic. Vomiting may occur.

biliary fistula an abnormal track conveying bile to the surface or to some other organ.

biliary tract the bile ducts and gallbladder. The pathway from the bile canaliculi in the liver, by way of the gallbladder, to the opening of the common bile duct into the duodenum at the hepatopancreatic ampulla (Figure B.5).

bilious *adj* **1.** a word usually used to signify vomit containing bile. **2.** a non-medical term, usually meaning 'suffering from indigestion'.

bilirubin *n* a red bile pigment mostly derived from haemoglobin during red blood cell breakdown. Unconjugated fat-soluble bilirubin, which gives an indirect reaction with

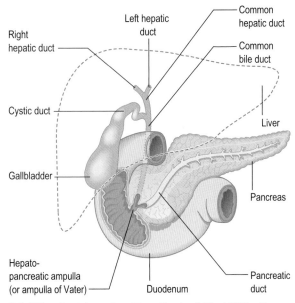

B.5 Biliary tract (reproduced from Brooker & Nicol 2003 with permission).

Van den Bergh's test, is potentially toxic to metabolically active tissues, particularly the basal nuclei of the immature brain. Unconjugated bilirubin is transported to the liver in the blood attached to albumen to make it less likely to enter and damage brain cells. In the liver the enzyme glucuronyl transferase conjugates fat-soluble bilirubin with glucuronic acid to make it water-soluble, in which state it is relatively non-toxic (reacts directly with Van den Bergh's test) and can be excreted in the bile. ⊃ haemolytic disease of the newborn, jaundice, phototherapy.

bilirubinaemia *n* the presence of bilirubin in the blood. Sometimes used (incorrectly) for an excess of bilirubin in the blood. ⊃ hyperbilirubinaemia.

bilirubinometer instrument for measuring the serum bilirubin concentration.

bilirubinuria *n* the presence of the bile pigment bilirubin in the urine.

biliverdin *n* the green pigment formed by oxidation of bilirubin.

Billings' method (J & E Billings, Australian physicians, 20th century) a method of natural family planning that uses the changes in cervical mucus during the menstrual cycle to estimate the timing of ovulation. The mucus increases in amount and becomes clear, thinner, slippery and more elastic during the time around ovulation. ⊃ ferning, spinnbarkeit.

Billroth's operation (C Billroth, Austrian surgeon, 1829–1894) ⊃ gastrectomy.

bilobate *adj* having two lobes.

bilobular *adj* having two little lobes or lobules.

bimanual *adj* performed with both hands. A method of examination sometimes used in gynaecology whereby the internal genital organs are examined between one hand on the abdomen and one or two fingers of the other hand within the vagina.

bimanual compression of the uterus manoeuvre to arrest severe postpartum haemorrhage after delivery of the placenta when the uterus is atonic. The right hand is introduced into the vagina and closed to form a fist, which is pressed into the anterior vaginal fornix. The left hand, on the abdominal wall, pulls the uterus forwards, so that the anterior and posterior walls are pressed firmly together, enabling direct pressure to be applied to the placental site to stop the bleeding.

bimaxillary strictly, pertaining to the left and right maxilla. Loosely used (particularly in orthodontics) to describe an affectation, relationship or connection between the maxilla and the mandible.

bimaxillary protrusion a forward projection or prognathism of both jaws, the alveolar processes and the teeth, beyond normal limits in relation to the cranial base.

binangled describes hand instruments, such as some enamel chisels, in which the shank has two angles. The cutting edge is placed at right angles to the long axis of the handle.

binary a system of counting to base two, i.e. generating figures with only 0 or 1. For example, decimal 1, 2, 3, 4, 5, 6, 7 become 1, 10, 11, 100, 101, 110, 111. Used in digital computer processes.

binary digit ⊃ bit, byte.

binary fission a method of reproduction common among the bacteria and protozoa. The cell divides into two equal 'daughter' cells.

binasal hemianopsia hemianopsia in the nasal halves of the visual fields of both eyes. ⊃ bitemporal hemianopsia.

binaural *adj* pertaining to, or having two ears. Applied to a type of stethoscope.

binder in radiography, an agent used to suspend the phosphors in the phosphor layer of an intensifying screen; acetate acrylate is often used and contains a dye to control screen speed and unsharpness.

Binet's test (A Binet, French psychologist, 1857–1911) a test of mental capacity in children and young people. The answers given to a series of questions (standardized for mental capacity of normal children at different ages) are used to calculate the mental age of the child being tested.

binge-eating disorder an eating disorder characterized by a tendency to engage in episodes of binge eating which result in obesity. Similar to bulimia nervosa but without the accompanying compensatory behaviours such as self-induced vomiting and purging. ⊃bulimia, eating disorders.

binge–purge syndrome ⊃ bulimia, eating disorders.

binocular disparity ⊃ retinal disparity.

binocular fusion ⊃ sensory fusion.

binocular indirect ophthalmoscope (BIO) an indirect ophthalmoscope with a binocular viewing system for obtaining a magnified, inverted, stereoscopic image of the fundus. It consists of a light source mounted above and

between the examiner's eyes on a headset. This illuminates a hand-held condensing lens of high positive power close to the patient's eyes which forms an image of the patient's pupil in both of the examiner's pupils. An aerial image of the patient's fundus is formed between the condensing lens and the examiner (if the patient is emmetropic the image will be formed in the focal plane of the condensing lens). It appears inverted and stereoscopically through the oculars attached to the headset. Stereopsis is obtained by reducing the interpupillary distance by means of mirrors or prisms within the headset of the instrument. This ophthalmoscope allows examination of a wide area of fundus and perception of depressed and raised areas. ⊃ direct ophthalmoscope, indirect ophthalmoscope, ophthalmoscopy, scanning laser ophthalmoscope.

binocular microscope a microscope with two eyepieces thus enabling objects to be seen in perspective. ⊃ microscope.

binocular perception perception obtained through simultaneous use of both eyes.

binocular vision (BV) the condition in which both eyes contribute towards producing a percept which may or may not be fused into a single impression. ⊃ bar reading test, FRIEND test, hole in the hand test, monoblepsia, sensory fusion, Worth's classification of binocular vision, Worth's four dot test.

binovular *adj* derived from two separate ova. Binovular twins may be of different sexes. ⊃ uniovular *opp*.

BIO *abbr* binocular indirect ophthalmoscope.

bio- a prefix that means 'life', e.g. *biochemistry*.

bioassay *n* the measurement of biologically active compounds (e.g. hormones, vitamins and essential amino acids) by their ability to support growth of animals or micro-organisms.

bioavailability *n* the amount of a drug (or nutrient) that enters the circulation in the active form. It is dependent on the route of administration and the degree to which the drug is metabolized before it reaches the bloodstream. Drugs administered intravenously will have 100% bioavailability, whereas those given orally may not be fully absorbed and are subject to first-pass metabolism/effect in the liver. Some drugs are totally metabolized in the liver (e.g. glyceryl trinitate), so other routes of administration must be used such as sublingually or transdermally.

biochemical screening tests that screen for conditions or diseases, through analysis of biochemical markers. For example, in pregnancy maternal serum screening may be used to screen for fetal Down's syndrome or inherited metabolic disorders. The newborn blood-spot screening test relies on biochemical markers to identify newborns with conditions such as phenylketonuria, cystic fibrosis, hypothyroidism, etc. ⊃ neonatal screening.

biochemistry *n* the chemistry of life and organic molecules—**biochemical** *adj*.

biocytin the main form of the biotin (part of the B vitamin group) in most foods, bound to lysine an amino acid.

bioelectrical impedance (BEI) analysis a whole-body conductivity method for assessing body composition including the proportion of fat in the body. A small alternating current flowing between two electrodes passes more rapidly through hydrated fat-free body tissues and extracellular water than through fat or bone because of the greater electrolyte content (lower electrical resistance) of the fat-free component. Impedance to electric current flow can be related to total body water content and in turn to fat-free mass, body density and percentage body fat.

bioethics *n* the application of ethical principles to biological problems.

biofeedback *n* presentation of immediate visual or auditory information about usually unconscious body functions such as blood pressure, heart rate and muscle tension. Either by trial and error or by operant conditioning a person can learn to repeat behaviour which results in a satisfactory level of body functions. In optometry, the technique has been used in myopia control and in acuity improvement but the value of the technique in these conditions is still unproven. ⊃ small in large out (SILO) response.

biofilm *n* collection of micro-organisms and their extracellular polymeric substances, or sticky polymers, which hold the biofilm together. The biofilm is able to adhere to both inert or living surface, these include urinary catheters, water pipes, dental plaque and so on.

bioflavonoids *npl* ⊃ flavonoids.

biofortification improving the nutrient content of plants through genetic modification or selective plant breeding. For example, increasing the essential amino acid content of certain staple cereal crops.

biographical and health data a term usually applied to information collected at the initial assessment of a patient after admission to the healthcare service, whether hospital or the community. Most of the biographical data will not change but it will be helpful to all health professionals involved in care and treatment, enabling them to individualize contacts with the person. The health data, particularly those about dependence/independence for carrying out everyday living activities, may well change during the patient's contact with the healthcare service. All data will be useful when planning the person's discharge from the service.

biohazard *n* anything that presents a hazard to life. For instance, some specimens for the pathological laboratory are so labelled.

bioinformatics the application of computer technology and techniques to extract meaning from complex, multifaceted biological data.

biological body 'clock' an inherent timing mechanism that controls physiological processes and is not dependent on external factors.

biological débridement ⊃ débridement.

biological effect when a body is irradiated changes can occur which can include, skin reddening, loss of hair, radiation-induced cancers, genetic changes, changes in blood count and, if sufficiently high radiation dose is received to the whole body, death.

biological engineering designing microelectronic or mechanical equipment for external use by patients: for attachment to patients, or placement inside patients.

biological effective dose (BED) a comparison between the total radiation dose given during a fractionated treatment and a single dose of the same quantity of radiation. A quantity used in the radiobiology of radiotherapy to compare the effects of different fractionation schedules. The total dose given in very small fractions required to produce a particular effect.

biological half-life time taken by the body to eliminate 50% of the dose of any substance (e.g. a drug) by normal biological processes. ⊃ half-life ($t_{1/2}$).

biological response modifier (BRM) cancer treatment that manipulates the patient's immune response in order to destroy cancer cells. They include colony stimulating factors, interleukins and interferons.

biological value (BV) the quantity of absorbed nitrogen from food that is retained for body maintenance, repair and/or growth.

biological width collective term to describe the overall dimension of the junctional epithelium and dentogingival connective tissue attachment. Range 2–4 mm in health.

biology *n* the science of life, concerned with the structure, function and organization of all living organisms— **biological** *adj*, **biologically** *adv*.

bioluminescence ⊃ luminescence

biomaterials synthetic, pharmacologically inert and non-toxic substances designed for implantation and incorporation in the human body.

biomechanical analysis the analysis of forces and motions of the human body, it may be qualitative or quantitative. ⊃ qualitative biomechanical analysis.

biomechanics the study of the structure and function of biological systems relative to the methods of mechanics. The understanding of forces and their effects on (and by) the human body and implements.

biomedical model a model of health and disease that conceptualizes the body as a machine. The model is grounded in an understanding of anatomy and physiology and does not take into account psychological, sociological, cultural and spiritual influences.

biometry the application of statistical methods to analyse data/measurements obtained in biological research.

biomicroscope 1. an instrument designed for detailed examination of ocular tissues containing a magnifying system and usually used in conjunction with a slit-lamp. **2.** a term commonly used to describe a slit-lamp (although this is not strictly correct). ⊃ slit-lamp.

biophysical profile assessment of fetal wellbeing, based on fetal adaptations to declining placental function in the presence of fetal growth restriction or maternal disease, to assess fetal body or limb movements, tone, fetal breathing movements, amniotic fluid volume and cardiotocograph, each with a score of 0 or 1, a healthy fetus achieving a score of 5.

biopsy *n* removal of tissue to provide a sample for microscopic examination to establish a precise diagnosis, such as the type and degree of differentiation in a malignant tumour. A biopsy may be excisional or incisional. ⊃ excisional biopsy, incisional biopsy.

biopsychosocial *adj* relating to biological, psychological and social perspectives.

biorhythm *n* the cyclical patterns of biological functions unique to each person, e.g. sleep–wake cycles, body temperature, etc.—**biorhythmic** *adj*.

BIOS *abbr* basic input/output system.

biosensors *npl* non-invasive devices that measure the result of biological processes, e.g. skin temperature or blood oxygen saturation.

biotechnology *n* the use of biology in the scientific study of technology and vice versa—**biotechnical** *adj*, **biotechnically** *adv*.

bioterrorism describes the intimidation of civilians, military forces and their governments through the release of harmful organisms or toxins. In recent years there has been an increase in the incidence of terrorism through biological agents. These agents can be disseminated in innumerable ways—through contamination of food and water, dispersal through aerosols, and even detonators filled with harmful material. Potential micro-organisms and toxic agents that can be used in bioterrorism include (those marked * are considered to have the highest potential): (a) bacteria—anthrax (*Bacillus anthracis**), plague (*Yersinia pestis**), tularaemia (*Francisella tularensis**), Brucellosis (*Brucella* spp.), food safety threats (e.g. *Salmonella* spp., *Escherichia coli* 0157:H7, *Shigella*), glanders (*Burkholderia mallei*), melioidosis (*Burkholderia pseudomallei*), psittacosis (*Chlamydia psittaci*), Q fever (*Coxiella burnetii*), typhus fever (*Rickettsia prowazekii*), water safety threats (e.g. *Vibrio cholerae*); (b) viruses—smallpox (*Variola major*), viral haemorrhagic fevers (filoviruses, e.g. Ebola, Marburg and *arenaviruses*, e.g. Lassa, Machupo)*, viral encephalitis (alphaviruses, e.g. Venezuelan equine encephalitis, Eastern equine encephalitis, Western equine encephalitis), emerging infectious diseases such as Nipah virus and hantavirus; (c) toxins—botulism (*Clostridium botulinum* toxin), epsilon toxin of *Clostridium perfringens*, ricin toxin from *Ricinus communis* (castor beans), staphylococcal enterotoxin B. Outbreaks of an uncommon infectious disease in clusters, febrile illness associated with sepsis, pneumonia, respiratory failure or a rash, or a botulism-like syndrome with flaccid muscle paralysis, especially if occurring in otherwise healthy persons, should suggest a possible act of bioterrorism. Weapons-grade anthrax in the US postal system in 2001 resulted in 22 anthrax cases with five deaths. A rapid response to contain the threat is key to minimizing morbidity, mortality and terror. Steps such as rapid identification of the organism, prompt isolation and treatment of the victims, protection of care providers and post-exposure

chemoprophylaxis are important. Heightened surveillance, use of information technology to alert and educate the population, and strategic vaccination can successfully minimize and contain the threat. ⊃ anthrax, smallpox.

biotin *n* a member of vitamin B complex. Dietary sources are liver, soya flour, egg yolk, cereals and yeast. It is also synthesized by commensal bacteria in the colon. Deficiency is rare in humans; symptoms include fatigue, anorexia, muscle pains and dermatitis. ⊃ biocytin.

BIPAP *abbr* biphasic positive airways pressure.

biparietal diameter (BPD) measurement of the distance between the two parietal eminences of the fetal skull. Assessed in pregnancy with ultrasound to confirm gestational age; accurate to within a week. When the biparietal diameter (BPD) has passed through the maternal pelvic brim the head is engaged. Crowning occurs when the BPD distends the vulva during delivery and the fetal head no longer recedes between contractions.

biparous *adj* producing two offspring at one birth.

biphasic an electrotherapy term. A pulse with two oppositely charged phases. The two phases may be balanced (equal charges in the positive- and negative-going phases) or unbalanced (level of charge in each phase not equal). If balanced there is no ion buildup over time on skin, if unbalanced the skin will become more alkaline under the cathode and more acidic under the anode. These changes will manifest as skin irritation, typically, itchiness initially. ⊃ alternating current, phases, pulsed current.

biphasic positive airways pressure (BIPAP) mode of ventilatory (respiratory) support in which the airway pressure alternates between two levels. The higher pressure ventilates the patient or provides pressure support, whilst the lower pressure acts as positive end expiratory pressure/continuous positive airway pressure. Can be delivered non-invasively (without intubation) by mask to patients with chronic lung disease or as an aid to weaning from ventilatory support.

bipolar *adj* having two poles.

bipolar affective disorder (*syn* bipolar depression, manic-depressive illness) a disorder of mood that is characterized by repeated episodes of mania/hypomania and depression.

bipolar cell a retinal cell located in the inner nuclear layer connecting the photoreceptors with amacrine and ganglion cells.

bipolar construct a concept arranged along a single dimension with two opposite extremes, such as good–bad. Often used in self-report rating scales. For example, mood states are often assessed by asking respondents to rate their mood on a set of bipolar scales such as composed–anxious, agreeable–hostile, elated–depressed.

bipolar (electrotherapy) Involves two equal-sized electrodes usually placed at either end of a muscle or muscle group to be stimulated. For example, to stimulate quadriceps femoris muscle: two large, equal sized, electrodes are placed on the line running from the superomedial pole of the patella to the anterior superior iliac spine (ASIS). The proximal electrode is placed approximately 30% of the distance from the ASIS (over vastus lateralis and rectus femoris muscles) and the distal 90% (over vastus medialis and rectus femoris). ⊃ unipolar.

bird-fancier's lung a respiratory disease. It is a type of extrinsic alveolitis that is caused by inhaling avian protein allergens found in bird excreta and feathers. Can occur in individuals who keep birds such as pigeons. ⊃ extrinsic allergic alveolitis.

bird flu ⊃ avian influenza.

birefringence *n* double refraction, a characteristic of some natural substances, such as crystals of calcite (calcium carbonate) and some biological materials. As a ray of light passes through the material it is split into two light rays.

birth *n* the act of expelling the young from the mother's body; delivery; being born. *premature birth* one occurring between 24 and 37 weeks of pregnancy. ⊃ preterm birth.

birth canal the cavity or canal of the pelvis through which the fetus passes during labour.

birth centres a self-contained unit where the emphasis is on supporting normal births with reduced medical intervention in a more homely (less medical) environment. They may be sited within a hospital, adjacent to a hospital or completely separate from the hospital site.

birth certificate statement issued by the registrar for births, marriages and deaths for the district in which the baby is born, which certifies details of parentage, name and sex of child, date and place of birth. This certificate must be obtained by the parents, or failing them, anyone present at the delivery, within 42 days of birth in England (21 days in Scotland). It gives legal status to the child and is necessary before Child Benefit can be paid. A birth certificate is issued to any baby born alive, irrespective of the period of gestation. A stillbirth certificate is issued for babies of 24 weeks maturity or longer who did not breathe or show other signs of life after complete expulsion from the mother.

birth control prevention or regulation of conception by any means; contraception.

birth injury any injury occurring during parturition, e.g. fracture of a bone, subluxation of a joint, injury to peripheral nerve, intracranial haemorrhage, etc.

birth mark naevus.

birth mother the woman who gives birth to the baby, but not necessarily the genetic mother.

birth, notification of someone present or in attendance at a birth or within 6 hours afterwards, must notify the Director of Public Health within 36 hours (Public Health Act, 1936); usually undertaken by the midwife in attendance.

birth plan a plan prepared by the pregnant woman, usually in conjunction with her partner and midwife, which records her preferences for care during and after labour.

birth rate the *crude birth rate* is the number of births as a proportion of a population. It is expressed as the number of live births per 1000 population in 1 year. *refined birth rate* ratio of the total number of births to the female population

over a 1 year. *true birth rate* the ratio of total births to the female population of childbearing age (between 15 and 44 years).

birth, registration of either parent must register the birth within 42 days at the registrar's office in the district in which the birth took place (21 days in Scotland). Failure to do so incurs a fine. The responsibility rests with the midwife if the parents default.

birthing chair chair on which to give birth. It combines advantages of an upright position with good visibility and access for the midwife during delivery; some delivery beds convert into a chair. Disadvantages are a higher mean blood loss and increased incidence of postpartum haemorrhage, but tilting the chair to 40° to the vertical immediately before delivery and during the third stage of labour may reduce these risks.

birthing room room, usually for normal labour and delivery, furnished comfortably and in a home-like way.

BIS *abbr* behavioural inhibition system.

bisacromial diameter diameter measured between the acromion processes on the scapulae (shoulder blades). The fetal measurement is about 12 cm.

biscuit in dentistry, describes the state of porcelain (such as used for a restoration) after it has been baked in a furnace once before being glazed. ⊃ bake.

bisect to cut into two parts.

bisecting angle technique in dental radiology, a technique in which the beam of radiation is directed perpendicularly towards an imaginary line which bisects the angle formed by the plane of the film and the long axis of the tooth.

bisection also called hemisection. The division into two parts by cutting.

bisexual *adj* **1.** having some of the physical genital characteristics of both sexes; a hermaphrodite. When there is gonadal tissue of both sexes in the same person, that person is a true hermaphrodite. **2.** describes a person who is sexually attracted to both men and women.

Bishop's score (E H Bishop, obstetrician, 1913–1995) an assessment of the cervix used in induction of labour. The score is made up of the sum of individual scores of 0, 1 or 2 assigned for cervical effacement, consistency, dilatation and position along with a score for the station of the presenting part. A score of 4 or less suggests that induction may be difficult. ⊃ cervical effacement.

bisphenol-a-glycidyl methacrylate Bowen's resin. A short polymer commonly associated with dental restorative materials and dentine adhesives. It is an extremely viscous liquid and is thinned with diluent monomers.

bisphosphonates *npl* drugs that reduce bone turnover, e.g. alendronic acid. Used in the management of bone diseases such as osteoporosis and the hypercalcaemia associated with cancer. ⊃ Appendix 5.

bit the smallest unit of data in a computer, a contraction of **bi**nary dig**it**. A bit is represented by 1 or 0 and can be viewed as an electronic on/off switch. The are eight bits in a byte. ⊃ binary, byte.

bite 1. Loose term for occlusion. **2**. Registration of the occlusion by the use of wax or other material. **3**. in orthodontics, term describing various classifications of occlusion. The occusal record or relationship between the upper (maxillary) and lower (mandibular) teeth. ➲ anterior open bite, bite block, bite plane, check bite, check record, closed bite, cross bite, edge-to-edge bite, open bite, posterior open bite.

bite block deprecated term commonly used to describe a block of wax used to determine the occlusal relationship of the jaws during the construction of a prosthesis. The preferred term is occlusal rim. ➲ occlusal rim.

bite block (in radiotherapy) dental impression suspended from a gantry which the patient bites to enable accurate head position to be maintained during radiotherapy treatment.

bite guard *n* an appliance designed to cover the incisal and occlusal surfaces of the teeth. It provides stability for the teeth and/or to provide a flat platform for excursive movements of the the mandible and to prevent damage to the teeth during nocturnal grinding. Deprecated term for occlusal overlay appliance.

bite plane acrylic resin orthodontic appliance covering all of the upper teeth and retained by wire clasps.

bite raising appliance deprecated term for occlusal overlay appliance. ➲ occlusal overlay appliance

bite wax bite registration material, usually in the form of thin sheets, used to register the occlusion of upper and lower teeth.

bite wing (BW) radiograph *n* a type of intraoral dental radiograph which demonstrates the coronal parts of the upper teeth (maxillary) and the lower teeth (mandibular) and parts of the interdental septa on a single film. The film is held in position by a holder or tab, on which the patient closes the teeth during exposure. The developed radiograph shows the presence of caries, overhanging edges of restorations, calculus and the level of the alveolar bone crests.

bitemporal diameter diameter measured between the most distant points of the coronal suture. It measures 8.2 cm on the fetal skull.

bitemporal hemianopsia hemianopsia in the temporal halves of the visual fields of both eyes. ➲ binasal hemianopsia.

bitrochanteric diameter diameter measured between the greater trochanters of the femora. It is approximately 10 cm in the fetus.The diameter which engages in a breech presentation.

Bitot's spots (*syn* xerosis conjunctivae) (P Bitot, French surgeon, 1822–1888) localized area of thickened, keratinized epithelium, with micro-organisms, at the limbus of the cornea. A manifestation of vitamin A deficiency.

biuret test a chemical test for the amount of protein in food. Sodium hydroxide (alkali) and copper sulphate are added to the sample solution A positive result is indicated by a violet colour as copper sulphate reacts with the peptide bonds in the alkaline solution.

bivalent *n* **1**. in chemistry a substance with a valence of 2. Also called divalent. **2**. in genetics a pair of synapsed homologous chromosomes.

bivalve *adj* having two blades such as in a vaginal speculum. In orthopaedics, the division of a plaster of Paris splint into two portions—an anterior and posterior half.

bivariate statistics descriptive statistics that compare the relationship between two variables, such as correlations. Can be used to decide whether multivariate statistics are needed.

Bjerrum's screen ➲ tangent screen.

black body thermal radiator which absorbs completely all incident radiation, whatever the wavelength, the direction of incidence or the polarization. This radiator has, for any wavelength, the maximum spectral concentration of radiant flux at a given temperature.

black copper cement zinc phosphate type of cement containing black copper oxide which gives the cement its characteristic black colour. Formerly used in the restoration of deciduous teeth and in the cementation of metal splints and orthodontic bands.

blackhead *n* ➲ comedone.

black heel a discoloured area over the Achilles tendon due to the rupture of small blood vessels in the skin. It is associated with certain sports that include squash.

Black's classification of cavities historical classification of tooth cavities according to the site of origin of the carious process (Figure B.6). *Class 1*: any simple occlusal, palatal or lingual cavity in molar or premolar teeth such as carious pits and fissures. *Class 2*: simple—any mesial or distal carious cavity in molar and premolar teeth. compound—simple cavity but also involving another surface. *Class 3*: cavity in the mesial or distal surfaces of canines and incisors but not involving the incisal angle. *Class 4*: cavity in the mesial

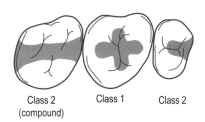

Class 2 (compound)　Class 1　Class 2

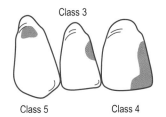

Class 3

Class 5　Class 4

Black's classification

B.6 Black's classification (reproduced from Heasman & McCracken 2007 with permission).

or distal surfaces of canines or incisors also involving the incisal angle. *Class 5:* cavity in the gingival third of the labial, buccal, lingual or palatal surface of any tooth. Does not classify recurrent or root surface lesions.

blackwater fever a serious complication of some forms of malaria where there is red blood cell haemolysis. The resultant haemoglobinuria causes dark coloured urine, jaundice and renal failure.

bladder *n* a membranous sac containing fluid or gas. A hollow organ for receiving fluid. ⊃ gallbladder, urinary bladder.

bladder augmentation an operation to increase the capacity of the urinary bladder.

bladder outflow obstruction pathophysiological obstruction to the lower urinary tract commonly due to benign prostatic enlargement in older males.

bladder retraining an intervention to prevent episodes of urinary incontinence and to reduce symptoms of frequency and urgency by gradually increasing the time interval between voiding. ⊃ incontinence.

Blake's universal gingivectomy knife a periodontal instrument.

Blalock–Taussig procedure (A Blalock, American surgeon, 1899–1964; H Taussig, American paediatric cardiologist, 1898–1986) a temporary measure to improve pulmonary blood flow in congenital heart abnormalities, such as tetralogy of Fallot. A shunt is constructed by anastomosing (joining) the subclavian artery to the pulmonary artery to divert blood from the systemic circulation to the lungs.

blanch to become pale or lose colour. It may affect a localized area exposed to pressure (e.g. a pressure area), or a more general loss of natural colour due to fear, cold, strong emotion or as a result of illness.

bland diet a diet that does not irritate or overstimulate the digestive tract. Generally avoiding pickles, spicey food, alcohol and strong tea or coffee.

blank lens a moulded piece of ophthalmic glass before completion of the surfacing processes. ⊃ glass, semi-finished lens, surfacing.

blast- a prefix that means 'immature cell', e.g. *blastoderm.*
-blast a suffix that means 'cell (immature)', e.g. *erythroblast.*

blastocyst *n* stage in early embryonic development in mammals that follows the morula, which becomes cystic and enfolds. Comprises a fluid-filled cavity and inner cell mass surrounded by an outer cell mass, or trophoblast. The inner cell mass is the source of embryonic stem cells from which all body structures are formed. The trophoblastic cells of the outer cell mass are involved in implantation of the blastocyst, and will eventually differentiate into two layers that form the chorion and placenta. ⊃ gastrula.

blastoderm *n* a cell layer of the blastocyst. Eventually becomes the three primary germ layers, ectoderm, endoderm and mesoderm, from which the embryo will form.

Blastomyces *n* a genus of pathogenic fungi. Species include *Paracoccidioides brasiliensis* in South America and *Blastomyces dermatitidis* in North America—**blastomycetic** *adj.*

blastomycosis *n* granulomatous condition caused by *Blastomyces dermatitidis*; infection usually affects the skin but it can involve the lungs, kidneys, nervous system, bones and joints. It is most common in the southeastern states of the United States and in Latin America—**blastomycotic** *adj.*

blastula (blastosphere) *n* an early stage in embryonic development in lower animals. It follows the morula and comprises a fluid-filled cavity (blastocoele) surrounded by a single layer of cells ⊃ blastocyst.

bleb *n* a large blister. ⊃ bulla, vesicle.

bleb-like dystrophy ⊃ Cogan's microcystic epithelial dystrophy.

bleaching 1. the physiological process of changing colour from the pink of a dark-adapted retina to a pale yellow colour after it has been exposed to light. This is due to the reaction of the rhodopsin pigment. The process is reversible if the healthy retina is allowed to remain in the dark. ⊃ rhodopsin, visual pigment. **2.** the process to remove a tint from organic lenses.

bleaching (of teeth) previous name for the removal of stains or discoloration from teeth. ⊃ teeth whitening. In dentistry, the elimination or reduction of discoloration of the crown of a tooth by the temporary application of bleaching agents such as hydrogen peroxide. The process may be accelerated by the action of heat or ultra-violet light.

bleeding on probing (BOP) index part of a full assessment of the extent and degree of periodontal disease present. Usually four or six surfaces (periodontal pockets) around each tooth are tested by gentle probing and the results recorded as a percentage. ⊃ index (dental).

'bleeding time' the time required for the spontaneous arrest of bleeding from a skin puncture: under controlled conditions this is assessed using the Ivy method.

blenno- a prefix that means 'mucus', e.g. *blennorrhoea.*

blennorrhagia *n* excessive discharge of mucus, such as from the urethra in urethritis. Also known as blennorrhoea.

blennorrhoea ⊃ blennorrhagia.

bleph- a prefix that means 'eyelid', e.g. *blepharitis.*
blephara ⊃ eyelids.

blepharitis *n* inflammation of the eyelids, particularly the lid margins, eyelash follicles and meibomian glands. There is redness, swelling and discharge that forms crusts—**blepharitic** *adj.*

blepharochalasis *n* a looseness of the eyelid skin that occurs as supporting tissues atrophy.

blepharoconjunctivitis *n* inflammation of the eyelids and the conjunctiva.

blepharon *n* the eyelid; palpebra—**blephara** *pl.*

blepharophimosis an abnormally narrow palpebral fissure, the gap or aperture between the eyelids.

blepharoplasty *n* tarsoplasty. Plastic surgery of the eyelid. An operation in which excess skin is removed from the eyelid.

blepharoptosis *n* ⊃ ptosis.

blepharospasm *n* spasm of the muscles in the eyelid. Excessive winking. A condition in which there is involuntary shutting of the eye, which can occur in isolation or be due either to local irritative lesions in the eye or to a movement disorder.

blighted ovum a failure of development. There are fetal membranes enclosing a fluid-filled cyst but no embryonic tissue.

blind abscess an abscess without an external opening or draining sinus.

blind loop syndrome a condition resulting from stasis in the small intestine leading to excessive bacterial growth, thus producing diarrhoea and malabsorption (e.g. due to surgical anastomosis or dysmotility).

blindness ➲ visual impairment.

blind sight a term used to indicate someone who is totally blind but yet is able, unconsciously, to locate an object on the basis of visual cues. It indicates a lesion which has destroyed the visual cortex but in which the retinotectal pathway to the superior colliculus remains unaffected. This pathway is not involved in conscious vision but receives some information from the retina. ➲ retintectal pathway.

blind spot the spot at which the optic nerve leaves the retina. Without any cones or rods it is insensitive to light. May also describe an abnormal gap in the visual field caused by pathology affecting the optic nerve or retina. ➲ optic disc.

blink a temporary closure of the eyelids (usually of both eyes). Blinks are usually involuntary but may be voluntary. The frequency of blinking is conditioned by a number of external and internal factors, e.g. glare, wind, emotion, attention, tiredness, etc. Normal blink rate is about 10 blinks per minute, although there are wide variations. The duration of a full blink is approximately 0.3–0.4 s. Blink rates are often altered with contact lens wear and in some diseased states (e.g. chalazion, Graves' disease). ➲ corneal reflex, tears.

blink mode the comparison of two images in quick succession to identify minute changes between the images.

BLISS *acron* **B**aby **LI**fe **S**upport **S**ystems.

blister *n* an elevated lesion of the skin containing fluid, usually serum. A blister can result from friction, burns, local allergic responses, e.g. stings, some skin conditions. Blisters are commonly associated with poor-fitting footwear or when exercise is of high intensity and long duration. ➲ bulla, vesicle.

blood *n* a fluid connective issue. It is the red fluid filling the heart and blood vessels (cardiovascular system). It consists of a colourless fluid, plasma, in which are suspended the red blood cells (erythrocytes), the white cells (leucocytes), and the platelets (thrombocytes). The blood transports: oxygen from the lungs to the tissues and carbon dioxide from the tissues to the lungs for excretion; nutrients from the alimentary tract to the tissues and cell wastes to the excretory organs, principally the kidneys; hormones secreted by endocrine glands to their target glands and tissues; heat produced in active tissues to other less active tissues; protective substances, e.g. antibodies; and coagulation (clotting) factors that coagulate blood, minimizing its loss from ruptured blood vessels. Blood makes up about 7–8% of body weight (about 5.6 litres in a 70-kg man). This proportion is less in women and considerably greater in children, gradually decreasing until the adult level is reached.

blood bank the area or department of a hospital responsible for the selection, testing and storage of blood for later transfusion to patients.

blood-borne viruses (BBV) viruses transmitted via blood to cause infection. They include: human immunodeficiency virus (HIV) and the hepatitis B and hepatitis C viruses. The secondary spread of viral haemorrhagic fevers (VHFs) such as Ebola, Lassa fever and Marburg disease can occur through direct contact with an infected patient's blood, or indirect contact with items contaminated with blood.

blood–brain barrier (BBB) the protective arrangement that prevents many substances crossing from the blood to the brain. It comprises the capillary endothelial cells and astrocytes (neuroglial cells) that ensure that the capillary wall is relatively impermeable. The barrier allows the passage of nutrients and metabolic waste. However, some drugs, alcohol and other toxic substances, e.g. lead in young children, can pass from the blood through this barrier to the cerebrospinal fluid.

blood coagulation ➲ coagulation.

blood count calculation of the number of red blood cells (erythrocytes), white blood cells (leucocytes) and platelets (thrombocytes) in a given volume of blood, using automated cell counting or a haemocytometer. ➲ differential blood count.

blood culture a sample of venous blood is incubated in a suitable medium at an optimum temperature, so that any micro-organisms can multiply and so be isolated and identified microscopically. ➲ septicaemia.

blood donor in the UK a healthy volunteer who donates blood or blood components for transfusion. The donation, processing and storage of blood in the UK is outlined in Colour section figure 23.

blood doping a prohibited ergogenic aid banned by the World Anti-Doping Agency (WADA). It is used illicitly by some athletes to increase aerobic performance and involves the administration of a blood transfusion to a sportsman or sportswoman in order to increase the oxygen-carrying capacity of the blood and as a result to improve performance. Most commonly, this involves removing up to a litre of the person's own blood and storing this while the body's normal mechanisms replace the loss of red blood cells. At a later date, usually just prior to competition, the stored blood is transfused into the circulation. Though banned, it is still used in some sports, such as athletics and cycling, as detection is difficult. The procedure is considered to be against the ethics of sport. The risks associated with blood doping include renal damage, circulatory overload and the transmission of infection if donor blood is used.

A

B

blood film the result of spreading a droplet of blood very thinly on a microscope slide. The blood can then be stained with dyes and examined for abnormalities under a microscope.

blood flow quantity of blood flowing through a vessel, region or organ in unit time. Dependent on the arterial blood pressure and the resistance to flow in the local vascular bed, determined by the state of constriction/dilatation mainly of the arterioles, influenced in turn by chemical (local and hormonal) and neural (sympathetic) effects on the vascular smooth muscle. ⊃ perfusion.

blood formation haemopoiesis.

blood gases ⊃ arterial blood gases.

blood glucose also known as blood sugar. The amount of glucose in the blood; varies within the normal range. Adult fasting values in venous blood are normally between 3.6 and 5.8 mmol/L. Neonatal values may be lower, between 2.2 and 5.3 mmol/L. Blood glucose is regulated by hormones that include insulin, glucagon, glucocorticoids, adrenaline (epinephrine) and growth hormone. In healthy people, blood glucose concentration is homeostatically controlled within the normal range; maintenance of the normal level is critical for the function, in particular of those tissues with an obligatory demand for glucose (brain, red blood cells, renal cortex, mammary gland and testis). When there is no uptake from the gut, about 8 g glucose per hour can be provided from the liver by breakdown of glycogen stores and by gluconeogenesis. During prolonged exercise glucose output from the liver closely matches the increased requirement, so that the blood concentration falls only when the liver glycogen store is depleted, close to exhaustion. ⊃ continuous glucose monitoring (CGM), gluconeogenesis, glycogen, glycogenolysis, hyperglycaemia, hypoglycaemia, self-monitoring of blood glucose (SMBG).

blood groups a way of classifying blood by the presence or not of certain genetically determined factors called antigens (agglutinogens) on the red blood cell membrane. There are many blood grouping systems including ABO, Rhesus, Duffy, Kell, Lewis, etc. The ABO and Rhesus are clinically significant in transfusion, maternal–fetal compatibility and transplantation. There are four groups in the ABO system— A, B, AB and O. The red cells of these groups contain the corresponding antigens (agglutinogens): group A has A; group B has B; group AB has both antigens; and group O has neither. In the plasma there are antibodies (agglutinins) which will cause agglutination (clumping) of any cell carrying the corresponding antigen. Group A plasma contains anti-B; group B plasma contains anti-A; group O plasma contains both anti-A and anti-B; and group AB plasma contains no agglutinins. This grouping is determined by (a) testing a suspension of red cells with anti-A and anti-B serum or (b) testing serum with known cells. Transfusion with an incompatible ABO group will cause a severe haemolytic reaction and death may occur unless the transfusion is promptly stopped. For most transfusion purposes, group A can receive groups A and O; group B can receive

Table B.1 ABO blood group compatibility

Recipient	Donor			
	A	**B**	**AB**	**O**
A	Yes	No	No	Yes
B	No	Yes	No	Yes
AB	Yes	Yes	Yes	Yes
O	No	No	No	Yes

Reproduced from Brooker & Nicol (2003) with permission.

groups B and O; group AB can have blood of any group; and group O can only have group O (Table B.1). The terms universal donor and recipient are outdated and confusing because of the many other blood groups that exist. *Rhesus blood group* a further three pairs of antigens coded for by genes designated the letters Cc, Dd and Ee are present on the red cells. The letters denote allelomorphic genes which are present in all cells except the gametes where, for instance, a chromosome can carry C or c, but not both. In this way the Rhesus genes and blood groups are derived equally from each parent. When the cells contain only the cde groups, then the blood is Rhesus negative (Rh−); when the cells contain C, D or E singly or in combination with cde, then the blood is Rhesus positive (Rh+). For general purposes, only the Dd antigens are of clinical significance. About 85% of the Caucasian population have the D antigen. In contrast to the ABO system, there are no preformed antibodies to the D antigen but these groups are antigenic and can, under suitable conditions, produce the corresponding antibody in the serum. Antibodies are formed if there is (a) transfusion of Rhesus positive blood to a Rhesus negative person, (b) immunization during pregnancy by Rhesus positive fetal red cells, with the D antigen, entering the maternal circulation where the women is Rhesus negative. This can cause haemolytic disease of the newborn (erythroblastosis fetalis). ⊃ ABO blood group system, anti-D, Rhesus incompatibility.

blood-letting venesection.

blood plasma ⊃ plasma.

blood pressure (BP) the pressure exerted by the blood on the blood vessel walls. Usually refers to the pressure within the arteries. Arterial blood pressure is usually measured in millimetres of mercury (mmHg). The arterial blood pressure fluctuates with each heart beat, having a maximum value (the systolic pressure) which is related to the ejection of blood from the heart into the aorta and the systemic arteries and a minimum value (diastolic pressure) when the aortic and pulmonary valves are closed and the heart is relaxed (Figure B.7). Usually values for both systolic and diastolic pressures are recorded (e.g. 120/70). The factors that contribute to blood pressure include: cardiac output, blood volume, blood viscosity, elasticity of the arterial walls, the venous return (the amount of blood returning to heart) and the peripheral resistance in the arterioles. The normal BP

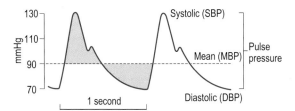

B.7 Arterial blood pressure as recorded over two cardiac cycles at heart rate 60 bpm (reproduced from Jennett 2008 with permission).

range varies with age; in healthy adults the normal BP is below 130 mmHg systolic and below 85 mmHg diastolic, and an optimum BP is below 120 mmHg systolic and below 80 mmHg diastolic. BP also varies during the 24 hour period and is influenced by factors, such as body position, physical activity, stress levels, etc. Arterial blood pressure is measured indirectly using a stethoscope with an anaeoid or mercury sphygmomanometer, or by using an automatic electronic device with a digital display. It may also be recorded directly in critical care situations by using an intra-arterial cannula with a pressure transducer. During pregnancy, the midwife should assess the woman's blood pressure at every antenatal appointment and refer to the obstetrician if the systolic pressure rises above 130 mmHg, or the diastolic pressure rises above 90 mmHg, or more than 15 mmHg above the first trimester baseline reading. ⊃ hypertension, hypotension, Korotkoff sounds, mean arterial blood pressure, pulse pressure.

blood sugar ⊃ blood glucose.

blood transfusion ⊃ blood donor, transfusion.

blood urea the amount of urea (the end product of protein metabolism) in the blood; varies within the normal range of between 2.5 and 6.5 mmol/L in adults. This is virtually unaffected by the amount of protein in the diet when the kidneys, which are the main organs of urea excretion, are functioning normally. When they are diseased the blood urea quickly rises. During pregnancy the normal range is between 2.3 and 5.0 mmol/L. ⊃ uraemia.

bloomed lens ⊃ coated lens.

Bloom's syndrome (D Bloom, American dermatologist, 20th century) a rare inherited disorder. It is transmitted as an autosomal recessive trait and mainly affects Ashkenazi Jews. Affected individuals have short stature, abnormalities of the capillaries in the arms and face, increased sensitivity to sunlight, recurrent infections and a higher than normal risk of leukaemia.

blow-out fracture fracture of the orbital wall due to blunt trauma.

BLS *abbr* basic life support.

blue visual sensation evoked by radiations within the waveband 450–490 nm. It is a primary colour and the complementary of yellow. ⊃ complementary colour, primary colours.

blue arcs entoptic phenomenon appearing as two bands of blue light arching from above and below the source towards the blind spot. This phenomenon is induced by a small

source of light (preferably red) stimulating the temporal side of the retina near the fovea. ⊃ entoptic image/phenomena.

'blue baby' cyanotic appearance at birth, often attributed to congenital cyanotic heart defects.

blue-based films in radiography, films that have a blue dye in the base and produce a slightly higher visual contrast.

blue blindness ⊃ tritanopia.

blue cataract ⊃ blue-dot cataract.

blue-dot cataract (*syn* blue cataract, punctate cataract) a developmental anomaly of the crystalline lens characterized by numerous small opacities in the outer nucleus and cortex which appear as translucent bluish dots. The condition is very common and does not usually affect acuity.

blue field entoptoscope an instrument enabling the visualization, especially by patients with a dense cataract, of the shadows of leucocytes flowing in the retinal capillaries and therefore providing a test of macular function. It consists of a very bright light source, an interference filter with a maximum transmission in the blue end of the spectrum, and a diffuser. The instrument is held close to the eye of the patient who is asked to describe his or her observations. The leucocytes appear as flying corpuscles and if many corpuscles (at least 15) are seen moving in the entire field the test is considered positive whereas if none or only a few corpuscles are seen the test is considered negative. Positive responses usually indicate that the patient has good macular function and negative responses usually indicate that the patient has poor macular function. This test is very useful in predicting central vision before cataract extraction. ⊃ angioscotoma, cataract extraction, clinical maxwellian view system, entoptic image/phenomena.

blue pus bluish/green discharge from a wound infected with *Pseudomonas aeruginosa*.

blue-yellow blindness ⊃ tritanopia

B-lymphocyte (B-cell) ⊃ lymphocyte.

B-mode brightness modulation in ultrasound techniques. When the ultrasound reflections are recorded as dots of varying brightness on an oscilloscope, which is converted into a grey scale picture by a scan converter and a two-dimensional image is formed showing a section through the organ being examined.

BM *abbr* bowel movement.

BMD *abbr* bone mineral density.

BME *abbr* benign myalgic encephalomyelitis.

BMI *abbr* body mass index.

BMR *abbr* basal metabolic rate.

BMT *abbr* bone marrow transplantation/transplant.

BMUS *abbr* British Medical Ultrasound Society.

BN *abbr* bulimia nervosa.

BNF *abbr* British National Formulary. ⊃ formulary.

BNR *abbr* beam nonuniformity ratio.

Boari flap method of extending one side of the bladder to compensate for a shortened/pathological distal ureter.

Boas' sign (I Boas, German gastroenterologist, 1858–1938) hyperaesthesia (increased sensitivity) of the skin overlying the wing of the right scapula, a feature of cholecystitis.

Bobath concept (pioneered by Berta and Karel Bobath) the concept of treatment of abnormal muscle tone and movement disorder, seen in children with cerebral palsy and adults after a stroke, and now widely applied to similar dysfunction caused by multiple sclerosis and other neurological conditions.

BOD *abbr* biochemical oxygen demand

body building the use of exercise and diet (and often, undesirably, also drugs) to enhance size and definition of skeletal muscles. ⊃ anabolic steroids, ergogenic aids, strength training.

body composition whole-body composition is of interest in the contexts of control of body weight, assessment of obesity, and sport and exercise. It comprises total body fat (essential fat plus storage fat) and fat-free body mass (FFM) (includes muscle, water and bone). From body density measurements, using established corrections and equations, the ratio of fat mass to fat-free mass can be calculated, based on the much lower density of the fat compartment. However, within the FFM, bone is more dense than muscle, so if there is either relative loss of bone density (osteoporosis) or increase in muscle mass (with training), fat percentage may be overestimated. Densitometry techniques include underwater (hydrostatic) weighing and air displacement plethysmography. Estimates can be made of lean body mass (LBM), body mass devoid of storage fat, but LBM does not exclude essential fat, so it is slightly higher than the FFM. ⊃ body density, body fat.

body density the density of lean body mass is 1.10, while that of body fat is 0.90. A calculation of the proportions of lean body tissue and fat can be made once density has been determinded. This is either by weighing in air and in water, or by measuring body weight and volume.

body discrepancy a person's perceived discrepancy between their actual and ideal body size.

body dysmorphic disorder (BDD) a disorder where individuals experience a pervasive feeling that they have a defect in their physical defect or in a specific part of the body when, in fact, they look normal and others confirm this. ⊃ muscle dysmorphic disorder.

body fat normal healthy values usually quoted for total body fat are 15% (12–19%) of body mass for young men and 27% (25–30%) for women, both increasing by about 5% from late teens to sixties. Essential fat in the tissues and organs (including bone marrow, nervous system and muscle) averages 3% body mass for men and 12% for women (extra related to reproductive function); it is not a labile energy reserve, but a vital component for normal structure and function. Storage fat represents the energy reserve that accumulates as adipose tissue beneath the skin and in visceral depots, averaging 12% body mass for men and 15% body mass for women. Methods most commonly used for estimating percentage fat are: measurement of skinfold thickness at prescribed sites, body density measurement, and bioelectrical impedance analysis. ⊃ bioelectrical

impedance (BEI) analysis, body composition, body mass index, obesity, skinfold thickness.

body fluids the total water in the body accounts for more than half of body mass (typically 40 kg in a 70-kg man). Around two-thirds of the total body water (28 L) is in intracellular fluid (ICF) and the remaining amount (12 L) in extracellular fluid (ECF)—all body fluids external to cells; of this, blood plasma accounts for ~2.5 L, interstitial fluid in the tissues and lymph for ~9.5 L. ⊃ fluid compartments.

body image the image present in an individual's mind of his or her own body. Distortions of this occur in anorexia nervosa. ⊃ mutilation.

body language non-verbal symbols that express a person's current physical, emotional and mental state. They include body movements, postures, gestures, facial expressions, spatial positions, clothes and other bodily adornments.

body mass index (BMI) also known as Quetelet's index. Used as an index of adiposity and obesity. It is calculated by dividing an individual's weight (kg) by their height (m) squared. Separate charts are available for adults and children; adult charts should not be used for children or pregnant women. A BMI of less than 18.5 is underweight, BMI 18.5–24.9 is normal weight (some authorities use 20–24.9), BMI 25–29.9 is overweight, BMI over 30 is obese, BMI greater than 35 is morbidly obese, and BMI over 40 is extreme obesity. BMI has some limitations, for example a high BMI can lead to an overestimation of fatness in relatively lean individuals with a disproportionately high muscle mass because of genetic make-up. It is also inaccurate in athletes with particularly well-developed muscle tissue due to their exercise training regimen; this applies, for example, to body builders, weightlifters or upper weight class wrestlers. ⊃ obesity, waist:hip ratio.

body protected areas an electrotherapy term. The level of electrical safety required when patients have contact with electromedical equipment. Less stringent than type used when direct connection to the heart may occur.

body temperature the balance between heat produced and heat lost in the body. It is maintained around 37°C throughout the 24 hours, but varies between 0.5 and 1.0°C during that period. Most heat is produced by metabolism, voluntary and involuntary muscular activities, and heat loss occurs through convection, conduction and evaporation of sweat; small amounts are lost during expiration, urination and defecation. *core body temperature* that in the organs of the central cavities of the body (cranium, thorax and abdomen). *shell body temperature* that outside the body core. Varies between sites, e.g. 36°C at the shoulder and 28°C at the forearm (Figure B.8).

body type, somatotype the physical appearance of the body. There are three basic types. ⊃ ectomorph, endomorph, mesomorph.

body weight a term in common use for what is properly called body mass and commonly, but incorrectly, referred to in units of mass, e.g. kilograms (kg), stones (st) and pounds (lb) or pounds. Strictly, body weight is the force

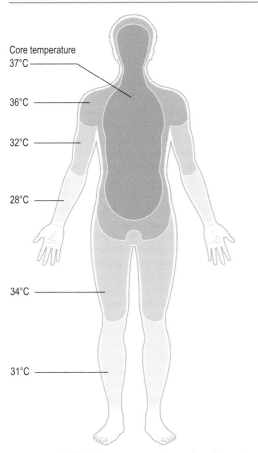

Core temperature
37°C
36°C
32°C
28°C
34°C
31°C

B.8 Core/shell body temperature (reproduced from Brooker & Nicol 2003 with permission).

due to the effect of gravity on body mass, expressed in newtons (N). ⊃ body composition, body mass index.

Boeck's disease (C Boeck, Norwegian dermatologist, 1845–1917) a form of sarcoidosis.

Bohler's angle two lines drawn on a lateral radiograph of a calcaneus (calcaneum, os calcis). Line one is from the posterior aspect of the calcaneus to its highest midpoint. The second line is from the highest midpoint to the highest anterior point. The normal angle is 25–40°, any other angle indicating an injury to the calcaneus.

Bohn's nodules tiny white nodules on the palate of the newly born.

Bohr effect (C Bohr, Danish physiologist, 1855–1911) the effect of hydrogen ion concentration (pH) on the oxygen dissociation curve. An increase in carbon dioxide in the blood or hydrogen ion concentration (i.e. a fall in pH) and also increased temperature causes the curve to 'shift to the right' and decreases the affinity of haemoglobin for oxygen. This means that more oxygen is unloaded to meta-bolically active tissues. The Bohr effect is particularly important in supplying oxygen to contracting muscle and in the placenta where oxygen passes from maternal to fetal vessels. ⊃ oxygen dissociation curve.

boil *n* (*syn* furuncle) an acute inflammatory condition, surrounding a hair follicle; often caused by *Staphylococcus aureus*. Usually attended by suppuration; it has one opening for drainage in contrast to a carbuncle.

boiling-out term used in the construction of dentures. The action of placing a flask in boiling water in order to separate it into two halves and thus enable the dental technician to wash out the melted wax leaving the denture teeth embedded in the plaster.

Bolam test the test laid down in the case of Bolam v. Friern HMC on the standard of care expected of a professional in cases of alleged negligence.

Bolivian haemorrhagic fever (BHF) (*syn* machupo haemorrhagic fever, machupo virus) a haemorrhagic fever caused by the Machupo virus (of the family *Arenaviridae*). It occurs in Central and South America. It is a zoonosis; the vector is a type of mouse. ⊃ viral haemorrhagic fever

bolus *n* **1.** a soft, pulpy mass of masticated food. **2.** a large dose of a drug given at the beginning of a treatment regimen to raise the blood concentration rapidly to a therapeutic level. **3.** a tissue equivalent material used in radiotherapy when irradiating irregular body shapes, to attenuate the primary beam and absorb scattered radiation to maintain accurate treatment dosage or to increase the dose to the skin when high-energy photon beams are used.

bonded crown jacket crown in which porcelain is fused to a platinum–gold matrix which forms the fitting surface of the dental restoration.

bonded retainer ⊃ retainer.

bonding *n* **1.** the emotional tie one person forms with another, making an enduring and special emotional relation-ship. There is a fundamental biological need for this to occur between an infant and its parents, particularly the mother. When newborn babies are cared for in an intensive care setting, special arrangements have to be made to encourage bonding between the parents and their new baby. **2.** binding together, e.g. porcelain to gold or other metal, or certain filling materials to tooth enamel.

bonding resin ⊃ resin.

bone *n* connective tissue in which salts, such as calcium carbonate and calcium phosphate, are deposited in an organic matrix to make it hard and dense. Bone tissue is of two types, hard dense *compact bone* (Figure B.9) and spongy *cancellous bone*. The separate bones make up the skeleton.

bone chisel single-ended dental chisel with longer handle and a square end which can be struck by a mallet.

bone-cutting forceps a dental instrument. Also known as bone shears. ⊃ forceps.

bone file in dentistry, a hand instrument, which is mostly double ended with serrated cutting blades. Used to smooth irregular bone edges.

bone graft the transplantation of a piece of bone from one part of the body to another, or from one person to another. Used to repair bone defects or to supply osteogenic tissue.

A
B

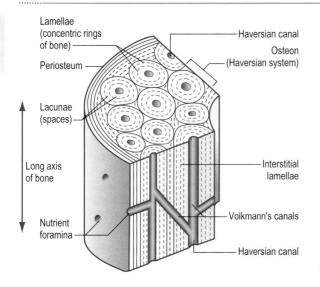

B.9   Bone tissue (reproduced from Brooker 2006A with permission).

bone marrow   the substance contained within bone cavities. At birth the cavities are filled with blood-forming *red marrow* but later in life, deposition of fat in the long bones converts the red marrow into *yellow bone marrow*.

bone marrow biopsy (sampling)   an investigation of blood cell production whereby a sample of marrow is obtained by aspiration or trephine. Usually the site used is the iliac crest or sometimes the sternum.

bone marrow transplantation (BMT) ➲ haemopoietic stem cell transplantation (HSCT).

bone mineral density (BMD)   a measure of bone density. It decreases as part of normal ageing and is changed with osteoporosis. Men and women who participate in strength and power activities have a bone mass as great as, or greater than, that of endurance athletes. On the other hand, the amenorrhoea that is prevalent among female athletes in weight-related sports is associated with a decrease in bone mass, leaving them at increased risk of osteoporosis and stress fractures despite competitive athletic participation. ➲ dual emission X-ray absorptiometry (DEXA), female athlete triad, osteoporosis, peak bone density.

bone nibbling forceps (rongeurs)   a dental instrument ➲ forceps.

bone-on-bone force   the force due to contact between two bones at a joint. Includes joint reaction force and muscle forces.

bone plate   perforated plates usually made out of titanium which are secured across the fracture line of a bone with screws in order to achieve fixation.

bone scan ➲ technetium (Tc) bone scan.

bone shears   a dental instrument, also known as bone cutting forceps. ➲ forceps.

bone wax   in dentistry, a wax used for filling sterile bone cavities.

Bonnet's capsule ➲ Tenon's capsule.

Bonnevie–Ullrich syndrome (K Bonnevie, Norwegian zoologist, geneticist, 1872–1948; O Ullrich, German paediatrician, 1894–1957). ➲ Noonan's syndrome, Turner's syndrome.

bony labyrinth ➲ labyrinth.

bony nasion   an anatomical landmark. The most anterior point of the frontonasal suture as seen on a lateral skull radiograph. ➲ nasion.

booking   the initial appointment of a pregnant woman with a midwife to arrange antenatal and labour care, discuss any issues of concern and begin to develop a working relationship. May be held in the woman's home, general practitioner's surgery, health centre or hospital antenatal clinic. A detailed history is taken of the woman's personal and family medical, surgical, obstetric and social history and baseline observations/measurement of weight, urinalysis and blood pressure are recorded. A sample of blood is taken for a variety of tests.

booking visit   first antenatal appointment to introduce the pregnant woman to the maternity service and to obtain information about the pregnancy and birth, as well as enabling the midwife to take a full personal, social, psychological and medical history, initiate relevant tests and investigations and discuss the parents' options for care.

BOOP *abbr* bronchiolitis obliterans organizing pneumonia.

boot   the start-up procedure that a personal computer follows as it runs some checks and loads the operating system when it is first switched on. ➲ operating system.

BOP *abbr* bleeding on probing (index).

borax ➲ disodium tetraborate.

borborygmi *npl* rumbling noises caused by the movement of gas in the intestines.

boredom   a feeling of tedium, dullness or monotony arising from an inability to engage with the activity being performed.

borderline substances *npl* foods and toiletries that possess the characteristics of medication for specified disorders. These may be supplied to patients as an NHS prescription in the UK. Examples of foods include gluten-free products for gluten-sensitive enteropathies, liquid feeds for short bowel syndrome, dysphagia, inflammatory bowel disease, etc. Toiletries include emollient bath oil for dermatitis, sunblocks/sunscreens for photodermatoses, etc.

border moulding   shaping of an impression material by the manipulation of the soft tissues adjacent to the borders of an impression.

border movement   movement of the mandible along the extremity of its range in any direction.

border seal ➲ seal.

Bordetella *n* (J Bordet, Belgian bacteriologist, 1870–1961) a genus of Gram negative coccobacilli bacteria. Species that are pathogenic to humans include *B. pertussis* which causes whooping cough (pertussis).

Borg dyspnoea scale   a validated scale (0–10) used by patients to quantify their perception of the severity of dyspnoea. The scale records no breathlessness at 0 up to maximal breathlessness at 10.

Borg (perceived exertion) scale a simple method of rating perceived exertion used by coaches to gauge an athlete's level of intensity in training and competition. The commonest used is a 15-point scale, using the numbers 6–20 to describe a range of levels of exertion from very, very light (6) to exhaustion (20). Research has shown that there is a correlation between an athlete's rate of perceived exertion (RPE) and their heart rate, lactate threshold and $\dot{V}O_{2max}$. Named after the Swedish scientist Gunnar Borg.

Bornholm disease (*syn* epidemic myalgia, epidemic pleurodynia) an epidemic pleurodynia usually associated with the B group of coxsackie viruses. It was first identified on Bornholm a Danish island. Incubation is 2–14 days. There is sudden onset of severe pain in lower chest and/or abdominal and/or lumbar muscles. Breathing may be difficult, because of the pain, and fever is common. May last up to one week. There is no specific treatment.

Borrelia (A Borrel, French bacteriologist, 1867–1936) a genus of coiled spirochaetes. Various species are responsible for louse-borne and tick-bourne relapsing fevers. Lyme disease is caused by the bacterium *Borrelia burgdorferi*.

BOS *abbr* bronchiolitis obliterans syndrome.

botulinum toxin an exotoxin produced by the bacterium *Clostridium botulinum*; it produces weakness in targeted muscles by blocking the release of acetylcholine at the neuromuscular junction. It is used in the treatment and management of focal plasticity. The effects lasts for up to 3 months and it should only be given as an adjunct to treatment.

botulism *n* an intoxication with the preformed exotoxin of *Clostridium botulinum*. Vomiting, respiratory, ocular and pharyngeal paralysis occur within 24–72 h of eating food contaminated with the spores, which require anaerobic conditions to produce the toxin. Associated with home preserving of vegetables and meat and improperly treated tinned food.

Bouchard's node (C Bouchard, French physician, 1837–1915) bony enlargement of the proximal interphalangeal finger joints. Characteristic of osteoarthritis. ⊃ Heberden's nodes

bougie *n* a cylindrical instrument made of gum elastic, metal or other material. Used in varying sizes for dilating strictures, e.g. oesophageal or urethral.

boundary layer microscopic layer of fluid (liquid or gas) next to the surface of a body or object moving relative to it, important in considering the drag force upon the object. ⊃ laminar boundary layer, turbulent boundary layer.

bounded saddle that portion of a prosthesis which is limited by a natural tooth at each end.

Bourneville's disease (D Bourneville, French neurologist, 1840–1909) ⊃ tuberous sclerosis

boutonneuse fever also known as Mediterranean Spotted Fever. A rickettsial infection caused by *Rickettsia conorii*, it is transmitted by tick bites. The infection is endemic in areas around the Mediterranean. The clinical features include the bite site turning black (tache noire), high fever,

chills, headache, photophobia, joint and muscle pain and a rash, which may become petechial.

boutonnière deformity a deformity of the finger occurring in rheumatoid arthritis. There is flexion of the proximal interphalangeal joint with hyperextension affecting the distal interphalangeal joint.

bovine *adj* relating to the cow or ox. *bovine tuberculosis* ⊃ tuberculosis

bovine somatotrophin (BST) a natural growth hormone of cattle. The administration of biosynthetic BST to dairy herds to increase milk production is prohibited in the European Union.

bovine spongiform encephalopathy (BSE) a fatal, infective (prion) neurological disease of cattle. ⊃ Creutzfeldt–Jakob disease.

bow orthodontic wire bent to the shape of the dental arch in the incisor region. May be labial or lingual. Usually has U-loops for adjustment of the tension of the bow.

bowel *n* the large intestine. ⊃ intestine.

bowel washout also called colonic washout. The washing out of the rectum and sigmoid colon with fluid, usually water. It may be used to remove faecal material to empty the bowel prior to a radiographic examination (e.g. barium enema), endoscopic examination (e.g. colonoscopy, sigmoidoscopy), or surgery involving the rectum or colon. The fluid is introduced through a tube by gravity and then returned by siphoning the fluid off. Used less often now that oral bowel cleanser preparations and disposable enemas are available for use.

Bowen's disease (J Bowen, American dermatologist, 1857–1940) intraepidermal carcinoma. A form of carcinoma in situ, which may progress to invasive malignancy, characterized by red-brown scaly or crusted lesions that resemble a patch of psoriasis or dermatitis. ⊃ intraepidermal carcinoma (Bowen's disease).

Bowen's resin ⊃ bisphenol-a-glycidyl methacrylate.

bowleg *n* ⊃ genu varum.

bowler's finger in sports medicine a colloquial term used to describe compression of the digital nerve on the medial aspect of the thumb leading to paraesthesia of the thumb.

Bowman's capsule (W Bowman, British anatomist, 1816–1892) glomerular capsule. The cup-like end of the renal tubule that encloses the glomerulus.

Bowman's layer ⊃ Bowman's membrane.

Bowman's membrane (W Bowman) (*syn* anterior limiting lamina, anterior limiting layer, Bowman's layer) thin layer of the cornea (about 12 mm) located between the anterior stratified epithelium and the stroma. This membrane is acellular; it is a modified superficial stromal layer found only in primates. It is composed of a randomly orientated array of fine collagen fibrils, primarily of collagen types I, III and V.

box in dentistry, that part of a compound cavity, excluding the occlusal portion, which has four cavity surfaces.

boxer's fracture in sports medicine a colloquial term used to describe a fracture of the fifth metacarpal bone secondary to a compressive force when the head of the metacarpal rotates over the neck leading to a flexion deformity.

boxing (of an impression) provision of a wall, usually of wax, to form a box around an impression to reduce time and effort in subsequently trimming and shaping plaster models. It is attached to the perimeter of the impression to contain the cast material until it has set.

boxing out in orthodontics, a recess created on the fitting surface of a removable appliance to allow for the movement of an active spring.

box impression tray ⊃ impression tray.

box technique in radiotherapy when two intersecting parallel pairs produce a uniform distribution of dose over the centrally placed volume enclosed by all four fields.

Boyd Gardner elevator ⊃ elevator (dental).

Boyle's anaesthetic machine apparatus for delivering anaesthetic agents mixed with oxygen and nitrous oxide or air. ⊃ pin index.

Boyle's law (R Boyle, English scientist, 1627–1691) a gas law that states that the volume of a quantity of a dry gas is inversely proportional to the pressure, if the temperature is constant.

BP *abbr* **1**. blood pressure. **2**. British pharmacopoeia.

BPD *abbr* **1**. biparietal diameter. **2**. bronchopulmonary dysplasia.

BPE *abbr* **1**. basic periodontal examination. **2**. benign prostatic enlargement.

BPF *abbr* bronchopleural fistula.

BPH *abbr* benign prostatic hyperplasia.

bpm *abbr* beats per minute.

B-point an orthodontic cephalometric landmark defined as the position of the deepest concavity on the anterior profile of the mandibular symphysis.

BPPV *abbr* benign paroxysmal positional vertigo.

brachial *adj* pertaining to the arm. Applied to vessels in this region and a nerve plexus at the root of the neck.

brachial artery the main artery of the upper arm. The brachial artery is a continuation of the axillary artery. It runs down the medial aspect of the upper arm, passes to the front of the elbow and extends to about 1 cm below the joint, where it divides into radial and ulnar arteries. The artery routinely used for the measurement of indirect blood pressure recording. ⊃ Colour Section Figure 9.

brachial plexus it is formed from the anterior rami of the lower four cervical nerves (C5–C8) and a large part of the first thoracic nerve (T1). The plexus is situated in the neck and shoulder above and behind the subclavian blood vessels and in the axilla. The branches of the brachial plexus supply the skin and muscles of the upper limbs and some of the chest muscles. Five large nerves and a number of smaller ones emerge from this plexus, each with a contribution from more than one nerve root, containing sensory, motor and autonomic fibres: axillary (circumflex) nerve—C5, 6; radial nerve— C5, 6, 7, 8, T1; musculocutaneous nerve—C5, 6, 7; median nerve—C5, 6, 7, 8, T1; ulnar nerve—C7, 8, T1; and the medial cutaneous nerve—C8, T1. The *axillary (circumflex) nerve* winds round the humerus at the level of the surgical neck. It then breaks up into minute branches to supply the deltoid muscle, shoulder joint and overlying skin. The *radial nerve* is the largest branch of the brachial plexus. It supplies the triceps muscle behind the humerus, crosses in front of the elbow joint then winds round to the back of the forearm to supply extensor muscles of the wrist and finger joints. It continues into the back of the hand to supply the skin of the thumb, the first two fingers and the lateral half of the third finger. The *musculocutaneous nerve* passes downwards to the lateral aspect of the forearm. It supplies the muscles of the upper arm and the skin of the forearm. The *median nerve* passes down the midline of the arm in close association with the brachial artery. It passes in front of the elbow joint then down to supply the muscles of the front of the forearm. It continues into the hand where it supplies small muscles and the skin of the front of the thumb, the first two fingers and the lateral half of the third finger. It gives off no branches above the elbow. The *ulnar nerve* descends through the upper arm lying medial to the brachial artery. It passes behind the medial epicondyle of the humerus to supply the muscles on the ulnar aspect of the forearm. It continues downwards to supply the muscles in the palm of the hand and the skin of the whole of the little finger and the medial half of the third finger. It gives off no branches above the elbow. The anterior and posterior branches of the *medial cutaneous nerve* supply the skin of the front, medial aspect and the back of the forearm. ⊃ Colour Section Figure 11.

brachial plexus sports injury brachial plexus injury is most common in sports with upper body contact such as rugby and American football (where it is called a 'stinger'), with forced lateral flexion, hyperextension or rotation of the neck. Symptoms include pain and burning sensation in the neck with paraesthesia, heaviness and weakness of the affected arm and can last from a few minutes to a few weeks. If symptoms persist, a formal neurological assessment including scanning is required, though in most cases complete resolution results.

brachial vein a deep vein of the arm. It follows the same course as the brachial artery, and drains blood into the axillary vein. ⊃ Colour Section Figure 10.

brachialis *n* a muscle of the upper arm. Its origin is on the humerus and it inserts on the coronoid process of the ulna. It is deep to the biceps brachii and flexes the forearm. ⊃ Colour Section Figure 4.

brachi/o- a prefix that means 'arm', e.g. *brachialis*.

brachiocephalic *adj* pertaining to the arm and head.

brachiocephalic (innominate) artery or trunk one of three large arteries branching from the aortic arch. It is about 4–5 cm long and passes obliquely upwards, backwards and to the right. At the level of the sternoclavicular joint it divides into the right common carotid artery and the right subclavian artery. ⊃ Colour Section Figure 9.

brachiocephalic (innominate) veins two large veins situated one on each side in the root of the neck. Each is formed by the union of the internal jugular and the subclavian veins. The left brachiocephalic vein is longer than the right and passes obliquely behind the manubrium of the sternum, where it joins the right brachiocephalic vein to form the superior vena cava. ⊃ Colour Section Figure 10.

brachioradialis *n* a superficial muscle of the forearm involved in forearm flexion. Its origin is on the lateral aspect of the distal humerus and it inserts on the styloid process of the radius. ⊃ Colour Section Figure 4.

brachium *n* the arm (especially from shoulder to elbow), or any arm-like appendage—**brachia** *pl*, **brachial** *adj*.

brachy- a prefix that means 'short', e.g. *brachydactylia*.

brachycephaly a congenital malformation that results in a short, broad skull.

brachydactylia abnormally short fingers.

brachygnathia also called micrognathia. There is under-development of the mandible.

brachytherapy *n* radiotherapy delivered from a sealed radioactive source placed in a body cavity, or inserted into tissue to deliver a large radiation dose to a tumour with a smaller dose to the surrounding tissue. The technique may be used to treat cancers of the anus, breast, uterine cervix, lung, oesophagus, prostate gland and the tongue.

bracing resistance to the horizontal components of masticatory forces.

bracing arm that portion of a partial denture designed to resist the action of lateral displacing force. Sometimes known as a lateral resistive arm.

bracket orthodontic attachment. The metal, plastic or ceramic orthodontic component welded to an orthodontic band or bonded (cemented) directly onto a tooth. Arch wires or other orthodontic wires may be attached to it.

bracket removing pliers ⊃ pliers.

Braden risk scale a pressure ulcer risk scale in which the lower the number scored, the higher the risk of developing a pressure ulcer. It scores risk factors that include activity, mobility, nutrition, sensory perception, moisture and friction and shear. ⊃ pressure ulcer risk scale.

Bradford frame (E Bradford, American surgeon, 1848–1926) a stretcher type of bed used for: (a) immobilizing the spine; (b) resting trunk and back muscles; (c) preventing deformity. It is a tubular steel frame fitted with two canvas slings allowing a 100–150 mm gap to facilitate personal care and elimination.

brady- a prefix that means 'slow', e.g. *bradykinesia*.

bradycardia *n* slow rate of heart contraction. Defined in adults at rest as a pulse rate less than 60 beats per minute. It is known as sinus bradycardia when it arises from the normal pacemaker in the heart (sinus node or sinoatrial node), e.g. the slow resting heart rate in trained athletes, when vagal tone is increased. Pathological causes include the action of some drugs, or hormonal or electrolyte abnormalities; a fixed slow rate can arise from an abnormal focus, when the spread of excitation from the sinus node (SA node) is prevented by heart block. In the fetus, a heart rate of less than 100 beats per minute.

bradyglossia abnormal slowness or deliberation in speech.

bradykinesia abnormally slow or retarded movement associated with difficulty initiating and then stopping a movement; typically seen in Parkinson's disease.

bradykinin a kinin. A polypeptide mediator of the inflammatory process. It causes vasodilation, increases blood vessel permeability, smooth muscle contraction and induces pain. ⊃ kinins.

bradyphagia very slow eating.

bradypnoea an abnormally slow respiratory rate.

Braille (L Braille, French teacher, 1809–1852) a printing system that produces a series of raised dots representing the alphabet. People with visual impairment are able to read by touch.

brain *n* the encephalon; the largest part of the central nervous system (CNS): it is contained in the cranial cavity and is surrounded by three membranes called meninges (from outside in—the dura mater, arachnoid mater and the pia mater). The cerebrospinal fluid inside the brain is contained in the ventricles, and outside in the subarachnoid space acts as a shock absorber to the delicate nerve tissue of the brain and spinal cord. The brain comprises the cerebral hemispheres, brainstem (midbrain, pons and medulla oblongata) and the cerebellum. ⊃ Colour Section Figure 1. The brainstem connects the cerebral hemispheres to the cerebellum and the spinal cord. The CNS comprises grey matter and white matter. Grey matter refers to regions and clusters consisting mainly of neuron cell bodies (forming the cortical layers and more deeply the various control centres and nuclei), whereas white matter is composed mainly of myelinated nerve fibres in the tracts that link neurons in the different parts of the brain to each other and to the spinal cord. Uppermost in the brain are the anatomically symmetrical left and right cerebral hemispheres with frontal, parietal, temporal and occipital lobes, the grey matter of the cerebral cortex forming the convoluted outermost layer. ⊃ Colour Section Figure 24. Below the hemispheres the medulla oblongata (the lowest part of the brainstem) is continuous with the spinal cord at the foramen magnum (an opening) in the base of the skull. The cerebellum, also with a cortex of grey matter, lies behind and alongside the brainstem, with connections to it, and relays up and down to other parts of the CNS.

brain death a situation where the brainstem is fatally and irreversibly damaged. The brainstem is responsible for maintaining vital functions including breathing. Strict criteria must be met before the patient is declared dead. These include testing certain reflexes, e.g. gag and pupillary, and the absence of factors that could depress brainstem activity. Suitable patients may become organ donors if this coincides with the wishes of the family and those of the patient if known. ⊃ death.

bran *n* the husk of grain. The coarse outer part of cereals, especially wheat, high in non-starch polysaccharide (NSP) and the vitamin B complex.

branchial *adj* relating to the gills. Embryonic clefts or fissures either side of the neck from which the nose, ears and mouth will eventually develop.

branchial cyst a cyst in the neck resulting from a developmental abnormality of the branchial clefts.

Brandt–Andrews method (T Brandt, Swedish obstetrician, 1819–1895; H Andrews, British obstetrician, 1871–1942) a method of delivering the placenta after separation and descent into the vagina during the third stage of labour. Now superseded by controlled cord traction. ⊃ controlled cord traction.

BRAO *abbr* branch retinal arterial occlusion.

Braun's frame a metal frame, bandaged for use, and equally useful for drying a lower leg plaster and for applying skeletal traction (Steinmann's pin or Kirschner wire inserted through the calcaneus) to a fractured tibia, after reduction.

Braxton Hicks contractions (J Braxton Hicks, British physician, 1823–1897) painless uterine contractions occurring during pregnancy. They facilitate uterine blood flow through the placenta, thereby promoting oxygen delivery to the fetus.

BRCA1, BRCA2 genes that normally protect against abnormal cell growth. A defective version of the gene does not prevent cell proliferation and the individual is at risk of developing breast or ovarian cancer.

break-bone fever ⊃ dengue.

break test an isometric contraction against manual resistance (provided by the examiner) with the joint in its mid-range position; used to determine the athlete's ability to generate a static force within a muscle or muscle group.

break-through bleeding loss of blood from the uterus not associated with menstruation.

break-up time (BUT) test a test for assessing the precorneal tear film. Fluorescein is applied to the bulbar conjunctiva and the patient is asked to blink once or twice and then to refrain from blinking. The tear film is scanned through the slit-lamp using a cobalt blue filter with a wide beam, while the examiner counts or records the time between the last blink and the appearance of the first dry black spot which indicates that the tear film is breaking up. In normal subjects, break-up times vary between 15 and 35 s (in Caucasians). A BUT of 10 s or less is abnormal and may be due to mucin deficiency and is often considered to be a negative factor for success in contact lens wear, especially soft lenses. However, this test has been shown to be flawed, because fluorescein can disrupt the tear film. ⊃ cobalt lens, mucin, non-invasive break-up time test, precorneal film.

breast *n* **1.** the anterior upper part of the thorax. **2.** the milk-secreting mammary gland.

breast awareness the activities undertaken by the woman in order to detect abnormal breast changes. These include change in breast size or shape, lumps in the breast or axilla, thickening, skin changes such as dimpling, nipple inversion, nipple discharge or itching, or pain.

breast board an immobilization device used to aid and maintain patient positioning during radiotherapy treatment. The patient's shoulders may be raised while providing arm support and/or handgrips.

breast bone colloquial term for the sternum.

breast cancer breast cancer is the commonest malignancy in the UK; about 1–2% of all breast cancers occur during pregnancy or lactation. Men may also be affected and about 1% of all breast cancers occur in men. It is generally a disease of older men and the presentation, diagnosis, prognosis and treatment are similar to those for women. The majority of breast cancers present as a lump. All lumps should be investigated, although the majority will not be malignant. Most breast cancers are painless at presentation, but around 20% of women will feel some discomfort or altered sensation. A locally invasive breast cancer may cause puckering or dimpling. Some breast cancers may present with an indrawn nipple or discharge. A small number of breast cancers present with an enlarged axillary lymph node. Lymphatic system involvement may be indicative of metastatic spread. The mammography screening programme will pick up very small, non-palpable tumours. Inflammatory cancers of the breast (locally advanced tumours) present with redness, swelling and breast pain. The skin resembles that of an orange with fine indentations and is referred to as *peau d'orange*. Whether a patient is diagnosed as a result of signs or symptoms, or through screening, the approach is the same. The assessment will involve a clinical history and examination that may help distinguish cyst from solid lump. Diagnostic mammography may identify malignant calcification or other features of concern, or the presence of a cyst. This may be complemented by ultrasound, and magnetic resonance imaging (MRI) may help if the findings are equivocal. Cytological examination of material obtained from fine needle aspirate (FNA) and/or histopathology from a core biopsy will include measurement of tumour grade, oestrogen receptor status and in some cases progesterone receptor and/or HER2 status. These can be performed (probably more accurately) on a definitive resection specimen (wide local excision or mastectomy). Once a diagnosis of invasive cancer is made, further staging is performed. Commonly this will include a chest X-ray, bone scan and liver ultrasound. However, less common or geographical variations may include bone marrow biopsy (sampling) and computed tomography (CT) of the chest and abdomen. Management depends upon the stage of the cancer and if it has spread and whether a woman is pre- or post-menopausal. The treatment modalities, which are used in various combinations, include: (a) surgery—'lumpectomy', simple mastectomy (usually with breast reconstruction), removal of lymph nodes; (b) radiotherapy; (c) chemotherapy— drugs such as cyclophosphamide, docetaxel, doxorubicin, epirubicin, 5-fluorouracil, methotrexate, etc. in various combinations; (d) hormonal treatments—tamoxifen (oestrogen receptor antagonist), aromatase inhibitors (e.g. letrozole), ovarian ablation, gonadotrophin-releasing hormone (GnRH) analogues, such as goserelin, inhibit the release of goadotrophins; (e) biological treatments—trastuzumab, lapatinib. ⊃ breast awareness, breast care nurse, human epidermal growth factor receptor-2 (HER2), mammography.

breast care nurse specialized nurses who provides care, counselling and support to patients (and their families) having investigations for breast disease and those with a diagnosis of disease including breast cancer. She/he provides nurse-led services (e.g. post-treatment follow up), information about various treatment modalities, breast reconstruction and the various prostheses available to women who have had a mastectomy.

breast jig a support which raises the patient's shoulders and provides arm support and/or handgrip to enable the patient to maintain the position during radiotherapy treatment.

breast milk substance secreted from the breasts via the nipple, consisting first of colostrum, then once lactation is established, of foremilk, a high volume of relatively low fat milk, followed by hindmilk, a lower volume of milk with up to five times more fat than foremilk. It contains fats, fatty acids, carbohydrate, proteins, vitamins, minerals and trace elements, plus a number of anti-infective factors including immunoglobulins, lysozymes, lactoferrin, bifidus, hormones and growth factors.

breast milk jaundice elevated unconjugated bilirubin in some breastfed babies due to presence of a steroid in the milk which inhibits glucuronyl transferase conjugating activity.

breast milk substitutes infant formulae, usually made from modified cows' milk, with strict regulations as to the permitted constituents specified in the Infant Formula and Follow-on Formula Regulations 1995. Infant formulae may be whey dominant in which the ratio of proteins approximates to the whey:casein ratio in human milk, or casein dominant which forms relatively indigestible curds in the stomach, intended to make the baby feel satisfied, but which places greater metabolic demands on the baby.

breast pump suction apparatus used to withdraw milk from the breast, with a vacuum created by hand pressure on a rubber bulb, or by an electrical pump.

breath-hold voluntary suppression of breathing movements. The breath-hold time is very variable between subjects and conditions. Starting from full lung volume, breathing air, less than one minute is usual, but longer after hyperventilation or after breathing oxygen. Although the unsuppressible stimulus to breathe at break-point (in healthy subjects) is related to rising carbon dioxide, interaction with other factors is complex, involving central respiratory rhythm, afferents from the diaphragm and decreasing lung volume. ➲ diving.

breath holding involuntary breath holding in otherwise healthy toddlers. They typically occur when the child is upset or startled, and starts to cry.

breathing the regular inflation and deflation of the lungs, serving the purpose of respiratory gas exchange. Breathing and its pattern—the depth and frequency of breaths—are controlled by a group of neurons in the brainstem, and vary in response to changes in afferent information from several sites, notably the chemoreceptors (sensitive to changes in oxygen, CO_2 and pH in arterial blood, and to the pH in the brain) and from muscles and joints (which signal changes in activity). Breathing consists of inspiration (involving effort), expiration (usually a passive phase using the energy

stored from inspiration) and rest (a time of no airflow) prior to the next inspiration. Air enters the lungs as a result of the pressure gradients generated by thoracic expansion and contraction. For breathing to be efficient, it must exceed the body's requirements for oxygen uptake and carbon dioxide removal. The output from the 'respiratory centre' regulates, via the phrenic nerves, the frequency and strength of contraction of the diaphragm, which accounts alone for breathing at rest. With increasing demand, the intercostal muscles contribute additional lung inflation/deflation by their action on the size and shape of the ribcage, assisted when breathing is deepest by the accessory muscles of respiration, including neck, chest and abdominal muscles. ➲ abdominal breathing, apnoea, dyspnoea, ventilation.

breathing ventilation The alternate cycle of inspiration and expiration as air is moved in and out of the lungs.

breathing frequency the number of breaths per minute. Also known as respiratory rate. At rest, varies among adults from about 10–20 per minute. In exercise, can rise to 40–50 per minute.

breathlessness dyspnoea. One of the four cardinal symptoms of respiratory disease. It is a subjective perception, related to life experience and is, therefore, a symptom reported and detailed by the patient. The clinician cannot fully appreciate nor judge the level of dyspnoea, as with other similar sensations, e.g. pain, fear, hunger, grief. It should not be confused with tachypnoea (a rapid respiratory rate). The sensation becomes distressing when the breathlessness perceived is greater than that expected for the activity undertaken. This symptom is thought to play a significant role in the deconditioning, which occurs through avoidance measures undertaken by patients suffering from chronic lung disease. ➲ Borg dyspnoea scale.

breath sounds the sounds generated in the larger airways, mainly during inspiration and for a short time during expiration. They can be heard using a stethoscope. Abnormal breath sounds include diminished, rhonchi (wheeze), a pleural rub and crepitations (crackles).

breath tests non-invasive investigations for gastrointestinal conditions such as the presence of *Helicobacter pylori* or malabsorption.

breech *n* the buttocks. ➲ buttock.

breech delivery the fetal dangers include intracranial haemorrhage, hypoxia, fractures, dislocations and soft tissue injuries. An episiotomy is performed in second stage before the anterior buttock is delivered to minimize compression on the aftercoming fetal head, the feet are guided over the perineum and a loop of cord is pulled down to prevent traction on the umbilicus. If the arms are flexed, the shoulders are delivered with the next contraction; extended arms are delivered using Løvset's manoeuvre. Once the trunk and shoulders are born, the infant is allowed to hang by his/her own weight (Burns-Marshall manoeuvre) for about one minute, to aid flexion and descent of the head. When the hair line appears at the vulva the infant is held firmly by the ankles and the trunk is raised in a wide arc up and over the

A
B

mother's abdomen. The Maurceau–Smellie–Veit manoeuvre is used when the head is extended and fails to descend. ⊃ Burns Marshall manoeuvre, Løvset's manoeuvre, Maurceau–Smellie–Veit manoeuvre.

breech presentation refers to the position of a infant in the uterus such that the buttocks, knee or foot would be born first (Figure B.10): the normal position is head first. Breech presentation is a longitudinal lie with fetal buttocks presenting in the lower uterine pole, due to pelvic, uterine, fetal or incidental causes; approximately 2.5% incidence at term. Abdominally the fetal head is palpated in the fundus; vaginally the buttocks, anal orifice, genitalia or feet are palpated; diagnosis is confirmed on ultrasound; changing the presentation with external version or moxibustion may be attempted.

bregma *n* anterior fontanelle, a kite-shaped membranous area in the head of the fetus and infant at the junction of the frontal, coronal and sagittal sutures. ⊃ fetal skull, fontanelle.

Bremsstrahlung radiation electromagnetic radiation produced by the rapid deceleration of an electron during a close approach to the atomic nucleus, e.g. the X-ray quanta produced when electrons from the filament of the X-ray tube interact with the nuclei of the target.

Breslow's depth (A Breslow, American pathologist, 1928–1980) the depth to which a malignant melanoma has infiltrated. ⊃ Clark's level.

bridge *n* in dentistry, a fixed prosthesis used for a restoration to replace one or more teeth using artificial crowns connected to natural teeth. It is soldered or otherwise attached to one or more retainers such as a metal wing, crown or gold inlay, themselves cemented to abutment teeth roots or implants. It is not intended to be removed by the patient. ⊃ adhesive bridge, bridge retainer, bridge span, bridge unit, cantilever bridge, fixed-fixed bridge, fixed-movable bridge, Maryland bridge, Rochette bridge, spring cantilever bridge, temporary bridge.

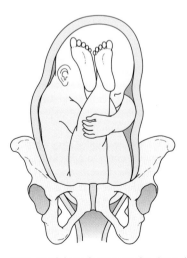

B.10 Frank breech presentation (reproduced from Fraser & Cooper 2003 with permission).

bridge retainer in dentistry, a restoration cemented to an abutment tooth which provides retention for a bridge. ⊃ bridge.

bridge span in dentistry, that part of a bridge between two abutments. ⊃ bridge.

bridge unit in dentistry, an individual part of a bridge such as a pontic or a retainer. ⊃ bridge.

bridle wire ⊃ wiring.

Brinell hardness scale or number (BHN) ⊃ hardness scale.

British sign language (BSL) a type of sign language (signing) used in the UK.

brittle bone disease ⊃ osteogenesis imperfecta.

brittle diabetes poor glycaemic control of diabetes mellitus. Blood glucose levels are unstable.

BRM *abbr* biological response modifier.

broad focus the selection of a large filament to enable a larger area of the anode to be bombarded with electrons.

broad ligaments lateral ligaments; not a ligament but a double fold of parietal peritoneum which hangs over the uterus and outstretched uterine (fallopian) tubes, forming a lateral partition across the pelvic cavity. Also called the mesometrium. ⊃ Colour Section Figure 17.

broad thumb syndrome Rubinstein–Taybi syndrome.

Broca's aphasia a disturbance of language where the person has difficulty speaking or repeating words, but has a good understanding. Named after the area of the brain that is damaged in this disorder. ⊃ Broca's area.

Broca's area (P Broca, French neurologist, 1824–1880) the motor speech area, situated in the dominant cerebral hemisphere (usually the left). Injury to this centre can result in a disturbance of language.

Brock's after-image test ⊃ after-image transfer test.

Brock's string (*syn* bead on string) a white string used to demonstrate physiological diplopia. One end of the string is placed against the bridge of the nose and the other end against a distant object (e.g. a doorknob). The subject should see two strings intersecting wherever the horizontal components of the visual axes meet. Red and green filters, one before each eye, enhance or facilitate the observation of the two strings. Several beads, each of a different colour, are usually threaded on the string so that they can be moved at will. One bead may be used for fixation while the other/s appear double; in crossed diplopia for the one closer to the eyes than the fixation bead, and in uncrossed diplopia for the one further away than the fixation bead. Brock's string is commonly used in visual training. The observation of physiological diplopia with Brock's string is often referred to as Brock's string test. ⊃ physiological diplopia.

Brodie's abscess (B Brodie, British surgeon, 1783–1862) chronic osteomyelitis occurring without previous acute phase. ⊃ abscess.

Brodmann areas (K Brodmann, German neurologist, 1868–1918) areas of the cerebral cortex that are associated with specific neurological functions such as movement (motor cortex) or vision (visual cortex), etc. Each area is distinguished histologically by the different staining characteristics of the neurons.

bromatology the science concerned with foods.

bromidrosis *n* a profuse, fetid perspiration, especially associated with the feet—**bromidrotic** *adj*.

bromism *n* chronic poisoning due to continued or excessive use of bromides.

bromopnoea bad breath. ⇨ halitosis.

bronch/i/o- a prefix that means 'bronchi', e.g. *bronchiolitis*.

bronchi *npl* the two tubes into which the trachea divides at its lower end—**bronchus** *sing*. ⇨ bronchus, Colour Section Figures 6, 7.

bronchial *adj* pertaining to the bronchi.

bronchial asthma ⇨ asthma.

bronchial cancer ⇨ non-small cell carcinoma, oat cell carcinoma.

bronchial tree network of bronchi and bronchioles as they subdivide within the lungs. The air passages leading from the trachea to the lung alveoli, via a left and a right main bronchus, the branches from these to the lobes of the lungs, and within the lungs the progressively smaller bronchioles, terminal bronchioles (~0.2 mm diameter) and finally the respiratory bronchioles which open into the alveolar ducts and the alveoli. All branches except the final, smallest ones have circular smooth muscle in their walls, which can change the diameter, varying the resistance to airflow. Cartilage stiffens the walls down to the bronchioles, forming C-shaped rings in the trachea, becoming less complete in the bronchi and their branches. ⇨ airways.

bronchiectasis *n* abnormal dilatation of the bronchi which, when localized, is usually the result of pneumonia or lobar collapse in childhood, but when generalized is due to some inherent disorder of the bronchial mucous membrane as in cystic fibrosis. Characterized by recurrent respiratory infections with profuse purulent sputum and digital clubbing. Eventually leads to respiratory failure. Mainstay of treatment is prompt treatment with appropriate antibiotics and regular physiotherapy to optimize sputum clearance—**bronchiectatic** *adj*.

bronchioles *n* the minute subdivisions of the bronchi which terminate in the alveoli (air sacs) of the lungs. The subdivisions of the bronchi commence five to 14 divisions below the segmental bronchi, usually 2 mm or less in diameter, containing no cartilage within their walls. The presence of bronchial smooth muscle enables changes in the diameter of the airways, with contraction resulting in bronchoconstriction (airway narrowing) and changes in airway resistance. The terminal bronchioles are smaller subdivisions and these terminate at the respiratory bronchioles prior to the alveolar ducts and alveoli. The bronchioles are held open by the outward traction pull of adjacent alveoli—**bronchiolar** *adj*.

bronchiolitis *n* inflammation of the bronchioles, usually due to an acute lower respiratory tract infection caused by the respiratory syncytial virus (RSV) in infants during the first year of life. The infant is breathless, with a wheeze and has respiratory distress—**bronchiolitic** *adj*.

bronchiolitis obliterans organizing pneumonia (BOOP) ⇨ cryptogenic organizing pneumonia.

bronchiolitis obliterans syndrome (BOS) progressive scarring and loss of function seen in the lungs, in part as a result of chronic rejection of a transplanted lung over time.

bronchitis *n* inflammation of the bronchi. *acute bronchitis* as an isolated incident is usually a primary viral infection occurring in children as a complication of the common cold, influenza, whooping cough, measles or rubella. Secondary infection occurs with bacteria, commonly *Streptococcus pneumoniae* or *Haemophilus influenzae*. Acute bronchitis in adults is usually an acute exacerbation of chronic bronchitis precipitated by a viral infection but sometimes by a sudden increase in atmospheric pollution. *chronic bronchitis* is defined as a cough productive of sputum for at least three consecutive months in two consecutive years. The bronchial mucus-secreting glands are hypertrophied with an increase in goblet cells and loss of ciliated cells due to irritation from tobacco smoke, or atmospheric pollutants. ⇨ chronic obstructive pulmonary disease (COPD), pulmonary emphysema—**bronchitic** *adj*.

bronchoalveolar lavage (BAL) endoscopic diagnostic irrigation of the lungs with small volumes of saline which are then aspirated and examined for cancer, infection and other abnormalities; occasionally large volume lavage may be therapeutic.

bronchoconstriction a narrowing of the bronchi due to contraction of the smooth muscle. This can occur through irritation of the respiratory tract in response to the inhalation of noxious substances, e.g. post aspiration, cigarette smoking, smoke inhalation and trauma. Symptoms include wheeze and dyspnoea.

bronchoconstrictor *n* any agent which constricts the bronchi.

bronchodilation a widening of the tracheobronchial tree through relaxation of the smooth muscle contained within the bronchial walls. This may result from stimulation of the sympathetic nervous system, but can also follow the administration of bronchodiator drugs.

bronchodilator *n* any agent which dilates the bronchi, e.g. the drug salbutamol. ⇨ beta (β)-adrenoceptor agonists, muscarinic antagonists. ⇨ Appendix 5.

bronchogenic *adj* arising from one of the bronchi.

bronchography *n* mainly obsolete radiological demonstration of the bronchial tree following the introduction of contrast agent via the trachea.

bronchomycosis *n* general term describing a variety of fungal infections of the bronchi and lungs, e.g. pulmonary candidiasis—**bronchomycotic** *adj*.

bronchophony *n* abnormal transmission of voice sounds heard over consolidated lung or over a thin layer of pleural fluid.

bronchopleural fistula (BPF) pathological communication between the pleural cavity and one of the bronchi. It occurs as a thoracic surgical complication, most commonly, post pneumonectomy (spillage of the space contents occurs into the opposite lung via the stump of the surgically removed lung). Bronchopleural fistula is more likely to occur when resections have been performed for tuberculosis or fungal infections and the severity of patient presentation varies with the size of the fistula.

bronchopneumonia *n* describes a type of pneumonia in which areas of consolidation are distributed widely around bronchi and not in a lobar pattern. Generally affects patients at the extremes of age, those who are debilitated or secondary to existing condition—**bronchopneumonic** *adj*.

bronchopulmonary *adj* pertaining to the bronchi and the lungs—**bronchopulmonic** *adj*.

bronchopulmonary dysplasia (BPD) a chronic condition that occurs in infants who required long term respiratory support with mechanical ventilation or oxygen. It is characterized by thickening of pulmonary blood vessels and scarring of lung tissue, resulting in a ventilation/perfusion mismatch.

bronchopulmonary segment subdivisions of the lobes of the lungs, each containing its own segmental bronchus.

bronchorrhoea *n* an excessive discharge of mucus from the bronchial mucosa—**bronchorrhoeal** *adj*.

bronchoscope *n* an endoscope used for examining, photographing and taking biopsies from the interior of the bronchi. Also used for removal of inhaled foreign bodies. Bronchoscopes are either flexible fibreoptic instruments or rigid tubes—**bronchoscopic** *adj*, **bronchoscopically** *adv*.

bronchoscopy *n* endoscopic examination of the tracheobronchial tree.

bronchospasm *n* sudden constriction of the bronchial tubes due to contraction of involuntary smooth muscle in their walls—**bronchospastic** *adj*.

bronchostenosis *n* narrowing of one of the bronchi—**bronchostenotic** *adj*.

bronchotracheal *adj* pertaining to the bronchi and trachea.

bronchus *n* the first division of the airways. The bronchi (left and right) arise from the trachea. The left bronchus is longer and more angled than the right, so that accidental inhalation of material enters the right lung more readily than the left. The bronchi has cartilaginous walls providing upper-airway stability during respiration. There are around 10 divisions of bronchi from the trachea—**bronchi** *sing*.

bronze diabetes ⊃ haemochromatosis.

Brook airway ⊃ airway.

Broselow™ paediatric resuscitation system designed in the USA for use during paediatric resuscitation. The Broselow tape measure, with its colour segments, is placed alongside the child. This provides the medical team with accurate information, from the colour segment that corresponds to the length of the child, regarding the correct size of equipment and appropriate drug doses to be used for that child. The equipment is stored in colour-coded packaging.

brought in dead (BID) describes a situation where the person has died prior to arriving at the hospital.

brow *n* the forehead; the region above the supraorbital ridge.

brow presentation cephalic presentation with the attitude of the fetal head midway between flexion and extension; presenting mentovertical diameter of 13.0–13.75 cm is larger than those of the average pelvis, leading to obstructed labour. The causes include: android pelvis, in which the biparietal diameter impacts in the sacrocotyloid diameter of the pelvis, causing head extension; fetal conditions e.g. hydrocephaly or anencephaly. Occurs in approximately one in 1000–1500 labours. Abdominally the fetal head will be high above the pelvic brim; vaginally the head will not be felt, but occasionally the bregma and orbital ridges can be felt. Caesarean section is usually required or if not feasible, vaginal manipulation to flex the head to a vertex presentation, or to extend it further into a face presentation, with forceps then being applied. Internal podalic version and breech delivery may also be attempted. ⊃ face presentation.

brown adipose tissue (brown fat) present in newborns and rarely in adults. It is metabolically highly active adipose tissue with a greater thermogenic activity than ordinary white fat. Provides the heat energy needed by infants to maintain body temperature.

Brown-Séquard syndrome (C Brown-Séquard, French physiologist, 1817–1894) a condition resulting from compression of one side of the spinal cord above the tenth thoracic vertebra. There is spastic paralysis on the same side of the body, loss of proprioception and loss of pain and temperature sensation on the other side.

Brucella *n* a genus of bacteria causing brucellosis (undulant fever in humans; contagious abortion in cattle). *Brucella abortus* is the bovine strain. *Brucella melitensis* the sheep/goat strain, both transmissible via infected milk.

brucellosis *n* (*syn* melitensis) a generalized infection in humans resulting from one of the species of *Brucella*: *B. abortus* in cattle, *B. suis* in pigs and *B. melitensis* in sheep and goats. It is transmitted by contaminated milk or contact with the carcass of an infected animal. High risk groups include farmers, abattoir workers and veterinary surgeons. There are recurrent attacks of continuous or undulating fever and low mood. It may last for months with relapses. The condition is also known as 'Malta fever', 'abortus fever', 'Mediterranean fever' and 'undulant fever'.

Bruce protocol (R Bruce, American cardiologist, 1916–2004) a protocol for exercise tests in which the intensity is increased incrementally at 3-minute intervals. Normally a treadmill test, with increments of gradient and speed, but can be adapted for a static cycle ergometer. Used commonly in the assessment of patients with known or suspected heart disease. The modified Bruce protocol has two initial stages at a lower intensity than in the standard test, allowing assessment of those who are symptomatic at lower levels of activity or less fit as a result of other diseases, such as arthritis or respiratory disease. ⊃ incremental exercise.

Bruch's membrane (K Bruch, German anatomist, 1819–1884) the innermost layer of the choroid. It is a thin (about 1.5 mm), shiny, non-vascular layer of the choroid located on the inner side next to the pigment epithelium of the retina.

It consists of two contiguous layers; the inner one called the *lamina vitrea* (or basement membrane of the pigment epithelium) and the outer one called the *lamina elastica*. ⊃ age-related macular degeneration, angioid streaks, choroid, retinal pigment epithelium.

Brudzinski's sign (J Brudzinski, Polish physician, 1874–1917) immediate flexion of knees and hips on raising head from pillow. Seen in meningitis.

bruise *n* (*syn* contusion, ecchymosis) a discolouration of the skin due to an extravasation of blood into the underlying tissues; there is no break of the skin. ⊃ contusion.

bruit *n* ⊃ murmur.

Brunner's glands (J Brunner, Swiss anatomist, 1856–1927) mucus-secreting glands of the small intestine.

Brunnstrom approach a technique developed by Brunnstrom for maximizing recovery after stroke. It is based on the idea that reflex activity and movement synergies are used as the basis for voluntary movement and a progression from gross proximal movement towards distal fine movement.

brush border microvilli present on the surface of absorptive cells in the small intestine and those in the proximal convoluted tubule of the nephron.

Brushfield's spots (T Brushfield, British physician, 1858–1937) white, grey or yellow spots on the iris of the eye. Typically associated with Down's syndrome but occasionally seen in other infants.

Bruton's agammaglobulinaemia (O Brunton, American physician, 1908–2003) a congenital condition in boys, in which B lymphocytes are absent but cellular immunity remains intact. ⊃ dysgammaglobulinaemia.

bruxism *n* the involuntary grinding or clenching of teeth. Often associated with stress or anxiety and frequently triggered by occlusal irregularities. Sequelae to bruxism may include abnormal tooth-wear patterns, joint or neuromuscular problems and periodontal breakdown.

BRVO *abbr* branch retinal vein occlusion.

Bryant's 'gallows' traction (T Bryant, British physician, 1828–1914) skin traction applied to the lower limbs; the legs are then suspended vertically (from an overhead beam), so that the buttocks are lifted just clear of the bed. Formally used for fractures of the femur in children up to 4 years. Now largely replaced with hoop traction.

BSE *abbr* 1. bovine spongiform encephalopathy. 2. breast self-examination.

BST *abbr* bovine somatotrophin.

bubo *n* enlargement of lymph nodes, especially in the groin. A feature of chancroid, lymphogranuloma venereum and bubonic plague—**bubonic** *adj*.

bubonic plague ⊃ plague.

buccal *adj* relating to or adjacent to the cheek or mouth. Term denoting the surfaces of premolars and molars facing towards the cheeks. ⊃ buccal cavity, buccal sulcus.

buccal cavity ⊃ mouth, oral cavity.

buccal drug administration a method where a drug, usually in tablet form, is dissolved between the cheek and gum or the top lip and gum. The buccal mucosa has a plentiful blood supply which allows the drug to be absorbed into the circulation thereby overcoming first pass metabolism/first pass effect in the liver. Sometimes a spray containing the drug is used. ⊃ sublingual.

buccal inlay ⊃ skin grafting vestibuloplasty.

buccal plate term used to describe the buccal cortex of alveolar bone.

buccal segment classificaion anteroposterior relationships of the jaws classified according to the relationship of the lower molar teeth to the upper molar teeth, with particular reference to the first molars. ⊃ Angle's classification.

buccal spring orthodontic wire spring working from the buccal aspect of a tooth.

buccal sulcus fold in the oral tissues, by mucous membrane and bounded externally by the cheeks and internally by the teeth.

buccal surface ⊃ surface.

buccal tube tube usually attached to the buccal aspect of an orthodontic appliance in the molar region, through which a wire may pass.

buccinator a thin flat cheek muscle, important in the mastication of food. Its origin is on the maxilla and mandible and it inserts onto the orbicularis oris muscle.

bucket handle tear a description given to a type of tear of the meniscus of the knee joint that extends along the length of the meniscus.

bucky a device for holding a cassette beneath an X-ray table which contains a grid which moves during the radiographic exposure.

Budd–Chiari syndrome (G Budd, British physician, 1808–1882; H Chiari, German pathologist, 1851–1916) a liver condition. Obstruction of the hepatic vein leads to hepatic portal hypertension.

Buerger's disease (*syn* thromboangiitis obliterans) (L Buerger, American physician, 1879–1943) a chronic obliterative vascular disease of peripheral vessels that results in ischaemia, intermittent claudication, skin changes and gangrene. The incidence is associated with the presence of human leucocyte antigens HLA-A9 and HLA-B5. It affects young and middle-aged men.

Buerger's exercises exercises designed to treat Buerger's disease (thromboangiitis obliterans). The legs are placed alternately in elevation and dependence to assist perfusion of the extremities with blood.

buffer *n* 1. substances that limit pH change by their ability to accept or donate hydrogen ions as appropriate. In biological systems they limit pH changes that would inhibit cell functioning. The important buffer systems in the body include: bicarbonate (hydrogen carbonate) system, hydrogen phosphates and proteins, e.g. haemoglobin. 2. any agent that reduces shock or jarring due to contact. 3. in radiographic film processing, in developer boric acid and sodium hydroxide are used to absorb the products of development and therefore maintain the pH of the solution. 4. in computing, an area which stores information at one rate and releases it at a slower rate to another device.

buffering agents substances which when ingested induce alkalosis and so counteract and limit reduction in pH during exercise. Important agents used in sport to improve performance are sodium bicarbonate and sodium citrate. ⊃ ergogenic aids.

bug a mistake in a computer system or program that causes it to crash competely or malfunction. ⊃ crash.

bulbar *adj* pertaining to the medulla oblongata.

bulbar conjunctiva ⊃ conjunctiva.

bulbar palsy or paralysis paralysis which involves the labioglossopharyngeal (lips, tongue and pharynx) region and results from degeneration of the motor nuclei in the medulla oblongata. There are problems with swallowing and speech. Individuals are at risk of inhaling fluids and food, with the development of pneumonia.

bulbar poliomyelitis ⊃ poliomyelitis.

bulbocavernosus muscles two perineal muscles surrounding the vaginal introitus, with a weak sphincter-like action.

bulbourethral (Cowper's) glands two mucus-secreting glands which open into the bulb of the male urethra. Their secretion is part of seminal fluid.

bulimia *n* literally 'ox hunger'. An eating disorder involving repeated uncontrolled consumption of large quantities of food. ⊃ anorexia nervosa (AN), bulimia nervosa, eating disorders.

bulimia nervosa (BN) (*syn* binge–purge syndrome) an eating disorder. Patients are usually at or near normal weight (unlike in anorexia nervosa), but display a morbid fear of fatness. Despite this they recurrently embark on eating binges, often followed by corrective measures such as self-induced vomiting, purging or restricted food intake. The prevalence is similar to or slightly greater than that of anorexia nervosa, but only a small proportion of sufferers reach treatment services. Bulimia nervosa (BN) usually begins later in adolescence than anorexia nervosa, and is even more predominantly a female malady. Diagnostic criteria include: (a) recurrent bouts of binge eating; (b) lack of self-control over eating during binges; (c) self-induced vomiting, purgation or dieting after binges; (d) weight maintained within normal limits. Physical signs of repeated self-induced vomiting include pitted teeth (from gastric acid), calluses on knuckles and parotid salivary gland enlargement. There are many associated physical complications including the dental and oesophageal consequences of repeated vomiting, as well as electrolyte abnormalities, cardiac arrhythmias and renal problems. ⊃ eating disorders. Cognitive behaviour (CBT) achieves short- and long-term improvements. Guided self-help and interpersonal psychotherapy may also be of value. There is also evidence for benefit from the selective serotonin reuptake inhibitor (SSRI) fluoxetine, although high doses (60 mg daily) and long courses (1 year) are required; this appears to be independent of the antidepressant effect. Bulimia does not carry the mortality associated with anorexia nervosa, and few sufferers 'cross over' to anorexia. At 10 years, approximately 10% are still unwell, 20% have a subclinical degree of BN, and the remainder have recovered. ⊃ anorexia nervosa (AN), binge-eating disorders, eating disorders.

bulk transport the transfer of particles too large to cross cell membranes occurs by pinocytosis or phagocytosis. These particles are engulfed by extensions of the cytoplasm which enclose them, forming a membrane-bound vacuole. When the vacuole is small, pinocytosis occurs. In phagocytosis larger particles, e.g. cell fragments, foreign materials, microbes, are taken into the cell. Lysosomes then adhere to the vacuole membrane, releasing enzymes which digest the contents. Extrusion of waste material by the reverse process through the plasma membrane is called exocytosis. Secretory granules formed by the Golgi apparatus usually leave the cell in this way, as do any indigestible residues of phagocytosis.

bulk-forming laxatives ⊃ laxatives. ⊃ Appendix 5.

BULL *acron* **B**uccal of **U**pper; **L**ingual of **L**ower (cusps).

bulla *n* (*syn* blister) a fluid-filled skin blister with a diameter greater than 5 mm. In dermatology, multiple bullae may suggest pemphigoid or pemphigus, but they occur sometimes in other diseases of the skin, e.g. in impetigo, in dermatitis herpetiformis, etc.—**bullae** *pl*, **bullate**, **bullous** *adj*.

bullous keratopathy a degenerative condition of the cornea characterized by the formation of epithelial blebs or bullae which burst after a few days. This condition may follow cataract surgery, corneal trauma, severe corneal oedema, glaucoma, iridocyclitis, etc. Soft contact lenses have often been found useful to relieve pain in this condition by protecting the denuded nerve endings. ⊃ cornea, cornea guttata, Fuchs' endothelial dystrophy, therapeutic soft contact lens.

bullous pemphigoid an immune-mediated blistering (bullous) skin condition. Typically affects people aged over 60 years. The blisters, which are tense, occur on the trunk (especially flexures) and the limbs. There is occasional mucous membrane involvement. Management includes the use of systemic corticosteroids and azathioprine. ⊃ Colour Section Figure 54.

bundle bone bone lining the tooth socket into which are inserted Sharpey's fibres. ⊃ alveolar bone, basal bone.

bundle branch block (BBB) a disorder affecting the conducting fibres of the heart. The cardiac impulses are not transmitted, leading to changes to the QRS complex. Commonly seen following an anterior myocardial infarction.

bundle of His (W His, Swiss anatomist, 1863–1934) atrioventricular bundle. Part of the cardiac conduction system. ⊃atrioventricular.

bunion *n* ⊃ hallux valgus.

buoyancy force the force due to fluid (liquid or gas) supporting an object, resulting from the different densities of the object and the fluid. Usually acts upwards. Also known as upthrust. ⊃ centre of buoyancy.

buphthalmos *n* (ox eye) enlarged eye, usually secondary to congenital glaucoma. ⊃ congenital glaucoma.

bur in dentistry, rotary milling tool with sharp blades of various shapes, designed to fit into handpieces. Term also used for small rotary diamond instruments. Consists of a cutting portion (the head), the shaft which attaches the bur to the handpiece and a generally tapering shank which joins the head to the shaft. Burs of various shapes and sizes are used to prepare cavities and trim dental restorations. They may have long smooth shanks to be used in straight handpieces, or latch type with shorter shafts. They are made of steel and some may have hardened blades made of tungsten carbide (*TC bur*). There are also smaller, smooth shaft burs which are retained in the head of high-speed handpieces by friction grip (*FG bur*). There are three main types: (a) *fissure bur* cylindrical or tapered with flat or rounded ends and their blades may be cross-cut, e.g. *flat fissure bur, X-cut fissure bur, round-ended fissure bur, tapered fissure bur*; (b) *inverted cone bur, round* or *(rosehead) bur*; (c) in addition there are *Curson cavity* and *restoration finishing burs* of various shapes. *Wheel bur, end-cutting bur* which has its cutting blades at its end only, used for cutting and smoothing shoulder preparations. *Diamond bur* round, cylindrical, tapered and a variety of other shapes. *Finishing bur* these burs have smaller and more numerous blades, made in various shapes and sizes, e.g. round, flame, barrel, pear. *Miniature bur* range of burs made to be used in miniature handpieces.

Burch colposuspension operation the vagina is suspended from the iliopectineal ligament. Carried out for severe stress incontinence of urine.

Burkitt's lymphoma (D Burkitt, British surgeon, 1911–1993) a highly malignant lymphoma frequently of the jaw but other sites as well. Most commonly diagnosed in areas of Africa and New Guinea where malaria is endemic.

burn *n* tissue damage (necrosis) due to chemicals, moist heat, dry heat, electricity, flame, friction or radiation; classified as partial or full thickness according to the depth of skin destroyed: the latter usually requiring skin graft(s). Analgesia, fluid replacement and the prevention of shock, infection and malnutrition are important aspects of treatment. ➲ Lund and Browder's charts, rule of nines, total burn surface area.

burning mouth a burning sensation that affects the oral mucosa associated with a number of pathological conditions such as lichen planus, sensitivity reactions, geographic tongue and pernicious anaemia. The burning sensation can affect otherwise clinically normal oral mucosa and is then labelled *burning mouth syndrome*.

burnisher in dentistry, hand instrument with rounded edges, used to polish or burnish the surface of metallic restorations by rubbing, e.g. *ball, beavertail, fishtail-shaped. Engine-driven bur* are also available.

burn-out 1. elimination, by heat, of a wax or acrylic pattern from an investment which has set hard to form a mould into which a molten metal may be cast. ➲ lost wax casting process. **2.** in radiography, an area of film with excessive blackening due to a relative overpenetration of the X-ray beam.

burnout syndrome a condition resulting from exposure to stressors. The stressors are often chronic and work-related including those experienced in sport, where prolonged, intensive training or overfrequent competition are stressors. Burnout may occur after exposure to an acute stressor and may also result from stressful family roles such as caring for a relative, or a combination. Health professionals are at particular risk of burnout because of their prolonged contact with ill people. It has been described as emotional exhaustion, isolation, becoming indifferent to others, and a lack of ability to deal with problems. The adverse effects may be physical, emotional, intellectual, social and spiritual, and may include anxiety, poor coping strategies, insomnia, inability to make decisions, appetite and weight changes, excessive tiredness, apathy, lack of motivation, relationship difficulties and possible misuse of alcohol and drugs. ➲ general adaptation syndrome, overtraining, stress, stressor.

Burns Marshall manoeuvre a manoeuvre used to deliver the aftercoming head in a breech presentation. Once the trunk is delivered, the infant hangs by his own weight to aid flexion and descent of the head; when the hair line appears at the vulva the head is at the outlet; it is delivered by raising the trunk, holding the infant's ankles and exerting slight traction, and carrying through a wide arc up and over the mother's abdomen. The perineum is retracted exposing the infant's nose and mouth, enabling clearing of the airway and oxygen administration. The birth of the head is completed slowly, usually with obstetric forceps applied to the aftercoming head.

burr *n* an attachment for a surgical drill which is used for cutting into tooth or bone.

burrow *n* a tunnel in the skin that may house an ectoparasite, e.g. acarus of scabies.

bursa *n* a fibrous sac lined with synovial membrane and containing a small quantity of synovial fluid. Bursae are found between (a) tendon and bone, (b) skin and bone, (c) muscle and muscle. Their function is to facilitate movement by reducing friction between these surfaces—**bursae** *pl*.

bursitis *n* inflammation of a bursa. ➲ olecranon bursitis, prepatellar bursitis, retrocalcaneal bursitis, trochanteric bursitis.

burst an electrotherapy term. A continuous series of biphasic pulses (train) followed by no pulses (i.e. an interburst interval) and then more bursts of pulses, depending on the burst frequency.

bus a semi-standard connector to the computer through which all data are passed to an external device.

Busacca's nodules (*syn.* floccules of Busacca) nodules often found in the iris stroma of an eye affected by granulomatous uveitis (up to about 30% of cases). ➲ iris nodules, Koeppe's nodules.

BUT *acron* break-up time (BUT) test.

butterfly rash an erythematous butterfly-shaped rash occurring over the cheeks, connected by a narrow area of rash over the nose. A feature of systemic lupus erythematosus.

buttock *n* nates. The two rounded projections posterior to the hip joints. Formed mainly of the gluteal muscles, gluteus maximus, gluteus medius and gluteus minimus. They arise from the surface of the ilium of the hip bone and cross the back of the hip joint to be inserted into the femur. The gluteus maximus, the largest, is crucial in the maintenance of the upright posture, as an extensor at the hips, and also in running, climbing and walking up steps. It also assists in keeping the leg straight at the knee, via a fibrous band attached to the tibia. The two smaller muscles (g. medius, g. minimus) mainly take part in abduction and rotation at the hip.

buttonholing a term applied to the appearance of the perineum as it is distended by the fetal head in the second stage of labour. The skin starts to tear along and within the perineal body indicating that a moderate to severe laceration will occur.

butyric acid a saturated fatty acid.

BV *abbr* **1.** biological value. **2.** bacterial vaginosis.

BVP *abbr* back vertex power.

BW *abbr* **1.** birth weight. **2.** bite wing radiograph. **3.** body weight.

Bx *abbr* biopsy.

BXO *abbr* balanitis xerotica obliterans.

bypass *n* describes a surgical procedure that usually diverts or provides a shunt for blood, other fluids or gastrointestinal contents. ➲ cardiac bypass operation, cardiopulmonary bypass, coronary artery bypass graft, extracorporeal membrane oxygenation.

byssinosis *n* an occupational disease caused by inhalation of flax, hemp or cotton fibres. Not all inhaled organic dusts cause interstitial infiltration. In byssinosis the initial lesion caused by cotton dust inhalation is acute bronchiolitis associated with symptoms and signs of generalized airflow obstruction, more in keeping with asthma (e.g. wheeziness, cough, dyspnoea and chest tightness). Initially, symptoms tend to recur after the weekend break ('Monday fever') but eventually become continuous. There is usually no radiological abnormality. Recovery usually follows removal from the dust hazard. Smokers have a greater incidence of byssinosis than non-smokers. Continued exposure to the dust will lead to fibrosis, chronic airways obstruction and pulmonary hypertension. Eventually this may lead to respiratory and cardiac failure.

byte a unit of computer data storage capacity. One byte contains eight bits, usually stores one character. Larger units include kilobyte (Kb) containing 1024 bytes, and the megabyte (Mb) which has 1048576 bytes. ➲ binary, bit.

C *abbr* **1.** Celsius (centigrade). **2.** coulomb.

CA-125 *abbr* cancer cell surface antigen 125, a glycoprotein. Levels in the blood may be used as a tumour marker for ovarian and other cancers.

CAB *acron* cellulose acetate butyrate.

CABG *abbr* coronary artery bypass graft.

CACG *abbr* chronic angle-closure glaucoma.

cachexia *n* a constitutional disorder, malnutrition and general ill health caused partly by inadequate food intake but mainly the effects of disease that lead to hypermetabolism and the breakdown of lean (protein) tissue. There is debility, muscle weakness and anaemia. The chief signs of this condition are emaciation, wasting, sallow unhealthy skin and heavy lustreless eyes. A feature of advanced disease such as cancer and AIDS—**cachectic** *adj*.

cacosmia *n* an abnormality of smell. There is a perception of a foul stench or odour which others do not notice. It may occur with disorders affecting the brain or olfactory nerve, or occur as an olfactory hallucination.

CAD *acron* **1.** **C**omputer-**A**ided **D**rawing. **2.** **C**oronary **A**rtery **D**isease.

cadaver *n* a corpse. In a medical context it implies a dead body which is dissected in a medical school, or in a mortuary at a postmortem examination.

cadaverine a molecule produced when protein breaks down during the putrefaction of animal tissue. It results from the decarboxylation of lysine an amino acid and has an extremely foul odour. ⟩ putrescine.

cadence the rhythm of a movement or the voice. In physiotherapy practice it also refers to the number of steps taken in a specific time period, frequently used as an outcome measure.

cadmium (Cd) a poisonous metallic element.

cadmium poisoning may occur as an occupational hazard. The inhalation of fumes during industrial processes such as welding or smelting can lead to lung damage and kidney disease. Ingestion of cadmium causes gastrointestinal effects that include vomiting.

caecostomy *n* a surgically established fistula between the caecum and anterior abdominal wall, usually to achieve drainage and/or decompression of the caecum. It is usually created by inserting a widebore tube into the caecum at operation.

caecum *n* the blind, pouch-like commencement of the colon in the right iliac fossa. To it is attached the vermiform appendix; it is separated from the ileum by the ileocaecal valve—**caecal** *adj*.

caesarean section, c-section (CS) delivery of the fetus through an abdominal incision, said to be named after Caesar, who is supposed to have been born in this way. An obstetric operation to extract the fetus from the uterus through an incision in the abdominal and uterine walls after 24 weeks of pregnancy, performed for cephalopelvic disproportion; grade III or IV placenta praevia; placental abruption to deliver a live fetus; first stage fetal distress; failure to progress, especially with malpresentation or malposition; serious maternal medical conditions; preterm delivery when the extrauterine environment is deemed to be safer for the fetus than the intrauterine environment. The midwife assists with pre- and postoperative care and observations; she/he may also be required to assist the anaesthetist, or attend the mother throughout the operation if regional anaesthesia is used; to act as the scrub practitioner or 'runner' in theatre; or to receive the infant and provide immediate resuscitative care as required. ⟩ lower segment caesarean section, classical caesarean section.

caesium-137 (^{137}Cs) *n* a radioactive substance which, when sealed in needles or tubes, can be used for interstitial and surface applications during radiotherapy. It can also be employed as a source for treatment by Selectron. Historically has been used for external beam therapy.

caesium iodide crystal a crystal previously used in the detector of a computed tomography (CT) scanner to detect any radiation passing through the patient. Now obsolete. ⟩ ceramic detectors.

café au lait spots pale brown (like milky coffee) patches or spots on the skin. Some isolated spots may be normal but the appearance of several spots my be indicative of neurofibromatosis.

caffeine *n* occurs naturally in the leaves, seeds or fruits of more than 60 different plants, including coffee beans, kola nuts (cola) and tea leaves, and is also added to some foods and soft drinks; there is also a closely related substance in cocoa beans (chocolate). It causes a diuresis, increases heart rate and may cause restlessness and difficulty sleeping. It has been given as a diuretic, but its main use is in analgesic preparations such as with codeine. Excess intake may result in caffeine poisoning with anxiety, tremor, nausea, tachycardia, cardiac arrhythmias and insomnia. Caffeine is often said to be the most widely used 'drug' in the world. It is one of the commonest ingredients in fat-loss supplements. By virtue of its stimulant action on the central nervous system, it is used in many sports to improve alertness, concentration and reaction time and to delay central fatigue. By promoting lipolysis, and therefore fat oxidation, caffeine acts as an aid to endurance but its diuretic action may enhance fluid loss and thus reduce hydration. ⟩ ergogenic aids, fatigue, lipolysis, methylxanthines.

115

Caffey's disease (J Caffey, American paediatrician, 1895–1978) ⊃infantile cortical hyperostosis.

CAH *abbr* congenital adrenal hyperplasia.

caisson disease ⊃ decompression sickness/illness.

caked breast a state of extreme engorgement of the breasts in which they become hard as the milk comes in and is not removed.

calamine *n* zinc carbonate with ferric oxide. Used in lotions and creams for the relief of itching; however, it is not generally effective.

calcaneal spur the formation of a bony spur, extending from the calcaneus into the plantar fascia.

calcaneum ⊃ calcaneus.

calcaneus (*syn* calcaneum, os calcis) the largest of the tarsal bones, it forms the heel bone. It articulates distally with the cuboid and proximally with the talus. ⊃ Colour Section Figure 3.

calcareous *adj* chalky. Relating to lime or calcium.

calc/i- a prefix that means 'chalk, calcium', e.g. *calcitonin*, or 'heel', e.g. *calcaneus*.

calcidiol *n* 25-hydroxycholecalciferol, a derivative of vitamin D. It is the main circulating and storage form of vitamin D in the body.

calciferol ⊃ ergocalciferol. Sometimes used as a general term for vitamins D_2 and D_3.

calcific barrier (*syn* dentine bridge) barrier or bridge of calcific material which may gradually form over an exposed pulp, or an open root-end in response to treatment. ⊃ apexification, direct pulp cap.

calcification *n* the process whereby calcium salts are deposited in specialized tissue. The condition may be physiological, as in the formation of teeth or bone, or pathological, as in hyperparathyroidism or its deposition in arteries. Acids formed by plaque, and acid etchants, decalcify enamel tissue—a reverse process to calcification.

calcifying epithelial odontogenic tumour uncommon new growth arising from odontogenic epithelium, and characterized by sheet-like arrangements of epithelium. Clinically it behaves like an ameloblastoma with regard to age, sex and distribution.

calcination to heat a substance in order to drive off any water, so leaving a calcined, dry powder, e.g. plaster of Paris.

calcinosis *n* the abnormal deposition of calcium salts in tissues and organs. Some cases are caused by an excessive intake of vitamin D.

calciol cholecalciferol (vitamin D_3), the naturally occurring form of vitamin D.

calcitonin *n* (*syn* thyrocalcitonin) hormone secreted by the thyroid gland. It has a fine-tuning role in calcium homeostasis. It opposes the action of parathyroid hormone and reduces levels of calcium and phosphate in the serum by its action on the kidneys and bone. It inhibits calcium reabsorption from bone and stimulates the excretion of calcium and phosphate in the urine. Calcitonin is released when the concentration of calcium in serum rises. Synthetic calcitonin is used in the management of metastatic bone cancer, Paget's disease and osteoporosis.

calcitriol *n* 1,25-dihydroxycholecalciferol. Formed in the kidneys from 25-hydroxycholecalciferol (calcidiol). It is the active form of vitamin D (vitamin D_3) concerned with calcium homeostasis. It controls calcium levels by increasing calcium absorption from the small intestine.

calcium (Ca) *n* a metallic element. The most abundant mineral in the body. Combined with phosphorus (as phosphate) in bones and teeth. The two minerals together represent about 75% of the body's total mineral content. Of the remaining calcium, approximately half exists in its ionized state (Ca^{2+}), while the other half is bound to plasma proteins, primarily albumin. Ionized calcium levels in the body are maintained within a narrow range (2.1–2.6 mmol/L). The level of calcium and phosphate in the blood is regulated through the influence of hormones, mainly parathyroid hormone with calcitonin playing a minor role, and vitamin D. Hormonal regulation is achieved through a complex interrelationship between the amount of calcium absorbed from the gut, the amount mobilized from the bones and the amount excreted by the kidney.The plasma pH exerts an influence on the ratio of ionized to protein-bound calcium in the blood. Acidaemic states increase plasma ionized calcium levels. Alkalotic states have the opposite effect, thus reducing ionized calcium levels. Another factor that influences this ratio is the serum albumin level. If this is low, then the proportion of ionized calcium increases. Ionized calcium (Ca^{2+}) plays a crucial role in all physiological functions including neuromuscular conduction (transmission of nerve impulses, muscle action); it is factor IV of blood coagulation where it is essential for the conversion of prothrombin to thrombin, and the activation of the factor XII, which stabilizes the fibrin clot; the activation of several enzymes; and transport across all cell membranes. Calcium is one of the most frequently inadequate nutrients in the diet of both athletes and non-athletes. Female dancers, gymnasts and endurance competitors are among those most prone to calcium dietary insufficiency. ⊃ bone, coagulation, excitation-contraction coupling, hypercalcaemia, hypocalcaemia, minerals, parathyroid glands, parathyroid hormone, tetany.

calcium carbonate (CaCO₃) a calcium salt used in many antacid medicines. When finely ground, it is used as an abrasive in toothpastes and polishing agents.

calcium channel blockers (antagonists) a group of drugs that block the flow of calcium ions in smooth muscle, e.g. nifedipine. They are negatively inotropic and may reduce myocardial contractility. ⊃ inotropes. ⊃ Appendix 5.

calcium chloride (CaCl₂) a calcium salt administered intravenously in the treatment of hypocalcaemic tetany. Also used during cardiopulmonary resuscitation.

calcium gluconate a calcium salt used orally to treat calcium deficiencies and disorders such as rickets. Used intravenously to treat hypocalcaemic tetany.

calcium hydroxide (Ca(OH)₂) a salt of calcium used to encourage the formation of reparative dentine. The powder may be mixed with water to form a paste, or it may be obtained ready mixed in tubes. It is placed in deep cavities as a seal and a protective lining, or in direct contact with the pulp in endodontic procedures. ⊃ apexification.

calcium pump one of many similar molecular complexes embodying ion-binding sites and an ATPase in the surface membrane of many cell types, including smooth and cardiac muscle, and in the membrane of the sarcoplasmic reticulum (SR) in skeletal muscle. The pumps actively transport calcium ions (Ca^{2+}) out of the cytoplasm; those in the surface membrane return them to the extracellular fluid, and those in SR membrane return them to within the SR. All use energy derived from hydrolysis of adenosine triphosphate (ATP).

calcium sulphate ($(CaSO_4)_2$) gypsum, plaster of Paris. A salt of calcium obtained by calcining naturally occurring gypsum. It yields two forms of hemihydrate: the alphahemihydrate forms the basis of artificial stone and the beta-hemihydrate forms plaster of Paris (POP). Both are used in the construction of dental models and as investing material.

calcium tungstate ($CaWO_4$) the main phosphor used in conventional intensifying screens now superseded by rare earth phosphors.

calculus *n* **1.** a stone. An abnormal concretion composed chiefly of mineral substances and formed in the passages which transmit secretions, or in the cavities which act as reservoirs for them. Examples include gallstones and renal calculi—**calculi** *pl*, **calculous** *adj*. ⊃dental calculus, gallstones, renal calculus. **2.** the use of small changes to calculate derivatives of equations. Includes differentiation (calculation of gradients) and integration (calculation of areas).

Caldicott guardian every NHS establishment, e.g. NHS Trust or Health Authority, must appoint a board member to take responsibility for the security and confidentiality of all patient-identifiable information. The guardian will be involved with approving and reviewing local protocols, and controlling the use and protection of patient-identifiable information. They also fulfil a strategic role, for example, in the development of confidentiality and security policies and representing confidentiality issues at Board level.

Caldwell–Luc operation (*syn* radical antrostomy) a radical operation previously used for sinusitis.

Caldwell–Moloy pelvic classification a system used for classifying the female pelvis as one of four types. ⊃ android pelvis, anthropoid pelvis, gynaecoid pelvis, platypelloid pelvis.

calf the twin 'bellies' of the gastrocnemius muscles are prominent in the upper half of the calf, e.g. when standing on tip-toe; this and the flatter soleus muscle in front of it (known together as the *triceps surae*) form the main bulk of the calf muscles; their tendons join to attach to the calcaneus (calcaneum or os calsis) via the Achilles tendon. Accessory to the gastrocnemius is the plantaris muscle. Deeper muscles include the flexors of the toes, with long tendons passing into the foot.

calibrated stepwedge a piece of equipment used in radiography. It is made up of different thickness of aluminium with a layer of copper on the base, wedges are calibrated so that when radiographed each step produces an exact increase or decrease in density on the film. ⊃ stepwedge.

caliper *n* **1.** a two-pronged instrument for measuring the diameter of a round body. Used chiefly in pelvimetry. **2.** a two-pronged instrument with sharp points which are inserted into the lower end of a fractured long bone. A weight is attached to the other end of the caliper, which maintains a steady pull on the distal end of the bone. **3.** *Thomas' walking caliper* is similar to the Thomas' splint, but the W-shaped junction at the lower end is replaced by two small iron rods which slot into holes made in the heel of the boot. The ring should fit the groin perfectly, and all weight is then borne by the ischial tuberosity. **4.** external orthosis used to assist patients to walk, by mechanically stabilizing joints and providing support for the intrinsic weight of the limb. They are commonly used by paraplegic patients.

callosity *n* a local hardening of the skin. ⊃ callus.

callus *n* **1.** the partly calcified tissue which forms about the ends of a broken bone during fracture healing and ultimately accomplishes repair of the fracture. When this is complete the bony thickening is known as *permanent callus*. **2.** (*syn* callosity, corn, keratoma, mechanically induced hyperkeratosis) a yellowish plaque of hard skin caused by pressure or friction. The stratum corneum becomes hypertrophied. Most commonly seen on the feet and palms of the hands. A painful, cone-shaped overgrowth and hardening of the epidermis, with the point of the cone in the deeper layers. Corns on the sole of the foot and over joints are often described as hard corns, and those occurring between the toes are described as soft corns.

calmodulins a group of intracellular calcium-binding proteins, they are important in mediating many biochemical processes including signalling functions within cells.

calor *n* heat: one of the five classic local signs and symptoms of inflammation—the others are dolor, loss of function, rubor and tumor.

caloric test irrigation of the outer/external ear canal with water at 30°C and then at 44°C to assess vestibular function by stimulating the lateral semicircular canals. Each ear is tested separately. When the ear is normal the test produces nystagmus, whereas nystagmus may not be produced if the ear is diseased.

calorie *n* a unit of heat. In practice the calorie is too small a unit to be useful and 1000 calories, the kilocalorie (kcal), is the preferred unit in studies in metabolism. A kcal is the amount of heat required to raise the temperature of 1 kg of water by 1°C. In medicine, science and technology generally, the calorie has been replaced by the joule (derived SI unit) as a unit of energy, work and heat. For approximate conversion 4.2 kJ = 1 kcal.

calorific *adj* describes any phenomena that relate to heat production.

calorimeter *n* an instrument used to measure the heat gain or loss occurring during physical and chemical changes.

A calorimeter is used to determine the amount of oxidizable energy in a specific food, by burning it in oxygen and measuring heat production.

calorimetry *n* in nutrition the measurement of energy expenditure by the body. *direct calorimetry* is the measurement of heat produced from the body, as an index of energy expenditure, and hence the individual's energy requirements. Heat loss is detected by using room-sized chambers. *indirect calorimetry* measures the heat produced during oxidation of nutrients through determining the consumption of oxygen, or by measuring the carbon dioxide and converting the values into a heat equivalent. For greater accuracy and information about the relative amounts of nutrients (carbohydrate, fat and protein) oxidized, carbon dioxide production is also measured and urea production estimated. ⊃ Douglas bag method.

calvaria *n* the superior part of the skull, the vault.

CAM *acron* **1.** cell adhesion molecule. **2.** complementary and alternative medicine.

CAMI *abbr* Carers Assessment of Managing Index.

cAMP *abbr* cyclic adenosine monophosphate.

Camper's line ⊃ ala-tragal line.

campimeter an instrument for the measurement of the visual field, especially the central region (usually within a radius of 30°). ⊃ Amsler chart, perimeter, tangent screen.

campimetry the measurement of the visual field with a campimeter.

Campylobacter *n* a genus of Gram-negative, non-spore-forming motile bacteria. They are spirally curved rods with a flagellum at either or both ends. *Campylobacter jejuni* is a common cause of bacterial food poisoning. It causes abdominal pain and bloodstained diarrhoea that may last for 10–14 days. The micro-organism is associated with raw meat and poultry, the fur of infected pet animals and unpasteurized milk. No reported person-to-person spread. *C. fetus* causes abortion in cattle. It is an opportunistic organism and causes bacteraemia in humans, this can lead to local infections, e.g. involving the meninges. Immunocompromised individuals and neonates may develop septicaemia, which, in rare cases, results in death.

canaliculus *n* a minute capillary passage. Any small canal, such as the passage leading from the edge of the eyelid to the lacrimal sac or one of the numerous small canals leading from the Haversian canals and terminating in the lacunae of bone—**canaliculi** *pl*, **canalicular** *adj*, **canaliculization** *n*.

canal of Petit a space between the posterior fibres of the zonule of Zinn and the anterior surface of the vitreous body (humour). ⊃ vitreous body (humour), zonule of Zinn.

canal of Schlemm (F Schlemm, German anatomist, 1795–1858) ⊃ glaucoma, scleral venous sinus, Colour Section Figure 15.

canals of Lambert collateral channels of ventilation between the terminal bronchioles and alveoli. They remain in an open state even during bronchial smooth muscle contraction and are around 30 μm in size.

canbra oil (canola oil) ⊃ canola oil.

cancellous *adj* resembling latticework; light and spongy; like a honeycomb. Describes a type of bone tissue (cancellous, spongy or trabecular). ⊃ bone.

cancer *n* a general term which covers any malignant growth in any part of the body. The growth is purposeless, parasitic, and flourishes at the expense of the human host. Characteristics are the tendency to cause local destruction, to invade adjacent tissues and to spread by metastasis. Frequently recurs after removal. Carcinoma refers to malignant tumours of epithelial tissue, sarcoma to malignant tumours of connective tissue—**cancerous** *adj*. ⊃ grading, staging.

cancer cell surface antigen 125 (CA-125) ⊃ CA-125.

cancerophobia *n* obsessive fear of cancer—**cancerophobic** *adj*.

cancrum oris gangrenous stomatitis of cheek in debilitated children. Often called noma. Associated with measles in malnourished African children. ⊃ noma.

candela (cd) one of the seven base units of the International System of Units (Système International d'Unités [SI]). Measures luminous intensity and is defined as the luminous intensity, in a given direction, of a source that emits monochromatic radiation of frequency 540×10^{12} hertz and that has a radian intensity in that direction of 1/683 watt per steradian. ⊃ Appendix 2.

candelilla wax naturally occurring wax used in dentistry to harden inlay casting wax obtained from the candelilla shrub.

Candida *n* (*syn Monilia*) a genus of fungi. They are widespread in nature. *Candida albicans* is a commensal of the mouth, gastrointestinal tract, vagina and skin in humans.

candidiasis *n* (*syn* candidosis, moniliasis, thrush) infections caused by a species of *Candida*, usually *Candida albicans*. Infection may involve the mouth, gastrointestinal tract, skin, nails, respiratory tract or genitourinary tract (vulvovaginitis, balanitis), especially in individuals who are debilitated, e.g. by cancer or diabetes mellitus, or immunosuppressed, and after long-term or extensive treatment with antibiotics, which upsets the microbial flora, and other drugs, e.g. corticosteroids. Candidiasis is also a feature of immunodeficiency conditions such as HIV disease. Oral infection can be caused by poor oral hygiene, including carious teeth and ill-fitting dentures. ⊃ Colour Section Figure 55.

canicola fever leptospirosis.

canine *adj* of or resembling a dog.

canine eminence ridge of bone on the maxilla covering the root of the canine tooth.

canine fossa depression on the external surface of the maxilla distal to the canine eminence.

canine guidance directional guidance provided by the upper canine during lateral excursions of the mandible.

canine protected articulation an arrangement of the canine teeth that prevents posterior tooth contact or lateral eccentric mandibular movements.

canine tooth a lay term for the upper permanent canine is 'eye tooth'. A single cusped tooth having a relatively long root and a pronounced cingulum in the permanent (secondary) dentition. In the primary dentition it lies distal to the lateral incisor and mesial to the first primary molar in each quadrant. In the permanent (secondary) dentition it lies distal to the lateral incisor and mesial to the first permanent premolar in each quadrant (Figure T.4b, p. 779). It is intended to tear and cut food. The permanent maxillary canine is the longest tooth. The crown of the lower canine is usually tilted lingually. The primary canines begin to calcify before birth, and erupt at about 18 months. Calcification is usually complete by 2½ years and the root starts to resorb at 7 years of age before being shed at 12 years. The permanent canines commence to calcify at 4–5 months and are complete on eruption at the age of 10–12.

canities *n* a loss of pigment, as in the greying of hair, or the formation of white streaks in the nails.

cannabinoids *npl* a group of antiemetic drugs derived from cannabis, e.g. nabilone. ⊃ Appendix 5.

cannabis (*syn* marihuana/marijuana, grass, pot, hashish, etc.) a psychoactive drug that produces euphoria and hallucinations. It is usually smoked. In the UK the cultivation, possession and supply of cannabis are criminal offences (⊃ Appendix 5). There is, however, considerable interest in possible medicinal uses and trials are ongoing. ⊃ marijuana.

cannula *n* a hollow tube, usually plastic, for the introduction, such as of intravenous fluids, or withdrawal of fluid from the body (Figure C.1). In some types the lumen is fitted with a sharp-pointed trocar to facilitate insertion, which is withdrawn when the cannula is in situ—**cannulae** *pl*.

cannulation *n* insertion of a cannula, such as into a vein to facilitate the administration of intravenous fluids or drugs.

canola oil (canbra oil) oil obtained from a variety of rapeseed, which is low in glucosinolates. Developed to contain no more than 2% erucic acid.

cans the container for the sodium iodide crystals of scintillation counters to prevent the absorption of moisture by the crystal which would make it cloudy.

canthoplasty plastic surgery to refashion either canthus or correct a defect.

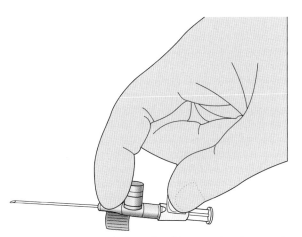

C.1 **Intravenous cannula** (reproduced from Nicol et al 2004 with permission).

canthus *n* palpebral commissure, The angle formed by the junction of the eyelids. The inner one is known as the *nasal*, or *medial canthus* and the outer as the *temporal* or *lateral canthus*—**canthi** *pl*, **canthal** *adj*. ⊃ epicanthus.

cantilever bridge in dentistry, a bridge in which the pontic has a bridge retainer or retainers at one end only. ⊃ bridge.

cap in dentistry, a protective covering. Colloquialism for a full or partial replacement of a natural crown.

cap splint ⊃ fixation (dentistry/maxillofacial surgery).

capacitance the amount of charge a body can hold per unit potential difference. In a sphere the capacitance is the ratio of the total charge on the body to its potential. If there are two surfaces the capacitance is the ratio of the total charge of one sign on the body to the potential difference between the surfaces. In electrotherapy, capacitance is increased by having larger capacitor plates, a higher dielectric of the material between them (e.g. water, kidney and fatty tissue all have a higher dielectric than bone marrow) and inversely reduced with increasing distance between the plates. Skin resistance is a combination of the capacitive reactance (mainly provided by the outer drier thicker skin layers) and resistance.

capacitance capacitor an electrical component consisting of two plates separated by a dielectric, when it receives a potential difference across the plates a charge is stored.

capacity potential to perform a task or activity to a satisfactory level.

CAPD *abbr* continuous ambulatory peritoneal dialysis.

CAPE *acron* Clifton Assessment Procedures for the Elderly.

capelline bandage (divergent spica) a bandage applied in a circular fashion to the head or an amputated limb.

Capgras syndrome (J Capgras, French psychiatrist, 1873–1950) characterized by a delusion, whereby the person belives that the other people around them have been replaced by doubles or imposters.

capillarization *n* a long-term adaptation to endurance exercise where the number and usage of blood capillaries in muscle tissue increases to meet the need for oxygenated blood. ⊃ aerobic adaptations.

capillary *n* (literally, hair-like) a tiny thin-walled blood vessel forming part of a network which facilitates rapid exchange of substances between the contained fluid and the surrounding tissues. For example the exchange of oxygen and waste carbon dioxide between the blood and the cells. The walls of capillaries consist of a single layer of epithelial cells known as endothelial cells which part at their junctions to allow leucocytes to pass through them during the inflammatory response. The tiny blood capillaries unite an arteriole and a venule. ⊃ capillary bed, capillary fragility, capillary refill time, lymph capillary.

capillary bed the network of capillaries between the arteriole and the venule (Figure C.2).

capillary blockade the injection of large radioactive particles (20–50 μm) that are unable to pass through capillaries and therefore block the first capillary bed they reach. Used in radionuclide imaging to see the vascular bed of the lungs.

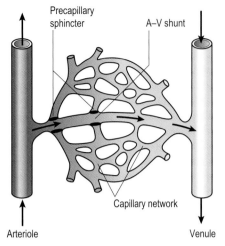

Precapillary sphincter

A–V shunt

Capillary network

Arteriole

Venule

C.2 **Capillary bed** (reproduced from Brooker 2006B with permission).

capillary fragility an expression of the ease with which blood capillaries may rupture.

capillary haemorrhage haemorrhage from capillaries; the blood is red (neither bright red nor dark red) and tends to ooze from the vessels, mucosae or wound.

capillary refill time used for the assessment of skin perfusion and cardiac output. Pressure is applied to a nail bed (peripheral area), or a central area such as the skin over the sternum if the patient has poor peripheral circulation or a low cardiac output. Normal skin colour should return within 2 seconds of the removal of pressure. A prolonged capillary refill time can indicate that the cardiac output is low. ⊃ nail blanch test.

capital budget financial allocation for the purchase of items, such as equipment, that will last longer than 12 months, or items that cost more than an agreed level. ⊃ revenue budget.

capitate *adj* shaped like a head.

capitate bone *n* one of the carpal bones of the wrist. It articulates with other carpal bones—scaphoid, lunate, hamate and trapezoid—and the second, third and fourth metacarpal bones.

capitation funding method of allocating money and other resources based on the number of people living in a geographical area. ⊃ weighted capitation

capitulum *n* a rounded prominence on the end of a bone where it articulates with another bone. For example the *capitulum humeri*, the prominence at its distal end that articulates with the radius at the elbow.

Caplan's syndrome a respiratory extra-articular manifestation of rheumatoid arthritis. It is a combination of rheumatoid nodules within the lungs and pneumoconiosis.

capnograph (carbon dioxide analyser) an instrument for measuring the level of carbon dioxide in expired air.

capnophilic describes micro-organisms which grow best in or may require for growth carbon dioxide at a concentration higher than that normally found in air.

capping in dentistry, the technique of covering an exposed pulp to protect against irritants and to encourage healing. A colloquialism for crowning. ⊃ cap.

capsaicin *n* an irritant chemical present in sweet peppers. It prevents the transmission of pain impulses. Used topically to relieve the pain of postherpetic neuralgia, which follows an attack of herpes zoster (shingles).

capsid the protein layer that encloses viral nucleic acid.

capsular glaucoma ⊃ pseudoexfoliation.

capsule *n* **1.** the ligaments which surround a joint. **2.** a gelatinous or rice paper container for a drug. **3.** the outer membranous covering of certain organs, such as the kidney, liver. **4.** the outer covering of certain bacteria. **5.** in dentistry, the container in which filling materials may be mixed mechanically—**capsular** *adj*.

capsule of the crystalline lens the transparent elastic capsule covering the crystalline lens of the eye. The thickness of the capsule varies; the anterior portion is thicker than the posterior and it is also thicker towards the periphery (or equator). This variation in thickness plays a role in moulding the lens substance, contributing to an increase in the curvature of the front surface, in particular, during accommodation. The capsule increases in thickness with age, and its modulus of elasticity decreases with age, which (besides flattening of the lens, and a hardening of the lens substance) contributes to presbyopia. Under electron microscopy the capsule appears to have a lamellar structure that disappears with age. The capsule receives the insertion of the fibres of the zonule of Zinn. ⊃ lens fibres, crystalline lens, Fincham's theory, modulus of elasticity, presbyopia, shagreen of the crystalline lens, zonule of Zinn.

capsule of the eyeball ⊃ Tenon's capsule.

capsule vibrator in dentistry a mechanical apparatus used to mix restorative materials in a capsule.

capsulectomy *n* the surgical excision of a capsule. Refers to a joint or lens; less often to the kidney.

capsulitis *n* inflammation of a capsule. Sometimes used as a synonym for frozen shoulder.

capsulotomy *n* incision of a capsule, usually referring to that surrounding the crystalline lens of the eye, which remains after modern cataract surgery. Usually created by a laser.

caput *n* the head.

caput medusae dilated knot of veins around the umbilicus, associated with hepatic portal hypertension.

caput succedaneum an oedematous swelling covering the fetal scalp at birth. Results from the pressure of the cervix on the fetal head during labour. The swelling is diffuse, not delineated by skull suture lines and resolves spontaneously after delivery. ⊃ cephalhaematoma, moulding.

Carabelli's cusp accessory cusp situated on the mesiopalatal aspect of some maxillary permanent first molars and deciduous second molars.

carat 1. the carat of an alloy refers to the parts of gold in an alloy in 24 parts. For example a 22 carat gold has 22 parts of gold and 2 parts of other metals; 24 carat being pure gold.

fineness (of alloy), gold. **2**. Measure of weight for precious stones (1 carat = 200 mg).

carbaminohaemoglobin *n* a compound formed between carbon dioxide and haemoglobin. Some carbon dioxide in the blood is normally carried in this form.

carbapenems *npl* a group of β-lactam antibiotics, e.g. imipenem. ➲ Appendix 5.

carbohydrate (CHO) *n* an organic compound containing carbon, hydrogen and oxygen. Formed in nature by photosynthesis in plants. Carbohydrates (CHO) are the major source of energy in most diets, on average 1 g of CHO is metabolized to produce 16 kJ energy. They include saccharides, starches, glycogen and cellulose, and are often classified in groups—monosaccharides (e.g. glucose, fructose, galactose), disaccharides (maltose, sucrose, lactose), polysaccharides (e.g. starch, glycogen) and non-starch polysaccharides (NSP) (e.g. cellulose). CHO is the most abundant and economic source of food energy in the human diet, comprising 40–80% of total energy intake in different populations. The recommended ideal is at least 50–55% and a high-carbohydrate diet is defined as one providing more than 55% of energy as CHO. Contained in breads, pasta, chapatti, noodles, sugar, jam, honey, cereals, fruits, vegetables, cakes, biscuits and pastry, and as sugars in soft drinks and dairy products. In Western diets about 60% of dietary CHO is in the form of polysaccharides of D-glucose, mostly starch, and about 25% 'free sugars', mainly sucrose. The quantity and quality of CHO consumed have an impact on energy balance, digestive function, insulin sensitivity and blood lipids. CHO is present in the blood as glucose and carbohydrate stores are in the form of glycogen in the liver and skeletal muscle and to a small extent in other tissues including, importantly, the brain. ➲ glycaemic index.

carbohydrate-electrolyte solutions ➲ sports drinks.

carbohydrate intake guidelines for athletes the International Olympic Committee (IOC) suggests that athletes with considerable and prolonged energy demands of training should have a high-carbohydrate diet, increasing carbohydrate (CHO) intake to 65–70% of dietary energy. However, due to the high total energy intake of athletes, population dietary guidelines that recommend a CHO component of at least 50–55% are in most cases appropriate also for the health needs and fuel requirements of athletes. For athletes, therefore, the recommended CHO intake is usually expressed in grams per day or grams per day per kg body mass, rather than as a percentage of the total.

carbohydrate loading (carboloading, glycogen loading) aims to maximize (supercompensate) muscle glycogen stores. This allows athletes to maintain a chosen pace for longer periods and also enhances the performance of a set amount of work (i.e. set distance) by preventing a decline in pace or work output associated with carbohydrate depletion. The procedure is popular with long-distance runners and other endurance-type athletes; it is an important nutritional strategy for events lasting more than 90 minutes, which would otherwise be limited by the depletion of muscle glycogen stores. In practice, loading is performed in two stages: a glycogen depletion stage and a carbohydrate loading phase, typically spread over 6–7 days, which entail a few days of minimal carbohydrate intake with initially high but then decreasing intensity of training, followed by a few days of high carbohydrate diet and minimal exercise.

carbol fuchsin a stain used in microbiology and to stain cell nuclei prior to microscopic examination.

carbolic acid ➲ phenol.

carbolized resin in dentistry, a sedative and antiseptic dressing used for the relief of pain due to an exposed pulp. Consists of a mixture of phenol, resin alcohol and, sometimes, zinc oxide and cotton wool fibres.

carboloading ➲ carbohydrate loading.

carbon *n* a non-metallic element found in all organic molecules and living matter. Carbon can bond with four other atoms and is able to form a huge number of complex molecules. Carbon is a constituent of important biochemical molecules including amino acids (proteins), carbohydrates, lipids, hormones, enzymes and nucleic acids.

carbon dioxide a gas; a waste product of many forms of combustion and metabolism, excreted via the lungs. Carbon dioxide retention occurs in respiratory insufficiency or failure, due for instance to alveolar hypoventilation, the carbon dioxide tension in arterial blood ($PaCO_2$) rises above normal levels and acid—base balance is adversely affected. ➲ hypercapnia. In its solid condition (*carbon dioxide snow*) it may be used as an escharotic and as a method of testing the vitality of teeth.

carbon dioxide narcosis full bounding pulse, muscular twitchings, confusion and eventual unconsciousness due to increased $PaCO_2$. ➲ hypercapnia.

carbonic anhydrase a zinc-containing enzyme involved in maintaining acid—base balance in the body. It increases the rate of transfer of carbon dioxide from tissues to blood and then to alveolar air in the lungs. This is achieved by reversibly catalysing the interconversion of carbon dioxide and water from the tissues to carbonic acid, which dissociates into bicarbonate and hydrogen ions. Once in the lungs the reactions are reversed, thereby facilitating the excretion of acid carbon dioxide by the lungs. The enzyme is involved in acid—base balance and the regulation of pH by the kidneys. For example, the conservation and reabsorption of bicarbonate (hydrogen carbonate) ions by the renal tubule in order to replenish the alkaline reserve, and the secretion of hydrogen ions.

carbonic anhydrase inhibitors drugs that reduce the production of aqueous humour, thereby reducing intraocular pressure, e.g. acetazolamide. They also have some diuretic effects. ➲ Appendix 5.

carbon monoxide (CO) a poisonous gas, it is odourless and colourless. Carbon monoxide is produced by the incomplete combustion (oxidation) of organic fuels in situations where there is limited oxygen. The gas is produced by the internal combustion engine and is present in exhaust fumes; by wood-burning stoves; faulty central heating boiler (furnace) and other heaters. It combines with haemoglobin to form a

121

stable compound. This blocks the normal reversible oxygen-carrying function and leads to hypoxia. The onset of hypoxia may be insidious but it is associated with confusion, headache, increasing respiratory rate, cherry-pink flushed appearance, changes in conscious level, seizures, cardiac arrhythmias and without treatment death. Exposure to carbon monoxide may occur intentionally during suicide attempts or accidently through inhalation of vehicle exhaust fumes or from a faulty central heating boiler.

carbon monoxide diffusing capacity test (DLCO) an investigation of lung function, which estimates the effectiveness of oxygen diffusion across the alveolar capillary membrane from alveoli to the blood. It measures the diffusion capacity for carbon monoxide in mL/min/mmHg rather than oxygen, which is difficult to measure.

carbon tetrachloride colourless volatile liquid used in dry cleaning and some types of antifreeze. Exposure may result in toxicity and liver damage.

carborundum in dentistry, abrasive powder containing silicon carbide bonded with clay or other material. Used in rotary grinding instruments.

carboxyhaemoglobin *n* a stable compound formed by the union of carbon monoxide and haemoglobin; the red blood cells thus lose their respiratory function. Large amounts are present in carbon monoxide poisoning but smaller amounts are also present in smokers' blood.

carboxyhaemoglobinaemia *n* carboxyhaemoglobin in the blood—**carboxyhaemoglobinaemic** *adj.*

carboxyhaemoglobinuria *n* carboxyhaemoglobin in the urine—**carboxyhaemoglobinuric** *adj.*

carboxylase *n* an enzyme that catalyses the reaction that adds carbon dioxide to a substance to create a carboxyl group (COOH).

carboxylation the process by which a carboxyl group (COOH) replaces a hydrogen atom.

carboxypeptidase a pancreatic enzyme, secreted as inactive procarboxypeptidase, which hydrolyses amino acids from the carboxyl end of proteins and polypeptides during digestion in the small intestine.

carbuncle *n* an acute inflammation (usually caused by *Staphylococcus*). There is a collection of boils causing necrosis in the skin and subcutaneous tissue. ⊃ Colour Section Figure 56.

carcin/o- a prefix that means 'cancer', e.g. *carcinogen*.

carcinoembryonic antigen (CEA) an oncofetal antigen. Its presence in the serum of adults can be a tumour marker for colorectal cancers and those of the stomach, pancreas, breast and lung; and for non-malignant conditions, such as liver cirrhosis caused by alcohol misuse and pancreatitis. ⊃ oncofetal antigens.

carcinogen *n* agent, substance or environment causing cancer—**carcinogenic** *adj*, **carcinogenicity** *n.*

carcinogenesis *n* the production of cancer—**carcinogenetic** *adj.*

carcinoid syndrome cluster of symptoms including flushing, palpitation, diarrhoea and bronchospasm from histological

(usually low grade) malignancy; often originates in the appendix or in the bronchial tree. ⊃ APUD cells, apudoma, argentaffinoma, 5-hydroxyindoleacetic acid.

carcinoma *n* a cancerous growth of epithelial tissue (e.g. mucous membrane) and derivatives such as glands.

carcinoma in situ (CIS) condition with cells closely resembling cancer cells. A very early cancer (premalignant) where the abnormal cell growth has not invaded the basement membrane. Well described in uterine cervix and endometrium, lip, oral mucosa, oesophagus, anus, prostate and bronchi. Previously called preinvasive carcinoma—**carcinomata** *pl*, **carcinomatous** *adj.*

carcinomatosis *n* widespread malignancy affecting many organs.

cardia *n* the oesophageal opening into the stomach.

cardiac *adj* **1.** pertaining to the heart **2.** pertaining to the cardia of the stomach.

cardiac arrest complete cessation of effective output (of blood) from heart activity. Failure of the heart action to maintain an adequate circulation. The clinical picture of cessation of circulation in a patient who was not expected to die at the time. There are several forms: asystole, pulseless electrical activity/electromechanical dissociation, pulseless ventricular tachycardia or ventricular fibrillation. ⊃ arrhythmia, Appendix 10.

cardiac bed one which can be manipulated so that the patient is supported in a sitting position.

cardiac bypass operation the bypassing of atheromatous vessels (coronary arteries) supplying heart muscle (myocardium). ⊃ coronary artery bypass graft.

cardiac catheterization a long plastic catheter or tubing is inserted into an artery or vein and moved under X-ray guidance until it reaches the heart. A catheter inserted into the brachial or femoral artery gives access to the left side of the heart and those inserted into the brachial or femoral vein can be guided into the right atrium, ventricle and the pulmonary artery. Cardiac catheterization can be used for: (a) recording pressures and cardiac output, ⊃ pulmonary artery occlusion pressure; (b) the introduction of radiopaque contrast agent for angiography; (c) treatments, such as angioplasty and stent insertion, ⊃ angioplasty.

cardiac cycle the rhythmic contraction (systole) and relaxation (diastole) of the heart as it fills with blood and pumps it around the body and to the lungs. The cycle provides an adequate output of blood from the heart. There are a series of stages that occur during a single heartbeat, which normally is completed in less than one second. Cycles follow on without pause to maintain a continuous flow of blood. The electrical cycle begins with discharge from the sinus (sinoatrial) node, spreading excitation through the atrial muscle then via the atrioventricular (A-V) node to the ventricular muscle; after this an isoelectric phase precedes the next cycle. The mechanical cycle begins with simultaneous contraction of the right and left atria (assisting filling of the ventricles); contraction of the ventricles (systole), raising pressure within them, which closes the atrioventricular and opens the aortic and pulmonary valves; ejection of blood; then relaxation (diastole) and refilling. ⊃ blood pressure, diastole, cardiac output, electrocardiogram, systole.

cardiac enzymes released from damaged myocardial cells. Abnormal levels found in the blood are suggestive of a diagnosis of myocardial infarction. Used to confirm or refute the diagnosis of myocardial infarction. The enzymes usually measured are cardiac troponins (I and T) and creatine kinase (CK). Elevated levels of troponins indicate myocardial damage from any cause and they are used to differentiate between chest pain caused by unstable angina and myocardial infarction. Aspartate aminotransferase (AST) and lactate dehydrogenase (LDH) may also be measured.

cardiac hypertrophy thickening of the myocardium, particularly the left ventricle. This may occur physiologically as a result of athletic training and is usually a uniform increase in thickness of the ventricular wall. Pathologically it may be the result of hypertension, secondary to outflow tract obstruction (e.g. aortic valve stenosis) or to congenital abnormalities. ⊃ athlete's heart, hypertrophic obstructive cardiomyopathy.

cardiac index (CI) the measure of cardiac output in relation to body surface area, i.e. $L/min/m^2$.

cardiac massage ⊃ cardiopulmonary resuscitation (CPR), chest compressions.

cardiac muscle a distinct muscle type that forms the myocardium. It has common features with both skeletal and smooth muscle. Its short branching fibres may have a single nucleus or two, are striated, but contraction is involuntary. The presence of an inherent 'pacemaker' produces rhythmic contractions that are modified to meet changing physiological needs by the autonomic nervous system and hormones. The boundaries between individual fibres, which are not well defined, are formed by intercalated discs; a feature that ensures that the wave of contraction passes easily across the myocardium, which behaves like a syncytium. ⊃ muscle.

cardiac nerve supply the heart is innervated by both sympathetic and parasympathetic fibres. Adrenergic nerves from the cervical sympathetic chain supply muscle fibres in the atria and ventricles and the electrical conducting system. Positive inotropic and chronotropic effects are mediated by β_1-adrenoceptors, whereas β_2-adrenoceptors predominate in vascular smooth muscle and mediate vasodilatation. Parasympathetic pre-ganglionic fibres and sensory fibres reach the heart through the vagus nerves (tenth cranial nerves). Cholinergic nerves supply the atrioventricular (AV) and sinus nodes (sinoatrial, SA node) via muscarinic (M2) receptors. Under resting conditions, vagal inhibitory activity predominates and the heart rate is slow. Adrenergic stimulation associated with exercise, emotional stress, fever and so on causes the heart rate to increase. In disease states the nerve supply to the heart may be affected. For example, in patients with heart failure the sympathetic system may be up-regulated, and in patients with diabetes the nerves themselves may be damaged so that there is little variation in heart rate. ⊃ cardiac cycle.

cardiac oedema gravitational oedema. Such patients secrete excessive aldosterone which increases excretion of potassium and conserves sodium and chloride. Antialdosterone (aldosterone antagonists) drugs may be useful, e.g. spironolactone. ⊃ oedema.

cardiac output (CO) the volume of blood ejected per minute from each ventricle of the heart simultaneously, i.e. to the lungs via the pulmonary artery, and to the rest of the body via the aorta (although often defined solely as the output from the left ventricle). The product of stroke volume (SV) and heart rate (HR): at rest, e.g. 70 mL × 70 beat per minute (bpm) = 4.9 L per min (4–6 L per min varying with body size). Increase in cardiac output (CO) in exercise involves increase in heart rate, accompanied by greater filling during diastole (by increased venous return to the heart), maintaining then increasing stroke volume, due to stretch of the ventricular muscle and to enhanced contractility from sympathetic stimulation; also the residual volume remaining in the ventricles after ejection decreases. Maximal CO in exercise increases with athletic training (by hypertrophy of ventricular muscle, with raised SV and lowered HR at rest, allowing a greater increase) exceptionally up to SV 200 mL × HR 200 bpm = 40 L per min, but a more modest maximum is typical. CO can be expressed as the cardiac index (CI), cardiac output divided by body surface area. ⊃ cardiac index, stroke volume.

cardiac pacemaker an electrical device for maintaining myocardial contraction by stimulating the heart muscle. A pacemaker may be permanent or temporary. They are programmed in a variety of modes. Nowadays pacemakers can be programmed to alter their rate in response to physical activity.

cardiac reflex an automatic neural process that alters heart rate. It functions through stretch receptors in the right side of the heart which respond to the volume of venous blood returning to the heart.

cardiac rehabilitation provided primarily for patients after a myocardial infarction or revascularization but also for those with angina or heart failure. The structured, planned programmes involve a multidisciplinary team (specialist nurse, exercise expert, dietitian, physiotherapist, occupational therapist and physician) and are likely to involve education about risk factor modification, exercise, counselling and psychological and social support. Designed to achieve and maintain the maximum degree of physical and psychological independence of which they are capable. The programme is exercise based, with a gradual increase in activity individually tailored to suit clinical status and level of symptoms. Educational (risk factor modification) and nutritional sessions are included for both patient and spouse/partner and the psychosocial aspects such as return to work, resumption of sexual activity, etc. are covered.

cardiac sphincter ⊃ lower oesophageal sphincter.

cardiac tamponade excessive fluid surrounding the heart, usually blood when the cause is traumatic. Can occur in surgery and penetrating wounds or cardiac rupture. Causes compression of the heart leading to heart failure from haemopericardium. ⊃ Beck's triad.

cardiac veins several small veins that carry most venous blood from the myocardium. They unite to form the coronary sinus.

cardialgia *n* literally, pain in the heart. Often used to mean heartburn (pyrosis).

cardi/a/o- a prefix that means 'heart', e.g. *cardiomegaly*.

cardinal ligaments two thickened bands of parametrium stretching from the uterine cervix to the lateral walls of the pelvis, which help to support the uterus; also known as transverse cervical or Mackenrodt's ligaments.

cardinal movements of labour the principal positions and movements of the fetus during its passage through the birth canal.

cardinal planes planes, normal to the optical axis, which pass through the cardinal points of a lens or optical system. They are the focal planes, the nodal planes and the principal planes. (Sometimes, this definition also includes the object and image planes.) ⊃ cardinal points.

cardinal points (*syn* gaussian points [although this term does not include the two nodal points, nor the object and image points]) the six points on the optical axis of a lens system or thick lens: the two principal foci, the two principal points and the two nodal points. (Sometimes, this definition also includes the axial object and image points.). ⊃ cardinal planes.

cardiogenic *adj* of cardiac origin, such as the shock that may be due to low cardiac output following an extensive acute myocardial infarction.

cardiograph *n* an instrument for recording graphically the force and form of the heart beat—**cardiographic** *adj*, **cardiogram** *n*, **cardiographically** *adv*. ⊃ electrocardiograph.

cardiologist *n* a medically qualified person who specializes in diagnosing and treating diseases of the heart.

cardiology *n* study of the structure, function and diseases of the heart.

cardiomegaly *n* enlargement of the heart.

cardiomyopathy *n* a disease of the myocardium associated with cardiac dysfunction. It is classified as dilated cardiomyopathy, hypertrophic cardiomyopathy, arrhythmogenic right ventricular cardiomyopathy or restrictive cardiomyopathy. Management includes treatment of the cause (if possible), treatment of heart failure and sometimes heart transplantation—**cardiomyopathic** *adj*. ⊃ hypertrophic obstructive cardiomyopathy.

cardiomyoplasty *n* a surgical procedure whereby ventricular contraction is augmented by the use of stimulated skeletal muscle.

cardiomyotomy *n* cutting or dissection of the muscular tissue at the gastro-oesophageal junction for achalasia.

cardiophone *n* a microphone strapped to a patient which allows audible and visual signal of heart sounds. By channelling pulses through an electrocardiograph, a graphic record can be made. Can be used for the fetus.

cardioplegia *n* **1.** paralysis of the heart. **2.** the use of an electrolyte solution to induce cardiac arrest. *cold cardioplegia* cardioplegia combined with hypothermia to reduce the oxygen consumption of the myocardium during open heart surgery.

cardiopulmonary *adj* pertaining to the heart and lungs. *cardiopulmonary bypass* used in open heart surgery. The heart and lungs are excluded from the circulation and replaced by a pump oxygenator (heart-lung machine)—**cardiopulmonic** *adj*.

cardiopulmonary resuscitation (CPR) the techniques used to maintain circulation and respiration following cardiopulmonary arrest. It involves (a) the maintenance of a clear airway, (b) rescue breaths (artificial respiration) using mouth-to-mouth or mouth-to-nose respiration, or with a bag and face mask, or by an endotracheal tube, and (c) maintenance of the circulation of blood by chest compressions (external cardiac massage). ⊃ resuscitation, Appendix 10.

cardiorenal *adj* pertaining to the heart and kidney.

cardiorespiratory *adj* pertaining to the heart and the respiratory system.

cardiorrhaphy *n* stitching of the heart wall: usually reserved for traumatic surgery.

cardiospasm *n* the failure of the lower oesophageal sphincter (gastro-oesophageal [cardiac] sphincter) between the oesophagus and stomach to relax and allow food or fluids through. A type of achalasia.

cardiothoracic *adj* pertaining to the heart and thoracic cavity. A specialized branch of surgery.

cardiotocograph *n* the instrument used in cardiotocography.

cardiotocography (CTG) *n* fetal monitoring. A procedure whereby the fetal heart rate is measured either by an external microphone or by the application of an electrode to the fetal scalp, recording the fetal ECG and from it the fetal heart rate. Fetal movements are also recorded. An external transducer placed on the woman's abdomen or an intrauterine catheter measures the frequency and strength of the uterine contractions. Used for the early detection of fetal distress caused by hypoxia and other depatures from normal. ⊃ fetal blood sampling, tocography.

cardiotomy 1. incision into the heart. **2.** surgical procedure in which the cardiac orifice of the stomach is incised.

cardiotomy syndrome pyrexia, pericarditis and pleural effusion following heart surgery. It may develop weeks or months after the operation and is thought to be an autoimmune reaction.

cardiotoxic *adj* describes any agent that has an injurious effect on the heart.

cardiovascular *adj* pertaining to the heart and blood vessels.

cardiovascular disease (CVD) includes disease affecting the heart and/or blood vessels, for example coronary heart disease, cerebrovascular accident (stroke), peripheral vascular disease, etc.

cardiovascular endurance the ability to sustain exercise without undue fatigue, cardiac distress or respiratory distress.

cardioversion *n* use of an electrical direct current (DC) countershock for restoring the heart rhythm to normal. Such as slowing a rapid heart rate or converting atrial fibrillation to sinus rhythm. It may be accomplished with either an external or an internal defibrillator implanted in the chest.

carditis *n* inflammation of the heart. A word seldom used without the appropriate prefix, e.g. endo-, myo-, peri-. Often more than one layer is involved. ⊃ endocarditis, myocarditis, pericarditis.

care pathway an integrated plan or pathway agreed locally by the multidisciplinary team for a specific patient/client groups or disorder. The agreed pathway is based on available evidence and guidelines. ⊃integrated care pathway.

care plan the document on which nursing information is recorded. In some instances, it is used as a collective term which includes: information from the initial patient assessment; statement of patient's actual and potential problems with everyday living activities which are amenable to nursing intervention; statement of the goals related to the problems to be achieved by the patient; and the plan of nursing interventions and their implementation, together with information from ongoing assessment and evaluation of whether or not the goals have been, or are being, achieved.

Care Programme Approach (CPA) developed to improve continuing care in the community of people with severe learning disabilities and mental health problems. The CPA is designed to ensure that people do not slip through the net by prescribing and monitoring essential requirements for good practice in their care and supervision. These are: (a) assessment of health and social care needs; (b) a written plan of care agreed with the user and carers; (c) a key worker appointed with responsibility for coordinating the care programme; (d) regular reviews with multidisciplinary professional and user/carer involvement.

Care Quality Commission (CQC) the single body formed from the merger of three separate regulatory bodies: the Health Care Commission, Mental Health Act Commission and the Commission for Social Care Inspection. The aims of the merger under the provisions of the Health and Social Care Act 2008 are to: provide a single regulator for health and adult social services; ensure service safety and quality; provide performance assessment of both commissioners and providers of health care and adult social services; monitor the functioning of the Mental Health Act; and make sure that the regulation and inspection processes for health and adult social services are co-ordinated and managed. (Department of Health (DH) 2008 Health and Social Care Act 2008. online www.dh.gov.uk/) ⊃ Health and Social Care Act 2008.

Caregiver Strain Index (CSI) used by mental health nurses and others to assess caregiver strain, using a simple questionnaire. Although unsophisticated, it has the benefit of being quick and simple.

carer *n* someone who takes the responsibility for caring for another (child, sick, disabled or older person). Usually describes unpaid family, friends and neighbours of vulnerable people in the UK, and not paid helpers such as care workers, nurses or social workers. ⊃ Caregiver Strain Index, Carers Assessment of Managing Index, Experience of Caregiving Inventory.

Carers Assessment of Managing Index (CAMI) used by mental health nurses and others to assess coping styles and management of stress by questionnaire. Important in that it assumes that carers have coping strategies, which can be enhanced.

caries *n* inflammatory decay of bone, usually associated with pus formation—**carious** *adj*. ⊃ dental caries.

caries-free or immune a person who shows no evidence of dental caries.

caries-prone a person who in spite of good oral hygiene and regular dental care exhibits a generally increased rate of dental caries.

carina *n* a keel-like structure exemplified by the keel-shaped cartilage at the bifurcation of the trachea into two bronchi—**carinal** *adj*.

cariogenic *adj* causing caries, by convention referring to dental caries. Examples include soft drinks with high levels of sugar and confectionary.

cariostatic agents such as the oils and fats in food that coat the teeth and prevent acids and sugars from forming plaque.

carious describes a tooth affected by caries.

carminative *adj*, *n* having the power to relieve flatulence and associated colic. They include cinnamon, nutmeg, peppermint.

carnauba wax naturally occurring wax obtained from the Brazilian wax palm and used in dentistry to harden inlay casting wax.

carneous mole a fleshy mass in the uterus comprising blood clot and a dead fetus or parts thereof that have not been expelled with miscarriage.

carnitine (L-carnitine) a short-chain nitrogen-containing carboxylic acid formed from the amino acid lysine, needed for the transport of fatty acids within cells prior to their oxidation. It is mainly located in skeletal and cardiac muscle cells. Over half the daily requirement is provided from meat and dairy products in a balanced diet; the remainder is synthesized in the liver. It has been hypothesized that supplementary ingestion of L-carnitine might upregulate the capacity to transport fatty acids into mitochondria matrix where they are metabolized and so increase their oxidation, thus benefiting both endurance athletes and those wishing to reduce their body fat. Research has not supported these claims. ⊃ ergogenic aids.

carnitine palmitoyltransferase (CPT) an inner mitochondrial membrane enzyme involved in lipid metabolism. It catalyses the reversible reaction that converts palmitoyl-CoA to palmitoylcarnitine.

carnitine palmitoyltransferase (CPT) deficiency an inherited disorder of lipid metabolism caused by a deficiency of the enzyme carnitine palmitoyltransferase. It gives rise to a myopathy characterized by muscle pain on prolonged exercise and myoglobinuria. Diagnosis is based on an elevated creatine kinase occurring during bouts of muscle pain (which is normal between) and muscle biopsy. ➲ carnitine palmitoyltransferase (CPT), inherited metabolic myopathy.

Caroli's disease II (J Caroli, French gastroenterologist, 1902–1979) congenital dilatation of the small intrahepatic bile ducts. It is associated with an increased risk of cholangitis (inflammation of the bile ducts), liver abscess and septicaemia.

carotenaemia, carotinaemia also called xanthaemia. Abnormally high amounts of carotene in the blood, which leads to yellow colouration of the skin. May be due to an excess intake of foods high in carotene such as carrots, or certain diseases.

carotenes *npl* a group of naturally occurring pigments within the larger group of carotenoids. They are fat-soluble and have antioxidant properties. Carotene occurs in three forms—alpha (α), beta (β) and gamma (γ). The β form is converted in the body to vitamin A; it is therefore a provitamin. ➲ beta (β)-carotene.

carotenoids *npl* a group of about 100 naturally occurring yellow to red pigments found mostly in plants, some of which are carotenes. Heating of foods before eating usually improves carotenoid availability.

carotid angiography the radiographic demonstration of the brain circulation by direct injection of a contrast agent into the carotid artery or via a catheter inserted in the femoral artery which is passed upwards in the arterial system to the carotid artery.

carotid arteries the principal arteries on each side of the neck supplying the head and neck. The *right common carotid artery* is a branch of the brachiocephalic artery. The *left common carotid artery* is one of three large arteries that arise directly from the arch of the aorta. The carotid arteries pass upwards on either side of the neck and have the same distribution on each side. The common carotid arteries are embedded in fascia, called the carotid sheath. At the level of the upper border of the thyroid cartilage each divides into an *internal carotid artery* and an *external carotid artery*. The internal carotid artery is a major contributor to the circulus arteriosus (circle of Willis), which supplies the greater part of the brain. It also has branches that supply the eyes, forehead and nose. It ascends to the base of the skull and passes through the carotid foramen in the temporal bone. The external carotid artery supplies the superficial tissues of the head and neck, via a number of branches. These include: superior thyroid artery; lingual artery; facial artery; occipital artery; temporal artery; maxillary artery and its branch the middle meningeal artery. ➲ carotid bodies, carotid sinuses, circulus arteriosus (circle of Willis), facial artery, lingual artery, maxillary artery, middle meningeal artery, occipital artery, superior thyroid artery, temporal artery, Colour Section Figure 9.

carotid bodies a collection of chemoreceptors associated with each common carotid artery at its bifurcation. They are sensitive to changes in the level of oxygen and carbon dioxide in the blood and stimulate the respiratory centre in the medulla oblongata to make the necessary respiratory adjustments.

carotid compression tonography ➲ tonography.

carotid sinuses a collection of baroreceptors sited at the bifurcation of each common carotid artery; they are sensitive to pressure changes and when blood pressure changes they signal the vasomotor centre in the medulla oblongata to make the necessary adjustments to blood pressure through, for example, peripheral vasodilation and reducing heart rate when blood pressure rises. ➲ baroreceptors.

carotid sinus massage firm rubbing over the area of carotid sinus is used to stimulate reflex vagal slowing of the heart. The technique can be used by a competent practitioner to slow the heart rate in certain supraventricular tachyarrhythmias.

carpal 1. *adj* pertaining to the wrist. **2.** *n* one of the eight bones of the wrist.

carpal tunnel syndrome nocturnal pain, numbness, weakness of the thumb and tingling in the area of distribution of the median nerve in the hand. Due to compression as the nerve passes through the carpal tunnel. Most common in middle-aged women.

carphology *n* involuntary picking at the bedclothes, as seen in exhaustive or febrile delirium.

carp/o- a prefix that means 'wrist', e.g. *carpal*.

carpometacarpal *adj* pertaining to the carpal and metacarpal bones.

carpopedal *adj* pertaining to the hands and feet. ➲ carpopedal spasm.

carpopedal spasm painful spasm of hands and feet in tetany. The hands in carpal spasm adopt a characteristic position. The metacarpophalangeal joints are flexed, the interphalangeal joints of the fingers and thumb are extended, and there is opposition of the thumb ('main d'accoucheur'). Pedal spasm is much less frequent. ➲ Chvostek's sign, hypocalcaemia, tetany, Trousseau's sign.

carpus *n* the wrist. Comprises eight bones: trapezium, trapezoid, capitate, hamate, scaphoid, lunate, triquetral and pisiform, in two rows. ➲ Colour Section Figure 2.

carrier *n* **1.** a person who, without manifesting an infection, harbours the micro-organism which can cause the overt infection, and who can transmit infection to others. **2.** a person who carries a recessive gene at a specific chromosome location (locus).

carrier molecule a cell membrane protein that assists the transfer of drugs, ions and nutrients into the cell.

Cartesian co-ordinate system ➲ co-ordinates.

cartilage *n* a dense connective tissue capable of withstanding pressure. There is relatively more cartilage in a child's skeleton but much of it has been converted into bone by adulthood. There are three basic types of cartilage each with a different function to fulfil. *fibrocartilage (white)* forms the pads between the vertebrae, ligaments, the semilunar cartilages in the knee and the rim or labrum that deepens the sockets of the shoulder and hip joints; *elastic fibrocartilage (yellow)* is found in the pinna of the ear, in the middle coat of blood vessels and in the epiglottis; and *hyaline cartilage* forms part of the larynx, trachea and bronchi, the costal cartilages that join the ribs to the sternum and covers the articular surfaces of long bones—**cartilaginous** *adj.*

cartilaginous joint amphiarthrosis. One of the three main classes of joint. A slightly movable joint where the two bones are connected by cartilage. There are two types, symphysis and synchondrosis. ⊃ symphysis, synchondrosis.

caruncle *n* a red fleshy projection. Hymenal caruncles surround the entrance to the vagina after rupture of the hymen ⊃ carunculae myrtiformes. The lacrimal caruncle is the fleshy prominence at the medial canthus (angle) of the eye.

carunculae myrtiformes small elevations of mucous membrane around the vaginal orifice; the remnants of the ruptured hymen.

carve in dentistry, to shape or model a filling material in its plastic condition, e.g. amalgam, wax.

carver hand instrument with a blade or nib used in dentistry to contour the surface of filling materials in their plastic state, waxes, models and patterns, e.g. Ward's, Frahm's, LeCron's.

carving wax coloured, high-melting point wax, used chiefly for instruction in tooth carving exercises.

case control study an epidemiological approach comprising a retrospective research study that compares outcomes for a group with a particular condition with those of a matched for age, gender, etc. control group who do not have the condition.

case mix database computerized record system which combines all the data received from patient administration and operational systems to provide comprehensive information about all treatment and services received by each patient during an episode of care; helps to develop expected care profiles for different groups, to analyse and compare different treatment regimens, to produce comparative costings for different treatments; may be used for medical audit.

case study research that studies data from one case, or a small group of cases.

caseation *n* the formation of a soft, cheese-like mass, as occurs in tuberculosis—**caseous** *adj.*

casein *n* a protein produced when milk enters the stomach. Coagulation occurs and is due to the action of rennin upon the caseinogen in the milk, splitting it into two proteins, one being casein. The casein combines with calcium and a clot is formed. Casein is known as paracasein in the United States.

casein hydrolysate predigested protein food derived from casein; can be added to other foods to increase the protein content.

caseinogen *n* the principal protein in milk. It is not soluble in water but is kept in solution in milk by inorganic salts. The proportion to lactalbumin is much higher in cows' milk than in human milk. In the presence of rennin it is converted into insoluble casein. Caseinogen is known as casein in the United States.

caseload midwifery a way of organizing midwifery practice where each midwife is responsible for the total care of a small group of women (usually between 35 and 40 per year). ⊃ continuity of care, team midwifery.

caseous degeneration cottage cheese-like tissue resulting from atrophy in a tuberculoma or gumma.

Casoni test intradermal injection of fresh, sterile hydatid fluid. A white papule indicates a hydatid cyst.

cassette in radiography, a piece of equipment to hold either an imaging plate or radiographic film. It may also contain intensifying screens and a grid. In dental radiography, it is used extra-orally. Contains a pair of intensifying screens, the unwrapped film being placed between them in a darkroom. A marker may be required to indicate whether the film relates to the patient's right or left side.

cast *n* **1.** material or exudate that has been moulded to the form of the cavity or tube in which it has collected. **2.** a rigid casing often made with plaster of Paris and applied to immobilize a part of the body. **3.** in dentistry, the reproduction obtained from an impression of oral or facial tissues, usually in plaster of Paris, which may be strengthened by the addition of other substances. **4.** to make a cast or casting, using an impression as a mould, in a heated investment material. *diagnostic (study) cast* a cast made especially for study, diagnosis and treatment planning. *investment cast* a cast made of a refractory material that will withstand high temperatures without disintegrating. *master cast* the accurately made cast on which dental restorations and prostheses are fabricated. *study cast* ⊃ diagnostic (study) cast.

cast crown a metal veneer crown, full or partial, and constructed entirely of a metal alloy by the casting process.

casting (in dental procedures) 1. shape, usually in metal, which has been formed in a mould. **2.** process of forcing molten metal into a mould to form a casting. ⊃ casting gold, casting machine, casting ring.

casting gold an alloy, mainly of gold, with small quantities of silver, copper and platinum. It is heated to the required temperature to become molten and then cast into a mould. Variations of the ingredients produce castings of different strength and hardness. ⊃ gold.

casting machine mechanism which injects, by centrifugal force, molten metal into a prepared preheated die by means of pressure, vacuum or centrifugal action.

casting ring metal tube containing a refractory investment material which forms a mould for casting of metal inlays, crowns, appliances and metal prostheses.

casting shrinkage ⊃ shrinkage.

casting wax (*syn* inlay wax) a mixture of waxes such as paraffin wax, beeswax, ceresin wax, carnauba wax and candelilla wax. Used for pattern making for metallic castings, such as inlays, and designed to leave no residue when burned out of investment materials. The working temperature, hardness, suppleness, expansion and contraction of casting wax are controlled by the ingredients. Blue or green in colour and obtainable in sticks, thin sheets and prefabricated shapes for clasps and bars. ⮑ wax.

castor oil a vegetable oil previously used as a stimulant laxative. ⮑ laxatives. Used with zinc ointment as a barrier cream for napkin and urinary rash.

castration *n* surgical removal of the testes in the male, or of the ovaries in the female. Castration can be part of the treatment for a hormone-dependent cancer—**castrated** *adj*, **castrate** *n, vt*.

CAT *acron* Computed Axial Tomography.

cat/a- a prefix that means 'down', e.g. *catalase*.

catabolic hormones natural or synthetic hormones that stimulate the breakdown of complex chemical substances in order to release energy. They include cortisol, adrenaline (epinephrine), glucagon and cytokines. Others, including the excitatory neuropeptides hypocretins (orexins), appear to be involved in balancing sleep–wake–activity cycles and hence the expenditure of energy by the body and appetite. Compare with anabolic hormones.

catabolism (or katabolism) *n* the series of chemical reactions in the living body whereby complex substances are broken down into simpler ones accompanied by the release of energy. This energy is needed for anabolism, heat production, work and the other activities of the body. ⮑ adenosine diphosphate, adenosine triphosphate, anabolism, hypercatabolism, metabolism—**catabolic** *adj*.

catagen *n* a short interval in the hair growth cycle between active growth and the resting stage. ⮑ anagen, telogen.

catalase *n* a cellular enzyme that catalyses the breakdown of hydrogen peroxide into oxygen and water.

catalysis *n* an increase in the rate at which a chemical reaction proceeds to equilibrium through the medium of a catalyst or catalyser. Reaction retardation is termed negative catalysis—**catalytic** *adj*.

catalyst *n* any substance that regulates or accelerates the rate of a chemical reaction without itself undergoing a permanent change.

cataplexy *n* a condition of muscular rigidity induced by severe mental shock or fear. The patient remains conscious—**cataplectic** *adj*.

cataract *n* a partial or complete loss of transparency of the crystalline lens substance or its capsule. Cataract may occur as a result of age, trauma, systemic diseases (e.g. diabetes mellitus), ocular diseases (e.g. anterior uveitis), ocular trauma, high myopia, long-term corticosteroid therapy, excessive exposure to infrared and ultraviolet light, heredity, maternal infections, Down's syndrome, etc. The incidence of cataract increases with age, amounting to more than 50% in the population over 82 years. It is also more prevalent in Africa, Asia and South America than in Europe and North America. The main symptom is a gradual loss of vision, often described as 'misty'. Some patients may also notice transient monocular diplopia, others fixed spots (not floaters) in the visual field and others better vision in dim illumination. Cataracts can easily be seen with the retinoscope, the ophthalmoscope and especially with the slit-lamp, although depending on the type, one instrument may be better than the other. At present the main treatment is surgical. Extraction is performed for one of three reasons: visual improvement, medical or cosmetic—**cataractous** *adj*. ⮑ blue-dot cataract, blue field entoptoscope, capsule of the crystalline lens, clinical maxwellian view system, crystalline lens, glare tester, hyperacuity, intraocular lens implant, leukocoria, lenticular myopia, persistent hyperplastic primary vitreous (PHPV), phacoemulsification, Colour Section Figure 57.

cataract extraction removal of the affected lens and usually the insertion of an intraocular lens. ⮑ extracapsular extraction, intracapsular extraction, phacoemulsification.

catarrh *n* chronic inflammation of a mucous membrane with constant flow of a thick sticky mucus. Usually applied to the inflammation of the nasal air passages and the trachea—**catarrhal** *adj*.

catastrophe theory a set of mathematical theorems employed in the modelling of discontinuities in the physical world, that result when gradually changing and interacting variables reach a critical point. Applied in sport psychology to the understanding of sudden decrements or increments in performance, incorporating changes in cognitive anxiety, physiological arousal and self-confidence.

catatonic schizophrenia a form of schizophrenia characterized by psychomotor disturbances (e.g. stupor, posturing, negativism, hyperkinesis). ⮑ schizophrenia.

catchlike current an electrotherapy term. The first few pulses in each on-time have a higher frequency, typically 80 Hz, than the later pulses, often 40 Hz. The aim is to reduce the muscle fatigue associated with using pulsed current.

catchment area the geographic area and its population served by a particular health provider or other organization, e.g. a health centre, school, NHS Trust.

cat cry syndrome ⮑ 'cri du chat' syndrome.

catecholamines *npl* a group of important physiological amines, such as adrenaline (epinephrine), noradrenaline (norepinephrine) and dopamine. They act as hormones and neurotransmitters and affect blood pressure, heart rate, respiratory rate and blood glucose (sugar). Released into the blood as hormones from the adrenal medulla, and as neurotransmitters at sympathetic nerve endings and within the central nervous system. Abnormally high levels are secreted by adrenal and other tumours and can be detected in the urine. ⮑ phaeochromocytoma.

categorical data data that can be categorized, e.g. hair colour. ⮑ nominal data, ordinal data.

catgut *n* a form of ligature and suture of varying thickness, strength and absorbability, prepared from animal tissue. The plain variety is usually absorbed in 5–10 days, whereas chromic catgut takes 10–21 days to be absorbed.

catharsis *n* in psychology, it describes the purging or outpouring of emotion through experiencing it deeply—**cathartic** *adj*.

cathepsins (kathepsins) group of intracellular enzymes that breakdown proteins. They function in the normal cellular turnover of tissue protein, and result in the changes that occur when meat and game are hung.

catheter *n* a hollow tube of variable length and bore, usually having one fluted end and a tip of varying size and shape according to function. Catheters are made of many substances including soft plastics and silicone with various coatings, soft and hard rubber, gum elastic, glass, silver and other metals, some of which are radiopaque. They have many uses including: insufflation of hollow tubes, cardiac catheterization, introduction of contrast agent for angiography, withdrawal of fluid from body cavities, e.g. urinary catheter and the administration of drugs, fluids and nutrients.

catheterization *n* insertion of a catheter, most usually referring to catheterization of the urinary bladder—**catheterize** *vt*. ⊃ cardiac catheterization.

cathetron *n* a high rate dose, remotely controlled, afterloading device for radiotherapy. Hollow steel catheters are placed in the desired position. They are then connected to a protective safe by hollow cables. The radioactive cobalt moves from the safe into the catheters. After delivery of the required dose, the cobalt returns to the safe, thus avoiding radiation hazard to staff. Currently superseded by units such as the Selectron.

cathode in electrotherapy, a conductor with a negative charge, attracting positively charged atoms or groups of atoms (cations). Usually is the black (or white) lead, attached to the distal electrode. Usually used as the stimulating electrode for motor stimulation with a monophasic or unbalanced pulse. In radiography, it is the assembly that contains the negatively charged filament, focussing cup, supporting wires and cathode support in an X-ray tube. ⊃ anode.

cathode rays streams of electrons coming from the heat filament or cathode.

cathode ray tube used in older computer monitors where an electron gun is focussed on a fluorescent screen, where electrons hit the screen light is produced and therefore an image is formed. ⊃ glass plasma display, liquid crystal display.

cation *n* an ion with a positive electrical charge, e.g. calcium (Ca^{2+}). These ions move towards the negative electrode (cathode) during electrolysis. ⊃ anion.

cation-exchange resin one of several high molecular, insoluble organic substances which exchange cations with other ions. ⊃ ion-exchange resin.

cat's eye reflex a whitish, bright reflection observed in the normally black pupil in several conditions, such as leukocoria, retinoblastoma, Coats' disease or persistent hyperplastic primary vitreous. It resembles the reflection from the tapetum lucidum of a cat when a light is shined at night. ⊃ Coats' disease, leukocoria, retinoblastoma, tapetum.

cat scratch fever a virus infection resulting from a cat scratch or bite. There is fever and lymph node swelling about a week after the incident. Recovery is usually complete, although an abscess may develop.

cauda *n* a tail or tail-like appendage—**caudal, caudate** *adj*. ⊃ cauda equina.

cauda equina lower part of the spinal cord where the nerves for the legs and bladder originate.

caudal anaesthesia injection of local anaesthetic into the epidural space at the level of the sacrum causing loss of sensation in the lower abdomen and pelvis.

caudate nucleus part of the basal nuclei (ganglia) involved in motor control.

caul *n* the amnion, instead of rupturing as is usual to allow the baby through, persists and covers the baby's head at birth.

cauliflower ear in sports medicine a colloquial term used to describe deformity of the pinna that may follow auricular haematoma (collection of blood between the perichondrium and cartilage of the outer/external ear) caused by repeated trauma sustained during contact sports that include boxing and rugby.

causalgia *n* ⊃ complex regional pain syndrome 2.

causality ⊃ locus of causality.

caustic *adj*, *n* **1**. the concentration of light in the caustic surface of a bundle of converging light rays which represents the focal image in an optical system uncorrected for spherical aberration. It appears as a hollow luminous cusp with its apex at the paraxial focus. ⊃ spherical aberration. **2**. corrosive or destructive to organic tissue; the agents which produce such results. Usually a strong alkali or acid, they are used to destroy over-abundant granulation tissue, warts or polyps. Carbolic acid, carbon dioxide snow and silver nitrate are most commonly employed.

cauterize *vt* to cause tissue destruction by applying a heated instrument, a cautery—**cauterization** *n*.

cautery *n* an agent or device, e.g. electricity, chemicals or extremes of temperature, which destroys cells and tissues. Uses include the prevention of blood loss during surgery, or to remove abnormal tissue.

cav- a prefix that means 'hollow', e.g. *cavitation*.

-caval a suffix that means 'pertaining to venae cavae', e.g. *portacaval*.

cavernous *adj* having hollow spaces.

cavernous sinus a channel for venous blood, on either side of the sphenoid bone. Contains many veins, several nerves, e.g. oculomotor (cranial nerve III), and the internal carotid artery. Its veins drain blood from the cerebral hemispheres, orbits and the bones of the skull. ⊃ cavernous sinus thrombosis.

cavernous sinus thrombosis acute infection, with thrombus formation, in the cavernous sinus. Often associated with oral sepsis draining into an air sinus, or infection around the eyes or nose. It is a very serious condition.

cavitation *n* the formation of a cavity, as in pulmonary tuberculosis or the process in which the hard tissues of a tooth crown are undermined by caries, causing them to cave in and form a cavity.

cavitation (electrotherapy) the formation of bubbles of a gas previously absorbed in a liquid. Can be stable (remain relatively unchanged) or unstable (tend to form and burst rapidly leading to release of heat). It can be produced by ultrasound. It is unlikely with therapeutic ultrasound applied to a living human body if the output is in the frequency range 0.8–3 MHz and the intensity 0–3 W/cm^2. Often described in explanations of how therapeutic ultrasound works but relevance to outcome is not clarified.

cavity *n* a hollow; an enclosed area. ⮌ abdominal cavity, buccal cavity, cavity (dental), cerebral cavity, cranial cavity, medullary cavity, nasal cavity, oral cavity, pelvic cavity, peritoneal cavity, synovial cavity, uterine cavity.

cavity (dental) in dentistry, a condition caused by caries, trauma, abrasion, erosion or attrition, resulting in the loss of hard tissue. Refers to such cavities only and should not be applied to a tooth preparation. *cavity base* cement lining placed in the depth of a tooth preparation to protect the pulp from thermal and chemical irritation, or trauma. *cavity floor* floor of a tooth preparation on which a restoration is placed. *cavity liner* a material, that may have adhesive properties, applied to the walls of a tooth preparation. Intended to seal the ends of the dentinal tubules and so protect them from irritants and the effects of micro-leakage. *cavity lining material* used as a lining beneath a restoration, to insulate the tooth against thermal or chemical irritation. May be used to reduce the bulk of a large restoration, e.g. zinc phosphate cement, zinc carboxylate cement and quick-setting zinc oxide cements. *cavity preparation (tooth preparation)* removal of diseased and weakened tooth tissue and the shaping of sound tooth tissue to permit the placing and retention of a temporary or permanent restoration. *cavity sub-base* material placed in the depth of a preparation before the insertion of a cavity base. May contain calcium hydroxide to promote the formation of reparative dentine. *cavity toilet* cleaning and removal of debris, and the drying of a tooth preparation by irrigation, spray and then compressed air. *cavity wall* one of the enclosing sides of a prepared cavity. *compound (complex) cavity* cavity involving two or more surfaces of the clinical crown, i.e. disto-occlusal or mesio-occlusal cavity.

cavity of the pelvis hollow within the pelvic walls, bounded by the pelvic brim (inlet) above and the outlet below. ⮌ pelvic cavity.

cavosurface angle angle formed between the surface of a tooth and a cavity wall.

cavosurface line angle ⮌ outline.

cavosurface margin ⮌ outline.

CBA *abbr* cost-benefit analysis.

CBC *abbr* complete blood count.

CBF *abbr* cerebral blood flow.

CBT *abbr* cognitive behaviour therapy.

C cells parafollicular cells in the thyroid gland. They produce a hormone calcitonin (thyrocalcitonin) which has a regulatory role in calcium and phosphate homeostasis.

CCK *abbr* cholecystokinin.

CCPNS *abbr* cell cycle phase non-specific.

CCPS *abbr* cell cycle phase specific.

CCU *abbr* coronary care unit. ⮌ high dependency unit, intensive care/therapy unit.

CD *abbr* 1. compact disc. 2. controlled drug.

CDC *abbr* Centers for Disease Control and Prevention.

CD4 cells denotes the immune helper T-cells (lymphocytes) which have the specific CD4 glycoprotein surface antigen. ⮌ delayed sensitivity T-cells, helper T-cells.

CD4/CD8 count the ratio of the CD4+ helper T-cells to the CD8+ cytotoxic or suppressor T-cells. It is used to monitor the immune system in people with viral infections such as HIV disease or following transplant. HIV disease and AIDS is associated with declining numbers of CD4+ helper T-cells.

CD8 cells denotes the immune cytotoxic/suppressor T-cells (lymphocytes) which have the specific CD8 glycoprotein surface antigen. ⮌ cytotoxic T-cells, suppressor-T cells.

CDH *abbr* congenital dislocation of the hip. ⮌ developmental dysplasia of the hip.

CDROM *abbr* compact disk read-only memory.

CDRW *abbr* compact disk re-writer.

CEA *abbr* 1. carcinoembryonic antigen. 2. cost-effectiveness analysis.

-cele a suffix that means 'tumour, swelling', e.g. *hydrocele*.

Celestin tube a soft intubation tube which is pulled through an oesophageal cancer by the use of a string or guidewire and is attached to the stomach with a suture. Used as a palliative measure to maintain a free passage of food and fluid, when the cancer is inoperable and or resistant to other treatment modalities.

cell *n* basic structural unit of living organisms. A mass of cytoplasm (protoplasm) and usually a nucleus within a plasma or cell membrane. Some cells, e.g. erythrocytes, are non-nucleated whereas others, such as voluntary muscle, may be multinucleated. The cytoplasm contains various subcellular organelles—mitochondria, ribosomes, etc. (Figure C.3)—that undertake the metabolic processes of the cell—**cellular** *adj*.

cell adhesion molecules (CAM) *npl* protein molecules located on the cell membrane, which either bind cells together or bind cells with the extracellular matrix. There

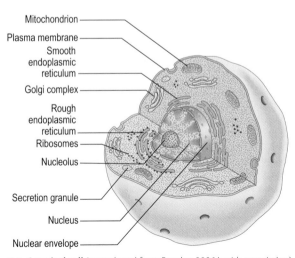

Mitochondrion
Plasma membrane
Smooth endoplasmic reticulum
Golgi complex
Rough endoplasmic reticulum
Ribosomes
Nucleolus
Secretion granule
Nucleus
Nuclear envelope

C.3 A typical cell (reproduced from Brooker 2006A with permission).

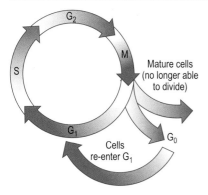

G₁ (gap1) variable-length period between mitosis and synthetic phase

S (synthetic) period of DNA replication and growth

G₂ (gap2) preparation for complete separation, growth and maturation

M (mitotic) phase when mitosis and cytokinesis occur

G₀ (quiescent) resting phase, but some cells rejoin the cell cycle when extra cells are required, e.g. liver cells following surgical resection

C.4 **Cell cycle** (reproduced from Brooker 2006A with permission).

are several types of molecules that facilitate cell adhesion, for example immunoglobulins.

cell cycle the events occurring within a cell from one mitotic division to the next. Comprises the dynamic course of division of normal and cancer cells incorporating phases of deoxyribonucleic acid (DNA) synthesis (S-phase), growth phases (G_1 and G_2), mitosis (M) and 'rest phase' (G0) (Figure C.4).

cell cycle phase non-specific (CCPNS) describes a cytotoxic drug that acts at any time in the cell cycle.

cell cycle phase specific (CCPS) describes a cytotoxic drug that acts during a specific phase of the cell cycle.

cell-mediated immunity cell mediated immunity is due to the T-lymphocyte-dependent responses which cause graft rejection, immunity to some infectious agents and tumour rejection. ⊃ immunity.

cell membrane ⊃ plasma membrane.

cell-surface molecules a diverse group of molecules present on the surface of cells. They facilitate and regulate cell functions and allow cells to communicate with each other and with the environment. They include cell recognition proteins; immune proteins; ion channels and other transport proteins for moving material in or out of the cell; receptors that respond to a specific ligand (e.g. hormone, growth factor, neurotransmitter or enzyme); and complexes of cell adhesion molecules forming desmosomes.

cellular streaming ⊃ microstreaming.

cellulitis *n* a diffuse acute inflammation of the skin and connective tissue, especially the loose subcutaneous tissue. Often caused by group A beta-haemolytic streptococci. When it occurs in the floor of the mouth it is called Ludwig's angina. ⊃ Colour Section Figure 58.

celluloid strip ⊃ strip.

cellulose *n* a carbohydrate forming the outer walls of plant and vegetable cells. A polysaccharide which cannot be digested by humans but supplies non-starch polysaccharides (NSP) for stimulation of peristalsis.

cellulose acetate in dentistry, a material used in the manufacture of matrix strips and crown forms.

cellulose acetate butyrate (CAB) is a transparent thermoplastic material which is used in the manufacture of gas permeable contact lenses as it transmits some oxygen. It is a copolymer with varying percentages of cellulose, acetyl and butyryl. CAB lenses vary in their characteristics depending on the percentages of the three components. It is also used to make spectacle frames. ⊃ oxygen permeability.

Celsius (A Celsius, Swedish scientist, 1701–1744) a temperature scale in which there are 100° Celsius between the melting point of ice (0°C) and the boiling point of water (100°C) recorded at sea level. ⊃ centigrade, Appendix 2.

cement any substance which sets to a hard mass on being mixed with water or other medium. In dentistry, term covering materials used for luting, lining and as a permanent (e.g. silicate, glass ionomer) or temporary (e.g. zinc phosphate, zinc oxide, etc.) filling. The components are mixed in their correct proportions to provide a plastic mass which sets in due course. ⊃ black copper cement, EBA cement (zinc oxide/EBA cement), glass ionomer cement, silicate cement, zinc oxide-eugenol cement, zinc phosphate cement, zinc polycarboxylate cement.

cementation in dentistry, a process of cementing a restoration in place by the use of a luting agent or cement.

cementoblast *n* the cell that forms the organic component of cementum.

cementocyte *n* the somewhat stellate-shaped cell with radiating thin processes. They are located within the lacunae of the cementum. They form from cementoblasts that are trapped during the formation of cementum.

cementoenamel junction line formed between the cementum and enamel at the anatomical neck of the tooth.

cementogenesis the formation of cementum by cementoblast cells.

cementoid the layer of matrix which has not yet calcified on the forming surface of cementum.

cementoma *n* generally benign proliferation of odontogenic connective tissue in the mandible or maxilla which produces cementum or cementum-like tissue. Often affects the apical part of the root of a tooth.

cementopathia *n* poor condition of the teeth due to diseased or deficient cementum. It is implicated in periodontal disease.

cementosis the laying-down of cementum.

cementum *n* the thin, calcified organic hard (bone-like) tissue forming on the surface of a root of a tooth, and providing attachment for the Sharpey's fibres. ⊃ tooth. *primary cementum* the acellular innermost layer of the cementum, that is later covered in the apical portion by cellular *secondary cementum*.

censor *n* term used by Freud to describe the resistance that prevents repressed material from easily re-entering the conscious mind from the subconscious (unconscious) mind.

Centers for Disease Control and Prevention (CDC) a federal agency in the US (Atlanta). Its functions include the investigation, identification, prevention and control of disease.

-centesis a suffix that means 'to puncture', e.g. *paracentesis*.

centi- a prefix that means a 'hundredth', e.g. *centile*.

centigrade *n* a scale with one hundred divisions or degrees. Most often refers to the thermometric scale in which the freezing point of water is fixed at 0° and the boiling point at 100°. It is usually called Celsius for medical and scientific purposes. ⊃ Celsius.

centile the numbered points that divide a set of scores into 100 points. ⊃ centile chart.

centile chart used to compare, for instance, a child's growth compared with children of the same sex and age. The chart shows the line for the average weight, height, etc. The individual child's measurements are charted on the appropriate centile and health professionals are able to predict the percentage of children of the same age and sex who would be bigger or smaller. For example, the 90th percentile would mean that 90% of children would be smaller and 10% of children would be bigger. Serial measurements will detect if a child's growth moves into another centile, or falls outside the 97th or 3rd centile which need further investigation.

central auditory processing disorder ⊃ auditory processing disorder.

central bearing device mechanical device, used intraorally, to record the position of the mandible in selected jaw positions.

central canal ⊃ hyaloid canal.

central corneal clouding diffuse, hazy appearance of the cornea due to oedema of the central region of the cornea, usually associated with the wearing of hard contact lenses (mainly PMMA), but it may also occur in keratoconus, Fuch's endothelial dystrophy or disciform keratitis. It is most easily seen with a slit-lamp using retroillumination against the pupil margin or sclerotic scatter illumination. This condition may give rise to Sattler's veil. ⊃ contact lens, cornea, cornea guttata, disciform keratitis, Fuch's endothelial dystrophy, keratoconus, retroillumination, Sattler's veil, sclerotic scatter illumination, slit-lamp.

central cyanosis ⊃ cyanosis.

central fatigue contribution of the central nervous system to the overall condition of fatigue in physical activity. Mainly significant in prolonged exercise, such as marathon running, where voluntary effort declines before muscle glycogen is exhausted and other peripheral indicators (heart rate, blood lactate, blood glucose, etc.) do not suggest particular stress. There is evidence that elevated 5-hydroxytryptamine (5-HT) and/or reduced dopamine levels in the brain are involved.

central limit theorem in research. Sampling distribution becomes more normal the more samples that are taken.

central line ⊃ central venous catheter/line.

central nervous system comprises the brain and spinal cord. ⊃ peripheral nervous system.

central pattern generators a network of neurons that can generate repetitive rhythmic output, e.g. stepping and breathing without sensory feedback. They are found in the spinal cord.

central processing unit (CPU) the chip which ultimately controls all elements of a personal computer.

central retinal artery a branch of the ophthalmic artery entering the optic nerve some 6–12 mm from the eyeball. It enters the eye through the optic disc and divides into superior and inferior branches and both these branches subdivide into nasal and temporal branches which course in the nerve fibre layer, supplying the capillaries feeding the bipolar and the ganglion cell layers of the retina (except for the fovea). ⊃ central retinal vein, cherry-red spot, retinal arterial occlusion, temporal arteritis.

central retinal arterial occlusion (CRAO) ⊃ retinal arterial occlusion.

central retinal vein a vein formed by the junction of the superior and inferior retinal veins at about the level of the cribriform plate of the sclera (lamina cribrosa) on the temporal side of the central retinal artery. After a short course within the optic nerve, it empties into the cavernous sinus, the superior ophthalmic vein and sometimes into the inferior ophthalmic vein. ⊃ central retinal artery, retinal vein occlusion.

central retinal vein occlusion (CRVO) ⊃ retinal vein occlusion.

central scotoma ⊃ scotoma.

central serous retinopathy (CSR) (*syn* central serous chorioretinopathy) an accumulation of serous fluid in the subretinal space which leads to a retinal detachment. It usually occurs in the central area of the retina and results in a sudden blurring and/or distortion of vision. The condition typically affects men between the ages of 20 and 45 years. It subsides by itself within a few months in most cases; otherwise photocoagulation may be necessary. ⊃ photocoagulation, retinal detachment.

central sterile supplies department (CSSD) designated area where packets are prepared containing the equipment and/or swabs and dressings necessary to perform activities requiring aseptic technique. ⊃ hospital sterilization and disinfection unit (HSDU).

central tendency statistic averages. The tendency for observations to centre around a specific value rather than across the entire range (Figure C.5). ⊃ mean, median, mode.

central venous catheter/line specialized intravenous cannula which is placed in a large vein (internal jugular, subclavian), or inserted into a peripheral vein in the arm. The cannula is advanced until the tip is in the superior vena cava or the right atrium of the heart. ⊃ Colour Section Figure 10. Used for the measurement of central venous pressure and central venous oxygen saturation (CVSO$_2$), and also for the administration of drugs and fluids. Also used for long

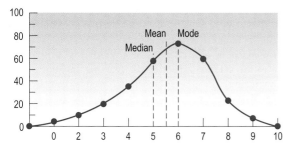

C.5 Central tendency statistic (reproduced from Gunn 2001 with permission).

term vascular access for the administration of drugs, blood products or nutritional support.

central venous pressure (CVP) central venous pressure (CVP) is commonly used as a guide to the circulating volume, by reflecting the right heart filling pressures. It is measured using a central venous line/catheter attached to a pressure transducer or occasionally a manometer is used. Serial readings are used in the assessment of circulatory function, circulating blood volume and to inform fluid replacement needs. It has significant limitations, partly as it is measuring a pressure (the right atrial pressure) which is then used to reflect a volume. Intracardiac pressures can be affected by a number of factors, including vascular tone, cardiac valve disorders, cardiac failure and pericardial tamponade. Consequently the measured pressure may change but may not necessarily indicate fluid imbalance. Access to the right atrium is gained via a central vein, such as the internal jugular or subclavian vein. After insertion, a chest X-ray is performed to check the position of the line/catheter and to check that a pneumothorax has not been inadvertently caused. Pneumothorax can occur during central line/catheter insertion if the pleura is punctured. A key responsibility for the medical/nursing team is to observe the patient closely for clinical signs of a pneumothorax until the chest X-ray has been checked. These signs include tachycardia, hypotension, hypoxia, dyspnoea, asymmetrical chest movement and a reduction in breath sounds to the affected lung. The normal CVP range (in the absence of any influencing factors, such as cardiac failure), when continuously measured using a transducer, is 3–10 mmHg. CVP can also be measured intermittently using a water manometer, the normal values then being 5–12 cmH$_2$O. When measuring the CVP using a manometer, it is important to ensure that the patient is always in the same position. Lying flat is best if the patient's condition will allow, and the point at which the manometer is level with the heart should be marked to ensure consistency. As with all types of invasive monitoring there are other factors to consider when making a decision to insert a CVP line/catheter. For example, a patient who is confused and breathless and requires a central venous catheter to assist with fluid balance estimation will be required to adopt a head-down position during insertion of the catheter. The breathless patient may not be able tolerate this position and the procedure may be more hazardous if the patient is confused. The benefits to be gained from the CVP information have to be balanced against the risks posed to the patient, the most significant of which is a pneumothorax. It may be necessary to wait until the patient is less breathless and more lucid and the risks are minimized to such an extent that the procedure is considered beneficial.

central vision vision of objects formed on the foveola or the macula. ⇒ foveola, macula, peripheral vision, sensory fusion.

central visual acuity visual acuity of the fovea and the macular area. ⇒ eccentric fixation, macula lutea.

centralized daylight system a system where the loading and unloading of a cassette or film magazine is directly linked to an automatic film processor.

centre of buoyancy imaginary point calculated by adding up the moments of the buoyancy forces of all segments of a body or object.

centre of gravity (CoG) imaginary point calculated by adding up the moments of the weights of all segments of a body or object. Usually the same as centre of mass (CoM), except where gravity varies within a body or object, as for example in a tall building—gravitational force would be very slightly different over the height of the building, so the centre of gravity (CoG) and the CoM would be very close but not in exactly the same place.

centre of gravity in pregnancy the mid-point or axis of rotation over which the weight of the body balances. In pregnancy the centre of gravity changes to accommodate the extra weight on the front of the abdomen; backache often results.

centre of mass (CoM) geometric centre of a body or object. Its position can be calculated by the segmental method from the position of the centre of mass (CoM) of each body segment and the mass of each segment. Usually the same as centre of gravity.

centre of percussion imaginary point on a pivoted object or body where translational forces are equal and opposite to rotational ones. Also known as the sweet spot. For example, if a shot with a cricket bat is hit from the centre of percussion then it 'feels good' because the translational forces and rotational forces are balanced.

centre of pressure 1. imaginary point calculated by adding up the moments of the fluid (liquid or gas) pressure, or drag, of all segments of a body or object. **2.** biomechanical term referring to the forces acting beneath the foot.

centre of rotation of the eye when the eye rotates in its orbit, there is a point within the eyeball which is more or less fixed relative to the orbit. This is the centre of rotation of the eye. In reality, the centre of rotation is constantly shifting but by a small amount. It is considered, for convenience, that the centre of rotation of an emmetropic eye lies on the line of sight of the eye 13.5 mm behind the anterior pole of the cornea when the eye is in the straight ahead position (or straightforward position), that is when the line of sight is perpendicular to both the base line and the frontal plane. ⇒ anteroposterior axis, base line, frontal plane, line of sight.

centres of ossification ⇒ ossification centres.

centric relating to, or situated at the centre.

centric jaw relation, centric relation ⊃ retruded jaw relation.

centric occlusion (*syn* intercuspal occlusion) position of centric jaw relationship in which there is maximum intercuspation of the teeth.

centrifugal *adj* literally, 'centre-fleeing'. Efferent. Having a tendency to move outwards from the centre, as the nerve impulses from the brain to the peripheral structures. ⊃ centrifugal acceleration, centrifugal force.

centrifugal acceleration apparent (inertial) acceleration of an object, imagined by a moving observer who is rotating. For example, if a hammer thrower is rotating, all objects in his surroundings appear to him to be moving, i.e. to have centrifugal acceleration, whilst the hammer itself appears to stay still, yet he is having to apply a centripetal acceleration to keep it moving in a circle. Therefore, by Newton's first law there must be a balancing (centrifugal) acceleration, but this is imaginary since due only to the rotation of the thrower himself, whilst the hammer is not actually stationary.

centrifugal force the apparent (inertial) force on an object. In dentistry, the principle of centrifugal force is used when introducing a paste into a root canal with a spiral root canal filler and in a casting machine.

centrifuge *n* an apparatus which subjects solutions to centrifugal forces by high-speed rotation, thereby separating substances of different densities into discrete bands within the liquid phase. It is usually used to separate ('spin down') particulate material (e.g. subcellular particles) from a suspending liquid.

centriole *n* a subcellular organelle that aids spindle formation during nuclear division. ⊃ meiosis, mitosis.

centripetal *adj* literally, 'centre-seeking'. Afferent. Having a tendency to move towards the centre, as the rash occurring in chickenpox. ⊃ centripetal acceleration, centripetal force.

centripetal acceleration a real acceleration towards the centre of a circle (or curve) due to change in the directional component of velocity.

centripetal force a real force towards the centre of a circle (or curve) equal to centripetal acceleration multiplied by mass.

centrocaecal scotoma ⊃ scotoma.

centromere *n* the structure that joins the double chromosome (2 chromatids) and eventually attaches to the spindle during nuclear division. ⊃ meiosis, mitosis.

centronics a type of standard interface between computer and peripheral.

centrosome *n* a region adjacent to the cell nucleus that contains the centrioles.

cephalalgia *n* pain in the head; headache.

cephalhaematoma *n* a collection of blood in the subperiosteal tissues of the scalp of an infant. It is usually caused by pressure on the scalp during a long labour. ⊃ caput succedaneum, moulding.

cephalic *adj* pertaining to the head; near the head.

cephalic vein *n* a superficial vein that drains blood from the arm. The cephalic vein begins at the back of the hand where it collects blood from a complex of superficial veins, many of which can be easily seen. It then winds round the radial side to the anterior aspect of the forearm. In front of the elbow it gives off a large branch, the median cubital vein, which slants upwards and medially to join the basilic vein. After crossing the elbow joint the cephalic vein passes up the lateral aspect of the arm and in front of the shoulder joint to end in the axillary vein. Throughout its length it receives blood from the superficial tissues on the lateral aspects of the hand, forearm and arm. ⊃ Colour Section Figure 10.

cephalic version turning the fetus so that the head presents. ⊃ version.

cephalin *n* a phospholipid present in nervous tissue—the white matter of the brain, spinal cord and nerves.

cephal/o- a prefix that means 'head', e.g. *cephalometry*.

cephalocele *n* hernia of the brain; protrusion of part of the brain through the skull.

cephalohaematoma *n* cephalhaematoma.

cephalometric analysis analysis of measurements of the skull taken from lateral and anteroposterior radiographs of certain fixed points of the skull. In orthodontic diagnosis various tracings are drawn from lines joining recognized points and their angles of intersection are measured.

cephalometric radiograph a lateral projection of the skull and mandible for making cranial measurements to estimate the degree of any facial abnormality.

cephalometrics the technique of obtaining a cephalometric radiograph and preparing a series of cephalometric tracings from which measurements can be made for the purpose of orthodontic diagnosis and/or anthropometric evaluation.

cephalometric tracing tracing, on drafting paper or film, of selected structures from a cephalometric radiograph.

cephalometry *n* measurement of the living human head. Used antenatally to measure the biparietal diameter to assess fetal maturity and growth, most accurately by ultrasonography. After birth the infant's head is measured with a tape measure.

cephalopelvic disproportion (CPD) disparity between the fetal head and the maternal pelvis, either because the head is too large or abnormally positioned, or because the pelvis too small or abnormally shaped. It is detected in the last 4 weeks of pregnancy by failure of the fetal head to engage, either spontaneously or on pressure, and confirmed on ultrasound. In severe CPD caesarean section will be needed, but in mild CPD uterine contractions in labour help to mould the fetal head through the pelvis, often with increased flexion; in anticipation of this the woman may undergo a trial labour. ⊃ symphysiotomy.

cephalosporins *npl* a large group of beta-lactam antibiotics, closely related to the penicillins, e.g. cefaclor. ⊃ Appendix 5.

cephalostat (craniostat) apparatus used to hold the head steady and at a standard angle during radiological examinations, thus ensuring precise, reproducible relationships between the X-ray tube, the subject and the film.

ceramic detector a modern device used in computed tomography (CT) scanning to measure the amount of radiation transmitted through a patient, giving a reduction in noise compared with earlier detectors and in chest scans there is said to be a reduction in beam hardening artefacts.

ceramics a general term for dental porcelain work.

cerclage 1. a technique used to correct a detached retina in which a taut band is applied around the sclera to restore the contact between the retina and choroid. **2.** a technique whereby a wire or metal band is used to secure the bone ends or fragments of certain fractures such as a fractured patella. ⊃ cervical cerclage

cereal the grains or edible seeds obtained from the grass family, e.g. rice, wheat, barley, oats, rye, maize and millet.

cerebellar gait a staggering, reeling, lurching unsteady, wide based walk seen in patients with damage to the cerebellum or its connections. ⊃ gait.

cerebellum *n* that part of the brain which is situated behind the pons and immediately below the posterior portion of the cerebrum occupying the posterior cranial fossa. It is ovoid in shape and has two hemispheres, separated by a narrow median strip called the vermis. Grey matter forms the surface of the cerebellum, and the white matter lies deeply. The cerebellum is concerned with the coordination of voluntary muscular movement, posture and balance. Cerebellar activity is not under voluntary control. The cerebellum controls and coordinates the movements of various groups of muscles ensuring smooth, even, precise actions. It coordinates activities associated with the maintenance of posture, balance and equilibrium. The sensory input for these functions is derived from the muscles and joints, the eyes and the ears. Proprioceptor impulses from the muscles and joints indicate their position in relation to the body as a whole, and those impulses from the eyes and the semicircular canals in the ears provide information about the position of the head in space. Impulses from the cerebellum influence the contraction of skeletal muscle so that balance and posture are maintained. The cerebellum may also have a role in learning and language processing. Damage to the cerebellum results in clumsy uncoordinated muscular movement, staggering gait and inability to carry out smooth, steady, precise movements—**cerebellar** *adj*. ⊃ Colour Section Figures 1, 11.

cerebral *adj* pertaining to the cerebrum.

cerebral aqueduct (*syn* aqueduct of Sylvius, aqueductus cerebri, sylvian aqueduct, ventricular aqueduct) the canal in the midbrain that conveys cerebrospinal fluid between the 3rd and 4th ventricles of the brain.

cerebral cavity the ventricles of the brain.

cerebral compression arises from any space-occupying intracranial lesion, for example tumour, swelling, haemorrhage, etc.

cerebral cortex the outer layer of cells (grey matter) of the cerebral hemispheres.

cerebral embolism the presence of an embolus impeding blood flow in a cerebral blood vessel resulting in cerebral ischaemia leading to cerebral infarction. The embolus can originate in the heart such as in atrial fibrillation. ⊃ cerebral infarction, cerebrovascular accident.

cerebral function monitor (CFM) equipment for continuous monitoring of brain wave activity, e.g. to detect seizures in sedated and paralysed patients.

cerebral haemorrhage bleeding from a cerebral blood vessel into the substance of the brain. It may arise from: degenerative disease affecting the vessel or from hypertension, as in a stroke (cerebrovascular accident); from the rupture of a congenital aneurysm or other vessel abnormality; or as a result of trauma. Traditional management of cerebral bleeding caused by an aneurysm was to clip the aneurysm to prevent further bleeding but newer and less invasive treatments are now available. Whereby a neuroradiologist inserts tiny platinum coils into the aneurysm through a microcatheter passed via the blood vessels in the groin through the body and into the aneurysm. The coils cause the blood in the aneurysm to clot, preventing it from rupturing. ⊃ cerebrovascular accident, embolization, extradural haematoma, intracerebral haemorrhage, subarachnoid haemorrhage, subdural haematoma.

cerebral hemisphere one side of the cerebrum, right or left.

cerebral infarction cerebral infarction is mostly due to thromboembolic disease secondary to atherosclerosis in the major extracranial arteries (carotid artery and aortic arch). About 20% of infarctions are due to embolism from the heart, and a further 20% are due to intrinsic disease of small perforating vessels (lenticulostriate arteries), producing so-called 'lacunar' infarctions. The risk factors for ischaemic stroke reflect the risk factors for the underlying vascular disease, this include: (a) fixed factors—age, gender (male > female, except in the very young and very old), race (African Caribbean > Asian > European), heredity, previous vascular event (e.g. myocardial infarction, stroke or peripheral embolism), high fibrinogen; (b) modifiable risks—high blood pressure, heart disease (atrial fibrillation, heart failure, endocarditis), diabetes mellitus, hyperlipidaemia, smoking, excess alcohol consumption, polycythaemia, oral contraceptives, social deprivation. Perhaps 5% are due to rare causes, including vasculitis, endocarditis and cerebral venous disease, e.g. cerebral venous sinus thrombosis (affecting the cavernous sinus, superior sagittal sinus, transverse sinus), cortical vein thrombosis and subdural haematoma.

cerebral palsy non-progressive brain damage that typically occurs at, or shortly after, birth resulting in a range of mainly motor conditions ranging from clumsiness to severe spasticity. The neurological deficit may result in spastic hemiplegia, monoplegia, diplegia or quadraplegia, athetosis or ataxia seizures, parathesia, along with varying degrees of learning disabilities, impaired speech, vision and hearing. Little's disease.

cerebral perfusion pressure (CPP) the pressure which drives blood through the brain. It is the difference between the mean arterial blood pressure (MABP) and the intracranial pressure (ICP). If CPP is too low the blood flow to the brain may be inadequate and the brain deprived of oxygen. ⟳ intracranial pressure, mean arterial blood pressure.

cerebral thrombosis the presence of a blood clot impeding blood flow in a cerebral vessel resulting in cerebral ischaemia leading to cerebral infarction. The clot forms within the cerebral blood vessel. ⟳ cerebral infarction, cerebrovascular accident.

cerebration *n* mental activity.

cerebr/i/o- a prefix that means 'brain', e.g. *cerebral*.

cerebroside *n* one of a group of glycolipids found in the brain and the myelin sheath covering nerves. ⟳ ganglioside, glycosphingolipids.

cerebrospinal *adj* pertaining to the brain and spinal cord.

cerebrospinal fluid the clear fluid found within the ventricles (cavities) of the brain, central canal of the spinal cord and beneath the cranial and spinal meninges in the subarachnoid space. Protects and nourishes the brain and spinal cord. It is formed by the choroid plexuses in the ventricles and circulates around the brain and spinal cord before being returned to the blood through the arachnoid villi/granulations, which project into the venous sinuses of the brain.

cerebrovascular *adj* pertaining to the blood vessels of the brain.

cerebrovascular accident (stroke)(CVA) in epidemiological studies, the term stroke is reserved for those events in which symptoms last more than 24 hours. There is interference with the cerebral blood flow due either to thromboembolic disease leading to cerebral infarction, or intracerebral haemorrhage. Of patients presenting with a stroke, 85% will have sustained a cerebral infarction due to inadequate blood flow to part of the brain. The remainder will have had an intracerebral haemorrhage. Brain imaging is required to distinguish these pathologies and to guide management. The combination of severe headache and vomiting at the onset of the focal neurological deficits increases the likelihood of a haemorrhagic stroke. Signs and symptoms vary according to the type of stroke, the time since it occurred, extent and site of tissue damage; there may be only a passing, inability to move a hand or foot; weakness or tingling in a limb; stertorous breathing; incontinence of urine and faeces; coma; paralysis of a limb or limbs; and speech deficiency (aphasia). ⟳ cerebral infarction, completed stroke, intracerebral haemorrhage, progressing stroke, transient ischaemic attack.

cerebrum *n* the largest and uppermost part of the brain. It occupies the anterior and middle cranial fossae and is divided by a deep cleft, the longitudinal cerebral fissure, into right and left cerebral hemispheres, each containing one of the lateral ventricles. Deep within the brain the hemispheres are connected by a mass of white matter (nerve fibres) called the corpus callosum. The falx cerebri, formed by the dura mater, separates the two hemispheres and penetrates to the depth of the corpus callosum. The superficial (peripheral) part of the cerebrum is composed of nerve cell bodies or grey matter, forming the cerebral cortex, and the deeper layers consist of nerve fibres or white matter.The cerebral cortex shows many infoldings or furrows of varying depth. The exposed areas of the folds are the gyri or convolutions and these are separated by sulci or fissures. These convolutions greatly increase the surface area of the cerebrum. For descriptive purposes each hemisphere of the cerebrum is divided into lobes which take the names of the bones of the cranium under which they lie: frontal, parietal, temporal, occipital. The boundaries of the lobes are marked by deep sulci (fissures). These are the central, lateral and parieto-occipital sulci. The surface of the cerebral cortex is composed of grey matter (nerve cell bodies). Within the cerebrum the lobes are connected by masses of nerve fibres, or tracts, which make up the white matter of the brain. The afferent and efferent fibres linking the different parts of the brain and spinal cord are: (a) association (arcuate) fibres—connect different parts of a cerebral hemisphere by extending from one gyrus to another, some of which are adjacent and some distant; (b) commissural fibres—connect corresponding areas of the two cerebral hemispheres (the largest and most important commissure is the corpus callosum); (c) projection fibres—connect the cerebral cortex with grey matter of lower parts of the brain and with the spinal cord, e.g. the internal capsule. The internal capsule is an important area consisting of projection fibres. It lies deep within the brain between the basal nuclei (previously named ganglia) and the thalamus. Many nerve impulses passing to and from the cerebral cortex are carried by fibres that form the internal capsule. Motor fibres within the internal capsule form the pyramidal tracts (corticospinal tracts) that cross over (decussate) at the medulla oblongata. The three main varieties of activity associated with the cerebral cortex are: (a) mental activities involved in memory, intelligence, sense of responsibility, thinking, reasoning, moral sense and learning are attributed to the higher centres; (b) sensory perception, including the perception of pain, temperature, touch, sight, hearing, taste and smell; (c) the initiation and control of skeletal (voluntary) muscle contraction—**cerebral** *adj*. ⟳ Colour Section Figures 1, 11, 24.

certified *adj* a redundant psychiatric term. In the UK patients detained under current mental health legislation are said to be formally detained or 'sectioned'.

ceruloplasmin *n* plasma protein involved in copper transport.

cerumen *n* ear wax, sticky brown secretion from glands in the external auditory meatus/canal. Traps dust and other particles entering the ear—**ceruminous** *adj*.

cervical *adj* 1. pertaining to the neck. 2. pertaining to the cervix (neck) of an organ, such as the uterine cervix. 3. in dentistry, the area where the tooth crown joins the root.

cervical amnioscopy ⟳ amnioscopy.

cervical burn out (cervical radiolucency) in radiography, is the radiolucency seen at the margin of a tooth and sometimes mistaken for caries.

cervical canal the lumen of the cervix uteri that reaches from the internal os to the external os.

cervical cerclage the insertion of a non-absorble purse-string suture (stitch) in the cervix to keep it from opening. It is indicated for women who have a cervix which does not fully close (incompetent cervix), which may lead to miscarriage or preterm birth. The suture is inserted at 14 weeks' gestation and removed at 38 weeks' gestation or sooner if labour commences.

cervical effacement thinning, softening and shortening of the cervix, as the internal os is taken up to become part of the lower uterine segment, and have contact with the forewaters and the presenting part. The cervical canal becomes a circular orifice with extremely thin edges (Figure C.6). Usually it occurs in the last two weeks before labour in a primigravida, and during labour in a multigravida.

cervical eversion (ectropion) erroneously called an erosion. It is caused by high levels of oestrogen during pregnancy that cause a proliferation of columnar epitheium in the cervical canal which encroaches over the squamous epithium which is normally present over the vaginal portion of the cervix. The junction where the two epithelial tissue types meet everts into the vagina. The eversion usually resolves after the birth.

cervical intraepithelial neoplasia (CIN) staging of cellular changes in the uterine cervix that occur prior to the development of carcinoma in-situ and invasive cancer. Abnormal cells are detected by a smear test and the diagnosis is confirmed by colposcopy and biopsy. CIN1, mild dysplasia; CIN2, moderate dysplasia; CIN3, severe dysplasia, carcinoma in-situ. ➲ conization.

cervical line in dentistry, the line around a tooth marking the junction of the enamel of the crown and the cementum of the root.

cervical margin in dentistry, That part of a preparation, or of a restoration, closest to the neck of a tooth.

cervical nerves the eight pairs of spinal nerves that arise from the cervical part of the spinal cord. The first nerve exits above the atlas (first cervical vertebra) and the others exit from below each of the seven cervical vertebrae. The cervical nerves C1–C4 innervate the head and neck, and cervical nerves C5–C8 innervate the arms, back and scalp.

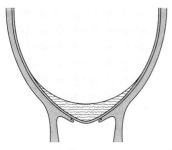

C.6 **Cervical effacement** (reproduced from Fraser & Cooper 2003 with permission).

cervical plexus the complex network of deep and superficial branches formed by the anterior rami of cervical nerves C1–C4. It lies opposite the first, second, third and fourth cervical vertebrae under the protection of the sternocleidomastoid muscle. These nerves supply the skin over the front of the neck, the back and side of the head, the neck muscles, and one branch the *phrenic nerve* supplies the diaphragm. The *superficial branches* supply the structures at the back and side of the head and the skin of the front of the neck to the level of the sternum. The *deep branches* supply muscles of the neck, e.g. the sternocleidomastoid and the trapezius. The *phrenic nerve* originates mainly from cervical root 4 with less important contributions from cervical roots 3 and 5. The nerve passes downwards through the thoracic cavity in front of the root of the lung to supply the muscle of the diaphragm with impulses which stimulate contraction. ➲ Colour Section Figure 11.

cervical rib an extension of the transverse process of the seventh cervical vertebra in the form of bone or fibrous tissue; this causes an upward displacement of the subclavian artery. ➲ thoracic outlet syndrome.

cervical smear microscopic examination of cells obtained from the surface of the cervix. ➲ cervical intraepithelial neoplasia, Papanicolaou test.

cervical spondylosis degenerative arthritis that affects the cervical spine.

cervical strap or neckstrap in orthodontics, is a type of headgear that fits around the neck only.

cervical vertebrae (spine) the first seven vertebrae. The first two are atypical: the first vertebra or *atlas* supports the skull and rotates around the odontoid process (dens) of the second vertebra or *axis*. The cervical part of the spinal cord passes through the cervical vertebrae from the brain to the thoracic part of the spine. Damage to the spinal cord at a high cervical level, where the phrenic nerves to the diaphragm originate, can paralyse breathing. Cervical cord damage in sport may result in tetraplegia (quadriplegia), seen in sports such as rugby (collapsed scrum), trampolining and horse riding. ➲ atlas, axis, spinal injury, vertebra (typical), Colour Section Figure 3.

cervical wall in dentistry, cavity surface bounded by the cavity floor and the cavosurface angle, and further qualified by its position, e.g. mesial, distal, etc.

cervicectomy *n* amputation of the uterine cervix.

cervicitis *n* inflammation of the uterine cervix.

cervic/o- a prefix that means 'neck', e.g. *cervicitis*.

cervix *n* a neck. *cervix uteri, uterine cervix* the neck of the uterus—**cervical** *adj*. ➲ Colour Section Figure 17.

cestode *n* tapeworm ➲ *Taenia*.

cetrimide *n* a disinfectant with detergent properties. Used for wound cleansing and skin preparation.

CF *abbr* cystic fibrosis.

CFA *abbr* cryptogenic fibrosing alveolitis.

CFC *abbr* chlorofluorohydrocarbons.

C fibres nerve fibres that are postganglionic and autonomic in nature, with temperature and pain sensation capabilities.

CFM *abbr* cerebral function monitor.

CFS/ME *abbr* chronic fatigue syndrome/myalgic encephalomyelitis.

CFT *abbr* complement fixation test.

CFTR *abbr* cystic fibrosis transmembrane regulator.

CGD *abbr* chronic granulomatous disease.

CGM *abbr* continuous glucose monitoring.

CH50 *abbr* classical haemolytic pathway 50.

Chadwick's sign dark purplish discolouration and congestion of vaginal membrane due to increased vascularity; a sign of pregnancy but occurs in any condition in which there is pelvic congestion.

Chagas' disease ⊃ trypanosomiasis.

chaining a skills training technique used for people with a learning disability. Each small step in a skilled task, such as dressing or making a sandwich, is taught in sequence. It may be *forward* where the skill is learnt from the beginning in the sequence it normally occurs with each step linking to the next. Or *backward* where the skill is learnt by working backwards from the final step of the finished task.

chalazion *n* a cyst in the eyelid caused by chronic inflammation of retained secretion of a meibomian gland.

chalcosis *n* a condition that results from an intraocular copper foreign body. The serious chemical reaction that occurs causes endophthalmitis and rapid visual impairment.

challenging behaviour behaviour which, by the nature of its character, frequency or severity, may seriously threaten the safety of the individual or other people, or behaviour that hinders the integration of the individual into the community by preventing his or her access to various facilities and activities, such as mainstream education. It may involve self-injurious behaviour, sexual behaviour or verbal or physical violence. Most often applied to the behaviour of people with a learning disability judged to be unacceptable by the social standards relevant to age and cultural background.

chalone *n* a substance that inhibits rather than stimulates, e.g. enterogastrone inhibits gastric secretions and motility.

chance a research term—random variation. Statistical methods are used to estimate the probability that chance alone has accounted for the difference in outcome.

chancre *n* the primary syphilitic ulcer developing at the site of infection with *Treponema pallidum*. It is associated with swelling of local lymph nodes. The chancre is painless, indurated, solitary and highly infectious. It heals spontaneously without treatment.

chancroid *n* (*syn* soft sore) a type of sexually transmitted infection prevalent in warmer climates. Caused by the bacillus *Haemophilus ducreyi*. Causes multiple, painful, ragged ulcers on the genitalia, often with bubo formation.

channel slice preparation tooth preparation for a cast-metal restoration in which the walls are tapered or sliced and tapering grooves are cut to increase retention.

character *n* **1.** the sum total of the known and predictable mental characteristics of an individual, particularly his or her conduct. **2.** a numeral, letter, symbol or any other mark that can be seen on the computer screen or printed.

character change denotes change in the form of conduct, to one foreign to the patient's natural disposition, e.g. violent or indecent behaviour.

characteristic curve in radiography, applies to a particular film or film/screen combination and is the curve which results when the density is plotted against the log of relative exposure. It is also called D log E curve, a Hurter and Driffield curve, a log It curve. The curve is used to determine the basic fog level, threshold, toe, straight line portion, shoulder and maximum density of the film. ⊃ basic fog, maximum density, shoulder, straight line portion, threshold.

characters per second a measure of the speed of data output.

charcoal *n* used therapeutically for its adsorptive and deodorant properties. Oral administration of activated charcoal is used for certain types of poisoning. It binds to some poisons in the gastrointestinal tract and prevents their absorption, and may also be used for active elimination techniques once the poison has been absorbed into the body. Activated charcoal when incorporated into dressings is used to reduce odour in malodorous discharging wounds.

Charcot's joint (J M Charcot, French neurologist, 1825–1893) complete disorganization of a joint associated with syringomyelia, diabetes mellitus, or advanced cases of tabes dorsalis (locomotor ataxia). The condition is painless.

Charcot's triad I (J M Charcot) sometimes seen as a manifestation of multiple sclerosis—nystagmus, intention tremor and scanning or staccato speech.

charge an electrotherapy term. A fundamental property of matter, measured in coulombs (C). For example, an electron has a negative charge and a particle or body that loses sufficient electrons (1 or more depending on the initial state) will become positively charged. ⊃ coulomb.

'Charge syndrome' syndrome characterized by defects of the eye, heart, ear, oesophageal atresia, growth retardation. It may be associated with choanal atresia. ⊃ choanal atresia.

charley horse a colloquial term used in sport for a haematoma of the quadriceps group of muscles as a result of trauma. Rarely it may develop areas of ossification, which prolong rehabilitation and may require surgery.

CHART *acron* continuous hyperfractionated accelerated radiotherapy. ⊃ accelerated fractionation.

chart (dental) in dentistry, a visual record or diagram of a patient's dentition and dental state.

charting (dental) in dentistry, recording of clinical details of a patient's dentition and surrounding tissues, personal details and medical history. Most dental charts have a diagrammatic representation of the teeth which is divided into quadrants. The Zsigmondy–Palmer or Chevron charting system is widely used in Europe and in the UK National Health Service.

CHD *abbr* **1.** congenital heart disease. **2.** coronary heart disease.

check bite (*syn* check record) thin wax rim used to record an occlusion. Often has a thin soft metal foil embedded in it. Warmed before use and chilled afterwards.

check ligament a strong band of connective tissue which leaves the surface of the sheath of the extraocular muscles and attaches to the surrounding tissues, so as to limit the action of the muscle. The medial rectus muscle is attached to the lacrimal bone (*medial check ligament*) and the lateral rectus muscle to the zygomatic bone (*lateral check ligament*). There are also check ligaments restricting the vertical movements but the expansions of these muscles are thinner and less distinct than those of the horizontal recti muscles. ⮑ lateral rectus, medial rectus muscle.

check record in dentistry, a method of verifying a previously taken interocclusal record by repeating the procedure. Sometimes referred to as a check bite. ⮑ interocclusal record.

Chediak–Higashi syndrome (A M Chédiak, Cuban physician, 20th century; O Higashi, Japanese physician, 20th century) an inherited autosomal recessive disorder of the immune system. The leucocytes are abnormal that results in chronic infection. There is decreased pigmentation in skin and eyes, neurological disease, photophobia and early death.

cheek biting damage to the buccal mucosa that results from malocclusion, poor chewing coordination, or habit.

cheek teeth collective (lay) term for molars and premolars.

cheek wire ⮑ wiring.

cheilitis *n* inflammation of the lip.

cheil/o- a prefix that means 'lip', e.g. *cheilosis*.

cheiloplasty *n* any plastic operation on the lip. Procedure to correct congenital, traumatic or other types of lip deformity.

cheilosis *n* maceration at the angles of the mouth; fissures occur later. May be due to riboflavin deficiency.

cheir/o, chir/o- a prefix that means 'hand', e.g. *cheiropompholyx*.

cheiropompholyx *n* symmetrical eruption of skin of hands (especially fingers) characterized by the formation of tiny vesicles and associated with itching or burning. On the feet the condition is called podopompholyx.

chelate a compound composed of a central metal ion and an organic molecule with multiple bonds, formed in a ring formation.

chelating agents soluble organic compounds that combine with certain metallic ions, such as iron, to form complexes that are safely excreted in the urine. For example desferrioxamine used for iron overload or poisoning. ⮑ DTPA, haemochromatosis, thalassaemia. ⮑ Appendix 5.

chelation in dentistry, chemical sequestration of calcium ions from tooth tissue.

chemical/medical débridement ⮑ débridement.

chemo- a prefix that means 'chemical', e.g. *chemoprophylaxis*.

chemokines small cytokines that induce chemotaxis and the recruitment and activation of leucocytes during the inflammatory response. They are released from many different cells in response to infection with bacteria or viruses and physical damage. Chemokines act upon cells of both innate and adaptive immunity. They attract leucocytes (neutrophils, monocytes and lymphocytes) to areas of damage or infection and some may stimulate the formation of new blood vessels (angiogenesis).

chemonucleolysis *n* injection of an enzyme, usually into an intervertebral disc, for dissolution of same—**chemonucleolytic** *adj*.

chemopallidectomy *n* the chemical destruction of a predetermined section of globus pallidus.

chemoprophylaxis *n* the prevention of disease (or recurrent attack) by administration of drugs such as antibiotics following some surgical procedures and for people exposed to infection, and antimalarial drugs. For example the administration of rifampicin to the contacts of patients with meningococcal meningitis—**chemoprophylactic** *adj*.

chemoradiation treatment that involves the administration of chemotherapy and radiotherapy at the same time.

chemoreceptor *n* a sensory nerve ending or a cell having an affinity, and capable of reacting to, a chemical stimuli, e.g. taste, oxygen levels in the blood. Usually refers to those which influence the respiratory and cardiovascular control centres in the brain stem: the medullary chemoreceptors, sensitive to pH changes in the cerebral extracellular fluid, and the arterial chemoreceptors which continually sense and respond to changes mainly in blood oxygen, carbon dioxide and pH, leading to appropriate reflex adjustments via afferent nerves to the brainstem control centres (e.g. increase in ventilation if arterial oxygen tension tends to fall and/or carbon dioxide to rise). ⮑ carotid bodies.

chemoreceptor trigger zone (CTZ) a vomiting centre in the medulla of the brain that is stimulated by chemical stimuli present in the blood, such as toxins; and impulses from the higher centres of the cerebral cortex, gastrointestinal tract and the vestibular apparatus and centres. ⮑ vomiting centre.

chemoresistant *adj* describes a tumour that does not usually shrink with chemotherapy.

chemosensitive *adj* describes a tumour that shrinks following chemotherapy administration.

chemosis *n* oedema or swelling of the bulbar conjunctiva—**chemotic** *adj*.

chemotaxis *n* movements of a cell (e.g. leucocyte) or a micro-organism in response to chemical stimuli; attraction is termed *positive chemotaxis*, repulsion is *negative chemotaxis*—**chemotactic** *adj*. ⮑ chemokines.

chemotherapy *n* chemical agents of various types; prescribed to delay or arrest growth of cancer cells through interruption/inhibition of cell cycle; usually given in combination rather than as single agents. They are non-selective and non-specific and therefore affect all cycling cells whether benign or malignant. Administration is by oral, intramuscular, intravenous, intracavitary or intra-arterial routes. ⮑ alkylating agents, antimetabolites, antitumour antibiotics, vinca alkaloids. ⮑ Appendix 5.

chenodeoxycholic acid a bile acid. It can be taken orally to dissolve certain types of gallstones.

cherry-red spot the bright red appearance of the macular area in an eye with occlusion of the central retinal artery,

Tay–Sachs disease or Niemann–Pick disease. In the case of central retinal artery occlusion the surrounding area is white due to ischaemia but the reddish reflex from the intact choroidal vessels beneath the fovea shows at that spot since the retina is thinnest there. There is a very marked, if not complete, loss of vision which appears suddenly. In cases of inherited lipid metabolic disturbance/storage disease (i.e. Niemann–Pick or Tay–Sachs), the area surrounding the fovea is artificially whitened and opaque, offsetting the normal pinkish colour of the fovea. ⊃ Niemann–Pick disease, retinal arterial occlusion, Tay–Sachs disease.

cherubism appearance of a child who is suffering from multilocular cysts of the jaws and thus has an expanded face likened to that of a cherub.

chest compressions external cardiac massage. Performed during cardiac arrest. With the person lying on his or her back on a firm surface, the lower part of the sternum (breastbone) is depressed to compress the heart and force blood into the circulation (Figure C.7). ⊃ basic life support. ⊃ Appendix 10.

chest drain/chest tube a tube inserted into the chest to drain off excess fluid or air, it usually incorporates a strip that is visible on X-ray. ⊃ haemothorax, intercostal chest drain, pneumothorax, underwater seal drain.

chest percussion 1. a respiratory assessment technique used in clinical examination. This technique enables the location of some key structures (e.g. the liver and heart) and enables evaluation of the transmission of air through the lungs. Percussion sounds should be compared on either side throughout the full length of the lungs. 'Dullness' of sounds is associated with poor aeration, e.g. pleural effusion, lung collapse, consolidation and, less commonly, an elevated diaphragm, tumour and thickened pleura. However, abnormalities, which lie deeper, may not be detected by changes in percussion resonance so its use is limited. **2.** a physiotherapeutic technique also known as clapping/cupping. Used to facilitate the clearance of excessive bronchial

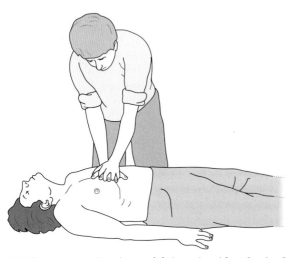

C.7 Chest compressions in an adult (reproduced from Brooker & Waugh 2007 with permission).

secretions. It has been demonstrated that the technique raises intrathoracic pressure. However, its efficacy has yet to be scientifically proven. The technique should be performed using a cupped hand (in order to trap air) that is struck over the chest wall (thus, causing a vibratory shock wave to pass through the chest wall and loosen secretions), but avoiding contact with bony structures.

Cheyne–Stokes respiration cyclical waxing and waning of breathing, characterized at one extreme by deep fast breaths and at the other by apnoea: it generally has an ominous prognosis.

CHF *abbr* congestive heart failure.

chi ⊃ Qi energy.

chiasma *n* an X-shaped crossing or decussation, such as the optic chiasma—**chiasmata** *pl*. ⊃ optic chiasma.

chiastopic fusion fusion obtained by voluntary convergence on two targets separated in space and such that the right eye fixates the left target and the left eye the right target. This is often facilitated by fixating a small mark above a single aperture placed in front of the two targets and then slowly shifting one's gaze to the targets. The procedure is aimed at improving positive fusional convergence. ⊃ fusional convergence, orthopic fusion.

chickenpox *n* (*syn* varicella) a generally mild, specific infection with varicella-zoster virus (VZV), a herpes virus, mainly affecting children. Non-immune (i.e. who have not had chickenpox, shingles or immunization) healthcare workers with patient contact are offered vaccination. Discussion continues regarding the addition of the varicella vaccine to the routine childhood programme in the UK. The incubation is 12–21 days. Successive crops of vesicles appear in a centripetal distribution, first on the trunk; they scab and usually heal without scars. The disease can be much more severe in adults, especially those who are immunocompromised such as those with HIV disease, or those having immunosuppression treatment, e.g. after transplant, when it may be fatal. Treatment with antiviral drugs is indicated. ⊃ herpes zoster, shingles, Colour Section Figure 59.

chief cells cells in the gastric mucosa that secrete pepsinogen, the inactive precursor of the digestive enzyme pepsin.

chignon large caput succedaneum seen on the head of an infant delivered by ventouse vacuum extraction. ⊃ vacuum extractor, Ventouse extraction.

chikungunya *n* a mosquito-transmitted haemorrhagic fever occurring in Africa.

chilblain *n* (*syn* erythema pernio) seasonal vasospasm (spasm of blood vessels) caused by cold. It mainly affects children and older people, and leads to congestion and swelling of the feet or hands. In the short, acute stage there is redness with severe itching and burning sensation. The chronic stage is characterized by dull redness and congestion in the affected area. The affected skin is easily damaged and healing is prolonged. ⊃ perniosis.

child abuse physical, sexual or emotional abuse or neglect of children by relatives, other carers or health and social care staff. ⊃ non-accidental injuries.

child protection register record of children at risk of, or suspected of being at risk of abuse. A keyworker, usually a social worker, is appointed to ensure the Child Protection Plan is carried out. Access to the register of named children is restricted to those with direct dealings with the children.

Child Support Agency (CSA) in the UK, a government agency set up under the Child Support Act 1991 to operate a scheme for child maintenance in cases where the parents are living apart. It is responsible for assessing each case where one parent has requested child maintenance, reviewing the situation at 2-yearly intervals and, if necessary, collecting the money from the absent parent.

Children Act 1989 the Act of Parliament which brings together the comprehensive law relating to children, defining their rights, identifying parental responsibilities and detailing procedures to protect children. Child welfare is paramount in all court decisions, which should be made with minimum delay and, where possible, take into account the child's wishes. The Court may issue a variety of orders, including a *contact order* which requires the person with whom the child lives to permit access to another named person; a *residence order* which settles arrangements over where a child lives; *care* and *supervision orders* to place a child in local authority care; a *child assessment order* to enable the child to remain in his normal residence whilst allowing access for assessment; and an *emergency protection order* to remove a child from potential harm, usually to local authority care.

children's dentistry ⊃ paedodontics or paediatric dentistry.

chin cup an orthodontic appliance used to attempt to restrict development of the mandible in growing children.

china clay naturally occurring hydrous aluminium silicate used as a filler in certain dental materials.

Chinese restaurant syndrome (Kwok's syndrome) postprandial disturbance once thought to be caused by eating the flavour enhancer monosodium glutamate, which is used as a food additive and to enhance flavours in Chinese cooking. It is characterized by flushing, headache, palpitations, numbness and abdominal symptoms. The cause is not known.

chip a piece of silicon or gallium arsenide which contains the microcircuitry which operates the computer. They control a range of functions from simple tasks to extremely complex procedures. ⊃ central processing unit.

chiropodist *n* ⊃ podiatrist.

chiropody *n* ⊃ podiatry.

chiropractic *n* a technique of spinal manipulation, based on the principle that defects in vertebral alignment may result in various problems caused by functional changes in the nervous system. In the UK chiropractic is subject to statutory regulation which means that practitioners must be registered with the General Chiropractic Council in order to practice.

chiropractor *n* a person who uses chiropractic techniques.

chisel (dental) in dentistry, the hand instrument used to remove hard tissues such as enamel or bone by chipping, cleaving or paring. The bevelled blade may be in line with the handle or at an angle to it. ⊃ bone chisel, Coupland chisel, enamel chisel.

chi-square statistic (χ^2) a statistical technique used to analyse the relationship between expected frequency and the actual frequency of data obtained. A test of statistical significance used to determine the probability of results occurring by chance. ⊃ non-parametric tests.

chi-square test a statistical test used to compare groups to see if the behaviour of one of the groups is significant. A chi-square table is used and the results must be equal to or greater than the value given in the table to be significant.

chlamydiae *npl* micro-organisms of the genus *Chlamydia*. They are intracellular parasites and have features common to both bacteria and viruses. *Chlamydia psittaci* infects birds and causes psittacosis in humans. ⊃ ornithosis. Subgroups of *Chlamydia trachomatis* cause genital tract infection in adults, and are sexually transmitted. In men, may be associated with urethritis, but infection is often symptomless; epididymitis may be a complication. In women, most infections are symptomless; about 20% of untreated women develop pelvic inflammatory disease with subsequent scarring of the uterine (fallopian) tubes with risk of infertility or of ectopic pregnancy. Reactive arthritis is an uncommon complication. Autoinoculation from the genital tract can cause conjunctivitis in adults. Chlamydial conjunctivitis and pneumonia in infants can result from infection during birth. Lymphogranuloma venereum is caused by a different subgroup of *Chlamydia trachomatis*. The micro-organism also causes trachoma. ⊃ adult inclusion conjunctivitis, trachoma.

chloasma *n* patchy brown discoloration of the skin, especially the face. Can appear during pregnancy and during use of the oral contraceptive. ⊃ melasma.

chlor/o- a prefix that means 'green', e.g. *chloropsia*.

chlorhexidine *n* a disinfectant solution which is effective against a wide range of bacteria. Used for general skin cleansing and disinfection, and hand decontamination, etc. It also inhibits bacterial plaque when used as a mouthwash in a 0.2% strength three times daily. Also incorporated in a toothpaste.

chloride *n* a salt of hydrochloric acid. A major anion in extracellular fluid.

chloride shift the movement of chloride ions into the red blood cells to restore electrical balance, as bicarbonate (hydrogen carbonate) ions move out into the blood during the transport of carbon dioxide.

chlorine *n* a greenish-yellow, irritating gaseous element. Powerful disinfectant, bleaching and deodorizing agent in the presence of moisture when nascent oxygen is liberated. Mainly used as hypochlorites, or other compounds which slowly liberate active chlorine.

chloroform *n* a heavy liquid, once used extensively as a general anaesthetic. Used as chloroform water as a flavouring and preservative in aqueous mixtures.

chlorolabe a pigment contained in one group of cones; responds to green light.

chloropsia an abnormality of vision where all objects are seen as green.

CHM *abbr* Commission on Human Medicines.

CHO *abbr* carbohydrate.

choanae *npl* funnel-shaped openings. ⊃ nares—**choana** *sing*, **choanal** *adj*.

choanal atresia membranous or bony obstruction of the posterior nares, which causes neonatal respiratory difficulty at or shortly after birth, leading to cyanosis.

chocolate cyst an endometrial cyst containing altered blood. The ovaries are the most usual site. ⊃ endometriosis.

choice reaction time ⊃ reaction time.

'choking' in sport psychology, a sudden inability to perform at one's normal standard. Associated with high levels of competitive sport anxiety.

cholagogue *n* a drug which increases the flow of bile into the intestine.

cholangiography *n* rarely performed radiographic examination of hepatic, cystic and bile ducts (biliary tract). Can be performed: (a) after oral or intravenous administration of contrast agent, (b) by direct injection at operation to detect any further stones in the ducts, (c) during or after operation by way of a T-tube in the common bile duct; or (d) percutaneously by means of an injection via the skin on the anterior abdominal wall and the liver. ⊃ endoscopic retrograde cholangiopancreatography, percutaneous transhepatic cholangiography (PTC).

cholangitis *n* inflammation of the bile ducts.

cholecalciferol *n* vitamin D_3. An essential precursor of the active forms of vitamin D.

chol/e, chol/o- a prefix that means 'bile', e.g. *choleic*.

cholecystectomy *n* surgical removal of the gallbladder. *laparoscopic cholecystectomy* removal of the gallbladder using minimally invasive surgical techniques.

cholecystenterostomy *n* literally, the establishment of an artificial opening (anastomosis) between the gallbladder and the small intestine. Specific terminology more frequently used.

cholecystitis *n* acute or chronic inflammation of the gallbladder, most often associated with the presence of gallstones.

cholecyst/o- a prefix that means 'gallbladder', e.g. *cholecystography*.

cholecystoduodenal *adj* pertaining to the gallbladder and duodenum as an anastomosis between them.

cholecystoduodenostomy *n* the establishment of an anastomosis between the gallbladder and the duodenum.

cholecystography *n* rarely performed radiographic examination of the gallbladder after administration of opaque contrast agent. Superseded by computed tomography (CT) and magnetic resonance imaging (MRI) scanning.

cholecystojejunostomy *n* an anastomosis between the gallbladder and the jejunum.

cholecystokinin (CCK) *n* a hormone that contracts the gallbladder and relaxes the sphincter of Oddi thus allowing bile into the duodenum, and stimulates the secretion of pancreatic enzymes. Secreted by the duodenal mucosa.

cholecystolithiasis *n* the presence of a gallstone or stones in the gallbladder.

cholecystostomy *n* a surgically established fistula between the gallbladder and the abdominal surface; used to provide drainage, in empyema of the gallbladder.

cholecystotomy *n* incision into the gallbladder.

choledoch/o- a prefix that means 'common bile duct', e.g. *choledocholithotomy*.

choledochoduodenal *adj* pertaining to the bile ducts and duodenum, e.g. *choledochoduodenal fistula*.

choledochography *n* cholangiography.

choledochojejunostomy *n* an anastomosis between the bile duct and the jejunum.

choledocholithiasis *n* the presence of a gallstone or gallstones in the extrahepatic bile ducts.

choledocholithotomy *n* surgical removal of a stone from the common bile duct.

choledochoscope *n* endoscopic instrument used to examine the lumen of the biliary tree (bile ducts).

choledochoscopy *n* endoscopic examination of the biliary tree.

choledochostomy *n* drainage of the common bile duct using a T-tube, usually after exploration for a gallstone.

choledochotomy *n* incision into the common bile duct.

cholelithiasis *n* the presence or formation of gallstones in the gallbladder or bile ducts.

cholera *n* acute enteritis occurring in Africa and Asia, where it is endemic and epidemic. At the time of writing an epidemic originating in Zimbabwe has caused over 1000 deaths. It is caused by the bacterium *Vibrio cholerae* and is associated with faecal contamination of water, overcrowding and insanitary conditions. There is diarrhoea (rice-water stools) accompanied by agonizing cramp and vomiting, resulting in dehydration, electrolyte imbalance and severe collapse. There are high mortality rates without adequate fluid and electrolyte replacement. The early adminstration of oral rehydration salts to replace fluids lost through diarrhoea is vital. Intravenous fluids may be needed in individuals with severe disease. Many strains of *Vibrio cholerae* have developed antibiotic resistence and this varies across regions. In situations where the organism is sensitive to the tetracyclines, therapy with single-dose doxycycline may be initiated.

choleric temperament one of the four classical types of temperament, hasty and with a propensity to emotional outbursts.

cholestasis *n* an obstruction to the flow of bile. It produces jaundice, dark urine, pale stools, metallic taste and pruritus. *extrahepatic cholestasis* caused by a blockage to a large duct, e.g. the common bile duct, by a gallstone or cancer involving the head of the pancreas. *intrahepatic cholestasis* caused by blockage of the small bile ducts within the liver, such as in hepatitis or due to cirrhosis—**cholestatic** *adj*. ⊃ intrahepatic cholestasis of pregnancy.

cholesteatoma *n* a benign encysted tumour containing squamous epithelial debris. Mainly occurs in the middle ear—**cholesteatomatous** *adj*.

cholesterol *n* a sterol found in many tissues. It is an important component of cell membranes and is the precursor of many biological molecules, such as steroid hormones, and is concerned with the absorption and transportation of fatty acids. High levels of low-density lipoprotein cholesterol in the blood are linked with the development of arterial disease and some types of gallstones. It is present in some foods, and is produced in and processed by the liver. Cholesterol circulates in the blood combined with high-density and low-density lipoproteins (HDL and LDL). HDL-cholesterol removes excess cholesterol from cells and transports it to the liver for excretion; LDL-cholesterol delivers cholesterol to cells of all organs and tissues. ⊃ hypercholesterolaemia.

cholesterosis *n* abnormal deposition of cholesterol.

cholic acid a bile acid produced from cholesterol in the liver.

choline *n* a chemical found in animal tissues as a component of phospholipids, e.g lecithin (phosphatidylcholine); has an important influence on the production of the neurotransmitter acetylcholine. Choline is involved in the transportation of fats and the entry of fats into cells. In sport, choline is promoted as an ergogenic aid to increase strength and/or decrease fat. No valid studies have confirmed these effects. ⊃ ergogenic aids.

choline salicylate dental paste anti-inflammatory, analgesic paste containing a soluble salicylate which may be applied to the affected mucosa three to four times daily.

cholinergic *adj* applied to nerves that release acetylcholine as the neurotransmitter at their synapases. They include the somatic motor nerves innervating voluntary skeletal muscle, all parasympathetic nerves (preganglionic and postganglionic), preganglionic sympathetic nerves and a few postganglionic sympathetic nerves (the innervation to some sweat glands and the blood vessels supplying the skin and skeletal muscle). ⊃ adrenergic.

cholinergic crisis severe muscle weakness, flaccid paralysis and respiratory failure caused by an excess of acetylcholine at the neuromuscular junction. It can result from overtreatment with the anticholinesterase drugs used to treat myasthenia gravis, or from organophosphate poisoning.

cholinergic receptors receptor sites on the effector structures innervated by parasympathetic and voluntary motor nerves. The receptors may be muscarinic or nicotinic depending on their response to acetylcholine. They may be excitatory or inhibitory depending on their location. Both muscarinic and nicotinic receptors are further subdivided. ⊃ edrophonium test.

cholinesterase *n* an enzyme that inactivates acetylcholine at nerve endings. It catalyses the reaction whereby acetylcholine is broken down into choline and water.

choluria *n* bile in the urine.

chondritis *n* inflammation of cartilage.

chondr/i, chondr/o- a prefix that means 'cartilage', e.g. *chondrocyte*.

chondroblast *n* a mesenchymal cell that produces cartilage. Particularly important in endochondrial ossification.

chondroblastoma *n* a benign tumour of the precursor cells of cartilage.

chondrocalcinosis an arthritic condition characterized by calcium deposits in joints, especially the knee. It usually affects people over 50 years of age.

chondrocostal *adj* pertaining to the costal cartilages and ribs.

chondroclast a cell involved in the reabsorption of cartilage.

chondrocyte a cartilage cell.

chondrodynia *n* pain in a cartilage.

chondrodystrophy *n* a group of conditions in which cartilage is converted to bone. Commonly occurs in the epiphyses of long bones. Affected individuals have short stature with shortened limbs and normal trunk size.

chondroectodermal dysplasia also known as Ellis–van Creveld syndrome. A rare genetic disorder transmitted by an autosomal recessive gene. It is characterized by polydactyly; acromelic dwarfism with abnormally short limb bones; congenital heart defects; defects affecting the nails and hair; and the upper and lower jaw and the teeth, which may be absent, erupt prenatally or defective.

chondrolysis *n* dissolution of cartilage—**chondrolytic** *adj*.

chondroma *n* a benign tumour of cartilage. It may be on the surface of the cartilage (ecchondroma) or within the cartilage (enchondroma)

chondromalacia *n* softening of cartilage.

chondromalacia patellae (CMP) the common name given to a collection of syndromes that result in softening of the cartilage on articular surface of the patella. Commonly seen in adolescents, young women and frequently associated with functional and biomechanical deficiencies of the patellofemoral joint such as an abnormal Q angle. It may be related to overuse, trauma and/or abnormal forces on the knee. It is more common in females. Symptoms include: knee tenderness; recurrent effusions and increased joint temperature; anterior knee pain that worsens after prolonged sitting; and a grating or grinding sensation under the patella on knee extension. ⊃ Clark's test, Q (quadriceps)-angle.

chondrosarcoma *n* malignant tumour of cartilage or its precursor cells—**chondrosarcomata** *pl*, **chondrosarcomatous** *adj*.

chondrosternal *adj* pertaining to the costal cartilages and sternum.

chordae tendineae structures that stabilize the atrioventricular valves; mitral (bicuspid) and tricuspid valves of the heart by attaching them to the papillary muscles.

chordee *n* angulation of the penis associated with hypospadias.

chordotomy ⊃ cordotomy.

chorea *n* describes irregular and jerky dance-like movements, beyond the patient's control. Chorea may follow childhood rheumatic fever, *Sydenham's chorea*, but usually results from a disorder or drug affecting the basal nuclei. In adults, chorea is a feature of the inherited condition Huntington's disease and the administration of drugs

C
D

including the phenothiazines and L-dopa used in parkinsonism—**choreal, choreic** *adj.* ◑dyskinetic movements.

choreiform *adj* resembling chorea.

chorioamnionitis inflammation of the chorionic and amnionic membranes as a result of bacterial invasion.

chorioangioma collection of fetal blood vessels in Wharton's jelly, forming a tumour on the placenta. It is of little clinical significance but may be associated with polyhydramnios.

choriocapillaris the layer of the choroid adjacent to the membrane of Bruch and consisting of a network of capillaries which supplies nutrients to the retina. ◑ Bruch's membrane, choroid.

choriocarcinoma *n* (*syn* chorionepithelioma) a malignant gestational trophoblastic tumour that may develop following normal pregnancy (rarely), miscarriage, ectopic pregnancy or following the evacuation of a molar pregnancy. The risk of persistent trophoblastic disease or choriocarcinoma is increased following a molar pregnancy, increasing maternal age (especially over 40 years of age) and is more common in Asian women. A sensitive (though not specific) tumour marker is human chorionic gonadotrophin (hCG). In the UK women are referred for treatment to one of three specialist centres (Dundee, London and Sheffield). Choriocarcinoma and persistent trophoblastic disease are treated with chemotherapy, the choice of drug depending on the stage of the disease and whether it has spread beyond the uterus or metastasized to distant sites such as the lung. Chemotherapy may be given as a single drug or as a combination of drugs. The drugs used include cisplatin, dactinomysin (actinomycin-D), etoposide, methotrexate, vincristine ◑ gestational trophoblastic tumour, molar pregnancy.

chorion *n* outer of the two membranes enclosing the fetus *in utero*, derived from the trophoblast. It is opaque and friable and sometimes retained after delivery—**chorial, chorionic** *adj.* ◑ chorion frondosum, chorionic villus sampling, chorion laeve.

chorion biopsy ◑ amnion, chorionic villus sampling.

chorionepithelioma ◑ choriocarcinoma.

chorion frondosum part of the chorion covered by villi in the early weeks of embryonic development before the placenta is formed.

chorion laeve non-villous, membranous part of the trophoblast which develops into the chorion.

chorionic *adj* pertaining to the chorion.

chorionic gonadotrophin ◑ human chorionic gonadotrophin.

chorionicity placental formation in multiple pregnancy. Monochorionic twins are connected to a single placenta and have an increased risk of fetofetal (twin-to-twin) transfusion syndrome. Whereas, dichorionic twins have two separate placentae, although they may fuse, but there is a lower risk of complications.

chorionic villi minute finger-like projections arising from the trophoblast and persisting in the chorion frondosum, having an outer syncytiotrophoblastic layer with multiple nuclei

and without cell membranes, and an inner cytotrophoblastic layer with cell membranes containing single nuclei. Fetal capillaries are embedded in mesoderm; oxygenated maternal blood spurts in cascades over the villi in the intervillous spaces, so that oxygen, nutrients, etc., may pass into the fetal circulation and carbon dioxide, etc., may pass out; after 24 weeks' gestation the cytotrophoblastic cell layer remains only in isolated areas.

chorionic villus sampling (CVS) also known as chorion or chorionic villus biopsy, or placental biopsy. A prenatal screening test for chromosomal (e.g. Down's syndrome) and inherited disorders (e.g. haemoglobinopathies, Tay-Sachs disease). Samples of fetal tissue are obtained under ultrasound control either via a needle or fine catheter passed through the cervix into the uterus (transvaginally) (Figure C.8) or through a transabdominal puncture (transabdominally). It can be performed after 11 weeks' gestation but earlier than amniocentesis, although interpretation of CVS results can sometimes be difficult. There is a procedure-induced, operator-dependent risk of miscarriage of 1–2%.

chorioretinal *adj* pertaining to the choroid and the retina.

chorioretinitis *n* (*syn* retinochoroiditis) inflammation involving both the choroid and retina. It may be an autoimmune disorder, or bacterial, viral, fungal, or parasitic in origin.

choroid *n* the middle pigmented, highly vascular coat of the posterior five-sixths of the eyeball, continuous with the iris in front. It lies between the sclera externally and the retina internally. The choroid is part of the uveal tract. Its main function is to nourish the retina. It is a thin membrane extending from the optic nerve to the ora serrata. It consists

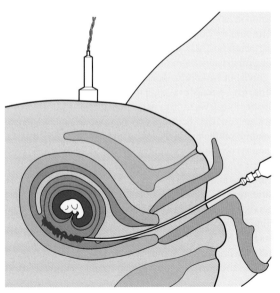

C.8 Transcervical chorionic villus sampling (reproduced from Rodeck & Whittle 1999 with permission).

of five main layers from without inward: the suprachoroid (or lamina fusca), the layers of vessels (Haller's layer and Sattler's layer), the choriocapillaris and the membrane of Bruch (or lamina vitrea)—**choroidal** *adj.* ➲ Bruch's membrane, choriocapillaris, choroiditis, ciliary body, epichoroid, fuscin, iris, Colour Section Figure 15.

choroidal pertaining to the choroid coat of the eye.

choroidal fissure ➲ optic fissure.

choroidal flush this is the first evidence of fluorescein dye reaching the eye during the method of fluorescein angiography. It occurs approximately 1 second before reaching the retinal circulation because the route from the ophthalmic artery to the choroidal circulation is shorter.

choroidal melanoma (*syn* malignant melanoma of the choroid) the most common primary malignant tumour in the eye in adults. It appears under ophthalmoscopic examination as a pigmented, elevated mass, usually brown in colour and sometimes with orange pigment. The tumour may cause a decrease in vision or a defect in the visual field, or be asymptomatic, depending on its size or location. The condition is typically unilateral. Differential diagnosis with retinal detachment or choroidal naevus is essential. Treatment may include radiotherapy or photocoagulation, or enucleation if the melanoma is large and vision irreversibly lost. ➲ choroidal naevus.

choroidal naevus a benign accumulation of melanocytes in the choroid. It affects some 10% of the population. Ophthalmoscopically it appears as a slate-grey lesion, flat or minimally elevated, oval or circular. With time drusen may also appear. ➲ choroid, choroidal melanoma, drusen, melanocytes.

choroidal neovascularization (CNV) the growth of new blood vessels in the choroid, such as occurs in wet age-related macular degeneration.

choroiditis *n* inflammation of the choroid layer of the eye. It causes blurring of vision.

choroid plexus an area of specialized capillaries surrounded by modified ependymal cells that line the cerebral ventricles. They produce cerebrospinal fluid (CSF) from blood. ➲ cerebrospinal fluid.

CHRE *abbr* Council for Healthcare Regulatory Excellence.

Christmas disease haemophilia B. ➲ haemophilias.

Christmas factor factor IX (or antihaemophiliac factor B) in the coagulation cascade. It is involved in the intrinsic coagulation system. Deficiency causes Christmas disease (haemophilia B).

chromaffin an affinity for staining with chromium salts, such as the cells of the adrenal medulla. ➲ chromaffin cells.

chromaffin cells neuroendocrine cells that form from the neural crest in the embryo. They are present in the adrenal medulla and sympathetic nervous system ganglia. The cells in the adrenal medulla release the catecholamines adrenaline (epinephrine) and noradrenaline (norepinephrine) when stimulated by the splanchnic nerve.

chromatic aberration the non-convergence of different coloured rays in a lens.

chromatic difference of magnification ➲ lateral chromatic aberration.

chromatic parallax apparent lateral displacement of two monochromatic sources (e.g. a blue object and a red object) when observed through a disc with a pinhole placed near the edge of the pupil. When the pupil is centred on the achromatic axis (in some people the pinhole may have to be placed away from the centre of the pupil), the two images appear superimposed. The relative displacement of the two images becomes reversed when the pinhole is on the other side of that axis. This phenomenon is attributed to the chromatic aberration of the eye. ➲ achromatic axis, chromostereopsis, longitudinal chromatic aberration.

chromatic stereopsis ➲ chromostereopsis.

chromaticity diagram (*syn* colour triangle) a plane diagram showing the results of mixtures of colour stimuli, each chromaticity being represented by a single point on the diagram. ➲ CIE standard illuminants, purple, spectrum locus, white light.

chromatid *n* one of the strands that result from the duplication of chromosomes during nuclear division.

chromatin *n* the threads of DNA and protein that form the substance of chromosomes.

chromatography *n* analytical methods used to separate and identify substances in a complex mixture based on their differential movement through a two-phase system. Include: gel filtration chromatography, gas chromatography and ion exchange chromatography.

chromatopsia a disorder of colour vision. It may be a type of colour blindness where people have abnormal perception of various colours. Or a condition in which colourless objects may appear to be tinged with a particular colour.

chrom/o, chromat/o- a prefix that means 'colour', e.g. *chromatopsia.*

chromoretinoscopy an objective method of measuring the longitudinal chromatic aberration of the eye by carrying out retinoscopy through various coloured filters (usually a red and a green filter). However, it is necessary to use a retinoscope source of high luminance (e.g. halogen). The difference in the retinoscopic value obtained with the two coloured filters represents the longitudinal chromatic aberration of the eye between these two dominant wavelengths. ➲ longitudinal chromatic aberration.

chromostereopsis (*syn* chromatic stereopsis, colour stereoscopy) a sensation of apparent depth among coloured objects placed at the same distance from the subject and viewed binocularly, when the pupils are eccentric to the achromatic axes or the visual axes do not coincide with the achromatic axes. This phenomenon is attributed to the retinal disparity created by the chromatic aberration of the eye. If the objects are red and blue (or green), the red appears closer than the blue (or green) in many people. Other people see the reverse impression and a few others do not see any apparent depth at all. The phenomenon can be enhanced, eliminated or reversed by using prisms or pinhole pupils placed in different regions of the pupil. If the pinhole pupils are decentred symmetrically temporally in front of the natural pupils the red object will appear closer than the blue (positive chromostereopsis) and if they are decentred nasally the blue object appears closer than the red (negative chromostereopsis). Apparent depth is eliminated when the pinholes are centred on the achromatic axes or when using prisms of appropriate power and direction. ⊃ lateral chromatic aberration, longitudinal chromatic aberration, stereopsis.

chromium (Cr) *n* **1.** an essential trace element required in very small amounts in the diet. It potentiates the action of insulin in carbohydrate, lipid and protein metabolism. Symptoms of chromium deficiency include impaired glucose tolerance. Hyperglycaemia has occurred in children suffering from protein-energy malnutrition (PEM), and rarely during long-term parenteral nutrition. **2.** a metal which is very resistant to corrosion. Used as an alloy in fixed and removable dental prostheses.

chromium oxide in dentistry, used as a fine polishing agent.

chromophore a chemical group, which when present gives colour to a compound.

chromosomal aberration loss, gain or exchange of genetic material in the chromosomes of a cell resulting in deletion, duplication, inversion or translocation of genes. ⊃ amniocentesis.

chromosome *n* the genetic material present in the nucleus of the cell. During the preparation for cell division chromosomes appear as microscopic threads. They contain strands of DNA molecules or genes. Each species has a constant number; humans have 23 pairs (46) in each somatic cell: 22 pairs of autosomes and 1 pair of sex chromosomes—males have XY (Figure C.9) and females have XX. Mature gametes, however, have half the usual number (haploid) which results from the reduction division during meiosis. The 23 unpaired chromosomes inherited from each parent unite to produce an embryo with 46 chromosomes (diploid). Genetic sex is determined by the male gamete and depends on whether the oocyte is fertilized by a sperm that contributes a Y chromosome (genetic male) or an X chromosome (genetic female). Some genetic material is also present in organelles, such as the mitochondria—**chromosomal** *adj*. ⊃ chromosomal aberration, meiosis, mitochondrial genes, mitosis.

chronaxie an electrotherapy term. A measure applied to a strength–duration graph to evaluate peripheral nerve function. Calculation based on the rheobase as is defined as the duration required for a minimally perceptible response (motor or sensory, depending on the test) at twice rheobasic intensity using a monophasic pulse and a frequency of approximately 1 Hz. Normal values vary whether constant current or constant voltage stimulator used.

chronic *adj* lingering, lasting, opposed to acute. The word does not imply anything about the severity of the condition—**chronicity** *n*, **chronically** *adv*.

chronic angle-closure glaucoma ⊃ angle-closure glaucoma.

chronic bronchitis ⊃ bronchits, chronic obstructive pulmonary disease.

chronic constipation ⊃ constipation.

chronic energy deficiency a term used to describe malnutrition occurring in adults. Generally defined by a body mass index below the normal range or wasting. ⊃ protein-energy malnutrition.

chronic exertional compartment syndrome often occurs with a particular predictable amount of strenuous activity, when increased muscle volume raises compartment pressure, impeding blood flow and causing pain which is relieved by rest. Many causes include repetitive overuse, muscle hypertrophy due to training, and foot conditions which alter lower limb biomechanics.

chronic fatigue syndrome/myalgic encephalomyelitis (CFS/ME) sometimes referred to as post-viral fatigue. A flu-like illness characterized by disabling fatigue, with varied signs and symptoms including dizziness, adenopathy, muscle fatigue and spasm, myalgia, joint pain, sore throat, headaches and other neurological pain, poor concentration and impaired memory. The cause is unclear but may be associated with a viral infection, or a poorly functioning immune system. Management is directed towards symptom relief including the use of complementary therapies. Cognitive behavioural therapy or physiotherapy can be helpful for some people.

chronic glaucoma ⊃ open-angle glaucoma.

chronic heart failure also known as congestive heart failure. A chronic inability of the heart to maintain an adequate output of blood from one (right- or left-heart failure) or both ventricles, resulting in pulmonary congestion and overdistension of certain veins and organs with blood, and in an inadequate blood supply to the body tissues.

chronic injury an injury with long onset and duration.

chronic leukaemia ⊃ leukaemia.

chronic mastitis ⊃ fibrocystic disease of breast.

chronic mountain sickness (Monge's disease) this occurs on prolonged exposure to altitude and has been

C.9 **Chromosomes—normal male** (reproduced from Brooker 2006A permission).

reported in residents of Colorado, South America and Tibet. Patients present with headache, poor concentration and other signs of polycythaemia. They are cyanosed and often have finger clubbing.

chronic obstructive pulmonary disease (COPD) also known as chronic airflow limitation or chronic obstructive airways disease. A group of obstructive lung diseases where airway resistance is increased with impaired airflow, e.g. pulmonary emphysema, chronic bronchitis. Some authorities include asthma in the COPD group. Defined on spirometric grounds as an FEV_1 <80% and an FEV_1:FVC ratio <70%. Usually seen as a long term sequela of smoking. Genetic factors include α_1-antitrypsin deficiency, and more recently, family clustering studies suggest other genetic susceptibility factors.

chronic pain pain that does not resolve, usually lasting longer than 3 months. Chronic pain can be subdivided into non-malignant pain (not life-threatening) such as that associated with arthritis or phantom limb pain, and malignant pain, which is associated with terminal diseases especially cancer. Chronic pain affects every aspect of a person's life and can lead to relationship problems, financial problems, social isolation, depression and in extreme cases suicidal ideation. ⊃ acute pain, neuropathic pain, nociceptive pain.

chronic pancreatitis ⊃ pancreatitis.

chronic progressive external ophthalmoplegia (CPEO) a mitochondrial myopathy syndrome. It is characterized by progressive ptosis and external oculomotor palsy, proximal myopathy ± deafness, ataxia and cardiac conduction defects. ⊃ Kearns-Sayre syndrome, mitochondrial myopathy syndromes.

chronic suppurative otitis media (CSOM) chronic inflammation of the middle ear. It is classified as either *tubotympanic*, a 'safe' condition that leads to fewer intracranial problems or *atticoantral*, which is classified as an 'unsafe' condition as it is associated with an increased risk of intracranial problems.

chronic wound a wound that is slow to heal and displays delayed healing, such as a venous leg ulcer. ⊃ acute wound, wound healing.

chronological age a person's age in years.

chronotherapy *n* the administration of treatment modalities, such as chemotherapy or radiotherapy, at the most effective time.

chuck in dentistry, the adjustable tool for holding rotary instruments. Used on a lathe or by hand. Also used in turbine hand-pieces to retain friction grip burs.

chunking *n* the organization and coding of 'chunks' of data/information that facilitates an increase in the effective capacity of short term memory, which can only store around seven items of information.

Churg–Strauss syndrome (CSS) (J Churg, American pathologist, 20th century; L Stauss, American pathologist, 1913–1985) an ANCA-associated vasculitis. The annual incidence is 1–3 per million in the UK. Most patients have a prodromal period for many years, characterised by allergic rhinitis, nasal polyposis and late onset asthma that is often difficult to control. The typical acute presentation is with a triad comprising skin lesions (purpura or nodules), asymmetric mononeuritis multiplex and eosinophilia on a background of resistant asthma. Pulmonary infiltrates and pleural or pericardial effusions due to serositis may be present. Up to 50% of patients have abdominal symptoms due to mesenteric vasculitis. Either c-ANCA or p-ANCA is present in around 40% of cases. ⊃ antineutrophil cytoplasmic antibodies - associated vasculitis.

Chvostek's sign (F Chvostek, Austrian surgeon, 1835–1884) spasm or twitching of the face on tapping the facial nerve seen with hypocalcaemia: a sign of tetany.

chyle *n* fatty, milky fluid formed from chylomicrons within the lymphatic lacteals of the intestinal villi—**chylous** *adj*.

chylomicron *n* tiny particles formed from triglycerides, lipoproteins and cholesterol within the intestinal mucosa following the absorption of digested fat. They form chyle within the lacteals.

chylothorax *n* leakage of chyle from the thoracic duct into the pleural cavity.

chyluria *n* chyle in the urine, which can occur in some nematode infestations, either when a fistulous communication is established between a lymphatic vessel and the urinary tract or when the distension of the urinary lymphatics causes them to rupture—**chyluric** *adj*.

chyme *n* partially digested food which passes from the stomach to the duodenum. Its acidity controls the pylorus to regulate the amount entering the duodenum.

chymotrypsin *n* the active proteolytic enzyme secreted as inactive chymotrypsinogen by the pancreas: it is activated by trypsin.

ci *abbr* curie.

CI *abbr* **1.** cardiac index. **2.** confidence interval.

Ciaccio's glands ⊃ Wolfring's glands.

cicatricial alopecia progressive alopecia of the scalp in which tufts of normal hair occur between scarred bald patches.

cicatricial pemphigoid (*syn* benign mucous pemphigoid) a rare, idiopathic, chronic systemic disease, most commonly affecting older adults and characterized by recurrent blisters and bullae of the skin and mucous membranes, with subsequent scarring and shrinkage. The disease may affect only the conjunctiva (ocular pemphigoid). In this case, the clinical picture is a conjunctivitis with hyperaemia, mucus discharge and small vesicles which on bursting result in ulceration, pseudomembranes, conjunctival subepithelial fibrosis and conjunctival shrinkage. The disease may give rise to the following complications: adhesion between the palpebral and bulbar conjunctiva (symblepharon), ankyloblepharon, xerophthalmia, keratoconjunctivitis sicca, entropion, trichiasis and dry eye with corneal ulcer. There is pain or irritation and blurred vision. Treatment includes corticosteroids, surgery for entropion and trichiasis, and keratoprosthesis if vision is affected. ⊃ pseudomembranous conjunctivitis.

cicatrix *n* ➲ scar.

-cide a suffix that means 'destructive, killing', e.g. *infanticide*.

CIE *abbr* Commission Internationale de l'Eclairage.

CIE standard illuminants the colorimetric illuminants A, B, C and D defined by the Commission Internationale de l'Eclairage (CIE) in terms of relative spectral energy (power distribution): *standard illuminant A* representing the full radiator at T = 2854 K; *standard illuminant B* representing direct sunlight with a correlated colour temperature of T = 4874 K; *standard illuminant C* representing daylight with a correlated colour temperature of T = 6774 K; and *standard illuminant D* representing daylight with a correlated colour temperature of T = 6504 K (CIE). ➲ chromaticity diagram, Macbeth lamp, white light.

cilia *npl* **1**. the eyelashes. **2**. microscopic hair-like projections from certain epithelial cells. Membranes containing such cells, e.g. those lining the trachea and uterine (fallopian) tubes, are known as ciliated membranes— **cilium** *sing*, **ciliary, ciliated, cilial** *adj*.

ciliary *adj* hair-like.

ciliary arteries branches of the ophthalmic artery which supply the whole of the uveal tract, the sclera and the edge of the cornea with its neighbouring conjunctiva. The ciliary arteries comprise: the short posterior ciliary arteries; the long posterior ciliary arteries; and the anterior ciliary arteries. The short posterior ciliary arteries are some 10–20 branches of the ophthalmic artery which pierce the eyeball around the optic nerve to supply the posterior choroid, the optic disc, the circle of Zinn, the cilioretinal and episcleral arteries. The long posterior ciliary arteries are two branches from the ophthalmic artery which pierce the sclera on either side of the optic nerve, further anteriorly than the short posterior ciliary arteries, and course in the perichoroidal space. They form, with the anterior ciliary arteries, the major arterial (or iridic) circle of the iris, which supplies the ciliary body, the anterior choroid and the iris. The anterior ciliary arteries are derived from the arteries to the four recti muscles and they anastomose in the ciliary muscle with the long posterior ciliary arteries to form the major arterial circle of the iris. They also give branches that supply the episclera (episcleral arteries), sclera, corneal limbus and conjunctiva (anterior and posterior conjunctival arteries). ➲ major arterial circle of the iris.

ciliary block glaucoma (*syn* malignant glaucoma) a secondary glaucoma which occurs when aqueous fluid becomes misdirected into the vitreous cavity. The accumulating fluid then produces a displacement of the lens and iris, causing a narrowing of the anterior chamber angle with resultant raised intraocular pressure. This condition occurs most commonly following intraocular surgery, especially glaucoma surgery after the cessation of cycloplegic medications. Treatment consists of medical intervention (cycloplegics, beta-adrenergic agents, carbonic anhydrase inhibitors and hyperosmotic agents) or puncture of the vitreous face with the Nd-YAG laser if medical treatment is unsuccessful. In phakic eyes, vitrectomy is sometimes required to open the anterior vitreous face.

ciliary body part of the uveal tract. It is anterior to the ora serrata and extending to the root of the iris where it is attached to the scleral spur. It comprises the ciliary muscle and the ciliary processes and is roughly triangular in sagittal section. The whole ciliary body forms a ring. The part just beyond the ora serrata is smooth and is thus known as pars plana (or orbiculus ciliaris). Anterior to this lies a region of ridges which are the ciliary processes; this region is called the pars plicata (or corona ciliaris). ➲ angle recession, choroid, ciliary muscle, ciliary processes, cyclitis, iridodialysis, iris, striae, Colour Section Figure 15.

ciliary flush ➲ ciliary injection.

ciliary ganglion (*syn* lenticular ganglion; ophthalmic ganglion) a small reddish-grey body about the size of a pinhead situated at the posterior part of the orbit about 1 cm from the optic foramen between the optic nerve (second cranial nerve) and the lateral rectus muscle. It receives posteriorly three roots: (a) the long, nasociliary or sensory root (or ramus communicans), which contains sensory fibres from the cornea, iris and ciliary body and some sympathetic postganglionic axons going to the dilator muscle; (b) the short (or motor root or oculomotor root) which comes from the Edinger–Westphal nucleus through the occulomotor nerve (third cranial nerve). It carries fibres supplying the sphincter pupillae and ciliary muscles; (c) the sympathetic root which comes from the cavernous and the internal carotid plexuses. It carries fibres mediating constriction of the blood vessels of the eye and possibly mediating dilatation of the pupil. The ciliary ganglion gives rise to 6–10 short ciliary nerves. ➲ Edinger–Westphal nucleus, oculomotor nerve, pupillary light reflex.

ciliary injection (*syn* ciliary flush) characterized by redness (almost lilac) around the corneal limbus of the eye caused by dilatation of the deeper small blood vessels located around the cornea. It occurs in inflammation of the cornea, iris and ciliary body, and in angle-closure glaucoma. Each of these conditions is associated with loss of vision and usually pain. ➲ glaucoma, iritis, keratitis, keratomycosis, pericorneal plexus, uveitis.

ciliary muscle the smooth (or unstriated and involuntary) muscle of the ciliary body. In a meridional section of the eye it has the form of a right-angled triangle, the right angle being internal and facing the ciliary processes. The posterior angle is acute and points to the choroid, the hypotenuse runs parallel with the sclera. Some of its fibres have their origin in the scleral spur at the angle of the anterior chamber, while other fibres take origin in the trabecular meshwork. The fibres radiate backward in three directions: (a) fibres coursing meridionally or longitudinally more or less parallel to the sclera and can be traced posteriorly into the suprachoroid to the equator or even beyond. They end usually in branched stellate figures known as muscle stars with three or more rays to each. These fibres represent Brücke's muscle. (b) other fibres course radially. These fibres lie deep in the longitudinal fibres from which they are distinguished by the reticular character of their stroma but are often very difficult to separate from the circular fibres. (c) the circular fibres (or Müller's muscle) occupy the anterior and inner portion of the ciliary body and run parallel to the corneal limbus. As a whole, these fibres form a ring. Innervation to the ciliary muscle (mainly parasympathetic fibres derived from the oculomotor nerve [third cranial nerve]) is provided through the short ciliary nerves and stimulation causes a contraction of the muscle. However, a small amount of sympathetic supply is also believed to act and relax the muscle. Blood supply to the ciliary muscle is provided by the anterior and long posterior ciliary arteries. Contraction of the ciliary muscle causes a reduction in its length thus causing the whole muscle to move forward and inward. Consequently the zonule of Zinn, which suspends the lens, relaxes. This leads to a decrease in the tension in the capsule of the lens allowing it to become more convex and thereby providing accommodation. ⊃ ciliary body, corneal limbus, Helmholtz's theory of accommodation, mechanism of accommodation, resting state of accommodation, zonule of Zinn.

ciliary processes about 70 ridges, some 2 mm long and 0.5 mm high, arranged meridionally and forming the corona ciliaris of the ciliary body. The ciliary processes consist essentially of blood vessels which are the continuation forward of those of the choroid. The region of the ciliary processes is the most vascular of the whole eye. The processes are involved in the secretion of aqueous humour.

ciliary sebaceous glands ⊃ Zeis' glands.

ciliary sulcus a groove situated between the posterior root of the iris and the ciliary body. It may be used, sometimes, as a site of fixation of an intraocular lens implant.

ciliary sweat glands ⊃ Moll's glands.

ciliated epithelium this is formed by columnar cells each of which has many microscopic, hair-like processes, called cilia (Figure E.7, p. 264). The cilia consist of microtubules inside the plasma membrane that extends from the free border (luminal border) of the columnar cells. The wave-like movement of many cilia propels the contents of the tubes, which they line in one direction only. Ciliated epithelium is found lining the uterine (fallopian) tubes and most of the respiratory passages. In the uterine tubes the cilia propel oocytes towards the uterus and in the respiratory passages they propel mucus towards the throat. ⊃ epithelium, goblet cells, mucociliary escalator/transport.

cilioretinal artery a small artery running from the temporal side of the optic disc to the macular area. It originates from the circle of Zinn and supplies the retina between the macula and the disc. This artery is present in only about a fifth, or less, of human eyes. If a patient possesses this artery central vision will be spared in case of occlusion of the central retinal artery. In some other eyes the cilioretinal artery supplies some other region of the retina. ⊃ circle of Zinn.

ciliosis spasmodic twitching of the eyelids.

cilium ⊃ cilia.

CILs *abbr* centres of integrated (or independent) living.

Cimex *n* a genus of insects of the family Cimicidae. *Cimex lectularius* is the common bedbug.

CIN *abbr* cervical intraepithelial neoplasia.

CINAHL *abbr* Cumulative Index to Nursing and Allied Health Literature.

cinchona *n* the bark from which quinine is obtained.

cinchonism *n* quininism.

cine- a prefix that means 'film, motion', e.g. *cinematography*.

cinematography in biomechanics, the use of cine film for analysis of human movement, now less common than video analysis.

cingulum bulge or ridge found on the palatal or lingual aspects of incisor and canine teeth, near to their cervical margins.

C1 inhibitor (C1 INH) an essential regulator of the classical complement pathway.

CIP *abbr* continuous inflating pressure.

circadian rhythm circadian means 'about a day'. Any rhythm with a periodicity of about 24 h, such as the sleep–wake cycle, body temperature, the secretion of some hormones including cortisol, urine output, etc. It is controlled by a 'clock' in the brain (nerve centres in the hypothalamus, with input from the eyes); normally synchronized to the light–dark cycle, but effective even in conditions without cues from light or time. Influenced by the hormone melatonin from the pineal gland. ⊃ jet lag, ultradian.

circinata *n* ⊃ tinea.

circinate *adj* in the form of a circle or segment of a circle, e.g. the skin eruptions of late syphilis, ringworm, etc.

circle of Haller ⊃ circle of Zinn.

circle of Willis (T Willis, English physician, 1621–1675) ⊃ circulus arteriosus.

circle of Zinn (J Zinn, German anatomist/botanist, 1727–1759) (*syn* circle of Haller) an anastomosing circle of short ciliary arteries which have pierced the sclera about the optic nerve. Branches pass forward to the choroid, inward to the optic nerve and backward to the pial network.

circuit training training that includes a number of specific exercises/activities targeted at working specific muscle groups and often the associated skills, involved in the target activity.

circulation *n* passage in a circle. Usually means circulation of the blood—**circulate** *vi, vt.* **circulatory** *adj.* ⊃ pulmonary circulation, systemic circulation.

circulation of bile ⊃ enterohepatic circulation.

circulation of blood the passage of blood from heart to arteries to capillaries to veins and back to heart. The flow of blood from the left side of the heart through the systemic circulation via the branching arterial system to the capillary beds in all tissues except the lungs, and returning in the veins to the right side of the heart; thence in the pulmonary circulation, via the pulmonary artery and its branches to the alveolar capillaries in the lungs, and carrying oxygenated blood back to the left side of the heart via the pulmonary veins (Figure C.10). The pulmonary circulation is characterized

C
D

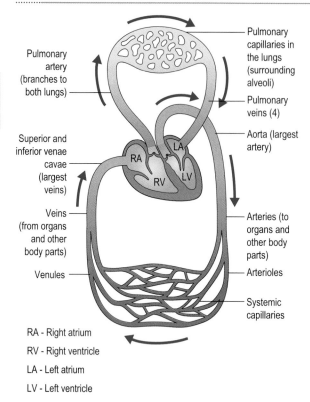

Pulmonary artery (branches to both lungs)

Pulmonary capillaries in the lungs (surrounding alveoli)

Pulmonary veins (4)

Aorta (largest artery)

Superior and inferior venae cavae (largest veins)

RA
LA
RV
LV

Veins (from organs and other body parts)

Arteries (to organs and other body parts)

Venules

Arterioles

Systemic capillaries

RA - Right atrium

RV - Right ventricle

LA - Left atrium

LV - Left ventricle

C.10 Systemic and pulmonary circulation (reproduced from Brooker and Waugh 2007 with permission).

by operating at lower pressure than in the systemic circulation.

circulation of cerebrospinal fluid takes place from the ventricles of the brain to the cisterna magna, whence the fluid bathes the surface of the brain and the spinal cord, including its central canal. It is absorbed into the blood in the cerebral venous sinuses.

circulation of lymph lymph is collected from the tissue spaces and passed in the lymphatic capillaries, vessels, nodes and ducts to be returned to the bloodstream.

circulus arteriosus circle of Willis. The circular arrangement of blood vessels formed by an anastomosis of the arteries supplying the greater part of arterial blood to the brain (Figure C.11). It is located at the base of the brain and is formed from the two internal carotid and two vertebral arteries. The vertebral arteries unite to form the basilar artery. Anteriorly there are two anterior cerebral arteries and an anterior communicationg artery. Posteriorly there are two posterior cerbral arteries and two posterior communicating arteries. This arrangement ensures that most of the brain receives sufficient blood if one of the arteries is occluded or otherwise damaged and during excessive movement of the neck and head.

circum- a prefix that means 'around', e.g. *circumduction*.

circumcision *n* excision of the prepuce or foreskin of the penis, usually for religious or cultural reasons. The operation is sometimes required for phimosis or paraphimosis. ⊃ female circumcision.

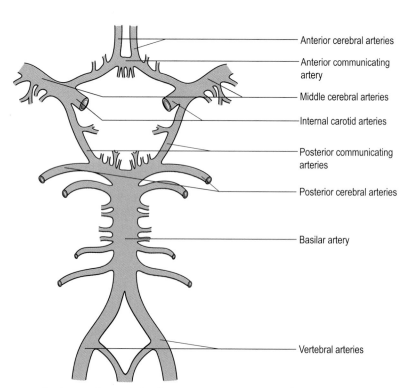

Anterior cerebral arteries

Anterior communicating artery

Middle cerebral arteries

Internal carotid arteries

Posterior communicating arteries

Posterior cerebral arteries

Basilar artery

Vertebral arteries

C.11 Circulus arteriosus (circle of Willis) (reproduced from Watson 2000 with permission).

150

circumcorneal *adj* (*syn* limbal) around the cornea.

circumduction the circular movement comprising abduction, flexion, extension and adduction, such as when the arm traces a cone in space.

circumferential clasp clasp which is continuous around a tooth.

circumferential epithelial radiofrequency ablation a technique being evaluated as a treatment for Barrett's oesophagus; it uses heat to destroy abnormal cells in the mucosal lining of the oesophagus. ⊃ Barrett's oesophagus.

circumferential wiring technique used in mandibular jaw fracture cases to immobilize the bone fragments. Stainless steel wire is passed round the lower border of the mandible from within the mouth under an anaesthetic. The ends are then tied over a splint or existing denture. ⊃ wiring.

circumoral *adj* surrounding the mouth—**circumorally** *adv*. ⊃ circumoral pallor.

circumoral pallor a pale appearance of the skin around the mouth, in contrast to the flushed cheeks. A characteristic of scarlet fever.

circumplex model any of a variety of models that have been applied to the understanding of personality, affect or other psychological domains whereby variables are arranged in two-dimensional space into a circular array and along two orthogonal axes (Figure C.12). Elements that lie close together on the circumference of the circle are more related than elements that lie further apart and elements lying in opposite positions on the axes are negatively related. For example, a popular model of exercise-induced affect conceptualizes affect as varying along two dimensions: valence (pleasant *vs* unpleasant feelings) and activation (aroused *vs* unaroused). Individuals can be located within the circumplex according to the combination of these two dimensions.

circumvallate *adj* surrounded by a raised ring or ridge, as the large circumvallate papillae at the base of the tongue.

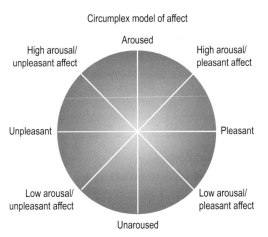

C.12 Circumplex model (reproduced from Jennett 2008 with permission).

circumvallate placenta one with a well-defined ring or edge on the fetal surface. It is formed from the chorion and amnion. ⊃ placenta circumvallata.

cirrhosis *n* hardening of an organ. There are degenerative changes in the tissues with resulting fibrosis—**cirrhotic** *adj*.

cirrhosis of liver increasing in prosperous countries, liver (hepatic) cirrhosis can occur at any age and often causes prolonged morbidity. It frequently manifests itself in younger adults and is an important cause of premature death. Damage to liver cells can be from: (a) alcohol misuse; (b) chronic viruses (hepatitis B or C); (c) non-alcoholic fatty liver disease; (d) immune—primary sclerosing cholangitis, autoimmune liver disease; (e) biliary—primary biliary cirrhosis, cystic fibrosis; (f) genetic—haemochromatosis, α_1-antitrypsin deficiency, Wilson's disease; and (g) crytogenic (unknown cause). World-wide, the most common causes of cirrhosis are viral hepatitis and prolonged excessive alcohol consumption. Clinical features vary greatly and include any combination of the following: hepatomegaly (although the liver may also be small), jaundice, ascites, circulatory changes (spider telangiectasia, palmar erythema, cyanosis), endocrine changes (loss of libido, hair loss; men may have gynaecomastia, testicular atrophy, erectile dysfunction; women may have breast atrophy, irregular menses, amenorrhoea), haemorrhagic tendency (bruises, purpura, epistaxis, menorrhagia), hepatic portal hypertension (splenomegaly, collateral vessels, oesophageal varices with bleeding, fetor hepaticus), hepatic encephalopathy, pigmentation, digital clubbing. Cirrhosis may be entirely asymptomatic; in life it may be found incidentally at surgery or may be associated with minimal features such as isolated hepatomegaly. Frequent complaints include weakness, fatigue, muscle cramps, weight loss and non-specific digestive symptoms such as anorexia, nausea, vomiting and upper abdominal discomfort. Otherwise, clinical features are due mainly to hepatic insufficiency and hepatic portal hypertension.

CIS *abbr* carcinoma in situ.

cis configuration means on the same side. In chemistry, describes an isomerism in which the two substituent groups are on the same side of a carbon–carbon double bond. ⊃ trans configuration.

cissa desire for extraordinary or abnormal foods. Also known as allotriophagy, cittosis and pica.

cisterna *n* any closed space serving as a reservoir for a body fluid—**cisternal** *adj*.

cisterna chyli the pear-shaped commencement of the thoracic duct. It receives lymph.

cisterna magna a subarachnoid space in the cleft between the cerebellum and medulla oblongata

cisternal puncture insertion of a special hollow needle with stylet between the occiput and atlas, into the cisterna magna. One method of obtaining cerebrospinal fluid but rarely used. ⊃ lumbar puncture.

cisternography an investigation that involves the injection of a radionuclide into the subarachnoid space via a lumbar puncture. The radionuclide concentrates in the ventricles of the brain and demonstrates communicating hydrocephalus, cerebrospinal fluid shunts and fistulae.

cistron the smallest fragment of DNA that codes for the amino acids needed for a particular polypeptide chain during the synthesis of proteins. A cistron is in effect a gene.

citizenship the range of human and civil rights and obligations expected in a democratic society. These include the right of participation in the selection of a legitimate government, the right of free speech and the right of religious freedom. Obligations include obeying the law and taking the needs of others into consideration.

citric acid an organic acid present in citrus fruit such as lemons and oranges and in soft fruit.

citric acid cycle ➲ Krebs' cycle.

citrullinaemia *n* an inborn error of metabolism in which the enzyme argininosuccinic acid synthetase is deficient. Untreated, the presence of citrulline and other metabolites in the blood results in seizures, poor development and learning disability. Management includes a low-protein diet, which still provides the essential nutrients.

citrulline an amino acid formed as a metabolic intermediate in the urea cycle. It is normally converted to arginine.

cittosis desire for extraordinary or abnormal foods. Also known as allotriophagy, cissa and pica.

City University test (CUT) ➲ pseudoisochromatic plates.

CIVD *abbr* cold-induced vasodilatation. ➲ ice/cold therapy.

civil action proceedings brought in the civil courts.

civil law law relating to non-criminal matters. Deals with the conduct and conflicts between people. A person (the claimant) who has suffered a perceived wrong can seek redress by bringing an action or claim in the civil courts. The claim may be settled with an award of financial compensation or damages, or an order (injunction) banning an unlawful act or an order that requires some action. The burden of proof in civil cases is lower than in criminal cases; the claimant must prove the facts 'on a balance of probabilities'.

civil wrong act or omission which can be pursued in the civil courts by the person who has suffered the wrong.

CJD *abbr* Creutzfeldt–Jakob disease.

CK *abbr* creatine kinase.

clamps a variety of instruments with locking handles used in surgical procedures. They can be used to grip, hold or compress vessels, ducts or organs. Used mainly to compress blood vessels to prevent bleeding (haemostasis).

clap *n* a slang term for gonorrhoea.

CLAPC *abbr* contact lens associated papillary conjunctivitis.

clapping/cupping ➲ chest percussion.

Clark level (W Clark, American dermatologist, b. 1924) vertical levels (anatomical landmarks) through the skin, used to determine the stage of a melanoma. ➲ Breslow's depth.

Clarke's test compression of the patella with simultaneous resisted knee extension. It is commonly used as a test of chondromalacia patellae.

clasp in dentistry, a metal holding device such as is used for partial dentures and orthodontic appliances, in the form of a cast-metal arm or wire which acts as a direct retainer and stabilizer by contacting and surrounding, or partially surrounding, an abutment tooth. ➲ Adams' arrowhead clasp, circumferential clasp, gingivally approaching clasp, occlusally approaching clasp, orthodontic clasp, reciprocal clasp.

clasp-knife phenomenon a pathological manifestation of the stretch reflex in which great resistance at the beginning of passive movement suddenly collapses; characteristic of spasticity.

class *n* the socioeconomic diversity between groups that explains the differences in their level of wealth and influence. ➲ social class.

classical caesarean section involves a vertical incision in the body of the uterus, the scar of which is more likely to rupture in subsequent pregnancies.

classical conditioning ➲ conditioning.

classical polyarteritis nodosa ➲ polyarteritis nodosa (PAN).

classical scattering ➲ coherent scattering.

classified person an employee who is likely to receive a dose of ionizing radiation which exceeds three-tenths of any relevant dose limit.

claudication *n* literally limping. Cramp-like pain caused by interference with the blood supply to the muscles of the legs. The cause may be arterial spasm or atheromatous disease of the vessels themselves. ➲ intermittent claudication, peripheral vascular disease.

claustrophobia *n* a fear of enclosed spaces—**claustrophobic** *adj*.

clavicle *n* the collar bone, an S-shaped long bone. It articulates with the manubrium of the sternum at the sternoclavicular joint and forms the acromioclavicular joint with the acromium process of the scapula. It provides the only bony link between the upper limb and the axial skeleton—**clavicular** *adj*. ➲ Colour Section Figure 2.

clavus *n* a corn. ➲ callus.

claw-foot *adj, n* ➲ pes cavus.

claw-hand *n* the hand is flexed and contracted giving a claw-like appearance; the condition may be due to injury or disease.

clean intermittent self-catheterization ➲ intermittent self-catheterization.

cleanser *n, adj* (describes) agents that have cleansing properties. Substances such as cetrimide are both disinfectant and cleansing. Used to remove dirt, grease, etc., from the skin or wounds, and for removing crusts and other debris from skin lesions.

clearance *n* the ability of the kidney to remove a specific substance from the blood. *renal clearance* used to measure glomerular filtration rate (GFR) and kidney function by calculating the volume of blood cleared of a substance such as creatinine or inulin, in a given time, usually one minute. ➲ creatinine, inulin.

clearance (dental context) in the UK a *full clearance* is the removal of all teeth from a patient's mouth. *upper clearance* the act of removing all the upper teeth. *lower clearance* the act of removing all the lower teeth. In the USA the term means to remove calculus from the teeth. ➲ scaling.

C
D

clear-based films in radiography, films that have no dye in the base and have a low base fog and are particularly suited for ultrasound imaging.

clearing time in radiography, the time taken in a fixer solution for the unexposed areas of the film to become transparent.

cleavage the mitotic divisions that occur immediately following fertilization of the oocyte (ovum). This converts the single-celled zygote into a ball of cells that will eventually develop into an embryo with the capability to differentiate into many different cell types.

cleft lip a congenital condition (sometimes involving the maxillary bone) in which there is a developmental defect along the normal lines of fusion of the lip tissues, causing a cleft or fissure. May be uni- or bilateral and is frequently associated with cleft palate. Gives rise to feeding problems. Treatment is by orthodontic therapy and/or surgery.

cleft palate congenital failure of fusion between the right and left palatal processes. May be partial or complete and is often associated with cleft lip. It gives rise to feeding, dental and speech problems. It is usually surgically repaired when the infant is around 6 months old. The child may need regular reviews and referral to a speech and language therapist and or an orthodontist as necessary.

cleidocranial dysostosis a rare congenital condition in which there is faulty ossification of the cranial bones and the partial or complete absence of the clavicles (collar bones). It is characterized by abnormalities of the skull, teeth, jaws and clavicle. Orally there is usually a high arched palate, underdeveloped maxilla and sinuses, and frequently a cleft palate. The shedding of the primary teeth is retarded with consequent delay in the eruption of the permanent teeth.

cleidotomy rare procedure involving division of the fetal clavicles with scissors to facilitate delivery of obstructed shoulders, e.g. in a large anacephalic fetus.

client-centred practice the process of collaboration between the therapist, the client and relevant others, in which therapeutic goals and interventions are negotiated and agreed.

client quality the client's/patient's view of how well the service or product provides what is expected by the clients or patients.

Clifton Assessment Procedures for the Elderly (CAPE) a series of tests which measure cognitive function in older people as well as behavioural aspects.

climacteric *n* the perimenopause and postmenopause. A period of time during which ovarian activity declines and eventually ceases. In most women it occurs between the mid forties to mid fifties. The cessation of menstruation is a single event during the climacteric. ➲ menopause.

climbing fibres the axon of an inferior olive neuron that innervates a Purkinje cell of the cerebellum. ➲ mossy fibre.

clinical *adj* pertaining to a clinic. Describes the practical observation and treatment of sick persons as opposed to theoretical study.

clinical audit critical and systematic analysis of the quality of clinical care and treatment. It includes diagnostic procedures, treatment, resource use and outputs including quality of life.

clinical crown an anatomical term for that part of a tooth which is visible above the gingival margin at any stage of eruption.

clinical dental technician a member of the dental team who, in addition to the remit of a dental technician, is able to provide clinically a range of removable dental appliances and complete dentures, without prior review by a dentist.

clinical directorate system of devolved management responsible for its own budgeting and use of resources, in which a clinical specialty such as obstetrics and gynaecology is headed by a director who is usually a medical practitioner and assisted by a senior midwife/nurse and a business manager.

clinical effectiveness the extent to which an intervention produces an overall health benefit in routine clinical practice.

clinical efficacy the extent to which an intervention achieves its desired effect when studied under controlled research conditions.

clinical governance the framework within which all NHS organizations are accountable for their services, and are required to operate an active programme of continuous quality improvement within an overall, coherent framework of cost-effective service delivery.

clinical guidelines systematically developed statements that help the practitioner and patient in making decisions about care. ➲ evidence-based practice.

clinical iceberg a way of illustrating the idea that most illness and disease is submerged and does not come to the attention of medical professionals.

clinical maxwellian view system an instrument designed to measure visual acuity by using a narrow beam or beams of light focused within the entrance pupil of the eye. The location of the beam or beams within the pupil can be controlled by the clinician. Such an instrument is valuable to assess acuity when part of the pupil is obstructed by a cataract or other opacity as the beam or beams of light can be directed to enter the eye through an area of the pupil where there is no opacity, thus providing an estimate of the visual acuity unaffected by optical image degradation. The results can contribute to the decision as to whether removal of a cataract will be beneficial. There are several types of these instruments: the Potential Acuity Meter (PAM) which focuses a single beam of light in the pupil and a letter chart onto the retina. Others focus two beams of light in the pupil and a grating which can be produced on the retina by interference (if the two sources are coherent). This method is called laser interferometry. Examples of these are the Lotmar Visometer and the IRAS Randwal Interferometer which are referred to as clinical interferometers. ➲ blue field entoptoscope, cataract, coherent sources, hyperacuity, interferometer.

clinical nurse specialist a nurse who develops skills in relation to a particular group of patients, e.g. those with a stoma, mental health problems, or with diabetes, or a particular area of nursing, e.g. infection control or intravenous therapy.

client quality the patient's view of how well the service or product provides what is expected by the patient.

clinical reasoning the range of cognitive processes and mental strategies that are used by the therapist (or other practitioner) in identifying, framing and solving problems and in making decisions about what course of action to take at each stage of an intervention.

clinical risk index for babies professional scoring tool used to assess initial neonatal risks and for comparing performance of one neonatal intensive care unit with another.

clinical root that portion of the anatomical root of a tooth attached to the alveolar bone by the periodontal ligament.

clinical supervision assists practitioners to develop skills, knowledge and professional values throughout their working life, and implies a requirement to reflect and measure risk. Increases the understanding of what it is to be an accountable practitioner and aims to achieve the delivery of high-quality healthcare.

clinical target volume the total treatment field in relation to the tumour in radiotherapy.

clinical thermometer previously, glass and mercury thermometers of various types were used. These have mostly been replaced by safer alternatives, such as electronic probes, e.g. tympanic membrane thermometers, and single-use thermometers.

clinician in medicine, nursing, midwifery and other health professions context, the word is used to designate those individuals who work with patients/clients as opposed to those who indirectly serve patients, e.g. managers and educators. Also used to describe all those involved directly with patient care, such as podiatrists, dentists, dieticians, doctors, medical laboratory scientific officers, optists, physiotherapists, radiographers and speech and language therapists, etc.

clinodactyly incurving of a finger, usually the fifth.

clip-on ⊃ clipover.

clipover (*syn* clip-on, fit-over, trial lens clip) an attachment holding an auxiliary lens or lenses (an add, a prism or a tint) in front of spectacles by spring action. There are many (albeit similar) types of clips which fit over one lens of a pair of spectacles (e.g. Bernell clip, Bommarito clip, Halberg clip, Jannelli clip). They are used extensively in the refraction of low vision patients.

clitoridectomy *n* the surgical removal of the clitoris. ⊃ circumcision.

clitoriditis *n* inflammation of the clitoris.

clitoris *n* a small erectile organ situated at anterior junction of the labia minora. Involved in the female sexual response. Homologous to the corpora cavenosa of the penis.

clitoromegaly an abnormal enlargement of the clitoris. It may lead to confusion regarding a newborn's gender. ⊃ congenital adrenal hyperplasia.

CLL *abbr* chronic lymphocytic leukaemia.

CLO *abbr* columnar-lined oesophagus.   ⊃   Barrett's oesophagus.

cloaca *n* in osteomyelitis, the opening through the involucrum which discharges pus—**cloacal** *adj.*

clone *n* a group of genetically identical cells or organisms derived from a single cell or common ancestor. ⊃ monoclonal.

clonic *adj* ⊃ clonus.

clonogenic cell a cell that can proliferate into a colony of genetically identical cells.

clonorchiasis infestation with the hepatobiliary (liver and biliary tract) fluke, *Clonorchis sinensis*. The adult fluke lives in the bile ducts and, while it may produce cholangitis, hepatitis and jaundice, it may be asymptomatic or be blamed for vague digestive symptoms. ⊃ fluke.

Clonorchis sinensis (*syn Opisthorchis sinensis*) the Chinese or Oriental fluke. A trematode fluke that infests the liver and biliary tract. It is caused by eating raw or partially cooked fish, or smoked, salted, or pickled fish. Can cause serious liver and biliary disease. ⊃ fluke.

clonus *n* a series of intermittent muscular contractions and relaxations. ⊃ tonic *opp*, ankle clonus—**clonic** *adj*, **clonicity** *n*. ⊃ myoclonus.

closed-angle glaucoma ⊃ angle-closure glaucoma(ACG).

closed bite a bite where there is a reduction in the occlusal vertical dimension.

closed chain exercise ⊃ closed kinetic chain.

closed fracture ⊃ fracture.

closed kinetic chain in sports medicine or physiotherapy describes a motion during which the distal segment of the extremity is weight bearing or otherwise fixed, e.g. a squat (lower limb) or a press up (upper limb) (Figure C.13). ⊃ kinematic chain exercises, open kinetic chain.

closed loop control in motor control, a movement in which sensory feedback is involved in its planning, execution and modification. For example, when catching a ball, visual information concerning its trajectory is used to guide one's grasp. ⊃ open-loop control.

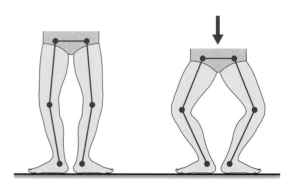

C.13 **Closed kinetic chain** (reproduced from Porter 2005 with permission).

closed manipulation a method of manually realigning broken bones under general anaesthetic without the use of surgery.

closed reduction ➲ fracture reduction.

closed skill ➲ skill.

closed urinary drainage system a means of draining urine via a self-retaining catheter into a drainage bag, which has a non-return valve at the inlet and may have a drainage tap as an outlet.

Clostridium n a genus of bacteria. They are large Gram-positive, spore-forming anaerobic bacilli of the Bacillaceae family. They are present as commensals in the gut of animals and humans and as saprophytes in the soil. Many species are pathogenic due to the production of exotoxins, e.g. *Clostridium botulinum* (botulism); *C. difficile* ➲ antibiotic-associated colitis (antibiotic-associated diarrhoea, pseudomembranous colitis); *C. perfringens*, previously known as *C. welchii* (gas gangrene); *C. tetani* (tetanus).

clotting time the time taken for blood to form a clot. Also called coagulation time. Mostly replaced by the activated partial thromboplastin time.

clotting/coagulation factors ➲ coagulation, factor.

cloverleaf pupil a cloverleaf-shaped pupil. It is associated with iritis (anterior uveitis) and the formation of posterior synechiae.

Cloward's spots areas of referred pain in the thoracic spine, close to the scapula, often found in association with degenerative cervical spine disorders.

CLPC *abbr* contact lens papillary conjunctivitis.

clubbing enlargement of the distal phalanges particularly of the fingers. There is thickening and broadening of the bulbous fleshy portion of the fingers under the nails. (Figure C.14). The cause is not known but it occurs in people who have reduced oxygen tension in the blood such as with chronic heart and/or some lung diseases. Also occurs in

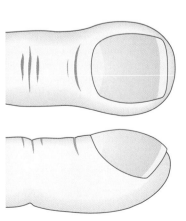

C.14 Finger clubbing (reproduced from Boon et al 2006 with permission).

other conditions, e.g. biliary cirrhosis, colitis, etc., and as a benign congenital abnormality.

club foot n a congenital malformation, either unilateral or bilateral. ➲ talipes.

clue cell epithelial cell to whose surface Gram-variable, Gram-negative and Gram-positive bacteria adhere. A microscopical feature of bacterial vaginosis.

clumping n agglutination.

clunk test a test used to diagnose a glenoid tear affecting the shoulder.

cluster headache an uncommon migraine varient, which occurs more often in men. There is intense unilateral pain, commonly around an eye. It may be accompanied by Horner's syndrome with nasal congestion and a watering eye. The attacks of excruciating pain occur in clusters and typically last for a short time (30–90 min).

Clutton's joints (H Clutton, British surgeon, 1850–1909) joints which show symmetrical swelling usually painless, the knees often being involved. Associated with congenital syphilis.

-clysis a suffix that means 'infusion, injection', e.g. *proctoclysis*.

CML *abbr* chronic myeloid leukaemia.

CMO *abbr* **1**. chief medical officer. **2**. cystoid macular oedema.

CMV *abbr* **1**. controlled mandatory ventilation. **2**. cytomegalovirus.

CNHC *abbr* Complementary and Natural Healthcare Council.

CNMES *abbr* chronic neuromuscular electrical stimulation.

CNO *abbr* chief nursing officer

CNS *abbr* **1**. central nervous system. **2**. clinical nurse specialist.

CNV *abbr* choroidal neovascularization.

CO *abbr* cardiac output.

co- a prefix that means 'together', e.g. *coalesce*.

coach's finger in sports medicine a colloquial term used to describe the dislocation of the proximal interphalangeal joint leading to a fixed flexion deformity of the finger.

coaction effects ➲ social facilitation.

coagulant a drug or other agent that causes blood to coagulate (clot).

coagulase n an enzyme produced by some staphylococci: it coagulates plasma and is used to classify staphylococci as coagulase-negative or coagulase-positive.

coagulate to become clotted or to cause coagulation.

coagulation the third of four overlapping processes involved in haemostasis. Coagulation (clotting) occurs through a series of complex reactions that use enzyme cascade amplification to start the formation of a fibrin clot to stop bleeding. There are two pathways/systems, intrinsic and extrinsic, which converge to follow a common final pathway. Coagulation starts when platelets break down, tissue is damaged and thromboplastins are released. Various factors are involved in coagulation: I, fibrinogen; II, prothrombin; III, thromboplastin (tissue factor); IV, calcium ions; V, labile factor (proaccelerin); VII, stable factor (proconvertin); VIII, antihaemophilic factor (AHF); IX, Christmas factor; X, Stuart–Prower factor; XI, plasma thromboplastin antecedent; XII, Hageman factor; and XIII, fibrin-stabilizing factor. During the final common pathway, inactive prothrombin is converted to thrombin, the active enzyme. Thrombin converts soluble fibrinogen to insoluble fibrin, which forms a network of fibres in which blood cells are caught to form the clot. ⊃ fibrinolysis, haemostasis, platelet plug, vasoconstriction.

coagulation time ⊃ clotting time.

coalesce *vi* to grow together; to unite into a mass. Often used to describe the development of a skin eruption, when discrete areas of affected skin coalesce to form sheets of a similar appearance—**coalescence** *n*, **coalescent** *adj*.

coal-miners/worker's pneumoconiosis ⊃ anthracosis.

coal tar obtained by the distillation of coal. Used in topical preparations for the treatment of psoriasis and eczema.

coarctation *n* contraction, stricture, narrowing; applied to a vessel or canal.

coarctation of the aorta congenital narrowing of the aorta, commonly affecting the area just after the origin of the left subclavian artery. ⊃ Colour Section Figure 25.

coarse tremor violent trembling.

coated lens (*syn* anti-reflection coated lens, bloomed lens) a lens upon which is deposited an evaporated film consisting of a metallic salt such as magnesium fluoride, about one-quarter as thick as a wavelength of light. This film reduces, by interference, the amount of light reflected by the surfaces and to some extent the amount of stray light reflected inside the lens. With multilayer coating the lens can selectively reflect radiations and increase transmission. All coated lenses show some residual colour. ⊃ antireflection coating, bandpass filter, coating, Fresnel's formula, ghost image.

coating (*syn* blooming) the process of depositing a thin film of transparent material on the surface of an optical element (e.g. lens, mirror, prism) for the purpose of decreasing or increasing reflection. Reflection from specific wavelengths can be reduced or eliminated by varying the thickness of the film and by multilayer coating. ⊃ antireflection coating, bandpass filter, coated lens, Fresnel's formula, white body.

coating weight the amount of phosphor per unit volume in a radiographic intensifying screen.

Coats' disease (G Coats, British ophthalmologist, 1876–1915) (*syn* exudative retinitis, retinitis exudativa externa) a progressive retinal exudative retinopathy/retinitis occurring predominantly in young males. It is characterized by retinal exudates and usually associated with malformation of retinal blood vessels and appears as a whitish fundus reflex. Subretinal haemorrhages are frequent and eventually retinal detachment may occur. The main symptom is a decrease in central or peripheral vision. ⊃ leukocoria.

cobalamins *npl* a group of molecules containing a cobalt atom and four pyrrole units. A constituent of substances having vitamin B_{12} activity. ⊃ cyanocobalamin.

cobalt (Co) *n* 1. an essential trace element, utilized as a constituent of vitamin B_{12} (cobalamins). Required for healthy red blood cell production and proper neurological function. 2. metallic element used to form many alloys and pigments. *cobalt chromium* an alloy of cobalt and chromium used in the construction of some partial dentures and other prostheses. The alloy is hard, resistant to corrosion and has a high melting point.

cobalt-60 (^{60}Co) a radioactive isotope of cobalt which is used as a source of radiation in teletherapy.

cobalt-blue glass ⊃ cobalt lens.

cobalt lens (*syn* cobalt-blue glass) a lens which absorbs the central region of the visible spectrum and only transmits the red and blue ends of the spectrum. It is sometimes used in the testing of ametropia, since a light source located at 1.4 m from the eye will form, in an emmetropic eye viewing it through a cobalt lens, two equal circles superimposed on the retina and the subject will report seeing a purple circle. A person with hypermetropia (hyperopia) will see a blue spot surrounded by a red annulus and a person with myopia will see a red spot surrounded by a blue annulus. An appropriate spherical lens placed in front of the eye which changes the appearance to a purple circle represents the spherical refractive correction. ⊃ duochrome test.

cobalt unit a radiotherapy machine housing the isotope cobalt-60, the resultant radiation delivers the maximum dose below the skin surface and therefore reduces the likelihood of skin reactions.

COC *abbr* combined oral contraceptive.

cocaine *n* a powerful local anaesthetic obtained from the leaves of the coca plant. It is a Class A controlled drug which is highly addictive and subject to considerable criminal misuse. Toxic, especially to the brain; may cause agitation, disorientation and convulsions. Cocaine is on the World Anti-doping Agency list of banned substances in sport. ⊃ crack cocaine, Appendix 5.

cocarcinogen a substance that potentiates the action of a carcinogen.

Coccidioides a genus of pathogenic fungi, such as *C. immitis*, that causes coccidioidomycosis and pneumonia.

coccidioidomycosis *n* infection caused by the fungus *Coccidioides immitis*. The infection is endemic in Central and South America, and the southern United States, and causes opportunistic infection in people with HIV disease. Inhalation of fungal spores leads initially to a flu-like illness but the secondary infection is characterized by dyspnoea, haemoptysis, fever, weight loss, skin lesions, and bone and joint pain.

coccobacilli *npl* rod-shaped bacteria which are slightly elongated. They include the genus *Brucella* and the bacterium *Haemophilus influenzae*.

coccus *n* a spherical bacterium, such as staphylococcus—**cocci** *pl*, **coccal**, **coccoid** *adj*.

-coccus a suffix that means 'spherical cell', e.g. *streptococcus*.

coccydynia *n* pain in the region of the coccyx, usually the result of a fall.

coccygeal nerves the last of the spinal nerves. ⊃ Colour Section Figure 11.

coccygeal plexus a small plexus formed by a branch of the fourth sacral nerve, the fifth sacral nerve (S4–S5) and the coccygeal spinal nerves (Co). The nerves from this plexus supply the skin in the area of the coccyx and the levators ani and coccygeus muscles of the pelvic floor and the external anal sphincter.

coccygectomy *n* surgical removal of the coccyx.

coccygeus one of two muscles arising from the ischial spines, inserted into the lateral borders of the sacrum and coccyx, and forming part of the pelvic floor. Also called ischiococcygeus.

coccyx *n* the last bone of the vertebral column. It is a small triangular bone composed of four or five rudimentary vertebrae, cartilaginous at birth, ossification and fusion being completed at about the 30th year. Its broad base articulates with the sacrum above—**coccygeal** *adj*. ⊃ vertebra (typical), Colour Section Figure 3.

cochlea *n* a spiral canal resembling the interior of a snail shell, in the anterior part of the bony labyrinth of the inner ear. It contains the organ of Corti (the organ of hearing)—**cochlear** *adj*. ⊃ Colour Section Figure 13.

cochlear aqueduct a tiny canal between the scala tympani of the inner ear and the subarachnoid space. Any perilymph within the aqueduct will drain into the cerebrospinal fluid.

cochlear implant the insertion of an electronic device into the cochlea of people who have profound deafness or severe hearing loss. It comprises an external microphone; a transmitter outside the skin; a receiver/stimulator inserted under the skin behind the ear; and electrodes that feed through to the cochlea from where impulses are conveyed to the brain.

Cochrane collaboration (A Cochrane, British epidemiologist, 1909–1988) a not-for-profit organization that provides accurate, authorative systematic literature reviews of healthcare interventions. Important in the provision of evidence-based practice. The major product of the Collaboration is the Cochrane Database of Systematic Reviews, published quarterly as part of The Cochrane Library. Those who prepare the reviews are mostly healthcare professionals who volunteer to work in one of the many Collaborative Review Groups, with editorial teams overseeing the preparation and maintenance of the reviews, as well as application of the rigorous quality standards for which Cochrane Reviews have become known.

Cochrane review (A Cochrane) a systematic review of the evidence relating to a particular health problem or healthcare intervention, produced by the Cochrane Collaboration. Available, via the internet, as part of the Cochrane Library.

Cockayne's syndrome (E Cockayne, British physician, 1880–1956) a condition with autosomal recessive inheritance. It is characterized by dwarfism, learning disability, retinal atrophy, hearing impairment and a type of epidermolysis bullosa. ⊃ epidermolysis bullosa.

Cockcroft–Walton generator utilizes a number of rectifiers and capacitors, connected in series to produce a fully rectified voltage with less than 0.2% ripple. A single unit can cover the low-energy therapeutic X-ray range but for medium energy radiotherapy machines two units are used back to back. A voltage multiplier circuit using diodes and capacitors used in some X-ray generator systems.

cockup splint a splint that immobilizes the wrist joint while leaving the fingers free.

code of conduct/practice the guidelines setting out how healthcare professionals should fulfil their roles, duties, obligations and responsibilities, such as those produced by the statutory bodies whose functions are to regulate the standards, registration and practice of healthcare professionals, e.g. Health Professions Council, General Medical Council.

codes of ethics guidelines that are produced by professional organizations that assist practitioners with ethical decision making and give guidance on duties, responsibilities and appropriate standards of behaviour. The guidance given is broad and general and does not absolve professionals from the responsibility of making ethical decisions. There is a tendency for ethical codes to mix genuine ethical issues with issues concerned with professional image and etiquette such as upholding the good name of the profession.

Codex Alimentarius part of the United Nations FAO/WHO Commission on Food Standards used since the early 1960s to simplify and integrate food standards for international adoption.

Codman's exercises (E Codman, American surgeon, 1869–1940) gentle exercises that aim to restore normal range of motion in the shoulders and arms.

codominance in genetics, a situation where both alleles of a pair are expressed in the phenotype of the heterozygous individual. For example, if the A and B blood group alleles are inherited the person will have type AB blood.

codon *n* in genetics, the three complementary bases carried by messenger RNA (mRNA) involved in protein synthesis (transcription stage). ⊃ anticodon.

coefficient of elasticity ⊃ modulus of elasticity.

coefficient of friction ⊃ friction.

coefficient of restitution dimensionless (no units) number representing the ratio of separation velocity to approach velocity after impact of two bodies or objects. Dependent on elasticity of the objects. For example, during impact of a golf ball on a golf club face, ball and club deform and then rebound, which means that the ball increases its velocity. Likewise with a ball and racquet strings.

coeliac *adj* relating to the abdominal cavity; applied to arteries and a nerve plexus.

coeliac disease (*syn* gluten-induced enteropathy) due to intolerance to the protein gluten in wheat and rye, the gliadin fraction being harmful. This results in subtotal villous atrophy of the mucosa of the small intestine and the malabsorption syndrome. Symptoms may become apparent at any age or patients may be asymptomatic. Treatment is with gluten-free diet.

coelom the body cavity in the embryo.

coenzyme *n* a non-protein enzyme activator, e.g. substances formed from the B vitamins.

coenzyme A a cofactor important in metabolism, it is a carrier molecule for acyl groups. ⊃ acetyl coenzyme A.

coenzyme Q10 ⊃ ubiquinone.

cofactor substances, such as metal ions and coenzymes, required for certain enzyme activation.

coffee ground vomit vomit containing blood, which in its partially digested state resembles coffee grounds. Indicative of slow upper gastrointestinal bleeding ⊃ haematemesis.

coffin spring in orthodontics, heavy gauge wire placed posteriorly between two separated sections of a removable orthodontic appliance to exert pressure causing expansion or contraction.

CoG *acron* centre of gravity.

Cogan's lid twitch sign (D Cogan, American opthalmologist, 1908–1993) a twitch of the upper eyelid in an eye with ptosis when the patient is asked to look in the primary position following a downward look. The eyelid then returns to its ptosis position. This condition occurs in myasthenia gravis. ⊃ myasthenia gravis, ptosis.

Cogan's microcystic epithelial dystrophy (D Cogan) (*syn* anterior membrane dystrophy, bleb-like dystrophy, epithelial basement membrane dystrophy, fingerprint dystrophy) a bilateral corneal dystrophy located in the corneal epithelium and occurring most commonly in females. It is characterized by variously shaped greyish-white microcysts and debris which vary in shape and location over time, coalescing with other microcysts, forming lines, and resembling a fingerprint pattern. Symptoms are minimal and vision is unaffected unless the lesions are in the central zone of the cornea. The condition may be associated with recurrent epithelial erosions which cause pain, lacrimation, photophobia and blurred vision. Management normally includes artificial tears, patching and antibiotics and occasionally therapeutic soft contact lenses for frequent or more severe types. ⊃ corneal erosion, therapeutic soft contact lens.

Cogan's syndrome (D Cogan) keratitis and iridocyclitis occurring with veritigo, tinnitus and sensorineural deafness. Also describes a form of oculomotor apraxia that occurs during childhood. ⊃ interstitial keratitis.

cognition *n* awareness; one of the three aspects of mind. A general term that describes all the psychological processes by which individuals gain awareness and knowledge about their environment. Includes perception, reasoning, understanding, making judgements, problem-solving—**cognitive** *adj*. ⊃ affection, conation.

cognitive anxiety the cognitive elements of anxiety including worrying thoughts, fear of failure and negative expectations about performance, also known as cognitive stress. ⊃ anxiety.

cognitive behaviour therapy (CBT) a form of psychotherapy combining elements of cognitive therapy and behaviour therapy which aims to modify dysfunctional patterns of thinking and self-talk in order to resolve a variety of mental and social health problems. Also known as cognitive behaviour modification.

cognitive dissonance a subjective state of psychological tension induced when a person holds two or more cognitions that are inconsistent. For example, a person might hold the cognition that they enjoy smoking whilst at the same time believing that smoking is harmful to their health. It is proposed that such dissonant states motivate one of three kinds of behaviour to reduce the dissonance: changing one of the cognitions (e.g. by changing the behaviour associated with it, such as giving up smoking); dismissing the importance of one of the cognitions (e.g. by telling oneself that smoking is not that bad for one's health); or by adding a justifying cognition (e.g. by telling oneself that one does not smoke too much).

cognitive interview a structured interview designed to facilitate recall of an event by the use of a variety of memory-enhancing techniques.

cognitive psychology the study of the development of intelligence, language, thought processes, and the acquisition, storage and use of knowledge.

cognitive restructuring ⊃ reframing.

cognitive skills ⊃ mental skills.

cognitive stress ⊃ anxiety, anxiety disorder.

cognitive therapy an approach to the psychological treatment of some mental health problems such as anxiety-related disorders. It is based on the assumption that some mental health problems are the result of faulty or distorted perceptions of oneself or the world. It concentrates on, and is effective through, modifying dysfunctional beliefs, correcting the individual's cognitive dysfunctions, such as errors in thinking and poor problem-solving. ⊃ cognitive behaviour therapy.

cogwheel rigidity a pathological pattern of resistance to passive movement of a limb which yields in a series of jerks, observed in people with Parkinson's disease, thought to be due to tremor superimposed on lead pipe rigidity.

coherent scattering when a photon interacts with an electron, is deflected from its path but does not lose energy. ⊃ elastic scattering.

coherent sources if light beams from two independent sources reach the same point in space, there is no fixed relationship between the phases of the two light beams and they will not combine to form interference effects. Such light waves are called *incoherent*. If, on the other hand, the two light beams are superimposed after reaching the same point by different paths but are both radiated from one point of a source, interference effects will be seen because the phase difference in the two beams is constant. The two virtual sources from which these two beams are apparently coming are called *coherent sources* and any rays in which there is a constant phase difference are called *coherent rays*. Prior to the advent of the laser, the only way in which one could obtain coherent rays was by dividing the light coming from a point source into two parts. ⊃ holography, interference, Young's experiment.

cohesion property exhibited by some materials whereby their constituent molecules are attracted to each other and resist separation.

cohesive gold foil ⊃ foil.

cohort *n* a group of people who have some common feature or characteristic, e.g. year group at university.

cohort study a longtitudinal research study in which the groups studied belong to a population that shares a common feature, such as occupation.

coil **1**. single or multiple loops of wire designed to produce (or transmit) a magnetic field when current flows through the wire or measure (or receive) an induced voltage in the loop caused by a changing magnetic field. ⊃ induction, transformer. **2**. an object wound in a spiral.

coil spring winder an orthodontic instrument consisting of a sleeved spindle around which a fine stainless steel wire is wound to form a coil spring.

coitus *n* insertion of the erect penis into the vagina; the act of sexual intercourse or copulation.

coitus interruptus removal from the vagina of the penis before ejaculation of semen as a means of contraception. The method is considered unsatisfactory as it is not only unreliable but can lead to sexual disharmony—**coital** *adj.*

col- a prefix that means either 'together', e.g. collateral or 'colon', e.g. *colonoscopy.*

col small depression in the inter-dental gingiva below the inter-proximal contact area between the buccal and lingual papillae.

cold abscess one occurring in the course of such chronic inflammation as may be due to *Mycobacterium tuberculosis*. ⊃ abscess.

cold agglutinin disease ⊃ autoimmune haemolytic anaemia.

cold curing resin ⊃ resin.

cold flow *n* ⊃ creep.

cold-induced vasodilatation (CIVD) ⊃ ice/cold therapy.

cold injury cellular damage and impaired function occurring as a result of exposure to cold environmental temperatures.

cold sore *n* oral herpes simplex.

cold spot a term used in radionuclide imaging when a lower than expected quantity of radiation is detected.

cold water processor in radiography, an automatic film processor that only has a cold water supply and is more energy efficient than processors that use hot and cold water.

colectomy *n* excision of part or the whole of the colon.

coli- a prefix that means 'bowel', e.g. *coliform.*

colic *n* severe pain resulting from periodic spasm in an abdominal organ—**colicky** *adj.* ⊃ biliary colic, intestinal colic, renal colic, uterine colic.

coliform *adj* describes any of the enterobacteria (intestinal bacteria) such as *Escherichia coli.*

colitis *n* inflammation of the colon. May be acute or chronic, and may be accompanied by ulcerative lesions. ⊃ inflammatory bowel disease, ulcerative colitis.

collagen *n* the main protein constituent of white fibrous tissue of skin, tendon, bone, cartilage and all connective tissue.

collagen diseases ⊃ connective tissue diseases.

collagen fibres found in connective tissue, the most common tissue in the body. They do not stretch.

collapse **1**. the 'falling in' of a hollow organ or vessel, e.g. collapse of lung from change of air pressure inside or outside the organ (pneumothorax). **2**. a vague term describing physical or nervous prostration.

collapsing pulse also known as Corrigan's pulse. The water-hammer pulse of aortic regurgitation with high initial upthrust which quickly falls away.

collar **1**. a band that encircles any neck-like structure. **2**. in dentistry, a narrow metal band that fits over an abutment or forms part of a post and core construction.

collar-bone *n* the clavicle.

collarette the line separating the pupillary zone and the ciliary zone which can be seen on the anterior surface of the iris. In the normal iris it is an irregular circular line lying about 1.5 mm from the pupillary margin. ⊃ Fuchs' crypts, iris, minor arterial circle of the iris.

collateral circulation an alternative route provided for the blood by secondary blood vessels when a primary vessel is blocked.

Colles' fracture (A Colles, Irish surgeon/anatomist, 1773–1843) a break at the lower end of the radius following a fall on the outstretched hand. The backward displacement of the hand produces the 'dinner fork' deformity (Figure C.15). A common fracture in older women and associated with osteoporosis.

collet in dentistry, that area of a prosthesis which serves as a collar round the neck of a tooth.

Collier's sign unilateral, or more commonly bilateral, eyelid retraction that exposes an unusual amount of the sclera of the eye above and below the iris; it gives the person a frightened or startled expression. It is due to a midbrain lesion. ⊃ Parinaud's syndrome.

collimate literally to make parallel. Restriction of the X-ray beam to a particular area. In computed tomography (CT) scanning this may be done pre-patient or pre and post patient. ⊃ post-patient collimation, pre-patient collimation.

collimation the restriction of the size of an X-ray beam to minimize radiation dosage.

collimator a device used in radiography and radiotherapy to reduce the size and shape of a beam of radiation, thereby reducing the scatter radiation. This enhances the quality of the radiographic image and deceases the radiation dose needed to investigate or treat a patient. ⊃ converging collimator, multi-leaf collimation, parallel-hole collimator, pinhole collimator, primary collimator, secondary collimators.

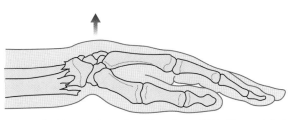

C.15 **Colles' fracture** (reproduced from Porter 2005 with permission).

collision in computing, a collision occurs if two computers access the network at the same time.

collision sport individual or team sports during which the participants use their bodies to deter or block opponents, thereby relying on the physical dominance of one athlete over another.

collodion *n* a solution forming a flexible film on the skin. Previously used as a protective dressing.

collodion baby an infant born with skin resembling a scaly paper-like membrane.

colloid *n* glue-like. A non-crystalline chemical; diffusible but not soluble in water; unable to pass through a semipermeable membrane. Some drugs can be prepared in their colloidal form.

colloid bodies ➲ drusen.

colloid degeneration that which results in the formation of gelatinous material, as in tumours.

colloid goitre enlargement of the thyroid gland caused by the presence of viscid, iodine-containing colloid within the gland.

colloid solutions ones containing large particles (solutes). When administered intravenously they stay in the blood because they are too large to pass through capillary membranes. Colloid solutions, such as human albumin solution or those containing gelatin or starch, are used to increase blood volume. ➲ crystalloid solutions.

collutorium, collutory a mouthwash or gargle.

coloboma *n* a congenital, pathological or operative anomaly in which a portion of the structure of the eye is lacking, e.g. coloboma of the choroid, coloboma of the eyelid, coloboma of the iris, coloboma of the lens, etc. Congenital colobomas are discontinuities in a layer of the eyeball caused by failure of closure of the optic fissure; they are usually located inferiorly (Figure C.16). *coloboma of the optic disc* is characterized by a glistening, white excavation, decentred inferiorly. It is sometimes confounded with glaucomatous cupping, especially when it is accompanied by a field defect. The condition is often associated with microphthalmia and several syndromes (e.g. Edward's syndrome, Patau's syndrome) —**colobomata** *pl*.

colon *n* the large bowel. Extends from the caecum to the rectum and anal canal. ➲ Colour Section Figure 18b. For descriptive purposes the colon is divided into the caecum, ascending colon, transverse colon, descending colon, sigmoid colon,

rectum and anal canal. The *caecum* is a dilated region which has a blind end inferiorly and is continuous with the ascending colon superiorly. Just below the junction of the two the ileocaecal valve opens from the ileum. The vermiform appendix is a fine tube, closed at one end, which leads from the caecum. It is usually about 13 cm long and has the same structure as the walls of the colon but contains more lymphoid tissue. The *ascending colon* passes upwards from the caecum to the level of the liver where it curves acutely across at the right colonic (hepatic) flexure to become the transverse colon. This is a loop of colon which extends across the abdominal cavity in front of the duodenum and the stomach to the area of the spleen where it forms the left colonic (splenic) flexure and curves acutely downwards to become the descending colon. The *descending colon* passes down the left side of the abdominal cavity then curves towards the midline. After it enters the true pelvis it is known as the *sigmoid colon*. This part describes an S-shaped curve in the pelvis then continues downwards to become the rectum. The *rectum* is a slightly dilated section of the colon about 13 cm long in an adult. It leads from the sigmoid colon and terminates in the anal canal. The anal canal is a short passage about 3.8 cm long in the adult and leads from the rectum to the exterior. Two sphincter muscles control the anus; the internal sphincter, consisting of smooth muscle fibres, is under the control of the autonomic nervous system and the external sphincter, formed by skeletal muscle, is usually under voluntary control from early childhood. ➲ flexure; *spasmodic colon* ➲ megacolon—**colonic** *adj*.

colonic washout/lavage the washing out of the colon with water or other fluid. ➲ bowel washout.

colonization *n* the installation of micro-organisms in a specific environment, such as a body site with only minimal or no response. There is no disease or symptoms, but colonization leads to the formation of a reservoir of micro-organisms that may be a source of infection—**colonize** *vt*.

colonoscopy *n* use of an endoscope to view, biopsy or photograph the colonic mucosa—**colonoscopic** *adj*, **colonoscopically** *adv*.

colony *n* a mass of bacteria resulting from the multiplication of one or more micro-organisms. Containing many millions of individual micro-organisms it may be visible to the unaided eye; its physical features are often characteristic of the species.

colony stimulating factors (CSF) growth factors, such as granulocyte colony-stimulating factor (G-CSF), which cause blood stem cells to produce a specific white blood cell line.

colorectal *adj* pertaining to the colon and the rectum.

colorimeter an instrument that uses colour intensity to measure the amount of a substance present. Can be used to determine the level of haemoglobin in the blood.

colostomy *n* a surgically established fistula between the colon and the surface of the abdomen; a type of stoma that discharges faeces. May be temporary, such as when an anastomosis (join) in the bowel is healing, or permanent when the colon and rectum have been removed.

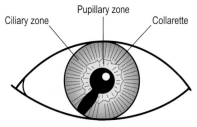

Ciliary zone Pupillary zone Collarette

C.16 Coloboma (reproduced from Millodot 2004 with permission).

colostrum *n* fluid secreted by the breasts during late pregnancy and in the 3 days following parturition. It is a rich source of maternal immunoglobulins, and has a different composition to true milk, i.e. more protein, but less fat and lactose.

colotomy *n* incision into the colon.

colour an aspect of visual perception, characterized by the attributes of hue, brightness and saturation, and resulting from stimulation of the retina by visible photopic light levels.

colour blindness a lay term for dysfunction in or absence of a photoreceptor subtype (cones) stimulated by red, green or blue light, leading to difficulty distinguishing between certain colours. ⊃ achromatopsia, chloropsia, chromatopsia, cyanopsia, defective colour vision, deuteranopia, dichromatic vision, erythropsia, hemichromatopsia, xanthopsia.

colour depth the maximum number of colours a computer monitor is able to display and is determined by the bit depth, with 16 giving good colour and 24 giving true colour.

colour flow Doppler the simultaneous ultrasound display of anatomical and flow information. Anatomy is shown as a grey scale image and blood flow in colour, for example, blood flowing towards the transducer is usually in red and away from the transducer is usually displayed in blue.

colour mixture the production of a colour by mixing two or more lights of different colours (additive colour mixture) or two or more pigments (subtractive colour mixture). ⊃ complementary colour, primary colours.

colour sensitizing in radiography, increasing the spectral sensitivity of the film by adding impurities to the film emulsion. ⊃ spectral sensitizing.

colour stereoscopy ⊃ chromostereopsis.

colour triangle ⊃ chromaticity diagram.

colour vision colour vision is dependent on the integrity of the retinal cone cell. The eye is stimulated by light of wavelengths between 400–750 nm and this represents an ability to recognize many separate hues. The short wavelengths of light are from the violet end of the spectrum and the long wavelengths are from the red end. The eye is not equally sensitive to the three primary light colours, and if blue light, green light and red light are matched for intensity, the red light is perceived as being the brightest and the blue light appears to be the dimmest. The difference in sensitivity to red light and green light is not very great, but the eye is considerably less sensitive to blue light. This difference may reflect differences in photopigment absorption properties, differences in amounts of photopigment contained in the three cone types, or differences in the numbers and distribution of the three cone types. It is known that blue cones are not found in some areas and therefore colour vision is dichromatic here. Furthermore, the pattern of distribution and connection of blue cones is more diffuse and shows greater convergence onto ganglion cells than that shown by the red and green cones. ⊃ cone, defective colour vision, Hering's theory of colour vision, visual pigment, Young–Helmholtz theory.

colour wool test ⊃ wool test.

coloured filter ⊃ interference filter.

colpalgia pain in the vagina.

colpitis *n* inflammation of the vagina.

colp/o- a prefix that means 'vagina', e.g. *colposcopy*.

colpocele *n* protrusion or prolapse of either the bladder or rectum so that it presses on either the anterior or the posterior vaginal wall.

colpocentesis *n* withdrawal of fluid from the vagina, as in haematocolpos.

colpocystitis inflammation of the vagina and urinary bladder.

colpohysterectomy *n* removal of the uterus through the vagina. ⊃ hysterectomy.

colpoperineorrhaphy *n* the surgical repair of vaginal injury and deficient perineum.

colpophotography *n* filming the cervix using a camera and colposcope.

colporrhaphy *n* surgical repair of the vagina. An anterior colporrhaphy repairs a cystocele and a posterior colporrhaphy repairs a rectocele.

colposcope *n* a binocular instrument used to obtain a high power view of the cervix in cases of abnormal cervical smears. Used for diagnostic procedures and local treatments to the cervix—**colposcopy** *n*, **colposcopically** *adv*.

colposuspension *n* surgical procedure involving placement of sutures between the vaginal fornices and the pectineal ligaments for genuine stress incontinence.

colpotomy *n* incision of the vaginal wall. A posterior colpotomy drains an abscess in the rectovaginal pouch (pouch of Douglas) through the vagina.

columnar epithelium this is formed by a single layer of cells, rectangular in shape, on a basement membrane (Figure E.7, p. 264). It is found lining the organs of the alimentary tract and consists of a mixture of cells; some absorb the products of digestion and others secrete mucus. Mucus is a thick sticky substance secreted by modified columnar cells called goblet cells. ⊃ epithelium, goblet cells.

CoM *abbr* centre of mass.

com- a prefix that means 'together', e.g. commissure .

coma *n* **1.** a state of unrousable unconsciousness, the severity of which can be assessed by corneal and pupillary reflexes and withdrawal responses to painful stimuli. ⊃ Glasgow Coma Scale—**comatose** *adj*. **2.** a monochromatic aberration of an optical system produced when the incident light beam makes an angle with the optical axis. The image appears like a comet with the tail pointing towards the axis. ⊃ aplanatic lens, monochromatic aberration, optical aberration, sine condition.

combination lens a lens made from two different materials; usually a rigid centre portion made from gas-permeable material surrounded by a soft peripheral flange of hydroxyethyl methacrylate (HEMA) material. It is used in the management of keratoconus, irregular astigmatism, etc. Few such lenses exist at present. ⊃ piggyback lens.

combination therapy in physiotherapy practice, the simultaneous application of ultrasound with electrical stimulation is the most commonly applied form of combination therapy, though the term is not exclusive to this combination. The most frequently combined modalities are ultrasound with interferential therapy, or sometimes ultrasound with diadynamic current.

combined B- and T-lymphocyte immune deficiencies ⊃ severe combined immunodeficiency.

combined oral contraceptive (COC) pill is very widely used and the most effective method of preventing conception. It is a combination of an oestrogen and a progestogen and acts in several ways. The oestrogens used are ethinylestradiol or mestranol (a few). The progestogens used are desogestrel, gestodene, ethynodiol, levonorgestrel or norethisterone. The mechanism of action is: (a) the oestrogen inhibits the release of follicle stimulating hormone (FSH) by a negative feedback effect, thus inhibiting follicular development; (b) the progestogen inhibits the release of luteinizing hormone (LH), so that ovulation cannot occur. Together, the two chemicals render the endometrium hostile to implantation; (c) both chemicals may upset the coordinated contractions of the uterine (fallopian) tubes, uterus and cervix. Usually the composition of the pill is unaltered throughout the monthly course, but there are a few preparations in which pills of varying composition are given sequentially: namely the *biphasic* and *triphasic* preparations. Of the many preparations now available the most effective and widely used are those in which both an oestrogen and a progestrogen are given throughout the course, with a failure rate of less than 0.5 per 100 women years.

combined test first trimester Down's syndrome screening test performed via assessment of maternal blood for pregnancy associated plasma protein (PAPP-A) and nuchal translucency (NT) ultrasound scan. The results are combined with the maternal age-related Down's syndrome risk to produce an overall result, which gives improved sensitivity and specificity over that of NT or PAPP-A screening alone. ⊃ nuchal translucency, pregnancy associated plasma protein.

comedone, comedo *n* a worm-like cast formed of sebum which occupies the outlet of a hair follicle in the skin, a feature of acne vulgaris. Open comedones have a black colour because of pigmentation (blackheads). Closed comedones are closed cysts (whiteheads)—**comedones** *pl*.

comet tail artefact multiple reflections of ultrasound usually produced by small artefacts, usually in the gallbladder wall.

commensals *npl* parasitic micro-organisms adapted to grow on the skin and mucous surfaces of the host, forming part of the normal flora. Some commensals are potentially pathogenic, e.g. bowel commensals that include *Escherichia coli* cause urinary tract infection.

comminuted fracture ⊃ fracture.

Commission for Health Improvement ⊃ Healthcare Commission, Care Quality Commission.

Commission on Human Medicines (CHM) established in 2005, it combines the functions and roles of the Committee on Safety of Medicines and the Medicines Commission.

The Commission advises ministers and the licensing authority about the safety, quality and efficacy of human medicines; promotes the collection and investigation of information about adverse drug reactions; and considers representation from applicants or licence holders. ⊃ adverse drug reactions, European Medicines Agency, yellow card reporting.

commissioning *n* a complex process that aims to ensure that a specific population has an appropriate level of service provision. The stages include a needs assessment that is used to determine priorities, taking into account the overall national policy guidance from government. On completion of this process, an appropriate range of services are purchased from relevant providers. The final stage is evaluation.

commissioning tests (radiotherapy) checks made on new radiotherapy equipment to ensure that it is safe to treat patients; tests include radiation protection, leakage, accuracy of beam direction devices, beam modalities and output dose calibration.

commissure 1. the site at which two anatomical structures unite, such as the labia. **2.** a connecting structure such as the band of nervous tissue connecting the two sides of the brain, the corpus callosum, or the spinal cord.

committed dose the absorbed dose of radiation an individual receives as the result of the intake of radioactive material.

Committee on Safety of Medicines (CSM) in the UK the body that previously monitored drug safety and advised the licensing authority regarding the safety, efficacy and quality of medicines. ⊃ Commission on Human Medicines.

common bile duct the bile duct formed by the merging of the right and left hepatic ducts and the cystic duct. It conveys bile to the duodenum. It is joined by the pancreatic duct at the opening into the duodenum (hepatopancreatic ampulla). ⊃ Colour Section Figure 18b.

common law case law. Law made by judges rather than by statute.

common peroneal nerve ⊃ peroneal nerve.

common variable immunodeficiency (CVID) one of the primary antibody deficiency syndromes, presenting in children or adulthood and associated with recurrent infections, autoimmunity and an increased risk of malignancy.

common warts are due to human papilloma virus (HPV) and usually occur on the hands or feet.

communal hygiene embraces all measures taken to supply the community with pure food and water, good sanitation, housing, etc.

communicable *adj* transmissible directly or indirectly from one person to another, such as an infectious disease.

communicating *n* the exchange of information between at least two individuals. Most often accomplished by the use of language: verbal, which can be spoken, hand written, word processed/typed, printed or displayed on a screen; or non-verbal, which allows the transmission of attitudes, values and beliefs that are appropriate and relevant to the information exchanged.

community *n* a social group defined by geographical boundaries and/or common values and interests. Also implies shared relationships, lifestyles, and a greater frequency and intimacy of contact among those who live in a community.

community care the care and support of individuals in community settings. Such care is delivered by health and social care professionals and unpaid carers such as family and neighbours. The community or primary care setting is increasingly important in the development and delivery of health services. ⊃ Primary Care Trust.

community dentistry dental public health. That branch of dentistry that is concerned with the prevention and control of dental diseases and the promotion of oral health.

community development 1. whole-community initiatives that enable individual communities to assess their particular needs, such as for health care, and decide on what action should be taken by the community. In the broadest sense, community care services could be provided by the 'community' on a voluntary basis, or by statutory organizations in residential settings or by professionals working in the community. For example, the development of adequate provision of (community) care services such as the treatment of long term sick and frail people in their own homes. This can be interpreted to cover personal, domiciliary and social care as well as medical or nursing care. The community includes family, friends and community self-help. 2. an approach to intervention in which the therapist works in partnership with the community to bring about change.

community nurse generic term which describes those nurses based in the community and concerned with the health, well-being and care of people in their homes and other community settings. Community nurses include district nurses, community psychiatric (mental health) nurses (CPN) or learning disability nurses, community children's nurses, school nurses, practice nurses or family planning nurses. ⊃ specialist community public health nurse.

community periodontal index of treatment needs (CPITN) ⊃ index (dental).

community therapists therapists including occupational therapists, physiotherapists and speech and language therapists who work in community settings, for example based in a health centre or attached to a primary care team. They visit clients in their own homes, schools, care homes, etc., to undertake assessments or to provide professional services such as the provision of adaptive equipment and adaptations to the environment.

comorbidity *n* coexistence of two or more diseases.

compact disk (CD) a 120-mm sheet of aluminium covered with a layer of acetate and with a polycarbonate backing. Used in computing to store data in digital form which can be read by a laser.

compact disk read-only memory (CDROM) an object for storing computer data; once the data have been stored they cannot be changed.

compact disk re-writer (CDRW) an object for storing computer data; the data can be re-written if required.

compactor in dentistry, 1. a condenser; an instrument that aids the process of joining or packing a material, e.g. in gold foil restorations. 2. in endodontics, a small, engine-driven instrument, akin to a Hedstroem file but with reverse flutes, used to feed in, plasticize and compact gutta percha in a root canal. Sometimes called a McSpadden Compactor® after its inventor.

comparative study research study that compares two separate populations.

compartment syndrome 1. if muscles become damaged or inflamed at the time of injury and intramuscular pressure builds up with no means of release, necrosis (death) of the tissues from ischaemia (lack of blood supply) may result. It is defined as the condition in which high pressure within a closed fascial sheath reduces capillary blood perfusion below the level necessary for tissue viability. Compartment syndrome is seen most commonly in the anterior tibial muscles or forearm muscles. It may follow traumatic injury, or compression caused by bandages or plaster casts. The signs and symptoms of the affected limb are: pallor, pain, pulseless, paraesthesiae and paralysis (known as the '5Ps'). Treatment revolves primarily around accurate diagnosis, by observing limb colour, sensation and movement after any injury or surgery; and elevation and cooling of the limb. Surgical decompression (fasciotomy) may be necessary as an emergency procedure. ⊃ anterior compartment syndrome, lateral compartment syndrome, posterior compartment syndrome, Volkmann's ischaemic contracture. 2. in sports medicine a term used to describe a condition where increased intramuscular pressure brought on by activity impedes blood flow and function of the tissues within that intermuscular compartment. ⊃ chronic exertional compartment syndrome.

compatibility *n* suitability; congruity. The ability of a substance to mix with another without unfavourable results, e.g. two medicines, blood plasma and cells—**compatible** *adj*.

compensated glaucoma ⊃ open-angle glaucoma.

compensated heterophoria any heterophoria which does not give rise to symptoms or to suppression. ⊃ uncompensated heterophoria.

compensating curve curvature of the plane of dentures made to compensate the effects of the movements of the condyles of the mandible and to obtain a balanced occlusion.

compensating extraction removal of a tooth from one quadrant following the extraction of a tooth from the opposing quadrant in order to preserve buccal occlusion and prevent the development of a malocclusion.

compensating prism ⊃ associated heterophoria, relieving prism.

compensation *n* 1. a mental mechanism, employed by a person to cover up a weakness, by exaggerating a more socially acceptable behaviour trait. 2. the state of counterbalancing a functional or structural defect, e.g. cardiac compensation, where the heart muscle enlarges by hypertrophy to maintain cardiac output in chronic heart failure.

compensatory techniques adaptive techniques using relatively intact skills to compensate for physical or cognitive deficits in performance. This might include the provision of adaptive equipment, adaptations to the environment, or new methods of performing tasks.

competence ability to perform a task or activity skilfully.

competent lips lips which provide a seal when the mandible and the facial muscles are at rest.

competitive sport anxiety the anxiety response to competitive sporting situations or to sport competition in general. ⊃ anxiety.

complement *n* a system of over 20 serum proteins involved in cytolysis, opsonization, phagocytosis and anaphylaxis. Several cascading systems, including the classical pathway (antibody mediated), alternate pathway and a third pathway, converge resulting in the formation of a multimeric (composed of multiple parts) membrane attack complex capable of lysing cells. The system is regulated by numerous proteins and cell surface receptors.

complement fixation test (CFT) a test in which complement fixation is found. It indicates the presence of a particular specific antigen.

complement pathway deficiencies genetic deficiencies of almost all the complement pathway proteins have been described. The major feature of deficiencies of the classical and alternative pathway components is recurrent infection with encapsulated bacteria, particularly *Neisseria* species. This reflects the importance of the complement membrane attack complex in defence against these bacteria. In addition, genetic deficiencies of the classical complement pathway (C1, C2 and C4) are associated with a high prevalence of autoimmune disease, particularly severe systemic lupus erythematosus (SLE). In contrast to other complement deficiencies, mannose-binding lectin deficiency is very common (5% of the population). Individuals with complete mannose-binding lectin deficiency have an increased incidence of bacterial infections if subjected to an additional cause of immune compromise, such as prematurity or chemotherapy. However, the importance of this deficiency in otherwise healthy individuals remains uncertain. Deficiency of the regulatory protein C1 inhibitor is not associated with recurrent infections, but causes recurrent angioedema. Complement C3 and C4 are the only complement components that are routinely measured. Screening for complement deficiencies is performed using functional tests of the complement pathway. The classical haemolytic pathway 50 (CH50), also known as total haemolytic complement (THC), involves adding the patient's serum to sheep red blood cells (SRBC) coated with anti-SRBC antibody. If the cells lyse, the serum contains all the components of the classical and membrane attack pathways. Absence of lysis indicates a complement deficiency and should be followed by measurement of individual components. However, complement proteins degrade rapidly at room temperature, and the most common cause of an absent CH50 is delay in transportation of the sample to the laboratory. There is no definitive treatment of complement deficiencies. Patients are at risk of meningococcal and other infections, and should be vaccinated with meningococcal, pneumococcal and *Haemophilus influenzae* B vaccines in order to boost their adaptive immune responses. Life-long prophylactic penicillin to prevent meningococcal infection is also recommended. At-risk family members should be screened for complement deficiencies with functional complement assays.

complemental air the extra air that can be drawn into the lungs during deep inspiration.

complementary and alternative medicine (CAM) health-related therapies that are not considered to be part of conventional (allopathic) medicine. Some therapies offered in conjunction with conventional medical interventions are described as complementary, e.g. aromatherapy. Whereas others, such as osteopathy, provide diagnostic information and are offered as an alternative to conventional medicine. ⊃ integrated medicine.

complementary colour one of a pair of colours which, when mixed additively, produce white or grey (that is to say an achromatic sensation). For example, green is the complementary colour of red-purple and yellow is the complementary colour of blue.

complementary feeds feeds given to a neonate in addition to a planned feeding regimen, whether breast or bottle feeds.

complementation describes a situation when a relative deficiency of an amino acid in one protein is compensated by a relative surplus from another protein consumed in the same meal.

complete abortion ⊃ complete miscarriage.

complete amelia absence of both arms and legs.

complete blood count (CBC) the calculation of the cellular elements of blood.

complete denture correct term for full denture which replaces the whole of the normal dentition in the dental arch with the exception of the third molars. Describes a denture replacing the entire maxillary or mandibular dentition.

completed stroke describes a stroke in which the focal deficit persists and is not progressing.

complete miscarriage the entire contents of the uterus are expelled.

complete mole ⊃ molar pregnancy.

complete partial seizure (*syn* psychomotor epilepsy, temporal lobe epilepsy) ⊃ epilepsy.

complex *n* a psychodynamic term meaning a series of emotionally charged ideas repressed because they conflict with ideas acceptable to the individual. ⊃ Electra complex, Oedipus complex.

complex cavity ⊃ cavity (dental).

complex composite odontome ⊃ odontome.

complex regional pain syndrome (CRPS) a chronic pain syndrome of which there are two types, 1 and 2.

complex regional pain syndrome (CRPS) 1 a chronic pain syndrome caused by a chronic nerve problem that follows an injury. It most often affects the arms or legs. Previously known as reflex sympathetic dystrophy.

complex regional pain syndrome (CRPS) 2 a chronic pain syndrome that causes excruciating pain, resulting from an identified injury to a cutaneous nerve. Previously known as algodystrophy, causalgia, Sudeck's atrophy.

compliance *n* **1.** the acceptance (understanding and remembering) of and following health (medical) advice or specific regimens of treatment. Two main models are proposed for health professionals to increase compliance when giving health (medical) advice: (a) the adherence model suggesting that there are patient centred factors that affect the process of following advice, such as locus of control, social support and disruption of life style; (b) the cognitive model where compliance is influenced by the level of understanding, satisfaction with and recall of the advice given. **2.** the ability to distend, such as the lungs. ⊃ concordance, lung compliance.

complicated fracture ⊃ fracture.

complication *n* in medicine, an accident or second disease arising in the course of a primary disease; may worsen the prognosis or can be fatal.

component vaccines ⊃ vaccines.

composite substance made up of separate parts.

composite odontome ⊃ odontome.

composite resin composite filling material. In dentistry, resin-based filling material consisting of an organic polymer resin matrix such as methyl methacrylate or polymer precursors to which has been added an inert inorganic filler material such as quartz, aluminium silicate or glass. Polymerization of the matrix may be initiated by chemical catalysts or visible light. A type of tooth-coloured resin used in restorative dentistry to fill defects in teeth. They are generally hard wearing, resistant to fractures and easy to polish. ⊃ filling material, hybrid composite resin, microfilled composite resin.

compos mentis of sound mind. Mentally competent is now the preferred term.

compound *n* a substance composed of two or more elements, chemically combined in a definitive proportion to form a new substance which displays new properties.

compound filters beam-hardening filters made of tin, copper and aluminium used in radiotherapy. To be effective the filters must be fitted in the correct order, with those of the highest atom number nearest the target and the lowest nearest the patient.

compound impression material ⊃ impression material.

compound (open) fracture ⊃ fracture.

compound presentation rare complication of labour in which more than one part of the fetus presents, e.g. head and hand; head and foot; breech, hand and cord.

comprehension *n* mental grasp of ideas, their meaning and relationships.

compress *n* usually refers to a folded pad of lint, gauze or other material used to arrest haemorrhage or apply pressure, cold, heat, moisture or medication. Used to reduce swelling or pain, such as a cold compress to ease a headache.

compression *n* the state of being compressed. Pressing or squeezing together. ⊃ intermittent pneumatic compression.

compression band in radiography, an immobilization device which also displaces body tissue laterally and therefore enables a reduction in radiographic exposure factors and as a result radiation dose to the patient.

compression bone plate perforated metal plate designed to exert a compressing force at the site of a fracture.

compression fracture ⊃ fracture.

compression garment these may be used following burns or other problems such as lymphoedema, they work by fitting the body very closely and exerting pressure on the tissues to limit build up of fluid.

compression therapy various types of bandaging technique, or compression hoisery used in the management of venous leg ulceration. The application of graduated linear compression to the lower limb reduces venous hypertension and increases venous return from the legs. Compression hosiery can be used to prevent venous leg ulcers occurring where there is venous insufficiency, or to reduce the risk of ulcer recurrence. ⊃ anti-embolism hoisery/stockings, venous ulcer.

compressive force a force applied along the length of a structure, causing the tissues to approximate one another. This force can be caused by muscular activity, weight bearing, gravity or external loading down the length of the bone. It is necessary for the development and growth of bone. If a large compressive force, which surpasses the stress limits of the structure, is applied, a fracture will occur.

compromise *n* in psychoanalysis, a mental mechanism whereby a conflict is evaded by disguising the repressed wish to make it acceptable in consciousness.

Compton scattering (effect) takes place when an X-ray photon collides with an electron and in doing so gives up some of its energy to the electron resulting in a decrease in the unit mass and an increase in the photon energy.

compulsion *n* an urge to carry out an act, recognized to be irrational. Resisting the urge leads to increasing tension which is only relieved by carrying out the act.

computed axial tomography (CAT) ⊃ computed tomography (CT).

computed radiography the use of digital imaging in imaging departments. ⊃ digital imaging.

computed tomography (CT) also known as computed axial tomography. Computer-constructed imaging technique of a thin slice through the body, derived from X-ray absorption data collected during a circular scanning motion.

computed tomography angiography contrast agent injected intravenously into an arm vein during CT scanning enhances the visualization of the relevant arterial system, e.g. the cerebral circulation.

computed tomography (CT) scanner computed tomography equipment now most commonly used to produce a volume of data which can provide multi-planar sectional images of the patient using a beam of radiation that rotates continuously around the patient as they move through the path of the beam. The image is produced by a computer which measures the attenuation of radiation in the body and reconstructs images on a monitor.

C
D

165

computed tomography (CT) simulator equipment for very accurate treatment planning prior to radiotherapy comprising a CT scanner, laser positioning aids and a virtual simulation treatment planning computer.

computer algorithms instructions within computer programs which translate the raw data into a usable form.

computer vision syndrome (CVS) a condition resulting from extensive viewing of computer screens or video display terminals (VDT) or visual display units (VDU). The person may complain of eyestrain, dry red eyes, headaches, transient blurred vision or diplopia, as well as neckache or backache. The ocular symptoms are caused by continuous accommodative demands produced by the pixels or tiny dots of the computer screen that are difficult to keep in focus, unlike print on a page. Other causes are frequent saccadic eye movements, convergence demands and position of the screen. Management includes exact correction for the distance at which the VDT appears, viewing it about 10°–20° below the straight-ahead position and special dispensing.

con- a prefix that means 'together', e.g. concrescence.

conation *n* the will, desire or volition. The conscious tendency to action. One of the three aspects of mind. ➲ affection, cognition.

concealed haemorrhage (*syn* internal haemorrhage) bleeding occurring within a body structure or cavity, such as into a joint, the chest cavity or into the bowel or uterus. It is not immediately obvious and cannot be seen but will, if blood loss is excessive, eventually cause deterioration in the condition of the individual and the vital signs. Bleeding may also be revealed by events such as the passage of altered blood rectally in the form of black tarry stools (melaena), or swelling of a joint, etc. ➲ haemorrhage.

concentric *adj* having a common centre or point.

concentric contraction concentric action. The 'true' form of contraction of a muscle in which it shortens against a load (which may be only that of gravity on the relevant body part), and so does positive work. Hence concentric exercise: that in which the principal agonists act concentrically. The shortening of a muscle to pull its attachments closer together and produce movement at a joint. For example, the quadriceps femoris muscle group of the anterior and lateral thigh work concentrically to straighten the knee. ➲ eccentric action, muscle contraction.

concept *n* the abstract idea or image of the properties of a class of objects. Results from the mental process of abstracting and recombining certain qualities or characteristics of a number of ideas.

conception *n* **1.** the creation of a state of pregnancy: impregnation of the oocyte by the spermatozoon. **2.** an abstract mental idea of anything—**conceptive** *adj*.

conceptional age the age of the fetus or embryo in weeks from conception rather than from the last menstrual period—usually 2 weeks less.

conceptual framework for nursing a group of concepts which are defined and organized in such a way that they describe the author's interpretation of the highly complex activity called nursing. The framework provides the matrix in which the selected concepts are related to each other, thus providing a way of 'thinking about nursing'.

conceptual model of practice in occupational therapy practice the theoretical understanding of the significance of occupation in human life. Conceptual models develop through research and often have associated assessment frameworks and instruments that have been developed along with the conceptual model and assist in the implementation of theory into practice.

conceptus *n* the product of conception. It comprises the developing embryo/fetus and the enclosing fetal membranes throughout the developmental stages from implantation to the birth of the infant.

concha *n* any shell-like structure—**conchae** *pl*. ➲ concha auris, nasal conchae

concha auris the external part of the ear surrounding the external auditory meatus/canal.

concomitant several things occurring simultaneously such as chemotherapy and radiotherapy.

concordance *n* **1.** the expression of one or more specific physical traits in both twins. **2.** an approach to prescribing medicines and other treatments which respects the beliefs and wishes of the patient/client in determining whether a treatment should be used and how it should be used. An agreement is reached through negotiation between the patient/client and the health professional.

concrescence a growing together of structures that are normally separate. In dentistry, the growing together of two teeth after eruption, or the fusion of the roots of adjacent teeth.

concretion *n* **1.** a deposit of hard material; a calculus, such as in the kidney, gallbladder, salivary gland, etc. **2.** a mass formed of parts pressed together.

concussion *n* **1.** a condition resulting from a blow to the head characterized by headache, nausea, confusion, amnesia and visual symptoms. ➲ Glasgow Coma Scale. **2.** in dentistry, minor injury to a tooth in which the tooth is not displaced or mobile and there is no rupture of periodontal ligament fibres.

condensation *n* the process of becoming more compact, e.g. the changing of a gas to a liquid.

condensation (in dentistry) compaction of material into a smaller space to increase density. In endodontics, to compact filling material into a root canal. *cold compaction* compaction of materials by pressure alone. *warm (thermoplastic) compaction* compaction of material after warming to improve material flow and adaptation.

condenser 1. in dentistry, a hand instrument designed to pack restorative materials into a prepared tooth cavity. *automatic* or *mechanical condenser* instrument designed to supply a controlled force during the condensation of restorative materials such as amalgam or gold foil. May be spring activated or pneumatically or electrically controlled. **2.** (*syn* condensing lens) an optical system with a large aperture and small focal length used in microscopes and projectors in order to concentrate as much light as possible onto an object.

condensing lens ⊃ condenser.

condensing osteitis localized, chronic, low-grade inflammation in which abnormally dense bone is produced. Associated with the apices of non-vital teeth or with the site of the apex after extraction of the tooth.

conditioned reflex a reaction acquired by practice or repetition. A reflex in which the response occurs, not to the sensory stimulus which caused it originally, but to another stimulus which the subject has learned to associate with the original stimulus: it can be acquired by training and repetition. In Pavlov's classic experiments, dogs learned to associate the sound of a bell with the sight and smell of food: even when food was not presented, salivation occurred at the sound of a bell (I Pavlov, Russian physiologist, 1849–1936).

conditioning *n* the encouragement of new (desirable) behaviour by modification of the stimulus/response associations. *classical conditioning* where the conditioned reflex occurs in response to a neutral stimulus, i.e. a conditioned reflex. *operant conditioning* the term used when there is a programme to reward (or withhold the reward) a response each time it occurs, so that given time, it occurs more (or less) frequently. ⊃ deconditioning.

conditioning (sport and exercise context) sport and exercise usage of the term 'conditioning' often refers broadly to physical training, particularly muscle conditioning.

condom *n* a latex sheath used as a male contraceptive. It also protects both partners against sexually transmitted infections (STIs). ⊃ female condom.

condom drainage used for males suffering urinary incontinence. A modified condom with a tube attached is affixed to the penis. Urine escapes into a body-worn drainage bag, which has a clamped outlet at its base to facilitate emptying. ⊃ closed urinary drainage system.

conduct disorder characterized by repetitive behaviour that is usually evident during childhood. The behaviour neither meets the prevailing social norms nor shows consideration for the feelings and rights of other people. The child may be physically aggressive or cruel to other people or animals; damage or destroy property; tell lies or steal; and seriously disregard rules or laws. It can progress to an antisocial personality disorder in adulthood.

conduction *n* the transmission of heat, light, or sound waves through suitable media; also the passage of electrical currents and nerve impulses through body tissues—**conductivity** *n*.

conduction band an area containing electrons which are free of the nucleus of the atom and are therefore free to move around. They therefore take part in electrical conduction through the material.

conductive hearing loss/deafness partial or total hearing loss due to interruption of the conduction of sound waves from the atmosphere to the inner ear. It is usually acquired but may be congenital. Congenital causes include fixed middle ear ossicles, faulty development of part or all components of the ear (microtia, anotia), or associated with various inherited syndromes, such as Goldenhar syndrome or Treacher-Collins syndrome. The causes of acquired conductive hearing loss include: excess ear wax, foreign bodies, stenosis of the external auditory meatus caused by chronic inflammation or following surgery, otitis media with effusion ('glue ear'), perforations and other conditions affecting the tympanic membrane such as sclerosis, cholesteatoma, disruption to the contact between ossicles, otosclerosis, etc.

conductor *n* a substance or medium which transmits heat, light, sound, electric current, etc. The degree of conductivity varies, some substances being good conductors, whereas others are non-conductors.

condylar relating to or involving a condyle.

condylar axis (dental) ⊃ intercondylar axis (dental), transverse condylar axis.

condylar guide that part of an anatomical articulator which attempts to guide the replica condyles into the true condylar path known as the condylar track.

condylar joint a synovial joint that allows flexion, extension and rotation, for example, the knee joint.

condylar path path travelled by the mandibular condyle during any mandibular excursions.

condyle *n* a rounded projection situated at the end of some bones, e.g. tibia, mandible.

condylectomy surgical removal of the whole of a condyle, such as that of the mandible.

condyle of the mandible knob-shaped process on the superior aspect of the posterior border of the ramus of the mandible. It has a narrow neck expanding upwards into a head which is relatively narrow anteroposteriorly and wide from side to side. It is smooth on the articular surface. Together with the condyle on the opposite side of the head, it forms the hinge part of the temporomandibular joint system, fitting into the glenoid fossa of the temporal bone. The lateral pterygoid muscle is attached to its neck anteriorly.

condyloid resembling a knuckle.

condyloma *n* papilloma—**condylomata** *pl*, **condylomatous** *adj*.

condylomata acuminata fleshy, viral warts, caused by the human papillomavirus (HPV), affecting the genital or anal areas.

condylomata lata wart-like lesions found in moist areas of the body during early syphilis (secondary stage) of syphilis.

condylotomy sectioning of the condylar neck of the mandible without removal of the condyle.

cone in radiology. The equipment slotted into the base of a light beam diaphragm to further collimate the emergent beam of radiation.

cone *n* the photoreceptor of the retina which connects with a bipolar cell and is involved in colour vision and high visual acuity and which functions in photopic vision. The outer segment of the cell is conical in shape, except in the fovea centralis where it is rod-like. In the outer segment (i.e. the part closest to the pigment epithelium) are contained hollow discs (or lamellae), the membranes of which are joined together and are also continuous with the boundary membrane of the cone cell. The visual pigments are contained in these discs. There are three types of cones, each containing a different pigment sensitive to a different part of the light spectrum. They are referred to as long-wave-sensitive (or L-cones), medium-wave-sensitive (or M-cones) and short-wave-sensitive (or S-cones). There are about six million cones in the retina, with the greatest concentration in the macular area. ⊃ colour vision, macula, photopic vision, retina, rods, visual pigment.

cone biopsy cone-shaped excision of the cervix, performed using a colposcope, for certain stages of cervical intra-epithelial neoplasia.

confabulation *n* a symptom common in delirium when there is impairment of memory for recent events. The gaps in the patient's memory are filled in with fabrications. ⊃ amnesic syndrome, dysmnesic syndrome, Korsakoff's (Korsakov's) syndrome.

confidence interval (CI) in statistics, a level, e.g. 95%, that indicates the level of confidence that the test result, such as a mean, will occur within a specified range.

confidentiality *n* a legal and professional requirement to protect all confidential information concerning patients/clients obtained in the course of professional practice, and make disclosures only with consent, where required by specific legislation, or a court order, or where disclosure in the wider public interest is justified.

conflict *n* in psychoanalysis, the presence of two incompatible and contrasting wishes or emotions. When the conflict becomes intolerable, repression of the wishes may occur. Mental conflict and repression form the basic causes of many mental health problems and distress.

confluence *n* becoming merged; flowing together; a uniting, as of adjacent lesions of a rash.

confluence of the dural venous sinuses the wide junction or point of merger of the superior sagittal, straight and occipital sinuses with the large transverse sinuses. In obstetric practice, trauma to the fetal head from forceps, assisted breech delivery or abnormal moulding may cause bleeding into the infant's brain and cerebral palsy may result.

confocal microscope a microscope which allows viewing of cells, organisms (such as bacteria or fungi) and other structures within various tissues, in living patients. The instrument has been used to investigate and diagnose corneal disease processes, including dystrophies and infectious keratitis, or to follow corneal healing after laser or traditional surgery. It is based on focusing on a single illuminated corneal plane while the out-of-focus light above and below the plane of focus is greatly reduced. In addition, the instrument scans the object of interest by varying the plane of focus to form an image in three dimensions, of higher contrast and resolution than provided by a specular microscope. ⊃ specular microscope.

conformal therapy radiotherapy techniques that try to ensure that the dosage given to the treatment area matches exactly the size and shape of the tumour while minimizing the dosage to healthy tissue. Employs the use of a multi-leaf collimator.

conformity *n* a propensity to alter views and/or behaviour to better match the prevailing social norms in response to social pressure.

confounding factors extraneous factors, apart from the variables already allowed for, that distort research findings. ⊃ variable.

confusion *n* being out of touch with reality—associated with a clouding of consciousness. Occurs in a wide variety of mental health problems, particularly organic disorders. Acute confusional states may have an acute medical cause, such as infection, electrolyte imbalance, anaemia, inappropriate medication, etc. Chronic confusion may have an insidious onset and be caused by an unnoticed chronic condition, e.g. hypothyroidism. ⊃ acute confusional state.

confusion colours in optometry, the colours that are confused by a dichromat. The colours confused by a deuteranope, a protanope and a tritanope are not the same. For example, the deuteranope will confuse reds, greens and greys, whereas the protanope will confuse reds, oranges, blue-greens and greys. ⊃ deuteranopia, protanopia, pseudo-isochromatic plates, tritanopia.

congenital *adj* of abnormal conditions, present at birth, often genetically determined ⊃ genetic. Existing before or at birth, usually associated with a defect or disease, e.g. developmental dysplasia of the hip (DDH) (previously known as congenital dislocation of the hip [CDH]). ⊃ congenital heart disease, developmental dysplasia of the hip (DDH).

congenital adrenal hyperplasia (CAH) a group of inherited conditions characterized by excessive secretion of adrenal androgen (male) hormones. It is caused by a deficiency of one of the enzymes needed to synthesize the hormones cortisol and aldosterone. Defects in the cortisol biosynthetic pathway result in insufficiency of hormones 'distal' to the block, with impaired negative feedback and increased adrenocorticotrophic hormone (ACTH) secretion. ACTH then stimulates the production of steroids 'proximal' to the enzyme block. This produces adrenal hyperplasia and a combination of clinical features that depend on the severity and site of the defect in biosynthesis. All of these enzyme abnormalities are inherited as autosomal recessive traits. The most common enzyme defect is 21-hydroxylase deficiency. This results in impaired synthesis of cortisol and aldosterone and accumulation of 17OH-progesterone, which is then diverted to form adrenal androgens (male sex hormones). In about one-third of cases this defect is severe and presents in infancy with features of glucocorticoid deficiency (e.g. weight loss, anorexia, nausea, vomiting, shock, hypoglycaemia, dilutional hyponatraemia, hypercalcaemia), mineralocorticoid deficiency (e.g. hypotension, shock, depletional hyponatraemia, hyperkalaemia) and androgen excess (i.e. ambiguous genitalia in girls). In the other two-thirds, mineralocorticoid secretion is adequate, but there may be features of cortisol insufficiency and/or ACTH and androgen excess (including precocious pseudo-puberty). Sometimes the mildest enzyme defects are not apparent until adult life, when females may present with amenorrhoea and/or hirsutism. This is called 'non-classical' or 'late-onset' congenital adrenal hyperplasia. Defects of all the other enzymes have been described, but are much rarer. Both 17-hydroxylase and 11β-hydroxylase deficiency may produce hypertension due to excess production of 11-deoxycorticosterone, a mineralocorticoid. On investigation high levels of plasma 17OH-progesterone are found in 21-hydroxylase deficiency. In late-onset cases this may only be demonstrated after ACTH administration. To avoid salt-wasting crises in infancy, 17OH-progesterone can be routinely measured in heel prick blood spot samples taken from all infants in the first week of life. In siblings of affected children, antenatal genetic diagnosis can be made by amniocentesis or chorionic villus sampling (CVS). This allows prevention of virilization of affected female fetuses by administration of dexamethasone to the mother. The management of CAH involves the replacement of deficient corticosteroids, and also the suppression of ACTH and hence adrenal androgen production. In contrast with glucocorticoid replacement therapy in other forms of cortisol deficiency, it is usual to give 'reverse' treatment, i.e. a larger dose of a long-acting synthetic glucocorticoid just before going to bed to suppress the early morning ACTH peak, and a smaller dose in the morning. A careful balance is required between adequate suppression of adrenal androgen excess and excessive glucocorticoid replacement resulting in features of Cushing's syndrome. In children, growth velocity is the most useful measurement since either under- or over-replacement with glucocorticoids suppresses growth. In adults, clinical features (menstrual cycle, hirsutism, weight gain, blood pressure) and biochemical profiles (plasma renin activity and 17OH-progesterone levels) provide a guide. Patients with late-onset 21-hydroxylase deficiency may not require corticosteroid replacement. If hirsutism is the main problem, anti-androgen therapy may be just as effective.

congenital epulis of the newborn benign tumour of soft tissue of the mandibular or maxillary area, present at birth.

congenital glaucoma (*syn* buphthalmos, hydrophthalmos, infantile glaucoma) glaucoma occurring with developmental anomalies that are manifest at birth and interfere with the drainage of the aqueous humour causing an increase in intra-ocular pressure (IOP). This in turn causes stretching of the elastic coats of the eye, enlargement of the globe as the sclera and cornea stretch, optic atrophy, marked cupping of the optic disc and loss of vision. Most noticeable is the enlargement of the cornea. Congenital glaucoma is inherited as an autosomal recessive condition with incomplete penetrance. Glaucoma occuring after the age of about 3 years is more often referred to as juvenile glaucoma as it follows a course similar to adult glaucoma without enlargement of the globe. ⊃ luxation of the lens, Colour Section Figure 60.

congenital haemolysis inherited red cell defects of structure or metabolism may result in a chronic haemolytic state. The principal pathologies are red cell membrane defects (hereditary spherocytosis or elliptocytosis), glucose-6-phosphate dehydrogenase (G6PD) deficiency and the haemoglobinopathies (sickle cell disease, thalassaemia).

congenital hearing loss/deafness hearing loss present at birth, such as that caused by maternal rubella in the early weeks of pregnancy. Early diagnosis is essential through the use of routine screening, thus allowing treatment to commence as soon as possible. ⊃ automated auditory brainstem response (AABR) testing, otoacoustic emission (OAE) testing.

congenital heart disease (CHD) developmental abnormalities in the anatomy of the heart, resulting postnatally in imperfect circulation of blood and often manifested by murmurs, cyanosis, breathlessness, poor feeding and sweating. Congenital heart disease usually manifests in childhood but may pass unrecognized and not present until adult life. Defects which are well tolerated, e.g. atrial septal defect, may cause no symptoms until adult life or may be detected incidentally on routine examination or chest X-ray. Congenital defects that were previously fatal in childhood can now be corrected, or at least partially corrected, so that survival to adult life is the norm. Such patients may remain well for many years and subsequently re-present in later life with related problems such as arrhythmia or ventricular dysfunction. Understanding the fetal circulation helps to understand how some forms of congenital heart disease occur. The fetus has only a small flow of blood through the lungs, as it obviously does not breathe in utero. The fetal circulation therefore allows oxygenated blood from the placenta to pass directly to the left side of the heart through the foramen ovale without having to flow through the lungs ⊃ Colour Section Figure 27. Congenital defects may arise if the changes from fetal circulation to the extrauterine circulation are not properly completed. *Atrial septal defects* occur at the site of the foramen ovale. A *patent ductus arteriosus* may remain if it fails to close after birth. Failure of the aorta to develop at the point of the aortic isthmus and where the ductus arteriosus attaches can lead to narrowing or *coarctation of the aorta*. In fetal development, the heart develops as a single tube which folds back on itself and then divides into two separate circulations. Failure of septation can lead to some forms of *atrial and ventricular septal defect*. Failure of alignment of the great vessels with the ventricles contributes to *transposition of the great arteries, tetralogy of Fallot* and *truncus arteriosus*. The incidence of haemodynamically significant congenital cardiac abnormalities is about 0.8% of live births; ventricular septal defects account for 30% of all CHDs. Maternal infection or exposure to drugs or toxins may cause congenital heart disease. Maternal rubella infection is associated with persistent ductus arteriosus, pulmonary valvular and/or artery stenosis, and atrial septal defect. Maternal alcohol misuse is associated with septal defects, and maternal lupus erythematosus with congenital complete heart block. Genetic or chromosomal abnormalities such as Down's syndrome may cause septal defects, and gene defects have also been identified as causing specific abnormalities, e.g. Marfan's and DiGeorge's (deletion in chromosome 22q) syndromes. Symptoms may be absent, or the infant/child may be breathless or fail to attain normal growth and development. All degrees of severity occur. Some defects are not compatible with extrauterine life, or only for a short time. Clinical signs vary with the anatomical lesion. Murmurs, thrills or signs of cardiomegaly may be present. In coarctation of the aorta, radiofemoral delay may be noted. Tall stature with long limbs and lens dislocation may be obvious in Marfan's syndrome. Features of other congenital conditions such as Down's syndrome, may also be apparent. Cerebrovascular accidents (strokes) and cerebral abscesses are complications of severe cyanotic congenital disease. Early diagnosis is important because many types of congenital heart disease are amenable to surgical treatment, but this opportunity may be lost if secondary changes such as pulmonary vascular damage occur. Central cyanosis of cardiac origin occurs when desaturated blood enters the systemic circulation without passing through the lungs (i.e. a right-to-left shunt). In the neonate, the most common cause is transposition of the great arteries, in which the aorta arises from the right ventricle and the pulmonary artery from the left. In older children, cyanosis is usually the consequence of a ventricular septal defect combined with severe pulmonary stenosis (tetralogy of Fallot) or with pulmonary vascular disease (Eisenmenger's syndrome). Prolonged cyanosis is associated with finger and toe clubbing. Growth retardation and learning difficulties may be a feature with large left-to-right shunts at ventricular or great arterial level, but can also occur with other defects, especially if they form part of a genetic syndrome. Major intellectual impairment is uncommon in children with isolated congenital heart disease; however, minor learning difficulties can occur and may also be the consequence of cardiac surgery. In the presence of increased pulmonary vascular resistance or severe left or right ventricular outflow obstruction, exercise may provoke syncope as systemic vascular resistance falls on exercise but pulmonary vascular resistance may rise, worsening right-to-left shunting and cerebral oxygenation. Persistently raised pulmonary flow (e.g. with left-to-right shunt) leads to increased pulmonary resistance followed by pulmonary hypertension. Progressive changes, including obliteration of distal vessels, take place in the pulmonary vasculature and, once established, the increased pulmonary resistance is irreversible. Central cyanosis appears and digital clubbing develops. The chest X-ray shows enlarged central pulmonary arteries and peripheral 'pruning' of the pulmonary vessels. The electrocardiogram (ECG) shows right ventricular hypertrophy. If severe pulmonary hypertension develops, a left-to-right shunt may reverse, resulting in right-to-left shunting and marked cyanosis (Eisenmenger's syndrome). This is more common with large ventricular septal defects or persistent ductus arteriosus than with atrial septal defects. Patients with Eisenmenger's syndrome are at particular risk from abrupt changes in afterload that exacerbate right-to-left shunting, e.g. vasodilatation, anaesthesia, pregnancy. During pregnancy, there is a 50% increase in plasma volume, a 40% increase in whole blood volume and a similar increase in cardiac output. Abnormalities causing severe outflow tract obstruction, such as aortic stenosis, are not well tolerated and are associated with significant maternal morbidity and mortality. However, most patients with surgically corrected congenital heart disease, and many with palliated or untreated disease, will tolerate pregnancy well. Pregnancy is particularly hazardous in the presence of conditions associated with cyanosis or severe pulmonary hypertension. For example, maternal mortality in patients with Eisenmenger's syndrome is more than 50% and sterilization is usually recommended in such patients. There is a 2–5% risk that the offspring of patients with congenital heart disease will be born with cardiac abnormalities; this is greater if the mother rather than the father is affected. ➲ aortic valve stenosis, atrial septal defect (ASD), coarctation of the aorta, Eisenmenger's syndrome/reaction, Fallot's tetralogy, patent/persistent ductus arteriosus, pulmonary valve stenosis, transposition of the great vessels, truncus arteriosus, ventricular septal defect.

congenital hypothyroidism ➲ hypothyroidism.

congenital megacolon ➲ Hirschsprung's disease, megacolon.

congenital nystagmus a motor nystagmus which is present at birth or soon after. It may be inherited as X-linked recessive or autosomal dominant, or induced in the uterus, and results from decreased vision due to corneal opacity, cataract, albinism, aniridia, macular disease or optic atrophy. It is typically a horizontal jerk nystagmus and it may be associated with abnormal head movement and decreases in intensity with convergence. The visual prognosis is reasonably good, but if the head turn is excessive, extraocular muscle surgery may be needed.

congenital syphilis ➲ syphilis.

congestion *n* hyperaemia. Passive congestion results from obstruction or slowing down of venous return, as in the lower limbs or the lungs—**congestive** *adj*, **congest** *vi, vt.*

congestive dysmenorrhoea ➲ dysmenorrhoea.

congestive glaucoma ➲ acute angle-closure glaucoma (AACG).

congestive heart failure ➲ chronic heart failure.

congruent *adj* when describing a visual field defect implies the defect affects the same area of the field in both eyes.

congruous hemianopsia hemianopsia in which the defects in the two visual fields are identical. ➲ incongruous hemianopsia.

conical cone shaped.

conical cornea ➲ keratoconus (KC).

conical tooth ➲ tooth.

coning a term describing the events that occur in brain swelling and increasing intracranial pressure. The raised intracranial pressure leads to brain shifts and eventual brain herniation down through the foramen magnum. This is a neurosurgical emergency.

conization *n* removal of a cone-shaped part of the cervix by knife or cautery.

conjoined twins identical twins where the normal separation during early development has not occurred. They may be joined, for instance, at the head, chest or abdomen. There may be sharing of vital organs such as the heart or liver. Surgical separation is undertaken successfully in some cases.

conjugate *n* a measurement of the bony pelvis. *diagonal conjugate* the clinical measurement taken in pelvic assessment, from the lower border of the symphysis pubis to the sacral promontory = 111–126 mm. It is 18.5 mm greater than *obstetrical conjugate*, the available space for the fetal head, i.e. the distance from the sacral promontory to the posterior surface of the top of the symphysis pubis = 108–114 mm. *true conjugate* the distance from the sacral promontory to the summit of the symphysis pubis = 110.5 mm.

conjugate distances an optical system will form an image of an object. As the path of light is reversible, the position of object and image are interchangeable. These pairs of object and image points are called conjugate points (or conjugate foci) and the distances of the object and the image from the optical surface are called the conjugate distances. When an eye is accurately focused for an object, object and retina are conjugate. ⮕ ametropia, emmetropia, Scheiner's experiment.

conjugate vaccines ⮕ vaccines.

conjugation *n* **1.** in microbiology, one of the sexual reproductive processes whereby unicellular organisms, such as some bacteria, are able to transfer or exchange genetic material (DNA) by means of sex pili. It allows the genes that confer antibiotic resistance to be passed between bacteria. ⮕ transduction, transformation. **2.** the joining together of molecules. It is an important physiological process, usually occurring in the liver, where toxic substances such as drug residues are conjugated with molecules that include glucuronic acid, glutathione, etc., to allow their safe excretion from the body.

conjunctiva *n* a thin transparent mucous membrane lining the posterior surface of the eyelids from the eyelid margin and reflected forward onto the anterior part of the eyeball where it merges with the corneal epithelium at the corneal limbus. It thus forms a sac, the conjunctival sac, which is open at the palpebral fissure and closed when the eyes are shut. The depths of the unextended sac are 14–16 mm superiorly and 9–11 mm inferiorly. The conjunctiva is divided into three portions: (a) the portion that lines the posterior surface of the eyelids is called the *palpebral conjunctiva*. It is itself composed of the *marginal conjunctiva* which extends from the eyelid margin to the *tarsal conjunctiva*; the tarsal conjunctiva which extends from the marginal conjunctiva to the *orbital conjunctiva*; and the orbital conjunctiva which extends from the tarsal conjunctiva to the fornix; (b) that part reflected over the anterior eyeball is the *bulbar conjunctiva*. It is itself composed of the *limbal conjunctiva* which is fused with the episclera at the corneal limbus and the *scleral conjunctiva* which extends from the limbal conjunctiva to the fornix; and (c) the intermediate part forming the bottom of the conjunctival sac, unattached to the eyelids or the eyeball and joining the bulbar and the palpebral portion is called the fornix (or conjunctival fold, or cul-de-sac)—**conjunctival** *adj*. ⮕ conjunctival glands, dyskeratosis, eyelids, lid eversion, subtarsal sulcus.

conjunctival concretions (*syn* conjunctival lithiasis) minute, hard, whitish spots of calcium present in the palpebral conjunctiva due to cellular degeneration. This condition occurs most commonly in older people or in people with prolonged conjunctivitis. They are asymptomatic but may be removed with a needle. ⮕ conjunctiva.

conjunctival follicle small localized aggregation of lymphocytes, plasma and other cells appearing as white or grey elevations on the palpebral conjunctiva (tarsal area) as a result of chronic irritation (allergic, viral or mechanical such as contact lenses). ⮕ follicular conjunctivitis.

conjunctival glands any gland which secretes a substance into the conjunctiva such as the lacrimal, meibomian, Krause and Wolfring glands or a goblet cell. ⮕ conjunctiva, goblet cells, tears.

conjunctival injection redness (bright red or pink) of the conjunctiva fading towards the corneal limbus due to dilatation of the superficial conjunctival blood vessels occurring in conjunctival inflammations. There is no loss of vision but ocular discomfort and no pain. ⮕ conjunctivitis, keratomycosis, pericorneal plexus.

conjunctival lithiasis ⮕ conjunctival concretions.

conjunctival vein one of many veins which drains the tarsal conjunctiva, the fornix, and the major portion of the bulbar conjunctiva.

conjunctivitis *n* inflammation of the conjunctiva. It may be acute, subacute or chronic. It may be due to an allergy, a bacterial infection (e.g. *Staphylococcus, Streptococcus, Haemophilus*, etc.), viral inflammation, an irritant (dust, wind, chemical fumes, ultraviolet radiation or contact lenses), or as a complication of gonorrhoea, syphilis, influenza, hay fever, measles, etc. Conjunctivitis is characterized by various signs and symptoms which may include conjunctival injection, oedema, small follicles or papillae, secretions (purulent, mucopurulent, membranous, pseudomembranous or catarrhal), pain, itching, grittiness and blepharospasm. The most common type of conjunctivitis is that due to a bacterium and in many cases is self-limiting and subsides without treatment. Treatment of that type includes irrigation of the lid and the use of topical antibiotics. ⮕ acute conjunctivitis, acute haemorrhagic conjunctivitis, allergic conjunctivitis, conjunctival concretions, conjunctival injection, contagious conjunctivitis, follicular conjunctivitis, giant papillary conjunctivitis, ligneous conjunctivitis, ophthalmia neonatorum, phlyctenular conjunctivitis, pseudomembranous conjunctivitis, Stevens–Johnson syndrome, trachoma, vernal conjunctivitis.

connective tissue the diverse group of tissue that includes adipose, areolar, bone, cartilage, blood and blood producing tissue, cells in the tissue interstices (e.g. macrophages), elastic, fibrous and lymphoid (reticular tissue). Connective tissue performs a variety of functions including support, protection and partitioning around and within body structures, and the functions performed by blood cells and blood producing tissues, and storage (e.g. energy stores in fat-containing adipocytes). The different types vary from delicate networks to tough bands and sheets. All have cells within some type of matrix, which they form, and which may be mainly fibrous, cartilaginous, bony or fluid, i.e. blood has a fluid matrix in which the blood cells are suspended. Bundles of white collagen fibres (containing the protein collagen), strong and only slightly extensible, provide a supporting network in organs and tissues everywhere in the body (except the central nervous system) and in the sheaths and membranes that surround or separate them, form the basis of tendons and ligaments and are components of cartilage and bone. Extensible elastic fibres (containing the protein elastin) form networks, e.g. in the walls of arteries and in the lungs, and are a component of flexible cartilage (such as in the nose and ears); reticular fibres form delicate networks, e.g. in the skin deep to the epidermis, and in the walls of small blood vessels. The cells associated with all these fibres are known as fibroblasts or, when inactive, as fibrocytes. Adipose tissue is a connective tissue with a fibrous stroma, widely distributed internally as well as subcutaneously; its cells, adipocytes, are closely related to fibrocytes; likewise the osteocytes in bone and chondrocytes in cartilage. ⊃ mesenchyme.

connective tissue massage manipulations that stretch the superficial and deep connective tissue in order to stimulate the circulation.

connective tissue diseases previously known as collagen diseases. A group of chronic inflammatory disorders often characterized by inflammation affecting collagen and elastin, the structural protein molecules found in connective tissue. ⊃ inherited connective tissue disease, mixed connective tissue disease, systemic connective tissue disease.

connector in dentistry, that part of a removable partial denture that joins components on one side of the arch to those on the other side. *minor connector* the connecting link between the *major connector* or the body of the partial denture and other units of the denture such as clasps, occlusal rests or indirect retainers. ⊃ labial bar, lingual bar, Kennedy bar, palatal bar.

Conn's syndrome (J Conn, American physician, 1907–1994) primary hyperaldosteronism caused by an aldosterone-secreting adenoma of the adrenal cortex. It results in hypertension, hypokalaemia, muscle weakness (proximal), polyuria and polydipsia. Conn's adenoma is the only cause of primary hyperaldosteronism which is usually treated by surgery. Abdominal computed tomography (CT) is often the only test required to localize the tumour, but it is important to recognize that non-functioning adrenal adenomas are present in about 20% of patients with essential hypertension, and adrenal CT should only be performed when the biochemistry supports the diagnosis of adrenal tumour. If the scan is inconclusive, then adrenal vein catheterization with measurement of aldosterone (and cortisol to confirm positioning of the catheters) or ^{131}iodo-norcholesterol scanning may be helpful. In patients with Conn's adenoma the mineralocorticoid receptor antagonist spironolactone is usually given for a few weeks to normalize whole-body electrolyte balance before unilateral adrenalectomy. This is valuable in treating both hypokalaemia and hypertension in all forms of mineralocorticoid excess. High doses of spironolactone may be required. Laparoscopic surgery cures the biochemical abnormality but hypertension remains in as many as 70% of cases, probably because of irreversible damage to the systemic microcirculation. ⊃ aldosteronism, primary hyperaldosteronism.

Conradi–Hünermann syndrome (E Conradi, German physician, 20th century; C Hünermann, German physician, 20th century) a skeletal dysplasia which is inherited as an autosomal dominant trait. Skeletal abnormalities are variable; they are present at birth. After the first few weeks, life expectancy is normal.

consanguinity *n* blood relationship. May be close (as between parent and child) or less so (as between cousins)—**consanguineous** *adj*.

conscientiousness one of the big five personality factors characterized by a tendency to be organized, thorough and reliable.

conscientious objection a legal recognition that an individual is not bound to take part in some specific activities such as termination of pregnancy. It may also apply to other strongly held beliefs that are not acknowledged by law.

consciousness *n* a complex concept which implies that a person is consciously perceiving the environment through the five sensory organs, and responding to the perceptions. ⊃ anaesthesia, sleep.

consent *n* patients are legally required to consent to treatment, surgery and any intervention that requires physical contact. Consent may be verbal, written or implied, i.e. by non-verbal communication. However, where there are likely to be risks or disputes, written consent is advisable. It is the responsibility of the healthcare professional undertaking the procedure to provide a full explanation to the patient prior to treatment or surgery about what is involved and any additional measures that may be required and to obtain written consent. Previously this was the doctor concerned, but increasingly other healthcare professionals are undertaking treatments, e.g. endoscopy by nurses. If the patient is a minor, or incapable of giving informed consent, the next-of-kin must sign the consent form.

consequentialist ethics an ethical theory that considers the consequences of actions or inactions.

conservation of mechanical energy in the absence of changes in all other sorts of energy, the total mechanical energy of an object or body will remain constant. ⊃ mechanical energy.

conservative dentistry the diagnosis, treatment and restoration of diseased or injured teeth. In the UK the term is restricted to that part of restorative dentistry which concerns itself with the restoration of individual teeth and includes endodontics, crowning and fixed bridgework. However, the dividing line between conservative and prosthetic dentistry is ill defined and, generally speaking, removable prostheses depending for their retention on precision attachments are considered to be within the province of conservative dentistry, while those relying on clasps for retention and stabilization belong to the field of prosthetic dentistry. ⮑ endodontics, prosthetic dentistry, prosthodontics (prosthetic dentistry).

conservative treatment aims at preventing a condition from becoming worse without using radical measures. For example, the use of drug therapy rather than surgery. ⮑ treatment.

consolidation *n* becoming solid, as, for instance, the state of the lung due to exudation and organization in lobar pneumonia.

CONSORT statement (consolidated reporting of clinical trials) recommendations for improving the reporting of randomized controlled trials in journals. A flow diagram and checklist allow readers to understand the conduct of the study and assess the validity of the results.

constant current an electrotherapy term. Current remains as set by the equipment operator. If set at 10 mA, the current output stays at 10 mA irrespective of changes in impedance or voltage. Ohm's law indicates that any changes to the resistance will, therefore, produce a change in the voltage. ⮑ constant voltage.

constant potential (CP) a constant voltage produced by smoothing a fully rectified voltage by using capacitors.

constant voltage an electrotherapy term. Voltage remains as set. If set at 20 V it stays set at 20 V irrespective of any changes in impedance or current. Ohm's law indicates that any changes to the resistance will, therefore, produce a change in the current. ⮑ constant current.

constipation *n* an implied chronic condition of infrequent and often difficult evacuation of faeces due to insufficient high fibre food or fluid intake, immobility, or to sluggish or disordered action of the bowel musculature or nerve supply, or to habitual failure to empty the rectum. Other causes include pain on defecation, inability to respond to the urge to defecate, hypokalaemia, drugs such as iron preparations, pregnancy (hormonal), depression, colorectal cancer (alternating with diarrhoea) and some systemic diseases. *Acute constipation* signifies intestinal obstruction or paralysis of the gut of sudden onset.

constituents of developer in radiography. Developing agents, preservative, accelerator, restrainer, buffer, sequestering agent, solvent, hardening agent, wetting agent, antifrothing agent, fungicide.

constituents of fixer in radiography, Fixing agent, acid, buffer, preservative, hardener and solvent.

constringence (*syn* Abbé's number, V-value) a positive number (*symbol*: V) which specifies any transparent medium. It is equal to

$$V = \frac{n_D - 1}{n_F - n_C}$$

where n_D, n_F and n_C are the refractive indices for the Fraunhofer spectral lines D (589.3 nm), F (486.1 nm) and C (656.3 nm). A material with a high constringence (e.g. V = 50) produces less chromatic aberration than one with a low constringence (e.g. V = 30). The reciprocal of the constringence is called the dispersive power. ⮑ dispersion, Fraunhofer's lines, longitudinal chromatic aberration, refractive index.

constructional apraxia an inability to arrange objects to a plan.

constructivism in the philosophy of science, the doctrine that people actively construct their reality on the basis of their beliefs and expectations. Also known as constructionism.

constructivist a person who espouses constructivism.

consultation in dentistry, a visit by a patient seeking advice on a specific dental and/or oral condition. It should include taking a full history (medical and dental), a full dental and oral examination, a careful assessment of the findings and a formulation and presentation of a treatment plan to the patient, preferably as a written report.

consumerism the practice of buying and selling goods in a free market and at a market price. Government reforms, for example the NHS and Community Care Act (1990), have sought to give patients and clients (often referred to as customers and consumers) more choice within health and social services. Their choice is, however, limited because of restricted resources and lack of control. The health and social care market can thus be considered a 'quasi-market'. ⮑ internal market.

consumption *n* **1.** act of consuming or using up. **2.** a once popular term for pulmonary tuberculosis, which 'consumed' the body—**consumptive** *adj*.

contact *n* **1.** direct or indirect exposure to infection. **2.** a person who has been so exposed.

contact angle (*syn* wetting angle) the angle formed by a surface and a tangent to a sessile drop of fluid (usually water) at the point where the drop meets the surface. This angle indicates the degree of wettability of that surface. The more wettable (or hydrophilic) the material, the smaller the angle, being equal to 0° for a completely hydrophilic material when water spreads evenly over that surface. Hydrophobic surfaces can have contact angles greater than 90°, e.g. silicone rubber in which the angle is about 120°. ⮑ sessile drop test, silicone rubber.

contact area the area of crown contact between two adjacent teeth, sometimes referred to as a *contact point*.

contact force the force due to contact between two objects or bodies.

contact lens a small lens of glass or usually plastic, worn under the eyelids in direct contact with conjunctiva or sclera and used to correct refractive errors of the eye, or for cosmetic reasons. There are many types of contact lenses. Lenses that rest on the sclera are called scleral (or haptic) contact lenses whereas lenses that rest on the cornea are called corneal contact lenses, or, more commonly, contact lenses. Lenses that are made of a hard plastic material which is impermeable to oxygen, such as those made of polymethylmethacrylate (PMMA), are called hard or rigid contact lenses. Hard contact lenses which transmit oxygen are called gas permeable contact lenses (GP, GPL, GPCL, HGP or RGP). Other lenses made of a soft plastic material which transmit a certain amount of oxygen are called soft (or hydrophilic or hydrogel or gel or flexible) contact lenses (SCL) whose water content varies; the greater the water content the more oxygen is transmitted (for equal thickness). Very high water content lenses are used for extended wear (EW). There are also bifocal contact lenses consisting of two segments with different focal powers which provide either simultaneous vision (light from both the distance and near portions enters the eye at the same time) or alternating vision (the lens must be moved to see through either portion). Other bifocal contact lenses have a zone of variable power between the two portions and others are diffractive in which light from both distance and near objects can be focused on the retina (without moving the lens) owing to diffraction produced by a series of rings in the centre of the back surface of the lens (the higher the near addition the greater the number of rings). There are also toric contact lenses in which the back optic surface is toroidal; they are used to improve the physical fit. Bitoric contact lenses are lenses in which both surfaces are toroidal; they are used to improve the physical fit and correct the induced astigmatism. Disposable contact lenses are worn for about 1 week continuously (or 2 weeks on a daily basis) and then discarded. ⊃ adherence lens, back toric contact lens, cast-moulding lens, ChromGen lens, cosmetic contact lens, extended wear lens, fenestrated lens, flare lens, flat lens, flexure lens, lathe-cut contact lens, liquid lens, piggyback lens, scleral contact lens, sealed scleral contact lens, silicone hydrogel lens, spin-cast contact lens, steep lens, therapeutic soft contact lens, water content (of lens), X-Chrom lens.

contact lens deposits an accumulation of materials on or into the matrix of contact lenses. They are mainly tear components (proteins, calcium, lipids, mucin) but other materials can be found, such as mercurial or iron deposits, nicotine, hand cream. Deposits reduce comfort, vision, patient tolerance and discolour and spoil the lenses. They may act as antigens for the development of giant papillary conjunctivitis. Most of these deposits can be removed with a surfactant, an enzymatic system and a calcium-preventing solution. ⊃ giant papillary conjunctivitis, surfactant.

contact sports individual or team sports in which contact between two players or opponents is an integral part and frequent factor of the game or sport, such as rugby and boxing.

contact surface ⊃ approximal surface.

contact tracer ⊃ health adviser.

contagious *adj* capable of transmitting infection or of being transmitted.

contagious conjunctivitis (*syn* epidemic conjunctivitis, epidemic keratoconjunctivitis, pink eye [colloquial]), acute conjunctivitis caused by *Haemophilus aegyptius*, adenovirus types 3 and 7 or 8 and 19, or a pneumococcal infection. It may be transmitted by respiratory or ocular infections, contaminated towels or equipment (e.g. tonometer heads). It is characterized by acute onset, redness, tearing, discomfort and photophobia. The condition is often self-limiting but keratitis is a common complication. ⊃ acute conjunctivitis.

containment isolation separation of a patient with any type of infection to prevent spread of the condition to others. ⊃ protective isolation, source isolation.

contaminants describes any undesirable chemicals present in food stuffs. These include, residues of agricultural chemicals, e.g. fertilizers, herbicides, pesticides, fungicides, etc., occurring during processing or caused by pollution, or the result of a malicious act.

context the relationships between the environment, personal factors and events that influence the meaning of a task, activity or occupation for the performer. (Reproduced with permission from the European Network of Occupational Therapy in Higher Education (ENOTHE) Terminology Project, 2008)

contiguous touching, close. In computed tomography (CT) scanning refers to slice reconstruction with no interslice spacing.

continent diversion surgical technique of bladder reconstruction by the creation of a pouch that can be emptied using a catheter.

continent ileostomy ⊃ ileostomy.

contingency fund an amount of money included in the costings of a project that would be used for some unplanned or unpredictable expense.

contingency screening method of antenatal Down's syndrome screening currently being developed. It includes first trimester biochemical screening (human chorionic gonadotrophin [hCG] and pregnancy associated plasma protein [PAPP-A]), which may be combined with nuchal translucency (NT) scan. Women at high risk are then offered more precise diagnostic investigations while those at low risk exit the screening programme. Those with mid-range risks proceed to second trimester biochemical screening to obtain results which combine first and second trimester values, improving detection rate and reducing the false positive rate.

continuing professional development (CPD) developing and improving skills and knowledge through a range of learning activities throughout a professional career in order to maintain the capacity to practise safely and effectively.

continuity equation used in ultrasound to assess the area of a heart valve using measurements of the velocity and mean pressure gradient of the blood flow through the valve and the width of the valve.

continuity of care term used to describe care given to one pregnant woman from booking until discharge to the health visitor, in which good communication from one appointment to the next and between all professionals ensures that there are no omissions or duplications in the care of that woman. Continuity does not necessarily mean that only one professional is in contact with the woman, as this would indeed be unrealistic. However, verbal and written communication between professionals should be comprehensive enough to avoid errors and to facilitate the woman's sense of security in the care she is receiving. Various schemes of care exist in an attempt to provide continuity of care. ⊃ caseload midwifery, team midwifery.

continuity theory a psychological theory of aging lying somewhere between the acitivity and disengagement theories. It describes a process whereby people, as they age, struggle to retain as many of the activities of their younger life as possible. Clearly, there is a wide range of experience amongst older people in terms of activity, which will be dictated by many factors such as ability, health status, motivation and financial status.

continuous ambulatory peritoneal dialysis (CAPD) peritoneal dialysis carried out every day, by patients needing renal replacement therapy, at home.

continuous glucose monitoring (CGM) use of a subcutaneous probe to monitor tissue glucose concentrations giving a continuous profile over 48 to 72 hours; useful for adjustment of insulin doses.

continuous inflating pressure (CIP) pressure of water used against an infant's spontaneous breathing in respiratory distress syndrome. Its purpose is to prevent hypoxaemia, apnoeic attacks or rising levels of carbon dioxide in the blood (PCO_2).

continous loop wire ⊃ wiring.

continuous passive motion (movement) (CPM) type of passive mobilization, it may be used to help the recovery of cartilage after knee surgery. The benefits include: (a) maintenance of synovial sweep and thus hyaline articular cartilage; (b) regular rhythmical motion can act as an analgesic, can stimulate circulation and may assist in reduction of swelling; (c) CPM has been used following anterior cruciate reconstruction particularly following patellar tendon graft—it is possible that this encourages more rapid revascularization and, therefore, strength of the donor graft; (d) it is possible to increase flexion/extension in a controlled manner that is immediately obvious to the patient and can assist in giving the patient a goal to strive for; (e) some units have counters so that the healthcare team can tell exactly for how long the patient has been using the unit; (f) CPM units are now available for shoulder, wrist and other joints; and (g) CPM units may now be used in the patient's home. There are, however, some disadvantages associated with the use of CPM. They include: (a) it is passive and, therefore, by definition will not build muscle strength. Some patients mistakenly neglect active movement exercises in the belief that they no longer need to undertake them. It is the responsibility of the physiotherapist

to ensure that this situation does not occur; (b) some patients are distressed by the appearance of and feel threatened by the unit (most units have a panic button so the patient can stop the unit for rest, meals, toiletting and so on); (c) the units can be bulky and expensive; (d) if incorrectly positioned they can cause pressure problems and be uncomfortable; and (e) they pose an infection risk if not properly cleaned and policies for their use followed. ⊃ passive movement.

continuous positive airways pressure (CPAP) the application of gas at a constant positive pressure, to the airway of a spontaneously breathing patient, via an endotracheal tube, a tightly fitting face mask that covers both the mouth and nose, or a nasal mask. It reduces alveolar collapse at the end of expiration and reduces the work of breathing; used at night in patients with sleep apnoea syndromes. CPAP is increasingly used to correct hypoxaemia.

continuous subcutaneous insulin infusion (CSII) the use of a pump to deliver insulin continuously, either with a fixed or variable basal rate, and with a facility for bolus dosing, to achieve almost physiological control of diabetes mellitus.

continuous wave Doppler when a fixed frequency ultrasound is transmitted continuously by one crystal and is received continuously by an adjacent crystal. Any motion within the beam will produce a measurable Doppler shift. It can measure very high flow velocities but has no range resolution. ⊃ Doppler shift.

continuous wave probe (CW probe) used in a Doppler scan where one half of the transducer head emits a continuous ultrasound beam and the other half continuously receives the reflected beam, for example, a pencil probe. ⊃ Doppler effect, Doppler scanner.

continuous loop wiring ⊃ wiring.

contour 1. a boundary or outline. 2. to sculpt or carve a material or restoration to a desired shape.

contouring device an aid to radiotherapy planning. The device accurately records the patient outline to facilitate accurate dose distributions to be planned. ⊃ adjustable template, lead strip, rotating jig.

contour lines of Owen microscopic lines sometimes seen in dentine representing co-incidence of the secondary curves of the dentinal tubules or accentuated deficiencies of mineralization.

contra- a prefix that means 'against', e.g. *contraception*.

contra-angle in dentistry, an instrument having two or more off-setting angles along its shank in order to bring the working end closer to the long axis of the handle.

contraceptive *n, adj* (describes) an agent used to prevent conception, e.g. condom, spermicidal vaginal pessary or cream, rubber cervical cap, intrauterine device. ⊃ combined oral contraceptive (COC) pill, emergency contraception, intrauterine device—**contraception** *n*.

contract *v* 1. draw together; shorten; decrease in size. 2. acquire by contagion or infection.

contracted pelvis pelvis in which any diameter of the brim, cavity or outlet is reduced to an extent where it interferes with the progress of labour.

contractile *adj* having the ability to shorten—usually following stimulation; a property of muscle tissue—**contractility** *n*.

contraction *n* shortening, e.g. in muscle fibres.

contraction stress test (CST) an artificial stimulation of contraction of the uterus using oxytocin and simultaneous electronic monitoring of the fetal heart, unrelated to labour. The fetal response is assessed as an indicator of its ability to withstand the rigours of labour.

contracture *n* shortening of scar or muscle tissue, causing deformity ⊃ Dupuytren's contracture, Volkmann's ischaemic contracture.

contraindication *n* any factor or condition indicating that a certain type of treatment (usually used for that condition) should be discontinued or not used. For example, a drug to which the person is allergic, or a therapy such as the use of shortwave diathermy within 3–5 m of a patient with an indwelling stimulator such as a pacemaker or applying ultra-violet radiation or laser light (Class 3B) without therapist and patient wearing wavelength specific protective goggles. ⊃ interactive effects.

contralateral *adj* on the opposite side—**contralaterally** *adv*. ⊃ homolateral, ipsilateral.

contrast in radiography, the difference in density between two adjacent areas on a film, the higher the contrast the more black and white the film, the lower the contrast the more shades of grey. ⊃ film contrast, gamma, radiographic contrast, subject contrast, subjective contrast.

contrast agent in radiography. Either positive substances (non-ionic iodine compounds or barium) or negative substances (air, water or carbon dioxide) which can be used to demonstrate organs, vessels or parts of the body more clearly during imaging investigations by changing the subject density.

contrast medium ⊃ contrast agent.

contrast sensitivity chart a chart designed to test contrast sensitivity. Such a test is useful with patients having low vision and in the early detection of diseases.

contrecoup *n* injury or damage at a point opposite the impact, resulting from transmitted force. It can occur in an organ or part containing fluid. For example the brain inside the skull; when a blow to the right side of the skull causes damage to the left side of the brain.

constriction ring a localized annular spasm of the uterine muscle at any level but often near the junction of the upper and lower uterine segments. In the first and second stages of labour it may form round the neck of the fetus and in the third stage forms an hourglass contriction of the uterus, causing a retained placenta. It may result from the use of oxytocic drugs in situations where the uterus has uncoordinated function, following early rupture of the membranes, and especially if intrauterine manipulation is carried out.

control group in research, the group that is not exposed to the independent variable, such as a therapeutic intervention or experimental drug. ⊃ experimental group, variable.

controlled area in radiology. An area where the dose rate exceeds a specific dose rate or an employee is likely to receive more than three tenths the relevant dose limit. Access is restricted to specific staff members and patients undergoing therapeutic or diagnostic procedures.

controlled cord traction method of delivering the placenta and membranes, in which, once the placenta is known to have separated, the midwife places the ulnar border of her left hand in the suprapubic region and pushes the contracted uterus upwards, while with her right hand she gains a firm hold on the cord and exerts gentle traction, following the curve of Carus. The membranes are eased out slowly and gently to avoid tearing them, which can lead to retained products. If an oxytocic drug is administered to facilitate separation of the placenta it is not necessary to await signs of separation and descent before attempting controlled cord traction. However, if the placenta has been allowed to separate physiologically it is imperative to await these signs to avoid risks to the woman of haemorrhage or even uterine inversion.

controlled delivery device in dentistry, a method of applying an antimicrobial preparation to a periodontal pocket. An adjunctive treatment method for periodontal disease. Designed to provide drug delivery for over 24 hours. For example a preparation containing chlorhexidine in a gelatine matrix; doxycycline in a polymer vehicle.

controlled-dose transdermal absorption of drugs application of a drug patch to the skin: gradual absorption gives a constant level in the blood. Examples include analgesics such as fentanyl, various types of hormone replacement, and nicotine for smoking cessation.

controlled drugs (CD) drugs that are subject to statutory control, e.g. barbiturates, cocaine, morphine. ⊃ Appendix 5.

controlled processing information processing that requires conscious attention, especially as in the execution of a novel or difficult task. ⊃ automatic processing.

Control of Substances Hazardous to Health (COSHH) regulations relating to obligatory risk assessment and action to be taken, such as during the use of certain anaesthetic agents.

contusion *n* a common injury especially in sport, the result of direct contact without the skin being broken. If superficial, it will result in visible bruising. If the injury is deep, a haematoma will develop within the affected tissue, commonly muscle. ⊃ bruise—**contuse** *vt*.

convection *n* transfer of heat from the hotter to the colder part; the heated substance (air or fluid), being less dense, tends to rise. The colder portion, flowing in to be heated, rises in its turn; thus *convection currents* are set in motion.

convenience form in dentistry, shaping of a cavity preparation to allow access and to facilitate the manufacture and insertion of a restoration.

conventional fractionation radiotherapy given once daily over a predetermined period of time.

convergence **1.** the movement of the eyes turning inward or towards each other to focus on near objects. **2.** characteristic of a pencil of light rays directed towards a real image point. ⊃ angle of convergence, vergence.

convergence accommodation 1. accommodation induced directly by a change in convergence. **2.** *syn.* vergence accommodation. That component of accommodation induced by the binocular disparity of the retinal images. ⊃ retinal disparity.

convergence insufficiency an inability to converge, or to maintain convergence, usually associated with a high exophoria at near and a relatively orthophoric condition at distance. It results in complaints of fatigue or even diplopia due to the inability to maintain (and sometimes even to obtain) adequate convergence for prolonged close work. Treatment includes orthoptic exercises (e.g. the pencil-to-nose exercise or pencil push-up in which the tip of a pencil is moved slowly towards the eyes while it is maintained singly for as long as possible and this procedure is repeated until the pencil can be brought within 10 cm before doubling occurs), or a reading addition sometimes with BI prisms. ⊃ accommodative insufficiency, exophoria, near point of convergence.

convergence-retraction nystagmus a jerk nystagmus which appears on attempted upward gaze and in which the fast phase brings the two eyes towards each other in a convergent movement with retraction of the globes into the orbit. It may result from a lesion affecting the tectum or dorsal midbrain or a pineal tumour, or form part of Parinaud's syndrome. ⊃ Parinaud's syndrome, tectum of the mesencephalon.

converging collimator gamma camera collimator where the piece of lead has holes which are shaped to focus the gamma rays on a single spot, the main use is in brain imaging.

conversion *n* a mental defence mechanism. A psychological conflict being expressed as a physical symptom.

conversion (radiography context) in an intensifying screen it is when energy is released from absorbed electrons in the form of light photons. In developer, when the chemical precipitates metallic silver from the silver salts in the film during processing. In the fixer when the unexposed, undeveloped silver halides are removed from the film to make the image stable.

conversion disorder an old term for dissociative disorders.

convolutions *npl* folds, twists or coils as found in the intestine, renal tubules and the surface of the brain—**convoluted** *adj.*

convulsions *npl* involuntary contractions of muscles resulting from abnormal electrical activity in the brain: there are many causes. They occur with or without loss of consciousness. ⊃ epilepsy, febrile seizures, seizures. *clonic convulsions* show alternating contraction and relaxation of muscle groups. *tonic convulsions* reveal sustained muscle rigidity—**convulsive** *adj.*

Cooley's anaemia (T Cooley, American paediatrician, 1871–1945) ⊃ thalassaemia.

Coombs' test (R Coombs, British immunologist, b.1921) a highly sensitive test designed to detect antibodies to red blood cells, such as those found in Rhesus incompatibility or haemolytic anaemia. The indirect method detects unbound antibodies in the serum, whereas the direct method detects those bound to the red cells. ⊃ direct Coombs' test, indirect Coombs' test.

co-ordinates numbers specifying the position of an object or body. *Cartesian co-ordinates* are specified on axes that are orthogonal (at right angles) to each other (usually X, Y and Z or i, j and k). *polar co-ordinates* are specified by an angle (degrees) and a distance from a fixed point.

coordination *n* moving in harmony. The body's ability to execute smooth, fluid, accurate and controlled movements.

COP *abbr* **1.** centre of pressure. **2.** cryptogenic organizing pneumonia.

copal resin obtained from tropical trees and used in a solvent as varnish.

COPD *abbr* chronic obstructive pulmonary disease.

coping *n* **1.** the way in which a person deals with a circumstance which can be either negative or positive. The coping response can be negative, e.g. reducing social activities because of failing sight, or the odour of a chronic wound; or it can be positive, e.g. increasing participation in sport although the person uses a wheelchair. **2.** in dentistry, a thin, cast-metal cap, without external undercuts, that is fitted over a preparation. *implant impression coping* a removable close fitting attachment for an implant fixture or abutment, usually held in place via a screw or by friction, they allow an accurate impression of an implant fixture or abutment to be recorded prior to construction of the definitive restoration. *transfer coping* a base metal or resin cap used to obtain precise relative locations during the taking of impressions of multiple preparations. ⊃ implant.

coplanar forces forces acting in the same plane.

copolymer a polymer made up of two or more different monomer units.

copper (Cu) *n* essential trace element widely distributed in the body tissues; an important component of metalloenzymes involved in protein synthesis. Copper deficiency can develop in preterm infants and full term infants who have been fed cows' milk instead of breast milk or infant formula milk. In young children it is characterized by microcytic hypochromic anaemia, poor growth, skeletal rarefaction and dermatosis.

copper-7 an intrauterine contraceptive device containing copper wire embedded in the plastic shape.

copper amalgam amalgam containing mainly copper and mercury and made plastic by heating, just prior to use, and trituration.

copper band ⊃ copper ring.

copper ring thin-walled copper tube used to contain and support impression material. Supplied in graded and numbered sizes. May be softened by annealing. Can also be used as a temporary crown or matrix band.

copper ring impression impression of a tooth preparation using a copper ring to contain the impression material. An overall impression may be necessary to demonstrate the contact areas to the technician.

copper sulphate blue crystalline substance used in solution to permit the deposition of copper in plating techniques. In powdered form has been used in the treatment of periodontal pockets.

coprolalia *n* the excessive use of obscene speech. Occurs as a sign most commonly in cerebral deterioration or trauma affecting frontal lobes of the brain. ⮑ Tourette's syndrome.

coprolith *n* faecalith.

coproporphyrin *n* nitrogenous substance derived from the breakdown of bilirubin produced when haemoglobin is decomposed, normally excreted in the faeces.

copulation *n* coitus, sexual intercourse.

copy film film used to produce exact copies of radiographs by direct contact printing.

COR *abbr* critical oxygen requirement.

cor the heart or pertaining to the heart.

coracobrachialis muscle a muscle of the upper arm which causes adduction and flexion of the humerus. Its origin is on the scapula and the insertion on the medial aspect of the humerus. ⮑ Colour Section Figure 4.

coracoid process beak-like process of the scapula, provides attachment for the pectoralis minor muscle and other muscles.

cord *n* a thread-like structure. *spermatic cord* that which suspends the testes in the scrotum. *spinal cord* a structure which lies in the spinal column, reaching from the foramen magnum to the first or second lumbar vertebra. It is a direct continuation of the medulla oblongata. *umbilical cord* attaching the fetus to the placenta. It contains two arteries and a vein. *vocal cord* the membranous bands in the larynx, vibrations of which produce the voice. ⮑ spermatic cord, spinal cord, vocal folds (cords).

cord presentation a situation where the umbilical cord is below the presenting part of the fetus.

cord prolapse an obstetric emergency occurring as a complication of a cord presentation. Once the fetal membranes rupture the umbilical cord may prolapse and the umbilical blood vessels become compressed between the presenting part and the cervix, thus depriving the fetus of oxygen and causing hypoxia.

cordectomy *n* surgical excision of a cord, usually reserved for a vocal cord.

cordocentesis percutaneous umbilical cord blood sampling; fetal blood sampling; funipuncture. An invasive antenatal investigation undertaken after 18 weeks' gestation to obtain a fetal blood sample, usually performed by entering the intrahepatic portal vein or placental cord insertion to reduce haemorrhage. Risks include miscarriage, fetal haemorrhage and infection. Fetal sedation achieved by administering maternal opiate drugs may reduce fetal movement during the procedure. Developments in chromosomal and genetic analysis from amniotic fluid and chorionic villus sampling mean that cordocentesis is less used now, but it remains useful to check fetal blood indices and to perform in-utero blood transfusion for haemolytic disease.

cordotomy *n* (*syn* chordotomy) division of the anterolateral nerves in the spinal cord to relieve intractable pain in the pelvis or lower limbs.

core *n* **1.** central portion, may be applied to the slough in the centre of a boil. **2.** in dentistry, correctly shaped and well-retained substructure to a partial or full veneer crown. May be part of a post and core system and may be cast or prefabricated. A core may also be constructed of a plastic material adhered to remaining tooth tissue or retained physically. ⮑ core porcelain.

core body temperature ⮑ body temperature.

core porcelain opaque porcelain laid on the platinum matrix which provides a strong and optically uniform base for jacket crown construction.

core skills competencies. The basics of professional practice which remain relatively constant. In occupational therapy practice they include therapeutic use of self assessment, environmental analysis and adaptation, and occupational analysis and adaptation.

core stability the ability to control the movement and position of the muscles of the central 'core' of the body which are responsible for posture and limb movement. These include the muscle groups of the lower back and abdomen. Good core stability will allow the sportsman/woman to maximize their sporting performance and minimize injury risk. A well-conditioned core will control and increase the power of muscle movement, resulting in more efficient and coordinated limb movement and limiting potential injury by excessive or abnormal loads. Core stability is improved through a regular and repeated exercise programme, which does not require any equipment.

corectopia (*syn* ectopia pupillae) the displacement of the pupil of the eye from the normal position in the centre of the iris. It may occur as a result of ocular surgery, trauma or from a congenital defect. ⮑ luxation of the lens, pupil.

coreometer ⮑ pupillometer.

Cori cycle (C Cori, American biochemist 1896–1984; G Cori, American biochemist, 1886–1957) a biochemical pathway that recycles lactate produced by muscle during anaerobic glycolysis. The lactate is released to the blood, taken up by the liver and converted back to glucose, which is released again to be used by muscle.

Cori's disease type III glycogen storage disease in which there is a deficiency of debrancher enzyme. It presents during childhood and is characterized by hepatomegaly and mild hypoglycaemia.

corium the dermis of the skin.

corn *n* ⮑ callus.

cornea *n* the transparent anterior portion of the fibrous coat of the globe of the eye. It has a curvature somewhat greater than the rest of the globe, so a slight furrow marks its junction with the sclera. Looked at from the front the cornea is about 12 mm horizontally and 11 mm vertically. It is the first and most important refracting surface of the eye, having a power of about 42D. The anterior surface has a radius of curvature of about 7.8 m, the posterior surface 6.5 mm, and the central thickness is about 0.5 mm. It consists of five layers, starting from the outside: (1) the stratified squamous epithelium; (2) Bowman's membrane; (3) the stroma (or substantia propria); (4) Descemet's membrane; and (5) the endothelium. The cornea is avascular, receiving its nourishment by permeation through spaces between the lamellae. The sources of nourishment are the aqueous humour, the tears and the limbal capillaries. The cornea is innervated by the long ciliary and other nerves of the surrounding conjunctiva which are all branches of the ophthalmic division of the trigeminal nerve (fifth cranial nerve). Innervation is entirely sensory. Within the cornea there are only unmyelinated nerve endings. The density of nerves in the cornea is very high, making it the most sensitive structure in the body. The cornea owes its transparency to the regular arrangement of the collagen fibres, but any factor which affects this lattice structure (e.g. swelling, pressure) results in a loss of transparency. The cornea contains some 78% water, some 15% collagen and some 5% of other proteins—**corneal** *adj.* ➲ Bowman's membrane, dellen, Descemet's membrane, deturgescence, dyskeratosis, glycosaminoglycan, Hudson-Stahli line, keratitis, keratometer, keratomycosis, limbus, Maurice's theory, microcornea, optical zone of cornea, pachometer, specular microscope, Colour Section Figure 15.

cornea guttata (*syn* corneal guttae, endothelial corneal dystrophy) dystrophy of the endothelial cells of the cornea which may result from corneal trauma, cataract surgery, keratic precipitates, tonography, ageing, continuous contact lens wear, or as part of the early stages of Fuch's endothelial dystrophy (a disease associated with ageing and with females more than males). It is seen clinically by slit-lamp examination as black spherules in the endothelial pattern. The condition is bilateral, although one eye may be affected more than the other. As the condition progresses the cornea becomes oedematous with a consequent loss of vision and eventually turns into bullous keratopathy. If the degenerated cells are located at the periphery of the cornea they are called Hassall–Henle bodies and are of no clinical significance except as an indication of ageing. ➲ bullous keratopathy, central corneal clouding, corneal endothelium, keratic precipitates, specular reflection illumination.

corneal *adj* pertaining to the cornea.

corneal abrasion an area of the cornea which has been removed by rubbing. The condition ranges from punctate staining with fluorescein to a total removal of the epithelium. Corneal abrasions may result from overwear of contact lenses, foreign bodies, fingernail scratches, etc. Symptoms may be pain, photophobia, tearing and blepharospasm. The condition usually heals quickly if not severe and if infection has not occurred. Treatment consists of removal of the foreign bodies, if any, usually by irrigation, tight patching of the eye and antibiotic ointment; if due to contact lenses, discontinue wear until full recovery. Local anaesthetics should not be used in the treatment as they tend to delay the regeneration of the corneal epithelium. ➲ fluorescein, overwear syndrome, rose bengal.

corneal apex the most anterior point of the cornea when the eye is in the primary position. It does not automatically coincide with any common reference point (e.g. line of sight). ➲ apical clearance, primary position (of the eye).

corneal arcus (*syn* arcus senilis, gerontoxon) a greyish-white ring (or part of a ring) opacity occurring in the periphery of the cornea, in middle and old age. It is due to a lipid infiltration of the corneal stroma. With age the condition progresses to form a complete ring. That ring is separated from the limbus by a zone of clear cornea. The condition can also appear in early or middle life and is referred to as *arcus juvenilis* (or *anterior embryotoxon*): it is somewhat whiter than corneal arcus. Arcus juvenilis is often associated with heart disease in men.

corneal cap ➲ optical zone of cornea.

corneal conjunctiva the stratified squamous epithelium of the cornea.

corneal endothelium the posterior layer of the cornea consisting of a single layer of cells, about 5 mm thick, bound together and predominantly hexagonal in shape. The posterior border is in direct contact with the aqueous humour while the anterior border is in contact with Descemet's membrane. The endothelium is the structure responsible for the relative dehydration of the corneal stroma. The endothelium receives most of its energy from the oxidative breakdown of carbohydrates via the Krebs' cycle. With age, disease or trauma the density of cells decreases but with disease or trauma this reduction may affect corneal transparency as some fluid then leaks into the cornea. ➲ cornea, cornea guttata, endothelial bedewing, endothelial blebs, endothelial polymegethism, specular microscope, specular reflection illumination, phacoemulsification.

corneal epithelium the outermost layer of the cornea consisting of stratified epithelium mounted on a basement membrane. It is made up of various types of cells; next to the basement membrane are the basal cells (columnar in shape), then two or three rows of wing cells and near the surface are two or three layers of thin surface squamous cells (or superficial cells). The outer surfaces of the squamous cells have projections (called microvilli and microplicae) which extend into the mucin layer of the precorneal tear film and are presumed to help retain the tear film. The epithelium in humans has a thickness of about 51 mm. Some dendritic cells of mesodermal origin are also normally present. The corneal epithelium receives its innervation from the conjunctival and the stromal nerves. The life cycle of epithelial cells is about a week. ➲ epikeratoplasty, mitosis, pachometer, palisades of Vogt.

corneal exhaustion phenomenon ➲ corneal exhaustion syndrome.

corneal exhaustion syndrome (*syn* corneal fatigue syndrome, corneal exhaustion phenomenon) an intolerance to continue wearing contact lenses after many years of wear, probably due to endothelial dysfunction as a result of chronic hypoxia and acidosis. It occurs primarily with PMMA lenses but also with other lenses with low oxygen transmissibility. Some of the signs associated with this syndrome are: endothelial polymegethism, corneal oedema, loss of corneal sensitivity, variations in corneal curvature and refractive error, blurred vision, lacrimation, hyperaemia and discomfort. Management usually consists in discontinuing contact lens wear. Refitting with lenses with high oxygen transmissibility is often successful. ⟳ corneal hypoxia, overwear syndrome.

corneal fatigue syndrome ⟳ corneal exhaustion syndrome.

corneal graft/transplant (*syn* keratoplasty) replacement of the cornea with a healthy cornea from a human donor. This can be done either over the entire cornea (total keratoplasty) or over a portion of it (partial keratoplasty). Two main techniques are used: the *penetrating keratoplasty* in which the entire thickness of the cornea is removed and replaced by transparent corneal tissue; or the *lamellar keratoplasty* in which a superficial layer is removed and replaced by healthy tissue. Common indications to perform keratoplasty are therapeutic (e.g. keratoconus, corneal ulcer) or cosmetic (e.g. removing an unsightly opacity). ⟳ eye bank, granular dystrophy.

corneal granular dystrophy ⟳ granular dystrophy.

corneal guttae ⟳ cornea guttata.

corneal hypoxia an inadequate supply of oxygen to the cornea. It may occur in some pathological conditions. For example, in longstanding diabetes mellitus there is corneal hypoxia (with consequent high epithelial fragility and some neovascularization). Corneal hypoxia, with consequent oedema, loss of sensitivity, etc., may also occur in contact lens wear. ⟳ corneal exhaustion syndrome, critical oxygen requirement, overwear syndrome, proliferative retinopathy, retinal hypoxia.

corneal infiltrates small hazy greyish areas (local or diffuse) located in the cornea typically near the corneal limbus. The adjacent conjunctiva is usually hyperaemic. They appear as a result of corneal inflammation, reaction to solution preservatives and some contact lens wear (especially extended wear) which causes prolonged corneal hypoxia. Management depends on the cause; for example, if due to contact lenses, cessation of wear is usually indicated. ⟳ keratitis, keratoconjunctivitis.

corneal limbus *n* (*syn* corneoscleral junction) often referred to as the limbus. The transition zone, about 1.5 mm wide, between the conjunctiva and sclera on the one hand, and the cornea on the other. ⟳ cornea, limbal blanching.

corneal reflex a reaction of blinking when the cornea is touched.

corneal topography a technique used to determine the exact shape of the cornea and its refractive power. Important in the surgical correction of refractive errors, such as with the use of lasers.

corneal ulcer a superficial loss of corneal tissue as a result of infection which has led to necrosis. It may be caused by a bacterium (e.g. *Pseudomonas aeruginosa, Streptococcus*

pneumoniae), by a virus (e.g. herpesvirus), or by a genus of fungi (e.g. *Candida, Aspergillus, Penicillium*). It causes pain and usually reduced visual acuity, especially if the ulcer occurs in the centre of the cornea. Corneal ulcers usually look dirty grey or white and are opaque areas of various sizes and a mucopurulent discharge may be present. If induced by contact lenses, especially extended wear lenses, patients must cease wearing their lenses immediately, and the appropriate therapy instituted: antibacterial, antifungal or antiviral agent. ⟳ dendritic ulcer, hypopyon, Colour Section Figure 61.

corneoscleral *adj* pertaining to the cornea and sclera

corneoscleral junction the circular junction between conjunctiva and sclera on the one hand, and the cornea. ⟳ corneal limbus.

cornu *n* a horn-shaped structure, such as the upper angles of the uterus where the uterine (fallopian) tubes join, or part of the thyroid cartilage—**coruna** *pl*, **corunal** *adj*.

cornual pregnancy a pregnancy which has implanted in the narrow section of the uterine (fallopian tube) as it enters the uterus. The pregnancy is not viable as the tube will rupture with severe bleeding by week 12—this is an emergency life-threatening situation requiring urgent surgery.

corona 1. a crown. 2. crown-like encircling structure or projection.

coronal *adj* in dentistry, relating to a crown of a tooth as opposed to the root. Also pertains to the crown of the head.

coronal discharge when electrons are forcibly removed from their orbits to create an electric spark.

coronal plane ⟳ frontal plane.

coronal seal protection against the ingress of fluids and microorganisms from the mouth.

corona radiata 1. the follicular cells surrounding the zona pellucida in the ovum. 2. a network of fibres associated with the internal capsule in the cerebral hemispheres and the fibres of the corpus callosum.

coronary *adj* crown-like; encircling, as of a vessel or nerve.

coronary angiography demonstration of the coronary arteries that supply the myocardium following the injection of a contrast agent.

coronary arteries those supplying the myocardium, the first pair of arteries to branch from the aorta as it leaves the left ventricle (Figure C.17). Spasm, narrowing or blockage of these vessels causes angina pectoris or myocardial infarction (heart attack). Diseased vessels may be cleared by balloon angioplasty, lasers or replaced with veins taken from the legs. ⟳ angioplasty, coronary circulation.

coronary artery bypass graft (CABG) a technique used to revascularize the myocardium thereby relieving anginal pain and decreasing the risk of myocardial infarction. A healthy portion of saphenous vein from the leg, or the mammary artery is grafted between the aorta and a point beyond the blockage in a coronary artery. Often more than one artery is bypassed. Increasingly the procedure is undertaken using minimally invasive techniques.

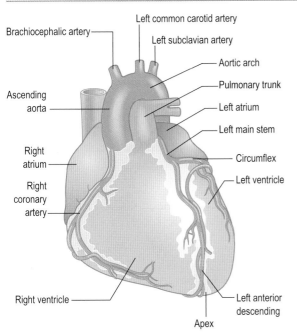

Left common carotid artery

Brachiocephalic artery

Left subclavian artery

Aortic arch

Pulmonary trunk

Ascending aorta

Left atrium

Left main stem

Right atrium

Circumflex

Right coronary artery

Left ventricle

Right ventricle

Left anterior descending

Apex

C.17 Coronary arteries (reproduced from Brooker & Nicol 2003 with permission).

coronary care unit (CCU) high dependency area in a hospital specialized in the care of patients with acute heart problems, particularly those with cardiac arrhythmias, unstable angina pectoris and after a myocardial infarction.

coronary circulation the left main and right coronary arteries arise from the left and right coronary sinuses, just distal to the aortic valve. Within 2.5 cm of its origin the left main stem (left main coronary artery) divides into the left anterior descending artery (LAD), which runs in the anterior interventricular groove, and the left circumflex artery (CX), which runs posteriorly in the atrioventricular groove. The LAD gives branches to supply the anterior part of the septum (septal perforators) and the anterior wall and apex of the left ventricle (LV). The CX gives marginal branches that supply the lateral, posterior and inferior segments of the LV. The right coronary artery (RCA) runs in the right atrioventricular groove, giving branches that supply the right atrium (RA), right ventricle (RV) and inferoposterior aspects of the LV. The posterior descending artery runs in the posterior interventricular groove and supplies the inferior part of the interventricular septum. This vessel is a branch of the RCA in approximately 90% of people (dominant right system) and is supplied by the CX in the remainder (dominant left system). The exact coronary anatomy varies greatly from person to person and there are many 'normal variants'. The right coronary artery supplies the sinus node (also known as sinoatrial [SA]) node in about 60% of individuals, and the atrioventricular (AV) node in about 90%. Proximal occlusion of the RCA therefore often results in sinus bradycardia, and may also cause electrical conduction block of the AV node. Abrupt occlusions in the RCA, due to coronary

thrombosis, result in infarction of the inferior part of the LV and often the RV. Abrupt occlusion of the LAD or CX causes infarction in the corresponding territory of the LV, and occlusion of the left main coronary artery is usually fatal. The venous system mainly follows the coronary arteries but drains to the coronary sinus in the atrioventricular groove, and then to the right atrium. An extensive lymphatic system drains into vessels that travel with the coronary vessels and then into the thoracic duct. ⊃ coronary arteries, coronary sinus.

coronary heart disease (CHD) also known as coronary artery disease and more rarely ischaemic heart disease. It includes angina pectoris, unstable angina and myocardial infarction. A deficient supply of oxygenated blood to the myocardium, causing central chest pain of varying intensity that may radiate to arms and jaws. The lumen of the blood vessels is usually narrowed by atheromatous plaques. If treatment with drug therapy is unsuccessful, percutaneous transluminal coronary angioplasty, or bypass surgery, may be considered. ⊃ acute coronary syndrome, angina pectoris, angioplasty, coronary artery bypass graft, myocardial infarction.

coronary ligament the ligament that attaches the anterior horn of the medial meniscus of the knee to the tibial plateau.

coronary sinus channel receiving most venous blood from the myocardium and opening into the right atrium.

coronary thrombosis occlusion of a coronary artery by a thrombus. The area deprived of blood becomes necrotic and is called an infarct. ⊃ acute coronary syndrome, coronary heart disease, myocardial infarction.

coronaviruses *npl* a group of RNA viruses responsible for acute respiratory infections such as the common cold.

coroner *n* in England and Wales, an officer of the Crown, usually a solicitor, barrister or doctor, who presides over the Coroner's Court responsible for establishing the cause of death in cases where violence may be a possibility or suspected. Where doubts exist about the cause of death the doctor should consult the coroner and act on his or her advice. The coroner must be notified if a patient dies within 24 hours of admission to hospital. In addition all theatre/anaesthetic deaths must also be reported. Any death where the deceased has not been seen by a doctor recently requires that a coroner's postmortem is undertaken. In Scotland, reports about such deaths are submitted to the Procurator Fiscal but a postmortem is normally only ordered if foul play is suspected. The Scottish equivalent of the Coroner's Inquest is the Fatal Accident Enquiry, presided over by the Sheriff.

coronoid fossa a fossa on the distal dorsal aspect of the humerus, it receives the coronoid process of the ulna when the elbow is bent to flex the forearm.

coronoid process 1. a process on the anterior superior margin of the ramus of the mandible, which provides attachment for the temporalis muscle. 2. a process at the proximal end of the ulna, it form part of the trochlear notch that articulates with the humerus at the elbow.

coronoidectomy surgical removal of the coronoid process of the mandible.

coronoidotomy sectioning of the coronoid process of the mandible.

cor pulmonale enlargement of the right ventricle and right-sided heart disease resulting from primary disease of the lung (emphysema, fibrosis, silicosis, etc.) or pulmonary blood vessels, which strains the right ventricle. It is often associated with severe chronic obstructive pulmonary disease and results from prolonged hypoxaemia due to the reflex response (to hypoxaemia) of pulmonary vasoconstriction. Other contributory and interactive factors to cor pulmonale include increased blood viscosity (with polycythaemia), myocardial hypoxia (causing poor ventricular contraction and function), destruction of the pulmonary vascular bed (in association with emphysematous lung disease changes) and acidosis (causing secondary retention of water and sodium).

corpus *n* a body, any mass of tissue which is easily distinguishable from its surroundings—**corpora** *pl*.

corpus albicans the white scar remaining on the ovary once the corpus luteum has degenerated.

corpus cavernosum one of two lateral columns of spongy erectile tissue in the penis and also the clitoris. ⊃ Colour Section Figure 16.

corpus luteum a yellow mass which forms in the ovary after ovulation. It secretes progesterone and persists to maintain pregnancy should it occur.

corpus spongiosum the single ventral column of erectile tissue in the penis. ⊃ Colour Section Figure 16.

corpus striatum part of the basal nuclei (basal ganglia).

corpuscle *n* outdated term for blood cells—**corpuscular** *adj*. ⊃ erythrocytes, leucocytes.

correction in optometry, 1. (*syn* refractive correction) the term used to designate the prescription of spectacle or contact lenses to compensate for ametropia. 2. the process whereby the aberrations of an optical system are minimized. ⊃ achromatic lens, aplanatic lens, doublet, metamorphopsia, refractive error, triplet.

corrective *adj, n* something which changes, counteracts or modifies something harmful.

correlation *n* in statistics. The relationship between variables, i.e. how one characteristic influences another, or in other words it is a measure of cause and effect. The two types of correlation are positive and negative (inverse). ⊃ negative correlation, positive correlation.

correlation coefficient (r) illustrates the degree of association between a pair of variables. Correlation coefficient values range between $+1$ (perfect positive) to -1 (perfect negative), with a value of 0 indicating that there is no linear relationship.

Corrigan's pulse (D Corrigan, Irish physician, 1802–1880) ⊃ collapsing pulse.

corroborating evidence generally, any evidence which tallies with the predictions of a hypothesis or theory. For the strict proponent of falsificationism, however, only a prediction unique to the theory concerned corroborates it. ⊃ falsificationism

cortex *n* the outer layer of an organ or structure beneath its capsule or membrane such as the cerebral cortex, adrenal cortex or renal cortex—**cortices** *pl*, **cortical** *adj*.

cortical *adj* pertaining to the cortex.

cortical magnification (*syn* magnification factor) the term referring to the fact that the amount of cortical area devoted to processing visual information from the central area of the retina far exceeds the amount devoted to the peripheral retina. It is estimated that about 25% of the cells in the visual cortex are devoted to processing the central 2.5° of the visual field. ⊃ visual area, visual pathway.

cortical mastoidectomy ⊃ mastoidectomy.

cortical plate hard bone covering the inner and outer surface of the alveolar process.

corticospinal tract a tract that originates in the cortex of the brain and terminates in the spinal cord and is involved in the control of voluntary movement.

corticosteroids *npl* hormones produced by the adrenal cortex. ⊃ glucocorticoids, mineralocorticoids, sex hormones. The word is also used for synthetic steroids such as prednisolone and dexamethasone. ⊃ Appendix 5.

corticotrophin *n* ⊃ adrenocorticotrophic hormone.

corticotrophin-releasing hormone (CRH) a polypeptide hormone produced by the hypothalamus. It stimulates the release of adrenocorticotrophic hormone (corticotrophin) from the anterior lobe of the pituitary gland.

cortisol *n* hydrocortisone, one of the principal adrenal cortical steroids. It is essential to life. There is decreased secretion in Addison's disease and increased amounts in Cushing's disease and syndrome.

cortisone *n* one of the hormones of the adrenal gland. It is converted into cortisol before use by the body. Used therapeutically as replacement in conditions that include Addison's disease.

corundum mineral form of aluminium oxide powder used as an abrasive in polishing.

Corynebacterium *n* a bacterial genus of Gram-positive, curved rod-shaped bacteria. Many strains colonize the upper respiratory tract, and some are pathogenic and produce exotoxins such as *Corynebacterium diphtheriae* that causes diphtheria.

coryza *n* the 'common cold'. Rhinoviruses, coronaviruses and adenoviruses cause an acute upper respiratory infection of short duration; highly contagious.

COSHH *abbr* Control of Substances Hazardous to Health.

cosmesis the use of cosmetics or surgery for preserving or enhancing self-image.

cosmetic *adj, n* aesthetic. (That which is) performed to improve the appearance or prevent disfigurement. ⊃ plastic surgery.

cosmetic contact lens a contact lens designed to improve the appearance of the eye, to conceal a disfigurement (e.g. a scar), or to change the colour of the eye. Examples include: a tinted lens; an opaque lens with an artificial pupil and iris. ⊃ aniridia, tinted lens.

cosmetic dentistry lay term to describe conservative dental procedure aimed at improving the aesthetics of the patient's dentition and general facial appearance.

cosmetic orthodontics limited orthodontic treatment which aims to improve appearance, such as the closing of a diastema (gap) between central incisors.

cosmetic prosthesis an appliance designed to improve a person's appearance.

costal *adj* pertaining to the ribs.

costal cartilages the cartilages which attach the ribs to the sternum and each other.

cost–benefit analysis (CBA) method of analysis used in the economic evaluation of healthcare interventions (programmes or procedures). Health outcomes are measured in monetary terms to enable comparisons between interventions from a variety of disciplines. There are problems with valuing life and health in monetary terms. So this method is not widely used.

cost centre a department, for example physiotherapy or catering, for which a budget covering staff and other resources has been set.

cost–effectiveness analysis (CEA) analytical technique used in the economic evaluation of healthcare interventions (programmes and procedures). A cost–effectiveness analysis is used when the outcomes of the procedures are not necessarily the same, but can be measured in the same natural units. For example, the outcomes may be measured in death rates, healthy years of life gained, symptom free days, or even blood pressures. The output of this type of analysis is 'cost per unit increase'. For example, cost of intervention against cost per life year gained. Health benefits are measured in natural units (e.g. mortality rates, survival rates) or final clinical outcomes (e.g. cost per life years gained, cost per days off sick reduced). Intermediate clinical outcomes are sometimes used (e.g. number of cancers detected in a screening programme) but this is not valid if a clear association between cancer detected and survival or quality of life cannot be demonstrated.

Costen's syndrome ⊃ temporomandibular joint dysfunction syndrome.

costive *adj* lay term for constipated. ⊃ constipation— **costiveness** *n*.

cost minimization analytic technique used in economic evaluation of healthcare interventions (programmes or procedures). A cost minimization analysis is used when the outcomes or consequences of the procedures are the same. A prerequisite for such a study is that there is evidence (preferably from a randomized clinical trial) that the different procedures are equally effective. A cost minimization analysis therefore solely consists of the analyses of costs. Common examples include comparisons of home and hospital care for chronic and terminal conditions.

costo- a prefix that means 'rib', e.g. *costochondral*.

costochondral *adj* pertaining to a rib and its cartilage.

costochondral junction the junction between the ribs and costal cartilages.

costochondritis *n* inflammation of the costochondral cartilage. ⊃ Tietze syndrome.

costoclavicular *adj* pertaining to the ribs and the clavicle.

costoclavicular syndrome a synonym for cervical rib and thoracic outlet syndrome. ⊃ thoracic outlet syndrome.

cost utility analysis (CUA) analytic technique used in economic evaluation of healthcare interventions (programmes or procedures). A cost utility analysis is used when the outcomes cannot be measured in natural units, so a utility or value scale has to be employed. This may be because the important outcomes of the procedures are not directly comparable or they are multi-faceted, e.g. a comparison of amputation against waiting for the treatment of a gangrenous foot— outcomes could be pain, mobility and/or survival. The commonly used utility scale is quality-adjusted life years (QALYs), which use survey tools such as the Nottingham Health Profile to allocate 'relative qualities' to different health states. However, different people value their health differently; therefore utility ratings are not unique. Research has provided 'average' utility. Cost utility analyses report results as 'costs per QALY (gained)'.

cot death ⊃ sudden unexpected death in infancy (sudden infant death syndrome).

cotton wool spot white swelling in the nerve fibre layer of the retina caused by microinfarction.

cotyledon *n* one of the subdivisions of the uterine surface of the placenta.

cough *n* explosive expulsion of air from the lungs. One of the four cardinal signs/symptoms of respiratory disease. It may be voluntary, or as protective reflex that expels a foreign body such as food or sputum. Cough is a feature of numerous respiratory and cardiac conditions. It can be defined as dry where no sputum is expectorated, or wet if sputum is present. ⊃ postural drainage.

coulomb (C) (C de Coulomb, French physicist, 1736–1806) the Système International d'Unités (SI) unit (International System of Units) of electrical charge equal to the quantity of electricity transferred in 1 second (s) by 1 ampere (A) of current. ⊃ charge.

count rate in radiology, the number of gamma ray detections made by a gamma camera per minute.

coumarins *npl* a group of anticoagulant drugs, e.g. warfarin. ⊃ Appendix 5.

Council for Healthcare Regulatory Excellence (CHRE) a UK-wide statutory body that oversees the regulation of healthcare professionals by several individual statutory regulatory bodies that include the General Medical Council, Health Professions Council, Nursing and Midwifery Council, etc.

Councilman bodies (W Councilman, American pathologist, 1854–1933) deposits of hyalin found in the liver in cases of yellow fever. ⊃ yellow fever.

counselling *n* a professional client-centred helping relationship with a client who is experiencing psychological problems. The counsellor listens actively and helps the client to identify and clarify the problems and supports the client in making a positive attempt to overcome the problems.

counterextension extension by means of holding back the upper part of a limb while pulling down on the other end.

counterirritant *n* an agent which, when applied to the skin, initiates a mild inflammatory response (hyperaemia) and relief of pain and congestion associated with deep-seated inflammation—**counterirritation** *n*.

countertraction *n* traction upon the proximal extremity of a fractured limb opposing the pull of the traction apparatus on the distal extremity.

counter transference the emotional response (unconscious or conscious) of a therapist to a client/patient, for example interacting with the client as if a close relative. Such responses are inappropriate in the therapeutic relationship.

Coupland chisel bone hand dental chisel or gouge with hollowed out blade attached to a pear-shaped hollow octagonal handle. Obtainable in several widths.

couple two moments applied in the same rotational direction to a rotating object or body. Also known as force couple.

coupling gel a gel put on a patient's skin during an ultrasound examination to exclude any air between the transducer and the skin surface to enable the transmission of ultrasound waves between the transducer and the patient.

couvades *n* exhibiting the symptoms of pregnancy and childbirth by the father. Common in some cultures.

Couvelaire uterus (A Couvelaire, French obstetrician, 1873–1948) 'uterine apoplexy'. Bruising and swelling due to bleeding into the uterine muscle associated with serious placental abruption (abruptio placentae).

cover screw a generic term used to describe a screw fixed to the exposed surface and internal thread of an implant fixture or implant abutment. It is placed to avoid tissue ingress or packing of debris inside the implant.

cover test (CT) (*syn* occlusion test, screen test) a test for determining the presence and the type of heterophoria or strabismus. The subject fixates a small letter or any fine detail at a given distance. Strabismus is usually tested first. The opaque cover or occluder is placed over one eye and then removed, while the examiner observes the other eye and then the same operation is repeated on the other eye (this is called the unilateral cover test). If neither uncovered eye moves the subject does not have strabismus. If the unoccluded eye moves when a cover is placed in front of the other, strabismus is present. In esotropia the unoccluded eye will move temporally to take up fixation, while in exotropia the unoccluded eye will move nasally, and an upward or downward movement indicates hypotropia or hypertropia, respectively. In alternating squint, in which either eye can take up fixation, the eye behind the cover will appear deviated when uncovered and will move as the cover is shifted to the other eye. The type of heterophoria can be detected by observing the eye behind the cover. If there is no movement of the eye behind the cover, the subject is orthophoric. If the eye behind the cover moves inward, and outward when the cover is removed, the subject has esophoria. If the eye behind the cover moves outward, and inward when the cover is removed, the subject has exophoria.

A similar procedure is used for hyperphoria and hypophoria. As it is difficult to view the eye behind the cover without allowing sufficient peripheral fusion to stop the eyes going to the phoria position, the observer usually watches for the recovery movement as the occluder is removed. By placing prisms of increasing power in front of one of the eyes until no movement is evoked, one can evaluate the approximate amount of the phoria. The cover test is the only objective method of measuring heterophoria. The determination of the magnitude of the deviation of the strabismus or heterophoria can also be done with the *alternate (or alternating) cover test* (ACT). The subject fixates a target and the cover is successively placed in front of one eye and then the other while watching the eye which has just been uncovered to see the direction of the deviation. The amount of deviation can be estimated by using prisms of appropriate strength and base direction until the movement of the eye is neutralized when the cover is alternated from one eye to the other (*prism cover test*). Although these tests are objective, they are sometimes used subjectively, i.e. the patient indicates the apparent movement of the fixation object. The alternate cover test is the most appropriate test for subjective testing. An apparent movement of the fixation object in the same direction as the cover indicates exophoria, while an apparent movement of the fixation object in the opposite direction to the cover indicates esophoria. An apparent downward movement of the fixation indicates hyperphoria of the eye from which the occluder is moved. Again prisms can be placed in front of the eyes until the apparent movement disappears, thus giving a measure of the heterophoria. This subjective perception of a movement of a stationary fixation object in people with heterophoria or strabismus is a particular example of the phi phenomenon. ⊃ heterophoria, strabismus.

Cowper's glands (W Cowper, English surgeon, 1666–1709) ⊃ bulbourethral glands.

cowpox humans in contact with infected cows develop large vesicles, usually on the hands or arms and associated with fever and regional lymphadenitis. The reservoir is thought to be wild rodents, and the virus also produces symptomatic disease in cats and a range of other animals.

cow's horn forceps ⊃ forceps.

cox- a prefix that means 'hip', e.g. *coxalgia*.

COX-2 *abbr* cyclo-oxygenase-2.

COX-2 inhibitors cyclo-oxygenase-2 inhibitors, e.g. celecoxib, are selective NSAIDs. They have a lower incidence of gastrointestinal disburbances, but there are serious worries regarding cardiovascular safety. ⊃ Appendix 5

coxa *n* the hip joint—**coxae** *pl*. ⊃ coxa valga, coxa vara.

coxa valga an increase in the normal angle between neck and shaft of femur.

coxa vara a decrease in the normal angle plus torsion of the neck, e.g. slipped femoral epiphysis.

coxalgia *n* pain in the hip joint.

Coxiella *n* a microbial genus closely related to *Rickettsia* including *Coxiella burnetii* which causes Q fever.

coxitis *n* inflammation of the hip joint.

coxsackievirus *n* one of the three groups of viruses included in the family of enteroviruses. Divided into groups A and B. Cause conditions that include: aseptic meningitis, herpangina, Bornholm disease, gastroenteritis and myocarditis.

CP 1. constant potential. **2.** creatine phosphokinase.

CPA *abbr* care programme approach.

CPAP *abbr* continuous positive airways pressure.

CPD *abbr* **1.** cephalopelvic disproportion. **2.** continuing professional development.

CPEO *abbr* chronic progressive external ophthalmoplegia.

c-peptide an inactive peptide formed when proinsulin is converted to insulin in the beta cells of the pancreas. The amount of c-peptide in the blood can be measured to give an indication of pancreatic beta cell function.

CPITN *abbr* community periodontal index of treatment needs. ⊃ index (dental).

CPK/CP *abbr* creatine phosphokinase ⊃ creatine kinase.

CPM *abbr* continuous passive motion (movement).

CPN *abbr* Community Psychiatric Nurse.

CPP *abbr* cerebral perfusion pressure.

CPR *abbr* cardiopulmonary resuscitation.

CPS *abbr* characters per second.

CPT *abbr* carnitine palmitoyltransferase.

CPU *abbr* central processing unit.

CQC *abbr* Care Quality Commission.

Cr *abbr* creatine.

crab louse phthirus pubis.

crack cocaine a highly potent and addictive form of cocaine (a Class A drug).

cracked nipple nipple damage occuring during breast-feeding due to the infant being incorrectly fixed on the breast, causing pressure leading to soreness and bleeding. It can be prevented by teaching the woman how to position the infant at the breast correctly. Treatment if the nipple is too sore to continue feeding involves mechanical milk expression to maintain lactation. Creams containing camomile or the application of moist camomile teabags may ease the discomfort and aid healing.

cracked tooth syndrome transient pain during eating can indicate a crack in a tooth. The cause is difficult to locate and is commonly due to a vertical tooth fracture or split extending across the marginal ridge, through the crown and into the pulp chamber. It may become visible by the use of disclosing dyes and by transillumination. Often occurs in people who crush ice or crack nuts with their teeth.

cradle cap *n* scaling of the scalp of infants, often due to atopic eczema or seborrhoeic dermatitis.

cramp *n* specific form of spasm: involuntary, sustained and painful muscle contraction, particularly in the legs, often associated with fatigue and usually relieved by stretching. ⊃ exercise-associated muscle cramp (EAMC), nocturnal cramp.

cranial *adj* pertaining to the cranium.

cranial cavity the rigid 'box' containing and protecting the brain. Its boundaries are formed by the bones of the cranium: anteriorly—1 frontal bone; laterally—2 temporal bones; posteriorly—1 occipital bone; superiorly—2 parietal bones; and inferiorly—1 sphenoid and 1 ethmoid bone and parts of the frontal, temporal and occipital bones.

cranial nerves twelve pairs of nerves that arise from the brain and exit through openings in the skull (Figure C.18). They have names and are designated by Roman

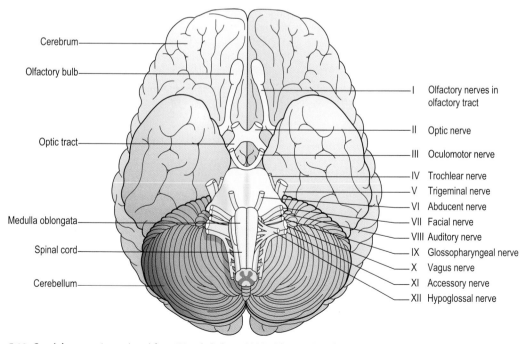

C.18 Cranial nerves (reproduced from Waugh & Grant 2006 with permission).

numerals—olfactory (I); optic (II); oculomotor (III); trochlear (IV); trigeminal (V); abducens (abducent) (VI); facial (VII); vestibulocochlear (auditory/acoustic) (VIII); glossopharyngeal IX; vagus X; accessory XI; hypoglossal XII.

crani/o- a prefix that means 'skull', e.g. *craniometry.*

craniodidymus a form of conjoined twins with two heads but fused bodies.

craniofacial *adj* pertaining to the cranium and the face.

craniofacial dysjunction fracture ⮑ Le Fort III fracture.

craniofacial dysostosis Crouzon's disease. Congenital disease of bone characterized by bossing of the frontal region, hypoplasia of the maxilla, mandibular prognathism and often cleft palate. Other bones may be involved as well as eye changes, often resulting in blindness.

craniomandibular fixation ⮑ fixation (dentistry/maxillofacial surgery).

craniomaxillary fixation ⮑ fixation (dentistry/maxillofacial surgery).

craniometry *n* the science which deals with the measurement of skulls.

craniopharyngioma *n* a tumour which develops between the brain and the pituitary gland.

cranioplasty *n* operative repair of a skull defect—**cranioplastic** *adj.*

craniosacral *adj* pertaining to the skull and sacrum. Applied to the outflow of the parasympathetic nervous system.

craniosacral therapy form of osteopathic treatment using very gentle manipulation of the cranium to release tensions within the skull, thought to cause various problems. Successfully used to treat infants fractious after difficult forceps or vacuum extraction deliveries, and colic and hyperactivity in older infants.

craniostat ⮑ cephalostat.

craniostenosis *n* a condition in which the skull sutures fuse too early and the fontanelles close. It may cause increased intracranial pressure requiring surgery.

craniosynostosis *n* craniostosis. Premature fusion of cranial sutures resulting in abnormal skull shape and craniostenosis. Deformities depend on which sutures are affected. Often associated with other skeletal abnormalities.

craniotabes *n* a thinning or wasting of the cranial bones occurring in infancy. May persist in infants/children who later have rickets—**craniotabetic** *adj.*

craniotomy *n* a surgical opening of the skull in order to remove a growth, relieve pressure, evacuate blood clot or arrest haemorrhage.

cranium *n* the part of the skull enclosing the brain. It comprises eight bones: the occipital, two parietals, frontal, two temporals, sphenoid and ethmoid—**cranial** *adj.*

crank test a test used to assess shoulder stability.

CRAO *abbr* central retinal arterial occlusion.

craquelé *adj* describes cracked skin resembling crazy paving. A term used in association with a certain type of eczema seen in older people.

crash a computer term that describes sudden and serious malfunction or complete loss of program. ⮑ bug.

crazing in dentistry, the pattern of minute hair-like cracks on the surface of porcelain and acrylic polymers. Also known as microcracks.

CRE *abbr* cumulative radiation effect.

C-reactive protein (CRP) an acute phase protein. Elevated amounts are present in the plasma in response to inflammation and tissue damage. It is a very sensitive progress indicator of many inflammatory conditions, such as infective endocarditis.

creatine (Cr) *n* a nitrogenous organic compound produced in the body, held primarily in skeletal muscle. Obtained from a normal diet (mainly in meat and eggs) and also synthesized from amino acids in the liver. In resting conditions, about 60% is in the phosphorylated form (the important form of high-energy phosphate), creatine phosphate (CrP). Creatine plus phosphorylated creatine constitute the creatine pool. Creatine is the fastest selling ergogenic aid among athletes; creatine supplementation aims to increase the CrP energy reserve, delaying CrP depletion and hence reducing requirement for anaerobic glycolysis; also facilitating CrP resynthesis between bouts of high-intensity exercise, enhancing performance during multiple repeats. When supplementation is combined with resistance training, leads to greater gain in muscle mass. A typical protocol involves daily Cr intake of 20–25 g for 5 days, then continued daily supplementation with 2–3 g. The response varies between individuals, with uptake inversely related to the initial muscle concentration, and ∼30% appearing to be 'non-responders'. ⮑ ergogenic aids.

creatine kinase (CK) (*syn* ATP:creatine phosphokinase [CPK, CP]) a cytoplasmic enzyme occurring as three isoenzymes; it catalyses the transfer of phosphate group from creatine phosphate to adenosine diphosphate (ADP), producing adenosine triphosphate (ATP) and creatine (Figure C.19). It is found in brain tissue, skeletal muscle, blood and myocardial tissue. The isoenzymes can be distinguished in the blood when either skeletal or cardiac muscle has been damaged. ⮑ muscle enzymes.

C.19 Creatine kinase (CK) reaction (reproduced from Jennett 2008 with permission).

creatine kinase test increased levels of the myocardial iso-enzyme in serum is indicative of acute myocardial infarction. If the test follows strenuous exercise, especially if it had a large eccentric component, distinction from the skeletal muscle isoenzyme is critical.

creatine phosphate (CrP) provides muscle with a reservoir of high-energy phosphate for the rapid rephosphorylation of adenosine diphosphate (ADP) to adenosine triphosphate (ATP) during high-intensity exercise. Other functions of CrP are the buffering of hydrogen ions produced during anaerobic glycolysis, and the transport of ATP, generated by aerobic metabolism, from mitochondria to cytoplasm where it can be utilized in contraction and other cellular processes. Also known as phosphocreatine (PCr).

creatinine *n* a by-product of the metabolism of creatine phosphate in muscle tissue. The amount produced daily is fairly constant and depends on the muscle mass, which is influenced by age, gender and body weight. Creatinine is normally cleared by the kidneys and excreted in the urine. Blood level of creatinine is related to muscle mass. Serum creatinine is raised in renal failure, hyperthyroidism and muscle wasting disorders, but the interpretation of the results must take account of age, gender and body weight. The measurement in blood and urine are used as an indicator of renal function.

creatinine clearance test measures the rate at which the kidneys clear creatinine from the blood. The relationship between age, gender, body weight and serum creatinine may be used to calculate the creatinine clearance rate, which can be used to provide an estimate of the glomerular filtration rate.

creatinuria excess amount of creatine present in the urine, as in situations where muscle protein is rapidly broken down.

creative activities activities that place demands on the individual or group to use imagination and skill in order to produce a new and worthwhile outcome.

creativity the ability to use imagination, to think and act independently in order to bring into being something new that has personal and/or social value. The creative product may be an object, a thought, a theory or a solution to a problem.

Credé's expression technique to aid separation and expulsion of a partially separated placenta in severe postpartum haemorrhage. It is intensely painful and can cause shock and is rarely used.

creep *n* **1.** (*syn* cold flow) the continued change in the size of the lumen of plastic tubing in intravenous giving sets after release of the clamp. It can change the rate of the fluid passing along the tube. **2.** to slowly change shape, as do heated metals and ceramics under load. Amalgam restorations may flow or creep under heavy masticatory forces.

crenation the shrinkage of red blood cells when they are placed in a hypertonic solution.

crepitation ➲ crepitus.

crepitus *n* **1.** (crepitation) grinding noise or sensation within a joint, as in osteoarthritis. A feature of fracture and overuse injury. **2.** crackling sound heard via stethoscope. **3.** crackling sound elicited by pressure on tissue containing air (surgical emphysema).

cresent sign ➲ meniscus sign.

cresol *n* yellowish liquid obtained from coal tar. Chemically related to phenol. Used in many general environmental disinfectants. In dentistry, sometimes used as an antiseptic and as a disinfectant. In combination with formaldehyde solution, formocresol is used in root canal therapy as a devitalizing agent and antiseptic.

crest in anatomy a narrow ridge or elevation generally used in the description of bones, e.g. nasal crest of the maxilla, iliac crest. Sometimes used to describe soft tissue, e.g. gingival crest.

CREST syndrome *acron* **C**alcinosis, **R**aynaud's phenomenon, (o)**E**sophageal dysfunction, **S**clerodactyly and **T**elangiectasis. A form of systemic sclerosis.

cretinism *n* obsolete term. ➲ hypothyroidism.

Creutzfeldt–Jakob disease (CJD) (H Creutzfeldt, German neurologist, 1885–1964; A Jakob, German neurologist, 1884–1931) a progressive dementia transmissible through prion protein. New variant vCJD, mainly affecting young adults, is possibly linked with the prion causing bovine spongiform encephalopathy (BSE). CJD follows a rapid degenerative course often with myoclonus and is usually fatal.

crevice narrow opening or fissure.

crevicular epithelium an extension of non-keratinized squamous cells into the crevice from the gingival crest epithelium.

CRF *abbr* chronic renal failure. ➲ renal failure.

CRH *abbr* corticotrophin-releasing hormone.

crib round wire clasp fitting round a tooth to provide retention for a prosthesis. Both ends of the wire are secured to the baseplate of a removable orthodontic appliance or a denture. ➲ Adams' clasp.

cribriform *adj* perforated, like a sieve.

cribriform plate that portion of the ethmoid bone allowing passage of fibres of olfactory nerve.

cribriform plate of the sclera (*syn* lamina cribrosa [although this term also refers to the striated portion of the bulbar optic nerve which includes the cribriform plate]) the part of the sclera which is situated at the site of attachment of the optic nerve, 3 mm to the inner side of and just above the posterior pole of the eye. There, the sclera is a thin sieve-like membrane through which pass fibres of the optic nerve. ➲ optic nerve.

cricoid *adj* ring-shaped. Applied to the cartilage forming the inferior anterior/posterior part of larynx. ➲ Colour Section Figure 6.

cricoid pressure (Sellick's manoeuvre) a manoeuvre in which manual pressure is applied over the cricoid cartilage to occlude the oesophagus to prevent regurgitation and aspiration of gastric contents during induction of anaesthesia.

cricothyroid membrane fibroelastic membrane that joins the cricoid and thyroid cartilages.

cricothyroidotomy *n* (*syn* cricothyrotomy) incision through the skin and cricothyroid membrane into the larynx to secure a patent airway for emergency relief of upper airway obstruction. ⇲ minitracheostomy, tracheostomy.

'cri du chat' syndrome caused by the partial deletion of one arm of chromosone number 5 leading to learning disability and shortened lifespan. There are certain physical abnormalities and a curious flat, toneless cat-like cry in infancy.

Crigler–Najjar syndrome (J Crigler, American paediatrician, b. 1919; V Najjar, American microbiologist, b. 1914) an inherited condition, in which the enzyme glucuronyl transferase is absent or deficient. There is jaundice and unconjugated hyperbilirubinaemia resulting in damage to the central nervous system.

criminal abortion ⇲ abortion.

criminal law deals with actions/behaviour regarded as wrong. Criminal offences relate to people and property and result in a prosecution and, if the defendant is convicted, usually result in punishment (discharge, fine, community penalty or a custodial sentence—suspended or immediate). The burden of proof in criminal cases requires that the prosecution prove the facts 'beyond reasonable doubt' to the court, either to the magistrates in the Magistrates' court or the jury in the Crown court. The offences heard in the criminal courts include criminal damage, child cruelty, common assault, drink driving, fraud, public order offences, manslaughter, murder, rape, robbery, theft and many others.

criminal wrong an act or omission that can be pursued in the criminal courts.

crisis 1. *n* the turning point of a disease—as the point of defervescence in fever. ⇲ lysis *opp.* **2.** muscular spasm in tabes dorsalis referred to as visceral crisis (gastric, vesical, rectal, etc.)—**crises** *pl.*

crista 1. an anatomical crest. **2.** the crista ampullaris, sensory structure in the ampulla of the semicircular canals within the inner ear. **3.** the infolding of the inner membrane of a mitochondrion.

cristobalite form of silica used with plaster of Paris as a refractory in investment materials. ⇲ investing.

critical angle 1. in optometry, that angle of incidence which results in the refracted ray travelling along the surface between the two media (angle of refraction equal to 90°). If the angle of incidence is greater than the critical angle, the ray is totally reflected. If, however, the angle of incidence is smaller than the critical angle, the ray is refracted (with some light reflected). ⇲ refractometer. **2.** in ultrasonography, when an incident beam of ultrasound strikes an interface at an angle equal to or greater than this angle, only reflection of the beam will occur.

critical appraisal the process of making an objective judgement regarding a research study. Includes research design, methodology, analysis, interpretation of results and the applicability of the study findings to a particular area of health care.

critical care (outreach) team in hospital the provision of an outreach team of specialist critical care practitioners with three objectives: to prevent admissions to critical care facilities; to share critical care skills with ward-based staff; and to facilitate timely discharges from critical care.

critical oxygen requirement (COR) (*syn* critical oxygen tension) in relation to a contact lens, the minimum oxygen pressure at the epithelial surface required to prevent corneal swelling during the day. This value was initially assumed to be between 11 and 19 mmHg but it is nowadays considered to be at least 74 mmHg near the centre of the cornea (or 10% equivalent oxygen pressure or a Dk/L of about 25×10^{-9} $(cm^2 \; mL \; O_2)/(s \; mL \; mmHg)$ at 25°C) for daily wear. This figure increases to at least 90×10^{-9} for overnight wear. ⇲ equivalent oxygen pressure, hypoxia.

critical oxygen tension ⇲ critical oxygen requirement (COR).

critical period (*syn* plastic period, [however, this term relates more specifically to the time course during which the visual system is still responsive to treatment. This may differ from the critical period of development], sensitive period) a time after birth during which neural connections can still be modified by interference with normal visual experience or lesion of the visual pathway. If a person has an anomaly (e.g. amblyopia), the treatment is most likely to be effective during the earliest part of the critical period. In humans it lasts up to about 8–10 years of age.

critical pH the pH below which tooth enamel is demineralized.

critical power if the tolerable duration of high-intensity exercise is plotted (horizontal axis) against a direct or indirect measure of power output (e.g. running speed: vertical axis), starting at the top end (maximum aerobic power, $\dot{V}O_{2max}$), a power output will be found at which endurance extends into a plateau. This is termed the critical power and in a trained endurance athlete may last several tens of minutes.

critique the academic process whereby a review is made of a piece of written or practical work.

CRL *abbr* crown–rump length.

crocodile shagreen (*syn* crocodile shagreen of Vogt) polygonal greyish-white corneal opacities separated by relatively clear spaces and located in the stroma, either near Bowman's membrane (anterior crocodile shagreen) or occasionally near Descemet's membrane (posterior crocodile shagreen). They are the result of an irregularity of the stromal collagen lamellae. The condition occurs in older people who are asymptomatic, with little or no effect on vision.

Crohn's disease (B Crohn, American physician, 1884–1983) a chronic recurrent granulomatous inflammation affecting any part of the bowel from mouth to anus. Inflammation may be discontinuous ('skip lesions') with normal bowel in between. May be complicated by fistulae and strictures. The ocular manifestations include acute iridocyclitis, scleritis, conjunctivitis and corneal infiltrates. ⇲ inflammatory bowel disease.

Crosby capsule a special tube which is passed through the mouth to the small intestine. Allows biopsy of jejunal mucosa. Endoscopic biopsy is often used in preference to this time-consuming investigation.

cross bite malocclusion of anterior or posterior teeth in which the labiolingual or buccolingual relationship of opposing teeth is the reverse of normal, i.e. a reverse horizontal overlap. Can be uni- or bilateral malocclusion involving one or more teeth in each dental arch.

cross-bridge the (actin-) myosin cross-bridge in muscle, strictly refers to the molecular structure consisting of a myosin head-group bound to an actin molecule. Widely, though loosely, also used for the head-group alone, particularly when seen as an ultrastructural component in a striated muscle fibre. ⊃ length–tension relationship, muscle contraction, myosin.

cross-bridge cycle the cycle of force-generating attachment/detachment interactions between myosin head-groups and actin, powered by the hydrolysis of adenosine triphosphate (ATP). ⊃ length–tension relationship, muscle contraction, myosin.

cross-cylinder lens (*syn* Jackson cross-cylinder lens) an astigmatic lens consisting of a minus cylinder ground on one side and a plus cylinder ground on the other side, the two axes being located 90° apart. The dioptric power in the principal meridians is equal. Usual cross-cylinder lenses are provided in three powers: ±0.25 D, ±0.37 D and ±0.50 D (higher values are also available for use with low vision patients). This lens is used in the subjective measurement of the power and axis of astigmatism, or to refine the cylindrical correction determined otherwise. ⊃ astigmatism, cross-cylinder test for astigmatism.

cross-cylinder method ⊃ cross-cylinder test for astigmatism.

cross-cylinder test ⊃ cross-cylinder test for astigmatism.

cross-cylinder test for astigmatism (*syn* cross-cylinder method, cross-cylinder test, Jackson crossed cylinder test) a subjective test for measuring the axis and the amount of astigmatism using a cross-cylinder lens. Having obtained the best visual acuity with a spherical lens, the cross-cylinder lens is placed before the eye being tested with its axes at 45° to the cylinder axis determined by retinoscopy. The person looks at a single circular target, often a letter (O or C or Verhoeff's circles), the cross-cylinder lens is then flipped and if one position provides a clearer image of the target, the axis of the correcting (minus) cylinder should be turned towards the minus axis of the cross-cylinder lens until vision is equally blurred in both positions of the cross-cylinder lens. That point indicates the correct axis of the correcting cylinder. The determination of the power of the correcting cylinder is carried out by placing the cross-cylinder lens with one of its axes parallel to the axis of the correcting cylinder. The cross-cylinder lens is flipped and the position which provides the clearer vision indicates whether to increase the cylinder power (when the minus axis of the cross-cylinder is parallel) or decrease the cylinder power (when the plus axis is parallel). The proper amount of cylinder correction is obtained when the vision is equally blurred in both positions of the cross-cylinder lens. ⊃ cross-cylinder lens, Verhoeff's circles.

crossed diplopia ⊃ heteronymous diplopia.

cross infection occurs when pathogens are transferred from one person to another. ⊃ infection.

cross-linking creates chemical bonds between molecular chains in a polymer, making the resin stronger and more rigid.

cross marking the practice of markers marking the same piece of student work, usually blinded and comparing marks in an attempt at standardization of marks.

cross-over effect in radiography, the amount of light transmitted to the opposite side of a film base expressed as a percentage.

cross-over studies a research study where the participants are exposed to both the experimental intervention and the placebo one after another.

cross-sectional study in research a survey of an entire population for the presence or absence of a disease and/or other variable in every member (or a representative sample) and the potential risk factors at a particular point in time or time interval.

cross-striations lines seen under the microscope which cross enamel prisms and are thought to indicate their daily growth.

croup *n* viral infection leading to laryngeal narrowing. The child has 'croupy', stridulous (noisy or harsh-sounding) breathing. Narrowing of the airway which gives rise to the typical attack with crowing inspiration may be the result of oedema or spasm, or both.

Crouzon's disease (L Crouzon, French neurologist, 1874–1938). ⊃ craniofacial dysostosis.

crowding malocclusion resulting from the disproportion in the combined mesiodistal dimension of the teeth and the size of the maxilla or mandible, leading to a displacement from the dental arch.

crown *n* the top part of a structure. **1.** that part of a tooth covered by enamel. ⊃ tooth. **2.** replacement (restoration) of part or all of the clinical crown of a tooth, cemented into place. May be made of metal, plastic, porcelain or a combination of these. Classified by extent, method of construction and materials used. ⊃ anatomical crown, basket crown, cast crown, clinical crown, crown lengthening, dowel crown, full veneer crown, jacket crown, partial veneer crown, polycarbonate crown, porcelain bonded crown, porcelain jacket crown (PJC), post crown, preformed metal crown, shell crown, strip crown, telescopic crown, temporary crown, temporary post crown.

crown glass glass characterized by low dispersion. The most commonly used crown glass in ophthalmic lenses, called ophthalmic crown or spectacle crown, has a refractive index $n = 1.523$ and a constringence or V-value of 59. There are other types of crown glass (e.g. dense barium crown $n = 1.623$, V-value 56; fluor crown $n = 1.485$,

V-value 70). ⊃ constringence, dispersion, doublet, Fresnel formula, triplet.

crown–heel length the distance from the crown of the head to the heel in the embryo, fetus and infant, equivalent to standing height.

crown lengthening a surgical procedure sometimes required to increase crown length and thus improve artificial crown retention.

crown of a tooth that part of the tooth covered with enamel. ⊃ tooth.

crown–rump length (CRL) the distance from the crown of the head to the breech in the embryo, fetus and infant, equivalent to sitting height. It can be measured by ultrasound imaging between 6 and 14 weeks' gestation to assess fetal maturity. It is accurate to within 3 to 4 days. ⊃ dating scan.

crown scissors ⊃ scissors.

crowning the time during the second stage of labour when the fetal head is visible at the vaginal introitus.

CrP *abbr* creatine phosphate.

CRP *abbr* C-reactive protein.

CRPS *abbr* complex regional pain syndrome.

CRS *abbr* (NHS) care record service.

CRT *abbr* cathode ray tube.

cruciate *adj* shaped like a cross such as the cruciate ligaments stabilizing the knee joint.

cruciate ligaments two intracapsular ligaments of the knee, forming an X-shape, linking the femur to the tibia, strong but not elastic, which are crucial for the stability of the knee joint (see Figure A.11, p. 49). The anterior cruciate ligament (ACL) runs upwards, backwards and laterally from the front of the upper end of the tibia to attach to the medial aspect of the lateral femoral condyle; it limits forward movement of the tibia relative to the femur and tightens with extension at the knee. It is short and thick with a poor blood supply. The posterior cruciate ligament (PCL) arises from the posterior intercondylar area of the tibia and runs forwards, upwards and medially to attach to the anterolateral surface of the medial femoral condyle. It limits backwards movement of the tibia relative to the femur and tightens with flexion at the knee.

cruciate ligament injury injury, especially to the anterior ligament, can result in a rapid accumulation of blood in the knee joint (haemarthrosis) and is often associated with damage to other structures, especially the medial meniscus. Treatment depends on the sport involved, the degree of instability and of other damage. In sportspeople complete rupture usually requires surgical repair, resulting in a lengthy (up to 9 months) rehabilitation programme, before return to sport. Disruption of only the posterior ligament may result in significant instability but may be hard to diagnose clinically. ⊃ anterior (PA) drawer test, Lachman's test (modified anterior drawer test), posterior (AP) drawer test.

crude birth rate ⊃ birth rate.

crural *adj* relating to the thigh.

crus *n* a structure which is leg-like or root-like. Applied to various parts of the body, e.g. crus of the diaphragm—**crura** *pl*, **crural** *adj*.

'crush' syndrome traumatic uraemia. Following extensive trauma to muscle, there is a period of delay before the effects of renal damage manifest themselves. There is an increase of non-protein nitrogen in the blood, with oliguria, proteinuria and urinary excretion of myohaemoglobin. Loss of blood plasma to damaged area is marked. Where hypotension has occurred the renal failure will be exacerbated by tubular necrosis.

crutch palsy paralysis of extensor muscles of wrist, fingers and thumb from repeated pressure of a crutch upon the radial nerve in the axilla.

CRVO *abbr* central retinal vein occlusion.

cryaesthesia *n* **1**. the sensation of coldness. **2**. exceptional sensitivity to a low temperature.

Cryer's elevator ⊃ elevator (dental).

cryo- a prefix that means 'cold', e.g. *cryopexy*.

cryoanalgesia *n* the relief of pain symptoms by blocking peripheral nerve conduction with extreme cold.

cryogenic *adj, n* produced by low temperature. Also used to describe any means or apparatus involved in the production of low temperature.

cryoglobulin *n* an immunoglobulin that precipitates on cooling, and redissolves on warming; associated with numerous pathological conditions including occlusion of peripheral blood vessels, ulceration and gangrene. *Type 1 cryoglobulins* are monoclonal and are associated with lymphoproliferative disorders. *Type 2 cryoglobulins* are monoclonal with reactivity against polyclonal immunoglobulins, i.e. they are rheumatoid factors. *Type 3 cryoglobulins* are polyclonal with rheumatoid factor activity.

cryokinetics *n* use of cold treatments prior to activity.

cryopexy *n* surgical fixation by freezing, of a detached retina.

cryoprecipitate a preparation of factor VIII obtained by rapid freezing and thawing of plasma. Used in the treatment of haemophilia.

cryoprobe *n* freezing probe which can be used to destroy tumours.

cryosurgery *n* the use of intense, controlled cold to remove or destroy diseased tissue.

cryothalamectomy *n* freezing applied to destroy groups of neurons within the thalamus in the treatment of Parkinson's disease and other hyperkinetic conditions.

cryotherapy *n* the use of cold for the treatment of disease. Includes the use of a local or general form of cooling. Most commonly used as part of RICE to reduce extent of acute pain or responses of the body to acute trauma. Local methods include applications of a crushed ice pack or pre-made cooled gel pack in damp covering or an inflatable cuff through which cooled water can circulate. Ice packs are usually used in conjunction with rest, compression and depending on the region affected, elevation. ⊃ ice/cold therapy.

crypt small blind recess or pocket. *dental crypt* cavity in the alveolar bone in which a tooth develops before eruption.

crypt/o- a prefix that means 'hidden, concealed', e.g. *cryptorchism*.

cryptococcosis *n* the disease resulting from infection with the yeast *Cryptococcus neoformans*, which is present in soil and pigeon excreta. It most commonly causes meningitis but may also affect the lungs, skin and bones. Immunocompromised individuals, such as those with AIDS, are at increased risk.

Cryptococcus *n* a genus of fungi. *Cryptococcus neoformans* occasionally causes disease in humans.

cryptodidymus conjoined twins, one being considerable smaller and developing within the body of the other.

cryptogenic *adj* of unknown or obscure cause.

cryptogenic fibrosing alveolitis (CFA) ⟳ idiopathic pulmonary fibrosis.

cryptogenic organizing pneumonia (COP) (*syn* bronchiolitis obliterans organizing pneumonia) one of the idiopathic interstitial pneumonias. It presents as clinical and radiological pneumonia. Systemic features and markedly raised erythrocyte sedimentation rate (ESR) are common. Finger clubbing is characteristically absent. The biopsy shows a florid proliferation of immature collagen (Masson's bodies) and fibrous tissue. The response to corticosteroids is classically dramatic.

cryptomenorrhoea *n* retention of the menses due to a congenital obstruction, such as an imperforate hymen or atresia of the vagina. ⟳ haematocolpos.

cryptophthalmos ⟳ Fraser syndrome.

cryptorchism *n* (*syn* undescended testes) a developmental defect whereby the testes do not descend into the scrotum; they are retained within the abdomen or inguinal canal— **cryptorchid, cryptorchis** *n*. ⟳ undescended testes.

cryptosporidiosis *n* infection caused by cryptosporidium species (protozoa). The organisms are present in the faeces of both domestic and farm animals, and transmission to humans occurs through contaminated water and food. Infection may be symptomless or result in profuse watery diarrhoea. Immunocompromised individuals may be seriously affected.

crystal defects imperfections within a crystal which create areas of low energy called 'electron traps' and 'holes'. ⟳ line defects, point defects.

crystalline *adj* like a crystal.

crystalline lens the lens of the eye. The biconvex, usually transparent body, situated between the iris and the vitreous body (humour) of the eye and suspended from the ciliary body by the zonular fibres (zonule of Zinn) which are attached to the equator of the lens. It separates the aqueous humour from the vitreous body (humour). The diameter of the lens is equal to 9–10 mm and its thickness 3.6 mm, being greater when the eye accommodates. The radii of curvature of the anterior and posterior surfaces are 10.6 mm and −6.2 mm, respectively in the unaccommodated eye, while maximum accommodation alters these values to about 6 mm and −5.3 mm, respectively. The crystalline lens displays a complex gradient of refractive index (averaging 1.42), and a power of 21 D. It consists of the capsule which envelops the lens, the anterior epithelium and the cortex which surrounds the nucleus, the latter two containing the lens fibres. With age, there is an increase in light scatter originating in the nucleus, as well as some light absorption and yellowing of the nucleus. ⟳ accommodation, capsule of the crystalline lens, capsulectomy, intraocular lens implant, lens paradox, lenticular myopia, optic fissure, phakic, shagreen, zonule of Zinn.

crystallins *npl* proteins forming the lens of the eye.

crystalloids *npl* substances in solution that will diffuse through a semipermeable membrane.

crystalloid solutions clear solutions containing small molecules that are able to pass through the capillary membrane thereby moving between the bloodstream and the tissue fluid. They are used intravenously to maintain hydration and electrolyte balance, for example 0.9% sodium chloride. ⟳ colloid solutions.

crystalluria *n* excretion of crystals in the urine— **crystalluric** *adj*.

crystal violet (*syn* gentian violet) a brilliant, violet-coloured, antiseptic aniline dye, used as 0.5% solution as a stain. It is only licensed for application to intact skin, the exception being marking the skin before surgery.

CS *abbr* caesarean section.

CSA *abbr* Child Support Agency.

CSF *abbr* 1. cerebrospinal fluid. 2. colony stimulating factor.

CSI *abbr* Caregiver Strain Index.

CSII *abbr* continuous subcutaneous insulin infusion.

CSM *abbr* Committee on Safety of Medicines.

CSOM *abbr* chronic suppurative otitis media.

CSR *abbr* central serous retinopathy.

CSS *abbr* Churg–Strauss syndrome.

CSSD *abbr* central sterile supplies department.

CSSU *abbr* central sterile supply unit.

CST *abbr* contraction stress test.

CT *abbr* 1. cerebral tumour. 2. computed tomography. 3. coronary thrombosis. 4. cover test.

CTG *abbr* cardiotocography.

CT number the number given to a pixel in a digital image to denote the calculated attenuation at that point of the image, expressed in Hounsfield units. ⟳ Hounsfield unit.

CT scanner ⟳ computed tomography (CT) scanner.

CT simulator ⟳ computed tomography (CT) simulator.

CTZ *abbr* chemoreceptor trigger zone.

CUA *abbr* cost-utility analysis.

cubital *adj* pertaining to the elbow, such as the *cubital fossa* in the front of the elbow.

cubital tunnel external compression syndrome ulnar paralysis resulting from compression of the ulnar nerve within the cubital tunnel situated on the inner and posterior aspect of the elbow—sometimes referred to as the 'funny bone'.

cubital vein (median cubital vein) a superficial vein at the front of the elbow. ⟳ Colour Section Figure 10.

cubitus *n* the forearm; elbow—**cubital** *adj*.

cuboid *adj* shaped like a cube. Lateral tarsal bone, it articulates with the lateral cuneiform bone, sometimes with the navicular, and with the fourth and fifth metatarsals to form the lateral longtitudinal arch of the foot.

cuboidal (cubical) epithelium this consists of cube-shaped cells fitting closely together lying on a basement membrane (Figure E.7, p. 264). It forms the tubules of the kidneys and is found in some glands. Cuboidal epithelium is actively involved in secretion, absorption and excretion. ⊃ epithelium.

cue *n* during communication, a verbal or non-verbal signal from another individual that is perceived by the observer to require sensitive exploration (by prompting or reflection) as to its meaning for the individual exhibiting it.

culdocentesis *n* aspiration of the rectovaginal pouch (pouch of Douglas) via the posterior vaginal wall.

culdoscope *n* an endoscope used via the vaginal route.

culdoscopy *n* a form of peritoneoscopy or laparoscopy. Passage of a culdoscope through the posterior vaginal fornix, behind the uterus to enter the peritoneal cavity, for viewing same—**culdoscopic** *adj*, **culdoscopically** *adv*.

-cule a suffix that means 'little', e.g. *saccule*.

Cullen's sign (T Cullen, American gynaecologist, 1868–1953) blue-black discoloration of the skin around the umbilicus, a sign seen in acute pancreatitis. ⊃ Grey Turner sign.

culture *n* the growth of micro-organisms on artificial media under ideal conditions. ⊃ medium.

Cumulated Index Medicus (CIM) ⊃ Index Medicus.

cumulative action when a dose of a slowly excreted drug is repeated too frequently, an increasing action occurs. This may lead to an accumulation of the drug in the system and toxic symptoms, such as with digoxin.

Cumulative Index to Nursing and Allied Health Literature (CINAHL) computerized database of literature relevant to nursing and allied health.

cuneiform bones three tarsal bones. All three articulate with the navicular bone and each one articulates with the corresponding metatarsal bone (first, second or third) to complete the medial longtitudinal arch of the foot.

cup arthroplasty the articular surface of the joint is reconstructed and covered with a vitallium cup.

cup-disc ratio the ratio of the horizontal diameter of the physiological cup to that of the horizontal diameter of the optic disc. It should be less than 0.5. If it exceeds that value, or if there is a difference in ratio between the two eyes, or if there is a progressive enlargement of the cup, glaucoma may be suspected. ⊃ glaucomatous cup.

cupped disc an enlarged and deepened excavation of the physiological cup. It may be physiological, or due to glaucoma (glaucomatous cup), or following atrophy of the optic nerve (as in papilloedema). ⊃ glaucomatous cup, papilloedema, physiological cup.

cupola *n* **1.** gelatinous material surrounding the 'hair' cells projecting from the ampulla of a semicircular canal. ⊃ crista. **2.** gelatinous material surrounding the 'hair' cells and otoliths in the maculae of the utricle and saccule in the inner ear.

cupping *n* space within the optic nerve head due to absence of nerve fibres, often due to glaucoma.

cupula ⊃ cupola.

curative treatment ⊃ treatment.

cure 1. to restore to health. **2.** in dentistry, the process whereby an acrylic resin is polymerized and thus hardened.

curettage *n* the scraping of unhealthy or exuberant tissue from a cavity. This may be treatment or may be done to establish a diagnosis after laboratory analysis of the scrapings. In dentistry, instrumenting the walls of a bony cavity by curette to remove chronically inflamed tissue and bone.

curette *n* a spoon-shaped instrument or a metal loop which may have sharp and/or blunt edges for scraping out (curetting) cavities.

curettings *npl* the material obtained by scraping or curetting and usually sent for histological examination.

curie (Ci) (M Curie, Polish-born chemist/physicist, 1867–1934; P Curie, French scientist, 1859–1906) a measure of radioactivity, equal to 3.7×10^{10} nuclear disintegrations per second, now replaced by the becquerel (Bq).

curing time the time necessary to attain a full cure in a thermosetting plastic or rubber.

Curling's ulcer (T Curling, British surgeon, 1811–1888) acute peptic ulceration which occurs either in the stomach or duodenum as a response to physiological stress. First identified after extensive burns but also occurs following other physiological stressors, such as severe haemorrhage and hypovolaemia.

current an electrotherapy term. A flow of charged particles (ions or electrons) per unit time. Clinically current is usually at the mA level. If using microcurrent, μA. ⊃ current density.

current density an electrotherapy term. Current per unit area of electrode. Measured clinically in mA/cm². ⊃ constant current.

curriculum vitae personal details, education, professional qualifications and attainment and employment experience. ⊃ Appendix 13.

curvature of field an aberration of an optical system due to the obliquity of the incident rays of light relative to the optical axis. The image corresponding to a plane object lies on a curved surface. This aberration does not usually affect the eye as the retina is itself curved. ⊃ optical aberration, Petzval surface.

curvature of a surface a measure of the shape of a curved surface. It is expressed in a unit called reciprocal metre, usually written as m^{-1}, which is equal to the reciprocal of the radius of curvature of a surface in metres. For example, if a surface has a radius of curvature r of $+0.5$ m, its curvature R will be $R = 1/r = 1/ + 0.5 = 2 \, m^{-1}$.

curve to bend without any angles. An arch. That which is bent.

curved array in ultrasound, a set of elements mounted in a curved line to give a wide field of view, for example, in obstetric scans.

curved lens ⊃ meniscus lens.

curve of Carus arc corresponding to the pelvic axis, the route taken by the fetus on its passage through the birth canal.

curve of Monson an occlusal curve on which artificial teeth are set up. All of the cusps should touch a curve of 102 mm in radius whose centre is at a smooth point between the eyebrows (glabella).

curve of Spee curve running from the condyle of the mandible along the superior surface of all mandibular teeth to the central incisors, having an arc of 6.5–7 mm when seen from the lateral skull view. ⊃ reverse curve of Spee.

curve of Stephan graph illustrating the 24-hour rise and fall of plaque acidity during and between meals, especially the increased rise due to intake of refined carbohydrates—particularly sweets and sweet drinks between meals.

CUS *abbr* continuous ultrasound.

Cusco's speculum a bivalve speculum used for inspection of the cervix and vagina and for holding the vaginal walls apart while taking high vaginal swabs and cervical smears.

cushingoid a description of the moon face, central obesity and facial plethora common in people with elevated levels of plasma glucocorticoids from whatever cause.

Cushing scalers ⊃ scalers.

Cushing's disease (H Cushing, American neurosurgeon, 1869–1939) a rare disorder, mainly of females, characterized principally by a cushingoid appearance, proximal myopathy, hyperglycaemia, hypertension and osteoporosis; due to excessive cortisol production by hyperplastic adrenal glands as a result of increased adrenocorticotrophin (ACTH) secretion by a tumour or hyperplasia of the anterior pituitary gland.

Cushing's reflex a rise in blood pressure and a fall in pulse rate; occurs in cerebral space-occupying lesions.

Cushing's syndrome clinically similar to Cushing's disease but including all causes: (a) adrenocortical hyperplasia, adenoma or carcinoma, which can be associated with hirsutism and hypokalaemia due to excess of other adrenal steroids; (b) ectopic ACTH secretion by tumours, e.g. small cell lung cancer, often associated with hyperpigmentation; (c) iatrogenic due to treatment with glucocorticoids.

cusp *n* a projecting point, such as the protrusion or eminence usually arising from the occlusal surface of a posterior tooth and canines. Also the segment of a heart valve. The cardiac tricuspid valve has three, the mitral (bicuspid) valve two cusps.

cusp angle the angle made by the slopes of a cusp with a plane at right angles to the long axis of the tooth.

cusp capping the inclusion of cusp (s) in the cavity preparation and their restoration to functional occlusion with a restorative material.

cusp of Carabelli ⊃ Carabelli's cusp.

cusp height the distance between the tip of a cusp and its base plane.

cuspal interference unwanted contact of any cusp with an opposing tooth which may deflect or prevent the normal occlusion of the rest of the teeth.

cuspid ⊃ canine (preferred name).

cuspidor in dentistry, a spittoon generally fitted with a water-flushing device.

custom tray ⊃ impression tray, tray.

CUT *acron* City University test.

cutaneous *adj* relating to the skin.

cutaneous nerve any mixed nerve supplying a region of the skin. ⊃ Colour Section Figure 12.

cutaneous ureterostomy the ureters are transplanted so that they open on to the skin of the abdominal wall.

cuticle *n* 1. the epidermis. 2. the eponychium. The epidermis or dead epidermis, which covers the proximal part of a nail—**cuticular** *adj*. ⊃ nail.

cut-off sensitivity in radiography. The electromagnetic wavelength that a film emulsion is no longer sensitive to.

cuttle in dentistry, a polishing agent made of ground cuttle fish bone and consisting mainly of calcium carbonate.

CV *abbr* curriculum vitae.

CVA *abbr* cerebrovascular accident.

CVD *abbr* cardiovascular disease.

CVID *abbr* common variable immunodeficiency.

CVP *abbr* central venous pressure.

CVS *abbr* 1. cardiovascular system. 2. chorionic villus sampling. 3. computer vision syndrome.

CVVH *abbr* continuous veno-venous haemofiltration. ⊃ haemofiltration.

CVVHD *abbr* continuous veno-venous haemodiafiltration (haemodialysis). ⊃ haemodiafiltration.

CW (probe) *abbr* continuous wave probe.

CX *abbr* circumflex artery.

CXR *abbr* chest X-ray.

cyan/o- a prefix that means 'blue', e.g. *cyanosis*.

cyanoacrylate adhesive rapid-setting acrylate-based adhesive employed in household, industrial and medical applications. Applications in dentistry include wound closure and retrieval of fractured instruments from root canals.

cyanocobalamin *n* the most stable form of vitamin B_{12}, which is produced commercially by bacterial fermentation. This synthetic form must be converted in the body to a naturally occurring form before it can be utilized by the body. ⊃ cobalamins.

cyanolabe a pigment contained in one group of cones; responds to blue light.

cyanopsia an abnormality of vision where all objects are seen as blue.

cyanosis *n* a bluish tinge manifested by hypoxic tissue, observed most frequently under the nails, lips and skin. It is always due to lack of oxygen, and the causes of this are legion—**cyanosed, cyanotic** *adj. central cyanosis* blueness seen on the warm surfaces such as the oral mucosa and tongue. It increases with exertion. *peripheral cyanosis* blueness of the limb extremities, the nose and the ear lobes.

cyclamate intense sweetener with approximately 50 times the sweetness of sucrose (beet or cane sugar). ⊃ sweetener.

cycle *n* 1. a regular series of movements or events; a sequence which recurs. ⊃ cardiac, menstrual—**cyclical** *adj*. 2. one complete waveform in alternating current, usually measured from zero to zero or from peak to peak.

cycle ergometer a fixed cycling machine used in fitness testing to estimate the exercise intensity (power output) from the rpm and the resistance to pedalling, which can be adjusted to vary the intensity.

cyclic adenosine monophosphate (cAMP) a metabolic molecule that acts as a 'second messenger' for many hormones and in processes where many reactions are occurring simultaneously (enzyme cascade).

cyclical syndrome an alternative term preferred by some people to that of premenstrual syndrome.

cyclical vomiting periodic attacks of vomiting in children, usually associated with ketosis and usually with no demonstrable pathological cause. Occurs mainly in highly strung children.

cyclist's nipples a colloquial expression used in sports medicine to describe the irritation of the nipple due to the combined effects of perspiration and windchill. ➲ jogger's nipples.

cyclist's palsy a colloquial expression used in sports medicine to describe the paraesthesia of the ulnar nerve distribution of the forearm and hand due to prolonged leaning on the handlebars when cycling.

cyclitis *n* inflammation of the ciliary body of the eye. ➲ iridocyclitis.

cyclodestruction *n* destruction of the ciliary body by heat (usually laser induced) or freezing.

cyclodialysis *n* the formation of a communication between anterior chamber and suprachoroidal space. May be used for the relief of glaucoma.

cyclo-oxygenase-2 inhibitors ➲ COX-2 inhibitors.

cyclophoria (*syn* periphoria) when binocular vision is dissociated (i.e. when stimuli to fusion are eliminated) one eye or both rotate about its/their respective anteroposterior axes to take up the passive position. If the upper portion of the eye rotates inward it is called *incyclophoria* and if it rotates outward it is called *excyclophoria*. It is usually caused by an anomaly of the oblique muscles. ➲ double prism test, Maddox rod test.

cycloplegia *n* paralysis of the ciliary muscle of the eye—**cycloplegic** *adj*.

cycloplegics *npl* drugs which paralyse the ciliary muscle of the eye, e.g. atropine, cyclopentolate. ➲ mydriatics.

cyclothymia *n* a tendency to alternating but relatively mild mood swings between elation and depression—**cyclothymic** *adj*.

cyclotron *n* a device to accelerate charged particles or ions which then bombard a target in which nuclear reactions result in the production of radionuclides (radioisotopes). These can then be used as a source of neutrons or protons for therapeutic radiopharmaceuticals.

cyesis *n* pregnancy. When there are signs and symptoms of pregnancy in a woman who believes she is pregnant, and this is not so, it is called pseudocyesis. ➲ phantom pregnancy.

cylinder axis **1.** a line of zero curvature on a cylindrical surface. **2.** that principal meridian of a planocylinder in which the power is zero. ➲ astigmatic lens.

cylindrical lens a lens in which one of the principal meridians has zero refractive power. It usually consists of one plano surface and one cylindrical surface. ➲ astigmatic lens.

cylindroma *n* a tumour of the endothelial element of apocrine tissue such as a sweat gland or a salivary gland. The supporting stroma is hyalinized.

cyst *n* a closed cavity or sac usually with an epithelial lining, enclosing fluid or semisolid matter—**cystic** *adj*.

cyst lining membrane soft tissue lining of a cyst, usually composed of epithelium.

cyst of dental origin cyst arising from proliferation of ectodermal tissue present in the formation of teeth. *dentigerous cyst* a cyst arising from the follicle surrounding the developing tooth. *developmental cyst* a cyst arising from abnormal development tissues. *eruption cyst* cyst arising from the follicle of an erupting tooth.

cyst pack in dentistry, pack of ribbon gauze impregnated with antiseptic, bismuth iodoform paraffin paste (BIPP) or Whitehead's varnish. Inserted post-operatively into a cyst cavity.

cyst plug in dentistry, plug of material such as acrylic resin used postoperatively to keep open a cyst cavity, allowing it to heal from the base upwards.

cystadenoma *n* an innocent cystic new growth of glandular tissue. Liable to occur in the female breast.

cystalgia pain in the urinary bladder.

cystathioninuria *n* inherited disorder of cystathionine metabolism marked by excessive excretion of cystathionine in the urine, an intermediate product in conversion of methionine to cysteine. Sometimes associated with learning disability.

cystectomy *n* usually refers to the removal of part or the whole of the urinary bladder. This may necessitate urinary diversion.

cysteine *n* a sulphur-containing conditionally essential (indispensable) amino acid. It is synthesized from the amino acids methionine and serine. Cysteine is needed for the synthesis of coenzyme A, glutathione and taurine.

cyst/i/o- a prefix that means 'bladder', e.g. *cystitis*.

cystic duct the bile duct that transports bile between the gallbladder and the common bile duct.

cysticercosis *n* infection of humans with cysticercus, the larval stage of the pork tapeworm (*Taenia solium*). After ingestion, the ova do not develop further, but form 'cysts' in subcutaneous tissues, voluntary muscle and the brain, where they cause seizures.

cysticercus *n* the larval form of *Taenia solium*.

cystic fibrosis (CF) (*syn* fibrocystic disease of the pancreas, mucoviscidosis) an autosomal recessive disorder affecting the exocrine glands; diagnosis may be confirmed by high levels of sodium in sweat. It is the commonest genetically determined disease in Caucasian populations. Meconium ileus in newborns may be an early physical effect. The affected glands produce viscous mucus which leads to blocked dilated ducts, stasis of mucus, infection and fibrosis. The lungs and pancreas are primarily affected giving rise to digestive problems including steatorrhoea and malabsorption, repeated chest infections and respiratory and cardiac deterioration leading ultimately to respiratory and cardiac failure. Current treatment involves physiotherapy, antimicrobial drugs and replacement of pancreatic enzymes, but advances in management include: heart/lung transplants, identification of the defective gene, antenatal testing, gene therapy and genetic counselling for affected couples. ➲ sweat test.

cystic fibrosis transmembrane regulator (CFTR) also known as cystic fibrosis membrane conductance regulator. A protein required for the transport of chloride ions across epithelial cell membranes in the respiratory tract, gastrointestinal tract, pancreas, the skin and the reproductive tract. The gene that encodes for the CFTR protein is located on chromosome number 7. Mutations occurring in the CFTR protein cause abnormal chloride channels that results in cystic fibrosis. Other mutations cause congenital absence of the deferent duct (vas deferens).

cystic hygroma multilocular cystic collection of lymphatic fluid due to abnormal lymphatic development, commonly at the back of the neck. Fetal cystic hygromas can be seen on ultrasound from 10–11 weeks' gestation and differentiated from enlarged nuchal translucency because they are septated. Associated with chromosomal abnormalities such as Turner's syndrome. Chorionic villus sampling or amniocentesis is offered to couples if cystic hydroma is seen on ultrasound.

cystine *n* a sulphur-containing amino acid, produced by the breakdown of proteins during the digestive process. It is readily reduced to two molecules of cysteine.

cystinosis *n* a recessively inherited metabolic disorder in which crystalline cystine is deposited in the body. Cystine and other amino acids are excreted in the urine.

cystinuria *n* metabolic disorder in which cystine and other amino acids appear in the urine. A cause of renal stones—**cystinuric** *adj*.

cystitis *n* inflammation of the urinary bladder; the cause is usually bacterial. The condition may be acute or chronic, primary or secondary to stones, etc. More frequent in females, as the urethra is short.

cystocele *n* prolapse of the posterior wall of the urinary bladder into the anterior vaginal wall (Figure C.20). ➲ colporrhaphy, procidentia, rectocele.

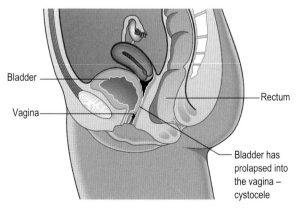

Bladder

Vagina

Rectum

Bladder has prolapsed into the vagina – cystocele

C.20 Cystocele (reproduced from Brooker & Nicol 2003 with permission).

cystodiathermy *n* the application of a cauterizing electrical current to the walls of the urinary bladder through a cystoscope, or by open operation.

cystography *n* radiographic examination of the urinary bladder. A catheter passed into the bladder via the urethra is used for the introduction of contrast agent—**cystographic** *adj*, **cystograph** *n*, **cystogram** *n*, **cystographically** *adv*.

cystoid macular oedema (CMO) oedema and cyst formation of the macular area of the retina. It may occur as a result of, or be associated with, systemic vascular disease, retinal vein occlusion, diabetic retinopathy, uveitis, retinitis pigmentosa and following some ocular surgery such as vitreoretinal, photocoagulation, glaucoma procedures and especially cataract surgery. When cystoid macular oedema follows cataract surgery it is called the Irvine-Gass syndrome and it is sometimes accompanied by intraoperative vitreous body (humour) loss or vitreous adhesion to the iris or to the corneoscleral wound. Visual acuity is affected initially but recovers in the majority of cases. In some cases antiinflammatory therapy may help in restoring visual acuity and in other cases the vitreous adhesion may be disrupted with a Nd-Yag laser.

cystolithiasis *n* the presence of a stone or stones in the urinary bladder.

cystometer *n* an apparatus for measuring the pressure under various conditions in the urinary bladder.

cystometrogram *n* a record of the changes in pressure within the urinary bladder under various conditions; used in the study and diagnosis of voiding disorders.

cystometry *n* the study of pressure changes within the urinary bladder—**cystometric** *adj*.

cystopexy surgical procedure to secure the urinary bladder in a sepecific position.

cystoplasty *n* surgical repair or augmentation of the urinary bladder.

cystosarcoma phylloides a malignant connective tissue of the breast. It is characterized by rapid growth and recurrence if surgical removal is incomplete.

cystoscope *n* an endoscope used to visualize the inside of the urinary bladder—**cystoscopic** *adj*, **cystoscopically** *adv*.

cystoscopy *n* use of a cystoscope to view the internal surface of the urinary bladder. Also used for biopsies, photographing areas of interest and for some treatments.

cystostomy *n* (*syn* vesicostomy) an operation whereby a fistulous opening is made into the urinary bladder via the abdominal wall. Usually the fistula can be allowed to heal when it is no longer needed.

cystotomy *n* incision into the urinary bladder via the abdominal wall.

cystourethritis *n* inflammation of the urinary bladder and urethra.

cystourethrogram *n* radiographic examination of the urinary bladder and urethra—**cystourethrographic** *adj*, **cystourethrograph** *n*, **cystourethrographically** *adv*. ➲ micturating cystourethrogram, vesicoureteric reflux.

cystourethropexy *n* operation used for some types of urinary incontinence. The bladder and upper urethra are fixed in a forward position. ⊃ Marshall–Marchetti–Krantz operation.

-cyte a suffix that means 'cell', e.g. *lymphocyte*.

cyto- a prefix that means 'cell', e.g. *cytogenetics*.

cytochemistry the study of the biochemical compounds within living cells and their action and function in cellular processes.

cytochromes *npl* a series of haem (heme) proteins containing iron or copper. They have a similar structure to haemoglobin and are involved in mitochondrial oxidation-reduction reactions (electron transport chain) that produce adenosine triphosphate (ATP). ⊃ oxidative phosphorylation.

cytochrome P$_{450}$ a family of liver enzymes important in the oxidation and clearance of a variety of compounds including cholesterol and lipid-soluble drugs. The drugs are made more water-soluble thereby allowing them to be safely excreted by the kidney. ⊃ P$_{450}$ enzymes.

cytodiagnosis *n* diagnosis by the microscopic study of cells—**cytodiagnostic** *adj*.

cytogenetics *n* the scientific study of cells; particularly of chromosomes, genes and their behaviour. Chromosomes can be studied by culture techniques, using either tissue such as skin or lymphocytes, or fetal cells obtained by chorionic villus sampling or amniocentesis—**cytogenesis** *n*.

cytoid bodies small, swollen white spots found on the retina resembling cells. They are due to degenerated retinal nerve fibres in which cellular components become trapped in the peripheral axons of the optic nerve blocking axonal flow. Collection of cytoid bodies are thought to represent the 'cotton-wool' spots found on or around the optic disc in papilloedema, retinal trauma, diabetic retinopathy, HIV/AIDS disease, systemic lupus erythematosus, etc. ⊃ exudate.

cytokine modulators/inhibitors monoclonal antibodies used to inhibit the action of certain cytokines including those involved in inflammation. For example, the monoclonal antibody infliximab used in the management of rheumatoid arthritis inhibits the cytokine tumour necrosis factor α responsible for augmenting inflammatory changes. Considerable research effort is in progress to develop further monoclonal antibodies for use in a wide range of diseases/conditions.

cytokines *npl* large group of proteins which act either on the cytokine-producing cell, or on other cells, via cell-surface receptors. The term is usually applied to proteins which act on immune cells (T cells, B cells, monocytes, etc.). Cytokines have many diverse effects on many different cell types. Examples include interleukins, (e.g. IL-1, IL-2), tumour necrosis factor, interferon-alpha and interferon-gamma. ⊃ cytokine modulators/inhibitors.

cytokinesis the division of the cell cytoplasm into two daughter cells following nuclear division. ⊃ meiosis, mitosis.

cytology *n* the microscopic study of cells. The term *exfoliative cytology* is used when the cells studied have been shed, or sampled, from the surface of an organ or lesion, such as from the uterine cervix—**cytological** *adj*.

cytolysis *n* the degeneration, destruction, disintegration or dissolution of cells—**cytolytic** *adj*.

cytomegalic inclusion disease infection caused by the cytomegalovirus. It is marked by nuclear inclusion bodies in large infected cells. In neonates the disease is characterized by hepatosplenomegaly, purpura, encephalitis and microcephaly with learning disability, or death. In adults it causes an illness similar to infectious mononucleosis (glandular fever) and pneumonia. ⊃ cytomegalovirus.

cytomegalovirus (CMV) *n* a herpesvirus. Can cause latent and asymptomatic infection. The virus is excreted in urine and saliva. It can be passed to the fetus in utero and may cause miscarriage, stillbirth or serious neonatal disease. It also affects adults and the virus is a serious threat to immunocompromised individuals. ⊃ cytomegalic inclusion disease, cytomegalovirus retinitis .

cytomegalovirus retinitis a rare chronic, diffuse infection of the retina caused by the cytomegalovirus (CMV). It affects people with an impaired immune system as a result of either HIV/AIDS disease, organ transplantation or chemotherapy, etc. The signs are whitish retinal lesions which look granular (not fluffy, cottonwool spots). These lesions progress into retinal necrosis with absolute visual field loss in that area. The lesions are usually accompanied by haemorrhages. Eventually the lesions coalesce and involve the entire fundus, resulting in complete visual loss. In the initial phase of the disease most people are usually asymptomatic while those with symptoms will complain of floaters, blurred vision, photopsia, scotomas, metamorphopsia, etc. In some cases, retinal detachment follows the disease. Treatment with antiviral drugs such as ganciclovir, valganciclovir or cidofovir (with probenecid) produces some regression of the disease.

cytometer a device for counting and measuring cells, such as blood cells.

cytoplasm *n* (*syn* protoplasm) the complex chemical compound constituting the main part of the living substance of the cell, other than the contents of the nucleus—**cytoplasmic** *adj*.

cytoplasmic energy state ⊃ phosphorylation potential.

cytoplasmic inheritance inheritance of diseases or traits through the genetic material present in mitochondria rather than that on the chromosomes.

cytoreduction the reduction of the size of a tumour using hormone therapy or cytotoxic drugs.

cytoscreening *n* the process of carefully evaluating cells on a cytological preparation for the detection of malignancy.

cytosine *n* a nitrogenous base derived from pyrimidines. With other bases, one or more phosphate groups and a sugar it is part of the nucleic acids DNA and RNA. ⊃ deoxyribonucleic acid, ribonucleic acid.

cytospin *n* process of centrifuging fluid in order to separate the cells for cytological evaluation.

cytostasis *n* arrest or hindrance of cell development—**cytostatic** *adj*.

cytotoxic *n, adj* any substance which kills cells.

cytotoxic drugs drugs used mainly for the treatment of malignant diseases, but sometimes for other conditions, e.g. methotrexate may be used for severe psoriasis. They work in different ways, but they all eventually cause cancer cell death by either disrupting DNA or causing apoptosis. Some are cell cycle phase specific (CCPS) whereas others work at any point in the cell cycle and are termed cell cycle phase non-specific (CCPNS). They also harm some normal cells and some have longer-term side-effects. ⊃ chemotherapy. There are five groups: (a) alkylating agents that disrupt DNA, e.g. busulfan, cyclophosphamide; (b) antimetabolites that disrupt DNA by blocking enzymes required for its synthesis, e.g. 5-fluorouracil, methotrexate; (c) antitumour antibiotics that disrupt DNA and the cell membrane, e.g. bleomycin; (d) vinca alkaloids and etoposide disrupt microtubules during cell division, e.g. vincristine; (e) miscellaneous group of antineoplastic drugs that work in a variety of ways, including: crisantaspase; platinum-containing drugs such as carboplatin; taxanes, e.g. paclitaxel; topoisomerase I inhibitors, e.g. irinotecan hydrochloride; and trastuzumab, etc. ⊃ Appendix 5.

cytotoxic T-cell T-lymphocytes that destroy certain cells, such as virus-infected cells. ⊃ CD8 cells, suppressor-T cells

cytotoxins *npl* antibodies which are toxic to cells.

cytotrophoblast also known as Langhan's cell layer. The inner cell layer of the trophoblast. ⊃ chorionic villi.

D

D log E curve in radiography. Applies to a particular film or film/screen combination and is the curve which results when the density is plotted against the log of relative exposure. ⊃ characteristic curve.

dacry/o- a prefix that means 'tear', e.g. *dacryocystitis*.

dacr(y)oadenitis *n* inflammation of a lacrimal gland. May occur in mumps.

dacryocystectomy *n* excision of any part of the lacrimal sac.

dacryocystitis *n* infective inflammation of the lacrimal sac.

dacryocystography *n* rarely used radiographic examination of the tear drainage apparatus after it has been rendered radiopaque. Superseded by computed tomography (CT) scans and magnetic resonance imaging (MRI) scans.

dacryocystorhinostomy (DCR) *n* an operation to establish drainage from the lacrimal sac into the nose when there is obstruction of the nasolacrimal duct.

dacryolith *n* a concretion in the lacrimal passages.

dactyl *n* a digit, finger or toe—**dactylar, dactylate** *adj*.

dactyl/o- a prefix that means 'finger', e.g. *dactylology*.

dactylitis *n* inflammation of finger or toe. The digit becomes swollen due to periostitis. Associated with congenital syphilis, tuberculosis, sarcoid.

dactylology *n* finger spelling. Used in conjunction with British sign language to communicate with hearing impaired people. ⊃ British sign language, Makaton.

DAD *acron* diffuse alveolar damage.

DADL *abbr* domestic activities of daily living.

D and C *abbr* dilatation and curettage.

D and E *abbr* dilatation and evacuation.

dai ⊃ traditional birth attendant.

Dakin's solution ⊃ sodium hypochlorite.

Dalrymple's sign (J Dalrymple, British ophthalmologist, 1803–1852) retraction of the eyelids causing an abnormally widened palpebral fissure, in primary gaze; one of the signs occurring in Graves' hyperthyroid disease. The person appears to stare and to be frightened as some white sclera may be seen above the upper limbus. ⊃ Graves' ophthalmopathy.

dalton (J Dalton, British chemist/mathematician, 1766–1844) unit (kilodaltons) used to express the molecular weight of important biological molecules, such as nucleic acids and proteins. Also used as a unit for atomic mass. ⊃ atomic mass unit.

daltonism (J Dalton) a form of inherited red-green colour blindness. ⊃ defective colour vision, deuteranopia, dichromatism, protanopia.

Dalton's law of partial pressures a gas law that states that the pressure of a mixture of gases is the sum of the partial pressures that each gas would exert if it alone completely filled the space.

dam ⊃ posterior palatal seal (post dam), rubber dam.

dandruff *n* (*syn* scurf) the common scaly condition of the scalp. May be the forerunner of skin diseases of the seborrhoeic type, such as seborrhoeic dermatitis, or psoriasis.

dandy fever ⊃ dengue.

Dandy–Walker syndrome (W Dandy, American neurosurgeon, 1886–1946; A Walker, Canadian/American surgeon, 1907–1995) a congenital brain malformation of the cerebellum and the fourth ventricle leading to hydrocephalous.

Dane particle the complete hepatitis B virus particle.

dappen pot small glass or plastic receptacle for drugs and liquids used in dentistry.

Darier's disease (*syn* keratosis follicularis) (F-J Darier, French dermatologist, 1852–1938) an autosomal dominant condition characterized by greasy scaled papules on the flexures, trunk and face.

dark accommodation ⊃ resting state of accommodation.

dark adaptation adjustments made by the eye in reduced light or darkness. The pupils dilate, cone function ceases, rhodopsin is formed and the rod activity increases. ⊃ hemeralopia, light adaptation.

dark focus ⊃ resting state of accommodation.

dark room test ⊃ provocative test.

dark vergence ⊃ tonic vergence.

DAS *abbr* disease activity score.

DAT *abbr* direct antiglobulin test.

data *npl* items of information, usually collected for a specific purpose, for example to be used in the analysis of a problem or to study trends, or plan services. In clinical settings, data which are requested on the patient assessment form are collected at an initial interview with the patient. Other data are collected by ongoing assessment and evaluation—**datum** *sing*.

data analysis describes statistical analyses on data.

database software designed to store information (e.g. a mailing list), in a systematic way, and at the same time to allow easy retrieval and manipulation of all data. Each record contains a number of fields.

data collection data can be collected by interviewing, during which a structured form, such as a patient assessment form, may be used. In some circumstances an unstructured interview might be appropriate. The data are referred to as subjective or soft data. The practitioner (e.g. nurse), as a skilled interviewer, prompts and reflects so that the patient describes his/her condition as factually as possible. Other data are the result of measurement, e.g. the amount of urine passed in 24 h, and yet others are the result of testing, e.g. urine, and these are called objective or hard data. ⊃ confidentiality, data protection.

data compression in computing, the reduction in size of information to decrease transferred film size.

data processing storage, sorting and analysis of data, usually electronically with specific computer software.

data protection rules relating to information held about individuals. ⊃ Caldicott guardian, data protection legislation.

data protection legislation various pieces of legislation passed during the 1980s and 1990s that set out the duties and obligations of people/organizations who hold data about people, and the rights of individuals to know what information is held about them on computer, including health-related records. The Data Protection Act (1984) gives clients/patients access to their electronically held health records. ⊃ Access to Health Records Act (1990). Furthermore, the Data Protection Act (1984) regulates the storage and protection of patient/client information held electronically. The provisions of the Data Protection Act (1998) balance the right of individuals to privacy and the rights of those people/organizations who have valid reasons for holding and using personal data, such as healthcare professionals. This Act provides people with some rights about data held about them but also sets out certain duties/obligations for the people/organizations that collect, hold and process such information.

data set the data relating to a specific group such as a particular age group.

dating scan an ultrasound scan usually taken between 11 and 14 weeks' gestation, using the crown–rump length to accurately age the fetus.

daughter radionuclide a nucleus after it has decayed. ⊃ radioactive decay.

dawn phenomenon experienced by some people with type 1 diabetes, there is an increase in blood glucose during the early hours of the morning caused by increased secretion of growth hormone and cortisol during the night.

day case surgery ⊃ ambulatory surgery.

day hospital a centre which people attend on a daily basis or for some days in the week. Recreational and occupational therapy and physiotherapy are often provided. Greatest use is in the services for older people and those with learning disability or mental health problems. The day hospital provides vital respite for family, neighbours and other carers.

daylight systems a system which enables the loading and unloading of radiographic film without the use of a darkroom. ⊃ centralized daylight system, dispersed daylight system.

daylight vision ⊃ photopic vision.

DBP *abbr* diastolic blood pressure.

DC *abbr* direct current.

DCIS *abbr* ductal carcinoma in situ.

DCP *abbr* dental care professional.

DCR *abbr* dacryocystorhinostomy.

DCSS *abbr* diffuse cutaneous systemic sclerosis.

DDE index *abbr* developmental defects of enamel index. ⊃ index (dental).

DDH *abbr* developmental dysplasia of the hip.

de- a prefix that means 'away, from, down, off of, reversing', e.g. decompression.

dead fetus syndrome a dead fetus is retained in utero; if delivery does not occur the decomposition of the fetus may lead to blood coagulation disorders and severe haemorrhage at delivery.

dead space the air present within the respiratory tract that is not involved directly in gas exchange, it is usually about 150 mL in adults.

dead tooth ⊃ tooth.

dead tract dark tract in dentinal tubules seen in ground section under a microscope. The tubules appear dark because they contain air and not dentinal processes.

deaf-blind describes a person who has a severe hearing loss in addition to a visual defect. It is usually congenital but it may result from ageing or some systemic disease or as part of a syndrome (e.g. Usher's syndrome which accounts for about half of all cases of deaf-blind people). ⊃ rubella, Usher's syndrome.

deafferentation total or partial loss of the afferent nerve supply or sensory input derived from a particular body area.

deafness/hearing loss *n* a partial or complete loss of hearing. It may be congenital or acquired, and may be conductive, sensorineural or mixed hearing loss/deafness ⊃ conductive hearing loss/deafness, congenital hearing loss/deafness, hearing impairment, mixed hearing loss/deafness, noise induced hearing loss (NIHL)/deafness, sensorineural hearing loss (SNHL)/deafness.

deamination *n* removal of an amino group (NH_2) from organic compounds such as excess amino acids.

Dean's index ⊃ index (dental).

death *n* irreversible cessation of vital functions usually assessed by the absence of heart beat and breathing. Mechanical ventilation may maintain vital functions despite the fact that the brainstem is fatally and irreversibly damaged. Consequently stringent tests are necessary to diagnose death in such cases. Death may be expected and occurs when the failure of one or more organs and/or systems fails to maintain homeostasis. This may be due, for example, to cancer, chronic heart failure or chronic respiratory diseases. Sudden death occurs when the flow of blood to the brain ceases. This might be due to serious haemorrhage such as following a road traffic accident or other trauma, severe acute illness, cerebrovascular accident, myocardial infarction, cardiac arrest or suicide. ⊃ brainstem death, coroner.

death certificate official document, issued by the registrar of deaths to relatives or other authorized person, that allows for the disposal of the body. It is issued after a notification of probable cause of death is completed by the doctor in attendance upon the deceased or the appropriate documentation from the coroner.

debility *n* a condition of weakness with lack of muscle tone.

debonding the removal of bonding resin and brackets previously bonded to the teeth during orthodontic treatment. The surface of the teeth are restored to their pre-treatment condition.

débridement *n* the removal of foreign matter and contaminated or devitalized tissue from or adjacent to a wound. Required before wound healing can progress. *biological débridement* using larval (maggot) therapy for wound débridement. ⊃ larval therapy. *chemical/medical débridement* is accomplished by the external application of enzymes, e.g. streptokinase. *moist wound environment débridement* through using certain dressings, e.g. hydrocolloids, which augment natural débridement processes. *sharp débridement* using scalpel and scissors. *surgical débridement* more extensive procedure that is accomplished in theatre.

debris in dentistry, an accumulation of unwanted fragments such as food, pieces of tooth, drill dust and caries.

debugging the correction and, much more importantly, the finding of errors or bugs in a computer program.

debulking *n* removal of a significant proportion of a pathological mass. As in the reduction of tumour bulk prior to chemotherapy or radiotherapy.

deca- a prefix that means 'ten', e.g. *decade*.

decalcification *n* the removal of mineral salts, as from teeth in dental caries, bone in disorders of calcium metabolism.

decannulation *n* the removal of a cannula such as an intravenous cannula.

decapsulation *n* the surgical removal of a capsule.

decay *n* **1.** a psychological term that describes the loss of information from the memory that occurs spontaneously over time. **2.** gradual chemical decomposition of organic matter when exposed to the atmosphere. **3.** in dentistry, a deprecated term for caries. **4.** process of radioactive substance disintegration.

deceleration a change in motion of an object or body usually understood as the rate of reduction in speed (although it can also refer to a change in direction). A negative acceleration. ⊃ fetal heart deceleration.

deceleration time used in cardiac ultrasound studies to measure the function of a mitral (or left atrioventricular) valve, for example, a long mitral E wave deceleration time indicates diastolic dysfunction.

decerebrate *adj* without cerebral function; a state of deep unconsciousness.

decerebrate posture/rigidity a condition of the usually unconscious patient in which all four limbs are spastic and extended and which indicates severe damage to the cerebrum. The jaw is clenched and the neck retracted. There is hypertonus of the extensor muscles in both upper and lower limbs following severe decerebrating brain injury. ⊃ decorticate posture/rigidity, Glasgow coma scale, opisthotonos.

deci- a prefix that means 'tenth', e.g. decilitre.

decibel (dB) a unit of sound intensity (loudness).

decidua *n* the specialized endometrial lining of the uterus thickened and altered for the potential reception of the fertilized ovum. It is shed at the end of pregnancy—**decidual** *adj*. ⊃ decidua basalis, decidua capsularis, decidua vera.

decidua basalis that part of the decidua which lies under the embedded ovum and forms the maternal part of the placenta.

decidua capsularis that part of the decidua which lies over the developing ovum.

decidua vera the decidua that is not involved with the embedded ovum; the decidua that lines the rest of the uterus.

decidual cast expulsion of the decidua intact, in the shape of the uterine cavity, following death of the ovum in an ectopic pregnancy. ⊃ ectopic pregnancy.

deciduous *adj* shed periodically. By convention refers to the 20 teeth of the primary dentition. ⊃ primary detention.

decompensated heterophoria ⊃ uncompensated heterophoria.

decompensation *n* a failure of compensation usually referring to heart failure.

decompression *n* removal of pressure or a compressing force.

decompression (of bladder) in cases of chronic urinary retention, by continuous or intermittent drainage via catheter inserted per urethra.

decompression (of brain) achieved by the removal of a circular portion of the skull by trephining in order to evacuate clot.

decompression sickness/illness results from sudden reduction in atmospheric pressure, as experienced by divers on return to surface, or less commonly, exposure to rapid reduction in pressure in ascent from sea level in unpressurized aircraft. The condition is largely preventable by proper and gradual decompression technique. Variously described as 'bends, chokes and creeps' depending on the symptomatology. Originally called caisson disease when identified as a hazard for divers. Later recognized as a complication of high altitude. Symptoms range from pains in the joints, chest and back, weakness or sensory loss, to paralysis and loss of consciousness; severe neurological symptoms can be life-threatening. There are two main causes: (a) damage to the lungs by expansion of the gas in them if a diver does not freely exhale when surfacing. Gas can leak into the circulating blood (air embolus) or into the pleural cavity (pneumothorax); (b) release in the tissues (e.g. around joints or in the spinal cord) of bubbles of nitrogen that was dissolved in body fluids whilst at the higher pressure. Avoided or minimized by using computed tables to control speed of ascent and frequency of pauses, in relation to the duration and depth of the dive. All types of decompression illness require oxygen breathing as a first aid measure, and urgent treatment for all but the mildest by recompression to the initial higher pressure in a hyperbaric chamber, so that nitrogen is redissolved in body fluids, then more gradually released and exhaled as pressure is allowed to fall. ⊃ diving hazards.

deconditioning *n* eliminating an unwanted particular response to a particular stimulus ⊃ aversion therapy, conditioning.

decongestants *npl* agents which decrease congestion, usually referring to nasal congestion, e.g. ephedrine hydrochloride locally. Administered orally, or locally as drops or sprays. ⊃ Appendix 5.

decongestion *n* relief of congestion—**decongestive** *adj*.

decontamination in radiology, the method of removing foreign material such as radioactive substances for the safety of the individual.

decorticate posture/rigidity a condition of the unconscious patient in which there is marked extension of the lower limbs and body, and flexion of the upper limbs (wrists and elbows). It results from a severe brain injury. ⊃ decerebrate posture/rigidity, Glasgow coma scale.

decortication *n* surgical removal of cortex or outer covering of an organ such as the lung or kidney.

decubitus *n* the recumbent position; lying down. *decubitus ulcer* ⊃ pressure ulcer—**decubiti** *pl*, **decubital** *adj*.

decussation *n* intersection; a crossing of nerve fibres at a point beyond their origin, as in the optic and pyramidal tracts.

deep tendon reflexes also referred to as tendon reflexes. All muscles have a deep tendon reflex, when the muscle or tendon is briskly hit, a reflex contraction occurs. The stimulus is a rapid stretch of muscle and the response is a contraction of muscle that is checked by reciprocal stretch of antagonistic muscle, e.g. in the knee jerk, contraction of the quadriceps group of muscles (agonists) is checked by contraction of the hamstring muscles (antagonists). They are short latency reflexes often used to examine spinal cord function. They are: biceps jerk (tests cervical nerves 5 and 6, C5, C6), supinator jerk (tests C5, C6), triceps jerk (C7), finger jerk (C8), knee jerk (tests lumbar nerves 3 and 4, L3, L4) and the ankle jerk (tests sacral nerves 1 and 2, S1, S2). A diminished or absent reflex could indicate a problem in the lower motor neuron such as compression of a nerve. Hyperactive or exaggerated reflexes could indicate a problem affecting the upper motor neurone component, for example following a stroke. Reflex disturbance cannot be used as complete evidence of abnormality of the nervous system, but should be used along with other objective neurological findings. ⊃ reflex, reflex action.

deep transverse arrest obstruction of the fetal head during the second stage of labour, resulting from a first stage occipitoposterior position in which the fetus has attempted to turn anterioriorly (long rotation) but the head becomes caught between the ischial spines of the pelvic outlet, especially if they are prominent. Keilland's forceps delivery or manual rotation followed by Wrigley's forceps delivery is required to release the obstructed head. The baby may have excessive moulding leading to possible intracranial damage.

deep transverse friction (DTF) a technique pioneered by James Cyriax, it involves small amplitude massage to soft tissues. It has been suggested that they may have a local anaesthetic effect. Selective stimulation of mechanoreceptors by rhythmical movement over the affected area may close the pain gate. Another mechanism through which reduction in pain may be achieved is release of endogenous opiates. Friction massage may have a beneficial effect on all three phases of repair. Gentle transverse friction, applied in the early inflammatory phase, might enhance the mobilization of tissue fluid and, therefore, increases the rate of phagocytosis. During maturation, scar tissue is reshaped and strengthened by removing, reorganizing and replacing cells and matrix. Internal and external mechanical stress applied to the repair tissue is the main stimulus for remodelling immature and weak scar tissue with fibres oriented in all directions and through several planes into linearly rearranged bundles of connective tissue. As transverse friction aims basically to achieve transverse movement of the collagen structure of the connective tissue adhesion formation may be prevented. Friction induces a traumatic hyperaemia or increased bloodflow to the area that may facilitate the removal of chemical irritants and increases the transportation of endogenous opiates.

deep vein thrombosis (DVT) thrombus forming in a deep vein such as those in the legs or pelvis. It is associated with the slowing of blood flow, abnormal or inappropriate coagulation processes, or damage to veins (known collectively as Virchow's triad). A thrombus may break off to form an embolus that travels in the venous circulation, through the heart to the lungs. Factors increasing the risk of DVT include obesity, >40 years of age, smoking, previous DVT, and pregnancy and during the puerperium, etc. ⊃ pulmonary embolus, thromboembolic deterrents, venous thromboembolism (VTE).

deep veins of lower limb include the femoral vein, popliteal vein, tibial veins.

deep veins of upper limb include the axillary vein, brachial vein, deep palmar arch, radial vein, subclavian vein, ulnar vein.

DEF index *abbr* decayed, extracted, filled index applied to the primary dentition (deciduous) in order to classify the overall condition. Missing teeth are not included in this index because they may have come out naturally. ⊃ DMF index, index (dental).

defecation *n* voiding of faeces from the colon, through the rectum and anal canal. Involuntary, reflex or automatic defecation occurs in infancy because the infant has not yet developed voluntary control of their external anal sphincter. It is usual in the second or third year of life, for the child to develop the ability to override the defecation reflex. The rectum is normally empty, and the defecation reflex is initiated, when faeces moves into it, causing stretching of the rectal walls. The defecation reflex is mediated through the spinal cord and causes the walls of the sigmoid colon and the rectum to contract and the anal sphincter to relax, allowing faeces to pass into the anal canal. These contractions bring with them a feeling of fullness. Once control of defecation has been achieved it is usually possible to delay the opening of the external anal sphincter (controlled through the pudendal nerve). Defecation is aided by voluntary contraction of the diaphragm and abdominal muscles to increase intra-abdominal pressure and force faeces down. This is achieved by the Valsalva manoeuvre–a forced expiration against a closed glottis (opening between the vocal cords). If defecation is delayed the feeling of fullness will diminish as the rectal walls relax, until the next defecation reflex is initiated. Reflex defecation may occur after a stroke, or with sacral spinal cord damage or damage to the pudendal nerve—**defecate** *vi*.

defective colour vision a marked departure of an individual's colour vision aptitude from that of a normal observer. This is indicated by various tests, e.g. anomaloscope, pseudoisochromatic plates, Farnsworth test. The following types of defective colour vision are usually recognized: anomalous trichromatic vision or anomalous trichromatism; dichromatic vision or dichromatism; monochromatic vision or monochromatism (total colour blindness), anomaly of vision in which there is perception of luminance but not of colour. Both anomalous trichromatism and dichromatism occur in three distinct forms called respectively protanomalous vision and protanopia, deuteranomalous vision and deuteranopia, tritanomalous vision and tritanopia. The causes of defective colour vision may be an impairment of a cone pigment or a reduced number of cone cells. The majority of cases of defective colour vision are inherited. Acquired defects are rare and mostly tritanopic. They may be due to glaucoma, retinal or optic nerve disease, drug or chemical toxicity, diabetes, retinitis pigmentosa, etc. The inherited type occurs as a sex-linked disorder in which the defective gene is on the X chromosome. Since males have only one X chromosome while females have two, sex-linked disorders (most being X-linked recessive) affect mainly males who inherit the genetic defect from their mother. For women to show the defect, both of their X chromosomes have to carry the defective gene, a rare occurrence. Defective colour vision occurs in about 8% of the male population and 0.5% of the female population. ➲ achromatopsia, anomaloscope, daltonism, deuteranomaly, deuteranopia, Edridge–Green lantern, Farnsworth test, Kollner's rule, lantern test, monochromat, protanomaly, protanopia, pseudoisochromatic plates, tritanomaly, tritanopia, visual pigment, wool test.

defence mechanisms 1. the general protective measures by which the body is defended against a huge range of potentially harmful agents, e.g. viruses, bacteria, cancer cells, foreign cells. The measures are divided into two broad groups: (a) non-specific (innate), e.g. intact skin and mucous membranes, natural antimicrobial substances, the inflammatory response, and phagocytosis. (b) specific (adaptive) measures which are known as immunity, i.e. humoral immunity (antibody-mediated) or cell-mediated immunity. **2**. the unconscious processes by which the ego can prevent disturbing or unpleasant emotions from troubling the conscious mind. They all involve some degree of self-deception, distort the real situation, and can only provide a temporary relief from the problem. They include compensation, conversion, denial, displacement, identification, intellectualization, projection, rationalization, reaction formation, regression, repression, sublimation, suppression, withdrawal.

deferent duct (*syn* vas deferens) the excretory duct of the testis. A thick-walled muscular tube continuous with the epididymis. It carries spermatozoa to the ejaculatory ducts. It passes upwards from the testis to enter the abdomen through the inguinal canal and ascends medially towards the posterior wall of the bladder where it is joined by the duct from the seminal vesicle to form the ejaculatory duct. ➲ Colour Section Figure 16.

defervescence *n* the time during which a fever is declining. If the body temperature falls rapidly it is spoken of as crisis; if it falls slowly the term lysis is used.

defibrillation *n* the application of a direct current (DC) electric shock to correct ventricular fibrillation of the heart and restore normal cardiac rhythm (Figure D.1)— **defibrillate** *vt*.

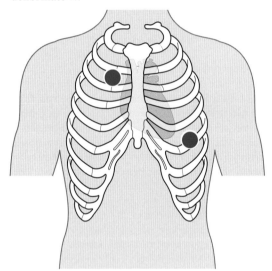

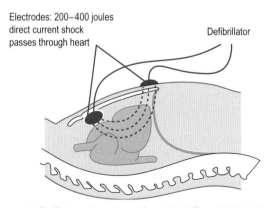

Electrodes: 200–400 joules direct current shock passes through heart

Defibrillator

D.1 Defibrillation (reproduced from Hinchliff et al 1996 with permission).

defibrillator *n* equipment for the application of DC electric shock to the heart. ➲ automatic implantable cardioverter defibrillator, automated external defibrillator, implantable defibrillator.

defibrinated *adj* rendered free from fibrin. A necessary process in the preparation of serum from whole blood. ➲ blood—**defibrinate** *v*.

deficiency disease disease resulting from deficiency of any essential nutrient. Can be caused by a diet that is deficient in a particular nutrient, e.g. iron, or because the nutrient present in the diet cannot be absorbed and metabolized by that individual.

definition 1. in optics and radiography, the sharpness, distinctiveness and clarity of a projected image. **2**. in microscopy, the clarity with which an object is viewed.

deflashing in dentistry, the finishing process of removing the flash or rind produced by spaces between mould cavity edges.

deflection when an ultrasound beam is refracted and therefore causes objects to appear to be in a different location from where they actually occur.

deflective occlusal contact tooth-to-tooth contact that alters the direction of mandibular movement during closure.

deflexion attitude of the fetus in which the head is not flexed, or only partially flexed, as may occur in occipitoposterior position.

DEFS index similar to DEF index but filled surfaces rather than filled teeth are counted and added to the decayed and extracted score. ➲ index (dental).

degaussing a method of demagnetizing a cathode ray tube if the shadow mask becomes magnetized.

degeneration *n* deterioration in quality or function. Regression from more specialized to less specialized type of tissue—**degenerative** *adj*, **degenerate** *vi*.

degenerative joint disease (DJD) ➲ osteoarthritis.

degloving 1. the tearing off, by injury, of the skin of a hand or a foot in a manner comparable to the removal of a glove. **2**. in dentistry, term used to describe the reflection of a mucoperiosteal flap from bone, in order to expose a larger area of bone.

deglutition *n* swallowing, a complex process that is partly voluntary, partly involuntary. ➲ swallowing.

dehiscence *n* the process of splitting or bursting open, as of a wound. Usually associated with wound infection.

dehydration *n* loss or removal of fluid. In the body this condition arises when the fluid intake fails to replace fluid loss. This is liable to occur when there is bleeding, diarrhoea, excessive exudation from a raw area as in burns or in some skin conditions, excessive sweating, polyuria, vomiting, or inadequate fluid intake for any number of reasons. It is accompanied by disruption to the electrolyte balance. If suitable fluid replacement cannot be achieved orally, then other routes must be used. These include subcutaneous infusion (hypodermoclysis), rectal infusion (proctoclysis), or by the intravenous route—**dehydrate** *vt*, *vi*.

7-dehydrocholesterol *n* a sterol found in the skin. It is converted to a form of vitamin D by the action of ultraviolet radiation from exposure to sunlight.

dehydroepiandrosterone (DHEA) a steroid hormone produced by the adrenal glands, the ovaries/testes, the brain and fatty tissue; the precursor of all the sex hormones, e.g. oestrogens, testosterone. The secretion of dehydroepiandrosterone varies across the lifespan. Secretion is high before birth, low during infancy and early childhood until it increases again from 6–8 years of age to peak in the mid twenties. Thereafter declining until it reaches very low levels in older people. ➲ adrenarche.

déjà vu phenomenon occurs in epilepsy involving temporal lobes of the brain and in certain epileptic dream states. An intense feeling of familiarity as if everything had happened before.

DEL *abbr* dose-equivalent limit.

delay in labour unusual prolongation of labour. Most common in the first stage in which the partogram shows if the rate of cervical dilatation is slower than expected (active phase rate of 1 cm per hour in a primigravida, or 1.5 cm per hour in a multipara), a delay of two hours or more may require augmentation of labour. Second stage delay is technically defined as more than 30–120 minutes in a nullipara and 10–60 minutes in a multipara, but in practice, as long as the fetal and maternal conditions remain satisfactory and gradual progressive descent of the presenting part is made, no action is taken. A physiological third stage of more than 2 hours, or an actively managed third stage of more than 30 minutes, in which there is delay in separation and expulsion of the placenta may require manual removal of the placenta and membranes. ➲ augmentation of labour.

delayed hypersensitivity T-cell a T-lymphocyte involved with macrophages and other T-cells in cell-mediated delayed hypersensitivity and chronic inflammation. ➲ CD4 cells.

delayed onset muscle soreness (DOMS) appears 24–48 hours after exercise; may be caused by severe, unaccustomed exercise, particularly that involving eccentric muscle action. ➲ reactive oxygen species.

delayed union longer than expected healing of a fracture. It may occur if the gap between the bone ends is too big, blood supply is poor (especially in the lower third of the tibia), the area is infected, or if internal fixation is used (this sometimes removes the stimulus for callus formation).

deletion in genetics, a mutation involving the loss of part of a chromosome or a sequence of genetic material. An example of a condition caused by chromosome deletion is cri du chat syndrome, which results from a deletion affecting chromosome number 5.

Delhi boil ➲ oriental sore.

deliberate self-harm (DSH) wilful non-fatal act(s) carried out in the knowledge that it was potentially harmful. Examples include self-poisoning (overdose), self-cutting and self-mutilation.

deliquescent *adj* capable of absorption, thus becoming fluid.

delirium *n* abnormal mental condition based on hallucinations or illusion. May occur in high fever, in mental health problems, or be toxic in origin.

delirium tremens (DTs) acute psychosis usually associated with the withdrawal of alcohol after a period of excessive intake over a considerable time. It is characterized by terror, hallucinations, confusion, disorientation and tremor—**delirious** *adj*.

delivery natural expulsion or extraction of the infant, placenta and fetal membranes at birth. *abdominal delivery* delivery of the infant through an incision made into the uterus via the abdominal wall (caesarean section). *instrumental delivery* delivery facilitated by the use of instruments, particularly forceps. *spontaneous delivery* delivery occurring without assistance of forceps or other mechanical aid. *vaginal delivery* complete expulsion of the infant, placenta and membranes via the birth canal, usually head-first presenting by the vertex; breech delivery is also possible.

dellen *npl* small areas of reduced thickness in the cornea. A transient shallow depression in the cornea near the limbus which is caused by a local dehydration of the corneal stroma leading to a compression of its lamellae. It can occur as a result of strabismus surgery, cataract surgery, swelling of the limbus (as in episcleritis or pterygium), rigid contact lens wear or increasing age. ⊃ keratitis sicca.

Delphi technique a research method where a consensus of expert opinion is obtained during a multiple-step process where the contributors are asked to rate a number of items, e.g. research priorities, in order of importance.

deltoid *adj* triangular.

deltoid ligament another name for the medial collateral ligament of the ankle joint, triangular in shape, hence its name. Much stronger than the lateral collateral ligaments; in fact, so strong that it is common for eversion injuries to cause fracture of the tip of the malleolus rather than rupture of the ligament itself.

deltoid muscle a thick muscle acting at the shoulder. Arises from the shoulder girdle, in continuity from the outer third of the front of the clavicle, the acromion of the scapula above the shoulder and the spine of the scapula behind it. From here the fibres converge to be inserted into the deltoid tuberosity on the outer side of the humerus. It is the prime mover of arm abduction when the main part of the muscle contracts. The anterior fibres cause flexion and the posterior fibres extend and cause lateral rotation of the shoulder. ⊃ Colour Section Figures 4, 5.

delusion *n* a fixed, usually false belief, inconsistent with an individual's culture and intelligence, which cannot be altered by argument or reasoning. A type of psychotic symptom.

DEM *abbr* developmental eye movement (DEM) test.

demand feeding feeding when the infant appears hungry and not according to a fixed timetable; also called 'on demand' feeding or baby-led feeding.

demarcation *n* an outlining of the junction of diseased and healthy tissue, often used when referring to gangrene.

dementia *n* (*syn* organic brain syndrome—OBS) an irreversible organic brain disease characterized by a loss of previously acquired intellectual function in the absence of impairment of arousal. There is progressive disturbance of memory and disintegration of personality, deterioration in personal care, impaired cognitive ability and disorientation. There are many potential causes of dementia but Alzheimer's disease and diffuse vascular disease are the most common. Causes include: (a) vascular—diffuse small-vessel disease, amyloid angiopathy, multiple emboli and rarely cerebral vasculitis; (b) degenerative or inherited—Alzheimer's disease, leucodystrophies, Huntington's disease, Wilson's disease, Pick's disease, myotonic dystrophy (dystrophia myotonica), cortical Lewy body disease, progressive supranuclear palsy and rarely mitochondrial encephalopathies; (c) malignancy—secondary deposits (common cause), primary cerebral tumour and rarely paraneoplastic syndrome; (d) inflammatory—multiple sclerosis and rarely sarcoidosis; (e) traumatic—chronic subdural haematoma, post-brain injury (both common traumatic causes), 'punch-drunk' syndrome; (f) hydrocephalus—communicating/non-communicating hydrocephalus, 'normal pressure' hydrocephalus; (g) toxic/nutritional—excess alcohol consumption (common toxic cause), vitamin B_1 thiamin(e) deficiency, vitamin B_{12} cobalamins deficiency and rarely anoxia/carbon monoxide poisoning, heavy metal poisoning; (h) infective—syphilis, HIV disease and rarely following encephalitis, Whipple's disease, subacute sclerosing panencephalitis (SSPE); (i) prion disease—sporadic Creutzfeldt-Jakob disease (CJD) and rarely variant CJD, kuru, Gerstmann–Sträussler–Scheinker disease. The distinction of senile from pre-senile dementia is unhelpful. However, rarer causes of dementia should be more actively sought in younger patients and those with short histories. When a patient presents with disturbance of personality or memory dysfunction, the first step is to exclude a focal lesion by determining that there is cognitive disturbance in more than one area. A careful history is, of course, essential and it is important to interview not just the patient but a close family member too. Simple 'bedside tests' such as the Mini-Mental State Examination (MMSE) are useful in assessing the cognitive deficit, but more formal help from clinical psychology may be required. General history and examination may give further clues to aetiology. Dementias are broadly divided into 'cortical' and 'subcortical' types, depending upon their clinical features. Many of the primary degenerative diseases that cause dementia have characteristic features that may allow a specific diagnosis during life. Creutzfeldt–Jakob disease is usually relatively rapidly progressive (over months), is associated with myoclonus, and there may be characteristic abnormalities on electroencephalogram

(EEG). Of the more slowly progressive dementias, Pick's disease presents with rather focal (temporal or frontal lobe) dysfunction often affecting language function early, and Lewy body dementia may present with visual hallucinations. However, it is often difficult to distinguish these dementias from each other or from Alzheimer's disease during life. The aim of investigations is to discover a treatable cause, if present, and to try to give an idea of prognosis. A standard set of investigations include: (a) imaging of the head—computed tomography and or magnetic resonance imaging; (b) blood tests—full blood count, urea and electrolytes, glucose, calcium, liver function tests, thyroid function tests, vitamin B_{12}, Venereal Disease Research Laboratory (VDRL) test, antinuclear antibody (ANA), anti-double-stranded DNA (anti-dsDNA); (c) chest X-ray; (d) electroencephalogram (EEG). In selected patients investigations including lumbar puncture, HIV serology and brain biopsy may be undertaken. Imaging of the brain is important to exclude potentially treatable structural lesions such as hydrocephalus, cerebral tumour or chronic subdural haematoma, though often the only abnormality seen is generalized atrophy. If the initial tests fail to yield an answer, more invasive tests such as lumbar puncture or, rarely, brain biopsy may be indicated. If there is concern that the memory disturbance may be a manifestation of depressive illness, formal neuropsychological evaluation is helpful. The management of dementia is directed at removing correctable causes, and providing support for patient and carers if no specific treatment exists. Anticholinesterase drugs, such as donepezil, rivastigmine and galantamine, or NMDA (N-methyl-D-aspartate receptor antagonists [memantine]) appear to improve cognitive function to some extent in Alzheimer's disease. ⊃ Alzheimer's disease, Creutzfeldt–Jakob disease, Huntington's disease, Lewy bodies, multi-infarct dementia, Pick's disease, Wilson's disease.

demographic indices such as age distribution, birth and mortality rates, occupation and geographical distribution. They are used to obtain a profile of a given population, compare different areas and plan services to meet specific needs. For example, an area with a large population of retired people will, along with other priorities, need to plan and provide services for degenerative conditions more common in an ageing population, and specific health promoting activities such as falls prevention.

demography *n* the study of population, such as gender and age distribution—**demographic** *adj*.

demulcent *n* a slippery, mucilaginous fluid that alleviates irritation and inflammation, especially of mucous membranes.

demyelination *n* destruction of the myelin sheaths surrounding nerve fibres. Can occur in the peripheral nerves (e.g. Guillain–Barré syndrome), or in the central nervous system (e.g. multiple sclerosis).

denatured alcohol ethyl alcohol to which certain denaturants have been added to render it unfit for human consumption or to adapt it for industrial uses.

denaturation a change in the basic structure or nature of a substance. As in proteins exposed to acids, alcohols, radiation or heat, such as the change in egg albumen (white of the egg) during cooking.

denaturation test Singer's test. A blood test used to distinguish fetal from maternal blood.

dendrite *n* (*syn* dendron) one of the branched filaments which are given off from the body of a nerve cell. That part of a neuron which transmits an impulse to the nerve cell—**dendritic** *adj*.

dendritic cell an antigen-presenting cell that presents a processed antigen to B and T lymphocytes bearing antigen-specific receptors. They are thought to be the cells important in determining the type of immune response generated against an antigen. ⊃ antigen-presenting cell.

dendritic keratitis an acute and chronic corneal inflammation that occurs in a person who has had a primary infection with herpes simplex virus type 1 (HVS-1). Some cases occur with other types of herpes viruses. It is characterized by the formation of small vesicles that break down and coalesce to form dendritic ulcers. ⊃ corneal ulcer, dendritic ulcer.

dendritic ulcer a linear corneal ulcer that sends out tree-like branches. Usually caused by herpes simplex virus.

dendron *n* ⊃ dendrite.

denervation *n* the means by which a nerve supply is cut off. Usually refers to incision, excision or blocking of a nerve.

dengue *n* (*syn* 'break-bone fever') a mosquito-transmitted viral haemorrhagic fever. The dengue flavivirus is a common cause of fever in and from the tropics. It is endemic in Southeast Asia and India and is also seen in Africa; there have been recent large epidemics in the Caribbean and Americas. The principal vector is the mosquito *Aedes aegypti*, which breeds in standing water; collections of water in containers and tyre dumps are a particular risk in large cities. *Aedes albopictus* is a vector in some Southeast Asian countries. There are four serotypes of dengue virus, all producing a similar clinical syndrome; homotypic immunity is life-long but heterotypic immunity between serotypes lasts only a few months. The incubation period from being bitten by an infected mosquito is usually 2–7 days. The disease varies in severity. The clinical features include: (a) prodrome—2 days of malaise and headache; (b) acute onset—fever, backache, arthralgias, headache, generalized pains ('break-bone fever'), pain on eye movement, lacrimation, anorexia, nausea, vomiting, relative bradycardia, prostration, depression, lymphadenopathy, scleral injection; (c) fever—continuous or 'saddle-back', with break on fourth or fifth day (usually lasts 7–8 days; (d) rash—transient macular in first 1–2 days. Maculopapular, scarlet morbilliform from 3–5 days on the trunk, spreading centrifugally and sparing the palms and soles. The morbilliform rash characteristically blanches under pressure. May desquamate on resolution. The convalescence is slow. Asymptomatic infections are common. *dengue haemorrhagic fever or dengue shock* *syndrome* occurs mainly in children in Southeast Asia. In mild forms there is thrombocytopenia and haemoconcentration. In the most severe form, after 3–4 days of fever, hypotension and circulatory failure develop with features of a capillary leak syndrome. Minor (petechiae, ecchymoses, epistaxis) or major (gastrointestinal bleeding) haemorrhagic signs may occur. The pathogenesis is unclear but preexisting immunity to a dengue virus serotype, heterotypic to the one causing the current infection, predisposes to the syndrome. In vitro such heterotypic antibody causes enhanced virus entry and replication in monocytes; it is believed that enhancing antibody from previous dengue infection with a different serotype, or from acquired maternal antibody in infants, facilitates development of a very heavy viral load. Disseminated intravascular coagulation (DIC), complement activation and release of vasoactive mediators may contribute to the pathogenesis of the syndrome, possibly triggered by immunopathological mechanisms. Cytokine release is thought to be the cause of vascular damage at the site of post-capillary endothelial junctions. Even with good treatment the case fatality may be up to 10%. Adults rarely have classical dengue shock syndrome but may have a stormy and fatal course characterized by elevated liver enzymes, haemostatic abnormalities and gastrointestinal bleeding. The diagnosis of dengue is easier in an endemic area when a patient has the characteristic symptoms and signs. However, mild cases may have a similar presentation to other viral infections. Leucopenia is usual and thrombocytopenia common. The diagnosis is confirmed by either a fourfold rise in IgG antibody titres, isolation of dengue virus from blood or detection of dengue virus genomic sequences by real-time polymerase chain reaction (PCR). Serological tests may detect cross-reacting antibodies from other flaviviruses, including yellow fever vaccine. There is no specific treatment. The severe pains can be relieved by paracetamol. Aspirin should be avoided. Volume replacement, blood transfusions and management of shock are indicated in the capillary leak syndrome. Corticosteroids have not been shown to help. No existing antivirals are effective. Breeding places of *Aedes* mosquitoes should be abolished and the adults destroyed by insecticides. There is as yet no vaccine and in any case a tetravalent vaccine would be needed to cover all four serotypes. Until the *Aedes* mosquito can be controlled or a cost-effective vaccine developed, the incidence of dengue can be expected to continue to escalate.

denial *n* a complex unconscious defence mechanism in which difficult situations, or unacceptable or distressing facts, are not acknowledged, so as to avoid distress, anxiety and emotional conflict. It may occur in response to drastically changed circumstances, e.g. sudden incapacitating illness, or terminal illness.

denidation degeneration and expulsion during menstruation of certain epithelial elements, potentially the nidus of an embryo and the intended shedding of uterine lining when postcoital hormonal contraception is used.

Dennis Browne splints (D Browne, Australian surgeon, 20th century) splints used to correct congenital talipes equinovarus (club foot).

denominator in obstetrics, a particular point on the presenting part of the fetus used to indicate its position in relation to a particular part of the women's pelvis. Includes the occiput in a vertex presentation, the sacrum in breech presentation or the mentum (chin) in a face presentation.

dens a tooth or tooth-like structure. Also the odontoid process of the second cervical vertebra (axis).

dens in dente an anomaly of teeth charaterized by invagination of the enamel. This gives a radiographic appearance suggestive of a 'tooth within a tooth'.

dens invaginatus developmental tooth anomaly in which there is a deep invagination on the lingual or palatal surface of incisor teeth, generally maxillary laterals. The invagination may be wholly or partially lined with enamel.

densitometer in radiography, an instrument for measuring the relative density of different steps on a film. ⊃ sensitometry.

density 1. the ratio of mass to volume. An indication of the compactness of a substance. Measured in kilograms per cubic metre ($kg \cdot m^{-3}$). In optometry, this property is usually given by lens manufacturers, the greater the density of a material, the greater its weight, all other factors being equal. 2. in radiology, the amount of blackening on a radiographic or photographic film and is the log of the opacity.

dent/a, dent/i, dent/o- a prefix/combining form that means 'tooth', e.g. *dentate*.

dental *adj* relating to teeth.

dental abrasion loss by wear of tooth substance or a restoration, caused by factors other than tooth contact, e.g. incorrect tooth brushing.

dental amalgam a compound of a basal alloy of silver and tin with mercury, used for restoring teeth. ⊃ amalgam.

dental ankylosis solid fixation of a tooth owing to fusion of cementum and alveolar bone, the periodontal ligament being obliterated.

dental arch describes the curved structure comprising the teeth and the alveolar ridge in each jaw. The bow-shaped arrangement of the mandibular and maxillary teeth.

dental-associated collagen fibres the bundles of collagen fibres found deep in the mucogingival complex are grouped according to their position. They are oblique—the majority group running obliquely downwards from the socket wall to the cementum of a tooth root; transeptal; circular; lontitudinal; alveologingival; and dentogingival.

dental attrition non-carious, mechanical wearing of teeth, either through normal mastication or as a result of parafunctional habits, e.g. bruxism.

dental calculus previously known as tartar (lay term) or calcarous deposit. A deposit of calcified dental plaque, containing calcium carbonate and phosphate, which forms on the surface of the teeth. Its presence is associated with periodontal disease and gum recession, which may lead to the loss of teeth. Depending on its location, relative to the gingival margin, it is described as *supragingival calculus* or *subgingival calculus*, and, rarely as *sub-* or *supra-marginal calculus.*

dental care professional (DCP) a member of the dental care team recognized and registered by the appropriate authority (the General Dental Council in the United Kingdom) and entitled to carry out certain dental procedures (clinically or in the laboratory). Team members include clinical dental technicians; dental hygienists; dental therapists; dental nurses; dental technicians; and orthodontic therapists.

dental caries said to be the most common human afflication. A microbial disease of the calcified tissues of the teeth, characterized by demineralization of the inorganic portion and destruction of their organic substance, cavitation and breakdown of calcified dental tissue. ➲ approximal caries, arrested caries, caries-free or immune, caries-prone, early childhood caries, insipient caries, radiation caries, rampant caries, recurrent caries, residual caries, root caries.

dental cavity ➲ cavity (dental).

dental cement substances used in dentistry to effect temporary restorations prior to longer term solutions.

dental dam device placed in the mouth during dental treatment to prevent the passage of saliva or water. Used to keep a tooth or teeth dry during treatment. ➲ rubber dam.

dental enamel the hard outer covering of the anatomical crown of a tooth, consisting of highly calcified, acellular, generally prismatic tissue of ectodermal origin. It is the hardest tissue in the body, composed of rods and prisms, has 96% inorganic content and is not sensitive. *decalcified enamel* enamel from which calcium has been removed. ➲ white spot. *enamel crystallites* crystals of biological apatites which occur in human enamel. *enamel cuticle* organic film found on the surface of enamel. *enamel fluid* aqueous solution found in the pores of the solid phase of enamel. *enamel hatchet* ➲ hatchet. *enamel lamella* thin sheets of imperfectly calcified organic material extending from the surface for a variable distance through the enamel. *enamel matrix* organic base, secreted by ameloblasts, within which inorganic crystallites are laid down and grow. *enamel organ* derived from the surrounding ectodermal tissues, the dental lamina and the tooth bud. Responsible for the formation of tooth enamel during development. *enamel pearl* enameloma. A small bead of enamel formed apically to the cement–enamel junction and resembling a pearl. Often found in the furcation of molars. *enamel porcelain* translucent, lightly pigmented outer covering of a porcelain jacket crown restoration used to simulate the translucency of a natural tooth. *enamel prism* basic morphological unit of enamel running from the amelo-dentinal junction to the enamel surface. *enamel protein* protein which forms a large part of the enamel organic material and is a product of the ameloblasts. *enamel spindles* extensions of the dentinal tubules which can be seen under the microscope to be running across (for a short distance) the amelo-dentinal junction into the enamel. *enamel striae of Retzius* incremental brown growth lines seen in enamel under the microscope running obliquely across the long axis of the enamel prism. *enamel tuft* area of unmineralized enamel matrix extending from the amelo-dentinal junction a short way into the enamel. *mottled enamel* enamel with white, yellow or brown areas—sometimes pitted—due to excessive ingestion of fluoride during enamel formation.

dental engine in dentistry, the rotary electric or foot-driven machine driving rotary instruments by means of a handpiece through a pulley or cable drive, or directly.

dental erosion non-carious wearing away of the surfaces of the teeth. There is irreversible loss of dental hard tissue by a chemical process that does not involve bacteria. Dissolution of mineralized tooth tissue occurs upon contact with intrinsic acid, such as caused by gastro-oesophageal reflux disease (GORD) or extrinsic acids. ➲ tooth surface loss.

dental examination an inspection and/or an investigation to evaluate the state of health or of a disease. In dentistry, a full examination should include a medical and dental history, a visual intra- and extraoral inspection including palpation, auscultation, measurement of tooth mobility and gingival pocket depth, pulp tests as well as various radiographic and laboratory procedures.

dental floss/tape waxed or unwaxed thread or tape used for removing plaque and food debris from interproximal surfaces and contact areas of the teeth. Regular use promotes oral hygiene and reduces the risk of dental caries and periodontal disease.

dental follicle fibrocellular layer of tissue surrounding a developing tooth before it erupts.

dental formulae a method of identifying individual teeth: adult teeth (permanent [secondary] dentition) are numbered and children's teeth (primary dentition) have letters. ➲ charting (dental).

dental gubernaculum a guiding pathway that leads from the developing tooth follicle to the surface of the gingiva.

dental hygienist a member of the dental team qualified to practise preventive and certain therapeutic aspects of dentistry, including plaque control measures, removal of deposits from the teeth, application of fissure sealants and topical fluoride, and instruction in oral hygiene measures. The treatment must be prescribed by a dentist.

dental hypoplasia defective formation of dentine due to illnesses such as measles or due to malnutrition or starvation.

dental implant a device, usually made from titanium, inserted in the jawbone to provide an abutment to support a crown, denture or a bridge.

dental jurisprudence forensic dentistry. The science that deals with the application of dental science to the civil and criminal law.

dental/maxillofacial splinting in dentistry and maxillofacial surgery, **1.** stabilizing one or more loose teeth by splinting them to firm adjacent teeth by means of wires, bands or cast splints made of metal or plastic. ➲ flexible splinting, rigid splinting. **2.** immobilization of fractured bone ends by wiring, pinning or splinting. ➲ fixation.

dental nurse a member of the dental team who provides close support for the dental surgeon and is responsible for the cleanliness and tidiness of surgery equipment, instruments and materials. The dental nurse should have a general understanding and working knowledge of the sterilization and disinfection of surgical instruments and equipment—and be responsible for the preparation of the dental surgery for all dental procedures. Training includes: the recording of dental charting; maintenance of dental treatment records; assisting at the chairside during all dental procedures; assisting in the care of the patient before, during and after an anaesthetic; oral hygiene instruction and advising patients on what actions to take following certain dental procedures; the taking, processing, mounting and filing of radiographs; upholding the ethical standards of the dental profession; reception and administration procedures.

dental opacity a tooth surface defect due to increased subsurface porosity of enamel or dentine.

dental pantomogram (DPT) a radiograph that includes the teeth in both jaws.

dental pantomography *n* panoramic radiography that gives a view of all the teeth in both jaws on a single radiograph.

dental papilla tissue partially enclosed by the enamel organ, which forms the dentine of a tooth and later becomes the pulp.

dental plaque a specific but highly variable and tenacious film composed of micro-organisms and cellular debris that rapidly forms on the surface of a tooth in the absence of effective oral hygiene. Clinically it occurs supragingivally and subgingivally and may also be found on other solid surfaces such as restorations and oral appliances. The causal factor of dental caries and periodontal disease when in combination with other factors over a period of time. ⮑ index (dental).

dental plaque control the removal of plaque by brushing and the use of floss, silk, tape, interdental brushes and other instruments to maintain oral hygiene and cleanliness.

Dental Practitioners' Formulary (DPF) a section of the British National Formulary that outlines the drugs that dental practitioners can prescribe within the National Health Service. In England the precription must be presented on the form FP10D, in Scotland (form GP14) and in Wales (form WP10D).

dental prop instrument used intraorally to maintain the mouth in an open position, e.g. Hewitt, McKesson, Brunton and Lane (centre prop). ⮑ mouth prop.

dental prophylaxis the procedure for removing dental plaque, acquired pellicle and stains from the teeth by the use of polishing paste on a rotating brush or flexible polishing cup.

dental prosthesis a fixed or removable artificial replacement for one or more teeth and their associated structures. Constructed by the dental technician using acrylic resin or a combination of metal and acrylic resin.

dental prosthetics a branch of dental science dealing with the artificial replacement of one or more natural teeth or associated structures by a denture or bridge.

dental prosthetist ⮑ prosthodontist.

dental public health ⮑ community dentistry.

dental pulp the fibrocellular, jelly-like tissue consisting of cell bodies, odontoblasts, blood vessels, nerves, lymphatics and connective tissue that occupies the core of the crown and the root canal(s) of a tooth. ⮑ pulp.

dental restoration the process of replacing part or all of a tooth by artificial means; also the term given to the type of replacement used, e.g. filling, crown, bridge.

dental scaling the removal of calculus, using special instruments, from the surfaces of the teeth.

dental stone. 1. a general term for model and die material. 2. the rotary abrasive instrument used for grinding and polishing.

dental tape ⮑ dental floss.

dental technician a member of the dental team who constructs dentures, crowns, inlays, bridges, orthodontic appliances, splints, etc. to the prescriptions of dentists.

dental therapist a member of the dental team who is trained to carry out certain dental treatments to the prescription of a dentist. They are permitted to carry out simple fillings in primary and permanent teeth, apply preventive solutions, gels and sealants to the teeth, give plaque control instruction at the chairside and to provide dental health education.

dental treatment plan following history taking, examination and diagnostic procedures, the setting out of what treatment is to be undertaken for a patient, in what order and at what intervals of time.

dental unit the combination of dental equipment in one unit. Formerly fixed and now mostly mobile. Combines high- and low-speed handpiece drivers, three-in-one air/water syringes and sometimes an ultrasonic or sonic scaler. Other appliances such as a cuspidor, dental operating light, bracket table and an X-ray machine may form part of the same dental unit.

dentate *adj* having natural teeth present.

denticle (pulpstone) the deposit of amorphous calcific material occurring around the pulpal vessels in an otherwise normal tooth. May be found in pulps which have been mildly irritated over a period of time.

dentiform shaped like a tooth.

dentifrice the collective term encompassing several kinds of tooth cleansers: tooth pastes, tooth powders, tooth 'whiteners' and mouthwashes.

dentigerous containing teeth or tooth-like structures.

dentigerous cyst ⮑ cyst of dental origin.

dentinal relating to dentine.

dentinal process ⮑ odontoblast process.

dentinal tubules the microscopic tubules within the dentine of a tooth running from the dental pulp to the amelo-dentinal junction. Contains the odontoblast process.

dentine the sensitive calcified tissue forming the bulk of a tooth and surrounding the pulp. The dentine itself is covered by enamel in the crown and by cementum in the root. Consists of about 70% of inorganic salts by weight, and

30% of water plus collagen fibres. Microscopically shows a vast number of S-shaped tubules, running outwards from the pulp, which house the long, slender processes of the odontoblast cells in the pulp and are responsible for the formation of dentine. When odontoblast cells have laid down the bulk of the dentine (the *primary dentine*) and the tooth is fully formed, they continue to lay down further regular *secondary dentine* throughout the time that the tooth remains vital. In response to any stimulus such as caries or abrasion, the odontoblast cells lay down secondary dentine at a more rapid rate. This type of dentine is known as *reparative secondary dentine*. *dentine pin* ⊃ pin. *dentine porcelain* (or *body porcelain*) the pigmented, translucent porcelain which is used to give the overall shape and shade to a jacket crown restoration or facing. *dentine screw* threaded length of wire inserted into the dentine to provide extra retention for a restoration, e.g. dentatus screw. *hypoplastic dentine* ⊃ dental hypoplasia. *sclerotic* or *translucent dentine* areas of dentine whose tubules have become occluded.

dentine adhesive resin based adhesive used to bond restorative materials to tooth substance.

dentino-enamel junction ⊃ amelo-dentinal junction.

dentinogenesis the production of dentine by the odontoblasts during tooth development.

dentinogenesis imperfecta **1.** localized mesodermal dysplasia that disrupts dentine formation. It may be inherited. **2.** an inherited disorder where the dentine is defective but the enamel is normal. **3.** a genetic disorder of dentine, in which there is early calcification of the root canals and pulp chambers, excessive wear and a characteristic grey-brown hue to the teeth. Often accompanied by a similar disturbance in bone.

dentinoma a rare tumour, arising from odontogenic mesenchymal tissue composed mainly of an irregular mass of dentine-like tissue.

dentist *n* any person who practises dentistry, and is qualified and licensed to do so.

dentistry *n* profession concerned with the prevention, diagnosis and treatment of diseases of the teeth, their supporting tissues and other oral tissues, including their restoration and replacement. Restores to normal function carious, fractured or badly worn teeth by means of fillings, inlays, crowns or bridges. Replaces missing teeth and other tissues by bridges and prostheses and treats dental abnormalities, diseases, traumatic injuries, and also provides preventive measures for caries and periodontal disease. ⊃ aesthetic dentistry, community dentistry, conservative dentistry, cosmetic dentistry, endodontics, forensic dentistry, four-handed dentistry, orthodontics, paediatric dentistry, paedodontics, periodontics, preventive dentistry, prosthetic dentistry, prosthodontics, restorative dentistry.

dentition the natural teeth in the dental arches. In humans consists of 20 primary teeth erupting from the age of 6 months onwards. Later gradually replaced and added to by 32 permanent teeth.

dentoalveolar abscess a 'gumboil'. Localized collection of pus within the alveolar bone, of dental origin.

dentoalveolar disproportion disproportion between the size of the teeth and the space available for them in the dental arch. May lead to either crowding or spacing between teeth.

dentofacial deformity any malformation involving the dentofacial complex—the mouth and jaw. Examples include cleft lip and palate, malocclusion, other skeletal anomalies.

dentogenesis ⊃ dentinogenesis.

dentogingival complex ⊃ mucogingival complex.

dentogingival junction ⊃ junctional epithelium.

dentulous having natural teeth.

denture *n* a removable dental prosthesis. An artificial substitute for missing teeth and their associated structures. May be partial or complete (replacing some, or all, of the teeth in either jaw respectively) and is generally constructed of acrylic resin alone or in conjunction with various metals. ⊃ acrylic denture, complete denture, denture base, denture bearing area, denture border, denture granuloma, denture hyperplasia, denture space, duplicate denture, hybrid denture, immediate replacement denture, implant supported denture, interim denture, over-denture, partial denture, sectional denture, skeletal denture, spoon denture, trial denture.

denture adhesive used to retain ill-fitting dentures, e.g. gum tragacanth.

denture base either that part of the denture which rests on the denture-bearing area of the oral mucosa, or material, generally acrylic resin, used in the construction of dentures and other appliances by the dough moulding and curing technique.

denture bearing area that portion of the edentulous ridge and the surface of the teeth that are covered by a denture.

denture border the border of the denture base.

denture granuloma a deprecated term for denture hyperplasia.

denture hyperplasia area of hyperplastic fibroepithelial tissue resulting from chronic irritation from a denture.

denture space irregular space in the mouth, bounded by the cheeks, lips, tongue and floor of the mouth, and within which a denture should lie.

denturist also called Clinical Dental Technician (UK). An accredited dental technician licenced to make and supply removable dentures to the general public.

Denver II previously known as the Denver Developmental Screening Test (DDST). A tool for assessing an infant's/child's developmental progress by comparing their behaviours with those shown by the majority of their age group. Comparative grids are used to assess milestones, which are arranged in four categories: personal and social; fine motor—adaptive; language; and gross motor.

deodorant *n, adj* a substance which destroys or masks an (unpleasant) odour. Deodorants are used for personal hygiene and within the environment. Topical antibiotics and charcoal dressings can be used to deodorize malodorous infected wounds—**deodorize** *vt*.

deontological *adj* ethical theory based on the science of deontology that supports the view that there is a duty to act within certain universal rules of morality. A theory associated with the work of Immanuel Kant. ⊃ utilitarianism.

deorsumvergence ⊃ infravergence.

deoxycholic acid a bile acid produced by the liver. It emulsifies fats in the small intestine and aids their absorption. Ursodeoxycholic acid is rarely used to dissolve gallstones.

deoxygenation *n* the removal of oxygen—**deoxygenated** *adj*.

deoxyribonucleases (DNase) enzymes that cleave deoxyribonucleic acid linkages at particular points on the strand. *recombinant human deoxyribonuclease* (rhDNase) a genetically engineered form of the natural enzyme called dornase alfa. It is administered, by jet nebulizer, to improve lung function in some people with cystic fibrosis.

deoxyribonucleic acid (DNA) a double-strand nucleic acid molecule found in the chromosomes of all organisms (except some viruses). Each strand is closely linked to another in a double helix. DNA (as genes) carries the coded instructions for passing on hereditary characteristics. DNA is a polymer formed from many nucleotides. These consist of the sugar deoxyribose, phosphate groups and four nitrogenous bases: adenine (A), guanine (G), thymine (T) and cytosine (C). Adenine and guanine are purine bases, and thymine and cytosine are pyrimidine bases. The nucleotide units are bound together to form a double helix with the adenine of one strand opposite the thymine of the other and the same for guanine and cytosine. ⊃ mitochondrial disorders, mitochondrial genes, Colour Section Figure 26.

dependence the condition of needing support in order to be able to perform everyday activities to a satisfactory level. (Reproduced with permission from the European Network of Occupational Therapy in Higher Education (ENOTHE) Terminology Project, 2008.)

dependency the state of needing help from others to meet physical and or emotional needs.

dependency culture a sociological term that describes the opinion that unlimited state welfare provision may reduce individuals' ability to be assertive and support themselves.

dependent variable ⊃ variable.

depersonalization *n* a subjective feeling that one no longer feels that one is real or exists. Occurs in a wide range of disorders including depressive states, anxiety disorder, with psychoactive substance misuse, etc.

depilate *vt* to remove hair from—**depilatory** *adj, n*, **depilation** *n*.

depilatories *npl* substances usually made in pastes (e.g. barium sulphide) which remove excess hair only temporarily; they do not act on the papillae, consequently the hair grows again. ⊃ epilation—**depilatory** *sing*. *Preoperative depilation* lessens the risk of wound infection because it is non-abrasive, unlike shaving the skin.

depolarization *n* in excitable cells the inside of the membrane becomes electrically positive with respect to the outside. A reduction of the normal voltage difference between the inside and the outside of a cell. Occurs during the transmission of a nerve impulse. ⊃ action potential, membrane potential, polarized.

depolished glass ⊃ ground glass.

depot *n* a body area where a drug is deposited or stored, and from where it can be released and distributed, such as hormone therapy.

depot injection drugs, usually psychotropic, that are given by deep intramuscular injections. Used when clients are unable (for a variety of reasons) to take their drugs on a regular basis.

depressed fracture ⊃ depressed skull fracture, fracture.

depressed skull fracture the skull fractures and forms a dent in the skull, which can be open (compound) or closed (simple). Although the patient may not exhibit any signs or symptoms, it can require neurosurgery to correct and internal trauma may be present. Usually, the result of someone being hit on the head by an object.

depression *n* **1.** a hollow place or indentation. **2.** a downward or inward movement or displacement. **3.** diminution of power or activity. **4.** a mental health disorder characterized by feelings of profound sadness. May be classified by severity (mild/moderate/severe), by the presence of somatic symptoms (anorexia, weight loss, impaired libido, sleep disturbance, etc.) and by the presence or absence of psychotic symptoms. Recognized cognitive symptoms include hopelessness, helplessness, guilt, low self-esteem and suicidal ideation. The previous description of reactive versus endogenous depression is outdated and not thought to be relevant to treatment or prognosis. **5.** in orthodontics, the adjustment of the vertical level of teeth that have overerupted beyond the general occlusal level of the dental arch.

deprivation indices a set of census variables and weightings used to assess levels of deprivation within a specific community or population. They include: levels of unemployment, lone-parent households, pensioners living alone and households without a car. ⊃ Jarman index, Townsend index.

depth of field for a given setting of an optical system (or a steady state of accommodation of the eye) it is the distance over which an object may be moved without causing a sharpness reduction beyond a certain tolerable amount. Depth of field increases when the diaphragm (or pupil) diameter diminishes as, for example, in older eyes. For example: viewing at infinity, the depth of field varies between infinity and about 3.6 m for a pupil of 4 mm in diameter; and between infinity and about 2.3 m for a 2 mm pupil. At a viewing distance of 1 m, the depth of field ranges from about 1.4 m to 80 cm with a 4 mm pupil; and from about 1.8 m to 70 cm with a 2 mm pupil.

depth of focus for a given setting of an optical system (or a steady state of accommodation of the eye) it is the distance in front and behind the focal point (or retina) over which the image may be focused without causing a sharpness reduction beyond a certain tolerable amount. (The criterion could be as much as a line of letters on a Snellen chart.) The depth of focus is represented by the total distance in front and behind. As with depth of field, it is inversely proportional to the diameter of the diaphragm (or pupil).

depth perception (*syn* spatial vision) perception of the distance of an object from the observer (absolute distance) or of the distance between two objects (relative distance). Our ability to judge the latter is much more precise than the former. There are many factors which contribute to depth perception. Most importantly is the existence on the two retinae of different images of the same object (called binocular disparity or retinal disparity). There are also many other contributing factors, such as the characteristics of the stimulus (called cues), binocular parallax and, to a smaller extent, the muscular proprioceptive information due to the efforts of accommodation and convergence. Depth perception is more precise in binocular vision but is possible in monocular vision using cues that include: interposition, relative position, relative size, linear perspective, textural gradient, aerial perspective, light and shade, shadow and motion parallax. ⊃ stereopsis, stereoscopic visual acuity.

De Quervain's tenosynovitis (F De Quervain, Swiss surgeon, 1868–1940) inflammation of the tendons and sheath of abductor pollicis longus and extensor pollicis brevis.

De Quervain's thyroiditis *n* (F De Quervain) an inflammatory condition of the thyroid gland. Often follows a viral infection of the upper respiratory tract. It is characterized by tenderness and swelling of the thyroid gland, pyrexia, neck pain and dysphagia.

Derbyshire neck goitre.

derealization *n* feelings that people, events or surroundings have changed and are unreal. These sensations may occur in normal people during dreams, in states of fatigue or after sensory deprivation. May sometimes occur in schizophrenia and depressive states. Also experienced with the use of hallucinogenic drugs.

dereistic *adj* of thinking, not adapted to reality. Describes autistic thinking.

derivative the result of the calculation (usually with calculus) of the change of one variable with respect to another. Also alludes to the number of 'steps' of calculus required (e.g. acceleration is the second derivative of displacement with respect to time). ⊃ differentiation.

derma, dermat/o, dermo- a prefix that means 'skin', e.g. *dermatitis*.

-derm/a, -dermia, -dermic a suffix that means 'skin', e.g. *hypodermic*.

dermabrasion *n* removal of superficial layers of the skin by abrasive methods.

dermatitis *n* inflammation of the skin (by custom limited to an eczematous reaction). ⊃ atopic eczema, dermatitis herpetiformis, eczema, industrial dermatitis.

dermatitis herpetiformis an intensely itchy blistering skin eruption of immune-mediated aetiology. It affects young people and is associated with coeliac disease (gluten-induced enteropathy). The eruption occurs on the elbows,

lower back and the buttocks. Treatment involves dapsone and a gluten-free diet.

dermatochalasia *n* loose, superfluous eyelid skin which causes the eyelid to droop. A feature of normal ageing, it occurs in older people.

dermatofibroma a small round, painless lump usually found on the extremities.

dermatoglyphics *n* study of the ridge patterns of the skin of the fingertips, palms and soles to identify certain chromosomal anomalies.

dermatographia *n* ⊃ dermographia.

dermatologist *n* medically qualified individual who studies skin diseases and is skilled in their treatment. A skin specialist.

dermatology *n* the science which deals with the skin, its structure, functions, diseases and their treatment— **dermatological** *adj*, **dermatologically** *adv*.

dermatome *n* **1.** an instrument for cutting slices of skin of varying thickness, usually for grafting. **2.** the area of skin supplied by a single spinal nerve (Figures D.2, D.3).

dermatomycosis *n* a superficial fungal infection of the skin—**dermatomycotic** *adj*.

dermatomyositis *n* an idiopathic inflammatory myopathy (IIM). The muscle manifestations are identical to polymyositis, but occur in combination with characteristic cutaneous manifestations. Gottron's papules are scaly erythematous/violaceous plaques or papules occurring over the extensor surfaces of the proximal and distal interphalangeal joints. The heliotrope rash is a violaceous discoloration of the eyelid in combination with periorbital oedema. ⊃ Colour Section Figure 62. Similar rashes occur on the upper back,

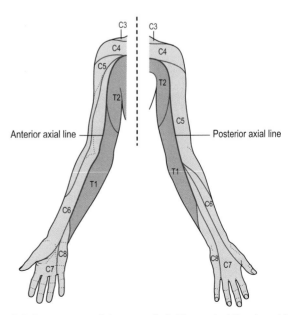

D.2 Dermatomes of the upper limb (C = cervical, T = thoracic) (reproduced from Porter 2005 with permission).

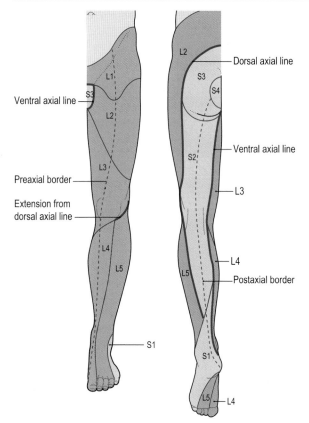

Ventral axial line

Preaxial border

Extension from
dorsal axial line

Dorsal axial line

Ventral axial line

Postaxial border

D.3 Dermatomes of the lower limb (L = lumbar, S = sacral) (reproduced from Porter 2005 with permission).

chest and shoulders ('shawl' distribution). Periungual nail-fold capillaries are often abnormal. Other systemic manifestations include arthralgia, weight loss and fever. Can be associated with an underlying malignancy in older people—a paraneoplastic syndrome. ⊃ collagen, connective tissue diseases, idiopathic inflammatory myopathies (IIMs), polymyositis.

dermatophytes *npl* a group of fungi (*Epidermophyton*, *Microsporum* or *Trichophyton*) that cause superficial infections of skin, hair and nails.

dermatophytosis *n* infection of the skin caused by one of the dermatophyte species—*Epidermophyton*, *Microsporum* or *Trichophyton*.

dermatosis *n* generic term for skin disease—**dermatoses** *pl*.

dermis *n* the true skin; the cutis vera; the layer below the epidermis—**dermal** *adj*. ⊃ Colour Section Figure 12.

dermoepidermal junction the basement membrane zone between the epidermis and dermis. ⊃ epidermis, skin.

dermographia *n* (*syn* dermatographia, factitial urticaria) a condition in which weals occur on the skin after a blunt instrument or fingernail has been lightly drawn over it. Seen in vasomotor instability and urticaria—**dermographic** *adj*.

dermoid *adj* pertaining to or resembling skin.

dermoid cyst a cyst which is congenital in origin and usually occurs in the ovary. It contains elements of ectodermal origin such as hair, nails, skin, teeth, etc. May also be present in skin, floor of the mouth and the upper neck.

Descartes' law ⊃ law of refraction.

Descemet's membrane (J Descemet, French physician, 1732–1810) (*syn* posterior elastic lamina, posterior limiting layer) the deepest layer of the corneal stroma, it is in contact with the endotheium. It is a strong, resistant, thin (about 8 mm) layer of the cornea located between the endothelium (from which it is secreted) and the stroma. It is practically the last corneal structure to succumb to disease processes and it can regenerate after injury. ⊃ descemetocele, Kayser–Fleischer ring.

descemetocele (*syn* keratocele) a forward bulging of Descemet's membrane due to either trauma or a deep corneal ulcer which has eroded the overlying stroma. ⊃ Descemet's membrane.

descending colon that part of the colon from the left colonic (splenic) flexure that passes down the left side of the abdominal cavity then curves towards the midline. After it enters the true pelvis it is known as the sigmoid colon. ⊃ Colour Section Figure 18b.

descent downward movement. In obstetrics, the descent of the fetus during labour through the brim, cavity and outlet of the pelvis. Descent is assessed by abdominal examination described in fifths.

descriptive epidemiology the retrospective analysis of the relationship between disease and suspected cause of the disease.

descriptive statistics that which describes or summarizes the observations of a sample. ⊃ inferential statistics.

desensitization *n* **1.** process of reducing subsequent immediate-type hypersensitivity reactions to venoms and other allergens by repeated injection of minute quantities of allergen in order to modulate the immune response away from the harmful allergic type reaction to a less pathological response. **2.** a behavioural therapy used for phobias where people are helped to overcome their irrational fear. In general there is a gradual exposure in a safe environment to the object, situation or stimulus that causes them acute anxiety or other negative reaction through imagining the object, looking at pictures or by eventually confronting the real thing. The aim being for the person to be able to tolerate the event without becoming dysfunctional. The anxiety-provoking stimulus is repeatedly paired with a relaxation response, either in the imagination or in real life (the latter known as *in vivo* desensitization), in order to eventually eliminate the anxiety response and replace it with the relaxation response. In systematic desensitization a hierarchy of increasingly anxiety-provoking stimuli is established and each stimulus is paired with the relaxation response in turn, beginning with the least feared and working towards the most feared. Also known as reciprocal inhibition therapy. **3.** with reference to repeated dose of a drug, a progressive decline in its effects —**desensitize** *vt*.

desensitizing agent in dentistry, a preparation for topical application to sensitive areas of a tooth surface. May be in the form of a solution, gel or varnish, e.g. 2% zinc chloride solution and proprietary preparations.

desiccation *n* drying out. As in desiccation of the nucleus pulposus, thus diminishing the cushioning effect of a healthy intervertebral disc.

designated area an area where radiation is being used and therefore there are restrictions placed on who can be present in the area. Areas are described as being controlled or supervised.

designer foods ⮌ functional foods.

-desis a suffix that means 'to bind together', e.g. *arthrodesis*.

desloughing the process of removing slough from a wound. ⮌ débridement.

desmoid tumour a benign tumour of fibrous connective tissue. Occurs on the neck, arms, legs and within the abdomen.

desmosines compounds forming the cross-linkages between chains of elastin, the structural protein of connective tissue.

desmosome also known as macula adherens. A complex junction that aids adhesion between cells. They are composed of proteins that span the gap between squamous epithelial cells such as those in the skin. Desmosomes are able to prevent structural damage from shearing forces.

desquamation *n* shedding; flaking off; casting off, as of the skin—**desquamate** *vi, vt*.

desquamative gingivitis chronic, diffuse inflammation of the gingiva characterized by desquamation of the gingival epithelium.

desquamative interstitial pneumonia (DIP) one of the idiopathic interstitial pneumonias. It is more common in men and smokers. It presents in the forties or fifties with an insidious onset of dyspnoea. Clubbing of the fingers is present in 50% of patients. A biopsy shows increased macrophages in the alveolar spaces, septal thickening and type II pneumocyte hyperplasia. The prognosis is generally good.

detached retina separation of the neurosensory retina from the pigment epithelium. May be caused by retinal tears or holes, fibrous traction on the retina, or by exudation of fluid under the neurosensory retina. ⮌ retinal detachment.

detained patient a person with a mental disorder who has been detained under the relevant legislation such as the Mental Health Act in England and Wales, or in Scotland the Mental Health (Care and Treatment) (Scotland) Act. ⮌ informal patient.

detected quantum efficiency (DQE) in radiology, it is the relationship between the density of useful quanta of light and the density of radiation quanta falling on the detector. Ideally this should be as near to 100% as possible.

detection acuity the ability of an individual to see the presence of small objects.

detector a device used to measure the amount of radiation transmitted through a patient. Modern computed tomography

(CT) units typically use solid state ceramic detectors. ⮌ scintillation detector.

detergent *n, adj* (describes) a cleansing agent. ⮌ cetrimide.

deterioration *n* progressive impairment of function: worsening of the patient's condition.

determinants of health factors that may influence the health of an individual, or differences in health between individuals, apart from age, sex and constitution (physiological, genetic factors). These could be social and economic, environmental or psychological factors that increase the risk of ill health or disease (e.g. heart disease, cancers, diabetes). These determinants, or indicators, are associated with better or worse health of populations as measured by mortality (standardized mortality ratios), valid measures of morbidity or self-reported health status (e.g. health surveys, census, standardized illness ratios). For example, higher infant mortality may be associated with environmental factors, healthcare provision, social and community support, maternal deprivation and poverty. There may also be a cultural and behavioural perspective. ⮌ morbidity, mortality.

deterministic effect an effect that always occurs; with radiation dose it is an effect which occurs above a specific dose, skin reddening, hair loss, temporary depression of blood count, death. ⮌ stochastic effect.

detoxication *n* the removal of the poisonous property of a substance—**detoxicant** *adj, n*, **detoxicate** *vt*.

detritus *n* matter produced by detrition; waste matter from disintegration.

detrusor *n* an expelling muscle such as that of the urinary bladder.

detrusor instability (*syn* urge incontinence) failure to inhibit reflex detrusor contraction. ⮌ incontinence.

detumescence *n* subsidence of a swelling.

deturgescence the state of relative dehydration maintained by the normal cornea which is necessary for transparency. It is maintained by the epithelium which, to a large extent, is impermeable to water, and also by a metabolic transport system in the endothelium.

deutan a person who has either deuteranomaly or deuteranopia.

deuteranomal a person who has deuteranomaly.

deuteranomalous trichromatism ⮌ deuteranomaly.

deuteranomalous vision ⮌ deuteranomaly.

deuteranomaly (*syn* deuteranomalous trichromatism, deuteranomalous vision, green-weakness) a type of anomalous trichromatism in which an abnormally high proportion of green is needed when mixing red and green light to match a given yellow. This is the most common type of colour vision deficiency occurring in about 4.6% of males and 0.35% of the female population. ⮌ anomaloscope, defective colour vision, pseudoisochromatic plates, trichromatism.

deuteranope a person who has deuteranopia.

deuteranopia a rare form of colour blindness. A type of dichromatism in which red and green are confused, although their relative spectral luminosities are practically the same as

213

in normal individuals. In the spectrum, the deuteranope only sees two primary colours, the long wavelength portion of the spectrum (yellow, orange or red) appears yellowish and the short wavelength portion (blue or violet) appears bluish. There is, in between, a neutral point which appears whitish or colourless, at about 498 nm. It occurs in slightly over 1% of the male population and only rarely in females. Also called green blindness (although this term is incorrect as green lights appear to a deuteranope as bright as to a normal observer). ⊃ defective colour vision, dichromatism, neutral point, pseudoisochromatic plates.

developer in radiography, a chemical which reacts with exposed film and reduces exposed silver bromide crystals to black metallic silver by donating electrons to the crystals. Developer has a pH of 9.6–10.6.

developing agent in radiography, the chemical which reduces exposed silver bromide crystals to metallic silver, for example, a combination of phenidone and hydroquinone.

developmental cyst ⊃ cyst of dental origin.

developmental dysplasia of the hip (DDH) also known as congenital dislocation of the hip (CHD). The term DDH is useful in describing the varying causes and severity of the condition. There is poor development of the acetabulum, femoral head and surrounding tissues, which allows the head of the femur to dislocate. Occurs more commonly if there is a family history, if the fetus has presented by the breech, and in female infants. About 1–2% of neonates have dislocated or dislocatable hips, usually found as part of the routine examinations performed by midwives and paediatricians in the first 24 hours of life and confirmed on ultrasound. ⊃ Barlow's sign/test, Ortolani's sign/test.

developmental eye movement (DEM) test an indirect test for saccadic eye movements in which the subject reads numbers placed in four vertical columns (total of 80 numbers) and 16 horizontal rows (total of 80 numbers). The lengths of time taken to perform the horizontal and the vertical subtests are measured independently and assessed as a ratio, as well as the number of errors (omissions, additions, transpositions or substitutions). All results are compared to test norms for the age of the subject. The vertical array mainly gives an indication of visual-verbal number skills (automaticity), whereas the horizontal array provides additional information on oculomotor function.

developmental milestones the skills or competencies usually attained by the infant or child by a given age, e.g. walking by 18 months. The skills are usually grouped in categories—fine motor, gross motor, personal and social and language. ⊃ Denver II.

deviance *n* a variation from normal. A sociological term that describes a change from the accepted social norm.

deviation abnormal position of the eyes, for example both eyes deviated to right or left when the person is facing to the front. May be a feature of some neurological disorders. ⊃ sexual deviation.

devitalize to kill or remove living tissue or cells. In endodontics *devitalize a pulp* to apply a chemical agent to kill pulp tissue. *devitalize a tooth* to remove vital pulp tissue from a tooth.

devitalizing/mummifying paste (or compound) material, usually containing formaldehyde and various other antiseptic ingredients, which when placed in contact with an exposed pulp coagulates the protein of pulp with which it is in contact, allowing further pulp therapy at a later visit. Sometimes referred to as Easlick's Devitalizing Paste. ⊃ devitalizing (mummifying) pulp therapy.

devitalizing (mummifying) pulp treatment a method of devitalizing the pulp of primary teeth prior to their removal followed by preservation of the remaining radicular pulp in an aseptic state until the tooth is shed normally. Rarely used in the permanent (secondary) dentition.

DEXA *abbr* dual-energy X-ray absorptiometry.

dexamethasone suppression tests tests using different doses and durations of dexamethasone treatment to identify patients with Cushing's syndrome.

dextral *adj* referring to the right-hand side.

dextran *n* a colloid solution obtained by the action of a specific bacterium on sugar solutions. Previously used for replacing fluids in hypovolaemia. It is no longer routinely used as a colloid. Dextran may cause allergic reactions. It also affects clotting and interferes with blood cross-matching. ⊃ colloid solutions.

dextrin *n* a soluble polysaccharide resulting from the hydrolysis of starch.

dextr/o- a prefix that means 'to the right', e.g. *dextrocardia*.

dextrocardia *n* transposition of the heart to the right side of the thorax—**dextrocardial** *adj*.

dextrose *n* (*syn.* glucose) a soluble carbohydrate (monosaccharide) widely used in intravenous infusion solutions. Also given orally as a readily absorbed sugar in rehydration fluids for fluid and electrolyte replacement, and for hypoglycaemia.

DHA *abbr* docosahexaenoic acid.

DHEA *abbr* dehydroepiandrosterone.

dhobie itch tinea cruris.

DHS *abbr* dynamic hip screw.

dia- a prefix that means 'through, across, between, apart', e.g. *diapedesis*.

diabetes *n* a disease characterized by polyuria, with consequent polydipsia; used without qualification implies diabetes mellitus—**diabetic** *adj*, *n*.

diabetes insipidus diabetes caused by disordered water homeostasis. It may be *cranial* due to deficiency of antidiuretic hormone (ADH), either idiopathic or due to trauma, tumour or inflammation affecting posterior pituitary lobe function, or *nephrogenic* due to renal tubular resistance to the action of ADH.

diabetes mellitus diabetes due to glycosuria and osmotic diuresis resulting from hyperglycaemia; defined as fasting plasma glucose ≥7.0 mmol/L, or a glucose level 2 hours following 75 g glucose load (oral glucose tolerance test)

≥ 11.1 mmol/L. Diabetes mellitus is classified as: *type 1* due to autoimmune destruction of insulin producing cells in the pancreatic islets, uncontrolled it leads to ketoacidosis; *type 2* due to varying degrees of insulin resistance, often due to obesity, and impaired insulin secretion, if uncontrolled leads to hyperglycaemic hyperosmolar non-ketotic coma (HHNK)/ hyperosmolar non-ketotic coma (HONK); may also be *secondary* to other diseases, e.g. pancreatitis, Cushing's syndrome, haemochromatosis; or *genetic*, e.g. maturity onset diabetes of the young (MODY), mitochondrial diabetes; or *gestational diabetes* ⊃ gestational diabetes.

diabetic amyotrophy a complication of poorly controlled diabetes. A mononeuropathy affecting the lower limb caused by pathology affecting the tiny blood vessels that supply the femoral nerve and the lumbar plexus. It typically occurs in one leg and causes tenderness, weakness and wasting of the anterior thigh muscles (quadriceps femoris) and absence of the knee-jerk reflex. Slow recovery and improvement can occur if diabetic control improves.

diabetic 'honeymoon' period a phenomenon occurring, in some people, soon after the diagnosis of type 1 diabetes. It occurs because there are often a few beta cells remaining in the pancreas and these can recover sufficiently after insulin therapy is started so that they produce insulin again. Some people need less insulin and more uncommonly other people need no insulin for a variable time period. However long this period lasts, all those who have a 'honeymoon' period will require larger doses of insulin in the future.

diabetic ketoacidosis ⊃ ketoacidosis.

diabetic nephropathy a long-term microvascular complication of diabetes characterized by glomerulosclerosis caused by damage to the glomerular capillaries. There is microalbuminuria, hypertension, and eventually loss of glomeruli and end-stage renal failure in some cases.

diabetic neuropathy a long-term microvascular complication of diabetes characterized by damage to nerves (motor, sensory and autonomic). It may present as a sensorimotor neuropathy in the lower limbs ('stocking' distribution); neuropathic foot ulcers; mononeuropathies, such as diabetic amyopathy; and nerve compression, e.g. carpal tunnel syndrome. The effects of autonomic nerve damage depend on the structures affected and can cause erectile dysfunction, sweating after eating, gastroparesis, diarrhoea, constipation, incomplete bladder emptying and postural hypotension.

diabetic retinitis ⊃ diabetic retinopathy (DR).

diabetic retinopathy (DR) *syn* diabetic retinitis, proliferative diabetic retinopathy [PDR]. Retinal changes occurring in longstanding cases of diabetes mellitus. It is the most common retinal vascular disease. In general, the severity of the retinopathy parallels the duration of the diabetes. The retinopathy is characterized by the presence of new blood vessels (neovascularization) which proliferate on or near the optic disc on the surface of the retina, microaneurysms (small round red spots) and sharply defined white or yellowish waxy exudates. Vitreous detachment is a likely

outcome. If the vessels bleed there can be a preretinal haemorrhage with visual loss. Both eyes are usually involved although to different degrees. Visual acuity may be unaffected unless the fovea is involved. After the condition has reached the stage of proliferative retinopathy, the principal treatment is with laser photocoagulation which reduces the risk of further visual loss. Low vision aids may be needed afterward. ⊃ exudate, fluorescein angiography, microaneurysm, photocoagulation, proliferative retinopathy.

diagnosis *n* the art or act of distinguishing one disease from another—**diagnoses** *pl*, **diagnose** *vt*. ⊃ differential diagnosis.

diagnostic *adj* **1**. pertaining to diagnosis. **2**. serving as evidence in diagnosis—**diagnostician** *n*.

***Diagnostic and Statistical Manual of Mental Disorders* (DSM-IV)** a manual that lists the official classification of mental disorders. It is published by the American Psychiatric Association. ⊃ *International Classification of Diseases* (ICD).

diagnostic injection or analgesia in dentistry, an aid to diagnosis whereby a local analgesic is injected into a specific area in order to eliminate pain, and thus prove that the pain arises from the specific site. Careful serial intraligamental injections are now used to refine this diagnostic test.

diagnostic positions of gaze a method of evaluating the integrity of the extraocular muscles by testing the primary, the four secondary and the four tertiary positions of gaze, monocularly or binocularly.

diagnostic ultrasonography information is derived from echoes which occur when a controlled beam of sound energy crosses the boundary between adjacent tissues of differing physical properties.

diagonal conjugate ⊃ conjugate.

dialysate *n* exogenous fluid used in dialysis to promote diffusion and removal of waste products.

dialyser *n* (*syn* artificial kidney) used in haemodialysis; consists of blood and dialysate compartments separated by a semipermeable membrane.

dialysis a renal replacement therapy. The process by which solutes are removed from solution by diffusion across a porous membrane; requires the presence of a favourable solute gradient. ⊃ haemodialysis, peritoneal dialysis—**dialyses** *pl*, **dialyse** *vt*.

diamagnetic a substance that will slightly reduce the strength of the magnetic field in which it is placed, the magnetic field induced is opposed to that of the surrounding magnetic field and has negative magnetic susceptibility. ⊃ ferromagnetic, paramagnetic, superparamagnetic.

diamagnetism the influence of an applied magnetic field on the electrons orbiting the nuclei within the substance is rarely permanent. ⊃ ferromagnetism, paramagnetism.

diamond crystalline form of carbon, harder than any other naturally occurring substance. *diamond instrument* a rotary instrument, such as a bur or wheel, used as an abrasive cutting tool having commercial or synthetic diamond grit embedded in its metal surface.

diapedesis *n* the passage of cells from within blood vessels through the vessel walls into the tissues, such as during the inflammatory response—**diapedetic** *adj*.

diaphoresis *n* perspiration.

diaphoretic *adj*, *n* (*syn* sudorific) an agent which induces diaphoresis (sweating).

diaphragm *n* **1**. the dome-shaped musculotendinous partition between the thoracic cavity above and the abdominal cavity below. It is the major inspiratory muscle constructed of a mix of different types of muscle fibres enabling fast, strong, prolonged low-tension contractions. It is attached at the crural portion to the upper lumbar vertebrae and at the costal portion to the inner aspect of the lower six ribs. On contraction (i.e. on inspiration), the diaphragm descends against the abdominal contents (pushing the abdominal wall outwards) so using the abdomen as a fulcrum on which to elevate the thoracic cage, causing a rise in intra-abdominal pressure. An abundant blood supply and high oxidative capacity enable the diaphragm to sustain the major increase in the work of breathing during exercise, but at high intensity its demand for blood competes with that of the exercising muscles. Fatigue of the diaphragm (and of other respiratory muscles) has been shown to contribute to exercise limitation. Unique among skeletal muscles in maintaining its activity continuously for a lifetime under involuntary control, yet which can, within limits, be voluntarily overridden. Inward movement of the diaphragm on inspiration (paradoxical movement) is indicative of diaphragmatic fatigue/weakness/paralysis. Higher lung volumes will reduce the resting length of the diaphragm and, therefore, provide a mechanical disadvantage to tension generation (as with hyperinflated states such as chronic airflow obstruction. These may result in an increased work of breathing and predispose diaphragmatic fatigue and respiratory muscle pump failure). **2**. any partitioning membrane or septum. **3**. a cap which encircles the cervix to act as a barrier contraceptive. Reliable when correctly fitted and used with a spermicidal chemical. **4**. in restorative dentistry, the thin veneer of metal extended from the core of a post-crown to some or all of the margins of the prepared root face— **diaphragmatic** *adj*.

diaphragmatic hernia ⇨ hiatus hernia.

diaphysis *n* the shaft of a long bone—**diaphyses** *pl*, **diaphyseal** *adj*. ⇨ epiphysis.

diarrhoea *n* deviation from established bowel habit characterized by an increase in frequency and fluidity of the stools. May cause dehydration, hypokalaemia, acidosis (metabolic), malabsorption of nutrients and perianal soreness. Causes include, infection, food sensitivity, laxative misuse, drugs such as antibiotics, dietary change or indiscretion, anxiety, inflammatory bowel disease, colorectal cancer (alternating with constipation) and some systemic diseases. ⇨ spurious diarrhoea.

diarthrosis *n* a synovial, freely movable joint—**diarthroses** *pl*, **diarthrodial** *adj*.

diastasis *n* **1**. the forcible separation of bones without fracture. **2**. the separation of two muscles. For example the rectus muscles. ⇨ diastasis recti abdominis.

diastasis recti abdominis separation of the two rectus muscles. It can occur following pregnancy, especially after multiple births or multiple pregnancies. In neonates it is caused by a developmental abnormality.

diastasis symphysis pubis ⇨ symphysis pubis dysfunction.

diastema *n* a naturally occurring, but abnormally large space between two teeth.

diastole *n* the relaxation filling period of the cardiac cycle, usually refers to ventricular filling—**diastolic** *adj*. ⇨ systole.

diastolic blood pressure the lowest blood pressure measured between cardiac contractions, i.e. when the aortic and pulmonary valves are closed and the heart is relaxed. ⇨ systolic blood pressure.

diathermy *n* the passage of a high frequency electric current through the tissues whereby heat is produced. When both electrodes are large, the heat is diffused over a wide area according to the electrical resistance of the tissues. In this form it is widely used in the treatment of inflammation, especially when deeply seated (e.g. sinusitis, pelvic cellulitis). When one electrode is very small the heat is concentrated in this area and becomes great enough to destroy tissue. In this form (surgical diathermy) it is used to stop bleeding at operation by coagulation of blood, or to cut through tissue (Figure D.4).

diatomaceous (Kieselguhr) earth a form of finely divided silica used as a filler and polishing agent.

diatoric tooth ⇨ tooth.

dibenzodiazepines *npl* a group of atypical antipsychotic drugs (neuroleptics), e.g. clozapine. ⇨ Appendix 5.

DIC *abbr* disseminated intravascular coagulation.

dicephalous *adj* two-headed.

dichorionic twins twins who have separate chorions.

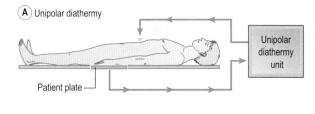

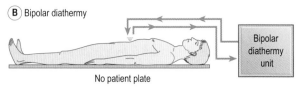

D.4 Unipolar and bipolar diathermy (reproduced from Brooker & Nicol 2003 with permission).

dichotomous question in research, a question which enables a respondent to give one of two answers, e.g. yes/no, true/false.

dichromatic vision dichromatopsia. A defect of colour vision in which the person can only perceive two of the three primary colours. ⊃ dichromatism.

dichromatism (*syn* daltonism, dichromatopsia, dichromatic vision) a form of colour vision deficiency in which all colours can be matched by a mixture of only two primary colours. The spectrum appears as consisting of two colours separated by an achromatic area (the neutral point). There are several types of dichromatism: deuteranopia, protanopia and tritanopia. ⊃ defective colour vision, deuteranopia, protanopia, tritanopia, visual pigment.

dichromatopsia ⊃ dichromatism.

Dick test (G F Dick, 1881–1967; G R Dick, 1881–1963; American physicians) a skin test used to determine whether an individual is sensitive to the toxin produced by the group A streptococci that cause scarlet fever.

DICOM *abbr* **d**igital **i**maging and **co**mmunications in **m**edicine.

dicoria (*syn* diplocoria) a condition in which there are two pupils in one iris. It may be congenital or the result of surgery or injury. ⊃ polycoria.

dichroic fog in radiography, used to be seen when a film was manually processed and was caused by development continuing in the fixer, it appears as a pink stain if viewed by transmitted light and greenish blue when viewed by reflected light.

dicrotic *adj, n* (pertaining to, or having) a double beat, as indicated by a second expansion of the artery during diastole. ⊃ anacrotic.

dicrotic notch the second rise in the arterial tracing caused by the closure of the aortic valve (that between the left ventricle and the aorta).

didactylism an condition in which there are only two digits on each hand.

didelphia a double uterus.

di-/dip- a prefix that means 'twos, double', e.g. *diploid*.

DIDMOAD syndrome *abbr* **d**iabetes **i**nsipidus, **d**iabetes **m**ellitus, **o**ptic **a**trophy and **d**eafness. ⊃ Wolfram syndrome

die in dentistry, the positive reproduction of a prepared tooth or teeth in a suitable hard material such as amalgam, stone or plaster. *die lubricant* a separating medium applied to the die so that the wax pattern may be withdrawn without sticking to the die.

dielectric a substance that acts as an electrical insulator and can contain an electric field.

dielectric constant (K) the ratio of the capacitance of the capacitor with the dielectric to the capacitance with a vacuum between the plates of the capacitor.

diembryonic *adj* relating to two embryos. For example, the formation of two embryos from a single ovum.

diencephalon the part of the brain between the mesencephalon and telencephalon. It contains the third ventricle, thalamus, hypothalamus and epithalamus.

diet 1. the foods and drink normally consumed by a person. **2**. the nutrient intake prescribed or restricted (type and amount) for treatment or management of conditions. For example a low salt intake for hypertension.

diet-induced thermogenesis increase in heat production in the body after consuming food. It is caused by the metabolic energy used during digestion and the energy used in forming glycogen and fat, etc. It is around 10% of the energy intake but this depends on the type of foods eaten. Also known as thermic effect of food. Fats have relatively little thermic effect and proteins the most.

dietary fibre ⊃ non-starch polysaccharides.

dietary reference intakes (DRI) used in the United States for dietary reference values.

dietary reference values (DRVs) in the UK a set of tables that estimate a range of nutritional requirements for different groups of the population (healthy individuals). Usually three values are given—estimated average requirement (EAR), lower reference nutrient intake (LRNI) and reference nutrient intake (RNI). ⊃ estimated average requirement, lower reference nutrient intake, reference nutrient intake.

dietary supplementation a term in sports medicine used to describe the food supplements (above what is required to ensure the intake of nutrients for a balanced diet) taken as an ergogenic aid. For example carbohydrate loading, creatine supplements and isotonic sports drinks.

dietetic foods foods specially prepared or modified to meet specific nutritional needs. Such as, for people who cannot digest or metabolize a food/nutrient, e.g. gluten free foods, or those who need to have a controlled intake of certain foods/nutrients, e.g. low fat foods.

dietetics *n* the interpretation and application of the scientific principles of nutrition to feeding in health and disease.

dieting any type of eating plan that aims at reducing body mass and body fat, and requires one to eat and drink sparingly or according to prescribed rules. Weight or fat reduction in athletes is generally motivated by a desire either to achieve a predesignated weight in order to compete in a specific weight class or category (e.g. horse racing, boxing) or to optimize performance by improving power to weight ratio (e.g jumping events, distance running).

dietitian *n* one who applies the principles of nutrition to the feeding of an individual or a group of individuals. Dietitians are employed in a range of hospital and community settings, the food industry, by local authorities and by national and international agencies, e.g. World Health Organization (WHO).

Dietl's crisis (J Dietl, Polish physician, 1804–1878) sudden severe pain in the kidney, due to distension of the renal pelvis, or ureteric obstruction such as kinking of the ureter.

Dieulafoy's lesion (P Dieulafoy, French physician, 1839–1911) an abnormality of small blood vessels (arterioles) in the gastric mucosa, which usually occur in the area adjacent to the gastro-oesophageal junction but they can occur elsewhere in the digestive tract. An uncommon cause of gastrointestinal bleeding. Treatment is usually by endoscopic coagulation techniques, sclerotherapy or banding.

C
D

difference threshold in psychophysics, the smallest difference between two sensory inputs that can be detected. Also known as difference limen, discrimination threshold or just noticeable difference. ➲ absolute threshold.

differential blood count the estimation of the relative proportions of the different white blood cells (leucocytes) in the blood. A normal differential count is: neutrophils (polymorphonuclear cells) 65–70%, lymphocytes 20–25%, monocytes 5%, eosinophils 0–3%, basophils 0–0.5%. In childhood the proportion of lymphocytes is higher. ➲ blood count.

differential diagnosis is the term used when making a correct decision between diseases presenting a similar clinical picture. ➲ diagnosis.

differential intraocular pressure test a test for differentiating between a muscle paresis and a mechanical restriction of the eye. The intraocular pressure is measured in the primary position and then again with the person turning his or her eyes in the direction of action of the suspected paretic muscle. An increase in intraocular pressure of 6 mmHg or more indicates a mechanical restriction (e.g. a fracture of the orbital floor), whereas no change in pressure suggests a muscle paresis. This test produces less discomfort to the person than some other tests.

differentiation *n* the process whereby cells and tissues expand the ability to perform specialized functions that distinguish them from other cell types. Cancer cells are graded by their degree of differentiation.

differentiation in mathematics the use of calculus to compute the change of one variable with respect to another. Equal to the gradient (slope) of a graph of the one plotted against the other.

differentiation test tests that help to determine the source of the patient's symptoms by objectively assessing different structures that may be the cause of the patient's complaint.

diffraction the deviation of the direction of propagation of a beam of light which occurs when the light passes the edge of an obstacle such as a diaphragm, the pupil of the eye or a spectacle frame. There are two consequences of this phenomenon. First, the image of a point source cannot be a point image but a diffraction pattern. This pattern depends upon the shape and size of the diaphragm as well as the wavelength of light. Second, a system of close, parallel and equidistant grooves, slits or lines ruled on a polished surface can produce a light spectrum by diffraction. This is called a diffraction grating. ➲ diffraction fringes, Maurice's theory.

diffraction fringes a pattern of alternate dark and light bands produced by diffracted light passing the edge of an opening. ➲ diffraction.

diffuse idiopathic skeletal hyperostosis (DISH) a disease of older men characterized by ligamentous ossification and large osteophytes that bridge across the vertebrae.

diffuse parenchymal lung disease (DPLD) the diffuse parenchymal lung diseases (DPLDs) are a heterogeneous group of conditions associated with diffuse thickening of the alveolar walls with inflammatory cells and exudates,

(e.g. the acute/adult respiratory distress syndrome—ARDS), granulomas (e.g. sarcoidosis), alveolar haemorrhage (e.g. anti-GBM disease), and/or fibrosis (e.g. fibrosing alveolitis). Lung disease may occur in isolation, or as part of a systemic connective tissue disorder—for example, in rheumatoid arthritis and systemic lupus erythematosus (SLE). The DPLDs are rare and poorly understood. However, although the presentation and natural history differ, they are frequently considered collectively as they share similar symptoms, physical signs, radiological changes and disturbances of pulmonary function. Establishing a diagnosis is important because: (a) there are prognostic implications—e.g. sarcoidosis is frequently self-limiting, whereas idiopathic pulmonary fibrosis (IPF) is most often fatal; (b) establishing a specific diagnosis will avoid inappropriate treatment—e.g. the powerful immunosuppressive regimens used for some cases of IPF would be undesirable if the underlying condition was asbestosis or hypersensitivity pneumonitis; (c) some DPLDs can be expected to respond better than others to treatment, e.g. a good symptomatic response to corticosteroids could be predicted in sarcoidosis, whereas the prognosis would need to be more guarded in IPF; (d) a lung biopsy taken when the patient is already established on empirical immunosuppressive therapy is not only associated with a higher morbidity and mortality, but the interpretation of the tissue obtained is more difficult. It is desirable, therefore, to be confident about the diagnosis before starting any therapy. Diagnosis often presents a considerable clinical challenge, necessitating meticulous attention to the history and physical signs and a cooperative approach from teams of clinicians, radiologists and pathologists. The duration of disease may sometimes be difficult to ascertain. Gradually progressive shortness of breath on exertion may be the only symptom, and hence the patient may not present clinically until there is extensive lung pathology. History-taking should include a thorough and comprehensive search for exposure to organic and inorganic dusts. A 'lifetime' occupational history is essential and should include hobbies that may involve similar exposures. Contact with birds at home or in the working environment is the cause of the most common form of hypersensitivity pneumonitis (HP). The smoking status should be recorded and a drug history that includes over-the-counter medicines should be obtained. A history of rashes, joint pains or renal disease may suggest an underlying connective tissue disorder or vasculitis. The presence of any comorbid disease should be ascertained such as collagen vascular disease, immunodeficiency, HIV disease or malignancy. In exceptional cases there is a family history of DPLD. In many cases, especially in early disease, there are few, if any, physical signs. In advanced disease, tachypnoea (increased respiratory rate) and cyanosis may be evident at rest and there may be signs of pulmonary hypertension and right heart failure. Finger clubbing may be prominent, particularly in IPF or asbestosis. There may be restriction of lung expansion and showers of end-inspiratory crackles. Extrapulmonary signs, including lymphadenopathy or uveitis, may be present in sarcoidosis and arthropathies or rashes may occur when a DPLD is a manifestation of a connective tissue disorder. Some blood tests may be useful in indicating systemic disease or providing crude indices of disease activity, for example lactate dehydrogenase (LDH), full blood count (FBC), erythrocyte sedimentation rate (ESR) or C-reactive protein (CRP), etc. Pulmonary function tests typically show a restrictive pattern with diminished lung volumes and a reduced gas transfer, although an elevated gas transfer may be seen in cases of alveolar haemorrhage. The chest X-ray typically shows some changes. However, plain radiography is insensitive and may not appear abnormal until disease is advanced. High-resolution computed tomography (HRCT) is more sensitive and specific and has become extremely valuable in detecting early interstitial lung disease, assessing the extent and type of involvement and guiding further investigations and management. Bronchoscopy is useful in certain circumstances. Increased numbers of lymphocytes in the bronchoalveolar lavage (BAL) may suggest either sarcoid or hypersensitivity pneumonitis, whereas a neutrophilia is more suggestive of IPF. Analysis of BAL may suggest important differential diagnoses such as infection or malignancy. Transbronchial biopsies may establish the diagnosis in sarcoidosis and in some conditions which mimic ILDs, such as lymphatic carcinomatosis and certain infections. However, it is less specific in heterogeneous disorders such as IPF where videoassisted thoracoscopy (VATS), or a limited thoracotomy, may be required to obtain a more representative sample.

diffuse periostitis ⊃ periostitis.

diffusion *n* **1.** the process whereby gases and liquids of different concentrations mix when brought into contact, until their concentration is equal throughout. ⊃ active transport, filtration, osmosis. **2.** dialysis. **3.** the scattering of light passing through a heterogeneous medium, or being reflected irregularly by a surface, such as a sand blasted opal glass surface. Diffusion by a perfectly diffusing surface occurs in accordance with Lambert's cosine law. In this case, the luminance will be the same, regardless of the viewing direction.

diffusion (in radiology) when water and other small molecules in tissue undergo random microscopic, parallel movement which can be measured by magnetic resonance imaging (MRI) techniques, for example, distinguishing cysts from solid tumours, strokes, and cerebrospinal fluid dynamic studies.

diffusing capacity refers to that of the lungs. The volume of a gas that moves across from the alveoli into the blood per minute, per unit partial pressure difference for that gas over the lungs as a whole. Depends, for any gas, on the total area and average thickness of the alveolar–capillary membrane. Of most interest for oxygen, since it determines the efficacy of oxygen intake, but usually estimated in terms of the diffusing capacity for carbon monoxide which is more straightforward to measure. Increased in exercise as greater

lung expansion both enlarges the area and decreases the thickness of the gas exchange surface.

digastric having two bellies, e.g. digastric muscle.

digastric muscle a muscle contributing to movement of the mandible and mouth during mastication. It has two bellies of muscle separated by a tendon, which runs through a pulley of fibrous tissue attached to the hyoid bone. The posterior belly is attached to the temporal bone and the anterior belly is attached at the digastric fossa near the midline, lower border of the medial surface of the mandible. Contraction of the digastric muscle, when the hyoid bone is held steady, helps to open the mouth, but during deglutition the muscle action raises the hyoid.

DiGeorge's syndrome (A DiGeorge, American paediatrician, b.1921) also known as thymic-parathyroid aplasia. One of the primary T-lymphocyte deficiencies. An inherited condition that results from failure of development of the 3rd/4th pharyngeal pouch usually caused by a microdeletion affecting chromosome 22 (22q11). It is characterized by immunodeficiency, hypocalcaemia and various physical abnormalities. These include the absence of the thymus and parathyroid glands, congenital cardiac disease, cleft lip and palate, oesophageal atresia, tracheo-oesophageal fistulae, abnormal facies (facial dysmorphism) with small mouth, low set ears and hypertelorism.There are very low numbers of mature T cells despite normal development in the bone marrow. Death, caused by an infection, usually occurs during early childhood. ⊃ primary T-lymphocyte deficiencies.

digestion *n* the processes which break down ingested food to substances that are absorbed from the gastrointestinal tract (alimentary canal) into the blood or lymph. Catalysed by the digestive enzymes in the saliva, gastric juice, pancreatic juice and those secreted from the lining of the small intestine. These juices together add up to a total of about 10 litres per day entering the gut. Apart from those that occur in the lumen of the gut, some further digestive processes are effected by the enterocytes, the cells in the lining of the small intestine. Depends also on other chemical processes, including for example emulsification of fats by bile produced by the liver—**digestible, digestive** *adj*, **digestibility** *n*, **digest** *vt*.

digestibility the fraction of a foodstuff that is absorbed from the gastrointestinal tract to enter the bloodstream. It is the difference between the food intake and faecal output, minus that part of faeces that is not derived from undigested food residues, such as micro-organisms, intestinal cells and digestive juices.

digestive system comprises the structures of the gastrointestinal tract (alimentary tract) and the accessory organs. The mouth, oesophagus, stomach, and small and large intestine; and the salivary glands, the pancreas and the liver and biliary tract. The digestive system is concerned with ingestion, propulsion, digestion, absorption and elimination. ⊃ Colour Section Figure 18b.

digit *n* a finger or toe—**digital** *adj*.

digital literally to do with numbers, now refers to the electronic production of films and computer images. In computing, represents a quantity changing in steps which are discrete. ⊃ analogue.

digital compression pressure applied by the fingers, usually to an artery to stop bleeding.

digital imaging and communications in medicine (DICOM) a project to bring manufacturers together to agree standardization in computerized image transfer and communications so that clinical information can be communicated among all specialities.

digital imaging system the production of a digital radiographic image by reading an imaging plate and then displaying an image on a computer screen (digital radiography) or reading the signal from a television camera attached to an image intensifier (digital fluoroscopy) (Figure D.5).

digitally reconstructed radiograph the electronic capture, manipulation and storage of X-rays to form a two- or three-dimensional radiographic image. In radiotherapy, computer reconstructions of radiographs from computed tomography (CT) slices made to imitate the divergent X-ray beam.

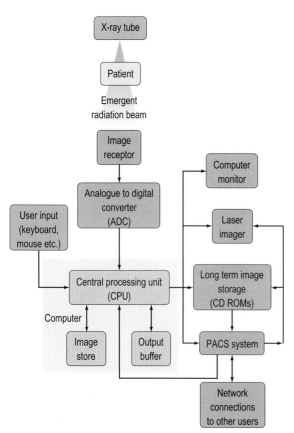

D.5 Major components of a digital imaging system (reproduced from Graham 1996 with permission).

digital pulp the tissue pad of the finger tip.

digital radiography (DR) the production of a digital radiographic image by reading an imaging plate and then displaying an image on a computer screen.

digital scanner equipment used to produce a digital image from a conventional radiographic film by passing light through the image and recording the intensity of the light.

digital signal the measurement of a signal in terms of numbers rather than a continuously varying value producing higher-quality image transfer to computers and television monitors.

digital subtraction an advanced technique that uses digital technology to produce radiographic images, especially of blood vessels. It can also be used to locate tumours of the parathyroid glands.

digital subtraction angiography (DSA) a method of increasing the contrast between vessels containing radiographic contrast agent and the background. An image (the mask) taken prior to the administration of contrast agent is digitized. Contrast is then introduced into the blood vessel and further images are obtained and digitized. Computer software subtracts the mask from the post-contrast images. Thus leaving an enhanced image of only those vessels that contain contrast agent.

digital verification the use of either silicon diodes or ionization chambers placed in the exit beam during radiotherapy treatment to confirm the correct dose of radiation is being administered to the patient.

digital versatile disk (DVD) a 120-mm sheet of aluminium covered with a layer of acetate and an outer layer of metal and with a polycarbonate backing. Used in computing to store data in digital form which can be read by a laser. Used to record information from a computer using a laser to burn the surface of a disk.

dihydrate a compound possessing two molecules of water.

direct video interface (DVI) a specialist computer connector for flat-panel computer monitors.

digitalis *n* leaf of the common foxglove containing glycosides, such as digoxin. ⊃ glycosides.

digitalization *n* physiological saturation with digitalis to obtain optimum therapeutic effect.

digiti minimi quinti varus (*syn* congenital overlapping fifth toe) the smallest toe lies on the dorsum of the base of the fourth toe in a medially deviated position. It may be bilateral or unilateral.

digitization the conversion of an analogue variable to a digital one, i.e. a continuous variable into a set of numbers. Used in biomechanics to describe the derivation of co-ordinate data from video (or cine) pictures, e.g. plotting the co-ordinates of markers on the body.

diglyceride diacylglycerol. A lipid substance that comprises a glycerol molecule and two fatty acids. Produced during the digestion of triglycerides (triacylglycerols).

dilaceration distortion occurring during the development of a tooth which disrupts the normal axial relationship between the crown and the root.

dilatation *n* stretching or enlargement. May occur physiologically, pathologically or be induced artificially.

dilatation and curettage (D and C) by custom refers to dilating the uterine cervix to obtain an endometrial sample by curettage. ⇌ hysteroscopy.

dilatation and evacuation (D and E) dilatation of the cervix and evacuation of the products of conception under anaesthetic for therapeutic termination of pregnancy or for the removal of a dead fetus in the second trimester of pregnancy.

dilator pupillae muscle smooth (unstriated), involuntary muscle whose fibres constitute the posterior membrane of the iris. This muscle extends from the ciliary body close to the margin of the iris where it fuses with the sphincter pupillae muscle. Contraction of the dilator pupillae muscle draws the pupillary margin towards the ciliary body and therefore dilates the pupil. This muscle is supplied by the sympathetic fibres in the long ciliary nerves and by a few parasympathetic fibres. ⇌ iris, mydriasis, mydriatic, sphincter pupillae muscle.

dilution analysis when a known quantity of radioactive material is introduced into a space or cavity in a patient to enable the volume of the space to be calculated in radionuclide imaging.

dimercaprol (BAL) *n* an organic compound used as an antidote for poisoning by heavy metals such as arsenic, bismuth, gold and mercury. It forms soluble but stable compounds with the metals, which are then rapidly excreted by the kidneys.

dimetria condition characterized by a double uterus.

dimorphism quality of existing in two distinct forms. ⇌ sexual diamorphism.

dinner fork deformity the typical deformity following a Colles' fracture where the hand is displaced posteriorly in relation to the forearm bones. ⇌ Colles' fracture.

diode a device containing an anode and a cathode in a vacuum and allows electrons to flow in one direction only, from the cathode to the anode.

diode laser a laser used in the treatment of retinal diseases.

diodontic implant in dentistry, a historical term used for a sterile metal rod placed in a root canal and extending through the root apex with the intention of stabilizing a tooth, especially one with a short root. Has also been known as endodontic implant.

Diogenes syndrome gross self-neglect. Most frequently seen in older people who are living in appalling conditions of squalor, sometimes with many companion animals or other livestock. The person concerned usually rejects offers of help, and strenuously resists any measures to change the situation.

dioptre (D) *n* **1.** a unit proposed by Monoyer to evaluate the refractive power of a lens or of an optical system. It is equal to the product of the refractive index (index of refraction) in the image space and the reciprocal of the focal length in metres. (*Symbol*: D.) Thus a lens with a focal length (in air) of 1 m has a power of 1D, one with a focal length of ½ m, has a power of 2D, etc. **2.** it is also incorrectly used to represent a unit of curvature, being equal to the reciprocal of the radius of curvature expressed in metres. ⇌ curvature of a surface, myodioptre, paraxial equation (fundamental), refractive error, refractive power, vergence.

dioptric power ⇌ refractive power (*F*).

dioxide *n* oxide containing two atoms of oxygen in each molecule, e.g. CO_2.

DIP *acron* desquamative interstitial pneumonia.

dipeptidases *npl* digestive enzymes that split dipeptides (paired amino acids) into individual amino acids.

dipeptide *n* a pair of amino acids linked by a peptide (dehydration) bond.

dipeptidyl peptidase 4 inhibitors (DPP-4 inhibitors) *npl* a group of oral hypoglycaemic drugs, e.g. sitagliptin. ⇌ Appendix 5.

2,3-diphosphoglycerate (2,3-DPG) *n* substance present in red blood cells that decreases the affinity of haemoglobin for oxygen, thus allowing oxygen to be released to the tissues. In the 'open' deoxygenated state, 2,3-diphosphoglycerate (2,3-DPG), a product of red cell metabolism, binds to the haemoglobin molecule and lowers its oxygen affinity. These complex interactions produce the sigmoid shape of the oxygen dissociation curve. The position of this curve depends upon the concentrations of 2,3-DPG, hydrogen ions and carbon dioxide; increased levels shift the curve to the right and cause oxygen to be released more readily. Tissue hypoxia increases all three and favours increased availability of oxygen from the red cell. Haemoglobin F (fetal haemoglobin) is unable to bind 2,3-DPG and has a left-shifted oxygen dissociation curve; this increased affinity, together with the low pH of fetal blood, ensures fetal oxygenation. ⇌ oxygen dissociation curve.

diphtheria *n* an acute, specific, infectious notifiable disease caused by the Gram-negative bacterium *Corynebacterium diphtheriae*. In many parts of the developing world diphtheria remains an important cause of illness. It was eradicated from much of the developed world by mass vaccination in the mid-20th century. Recent outbreaks have occurred in the Russian Federation (former Soviet Union) and continue to occur in Southeast Asia. The disease is notifiable in all countries of Europe and North America and international guidelines have been issued by the WHO for the management of infection. Infection with *Corynebacterium diphtheriae* occurs most commonly in the upper respiratory tract, and sore throat is frequently the presenting feature. The disease is usually spread by droplet infection from cases or carriers. The micro-organisms remain localized at the site of infection and serious consequences result from the absorption of a soluble exotoxin which damages the heart muscle and the nervous system. Infection may occur rarely on the conjunctiva or in the genital tract, or may complicate wounds, abrasions or diseases of the skin, especially in chronic lesions and those who misuse alcohol. The average incubation period is 2–4 days. Cases must be isolated until cultures from three daily nose and throat swabs are negative. The disease begins insidiously. Fever is seldom significant although tachycardia is usually marked. The diagnostic feature is the 'wash-leather' elevated greyish-green membrane

C
D

on the tonsils. It has a well-defined edge, is firm and adherent, and is surrounded by a zone of inflammation. There may be swelling of the neck ('bull-neck') and tender enlargement of the lymph nodes. In the mildest infections, especially in the presence of a high degree of immunity, a membrane may never appear and the throat is merely slightly injected. With anterior nasal infection there is nasal discharge, frequently blood-stained. In laryngeal diphtheria a husky voice and high-pitched cough signal potential respiratory obstruction requiring urgent tracheostomy. If infection spreads to the uvula, fauces and nasopharynx, the patient is gravely ill. Death from acute circulatory failure may occur within the first 10 days. Late complications occur as a result of toxin action on the heart or nervous system. About 25% of survivors of the early toxaemia may later develop myocarditis with arrhythmias or cardiac failure. These are usually reversible with no permanent damage other than heart block in survivors. Neurological involvement occurs in 75% of cases. After tonsillar or pharyngeal diphtheria it usually starts after 10 days with palatal palsy. Paralysis of accommodation often follows, manifest by difficulty in reading small print. Generalized polyneuritis with weakness and paraesthesia may follow in the next 10–14 days. Recovery from such neuritis is always ultimately complete. A clinical diagnosis of diphtheria must be notified to the public health authorities and the patient sent urgently to a hospital for infectious diseases. Treatment should begin once appropriate swabs have been taken before waiting for microbiological confirmation. Three main areas of management are: (a) administration of diphtheria antitoxin; (b) administration of antibiotics; (c) strict isolation procedures. Antitoxin has no neutralizing effect on toxin already fixed to tissues so must be injected intramuscularly without awaiting the result of a throat swab. However, since the antitoxin is hyperimmune horse serum, undesirable reactions to this foreign protein may occur. A potentially lethal immediate anaphylactic reaction with dyspnoea, pallor and collapse is recognized. 'Serum sickness' with fever, urticaria and joint pains may occur 7–12 days after injection. A careful history of previous horse serum injections or allergic reactions should alert the physician. A small test injection of serum should be given half an hour before the full dose in every patient. Adrenaline (epinephrine) solution must be available to deal with any immediate type of reaction (0.5–1.0 ml of 1/1000 solution i.m.). An antihistamine is also given. In a severely ill patient the risk of anaphylactic shock is outweighed by the mortal danger of diphtheritic toxaemia and up to 100 000 units of antitoxin are injected intravenously if the test dose has not given rise to symptoms. For disease of moderate severity, 16 000–40 000 units i.m. will suffice, and for mild cases 4000–8000 units. Penicillin 1200 mg 6-hourly i.v. or amoxicillin 500 mg 8-hourly should be administered for 2 weeks to eliminate *C. diphtheriae*. Patients allergic to penicillin can be given erythromycin. Due to poor immunogenicity all sufferers should be immunized with diphtheria toxoid following recovery. Patients must be managed in strict isolation attended by staff with a clearly documented immunization history until three swabs 24 hours apart are culture-negative. Diphtheria is prevented by active immunization which should be given to all children as part of the routine immunization schedule. If diphtheria occurs in a closed community, contacts should be given erythromycin, which is more effective than penicillin in eradicating the microorganism in carriers. All contacts should also be immunized or given a booster dose of toxoid. Booster doses are required every 10 years to maintain immunity. Low-dose toxoid should be given to prevent severe reactions—**diphtheritic** *adj*.

diphyllobothriasis *n* infestation with the fish tapeworm *Diphyllobothrium latum*.

Diphyllobothrium a genus of large tapeworm that parasitizes the intestine. Human infestation is often with the *Diphyllobothrium latum* present in fish. Infestation occurs through eating raw fish, and is common in certain countries, the Baltic states, Scandinavia, parts of Russia, and the northwest states of the USA. Infestation may lead to gastrointestinal symptoms, such as diarrhoea and malabsorption of vitamins.

diplacusis a condition in which a single sound is heard as two.

diplegia *n* symmetrical paralysis of legs, usually associated with cerebral damage—**diplegic** *adj*.

diplococcus *n* a coccal bacterium that occurs in pairs. *Diplococcus* may be used in a binomial to describe a characteristically paired coccus, e.g. *Diplococcus pneumoniae* (*Streptococcus pneumoniae* or pneumococcus).

diplocoria ⊃ dicoria.

diploë the layer of cancellous bone sandwiched between two layers of compact bone in the skull.

diploid (2n) *adj* describes a cell with a full set of paired chromosomes. In humans the diploid number is 46 chromosomes (44 autosomes and 2 sex chromosomes) arranged in 23 pairs in all cells except the gametes. ⊃ haploid.

diplopagus conjoined twins who are equally developed.

diplopia *n* the seeing of two objects when only one exists (double vision). ⊃ mononuclear diplopia.

diplopia test 1. (*syn* displacement test, prism dissociation test) a test for measuring heterophoria in which the fusion reflex is prevented by displacing the retinal image of one eye with a prism as in the von Graefe's test in which the magnitude of the phoria is estimated by the amount of prism necessary to align the two images. To measure lateral phorias the images are displaced vertically and aligned one above the other, whereas to measure vertical phorias the images are displaced horizontally and realigned horizontally (if a phoria is present). **2.** a test to investigate the integrity of the extraocular muscles in strabismus, in which the patient is required to view a light source in the dark with a red filter in front of one eye and a green filter in front of the other, to produce diplopia (prisms are sometimes necessary). The direction and extent of diplopia are evaluated relative to the size and direction of the angle measured with the cover test at the same distance. ⊃ hetero-phoria, red-glass test.

diplosomatia a condition in which complete twins are joined at some of their body parts.

dipsesis dipsosis. Experiencing extreme thirst, such as wanting abnormal fluids.

dipsetic tending to cause thirst.

dipsogen any agent such as food or drug that causes thirst.

dipsomania an uncontrollable morbid craving for alcohol.

Dipylidium *n* a genus of tapeworm. Dogs and cats are the definitive host of *Dipylidium caninum*, which can cause dis-ease in humans.

direct antiglobulin test (DAT) also known as the direct Coombs' test. Used to detect Rhesus haemolytic disease of the newborn. ⊃ direct Coombs' test.

direct attachment ⊃ direct bonding.

direct bonding the bonding of a fixed orthodontic bracket directly to a tooth surface by means of an adhesive tech-nique, most commonly using acid etch and composite adhesive.

direct bone wire ⊃ wiring.

direct Coombs' test also known as the direct antiglobulin test (DAT). The test detects maternal antiglobulin antibodies coating the infant's red blood cells. If the test is positive, haemolytic disease of the newborn may develop and the infant's serum bilirubin levels should be checked. ⊃ indirect antiglobulin test, indirect Coombs' test.

direct cost a cost that can be directly attributed to the bud-get of a specific department, for example pharmacy costs in a given department.

direct current an electrotherapy term. One of three recognized categories of therapeutic currents (pulsed, direct and alternating currents). Current with a continuous (defined variously as in excess of 100 ms or 1 s duration) unidirec-tional flow of charge (electrons). The direction is tradition-ally described as being from the negative (cathode) to the positive (anode) electrode. Used clinically in defibrillation, cadioversion, iontophoresis and, if interrupted, to stimulate denervated muscle.

direct exposure films films used without intensifying screens, for example, for intraoral dental films.

direct fracture a fracture occurring at the site of injury.

direct inlay technique in dentistry, the method of construc-tion of an inlay or casting by using a wax pattern taken directly from a tooth preparation and not from a model. Used in the lost wax casting technique.

direct interdental wiring ⊃ fixation (dentistry/maxillofa-cial surgery).

directly observed treatment (DOT) may be used in situations where patient compliance with a drug therapy may be poor. For example, the treatment of tuberculosis in rough sleepers.

direct ophthalmoscope an instrument that uses a perforated illuminated mirror to visualize eye structures directly. A direct ophthalmoscope provides a virtual, erect image with a magnification of about x15 of the fundus,

formed by the patient's eye in combination with whatever focusing lenses are needed to correct for the refractive errors of the observer and patient. The instrument is held at close range to the patient's eye and the field of view is small (less than 10°). ⊃ binocular indirect ophthalmoscope, indirect ophthalmoscope, ophthalmoscopy, scanning laser ophthalmoscope.

direct reflection ⊃ regular reflection.

direct retainer in dentistry, the part of a partial prosthesis designed to resist dislodgement along its path of insertion.

direct retention in dentistry, the retention obtained in a partial prosthesis by the use of direct retainers.

direct technique ⊃ direct inlay technique.

dis- a prefix that means 'separation, reversal, opposite', e.g. *disease*.

disability the limitations experienced by a person with an impairment, (e.g. chronic lung disease) when undertaking their normal functions. Disability can be defined from an individual model (including medical and tragedy models) or a social model. The individual model is dominant and assumes that the difficulties faced by people with a disability are a direct result of their individual impairments and loss or lack of functioning. The social model of disability recognizes the social origins of disability in a society geared by and for non-disabled people. The disadvantages or restrictions, often referred to as barriers, permeate every aspect of the physical and social environment. Disability can, therefore, be defined as a form of social oppression. ⊃ International Classification of Functioning, Disability and Health.

disabled role a role that people with disabilities are fre-quently expected to play that denies their own interests. It involves striving for 'normality' and 'independence' and 'adjusting' to and 'accepting' their situation within a dis-abling society. In this way the status quo is maintained and people with disabilities are kept in their disadvantaged position within society.

disablism stereotyped, negative beliefs about people with disabilities that may lead to discrimination. Disablism fre-quently leads to the denial of appropriate services and a lack of equal opportunities in comparison with other citizens.

disaccharidases enzymes that catalyse the hydrolysis reactions whereby disaccharides are split into their constitu-ent monosaccharides within the intestinal mucosa. They include lactase, sucrase and maltase.

disaccharide *n* a carbohydrate made up of two monosaccha-ride molecules, e.g. lactose, sucrose, maltose, which yields two molecules of monosaccharide on hydrolysis.

disarticulation *n* amputation at a joint.

disc 1. a flat, circular fibrocartilaginous structure separating the opposing surfaces of a joint, e.g. temporomandibular articular disc. **2**. in dentistry, a metal, plastic or cardboard disc having one surface carrying an abrasive, glued or bonded to it. Mounted on a mandrel, it may be used to abrade or polish restoration surfaces or to sharpen instruments.

discectomy *n* surgical removal of a disc, usually an intervertebral disc.

disc guard in dentistry, a protective metal shield placed partially round a rotary disc.

disc herniation/protrusion disruption to the normal integrity of an intervertebral disc, causing the nucleus pulposus to breach the annulus fibrosus. There are varying degrees, from minor bulging, which may be asymptomatic, to bursting through the outer annular fibres into the spinal canal causing severe leg pain and nerve compression. ➪ annulus fibrosis, intervertebral disc, nucleus pulposus.

disciform keratitis a deep localized keratitis involving the stroma usually characterized by a disc-shaped grey area (Wessley's ring) that may spread to the whole thickness of the cornea. It is due to a viral infection or to an immune reaction, or it may also occur as a sequel to trauma. It may heal without residue or may cause scarring and vascularization of the cornea. ➪ central corneal clouding, Wessley's ring.

disclosing agent non-toxic vegetable dye, such as erythrocin, used to reveal plaque and other deposits on a tooth surface. May be in gel, solution, capsule or tablet form.

discogenic *adj* arising in or produced by a disc, usually an intervertebral disc.

discography the introduction of a radiographic contrast agent into the nucleus of an intervertebral disc.

discoid having the shape of a hollow disc, e.g. the blade of a dental excavator.

discoid eczema a common form of eczema recognized from discrete coin-shaped lesions of eczema seen on the limbs of young men in association with alcohol excess, and of older men. It can occur in children with atopic eczema and tends to be more stubborn to treat.

disconjugate movements ➪ disjunctive eye movements.

discrete *adj* distinct, separate, not merging. For example used to describe some types of skin lesions.

discrete wedges individual wedges produced with a limited range of angles, usually 15°, 30°, 45°, and 60° which are fitted to the light beam diaphragm during radiotherapy treatment.

discrimination reaction time ➪ reaction time.

discus proligerus compact mass of follicular cells surrounding the oocyte before it is expelled from the Graafian follicle.

disease *n* any deviation from or interruption of the normal structure and function of any part of the body. It is manifested by a characteristic set of signs and symptoms and in most instances the aetiology, pathology and prognosis is known.

disease activity score (DAS) a tool used to measure disease activity in rheumatic joint disease on a scale between 1–10, depending on the erythrocyte sedimentation rate (ESR) and the number of tender, swollen joints.

disease modifying antirheumatic drugs (DMARD) a group of drugs that influence the immune response, which may be used to suppress the disease process in rheumatoid arthritis and other conditions. They include chloroquine, gold, penicillamine and sulfasalzine.

disease prevention reducing the risk of a disease process, illness, injury or disability. Includes preventive services, e.g. immunization and screening, preventive health education, e.g. advice about sensible alcohol intake, and preventive health protection, e.g. taxing tobacco and fluoridating water. Preventive activities are classified as primary, secondary or tertiary prevention. ➪ primary disease prevention, secondary disease prevention, tertiary disease prevention.

disengagement theory a psychosocial theory of ageing. It describes a process whereby older people gradually disengage from social life and physical activity as they become older. For example, a person may retire from employment and thereby have less involvement with the lives of the people who were also employed in the same company. ➪ activity theory, continuity theory.

DISH *acron* diffuse idiopathic skeletal hyperostosis.

disimpaction *n* separation of the broken ends of a bone that have been driven into each other during the impact which caused the fracture. Traction may then be applied to maintain the bone ends in good alignment and separate.

disinfectants *npl* the term usually reserved for liquid, chemical germicides that are too corrosive or toxic to be applied to tissues, but which are suitable for application to inanimate objects. They are used to destroy most or all pathogenic micro-organisms but not bacterial spores.

disinfection *n* the removal or destruction of pathogenic micro-organisms but not usually bacterial spores. It is commonly achieved by using heat or chemicals.

disinfestation *n* eradication of an infestation, especially of lice (delousing).

disinhibition a person loses the usual social inhibitions and as a result is inappropriate in the way they behave and what they say. It is associated with injury to the frontal lobes. For example, a patient may behave in a sexually inappropriate way.

disjugate eye movements ➪ disjunctive eye movements.

disjunction in genetics, the separation of paired homologous chromosomes during the first meiotic division, or the separation of the chromatids of a chromosome during mitosis and the second division in meiosis. ➪ nondisjunction.

disjunctive eye movements (*syn* disconjugate movements, disjugate eye movements) the movements of the two eyes in which the eyes move in opposite directions, as in convergence or divergence. They are known as vergence movements. ➪ vergence.

disk a general term describing various types of storage medium which permanently store computer data files. Most work by recording data by magnetic means, but some, such as CD-ROM and DVD, operate optically. *floppy disk* so called because it uses flexible magnetic material. It is removable from the computer which allows the physical transfer of data (maximum around 2 megabytes Mb) to another location. *hard disk* so called because it uses several metal platters. It is usually a fixed device in the computer and is capable of storing very large amounts of data. Often referred to as drive C. ➲ byte, CD-ROM, drive, DVD.

disk operating system (DOS) software which controls the way in which data is stored on a computer disk drive.

dislocation *n* displacement of organs, or the articular surfaces of joints, so that all apposition between them is lost. The disruption of the joint is such that the bony components no longer form a working joint. It may be congenital, spontaneous, traumatic, and dislocation may be recurrent. In sport, dislocations of fingers and the shoulder are the most common, as the result of collision with either an opponent or an object such as the ground or goal post. Replacement in position (reduction) may be spontaneous but if not, it should be attempted early and only by a skilled operator. Treatment of dislocation may include reduction under anaesthetic—**dislocated** *adj*, **dislocate** *vt*. ➲ subluxation.

disobliteration *n* rebore. Removal of that which blocks a vessel, most often intimal plaques in an artery. ➲ endarterectomy.

disobliterative endarterectomy ➲ endarterectomy.

disodium tetraborate common name borax. In dentistry, a substance used in fluxes for soldering, or to retard the setting time of plaster of Paris.

disorientation *n* loss of orientation. The person is disorientated to time, place and person, sometimes seen following neurological injury, can be transient or long term.

disparate retinal points non-corresponding retinal points. ➲ retinal corresponding points, retinal disparity.

disparity vergence ➲ motor fusion.

Disparometer a tradename for a clinical instrument designed to measure fixation disparity at near. The target does not have a binocular fixation point and the fusion lock is parafoveal. The instrument fits on the near point rod of a standard phoropter. The Disparometer has two stimuli: one for vertical disparity measurement and the other for horizontal disparity measurement. The test consists of successive pairs of vernier lines of increasing angular separation within a structureless field, each line being viewed by one eye through polarizing filters. The edge of the field provides a peripheral fusion stimulus. Fixation disparity is measured when the vernier lines appear to be aligned and the amount is given by the angular separation (in minutes of arc) of the lines indicated on the back of the instrument. A fixation disparity curve can be obtained by determining the fixation disparity for various amounts of prism power placed in front of the eyes. ➲ associated heterophoria, Mallett fixation disparity unit, retinal disparity.

dispensing practice a general practice where prescribed medications are dispensed by the practice, rather than patients taking their prescription to a local pharmacy. May be used in rural areas.

dispersed daylight system in radiography, a number of units of different sizes that are used to load films into cassettes and a cassette unloader that is fixed to an automatic film processor.

dispersion the phenomenon of the change in velocity of propagation of radiation in a medium, as a function of its frequency, which causes a separation of the monochromatic components of a complex radiation. All optical media cause dispersion by virtue of their variation of refractive index with wavelengths. Dispersion is specified by the difference in the refractive index of the medium for two wavelengths. The difference between the blue F (486.1 nm) and the red C (656.3 nm) spectral lines is called the mean dispersion, i.e. $n_F - n_C$. Dispersion is usually represented by its dispersive power ω or relative dispersion which is equal to the mean dispersion divided by the excess refractive index of the sodium D (589.3 nm) spectral line (n_D–1), often called the refractivity of the material,

$$\omega = \frac{n_F - n_C}{n_D - 1}$$

The reciprocal of the dispersive power is called the Abbé's number or constringence. ➲ achromatic axis, achromatic prism, chromatic aberration, constringence, Fraunhofer's lines, lateral chromatic aberration, longitudinal chromatic aberration, refractive index.

displacement *n* **1.** change in position of a body or object, including size (magnitude) and direction of change, i.e. a vector quantity. (Displacement must be distinguished from 'distance moved' which includes only magnitude and not direction.) ➲ angular displacement, linear displacement. **2.** the volume of fluid (usually water) that is moved when a body or object is immersed in it. **3.** a mental defence mechanism whereby a painful emotion is transferred to another person or object. **4.** describes the loss of pieces of information from short term memory as new information is added.

displacement test ➲ diplopia test.

disposable soma theory a theory of ageing attributed to Tom Kirkwood that posits that reproductive potential in early years is maximized at the expense of ageing in later years.

disposition a relatively enduring tendency to behave or respond to situations in a typical way—**dispositional** *adj*.

dissecting forceps ➲ forceps.

dissection *n* separation of tissues by cutting. When a group of lymph nodes are totally excised it is referred to as a *block dissection of nodes*: it is usually part of the treatment for cancer.

disseminated widely spread or scattered.

disseminated intravascular coagulation (DIC) an abnormal overstimulation of coagulation processes characterized by a rapid consumption of clotting factors which leads to microvascular thrombi and bleeding. It is associated with conditions leading to inadequate organ perfusion, such as hypovolaemia and/or sepsis. DIC can be initiated by a variety of different mechanisms in a number of diverse but distinct clinical situations. For example: (a) infection—caused by *Escherichia coli*, *Neisseria meningitidis*, *Streptococcus pneumoniae* or malaria; (b) cancers—lung, pancreas or prostate; (c) obstetric events—placental abruption, retained dead

225

fetus, pre-eclampsia or amniotic fluid embolism. Endothelial damage, due to many causes—e.g. endotoxaemia due to Gram-negative septicaemia—results in tissue factor expression, which leads to activation of the coagulation cascade through the extrinsic pathway. Intravascular coagulation takes place with consumption of platelets, factors V and VIII, and fibrinogen. This results in a potential haemorrhagic state, due to the depletion of haemostatic components, which may be exacerbated by activation of the fibrinolytic system secondary to the deposition of fibrin. DIC should be suspected when any of the clinical conditions described above are present. Definitive diagnosis depends on the finding of thrombocytopenia, prolongation of the prothrombin time (due to factor V and fibrinogen deficiency) and activated partial thromboplastin time (due to factors V, VIII and fibrinogen deficiency), a low fibrinogen concentration and increased levels of D-dimer (cleaved from fibrin by plasmin, establishing evidence of fibrin lysis). Therapy should be aimed at treating the underlying condition causing the DIC, e.g. intravenous antibiotics for suspected septicaemia. Exacerbating factors such as acidosis, dehydration, renal failure and hypoxia should be corrected. If the patient is bleeding, blood products such as platelets and/or fresh frozen plasma should be given to correct identified abnormalities. It may also be reasonable to treat severe coagulation abnormalities in the absence of frank bleeding to prevent sudden catastrophic haemorrhage such as an intracranial bleed or massive gastrointestinal haemorrhage. ⊃ multiple organ dysfunction syndrome, systemic inflammatory response syndrome.

dissociated heterophoria any heterophoria which is revealed by methods which produce complete dissociation such as the cover test, the Maddox rod test, the Thorington test, the von Graefe's test, etc. ⊃ associated heterophoria, diplopia test, Maddox rod, Thorington test.

dissociation *n* **1.** separation of complex substances into their components. **2.** ionization; when ionic compounds dissolve in water they dissociate or ionize into their ions.

dissociative disorder formerly known as conversion/hysteria disorders. Loss of conscious integration between control of body movement, sensory perceptions, self-identity and memory. Generally considered to be of 'psychogenic' aetiology. Usually of sudden onset/termination and short duration. Often associated with striking denial.

dissociative strategy in sport psychology, a strategy used by athletes in which they focus attention externally in order to distract themselves from feelings of pain or fatigue. Also known as dissociation. ⊃ associative strategy.

distal *adj* in anatomy, farthest away from some reference such as the head or source. For example, in a limb, further from the trunk—the wrist is distal to the forearm; the abdominal aorta divides distally into the two iliac arteries. ⊃ proximal *opp*—**distally** *adv*.

distal end cutter an orthodontic wire cutter with blades set at right angles to the handles and used to cut the distal ends of archwires.

distal radioulnar joint a pivot joint in which the distal extremity of the radius articulates with the head of the ulna.

distal surface that surface most distant from the midline. ⊃ surface

distal tibiofibular joint also called inferior tibiofibular joint. A fibrous joint between the distal ends of the tibia and fibula.

distichiasis *n* extra eyelashes at the posterior lid margin, which turn inwards against the eye.

distomolar a supernumerary fourth molar.

distortion **1.** an aberration of an optical system resulting in an image which does not conform to the shape of the object, somewhat resembling the image viewed through a cylindrical lens. This is due to an unequal magnification of the image. Distortion can be barrel-shaped (*barrel-shaped distortion*) in which the corners of the image of a square are closer to the centre than the middle part of the sides; or pincushion (*pincushion distortion*) in which the corners of the image of a square are farther from the centre than the middle part of the sides (Figure D.6). An example of barrel-shaped distortion is: a square object seen through an uncorrected negative spectacle lens. An example of pincushion distortion is: a square object seen through an uncorrected positive spectacle lens. ⊃ correction, fisheye lens, optical aberration, sine condition. **2.** in dental radiology, the distortion of the radiographic image from the true outline or shape of the object being radiographed. Generally due to incorrect angulation of the central beam, or to bending of the radiographic film.

distractibility *n* a mental health disorder of the power of attention when it can only be applied momentarily.

distraction osteogenesis a surgical procedure designed to increase bone dimensions. A fracture is surgically created in a bone and a mechanical device is then used to slowly move the ends of the fracture apart in order to achieve bony growth in the gap thereby achieving elongation of the bone hopefully without the need for a bone graft. Its origins are traced to G Ilizarov a Soviet orthopaedic surgeon (1921–1992). ⊃ external fixation, Ilizarov frame/method.

distraction test a crude test of hearing used to screen infants for hearing impairment. While the infant is distracted by a parent, the health professional makes a sound to the side/behind the infant and observes whether the infant turns toward the sound. Increasingly superceded by tests using more sophisticated computer-based equipment. ⊃ automated auditory brainstem response, otoacoustic emission testing.

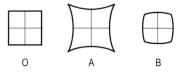

D.6 Distortion (O, object; A, pincushion distortion; B, barrel-shaped distortion) (reproduced from Millodot 2004 with permission).

distractor in experimental psychology, a stimulus that diverts a participant's attention away from another stimulus that they are required to detect or respond to.

distress ⊃ stress.

distribution server in a picture archiving communications system (PACS) a method of storing and sending images to an external user, the images can be encrypted to prevent unauthorized viewing.

district nurse registered nurses holding a specialist qualification who are employed to provide skilled nursing for patients in the community. They are qualified and accountable for assessing, prescribing and evaluating the nursing plan for such patients.

disuse atrophy loss of muscle mass due to inactivity. May follow a period of immobilization, e.g. bed rest or with a plaster cast. Prolonged disuse results in fibrous tissue replacing muscle tissue, limiting the extent of full rehabilitation.

ditch in dentistry, describes a long narrow trench.

ditching characteristic effect seen at the periphery of an amalgam restoration at its junction with the enamel of the tooth.

diuresis *n* increased production/secretion of urine.

diuretics *npl* substances that increase the secretion of urine by the kidney. They are contained in food and drink (e.g. caffeine). Several groups of diuretic drugs are used in the treatment of conditions that include hypertension (high blood pressure), chronic heart failure, pulmonary oedema. In sport the use of diuretics for two main purposes is banned: as a means of losing fluid, and thus weight, in sports such as boxing and weight lifting, which have weight categories or in an attempt to increase the production of urine and thus the excretion of a banned drug, to avoid detection. ⊃ caffeine, carbonic anhydrase inhibitors, loop diuretics, osmotic diuretics, potassium sparing diuretics, thiazide diuretics. ⊃ Appendix 5.

diurnal rhythm a process that follows a daily pattern, such as the sleep–wake cycle. ⊃ circadian rhthym. Also relates to a daily process, or a process occurring during daylight.

diurnal variation the changes that occur during a usual average day, such as changes in body temperature and the level of certain hormones.

diurnal variations (intraocular pressure) normal intraocular pressure (IOP) varies throughout the day within a range of about 4 mmHg, being higher in the morning than in the evening. In people with primary open-angle glaucoma this range is greater. This variation must be taken into consideration when measuring intraocular pressure. ⊃ intraocular pressure.

diurnal vision ⊃ photopic vision.

divagation discursive, digressing, rambling speech. The speaker is unable to stick to the main topic. May be present in a variety of serious mental health problems.

divalent bivalent. Having a valency of two.

divarication *n* separation of two points on a straight line.

divergence (*syn* negative convergence) **1**. the movement of the eyes turning away from each other. **2**. a characteristic of a pencil of light rays, as when emanating from a point source. ⊃ convergence, vergence.

diversional activity an activity chosen by the therapist for its potential to engage the client's interest and hold his attention in order to distract his mind and bring relief from disordered and distressing thoughts and feelings.

divers' paralysis ⊃ decompression sickness/illness.

diverticular disease the presence of small pouch-like sacs (diverticula) in the wall of the colon (Figure D.7). It is common in developed countries where the diet is highly refined and lacks dietary fibre (non-starch polysaccharides). The incidence increases with age and is associated with chronic constipation. It may be asymptomatic, cause bleeding, or become inflamed to cause diverticulitis, or the colon may perforate causing faecal contamination and peritonitis.

diverticulitis *n* inflammation of a diverticulum. Faecal contamination can cause abscess formation around the bowel (pericolic). Repeated attacks of inflammation can lead to fistula formation, or scarring and narrowing of the lumen of the colon which eventually leads to intestinal obstruction.

diverticulosis *n* a condition in which there are many diverticula, especially in the colon. Colonic diverticula increase in frequency with age. ⊃ diverticular disease.

diverticulum *n* a pouch or sac protruding from the wall of a tube or hollow organ. May be congenital or acquired—**diverticula** *pl*.

diving hazards various hazards are associated with the diverse sport of diving. **1**. diving in swimming pools carries the potential hazard of neck injury, if the dive is too steep relative to the depth of the water; **2**. in scuba diving the diver breathes compressed air from a cylinder, through a face mask and a closed system of tubes (self-contained underwater breathing apparatus). Pressure increases by 1 atmosphere (1 bar) per 10 metres of depth. Below 30 m the intoxicating effect of nitrogen narcosis is a danger, avoided by the use of

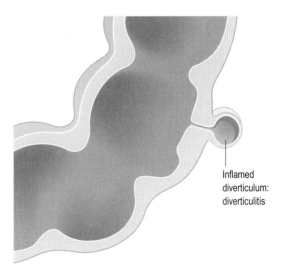

Inflamed diverticulum: diverticulitis

D.7 Diverticular disease (reproduced from Brooker 2008 with permission).

helium–oxygen mixtures. Hypothermia is also a hazard in cold climates; **3**. in breath-hold diving the duration of immersion can be increased if the dive is preceded by vigorous hyperventilation. This depletes carbon dioxide in the body so that it will take longer to rise to the level which would normally trigger the break-point, but importantly the oxygen in the lungs and the blood can be depleted to the point of threatening consciousness. ➲ barotrauma, cervical spine, decompression illness/sickness, nitrogen narcosis.

diving reflex a series of reflex changes to cardiovascular function and metabolic processes that occur if the face (mouth and nose) is immersed in water. The reflex adaptations operate in many species including birds, reptiles, and mammals. The cardiovascular adaptations, which conserve oxygen, include reduced heart rate and reduced blood flow to some areas of the body while ensuring sufficient oxygenated blood reaches the brain.

dizygotic relating to two zygotes. Describes non-identical twins that develop from two separate zygotes. ➲ monozygotic *opp.*

dizziness *n* a feeling of unsteadiness, usually accompanied by anxiety.

DJD *abbr* ➲ degenerative joint disease.

DLCO ➲ carbon monoxide diffusing capacity test.

DM1 ➲ myotonic dystrophy.

DM2 ➲ proximal myotonic myopathy (PROMM).

DMARD *abbr* disease modifying antirheumatic drug.

D Max *abbr* maximum density.

DMD *abbr* Duchenne muscular dystrophy.

DMF index *abbr* decayed, missing, filled index. An index giving the total number of decayed, missing and filled permanent teeth. Used to show the caries experience of an individual or an average group. A way used to manage statistically the numbers of decayed, missing or teeth with fillings in the mouth. ➲ DEF index, index (dental).

DMFS index *abbr* decayed, missing and filled surfaces index. An index giving the total number of decayed, missing and filled surfaces of permanent teeth. Used to show the caries incidence of an individual or an average group.

DMS *abbr* Director of Medical Services.

DNA *abbr* deoxyribonucleic acid.

DNA polymerase an enzyme that catalyses the reactions needed to form double-stranded deoxyribonucleic acid from the single-stranded template.

DNAR *abbr* do not attempt resuscitation.

DNase *abbr* deoxyribonuclease.

DNR *abbr* do not resuscitate.

DO$_2$ *abbr* oxygen delivery.

docosahexaenoic acid (DHA) a 22-carbon, omega-3 polyunsaturated fatty acid. It is present in oily fish and can also be made in the body from alpha-linolenic acid.

docosanoids a group of polyunsaturated fatty acids with 22 carbon atoms in their structure.

docosapentaenoic acid a 22-carbon polyunsaturated fatty acid.

doctor 1. title given to the recipient of a university degree (usually a PhD) higher than a Master's degree. **2.** a courtesy title given to medical practitioners and, in some countries, to dental surgeons.

documentation of nursing documentation usually reflects the phases of the process of nursing—assessing, planning, implementing and evaluating. Nursing records and documentation are required for day-to-day communication and may be needed for the investigation of complaints, disciplinary or professional conduct proceedings, an inquiry, litigation for damages or a criminal prosecution.

Döderlein's bacillus (A Döderlein, German obstetrician/gynaecologist, 1860–1941) a non-pathogenic Gram-positive rod normally part of the vaginal flora in women of reproductive age. It contributes to the protective acidic environment by the production of lactic acid. ➲ lactobacillus.

Doering rule the first fertile day of a woman's menstrual cycle is calculated from the earliest previous temperature change. Used as a back up check for recognizing the start of the fertile days.

Dolder bar metal bar of various shapes, soldered or screwed to a crown or post and core of abutment teeth or an asseointegrated implant abutment. Provides retention for a prosthesis by means of a clip on the fitting surface of the prosthesis.

dolichocephaly an abnormally long skull. ➲ scaphocephaly.

Doll's eye reflex oculocephalic reflex. A normal reflex present in newborns. The eyes remain stationary when the infant's head is moved from side to side. It normally disappears when ocular fixation is achieved by the infant. It may be present in children and adults with probems affecting the brain, vestibular apparatus, the cranial nerves III, VI, extraocular/extrinsic eye muscles, etc.

dolor *n* pain; usually used in the context of being one of the five classical signs and symptoms of inflammation—the others being calor, loss of function, rubor and tumor.

domain an internet address.

domain name used to locate an organization or individual on the internet.

Doman delecato technique a paediatric therapy technique. Repeated passive patterning accompanied by reverse hanging and developmental sequence of movement facilitates use of dormant pathways in central nervous system.

domestic activities of daily living (DADL) the things that a person does every day to maintain the living environment and contribute to the running of a household, such as cleaning and cooking.

domiciliary (dental) kit a portable basic dental kit comprising the equipment required for the treatment of patients confined to bed or patients with a disability in their own home, residential or care home, or in hospital.

dominant *adj* describes a gene with the ability to override the expression of other recessive genes. Dominant genes are expressed in both the homozygous state and the heterozygous state. Examples of dominant gene expression include: normal skin and hair pigmentation and Huntington's disease. ⊃ Mendel's law, recessive trait.

dominant hemisphere on the opposite side of the brain to that of the preferred hand. The dominant hemisphere for language is the left in most right-handed and around a third of left-handed people.

domino booking a maternity care plan in which a woman gives birth in a consultant unit, cared for by the community midwife, and returning home any time after 6 hours following delivery. It is derived from **dom**iciliary midwife **in** and **out**.

DOMS *abbr* delayed onset muscle soreness.

Donders' method ⊃ push-up method.

donor *n* a person who gives blood for transfusion, or semen for AID, or donates tissue for transplantation.

Donovan bodies (C Donovan, Irish physician, 1863–1951) Leishman–Donovan bodies.

donovanosis *n* chronic granulomatous ulceration of the genitalia or anal region, caused by *Klebsiella granulomatis*. Prevalent in warmer climates.

dopa *n* a compound formed in an intermediate stage during the synthesis of catecholamines, e.g. adrenaline (epinephrine), from tyrosine.

dopamine *n* a monoamine neurotransmitter. It functions in the central nervous system, especially the basal nuclei (basal ganglia) of the brain in pathways related to the co-ordination of movement and to behaviour and emotion; deficiency of dopamine in the brain is associated with Parkinson's disease. It is also secreted by nuclei in brain into the hypophyseal portal blood vessels; it inhibits prolactin secretion from the anterior pituitary gland. Also, in the adrenal medulla it is a precursor of adrenaline (epinephrine) and noradrenaline (norepinephrine), and is itself released as a neurohormone. Used intravenously in some types of shock to increase cardiac output and blood flow to the kidneys.

dopants impurities introduced into a crystal structure to control its characteristics. ⊃ activator, killers.

doping the addition of impurities to a substance, in extrinsic semiconductors impurities are added to the silicon or germanium to increase the electrical conductivity.

doping (in sport) the use of banned substances or methods, as defined and listed by the World Anti-doping Agency (WADA), in sport in an attempt to gain an unfair advantage. Considered to derive from the South African word 'dop' for a stimulant drink first given to racehorses. The WADA list is an agreed table of both synthetic and naturally occurring substances considered to offer an advantage when taken during training and competition. Sportsmen and women take performance-enhancing substances for a number of reasons. These include the physical effects of the drug itself (anabolic steroids will allow the athlete to train harder, faster and for longer), the pressure on the athlete to succeed (from coach, family, sponsors, media and general public) and the direct effect on athletes themselves (to boost confidence, lessen anxiety, etc.). ⊃ banned substance.

Doppler effect when ultrasound echoes are reflected from a moving structure they are changed in frequency, the amount and direction depends on the velocity, the direction of the moving interface and the position of the observer. Moving towards an object produces an increase in the reflected frequencies and moving away from the object produces a decrease infrequency.

Doppler scanner equipment used in ultrasound imaging to monitor a moving substance, for example, the flow of blood or the beating heart.

Doppler scanning an imaging technique that combines ultrasonography with pulse echo. Doppler ultrasound technique can be used to calculate cardiac output and stroke volume by measuring blood flow in the aorta via a probe passed into the oesophagus. Used to monitor haemodynamic status and response to treatment.

Doppler shift a measurement obtained by subtracting the known frequency of the original transmitted ultrasonic waveform from the reflected waveform.

Doppler technique (C Doppler, Austrian physicist and mathematician, 1803–1853) can be used to measure the velocity of blood flow through a vessel to determine the degree of occlusion or stenosis.

Doppler ultrasound technique is widely used to assess the arterial blood flow to the lower limb in patients with leg ulcers. ⊃ ankle-brachial pressure index. It can be used to calculate cardiac output and stroke volume by measuring blood flow in the aorta via a probe passed into the oesophagus. Used to monitor haemodynamic status and response to treatment. In obstetrics, it is used to detect blood flow, e.g. in the fetal umbilical artery (to assess placental function), middle cerebral artery (to assess placental failure and fetal anaemia) and ductus venosus (to detect hypoxia). The returning echoes from moving blood, which differ from those of surrounding stationary tissue, are reflected as sound waves and used to estimate speed and direction of blood flow; colour flow imaging helps to determine which vessels are being measured.

dorsal *adj* pertaining to the back, or the posterior part of an organ, referring to the embryological history of the surfaces. In the anatomical position the palms face forward and dorsal applies to the back of the hands and arms. ⊃ ventral *opp*.

dorsal column the routes by which sensory afferents travel to the brain. Includes receptors for vibration, touch and proprioceptors.

dorsal decubitus radiograph patient is supine and the central ray passes through the body from side to side.

dorsal horn the dorsal region of the spinal cord that contains cell bodies.

dorsal midbrain syndrome ⊃ Parinaud's syndrome.

dorsal root a group of sensory axons from the spinal nerve and attaching to the dorsal side of the spinal column.

dorsal root ganglia ⊃ ganglion.

dorsalis pedis artery *n* an artery passing over the dorsum of the foot; supplying blood to the muscles of the foot and toes. The dorsalis pedis pulse, which can be palpated on the top of the foot, is used to check blood flow to the foot, such as when arterial obstruction is suspected or following arterial surgery. ➲ Colour Section Figure 9.

dorsiflexion *n* movement at the ankle joint that points the foot up towards the leg, or movement of the toes that lifts them away from the sole of the foot. In the case of the great toe—upwards (compare plantar flexion). ➲ Babinski's reflex or sign.

dorsipalmar radiograph a radiograph of the hand with the palm in contact with the cassette.

dorsiplantar radiograph a radiograph of the foot with the sole in contact with the cassette.

dorsocentral *adj* at the back and in the centre.

dors/o, dors/i- a prefix that means 'dorsal, back posterior', e.g. *dorsiflexion*.

dorsolumbar *adj* pertaining to the lumbar region of the back.

dorsoventral *adj* pertaining to the dorsal (back) and the ventral (front) surfaces.

dorsum *n* the back of the body or the upper surface of a body part, such as the foot.

DOS *abbr* disk operating system.

dosage in electrotherapy, the general dosage parameters include: intensity, wavelength, duration and frequency of treatments, location of application. It is important to record all relevant parameters after every treatment—this enables appropriate modifications to repeat treatments and also helps in audits investigating the contribution of an electrophysical agent to an outcome.

dose build-up each layer of tissue produces recoil electrons which in turn deposit their kinetic energy through several other layers of tissue. The energy in each layer will be determined by the number of electrons passing through the layer plus the absorbed kinetic energy.

dose-equivalent limits the maximum dosage of radiation an individual can receive over a specific period of time in sieverts.

dose volume histogram a graphical representation of dose distribution in a specific anatomical structure.

dosimeter, dosemeter *n* a device worn by personnel or placed within equipment to measure incident X-rays or gamma rays. Thermoluminescent dosimeters, using lithium fluoride powder impregnated into plastic discs, are used in personnel monitoring, as part of health and safety requirements. Previously, photographic film in a special filter holder was used. ➲ film badges, Geiger–Müller counter, solid state radiation detector, thermoluminescent dosimeters.

DOT *acron* **D**irectly **O**bserved **T**reatment.

dots per inch a measure of image quality, the higher the number the better the image quality.

double blind study a randomized controlled trial in which neither the subjects (experimental and control) nor the investigators know which group is having the drug/treatment being investigated, or the placebo.

double contrast in radiology, the use of two contrast agents to produce the image. For example, the use of barium sulphate and air during a barium enema to produce a detailed image of the mucosal lining of the colon.

double prism test a test for determining the presence of cyclophoria, in which a double prism (a pair of prisms set base to base) with the base line horizontal is placed before one eye. The person is requested to fixate a horizontal line (or row of letters) which through the double prism appears as two lines (or two rows) vertically separated. On uncovering the other eye, the patient sees three lines (or rows). If there is no cyclophoria, all three lines (or rows) will appear parallel, but lack of parallelism indicates cyclophoria. The double prism used in this test consists of two weak prisms (about 4 or 5 Δ): this clinical type of double prism is commonly called a Maddox double prism. ➲ cyclophoria, Fresnel's bi-prism, Maddox rod test.

double uterus abnormal uterine development due to failure of fusion of the Müllerian ducts, producing two uterine bodies with or without duplication of the cervix and vagina, which may cause repeated miscarriages. Very occasionally two independent conceptions occur and implant into the two sections of the uterus; preterm labour is common.

double vision ➲ diplopia.

doublet a combination of two lenses usually cemented to each other used to correct chromatic aberration. Typically it consists of a positive crown lens and a negative flint lens. ➲ achromatizing lens, crown glass, flint glass, triplet.

doubling time time over which a tumour will double in size. A mark of tumour virulence and occasionally an indicator of chemoresponsiveness (faster doubling time often associated with high growth fraction and occasionally with higher chemoresponsiveness).

douche *n* a stream of fluid directed against the body externally or into a body cavity.

doughing time in dentistry, the time elapsing after mixing a material and before it is ready for manipulation. Used in connection with denture base resins. ➲ manipulation time, mixing time, working time.

Douglas bag method used for measurements of pulmonary ventilation and respiratory gas exchange and hence estimation of energy expenditure (indirect calorimetry). The subject breathes via a mouthpiece or face mask and one-way valve, so that the expired gas is collected in a large bag over a recorded period of time; the volume is then measured and the gas analysed for oxygen and carbon dioxide content; the differences from inspired air allow calculation of the rates of O_2 uptake and CO_2 output. Described in 1911 by Oxford physiologist C.G. Douglas. ➲ calorimetry.

doula from the Greek word meaning 'woman who serves other women'; in maternity care, one who provides emotional and practical support, most commonly during pregnancy and labour, but occasionally postnatally.

dovetail (keyway) in dentistry, a type of cavity retention lock which is wider at its extremity and narrower at its neck where it joins the main cavity. It provides a mechanical lock to aid retention of a restoration.

dowagers hump colloquial expression describing a curve on the upper spine. Often a sign of osteoporosis.

dowel crown a crown with a prefabricated post.

download to transfer information from one computer to another.

downregulation 1. in assisted conception, a phase in an IVF cycle. Whereby drugs are used to suppress the release of the hormone that stimulates oocyte production in order to establish a baseline prior to the drug-induced stimulation of the ovaries. **2.** in genetics, the processes that regulate gene activity.

Down's syndrome (J Down, British physician, 1828–1896) a genetic condition in which there is a mild to moderate learning disability and facial characteristics that include: oval tilted eyes, squint and a flattened occiput. The chromosome abnormality is of two types: (a) primary trisomy, caused by abnormal division of chromosome 21 (at meiosis). This results in an extra chromosome instead of the normal pair: the infant has 47 chromosomes and is often born of an older mother. (b) structural abnormality involving chromosome 21, with a total number of 46 chromosomes, one of which has an abnormal structure as the result of a special translocation. Such infants are usually born of younger mothers and there is a higher risk of recurrence in subsequent pregnancies.

DPF *abbr* Dental Practitioners' Formulary.

2,3-DPG *abbr* 2,3-diphosphoglycerate.

DPLD *abbr* diffuse parenchymal lung disease.

DPT *abbr* dental pantomogram.

DQE *abbr* detected quantum efficiency.

DR *abbr* **1.** diabetic retinopathy. **2.** digital radiography.

dracontiasis *n* infestation with *Dracunculus medinensis* common in Africa, Middle East and Asia. It is transmitted through contaminated drinking water. The female worm moves from the intestine to emerge through the skin surface in order to deposit larvae. There is inflammation, thickening and ulceration.

Dracunculus medinensis (*syn* Guinea worm) a nematode parasite (tissue-dwelling) that infests humans.

drag force a retarding force, acting opposite to the direction of motion of a body or object. Often caused by air resistance or friction. ⊃ form drag, propulsive drag force, surface drag.

drain *n* ⊃ wound drains.

drainage in dentistry, the channel created in soft tissues through which accumulated exudate and gases may be released. The creation of drainage from a pulp chamber or apical soft tissue.

drainage angle ⊃ angle of the anterior chamber.

Draper's law (*syn* Grotthus' law) an effect is produced in a medium, only by that portion of the spectrum which is absorbed by the medium. The effect may be thermal, chemical or the production of fluorescence.

drawer tests tests that elicit a clinical sign that describes the movement of the tibia relative to the femur and is positive if the relevant cruciate ligament is torn. The cruciates provide the primary stability of the knee joint. Disruption of the anterior cruciate will allow excess anterior movement of the tibia relative to the femur and posterior movement is a sign of posterior cruciate damage. ⊃ anterior (PA) drawer test, posterior (AP) drawer test.

dreaming altered state of consciousness where fantasies and remembered events are confused with reality.

D_2-receptor antagonists a group of antiemetic drugs that act by blocking the dopamine receptors, e.g. metoclopramide. ⊃ Appendix 5.

dressing in dentistry, a provisional restoration, often placed in an emergency situation. In endodontics, ⊃ root canal (dental procedures).

dressings *npl* ⊃ wound dressings.

Dressler's syndrome (W Dressler, American physician, 1890–1969) ⊃ postmyocardial infarction syndrome.

Drew–Smythe cannula S-shaped metal catheter used in obstetric practice to puncture the hindwaters when the fetal head is not engaged; rarely used now, as it can cause placental separation.

DRI *abbr* dietary reference intakes.

drill in dentistry, a rotating cutting device for making holes in hard substances.

drill biopsy in dentistry, a biopsy of hard tissues obtained by means of a hollow drill.

drillers' disease (vibration syndrome) caused by using vibrating machinery, resulting in cysts in the bones of the wrist and sometimes the hand. ⊃ hand-arm vibration syndrome, prescribed diseases, vibration-whole body.

drive 1. a compelling urge to satisfy a need. It may be an innate primary drive which is concerned with homeostasis, such as thirst. Secondary drives involve a wider range of human activities that evolve during growth and development, such as social activities. ⊃ drive theory. **2.** in computing, that part of a computer that writes to and reads from a disk. ⊃ disk.

drive theory a theory of learning developed by American psychologist Clark Leonard Hull (1884–1952) which proposes that deficits in physiological needs create a state of arousal that motivates the organism to engage in a behaviour to satisfy the need in order to reduce the arousal. For example, hunger motivates the organism to seek food. The linking of the drive state with the response that leads to the reduction in arousal produces learning of that response.

drive wire a wire used to hold a single radioactive source and cause it to oscillate over a prescribed length of a catheter.

drop attacks periodic falling because of sudden loss of postural control of the lower limbs, without vertigo or loss of consciousness. Usually followed by sudden return of normal muscle tone, allowing the person to rise, if uninjured. ⊃ vertebrobasilar insufficiency.

drop-out cast where part of a cast is cut away to allow the patient to undertake a movement while preventing movement in the opposite direction. Commonly used for the correction of contractures as it enables the patient to strengthen the opposing muscle group to the contracture. In the arm, if the arm is contracted into flexion, then the posterior part of the splint is cut away above the elbow so that the arm can extend, but cannot flex any further due to the cast. In the leg contracted into flexion, the anterior part of the splint is cut away below the knee so that the knee can extend, but cannot flex any further due to the cast.

droplet infection pathogen transmission in droplets of moisture such as during coughing or talking.

dropped beat refers to the loss of an occasional ventricular beat as occurs in extrasystoles.

dropsy *n* ⊃ oedema—**dropsical** *adj*.

drug *n* the generic name for any substance used for the prevention, diagnosis and treatment of diagnosed disease and also for the relief of symptoms. The term 'prescribed drug' describes such usage. ⊃ prescription only medicine (POM). The word medicine is usually preferred for therapeutic drugs to distinguish them from the addictive drugs which are misused illegally. For alleviating unpleasant symptoms of self-limiting illnesses, any remedy which does not require a medical prescription is termed an 'over-the-counter' (OTC) medicine. ⊃ general sales list (GSL).

drug dependence a state arising from repeated administration of a drug on a periodic or continuous basis (WHO, 1964). Now a preferable term to drug addiction and drug habituation.

drug errors are described as preventable prescribing, dispensing or administration mistakes.

drug eruptions cutaneous drug reactions are common and almost any drug can cause them. Drug reactions may reasonably be included in the differential diagnosis of most skin diseases. Although the mechanisms are poorly understood, drug eruptions may be classified as either: (a) non-immunological (non-allergic)—unwanted pharmacological effect (e.g. striae due to corticosteroids), drug overdose or failure to metabolize or excrete the drug (e.g. morphine rashes in patients with liver disease), drug interaction (e.g. warfarin toxicity when coadministered with aspirin or phenylbutazone), idiosyncratic reaction which may be genetically determined and is peculiar to the individual (e.g. drug induced variegate porphyria), phototoxic reaction (e.g. chlorpromazine-induced light reaction), altered skin ecology (e.g. tetracyclines and vaginal candidiasis), exacerbation of pre-existing skin conditions (e.g. lithium and beta-blocker worsening of psoriasis); (b) or immunological (allergic)—immediate hypersensitivity (e.g. penicillin-induced urticaria), immune complex reaction (e.g. drug-induced vasculitis or erythema multiforme), delayed hypersensitivity (e.g. drug-induced exfoliative dermatitis or photo-allergic reaction) (Table D.1). It is important to consider the possibility of a drug eruption when faced with a rash which is atypical of a known skin disease. There are no specific investigations which help. Prick tests and in vitro tests for allergy are too unreliable for routine use. Readministration, as a diagnostic test, is usually unwise

unless the reaction is mild and there is no suitable alternative drug. The first step in managing the eruption is to withdraw the suspected drug(s) (except in the case of suspected drug-induced photodermatoses where if possible phototesting can be carried out when the patient is on the drug and then again at a later date when the drug has been withdrawn). Drug withdrawal, however, may not be easy, or even possible, if there is no alternative available. The decision will depend on many factors, including the severity and nature of the drug reaction, its potential reversibility and the probability that the drug caused the reaction. Supportive treatment with antihistamines or a tailored course of systemic corticosteroids may be indicated, depending on the type of skin reaction. ⊃ adverse drug reactions, anaphylaxis.

drug induced teratogenesis a congenital abnormality resulting from the absorption of a certain substance which alters genetic coding and cellular development in the embryo and fetus.

drug interaction occurs when the action of one drug is affected by another drug, beverage or food taken previously or simultaneously.

drug misuse a term increasingly used to describe the illegal use of drugs and the inappropriate use of prescription or over-the-counter drugs. Substance misuse includes solvents and alcohol, as well as drugs such as cocaine or heroin.

drug reaction ⊃ adverse drug reactions.

drug resistance the increasing problem caused by the ability of many micro-organisms to develop resistance to certain antibiotics, e.g. vancomycin-resistant enterococci and meticillin (methicillin)-resistant *Staphylococcus aureus*.

drug tolerance a situation where the therapeutic effects of a drug lessen over time, which necessitates the administration of a larger dose to achieve the same benefit.

drug trials several levels of testing occurring during the development of new drugs. (a) Phase I trials where small numbers of healthy volunteers (usually male) are given small doses and monitored for adverse reactions. Blood samples are tested to determine drug distribution and excretion. (b) Phase II trials involve patients, and the new drug's efficacy is compared with existing treatments. (c) Phase III trials involve large multiple centre studies carried out before the drug is approved and licensed for use by the appropriate bodies. ⊃ Commission on Human Medicines, Committee on Safety of Medicines, Medicines and Healthcare Products Regulatory Agency. (d) Phase IV trials take place after the drug has been approved for clinical use. Aim to monitor and report adverse and idiosyncratic reactions not seen earlier.

drusen *npl syn* colloid bodies, hyaline bodies. Small, circular, yellow or white dots located throughout the fundus but more so in the macular region, around the optic disc or the periphery. They consist of deposits lying between the basement membrane of the retinal pigment epithelium and Bruch's membrane. Although they may be found in young people, they almost universally occur with ageing but also with retinal and choroidal degeneration (e.g. age-related macular degeneration [maculopathy], retinitis pigmentosa,

Table D.1 Drug eruptions and some drugs which may cause them

Reaction pattern	Clinical features	Drugs which commonly cause reactions
Toxic erythema	Erythematous plaques Morbilliform, sometimes with urticarial or erythema multiforme-like elements	Antibiotics (especially ampicillin) Sulphonamides, thiazide diuretics, phenylbutazone, para-aminosalicylic acid (PAS)
Urticaria	Itchy weals, sometimes accompanied by angioedema	Salicylates, codeine, antibiotics, dextran and ACE inhibitors
Erythema and scaling	Small, scaly, pink papules to large, scaly, red papules	Antibiotics (especially penicillins and sulphonamides), anticonvulsants, ACE inhibitors, barbiturates, gold and penicillamine
Allergic vasculitis	Painful, palpable purpura followed by necrotic ulcers	Sulphonamides, phenylbutazone, indometacin, phenytoin and oral contraceptives
Erythema multiforme	Target-like lesions and bullae on the extensor aspects of the limbs	Sulphonamides, phenylbutazone and barbiturates
Purpura	Widespread purpura not due to thrombocytopenia or a coagulation defect	Thiazides, sulphonamides, phenylbutazone, sulphonylureas, barbiturates and quinine
Bullous eruptions	May be associated with erythema and purpura May occur at pressure sites in drug-induced coma	Barbiturates, penicillamine, nalidixic acid
Exfoliative dermatitis	Universal redness and scaling, shivering	Phenylbutazone, PAS, isoniazid and gold
Fixed drug eruptions	Round, erythematous and sometimes bullous plaques develop at the same site every time the drug is given Pigmentation left in wake	Tetracyclines, quinine, sulphonamides and barbiturates
Acneiform eruptions	Rash resembles acne	Lithium, oral contraceptive, androgenic or glucocorticoid steroids, antituberculosis and anticonvulsant drugs
Toxic epidermal necrolysis	Rash resembles that of scalded skin	Barbiturates, phenytoin, phenylbutazone and penicillin
Hair loss	Diffuse	Cytotoxic agents, acitretin, anticoagulants, antithyroid drugs and oral contraceptives
Hypertrichosis		Diazoxide, minoxidil and ciclosporin
Photosensitivity	Rash limited to exposed skin	Thiazides, tetracyclines, phenothiazines, sulphonamides, nalidixic acid and psoralens
Pigmentation	Irregular melanin pigmentation on face Slate-grey colour of exposed skin Diffuse yellow coloration of skin Streaky depigmentation of hair	Oral contraceptives Phenothiazines Mepacrine Chloroquine

Reproduced from Boon et al (2006) with permission

angioid streaks) and primary dystrophy. There are several main types of drusen: (a) hard (or nodular) drusen are small, round and discrete. They are deposits of granular material as well as of abnormal collagen. They are the most common type and are usually innocuous. (b) soft (or diffuse or granular) drusen are often large with indistinct edges and with time they may enlarge, coalesce and increase in number. They are due to either a focal thickening of the inner layer of Bruch's membrane or to amorphous material located between that thickened, detached part and the rest of Bruch's membrane. They represent an early feature of age-related macular degeneration (maculopathy). (c) cuticular (or basal laminar) drusen are small subretinal nodular thickening of the basement membrane of the pigment epithelium. They occur in younger people more often than hard or soft drusen. (d) with time, the above drusen may calcify (calcific drusen) and take on a glistening appearance. Drusen rarely produce any symptoms and if there is a visual loss it is usually due to an accompanying macular haemorrhage. ➲ age-related macular degeneration (maculopathy).

DRVs *abbr* dietary reference values.

DRVVT *abbr* dilute Russell viper venom time.

dry eye keratitis sicca. An eye in which there is a minimum of moisture which causes damage to the interpalpebral ocular surface. It may result from tear deficiency, excessive tear evaporation, meibomian gland dysfunction, abnormal blink reflex, damage to the conjunctival or corneal surface or lacrimal apparatus, soft contact lens wear, Sjögren's syndrome, hormone changes during the climacteric, etc. Symptoms are irritation, foreign body sensation and sometimes transient blurring of vision. It often leads to keratitis sicca. Management consists mainly of artificial tears and frequent blinking exercises. ⇒ artificial tears, keratitis sicca, meibomian gland, mucin, Norn's test, phenol red cotton thread test, Schirmer's test, Sjögren's syndrome, tear meniscus, tears, xerophthalmia.

dry gangrene occurs when the drainage of blood from the affected part is adequate; the tissues become shrunken and black. ⇒ gangrene.

dry labour a colloquial term used to describe labour when there is no leakage of liquor amnii, the membranes having ruptured before the onset of labour.

dry socket ⇒ localized alveolar osteitis.

DSA *abbr* digital subtraction angiography.

DSH *abbr* deliberate self-harm.

DSM *abbr* Diagnostic and Statistical Manual of Mental Disorders.

DTPA diethylenetriamine-pentaacetic acid. A chelating agent used to remove the radioactive substances americium, curium and plutonium. Calcium-DTPA or zinc DTPA are administered following internal contamination with the radioactive materials. They bind to the radioactive material prior to its excretion by the kidney.

DTs *abbr* delerium tremens.

dual dosemeter two independent ionization chambers, that measure the integrated dose at the isocentre and feed signals to two independent dosimeters each capable of terminating a radiotherapy treatment exposure at a predetermined level. It provides a system of fail safe dose delivery control.

dual-energy X ray absorptometry (DEXA) an imaging technique that is currently the most widely used method of measuring bone mineral density. Used in the diagnosis of osteoporosis and to assess response to treatment. The person lies on a table and the scanner directs X-ray energy from two sources (increasing the accuracy) at the bone being examined. The greater the bone mineral density, the greater the signal picked up by the photon counter. Dual-energy X ray absorptometry (DEXA) scanning is more accurate than other methods (e.g. plain X-ray): quick, non-invasive, exposes the person to less radiation and is relatively inexpensive. Estimation of bone mineral density is a good predictor of fracture risk and DEXA can be used to screen those most at risk (postmenopausal women, previous fracture victims, smokers and those prescribed long-term corticosteroid therapy). DEXA can also be used for a three-compartment assessment of body composition, estimating lean body mass, fat mass and bone mass. ⇒ osteoporosis.

dual filament two filaments in an X-ray tube to enable either broad or fine focus to be selected.

dualism *n* in psychology, a view that mind and body are separate.

Duane retraction syndrome (DRS) ⇒ Duane's syndrome.

Duane's phenomenon ⇒ Duane's syndrome.

Duane's syndrome (A Duane, American ophthalmologist, 1858–1926) (*syn* Duane retraction syndrome (DRS), Duane's phenomenon, retraction syndrome, Stilling–Turk–Duane syndrome, Turk's disease) an autosomal dominant disorder characterized by limitation of eye movement. A complex disorder found in about 1% of patients with strabismus, it occurs in three different types. All three types are characterized by retraction of the globe of the eye into the orbit and by narrowing of the eyelids (palpebral fissure) on attempted adduction. The left eye is affected more often than the right eye and the condition is bilateral in about 20% of patients. In addition, each type presents an abnormal pattern of ocular motility. Type I, the most common affecting over three-quarters of all cases, presents limited or absent abduction and slight esotropia in the primary position, and typically a head turn towards the involved side. Type II presents limited adduction, slight exotropia and relatively normal or slightly limited abduction, and usually a head turn away from the involved side. Type III, the rarest (about 1% of all cases), presents limited abduction and adduction. The aetiology is believed to be a congenital absence of the sixth cranial nerve and its nucleus (partial absence in type II) and fibres from the third cranial nerve innervate the lateral rectus so that innervation results in contraction of both the lateral and medial recti muscles (co-contraction) and the degree of this paradoxical innervation determines the severity of the disorder. Management is frequently surgical especially in types II and III, but prismatic corrections have been found to be beneficial in selected cases.

DUB *abbr* dysfunctional uterine bleeding.

Dubowitz score (V Dubowitz, South African paediatrician, b. 1931) assesses gestational age, using physical and neurological characteristics, such as ankle dorsiflexion, posture, etc. ⇒ New Ballard Score.

Duchenne muscular dystrophy (DMD) (G Duchenne, French neurologist, 1806–1875) an X-linked recessive disorder affecting only boys; there are deletions in the dystrophin gene. A direct gene test is routinely available. The disorder usually begins to show between 3 and 5 years. It is characterized by progressive muscle weakness affecting the proximal muscles and limb girdle with loss of locomotor skills. There is cardiomyopathy and pseudohypertrophy of the calf muscles. With increasingly sophisticated management by a multidisciplinary team, death now usually occurs during the third decade (from respiratory or cardiac failure). ⇒ muscular dystrophies.

Ducrey's bacillus (A Ducrey, Italian dermatologist, 1860–1940) *Haemophilus ducreyi*.

duct *n* a tube for carrying away the secretions from a gland. For example the bile ducts carry bile away from the liver.

ductal carcinoma insitu (DCIS) a precancerous condition confined to the lactiferous (milk) ducts in the breast.

ductile able to be drawn out in fine strands or wires.

ductless glands endocrine glands.

ductus arteriosus a fetal blood vessel connecting the left pulmonary artery to the aorta, to bypass the lungs in the fetus. At birth the duct closes, but if it remains open it is called *persistent or patent ductus arteriosus*, a congenital heart defect. ⮑ persistent or patent ductus arteriosus.

ductus venosus a vessel of the fetal circulation. It allows blood to bypass the fetal liver by shunting blood from the umbilical vein to inferior vena cava. Closes at birth.

Dukes' staging (C Dukes, British pathologist, 1890–1977) a system for the staging of colorectal cancer. It has four categories A–D, and is based on the degree of tissue invasion and metastasis.

dulac technique positioning the patient so that the area of interest is in the centre of a sphere.

dumbness *n* ⮑ mutism.

'dumping syndrome' the name given to the symptoms of epigastric fullness, diarrhoea and a feeling of faintness and sweating after meals that sometimes follow gastric surgery such as partial gastrectomy or vagotomy. Rapid movement of hypertonic gastric contents into the duodenum causes fluid to move from the blood to the bowel lumen. Rapid absorption of glucose leads to rebound insulin secretion and hypoglycaemia. Autonomic reflexes release a range of gastrointestinal hormones which lead to the vasomotor effects such as flushing, palpitations, sweating, tachycardia and hypotension. Those affected are advised to avoid large meals with a high carbohydrate content.

Duncan disease/syndrome named for the original family in which the condition was described. ⮑ X-linked lymphoproliferative syndrome.

dunken ⮑ traditional birth attendant.

duochrome method ⮑ duochrome test.

duochrome test (*syn* bichrome test, duochrome method) a subjective refraction test in which the subject compares the sharpness of black targets (e.g. Landolt rings) of similar sizes, on a red background on one side and on a green background on the other side (blue is sometimes used) of a chart. In under-corrected myopia or overcorrected hyperopia, the letters on the red background will appear more distinct, while in overcorrected myopia or undercorrected hyperopia the letters on the green background will appear more distinct, and in emmetropia or corrected ametropia the letters should appear equally distinct on both sides. The test makes use of the chromatic aberration of the eye and assumes that when the eye is looking at distant objects it is focused on the yellow part of the visible spectrum. ⮑ chromatic aberration, cobalt lens, Verhoeff's circles.

duodenal intubation a double lumen tube is passed as far as the pyloric antrum under fluoroscopy. The inner tube is then passed along to the duodenojejunal flexure.

duodenal ulcer a peptic ulcer occurring in the duodenal mucosa. The majority are associated with the presence of the bacterium *Helicobacter pylori* in the stomach. Other factors include NSAIDs, smoking and genetic factors. Epigastric pain may occur some time after meals or during the night. The pain may be relieved by food, antacids and vomiting. The ulcer can bleed, leading to haematemesis and/or melaena, or it can perforate causing peritonitis. Severe scarring following chronic ulceration may produce pyloric stenosis and gastric outlet obstruction (GOO). Management includes: (a) general measures; smoking cessation, avoiding foods that cause pain, avoiding aspirin and NSAIDs; (b) eradication of *H. pylori*; (c) drugs to reduce gastric acid; H_2 receptor antagonists, e.g. ranitidine, proton pump inhibitors, e.g. omeprazole, antacids based on calcium, magnesium or aluminium salts; (d) rarely surgical treatment, e.g. after perforation.

duodenitis *n* inflammation of the duodenum.

duodenojejunal *adj* pertaining to the duodenum and jejunum.

duodenopancreatectomy *n* ⮑ pancreaticoduodenectomy.

duodenoscope *n* a side-viewing flexible fibreoptic endoscope—**duodenoscopic** *adj*, **duodenoscopy** *n*.

duodenostomy *n* a surgically made fistula between the duodenum and another cavity, e.g. cholecystoduodenostomy.

duodenum *n* the fixed, curved, first portion of the small intestine, connecting the stomach above to the jejunum below. The pyloric sphincter at the lower end of the stomach controls the amount of partially digested food entering the duodenum. The common bile duct and the pancreatic duct unite and enter the duodenum at the hepatopancreatic ampulla—**duodenal** *adj*. ⮑ Colour Section Figure 18b.

duplex scan a method of using real time imaging, colour and Doppler at the same time to demonstrate heart, blood vessels and in obstetrics.

duplicate denture an exact replica of an existing denture.

duplicating film film used to produce exact copies of radiographs by direct contact printing.

duplicating material the material used in dental laboratories to produce accurate duplication of models, casts, etc.

duplitized films radiographic films in which the emulsion is coated on both sides of the base.

Dupuytren's contracture (G Dupuytren, French surgeon, 1777–1835) painless, chronic flexion of the digits of the hand, especially the third and fourth, towards the palm. The aetiology is uncertain but some cases are associated with hepatic cirrhosis. Minor trauma and genetic predisposition may play a role. There is a fibrous contraction that occurs in the palmar fascia of the hand that may produce a flexion deformity of the metacarpophalangeal and proximal interphalangeal joints common in those of Anglo Saxon descent. One or both hands may be affected. The ring finger is affected most often, followed by the little, middle and index fingers. A nodule develops within the connective tissue and eventually develops into a cord-like band. Finger extension becomes limited. The condition becomes more common after the age of 40 years and it is commoner in men than women.

dural venous sinuses sinuses or channels enclosed by layers of dura mater that drain venous blood from the different parts of the brain. They include the cavernous, occipital, superior and inferior petrosal, superior and inferior sagittal, sigmoid, straight and transverse sinuses. ⊃ confluence of sinuses.

dura mater the fibrous outer meningeal membrane covering the brain and spinal cord. ⊃ falx cerebri, falx cerebelli, meninges, tentorium cerebelli—**dural** *adj*.

duration of pregnancy the duration of pregnancy averages 266 days from conception to delivery; and 280 days (40 weeks) from the first day of the last normal menstrual period to delivery. To calculate the estimated date of delivery (EDD) add 9 months and 7 days for an average 28-day menstrual cycle. If the menstrual cycle is less or more than 28 days, it is necessary to substract or add the number of days. The EDD is only a guide and women should be advised not to depend on the precise date. Normal labour may commence any time between 37 and 43 weeks of pregnancy; preterm labour is usually classified as occurring before 37 weeks' gestation, but in the case of pregnancy persisting more than 10 days past the EDD medical intervention may be advocated to expedite delivery.

duty of care the legal responsibility in the law of negligence that a person must take reasonable care to avoid causing harm.

duty cycle an electrotherapy term that indicates the percentage of time for which there is an output. On and off times are usually measured in seconds. Used most commonly for electrical stimulation and pulsed ultrasound and pulsed shortwave diathermy.

DVD *abbr* digital versatile disk.

DVI *abbr* direct video interface.

DVT *abbr* deep vein thrombosis.

dwarf *n* person of stunted growth. May be due to growth hormone deficiency. Also occurs in untreated congenital hypothyroidism and juvenile hypothyroidism, achondroplasia and other conditions.

dwarfism *n* arrested growth and development as occurs in congenital hypothyroidism, and in some chronic diseases such as intestinal malabsorption, renal failure and rickets.

dwell time the positioning of a radioactive source within a catheter for different intervals of time.

DWSIs *abbr* dentists with special interests.

dye sensitizing in radiography. Increasing the spectral sensitivity of the film by adding impurities to the film emulsion, because it is done by adding coloured dyes can be called spectral sensitizing.

dynamic computed tomography (CT) in early CT scanners when a number of scans were performed in rapid succession to demonstrate blood flow, now no longer used.

dynamic contraction muscle shortening which results in movement.

dynamic exercise exercise in which recurrent and substantial body movements predominate.

dynamic friction ⊃ friction.

dynamic flexibility active range of motion exercises used to increase flexibility.

dynamic hip screw (DHS) an orthopaedic procedure undertaken on some femoral neck fractures. It involves placing a plate on the femoral shaft and a screw that pierces the femoral head, the arrangement is such that when the person gets up to mobilize, there is some movement between the metal components and hence compression (and stimulation of bone healing) at the fracture site.

dynamic imaging the monitoring of the change in radioactive uptake over time in radionuclide imaging.

dynamic incremental computed tomography (CT) in early CT scanners, when a number of dynamic CT scans were performed at different levels in the body, now no longer used.

dynamic psychology a psychological approach which stresses the importance of (typically unconscious) energy or motives, as in Freudian or psychoanalytic theory.

dynamic range in ultrasound imaging the difference between the maximum and minimum values in a set of data, that is how many degrees of black and white are found in the grey scale image.

dynamic retinoscopy retinoscopy performed with the patient fixating binocularly a near object such as a letter, a word, or a picture mounted on, or held close to, the retinoscope and wearing the distance correction. No working distance lens power is subtracted or added to the finding since the plane of regard is at the same distance as the retinoscopy. Also known as *book retinoscopy* when the patient is reading a text; *cognitive retinoscopy* when the patient fixates a single letter or reads some words *near point retinoscopy*. ⊃ retinoscope, static retinoscopy.

dynamics the branch of mechanics concerned with the effects of forces on the motion of physical bodies. ⊃ acceleration, force.

dynamic splinting the use of modified splints that provide active forces and facilitate some controlled movement that counteracts the unwanted forces of the splint.

dynamic strength generally, strength displayed during movement; quantitatively expressed in terms of limb or trunk torque at a specified angular velocity, almost always during concentric muscle action.

dynamic stretching involves gaining range by an active movement and should not be confused with ballistic stretching, which involves the use of repetitive, bouncing, dynamic, rhythmic movements performed at higher velocities. Dynamic stretching involves progressively increasing the range through successive movements until the end of range is reached. These exercises are especially useful when dealing with more advanced sports-related rehabilitation problems, they enhance dynamic function and neuromuscular control due to repetition and practice, thereby enhancing the movement memory. ⊃ static stretching, stretching.

dynamic wedge a wedge angle produced by the rapid movement of the beam collimators, which does not affect the beam quality.

dynamometer *n* a device used to measure strength of muscle contraction.

dynamometry measurement of external force production by a human subject in a specific exercise such as knee extension or hand grip; may be performed either statically or dynamically, the latter in either concentric or eccentric mode, at a specified angular velocity. ⊃ grip dynamometer, isokinetic dynamometer.

-dynia a suffix that means 'pain', e.g. *pleurodynia*.

dys- a prefix that means 'difficult, painful, abnormal', e.g. *dysuria*.

dysaesthesia *n* impairment of touch sensation.

dysarthria *n* a speech disorder that results from a problem in muscular control of the mechanisms of speech. It is caused by damage to either the central or the peripheral nervous system, or both. Loss of muscular control may involve incoordination and/or slowness and weakness. The problem may affect articulation, phonation, prosody, resonance and respiration—**dysarthric** *adj*.

dysbarism any condition caused by changes in atmospheric pressure. ⊃ decompression sickness/illness.

dyschezia painful defecation. Causes include constipation, anal fissure, haemorrhoids, etc.

dyschondroplasia *n* Ollier's disease. A disorder of bone growth resulting in normal trunk, short arms and legs.

dyscoria abnormality of the shape of the pupil. ⊃ pupil.

dyscrasia *n* an abnormality in the cellular composition of the blood, as in leukaemia, agranulocytosis, aplastic anaemia, etc.

dysdiadochokinesia *n* impairment of the ability to perform alternating movements, such as pronation and supination, in rapid, smooth and rhythmical succession; a sign of cerebellar disease but also seen in the so-called 'clumsy child' with minimal brain damage.

dysentery *n* inflammation of the bowel with evacuation of blood and mucus, accompanied by tenesmus and colic—**dysenteric** *adj*. *amoebic dysentery* is caused by the protozoon *Entamoeba histolytica* ⊃ amoebiasis. *Bacillary dysentery* is caused by bacilli of the genus *Shigella*: *S. dysenteriae*, *S. flexneri*, *S. boydii* or *S. sonnei* (the commonest cause in the UK). The organism is excreted by cases and carriers in their faeces, and contaminates hands, food and water, from which new hosts are infected.

dysfunction 1. in occupational therapy practice, a temporary or permanent inability to perform tasks and activities to a satisfactory level or to engage in the range of occupations expected or required in daily life. 2. a temporary, or permanent, inability to adapt to the demands of a normal situation in a normal environment. 3. abnormal functioning of a body part or organ.

dysfunctional uterine bleeding (DUB) heavy bleeding from the uterus for which no organic cause is found. ⊃ menorrhagia.

dysgammaglobulinaemia *n* impaired immunoglobulin production in terms of quantitative or qualitative humoral immunity. There are numerous primary and secondary causes including common variable immunodeficiency, X-linked agammaglobulinaemia, X-linked hyper-IgM syndrome, myeloma and transient hypogammaglobulinaemia of infancy.

dysgenesis *n* malformation during embryonic development—**dysgenetic** *adj*, **dysgenetically** *adv*.

dysgerminoma *n* ovarian tumour, benign or of low grade malignancy. It originates from primitive/undifferentiated gonadal cells.

dysgeusia *n* impaired or abnormal sense of taste. Impaired taste is associated with fluid deficits and poor oral/dental health. Changes during normal ageing diminish the sense of taste. Abnormal taste may be due to a drug side-effect, such as with ACE-inhibitors, anticancer drugs and metronidazole. Disease processes can alter taste—some people experience strange taste sensations during an aura that precedes an epileptic seizure, and gustatory (taste) hallucinations may occur in some mental health disorders.

dysgnathia an abnormality of the maxilla or mandible, or both.

dysgraphia *n* an acquired problem of written language caused by brain damage. The affected person's ability to spell familiar and/or unfamiliar words is altered in one or many modes, e.g. word-processing or handwriting. Several different types of dysgraphia are described—**dysgraphic** *adj*.

dyshidrosis *n* a vesicular skin eruption on the palms and soles, formerly thought to be caused by blockage of the sweat ducts at their orifice, histologically an eczematous process.

dyskaryosis *n* abnormality of nuclear chromatin, indicating a malignant or premalignant condition.

dyskeratosis abnormal keratin production by epithelial cells; may indicate malignancy. Abnormal process which, in the eye, results in hornification of the epithelial layer of the conjunctiva or cornea. It may be hereditary or due to irritation (e.g. radiation) or to prolonged drug administration in the eye. It appears as a dry white plaque (called leucoplakia or leucokeratosis). It may be benign or malignant, in which case it must be surgically excised. ⊃ pterygium.

dyskinesia *n* 1. (clumsy child syndrome) impairment of voluntary movement. 2. involuntary purposeless movement—**dyskinetic** *adj*. ⊃ dyskinetic movements, tardive dyskinesia.

dyskinetic movements types of dyskinetic movements include tremors of different types (e.g. rest, action and intention); myoclonus; chorea; and dystonia (generalized and hemidystonia). Causes include: Parkinson's disease, drug-induced parkinsonism, Wilson's disease, hyperthyroidism, Huntington's disease, alcohol, lesions affecting the basal nuclei (ganglia), and cerebellar disease.

dyslalia a disorder of articulation characterized by poor pronunciation or the replacement of one sound for another, for instance the 'g' is replaced by 'd'.

dyslexia *n* a disorder affecting the ability to read. There are a number of different types of dyslexia, for example, *deep dyslexia* and *surface dyslexia*. Many individuals with dyslexia may also exhibit dysgraphia—**dyslexic** *adj*.

dyslogia disordered speech, an inability to express thoughts in speech. May be due to dementia, mental health problem, or learning disability, etc.

dysmaturity *n* signs and symptoms of growth retardation at birth. ➲ low birthweight.

dysmegalopsia a condition in which the perceptual size of objects is abnormal. Objects may appear larger (macropsia) or smaller (micropsia). ➲ macropsia, micropsia.

dysmelia *n* limb malformation, including deficiency.

dysmenorrhoea *n* painful menstruation. It may be *spasmodic or primary dysmenorrhoea*, most often affecting young women a year or two after menstruation commences, once ovulation has become established, or *congestive or secondary dysmenorrhoea* usually affecting women in their late twenties and may be associated with pelvic pathology, such as fibroids or endometriosis. Painful periods can interfere with training programmes or affect performance in sport. Sportswomen often use the combined oral contraceptive pill to regulate or manipulate the timing of their periods (to avoid competitions) and control dysmenorrhoea and its symptoms. Moderate physical exercise can be helpful for relieving period pain, and may help prevent it.

dysmetria *n* difficulty in assessing and achieving the correct distance and range of movement causing undershooting or overshooting of a target and the appearance of homing in on it.

dysmnesic syndrome a disorder of memory characterized by an inability to learn basic new skills. The person, however, retains the ablity to perform high level skills learned before their illness. The patient may confabulate where they create false memory to fill the gaps in memory. It is caused by damage to those parts of the brain concerned with memory.

dysmorphogenic ➲ teratogen.

dysmorphophobia *n* **1**. a morbid fear of deformity of a body part. **2**. the fixed belief that a part of the body is deformed or appears repulsive to others.

dysmotility *n* abnormality of intestinal peristalsis.

dysostosis *n* a disorder caused by faulty ossification. ➲ cleidocranial dysostosis, craniofacial dysostosis.

dyspareunia *n* painful or difficult coitus, experienced by the woman.

dyspepsia *n* 'indigestion'. A collective term for any symptoms thought to originate from the upper gastrointestinal tract. Epigastric discomfort and feeling of fullness after eating with 'heartburn', often exacerbated by stressful situations. It encompasses many different symptoms and disorders, including some arising outside the digestive system. The causes include: (a) upper gastrointestinal disorders—peptic ulceration, acute gastritis, gallstones, chronic cholecystitis, motility problems (e.g. oesophageal spasm), 'functional' (e.g. non-ulcer dyspepsia, irritable bowel disease); (b) other gastrointestinal disorders—pancreatitis, pancreatic cancer, hepatitis, liver metastases, colorectal cancer; (c) systemic disease—renal failure, hypercalcaemia; (d) drugs—non-steroidal anti-inflammatory drugs (NSAIDs), iron and potassium supplements, corticosteroids, digoxin; (e) others—alcohol consumption, anxiety, low mood. Although symptoms often correlate poorly with the underlying diagnosis, a careful history is important to: elicit symptoms classical of specific disorders, e.g. peptic ulcer; detect 'alarm' features requiring urgent investigation (e.g. weight loss, haematemesis and/or melaena, anaemia, dysphagia, vomiting, palpable abdominal mass; and detect atypical symptoms more suggestive of other disorders, e.g. myocardial ischaemia. Dyspepsia is extremely prevalent, affecting up to 80% of the population at some time, and very often no abnormality is discovered during investigation, especially in younger patients. Patients with 'alarm' symptoms, those over 55 years old with new dyspepsia, and younger patients unresponsive to empirical treatment require prompt investigation to exclude serious gastrointestinal disease. Examination may reveal important findings such as evidence of anaemia, weight loss, lymphadenopathy, abdominal masses or signs of liver disease—**dyspeptic** *adj.* ➲ gastro-oesophageal reflux disease (GORD), heartburn, *Helicobacter pylori*.

dysphagia *n* difficulty in swallowing. It may coexist with heartburn or vomiting but should be distinguished from both globus sensation (in which anxious people feel a lump in the throat without organic cause) and odynophagia (pain during swallowing, usually from gastro-oesophageal reflux or candidiasis). The difficulty in swallowing may be experienced with fluids and/or solid food. Dysphagia has oropharyngeal and oesophageal causes. Oropharyngeal disorders result from neuromuscular dysfunction affecting the initiation of swallowing by the pharynx and upper oesophageal sphincter (e.g. bulbar or pseudobulbar palsy, myasthenia gravis, cerebral palsy, motor neuron disease, cerebrovascular accident and dementia). Patients with oropharyngeal dysphagia have difficulty initiating swallowing and develop choking, nasal regurgitation or tracheal aspiration. Drooling, dysarthria, hoarseness and cranial nerve or other neurological signs may be present. Oesophageal causes include: (a) stricture—benign (e.g. peptic, fibrous rings), malignant (e.g. cancer of the oesophagus or stomach, extrinsic compression for example from head and neck cancers); (b) dysmotility of the oesophagus—achalasia, non-specific motility disorder; (c) oesophagitis—peptic due to gastric reflux, candidiasis. Patients with oesophageal disease complain of food 'sticking' after swallowing, although the level at which this is felt correlates poorly with the true site of obstruction. Swallowing of liquids may be normal until strictures become extreme. Dysphagia implies significant disease and should always be promptly investigated. Endoscopy is the investigation of choice because it facilitates biopsy and dilatation of suspicious strictures. If no abnormality is found, then barium swallow, with videofluoroscopic swallowing assessment, will detect most motility disorders. In a few cases oesophageal manometry is required. Assessment and management of dysphagia is best conducted by a multidisciplinary team that may include a gastroenterologist, specialist nutrition nurse, dietitian, speech and language therapist. The composition of the team will be determined by the needs of the patient, the medical condition underlying the swallowing problem, whether surgery is indicated, the clinical setting and the aim of treatment (curative or palliative)—**dysphagic** *adj.*

dysphasia *n* also sometimes known as aphasia. Dysphasia is a disorder of language and has nothing to do with intelligence level or an intellectual disorder. It is most commonly associated with cerebrovascular accident affecting the left side of the brain, but can occur after a brain injury or brain surgery. Dysphasia can affect the ability to understand language and also the use of language for expression. The presentation of dysphasia varies greatly and those affected have very different skills and difficulties. It is important that detailed, individual consideration is given to their difficulties. The understanding of language includes understanding both what is said and what is written. Likewise, expression includes both verbal expression and written expression. Discrepancies between the level of understanding and expression of language are common. Most often, people with dysphasia have problems both in comprehension and in expression although the degree of impairment in each may vary. Assessment and treatment of dysphasia needs a detailed understanding and breakdown of language. Speech and language therapists can provide therapy to assist individuals and their carers to improve their communication. Dysphasia has a considerable impact on most areas of life such as relationships, work and leisure activities. Rehabilitation takes time and may last many months. People affected by dysphasia can become very withdrawn and isolated if they do not receive sufficient support. ⊃ aphasia.

dysphemia a disorder of speech. ⊃ stammering.

dysphonia *n* a voice production disorder, e.g. hoarseness. It may have a neurological, behavioural, organic or psychogenic cause.

dysphoria low mood characterized by profound feelings of depression, unrest and anguish.

dysplasia *n* developmental abnormality, often referring to a premalignant condition and graded according to severity—**dysplastic** *adj.*

dyspnoea *n* shortness of breath, often abbreviated to SOB, or short of breath on exertion (SOBOE). There is difficulty in, or laboured, breathing; can be mainly of an inspiratory or expiratory nature. Causes include respiratory disease, cardiovascular disease, anaemia, etc. Breathlessness or dyspnoea is a sensation perceived by an individual and should not be confused with tachypnoea (increased respiratory rate), hyperventilation (breathing which exceeds metabolic requirements) or hyperpnoea (increased breathing). The conscious awareness of breathing becomes an overwhelming sensation severely affecting the lives of some people with chronic lung diseases. Since the sensation is subjective and related to life experience, the clinician cannot fully appreciate nor judge the level of dyspnoea, as with other sensations, e.g. pain, fear, hunger and grief (Borg 1982)—**dysponoeic** *adj.* ⊃ orthopnoea. (Borg G 1982 Psychophysical basis of perceived exertion. Med Sc Sports Ex 14: 377–381)

dyspraxia *n* lack of voluntary control over muscles, particularly the orofacial ones—**dyspraxic** *adj.*

dysreflexia autonomic ⊃ autonomic dysreflexia.

dysrhythmia *n* ⊃ arrhythmia.

dyssynergia loss of fluency of movement; poor sequencing and timing of movements; loss of coordination of muscles that normally act in unison, particularly the abnormal state of muscle activity due to cerebellar disease.

dystaxia *n* difficulty in controlling voluntary movements—**dystaxic** *adj.*

dysthyroid eye disease ⊃ thyroid ophthalmopathy.

dystocia *n* difficult labour characterized by slow progress or failure to progress. Causes include ineffective dilatation of the cervix, uncoordinated uterine contraction and lack of expulsion, unfavourable presentation of the fetus and pelvic abnormalities.

dystonia *n* a movement disorder in which there is the abnormal posturing of a part of the body, such as spasmodic torticollis. Describes an abnormal movement where the agonist and antagonistic muscles contract isometrically and involuntarily, leading to contorted posturing. This often occurs when the patient tries to initiate movement. Present in some neurological conditions and can affect the whole body or any part. ⊃ dyskinetic movements.

dystrophia literally, difficult or abnormal growth.

dystrophy *n* defective nutrition of an organ or tissue, usually muscle. The word is applied to several unrelated conditions. ⊃ muscular dystrophy, Duchenne muscular dystrophy.

dysuria *n* painful micturition. Usually associated with bacterial infection, such as cystitis, urethritis and prostatitis, or bladder tumours or urinary calculi causing obstruction and gynaecological disorders—**dysuric** *adj.*

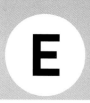

e⁻ *abbr* electron.

E *abbr* **1.** energy. **2.** exposure.

Eagle-Barrett syndrome ⊃ prune belly syndrome.

Eales' disease (H Eales, British ophthalmologist, 1852–1913) a condition affecting the retinal vessels, it is characterized by recurrent haemorrhages into the retina and the vitreous body (humour). It affects both eyes and causes sudden visual impairment.

EAMC *abbr* exercise-associated muscle cramp.

ear *n* the sensory organ concerned with hearing and balance. It has three parts, the outer (external), middle (tympanic cavity) and inner (internal) ear. The outer/external ear comprises the auricle (pinna) and the external auditory meatus/canal along which sound waves pass to vibrate the tympanic membrane which separates it from the middle ear. The middle ear cavity is air-filled and contains three tiny bones or ossicles: malleus, incus and stapes. The ossicles transmit the sound waves to the inner ear via the oval window. The middle ear communicates with the nasopharynx via the pharyngotympanic (eustachian or auditory) tube. The fluid-filled inner ear comprises the cochlea (organ of hearing) and the semicircular canals which are concerned with balance. The cochlea and semicircular canals contain the nerve endings of the cochlear and vestibular branches of the vestibulocochlear or auditory nerve (eighth cranial). ⊃ cerumen, cochlea, Colour Section Figure 13.

EAR *acron* **E**stimated **A**verage **R**equirement.

ear-bow an instrument, similar to a face-bow, that is centred on the external auditory meatus and records the relationship of the maxillary dental structures to the cranial structures and to the horizontal plane.

eardrum *n* the tympanic membrane at the end of the external auditory meatus/canal. The first auditory ossicle is attached to the inner surface. ⊃ Colour Section Figure 13.

ear injury usually refers to injury of the external ear, most commonly seen in contact sports such as rugby (especially in forwards) and boxing, and due to direct trauma. Lacerations and bruising are the most common. ⊃ cauliflower ear.

early childhood caries dental caries involving maxillary primary incisors within months after their eruption, which quickly spreads rapidly to involve other primary teeth. Previous known as rampant caries or baby bottle tooth decay/ caries.

early morning stiffness (EMS) this is a common feature of inflammatory conditions, particularly rheumatoid arthritis, and refers to slowness or difficulty moving the joints when getting out of bed or after being still in one position for too long, it usually gets better with movement.

ear wax ⊃ cerumen.

Eastman analysis an orthodontic cephalometric analysis undertaken by orthodontic tracing based on landmarks and use of A-point and B-point to define the skeletal relationship (ANB angle), measurement of maxilla plane and mandibular plane angles relative to the incisors and the angle of the maxilla and mandibular planes. ⊃ ANB angle.

eating disorders a term used to describe the conditions in which an individual's eating behaviour and nutrient intake is inappropriate for their needs. There are two well-defined eating disorders, anorexia nervosa (AN) and bulimia nervosa (BN), which share some overlapping features. The physical consequences of eating disorders are seen in all organ systems, they include: (a) cardiac—electrocardiogram (ECG) abnormalities (e.g. T wave inversion, ST depression and prolonged QT interval), arrhythmias (including profound sinus bradycardia and ventricular tachycardia); (b) haematological—anaemia, thrombocytopenia, leucopenia; (c) endocrine—pubertal delay or arrest, growth retardation and short stature, amenorrhoea, sick euthyroid state; (d) metabolic—electrolyte imbalance, uraemia, renal calculi, impaired bone mineralization, osteoporosis; (e) gastrointestinal—damage to teeth and oesophagitis caused by exposure to gastric acid during self-induced vomiting, constipation, abnormal liver function tests. Ninety per cent of cases are female. There is a much higher prevalence of abnormal eating behaviour in the population which does not meet diagnostic criteria for AN or BN, and a higher prevalence still of obesity, which is usually considered to be more a disorder of lifestyle or physiology than psychology. A complex mixture of social and psychological factors and life events predispose to and precipitate the development of eating disorders. Consequently they are best treated by a multidisciplinary team. ⊃ anorexia nervosa (AN), binge-eating disorder, bulimia nervosa (BN).

EB *abbr* epidermolysis bullosa.

EBA *abbr* **1.** epidermolysis bullosa acquista. **2.** ethoxybenzoic acid cement.

EBM *abbr* **1.** evidence-based medicine. **2.** expressed breast milk.

Ebola *n* a serious viral haemorrhagic fever that occurs sporadically in Africa. The first known outbreak occurred near the Ebola river in Zaire (now the Democratic Republic of the Congo). It is caused by a *Filovirus* and mortality rates can be as high as 90%. The mechanism for the primary infection is not known but secondary infection occurs through direct contact with infected body fluids, or by droplets. Initially there is high temperature, headache, muscle pain, etc., later there is a rash, diarrhoea and vomiting and internal bleeding that leads to shock and multiple organ dysfunction syndrome (MODS). Treatment is supportive only. ⊃ Marburg disease.

EBP *abbr* evidence-based practice.

Ebstein's anomaly (W Ebstein, German physician, 1836–1912) a congenital heart defect affecting the right atrioventricular (tricuspid) valve. There may be obstruction to filling and heart failure. Surgical correction may be necessary.

eburnation the act or process of becoming hard like ivory. **1.** the term for the polished appearance of articular cartilage affected by osteoarthritis. It refers to the dense, sclerotic appearance that the cartilage takes on in an attempt to remodel and deal with the extra stresses, it resembles ivory in that it is white and dense. **2.** in dentistry, the change in carious dentine from a soft decalcified mass to a hard, polished, black-to-brown state.

EBV *abbr* Epstein–Barr virus.

ecbolic *adj* describes any agent that causes contraction of the gravid uterus and accelerates expulsion of its contents, e.g. oxytocin used to induce and or augment labour. ⊃ oxytocic.

ecboline an abortifacient or substance used for accelerating labour.

ECCE *abbr* extracapsular cataract extraction.

eccentric *adj* positioned off centre.

eccentric action active resistance by a muscle to lengthening, e.g. during controlled descent of a hill or stairs. Also referred to, paradoxically and unwisely, as 'eccentric contraction' or even 'lengthening contraction'. Unlike a spring in the equivalent situation, a muscle expends energy even during such passive extension, as both excitation and cross-bridge cycling must continue, although this is a fraction of the energy cost of concentric actions generating the same force at the same absolute velocity. *eccentric exercise* involves the principal muscles in eccentric action. Because most (though not all) muscles can produce higher forces in this mode of action than in isometric or concentric exercise, greater training effects are widely considered to result, though greater muscle damage and delayed-onset muscle soreness (DOMS) may ensue in unaccustomed subjects. ⊃ concentric contraction, force–velocity relationship, muscle contraction, work.

eccentric fixation (*syn* anomalous fixation) a monocular condition in which the image of the point of fixation is not formed on the foveola. In this condition, the patients feel that they are looking straight at the object stimulating the nonfoveolar retinal area and the visual acuity of that eye is reduced. The condition occurs most commonly in strabismic amblyopia but can also occur when the fovea has been destroyed by some pathological process. ⊃ after-image transfer test, amblyopia, central visual acuity, eccentric viewing, occlusion treatment, penalization, pleoptics, Visuscope.

eccentric muscle work ⊃ eccentric action.

eccentric force a force applied at a distance away from an axis of rotation, therefore a force causing a rotational moment (torque). Applies to all muscle actions at joints, whether the muscle itself is acting eccentrically or concentrically. ⊃ concentric contraction, eccentric action.

eccentric jaw relationship any jaw relation which is lateral or protrusive to the retruded mandible relationship.

eccentric occlusion any lateral, protrusive or retrusive occlusion other than centric.

eccentric viewing fixation in which the eye moves so as to place the image of an object outside the fovea. The object is perceived by the patient as looking 'past' it and not directly at it as in eccentric fixation. Eccentric viewing is often applied by people with low vision suffering from macular degeneration to improve reading a letter or a word by looking slightly above, below or to the side of it. ⊃ eccentric fixation, low vision.

eccentric vision ⊃ peripheral vision.

ecchondroma *n* a benign tumour composed of cartilage which protrudes from the surface of the bone in which it arises—**ecchondromata** *pl*.

ecchymosis *n* ⊃ bruise—**ecchymoses** *pl*.

eccrine *adj* describes the most abundant type of sweat gland. ⊃ apocrine glands.

ecdemic *adj* describes an occurrence, such as a disease, which is not normally present in a population, i.e. it is not endemic.

ecdysis the shedding or 'moulting' of the outer skin layer. ⊃ desquamation

ECF *abbr* extracellular fluid.

ECG *abbr* electrocardiogram ⊃ electrocardiograph.

echinocacciasis infestation with the larval stage of a tapeworm of the genus *Echinococcus*. ⊃ hydatid cyst.

Echinococcus *n* a genus of cestodes, tapeworms, e.g. *Echinococcus granulosa*; the adult worms infest dogs and other canines as the primary host. The larval stage can infect humans through contaminated drinking water or handling affected dogs. The encysted larvae cause hydatid disease in humans and animals such as cattle and sheep who are secondary hosts. ⊃ hydatid cyst.

echo the reflection of an ultrasound wave back to the transducer when the beam hits a surface at right angles.

echocardiogram an ultrasound-produced image of the movements that take place in the heart.

echocardiography *n* ultrasound cardiography. The use of ultrasound for studying the structure and motion of the heart. Useful for measuring the ventricles, cardiac output, myocardial contraction and ejection fraction, and in the diagnosis of pericardial effusion, endocarditis, septal defects and other congenital defects, valve dysfunction and checking prosthetic valves. It can be performed through the chest wall as a noninvasive procedure (transthoracic echocardiography) by placing the ultrasound probe (transducer) on the chest, or by passing the ultrasound probe into the oesophagus (transoesophageal echocardiography). The transoesophageal route produces clearer images of some structures, e.g. heart valves and the atria.

echoencephalography *n* passage of ultrasound waves across the head to investigate intracranial structures. Can detect midline shift caused by space occupying lesions such as an injury, abscess, tumour or blood clot, etc., within the brain. Mostly superseded by magnetic resonance imaging (MRI) and computed tomography (CT) imaging.

echogenicity a characteristic of an ultrasound image, for example, benign masses are often homogeneous and malignant masses are often heterogeneous or fluid is black and solid areas appear white.

echolalia *n* repetition, almost automatically, of words or phrases heard. Occurs most commonly in people who have schizophrenia and dementia and sometimes in delirium—**echolalic** *adj*.

echopraxia the copying or repetition of the body movements of another person. Can be a feature of schizophrenia.

echo rephrasing the re-establishment of a magnetic resonance signal by either using a 180° radio frequency pulse or by gradient switching.

echo time (TE) the time between the centre of the excitation pulse and the peak of the echo.

echo train length (ETL) the number of echoes that are individually phase encoded for a fast spin-echo sequence and corresponds to the number of lines of K-space measured per repetition time interval, they range from 3 to 128 depending on the type of pulse sequence. ⊃ K-space, repetition time.

echoviruses *npl* name originates from **E**nteric **C**ytopathic **H**uman **O**rphan. A group of RNA viruses of the genus enterovirus that cause conditions that include: gastroenteritis, respiratory infection, aseptic meningitis, encephalitis and rashes.

echoxia *n* involuntary mimicking of another's movements.

ECI *abbr* Experience of Caregiving Inventory.

eclampsia *n* the commencement of convulsions in a pregnant woman or postpartum, which is not related to other cerebral conditions, occurring in a woman with pre-eclampsia. It is a rare but extremely serious complication of pre-eclampsia, characterized by epileptiform convulsions (seizures) occurring towards term, during or shortly after labour. The midwife should summon medical assistance urgently, position the woman on her side, insert an airway if possible, administer oxygen until breathing resumes, check reflexes regularly and prevent the woman from harming herself. Intravenous magnesium sulphate, or sometimes phenytoin, is used to control convulsions (seizures); the administration of ergometrine is contraindicated. The woman may start spontaneous labour and the use of sedating drugs, such as diazepam, may lead to misinterpretation of distress from contraction pain as the onset of further convulsions (seizures). Repeated convulsions (seizures) can cause cerebral haemorrhage, pulmonary oedema, renal or hepatic failure, or pneumonia from inhalation of secretions or gastric contents. The risks to the fetus include hypoxia and death *in utero*, especially during apnoeic phases. Prompt recognition and early treatment of pre-eclampsia should prevent all except the rare cases of sudden fulminating pre-eclampsia, with impending eclampsia—**eclamptic** *adj*. ⊃ HELLP syndrome, pre-eclamsia.

ECM *abbr* extracellular matrix.

ecmnesia *n* impaired memory for recent events with normal memory of remote ones. Common in older adults and in early cerebral deterioration.

ECMO *abbr* extracorporeal membrane oxygenator.

ECoG *abbr* electrocochleography.

ecological study a research study where a particular group of individuals rather than an individual, e.g. schools, towns, etc., form the unit being observed.

economy *n* describes spending or using as little as possible whilst still maintaining quality services. One of the three 'Es' of value for money. ⊃ effectiveness, efficiency, value for money.

Ecstasy *n* colloquial term for an amphetamine derivative methylenedioxymethamfetamine (MDMA) that causes euphoria and hallucinations. Recreational use is widespread at 'raves' and clubs. It is considered by many users to be safe, but serious effects from excessive physical activity and dehydration which leads to hyperpyrexia and possibly death have occurred. In the UK it is classified as a class A drug (Misuse of Drugs Act 1971). Currently there is debate as to whether the drug should be reclassified as a class B drug. It is considered, by some authorities, to be less harmful than other class A drugs.

ECT *abbr* electroconvulsive therapy.

-ectasis a suffix that means 'dilation, extension', e.g. *lymphangiectasis*.

ectasis, ectasia dilatation, bulging or distension of a hollow organ, duct or tube. For example, ectasia of the cornea or sclera.

ecthyma *n* a purulent skin infection caused by either *Staphylococcus* or *Streptococcus* and characterized by ulceration under an exudative crust. It is associated with poor hygiene and malnutrition, and minor trauma can predispose to development of the lesions. It affects any age group and is commonly seen in people who misuse drugs.

ecto- a prefix that means 'outside, without, external', e.g. *ectoparasite*.

ectoderm *n* the outer of the three primary germ layers of the early embryo. It gives rise to some epithelial and nervous tissues, e.g. skin structures, inner ear, mammary glands, pituitary gland, the central nervous system, cranial, spinal and autonomic nerves, adrenal medulla and the lens and retina of the eye—**ectodermal** *adj*. ⊃ endoderm, mesoderm.

ectodermal dysplasia a hereditary condition characterized by defects in the skin, teeth, hair and other organs.

ectogenesis *n* the growth of the embryo outside the uterus (in vitro fertilization).

ectomorph a frail body type (physique) in which the person is slender—**ectomorphic** *adj*. ⊃ endomorph, mesomorph.

-ectomy a suffix that means 'removal of', e.g. *cholecystectomy*.

ectoparasite *n* a parasite that lives on the exterior surface of its host, such as head lice—**ectoparasitic** *adj*.

ectopia *n* malposition of an organ or structure, usually congenital—**ectopic** *adj*. ⊃ corectopia, ectopia vesicae.

ectopia pupillae ⊃ corectopia.

ectopia vesicae an abnormally placed urinary bladder which protrudes through or opens on to the abdominal wall.

ectopic beat ⊃ extrasystole.

ectopic pregnancy (*syn* tubal pregnancy) extrauterine gestation, the uterine (fallopian) tube being the most common site (Figure E.1). Other, less common sites include the ovary, external os of the cervix and the abdominal cavity.

ectrodactyly, ectrodactylia *n* congenital absence of one or more fingers or toes or parts of them. ⊃ Colour Section Figure 63.

ectromelia a congenital abnormality in which there is gross hypoplasia or aplasia of one or more long bones of one or more limbs—**ectromelic** *adj*.

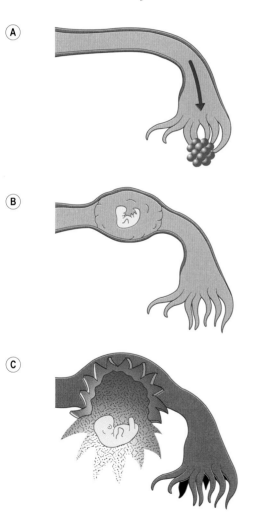

E.1 Possible outcomes of tubal pregnancy A. tubal abortion; B. tubal mole; C. tubal rupture (reproduced from Fraser & Cooper 2003 with permission).

ectropion *n* an eversion or turning outward, especially of the lower eyelid. It may be due to age-related tissue changes, trauma to the eyelids, facial nerve damage, or Bell's palsy. The eyelids do not close fully, which exposes the eyeball and disrupts the tear film. The tears cannot drain into the punctum and the eye waters. ⊃ entropion, Colour Section Figure 64.

ectropion uveae an ectropion affecting the iris and characterized by a portion of the posterior pigment epithelium of the iris growing or being drawn around the pupillary margin onto the anterior iris surface. It may be acquired (e.g. following iris neovascularization, neovascular glaucoma) or congenital (e.g. neurofibromatosis). ⊃ iris, neovascular glaucoma, von Recklinghausen's disease.

ectrosyndactyly a congenital condition in which some digits are absent; the remaining ones are webbed

ECV *abbr* external cephalic version.

eczema *n* the terms 'eczema' and 'dermatitis' are frequently used synonymously. They refer to distinctive reaction patterns in the skin, which can be either acute or chronic and are due to a number of causes. Some authorities, however, limit the word 'eczema' to the cases with internal (endogenous) causes while those caused by external (exogenous) contact factors are called *dermatitis*. In the acute stage of eczema, oedema of the epidermis (spongiosis) progresses to the formation of intra-epidermal vesicles, which may enlarge and rupture. In the chronic stage there is less oedema and vesiculation but more thickening of the epidermis (acanthosis); this is accompanied by a variable degree of vasodilation and T-cell lymphocytic infiltration in the upper dermis. There are several patterns of eczema—atopic, seborrhoeic, discoid, irritant, allergic, asteatotic, gravitational, etc.; some of these have identifiable environmental causes whereas others are more complex. The clinical signs are similar in all types of eczema and vary according to the duration of the rash. Acute eczema is characterized by redness and swelling, usually with ill-defined margins; papules, vesicles and more rarely, large blisters; exudation and cracking; scaling. Whereas, chronic eczema may show the signs associated with the acute condition (usually less vesicular and exudative); lichenification, a dry leathery thickening with increased skin markings, secondary to rubbing and scratching; fissures and scratch marks; pigment changes. The skin of patients with eczema may be colonized or infected with *Staphylococcus aureus*. ⊃ allergic eczema, asteatotic eczema, atopic eczema, dermatitis, discoid eczema, gravitational eczema, irritant eczema, lichen simplex, pompholyx, seborrhoeic eczema—**eczematous** *adj*.

eczema herpeticum also known as Kaposi's varicelliform eruption. A serious condition that occurs when the herpes simplex virus (HSV-1) infects existing eczema. There are clusters of small vesicles on areas of eczema and normal skin. It is accompanied by systemic effects and patients may feel very unwell. Management includes the administration of antiviral drugs, and in severe cases the person is hospitalized for intravenous administration. Patients are isolated as eczema herpeticum is infectious. ⊃ Colour Section Figure 65.

eczematous conjunctivitis ⊃ phlyctenular conjunctivitis.

E
F

ED *abbr* erectile dysfunction.

EDB *abbr* estimated date of birth.

EDD *abbr* expected date of delivery.

eddy currents are induced electric currents in a transformer core and oppose the direction of the current in the windings of a transformer resulting in a power loss in the transformer, they can be reduced by laminating the core. In magnetic resonance imaging (MRI) they are induced in the gradient coils or the structure of the magnet and degrade the image unless compensated for or eliminated.

edentate having no natural teeth.

edentulous *adj* toothless. Without natural teeth in the mouth, as when born or following total tooth clearance.

edge-to-edge articulation articulation of the anterior teeth along their incisal edges.

edge-to-edge bite a malocclusion in which the mandibular and maxillary incisors occlude along their incisal edges and do not overlap.

edge-to-edge occlusion an occlusion in which the anterior teeth of the jaws meet along their incisal edge when the teeth are in centric occlusion.

edgewise appliance ⊃ orthodontic appliance.

edgewise bracket an orthodontic bracket used in fixed orthodontic appliances having a horizontal channel or slot, most commonly 0.018 or 0.022 inch wide. Designed to receive a rectangular, square or round wire.

Edinger–Westphal nucleus (*syn* accessory oculomotor nucleus, accessory parasympathetic nucleus) part of the oculomotor nucleus, it is situated posterior to the main nucleus and contains the parasympathetic component of the complex. Axons from the Edinger–Westphal pass out along the oculomotor nerve (third cranial nerve) to synapse in the ciliary ganglion. Postganglionic fibres pass through the short ciliary nerves to the sphincter pupillae and ciliary muscles. The nucleus also receives fibres concerned with accommodation and fibres from the pretectal nucleus dealing with pupillary light reflexes. ⊃ ciliary ganglion, ciliary muscle, oculomotor nerve, pupillary light reflex, sphincter pupillae muscle.

EDRF *abbr* endothelium-derived relaxing factor. ⊃ nitric oxide.

Edridge–Green lantern an occupational colour vision test which consists of small round and variable sized coloured lights produced by coloured and neutral density filters. ⊃ defective colour vision, lantern test.

edrophonium test a test for myasthenia gravis, a small intramuscular dose of edrophonium chloride will immediately relieve symptoms, albeit temporarily, while quinine sulphate will increase the muscular weakness. Resuscitation drugs and equipment must be available, as respiratory depression may occur.

EDSS *abbr* expanded disability status scale.

EDTA *abbr* ethylene diamine tetra-acetic acid.

EDV *abbr* end diastolic volume.

Edwards' syndrome (J Edwards, British medical geneticist, b.1928) (*syn* trisomy 18) an autosomal trisomy of chromosome number 18 resulting in cells with 47 chromosomes. It is associated with characteristic skull and facial appearance (e.g. low-set ears, small eyes and micrognathia), frequent malformations of the heart, kidneys and other organs, growth retardation and learning disability.

EEG *abbr* electroencephalogram ⊃ electroencephalograph.

EFAs *abbr* essential fatty acids.

EFSA *abbr* European Food Safety Authority.

effacement of cervix ⊃ cervical effacement.

effective current the value of current flowing for the same time that would produce the same electrical energy in a circuit as the equivalent alternating current.

effective dose 1. the amount of a drug that can be expected to initiate a specific intensity of effect in people taking the drug. **2.** a calculation to determine that amount of radiation received by a patient, for radiation protection purposes, which is weighted for each organ because different organs in the body show different sensitivity to radiation.

effective half-life the time taken for a combination of radioactive decay and biological processes for the activity of a radionuclide in an organ to be reduced to half its original activity. ⊃ half-life ($t_{1/2}$)

effectiveness *n* describes using the available resources to achieve the required outcomes. One of the three 'Es' of value for money. ⊃ economy, efficiency, value for money.

effective photon energy the energy of a homogeneous beam of photons having the same half value layer as the X-ray beam being evaluated.

effective power the power of a lens or surface measured in a plane other than the principal plane and usually remote from the lens or surface. If a thin lens or surface of power F is illuminated by parallel incident light, the effective power F_x of another lens placed at a distance d from the original lens and forming an image in the same position, is given by the equation:

$$F_x = \frac{F}{1 - dF}$$

where d is in metres and positive when measured from left to right. ⊃ principal plane, refractive error, vertex distance.

effective voltage the value of voltage flowing for the same time that would produce the same electrical energy in a circuit as the equivalent alternating voltage.

effector *n* a motor or secretory nerve ending in a muscle, gland or organ. They stimulate muscle contraction or glandular secretion.

efferent *adj* 'going away'. Carrying, conveying, conducting away from a centre, such as motor nerves that carry nerve impulses away from the brain and spinal cord (central nervous system) to muscles or glands. Also describes blood or lymph vessels in which flow is away from some point of reference, e.g. efferent arterioles leaving the glomeruli of the kidney. ⊃ afferent *opp*.

efferent fibre a nerve fibre conducting impulses from the brain or spinal cord.

effervescent material used in radiotherapy to make an immobilizing device by placing the patient on an empty polythene bag, introducing the self hardening material and producing an impression of the patient's position, the impression can then be used during treatment to exactly replicate the patient position.

efficiency *n* **1.** the ratio of energy (or work) output by a body or device to the energy input required. ⟿ mechanical efficiency. **2.** describes the use of minimum resources to achieve the maximum outcomes. One of the three 'Es' of value for money. ⟿ economy, effectiveness, value for money.

effleurage *n* a massage manipulation, using long, whole-hand strokes in the direction of venous and lymphatic drainage, that aims to help venous return to the heart and the reduction of oedema. Deep effleurage causes dilatation of the arterioles by stimulating the axon reflex.

effort continua subjective response that occurs to an exercise stimulus that involves the three elements—physiological, perceptual and performance.

effort syndrome a form of anxiety disorder, manifesting itself in a variety of cardiac symptoms including chest pain, palpitations, dizziness, for which no pathological explanation can be discovered.

effusion *n* extravasation of fluid into body tissues or cavities, such as a pleural effusion, or into joints where it causes swelling. In sport a joint effusion is a sign of significant damage to the joint. A knee filled with blood, rather than with joint (synovial) fluid, is called a haemarthrosis, an injury requiring immediate care (e.g. cruciate ligament damage in the knee).

EFM *abbr* electronic fetal monitor.

EGF *abbr* epidermal growth factor.

ego *n* one of the three main aspects of the personality (the others being the id and superego); refers to the conscious self, the 'I', which according to Freud, deals with reality; is influenced by social forces and controls unconscious instinctual urges. ⟿ id, superego. ⟿ Freud, Sigmund.

ego involvement a state in which the individual's goal is to demonstrate ability relative to that of others. ⟿ task involvement.

ego orientation a dispositional tendency to feel most successful in an activity only when one demonstrates one's ability relative to that of others, such as when one outperforms an opponent. ⟿ achievement goal orientation, task orientation.

ego strength the ability of the ego to deal with the demands of the id as well as the real world constraints. Traits, such as tolerance of disappointment and loss, forgiveness, compassion, being able to defer gratification, flexibility, perseverance, etc., are condidered to contribute to good mental health.

ego support the defences utilized by the ego to ensure that inner conflicts are resolved without overwhelming.

EHEC *abbr* enterohaemorrhagic *Escherichia coli*.

Ehlers–Danlos syndrome (E Ehlers, Danish dermatologist, 1863–1937; H Danlos, French physician, 1844–1921) a group of inherited conditions affecting connective tissues. It is inherited as a dominant autosomal trait. It may result from mutations in several genes including *COLIA2*, lysyl oxidase, fibronectin and elastin. Abnormal collagen production leads to skin that is very elastic with increased laxity, fragile and easily damaged. There is joint hypermobility that leads to joint injuries—sprains, dislocation and joint effusion. There is scoliosis and short stature and visceral vascular catastrophes. The ocular signs include blue sclera, eye elongation and myopia, angioid streaks, ectopia lentis, keratoconus and retinal detachment.

EIA *abbr* exercise induced asthma. ⟿ asthma.

eicosanoids a variety of compounds formed from long-chain polyunsaturated fatty acids, e.g. arachidonic acid. They include prostaglandins, prostacyclins, thromboxanes and leukotrienes. They are all important as intercellular signalling molecules and for platelet aggregation, inflammation, and many other physiological processes.

eicosapentaenoic acid (EPA) a 20-carbon long-chain omega-3 polyunsaturated fatty acid. Present in fish oils.

eicosenoic acids a group of 20-carbon long-chain polyunsaturated fatty acids.

eidetic image a vivid image, usually visual but it can be auditory. The image, which is very detailed, is very close to actual perception. The person is still able to scan a visual display even after the display is no longer present. The image may be recalled with photographic accuracy, long after the original experience. It is one form of illusion. ⟿ illusion, pareidolic

EIEC *abbr* enteroinvasive *Escherichia coli*.

Eisenmenger's complex (V Eisenmenger, German physician, 1864–1932) congenital heart defect with an abnormal shunt between the left and right sides of the heart, malposition of the aorta and an abnormal pulmonary artery.

Eisenmenger's syndrome/reaction (V Eisenmenger) a syndrome associated with a ventricular septal defect or Eisenmenger's complex. The increased blood flow through the left-to-right shunt damages the pulmonary blood vessels, changes pulmonary vascular resistance and leads to pulmonary hypertension. This eventually leads to back flow that increases the pressure in the right side of the heart. At a certain point the shunt is reversed to a right-to-left shunt. Affected individual will also develop polycythaemia.

EIT *abbr* electrically initiated torque.

ejaculation *n* sudden emission of semen from the penis at the moment of male orgasm. ⟿ retrograde ejaculation.

ejaculatory ducts two ducts formed from the combining of the deferent duct (vas deferens) and the duct from the seminal vesicle. They go through the prostate gland, conveying seminal fluid containing spermatozoa to the urethra. ⟿ Colour Section Figure 16.

ejection fraction the fraction or percentage of the total ventricular filling volume of blood that is pumped out in each ventricular contraction. A reduced ejection fraction may indicate systolic heart failure.

ejector that which removes or expels, e.g. saliva ejector used to remove fluids from the mouth.

elastic capable of recovering normal shape and size after having been stretched.

elastic band used in orthodontics to produce tooth movement. ➲ intermaxillary elastic band, intramaxillary elastic band.

elastic collisions the mutual attraction of atoms, molecules etc. when the total energy is unchanged after the collision. ➲ inelastic collisions.

elastic fibre a basic constituent of loose connective tissue, elastic cartilage and skin dermis.

elastic fibrocartilage (yellow) one of the three types of cartilage. Comprises yellow fibres in a solid matrix. It is flexible and is present in the pinna of outer/external ear, the middle coat of blood vessels and in the epiglottis, where it supports and maintains shape. ➲ cartilage.

elastic potential energy the energy due to changes in the distance between molecules of a body or object, usually when it is compressed (e.g. a spring) or stretched (e.g. an elastic band). In animal (human) movement, important sources of such energy are muscles and tendons.

elastic scattering when a photon interacts with an electron, is deflected from its path but does not lose energy. ➲ coherent scattering.

elasticity the ability of a material to be compressed or stretched, and to return to its original state.

elastin *n* the strutural protein forming the principal constituent of elastic tissue. A class of connective tissue fibres that can be readily stretched. Elastin gives tissues and organs elasticity. It is present in the walls of distensible vessels and organs, e.g. veins, bladder, etc. It is found in arteries, lungs, intestines and skin. In function it complements collagen, whereas collagen provides rigidity, elastin allows connective tissues to stretch and then recoil.

elastomer a polymer with rubber-like elastic properties.

elastomeric impression material impression material based on a non-aqueous polymeric system and which exhibits rubber-like elastic properties. e.g. the polysulphide, polyether and silicone impression materials. ➲ impression material.

elbow joint a hinge joint, allowing only flexion and extension, between the distal end of the humerus and the upper ends of the ulna and radius. The muscles involved are the biceps brachii and brachialis (flexion), and the triceps (extension). The joint is formed by the trochlea and the capitulum of the humerus and the trochlear notch of the ulna and the head of the radius. It is an extremely stable joint because the humeral and ulnar surfaces interlock, and the capsule is very strong. Extracapsular structures consist of anterior, posterior, medial and lateral strengthening ligaments, which contribute to joint stability. The prominent medial and lateral epicondyles of the humerus provide attachment for the major ligaments on the two sides of the joint: on the inside to the margin of the concave notch on the ulna, and on the outside to the ligament around the head of the radius. ➲ lateral epicondylitis (tennis elbow), medial epicondylitis (golfer's elbow, javelin thrower's elbow).

elder abuse physical (including neglect), sexual, psychological, pharmacological or financial abuse of older people. May be carried out by family and other carers, neighbours, or by health and social care staff.

elderly primigravida colloquial term describing a woman over the age of 35 years in her first pregnancy; carries little real meaning in clinical terms except that ascribed to it by some practitioners.

elective surgery planned surgery rather than that undertaken as an emergency.

Electra complex excessive emotional attachment of daughter to father. The name is derived from Greek mythology.

electrically initiated torque (EIT) a term used in electrotherapy. The torque produced by stimulating a muscle electrically. EIT is usually less than the maximal voluntary torque (MVT), but can be greater. Developed as a way of comparing the comfort and effectiveness of different types of currents, e.g. pulsed versus alternating currents with a range of parameters. Used as a ratio with maximal voluntary torque to indicate change in fatigue and effectiveness of electrode positioning, but not a reliable measure (EIT/MVT). ➲ maximal voluntary torque.

electrical potential at a point is the measure of the work required to bring a unit positive charge from infinity to that point.

electric circuit the diagrammatic representation of electron flow through an electrical device.

electric current the rate of flow of electrons in a material. An electric current of one ampere flows at a point if a charge of one coulomb flows past the point per second.

electric field the area surrounding an electrical charge, if an electric charge is placed inside the field a noticeable force will be exerted on it.

electric pulp tester in dentistry, an instrument used to help determine the vitality of teeth. When the patient indicates that he or she can appreciate small amounts of current applied to a tooth, then the degree of vitality is noted. Should always be used in combination with other diagnostic tests before a tooth is pronounced pulpless.

electric shock shock caused when an electric current passes through the body, usually caused by accidental contact with an electric supply.

electro- a prefix that means 'electricity', e.g. *electrocautery*.

electrocardiogram (ECG) *n* a recording of the electrical activity of the heart muscle during the cardiac cycle made by an electrocardiograph. The normal heart produces a typical waveform, sinus rhythm, which consists of five deflection waves, known universally as P-QRS-T. ➲ ambulatory electrocardiogram (Holter monitoring), exercise tolerance test (ETT), P-QRS-T complex.

electrocardiograph *n* an instrument that records the electrical activity of the heart from electrodes placed on the limbs, and on several positions on the chest (Figure E.2) — **electrocardiographic** *adj*, **electrocardiography** *n*, **electrocardiographically** *adv*.

electrocardiophonography a combined investigation that stimultaneously records heart sounds during the cardiac cycle, and the electrical activity with an electrocardiogram.

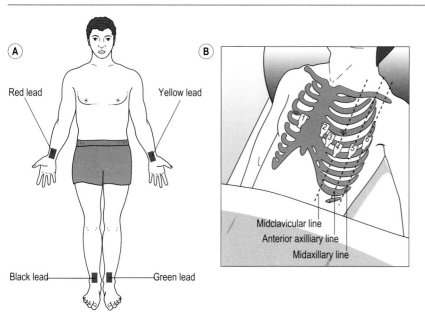

E.2 Electrocardiograph Position of (A) Limb leads (B) chest leads for 12-lead ECG (reproduced from Nicol et al 2004 with permission).

electrocautery a wire loop heated electrically to red heat and used to cauterize tissue.

electrocoagulation *n* technique of surgical diathermy. Coagulation, especially of bleeding points, by means of electrodes.

electrocochleography (ECoG) *n* direct recording of the action potential generated following stimulation of the cochlear nerve. ⊃ vestibulocochlear nerve.

electroconvulsive therapy (ECT) a physical treatment used in psychiatry, mainly in the treatment of severe/life-threatening depression or psychotic states. A device is used that delivers a definite electrical voltage for a precise fraction of a second to electrodes placed on the head, producing a convulsion. The convulsion is modified by use of an intravenous anaesthetic and a muscle relaxant prior to treatment. *unilateral ECT* avoids the sequela of amnesia for recent events. Memory for recent events is probably in the dominant cerebral hemisphere. ECT is therefore applied to the right hemisphere to reduce memory disturbance.

electrode *n* in medicine or therapy, a conductor in the form of a pad or plate, whereby electricity enters or leaves the body. In electrotherapy—means of applying the output current from a machine to the part of the body to be treated by electrical stimulation or for when amplifying bioelectrical signals, e.g. electromyogram (EMG), electroencephalogram (EEG), electrocardiogram (ECG). *types of electrode* for electrical stimulation include: reusable carbon rubber with purpose designed electrical stimulation gel or gel pads; metal (including aluminium and lead) used with moistened sponge or lint; self-adhesive; task-specific bare metal electrodes (e.g. anal or vaginal). *size of electrode* varies according to the aims and area being treated, whether both are the same or different sizes also depends upon the type of current and the aims; size affects current density, so if it is too small with a high average current, there is a high risk of skin burns. The location will vary with the aims of treatment. *number of electrodes* at least two per electrical circuit, four may be used (interferential or 2-channels concurrently) or, if using high-voltage pulsed stimulation (HVPS), may have one anode and two or more cathodes (bifurcated). *electrodes for amplification* the type, number and locations are usually quite different for EMG, EEG and ECG than for electrical stimulation. For example, for EMG biofeedback three small electrodes are typically used (one ground, two active along the line of the fibres). They may be separate or comprise a single tri-electrode pre-amplifier. ⊃ high-voltage pulsed stimulation.

electrodesiccation *n* fulguration. A technique of surgical diathermy. There is drying and subsequent removal of tissue. Used to remove superficial skin growths.

electrodiagnosis recording the electrical activity of electrically excitable body structures (spontaneous activity or following stimulation), as an aid to diagnosis, e.g. electrocardiography, electroencephalography, nerve conduction tests and evoked potentials (EP).

electrodiagnostic procedures (in optometry) methods such as the electroretinogram, the electro-oculogram and the visually evoked cortical potentials which are used to facilitate the diagnosis of some ocular diseases (e.g. retinitis pigmentosa) or the objective measurement of some visual functions (e.g. refractive error, visual acuity). ⊃ electro-oculography, electroretinography, visual-evoked cortical potential (VECP).

electroencephalogram (EEG) *n* a graphic recording of the various types of electrical activity occurring in the brain, made by an electroencephalograph. The device produces a trace of the brain waves—alpha, beta, delta and theta rhythms. It is used to investigate seizures and sleep disorders.

electroencephalograph *n* an instrument by which electrical activity derived from the brain can be amplified and recorded, in a fashion similar to that of the electrocardiograph. Electrodes are applied to various parts of the scalp—**electroencephalographic** *adj*, **electroencephalography** *n*, **electroencephalographically** *adv*.

electrogoniometer a device for measuring angles (usually joint angles) directly, giving an electrical output (often interfaced to a computer).

electroluminescence ⊃ luminescence.

electrolysis *n* **1.** chemical decomposition by electricity, with ion movement shown by changes at the electrodes. **2.** term used for the destruction of individual hairs (epilation), removal of moles, spider naevi, etc., using electricity.

electrolyte *n* a solution of a substance, such as sodium chloride, which dissociates into ions with an electrical charge—anions (negative charge) and cations (positive charge). Applies to those in the body fluids, where dissociated sodium chloride is the major electrolyte in extracellular fluids ([Na^+] and [Cl^-]), and potassium [K^+], with organic anions, in intracellular fluids. Other physiologically important cations are calcium and magnesium, and the anions bicarbonate (hydrogen carbonate) and phosphate. Normal electrolyte concentrations are essential for normal cellular function. Movements of ions are crucial in the maintenance of potential differences across cell membranes and, for example, in the generation and transmission of nervous impulses, neuromuscular and synaptic transmission, and all secretory function—**electrolytic** *adj*.

electrolyte balance the balance of relative amounts of electrolytes, e.g. potassium, sodium, magnesium, calcium, chloride, bicarbonate and phosphate in blood, other fluids and tissues. The balance between ions with a positive charge (cations), e.g. potassium, and those with a negative charge (anions), e.g. chloride, ensures overall electrical neutrality in the body. Many conditions and diseases cause electrolyte imbalance, which is often associated with loss of fluid and pH homeostasis. Exercise-induced disturbances in electrolyte balance are mainly related to either increase or decrease in concentration of sodium [Na^+], the most abundant cation in the extracellular fluids. Increase in plasma [Na^+] (hypernatraemia) is associated with depletion of blood volume by severe sweat loss and is common in athletes at the end of long-distance races. Exercise-associated decrease in plasma [Na^+] (hyponatraemia) is not uncommonly seen after prolonged activity such as a marathon where runners, aware of the importance of adequate fluid intake and rehydration, overcompensate with low-sodium drinks or excessive plain water (water intoxication). This can result in significant hyponatraemia, leading at worst to cardiovascular collapse and death. ⊃ anion, anion gap, cation, hydration status of athletes, sports drinks.

electrolytic polishing a process in which a metal is placed in an electrolytic solution and an electric current passed through it. Very minute particles of the surface of the metal are removed by electrolysis so leaving a polished surface.

electrolytic silver recovery a method for recovering silver from radiographic fixer solution using a carbon anode and a stainless steel cathode, a direct current is passed between the two and the positively charged silver ions are attracted to the cathode where they are neutralized and form metallic silver, either a low or a high current density is used.

electromagnet is formed when a piece of soft iron is placed inside a solenoid resulting in induced magnetism within the iron bar.

electromagnetic radiation waves of energy that are caused by the acceleration of charged particles.

electromagnetic spectrum the ordering of electromagnetic radiation into the various wavelengths and frequencies. It extends from the longest radio waves of some thousands of metres in wavelength through radar, microwave, infrared rays, visible rays (between wavelengths 780 nm and 380 nm) to ultraviolet rays, X-rays, gamma rays and cosmic rays with wavelengths as short as 8×10^{-12} mm. All these electromagnetic waves differ only in frequency (and wavelength) but have the same speed as light in a vacuum. ⊃ infrared radiations/rays (IRR), ultraviolet (UV) rays, wavelength.

electromechanical dissociation (EMD) older term for pulseless electrical activity (PEA). ⊃ cardiac arrest, pulseless electrical activity.

electromotive force (EMF) measures the force needed for an electric current to flow between two points. A derived Système International d'Unités (SI) unit (International System of Units), the volt (V), is used. ⊃ Appendix 2.

electromyography (EMG) *n* the use of an instrument which records electric currents generated in contracting muscle. The recording of electrical activity of muscle either percutaneously, with adhesive pad electrodes (more common but can only be applied to superficial muscles), or intramuscularly, through fine wires, usually of platinum, insulated except at their tips (records from a smaller domain within a muscle, but not necessarily a superficial one). Electromyography (EMG) is used in both normal and pathophysiology to study the timing of muscle activation, as well as its extent, to which the resultant force generation is approximately proportionate. The trace recorded is the electromyogram. *integrated EMG* electronically processed modification of the direct signal from the electrodes. As muscle action potentials pass under the electrodes they will each go positive and negative by turns, making a 'biphasic' (AC) signal; to integrate this, the signal is first rectified and then smoothed with a time constant such that the trace produced looks similar in form to a mechanical record of the resulting contraction (Figure E.3)—**electromyographical** *adj*, **electromyogram** *n*, **electromyograph** *n*, **electromyographically** *adv*.

electromyography biofeedback an electrotherapy term. The use of amplified bioelectrical signals from motor unit activity as a form of feedback. Used to increase or decrease level of motor unit activity. For example, used to retrain

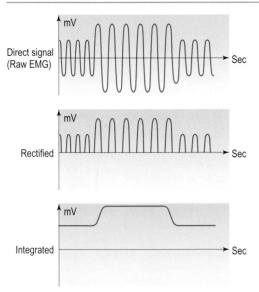

E.3 Electromyogram (diagrammatic) (reproduced from Jennett 2008 with permission).

movement after stroke and to decrease muscle activity associated with headaches. ⊃ electrode.

electromyogram the trace that is recorded during electromyography (EMG). *integrated EMG* electronically processed modification of the direct signal from the electrodes. As muscle action potentials pass under the electrodes they will each go positive and negative by turns, making a 'biphasic' (AC) signal; to integrate this, the signal is first rectified and then smoothed with a time constant such that the trace produced looks similar in form to a mechanical record of the resulting contraction.

electron *n* a negatively charged subatomic particle.

electron capture the capture of an electron by the nucleus of an atom, the electron combines with a proton to form a neutron and a neutrino which is ejected from the nucleus.

electron gun a piece of equipment that produces electrons by heating a spiral filament and then focussing them to form an electron beam.

electronically evoked twitch an investigation that involves the application of an electrical stimulus to a motor nerve adjacent to the muscle. Used to provide information about the maximal inherent muscle force.

electronic apex locator ⊃ apex locator.

electronic bibliography software many undergraduate and postgraduate students now choose electronic reference management systems such as EndNote®, Reference Manager® or ProCite® to help them search Internet libraries to capture relevant references to create their own personal databases and automatically generate and format in-text citations and bibliographies within their word processed papers. Rather than spending hours finding and managing references using traditional methods or creating and editing bibliographies manually, students may now turn to reference-management tools to save time, improve their accuracy

and streamline the whole writing process. For those already using bibliographic software, reference management has now been taken one step further with RefViz™: a new text analysis and visualization software package that lets the user visually evaluate the relevance of references. If documents feature technical or scientific content, it is worth considering investing in sciPROOF™: the scientific author's proofreading tool.

electronic callipers a method of measurement used to calculate the distance between two points identified during ultrasound imaging.

electronic collimation used in positron emission tomography (PET) cameras when an image is only recorded when two detectors simultaneously detect a photon of energy. ⊃ positron emission tomography.

electronic fetal monitor (EFM) a method of recording fetal heart activity by applying an electrode to the scalp. Uterine activity is recorded at the same time. The machine to which the electrode is attached can make the pulse audible and transmit it as a graphic record on paper.

electronic health record a computerized summary of a patient's health record showing all their interactions with general practitioners and primary care healthcare workers.

electronic patient record a computerized summary of all a patient's healthcare both in a primary and secondary care setting including written records, test results and medical images, for example, radiographs, scans, photographs, etc.

electronic portal imaging (EPI) a method of capturing an image digitally in real time and the image is superimposed on the original radiotherapy simulation film or image to verify the accuracy of the field placement.

electronic timer ⊃ timer.

electron microscope a microscope in which a beam of electrons replaces the beam of light of a simple microscope, enabling magnification up to 500 000 times to be achieved. ⊃ electron microscopy, microscope.

electron microscopy the use of a beam of electrons to visualize very small structures, such as virus particles. It may involve a *transmission electron microscope* or a *scanning electron microscope* (SEM). ⊃ microscope.

electron shells the orbits round the nucleus of an atom where the electrons are found in discrete levels, K is the nearest orbit to the nucleus and they are then labelled M, N, O, P etc.

electron transfer/transport chain a series of mitochondrial oxidation-reduction reactions that transfer electrons in order to generate cellular energy as adenosine triphosphate (ATP). A group of specific carrier molecules in the inner mitochondrial membrane transfer electrons from hydrogen to oxygen. The electrochemical energy generated via the electron transport is transferred to adenosine diphosphate (ADP) to reform ATP. ⊃ Krebs' cycle, oxidative phosphorylation.

electron trap an area of low energy within a crystal which has the ability to catch and hold an electron for a period of time before it acquires the energy to escape.

electro-oculography *n* the use of an instrument which records eye position and movement, and potential difference between front and back of the eyeball using electrodes placed on the skin near the eye. Can be used as a diagnostic test of retinal function—**electro-oculogram (EOG)** *n*.

electrophoresis *n* a technique where charged particles are separated in a liquid medium by their characteristic speed and direction of migration in an electrical field.

electrophysical agents (EPAs) an electrotherapy term. The methods of treatment using electrical stimulation or physical agents such as heat, cold, ultrasound, laser and ultraviolet radiations. Two agents also used diagnostically with appropriate equipment: ultrasound (for visualization of subcutaneous tissues) and ultraviolet radiations (for diagnosis of some skin conditions).

electroretinography *n* the use of an instrument to measure electrical currents generated in the retina stimulated by light—**electroretinogram (ERG)** *n*.

electrosurgery *n* the use of electrical devices that work on high-frequency electrical current during surgical procedures. ⊃ electrocoagulation, electrodesiccation.

electrotherapy *n* in physiotherapy. The use of electrophysical agents (EPAs), each producing different frequencies and waveforms, in treatments, e.g. short-wave diathermy, transcutaneous electrical nerve stimulation, interferential therapy, or laser may be used for musculoskeletal problems. Used in the treatment of injury, for the relief of pain or other therapeutic applications to stimulate tissue healing and restore function. Though the exact mechanism of action remains unclear, electrotherapy is used in physiotherapy to enhance natural healing. The various forms are used, as appropriate, to treat injury to different tissue types and at different stages. Electrical stimulation has been shown to block transmission of pain and promote endorphin release. In the USA the term refers to the use of electrical stimulation only.

element *n* a substance that cannot be broken down by chemical means into any other substance, each atom in the element contains a specific number of protons in the nucleus, a variable number of neutrons in the nucleus and a given number of electrons outside the nucleus. One of the constituents of a compound. The elements (e.g. carbon, sodium, iron and so on) are the primary substances which in pure form, or in combinations as compounds, constitute all matter.

elephantiasis *n* the swelling of a limb, usually a leg, as a result of lymphatic obstruction (lymphoedema), followed by thickening of the skin (pachyderma) and subcutaneous tissues. A complication of filariasis in tropical countries. ⊃ *Filaria*, filariasis, lymphoedema.

elephantiasis gingivae also known as gingival fibromatosis, idiopathic gingival hyperplasia ⊃ fibromatosis.

elevate to remove, by elevating or lifting. Such as, teeth or roots from the alveolus using an elevator. ⊃ elevator (dental).

elevated post-exercise oxygen consumption (EPOC) also known as excess post-exercise oxygen consumption.

Estimates the post-exercise elevation in resting metabolic rate. The duration and rate of EPOC depend on duration and intensity of the preceding exercise, training status, environmental circumstances, gender and other variables. Although the contribution of EPOC to daily energy expenditure is negligible, it may contribute to the regulation of energy balance and play a role in body mass reduction or maintenance. ⊃ oxygen debt.

elevation *n* an upward movement such as the scapulae when the shoulders are lifted. Or the positioning of a body part, such as a limb to reduce swelling.

elevator (dental) an instrument to lever tissues from each other. *apical elevator* a set of three elevators—right, left and straight—having hollow handles, small blades and long shanks. *Boyd Gardner elevator* right and left elevators with hollow handles. *Cryer's elevator* right and left elevators with triangular sharp-pointed blades and hollow handles. *Hospital pattern (Coleman) elevator* left, right, and straight serrated broad-bladed instruments with heavy serrated hollow handles. *Warwick James elevator* small-bladed, left, right, and straight elevators with flat, smooth handles. *Winter elevator* a set of paired levers, with corkscrew handles and various shaped blades. All elevators must be sterile when used and their pointed blades kept sharp for each operation. Hollow-handled elevators should not be placed in a dry heat sterilizer.

elimination *n* the passage of waste from the body—urine and faeces—**eliminate** *vt*.

ELISA *abbr* enzyme-linked immunosorbent assay.

elite athlete world-class performer in any physical sport.

elixir *n* a sweetened, aromatic solution of a drug, often containing alcohol.

ellipsoid joint a synovial joint that allows flexion, extension, abduction and adduction, for example, wrist joint.

elliptocytosis (ovalocytosis) *n* elliptical red blood cells. Characteristic of hereditary elliptocytosis, a rare congenital haemolytic anaemia. Also a feature of some anaemias, and a few ($<15\%$) may be present in normal blood. ⊃ hereditary elliptocytosis.

Ellis–van Creveld syndrome (R Ellis, British paediatrician, 1902–1966; S van Creveld, Dutch paediatrician, 1894–1971). ⊃ chondroectodermal dysplasia.

elongation in radiography, a distortion of an image in which the teeth appear longer than their true size, caused by incorrect angulation of the central beam in the bisecting angle technique. ⊃ bisecting angle technique.

eluting solution a liquid used to remove another substance by washing, used in a technetium generator where the eluting solution, saline, washes out the pertechnetate as sodium pertechnetate solution.

Ely's test a musculoskeletal test. Performed in cases of suspected rectus femoris tightness, the patient lies prone while the physiotherapist passively flexes the knee. If passive full knee flexion is attained the physiotherapist then passively moves the hip into extension, if during this the patient simultaneously flexes their hip then the rectus femoris is tight.

em- a prefix that means 'in', e.g. empyema.

emaciation *n* excessive leanness, or wasting of body tissue, such as that caused by malnutrition or widespread cancer—**emaciate** *vt*.

emancipation the politics of eliminating or reducing oppression, inequality, injustice and exploitation. It is the liberation of individuals and groups from the constraints and unequal power relations that limit their life chances and quality of life.

emasculation *n* castration.

Embden–Meyerhof pathway (G Embden; O Meyerhof) an important metabolic pathway in which a sequence of reactions convert glucose to pyruvate to generate adenosine triphosphate (ATP). Usually known as glycolysis.

embed in histology, the technique of fixing friable tissue in some rigid material, such as wax, so that thin sections may be prepared for microscopic examination.

embolectomy *n* surgical removal of an embolus from an artery, such as a limb artery, carotid artery, the aorta or pulmonary artery. Usually a fine balloon (Fogarty) catheter is used to extract the embolus, or the artery is opened during arteriotomy to faciltate removal of the obstruction.

embolic *adj* pertaining to an embolism or an embolus.

embolism *n* obstruction of a blood vessel by a body of undissolved material. Usually caused by a thrombus (clot), but other causes include cancer cells, fat, amniotic fluid, gases, bacteria and parasites. Rarer emboli, such as fat, may follow long bone fractures, air may enter the circulation via a penetrating chest wound or during surgery, and amniotic fluid during labour. The most common type is a thromboembolus that originates in the deep veins of the legs or pelvis, which travels in the veins, through the right side of the heart to lodge in a pulmonary artery—a pulmonary embolus. *arterial (systemic) embolism*, originating from the left side of the heart, such as with atrial fibrillation, or as a result of arterial disease, may travel to various sites including brain, bowel or a limb; the effects dependent on the size of vessel affected and site, e.g. gangrene of a limb or a portion of bowel. ⊃ cerebrovascular accident, deep vein thrombosis, fat embolism, pulmonary embolism.

embolization *n* therapeutic occlusion of a blood vessel using a foreign substance, such as polyvinyl alcohol or tiny coils. The minimally invasive technique is used to reduce menorrhagia caused by uterine fibroids, treat severe or recurrent epistaxis, aneurysms and arteriovenous malformations.

embologenic *adj* capable of producing an embolus.

embolus *n* solid body or gas bubble transported in the circulation. ⊃ embolism—**emboli** *pl*.

embouchure the position and use of the tongue, lips and teeth in the playing of wind instruments.

embrasure an opening, such as that between the proximal surfaces of the teeth.

embrocation *n* a liquid applied topically by rubbing.

embryo *n* developmental stage starting two weeks after fertilization until the end of week eight of gestation. The stage marked by rapid increase in size, cell differentiation and organ formation (organogenesis)—**embryonic** *adj*.

embryo/fetal reduction a number of healthy, embryos/fetuses in a multiple pregnancy are destroyed (but remain in the uterus until the end of pregancy) in order to increase the chances of survival for the one, two or three embryos left in place. It may be offered to couples who have conceived triplets or more, either naturally or after assisted conception treatments.

embryology *n* study of embryonic development—**embryological** *adj*, **embryologically** *adv*.

embryoma *n* ⊃ teratoma.

embryonic fissure ⊃ optic fissure.

embryonic plate part of inner cell mass of the blastocyst from which the embryo is formed.

embryopathy *n* abnormality or disease of the embryo—**embryopathic** *adj*.

embryoscopy *n* visualization of the embryo around the 9th weeks of gestation. It uses a small, specialized fibreoptic endoscope to examine the embryo through the intact sac of membranes. The endoscope may be inserted transabdominally, or transcervically. Usually used for couples from families who suffer from genetic disorders that can be identified from the appearance of the embryo. ⊃ fetoscopy.

embryotomy *n* a procedure that involves the destruction of the fetus to facilitate delivery. Very rarely performed.

EMD *abbr* electromechanical dissociation.

EMEA *abbr* European Medicines Agency.

emergency contraception postcoital contraception. Popularly referred to as the 'morning after' pill. A single dose of levonorgestrel (available without prescription) administered orally within 72 hours of unprotected intercourse, or the insertion of a copper-containing intrauterine contraceptive device within 5 days.

emergency obstetric unit emergency team from a consultant maternity unit comprising obstetrician, midwife, anaesthetist and/or paediatrician, who go by ambulance to emergencies in the home or small maternity hospitals. They take emergency equipment such as O Rhesus-negative blood, equipment for blood transfusion, operative delivery, manual removal of the placenta, anaesthesia (if required) and maternal and neonatal resuscitation.

Emergency Protection Order (EPO) an order issued by the court when they believe that a child may suffer significant harm. It transfers parental responsibility rights and allows for the child's removal to a safe place.

emery an abrasive powder, containing aluminium oxide and magnetite, used to smooth and polish metals. An impure form of corundum.

Emery–Dreifuss muscular dystrophy (A Emery, British geneticist, b.1928; F Dreifuss, British neurologist, 1926–1997) a muscular dystrophy inherited as an X-linked recessive condition; there are mutations in the emerin gene. The onset occurs between the ages of 4–5 years. Muscles affected are humero-peroneal and later proximal limb girdle. There is early development of contractures. Cardiac involvement leads to sudden death.

emesis *n* vomiting.

emetic *n* any agent used to produce vomiting.

emetogenic *adj* term that describes substances that cause vomiting, such as ipecacuanha used after certain types of poisoning, or may do so, e.g. cancer chemotherapy.

EMF *abbr* electromotive force.

EMG *abbr* electromyogram.

eminence *n* a rounded projection on a bone, such as the iliopectineal eminence on the hip bone.

emissary veins *npl* veins that connect the venous sinuses in the dura mater to veins on the outside of the skull.

emission *n* **1.** an ejaculation or sending forth, especially an involuntary ejaculation of semen. **2.** in physics, all bodies emit electromagnetic radiation but a black body is the most efficient. In an intensifying screen when the light photons leave the screen and expose the film emulsion.

EMLA *abbr* eutectic mixture of local anaesthetics.

emmenagogue any substance which may induce vaginal bleeding—**emmenagoguic** *adj*.

emmetropia *n* normal refractive power of the eye, such that light from a distant object forms a clear image on the retina without accommodative effort—**emmetropic** *adj*.

Emmet's operation surgical repair of a perineal or cervical tear.

emollient *adj, n* (an agent) which moisturizes and soothes skin or mucous membrane. Emollients are oil-based substances that are used when dry skin is a problem, such as in some skin diseases (e.g. eczema) and that resulting from normal age changes. The emollient replaces the natural substances that normally waterproof the skin and minimize water loss from the skin surface.

emotion *n* the tone of feeling recognized in ourselves by certain physiological changes, and in others by tendencies to certain characteristic behaviour. Aroused usually by ideas or concepts. A short-term positive or negative affective state. Typically differentiated from mood in that an emotion is of shorter duration and evoked in response to a specific event, such as anger.

emotional *adj* characteristic of or caused by emotion.

emotional bias tendency of emotional attitude to affect logical judgement.

emotional intelligence ability to effectively manage one's emotional life and to read and respond appropriately to other people's emotions.

emotional lability ⊃ lability.

emotional state effect of emotions on normal mood, e.g. agitation, depressed mood.

empathy *n* identifying oneself with another person or understanding the meaning and significance of the actions of another person. Having some understanding of their situation, feelings and experiences. Described as having awareness of and insight into the biopsychosocial experiences of another person. A vital component of a therapeutic relationship—**empathic** *adj*.

emphysema *n* gaseous distension of the tissues. ⊃ crepitation, pulmonary emphysema, surgical emphysema—**emphysematous** *adj*.

empirical *adj* describes treatment or management based on observation and experience rather than on scientific reasoning.

empirical treatment ⊃ treatment.

empowerment the acquisition of knowledge and skills that leads to personal development and growth. The enabling processes whereby people increase the control, authority and power that they have over decisions that influence how they live. Such as, when a person with a learning disability acquires the skills needed to live independently, or make individual decisions about, for example, what clothes they select to wear. Another example is the philosophy that women should be empowered during pregnancy, labour and the puerperium to take control over their own care and to work in partnership with maternity care providers.

empty follicle syndrome a condition in which there are no oocytes in a Graafian follicle.

empyema *n* pus in the pleural cavity.

EMRSA *abbr* epidemic meticillin (methicillin)-resistant *Staphylococcus aureus*.

EMS *abbr* early morning stiffness.

empty can test also known as supraspinatus test. Performed in sitting or standing 90° of shoulder abduction bilaterally, full available medial rotation and 30° horizontal flexion. The supraspinatus muscle is the main support for the suspended arm in this position. The physiotherapist resists abduction of the shoulder. Pain on resistance is a positive test for a lesion of the supraspinatus muscle or tendon.

emulsifying agents substances soluble in both water and fat. They facilitate the formation of an emulsion as fat is uniformly dispersed in water.

emulsion *n* **1.** the mixture of two immiscible liquids, e.g water and fat. The uniform suspension of fat or oil particles in an aqueous continuous phase (*O/W emulsion*) or aqueous droplets in an oily continuous phase (*W/O emulsion*). **2.** in radiography, the part of a radiographic film formed by light-sensitive salts, for example silver halides in a gelatine binder, that records the radiographic image. **3.** the sensitivity of a radiographic film to radiation exposure.

en- a prefix that means 'in, into, within', e.g. *encysted*.

enablement the process of creating opportunities for individuals and communities to develop effective coping strategies, to achieve what is important to them and to participate more fully in life situations through activity.

enamel *n* hard, acellular calcified tissue covering the anatomical crown of a tooth. ⊃ dental enamel, tooth.

enamel chisel a dental chisel usually single ended, except for marginal trimmers.

enamel rod a near-parallel rod or prism forming tooth enamel.

enarthrosis *n* a ball and socket joint in which the head of one bone articulates in a depression on another. For example, the head of femur articulates in the cup-like acetabulum of the pelvis. A type of freely movable joint or diarthrosis, which allows the greatest range of motion.

encapsulated enclosed within a capsule.

encapsulated alloy proportioned quantities of alloy and mercury separated in a capsule, the mercury being contained beneath a foil which is broken to allow mechanical mixing, so producing a standard property amalgam. ⊃ alloy.

encapsulated amalgam alloy preproportioned amalgam alloy and mercury supplied in a capsule which provides a standard mix.

encapsulation *n* enclosure within a capsule, such as an organ, a cancer, or a micro-organism.

encephalins *npl* ⊃ enkephalins.

encephalitis *n* inflammation of the brain; usually viral but can be bacterial. It may follow an infectious illness such as measles or influenza. A serious condition in which severe inflammation can result in neurological sequelea such as seizures or even death.

encephalitis lethargica also known as epidemic encephalitis or 'sleepy/sleeping sickness'. A worldwide pandemic (1917–1928) killed many millions of people and left others with severe neurological problems including postencephalitic Parkinson's disease. Sporadic cases still occur.

encephalocele *n* protrusion of brain substance through a congenital defect in the skull. Also associated with hydrocephalus when the protrusion occurs at a suture line. ⊃ neural tube defect.

encephalography *n* a general term for techniques used to examine the brain. ⊃ echoencephalography, electroencephalography, pneumoencephalography, ventriculography—**encephalogram** *n*.

encephaloid *adj* resembling brain tissue.

encephalomalacia *n* softening of the brain.

encephalomyelitis *n* inflammation of the brain and spinal cord. ⊃ encephalitis.

encephalomyelopathy *n* disease affecting both brain and spinal cord—**encephalomyelopathic** *adj*.

encephalon *n* the brain and its component parts—cerebrum, cerebellum, pons and medulla oblongata.

encephalopathy *n* any disease of the brain causing reduced levels of arousal and cognitive function, such as Wernicke's encephalopathy—**encephalopathic** *adj*.

encephalotrigeminal angiomatosis ⊃ Sturge–Weber syndrome.

enchondroma *n* a benign tumour of cartilage—**enchondromata** *pl*.

encopresis *n* the repeated involuntary or voluntary passage of faeces in inappropriate places, such as faecal soiling of clothing, or on the floor, by a child over 4 years of age who was previously continent. In many cases it is associated with prolonged constipation, with faecal impaction and leakage of liquid faeces. It may also be associated with neurological problems, surgery, or psychological disorders that include conduct disorder or oppositional defiant disorder—**encopretic** *adj, n*.

encounter group a form of psychotherapy. Small groups of individuals focus on becoming aware of their feelings and developing the ability to express them openly, honestly and with clarity. The objectives are to increase self-awareness, promote personal growth and improve interpersonal skills.

encryption a method of encoding computer data to prevent unauthorized people having access to the information.

encysted *adj* contained within a cyst or capsule.

endarterectomy *n* the surgical removal of an atheromatous core from an artery, along with the intimal lining sometimes called disobliteration or 'rebore'. It may be a *disobliterative endarterectomy,* or carbon dioxide gas can be used to separate the occlusive core in a *gas endarterectomy.*

endarteritis *n* inflammation of the intima or inner lining coat of an artery.

endarteritis obliterans the new intimal connective tissue obliterates the lumen.

end artery a terminal artery. An artery that does not join another blood vessel, it terminates in a body structure or organ, e.g. the retinal artery, which is completely dependent on the artery for its blood supply. Occlusion of an end artery leads to tissue damage due to ischaemia.

end-diastolic volume (EDV) the volume of blood in the cardiac ventricles at the end of diastole. ⊃ stroke volume.

endemic *adj* recurring in an area, particularly a disease that is always present in an area, e.g. a particular communicable disease such as the common cold. ⊃ epidemic *opp*.

endemic syphilis also known as non-veneral syphilis. Usually found in children, the infection is spread by skin-to-skin contact or from contaminated drinking vessels. Features similar to those of syphilis. ⊃ bejel, endemic treponematoses, pinta, yaws.

endemic treponematoses the non-venereal treponemal diseases—endemic (non-venereal) syphilis (bejel), yaws and pinta are caused by treponemes morphologically indistinguishable from *Treponema pallidum* that cannot be differentiated by serological tests. A Veneral Diseases Research Laboratory (VDRL) or rapid plasma regin (RPR) test may help to elucidate the correct diagnosis because adults with late yaws usually have low titres. They generally affect people living in rural communities in underdeveloped countries. Transmission occurs by skin contact in childhood. ⊃ bejel, pinta, yaws.

endemiology *n* the special study of endemic diseases.

end, endo, ent, ento- a prefix that means 'inner, within', e.g. *endoderm.*

end feel during passive movements, the end feel is noted. Different joints and different pathologies have different end feels. The quality of the resistance felt at the end of range was categorized by Cyriax (1982): (a) bony block to movement or hard feel is characteristic of arthritic joints; (b) an empty feel or no resistance offered at the end of range may be due to severe pain associated with infection, active inflammation and tumours; (c) a springy block is characterized by a rebound feel at the end of range and is associated with torn meniscus blocking knee extension; (d) spasm is experienced as sudden, relatively hard feel associated with muscle guarding; and (e) capsular feel:

E
F

a hardish arrest of movement. (Cyriax J 1982 Illustrated manual of orthopaedic medicine. Butterworth Heinemann, Oxford).

endobronchial tube plastic double-lumen tube introduced via the mouth into either of the two main bronchi in thoracic anaesthesia.

endocardial mapping the recording of electrical potentials from various sites on the endocardium to determine the origin of cardiac arrhythmias.

endocarditis *n* inflammation of the inner lining of the heart (endocardium) and heart valves due to infection by microorganisms (bacteria, fungi or *Rickettsia*), or to rheumatic fever. There may be temporary or permanent damage to the heart valves. ⊃ infective endocarditis.

endocardium *n* the smooth layer of flattened endothelial cells that line the chambers of the heart. In health the smoothness of the endocardium prevents turbulence, which could lead to the formation of blood clots. It is continuous with the endothelium lining the blood vessels that carry blood to and from the heart.

endocervical *adj* pertaining to the inside of the cervix uteri.

endocervicitis *n* inflammation of the mucous membrane lining the cervix uteri.

endochondral *adj* relating to the tissue within the cartilage.

endocrine *adj* secreting internally. ⊃ autocrine, exocrine *opp*, paracrine—**endocrinal** *adj*.

endocrine glands the ductless glands that produce hormones which pass directly into the blood or lymph to influence distant structures. They include the hypothalamus, pineal body (gland), pituitary, thyroid, parathyroids (4), thymus, adrenal cortex and medulla (2), ovaries (2), testes (2) and pancreas (has both endocrine and exocrine function). Other structures also produce hormones, e.g. placenta, gastrointestinal tract, kidneys and the heart.

endocrinology *n* the study of the endocrine structures and their internal secretions.

endocrinopathy *n* abnormality of one or more of the endocrine glands or their secretions. For example, an overactive thyroid gland—hyperthyroidism.

endocytosis a term for the bulk transport of large molecules into cells. ⊃ bulk transport, exocytosis *opp*, phagocytosis, pinocytosis.

endoderm *n* inner layer of the three primary germ layers of the early embryo. It gives rise to some epithelial tissue, e.g. that of the pharynx, middle ear, respiratory tract, gastrointestinal tract and bladder. ⊃ ectoderm, mesoderm.

endodontics *n* branch of clinical dentistry concerned with the prevention, diagnosis and treatment of diseases of the dental pulp and periapical tissues.

endodontic stop (*syn* rubber stop). A device to fix the depth to which an endodontic instrument is introduced into a root canal. Usually a moveable silicone ring whose position is set with the aid of a ruler.

endodontology the study of the dental pulp, its form function and behaviour in health, and the prevention, diagnosis and treatment of its diseases and their sequela.

end-of-life care the care given at the very end of life, during the last week, days and hours before death. Appropriate and effective care requires several members of the multidisciplinary team (MDT) to be involved in the care and support of patients with advanced disease, their families and friends. End-of-life care is part of the much broader palliative care provided for people with life-limiting diseases, such as heart failure and cancer.

endogenous *adj* originating within the organism. ⊃ ectogenous, exogenous *opp*.

endolymph *n* the fluid within the membranous labyrinth of the inner ear. ⊃ perilymph

endolymphatic duct *n* the duct that connects the endolymphatic sac to the saccule and utricle.

endolymphatic hydrops excess endolymph in the endolymphatic system. Distension of the endolymphatic system is associated with Ménière's disease.

endolymphatic sac *n* the dilated part of the endolymphatic duct.

endometrial *adj* pertaining to the endometrium.

endometrial ablation/destruction transcervical destruction of the basal layer of the endometrium by resection, laser ablation, microwaves, radio-frequency, or by using heat. Frequently used instead of hysterectomy in the treatment of menorrhagia. ⊃ embolization.

endometrial hyperplasia abnormal overgrowth of the endometrium resulting from prolonged contact with unopposed oestrogens, i.e without the controlling influence of progesterone. These may be endogenous oestrogens, such as occurs in anovulatory cycles, or exogenous if oestrogen-only hormone relacement therapy (without progesterone) is prescribed for women with an intact uterus. It may progress to endometrial cancer.

endometrioma *n* a tumour of misplaced endometrium ⊃ chocolate cyst—**endometriomata** *pl*.

endometriosis *n* the presence of endometrium in abnormal sites, i.e. outside the uterus. The tissue outside the uterus is influenced by hormones during the menstrual cycle, resulting in bleeding and the formation of adhesions. The commonest sites are the peritoneum of the rectovaginal pouch (pouch of Douglas), ovary, sigmoid colon, broad ligament and uterosacral ligament, but it can affect other pelvic structures, such as the bladder. The cause is unknown but two theories suggest that either endometrium travels along the uterine (fallopian) tubes during menstruation instead of being lost through the cervix, or that peritoneal mesothelium is transformed into tissue similar to endometrium. Signs and symptoms vary considerably, but commonly there is pelvic pain, which can be associated with menstruation or can occur at any other time due to adhesions. Treatment options include the use of drugs to reduce oestrogen secretion or oppose its action, or laporoscopic destruction of the ectopic endometrium. ⊃ chocolate cyst.

endometritis *n* inflammation of the endometrium.

endometrium *n* the specialized lining mucosa of the uterus. It contains many blood vessels and glands. During the

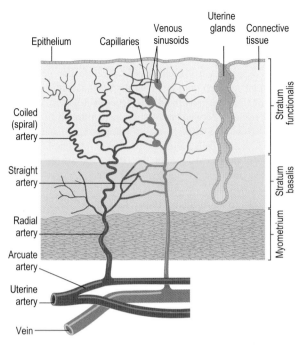

Epithelium | Capillaries | Venous sinusoids | Uterine glands | Connective tissue

Coiled (spiral) artery

Straight artery

Radial artery

Arcuate artery

Uterine artery

Vein

Stratum functionalis | Stratum basalis | Myometrium

E.4 Endometrium (reproduced from Brooker & Nicol 2003 with permission).

reproductive years the endometrium undergoes cyclical changes in response to ovarian hormones. This prepares the endometrium to receive an embryo should fertilization occurs. The endometrium comprises two layers: the permanent stratum basalis, and the stratum functionalis which regenerates after being lost every 28 days or so during menstruation (Figure E.4)—**endometrial** *adj.*

endomorph a soft, round body type (physique), with large thighs and trunk, and fat accumulation—**endomorphic** *adj.* ⊃ ectomorph, mesomorph.

endomyocardial *adj* relating to the endocardium and myocardium—**endomyocardium** *n.*

endomyocarditis *n* inflammation involving both the endocardium and myocardium.

endomysium *n* thin, inner connective tissue surrounding the muscle fibres. ⊃ epimysium, perimysium.

endoneurium *n* the delicate, inner connective tissue surrounding the nerve fibres. ⊃ epineurium, perineurium.

endoparasite *n* any parasite living within the host, such as threadworms—**endoparasitic** *adj.*

endopeptidase *n* an enzyme that catalyses the breakdown of internal peptide bonds between amino acids in a polypeptide or protein.

endophthalmitis *n* enophthalmia. A serious inflammation (bacterial or fungal) of the internal eye involving the anterior chamber and vitreous body (humour) and the layers of the wall of the eye. Rarely it may follow eye trauma or eye surgery. Urgent treatment to prevent blindness involves intensive use of topical and intravenous antibiotics. Antibiotics may also be injected into the eye (intracameral route).

endoplasmic reticulum (ER) part of the endomembrane system comprising interconnected membranous tubules within the cell cytoplasm. There are two distinct types: rough ER which have associated ribosomes and smooth ER without ribosomes. They are concerned with the synthesis of proteins, lipids and other macromolecules and their transport within the cell.

end organ a specialized encapsulated nerve ending in a structure such as the taste buds on the tongue

endorphins *npl* a group of opioid-like neuropeptides. Found in the brain, pituitary gland and the gastrointestinal tract; they have neurotransmitter or neurohormone properties. Released in strenuous exercise and in stressful or painful situations they bind to and activate opioid receptors of other cells (where opioid drugs also act). The three subtypes are alpha, beta and gamma. The subgroups have varied and widespread actions, diminishing the sensation of pain, inducing euphoria (e.g. 'runner's high') and interacting with the immune system. ⊃ enkephalins.

endoscope *n* instrument for visualization of the interior of hollow tubular structures such as the urinary, respiratory and gastrointestinal tracts, or body cavities, e.g. abdominal cavity and joints. The older ones were rigid metal tubes. Modern ones use fibreoptic technology: light is transmitted by means of very fine glass fibres along a flexible tube (Figure E.5). It permits examination, photography, biopsy and treatment of the cavities or organs of a relaxed (sedated) conscious person—**endoscopic** *adj*, **endoscopy** *n.*

endoscopic retrograde cholangiopancreatography (ERCP) introduction of a contrast agent into the pancreatic and bile ducts via a catheter from an endoscope located in the duodenum.

endoscopy visualization of hollow organs or structures by use of the appropriate endoscope. ⊃ amnioscopy, antroscopy, arthroscopy, bronchoscopy, choledochoscopy, colonoscopy, culdoscopy, cystoscopy, duodenoscopy, embryoscopy,

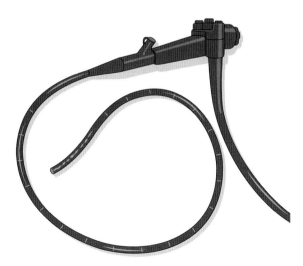

E.5 Endoscope (reproduced from Brooker & Nicol 2003 with permission).

fetoscopy, hysteroscopy, laparoscopy, laryngoscopy, mediastinoscopy, oesophagogastroduodenoscopy, proctoscopy, sigmoidoscopy, ureteroscopy.

endospore *n* a bacterial spore that has a solely vegetative function. It forms during adverse environmental conditions, such as drying. Its metabolism is minimal, thus allowing the micro-organism to resist heat, desiccation and disinfectants. Endospores can remain dormant for long periods and can become active when environmental conditions are suitable for growth and reproduction. The only genera which include spore-forming pathogenic species are *Bacillus* and *Clostridium*.

endosseous (endosteal) implant ⊃ implant.

endosteum *n* the membrane that lines the medullary cavity of a long bone. ⊃ periosteum.

endothelial bedewing a cluster of inflammatory cells deposited on the posterior surface of the corneal endothelium. They have been noted with anterior eye inflammation and contact lens wear. The symptoms may include slight stinging sensation, some interference with vision and intolerance to contact lens wear. Reduction of wearing time is usually indicated and in severe cases contact lens wear must be ceased. ⊃ corneal endothelium, endothelial blebs.

endothelial blebs oedema of some cells of the corneal endothelium which bulge towards the aqueous humour. With specular microscopy or with high magnification biomicroscopy the cells appear as black areas as they do not reflect light towards the observer. Blebs occur within minutes of inserting a contact lens on the eye and disappear within hours after insertion. They may result from a local acidic pH shift at the endothelium. ⊃ corneal endothelium, endothelial bedewing, specular reflection illumination.

endothelial corneal dystrophy ⊃ cornea guttata.

endothelial pleomorphism ⊃ endothelial polymorphism.

endothelial polymegethism the variation in the size of the endothelial cells of the cornea as a result of disturbed metabolism. It may be induced by contact lens wear, surgery, trauma or disease processes. Endothelial polymegethism is detected by observation with a specular microscope or a high magnification slit-lamp. If the condition is caused by contact lens wear, management consists of refitting the person with daily wear contact lenses of higher oxygen transmissibility. ⊃ corneal endothelium, endothelial polymorphism, specular microscope.

endothelial polymorphism (*syn* endothelial pleomorphism) the presence of many cell shapes which accompanies polymegethism. ⊃ endothelial polymegethism.

endothelin *n* a naturally occurring peptide that causes vasoconstriction, found in the smooth muscle of blood vessels. It is important, along with other vasoconstrictor substances, and vasodilators (e.g. prostacyclins, nitric oxide), in the balance between vasoconstriction and vasodilation. Abnormal activity of endothelin is associated with conditions that include pulmonary arterial hypertension. Drugs, such as bosentan, which act as endothelin receptor antagonists, can be used for patients with pulmonary arterial hypertension.

endothelioid *adj* resembling endothelium.

endothelioma *n* a tumour derived from endothelial cells.

endothelium *n* a type of specialized epithelial tissue with flat cells. A single layer of endothelium lines the heart, all blood vessels and lymph vessels. Endothelial cells are important in vasocontriction/vasodilation, haemostasis, the inflammatory response and angiogenesis (growth of new blood vessels). Movement of substances through the capillary walls is facilitated by a wall comprising a single layer of endothelial cells. Highly specialized endothelial cells are part of the blood–brain barrier (BBB) and the glomerular filtration membrane in glomerulus of the nephron—**endothelial** *adj*.

endothelium-derived relaxing factor (EDRF) ⊃ nitric oxide.

endothermic *adj* describes a chemical reaction in which there is heat absorption. ⊃ exothermic.

endotoxin *n* a toxin found within the cell wall of certain bacteria, e.g. *Neisseria meningitidis*. Specifically lipopolysaccharide, of Gram-negative bacterial cells walls liberated after the cell wall is destroyed. Endotoxin is a powerful mediator of the inflammatory response. ⊃ exotoxin—**endotoxic** *adj*.

endotracheal *adj* within the trachea.

endotracheal anaesthesia the administration of an anaesthetic through an endotracheal tube.

endotracheal intubation the introduction of an endotracheal tube into the trachea, either by way of the mouth or the nose.

endotracheal tube (ET) a plastic tube introduced via the nose or mouth into the trachea to maintain an airway during general anaesthesia and to facilitate short term intermittent positive pressure ventilation.

endovascular *adj* intraluminal (within the lumen) surgical approach to correction of vascular abnormalities, e.g. *endovascular stenting* of an abdominal aortic aneurysm.

end-plate also known as myoneural junction. The junction between the axon membrane of a motor nerve and the membrane of the muscle fibres. ⊃ motor end-plate.

end-stage renal disease/failure (ESRD) the deterioration of chronic renal failure (CRF) to the point of irreversible loss of renal function. Patients with CRF may or may not need renal replacement therapy, but once ESRD is reached they must have replacement therapy, such as haemodialysis, to survive. The causes of ESRD include any condition that disrupts normal kidney structure and function, e.g. diabetes mellitus, reflux nephropathy (chronic pyelonephritis), glomerulonephritis, adult polycystic kidney disease and hypertension.

end-systolic volume (ESV) the volume of blood remaining in the cardiac ventricles at the end of systole. Usually about 60 mL. ⊃ stroke volume.

end-tidal carbon dioxide (ETCO$_2$) partial pressure of carbon dioxide measured in the breath at the end of expiration. Used to monitor the adequacy of ventilation in mechanically ventilated patients.

endurance in general, the ability to perform physical work for a long time; quantitatively, the maximum duration for which an individual can sustain a specific activity, preferably also at a specified intensity. Used in isolation, the word usually implies whole-body endurance, considered in terms of many minutes or hours (long-term endurance) which is principally limited by cardiovascular fitness and muscle glycogen storage. ➲ anaerobic endurance, local muscle endurance.

endurance capacity loosely, equivalent to endurance. Also used to mean aerobic power or $\dot{V}O_{2max}$.

endurance performance in simple terms, continuous physical activity that lasts between 5 minutes and 4 hours. Although this includes a huge range of physical activities and sports most of the adenosine triphosphate (ATP) is produced by aerobic processes.

endurance training prolonged training at relatively low intensity, aimed at enhancement of cardiorespiratory function, together with aerobic capacity of the exercised muscles.

enema *n* the introduction of a liquid into the bowel via the rectum, to be returned or retained. The word is usually preceded by the name of the liquid used. It can be further designated according to the function of the fluid. The evacuant enemas are usually prepared commercially in small bulk as a disposable enema: the chemicals attract water into the bowel, promoting cleansing and peristaltic contractions of the lower bowel. The enemas to be retained are usually drugs, the most common being corticosteroids for the treatment of inflammatory bowel disease. ➲ barium enema, laxatives.

energy the capacity to undertake vigorous physical activity or to do work. The SI unit of energy is the joule (J), but in nutrition the kilojoule (kJ) or megajoule (MJ) is more appropriate. The amount of work done, measured in joules (J), for example, for low level laser that also uses energy density: = Power density (W/cm^2) × Time (s) = J/cm^2.

energy balance the condition when energy intake equals energy expenditure, so that there is neither increase nor decrease in body mass. ➲ energy requirement.

energy charge the ratio: [ATP] + ½ [ADP]/[ATP] + [ADP] + [AMP] proposed by Atkinson in 1977 as an index of cellular energy status. ➲ adenosine mono-, di- and triphosphates (AMP, ADP, ATP), phosphorylation potential.

energy conservation the use of techniques such as time management, problem solving and lifestyle planning to enable an individual to make the best use of limited energy.

energy expenditure the amount of energy, measured in kilocalories or kilojoules, that an individual uses in a given time. 24-h energy expenditure can be divided into three components: basal metabolic rate (BMR), energy expenditure of physical activity or thermic effect of activity (TEA), and the thermic effect of food (TEF). ➲ diet-induced thermogenesis, metabolic equivalent, metabolic rate.

energy metabolism a general term for the chemical reactions involved in the oxidation of metabolic fuels (mainly carbohydrates, fats and proteins under certain circimstances), which provide energy in the form of adenosine triphosphate for body processes.

energy requirement the energy intake that balances energy expenditure and thus in adults provides body mass stability. In children additional energy is needed for growth; also during pregnancy, for the growth of the uterus and the fetus, and in lactation for production of milk. In elite athletes, requirement is higher than in sedentary individuals since they easily expend 4100–8300 kJ/day (1000–2000 kcal/day) in sport-related activities. ➲ balanced diet.

energy resolution the ability to distinguish between two different energy values. In a gamma camera, the width of the absorption peak at half the maximum count rate observed at the peak.

energy systems those related to metabolic processes which yield energy for synthesis of adenosine triphosphate (ATP). These processes include creatine phosphate hydrolysis; glycolysis, which involves breakdown of blood-borne glucose or of muscle glycogen to either pyruvate (in aerobic conditions, when aerobic metabolism is possible) or lactate (when aerobic metabolism is not possible) and produces ATP by substrate-level phosphorylation reactions; oxidative phosphorylation, which involves oxidation within mitochondria of products of carbohydrate, fat, protein and alcohol metabolism to carbon dioxide and water.

enervation *n* **1.** the surgical removal of an entire nerve, or a part of a nerve. **2.** lack of strength, weakness, lassitude.

engagement *n* in obstetrics, it is when the widest transverse diameter of the presenting part passes through the pelvic brim. In a vertex (head first) presentation this will be the biparietal diameter, and the bitrochanteric diameter in a breech presentation. In a primigravida, the infant's head normally engages any time after the 36th week of gestation, whereas in multiparous women enagement may not happen until they are in labour.

engagement (occupational therapy) a sense of involvement, choice, positive meaning and commitment while performing an occupation or activity. (Reproduced with permission from the European Network of Occupational Therapy in Higher Education (ENOTHE) Terminology Project, 2008.)

engine mallet a dental engine-powered mallet sometimes used in the condensation of gold foil and amalgam.

engorgement a state of being overfilled.

engorgement of the breasts painful accumulation of secretion in the breasts, often accompanied by oedema and lymphatic and venous stasis at the onset of lactation which can be avoided by early on-demand breastfeeding with the baby correctly positioned at the breast. A firm supporting brassiere or breast binder may be helpful but care should be taken not to create pressure on the oedematous tissue.

enhanced computed tomography (CT) the use of a contrast agent to demonstrate more clearly vessels or organs of similar density to the surrounding tissue.

enhancement in radiography, the intensification of detail, making a radiograph more easily interpreted.

enkephalins *npl* (*syn* encephalins) peptides present in the central nervous system, and also present in the pituitary gland and gastrointestinal tract. They have opioid-like analgesic effects. ⊃ endorphins, neuropeptides.

enophthalmos *n* sunken position of an eyeball within its socket.

enostosis bony growth proliferating within a bone.

enrichment enriching foods by adding nutrients, e.g. cream or milk powder to soups, in order to increase the amount of nutrients present. Often used interchangeably with the term fortification.

ensiform *adj* sword shaped; xiphoid.

ENT *abbr* ear, nose and throat.

Entamoeba *n* (*syn* Endamoeba) a genus of protozoon parasites, there are three species infesting humans. Two are non-pathogenic: *Entamoeba coli* in the intestinal tract and *E. gingivalis* in the mouth, whereas *E. histolytica* is pathogenic causing amoebic dysentery.

enteral *adj* within the gastrointestinal tract.

enteral diets those which are taken by mouth or through a nasogastric tube; low residue enteral diets can be whole protein/polymeric, or amino acid/peptide.

enteral feeding method of providing nutrition when there is some gastrointestinal tract function. Includes via nasogastric and nasoduodenal tubes or via gastrostomy or jejunostomy tubes. Enteral feeding can be administered by bolus, gravity or pump controlled methods. ⊃ parenteral feeding, percutaneous endoscopic gastrostomy (PEG).

enterectomy excision of part of the intestine.

enteric *adj* relating to the small intestine.

enteric coating a coating applied to a pill that prevents drug release until it reaches the small intestine. Crushing tablets can alter the way in which the drug is absorbed and metabolized with deleterious effects. A liquid preparation of the drug should always be prescribed in situations where swallowing is difficult.

enteric fevers includes typhoid and paratyphoid fever.

enteritis *n* inflammation of the intestinal mucosa.

entero, enter a prefix that means 'intestine', e.g. *enteropathy*.

enteroanastomosis *n* intestinal anastomosis, a surgical join.

Enterobacter *n* a genus of Gram-negative bacilli of the family Enterobacteriaceae, they are facultative anaerobes. Includes two species, *Enterobacter aerogenes* and *Enterobacter cloacae*. They cause infection in hospital, especially of wounds, urinary and respiratory tract. They may cause opportunistic infection in immunocompromised individuals.

Enterobacteriaceae a family of coliform bacteria that include *Enterobacter* spp., *Escherichia* spp., *Klebsiella* spp., *Proteus* spp., *Salmonella* spp., *Serratia* spp., *Shigella* spp., *Yersina* spp.

enterobiasis (oxyuriasis) *n* infestation with *Enterobius vermicularis* (threadworm, pinworm). Because of the autoinfective life cycle, treatment aims at complete elimination. Everyone in the household is given an anthelmintic, mebendazole or less commonly piperazine citrate, and hygiene measures, such as handwashing, not sharing towels or flannels, etc., are also necessary to prevent reinfestation during treatment.

Enterobius a genus of parasitic nematode worms. Includes *Enterobius vermicularis* (threadworm, pinworm) which infests the small and large intestine.

enterocele *n* prolapse of intestine. Can prolapse into the upper third of vagina.

enteroclysis *n* the introduction of fluid into the intestine, such as contrast agent. ⊃ proctoclysis.

Enterococcus *n* a genus of Gram-positive cocci commensal in the bowel, e.g. *Enterococcus faecalis*, *E. faecium*. They are facultative anaerobes. They cause urinary tract infection and wound infection and occasionally meningitis in neonates. It is increasingly common as a cause of healthcare-associated infection, and many strains are developing resistance to antibiotics. ⊃ vancomycin-resistant enterococci (glycopeptide-resistant enterococci).

enterocolitis *n* inflammation of the small intestine and colon. ⊃ necrotizing enterocolitis.

enterocystoplasty *n* an operation to increase the capacity of the urinary bladder by using part of the small intestine.

enteroglucagon one of the glucagon-like peptides, e.g. oxyntomodulin, glicentin, produced by special intestinal cells. They are released in response to the intake of food and are hyperglycaemic.

enterohepatic circulation the recycling of bile salts and other substances including drugs that are secreted into bile. They are absorbed from the intestine and returned to the liver via the hepatic portal vein. The returning bile salts stimulate more bile and bile acid production, but recycled drugs, such as morphine, create a pool of active drug that prolongs drug activity and can lead to toxic levels.

enterokinase *n* (*syn* enteropeptidase) a proteolytic (protein-splitting) enzyme produced by duodenal mucosa. It converts inactive trypsinogen (pancreatic enzyme) into active trypsin.

enterolithiasis *n* the presence of intestinal stones known as enteroliths.

enteron *n* the gut.

enteropathy *n* any disorder affecting the small intestine, such as gluten-induced enteropathy (coeliac disease).

enteropeptidase *n* ⊃ enterokinase.

enteroscope *n* an endoscope for visualization of the small intestine—**enteroscopically** *adv*.

enterostomy *n* a surgically established fistula between the small intestine and some other surface. ⊃ gastroenterostomy, ileostomy, jejunostomy—**enterostomal** *adj*.

enterotomy *n* an incision into the small intestine.

enterotoxin *n* a toxin which has its effect on the gastrointestinal tract, causing vomiting, diarrhoea and abdominal pain.

enterovesical *adj* pertaining to the intestine and the urinary bladder.

enterovesical fistula an abnormal communication between the intestine and the urinary bladder. Also called vesicoenteric.

enteroviruses *npl* a group of picornaviruses that enter the body by the gastrointestinal tract. Comprise the polioviruses, echoviruses and coxsackieviruses.

enthesis the point at which a tendon inserts into a bone.

enthesopathy inflammation at the site of attachment of ligament or tendon to bone.

Entonox® *n* proprietary name for a gaseous mixture of oxygen and nitrous oxide in equal measures that is inhaled by the patient to provide analgesia, e.g. in obstetrics, during painful procedures and in intensive care.

entoptic image/phenomena visual phenomena that arise from within the eye itself, such as 'floaters' or flashes but perceived as in the external world. For example muscae volitantes or phosphene. ⊃ angioscotoma, blue arcs, blue field entoptoscope, floaters, Haidinger's brushes, Maxwell's spot, muscae volitantes, phosphene.

entrance dose (skin dose) the quantity of radiation (or dose) absorbed at the site of entry of the X-ray beam.

entrance maze a structure to prevent primary radiation and first scattered photons reaching the room door, used in radiotherapy treatment rooms so that lighter doors can be used and darkrooms so that people can enter while a film is being processed.

entropion *n* inversion of an eyelid, usually the lower, so that the lashes are in contact with the globe of the eye. It may be caused by spasm of the muscle that normally closes the eyelids (obicularis oculi), or trauma or disease affecting the conjunctiva or eyelids. Irritation by the eyelashes cause discomfort and tearing (watering). Untreated it can cause corneal ulceration. Treatment is either surgical or the repeated injection of botulinum toxin to relieve the muscle spasm. ⊃ ectropion, Colour Section Figure 66.

enucleation *n* the removal of an organ or tumour in its entirety, as of an eyeball from its socket, the complete removal of a cyst lining and contents, or of a tooth germ from its surrounding structures.

E-numbers identification numbers used in the European Union for permitted food additives. The categories include: (a) antioxidants (e.g. E300 ascorbic acid); (b) colours (e.g. E102 tartrazine); (c) emulsifiers, gelling agents, stabilizers and thickeners (e.g. E460 cellulose); (d) preservatives (e.g. E211 sodium benzoate); (e) sweeteners (e.g. E951 aspartame); (f) others such as E570 fatty acids. The food additive may be identified by name or E number on food labelling.

enuresis *n* incontinence of urine, especially bed-wetting. ⊃ nocturnal enuresis.

envelope of motion the three-dimensional space within which the mandible moves during its normal excursions.

environment *n* external surroundings. Living organisms are influenced by the physical and chemical conditions of the environment external to them, and by those within the organism—**environmental** *adj*.

environment (occupational therapy) external factors that demand and shape occupational performance. These factors are physical, sociocultural and temporal. (Reproduced with permission from the European Network of Occupational Therapy in Higher Education (ENOTHE) Terminology Project, 2008.)

environmental adaptation changes that the therapist makes to the client's physical or social environment to facilitate the performance of tasks, activities and occupations.

environmental assessment a process of collecting and interpreting information about the client's physical and social environments in order to identify risks or potential problems.

environmental monitoring a mechanism for ensuring that the protective barriers in radiology/radiotherapy departments provide a safe working environment for all staff and the general public.

environmental press the influence of the environment on the performance of tasks, activities and occupations.

enzyme *n* a protein that functions as a catalyst for specific intra- and extracellular biochemical reactions involving specific substrates. Many reactions in the body would proceed too slowly without an enzyme, e.g. waste carbon dioxide would not be removed from the tissues without the enzyme carbonic anhydrase. Each enzyme catalyses a specific biochemical reaction involving a specific substrate, most but not all within the cells themselves. Others are secreted by cells for external action, e.g. the digestive enzymes released into the gut. Enzyme names usually reflect their function or their substrate, e.g. dehydrogenases catalyse the removal of hydrogen in oxidative reactions and ATPases, the conversion of ATP to ADP. *rate-limiting enzymes* those acting within a complex chain or cycle, but having very much greater sensitivity than others to excitatory and inhibitory influences, thus effectively controlling flux in the whole pathway. *isoenzymes (isozymes)* multiple forms of enzymes that catalyse the same reaction, but with some different properties. ⊃ cardiac enzymes, muscle enzymes.

enzyme activation assays techniques used to assess the level of certain vitamins, for example vitamins B_1, B_2 and B_6.

enzyme induction the ability of some chemicals, e.g. alcohol, environmental chemicals and drugs, to increase the secretion of liver enzymes. ⊃ cytochromes. The increase in enzyme production can speed up the rate at which the inducer drug and others are metabolized and excreted. There is loss of drug effectiveness, e.g. the oral contraceptive is inactivated by rifampicin (antituberculosis drug). In some situations the induction of enzyme production may increase drug effects such as the toxic metabolites formed in paracetamol overdose.

enzyme inhibitors chemicals, including many drugs that inhibit specific enzymes in the body. The inhibition may be reversible or irreversible. Some inhibitors are false substrates (very similar to the normal substrate of the enzyme) and act as competitive inhibitors, e.g. some cytotoxic drugs inhibit the enzyme needed by cancer cells for folic acid use. Others inhibit liver enzymes and increase the effects of other drugs. For example, aspirin inhibits the enzymes needed to metabolize oral anticoagulants, which causes increased anticoagulation with the risk of bleeding.

enzyme-linked immunosorbent assay (ELISA) an assay technique for measuring soluble substances based on recognition of the target antigen by specific antibodies, linked to an enzyme which causes a colour change in a substrate solution. The degree of colour change is proportional to the concentration of the substance being examined. It is used to test for the presence of antibodies to HIV. All positive tests for HIV are confirmed by the more precise Western blot test before HIV infection is established.

EOG *abbr* electro-oculogram.

EOP *abbr* equivalent oxygen pressure.

eosin *n* a red staining agent used in histology and laboratory diagnostic procedures. It is crystalline stain (dye) derived from coal tar.

eosinopenia a reduction in the number of eosinophil leucocytes in the blood.

eosinophil *n* **1.** cells having an affinity for eosin. **2.** a type of polymorphonuclear leucocyte containing eosin-staining granules. It is associated with immune responses that involve allergies and immunoglobulin (IgE)—**eosinophilic** *adj*.

eosinophilia *n* increased number of eosinophils in the blood. Indicative of an allergic condition, a parasitic infestation and a rarer form of leukaemia.

eosinophilic granuloma a granuloma composed of eosinophils and histiocytes occurring in bone or soft tissue. ⊃ granuloma.

EOT *abbr* extraoral traction.

EP *abbr* evoked potentials.

EPA *abbr* **1.** eicosapentaenoic acid. **2.** electrophysical agent.

EPEC *abbr* enteropathic *Escherichia coli*.

ependymal cells part of the macroglia. A type of neuroglial cell that lines the fluid-filled cavities of the central nervous system (cerebral ventricles and the central canal of the spinal cord).

ependymoma *n* neoplasm arising in the lining of the cerebral ventricles or central canal of spinal cord. Occurs in all age groups.

ep, epi- a prefix that means 'on, above, upon', e.g. *epidermis*.

ephebiatrics a branch of medicine that specializes in the care of older children and adolescents.

ephelides *npl* freckles caused by an increase in pigment granules with a normal number of pigment cells. ⊃ lentigo—**ephelis** *sing*.

EPI *abbr* electronic portal imaging.

epicanthus *n* epicanthal or epicanthic fold. The congenital occurrence of a variable-size fold of skin that obscures the inner canthus of the eye. A normal feature in some racial groups in Asia, may also be seen abnormally in infants with Down's syndrome—**epicanthal** *adj*.

epicardium *n* the visceral layer of the pericardium—**epicardial** *adj*.

epichoroid another term for the suprachoroid (lamina fusca). ⊃ sclera.

epicondyle *n* an eminence on some bones situated above the condyles, e.g. femoral and humeral epicondyles. The epicondyles on the sides of the lower end of the femur and of the humerus, provide attachment for tendons around the knee and elbow joints. ⊃ epicondylitis

epicondylitis *n* inflammation of the muscles and tendons around the elbow. Can occur if the structures are subjected to excess or repetitive stress. It may affect the structures at the lateral (outer) or medial (inner) aspect of the elbow. Lateral epicondylitis (*syn* tennis elbow) may be associated with tennis, other racquet sports and weight training. Medial epicondylitis (*syn* golfer's elbow, javelin thrower's elbow) is primarily an overuse injury that may be associated with golf and poor lifting techniques. ⊃ bursitis, lateral epicondylitis, medial epicondylitis.

epicranium *n* the structures comprising the scalp—muscles, aponeuroses and the skin.

epicritic *adj* describes cutaneous nerve fibres which are sensitive to fine variations of touch and vibration. Concerned with proprioception and two-point discrimination. ⊃ protopathic *opp*.

epidemic *n* a disease, such as measles, influenza, simultaneously affecting many people in an area (more than the expected number). ⊃ endemic *opp*.

epidemic keratoconjunctivitis due to an adenovirus. Presents as an acute follicular conjunctivitis with preauricular and submandibular adenitis. ⊃ contagious conjunctivitis.

epidemic myalgia, epidemic pleurodynia ⊃ Bornholm disease.

epidemiology *n* the scientific study of the distribution of diseases, the risk factors and determinants. It is concerned with the incidence, distribution and control of disease—**epidemiological** *adj*, **epidemiologically** *adv*.

epidermal growth factor (EGF) a protein growth factor that promotes cell growth and differentiation. Its role is important during embryonic development and in wound healing. ⊃ transforming growth factor.

epidermal growth factor receptors some cancers produce epidermal growth factor, e.g. some metastatic colorectal cancers. A monoclonal antibody cetuximab is used, in some cases, to 'block' the epidermal growth factor receptors, thereby preventing EGF from stimulating further abnormal cell growth. ⊃ human epidermal growth factor receptor-2.

epidermis *n* the outermost layer of the skin composed of stratified keratinized squamous epithelium. The epidermis is cellular, avascular (without a blood supply) and varies in thickness. The epidermis is thicker in areas which are subject to greater levels of stress and require more protection, e.g. the palms of the hands and soles of the feet. A layer of epidermal cells lines the hair follicles, and sweat and sebaceous glands. In a healthy young adult, the epidermis is replaced approximately every 3 weeks, but the time for renewal increases with age. Within the epidermis there are five differentiated layers: (a) stratum corneum—the outermost layer composed of dead keratinocytes, which are thin, flattened cells filled with keratin, a fibrous protein which is insoluble and resistant to enzymatic digestion and changes in pH and temperature. Keratin is capable of absorbing large amounts of water and it is this capacity to absorb fluid which may lead to skin maceration and eventual breakdown with continuous exposure to moisture, e.g. in loss of continence; (b) stratum lucidum—the second layer of the epidermis which is not always present. In areas where the epidermal covering is very thin, e.g. the eyelids, it is usually absent. This layer is transparent and made up of dead cells with no visible nuclei. It serves a mainly protective function—hence its presence on areas such as the soles of the feet; (c) stratum granulosum—the middle layer of the epidermis is between one and three cells thick. It contains flattened cells which have all the organelles necessary for active metabolic functioning. The thickness of this layer is proportional and varies according to the thickness of the stratum corneum; (d) stratum spinosum—contains living cells. They have spiny processes called desmosomes along their edges which form the area of contact between cells and are important in maintaining epidermal integrity. Their contact with other cells is what prevents the cells from being torn apart when subjected to normal stresses and strains; (e) stratum basale—the innermost layer of the epidermis. This layer is sometimes grouped with the stratum spinosum and called the stratum germinativum (or germinative layer) as together they are responsible for producing new cells by constant mitotic activity. The stratum basale is only one cell thick and as the epidermis is avascular receives its supply of oxygen and nutrients via the dermal blood supply. Situated between the epidermis and the dermis is an acellular layer referred to as the basement membrane zone or dermoepidermal junction. It has two layers, the lamina lucida and the lamina densa (these names simply refer to their visibility under an electron microscope). The basement membrane is a semi-permeable membrane with two main functions: it regulates the transfer of materials, particularly proteins, between the dermis and the epidermis and also acts as a mechanical supporting layer for the epidermis with anchoring fibrils which extend in to the dermis. ⊃ skin.

epidermoid carcinoma a malignant tumour of a salivary gland.

epidermolysis bullosa (EB) a group of inherited diseases where the skin is very fragile and even very minor trauma results in bulla or blister formation. The types of epidermolysis bullosa include: (a) simple—inherited as an autosomal dominant trait in which the epidermal basal cells are affected. There is abnormal keratin (keratins 14 and 15). Usually the blisters are limited to the palms and soles. There is no scarring, the nails are normal and there is no oral involvement. There is a rare recessive type associated with muscular dystrophy (plectin mutation); (b) junctional—inherited as an autosomal recessive trait in which the lamina lucida is affected. There is abnormal laminin-5 and $\alpha_6 \beta_4$ integrin. There are large, raw areas and flaccid blisters at birth. These are commonly present around the mouth and anus, and are slow to heal.The nails and oral mucosa are also involved. The condition, which is often lethal, may be

diagnosed prenatally by chorionic villus sampling; (c) dystrophic—one type is inherited as an autosomal dominant trait in which the dermis below lamina densa is affected. There is abnormal collagen VII. There are blisters on the knees, elbows and fingers that heal with scarring. The nails may be involved but the mouth is seldom affected. The other type is inherited as an autosomal recessive trait. It too affects the dermis below the lamina densa and has abnormal collagen VII. There are blisters, often present at birth, seen on the hands, feet, elbows and knees. The blisters heal with scarring which is so severe that digits may be lost. There is oral and oesophageal blistering leading to scarring and stricture formation. The teeth are abnormal. Affected individuals have an increased incidence of cutaneous squamous cell carcinoma (SCC) during early adulthood. ⊃ Cockayne's disease, epidermolysis bullosa acquisita.

epidermolysis bullosa acquisita an acquired blistering condition that is associated with inflammatory bowel disease, multiple myeloma and lymphoma. These conditions should therefore be excluded.

Epidermophyton *n* a genus of fungi affecting the skin and nails. ⊃ dermatophytes, tinea.

epidermophytosis *n* infection with fungi of the genus *Epidermophyton* such as ringworm.

epididymectomy *n* surgical removal of the epididymis.

epididymis *n* a small oblong body attached to the posterior surface of the testes. It consists of the seminiferous tubules which carry the spermatozoa from the testes to the deferent ducts (vas deferens). ⊃ Colour Section Figure 16.

epididymitis *n* inflammation of the epididymis. It is a bacterial infection usually caused by *Escherichia coli* or *Chlamydia trachomatis*; there is acute pain and swelling. Rarely due to tuberculosis and possibly secondary to urological surgery. It is vital to differentiate between epididymitis and testicular torsion, as the latter requires urgent surgical correction.

epididymo-orchitis *n* inflammation of the epididymis and the testis.

epididymovasostomy an operation to join the epididymis to the deferent duct (vas deferens) in order to bypass a mechanical blockage in a man with azoospermia, and occasionally to reverse a vasectomy.

epidural *adj* upon or external to the dura mater (outer meningeal membrane).

epidural anaesthesia or block local anaesthetic (e.g. bupivacaine) injected into the space external to the dura (epidural space) either by single injection or intermittently via a catheter, causing loss of sensation in an area determined by the site of the injection and volume of local anaesthetic used (Figure E.6). It is used extensively during and after surgery and in obstetrics.

epidural anaesthesia in obstetric practice during labour the injection into the epidural space to block the spinal nerves, is either caudal, approached through the sacrococcygeal membrane covering the sacral hiatus, or lumbar, through the intervertebral space and ligamentum flavum.

261

E
F

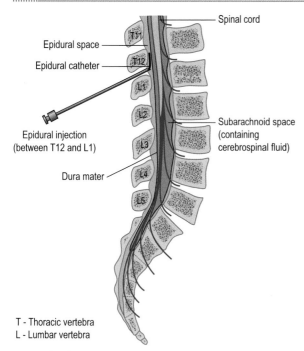

Spinal cord

Epidural space

Epidural catheter

T11
T12
L1
L2

Epidural injection
(between T12 and L1)

Subarachnoid space
(containing
cerebrospinal fluid)

L3

Dura mater

L4

L5

T - Thoracic vertebra
L - Lumbar vertebra

E.6 **Epidural** (reproduced from Brooker & Waugh 2007 with
permission).

Epidural anaesthesia is used in prolonged labour, occipito-posterior position, breech presentation; forceps delivery, to reduce hypertension in pre-eclampsia or eclampsia; for multiple or preterm delivery; caesarean section; maternal cardiac or respiratory disease; client preference. The dangers include sudden hypotension leading to fetal hypoxia; spinal or dural tap; toxic reactions to the drug; neurological sequelae from injury or haematoma; higher risk of instrumental delivery due to poor fetal head flexion as a result of the relaxed pelvic floor; infection. An intravenous cannula is inserted to provide vascular access should immediate treatment in the event of a problem be required. The woman should be positioned carefully to avoid hypotension. The midwife monitors maternal blood pressure and fetal heart rate frequently, especially after the first dose of bupivacaine which is given by the anaesthetist who inserts the epidural cannula, and after each 'top up', which midwives may be trained to administer. ➲ mobile epidural, patient controlled analgesia, spinal anaesthetic.

epidural blood patch treatment employed in the management of a dural puncture sustained during epidural catheterization. A small volume of the patient's blood is injected into the dural space; the clot which forms seals the breach and prevents further leakage of cerebrospinal fluid.

epidural space the region through which spinal nerves leave the spinal cord. It can be approached at any level of the spine, but the administering of anaesthetic is commonly done at the lumbar level or through the sacral cornua for caudal epidural block.

epigastrium *n* the upper, central abdominal region lying directly over the stomach—**epigastric** *adj.* ➲ Colour Section Figure 18a.

epigastrocele epigastric hernia. The protrusion of internal structures through the linea alba.

epiglottis *n* the thin leaf-shaped flap of cartilage attached to the top of the larynx which, during the act of swallowing, covers the opening leading into the larynx. Thus preventing food or fluids entering the larynx and trachea. ➲ Colour Section Figure 6.

epiglottitis *n* inflammation of the epiglottis. Acute epiglottitis, caused by the bacterium *Haemophilus influenzae* type B, is a serious condition that usually affects young children. There is fever, sore throat, croupy cough and inspiratory stridor. Swelling of the epiglottis may compromise the airway necessitating an emergency tracheostomy. ➲ Hib vaccine.

epikeratophakia ➲ epikeratoplasty.

epikeratoplasty (*syn* epikeratophakia, refractive keratoplasty and keratorefractive surgery [both terms also include keratomileusis, keratophakia and radial keratotomy]). A surgical procedure on the cornea aimed at curing ametropia. The person's corneal epithelium is removed and a donor's corneal disc (or lenticule) which was previously frozen and reshaped to produce a new anterior curvature is rehydrated and sutured to Bowman's membrane. The lenticule can be removed and exchanged to provide a different power. There are many problems associated with this procedure, in particular the surface re-epithelialization. ➲ Intacs, keratomileusis, keratophakia, LASIK, lenticule, radial keratotomy.

epilation *n* extraction or destruction of hair roots, e.g. by coagulation necrosis, electrolysis or forceps. ➲ depilation—**epilate** *vt.*

epilatory *adj, n* (describes) an agent which produces epilation.

epilepsy *n* correctly called the epilepsies, a group of conditions resulting from disordered electrical activity in the brain and manifesting as epileptic seizures or 'fits'. The seizure is caused by an abnormal electrical discharge that disturbs cerebration and results in a generalized or partial seizure, depending on the area of the brain involved. (a) *Generalized seizures* may be: *tonic-clonic (grand mal)* the commonest type of epileptic seizure with loss of consciousness and generalized convulsions. *absences (petit mal)* where there is a brief alteration in consciousness. (b) *Partial seizures* occur when the electrical disturbance is limited to a particular focus of the brain and are manifested in a variety of ways, including motor problems characterized by limb twitching that may spread, known as Jacksonian epilepsy. In *complex partial seizures* (also known as *psychomotor epilepsy or temporal lobe epilepsy*) there may be altered consciousness, paraesthesia, visual hallucinations, such as coloured patterns, and psychomotor seizures where there are changes to mood, behaviour, perception and memory with more complex hallucinations and physical manifestations, such as nausea. ➲ uncinate epilepsy. *Secondary generalized seizures* occur when partial seizure activity spreads to involve other areas of the brain and awareness is lost. ⊃ status epilepticus, uncinate epilepsy.

epileptic 1. *adj* pertaining to epilepsy. **2.** *n* a person with epilepsy.

epileptic aura premonitory subjective phenomena (tingling in the hand or visual or auditory sensations) that precede an attack of major epilepsy. ⊃ aura.

epileptiform *adj* resembling epilepsy.

epileptogenic *adj* capable of causing epilepsy.

epiloia *n* ⊃ tuberous sclerosis.

epimenorrhoea *n* reduction of the length of the menstrual cycle.

epimysium outer fibrous coat surrounding an entire muscle. ⊃ endomysium, perimysium.

epinephrine *n* ⊃ adrenaline (epinephrine).

epineurium *n* outer fibrous coat enclosing a nerve trunk. ⊃ endoneurium, perineurium.

epiphora *n* tearing. The pathological overflow of tears on to the cheek.

epiphysis *n* the end of a bone. During growth the epiphysis is separated from the shaft (diaphysis) by the epiphyseal plate (cartilage); from which growth in length occurs. The epiphyseal plate is replaced with bone (ossification) when growth ceases—**epiphyses** *pl*, **epiphyseal** *adj*. ⊃ diaphysis.

epiphysitis *n* inflammation of an epiphysis; can cause abnormal bone growth and deformity.

epiretinal membrane ⊃ preretinal macular fibrosis.

episclera *n* a loose connective and elastic tissue which covers the sclera and anteriorly connects the conjunctiva to it. It is a vascularized tissue whose deeper layers merge with the scleral stroma. It sends connective tissue bundles into Tenon's capsule. The episclera becomes progressively thinner towards the back of the eye—**episcleral** *adj*. ⊃ episcleritis, sclera, Tenon's capsule.

episcleritis inflammation of the episclera. It is a benign, self-limiting, frequently recurring condition that typically affects adults. The disease is characterized by redness (usually in one quadrant of the globe) and varying degrees of discomfort. There are two types of episcleritis: simple which is the most common and nodular which is localized to one area of the globe forming a nodule. Simple episcleritis usually subsides spontaneously within 1–2 weeks while the nodular type usually takes longer. If the discomfort is intense topical corticosteroids may be used. ⊃ dellen, episclera, scleritis.

episiorrhaphy *n* surgical repair of an episiotomy or lacerated perineum.

episiotomy *n* a mediolateral or median incision made in the thinned-out perineum during the birth of an infant to enlarge the vaginal outlet. The procedure is performed under local anaesthetic using lidocaine (lignocaine) at an appropriate strength. It may be performed to avoid maternal trauma with tearing of the perineum; to hasten the delivery if the fetus is distressed; before a forceps delivery or ventouse extraction; or to reduce risk of intracranial damage in preterm or breech delivery. Appropriately trained and competent midwives are permitted by the Nursing and Midwifery Council to infiltrate the perineum with local anaesthetic, perform an episiotomy and repair perineal trauma.

episodic memory the part of long-term memory responsible for storing personal experiences. It is organized with respect to when and where the experience occurred, e.g. an episode from the last performance review interview.

epispadias *n* a congenital opening of the urethra on the dorsal aspect of the penis, often associated with ectopia vesicae. ⊃ hypospadias.

epistasis a particular interation between genes. One gene modifies the action of a gene at a different locus. It may, for instance, suppress the expression of that gene.

epistaxis *n* bleeding from the nose. Local causes include nasal trauma such as from a punch or nose picking, tumours, nasal infections and sudden changes in atmospheric pressure. Bleeding from the nose may be a feature of coagulation disorders, hypertension, arteriosclerosis and anticoagulant drugs—**epistaxes** *pl*. ⊃ Little's area.

epistemology *n* theory of the grounds of knowledge. The discussion about knowledge and 'truth' and how it varies between different disciplines.

epithalamus part of the diencephalon. It is above and behind the thalamus. Contains the pineal body (gland) and forms part of the third ventricle.

epithelialization *n* the growth of epithelium over a raw area; a stage of wound healing.

epithelioma *n* a tumour arising from any epithelium.

epithelium *n* one of the four basic tissues. It lines body cavities and tubes, covers the body and forms glands. The structure of epithelium is closely related to its functions which include: the protection of underlying structures from, for example, dehydration, chemical and mechanical damage; secretion; and absorption. The cells are very closely packed and the intercellular substance, called the matrix, is minimal. The cells usually lie on a basement membrane, which is an inert connective tissue. It is classified according to the arrangement and shape of the cells it contains (Figure E.7). It may be *simple*, with a single layer of squamous (pavement), cuboidal, columnar or ciliated cells, or *stratified* with several cell layers, e.g. stratified or transitional—**epithelial** *adj*. ⊃ ciliatated epithelium, columnar epithelium, cuboidal epithelium, simple epithelium, squamous (pavement) epithelium, stratified epithelium, transitional epithelium.

epithelial referring to or composed of epithelium.

epithelial attachment ⊃ junctional epithelium.

epithelial basement membrane dystrophy ⊃ Cogan's microcystic epithelial dystrophy.

epithelial cell rests of Malassez cells of the epithelial root sheath of Hertwig, seen under the microscope as remains of the periodontal ligament.

epithelial cuff ⊃ junctional epithelium.

epithelial inlay ⊃ skin grafting vestibuloplasty.

epithelial microcysts (*syn* microepithelial cysts) very small, round vesicles containing fluid and cellular debris observed on the surface of the cornea under slit-lamp examination in some types of corneal dystrophy and in wearers of

E.7 Types of simple epithelium (reproduced from Watson 2000 with permission).

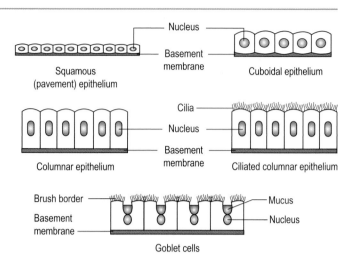

Squamous (pavement) epithelium

Nucleus

Basement membrane

Cuboidal epithelium

Columnar epithelium

Cilia

Nucleus

Basement membrane

Ciliated columnar epithelium

Brush border

Basement membrane

Mucus

Nucleus

Goblet cells

extended wear contact lenses, due to chronic hypoxia. They appear to originate in the basal layer of the corneal epithelium as a result of cellular necrosis. They can be seen by slit-lamp examination using a magnification of at least × 20. If caused by extended wear contact lenses, the person should be advised to change to daily wear contact lenses of high oxygen transmissibility. ⊃ extended wear lens, slit-lamp.

epithelial root sheath of Hertwig seen under the microscope as an extension of the enamel organ which, as it grows, forms the shape of the tooth root.

epitope *n* also known as antigenic determinant. The part (or region) of an antigen recognized by a specific antibody or T cell receptor. The location at which the paratope of the antibody binds to and acts on the antigen. ⊃ paratope.

Epley manoeuvre particle repositioning manoeuvre. A specific cycle of positions and movements used to relieve benign paroxysmal positional vertigo. The aim is to move debris in the semicircular canals to a more favourable location.

EPO *abbr* erythropoietin.

EPOC *abbr* elevated or excess post-exercise oxygen consumption.

eponychium the cuticle of the nail. It covers the thickened proximal edge of the nail the lunula.

eponym a place, anatomical structure, biochemical process, micro-organism, sign, a species or a disease/condition, etc., named after a person. For example Bartholin's glands, Cori cycle, *Borrelia*, Cullen's sign, Addison's disease, etc. Increasingly replaced by a standard descriptive nomenclature, for example, Bartholin's glands are the greater vestibular glands—**eponymous** *adj*.

epoophoron *n* vestigial remains of the embryonic mesonephric duct located between the ovary and uterine tube. ⊃ paraoophoron.

epoxy resin a synthetic resin used in die material and for applications using its adhesive properties.

EPP *abbr* equal pressure point.

EPR *abbr* electronic patient record.

EPROM *abbr* erasable programmable read only memory.

Epsom salts ⊃ magnesium sulphate.

EPSP *abbr* excitatory post-synaptic potential.

Epstein–Barr virus (EBV) (M Epstein, British pathologist and virologist, b.1921; Y Barr, British pathologist and virologist, b. 1932), a herpesvirus, the causative agent of infectious mononucleosis (glandular fever). Also linked with the formation of some malignant tumours, including Burkitt's lymphoma and nasopharyngeal cancer.

Epstein's pearls (Bohne's nodules) small yellowish-white nodules found on the palate and the crest of the alveolar ridges in the newborn infant. They generally disappear spontaneously after 2–3 months.

epulis *n* any localized enlargement of the gingiva. A tumour growing on or from the gums. A benign fibroid tumour of the gingiva may be associated with pregnancy and resolves following parturition.

equal energy spectrum a spectrum in which all wavelengths have about the same amount of energy. ⊃ achromatic, white light.

equality of opportunity equal access to opportunities for decent housing, education, a job, health care, etc., regardless of age, gender, race, religion, ability or social class.

equalization test ⊃ balancing test.

equal opportunity policy sets of practices and procedures within organizations and institutions designed to ensure that certain groups of people, such as women and people with disabilities, are not disadvantaged in terms of employment, housing, access to services and so on. Unless equal opportunity policies are robust they may serve as a 'smokescreen' to obscure discrimination.

equal pressure point (EPP) the point within the airways where the pleural and airway pressures are equal. ⊃ forced expiration technique.

equilibration the maintenance or restoration of a body into a state of equilibrium. ➲ occlusal adjustment, correction or equilibration.

equilibrium 1. in mechanics, a state when the force and moments on a body or object at rest or moving with constant velocity are balanced (i.e. the net force and net moment are zero). **2.** in chemistry, the condition when there are no net changes in the concentrations of reacting substances and their products.

equilibrium reactions these are small involuntary changes in tone or movements that occur to enable balance. For example, when lifting the arm there is increased activity in the back extensors to stabilize the trunk. They are often impaired in neurological conditions.

equinovarus a foot deformity in which the foot points down and inwards. Otherwise known as club foot or talipes equinovarus.

equinus *n* a condition in which the toes point down and the person walks on tiptoe. ➲ talipes.

equity *n* fairness of distribution of resources such as health care. Access to resources is based on need and the ability to benefit. The ability of a healthcare system to provide a comparable level of health care across the entire population. Covers the following dimensions: need for health care in the population (dependent on epidemiology of disease, determinants of health); availability, accessibility of healthcare resources; distribution of healthcare resources; use (utilization) of healthcare resources; geographic variation in need and healthcare utilization.

equivalent dose a unit of dose that allows for the fact that different types of radiation will deposit different types of energy depending on the specific mass and charge.

equivalent focal length in an optical system composed of more than one lens, it is the linear distance separating the principal focus from the corresponding principal point. It is usually the most important quantity in the specification of an optical system as in objectives, eyepieces, etc. ➲ equivalent power, principal focus.

equivalent oxygen pressure (EOP) a percentage value of the assumed oxygen pressure existing behind a contact lens. The oxygen pressure in the air corresponds to about 20.9% (or about 159 mmHg; that value is actually close to 155 mmHg because of the presence of water vapour) and each percentage point is equal to a pressure of about 7.4 mmHg.

equivalent power (*syn* true power) the refractive power of a lens or an optical system expressed with reference to the principal points. It corresponds to the refractive power of a thin lens placed in the second principal plane which would form an image of a distant object of the same size as that produced by the system that it replaces. It is equal to

$$F_e = \frac{n'}{f'} = -\frac{n}{f}$$

where n and n' are the refractive indices of the object and image space, respectively, f and f' the distances (in metres) between the first and second principal points and the first

and second principal foci, respectively. The equivalent power (symbol F_e) is in dioptres. It is also equal to

$$F_e = F_1 + F_2 - \left(\frac{d}{n}\right)F_1 F_2$$

where F_1 and F_2 are the powers of the lenses or surfaces comprising the system, d is the distance between the two and n the refractive index of the intervening medium. ➲ equivalent focal length, nominal power, principal plane, principal points.

equivalent square a square which produces the same percentage scatter as an elongated or circular field, used to calculate depth dose in radiotherapy.

equivalent wavelength the quality of a radiation beam by calculating Planck's constant times velocity over the maximum kilovoltage (Duane-Hunt's law).

ER *abbr* endoplasmic reticulum.

ERA *acron* **E**ffective **R**adiating **A**rea.

erasable optical disks (Magneto-optical disks or MO disks) read *and* write optical disks which combine magnetic and optical techniques.

erasable programmable read only memory (EPROM) a memory store which can be programmed and then erased by ultraviolet (UV) light.

Erb's palsy (W Erb, German neurologist, 1840–1921) paralysis involving the shoulder and arm muscles from a lesion of the fifth and sixth cervical nerve roots. The arm hangs loosely at the side with the forearm pronated ('waiter's tip position'). Most commonly caused by a birth injury.

ERCP *abbr* endoscopic retrograde cholangiopancreatography.

erectile *adj* upright; capable of being elevated.

erectile dysfunction (ED) erectile dysfunction (ED) is a common condition that is thought to have an annual incidence in men of between 15 and 20%. It can be defined as the inability of a man to gain an erection of sufficient quality for intercourse. This definition supersedes the older term, impotence, although such a definition is still used by the lay public. Historically, the causes of ED have been divided into organic and psychogenic factors, i.e. conditions known to affect nerve or blood supply and those where 'stress' can cause failure. The aetiology and associated risk factors are often multiple, with psychological, neurological, endocrinological, vascular, traumatic and iatrogenic components (e.g. drugs used to treat hypertension, some antidepressants, or following prostate surgery). The exact role played by lifestyle/medical events has yet to be fully elucidated, although smoking, hypertension, hyperlipidaemia, diabetes mellitus and the presence of vascular disease have been proposed as potential risk factors. Psychogenic ED is self-perpetuating: each failure increases the associated anxiety levels and can lead to the continual failure to have erections. This is the commonest cause of intermittent ED in young men, although it is usually secondary to organic dysfunction from middle age onwards. Up until the 1980s, psychogenic causes were attributed as the aetiology in up to 90% of cases of ED. Opinion now favours changes in blood flow as the key factor in ED, with alterations in blood flow to and from the penis the single most important cause. Evidence suggests that there is a marked delay (up to 5 years) between onset of symptoms and seeking treatment. Publicity about solutions to sexual problems such as sildenafil (Viagra®) has enabled men to seek help. Where there is a regular partner, it is also important to explore that person's situation and feelings about the sexual relationship. Irrespective of the cause of ED, there are only a limited number of treatments available. These include drugs, vacuum devices, surgery and psycho-sexual therapy: (a) drug treatment—*apomorphine hydro-chloride* which acts on dopaminergic receptors to increase the blood flow to the penis, *sildenafil citrate* is a phosphodi-esterase type V inhibitor and increases blood flow to the penis, *alprostadil* (prostaglandin E_1) increases blood flow to the penis. Intraurethral alprostadil such as 'Medicated ure-thral system for erections' (MUSE) may be used. Intraca-vernosal injection of alprostadil, e.g. Caverject®, Caverject dual chamber® or Viridal Duo®, is also used; (b) vacuum devices—work non-pharmacologically by drawing blood into the corpus cavernosum under pressure. Blood is held in place by a constriction band; (c) surgery (prostheses)—various prostheses are available. The prosthesis is implanted completely into the body, replacing the corpus cavernosum; (d) psychosexual therapy—a behavioural programme with counselling of underlying issues. It involves weekly or regu-lar attendance, with 'homework' that breaks the pattern of failure, removes anxiety and restores confidence. Not all patients can be treated by NHS prescription. In the UK the government has restricted NHS prescriptions to certain conditions and circumstances (e.g. diabetes mellitus, multi-ple sclerosis, prostate surgery, men receiving dialysis for renal failure, following renal transplant, spinal cord injury, etc.). Those men who do not 'fulfil' these criteria must seek a private prescription from their general practitioner.

erectile tissue vascular tissue, which, under stimulus, becomes rigid and erect from hyperaemia.

erection *n* the state accomplished when erectile tissue is hyperaemic.

erector *n* a muscle which achieves erection of a part.

erector spinae three muscles of the back—iliocostalis, longissimus and spinalis. Their actions are complex. The extensor muscles of the spine may be able to control individ-ual vertebral movements and it seems likely that the erector spinae complex works in complex patterns to resist the ten-dency of the spine to flex in various postures. ⊃ Colour Sec-tion Figure 5.

ERG *abbr* electroretinogram.

ergocalciferol *n* vitamin D_2 obtained from the diet. It is formed from the plant sterol ergosterol.

ergogenic *adj* a propensity to increase the output of work.

ergogenic aids agents that can enhance work output, particu-larly as it relates to athletic performance; often taken as dietary supplements, with the aim of improving performance beyond that associated with the typical balanced diet. They primarily serve to increase muscle mass, muscle energy supply and the rate of energy production in the muscle, but the effects claimed for many of them are not supported by sound evidence. Some aids may be allowed within the rules of the sport but others may be prohibited. The methods include mechanical, dietary supplementation, pharmaceuti-cal, hormonal and psychological. ⊃ anabolic steroids, blood doping, caffeine.

ergolytic agent one that decreases work output. Sometimes what is thought to be ergogenic for physical performance may actually be ergolytic. For example, depression of nervous system function by alcohol can profoundly impair performance in sports which require balance, hand-eye co-ordination, fast reaction time and in general any rapid processing of information.

ergometrine active alkaloid principle of ergot; an oxytocic drug effective in preventing or controlling postpartum haemorrhage and commonly used in conjunction with oxytocin as Syntometrine®. Acts within 45 seconds when given intrave-nously, within 7 minutes if administered intramuscularly, and gives a sustained uterine contraction. Oral ergometrine is used to treat secondary postpartum haemorrhage due to retained products of conception.

ergometry *n* measurement of work done by muscles—**ergometric** *adj*.

ergonomics *n* the study of the work environment and effi-cient energy use.

ergosterol *n* a sterol provitamin found in plants and fungi, particularly yeast. It is converted to ergocalciferol (vitamin D_2) by ultraviolet radiation, which is used to fortify foodstuffs with vitamin D.

ergot *n* a fungus, *Claviceps purpurea*, which infects rye. There are two important derivatives: (a) ergometrine, used to stimulate uterine contraction thus preventing or minimizing postpartum haemorrhage, and (b) ergotamine, which may occasionally be used for the treament of migraine. It has been mostly replaced by simple analgesics or specific and more effective medications. ⊃ 5-HT$_1$ agonists.

ergotism *n* poisoning by ergot, which may cause gangrene, particularly of the fingers and toes.

erosion 1. a gradually wearing away of a surface caused by chemical processes or physical events. **2.** a shallow ulcer. **3.** progressive loss of hard dental tissues by a chemical pro-cess without bacterial action. For example, erosion of the tooth enamel from acidic foods and beverages.

ERPC *abbr* evacuation of retained products of conception.

error scores in motor control and learning studies involving the performance of multiple trials to attain a criterion such as hitting a target or producing a given force, error scores are used to quantify the deviations of attempts around the target. *absolute error* the mean deviation of the attempts from the target, disregarding the direction of the errors, used as a measure of accuracy; *constant error* the distance from the target to the mean of the attempts, taking into account the direction of the error, used as another measure of accuracy; *variable error* the standard deviation of scores, used as a measure of consistency.

errorless learning methods of learning in which trial and error and hence the making of mistakes is avoided.

erubescence flushing or blushing—a reddening of the skin.

erucic acid a toxic fatty acid, found in rapeseed and mustard seed oils. Varieties of rapeseed (canola) with low levels of erucic acid have been developed for food use. ⊃ canola.

eructation belching. The bringing up air from the stomach, with a characteristic sound. ⊃ aerophagia.

eruption *n* **1.** the process by which a tooth emerges through the alveolar bone and gingivae. *active eruption* the normal movement of a tooth into or towards the oral cavity from its developmental position in the alveolar bone. *eruption haematoma* eruption or dentigerous cyst associated with erupting deciduous or permanent teeth. A dilatation of the normal follicular space around the crown of the tooth caused by the accumulation of blood or tissue fluid. **2.** the rapid formation of skin lesions, such as a rash occurring following the administration of a drug.

eruption cyst ⊃ cyst of dental origin.

ERV *abbr* expiratory reserve volume.

erysipelas *n* superficial inflammation, usually infective, of subcutaneous tissue and the lower dermis. The distinction between erysipelas and cellulitis can be difficult. The most common organism causing both these conditions is group A streptococcus. The clinical features include fever, and the associated findings, such as a raised white cell count, usually allow a firm diagnosis. There is often a predisposing cause such as a portal of entry for infection, e.g. tinea pedis, or underlying predisposition to infection such as a leg ulcer or diabetes. Erythema, heat, swelling and pain are constant clinical features. Erysipelas has a characteristic raised erythematous edge, indicating involvement of the dermis. It usually affects the face or the legs. Cellulitis most commonly involves the legs. Blistering occurs in both conditions. Treatment is with an appropriate antistreptococcal agent such as phenoxymethylpenicillin, or in cases of penicillin sensitivity, erythromycin or ciprofloxacin. In severe cases intravenous antibiotics are indicated. ⊃ Colour Section Figure 67.

erysipeloid *n* a skin condition resembling erysipelas. It occurs in butchers, fishmongers or cooks. The infecting organism is *Erysipelothrix rhusiopathiae (E. insidiosa)*, which causes a type of erysipelas that affects pigs, sheep, birds, reptiles and fish, etc.

Erysipelothrix a genus of parasitic bacteria that includes *Erysipelothrix rhusiopathiae (E. insidiosa)*.

erythema *n* reddening of the skin due to vascular congestion. In addition to diseases, reddening follows a therapeutic application of ultraviolet radiation (UVR) or heating or cooling. This is used as the basis for dosage of UVR. The level of UVR required to produce minimal perceptible (E1) grade of erythema. This is established in a test prior to UVR treatment. Grades are E1 to E4 and based on depth of reddening, time until skin becomes red and for which it remains red, degree of subsequent pigmentation and any desquamation—**erythematous** *adj*.

erythema induratum ⊃ Bazin's disease.

erythema infectiosum ⊃ human erythrovirus 19.

erythema multiforme a form of acute toxic or allergic eruption. The lesions are in the form of target-like papules often on the hands. A severe form called Stevens–Johnson syndrome may involve mucous membranes. ⊃ Stevens–Johnson syndrome. ⊃ Colour Section Figure 68.

erythema neonatorum patchy redness of variable size and shape on the body of a neonate. May be caused by heat, irritants or drugs but usually disappears after several days.

erythema nodosum an eruption of painful red nodules on the front of the legs. It may be a symptom of internal disease including tuberculosis and sarcoidosis.

erythema pernio ⊃ chilblain.

erythrasma a skin infection caused by the bacterium *Corynebacterium minutissimum*. It tends to occur in the axilla and the groin.

erythritol a bulk sweetener with approximately 0.7 times the sweetness of sucrose (beet or cane sugar) ⊃ sweetener.

erythr/o- a prefix that means 'red', e.g. *erythrocyte*.

erythroblast *n* a nucleated erythrocyte precursor found in the red bone marrow—**erythroblastic** *adj*.

erythroblastosis the abnormal presence of nucleated erythrocyte precursors in the blood. This may occur in situations when erythropoiesis (production of erythrocytes) is increased, such as in severe anaemia or when the bone marrow is affected by leukaemia or secondary cancer.

erythroblastosis fetalis ⊃ haemolytic disease of the newborn.

erythrocyanosis *n* a mottled red or purplish discoloration and swelling of the legs, particularly in cold weather. It commonly affects children, adolescents and older women.

erythrocyte glutathione reductase an enzyme present in erythrocytes. It is used for an enzyme activation assay to determine riboflavin (vitamin B_2) status.

erythrocyte sedimentation rate (ESR) citrated blood is placed in a narrow tube. The erythrocytes (red cells) fall, leaving a column of clear supernatant serum, which is measured at the end of an hour and reported in millimetres. It varies according to age and gender. Inflammation and tissue destruction cause an elevation in the ESR.

erythrocytes *npl* red blood cells. Non-nucleated red cells of the circulating blood. They carry oxygen and some carbon dioxide, and buffer pH changes in the blood. They are highly specialized for transporting oxygen from the lungs to the tissues and cells. Without a nucleus they are full of haemoglobin. In addition erythrocytes have no mitochondria (or other organelles) and rely on anaerobic glycolysis for energy production and therefore do not use the oxygen, which they carry. Mature erythrocytes are biconcave discs with a diameter of 7.0 μm and 2.2 μm thick (Figure E.8). Their surface area to volume ratio optimizes the transport of oxygen and carbon dioxide to and from the cells. Various genetically-determined antigens are present on the surface of the erythrocytes, including those for the ABO blood groups—**erythrocytic** *adj*.

E
F

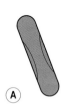 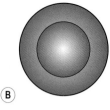

(A) (B)

E.8 Mature erythrocytes (reproduced from Watson 2000 with permission).

erythrocytopenia *n* deficiency in the number of erythrocytes (red blood cells)—**erythrocytopenic** *adj*.

erythrocytosis ⊃ polycythaemia.

erythroderma *n* excessive redness of the skin, typically involving more than 90% of the skin surface.

erythroedema polyneuropathy (*syn* acrodynia, pink disease) a condition of infancy characterized by red, swollen extremities, generalized skin rash, photophobia and irritability. May be caused by mercury poisoning.

erythrolabe a pigment contained in one group of cones; responds to light at the red end of the spectrum.

erythropoiesis *n* the production of erythrocytes (red blood cells) by the bone marrow. ⊃ erythropoietin, haemopoiesis.

erythropoietin (EPO) *n* a glycoprotein hormone/growth factor secreted mainly by kidney cells in response to reduced oxygen content in the blood, and also secreted by fetal liver cells. It acts on the bone marrow, stimulating erythropoiesis. A recombinant human form is used therapeutically to treat anaemia associated with chronic renal failure and platinum-containing chemotherapy.

erythropsia an abnormality of vision where all objects are seen as red.

erythropsin ⊃ rhodopsin.

eschar *n* a slough, as results from a burn, application of caustics, diathermy, etc.

escharotic a caustic or corrosive agent that may be used to produce a dry scab when applied to the skin.

escharotomy surgical incision into eschar to relieve restriction around a limb that could compromise the blood supply, or the chest to allow chest expansion.

Escherichia *n* (T Escherich, German physician, 1857–1911) a genus of bacteria of the family Enterobacteriaceae. Motile, Gram-negative bacilli that are widely distributed in nature. *Escherichia coli* is part of the normal flora in humans. Some strains are pathogens, causing gastroenteritis, peritonitis and wound infections, meningitis and urinary tract infections. The serotypes responsible for gastroenteritis are: (a) enterohaemorrhagic *E. coli* (EHEC), e.g. *E. coli* 0157, a virulent micro-organism that produces a toxin (verocytotoxin) and causes a variety of effects from mild diarrhoea to severe haemorrhagic bowel inflammation. It may cause life-threatening haemolytic uraemic syndrome; (b) enteroinvasive *E. coli* (EIEC), which causes bloodstained diarrhoea; (c) enteropathic *E. coli* (EPEC), which causes serious diarrhoea in babies, especially in developing countries; (d) enterotoxigenic *E. coli* (ETEC), responsible for outbreaks of gastroenteritis in developing countries. Leads to watery diarrhoea with fluid and electrolyte imbalance.

Esmarch's bandage (J von Esmarch, German surgeon, 1823–1908) a rubber roller bandage sometimes used to procure a bloodless operative field in the limbs.

esophoria *n* latent convergent strabismus.

esotropia *n* manifest convergent strabismus.

ESP *abbr* **1.** extended scope physiotherapy practitioner. **2.** extrasensory perception.

espundia *n* ⊃ leishmaniasis.

ESR *abbr* erythrocyte sedimentation rate.

ESRD/F *abbr* end-stage renal disease/failure. ⊃ renal failure.

essence a solution of an essential oil dissolved in alcohol.

Essence of Care Benchmarks in England, a series of patient/client/carer-focused benchmarks used to improve healthcare practice and for clinical governance. Currently the Department of Health have published eleven benchmarks covering the following areas of care: Personal and oral hygiene; Continence and bladder and bowel care; Food and nutrition; Pressure ulcers; Privacy and dignity; Record keeping; Safety of clients with mental health needs in acute mental health and general hospital settings; Principles of self-care; Communication; Promoting health, and most recently the Care environment in 2007.

essential amino acids also known as indispensable. The amino acids that cannot be synthesized in the body and therefore have to be provided by the diet. They are isoleucine, leucine, lysine, methionine, phenylalanine, threonine, tryptophan and valine in adults. Infants need these amino acids plus histidine and arginine. Other amino acids are considered to be conditionally essential because they become essential if the diet does not contain enough of the precursor amino acid from which they are synthesized: arginine, cysteine, glycine and tyrosine. ⊃ amino acids.

essential fatty acids (EFAs) the linoleic and alpha (α)-linolenic families of fatty acids. Polyunsaturated fatty acids (PUFAs) that cannot be synthesized in the body so must be supplied by the diet. Arachidonic, eicosapentaenoic and docosahexaenoic acids can all be synthesized from linoleic and α-linolenic acids, and become essential if linoleic and α-linolenic acids are in short supply. They have diverse functions, which include being the precursors for many regulatory lipids, e.g. prostaglandins; they fulfil an important role in lipid metabolism and are required for the integrity of cell membranes. They are present in oily fish and natural vegetable and seed oils.

essential oil the undiluted oil extracted from plants, usually diluted in a carrier oil prior to use during aromatherapy. Many essential oils are contraindicated in pregnancy, labour and during breast feeding.

Essix retainer ⊃ retainer.

establishment *n* describes the planned staffing levels in a particular area. Usually described as the number of whole time equivalents (WTEs).

ester an organic compound (a 'salt') formed from an organic acid and an alcohol. For instance, acetates are formed when the acid is acetic acid.

esterase an enzyme that splits esters into an acid and an alcohol.

estimated average requirement (EAR) one of the UK dietary reference values. It estimates the average requirement for a group of people, usually for energy requirements. It follows that 50% of people in the group will need more and 50% will need less. ⊃ dietary reference values.

estimated date of birth (EDB) a projected estimate of the date on which the infant will be born; only 3–4% of babies are born on the date calculated. It is estimated using Nägele's rule, and calculations may be adjusted to take into account personal factors such as menstrual history. ⊃ Nägele's rule.

estradiol *n Am* ⊃ oestradiol.

estrogen *n Am* ⊃ oestrogen.

ESWL *abbr* extracorporeal shock-wave lithotripsy.

ESV *abbr* end-systolic volume.

ET *abbr* endotracheal tube.

etching the selective dissolution of a surface by an acid or other agent. ⊃ acid etching.

ETCO$_2$ *abbr* end-tidal carbon dioxide.

ETEC *abbr* enterotoxigenic *Escherichia coli*.

ethanol *n* ethyl alcohol. The alcohol in alcoholic beverages.

ether *n* early volatile anaesthetic agent now rarely used.

ethernet a method of connecting a computer to a network to enable communication with other computers.

ethical reasoning the range of cognitive processes and mental strategies used by the therapist when identifying and thinking about the moral dimension of a situation in order to reach a decision on the best course of action.

ethics *n* a code of moral principles derived from a system of values and beliefs. It is concerned with rights and obligations.

ethics committees bodies that operate in academic institutions, Health Authorities and NHS Trusts to consider proposals for research projects. The approval of the appropriate ethics committee is usually a prerequisite for obtaining a research grant.

ethmoid *n* a spongy bone that occupies the anterior part of the base of the skull and helps to form the orbital cavity, the nasal septum and the lateral walls of the nasal cavity. On each side are two projections into the nasal cavity, the upper and middle conchae or turbinates (turbinated processes). It is a very delicate bone containing many ethmoidal air sinuses lined with ciliated epithelium and with openings into the nasal cavity. The horizontal flattened part, the cribriform plate, forms the roof of the nasal cavity and has numerous small foramina through which nerve fibres of the olfactory nerves (first cranial nerves, sense of smell) pass upwards from the nasal cavity to the brain. There is also a very fine perpendicular plate of bone that forms the upper part of the nasal septum. ⊃ cribriform, inferior nasal conchae.

ethmoidectomy *n* surgical removal of a part or all of the ethmoid bone.

ethnic *adj* relating to a social group who have common customs and culture. Frequently used incorrectly to describe race.

ethnocentrism the belief that one's own culture and lifestyle is superior to those of other groups. Often makes the assumption that the beliefs, values, priorities and views of one's culture are universal.

ethnography *n* a study of individuals in their usual surroundings. Used in qualitative research by anthropologists to describe customs, culture and social life through observation, informal interviews, etc.

ethnology *n* a branch of anthropology that studies mainly the cultural differences between social groups, particularly the beliefs, attitudes and values pertaining to life events that include birth, marriage, health care, death, etc.—**ethnological** *adj*, **ethnologically** *adv*.

ethoxybenzoic acid (EBA) cement (zinc oxide/EBA cement). Reinforced zinc oxide-eugenol cement in which some of the eugenol is replaced by 2-ethoxybenzoic acid. The zinc oxide is reinforced by the addition of inorganic fillers such as alumina and silica together with rosin. ⊃ cement.

ethyl chloride a volatile liquid used to test the onset of regional anaesthesia by reason of the intense cold sensation produced when applied to the skin.

ethylene diamine tetra-acetic acid (EDTA) a chelating agent that binds to metals such as calcium, mercury, iron, lead, etc. Used to treat severe hypercalcaemia and occasionally for mercury poisoning. Used in food processing and in many other industrial applications. *ethylene diamine tetra-acetic acid solution* in dentistry, used in root canal therapy to soften dentine and facilitate its removal from root canal walls by means of reamers and files.

ethylene oxide a gas used to sterilize delicate equipment that would be damaged by high temperatures.

ETL *abbr* echo train length.

ETT *abbr* exercise tolerance test.

eu- a prefix that means 'well, normal', e.g. *eutocia*.

EUA *abbr* examination under anaesthetic.

Eubacterium a genus of Gram-positive anaerobic bacteria with rigid cell walls, they are normally present in water and soil. They are of low pathogenicity but do sometimes cause soft tissue infections and may be implicated in periodontal disease.

eugenics *n* the study of genetics aimed at improving future generations—**eugenic** *adj*.

eugenol essential oil of oil of cloves. Liquid component of zinc oxide-eugenol cements and has sedative and obtundent properties. Classified as an antiseptic.

eugnathia a normal jaw, one in which the maxilla and mandible are in correct alignment.

euhydration a term used in sports medicine meaning normal state of body water. ⊃ hydration status of athletes, water balance.

eunuch *n* a human male from whom the testes have been removed; a castrated male.

eupepsia normal digestion.

euphoria *n* in psychiatry, an exaggerated sense of well-being—**euphoric** *adj*.

euploidy *n* having a deviation in chromosome number, which is a precise multiple of the haploid (n) number.

European Food Safety Authority (EFSA) the agency in the European Union that assesses risks to food safety and issues independent scientific advice about food safety. Their remit covers the entire food chain.

European Medicines Agency (EMEA) an agency of the European Union tasked with protecting and promoting the health of people and animals by evaluating and supervising human and veterinary medicines.

eustachian tube (B Eustachio, Italian anatomist, 1524–74). ⊃ pharyngotympanic (auditory) tube.

eustress ⊃ stress.

eutectic describes a mixture of two or more constituents that melts and resolidifies without separation of its constituents.

euthanasia *n* literally an 'easy death'. Inferring a painless death. Frequently interpreted as the act of causing a painless and planned death, such as relieving a person's extreme suffering from an incurable disease. Presently illegal in UK and opposed by many professional groups, it is regulated and practised legally in some European countries. ⊃ homicide.

euthyroid state denoting normal thyroid function.

Euthyscope ⊃ Visuscope.

eutocia *n* a natural and normal labour and childbirth without any complications.

eutrophia normal nutrition.

EV *abbr* exposure value.

evacuant *n* an agent which initiates an evacuation, such as of the bowel. ⊃ enema, laxatives.

evacuation *n* the act of emptying a cavity; generally refers to the discharge of faecal matter from the rectum. *manual evacuation* digital removal of faeces from the rectum.

evacuation of retained products of conception (ERPC) emptying the uterus following an incomplete miscarriage.

evacuator *n* an instrument for procuring evacuation, e.g. the removal from the bladder of a stone, crushed by a lithotrite.

evaluation (nursing) *n* in the United Kingdom, commonly accepted as the fourth stage of the nursing process. Care is evaluated to assess whether the stated patient/client goals have been or are being achieved. Although it is the final step in the nursing process, it should occur continuously from the first assessment to the patient's discharge from the healthcare system—**evaluating** *v*. ⊃ assessment, implementation, planning.

evaluation a process of obtaining, interpreting and appraising information in order to prioritize problems and needs, to plan and modify interventions and to judge the worth of interventions. (Reproduced with permission from the European Network of Occupational Therapy in Higher Education (ENOTHE) Terminology Project, 2008.)

evaporate *vt, vi* to convert from the liquid to the gaseous state by the application of heat.

evaporating lotion one which, applied as a compress, absorbs heat in order to evaporate and so cools the skin.

even echo rephrasing in magnetic resonance imaging (MRI), the re-establishment of spin-echo coherence of moving spins on symmetric even echoes in multiecho sequences as a result of sequential integration of signal phase shifts adding to zero.

evening primrose oil a source of γ-linolenic acid. Sometimes used to relieve the symptoms of premenstrual syndrome.

eventration the protrusion of the intestines through a wound in the abdominal wall. ⊃ dehiscence.

eversion *n* **1.** a turning outwards, as of the upper eyelid to expose the palpebral conjunctiva. **2.** turning the sole of the foot outwards (laterally). ⊃ inversion *opp*.

eversion injury damage to the medial structures of the ankle joint, by outward turning of the foot; the relative strength of the medial (deltoid) ligament may result in a fragment of bone being pulled off (avulsion fracture) rather than tearing of the ligament, and also accounts for it being less common than inversion injury.

evidence-based medicine (EBM) practice (EBP) describes the practice of medicine or delivery of healthcare interventions that are based on systematic analysis of information available in terms of effectiveness in relation to cost-effective health outcomes. The highest level of evidence (based on the robustness of the research methodology) is that gained from meta-analysis of randomized controlled trials (RCTs). Sometimes this level of evidence is not available and at the lowest level may be based on evidence from expert committee reports or opinions and/or clinical experience of respected practitioners.

evisceration *n* removal of internal organs. Also, describes the removal of the inner contents of the eye with the exception of the sclera. It is usually performed when there is intraocular suppuration. ⊃ enucleation.

evulsion *n* forcible tearing away of a structure.

EW *abbr* extended wear (contact lens).

Ewing's tumour (J Ewing, American pathologist, 1866–1943) sarcoma involving a long bone, usually diagnosed in a child or young adult.

exacerbation *n* increased severity, as of symptoms.

exanthema *n* a skin eruption—**exanthemata** *pl*, **exanthematous** *adj*.

excavation the process of scooping out. In dentistry, the removal of a softened dentine from a carious tooth.

excavator a hand-held cutting instrument used primarily to excavate softened dentine from a carious tooth. It has a sharp blade which may be circular, oval or spoon shaped. Usually double ended.

excess post-exercise oxygen consumption (EPOC) ⊃ elevated post-exercise oxygen consumption, oxygen debt.

excision *n* removal of a part by cutting—**excise** *vt*.

excitability *n* rapid response to stimuli; easily irritated such as nerve and muscle cells—**excitable** *adj*.

excitation *n* **1.** the act of stimulating an organ or tissue. **2.** the process of moving an electron in an atom into a higher orbit.

excitation–contraction coupling the link between excitation of muscle membrane and initiation of force generation at cross-bridges, producing muscle contraction. In all types of muscle this involves a rise in cytoplasmic ionized calcium $[Ca^{2+}]$ concentration but mechanisms for this rise differ substantially. In healthy skeletal muscle the sarcoplasmic reticulum (SR) is the sole effective source of $[Ca^{2+}]$, which within normal physiological function can only be released from the SR by a muscle action potential, triggered via the motor nerve. In cardiac muscle, the action potential is spontaneously initiated in cardiac pacemaker cells rather than by nerves, and $[Ca^{2+}]$ release from the SR is triggered by $[Ca^{2+}]$ itself, entering the cell from the extracellular fluid during the action potential. In certain smooth muscle masses, neural control mechanisms analogous to those of skeletal muscle operate but more commonly, hormones and/or other chemicals are involved; the $[Ca^{2+}]$ comes from both the SR and the extracellular fluid, as it does in cardiac muscle, but mediated largely by different mechanisms.

exchange list food portions which contain the same amount of energy, carbohydrate, fat and/or protein. Used to simplify meal, snack and diet planning for people with special dietary requirements.

exchange transfusion ⮕ transfusion.

excimer laser a gas laser which emits pulses of light in the ultraviolet region (at 193 nm). All the energy is absorbed by the superficial layers (e.g. the corneal epithelium) which are then exploded away or ablated without any change to the underlying or adjacent tissue or material. It is used to treat certain corneal pathologies, and in the surgical correction of refractive errors. ⮕ LASIK, radial keratotomy.

excision arthroplasty the gap in the joint is filled with fibrous tissue as in Keller's operation for hallux valgus.

excisional biopsy the complete removal of a lesion or abnormal tissue for histological examination.

excitatory post synaptic potential (EPSP) a physiological term that refers to the effect that is produced when excitatory input to a neuron causes brief depolarization that spreads to the axon hillock, the balance between this and the inhibitory post synaptic potential determine the final output from the neuron. ⮕ inhibitory post synaptic potential.

exclusion criteria a research term. The criteria by which members of the population of the sample will be excluded, for example in a study of heart rate, people with a history of cardiac problems would be excluded.

exclusion diet excluding foods that commonly cause food intolerance, then adding specific foods in order to test for intolerance.

exclusion isolation ⮕ protective isolation.

excoriation *n* ⮕ abrasion.

excrement *n* faeces.

excrescence *n* an abnormal protuberance or growth of the tissues.

excreta *n* the waste material that is normally cleared from the body, particularly urine and faeces.

excretion *n* the elimination of waste material from the body, and also the eliminated material—**excretory** *adj*, **excrete** *vt*.

excretion urography the radiographic investigation of the kidneys, ureters and bladder following the injection of a contrast agent.

excursion the movement of the mandible laterally, protrusively or retrusively.

excursive movements the movement occurring when the mandible moves away from the intercuspal position.

excyclophoria ⮕ cyclophoria.

executive dysfunction a loss of the normal high-level cognitive (executive) functions, due to brain injury. Patients can present as lethargic, poorly motivated, disinterested and with poor planning and organizational skills, however, superficially this deficit may not be immediately apparent unless the patient is asked to undertake complex tasks. They often also have disinhibition and so in social situations have great difficulties of which they are often not aware.

exenteration *n* removal of the viscera from its containing cavity, e.g. the eye from its socket, the pelvic organs from the pelvis.

exercise physical activity that aims to improve or maintain health, increase mobility during rehabilitation, improve strength, stamina and suppleness, and physical performance. ⮕ aerobic exercise, anaerobic exercise, exercise during pregnancy, isometric exercise, isotonic exercise.

exercise-associated muscle cramp (EAMC) occurs mainly during or after prolonged or high-intensity running; formerly blamed on salt and/or water deficiency or overheating, but more recently attributed to fatigue-enhanced input from muscle spindles that overactivates spinal motor neurons, whilst suppressing the Golgi tendon organs which are normally inhibitory. ⮕ cramp.

exercise dependence a dependency on engaging in exercise characterized by excessive amounts of exercising, often to the exclusion of other normal life activities, and feelings of guilt and negative moodstates when the exercise schedule is not adhered to. Also known as exercise addiction and compulsion to exercise.

exercise during pregnancy most women feel and look better if they exercise while pregnant and it helps to alleviate backache and maintain posture, ease joint discomfort, allow better sleep and minimize excessive weight gain. Pregnancy confers physiological benefits to exercise and possibly performance during the first trimester (3 months), especially by virtue of changes in the cardiorespiratory systems. Modern thinking is that exercise is generally safe and should be encouraged, if comfortable, until well into the last trimester, provided that there are no complications of pregnancy (bleeding, hypertension, multiple pregnancy, placenta praevia, etc.). Walking, cycling, dance and water-based activity are popular with pregnant women. Exercise should be symptom-limited and should stop if the woman becomes dizzy or breathless. Contact sports such as boxing and those where a fall is likely, such as horse riding, climbing and trampolining, are not recommended in case of damage to the fetus.

exercise economy the oxygen uptake needed to generate a specific speed or power output.

exercise induced asthma bronchospasm caused by exercise in a cold, dry climate.

exercise physiology involves the description and explanation of functional changes in the body brought about by either a single or repeated exercise sessions.

exercise (stress) test ⮕ exercise tolerance test (ETT).

exercise tests these tests provide valuable information concerning the cardiorespiratory system's abilities to meet increased demands for gas exchange and oxygen transport during raised activity levels, the ability of the musculoskeletal system to generate effort and muscular activity and the ability to endure additional requirements over time. The tests may take a number of formats including treadmill and cycle ergometry tests, field walk tests, such as the 6- and 12-min walk tests, shuttle walk test and shuttle runs, etc. The tests are aimed at detecting limitations to activity, identify levels of activity producing signs and symptoms, provide baseline values to enable reassessment and progression or decline in response to an intervention and form the basis for an individualized exercise prescription.

exercise tolerance exercise undertaken without marked dyspnoea or pain. American Heart Association's classification of functional capacity: Class I—no symptoms with ordinary effort; Class II—slight disability with ordinary effort (usually subdivided into Class IIa—able to carry on with normal housework under difficulty—and Class IIb—cannot manage shopping or bedmaking except very slowly); Class III—marked disability with ordinary effort which precludes any attempt at housework; Class IV—symptoms at rest or heart failure.

exercise tolerance test (ETT) also known as exercise (stress) test. It is performed during increasing levels of exertion to detect arrhythmias or ischaemic changes caused by physical stress. Frequently used for the diagnosis or prognosis of heart disease or to guide cardiac rehabilitation, or as part of an athletic fitness assessment. In sport, used primarily as a simple and inexpensive screening tool for potential causes of sudden death. A 12-lead ECG is recorded during exercise on a treadmill or static cycle ergometer. The limb leads are placed on the shoulders and hips rather than the wrists and ankles. The Bruce protocol has been well validated and is the most widely used test format for treadmill testing. Blood pressure is recorded and symptoms assessed regularly throughout the test. Common indications for exercise testing in cardiology include: (a) to confirm a diagnosis of angina; (b) to evaluate stable angina; (c) to assess prognosis following myocardial infarction; (d) to assess outcome after coronary revasculaization, e.g. coronary angioplasty; (e) to diagnose and evaluate the treatment of exercise-induced arrhythmias. A test is 'positive' if

anginal pain occurs, blood pressure falls or fails to rise, or there is ST segment shifts of > 1 mm. The results of an exercise tolerance test are not always conclusive. Some patients with a negative test will have underlying coronary disease (false negative) and, conversely, some with a positive test will not have coronary disease (false positive). Exercise testing is an unreliable population screening tool because in low-risk individuals (e.g. asymptomatic young or middle-aged women) an abnormal response is more likely to represent a false positive than a true positive test. In patients with symptoms suggestive of angina, exercise testing has much better sensitivity and specificity, and is clinically very useful. High-risk findings include: (a) low threshold for ischaemia (i.e. within stage 1 or 2 of the Bruce protocol); (b) a fall in blood pressure on exercise; (c) widespread, marked or prolonged ischaemic ECG changes; (d) exercise-induced arrhythmia. Exercise testing is not infallible and may produce false positive results in the presence of digoxin therapy, left ventricular hypertrophy, left bundle branch block or Wolff–Parkinson–White syndrome. The predictive accuracy of exercise testing is lower in women than men. The test should be classed as inconclusive (and not negative) if the patient cannot achieve an adequate level of exercise because of locomotor or other non-cardiac problems. Stress tests are contraindicated in the presence of unstable angina, decompensated heart failure and severe hypertension. ⮕ Bruce protocol.

ex, exo- a prefix that means 'away from, out, outside, outward, out of', e.g. *exogenous.*

exfoliation *n* 1. the scaling off of tissues in layers. 2. the shedding of the primary teeth—**exfoliative** *adj.*

exfoliation syndrome ⮕ pseudoexfoliation (PXF).

exfoliative cytology the cytological examination of cells shed, or sampled, from the surface of an organ or lesion, such as from the uterine cervix, or present in urine or sputum, etc. ⮕ cervical smear.

ex gratia as a matter of favour, e.g. without admission of liability, of payment offered by a NHS Trust to a claimant.

exhalation expiration, breathing out.

exhaustion ⮕ fatigue.

exhibitionism *n* 1. any kind of 'showing off'; extravagant behaviour to attract attention. 2. a psychosexual disorder confined to males and consisting of repeated exposure of the genitalia to a stranger who is usually an adult female or a child. The act of exposure is sufficient and usually no further contact is sought with the victim—**exhibitionist** *n.*

exit port (aperture or window) in radiography, the opening in the tube head through which X-rays leave.

exocrine *adj* describes glands from which the secretion passes via a duct; secreting externally, e.g. sweat glands. ⮕ endocrine *opp*—**exocrinal** *adj.*

exocytosis a term for the process by which some molecules, e.g. some hormones and mucus, leave cells. ⮕ bulk transport, endocytosis *opp.*

exodontics exodontia. The subject of and techniques used in the extraction of teeth or parts of them from the mouth.

exoenzyme an enzyme that acts outside the cell from which it was secreted, e.g. pepsin.

exogenous *adj* of external origin. ◔ endogenous *opp*.

exolever an elevator for extracting whole or parts of teeth.

exomphalos *n* (*syn* omphalocele) a condition present at birth and due to failure of the gut to return to the abdominal cavity during fetal development. The intestines and sometimes other structures, including the liver, protrude through a defect in the abdominal wall around the umbilical cord.

exon a gene segment that is represented in the messenger RNA product. It is involved in protein production, with each exon coding a specific part of the finished protein. ◔ intron.

exophytic tendency to grow outwards, such as a tumour that grows into the lumen of a hollow organ rather than into the wall.

expanded disability status scale (EDSS) a classification scheme (rating scale) that insures all participants in clinical trials are in the same class, type, or phase of multiple sclerosis. It is also used to follow the progression of disability and evaluate treatment results.

exopeptidase an enzyme that catalyses the breaking of the terminal peptide bonds between amino acids in a polypeptide or protein.

Experience of Caregiving Inventory (ECI) used by mental health nurses and others to assess both burden and coping. Comprises 66 questions which cover 10 areas. Eight areas described as 'negative', e.g. difficult behaviours; two areas described as 'positive', e.g. positive personal experiences.

expert witness a person with specific qualifications, a great deal of experience and knowledge in a particular area who is able to testify or give evidence in a court of law.

exophoria *n* latent divergent strabismus.

exophthalmometer/proptometer an instrument that measures the degree of exophthalmos.

exophthalmos *n* protrusion of the eyeball—**exophthalmic** *adj*.

exostosis *n* an overgrowth of bone tissue from the surface of a bone forming a benign tumour. May be due to chronic inflammation, constant pressure on the bone or tumour formation. In dentistry, it may influence the positioning of a prosthesis.

exothermic *adj* **1.** describes a chemical reaction in which there is release of heat. Found in the setting process of various cements and acrylic resin as a result of chemical reactions. **2.** relating to the temperature of the external body surface. ◔ endothermic.

exotoxin *n* a toxin released through the cell wall of a living bacterium, e.g. *Clostridium tetani*. They have extensive systemic effects, which include muscle spasm. ◔ endotoxin—**exotoxic** *adj*.

exotropia *n* manifest divergent strabismus.

expansion in dentistry, the movement of teeth by an orthodontic appliance in order to correct a malocclusion.

expectancy–value theory in psychology, the theory that behaviour is a function of the interaction between a person's expectancies about the outcomes of actions and the value they place on those outcomes. For example, a person might engage in regular exercise because they believe that exercise is good for their health and they also value good health.

expected date of delivery (EDD) usually calculated as 280 days from the first day of the last normal menstrual period.

expectorant *n* a drug which may promote expectoration.

expectoration *n* **1.** the elimination of secretions from the respiratory tract by coughing. **2.** sputum—**expectorate** *vt*.

experimental epidemiology the study of the effect of controlling the relevant suspected factors in the cause of a disease such as stopping cigarette smoking.

experimental group a research term that describes the group exposed to the independent variable (the intervention or experimental agent such as a drug). ◔ control group, variable.

expiration *n* the process of breathing out air from the lungs—**expiratory** *adj*, **expire** *vt*, *vi*.

expiratory reserve volume (ERV) a lung volume. It is the volume of air additional to the tidal volume that can be expired during a maximum expiration.

explorer ◔ probe (dental).

exponential law the decay or growth of a substance in which each step is half the value or double the value of the preceding step.

exposure **1.** the measure at a particular point in a beam of X or γ rays and is the total charge of one sign over a small volume of air, unit coulombs per kilogram, now replaced by the kerma. **2.** the act of laying open, as in a surgical exposure. **3.** subjection to infection, thermal changes, radiation, etc. **4.** in dentistry, a defect in the wall of a tooth pulp cavity leading to exposure of pulp tissue. This may be the result of instrumentation (*traumatic*) or of caries (*carious*).

exposure factors the settings used to produce the optimum radiographic image quality with the minimum radiation dose to the patient. The settings include the kilovoltage (kVp), milliamperes per second (mAs), source to image distance (SID), object to image distance (OID), source to object distance (SOD), the use of a secondary radiation grid, collimation and the type of film–screen combination used.

exposure rate the measure of the intensity of a beam in unit time.

expressed emotion a research concept that sought to establish how certain environments might influence the course of schizophrenia.

expression *n* **1.** expulsion by force as of the placenta from the uterus; milk from the breast, etc. **2.** a genetic term for the appearance of a particular trait or characteristic. **3.** facial disclosure of feelings, mood, etc.

expressive motor aphasia a type of aphasia where there is difficulty in language production. Those affected have word finding difficulties and may have problems producing sentence structures. May coexist with receptive aphasia.

exsanguination *n* the process of rendering bloodless—**exsanguinate** *vt*.

exsiccation ◔ desiccation.

exstrophy a congenital anomaly in which the interior surface of an organ, such as the bladder, communicates with the outside. In this situation the abdominal wall and the anterior wall of the bladder are absent and the inside of the bladder is exposed on the surface of the abdomen.

extended family the wider group of family relations including grandparents, aunts, uncles, cousins, etc. ⊃ nuclear family.

extended focus-to-skin distance techniques radiotherapy treatment techniques where the focus to skin distance (FSD) is greater than 100 cm.

extended scope physiotherapy practitioner (ESP) a specialist physiotherapist whose role has been extended to include assessment, ordering certain investigations, making referrals, etc. Practise in areas that include orthopaedics, rheumatology and with neurosurgical patients.

extended wear lens a contact lens designed to be worn continuously for more than one day and, usually, no more than seven days before cleaning and sterilization. It is, typically, a soft lens, with high oxygen transmissibility. ⊃ cornea guttata, corneal infiltrates, corneal ulcer, epithelial microcysts, oxygen transmissibility, pannus, silicone hydrogel lens, specular microscope.

extension *n* **1.** traction upon a fractured or dislocated limb. **2.** the straightening of a flexed limb or part. A movement at a joint that increases the joint angle, e.g. straightening the leg at the knee or the arm at the elbow, moving the hand backwards at the wrist; or one involving several joints that brings dorsal surfaces nearer together, e.g. extending the neck to tilt the head backwards or curving the spine backwards. ⊃ extensor, flexion *opp*.

extension-cone paralleling technique (XCP) paralleling technique using a long cone measuring about 40 cm. ⊃ paralleling technique.

'extension for prevention' a technique previously used. The extension in the course of preparation of a cavity, to include adjacent areas of sound tissue which are judged likely to become carious, i.e. pits and fissures. Now considered to be over-preparation of tooth tissue in view of current adhesive materials and concepts of caries management.

extensor *n* a muscle which on contraction extends or straightens a part, e.g. extensor carpi ulnaris, the triceps acting at the elbow and the quadriceps group acting at the knee. flexor *opp*. ⊃ Colour Section Figures 4, 5.

extensor carpi radialis brevis a superficial, posterior muscle of the forearm. Its origin is on the lateral epicondyle of the humerus and it inserts on the third metacarpal. It functions with the extensor carpi radialis longus to stabilize the wrist during flexion movements of the fingers, and abducts and extends the wrist. ⊃ Colour Section Figures 4, 5.

extensor carpi radialis longus a superficial, posterior muscle of the forearm. Its origin is on the humerus above the lateral epicondyle and it inserts on the second metacarpal. It functions to abduct and extend the wrist. ⊃ Colour Section Figures 4, 5.

extensor carpi ulnaris a superficial, posterior muscle of the forearm. Its origin is on the back of the ulna and the lateral epicondyle of the humerus and it inserts on the fifth metacarpal. It functions with the flexor carpi ulnaris to adduct and extend the wrist. ⊃ Colour Section Figures 4, 5.

extensor lag if a joint will extend passively but not actively, the resulting droop of the joint is known as an extensor lag.

extensor response a response initiated by contact of the back of the head with a supporting surface with the result that the body and limbs extend. Normally seen in severe brain injury or multiple sclerosis, this posturing is seen more markedly in supine lying.

extensor thrust a compensatory response where the patient thrusts backwards into extension in an attempt to gain activity against gravity.

exterioration a surgical procedure whereby an internal structure is repositioned on the body surface, such as the ileum or colon, to form a stoma.

external auditory meatus/canal the canal between the pinna and eardrum. ⊃ Colour Section Figure 13.

external bevel incision incision designed to reduce the thickness of gingiva from the external surface.

external cephalic version (ECV) the conversion of a breech to a cephalic presentation by manipulation through the abdominal wall. The technique is safer with the use of ultrasound and tachographic monitoring. ⊃ version.

external fixation a method of fracture immobilization by inserting pins above and below the fracture. External rods are used to secure the pins. The tension on parts of the device can be adjusted during healing. ⊃ Ilizarov frame/method.

external haemorrhage (*syn* revealed haemorrhage) ⊃ haemorrhage, revealed haemorrhage.

external haemorrhoids ⊃ haemorrhoids.

external imagery ⊃ imagery.

external jugular vein ⊃ jugular veins.

external (lateral) rotation a limb or body movement where there is rotation away from the vertical axis of the body. A movement at a joint that causes rotation of a limb or part of a limb around its long axis away from the midline of the body, e.g. external rotation at the elbow turns the forearm outwards, bringing the palm of the hand to face forwards, or the whole arm can be externally rotated at the shoulder; the whole leg can be externally rotated from the hip but the knee does not allow external rotation of the lower leg alone. ⊃ internal rotation *opp*.

external malleolus ⊃ malleolus.

external oblique muscle paired muscle of the anterior abdominal wall. ⊃ abdominal muscles.

external oblique ridge a smooth ridge on the buccal surface of the body of the mandible that extends from the anterior border of the ramus to the region of the mental foramen.

external or communicating hydrocephalus describes hydrocephalus where the excess of fluid is mainly in the subarachnoid space. ⊃ hydrocephalus.

external os ⊃ os.

external respiration is the exchange of gases between alveolar air and pulmonary capillary blood. Oxygen in the alveolar air moves into the blood, and carbon dioxide moves from the blood into the air in the lungs for excretion. ⊃ internal or tissue respiration.

external work ⊃ work.

exteroceptive receptors stimulated from the stimuli arising in the external environment.

extinction in psychology. The decline, over time, of a conditioned response unless it is reinforced.

extirpation *n* complete removal or destruction of a part. In endodontics, commonly used to describe the complete removal of vital dental pulp.

extra-articular *adj* outside a joint. An anatomical term referring to something that is external to a joint. For example, an extra-articular feature of rheumatoid arthritis may be anaemia.

extracapsular *adj* outside a capsule. ⊃ intracapsular *opp*.

extracapsular cataract extraction (ECCE) a surgical procedure for the removal of a crystalline lens affected by cataract. The anterior capsule is excised, the lens nucleus is removed and the residual equatorial cortex is aspirated. The posterior capsule may be polished. An intraocular lens implant may then be inserted. ⊃ capsule of the crystalline lens, capsulectomy, intraocular lens (IOL) implant, phacoemulsification.

extracardiac *adj* outside the heart.

extracellular *adj* outside the cell membrane.

extracellular fluid (ECF) that fluid outside the cells such as plasma, interstitial fluid, lymph, gastrointestinal secretions and CSF. In an adult with an ideal weight of 70 kg there will be around 12 L of plasma and interstitial fluid. ⊃ intracellular *opp*.

extracellular matrix (ECM) the material outside the cells, which supports cells and influences intercellular communication. It contains many different substances including elastin, collagen, hyaluronic acid, etc. ⊃ fibronectin.

extracellular polysaccharides (EPS) polysaccharides either produced outside the cell or produced inside the cell and then transported to the outside. In dentistry, the term refers to a variety of polymers of glucose or fructose produced extracellularly by a mixture of different enzymes using sucrose as the substrate. Fructan and levan are polymers of fructose, glucan and dextran are polymers of glucose. Extracellular polysaccharides have a variety of functions within dental plaque and are thought to contribute to plaque pathogenicity.

extracoronal outside the crown of a tooth. Describes a restoration which envelops the remaining natural crown.

extracoronal attachment a precision attachment which is attached to a restoration but situated outside the coronal contours of an abutment tooth.

extracorporeal *adj* outside the body.

extracorporeal circulation blood is taken from the body, directed through a machine ('heart–lung' or 'artificial kidney') and returned to the general circulation. ⊃ cardiopulmonary bypass, extracorporeal membrane oxygenation (ECMO), haemodialysis.

extracorporeal membrane oxygenation (ECMO) a cardiopulmonary bypass device which uses a membrane oxygenator (artificial lung). Venous blood from the patient circulates through the device. A fresh flow of oxygen into the device passes through a semipermeable membrane that allows the diffusion of oxygen whilst simultaneously removing carbon dioxide and water. Once the blood is oxygenated it is returned to the patient through an artery or a vein.

extracorporeal shock-wave lithotripsy (ESWL) the use of shock-waves produced by a lithotriptor to fragment renal calculi or gallstones. ⊃ lithotriptor.

extract *n* a preparation obtained by evaporating a solution of a drug.

extraction *n* commonly applied to the removal of a tooth.

extraction forceps ⊃ forceps.

extraction of lens surgical removal of the lens from the eye. It may be *extracapsular extraction*, when the capsule is ruptured prior to delivery of the lens and preserved in part, or *intracapsular extraction*, when the lens and capsule are removed intact.

extradural *adj* external to the dura mater.

extradural haematoma a collection of blood external to the dura mater (Figure E.9). This is caused by a bleed between the dura (the outer membrane of the meninges) and the skull following head injury. As there is nowhere for the blood to be absorbed it is very serious and rapidly leads to compression of the brain and death unless emergency neurosurgery is undertaken to stop the bleeding and remove the clot. Patients who receive neurosurgery in the early stages can make a full recovery and so it is essential that correct and frequent observations be undertaken on all head-injured patients to detect any deterioration.

extra, extro- a prefix that means 'outside, in addition to, beyond', e.g. *extradural*.

extrafoveal vision ⊃ peripheral vision.

extrafusal fibres the skeletal muscle fibres innervated by alpha (α)-motor neurons outside muscle spindle. ⊃ intrafusal fibres.

extrafusal muscle striated muscle fibre found outside the muscle spindle.

extrahepatic *adj* outside the liver.

extrahepatic cholestasis obstruction to the flow of bile occurring outside the liver. Caused by a blockage to a large bile duct, e.g. the common bile duct, by a gallstone or a tumour, or a tumour involving the head of the pancreas. ⊃ intrahepatic cholestasis.

extramural *adj* outside the wall of a structure—**extramurally** *adv*.

extraocular *adj* outside the eyeball.

extraocular muscles of the eye also called extrinsic muscles. Six muscles that move the eye. The muscles are attached at one end to the eyeball and at the other to the walls of the orbital cavity. There are four rectus (straight) muscles (medial, lateral, superior and inferior) and two

E
F

275

E.9 Extradural haematoma (reproduced from Parsons & Johnson 2001 with permission).

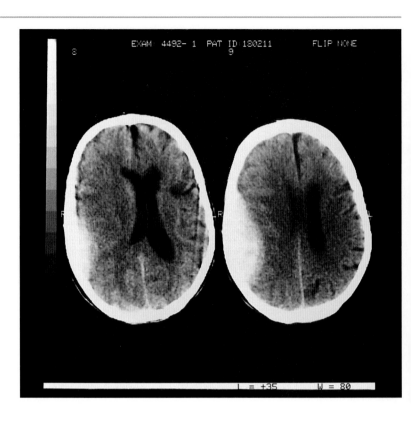

oblique muscles (superior and inferior). Moving the eyeballs to look in a particular direction is under voluntary control, but the coordination of movement, needed for convergence and accommodation to near or distant vision, is under autonomic (involuntary) control. Three separate cranial nerves supply the six extraoccular muscles: the oculomotor nerves (third pair of cranial nerves); the trochlear nerves (fourth pair of cranial nerves); and the abducens (abducent) nerves (the sixth pair of cranial nerves). ⏎ inferior oblique muscle, inferior rectus muscle, lateral rectus muscle, medial rectus muscle, superior oblique muscle, superior rectus muscle.

extraoral outside the mouth.

extraoral anchorage an anchorage obtained from outside the oral cavity. A type of orthodontic anchorage with apparatus using the top or back of the head or neck to achieve anchorage—headgear, cervical headgear or halo.

extraoral radiograph a radiograph in which the film is placed outside the mouth during exposure, e.g. panoramic radiographs, always housed in cassettes to reduce the amount of radiation used.

extraoral tracing ⏎ tracing.

extraoral traction (EOT) the use of extraoral apparatus to apply force to the teeth in orthodontic treatment.

extraperitoneal *adj* outside the peritoneum—**extraperitoneally** *adv.*

extrapleural *adj* outside the pleura, i.e. between the parietal pleura and the chest wall—**extrapleurally** *adv.*

extrapyramidal *adj* outside the pyramidal tracts.

extrapyramidal effects/disturbances include the tremor and rigidity seen in parkinsonism and Parkinson's disease and the side-effects of drugs, such as phenothiazine antipsychotic drugs (neuroleptics), which may cause a parkinsonian-like syndrome. ⏎ tardive dyskinesia.

extrapyramidal tracts motor pathways that pass outside the internal capsule. They modify pyramidal tract motor functions and influence coarse voluntary movement and affect posture, coordination and balance.

extrarenal *adj* outside the kidney—**extrarenally** *adv.*

extrasensory *adj* outside the normally accepted senses.

extrasensory perception (ESP) response to an external stimulus without what is generally accepted as normal contact or communication.

extrasystole *n* premature beats (ectopic beats) in the pulse rhythm: the cardiac impulse is initiated by an abnormal focus.

extrathoracic *adj* outside the thoracic cavity.

extrauterine *adj* outside the uterus.

extrauterine pregnancy ⏎ ectopic pregnancy.

extravasation *n* an escape of fluid from its normal enclosure into the surrounding tissues. It can result in tissue necrosis, such as following extravasation of chemotherapy drugs. ⏎ Colour Section Figure 69.

extraversion one of the big five personality factors characterized by a tendency to be sociable, outgoing and assertive.

extremophiles a general term for micro-organisms that can grow and reproduce in extreme environmental conditions, e.g. high temperature, extreme cold, extremes of pH, high pressure and high salt concentrations. ⮌ halophiles, osmophiles, psychrophiles, thermophiles.

extrinsic *adj* developing or having its origin from without; not internal.

extrinsic allergic alveolitis (*syn* hypersensitivity pneumonitis) an inflammatory response in the lungs to the inhalation of organic dusts, (e.g. farmer's lung or bird fancier's lung). The two main causes are microbial spores present in vegetable produce such as mouldy hay and animal proteins most commonly from pigeons and budgerigars. In an acute attack flu-like symptoms and breathlessness develop several hours after exposure; the symptoms generally subside spontaneously. If exposure continues a chronic condition with pulmonary fibrosis will develop. ⮌ hypersensitivity pneumonitis.

extrinsic factor vitamin B$_{12}$, essential for the maturation of erythrocytes and nerve function, cannot be synthesized in the body and must be supplied in the diet, hence it is called the extrinsic factor. Its absorption in the terminal ileum requires the presence of the intrinsic factor secreted by the stomach.

extrinsic injury one which results from factors external to the body. Extrinsic factors include equipment, footwear, opponents or environmental factors (such as the sporting surface and weather), poor training methods (such as dramatic changes in intensity or duration or excessive load), poor technique and lack of warm-up.

extrinsic motivation the drive to satisfy needs and avoid harm. ⮌ motivation (in sport).

extrinsic muscles of the eye ⮌ extraocular.

extrinsic semiconductors semiconductors that have impurities added to improve electrical conductivity. ⮌ intrinsic semiconductors.

extrinsic sugars sugars, such as lactose in milk and sucrose as the sugar used to sweeten food and beverages, that are not contained within cell walls.

extroversion *n* turning inside out. In psychology, the direction of thoughts to the external world.

extroversion of the bladder ⮌ ectopia vesicae.

extrovert (extravert) *adj* Jungian description of an individual whose characteristic interests and behaviour are directed outwards to other people and the physical environment. ⮌ introvert *opp*.

extrusion 1. condition of being forced or thrust out of a normal position. **2.** in dentistry, the movement of a tooth to a new position beyond its normal alignment. This may be caused by trauma, as part of an orthodontic treatment plan or by the absence of an opposing occlusal force (overeruption).

extubation *n* removal of an endotracheal tube.

exudate *n* the product of exudation; a liquid or semisolid which has been discharged through the tissues to the surface or into a cavity—**exudates** *pl*. Wound exudate is a protein-rich fluid produced during healing. It bathes the wound, keeps it moist and transports substances required for healing. ⮌ retinal exudates.

exudation *n* the oozing out of fluid through the capillary walls in situations, such as inflammation, which increase vessel permeability—**exude** *vt, vi*.

exudativa externa retinitis ⮌ Coats' disease.

exudative retinitis ⮌ Coats' disease.

exude to ooze through a tissue or opening.

eye *n* (*syn* organ of sight, visual organ) the peripheral organ of vision, in which an optical image of the external world is produced and transformed into nerve impulses. It is a spheroidal body approximately 24 mm in diameter with the segment of a smaller sphere (of about 8 mm radius), the cornea, in front. It consists of an external coat of fibrous tissue, the sclera and transparent cornea; a middle vascular coat, comprising the iris, the ciliary body and the choroid; and an internal coat, the retina, which includes the cones and rods photoreceptors. Within the eye, there are the aqueous humour located between the cornea and the crystalline lens, the crystalline lens held by the zonule of Zinn and the vitreous body (humour) located between the crystalline lens and the retina. The movements of the eye are directed by six extraocular muscles. ⮌ Colour Section Figure 15.

eyeball the globe of the eye.

eye bank an organization that collects, evaluates, stores and distributes eyes from donors. The eyes are used for corneal grafts/transplants and research. ⮌ corneal grafts/transplants.

eyebrows the supraorbital margin of the frontal bone and the hairs projecting from the overlying skin. They help to protect the eye from foreign bodies and sweat.

eye contact looking at the face of the person to whom one is talking. In many instances, it is a reciprocal activity and is such an important part of most cultures' non-verbal language that blind people are advised to turn their faces in the direction of the voice being heard. In some cultures, however, it may be perceived as bad manners or offensive to make or maintain eye contact during conversation, or when acknowledging a person.

eyeglass ⮌ eyepiece.

eye injuries sport is the commonest context for injury to the eyes, most commonly those such as football, rugby, boxing where opponents' fingers or elbows may come into contact with the eyes or those where small balls or the implements for hitting them may do the damage (squash, hockey, golf). Wearing protective glasses can reduce the incidence of injury.

eyelashes the row of hairs on each eyelid. They protect the eye from foreign bodies and injury.

eye lens ⮌ eyepiece.

eyelet wiring ⮌ interdental.

eyelids (*syn* blephara, lids, palpebrae) a pair of movable folds of skin which act as protective coverings of the eye. The upper eyelid extends downward from the eyebrow. It is the more moveable of the two, due to the action of a levator palpebrae muscle. When the eye is open and looking straight ahead, it just covers the upper part of the cornea; when it is closed, it covers the whole cornea. The lower eyelid reaches just below the cornea when the eye is open and rises only slightly when it shuts. Each eyelid consists of the following layers, starting anteriorly: (a) the skin; (b) a layer of subcutaneous connective tissue; (c) a layer of striated muscle; (d) the submuscular connective tissue; (e) the fibrous layer, including the tarsal plates; (f) a layer of smooth muscle; (g) and the palpebral conjunctiva. ⊃ ablepharia, blepharitis, ciliosis, Cogan's lid twitch sign, ectropion, entropion, epicanthus, hordeolum, inferior palpebral sulcus, lagophthalmos, lid eversion, myokymia, orbicularis oculi, palpebral ligament, superior palpebral sulcus, tarsorrhaphy, tarsus, xanthelasma.

eyepiece (*syn* eye lens, eyeglass, ocular) the lens or combination of lenses in an optical instrument (microscope, telescope, etc.) through which the observer views the image formed by the objective. The most common eyepieces are composed of two single lenses or two doublets: the lens or doublet nearer the eye is called the eye lens and the one nearer the objective is called the field lens. The role of the eyepiece is to magnify the image and to reduce the aberrations of the image formed by the objective.

eyestrain ⊃ asthenopia.

eye teeth *n* lay term for the canine teeth in the upper jaw.

F

F *abbr* **1.** farad. **2.** field size.

f *abbr* frequency of radiation.

fabella *n* a sesamoid bone sometimes present in the lateral head of the gastrocnemius muscle. It may resemble a loose body on a lateral knee radiograph.

Faber test also known as a figure 4 or four test. A test for problems affecting the sacroiliac joint/ligaments. It comprises **F**lexion, **Ab**duction and **E**xternal **R**otation of the hip: the patient lies supine, the foot of the affected side is placed across the opposite knee, the physiotherapist presses down on the flexed knee and the opposite anterior superior iliac crest. A positive result is pain in the sacroiliac area, which indicates a problem with the sacroiliac joint/ligaments.

Fabry's disease (J Fabry, German dermatologist, 1860–1930). ⊃ angiokeratoma corporis diffusum.

Face Arm and Speech Test (FAST) a diagnostic tool for the early identification of a cerebrovascular accident (stroke). The test assesses three symptoms of stroke: (a) facial weakness; (b) arm weakness; (c) speech problems. It is used by paramedics and other emergency healthcare professionals, and familes to make an accurate and early diagnosis that ensures that patients are admitted to hospital where they can receive prompt investigation and treatment in a specialist stroke unit.

face-bow **1.** instrument used in prosthetics to record the relationship of the maxilla to the transverse horizontal axis (hinge axis) of rotation of the mandible. This can then be transferred to an anatomical articulator. ⊃ articulator. **2.** in orthodontics, a wire frame used to transmit extraoral forces from a headgear to an orthodontic appliance.

face presentation a cephalic presentation with the fetal spine and head extended and the face lowest in the pelvis; occurs in about 1:500–600 deliveries. It may result from occipitoposterior position with insufficient flexion, causing the biparietal diameter to be caught in the sacrocotyloid diameter, extending the head, possibly due to android pelvis. Anencephaly is a less common cause now that ultrasound scans diagnose this early in pregnancy. The denominator is the mentum (chin): labour may be uncomplicated with spontaneous delivery in a mentoanterior position, especially in a multipara with a small baby; spontaneous delivery is unlikely in mentoposterior position unless the chin rotates anteriorly, but there is a risk of persistent mentoposterior position with obstructed labour, when caesarean section is necessary. The baby's face will be bruised and oedematous at delivery.

face to pubes persistent occipitoposterior position, in which the attitude of the head is military, neither flexed nor extended, and the sinciput, meeting the pelvic floor first, has rotated forwards bringing the occiput to the hollow of the sacrum. First and second stage delay is common. Maternal squatting may enlarge the pelvic outlet sufficiently to facilitate vaginal delivery but severe stretching and laceration of the pelvic floor often occurs. Forceps delivery is sometimes necessary. ⊃ persistent occipitoposterior position.

face to pubes delivery occurs with a cephalic presentation, usually when the head is not fully flexed and has passed through the pelvis in an occipitoposterior position. As crowning occurs the brow will be seen under the symphysis pubis. The occipit sweeps (stretches excessively and tears) the perineum as it is born by flexion. It will probably be born before the face has completely emerged from under the symphysis pubis.

facet *n* **1.** a face or front. **2.** in anatomy, a small, smooth, flat surface of a bone, especially on a surface of articulation. Also a face or flat surface on a calculus. **3.** in dentistry, a smooth worn area on a tooth surface made by movement of another tooth upon it.

facet joint ⊃ zygapophyseal joint.

facial *adj* pertaining to the face.

facial artery a branch of the external carotid artery. It passes outwards over the mandible just in front of the angle of the jaw and supplies the muscles of facial expression and structures in the mouth. The pulse may be felt where the artery crosses the jaw bone.

facial bones the group of skull bones about the eyes and nose, cheeks and the upper and lower jaw which form the architecture of the face. They are the 2 zygomatic (cheek) bones, 2 nasal bones, 2 lacrimal bones, vomer, maxilla, mandible, 2 palatine bones and 2 inferior conchae. In addition the frontal bone of the cranium forms the forehead and part of the orbital cavities.

facial hemiatrophy wasting of the soft tissues affecting one side of the face. It may be a congenital condition, or a manifestation of systemic sclerosis in which the structures on one side of the face are shrunken.

facial hemihypertrophy a congenital condition causing enlargement of one side of the face.

facial injury injuries to the structures in and around the face including the facial bones; abrasions and lacerations, septal and auricular haematomas and other injuries around the nose, ears and eyes. Sport accounts for up to 25% of facial injuries. They can result from direct contact with another person, with equipment such as a squash racquet, a goalpost or the ground. Common in contact sports such as rugby and boxing. The incidence can be reduced by the use of protective equipment, e.g. hockey goalkeeper's face protector.

facial myokymia twitching of facial muscles. It may result from long term use of the phenothiazine group of drugs; has also been observed in patients with multiple sclerosis.

facial nerve seventh pair of cranial nerves. They supply branches to the facial muscles, the salivary (sublingual and submandibular), lacrimal and nasal glands, and to the anterior two-thirds of the tongue. Damage or disease affecting the facial nerves results in paralysis of facial muscles. ⇒ Bell's palsy.

facial neuralgia a pain syndrome, generally of obscure aetiology, characterized by pain in any region of the face, teeth, tongue and often in the shoulder area. The pain is intermittent and may last for minutes or for days and is not characterized by a trigger zone.

facial palsy ⇒ Bell's palsy, facial paralysis.

facial paralysis paralysis of muscles supplied by the facial nerve.

facial plane the transverse plane through the skull represented on a lateral skull radiograph by a line joining the nasion and the pogonion.

facial seal in prosthetics, seal created by the contact of the lips and cheeks with the polished surface of a denture. The seal is effected by a salivary meniscus which prevents the entry of air.

facial surface in dental anatomy, the surface of a tooth directed towards the lips or cheeks (buccal or labial surfaces).

facial transfixation ⇒ fixation (dentistry/maxillofacial surgery).

-facient a suffix that means 'making', e.g. *rubefacient*.

facies *n* the appearance or the expression of the face. ⇒ adenoid facies, Parkinson facies.

facilitated diffusion process whereby larger non-fat-soluble molecules such as glucose pass into the cell by using a protein carrier molecule. No energy is required but there must be a concentration gradient.

facilitation 1. hastening or assistance of a natural process or the increased excitability of a neuron after stimulation. **2.** in occupational therapy, the action by the therapist that assists the client to practise a skill, to perform a task or activity or to engage in an occupation. **3.** in physiotherapy, facilitatory techniques can be used to either excite or inhibit activity. For example, a slow, smooth stretch to a muscle will tend to be inhibitory whereas a rapid sudden stretch would be excitatory. Techniques that can be considered as facilitatory are: brushing, ice, tapping, passive stretching, joint compression (approximation), vibration and vestibular stimulation.

facing in dentistry, a veneer applied to the visible surface of a restoration to improve its appearance.

faci/o- a prefix that means 'face', e.g. *facies*.

facioscapulohumeral muscular dystrophy (FSH) a muscular dystrophy inherited as an autosomal dominant condition; there is tandem repeat deletion chromosome 4q.

The onset occurs between the ages of 7–30 years. It affects the muscles of the face and upper limb girdle and pain in the shoulder is common. ⇒ muscular dystrophies.

factitious disorder a disorder of illness behaviour in which an individual feigns symptoms repeatedly and consistently. As a result there are often repeated investigations and treatment (including surgery) in spite of repeated negative findings. ⇒ Munchausen syndrome.

factor I a factor in the blood coagulation cascade. ⇒ fibrinogen.

factor II a factor in the blood coagulation cascade. ⇒ prothrombin.

factor III thromboplastin (tissue factor). A factor in the blood coagulation cascade. ⇒ thromboplastin.

factor IV calcium ions. A factor in the blood coagulation cascade. ⇒ calcium.

factor V a factor in the blood coagulation cascade. ⇒ labile factor (proaccelerin).

factor VII a factor in the blood coagulation cascade. ⇒ stable factor (proconvertin).

factor VIII a factor in the blood coagulation cascade. ⇒ antihaemophilic factor A, haemophilias.

factor IX Christmas factor, antihaemophilic factor B. A factor in the blood coagulation cascade. ⇒ Christmas factor, haemophilias.

factor X a factor in the blood coagulation cascade. ⇒ Stuart–Prower factor.

factor XI a factor in the blood coagulation cascade. ⇒ plasma thromboplastin antecedent.

factor XII a factor in the blood coagulation cascade. ⇒ Hageman factor.

factor XIII a factor in the blood coagulation cascade. ⇒ fibrin-stabilizing factor.

factor V Leiden factor V Leiden is associated with venous thrombosis. The genetic abnormality resides with the coagulation/clotting factor Va; a substitution of arginine by glutamine at position 506 prevents its cleavage and hence inactivation. Factor Va will therefore persist, resulting in a tendency to venous thrombosis. The mutation has been identified in about 3–5% of healthy individuals in Western Europe and North America, and in about 20–40% of those with a history of venous thrombosis at a young age. The risk of venous thrombosis is substantially increased if the patient is homozygous for the mutation or has a second plasma abnormality, e.g. a lupus anticoagulant. ⇒ venous thromboembolism.

facultative *adj* conditional; having the power of living under different conditions.

facultative aerobes micro-organisms that can grow within an anaerobic environment but grow more quickly if aerobic conditions prevail.

facultative anaerobes micro-organisms that can grow if molecular oxygen is present in the environment. Examples include *Escherichia coli*, staphylococci. ⇒ anaerobe.

FAD/FADH$_2$ *abbr* flavin adenine dinucleotide (oxidized and reduced forms respectively).

faecal impaction severe constipation caused by a mass of dried hardened faeces in the colon and rectum. May lead to faecal incontinence.

faecal incontinence simply defined as the leakage of liquid faeces. There is a lack of consensus about a precise definition but it is involuntary or inappropriate defecation. There may be faecal soiling of clothing such as when passing flatus, or being unaware of the urge to defecate. Constipation and impaction of faeces are common causes of incontinence.

faecalith *n* a concretion formed in the bowel from faecal matter: it can cause obstruction and/or inflammation.

faecal occult blood (FOB) a test used to detect minute amounts of blood in faeces that occurs as a result of bleeding in the gastrointestinal tract. It is used as a screening test for colorectal cancers in certain older age groups. People who have a positive FOB test are invited to have a diagnostic colonoscopy. ⊃ occult blood test.

faecal–oral route describes the ingestion of microorganisms from faeces which can be transmitted directly or indirectly. Often results in diarrhoeal disease.

faecal softeners ⊃ laxatives. ⊃ Appendix 5.

faeces *n* the waste material eliminated from the bowel, consisting mainly of indigestible cellulose, unabsorbed food, intestinal secretions, water, electrolytes and microorganisms, etc.—**faecal** *adj*.

Fahrenheit *n* (D Fahrenheit, German physicist, 1686–1736), a thermometric scale; the freezing point of water is 32° and its boiling point 212°.

failure to thrive failure to develop and grow at the expected rate for age and gender, ascertained by consistent measurement of height and weight plotted on a growth chart. It may result from an organic disorder, such as metabolic diseases, acute illness, kidney disease, or have non-organic causes, such as poor feeding, maternal deprivation or psychological problems. Careful investigation is required to establish the cause.

faint *n* (*syn* syncope) a temporary loss of consciousness— **faint** *vi*. ⊃ syncope.

falciform *adj* sickle-shaped.

falciform ligament also called the broad ligament of the liver. The fold of peritoneum between the right and left lobes of the liver, which helps to support the liver in position.

fallopian tubes ⊃ uterine tubes.

Fallot's tetralogy (E-L Fallot, French physician, 1850–1911) also known as tetralogy of Fallot. A cyanotic congenital heart defect comprising a ventricular septal defect, narrowing of the right ventricular outflow tract (subvalvular pulmonary stenosis), right ventricular hypertrophy and malposition of the aorta overriding the ventricular septum. Amenable to corrective surgery. ⊃ Colour Section Figure 28.

false ankylosis inability to open the mouth due to trismus rather than to disease of the temporomandibular joint.

false image ⊃ ghost image.

false labour painful uterine contractions simulating labour, but without cervical dilatation, possibly due to increasing muscle contractility but without normal uterine fundal dominance. ⊃ fundal dominance.

false pelvis the wide expanded part of the pelvis lying above the brim bounded by the iliac fossae laterally, lumbar spine posteriorly and abdominal wall anteriorly, of little importance in obstetrics.

false pocket a deprecated term for periodontal pocket due to gingival enlargement.

false positive reaction a research term. A mistakenly positive response. Positive test results found in subjects who do not possess the attribute for which the test is conducted.

false substrate chemicals, including some drugs, that compete with the normal substrate in a metabolic pathway. The pathway is disrupted. ⊃ enzyme inhibitors.

falsificationism also known as refutationism. A view, propounded by the philosopher Popper and coming to prominence in the English-speaking world in the 1950s, that the hallmark of good science is to challenge every hypothesis or theory ('conjecture') by actively identifying and testing predictions which follow only from it, not from competing theories, one criterion of a good theory being that it gives rise to many such explicit, unique and so 'vulnerable' predictions. Failure of the prediction will then falsify or refute the theory; on the other hand, success of a prediction can be regarded as corroborating evidence but not as irrefutable proof, which is never possible.

falx *n* a sickle-shaped structure.

falx cerebelli the portion of dura mater between the hemispheres of the cerebellum.

falx cerebri that portion of the dura mater separating the two cerebral hemispheres.

FAM *abbr* Functional Assessment Measure

familial *adj* relating to the family, as of a condition such as Huntington's disease that affects several members of the same family.

familial adenomatous polyposis a dominantly inherited condition in which multiple polyps occur throughout the large bowel and which invariably leads to colon cancer. Polyps also occur in the stomach and duodenum. ⊃ Gardner's syndrome, Peutz–Jeghers syndrome, Colour Section Figure 70.

familial amyloidosis ⊃ amyloidosis.

familial autonomic dysfunction ⊃ Riley–Day syndrome.

familial hypercholesterolaemia (FH) an inherited polygenic disorder of blood lipoproteins. It is usually caused by an autosomal dominantly inherited mutation, but there are other causes. It causes an excess of low density-lipoprotein (LDL) in the plasma. There is an increased risk of cardiovascular disease at an earlier age than in the general population. ⊃ hyperlipaemias.

familial Mediterranean fever a rare genetic disease. It is inherited as an autosomal-recessive trait. It usually affects Sephardic Jews and Armenians and is characterized by episodes of inflammatory arthritis, pyrexia, pleurisy and peritonitis. There may be secondary amyloidosis. Should not be confused with boutonneuse fever (Mediterranean spotted fever) caused by a rickettsial infection.

familial multicystic disease ⊃ cherubism.

Family Health Services (FHS) community-based services provided by family doctors, dentists, opticians and pharmacists as independent contractors. They are not directly employed by the NHS, but have contractual arrangements to practise in the NHS.

family planning the methods used to space or limit the number of children born to a couple, or for enhancing conception.

family therapy in psychotherapy, a therapy that focuses on the family relationships and communication between individuals in order to understand the problems experienced by a single member. The aims being to clarify issues and help the familty to modify their interactions with each other.

Fanconi anaemia (G Fanconi, Swiss paediatrician, 1892–1979) a rare autosomal-recessive disorder with the insidious onset of aplastic anaemia during childhood. Other abnormalities include short stature, polydactyly, abnormal kidneys, etc. Affected children may develop cancers including leukaemia. A haemopoietic stem cell transplantation may be a treatment option for some people. But most patients will die.

Fanconi syndrome an inherited or acquired dysfunction of the proximal renal tubules. Large amounts of amino acids, phosphates and glucose are excreted in the urine, and there is proximal renal tubular acidosis. Adults may develop osteomalacia, and children have rickets and fail to grow properly.

fantasy, phantasy *n* a 'day dream' in which the person's conscious or unconscious desires and impulses are fulfilled. May be accompanied by feelings of unreality. Occurs pathologically in schizophrenia.

farad (F) (M Faraday, British scientist, 1791–1867) the SI unit of capacitance. An electrical system has a capacitance of 1 farad if a charge of 1 coulomb held by the body results in a potential of 1 volt.

Faraday's laws of electromagnetic induction (M Faraday) *First law* a change in the magnetic flux linked with a conductor induces an electromotive force in the conductor. *Second law* the size of the induced electromotive force is proportional to the rate of change of the magnetic flux linkage.

faradic current (M Faraday) an electrotherapy term. It is used by some electromedical manufacturers to indicate a current designed for motor stimulation. Typically means a pulsed current with biphasic pulses, with a duration of less than 1 ms and a frequency between 30 Hz and 70 Hz. Variations include the use of monophasic pulses. 'Faradic' is not a helpful term as it was coined on equipment producing parameters no longer in use and, does not have a universally agreed definition.

Farber test microscopic examination of the meconium to detect lanugo, cells and ingested substances, the absence of which suggests intestinal obstruction. ⊃ meconium.

farmer's lung ⊃ extrinsic allergic alveolitis.

Farnsworth test (*syn* Farnsworth–Munsell 100 Hue test, FM 100 Hue test) a colour vision test consisting of 85 small discs made up of Munsell colours of approximately equal chroma and value, but of different hue for normal observers. The examinee must place the discs so that they appear in a continuous and smooth series. Errors are scored and a diagnosis of the type and severity of the colour defect can be made. A smaller version of the Farnsworth test called the Farnsworth D-15 exists. It consists of only 15 small discs and the procedure is the same but it is a more rapid test which does not give as much information as the large version. However, it has been found to be very valuable for detecting severe colour vision defects, including tritanopia. There exist also some versions of this test in which the colour samples are less saturated than the standard ones. These include: the L'Anthony desaturated D-15 test in which the colour samples are less saturated by 2 units of Munsell chroma but also lighter by 3 units of Munsell value than the standard D-15 test, and the Adams desaturated D-15 test in which only the saturation (or chroma) has been reduced by 2 units. These desaturated D-15 tests are more effective in detecting mild colour vision deficiencies than the standard D-15 test. ⊃ defective colour vision, Munsell colour system.

Farnsworth–Munsell 100 Hue test ⊃ Farnsworth test.

F(A)ROM *abbr* full (active) range of motion.

far point of the eye ⊃ far point of accommodation.

far point of accommodation (*syn* far point of the eye, punctum remotum) the point in space conjugate with the retina (more specifically the foveola) when the accommodation is relaxed. In emmetropia, the far point is at infinity; in myopia, it is at a finite distance in front of the eye; in hypermetropia, it is a virtual point behind the eye.

far point of convergence the farthest point where the lines of sight intersect when the eyes diverge to the maximum.

far point of the eye ⊃ far point of accommodation.

FAS *abbr* fetal alcohol syndrome.

fascia *n* a connective tissue sheath consisting of fibrous tissue and fat which unites the skin to the underlying tissues. It also surrounds and separates many of the muscles, and, in some cases, holds them together—**fascial** *adj*.

fascia bulbi ⊃ Tenon's capsule.

fasciculation *n* a localized contraction of muscles, that can be observed through the skin as a flickering or twitching, they represent a spontaneous discharge of a number of fibres innervated by a single motor nerve filament. Can occur in the upper and lower eyelids. It is common in motor neuron disease.

fasciculus *n* a little bundle, as of muscle or nerve—**fascicular** *adj*, **fasciculi** *pl*.

fasciitis inflammation of fascia (connective tissue). It may be caused by micro-organisms, such as streptococci, or be part of an inflammatory condition. ⊃ Fournier's gangrene, necrotizing fasciitis.

Fasciola *n* a genus of liver flukes, such as *Fasciola hepatica*. ⊃ Flukes.

fascioliasis *n* infestation with *Fasciola hepatica*. The ova of the fluke is present in the faeces of sheep and cattle, and snails are an intermediate host. Human infestation occurs through eating contaminated aquatic plants such as watercress. Infestation causes serious hepatobiliary disease, there is fever, malaise, a large tender liver and eosinophilia.

fasciolopsiasis *n* infestation with *Fasciolpsis buski*. It is prevalent in Asia and the Indian subcontinent. It affects humans and pigs and is acquired from ingesting contaminated aquatic plants. There is abdominal pain, diarrhoea, constipation, oedema and associated eosinophilia.

Fasciolopsis *n* a genus of large intestinal flukes, such as *Fasciolopsis buski*. ⮑ flukes

fasciotomy *n* incision of muscle fascia. ⮑ compartment syndrome.

FAST *acron* **F**ace **A**rm and **S**peech **T**est.

fast motor unit a motor unit containing an alpha (α)-motor neuron, which innervates quickly contracting and fatiguing muscle fibres.

fast-twitch muscle fibres skeletal muscle fibres adapted for fast response. They contract rapidly and strongly for a short period and fatigue quickly. Contain an extensive network of sarcoplasmic reticulum and a high level of glycogen. Metabolism to produce energy is mainly anaerobic but some subtypes also have aerobic metabolism ⮑ muscle fibre types, slow-twitch muscle fibres.

fast two-dimensional sequence ⮑ image acquisition time.

fastigium the summit, such as the highest temperature occurring in a fever.

fat *n* **1.** complex organic molecule composed of carbon, hydrogen and oxygen atoms, belonging to the broad category of lipids. Fats are formed by the combination of one molecule of glycerol with three fatty acids forming a triacylglycerol (triglyceride). May be of animal or vegetable origin, and may be fats or oils. Vegetable fats with polyunsaturated and monounsaturated fatty acids are liquids (oils) whereas the animal fats, e.g. on a lamb chop, contain more saturated fatty acids and are solid. The term 'fats' is sometimes used loosely to include other lipids. ⮑ adipose, body composition, body fat, brown adipose tissue, fatty acid, glycerol, kilojoule, triacylglycerol. **2.** adipose tissue, which acts as a reserve supply of energy and protects some organs—**fatty** *adj*.

fat embolus the release of fat from the bone marrow into the circulation. Can follow long bone fractures or crush injuries, diagnosed by increasing confusion, decreased oxygen saturation in the blood and occasionally petechial haemorrhages on the arms and chest, this can be fatal. ⮑ embolism.

fat-soluble vitamin vitamins A, D, E and K are fat-soluble. ⮑ water soluble vitamins

Fatal Accident Enquiry ⮑ coroner.

fatigue *n* weariness. Physiological term for diminishing muscle reaction to stimulus applied. A general affective disturbance resulting in tiredness and lethargy. General fatigue is difficult to quantify and assess. It is common in many chronic diseases, cancer, multiple sclerosis for example, in which advice on energy conservation may be needed.

fatigue fracture ⮑ stress fracture.

fatigue index (FI) the decline in power divided by the time (in seconds) interval between maximum (peak) and minimum power, recorded during an anaerobic power exercise test.

fatigue (in sport) in sports medicine, describes the reduced ability to sustain a physical or mental function as a consequence of the intensity and/or duration of the effort. Fatigue can last for periods ranging from a few tens of seconds to several days, its duration broadly correlating with that of the fatiguing activity, e.g. recovery from a 60 m sprint takes only a few minutes but few people would wish to run competitive marathons less than 7–10 days apart. Also describes the failure of muscle(s) to maintain force (or power output) during sustained or repeated contractions—**fatigability** *n*. ⮑ central fatigue, glycogen, muscle fatigue.

fatty acid the hydrocarbon component of fat and other lipids, which may be unsaturated (monounsaturated or polyunsaturated) or saturated depending on the number of double chemical bonds in their structure. Comprising straight hydrocarbon chains with the number of carbon atoms ranging from 4 to more than 20, although chains of 16 and 18 are the most prevalent. All fat-containing foods, and all fat or lipid in the human body, consist of a mixture of different proportions of saturated fatty acids (SFAs), monounsaturated fatty acids (MUFAs) and polyunsaturated fatty acids (PUFAs). ⮑ essential fatty acids, free fatty acids, monounsaturated fatty acids, omega-3 fatty acids, omega-6 fatty acids, omega-9 fatty acids, polyunsaturated fatty acids, saturated fatty acids.

fatty degeneration tissue degeneration that leads to the appearance of fatty droplets in the cytoplasm; found especially in disease of heart, liver and kidney.

fatty liver accumulation of fat in the liver, an indication of diffuse liver disease or benign changes, demonstrated using grey scale ultrasound.

fat/water suppression a method that suppresses signal within the imaging volume from either fat or water protons by applying a frequency selective, saturation, radio frequency pulse in magnetic resonance imaging (MRI).

fauces *n* the opening from the mouth into the pharynx, bounded above by the soft palate, below by the tongue and by four folds of mucous membrane that form two membranous arches; the palatopharyngeal arch and the palatoglossal arch (previously known as the pillars of the fauces). The two arches (anterior and posterior) lie laterally and surround a mass of lymphoid tissue known as the palatine tonsil—**faucial** *adj*. ⮑ palatoglossal arch, palatopharyngeal arch.

favism *n* increased breakdown of erythrocytes (red blood cells) precipitated by eating broad beans, in individuals deficient in the enzyme G6PD (glucose-6-phosphate dehydrogenase).

favus *n* a type of ringworm not common in Britain; caused by *Trichophyton schoenleini*. Yellow cup-shaped crusts (scutula) develop, especially on the scalp.

FB *abbr* foreign body.

FBC *abbr* full blood count.

FBS *abbr* **1.** fasting blood sugar. **2.** fetal blood sampling.

FDD *abbr* **1.** floppy disk drive. **2.** focus to diaphragm distance.

FDDI *abbr* fibre distribution data interface.

283

FDP(s) *abbr* **1.** fibrin degradation products. **2.** frequency doubling perimetry.

fear *n* an intense emotional state involving a feeling of unpleasant tension, and a strong urge to escape, which is a normal and natural response to a threat of danger but is abnormal when it exists without danger or is a continuous state. ⊃ anxiety, general adaptation syndrome.

fear–tension–pain syndrome a related phenomenological cycle first described by Grantly Dick Read as intensifying the pain of labour.

febrile *adj* feverish; accompanied by fever.

febrile seizures (convulsions) occur in children who have an increased body temperature; they do not usually result in permanent brain damage. Most common between the ages of 6 months and 5 years. ⊃ convulsions, seizures.

fecundation *n* impregnation. Fertilization. ⊃ superfecundation.

fecundity *n* the power of reproduction; fertility.

feedback *n* a homeostatic control mechanism. It is usually *negative feedback* in which a physiological process is slowed or 'turned off' by an increasing amount of product, e.g. hormone secretion, temperature control (Figure F.1). Much more rarely in *positive feedback* the process is speeded up by high levels of the product, e.g. normal blood clotting, the events of labour. *feedback treatment* ⊃ biofeedback.

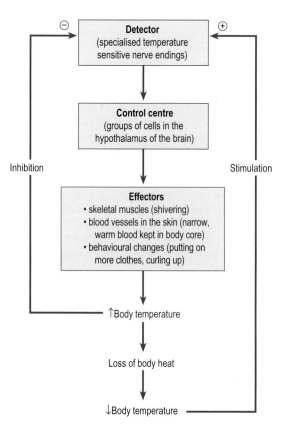

F.1 Negative feedback – temperature (reproduced from Waugh & Grant 2006 with permission).

FEF *abbr* forced expiratory flow.

feldspar (felspar) a crystalline mineral of aluminium silicate containing potassium, sodium, barium or calcium. An important constituent of dental porcelain.

Felty's syndrome (A Felty, American physician, 1895–1963) enlargement of the spleen and low white blood cell count (leucopenia) associated with rheumatoid arthritis in adults.

female athlete triad a syndrome comprising amenorrhoea, eating disorders and osteoporosis. It results from a reduction in energy intake such as decreasing food intake or an increase in energy use by extra training or exercise. The signs may be hidden by the athlete, making the diagnosis difficult, though early recognition can be achieved through risk factor assessment and screening questions. Risk factors include being a competitive athlete, taking part in sports in which low body weight is an advantage (such as gymnastics) or endurance sports (such as distance running). More common in those whose sport takes up all of their free time, and who may be under pressure from parents or coach. Features include amenorrhoea for more than 3 months, fainting, loss of weight to more than 10% below ideal. Decreased bone mineral density can result in recurrent premature osteoporotic stress fractures, with normal density never regained. There is also low self-esteem, anxiety, excessive exercise and a preoccupation with food and weight management. Management requires involvement of the athlete, her parents, coach, doctor and nutritionist, and includes appropriate diet, exercise modification and psychological support and counselling.

female circumcision excision of the clitoris, labia minora and labia majora. The extent of cutting varies from country to country. The simplest form is clitoridectomy; the next form entails excision of the prepuce, clitoris and all or part of the labia minora. The most extensive form, infibulation, involves excision of clitoris, labia minora and labia majora. The vulval lips are sutured together but total obliteration of the vaginal introitus is prevented by inserting a piece of wood or reed to preserve a small passage for urine and menstrual fluid.

female condom a polyurethane tube that fits inside the vagina to provide contraception and protection against sexually transmitted infections (STIs).

feminization 1. normal development of female secondary sexual characteristics during puberty. **2.** the presence of female sexual characteristics in a male. May be due to a faulty production of, or an inability to respond to testosterone. Males with chromosomal anomalies, such as Klinefelter's syndrome, have breast development. Others causes include oestrogen-secreting adrenal tumours; certain testicular tumours; treatment with female hormones for some cancers; drugs, e.g. spironolactone; and when a diseased liver fails to metabolize natural endogenous oestrogens.

femoral *adj* pertaining to the femur or thigh.

femoral arteriography a contrast agent is injected via a catheter in the femoral artery to demonstrate the arterial circulation of the leg.

femoral artery the large artery begins at the midpoint of the inguinal ligament and extends downwards in front of the thigh; then it turns medially and eventually passes round the medial aspect of the femur to enter the popliteal space where it becomes the popliteal artery. It supplies blood to the structures of the thigh and some superficial pelvic and inguinal structures. The *femoral pulse* may be palpated in the inguinal area (groin); midway between the symphysis pubis and the anterior superior iliac spine. ⊃ Colour Section Figure 9.

femoral hernia protrusion through the femoral canal, alongside the femoral blood vessels as they pass into the thigh.

femoral nerve one of the largest branches arising from the lumbar plexus (lumbar nerve roots 2, 3, 4). It passes behind the inguinal ligament to enter the thigh in close association with the femoral artery. It divides into cutaneous and muscular branch to supply the skin and muscles of the anterior thigh. One branch, the saphenous nerve, supplies the medial aspect of the leg, ankle and foot. ⊃ lumbar plexus.

femoral nerve stretch the patient lies prone. The physiotherapist flexes the person's knee and then extends the hip. Pain in the back or distribution of the femoral nerve indicates femoral nerve irritation. Comparison is made with the other side. ⊃ neurodynamics.

femoral triangle also known as Scarpa's triangle. An area at the top, inner part of the thigh. It is bounded by the inguinal ligament, the sartorius and adductor longus muscles, and contains the femoral artery, vein and nerve.

femoral vein the large vein that ascends in the thigh to the level of the inguinal ligament where it becomes the external iliac vein. It conveys blood from the deep veins of the leg and the small (short) saphenous vein (a superficial vein) via the popliteal vein, and from the great (long) saphenous vein (a superficial vein) which joins the femoral vein just below the inguinal ligament. ⊃ Colour Section Figure 10.

femoropopliteal *adj* usually, referring to the femoral and popliteal vessels.

femur *n* the thigh bone; the longest and strongest bone in the body. The femoral head articulates in the acetabulum to form the hip joint, and the femoral condyles articulate with the tibia and patella to form the knee joint—**femora** *pl*, **femoral** *adj*. ⊃ Colour Section Figures 2, 3.

fenamates *npl* a group of non-steroidal anti-inflammatory drugs. ⊃ Appendix 5.

fenestra *n* a window-like opening.

fenestra ovalis an oval opening between the middle and inner ear. ⊃ oval window.

fenestra rotunda a round opening that lies below the fenestra ovalis. ⊃ round window.

fenestration *n* 1. a perforation, opening or pore. The glomerular capillaries of the nephron, which form part of the filtration membrane, are adapted for permeability and filtration by the presence of fenestrations. 2. a surgical opening (or fenestra) in the inner ear to ease the deafness caused by otosclerosis.

FER *abbr* forced expiratory ratio.

Ferguson's reflex (J Ferguson, Canadian physiologist, b.1907) an important reflex involved in labour. A surge of oxytocin is released, which increases uterine contractions, when the cervix and upper vagina are stimulated by the presenting part. The contractions become expulsive and the woman experiences an uncontrollable need to bear down and push.

fermentation *n* the process whereby microbial (yeasts and bacteria) enzymes break down sugars (glycolysis) and other substrates. For example in the production of bread, cheese, alcohol and vinegar.

ferning aborization. A charateristic of cervical mucus containing high levels of oestrogen, the dried mucus forms a fern-like pattern on a slide. May be used to ascertain when ovulation occurs. ⊃ spinnbarkeit.

ferric *adj* relating to trivalent iron and its salts. Ferric iron is converted to the ferrous state by gastric acid.

ferric oxide an impure form of naturally occurring red oxide of iron, commonly called rouge. Used in dentistry as a polishing and colouring agent in synthetic teeth, ceramics and filling materials.

ferric sulphate in dentistry, a pulp medicament. It is increasingly being used in primary molar pulp therapy as an alternative to formocresol.

ferritin *n* an iron-protein (apoferritin) complex. It is a storage form of iron found in the liver, spleen and bone marrow. The level of ferritin in serum can indicate the total amount of iron stored in the body. Ferritin levels may be raised in disease processes, such as inflammation, which are linked to the synthesis of acute-phase proteins.

ferro, ferr, ferri- a prefix that means 'iron', e.g. ferrous.

ferromagnetic a substance that if placed in a magnetic field becomes magnetized and once the magnetic field is removed it retains its magnetism, for example iron, cobalt or nickel. ⊃ diamagnetic, paramagnetic, superparamagnetic.

ferromagnetism if an external magnetic force is applied to the material all the magnetic domains align in the same direction forming a strong magnet.

ferrous *adj* pertaining to divalent iron, as of its salts and compounds. *Ferrous carbonate, ferrous fumarate, ferrous gluconate, ferrous succinate* and *ferrous sulphate* are prescribed orally in the treatment of iron deficiency anaemias.

fertility rate known as the general fertility rate. A rate obtained by dividing the number of live births by the number of women of child-bearing age (15 to 44 years). Typically expressed as live births per 1000 women. ⊃ total fertility rate.

fertilization *n* the penetration of an oocyte by a spermatozoon.

FES *abbr* functional electrical stimulation.

FESS *abbr* functional endoscopic sinus surgery.

fester *vi* to become inflamed; to suppurate.

festinating gait rapid, short shuffling steps continuing until stopped by an object that gets in the way. Caused by lack of control of forward tilt of the pelvis with appearance of feet 'catching up' with centre of gravity that is too far ahead,

E
F

285

instead of over, them. Typically exhibited by a person with Parkinson's disease. Patients may lean too far forward and appear to be chasing their own centre of gravity.

FET *abbr* forced expiration technique.

fetal alcohol syndrome (FAS) a range of problems that include stillbirth, fetal abnormality and learning disability due to intrauterine growth restriction/retardation caused by excessive maternal alcohol consumption during pregnancy. Infants with fetal alcohol syndrome have typical facial features, and may have neurological problems and cardiac defects.

fetal blood sampling (FBS) 1. blood taken from the fetus during pregnancy to test for abnormalities, mostly superceded by newer diagnostic methods. Or to check fetal haemoglobin (HbF) levels in rhesus incompatibility to determine whether an intrauterine transfusion is required. **2.** blood from a fetal scalp vein obtained during labour is tested to detect acidosis if the fetal heart rate pattern is abnormal. The presence of acidosis indicates that the baby should be delivered. ⊃ cardiotocography

fetal circulation circulation adapted for intrauterine life. Extra shunts and vessels (ductus venosus, ductus arteriosus, foramen ovale and umbilical vein) allows blood to largely bypass the liver, gastrointestinal tract and lungs, as their functions are covered by maternal systems and the placenta. ⊃ Colour Section Figure 27 a, b.

fetal distress clinical manifestation of fetal hypoxia. Maternal medical causes include disturbances of respiration (e.g. eclampsia or epilepsy), inadequate circulation (e.g. cardiac failure, severe anaemia, hyper- or hypotension), diabetes mellitus, infection; uterine causes include hypertonicity, or excessive retraction in obstructed labour; and partial placental separation or placental insufficiency. Fetal causes include intracranial birth trauma, severe Rhesus incompatibility with gross anaemia, congenital abnormality, intrauterine infections, multiple pregnancy, malpresentation and malposition, cord prolapse, true knots, or traction on the cord. Diagnosis is made from abnormal fetal heart rate and regularity, meconium-stained amniotic fluid and excessive fetal movements. Delivery is expedited either by instrumental delivery or caesarean section ⊃ cardiotocography.

fetal heart deceleration slowing down. The fetal heart rate falls to below 90 beats per minute (b.p.m.) from a normal baseline rate of 120–150 b.p.m.

fetal movements movements made by the fetus in utero. These are present from the beginning of pregnancy but cannot be felt by the woman before the 16th to 19th week of gestation. Normally, the mother should feel at least 10 movements in a 12-hour period. ⊃ kick chart.

fetal reduction ⊃ embryo/fetal reduction.

fetal skull fetal bony head structure. The vault contains the brain and is composed of 2 frontal bones divided by a frontal suture, 2 parietal bones divided by the sagittal suture and separated from the frontal bones by the coronal suture, and 1 occipital bone separated from the parietal bones by the lambdoidal suture. The membranous junction of three or

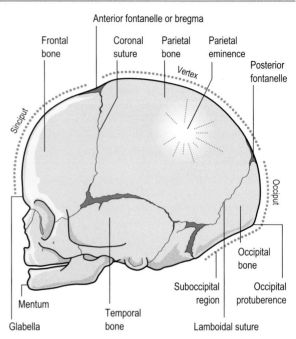

F.2 **Fetal skull** (reproduced from Fraser & Cooper 2003 with permission).

more sutures forms the anterior fontanelle or bregma and the posterior fontanelle or lambda (Figure F.2). Sutures and fontanelles felt on vaginal examination enable the midwife to determine the position of the fetal head in a cephalic presentation. The base of the skull is composed of 2 temporal, 1 ethmoid, 1 sphenoid and part of the occipital bone, and contains an opening called the foramen magnum through which passes the spinal cord. The face is composed of 14 fused bones. Diameters of the skull are assessed to estimate progress in labour, and are taken longitudinally or transversely; circumferences may also be assessed. Within the skull are the brain and intracranial membranes, the falx cerebri and the tentorium cerebelli carrying the venous sinuses by which venous blood is drained from the brain. The venous sinuses are: the superior and inferior longitudinal sinuses, the straight sinus, the transverse sinus and the great vein of Galen. If the delivery is difficult or moulding is excessive the intracranial membranes and sinuses may be torn, causing intracranial haemorrhage. ⊃ moulding.

feticide the deliberate destruction of a fetus. Medically it is used during fetal reduction or late termination. It may be achieved by injecting potassium chloride or saline into the fetal thorax.

fet/i, fet/o- a prefix that means 'fetus', e.g. *feticide*.

fetishism *n* a condition in which a particular material object is regarded with irrational awe or a strong emotional attachment. Can have a psychosexual dimension in which such an object is repeatedly or exclusively used in achieving sexual excitement.

fetofetal transfusion syndrome also called twin-to-twin transfusion syndrome. Blood from one monozygotic twin transfuses into the other twin through the placental blood vessels. A haemodynamic imbalance between monochorionic twins with chronic inter-fetal transfusion, resulting in discordant growth. In severe cases, the larger twin develops polycythaemia and polyhydramnios and the smaller twin becomes anaemic with oligohydramnios. Previously untreatable, contemporary management now includes methods to reduce amniotic fluid volume in the larger sac, septostomy to allow free passage of amniotic fluid between the two sacs or laser ablation of the inter-linked placental vessels. Pregnancies with monochorionic twins should be monitored closely between 14–26 weeks' gestation to ensure early detection and treatment of the syndrome.

fetor *n* offensive odour, stench. *fetor oris* bad breath.

fetoscopy *n* direct visual examination of the fetus by using an appropriate fibreoptic endoscope. It is performed transabdominally after the 11th week of gestation. The examination may be used to confirm possible abnormalities detected using ultrasound. It can be combined with amniocentesis, and increasingly for other interventions such as biopsies of abnormal tissue. ⮑ embryoscopy.

fetus *n* the developmental stage from the eighth week of gestation until birth—**fetal** *adj*.

fetus-in-fetu an abnormality in which the parts of one monozygotic twin are within the other twin.

fetus papyraceus a dead fetus, one of a twin which has become flattened and mummified.

fetus sanguinolentis a fetus that has died and started to decompose and is born with dark blood patches visible beneath the skin.

Feulgen stain (R Feulgen, German biochemist, 1884–1955) a stain used in histology to identify deoxyribonucleic acid or chromosomal material in specimens.

FEV *abbr* forced expiratory volume. ⮑ respiratory function tests, spirometry.

fever *n* (*syn* pyrexia) an elevation of body temperature above normal. Designates some infectious conditions, e.g. *paratyphoid fever, scarlet fever, typhoid fever*, etc.

FFA *abbr* free fatty acid.

FFD *abbr* focus to film distance.

FFM *abbr* fat-free body mass.

FH *abbr* **1.** familial hypercholesterolaemia. **2.** family history. **3.** fetal heart.

FHS *abbr* Family Health Services.

FI *abbr* fatigue index

fibre *n* a thread-like structure—**fibrous** *adj*. ⮑ non-starch polysaccharide. *afferent fibre* a nerve fibre conducting impulses to a nerve centre or spinal cord. *collagen fibre* a white, flexible but inelastic fibre which forms the chief constituent of connective tissue. *efferent fibre* a nerve fibre conducting impulses from the brain or spinal cord. *elastic fibre* a basic constituent of loose connective tissue, elastic cartilage and skin dermis. *principal fibre* the main group of collagen fibres which make up the periodontal ligament.

Sharpey's fibre connective tissue fibre that passes from the exterior into the cortex of bone. In dental anatomy, the extension of collagen fibres of the periodontal ligament embedded in the alveolar bone and cementum and which contribute greatly to the anchorage of a tooth in its socket.

fibre distribution data interface (FDDI) in computing a system similar to a token ring which uses fibreoptic cables to inform nodes when they can write to the network. ⮑ node, token ring.

fibreoptics *n* light is transmitted through flexible glass fibres which enable the user to 'see round corners'. The technology utilized in modern fibreoptics endoscopic equipment. In dentistry, it is commonly used as a light source attached to a handpiece.

fibril *n* a component filament of a fibre; a small fibre.

fibrillation *n* **1.** uncoordinated quivering contraction of muscle; referring usually to myocardial muscle (myocardium). ⮑ atrial fibrillation, cardiac arrest, ventricular fibrillation. **2.** the term for minute cracks that are seen in the early stages of osteoarthritis.

fibrin *n* the insoluble matrix on which a blood clot is formed. Produced from soluble fibrinogen by the action of thrombin—**fibrinous** *adj*.

fibrinogen *n* factor I of blood coagulation. A soluble plasma protein that is converted to fibrin by the action of the proteolytic enzyme thrombin.

fibrinolysin *n* ⮑ plasmin, plasminogen.

fibrinolysis *n* the last of the four overlapping processes of haemostasis. The dissolution of the fibrin clot by the proteolytic enzyme plasmin. There is normally a balance between blood coagulation and fibrinolysis in the body. ⮑ coagulation, platelet plug, thrombolytic, vasoconstriction, Colour Section Figure 29.

fibrinolytic drugs a group of drugs that disperse thrombi by acting as thrombolytics, e.g. alteplase. ⮑ Appendix 5, thrombolytic therapy.

fibrin-stabilizing factor an enzyme that causes polymerization leading to the formation of the insoluble stabilizing network within the fibrin clot. It is activated by thrombin in the presence of calcium ions that act as a cofactor. Factor XIII in the blood coagulation cascade.

fibr/o- a prefix that means 'fibre, fibrous tissue', e.g. *fibroblast*.

fibroadenoma *n* a benign tumour containing fibrous and glandular tissue, such as in the breast.

fibroblast *n* (*syn* fibrocyte) a blast cell that forms connective tissues. It secretes procollagen, fibronectin and collagenase, and is involved during growth and tissue repair—**fibroblastic** *adj*.

fibrocartilage (white) *n* one of the three types of cartilage. It comprises white collagen fibres within a matrix. It is a strong and slightly flexible tissue that provides support in a variety of locations. These include the intervertebral pads, ligaments between bones, the semilunar cartilages in the knee and deepening the sockets of the shoulder and hip joints—**fibrocartilaginous** *adj*.

fibrocaseous *adj* a soft, cheesy mass infiltrated by fibrous tissue, formed by fibroblasts.

fibrochondritis *n* inflammation of fibrocartilage.

fibrocyst *n* a fibroma which has undergone cystic degeneration.

fibrocystic *adj* pertaining to a fibrocyst.

fibrocystic disease of bone cysts may be solitary or generalized. If generalized and accompanied by decalcification of bone, it is symptomatic of hyperparathyroidism.

fibrocystic disease of breast the breast feels lumpy due to the presence of cysts, usually caused by hormone imbalance.

fibrocystic disease of pancreas ⊃ cystic fibrosis.

fibrocyte *n* ⊃ fibroblast—**fibrocytic** *adj*.

fibroid 1. *adj* having fibres. **2.** *n* fibromyoma, leiomyoma, uterine fibroid. A fibromuscular benign tumour usually found in the uterus. It may be on a stalk (penduculate). The location of uterine fibroids can be described as *intramural* (embedded in the wall of the uterus), *subserous* (protruding from the serosal surface into the peritoneal cavity) or *submucous* (protruding into the endometrial surface). Common pathology in women between 35 and 45 years of age. They cause menorrhagia, dysmenorrhoea, subfertility, problems if pregnancy does occur, such as miscarriage and preterm labour, large fibroids cause abdominal swelling and may cause urinary frequency. The fibroid may become twisted on its stalk, bleed, degenerate or rarely become malignant. ⊃ embolization, hysterectomy, myomectomy.

fibroma *n* a benign tumour composed of fibrous tissue—**fibromata** *pl*, **fibromatous** *adj*.

fibromatosis an abnormal proliferation of fibrous tissue

fibromatosis gingivae also known as gingival hyperplasia, idiopathic fibromatosis, idiopathic gingival hyperplasia, elephantiasis gingivae. A rare condition which may be associated with either the primary or the secondary dentition. The gingival enlargement may cover the teeth and may be hereditary, idiopathic or drug-induced.

fibromuscular *adj* pertaining to fibrous and muscle tissue.

fibromyalgia *n* a condition characterized by widespread pain and tender points. Many patients also complain of tiredness and of waking feeling unrefreshed.

fibromyoma *n* a benign tumour consisting of fibrous and muscle tissue—**fibromyomata** *pl*, **fibromyomatous** *adj*.

fibromyositis *n* general term for inflammation of fibrous and muscle tissue.

fibronectin *n* a glycoprotein present in the plasma, it occurs in several forms. It is important in the integrity of the extracellular matrix, proliferation of new epithelial cells, cell migration and adhesion. Thus, of importance in embryonic development and wound healing. Also involved with platelet aggregation during haemostasis and as part of the body's host defences.

fibroplasia *n* the production of fibrous tissue which is a normal part of healing. *retrolental fibroplasia* older term for retinopathy of prematurity.

fibrosarcoma *n* a form of sarcoma. A malignant tumour derived from fibroblastic cells—**fibrosarcomata** *pl*, **fibrosarcomatous** *adj*.

fibrosing alveolitis an inflammatory condition starting with diffuse alveolar damage and resulting in fibrosis commonly seen in collagen-vascular diseases.

fibrosis *n* the formation of excessive fibrous tissues in a structure. Such as pulmonary fibrosis caused by radiation, certain cytotoxic drugs and pneumoconiosis—**fibrotic** *adj*.

fibrositis *n* a lay term (now seldom used) that denotes non-specific soft-tissue pain. A benign, intermittently recurring and protracted disease process, with a lack of underlying pathology. The condition is often associated with muscular pain and stiffness. ⊃ fibromyalgia.

fibrous dysplasia *n* an abnormality of bone, whereby bone tissue is replaced by fibrous tissue. The onset generally occurs during childhood. There are several types and sometimes there are associated endocrine abnormalities. The effects include pain, pathological fractures and bony deformities. ⊃ Albright's syndrome.

fibrous joint one of the three main classes of joints. Usually an immovable joint or synarthrosis, e.g. the sutures of the skull. A joint, e.g. a tooth in the jaw, in which a tiny amount of movement occurs is called a gomphosis. Those joints where an interosseous ligament connects two bones is termed a syndesmosis, e.g. tibiofibular joint, they allow some 'give'.

fibrous tissue tissue that is made up mainly of closely packed bundles of collagen fibres with very little matrix. Fibrocytes (old and inactive fibroblasts) are few in number and are found lying in rows between the bundles of fibres. Fibrous tissue is found forming the ligaments, which bind bones together; as an outer protective covering for bone, called *periosteum*; as an outer protective covering of some organs, e.g. the kidneys, lymph nodes and the brain; and forming muscle sheaths, called *muscle fascia*, which extend beyond the muscle to become the tendon that attaches the muscle to bone.

fibrovascular *adj* relating to fibrous tissue which is well supplied with blood vessels.

fibula *n* one of the longest and thinnest bones of the body, situated on the outer side of the leg and articulating at the upper end with the lateral condyle of the tibia and at the lower end with the lateral surface of the talus (astragalus) and tibia. It is non-weight-bearing, but assists in stabilizing the ankle, and provides a surface for muscle attachments, e.g. soleus, peroneus longus and brevis—**fibular** *adj*. ⊃ Colour Section Figures 2, 3.

FID *abbr* free induction decay.

field an electrotherapy term. It is the force surrounding a charged particle or object. The size, distribution and magnitude of a field are represented by field lines around an object or between objects (e.g. capacitor plates used for shortwave diathermy). The magnetic field is the force surrounding a wire carrying an electric current. It depends on the magnitude of the current and the distance between adjacent loops of wire carrying current.

field defining wires metal wires attached to the light beam diaphragm, which can be adjusted to outline the exact treatment area on the subsequent radiograph produced in the simulator.

field notes/fieldwork diary a research term. The records or reflections kept by the researcher that act to enrich the data obtained or put them into some sort of context, commonly used in qualitative research.

field of view the area of the scanned plane which may be included in the computed tomography (CT) image.

field of vision ➲ visual field.

field size the size and shape of the X-ray beam. The maximum field of view of a gamma camera, usually between 25 and 50 cm.

fifth disease (erythema infectiosum) ➲ human erythrovirus 19.

FIGLU *abbr* formiminoglutamic (FIGLU) acid, an intermediate metabolite in histidine metabolism.

FIGLU test a test for folic acid deficiency, vitamin B_{12} deficiency, or the absence of an enzyme, which are all needed for histidine metabolism. Following a dose of histidine, the urine is tested for formiminoglutamic (FIGLU) acid and its presence in the urine indicates that either of the vitamins or the enzyme may be deficient.

FIGO the International Federation of Gynaecology and Obstetrics provides a classification staging cancer of the cervix from 0 (pre-invasive disease) to IVb (distant metastasis). A similar staging classification, based on locality and extent of disease, is available for ovarian and uterine cancer.

filament a fine, threadlike structure, such as the filaments of contractile proteins in muscle fibres.

filament (in radiology) a thin, coiled, tungsten wire that when heated produces electrons in an X-ray tube.

filamented swab a piece of gauze with a radiopaque strip. Used in the operating theatre for internal swabbing as it can be traced radiographically if unaccounted for during the last stages of an operation when final swab counts are undertaken.

filamentous composed of long thread-like structures.

Filaria *n* a genus of parasitic, thread-like nematode worms found mainly in the tropics and subtropics. They include *Brugia malayi*, *Loa loa*, *Onchocerca volvulus* and *Wuchereria bancrofti*. ➲ filariasis.

filariasis *n* infestation with *Filaria*. The adult worms may live in the lymphatics, connective tissues or mesentery, where they may cause obstruction, but the microfilariae migrate to the bloodstream and some infiltrate the eye, skin or pulmonary capillaries. The completion of the life cycle of some types is dependent upon passage through a mosquito. ➲ elephantiasis, loiasis, onchocerciasis.

filaricide *n* an agent, such as ivermectin and diethylcarbamazine, which destroys *Filaria*.

filariform hair-like, thread shaped.

file 1. a means of storing information or records. **2.** a metal hand instrument used in a rubbing action to reduce and smooth a surface, e.g. bone file. ➲ root canal file.

filiform *adj* thread-like.

filiform papillae small projections ending in several minute processes; found on the tongue.

filled resin ➲ composite resin.

filler in dentistry, substance or material used to fill a gap or to increase the strength of a substance.

filling 1. lay term for a dental restoration. **2.** in dentistry, the material placed in a preparation or cavity in order to fill it. ➲ retrograde filling, root canal, temporary filling. *root canal filling* ➲ root canal (dental procedures).

filling material suitable material inserted into a tooth preparation or cavity in an attempt to restore form or function, e.g. amalgam or composite. ➲ amalgam, composite resin.

film 1. a thin layer or coating. **2.** a thin sheet of material such as cellulose acetate which has been treated for use in photography or radiography.

film badge a badge worn by radiation workers which contains film, which when processed can be used to determine the amount of radiation received by that person.

film contrast in radiography, this is defined as the average gradient of the film. ➲ characteristic curve.

film development the chemical reaction in reducing the latent image in the emulsion of an exposed photographic or radiographic film in order to produce a stable image composed of minute grains of metallic silver.

film entry system the part of a radiographic film processor where the film enters the unit, it comprises a pair of rollers and a microswitch which determines the length of time the film is between the rollers and can be linked to the replenisher system to ensure accurate replenishment.

film fixation the chemical removal of metallic salts from the emulsion of an exposed film to produce a stable, permanent image.

film grain formed by the coarse structure of the crystals in a radiographic film forming an overall density in the emulsion.

film hanger a device to hold radiographic films during processing.

film holder a device to hold and stabilize a radiographic film in the mouth.

film packet a lightproof and moisture-resistant sealed packet or envelope containing one or more radiographic films for use in intra-oral radiography.

film processing the chemical transformation of a latent image, produced by exposure to either light or radiation, on the film emulsion, into a stable permanent image.

film speed the ability of the film to respond to exposure, the faster the film, the less exposure will be required to produce a comparable image, on a characteristic curve; generally, the nearer the curve is to the vertical axis the faster the film. ➲ characteristic curve.

filter *n* a device designed to remove particles over a certain size or rays of specific wavelength while allowing others to pass through. Examples include intravenous fluid filters and optical filters. **1.** a device consisting of a membrane or other permeable material (e.g. filter paper) which prevents the passage of some of the components of a mixture. **2.** in radiography, a device placed in the path of an X-ray beam to reduce selectively the intensity of certain undesirable wavelength components. **3.** in sound physics, a device to reduce the intensity of undesirable frequencies. **4.** the material or device used to absorb or transmit light of all wavelengths equally (neutral density filter) or selectively, such as the coloured filters (blue filter transmits only blue light, green filter transmits only green light, etc.). ➲ absorptive lens, green filter, interference filter, optical density, red filter, wavelength.

filtrate *n* substance that passes through the filter.

filtration *n* the process of straining through a filter under gravity, pressure or vacuum.

filtration (in radiology) the changes which occur in the X-ray beam when it passes through an object, it can reduce the amount of radiation and improve the quality of the beam by removing the low-energy photons.

filtration under pressure occurs in the nephron due to high pressure blood in the wide-bore afferent arteriole of the glomerulus. ➲ active transport, diffusion, osmosis.

filum *n* any filamentous or thread-like structure.

filum terminale a strong, fine cord blending with the spinal cord above, and the periosteum of the sacral canal below.

FIM *abbr* Functional Independence Measure.

fimbria *n* a fringe, e.g. of the uterine (fallopian) tubes— **fimbriae** *pl*, **fimbrial, fimbriated** *adj*. ➲ Colour Section Figure 17.

final impression also called master, major, working or second impression. In dentistry, the impression used to construct the master cast. ➲ impression.

Fincham's theory a theory of accommodation which attributes the increased convexity of the front surface of the crystalline lens, when accommodating, to the elasticity of the capsule and to the fact that it is thinner in the pupillary area than near the periphery of the lens. ➲ accommodation, capsule, crystalline lens, Helmholtz's theory of accommodation.

fine focus the selection of a small filament to enable a small area of the anode to be bombarded with electrons and help reduce the unsharpness on the subsequent radiograph.

fine motor control the specific control of the muscles allowing for completion of small, delicate tasks, such as picking up a pin.

fine motor skill ➲ motor skill.

fine-needle aspiration (FNA) a diagnostic test whereby a thin needle is used to obtain a tissue sample for examination. For example, it may be used to determine whether a breast lump or a thyroid swelling is benign or malignant.

fineness (of alloy) a method of rating the gold content of a gold alloy. The fineness of gold is the parts per thousand of pure gold, e.g. pure gold is 1000 fine. A gold alloy containing 800 parts gold and 200 parts of other metals is 800 fine. ➲ carat, gold.

fine tremor slight trembling as seen in the outstretched hands or tongue of a patient suffering from hyperthyroidism.

finger *n* a digit. ➲ clubbed finger.

finger-nose test the person is asked to touch the tip of their nose with an extended index finger. It tests voluntary eye-motor coordination and may be used to check cerebellar function.

fingerprint dystrophy ➲ Cogan's microcystic epithelial dystrophy.

finger spelling communication by spelling words using the fingers to make the letters of the alphabet. It may be either one-handed or two-handed finger spelling.

finger spring a palatal spring or retractor. A cantilever spring attached to the fitting surface of a removable orthodontic appliance.

finger-sucking a common habit in young children which, if it persists, can lead to various occlusal discrepancies such as anterior open bite, proclination of maxillary incisors and retroclination of mandibular incisors.

finished lens (*syn* uncut lens) a spectacle lens that has been surfaced on both sides to the required power and thickness and is still in uncut form. ➲ semi-finished lens, surfacing.

finishing in denture construction, the term is used to describe the final stages of denture construction. After the denture has been processed, the flask is opened and the denture cut out of the plaster. It is then cleaned of plaster, trimmed and polished, and thus made ready for insertion in the mouth. *finishing bur* ➲ bur. *finishing strip* ➲ strip.

finishing line in dental cavity preparation the line of demarcation between prepared tooth substance and tooth substance untouched by instruments.

Finkelstein's test (H Finkelstein, American surgeon, 1865–1939) the test for de Quervain's tenosynovitis, whereby the patient clenches his or her fingers over the thumb and performs ulnar deviation. Pain in the region means a positive result.

FiO$_2$ *abbr* fractional inspired oxygen concentration.

firewall either a programme or a dedicated computer used to protect a specific computer from external, unauthorized people accessing or changing information held on the computer.

firmware software, but stored on a chip.

first aid the immediate treatment or assistance given to a person after injury or sudden illness prior to the arrival of a qualified healthcare professional, e.g. paramedic. First aid aims are to preserve life, stop deterioration and encourage recovery.

first-class levers have the force and resistance on opposite sides of the fulcrum.

first degree tear ➲ perineal tear.

first heart sound (S1) the 'LUB' sound heard on the closure of the mitral (bicuspid) and tricuspid valves (left and right atrioventricular valves) at the onset of systole. ➲ heart sounds.

first intention ➲ primary intention, wound healing.

first order optics ➲ paraxial optics.

first order theory ➲ gaussian theory.

first pass metabolism (first pass effect) occurs when orally administered drugs are rapidly metabolized in the liver. This leads to a situation where the amount of the active drug reaching the circulation is insufficient to produce a therapeutic effect, such as with glyceryl trinitrate. Other routes of administration are used to overcome the problem, e.g. transdermal, or tablets or sprays that can be absorbed through the buccal, sublingual or nasal mucosa.

first stage of labour from onset of painful regular uterine contractions and dilatation of the cervix until full dilatation of the cervix.

FISH *acron* **F**luorescence **I**n **S**itu **H**ybridization.

Fish gingivectomy knife ➲ periodontal instruments.

fission *n* the act of splitting, such as occurs during radioactive decay when the nucleus of an atom elongates and breaks into two pieces. ➲ binary fission.

fissural (inclusion) cyst a cyst arising in the lines of junction of the embryonic processes forming the jaws.

fissure *n* a split or cleft. Can be moist or dry cracks in the epidermis or mucosa. They usually develop at 90° to the direction of the tension stress. Common sites include the anal mucosa and interdigitally for moist fissures, and the heel margins for dry fissures. ➲ anal fissure, palpebral fissure.

fissure (dental) in dentistry, a small groove or trough in the enamel of a tooth. An unfolding of the enamel between cusps and ridges. Fissure burs are designed to cut along the fissure.

fissured tongue ➲ tongue.

fissure sealant hard insoluble substance (usually unfilled composite resin) used in liquid form to seal the vulnerable pits and fissures in teeth against bacterial plaque and food debris. May be self-processing or require a curing light to activate setting (polymerization).

fistula *n* an abnormal communication between two epithelial surfaces (e.g. enterovesical between bowel and bladder). May occur in conditions such as Crohn's disease, diverticulosis and cancer—**fistulae** *pl*, **fistular, fistulous** *adj*. ➲ anal fistula, arteriovenous fistula, biliary fistula, bronchopleural fistula, enterovesical, oroantral fistula, tracheo-oesophageal fistula, vesicocolic, vesicovaginal.

fistulotomy *n* incision of a fistula.

fitness *n* general term used to describe a person's ability to undertake a series of different physical exercises.

fitness test test performed to assess an individual's physical ability to undertake a specific activity, e.g. after recovery from injury.

fit-over ➲ clipover.

fits ➲ convulsions, seizures.

fitted labial bow a wire closely adapted to the labial surfaces of a number of anterior teeth in orthodontic treatment. Usually has one or two small loops to allow for adjustment.

fitting (tissue) surface ➲ tissue surface.

fixation *n* **1.** in optics, the direct focusing of one or both eyes on an object so that the image falls on the fovea centralis. **2.** the point on the retina used to look directly at an object of interest, usually the fovea centralis. **3.** as a psychoanalytical term, an emotional attachment, generally sexual, to a parent, causing difficulty in forming new attachments later in life.

fixation (dentistry/maxillofacial surgery) in dentistry and/or maxillofacial surgery, the term can relate to the means by which a prosthesis or orthodontic appliance is kept in position, or the maintenance, in correct position, of the displaced fragments of a fractured bone. *arch bar fixation* surgical technique for immobilizing a fractured mandible or maxilla, by bending a metal bar to conform to the buccal and labial surfaces of the teeth and attaching the bar to the teeth by soft stainless steel wire ligatures passed around the necks of the teeth. *cap splint fixation* (archaic) a cast-metal or acrylic resin splint used in oral surgery to immobilize fractured bone ends. May be cast in silver alloy or other metals, to be a close fit over the crowns of the existing teeth, extending to the gingival margins. It is cemented in place and usually retained for at least 8 weeks to immobilize a fractured jaw. *craniomandibular fixation* (archaic) the fixation of the mandible to the cranium with rods connected either to bone pins or to a head frame and denture splints. The fixed mandible then being used to reposition and stabilize the fractured maxilla. *craniomaxillary fixation* (archaic) external metal rods or wires, running from a cast maxillary splint to a plaster of Paris head cap or metal halo, used to immobilize fragments of a fractured maxilla. *direct interdental wiring fixation* method of wiring the teeth together, generally in fracture cases, in which wires are passed round the necks of the teeth in both dental arches and their ends twisted together. Such ends are then themselves twisted together. *facial transfixation* (archaic) method of immobilizing maxillary fractures by passing pins, e.g. Steinmann pin, or wires, e.g. Kirschner wire, through the face and bone fragments, and the non-fractured zygomatic arch bones. *Gunning type fixation* used in edentulous fracture cases where existing dentures, or an acrylic resin splint, are wired circumferentially to the maxilla and the mandible and then wired together. *intermaxillary fixation* fixation of the lower to the upper jaw by means of splints or wiring. *internal skeletal fixation* stabilization of a fractured bone by internal or direct wiring, by bone plate and screws, or by transfixation by medullary pins. *intramedullary fixation* surgical technique in which a metal pin is inserted into the interior of the bone (in the medulla) across the line of fracture. *open reduction internal fixation (ORIF)* in dentistry/maxillofacial surgery, the facial skeleton fracture is surgically exposed and reduced under direct vision using fixation appropriate to the bone involved e.g. mini titanium plates and screws for a mandible or maxilla. *pin fixation* (archaic) immobilization of bone fragments in fracture cases by the use of steel pins inserted from the external surface of the face. The protruding pins are connected together by a system of rigid bars and universal joints. ➲ wiring.

fixation movements (*syn* involuntary eye movements, physiological nystagmus) the involuntary movements of the eye occurring when actually fixating an object. Three types of movements have been observed: the drifts, the micronystagmus (or tremors or microsaccades) and saccadic movements (saccades). These movements are too subtle to be seen by direct observation. The drifts are characterized by a small amplitude (1–7 minutes of arc) and a low frequency (2–5 Hz). The micronystagmus movements are characterized by a very small amplitude (10–20 seconds of arc) and a higher frequency (30–100 Hz) and the saccadic movements by a small amplitude (1–25 minutes of arc) and low frequency (0.1–1 Hz). ⊃ extraocular muscles, hypermetria, saccadic eye movement, stabilized retinal image.

fixed appliance orthodontic appliance involving the use of attachments, either bands or bonds, to one or more teeth. It cannot be removed by the patient and at the completion of the treatment is removed by the operator. Unlike removable appliances, its action is constant and achieves all orthodontic tooth movements including moving teeth bodily and not just by tilting. Oral hygiene including plaque control is rendered more difficult by these appliances.

fixed costs the costs incurred regardless of the level of activity, e.g. related to the buildings and land, equipment maintenance.

fixed-fixed bridge in dentistry, a one piece bridge, the pontic or pontics being integral with the retainers at both ends. ⊃ bridge.

fixed-movable bridge in dentistry, the pontic (that part which replaces the missing tooth or teeth) is integral with a bridge retainer at one end only. At its other end it has a limited degree of movement controlled by the retainer at that end. Often called fixed-free bridge (deprecated). ⊃ bridge.

fixer in radiography, a solution that converts and removes unexposed, undeveloped silver bromide into water-soluble silver complexes from the radiographic film during processing. Fixer has a pH of 4.2–4.9.

fixing agent a chemical, ammonium thiosulphate, that converts unexposed, undeveloped silver bromide into water-soluble silver complexes that can be removed from the radiographic film by the solvent in the fixer solution.

FL *abbr* femur length.

flaccid *adj* soft, flabby, not firm.

flaccidity *n* loss of muscle tone due to disturbance of the lower motor neuron, with varying degrees of paralysis depending on the extent of loss of motor supply to the muscles and associated with weakness due to lack of use. There is a lack of resistance to passive movement.

flagellate a protozoon that has flagella for propulsion. Examples include *Giardia*, *Leishmania* and *Trichomonas*.

flagellation *n* the act of whipping oneself or others to gain sexual pleasure. Can be a component of masochism and sadism.

flagellum *n* a fine, hair-like appendage capable of whip-like movements that moves the cell through fluid. Characteristic of spermatozoa, certain bacteria and protozoa—**flagella** *pl*.

flags refers to information obtained during patient assessment that highlights findings that need monitoring and/or referral to a medical consultant (red flags) and determines a method of specific physiotherapy management (yellow flags). *red flags* are findings from both subjective and objective examination that could indicate serious pathology such as fracture, tumour or infection and possible cauda equina syndromes. Subjective findings would include: (a) mode of onset—major trauma, road-traffic accident (RTA), sudden onset of severe symptoms, such as acute unremitting pain or bilateral weakness of the lower limbs; (b) history suggestive of tumour or infection, anyone aged over 50 years or under 20 years, history of cancer, unexplained weight loss, recent fever, frequent urinary tract infections, history of drug misuse or HIV disease; (c) possible cauda equina syndrome—bladder disturbance, such as urinary retention, increased frequency or overflow incontinence and bowel dysfunction such as unexpected laxity of the anal sphincter, saddle anaesthesia (numbness in the saddle region), bilateral parasthesia and/or weakness of the lower limb. The objective findings include: limping or coordination problems; neurological signs such as diminished or brisk reflexes, positive Babinski and clonus. *yellow flags* include: (a) psychological factors, such as maladapted attitudes and beliefs about pain, behaviours including reduced activities, poor compliance with physical exercise, extended rest periods, lack of satisfaction from previous interventions and avoidance of normal activity; (b) social factors including prolonged absence from work, withdrawal from hobbies/social activities and overly dependent on family.

flail chest unstable thoracic cage and chest wall due to multiple rib fractures. This occurs through thoracic trauma involving multiple rib fractures resulting in a destabilized segment of thoracic cage with paradoxical movement during breathing, i.e. the segment moves in during inspiration and outwards on expiration. Pulmonary contusion, haemothorax and pneumothorax frequently accompany this type of injury. ⊃ paradoxical respiration.

FLAIR *acron* **fl**uid **a**ttenuation **i**nversion **r**ecovery.

flame haemorrhage ⊃ preretinal haemorrhage.

flange a projecting flat rim. In dentistry, some saliva ejector attachments have flanges to control and protect the tongue, and reflect light during dental procedures. Also applies to that part of a denture base that lies in a sulcus.

flap *n* a unit of skin and other subcutaneous tissues that maintains its own blood and nerve supply, used to repair defects in other parts of the body. Common in plastic surgery to treat burns and other injuries; skin flaps used to cover amputation stumps. The flap may be partially severed from their bed or deeper surroundings. The blood supply can be preserved by keeping intact one of the margins, usually referred to as the base of the flap or in the case of free tissue transfer reconstruction, may be dissected free from the donor site and reanastomosed at the recipient site, e.g. radial forearm free flap.

flare *n* 1. skin redness at the periphery of an urticarial hypersensitivity reaction. 2. a sudden escalation of an existing condition. 3. expanding reddening of the skin around an area of irritation, or an infective lesion.

flashback involuntary phenomenon whereby people relive past traumatic events, or the abnormal perceptions, such as hallucinations, associated with previous use of hallucinogenic drugs. ⊃ derealization, hallucination, post traumatic stress disorder.

flash method of pasteurization ⊃ pasteurization.

flask in dentistry, **1.** sectional metal case containing and supporting the mould in which dentures are formed. **2.** also used to describe the action of investing a pattern in the flask.

flasking in dentistry, investing a wax denture or pattern in a flask.

flat back posture posture typified by cervical spine extension, upper thoracic spine flexion, an absent lumbar lordosis, posterior pelvic tilt, hip extension and slight ankle plantar-flexion. ⊃ sway back posture.

flat bone bones that have a thin layer of cancellous bone enclosed by two layers of compact bone, they either protect underlying structures, for example, in the bones of the skull, or are for muscle attachment, for example, the scapula.

flat foot *n* ⊃ pes planus.

flat pelvis (platypelloid) a pelvis in which the anteroposterior diameter of the brim is reduced.

flat screen monitor in radiography, a form of imaging monitor using a liquid crystal display to produce the image.

flattening filter a metal filter, conical in section being thick at the centre and thinning towards the edges, used to reduce the intensity of the central beam and ensure that during radiotherapy the central 80% of the beam does not vary more than plus or minus 3% at maximum density.

flat worm platyhelminth. Includes the cestodes (tapeworms) and trematodes (flukes).

flatulence *n* gastric and intestinal distension with gas—**flatulent** *adj*.

flatus *n* gas in the gastrointestinal tract.

flav- a prefix that means 'yellow', e.g. *flavonoids*.

flavin adenine dinucleotide (FAD/FADH₂) coenzyme synthesized from riboflavin. One of the major electron carrier/transfer molecules in the oxidation of fuel molecules in the mitochondria. ⊃ electron transfer chain.

flavin mononucleotide (FMN/FMNH₂) coenzyme synthesized from riboflavin. An electron carrier/transfer molecule involved in the oxidation of fuel molecules in the mitochondria. ⊃ electron transfer chain.

Flavivirus *n* a genus of RNA viruses that include those that cause dengue, St Louis encephalitis and West Nile fever.

flavonoids *npl* also known as bioflavonoids. A large group of plant pigments (e.g. yellow, red) that occur naturally in many vegetables and fruit (e.g. tomatoes, broccoli, cherries, plums, etc.). Bioflavonoids are also present in dark chocolate, tea and wine. Many are antibacterial, some others have antioxidant properties and may offer protection against heart disease and cancer, and others are phyto-oestrogens.

flavoproteins *npl* proteins combined with either flavin adenine dinucleotide or flavin mononucleotide. They function in the mitochondrial processes in which energy is produced from the oxidation of fuel. ⊃ cytochrome, electron transfer chain, oxidative phosphorylation.

flea *n* a blood-sucking wingless insect; it operates as a host and can transmit disease. Its bite provides an entry point for infection. *Pulex irritans* is the human flea. The rat flea *Xenopsylla cheopis*, is a transmitter of plague.

Fleischer ring (B Fleischer, German ophthalmologist, 1874–1965) a green/brown line around the cone of the cornea in keratoconus.

Fleming's left hand rule (J A Fleming, British physicist and engineer, 1849–1945) the direction of force in a conductor placed in a magnetic field is at right angles to both the current and the magnetic field. This can be predicted by holding the thumb, first and second fingers of the left hand at right angles to each other, thu*M*b = motion, *F*irst = force and se*C*ond = current.

Fleming's right hand rule (J A Fleming) the direction of force in a conductor placed in a magnetic field is at right angles to both the electron flow and the magnetic field. This can be predicted by holding the thumb, first and second fingers of the right hand at right angles to each other, thu*M*b = motion, *F*irst = force and s*E*cond = electron flow.

flexibilitas cerea literally waxy flexibility. A condition of generalized hypertonia of muscles found in catatonic schizophrenia. When fully developed, the patient's limbs retain positions in which they are placed, remaining immobile for hours at a time. Occasionally occurs in hysteria as hysterical rigidity.

flexibility *n* the range of movement possible around a joint or series of joints. Determined by the size and shape of the bones, the ability of tendons to stretch, the condition of the ligaments, normal joint mechanics, soft tissue mobility and extensibility of the muscles. Good flexibility is beneficial in sport especially, for example, gymnastics, and should be part of a sports-specific training programme and warm-up. However, flexibility training needs to be balanced with strength training to maintain joint stability. ⊃ hypermobility.

flexibility assessment an assessment can be made directly by measuring the angle of joint displacement using a goniometer, but this requires a skilful operator to achieve consistent results. More indirect measurements include the sit-and-reach or standing toe-touch tests.

flexible pes planus ⊃ pes planus.

flexible splinting the splinting used in avulsion and luxation injuries of teeth. The splint incorporates a flexible wire usually extending to one tooth either side of damaged tooth.

flexion *n* the act of bending by which the shafts of long bones forming a joint are brought towards each other, such as bending the elbow. A movement which decreases the joint angle between two ventral surfaces of the body, e.g. bending the elbow or knee, tilting the head forwards. ⊃ extension *opp*, flexor.

flexion reflex or withdrawal reflex the protective automatic withdrawal of an arm or leg that is exposed to a noxious stimulus. The flexor muscles contract and the extensor muscles simultaneously relax. If there is extension of the opposite limb it is described as a crossed extensor reflex (Davies et al 2001). (Davies A, Blackeley A, Kidd C 2001 Human physiology. Churchill Livingstone, Edinburgh.)

Flexner's bacillus (S Flexner, American pathologist and bacteriologist, 1863–1946). ⊃ *Shigella flexneri*.

flexor *n* a muscle which on contraction flexes or bends a part. For example, flexor carpi radialis, which flexes the hand and assists in hand abduction, biceps brachii acting at the elbow, hamstrings group acting at the knee, extensor *opp*. ⊃ Colour Section Figures 4, 5.

flexor carpi radialis a superficial, anterior muscle of the forearm. Its origin is on the medial epicondyle of the humerus and it inserts on the second and third metacarpals. It functions to flex the wrist, abduct the hand and is a synergistic muscle in flexion of the elbow. ⊃ Colour Section Figures 4, 5.

flexor carpi ulnaris a superficial, anterior muscle of the forearm. Its origin is on the medial epicondyle of the humerus, the back of the ulna and the olecranon process, and it inserts on the fifth metacarpal and the pisiform bone (a carpal bone). It functions to flex the wrist, works with the extensor carpi ulnaris to adduct the hand and stabilizes the wrist during extension movements of the fingers. ⊃ Colour Section Figures 4, 5.

flexor spasm a spasm (involuntarily contraction of the muscles) in the flexor muscle group, commonly seen in the lower limb with the result that the leg jumps up flexing at the hip and knee and dorsiflexing at the foot. Following the spasm the leg drops back down. Spasms can be painful and can lead to poor positioning and abnormal postures.

flexure *n* a bend, as in a tube-like structure, or a fold, as on the skin—it can be obliterated by extension or increased by flexion in the locomotor system—**flexural** *adj*. *left colic (splenic) flexure* is situated at the junction of the transverse and descending parts of the colon. It lies at a higher level than the *right colic* or *hepatic flexure*, the bend between the ascending and transverse colon, beneath the liver. *sigmoid flexure* ⊃ sigmoid colon.

flight of ideas succession of thoughts with no rational connection. A feature of manic disorders.

flint glass glass containing lead or titanium besides the usual ingredients and having a high dispersion compared to crown glass and a high refractive index ($n = 1.701$). It is, however, a softer and heavier material than crown. It is used in ophthalmic lenses of high power as it can be made much thinner than a crown glass lens of the same power. ⊃ constringence, dispersion, doublet, Fresnel formula, high index lens, refractive index, triplet.

flip angle the angle through which the magnetization vector moves relative to the longitudinal axis of the static magnetic field as a result of the application of a radio frequency pulse in magnetic resonance imaging (MRI). The variation in flip angle is used in gradient-echo imaging to obtain various tissue weighted images. A 10–30° flip angle produces a T_2 weighted image and a 90° flip angle provides a T_1 weighted image. ⊃ T_1 relaxation time, T_2 relaxation time, gradient echo.

flip lenses ⊃ lens flippers.
flipper bar ⊃ lens flippers.
flippers ⊃ lens flippers.
flip prisms ⊃ lens flippers.

floaters *npl* floating bodies in the vitreous body (humour) of the eye, which are visible to the person.

flocculation *n* the coalescence of colloidal particles in suspension resulting in their aggregation into larger discrete masses which are often visible to the naked eye as turbidity (cloudiness).

flocculent resembling tufts of wool. A fluid containing fluffy particles.

floccules of Busacca ⊃ Busacca's nodules.

flooding *n* **1.** a popular term to describe excessive bleeding from the uterus. **2.** a behavioural technique that may be used to reduce anxiety in people with phobias. The person is exposed to the particular stimulus that causes them anxiety while being being supported and encouraged to remain until the anxiety reduces and they feel calmer. Thus reducing the fear and consequent anxiety.

floppy baby syndrome may be due to nervous system or muscle disorder as opposed to benign hypotonia.

floppy disk ⊃ disk.

floppy disk drive (FDD) an electronic device that allows information to either be written on to or removed from a floppy disk using a magnetic field.

flora *n* used in microbiology to describe the colonization of various areas of the body by micro-organisms, e.g. *Staphylococcus epidermidis* on the skin. They are in most instances non-pathogenic, but can become pathogenic.

floss the waxed or unwaxed thread or cord used to remove plaque from the interproximal surfaces of the teeth. ⊃ dental floss/tape.

flossing mechanical cleaning of the interproximal tooth surfaces, by waxed or unwaxed thread (floss), or dental tape. Special floss is available for used with fixed orthodontic appliances.

flow 1. the volume of a fluid (liquid or gas) moving per unit time, e.g. blood flow to or through a region of the body, expressed in mL per minute. **2.** to circulate freely. To glide along. **3.** plastic deformation, under load, exhibited by some dental materials under certain conditions, e.g. amalgam, impression material, wax. **4.** in psychology, a state of complete involvement and focus on a task that occurs when there is a perfect match between one's skills and the demands of the task. **5.** a sense of exhilaration and pleasure that can arise from accepting challenges, participating fully in life and feeling in control of one's actions.

flowchart a diagrammatic representation of a computer program.

flow cytometer a laboratory instrument used to measure the proportions and absolute numbers of cell populations in, for example, blood. Cells of interest are stained with monoclonal antibodies against particular cell surface markers. The monoclonal antibodies are conjugated to fluorescent dyes and are detected once illuminated by a laser inside the flow cytometer. CD4+ T cell counts in HIV patients are commonly measured using flow cytometry.

flowmeter *n* a measuring instrument for flowing gas or liquid.

flow-related enhancement a process when the signal intensity of moving fluids can be increased compared with the signal from stationary tissue, when in-flowing, unsaturated, fully magnetized spins replace saturated spins within the imaging slice between successive radio frequency pulses in magnetic resonance imaging (MRI).

flow-volume loops graphical representation of the relation between inspiratory and expiratory airflow and the change in volume of the lungs; used in the assessment of lung function with respect to patency or obstruction of the airways, e.g. in the assessment of asthma.

fluctuation *n* a wave-like motion felt on digital examination of a fluid-containing tumour, e.g. abscess—**fluctuant** *adj*.

fluid balance ⊃ hydration status of athletes, water balance.

fluid compartments *npl* fluids in the body are either intracellular fluid (ICF) within the cells, or extracellular fluid (ECF) outside the cells, e.g. plasma, interstitial fluid, etc., (Figure F.3). In the adult about two-thirds of body water is intracellular. The remaining third is extracellular.

fluid displacement test a test performed by squeezing excess fluid out of the suprapatellar pouch, then stroking the medial side of the knee joint to displace any excess fluid to the lateral side of the joint. The procedure is repeated by stroking the lateral side of the joint. A positive finding is any excess fluid will be seen to move across the joint and distend the medial side.

fluid dynamics the study of motion (strictly accelerating motion) in or of a fluid medium (liquid or gas).

fluid lens ⊃ liquid lens.

fluid thrill a clinical sign indicative of fluid in the abdomen, such as ascites or an excess of amniotic fluid (polyhydramnios). A ripple or wave effect can be seen over the abdomen when one side is tapped.

fluke *n* a trematode worm of the order Digenea. Different flukes infest the hepatobiliary system, the lungs, blood and the intestine. The *hepatobiliary flukes Clonorchis sinensis* (Chinese fluke), *Opisthorchis viverrini* (Southeast Asia) are usually ingested with raw fish. ⊃ clonorchiasis, *Clonorchis sinensis,* opisthorchiasis, *Opisthorchis*. The *hepatobiliary fluke* present in Europe is the *European* or *sheep fluke (Fasciola hepatica),* which is usually ingested from watercress. ⊃ *Fasciola hepatica,* fascioliasis. The *lung fluke Paragonimus westermani* is usually ingested with raw crab and other shellfish in China and the Far East. ⊃ paragonimiasis, *Paragonimus*. The *blood fluke*s from the genus *Schistosoma* are present in Africa, the Middle East, the Philippines, Japan, Eastern Asia, the Caribbean and South America, they are *Schistosoma haematobium, S. japonicum* and *S. mansoni*. ⊃ *Schistosoma*, schistosomiasis. An example of an *intestinal fluke* is *Fasciolopsis buski,* it is endemic in Asia and tropical regions. ⊃ fasciolopsiasis, *Fasciolopsis buski*.

fluorescein *n* orange substance which fluoresces green when exposed to blue light. Used in dilute solution in the fitting of contact lenses and in the detection of corneal abrasions or other lesions. Also used in retinal angiography, by injection into a peripheral vein, to demonstrate the retinal and choroidal circulation, and chorioretinal disease. ⊃ fluorescein angiography.

fluorescein angiography a technique whereby fluorescein is injected intravenously (into a vein in the arm or hand) to demonstrate the retinal blood vessels and iris, any retinal pathology, the macula and optic disc and the presence of tumours of the choroid. Before the fluorescein is injected, the pupils of the eyes are dilated with a mydratic drug, such as tropicamide, to allow the fundus to be examined and photographs taken. It is a useful technique which facilitates the diagnosis of various retinal (e.g. diabetic retinopathy, retinal artery occlusion, retinal vein occlusion, age-related macular degeneration), choroidal (e.g. tumour of the choroid) and iris disorders. However, those of the choroid and iris are more difficult to observe. ⊃ choroidal flush, diabetic retinopathy.

fluorescein string test *n* used to detect the site of obscure upper gastrointestinal bleeding. The patient swallows a radiopaque knotted string. Fluorescein is injected intravenously and after a few minutes the string is withdrawn. If staining has occurred the site of bleeding can be determined.

fluorescence the property of a substance that, when illuminated, absorbs light of a given wavelength and re-emits it as radiations of a longer wavelength. For example fluorescein. ⊃ Draper's law, fluorescent lamp, luminescence, wavelength, Wood's light.

fluorescence in situ hybridization (FISH) a diagnostic chromosome test used to identify trisomy and sex chromosome aneuploides (but does not analyse the whole karyotype). It is performed on uncultured cells to obtain rapid results after chorionic villus sampling or amniocentesis, within 24–48 hours. The technique relies on coloured deoxyribonucleic acid (DNA) probes which attach to specific chromosome regions through hybridization. Fluorescent spots appear and the number of spots in each cell can then be counted. Two spots indicate normal diploid chromosomes; three spots indicate trisomy. ⊃ quantitative fluorescence-polymerase chain reaction (QF-PCR).

fluorescent agent (or pigment) material used in the fabrication of artificial teeth, crown and bridge porcelain and filling materials to impart fluorescence and thus simulate the fluorescence of natural teeth.

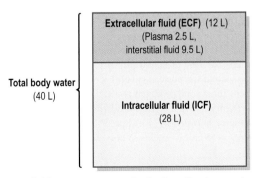

F.3 **Fluid compartments**—distribution of body water in a 70 kg adult male (reproduced from Brooker & Nicol 2003 with permission).

fluorescent antibody test *n* a technique for visualizing an antibody by coating it with a fluorescent dye which can then be viewed by use of a fluorescent microscope with a source of ultraviolet light. ⊃ immunofluorescence.

fluorescent lamp discharge lamp in which most of the light is emitted by a layer of fluorescent material excited by the ultraviolet radiation from the discharge (CIE). ⊃ fluorescence.

fluorescent treponemal antibody absorbed test (FTA-Abs) *n* a specific serological test for syphilis.

fluoridation *n* the adjustment of the amount of soluble fluoride in water supplies in order to reduce the incidence of dental caries. In temperate climates, the optimum level of the fluoride ion in the water supply is between 0.7–1.0 part per million (or 0.7–1.0 mg/litre). This has been found to reduce dental decay by as much as 40–50%. Naturally fluoridated water may contain a much higher fluoride ion concentration, especially in parts of Africa and Asia. Milk, salt and fruit juices may be artificially fluoridated for use in communities where water fluoridation is not possible. Excessive exposure to ingested fluoride may produce fluorosis of teeth. Minute traces of fluoride are found in most foods. ⊃ fluoride.

fluoride *n* an ion sometimes present in drinking water, toothpastes, tea, vegetables, sea food and other food stuffs. It can be incorporated into the structure of bone and teeth, where it provides protection against dental caries, but in gross excess it causes mottling of the teeth. Fluoride has an important influence on the prevention of dental caries, since it increases the resistance of the enamel to acid attack. If the water supply of a locality contains more than 1 part per million (ppm) of fluoride, the incidence of dental caries is low. Soft waters usually contain no fluoride, whilst very hard waters may contain over 10 ppm. The benefit of fluoride is greatest when it is taken before the permanent teeth erupt, while their enamel is being laid down. The addition of traces of fluoride (at 1 ppm) to public water supplies is now a widespread practice. Chronic fluoride poisoning is occasionally seen where the water supply contains > 10 ppm fluoride. It can also occur in workers handling cryolite (aluminium sodium fluoride), used in smelting aluminium. ⊃ fluorosis.

fluoride varnish ⊃ varnish.

fluorine (F) *n* halogen element.

fluoro computed tomography (CT) equipment allowing the acquisition and immediate display of multiple CT images per second, is used in minimally invasive microtherapy procedures.

fluoroquinolones *npl* a group of synthetic antibiotics, e.g. ciprofloxacin. ⊃ Appendix 5.

fluoroscopy *n* a real time radiographic examination of the human body, observed by means of an image intensifier and a television system.

fluorosis a condition caused by excessive intake of fluorine over a long period. Though water-borne fluorides at levels of 1 part per million are associated with significant immunity to dental caries, the presence of excessive quantities of fluoride in drinking water leads to a characteristic sequence of pathological changes in teeth, bone and periarticular tissues. A yellowish-brown mottling of teeth (permanent teeth being particularly affected) is an early and easily recognizable feature of chronic toxicity. This is important, as skeletal involvement may not be clinically obvious until advanced changes have taken place in bone. Radiological changes, however, are seen in the skeleton at an early stage and provide the only means of early diagnosis of relatively asymptomatic fluorosis. Such early cases are usually young adults who complain of vague pains in the small joints of the hands and feet and sometimes in the knees and spine. The changes in bone and periarticular tissues limit movement of the limbs and may cause back pain. Lesions may progress to cause serious disability, particularly kyphosis, due to progressive joint ankylosis. Changes in the bones of the thoracic cage may lead to rigidity that causes dyspnoea on exertion. In calcium-deficient children, the toxic effects of fluoride manifest even at marginally high exposures to fluoride. In endemic areas, such as Jordan, Turkey, Chile, India, Bangladesh, China and Tibet, fluorosis is a major public health problem. The maximum impact is seen in communities engaged in physically strenuous agricultural or industrial activities. Dental fluorosis is endemic in East Africa and some West African countries. ⊃ fluoride.

flux 1. the lines of force through a magnetic field. **2.** material used to prevent oxidation and facilitate the flow of solder.

FM *abbr* Fugel-Meyer.

FM 100 Hue test ⊃ Farnsworth test.

FMNH *abbr* fetal movements not felt.

FMN/FMNH$_2$ *abbr* flavin mononucleotide (oxidized and reduced form respectively).

FMPA *abbr* Frankfort mandibular plane angle.

FMRI *abbr* functional magnetic resonance imaging.

FNA *abbr* fine needle aspirate.

FOB *acron* faecal occult blood.

focal distance ⊃ focal length.

focal injuries those injuries that occur in a small concentrated area, usually due to a high velocity-low mass force, e.g. ice hockey puck making contact with an unguarded area of the player's body.

focal length *syn* focal distance. The linear distance separating the principal focal point (or focus) of an optical system from a point of reference (e.g. vertex, principal point, nodal point). The first (or anterior) focal length is the distance from the lens (or first principal point) to the first principal focus. The second (or posterior) focal length is the distance from the lens (or second principal point) to the second principal focus. Symbol: *f*. In a spherical mirror the focal length *f*, i.e. the distance between the focal point and the pole of the mirror, is equal to half its radius of curvature *r*,

$$f = \frac{r}{2}$$

⊃ refractive power, sign convention.

focal plane (plane of cut) in tomography, the selected plane that provides a clear image.

focal point ⊃ principal focus.

focal power ⊃ refractive power (*F*).

focal spot the area of the anode bombarded by electrons; due to the angle of the anode the real focal spot is larger than the apparent focal spot.

focal trough (image layer) in dental panoramic tomography, the depth of focus in which the selected layer provides a clear and distinct image.

focus 1. in optics, the point at which rays of light converge after passing through a convex lens to form a real image (real focus), or diverge from (virtual focus) after passing through a concave lens—**foci** *pl*. **2.** to adjust an optical system (e.g. camera or projector) in order to obtain a sharp image. Also known as focusing. **3.** the centre or starting point of a disease process; the main site of an infection. **4.** the area of the anode that is bombarded by electrons.

focus groups in research a method of obtaining data that involves interviewing people in small interacting groups. Groups of people who have been gathered together in order to gain some insight into their ideas and attitudes towards a particular subject. A useful technique used in conjunction with other research methods to achieve triangulation. The topic can then be pursued using research that is more quantitative in nature, they can help to clarify quantitative results or generate hypotheses for future research.

focus to film distance (FFD) in radiography, the distance from the focal spot to the film packet.

focusing coils produce magnetic fields to prevent divergence of the internal electron beam and therefore leakage of radiation from the equipment.

focusing cup part of the cathode in an X-ray tube that helps direct the electrons to land on the target.

foetor ⊃ fetor.

fog in radiography, the partial or complete darkening of a developed photographic or radiographic film due to sources other than the primary beam or to light exposure.

foil very thin sheet of metal such as tin, platinum or gold. *cohesive gold foil* 24 carat or 1000 fine pure gold, whose surface is completely pure so that it will cohere or weld at room temperature. *gold foil* pure gold rolled into extremely thin sheets and historically used in the restoration of teeth. *platinum foil* a precious metal foil with a high fusing point. In dentistry, it is most often used as the internal matrix onto which porcelain restorations are built up, prior to firing.

folate (*syn* pteroylglutamic acid) collective name for the B vitamin compounds derived from folic acid. Folates occur naturally in foods such as liver, yeasts and leafy green vegetables and are absorbed from the small intestine. They are coenzymes involved in many biochemical reactions in the body, e.g. purine and pyrimidine synthesis, and adequate amounts, along with vitamin B_{12}, are required for normal red cells and cell division generally. A deficiency results in a megaloblastic anaemia. It is recommended that supplements

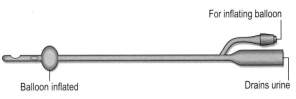

For inflating balloon

Balloon inflated   Drains urine

F.4 Self-retaining catheter (double-lumen Foley) (reproduced from Brooker & Waugh 2007 with permission).

are taken before and during the first weeks after conception, to reduce the risk of neural tube defects (NTDs) in the fetus.

fold-over (aliasing, wrap around) an artefact that occurs in magnetic resonance imaging (MRI) due to the image encoding process. It occurs when the field of view is smaller than the area being imaged.

Foley catheter a self-retaining urinary catheter (Figure F.4).

folic acid the molecule that gives rise to a large group of molecules known as folates that form part of the vitamin B complex. ⊃ folate.

folie à deux a rare psychiatric syndrome, in which one member of a close pair suffers a psychotic illness and eventually imposes his delusions on the other.

follicle *n* **1.** a small secreting sac. **2.** a simple tubular gland—**follicular** *adj*. ⊃ dental follicle.

follicle stimulating hormone (FSH) secreted by the anterior pituitary gland; it is trophic to the ovaries in the female, where it develops the oocyte-containing (Graafian) follicles; and to the testes in the male, where it stimulates spermatogenesis.

follicular carcinoma a malignant tumour of the thyroid gland which spreads via the blood stream and metastasizes to bone and lung.

follicular conjunctivitis conjunctivitis characterized by follicles (usually in one eye only) caused by adenoviruses or chemical or toxic irritation and frequently associated with lymphadenopathy. ⊃ conjunctival follicle, lymphadenopathy, trachoma.

folliculitis *n* inflammation of follicles, such as the hair follicles. ⊃ alopecia.

folliculitis decalvans is an alopecia of the scalp characterized by pustulation and scarring.

fomentation *n* a hot, wet application used to produce hyperaemia when applied to the skin.

fomites *npl* any article that has been in contact with infection and is capable of transmitting same, e.g. bed linen, surgical instruments.

fontanelle *n* a membranous space between the cranial bones. The diamond-shaped anterior fontanelle (bregma) is at the junction of the frontal and two parietal bones. It usually closes in the second year of life. The triangular posterior fontanelle (lambda) is at the junction of the occipital and two parietal bones. It closes within a few weeks of birth.

food allergy an abnormal immunological response to food that can be severe and life-threatening. Signs and symptoms include swelling of the mouth and throat, breathing

E
F

difficulties, skin rashes and gastrointestinal disturbances. The term is often used erroneously to describe any adverse reactions to food, whether or not the underlying mechanism has been identified. ⊃ allergy.

food impaction the forceful wedging of food interdentally.

food intolerance an abnormal reaction to a food that is not immunological in origin, e.g. the effects of lactose intake in a person with lactase deficiency. Symptoms can be chronic or acute, identification of the food can be difficult and may require an exclusion diet.

food poisoning a notifiable disease characterized by vomiting, with or without diarrhoea. It results from eating food contaminated with preformed bacterial toxin (e.g. from *Escherichia coli 0157*, *Staphylococcus aureus* and *Clostridium perfringens*) or multiplication of live micro-organisms in food (e.g. *Campylobacter jejuni*, *Salmonella typhimurium*, *Bacillus cereus* and viruses) or poisonous natural vegetation, e.g. berries, toadstools (fungi) or chemical poisons.

Food Standards Agency (FSA) in the UK a body set up by the government to over see food standards and safety.

foot *n* that portion of the lower limb below the ankle. As well as supporting the weight of the body, the foot works as a lever to move the body forwards. The many joints between the bones of the foot allow it to change shape to accommodate different and uneven surfaces. The skeleton of the foot comprises the seven tarsal bones, including the heel bone (calcaneus, calcaneum, or os calsis) and the talus which articulates with the leg bones at the ankle joint; beyond these, the five metatarsals and, in the toes, the phalanges. There are layers of small muscles in the sole, and tendons from the lower leg traverse the ankle to reach their various insertions in the sole and on the dorsum (upper part) of the foot.

foot angle also known as angle of gait. A biomechanical term describing the angle of foot orientation away from the line of progression during walking.

footballer's ankle also known as anterior impingement of the ankle. Occurs as a result of repeated injury to the joint capsule and ligaments. Overstretching allows excessive movement of the bones with local inflammation and the development of bony outgrowths at the front of the ankle where the capsule is attached. These may break off, becoming 'loose bodies' within the joint, resulting in pain and tenderness across the front of the ankle and on moving the foot up and down.

foot drop inability to dorsiflex the foot due usually to damage affecting the nerve supply to the foot. Can be a complication of bedrest. Paralysis or weakness of the ankle dorsiflexors may indicate several pathologies including: common peroneal nerve damage from a fracture or a plaster cast that is too tight around the neck of the fibula, an intervertebral disc prolapse in the lumbar spine or other neurological conditions. The tibialis anterior muscle primarily has the role of decelerating the foot following heel strike, so a person with a foot drop may slap the foot on the floor during walking or may adopt a high stepping gait in an attempt to ensure that the foot still clears the ground on swing through phase of gait.

foot drop splint a splint that is usually made to fit into a standard shoe. Can be trimmed or moulded with heat. They are used in cases of drop foot or gross instability at the ankle. ⊃ drop foot.

footling presentation a variation of the breech presentation in which one foot is presenting in front of the buttocks.

foramen *n* a hole or opening. Generally used with reference to bones where the foramen allows the passage of blood vessels, nerves and lymphatics—**foramina** *pl*.

foramen magnum the opening in the occipital bone through which the spinal cord passes.

foramen ovale 1. a fetal cardiac interatrial communication which normally closes at birth. **2.** the opening in the greater wing of the sphenoid bone which conducts the mandibular division of the trigeminal nerve and the small meningeal artery.

foramen rotundum the opening in the greater wing of the sphenoid bone through which passes the maxillary division of the trigeminal nerve.

forbidden energy gap an area between the top energy level of the valence band and the bottom level of the conduction band, electrons can pass through the gap but cannot exist within the band.

force an interaction between two bodies, objects or agents which changes (or tends to change) motion either by contact or by action at-a-distance. May be a 'push' or a 'pull'. Note that a force changes the state of motion (including change from zero) but does not itself maintain an existing state of motion. *net force* the mathematical result of all the forces applied to an object or body, taking into account the size and direction of the forces. Measured in newtons (N). ⊃ inertial movement.

force couple two moments applied in the same rotational direction to a rotating object or body. Also known as couple. For example, a single movement that is produced by the integrated activity of two or more muscles, such as rotation of the scapula.

force development, rate of the slope of a force–time graph, usually obtained from a force transducer (e.g. a force plate). May give information about how fast a muscle can develop forceful contraction. Can also be calculated as mass × jerk. Measured in newtons per second ($N . s^{-1}$).

force plate a device for measuring the force between a body or object and the ground (the ground reaction force). Often constructed from strain gauges or piezo-electric transducers. Also known as a force platform.

force–velocity relationship the relationship between force and velocity in a contracting muscle or isolated muscle fibre. In concentric contraction force is zero at maximum velocity and maximal at very low or at zero velocity (the latter being an isometric contraction). Between these extremes the force–velocity curve is approximately hyperbolic, as described by A.V. Hill in 1938. By contrast, in eccentric action, the form of the curve varies substantially between different muscles and in no case can it be adequately approximated mathematically. Thus in isolated, artificially stimulated muscles the force resisting extension rises well above the level in isotonic contraction as extension velocity increases, before falling off again at even higher velocities, (Figure F.5A) but in intact muscles the resisting force is less than this, to the extreme that the knee extensors (presumably because they act at a joint which is vulnerable in the face of high gravitational stress) show an almost flat curve in untrained people (Figure F.5B), and only a modestly convex one in those who are strength trained. Commonly plotted with force on the ordinate and velocity on the abscissa, even though this might more properly be called the 'velocity–force' relation. ⊃ torque–angular velocity relation.

forced-choice a test or experimental procedure where a respondent has to select a response from a limited set of choices.

forced expiration technique (FET) the forced expiration technique or huff is used to assist the expectoration of pulmonary secretions. The intrathoracic pressures produced during FET are less than those produced with a cough and, therefore, less exhausting. The technique is based on the

principle of the equal pressure point (EPP). The EPP is the point at which the airway and pleural pressures are equal. During a forced expiration, collapse and compression of the airways occurs toward the mouth, thus moving secretions in a peripheral direction as lung volume decreases. Hence, FET from low lung volumes will shift secretions from the more peripheral airways; while a huff at a high lung volume will clear secretions from the upper airways. ⊃ active cycle of breathing, equal pressure point.

forced expiratory flow (FEF) is measured spirometrically. This is used as a diagnostic tool in airflow obstruction, at different stages of the expired breath, e.g. through 25–75% (written as FEF_{25-75}).

forced expiratory ratio (FER) a spirometric term used to detail the ratio of the forced expiratory volume in one second (FEV_1) to forced expiratory volume (FVC). This ratio is diagnostic of restrictive, obstructive and combined lung diseases. Where the ratio is, 70%, airflow obstruction is diagnosed. ⊃ respiratory function tests, spirometry.

forced expiratory volume (FEV) volume of air exhaled during a given time (usually the first second: FEV_1). ⊃ respiratory function tests, spirometry.

forced vital capacity (FVC) the maximum gas volume that can be expelled from the lungs in a forced expiration. ⊃ respiratory function tests, spirometry.

forceps *n* surgical instruments with two opposing blades which are used to grasp or compress tissues, swabs, needles, many other surgical appliances and for the extraction of teeth, etc. The two blades are controlled by direct pressure on them (tong-like), or by handles (scissor-like). The many types adapted for specific functions include: *artery forceps* metal forceps with serrated, sometimes curved beaks and scissor-like handles with a ratchet device to maintain the grip until released. *bone-cutting forceps* two-handled instrument with knife- or chisel-shaped blades, also known as *bone shears. bone-nibbling forceps (rongeurs)* two-handled, pincer-like instrument used to cut away small portions of bone by means of cup-shaped beaks. *cow's horn forceps* forceps with cutting blades bearing resemblance to cow's horns in shape used to split and separate the roots of multi-rooted teeth. *dissecting forceps* tweezer-like instrument with curved, straight, serrated or rat-toothed jaws. Some are insulated for electrosurgery. *extraction forceps* pincer-like instruments for tooth extraction. Consist of handles, joints and beaks or blades, made in various shapes and widths. Classified by numbers stamped on the inner side of the handle by the makers, according to the shape of the beaks or handles or to their special uses. *lower molar forceps* forceps with both beaks set at right angles to the handles and arrow shaped to fit the bifurcation of the two roots of lower molars. *lower root forceps* straight-handled forceps with hollowed-out beaks in various widths, set at right angles to the handles. Used to extract lower incisors, canines, premolars and roots. *maxillary disimpaction forceps* instrument in which one blade passes into the nasal cavity and the other fits against the palate so that the displaced maxilla may be grasped,

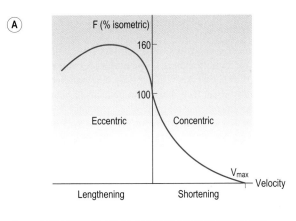

(A)

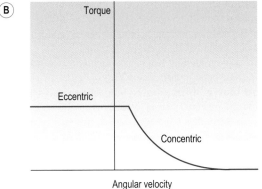

(B)

F.5 Force–velocity relationship (A) F–V curve including region of eccentric acitivity. (B) Torque–angular velocity curve for human knee extensors in both concentric and eccentric actions, obtained by isokinetic dynamometry (reproduced from Jennett 2008 with permission).

disimpacted and repositioned. *mosquito artery forceps* similar to Spencer Wells artery forceps but with fine beaks. *needle-holding forceps* instrument with scissor-type handles and often a ratchet device, to hold needles during suturing. *Spencer Wells artery forceps* original pattern of forceps used to clamp arteries. *tissue forceps* several types of fine-bladed forceps used to hold tissues. They have scissor handles with or without a ratchet device to hold their jaws together once closed. *upper anterior forceps* (*straight*) forceps with hollowed-out straight blades of various widths in line with the handles. *upper molar forceps* right and left instruments having one hollowed-out beak to fit the palatal root of upper molars and a pointed, spade-shaped beak to accommodate the bifurcation of the buccal roots. *upper root forceps* forceps with curved, hollowed-out beaks of various widths and curved handles (*Read's pattern*), one to fit into the palm of the hand and the other to provide a comfortable grip for the fingers. *upper root bayonet pattern forceps* having straight beaks set at an angle to the handles which may be curved (*Read's pattern*) or straight. Used for extraction of upper teeth and roots in the posterior part of the mouth. There are several other patterns including a range of smaller children's extraction forceps.

forceps delivery the use of various specialized obstetric forceps, e.g Wrigley's forceps, Kielland forceps, applied to the infant to facilitate delivery during the second stage of labour.

Forchheimer spots the petechial lesions appearing on the soft palate in rubella.

Fordyce's disease (J Fordyce, American dematologist, 1858–1925) a developmental anomaly consisting of enlarged sebaceous glands of the oral mucosa and genitals. Clinically it appears as a collection of small yellowish spots.

fore- a prefix that means 'before, in front of', e.g. *forewaters*.

forebrain the part of the brain comprising the cerebral hemispheres, basal nuclei and the structures of the diencephalon.

foregut the front part of the embryonic alimentary tract. It is endodermal tissue and will form the pharynx, oesophagus, stomach, some of the small intestine, the liver and pancreas. ➲ hindgut, midgut.

forensic dentistry dental jurisprudence. The examination, interpretation and presentation of dentally related evidence in a legal context.

forensic medicine (*syn* medical jurisprudence, or 'legal medicine'). The application of medical science to questions of law.

foreshortening in dental radiography, the decrease in length of the radiographic image of the tooth due to incorrect technique.

foreskin *n* the prepuce or skin covering the glans penis.

forewaters the sac of amniotic fluid situated in front of the fetal head. The pressure from the well-flexed head on the cervix creates a dam so that some amniotic fluid becomes trapped in front of the head. ➲ hindwaters.

-form a suffix that means 'having the form of', e.g. *epileptiform*.

formaldehyde *n* toxic gas used as a disinfectant. Dissolved in water (formalin), it is used mainly for disinfection and the preservation of histological specimens. In dentistry it may be mixed with cresol to be used as a root canal medication. ➲ formocresol.

formalin a 37% aqueous solution of the gas formaldehyde used to fix tissues for histological examination.

formants two major resonating frequencies determining the sound of a vowel.

form drag the resistance force caused by the shape of a body or object which is moving through a fluid medium. ➲ drag force, propulsive drag force, surface drag.

forme fruste **1.** an inherited condition in which there is only minimal expression of the faulty gene. **2.** a disease presentation which is atypical or incomplete and resolves earlier than is usual.

formication *n* a sensation as of ants running over the skin. Occurs in nerve lesions, particularly in the regenerative phase.

formiminoglutamic acid ➲ FIGLU test.

formocresol in dentistry, a pulp medicament, usually used in a 1:6 dilution. Used in primary molar pulp therapy to mummify or 'fix' pulpal tissue.

formula *n* a prescription. A series of symbols denoting the chemical composition of a substance, e.g. NaCl is the formula for sodium chloride—**formulae, formulas** *pl.*

formula diet a diet that requires only minimal digestion and is easily absorbed. It comprises amino acids or peptides, glucose and mono- and diglycerides.

formulary *n* a collection of formulas. The *British National Formulary* describes licensed pharmaceutical products available in the UK.

fornix *n* an arch; particularly referred to the vagina, i.e. the space between the vaginal wall and the cervix of the uterus—**fornices** *pl.*

Forster–Fuchs spot ➲ Fuchs' spot.

fortification the addition of specific nutrients to foods, such as vitamins A and D to margarine. Or, as in the United States, the addition of folic acid to all cereal products. Thus increasing intake levels in the population.

Fortran a programming language which is between BASIC and machine code in difficulty.

forward bias is when a battery is connected across a PN junction the potential barrier is lowered to allow current to flow. ➲ reverse bias *opp.*

forward parachute reflex ➲ parachute reflex.

fossa *n* an anatomical term for a depression, hollow or furrow—**fossae** *pl.*

fostering *n* placing a vulnerable child with a suitable family either as a short or long term measure. The aims are to provide a child with the security of a home environment, and to reunite the child with their natural family as soon as practical. Long term fosterings can be 'with a view to adoption'.

Fothergill's operation ◌ Manchester operation.

fourchette *n* a membranous fold connecting the posterior ends of the labia minora.

'four-day blues' ◌ postnatal depression.

four-dimensional ultrasound three-dimensional ultrasound with a real time, moving image.

four dot test ◌ Worth's four dot test.

four-handed dentistry dental surgeon and surgery assistant working together as a team on operative procedures.

Fourier analysis the method of dividing an image into the various spatial frequency areas and expressing them in mathematical terms.

Fourier transform used in electronic signal processing, a signal is analysed by taking a timed sample to identify its frequencies and their amplitudes and then to express them as a sum of frequencies multiplied by amplitude. This figure can then be electronically manipulated to improve the digital image.

Fournier's gangrene (J Fournier, French dermatologist, 1832–1914) a fulminating gangrene of the scrotum. ◌ fasciitis.

fourth degree tear ◌ perineal tear.

fourth heart (S4) an abnomal heart sound heard late in diastole may be present in severe left ventricular hypertrophy.

FOV *abbr* field of view.

fovea *n* a small depression or fossa. ◌ foveola.

fovea centralis (*syn* foveal pit, macula [term often used by clinicians]) a small area of the retina of approximately 1.5 mm in diameter situated within the macula lutea. At the fovea centralis, the retina is the thinnest as there are no supporting fibres of Mueller, no ganglion cells and no bipolar cells. These cells are shifted to the edge of the depression. The fovea centralis contains mainly cone cells, each one being connected to only one ganglion cell and thus contributing to the highest visual acuity of the retina. The visual field represented by the fovea centralis is equal to about 5°. ◌ foveola, macula lutea, visual acuity.

foveae palati the two pits situated near the junction of the hard and soft palate, one on either side of the midline.

foveal pit ◌ fovea centralis.

foveola (*syn* fovea [term often used by clinicians]) the foveola is the base of the fovea centralis with a diameter of about 0.4 mm (or about 1° of the visual field). The image of the point of fixation is formed on the foveola in the normal eye. The foveola contains cone cells only (rod-free area). The foveal avascular zone is slightly larger (about 0.5 mm in diameter).

FR *abbr* functional reach (test).

fractional inspired oxygen concentration (FiO₂) the concentration of oxygen in inspired gas, expressed as a fraction of 1 (e.g. FiO_2 0.6 equals 60% inspired oxygen concentration).

fractional utilization the percentage of maximum oxygen consumption/uptake (VO_{2max}) that can be sustained during exercise at competition/race pace. It is affected by the duration of exercise and the level of training.

fractionation *n* in radiotherapy it is the process of administering smaller doses of radiation over a period of time, excluding weekends, to minimize tissue damage. ◌ accelerated fractionation, conventional fractionation, hyperfractionation.

fracture *n* breach in continuity of a bone as a result of injury or disease (Figure F.6). ◌ Bennett's fracture, Colles' fracture. *closed fracture* there is no communication with external air. *comminuted fracture* a breach in the continuity of a bone which is broken into more than two pieces. *complicated fracture* a breach in the continuity of a bone when there is injury to surrounding organs and structures. *compression fracture* usually of lumbar or dorsal region of the spine; the anterior vertebral bodies are crushed together. *depressed fracture* the broken bone presses on an underlying structure, such as brain or lung. *impacted fracture* one end of the broken bone is driven into the other. *incomplete fracture* the bone is only cracked or fissured—called *greenstick fracture* when it occurs in children. *open (compound) fracture* there is a wound permitting communication of broken bone end with air. *pathological fracture* occurring in abnormal bone as a result of force which would not break a normal bone. *spontaneous fracture* one occurring without appreciable violence; may be synonymous with pathological

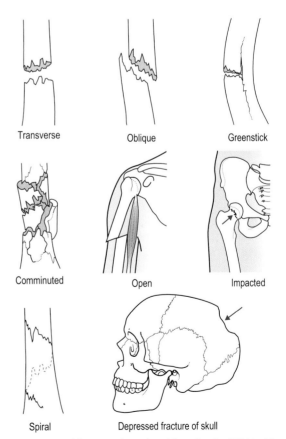

Transverse   Oblique   Greenstick

Comminuted   Open   Impacted

Spiral   Depressed fracture of skull

F.6 Types of fractures (reproduced from Brooker 2006A with permission).

fracture. ⊃ fracture-associated nerve injury, fracture reduction, intra-articular fracture, jaw fracture, march fracture, plaster of Paris, stress fracture.

fracture-associated nerve injury certain fractures, such as those involving the mid-shaft humerus, may lead to radial nerve palsy. If a plaster is too tight it may cause nerve damage, the common peroneal nerve is vulnerable to this if a plaster cast is moulded too tightly around the fibular head, resulting in foot drop as the tibialis anterior muscle is affected and unable to perform its function of decelerating the foot upon heel strike and permitting toe clearance during the swing through phase of gait.

fracture reduction the realignment of a fractured bone into the normal or as near normal anatomical position as possible. Reduction of a fracture may be either open or closed. *closed reduction* means that no surgical intervention is used; the fracture is manipulated by hand under local or general anaesthesia. *open reduction* means that the area has been surgically opened and reduced. Reduction may not always be necessary even when there is some displacement, e.g. fractures of the clavicle may heal with a bump that may only be a problem in the cosmetic sense.

Fraenkel appliances (Fraenkel, German orthodontist) myofuntional appliances used in orthodontic treatment. A Fraenkel 1 is used to correct Class II Division I malocclusions; a Fraenkel 2 to correct Class II Division II malocclusions; and a Fraenkel 3 to correct Class III malocclusions.

fraenotomy *n* frenotomy.

fraenum *n* ⊃ frenulum (frenum)—**fraena** *pl*, **fraenal** *adj*.

fragile X syndrome X-linked disorder mainly affecting males. During childhood there is relatively normal appearance, but some degree of learning disability. Physical features that include large ears and a long and narrow face, enlarged testes and in a smaller percentage very smooth skin, flat feet and mitral valve prolapse, which usually come to prominence after puberty.

fragilitas ossium ⊃ osteogenesis imperfecta.

Frahm's carver ⊃ carver.

framboesia *n* yaws.

frame of reference a number of theories that together provide a coherent conceptual foundation for practice.

frame rate the number of times an ultrasonic image is refreshed per second, a slow frame rate gives better resolution, a high frame rate better demonstrates movement.

framework in dentistry, the skeletal metal part of a partial denture to which the remaining denture components are attached.

Francisella (E Francis, American microbiologist, 20th century) a genus of Gram negative bacteria. The species *Francisella tularensis* causes tularaemia in humans. ⊃ tularaemia.

frank extended breech the fetus is presenting with the buttocks over the cervical os, the thighs are flexed and the legs are extended to lie alongside the shoulders.

Frankenhauser's plexus also known as Lee-Frankenhauser's plexus. A ganglion near the uterine cervix from which sympathetic and parasympathetic nerves supply the vagina, uterus and other pelvic viscera.

Frankfort mandibular plane angle the angle formed by the Frankfort horizontal plane and the mandibular plane.

Frankfort plane the plane passing through the lowest point in the floor of the left orbit (the orbitale) and the highest point of each external auditory meatus of the skull (the porion). It is horizontal when the head is in the normal upright position.

Frank–Starling relationship ⊃ Starling's law of the heart.

Fraser syndrome (G Fraser, American geneticist, b. 1932) a congenital absence of the opening between the eyelids. It is an autosomal recessive condition and is associated with other abnormalities that include abnormal eyeball development, cleft palate, heart problems, etc.

Fraunhofer's lines fine dark lines distributed throughout the length of the solar spectrum due to the absorption of specific wavelengths by elements in the atmosphere of the sun and the earth. Fraunhofer observed about 600 of these lines and denoted the most prominent ones by letters from A in the extreme red to K in the violet. *Examples*: A corresponds to 759.4 nm, C to 656.3 nm, D to 589.3 nm, F to 486.1 nm, etc. ⊃ constringence, refractive index.

FRC *abbr* functional residual capacity.

freckle small brown macules on the skin, especially after sun exposure. An inherited trait particularly common in people with red hair. ⊃ ephelis, lentigo.

free articulation condition where the dental articulation is not obstructed by any cuspal interference.

free body diagram a method of analysis of the force and motion characteristics of a body or object by drawing a simplified version of the external forces acting on it.

free cleansing in dentistry, improving the shape of a tooth surface or space between two teeth. This makes it easier to keep clean, by opening up the contact area, ensuring smooth margins on restorations or recontouring the tooth surface to discourage plaque build-up.

free end saddle a partial denture whose distal extension base terminates without support from a natural tooth or an implant.

free fatty acids (FFA) the fatty acids present in the circulating blood and within cells. Also known as non-esterified fatty acids (NEFA). Circulating free fatty acids (FFA) arise from triacylglycerol molecules of adipose tissue and triacylglycerol-rich lipoproteins. During endurance-type exercise a considerable amount of the energy released by contracting skeletal muscle is derived from oxidation of both circulating FFA and that provided by triacylglycerol stored in muscle. Theoretically, increasing FFA availability and utilization may reduce reliance on muscle glycogen and therefore delay onset of fatigue. There is therefore interest in strategies designed to enhance FFA oxidation (e.g. high-fat diets, caffeine, carnitine supplementation).

free-floating anxiety generalized pervasive anxiety with no link to a specific situation or object. The person feels persistent fear and unease.

free induction decay a brief signal that occurs as the transverse magnetism decays towards zero following the application of a radio frequency pulse in magnetic resonance imaging (MRI).

free radical reactive oxygen species, such as the superoxide ion and hydroxyl radical. They are extremely reactive chemicals produced during normal metabolism. Normally they are dealt with by complex antioxidant enzyme systems but they can cause oxidative damage to cells. ⮌ antioxidant nutrients, reactive oxygen species.

free text term in literature searching, a list of words that describe each part of the search question more fully. These may include alternative spellings (including American spelling), abbreviations, plurals and synonyms.

freeway space ⮌ interocclusal clearance.

freeze drying technique in which tissues for pathological examination, or dental materials such as the glass ionomer and carboxylate cements, are subjected to freezing and then dehydration in a high vacuum.

freezing *n* the sudden inability of a parkinsonian patient to take another step while walking until an external visual, auditory or cutaneous stimulus is appreciated. It is due to co-contraction of antagonistic muscle groups; a manifestation of dystonia.

Freiberg's infarction (A Freiberg, American surgeon, 1868–1940) an aseptic necrosis of bone tissue which most commonly occurs in the head of the second metatarsal bone. The aetiology is unknown: both traumatic and vascular causes have been suggested. Most common in athletic girls aged 10–15 in which it presents with pain and local tenderness. Changes may not be evident initially on X-ray, but can be visualized using magnetic resonance imaging (MRI).

fremitus a trembling vibration of a body structure, usually the chest wall. It can be palpated during examination or heard by ascultation when the patient speaks, breathes or coughs.

Frenkel defect the loss of an atom from a structure forming an interstitial ion or atom. ⮌ point defects.

Frenkel's exercises (H Frenkel, Swiss neurologist, 1860–1931) special repetitive exercises to improve muscle and joint sense.

frenectomy excision of a frenulum (frenum). The operation, sometimes carried out for orthodontic reasons, includes the removal of interdental fibrous tissue.

frenoplasty the surgical repositioning of attached frenulum (frenum).

frenotomy *n* surgical severance of a frenulum (frenum), particularly for tongue-tie.

frenulum or frenum *n* (*syn* fraenum) a small fold of mucous membrane that checks or limits the movement of an organ, e.g. tongue, prepuce of the penis. In the mouth it extends from the inner surface of the lip, cheek or tongue, to the alveolar process. *abnormal frenulum* an abnormal fold of mucous membrane which may obstruct the seating of a denture, or influence the periodontal attachment. *labial frenulum* a fold of mucous membrane in the midline, anterior to the upper central incisors, extending from the inner surface of the upper lip to the alveolar process. *lingual frenulum* a midline fold of mucous membrane extending from the inferior surface of the tongue to the floor of the mouth.

frequency 1. electromagnetic frequencies. The number of cycles per second, now measured in hertz (Hz). A parameter relevant to a number of electrophysical agents. For example, the frequency of ultrasound used therapeutically is usually between 0.8 and 3 MHz, and 1.5 MHz for fracture healing. For a twitch response to electrical stimulation (e.g. for strength duration testing), a frequency of 1 Hz is ideal. For a tetanic contraction (a fused response of individual motor units) a frequency of 30–50 Hz is required, depending on the muscle. Torque increases as the frequency of pulsed current is increased, peaks soon after 50 Hz and does not increase much after about 70 Hz. A carrier frequency is a frequency of alternating current pulses. ⮌ Russian current. **2.** the voiding of urine more often than is acceptable to the person, usually more often that previously experienced and in smaller volumes. **3.** the number of repetitions in a set time, e.g. respirations in 1 minute.

frequency distribution in statistics, the number of times (frequency) each value in a variable is observed.

frequency doubling perimetry (FDP) a method of testing the visual field based on the frequency doubling illusion and thus assessing the functional integrity of the large-diameter retinal ganglion M cells which are very susceptible to early glaucomatous damage. ⮌ open-angle glaucoma.

Fresnel's bi-prism (A Fresnel, French physicist, 1788–1827) an optical device consisting of two prisms of very small refracting power, set base to base and which forms two images of a single source. It is often used to produce interference fringes, double prism. ⮌ double prism test, interference fringes.

Fresnel's formula (A Fresnel) a formula used to determine the proportion of light lost by reflection at the interface between two transparent media. For example: the reflection from the two surfaces of a glass lens made of crown (n = 1.523) is equal to 8.6%. ⮌ high index lens, ghost image, reflection factor, refractive index, surface reflection.

Fresnel zone (A Fresnel) also called the near field. The area closest to the head of an ultrasound transducer. It is irregular in intensity but is generally the area which produces images with the best resolution, and the most beneficial therapeutic effects.

Freud, Sigmund (Austrian neurologist, 1856–1939) the originator of psychoanalysis and the psychoanalytical theory of the causation of neuroses. He first described the existence of the unconscious mind, censor, repression and the theory of infantile sexuality, and worked out in detail many mental mechanisms of the unconscious which modify normal, and account for abnormal, human behaviour.

Frey's syndrome (L Frey, Polish physician, 1889–1942) condition sometimes occurring as a sequel to operations involving the parotid salivary gland. Characterized by sweating and redness of the cheeks in the area of distribution of the auriculotemporal nerve on mastication.

E
F

friable *adj* easily crumbled; readily pulverized.

Fricke dosimeter a chemical dosimeter containing a solution of ferrous sulphate in sulphuric acid; when the chemical is irradiated ferric sulphate is produced. The quantity produced is assessed by measuring the optical density before and after irradiation.

friction *n* **1.** the force between the surfaces of two objects in contact, at least one of which is moving (or tending to move) relative to the other. *kinetic friction* friction due to motion of one object relative to another; also known as *dynamic friction*. The *coefficient of friction* is a dimensionless (no units) number representing friction between two bodies or objects. Calculated as the force parallel to the object or surface (tangential force) divided by the force perpendicular to the object or surface (normal force). **2.** rubbing. Can cause abrasion of skin, leading to a superficial pressure ulcer; the adhesive property of friction, increased in the presence of moisture, can contribute to a shearing force which can cause a more severe pressure ulcer.

friction murmur/rub heard through the stethoscope when two rough or dry surfaces rub together, as in pleurisy and pericarditis. ⊃ pleural rub.

frictions *npl* small, accurately localized, penetrating massage manipulations using the pads of the fingers and thumb. Used in a circular direction on connective tissue and muscle, or transversely across tendons, to mobilize tissues, for example to maintain and restore mobility of tissues at risk of developing adhesions following strain or injury.

Friedman's curve a curved line on pre-printed partograms which indicates the expected progress of labour (by medical definitions). If the woman's progress does not parallel the curve and deviates to the right by more than 2 hours, augmentation of labour may be offered.

Friedreich's ataxia (N Friedreich, German physician, 1825–1882) a recessively inherited progressive disease of childhood, in which there is sclerosis of the sensory and motor columns in the spinal cord, with consequent muscular weakness and staggering (ataxia). The heart may also be affected.

FRIEND test a subjective test for simultaneous binocular vision in which the word FRIEND printed with the letters FIN in green and RED in red is viewed through red and green filters, one before each eye. People with simultaneous binocular vision see all the letters, whereas those with suppression see only some of the letters. ⊃ suppression, Worth's four dot test.

frigidity *n* absence of normal sexual desire.

Frisby's stereotest (*syn* Frisby test) a stereoacuity test consisting of a square transparent plate on which four similar patterns (resembling a random-dot stereogram) are printed on one side. In the central part of one of the four patterns is a circular area which is printed on the other side of the plate and can appear in depth. The plate (made of plastic or glass) comes in three thicknesses: 6, 3 and 1 mm. By using the three plates and presenting them at different distances the test can produce a retinal disparity of the

circular area between 600 and 7 seconds of arc. In this test the patient's head must be kept still to avoid monocular cues. The plate can be turned upside down or rotated to alter the position of the pattern with relief. ⊃ random-dot stereogram.

Frisby test ⊃ Frisby's stereotest.

frit the material from which dental porcelain is made. It consists of partially or completely fused hot porcelain which is plunged into cold water. The mass cracks and fractures and is then pulverized into the correct grade of particle and packaged as dental porcelain.

frog plaster conservative treatment of developmental dysplasia of the hip (congenital dislocation of the hip), whereby the dislocation is reduced by gentle manipulation and both hips are immobilized in plaster of Paris, both hips abducted to 80° and externally rotated.

Fröhlich's syndrome (A Fröhlich, Austrian neurologist/pharmacologist, 1871–1953). ⊃ adiposogenital dystrophy.

Froin's syndrome (G Froin, French physician, 1874–1932) characterized by yellow cerebrospinal fluid which has an increased amount of protein.

Froment's sign (J Froment, French physician, 1878–1946) a test for ulnar nerve paralysis. The person grips a piece of paper between the thumb and index finger, the paper is pulled out and if the test is positive the interphalangeal joint of the thumb flexes.

frontal *adj* pertaining to the front of a structure.

frontal bone the cranial bone that forms the forehead and part of the orbital cavities.

frontal lobe the lobe of each cerebral hemisphere that lies under the frontal bone. Contains the primary motor area, the motor speech area and functions in higher mental activities.

frontal plane vertical plane running from head to foot. It divides the body into front and back parts and is at right angles to the median plane. Also called the coronal plane (Figure F.7).

frontal sinus the paranasal air sinus at the inner aspect of each orbital ridge on the frontal bone. ⊃ Colour Section Figure 14.

front pointer used in radiotherapy to indicate the central entry point of the radiation. ⊃ back pointer.

front power ⊃ front vertex power (FVP).

front vertex power (FVP) (*syn* front power) the symbol is F_v. The reciprocal of the front vertex focal length. It is equal to

$$F_v = \frac{n}{SF}$$

where n is the refractive index of the first medium, S is the point on the front surface through which passes the optical axis and F is the first principal focus. ⊃ effective power, equivalent power, vergence, vertex focal length.

frosted lens a lens made translucent by having one or both surfaces smoothed but not polished. ⊃ ground glass, surfacing, translucent.

frostbite *n* freezing of the skin and superficial tissues resulting from exposure to extreme cold. The lesion is

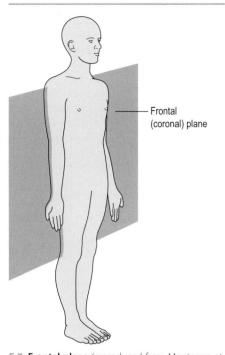

Frontal
(coronal) plane

F.7 Frontal plane (reproduced from Montague et al 2005 with permission).

similar to a burn and may become gangrenous with loss of fingers and toes, and other extremities. ➲ trench foot.

frozen shoulder also known as adhesive capsulitis. A condition of unknown aetiology, which results from shrinkage and scarring of the capsule in a previously normal joint. Symptoms include pain (lasting months) with stiffness, inflammation and significant restriction of movement (lasting months to years), making everyday activities, such as dressing and brushing hair, difficult. Most common in those aged over 50 years and may result from injury or be associated with a number of conditions, e.g. heart disease, thyroid disease or diabetes. Treatment includes adequate pain control and as pain subsides the introduction of a daily exercise programme, which is gradually intensified until full recovery is gained. Intra-articular corticosteroid injections and manipulation under anaesthetic are sometimes required.

fructan ➲ extracellular polysaccharide.

fructo-oligosaccharide a short chain of less than 10 fructose units.

fructosan general term for polysaccharides comprising fructose units, such as inulin.

fructose *n* (*syn* laevulose) fruit sugar, a monosaccharide found in some fruit and vegetables and in honey. Fructose is the sweetest of simple sugars. Some fructose is absorbed directly into the blood from the small intestine and the liver converts it to glucose; for this reason it is now being added to some energy drinks to provide a greater rate of carbohydrate uptake than can be achieved with glucose. Fructose can be converted to glycogen in the body, without the presence of insulin. Sucrose (beet or cane sugar) in the diet is digested to one molecule of fructose and one of glucose.

fructosuria presence of fructose in the urine. Caused by an enzyme deficiency.

fruitarian an extremely restrictive diet whereby the person will only eat fruit, nuts and seeds.

FSA *abbr* Food Standards Agency.

FSD *abbr* focus to skin distance.

FSH *abbr* **1.** facioscapulohumeral muscular dystrophy. **2.** follicle stimulating hormone.

FTA-Abs *abbr* fluorescent treponemal antibody absorbed test.

Fuchs' corneal endothelial dystrophy (E Fuchs, Austrian ophthalmologist, 1851–1930) an inherited degenerative condition of the eye characterized by progressive dystrophy of the corneal endothelium. It occurs more commonly in women than in men, usually in the fifth decade of life. It may be transmitted as an autosomal dominant trait. It is characterized by wart-like deposits on the endothelial surface. As the condition progresses there is oedema of the stroma and eventually of the epithelium and bullous keratopathy causing blurring of vision and pain. The stroma may also become vascularized. It is often associated with glaucoma and nuclear lens opacity. Treatment includes hypertonic agents (e.g. sodium chloride 5%), a bandage soft contact lens and in severe cases penetrating keratoplasty. ➲ bullous keratopathy, cornea guttata, keratoplasty.

Fuchs' crypts (E Fuchs) the pit-like depressions found near the collarette of the iris. ➲ collarette.

Fuchs' heterochromic cyclitis (E Fuchs) a disorder of the eye with the lighter coloured iris. There is uveitis of the lighter coloured iris, iridocyclitis and keratitic precipitates. Often there is cataract formation.

Fuchs' spot (E Fuchs) (*syn* Forster–Fuchs spot) a round or elliptical, pigmented spot, usually located in the macular or paramacular area. It occurs in patients who have pathological myopia. It is due to breaks in Bruch's membrane (called lacquer cracks) and to the development of a choroidal neovascular membrane followed by subretinal haemorrhage which has changed colour and has become pigmented. The patient may notice photopsia when the membrane breaks but eventually it causes a loss of vision with a central scotoma. ➲ photopsia.

Fuchs' spur (E Fuchs) a few fibres located about midway along the length of the sphincter muscle which join with a few fibres of the dilator muscle of the iris.

-fuge a suffix that means 'expelling', e.g. *taeniafuge*.

Fugel-Meyer (FM) an assessment used after a cerebrovascular accident (stroke) to assess sensorimotor recovery. It includes assessment of balance, sensation, pain, joint function and motor recovery. Does not assess fine or complex movement.

fugue state an apparently purposeful journey takes place with associated loss of memory. The behaviour of the person involved may appear normal or unspectacular to the casual observer. Occurs in dissociative disorder or postictally in some forms of epilepsy.

E
F

fulcrum the axis or pivot about which a lever system rotates (or could rotate).

Fulfield applicator a secondary beam collimator with lead-lined sides which form a cone and a 3-mm thick Perspex end.

fulgurate to flash as lightning. To destroy tissue by high-frequency electrical currents.

fulguration *n* destruction of tissue by diathermy.

full denture a complete denture. ➲ denture.

full mouth disinfection treatment method for periodontal diseases that involves the conventional removal of tooth surface deposits by scaling and root planing over 2 visits, usually within 24 hours. Various chlorhexidine preparations are also used to help eliminate oral pathogens from periodontal pockets and other 'infected' sites in the mouth such as the palatine tonsils and surface of the tongue. The aim is to reduce the likelihood of reinfection.

full-mouth radiological survey the complete radiographic examination of the teeth and surrounding bone, in which the film is positioned periapically in each tooth area. Normally consists of 10 films. Now superseded by panoramic techniques which subject the patient to less radiation and are usually extraoral.

full-mouth rehabilitation or full-mouth reconstruction the treatment intended to restore the integrity of the dental arches by the use of directly applied composite restorations, inlays, crowns, bridges, precision-attached prostheses, implants or partial prostheses.

full-term *adj* mature—describes a pregnancy that has lasted 40 weeks.

full-thickness flap a flap of mucosal tissue, including the periosteum, reflected from bone.

full-thickness graft (Wolfe) graft a free graft of the full thickness of skin removed from one part of the body and sutured in another part to repair a defect. ➲ skin graft.

full veneer crown a dental extracoronal restoration which covers the entire clinical crown of a tooth.

full-wave rectification ➲ rectified.

fulminant *adj* developing quickly and with an equally rapid termination.

fume cupboard in radiology, a cupboard with an external exhaust system to enable the handling of radioactive materials to prevent inhalation or ingestion of the dust or gaseous products.

fumigation *n* disinfection using the fumes of a vaporized disinfectant.

functio laesa loss of function; a fifth symptom/sign of inflammation added to the original four, i.e. rubor (redness), tumor (swelling), calor (heat/warmth) and dolor (pain).

function 1. the ability to adapt consistently and competently to the demands of any normal situation in any normal environment. **2.** describes the specific work done by a structure or organ in its normal state.

function (occupational therapy) 1. the underlying physical and psychological components that support occupational performance. (Reproduced with permission from the European Network of Occupational Therapy in Higher Education (ENOTHE) Terminology Project, 2008.) **2.** the capacity to use occupational performance components to carry out a task, activity or occupation. (Reproduced with permission from the European Network of Occupational Therapy in Higher Education (ENOTHE) Terminology Project, 2008.)

functional *adj* **1.** relating to function. **2.** of a disorder, of the function but not the structure of an organ. **3.** as a psychiatric term, describes a condition without primary organic disease.

functional appliance ➲ myofunctional appliance.

functional articulation the tooth contacts occurring between the maxillary and mandibular teeth during mastication and deglutition.

functional assessment the process of collecting and interpreting information about how the individual manages her/his normal range of occupations and daily life activities. Functional assessment enables the therapist and client to identify the client's main problem areas, strengths and resources.

Functional Assessment Measure (FAM) an outcome measure mainly used by teams working in rehabilitation. This was a further development from the Functional Independence Measure (FIM), and includes cognitive and speech items, and so is particularly useful for neurological patients. Each item has seven levels. With training and using the decision-tree manuals it has good reliability and so is used widely both clinically and for research studies. ➲ Functional Independence Measure.

functional bracing (cast bracing) functional braces have hinges to allow movement. The soft tissues of the limb squeeze against the inside of the brace and in conjunction with the use of a heel cup, permit weight to be taken through the substance of the brace. This has reduced many of the problems that were seen as a direct result of prolonged immobilization. Another benefit of allowing movement of joints, provided that it does not unduly stress the fracture site, is that it may promote union by improving the area's blood supply.

functional electrical stimulation (FES) functional electrical stimulation (FES) is a specific type of neuromuscular electrical stimulation (NMES) in which the aim is to enhance function rather than just muscle contraction. It has been argued that FES should be considered as a subgroup within NMES. Simple forms of FES include electrical stimulation of the ankle dorsiflexors following stroke or other central nervous system lesions. The stimulation is activated by some form of foot switch device located in the shoe. This enables the timely stimulation of the dorsiflexors, raising the toes and preventing a trailing foot during the swing phase and promoting a better heel strike (drop foot stimulators). More complex forms of FES include the standing and walking systems used for patients with more severe neurological deficits, such as people with paraplegia. These systems are usually multichannel stimulators, computer controlled and, in the more advanced systems, using implanted electrodes.

By stimulating numerous muscle groups in a carefully timed sequence, a pattern of stimulation can be achieved that mimics a functional activity, e.g. sit-to-stand or basic gait patterns. Recent advances in the computer control systems required to manage complex stimulation patterns together with significant advances in implanted electrode technology has moved these complex applications forward and they are becoming more widely used in specialist centres.

functional endoscopic sinus surgery (FESS) minimally invasive sinus surgery using a fine nasal endoscope.

functional equivalence the hypothesis that mental imagery functions in the same way as the physical perception. Thus, for example, if asked to scan between different objects within a mental image, it takes people longer to scan between objects close together than between objects further apart, just as it would if they were scanning between real objects in perception.

functional exercise in sports medicine the activity(ies) that mimic the stresses, demands and skills of a particular sport.

functional foods foods that have a high level of a nutrient, e.g. omega-3 fatty acids, or non-nutrients, which may confer health benefits if included in the diet.

functional impression ➲ impression.

functional incontinence erratic and involuntary urinary incontinence in the absence of physical problems in bladder, urethra or nervous system. It may be due to immobility or cognitive defects. ➲ incontinence,

Functional Independence Measure (FIM) a widely used outcome measure used in the multidisciplinary team for assessing a person's ability to function independently. The 18-item scale is used in rehabilitation settings, for example following a stroke, brain injury, spinal injury or after limb amputation. There is a paediatric version called the WeeFIM. More items have been developed leading to the Functional Assessment Measure (FAM) assessment, which is often preferred by teams treating neurological patients, as it has cognitive and speech items. ➲ Functional Assessment Measure.

functional limitations the inability to perform functional tasks.

functionally generated occlusal path the movement made by opposing cusp or cusps from centric occlusion to a number of eccentric positions.

functional magnetic resonance imaging (FMRI) A scanning technique, which can illustrate brain activity during functioning.

functional reach (FR) test a measure used to assess dynamic postural control, it is used clinically as a performance test to assess the postural responses to the patient reaching forwards. It is essential that the procedure be properly standardized for the data to be reliable. Mainly used in assessing neurological patients and patients with balance problems.

functional record ➲ record.

functional residual capacity (FRC) the volume of air remaining in the lungs following a normal expiration.

functional tests in sports medicine the assessment of the athlete's ability to move a body part actively, passively and against resistance. Also encompasses the normal activity of the internal and sensory organs.

functional tests (sport-specific) the use of activities and motions that closely represent the athlete's sport and position to assess a body part's readiness to return to competition.

fundal pertaining to the fundus of a structure or organ, e.g. of the uterus.

fundal dominance normal uterine contractions originate from a pacemaker in the fundus, the wave of contraction gradually weakening as it passes over the upper and lower segments of the uterus.

fundal pressure rarely used method of using the contracted fundus uteri as a piston to expel the placenta and complete the third stage of labour.

fundamental colours ➲ primary colours.

fundoplication *n* surgical folding of the gastric fundus to prevent reflux of gastric contents into the oesophagus. ➲ gastro-oesophageal reflux disease (GORD).

fundoscopy *n* examination of the fundus of the eye ➲ ophthalmoscope.

fundus *n* **1.** the basal portion of a hollow structure; the part which is distal to the opening, e.g. the uterine fundus. **2.** in anatomy, the inner surface of the eye (as viewed through the pupil using an ophthalmoscope) (Figure F.8) consisting of the retina, the retinal blood vessels and even sometimes the choroidal vessels when there is little pigment in the pigment epithelium (e.g. in people with albinism), the foveal depression, and the optic disc. The fundus appears red, owing mainly to the choroidal blood supply. The colour is lighter in fair skinned people than in darker skinned people and is dependent upon the amount of pigment in the pigment epithelium and in the choroid—**fundi** *pl*, **fundal** *adj*. ➲ fundus camera, melanin, ophthalmoscope, retina.

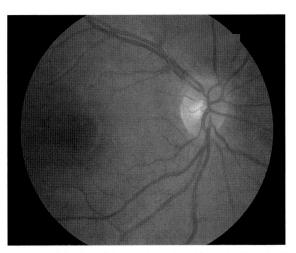

F.8 Normal fundus of the eye (reproduced from Kanski 1999 with permission).

fundus camera a camera attached to an indirect ophthalmo-scope aimed at photographing the image of the fundus of the eye. This image is produced by the objective of the ophthalmoscope at the first focal point of the objective of the viewing microscope (and of the camera) which forms an image on the film. A flip mirror within the optical path of the viewing microscope allows the observer to view the image of the fundus and focus it, thus ensuring that the image being photographed is as clear as that being viewed. Fundus cameras usually require a dilated pupil of about 4 mm and their fields of view extend up to 45°. They provide an objective photographic record of any condition in the fundus. They can also be used to take photographs of the anterior segment of the eye. ⊃ fundus, indirect ophthalmoscope, scanning laser ophthalmoscope.

fungi *npl* simple plants. Mycophyta, including mushrooms, yeasts, moulds and rusts, many of which cause superficial and systemic disease in humans, such as actinomycosis, aspergillosis, candidiasis and tinea—**fungus** *sing*, **fungal** *adj*.

fungicide *n* an agent that kills fungi—**fungicidal** *adj*. ⊃ antifungal.

fungiform *adj* resembling a mushroom, like the fungiform papillae of the tongue.

fungistatic *adj* describes an agent which inhibits the growth of fungi.

fungoid *adj* similar to a fungus in appearance, such as some cancers.

funic *adj* pertaining to the umbilical cord. *funic souffle* ⊃ souffle

funiculitis inflammation of a cord, including the spermatic cord.

funiculus *n* a cord-like structure.

funipuncture ⊃ cordocentesis.

funis umbilical cord.

funnel chest ⊃ pectus excavatum.

funnel pelvis a pelvis which narrows from above downwards, e.g. an android pelvis in which the outlet is smaller than the brim.

furcation an anatomical area where the root of a multirooted tooth divides. Known as a *bifurcation* in two-rooted teeth and *trifurcation* in three-rooted teeth. *furcation involvement* pathological condition involving the alveolar bone in the furcation of a multirooted tooth. *furcation tunnel procedure* a periodontal procedure where a mandibular molar, with bifurcation involvement and a wide U-shaped arch between the roots, is treated surgically by osteoplasty and odontoplasty in order to allow cleaning of the post-surgical site with an interdental brush. The horizontal furcation involvement may be classified as *grade I*, where there is incipient involvement in which the opening of the furcation is exposed with horizontal involvement of less than 1/3 the width of the tooth. *Grade II*, where the involvement extends beyond 1/3 the width of the tooth and *Grade III*, where there is a through-and-through involvement.

furnace a high temperature oven used in dentistry for firing ceramics, and in the preparation of an inlay pattern for casting. **1.** to produce a smooth, shiny surface on porcelain or composite filling materials. **2.** resinous material applied to the surface of a composite resin filling, to enhance its surface finish.

furuncle *n* a boil originating in a hair follicle. ⊃ boil.

furunculosis *n* an affliction due to boils.

fuscin a pigment present in granules in the pigment epithelium of the retina consisting of residual bodies ingested by lysosomes and sometimes fused with melanin granules. The residual bodies are thought to be mainly the undigested elements of disc membrane phagocytosis. In people with albinism the pigment granules are immature and colourless. ⊃ albinism, cone, melanin, retinal pigment epithelium, rod.

fusible able to be melted.

fusiform *adj* resembling a spindle with tapering ends.

fusiform aneurysm localized dilatation of an artery in which the circumference of the vessel is dilated. (Figure A.9, p. 42).

fusion area ⊃ Panum's area.

fusion field an area around the fovea of each eye within which the fusion reflex is initiated. If the disparate images fall within this area motor fusion will occur, but if the disparity is too great there will be no fusional movement. This field is much larger horizontally than vertically.

fusional convergence that component of convergence which is induced by fusional stimuli or which is available in excess of that required to overcome the heterophoria. It is usually a *positive fusional convergence*, but in some cases the eyes need to diverge to obtain fusion and this is called *negative fusional convergence*. An example is the movement of the eyes from the passive (one eye covered, the other fixating an object) to the active (both eyes fixating foveally the same object) position. However, as disparate retinal stimuli are a more powerful component of convergence than fusion, the concept of fusional convergence is being substituted by motor fusion (or disparity vergence). ⊃ accommodative convergence, initial convergence, motor fusion, orthopic fusion, proximal convergence, tonic vergence, vergence facility.

fusion reflex ⊃ motor fusion.

FVC *abbr* forced vital capacity.

FVP *abbr* front vertex power.

F v. West Berkshire Health Authority (1989) a professional who acts in the best interests of an incompetent person (incapable of giving consent) does not act unlawfully if he/she follows the accepted standard of care according to the Bolam test.

G

GABA *abbr* gamma aminobutyric acid.

gag *n* **1.** retching without vomiting. **2.** an instrument used to keep the mouth open.

gag reflex also known as pharyngeal reflex. The reflex causing contraction of the pharyngeal muscles and elevation of the palate to protect the airway when the soft palate or posterior pharynx is stimulated. An impaired gag reflex is a feature of many neurological diseases and is associated with dysphagia.

gain (swept gain) the amount of sound received back by an ultrasonic transducer, increasing the gain visualizes the organs further away from the probe.

gain correction a factor used to compensate for the variation in electrical signal for an absorbed intensity of radiation between detector channels in computed tomography (CT) scanning.

Gairdner headbox perspex box placed in the cot and over the infant's head into which a controlled amount of additional oxygen is provided in order to increase the oxygen concentration of inspired air.

gait *n* a manner or style of walking. A pattern of locomotion. Typically gait is divided into the following stages: (a) loading response: the initial double support stance; (b) midstance: from the time the opposite limb leaves the floor until body weight is aligned over the forefoot; (c) terminal stance: the time from heel rise until the other limb makes contact with the floor. During this phase body weight moves ahead of the forefoot; (d) pre-swing: from the time of initial contact with the contralateral limb to ipsilateral toe-off; (e) initial swing: from toe-off to when the swing limb foot is opposite the stance limb; (f) mid-swing: from the time the swing foot is opposite the stance limb to when the tibia is vertical; (g) terminal swing: from the time when the tibia is vertical to initial contact; and (h) push off: when there is an ankle plantar flexor moment. ⊃ ataxic gait, cerebellar gait, festinating gait, scissors gait, spastic gait, step length, stride, support, swing, tabetic gait.

galact/a, galact/o- a prefix that means 'milk', e.g. *galactocele*.

galactagogue *n* an agent inducing or increasing the flow of milk.

galactans *npl* polysaccharides. Polymers comprising many galactose units.

galactocele *n* a cyst containing milk, or fluid resembling milk.

galactorrhoea *n* excessive flow of milk. Usually reserved for abnormal or inappropriate secretion of milk.

galactosaemia *n* excess of galactose in the blood and other tissues. Normally the enzyme lactase in the small intestine converts lactose into glucose and galactose. In the liver another enzyme system converts galactose into glucose. Galactosaemia is an inherited autosomal recessive condition that results from a deficiency of the enzyme galactose-1-phosphate uridyltransferase. The infant has diarrhoea, vomiting, anorexia and fails to gain weight. There is hepatomegaly, cataract formation, and learning disability if diagnosis and treatment is delayed. Management centres on excluding lactose and galatose from the diet. Female carriers of the mutant gene should also exclude these substances from their diet during pregnancy. A milder form of the condition exists where individuals produce some of the enzyme, and may not experience ill effects—**galactosaemic** *adj*.

galactose *n* a monosaccharide that is produced by the digestion of the disaccharide lactose found in milk. ⊃ galactosaemia.

galactosuria the presence of galactose in the urine.

Galant reflex induced sideways flexion of the neonate's hips in the direction of contact when the lower back is stroked.

Galeazzi's fracture-dislocation (R Galeazzi, Italian surgeon, 1866–1952) a fracture of the distal radius and subluxation of the distal radioulnar joint.

gall *n* bile.

gallbladder *n* a pear-shaped, muscular sac/bag on the undersurface of the liver (see Figure B.5, p. 90). It concentrates and stores bile. ⊃ Colour Section Figure 18b.

gallipot *n* a small vessel for solutions and lotions.

gallium (Ga) a metallic element. Many gallium compounds are toxic.

gallium scan a radioactive isotope of gallium may be administered intravenously in a total body scan to detect metastatic spread, lymphomas, or a focus of infection.

gallop rhythm a heart rhythm with a third or fourth heart sound.

gallows traction ⊃ Bryant's 'gallows' traction.

gallstones *npl* concretions formed within the gallbladder or bile ducts; they are often multiple and faceted. They may contain cholesterol, bile pigments or both in varying proportions.

galvanic current an electrotherapy term. It is an old name for direct current, still often used by some electromedical manufacturers. Also have interrupted galvanic—unidirectional pulses that may be rectangular, trapezoidal, triangular, etc., in shape, with durations ranging from approximately 10 µs to 600 ms, a frequency of 1–1.5 Hz and used for strength-duration testing. ⊃ direct current.

galvanism in dentistry, the electrical effect produced when two dissimilar metals contact one another in the mouth. Most noticeable when a newly completed amalgam restoration contacts a gold restoration.

galvanometer *n* an instrument for measuring an electrical current.

Gamblers Anonymous an organization for compulsive gamblers.

gamekeeper's thumb (*syn* skier's thumb) a colloquial expression used in sports medicine to describe force abduction of the metacarpophalangeal joint whilst the thumb is extended, leading to rupture of the ulnar collateral ligament.

gamesmanship in sport, the use of unfair tactics or methods, which are not strictly against the rules of the sport, in order to obtain an advantage over one's opponent(s), such as feigning injury or engaging in other time-wasting strategies in order to delay the game.

gamete *n* a female or male reproductive cell with the haploid (n) chromosome number; oocyte or spermatozoon.

gamete intrafallopian tube transfer (GIFT) a technique used in assisted conception for couples where the woman has at least one patent uterine (fallopian) tube. The oocyte and sperm are placed in the uterine tube laparoscopically. Fertilization occurs as normal within the uterine tube and the ovum subsequently implants in the lining of the uterus.

gametogenesis *n* production of gametes (oocytes and spermatozoa) within the gonads (ovaries or testes). ⊃ oogenesis, spermatogenesis.

gamma in radiography, the measure of the slope of a characteristic curve, the higher the gamma the higher the contrast on the radiographic film. ⊃ average gradient, sensitometry.

gamma-aminobutyric acid (GABA) an inhibitory neurotransmitter present in the central nervous system.

gamma camera a large, stationary, scintillation counter, which records the activity over the whole field at the same time. It detects concentrations of gamma radiation in body locations following the introduction of a radionuclide (radioisotope) into the body. The device contains a crystal (the scintillator) in which scintillation events convert gamma rays to light. Used to detect pathologies where the physiology of the structure is changed. The image is viewed on a cathode ray tube

gamma-carboxyglutamate *n* a substance synthesized in the liver from the amino acid glutamic acid (glutamate) in reactions requiring vitamin K. It is an important component of proteins, e.g. osteocalcin, present in the bone matrix, and in blood coagulation factors, such as prothrombin.

gamma decay the emission of gamma rays from a nucleus which has excess energy.

gamma encephalography a small dose of a radioactive isotope (radionuclide) is given, which is concentrated in many cerebral tumours. The pattern of radioactivity is then measured.

gamma globulins *pl* a group of plasma proteins that have antibody activity, referred to as immunoglobulins (IgA, IgD, IgE, IgG and IgM). They are responsible for the humoral aspects of immunity.

gamma-glutamyltransferase (GGT, gamma-GT, γ-GT) an enzyme. Increased levels in the plasma reflect liver cell dysfunction, which may be indicative of liver and or biliary disease, but the level may be affected by the intake of alcohol and by some drugs.

gamma knife a method of treating tumours that are difficult to excise surgically by using multiple beams of radiation, focused at the tumour over a number of days.

gamma (γ)-linolenic acid (GLA) a polyunsaturated fatty acid ⊃ linolenic acids.

gamma (motor) system the component of the motor nerve outflow from the spinal cord which innervates intrafusal muscle fibres (the fibres within muscle spindles). The gamma (γ) motor neurons have smaller cell bodies and narrower-diameter axons than alpha (α) motor neurons, which innervate the main working fibres of the muscle (extrafusal fibres). ⊃ alpha (α) motor neurons, intrafusal fibres, muscle spindles.

gamma (γ) rays short wavelength, penetrating rays of the electromagnetic spectrum produced by disintegration of the atomic nuclei of radioactive elements. Used commercially to sterilize such single-use items as sutures, injection needles, scalpel blades and local analgesic cartridges.

ganglion *n* **1.** a small mass of nerve cell bodies in the peripheral nervous system, where synaptic connections relay afferent or efferent nerve impulses. *dorsal root ganglia* contain the cell bodies of sensory neurons, providing relay into the spinal cord, and there are equivalent afferent relays to the brainstem for sensory components of cranial nerves. *autonomic ganglia* provide efferent relay from nerve fibres from the central nervous system to the sympathetic and parasympathetic neurons that innervate relevant tissues throughout the body. ⊃ gasserian or trigeminal ganglion, otic ganglion, sphenopalatine ganglion, submandibular ganglion. **2.** localized cyst-like swelling near a tendon, sheath or joint, especially around the wrist. Sometimes occurs on the back of the wrist due to strain such as excessive use of a word processor keyboard. A ganglion is usually painless but they can increase in size to become tender, unsightly or large enough to restrict movement; treatment is not usually required but they can be surgically removed if troublesome—**ganglia** *pl*, **ganglionic** *adj*.

ganglion cell a retinal cell which connects the bipolar and other cells in the inner plexiform layer with the lateral geniculate body. The axons of the ganglion cells constitute the optic nerve fibres. There are many types of ganglion cells. The two major types are: the magno (or M or parasol) ganglion cells which project mainly to the magnocellular layers of the lateral geniculate bodies; and the parvo (or P or midget) ganglion cells which project to the parvocellular layers. They comprise about 10% and 80% of the retinal ganglion cells respectively.

ganglionectomy *n* surgical excision of a ganglion.

ganglioside a glycosphingolipid present in the brain and elsewhere in the nervous system. They belong to a group of cerebrosides that contain a sugar and have a basic composition of ceramide-glucose-galactose-*N*-acetylneuraminic acid. Important as a component of the cell membrane.

gangliosidosis ⊃ Tay–Sachs disease.

gangrene *n* death of part of the tissues of the body. Usually the results of inadequate blood supply, but occasionally due to direct injury (traumatic gangrene) or infection (e.g. gas gangrene caused by species of *Clostridium*). Deficient blood supply may result from pressure on blood vessels (e.g. tourniquets, tight bandages and swelling of a limb); from obstruction within healthy blood vessels (e.g. arterial embolism, frostbite where the capillaries become blocked); from spasm of the vessel wall (e.g. ergot poisoning); or from thrombosis due to disease of the vessel wall (e.g. arteriosclerosis in arteries, phlebitis in veins)—**gangrenous** *adj.* ⊃ dry gangrene, gas gangrene, moist gangrene.

gangrenous stomatitis ⊃ cancrum oris.

Ganser's syndrome (S Ganser, German psychiatrist, 1853–1931) a rare dissociative disorder characterized by 'approximate answers' to questions, disorientation/changes in consciousness, amnesia and pseudohallucinations. Sometimes associated with head injury.

gantry a structure or support, in computed tomography (CT) scanning a structure in which the X-ray tube, detectors and associated electronics are housed.

Gantt chart a project-planning tool. The anticipated timing of specific tasks within a project are identified. Project stages comprise the vertical column, dates run from left to right and each task is represented by a horizontal bar, the left end of which signifies the expected beginning of the task and the right end the planned completion date.

gap junction a junction between cells that contains pores or channels that allow the passage of ions and molecules, e.g. sugars, vitamins, amino acids, hormones. The passage of ions is particularly important in excitable tissues, such as the myocardium. ⊃ tight junction.

Garden classification a four part classification of fractures of the femoral neck. Type 1—inferior cortex not completely fractured; type 2—cortex fractured but without angulation; type 3—a degree of displacement and rotation of the femoral head; and type 4—complete displacement (Figure G.1). It is used to classify the severity of the fracture and to guide management.

Gardnerella vaginalis (F Gardner, American bacteriologist, b. 1919) a bacterium normally present in the vagina, but is found in increased concentrations in bacterial vaginosis. ⊃ bacterial vaginosis.

Gardner's syndrome (E Gardner, American physician, geneticist, 1909–1989) a type of familial adenomatous polyposis that affects the large bowel. Associated abnormalities include epidermal cysts, fibromas and osteomas.

gargle *n*, *vi* a solution used for washing the throat; to wash the throat.

gargoylism *n* mucopolysaccharidoses. A congenital disorder of mucopolysaccharide metabolism with either autosomal recessive or sex-linked inheritance. The polysaccarides chondroitin sulphate 'B' and heparitin sulphate are excreted in the urine. Characterized by skeletal abnormalities, coarse features, enlarged liver and spleen and a learning disability. ⊃ Hunter's syndrome, Hurler's syndrome.

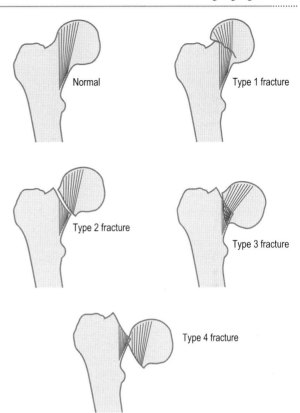

G.1 **Garden classification** (reproduced from Porter 2005 with permission).

garnet an abrasive powder composed of a crystalline silicate mineral. Used in dentistry, as a polishing material when bedded on rotary, plastic and card-board discs.

Garré's osteomyelitis (C Garré, Swiss surgeon, 1857–1928) a rare chronic, low-grade sclerosing osteitis or osteomyelitis due to infection. It is characterized by inflammation of the periosteum (periostitis) with thickening.

GAS *acron* general adaptation syndrome.

gas *n* one of the three states of matter, the others being solid and liquid. A gas retains neither shape nor volume when released—**gaseous** *adj.*

gas endarterectomy ⊃ endarterectomy.

gas exchange in the animal kingdom, the uptake of oxygen and excretion of carbon dioxide, exchanged between the body and the environment, also known as respiratory gas exchange. In human physiology pulmonary gas exchange refers to the diffusion of oxygen from the gas phase in the lung alveoli, through the thin alveolar-capillary membrane, into solution in the pulmonary capillary blood, and of carbon dioxide in the opposite direction, both driven by partial pressure gradients.

gas gangrene a serious wound infection caused by anaerobic organisms of the genus *Clostridium*, especially *Clostridium perfringens (welchii)*, a soil microbe often present in the intestine of humans and animals. It may follow traumatic

311

wounds or surgery. The wound is swollen and discoloured with necrotic tissue and there is foul discharge and gas formation. The systemic effects include fever, tachycardia and hypotension with circulatory collapse. Fatal without effective antibiotic and supportive therapy. ⇨ gangrene.

gasserian ganglion also known as the trigeminal or semilunar ganglion. It is deeply situated within the skull, on the sensory root of the trigeminal nerve (fifth cranial nerve), close to the brain on the anterior aspect of the petrous portion of the temporal bone. It is involved in trigeminal neuralgia and in severe cases the sensory nerve is sometimes cut at this point or the ganglion destroyed by injected drugs to obtain pain relief.

gastralgia *n* pain in the stomach.

gas transfer factor measure of the lung's ability to exchange gases. Particularly useful in the diagnosis and surveillance of interstitial lung diseases, sarcoidosis and emphysema.

gastrectasia abnormal dilation of the stomach. The causes include gastric outlet obstruction (GOO) due to pyloric stenosis, following gastrointestinal surgery or overeating. ⇨ acute dilatation of the stomach.

gastrectomy *n* removal of a part or the whole of the stomach. Usually for cancers but may occasionally be used for gastric ulcers that do not respond to drug therapy. *Billroth I gastrectomy* is a partial gastrectomy where the remaining portion of the stomach is anastomosed to the duodenum. *Polya partial gastrectomy* (known in the USA as *Billroth II gastrectomy*) involves removal of part of the stomach and duodenum and anastomosing the remaining part of the stomach to the jejunum. *total gastrectomy* a radical operation that may be performed for cancer in the upper part of the stomach. ⇨ Roux-en-y operation.

gastric *adj* pertaining to the stomach.

gastric aspiration or suction the intermittent or continuous aspiration of gastric contents via a nasogastric tube. It may be used to keep the stomach empty after some gastrointestinal or abdominal operations, when the bowel is obstructed, or to obtain samples.

gastric glands glands in the gastric mucosa containing different cells (chief, parietal [oxyntic]) that secrete pepsinogen (precursor of pepsin), rennin, hydrochloric acid (HCl), the intrinsic factor, water and salts; and mucus from goblet cells. ⇨ chief cells, parietal (oxyntic) cells.

gastric inhibitory peptide (GIP) a regulatory peptide hormone secreted by the small intestine mucosa when fatty acids and glucose are present in the duodenum. It inhibits gastric acid secretion and stimulates insulin secretion.

gastric juice approximately 2 L of acidic (pH 1.5–3) gastric juice are secreted by the gastric glands in the mucosa every day. Apart from hydrochloric acid, gastric juice contains water, protective mucus secreted by goblet cells, mineral salts, inactive enzyme precursors (pepsinogens) for the proteolytic pepsins, rennin (a milk curdling enzyme), which is important in milk-fed infants, and the intrinsic factor needed for the absorption of vitamin B_{12}. There is always a small

quantity of gastric juice present in the stomach, even when it contains no food (known as fasting juice). Secretion reaches its maximum level about 1 hour after a meal then declines to the fasting level after about 4 hours. There are three phases of secretion of gastric juice: (a) the cephalic phase in which a flow of juice occurs before food reaches the stomach and is due to reflex stimulation of the vagus (parasympathetic) nerves initiated by the sight, smell or taste of food; (b) the gastric phase which is stimulated by the presence of food. The enteroendocrine cells in the pyloric antrum and duodenum secrete gastrin, a hormone which passes directly into the circulating blood. Gastrin stimulates the gastric glands to produce more gastric juice. (c) the intestinal phase occurs when the partially digested contents of the stomach reach the small intestine. Two hormones, secretin and cholecystokinin, are produced by endocrine cells in the intestinal mucosa, which slows down the secretion of gastric juice and reduces gastric motility. By slowing the emptying rate of the stomach, the chyme become more thoroughly mixed with bile and pancreatic juice in the duodenum. This phase of gastric secretion is most marked when the meal has had a high fat content.

gastric ulcer a peptic ulcer in the gastric mucosa. The majority are associated with the presence of the bacterium *Helicobacter pylori* in the stomach. Other factors include a genetic predisposition, drugs such as non-steroidal anti-inflammatory drugs (NSAIDs) and smoking. The ulcer can bleed, leading to haematemesis and/or melaena, or it can perforate, constituting an abdominal emergency. Severe scarring following chronic ulceration may produce pyloric stenosis and gastric outlet obstruction (GOO). For management ⇨ duodenal ulcer.

gastrin *n* a local hormone. Polypeptide hormones secreted by special cells in the gastric mucosa of the antrum of the stomach, by fibres of the vagus nerve and to a lesser extent in the duodenum; stimulates the secretion of hydrochloric acid when food enters the stomach.

gastrinoma *n* a gastrin-secreting tumour of the pancreas or duodenum. ⇨ islet cell tumours, Zollinger–Ellison syndrome.

gastritis *n* inflammation of the stomach, such as that caused by an excessive intake of alcohol.

gastr/o- a prefix that means 'stomach', e.g. *gastritis*.

gastrocele *n* a hernia of the stomach.

gastrocnemius *n* the large two-headed superficial muscle of the calf. It has two origins, one on each femoral condyle, which join to form the inferior border of the popliteal fossa behind the knee. Together with its smaller accessory, the plantaris, and the soleus muscle (arising from the shaft of the tibia), it converges onto the Achilles (calcaneal) tendon, to be inserted into the back of the calcaneus (calcaneum) (see Figure A.1, p. 8). It acts to plantarflex the foot and raise the heel when walking. The gastrocnemius and plantaris also act as weak flexors at the knee. ⇨ Colour Section Figures 4, 5.

gastrocolic *adj* pertaining to the stomach and the colon.

gastrocolic reflex sensory stimulus arising on entry of food into stomach, resulting in strong peristaltic waves (mass movement) in the colon.

gastroduodenal *adj* pertaining to the stomach and the duodenum.

gastroduodenoscopy endoscopic examination of the stomach and duodenum.

gastroduodenostomy *n* a surgical anastomosis between the stomach and the duodenum.

gastrodynia *n* pain in the stomach.

gastroenteritis *n* food poisoning. Inflammation of mucous membranes of the stomach and the small intestine; usually due to micro-organisms, but may be caused by chemicals, poisonous fungi, etc. There is vomiting and diarrhoea due to either the multiplication of micro-organisms (invasive intestinal gastroenteritis) ingested in food or from bacterial toxins (intoxication). Microbial causes include: the bacteria *Bacillus cereus*, *Campylobacter jejuni*, *Clostridium perfringens* and *C. botulinum*, *Escherichia coli*, *Salmonella enteritidis*, *Staphylococcus aureus*, or viruses such as Norovirus (Norwalk-like virus), or rotavirus a common cause of gastroenteritis in infants. Gastroenteritis is generally transmitted by the faecal–oral route, either directly or indirectly. However, droplet spread is a feature of some viruses.

gastroenterology *n* study of the digestive tract, including the liver, biliary tract and pancreas and the associated diseases—**gastroenterological** *adj*, **gastroenterologically** *adv*.

gastroenteropathy *n* disease of the stomach and intestine—**gastroenteropathic** *adj*.

gastroenteroscope *n* an endoscope for visualization of stomach and intestine—**gastroenteroscopic** *adj*, **gastroenteroscopically** *adv*.

gastroenterostomy *n* a surgical anastomosis between the stomach and small intestine.

gastrointestinal *adj* pertaining to the stomach and intestine.

gastrojejunostomy *n* a surgical anastomosis between the stomach and the jejunum.

gastrolith *n* a solid 'stone' in the stomach, which forms around a mass of hair or vegetable matter. ⊃ bezoar.

gastro-oesophageal *adj* pertaining to the stomach and oesophagus.

gastro-oesophageal reflux disease (GORD) a condition caused by a malfunctioning lower oesophageal sphincter (gastro-oesophageal [cardiac] sphincter) which allows the acidic gastric contents to move into the oesophagus. This results in pain ('heartburn'), vomiting and potential complications that include oesophagitis, ulceration, scarring with stricture formation and Barrett's oesophagus. There is also the risk of aspiration pneumonia and dental erosion, particularly of the palatal aspects of the upper teeth. Reflux is associated with factors that include: gastric distension, increased abdominal pressure, e.g. during coughing, central nervous system disease, hiatus hernia, delayed gastric emptying and the presence of a gastrostomy. A fairly common condition in children, those at increased risk include children with asthma, cystic fibrosis, neurological conditions, or previous oesophageal surgery. Conservative treatment includes small frequent, thickened feeds for infants and frequent small meals for children and adults, sitting up after eating and elevating the head of the bed/cot at night. H_2-receptor antagonist drugs that reduce gastric acid, e.g. ranitidine, may be prescribed. Surgical treatment, such as a fundoplication, may be necessary if conservative measures fail, or if complications occur.

gastro-oesophageal sphincter the lower oesophageal sphincter, also known as the cardiac sphincter. A physiological sphincter that prevents the reflux of acidic stomach contents into the oesophagus. ⊃ lower oesophageal sphincter.

gastro-oesophagostomy *n* a surgical operation in which the oesophagus is joined to the stomach to bypass the natural junction.

gastroparesis delayed gastric emptying due to poor motility.

gastropathy *n* any disease of the stomach.

gastropexy *n* surgical fixation of a displaced stomach.

gastrophrenic *adj* pertaining to the stomach and diaphragm.

gastroplasty *n* previously any reconstructive operation on the stomach to repair damage or deformity. More recently it also includes surgical procedures, e.g. gastric banding, which seek to reduce stomach size as a treatment for morbid obesity.

gastroschisis *n* a congenital incomplete closure of the abdominal wall with consequent protrusion of the viscera uncovered by peritoneum.

gastroscope *n* a fibreoptics endoscope used to examine the inside of the stomach. ⊃ endoscope—**gastroscopic** *adj*, **gastroscopy** *n*.

gastrostomy *n* a surgically established fistula between the stomach and the external abdominal wall. A feeding tube is inserted either endoscopically, surgically or radiologically into the stomach. Allows feeding with liquid feeds. ⊃ percutaneous endoscopic gastrostomy.

gastrotomy *n* incision into the stomach during an abdominal operation for such purposes as removing a foreign body, securing a bleeding blood vessel, approaching the oesophagus from below to pull down a tube through a constricting growth.

gastrula *n* the stage following the blastocyst in embryonic development.

gastrulation *n* in early embryonic development the immense changes occurring as the blastocyst becomes the gastrula. The three primary germ layers are formed and cells move to their appointed locations in readiness for the start of structural development.

gate in computing, a gate performs a single logical operation when subjected to a number of inputs. It is the basis of all computer operations.

gate control theory a theory that proposes that there is active processing of pain sensation when it first enters the central nervous system at the dorsal horn of the spinal cord. The 'gate' in the spinal cord is opened or closed by a variety of ascending sensory impulses from the peripheral nerves and the descending impulses from the brain. Pain is reduced when the 'gate' is shut but increases when it is open.

gate-keeping a process whereby resources are rationed by restricting access to equipment or services. For example, general practitioners are the gate-keepers of specialist medical services and physiotherapists may be the gate-keepers of wheelchairs and other equipment.

Gaucher's disease (P Gaucher, French physician, 1854–1918) a rare inherited autosomal recessive disorder, there are three types of which types 1 and 3 mainly affect Jewish children. It is characterized by a disordered fat metabolism (lipid reticulosis) due to an enzyme deficiency, which leads to very marked enlargement of the spleen and liver, involvement of the bones and lymph nodes. Diagnosis follows biopsy of the bone marrow, liver or spleen. Abnormal histiocytes are found in the marrow. In type 2 of the disease the central nervous system is involved and the child has seizures and learning disability.

gauss an electromagnetic unit of magnetic induction now replaced by the tesla (1 tesla = 10 000 gauss).

gaussian optics ➲ paraxial optics.

gaussian points ➲ cardinal points.

gaussian space ➲ paraxial region.

gaussian theory (*syn* first order theory, paraxial theory) the theory that for tracing paraxial rays through an optical system, that system can be considered as having six cardinal planes: two principal planes, two nodal planes and two focal planes. The mathematical analysis can be carried out by the paraxial equation. ➲ Newton's formula, paraxial equation (fundamental), paraxial optics, paraxial ray.

gauze *n* a thin open-meshed absorbent material used in operations to dry the operative field and facilitate the procedure.

gavage *n* feeding liquids by a nasogastric tube directly into the stomach.

GBM *abbr* glomerular basement membrane.

GBS *abbr* Guillain–Barré syndrome

GCA *abbr* giant cell arteritis.

GCS *abbr* Glasgow Coma Scale.

G-CSF *abbr* granulocyte colony-stimulating factor.

GDC *abbr* General Dental Council.

GDP *abbr* general dental practitioner.

GDS *abbr* geriatric depression scale.

GE *abbr* gradient echo.

Geiger–Müller counter *n* (H Geiger, German physicist, 1882–1945; W Müller, German physicist, 20th century) a device for detecting and measuring radiation dosage, it has a glass envelope containing argon, a positively charged central electrode and a negatively charged mesh cylinder.

Geiger–Müller tube *n* (H Geiger) a radiation detector using an ionization chamber, used in personnel dosimetry and to detect the movement of gamma ray sources in brachytherapy.

gel 1. a semisolid or gelatinous colloidal suspension that has set to form a jelly. **2.** the water-soluble substance used to complete a circuit or to couple an output to the skin. Electrical stimulation gel: is used between the electrodes, if flexible reusable carbon rubber type and the skin to complete the circuit. Ultrasound gel enables ultrasound to pass from the applicator to the skin, not otherwise possible given the high acoustic impedance of air to MHz frequency ultrasound. Ultrasound gel is typically cheaper and with a higher resistance than electrical gel (usually labelled ECG gel or electrical stimulation gel) and should not be used as a replacement. **3.** in dentistry, gel containing fluoride used to harden and protect teeth.

gelatin(e) *n* the glue-like substance found in animal connective tissue, used in capsules, suppositories, culture medium and in food preparation. Alternative medicines may be needed for vegans, vegetarians and others who will not accept medicines containing gelatin—**gelatinous** *adj*.

gelatin(e) (in radiography) a complex compound used in the emulsion layer of a radiographic film to allow the absorption of water during chemical processing, keeping the silver halide grains in suspension, during manufacture to allow the grains to grow and bind the emulsion to the base of the film, it assists with forming and stabilizing the image during and after exposure to electromagnetic radiation.

gelatin(e) sponge an absorbable sponge made of gelatin(e) which may be placed in a tooth socket to reduce bleeding and promote clotting.

gelation the process wherein a colloid changes from a sol to a gel.

gelsolin an inhibitory protein released by macrophages. Once activated by calcium ions it breaks actin filaments. This action on the actin structure increases the motility of some types of cells.

gemellology scientific study of twins and twinning.

gemellus muscles a pair of muscles with origins one on the ischial spine and the other on the ischial tuberosity. The insertion is on the greater trochanter of the femur. They stabilize the hip and facilitate lateral rotation of the thigh. ➲ Colour Section Figure 5.

gemination a condition in which twin tooth forms develop from a single bud or follicle. They are rare, have only one pulp chamber and a dividing groove down their centre.

gender *n* more than just biological sex. The term encompasses the socially constructed views of feminine and masculine behaviour within individual cultural groups.

gender identity a person's sense of their biological sex.

gender role the set of behaviours, attitudes and other characteristics normally associated with masculinity and femininity within a given culture or social group; for example, certain sports are stereotypically viewed as reflecting a masculine role (e.g. basketball) whereas others reflect a feminine role (e.g. netball).

gene *n* a hereditary factor consisting of deoxyribonucleic acid (DNA) located at a specific locus of a specific chromosome. Each gene contains information in code that allows the cell to produce (almost always) a specific protein. ➲ dominant, performance genes, recessive.

gene expression all the processes whereby information encoded by a gene is converted to a physical manifestation of the trait, as observable in the phenotype, usually in the form of a protein.

gene therapy the techniques that deliver a normal version of a gene to replace the defective mutant gene, which cause diseases, such as cystic fibrosis. The process which is termed somatic-cell gene therapy aims to treat or cure the condition.

general adaptation syndrome (GAS) proposed by Hans Selye (Austrian/Canadian physician/endocrinologist, 1907–1982). It describes a three phase (triphasic) response of the body to a stressor. Comprising: alarm, resistance/adaptation and exhaustion. The alarm phase is the short-term immediate response involving activation of the sympathetic nervous system. The resistance/adaptation phase involves the activation of the body's defences against the stressor. If the stressor continues and cannot be adapted to, the exhaustion phase ensues in which resistance to the stressor and ability to resist disease collapses.

general anaesthesia loss of sensation with loss of consciousness. ⇨ anaesthetic.

general anaesthetic a drug that produces general anaesthesia by inhalation or injection.

General Dental Council (GDC) the statutory body that regulates the practice of dentistry in the UK. It oversees professional quality and continuing professional development standards for professional practice, discipline and conduct. It is responsible for the establishment and maintenance of a professional register for all dentists, dental therapists, dental hygienists, and from 2008, dental nurses and technicians working in the UK, and has the power to remove individuals from the register.

General Medical Council (GMC) the statutory body that regulates the practice of medicine in the UK. It oversees professional quality and continuing professional development standards for professional practice, discipline and conduct. It is responsible for the establishment and maintenance of a professional register for all doctors working in the UK, and currently has the power to remove individuals from the register in cases of professional misconduct, or in some cases to restrict practice or order specific training.

General Medical Services the medical services provided by family doctors.

general motion ⇨ motion.

general paralysis of the insane (GPI) a manifestation of neurosyphilis in which the brain is principally affected. ⇨ neurosyphilis.

general practice in the UK the services provided by generalist doctors in first contact health care. First defined in 1948 at the inception of the National Health Service. Provides general medical services as opposed to specialist services.

general refraction formula ⇨ paraxial equation (fundamental).

general sales list (GSL) in the UK. Drugs on sale, without prescription, to the public through various retail outlets such as supermarkets. Example include paracetamol, ibuprofen.

generalizability the extent to which research findings from a study of a patient/client group can be valid for another group, or within a different context. For example, can research carried out with a nursing home population be applicable to people living in their own homes or to patients in an acute hospital.

generalization in occupational therapy, the ability of clients to transfer knowledge and skills learned during therapy to a number of similar situations.

generalized anxiety disorder a state characterized by excessive and persistant generalized anxiety and worry. People may feel apprehensive, tense, indecisive and tired with a low mood. There may be physical manifestations such as rapid heart rate, sweating, breathlessness, changes in appetite and insomnia.

generalized motor programme ⇨ motor programme.

generalized seizure ⇨ epilepsy.

generative *adj* pertaining to reproduction.

generic denoting a drug name not protected by brand name or manufacturer. ⇨ Recommended International Non-proprietary Name.

generic descriptor a term that includes the different chemical forms of a vitamin, all with same biological activity.

-genesis a suffix that means 'formation, origin', e.g. *teratogenesis*.

genetic *adj* that which relates to heredity. For example, disorders the basis of which resides in abnormalities of the genetic material, genes and chromosomes. ⇨ congenital.

-genetic a suffix that means 'formation, origin', e.g. *oogenetic*.

genetic code the arrangement of genetic material stored as nucleotides in the DNA molecule (a double-stranded helix) of the chromosome. It is in this coded form that the information contained in the genes is transmitted to individual cells during transcription and translation. Transcription involves the encoding of the nucleotide sequence onto single-strand messenger RNA (mRNA) using the DNA as a template. The mRNA then conveys the code to the ribosomes. During translation the tranfer RNA (tRNA) and ribosomal RNA (rRNA) translate the code for the specific amino acid sequences needed for the ribosomes to synthesize the proteins that control cell activity. ⇨ anticodon, codon, transcription, translation.

genetic counselling the specialist multidisciplinary services provided for individuals, couples and families with a history of genetic diseases. They provide information about the genetic disease, its implications and the risk of having affected children. The service also provides information about genetic screening to identify carriers of a recessive mutant gene, prenatal diagnosis, termination of pregnancy and the assisted conception techniques such as the use of donated sperm and eggs.

genetic drift the random changes in allele frequency that occur in a finite population over time.

genetic engineering ⇨ recombinant DNA technology.

genetic potential also known as genetic endowment. Theoretical optimum performance capability which an individual could achieve in a specific activity, after an ideal upbringing, nutrition and training. In real terms it may be assumed that the finalists in a world championship are among the human beings whose performance comes closest to their genetic potential. ⊃ performance genes.

genetic profiling ⊃ performance genes.

genetics *n* the science of heredity and variation, namely the study of the genetic material, its transmission and its changes (mutations).

genetic screening 1. testing individuals for the presence of an abnormal gene, such as when a relative has the disease, or for carriers of a recessive gene, or where they belong to a group who have a high incidence of a particular genetic disease, e.g. thalassaemia in people from around the Mediterranean, or Tay–Sach's disease in Ashkenazic Jews. **2.** testing a specific population for the presence of a genetic disease, for example testing neonates for cystic fibrosis, congenital hypothyroidism, galactosaemia (in some countries), phenylketonuria, sickle-cell diseases and thalassaemia, and medium chain acyl-CoA dehydrogenase deficiency (MCADD).

genial relating to the chin.

genial tubercle one of two raised nodules of bone, one above the other, on each half of the lower border of the mandible near to the symphysis menti to which muscles are attached.

-gen, genic a suffix that means 'capable of causing', e.g. *pathogenic*.

geniculocalcarine tract ⊃ optic radiations.

genioglossus muscle a tongue muscle and the main protruder of the tongue. It arises from the inner surface of the mandible near the symphysis and is inserted in the body of the hyoid bone.

geniohyoid muscle a muscle arising from the inner surface of the mandible near the symphysis and is inserted into the anterior surface of the hyoid bone.

genioplasty also called mentoplasty. A surgical procedure to improve the size or shape of the chin. It may involve bone removal, or the use of bone grafts or implants to increase the size.

genital *adj* pertaining to the organs of generation.

genital herpes ⊃ herpes.

genital warts a very common disease caused by certain types of the human papillomavirus (HPV). Cauliflower-like lesions develop in the genital area or in the perianal region after a prepatent period that varies from several weeks to even years. Some strains of HPV are associated with the development cervical cancer.

genitalia *n* the external organs of generation.

genit/o- a prefix that means 'genitals, reproductive', e.g. *genitalia*.

genitocrural *adj* pertaining to the genital area and the legs.

genitofemoral nerve a nerve that arises from the lumbar plexus. It supplies the muscles and skin of the lower abdomen, upper and medial aspects of the thigh and the inguinal region. ⊃ lumbar plexus.

genitourinary *adj* pertaining to the reproductive and urinary organs.

genitourinary medicine (GUM) specialty concerned with the management of sexually transmitted infections and other medical conditions of the genital tract.

genome *n* the basic set of chromosomes and the genes, equal to the sum total of gene types possessed by different organisms of a species.

genotype *n* the total genetic information encoded in the chromosomes of an individual (as opposed to the phenotype). Also, the genetic make-up of a person at a specific locus, namely the alleles present at that locus. ⊃ phenotype.

gentian violet ⊃ crystal violet.

genu *n* the knee.

genupectoral position the knee-chest position, i.e. the weight is taken by the knees, and by the upper chest, while the shoulder girdle and head are supported on a pillow in front.

genu recurvatum abnormality of the legs due to hyperextending knees.

genu valgum (knock knees) abnormal incurving of the legs so the knees knock together during walking. The feet are widely separated.

genu varum (bowleg) abnormal outward curving of the leg(s) so that there is a gap between the knees when the feet are together.

genus *n* a classification ranking between the family and species.

geographic tongue a condition in which smooth, red depapillated patches on the superior aspect of the tongue are said to resemble a map.

geometric unsharpness blurring of a radiographic image due to the size of the focal spot on the anode, and can be reduced by increasing the focus to film distance and the object film distance.

geophagia *n* the habit of eating clay or earth.

Gerber attachment ⊃ precision attachment.

Gerdy's tubercle the lateral tubercle at upper end of tibia, the site of partial insertion of iliotibial band. Common site of pathology due to friction of iliotibial band on bone.

geriatric depression scale (GDS) a test of depression for use with older people.

geriatrician *n* one who specializes in geriatrics; the medical care of older people.

geriatrics *n* the branch of medical science dealing with old age and its diseases together with the medical care and nursing required by older people.

germ *n* colloquial term for a micro-organism, especially a pathogen.

German measles ⊃ rubella.

germ cell refers to a reproductive cell during any stage of gametogenesis (formation of gametes, oocytes or spermatozoa), e.g. gametogonia, gametocytes, or to the gametes themselves. A germ line cell rather than a somatic (body) cell. ⊃ gamete, gametogenesis, oogenesis, spermatogenesis.

germicide *n* any agent capable of killing micro-organisms (germs)—**germicidal** *adj*.

germinal *adj* pertaining to a germ cell, or to the first stages in embryonic development.

germinal epithelium the outer epithelial layer of the ovary. So called because it was previously thought to be the site of oogonia formation.

G
H

germ layers the three primordial cell layers responsible for every cell type in the body. The ectoderm, endoderm and mesoderm develop during gastrulation in very early embryonic development. Each layer differentiates into different cell types.

germ line the genetic material passed from the parents to their offspring through the oocyte and spermatozoa (gametes).

gerodontics the prevention and treatment of dental problems and diseases peculiar to ageing persons.

gero, geronto- a prefix that means 'old age', e.g. *gerontology*.

gerontology *n* the scientific study of ageing—**gerontological** *adj*.

gerontoxon ⊃ corneal arcus.

Gerstmann's syndrome (J Gerstmann, Austrian neurologist, 1887–1969) includes right-left disorientation, an inability to identify the fingers (finger agnosia), constructional apraxia, acalculia and agraphia. It may occur after damage to the parietal lobe of the brain, or following a stroke.

Gerstmann–Sträussler–Scheinker disease (J Gerstmann; E Sträussler, Austrian neurologist/psychiatrist, 1872–1959; I Scheinker, Russian neurologist, 1902–1954) an extremely rare inherited transmissible spongiform encephalopathy (TSE); it leads to ataxia and dementia.

gestagen hormones with progestational activity.

Gestalt theory a German word meaning 'organized whole'. A theory of behaviour developed early in the twentieth century. It contends that perception and learning are active, creative processes that are part of an 'organized whole'.

gestation *n* ⊃ pregnancy—**gestational** *adj*.

gestational diabetes also known as impaired glucose tolerance during pregnancy. Diabetes mellitus that develops, or is first observed during pregnancy. It is due to an intolerance to carbohydrate that leads to hyperglycaemia. The increased metabolic workload and insulin resistance, especially in women with a family history of type 2 diabetes, increasing age, or those with predisposing factors such as a previous baby weighing more than 4.5 kg, previous unexplained stillbirth or neonatal death, triggers a temporary diabetic state. The cause is unknown but the hormones of pregnancy may decrease the response to insulin. Possible complications include maternal infections, hypertension, polyhydramnios, ketoacidosis, fetal abnormalities, death or hypoxia, cephalopelvic disproportion and birth trauma, and neonatal hypoglycaemia or respiratory distress syndrome. Care is usually undertaken by a multidisciplinary team that includes: obstetrician, midwife, physician, specialist diabetic nurse and dietician for close monitoring of materno-fetal and diabetic conditions. It may be managed by diet alone, or with diet and insulin. The woman should be delivered in hospital, with careful observation of the blood glucose levels; caesarean section may be necessary. Blood glucose monitoring continues postnatally when the diabetic state resolves and the woman's insulin requirements fall

sharply. Extra carbohydrate is required if the mother is breastfeeding. An oral glucose tolerance test should be undertaken 6 weeks after the birth. Although, the diabetes resolves following the birth of the infant, affected women have a greater risk than normal of developing both type 1 and type 2 diabetes.

gestational trophoblast tumour (GTT) disease a general term covering a spectrum of conditions—molar pregnancy (hydatidiform mole), invasive mole, persistent trophoblastic disease, choriocarcinoma and the very rare placental site trophoblastic tumour (PSTT). ⊃ choriocarcinoma, invasive mole, molar pregnancy, placental site trophoblastic tumour.

gestation sac volume the volume of the sac which contains the embryo/fetus during pregnancy. Usually measured at 3–6 weeks' gestation using ultrasound.

GFR *abbr* glomerular filtration rate.

GGT, gamma-GT, γ-GT *abbr* gamma-glutamyltransferase.

GH *abbr* growth hormone.

GHb *abbr* total glycated (glycosylated) haemoglobin.

Ghon's focus/complex (A Ghon, Czechoslovakian pathologist, 1866–1936) ⊃ primary complex.

ghost image (*syn* false image) **1.** an unwanted image as may be formed by internal reflection in a lens or an optical system. These images are sometimes annoying to spectacle wearers, and even to observers as they detract from the appearance of the spectacle lens or hide the wearer's eyes behind a veil. The intensity of ghost images is diminished by antireflection coatings. **2.** the faint image seen in monocular diplopia. ⊃ antireflection coating, Fresnel formula, lens flare, monocular diplopia, stray light.

ghosting in ultrasound a mirror image which is produced when the gain is too high or when imaging objects with high acoustic reflections.

ghrelin an appetite-stimulating peptide hormone secreted by cells in the stomach and duodenum. It stimulates the secretion of growth hormone and regulates food intake and energy balance through its effects on the hypothalamus.

GHRH *abbr* growth hormone releasing hormone

GHRIH *abbr* growth hormone release inhibiting hormone.

GI *abbr* **1.** gastrointestinal. **2.** gingival (Loe and Silness) index. ⊃ index (dental). **3.** glycaemic index.

giant cell arteritis (GCA) a large vessel vasculitis predominately affecting branches of the temporal and ophthalmic arteries. The mean age of onset is 70 years with a 4:1 female:male ratio. The onset of symptoms may be abrupt but is often insidious over the course of several weeks or months. The most important clinical features are: (a) headache—usually the first symptom and is often localized to the temporal or occipital region, with scalp tenderness; (b) jaw pain—brought on by chewing or talking and is due to ischaemia of the masseters; (c) visual disturbance—the optic nerve head is supplied by the posterior ciliary artery, vasculitis of which leads to occlusion and acute anterior ischaemic optic neuropathy. Damage to the optic nerve results in loss of visual acuity and field, reduced colour perception and pupillary defects. Sudden visual symptoms in one eye, leading rapidly to blindness, constitute the most common pattern. On fundoscopy the optic disc may appear pale and swollen with haemorrhages, but these changes may take 24–36 hours to develop. Once blindness has occurred corticosteroids have a negligible effect but are indicated to prevent blindness in the other eye. There may be associated constitutional symptoms of anorexia, fatigue, weight loss, fever, depression and general malaise. Occasionally presentation is with neurological complications that include transient ischaemic attacks, brainstem infarcts and hemiparesis. The erythrocyte sedimentation rate (ESR) and C-reactive protein (CRP) are elevated. Ideally, a temporal artery biopsy should also be obtained. However, corticosteroid treatment should not be delayed; diagnostic information will still be present on biopsies taken a week later. Characteristic biopsy findings are fragmentation of the internal elastic lamina with necrosis of the media in combination with a mixed inflammatory cell infiltrate (lymphocytes, plasma cells and eosinophils). However, 'skip' lesions are common and a negative biopsy does not exclude the diagnosis. If GCA is suspected, systemic corticosteroid should be started immediately to prevent visual loss. Corticosteroid reduction should be guided by symptoms and ESR. Patients with known GCA should be advised to take 60 mg prednisolone and seek prompt medical advice should they experience any recurrence of headache or visual disturbance. Maintenance therapy is required for at least 1 year, and occasionally for the rest of the patient's life. Relapse occurs in 30%, and is an indication to restart high-dose corticosteroids with additional immunosuppressive agents, typically azathioprine or methotrexate. ➲ systemic vasculitis, temporal arteritis.

giant cell granuloma a granuloma or lesion of unknown aetiology but thought to be associated with an exaggerated inflammatory response. Consists of a vascular connective tissue with many giant cells. The lesion may grow to a large size and show aggressive neoplastic behaviour. ➲ granuloma.

giant papillary conjunctivitis (GPC) conjunctivitis, characterized by the appearance of 'cobblestones' (large papillae of 0.5 mm or more) on the tarsal conjunctiva of the upper eyelid (and sometimes the lower eyelid). Signs and symptoms include itching, discomfort, discharge of mucus and poor vision due to the presence of mucus. The condition may be induced by contact lens wear, ocular prosthesis, or exposed sutures following surgery. This conjunctivitis closely resembles vernal conjunctivitis and is also believed to be an allergic condition. In its early stages as a contact lens-induced condition, it is often referred to as contact lens papillary conjunctivitis (CLPC) or contact lens associated papillary conjunctivitis (CLAPC). In these cases the regular use of surfactant and protein removal tablets as well as frequent lens replacement reduce the incidence of this condition which is less prevalent with the wear of rigid gas permeable than soft contact lenses. Management may also include sodium cromoglicate or antihistamines such as antazoline and cessation of lens wear. ➲ contact lens deposits, vernal conjunctivitis, Colour Section Figure 128.

Giardia (A Giard, French biologist, 1846–1908) a genus of flagellate protozoans. They are parasites that infect the gastrointestinal tract where they cause inflammation in the duodenum and jejunum. In some individuals they may be commensals. Hosts include cats, dogs, cattle and sheep.

giardiasis *n* (*syn* lambliasis) infection with the flagellate *Giardia intestinalis*. May be symptomless, especially in adults. Causes crampy pain, bloating, vomiting, anorexia, foul-smelling diarrhoea with steatorrhoea and flatulence. Occurs worldwide but more common in tropical regions. It particularly affects children, people travelling to other areas and those who are immunocompromised.

gibbus an abnormal convex spinal curvature. It may be associated with vertebral body collapse, such as that occurring in tuberculosis affecting the spine.

GIF *abbr* graphics interchange format.

GIFT *abbr* gamete intrafallopian transfer.

gigabyte one billion (10^9) bytes, a measure of the size of a computer hard disk and denotes the quantity of information that can be stored on the system.

gigantism *n* abnormal overgrowth, especially in height, due to excess growth hormone in childhood prior to fusion of the epiphyseal plates in the long bones. Almost always due to a pituitary tumour.

Gigli's wire saw flexible toothed wire used to transect bone.

Gilles de Tourette syndrome (G Gilles de Tourette, French neurologist, 1857–1927) ➲ Tourette's syndrome

Gillick competence concerns the decision-making competence of children and young people and their capacity to give valid consent for medical treatment. It arises from the case of Gillick v West Norfolk and Wisbech Health Authority in which the House of Lords ruled that children under 16 years of age can give legally effective consent to medical treatment providing they can demonstrate sufficient maturity and intelligence to understand fully the treatment planned. The capacity to make a decision, which is judged by the health professional, is subject to certain guidelines. For example, that the treatment is in the best interests of the young person. The case in question centred on the provision of contraceptive advice and treatment in a female under 16 years of age.

Gillies' approach surgical approach to the zygomatic arch area through an incision in the temporal region, above the hairline.

gingiva *n* fibrous connective tissue, covered by epithelium, that surrounds and is attached to the tooth and alveolar bone and extends to the mucogingival junction. On the palatal aspect it is a rim of tissue that merges with the masticatory mucosa of the hard palate. Referred to in lay terms as the gum—**gingivae** *pl*, **gingival** *adj*. *attached gingiva* in health, salmon- or coral-pink-coloured tissue, stippled like orange peel, situated between the gingival crest and the mucogingival junction. It is attached to the underlying cementum and bone.

gingival relating to the gingiva.

gingival cleft narrow, V-shaped split in the marginal gingiva.

gingival col depression or valley in the interdental papilla.

gingival contouring the carving on the base material of a denture to simulate the natural curved gum outline about the necks of the teeth.

gingival corium the lamina propria of the gingiva.

gingival crater concave shape of the gingival papilla resulting from necrosis.

gingival crest the coronal border of the gingiva.

gingival crevice ⊃ gingival sulcus.

gingival crevicular fluid transudate of blood plasma found in the gingival sulcus due to leakage of plasma from blood capillaries in the free gingiva.

gingival fibres network of fibres that produce close apposition of the marginal gingiva to the tooth.

gingival fibromatosis dense overgrowth of gingival tissue.

gingival graft gingival tissue that has been completely detached and replaced on a different site.

gingival groove shallow, V-shaped groove sometimes seen on the outer aspect of the marginal gingiva.

gingival (Loe and Silness) index (GI) ⊃ index (dental).

gingivally approaching clasp (*syn* Roach clasp) denture-retaining clasp, the arm of which passes adjacent to the soft tissues and approaches its point of contact on a tooth from the gingival margin.

gingival margin that part of the gingiva surrounding the tooth and nearest to its crown. The crest of the free gingiva.

gingival margin trimmer hand instrument similar to a hatchet chisel but having its sharp blade curved in its length. Used to trim the cervical margin of a tooth preparation.

gingival morphology shape, contour and profile of the gingiva.

gingival papilla that part of the gingiva which occupies the interproximal space between the teeth.

gingival recession loss of gingiva over the root of a tooth on the vestibular or oral aspect.

gingival retraction process of temporarily expanding the gingival sulcus by displacing the gingival tissues to allow visualization of the margins of a restoration, e.g. crown preparation. May be undertaken with the use of gingival retraction cord soaked in an astringent solution. More recently expandable 'putty' materials have been brought to market that are injected into the gingival sulcus.

gingival stippling minute depressions on the attached gingival surface.

gingival sulcus previously known as the *gingival crevice*. A shallow invagination lying between the gingival crest and the neck of a tooth, extending from the margin of the free gingiva to the junctional epithelium. This may deepen, due to pathological processes, to produce a periodontal pocket. In health the sulcus may be up to 2 mm in depth. ⊃ index (dental).

gingivectomy surgical excision of infected or otherwise diseased gingiva. Such as for severe periodontal disease.

gingivectomy knife ⊃ periodontal instruments.

gingivitis *n* inflammation of the gingivae. Characterized by local and generalized redness of the gingivae, bleeding of the gingivae on brushing or spontaneously in severe cases and swollen gingivae. ⊃ desquamative gingivitis, necrotizing ulcerative gingivitis (NUG), pregnancy gingivitis.

gingivoplasty a periodontal procedure by which gingival deformities, not accompanied by pocketing, are reshaped to create a correct anatomical form.

gingivostomatitis inflammation of both oral mucosa and the gingivae.

ginglymus a hinge joint. A type of freely movable joint that has angular movment in one plane, such as the elbow.

ginseng name commonly used for several species of *Panax* herbs. A naturally occurring substance, not banned in sport, ginseng has been suggested to have performance-enhancing properties, though these have not been scientifically proven. In addition, several preparations of ginseng have been found to be contaminated with banned substances. Side effects include insomnia, depression and high blood pressure.

GIP *abbr* gastric inhibitory peptide.

girdle *n* usually a bony structure of oval shape such as the shoulder and pelvic girdles.

Girdlestone arthroplasty an excision arthroplasty of the hip.

GLA *abbr* gamma (γ)-linolenic acid.

glabella the flat triangular part of the frontal bone between the two superciliary ridges.

gland *n* an organ or structure capable of making an internal or external secretion. ⊃ endocrine, exocrine—**glandular** *adj*.

glanders *n* a contagious, febrile, ulcerative disease communicable from horses, mules and asses to humans. Caused by the bacterium *Burkholderia mallei* (previously called *Pseudomonas mallei*). The disease is characterized by skin nodules and ulceration of the respiratory mucosa. It is endemic in Central and South America, Asia, Africa and the Middle East.

glands of Ciaccio ⊃ Wolfring's glands.

glandular fever ⊃ infectious mononucleosis.

glans *n* the bulbous termination of the clitoris and penis. ⊃ Colour Section Figure 16.

glare a visual condition in which the observer feels either discomfort and/or exhibits a lower performance in visual tests (e.g. visual acuity or contrast sensitivity). This is produced by a relatively bright source of light (called the glare source) within the visual field. A given bright light may or may not produce glare depending upon the location and intensity of the light source, the background luminance, the state of adaptation of the eye or the clarity of the media of the eye.

glare tester an instrument for measuring the effect of glare on visual performance. There exist several (e.g. Brightness Acuity Tester, Miller–Nadler Glare Tester, Optec 1500 Glare Tester). Glare testing is valuable in patients with corneal and lenticular opacities before and after surgery and in older adults in whom adaptation to glare is usually more difficult. ➲ dark adaptation.

Glasgow Coma Scale (GCS) a reliable rating scale of conscious level for trauma and neurological patients that assesses their best motor, verbal and eye opening response (Table G.1). Used, for example, following brain/head injury and neurosurgery. The lowest score is 3 (1 in each category). A GCS score of 8 or less indicates severe injury, 9–12 moderate injury and 13–15 a mild injury. A modified scale is available for use with preverbal children.

glass 1. the material from which lenses and optical elements may be made. It is hard, brittle and lustrous and usually transparent. It is produced by fusing sand (silica) at about 1400°C with various oxides (potassium, sodium, etc.) and other ingredients such as lead oxide, lime, etc. Glass may be produced in various colours by the addition of different substances (e.g. metal oxides). **2.** a lens. ➲ blank lens, refractive index, striae, surfacing.

glass bead sterilizer ➲ sterilizer.

glass ionomer cement semitranslucent, tooth-coloured, fluoride releasing cement used to restore anterior teeth, especially labial cavities, pits and fissures. Also used to lute, line tooth preparations and act as a fissure sealant. Must be used in dry conditions and be protected by varnish after

being placed. By virtue of its molecular make-up, it has the unique ability of forming adhesive bonds with enamel and dentine. *resin modified glass ionomer cement* contain resin monomers, setting by acid base reaction and resin polymerization. Possesses properties that are generally considered superior to conventional glass ionomer cement.

glass plasma display the technology used for early flat screen computer monitors composed of neon gas cells between two electrodes. When the electrodes are activated the gas glows therefore forming an image.

glaucoma a group of eye diseases characterized by an elevated or unstable intraocular pressure (IOP) which cannot be sustained without damage to the eye's structure or impairment to its function. The increased pressure may cause optic atrophy with excavation of the optic disc as well as characteristic loss of visual field. Glaucoma is usually divided into *open-angle* and *angle-closure* types. If the cause of the glaucoma is a recognized ocular disease or injury (e.g. corneal laceration), it is called secondary, whereas if the cause is unknown it is called primary—**glaucomatous** *adj.* ➲ acute angle-closure glaucoma (AACG), ancampimetry, angle-closure glaucoma (ACG), cup-disc ratio, frequency doubling perimetry, glaucomatous cup, hyphaemia, intraocular pressure, iridectomy, neuroprotection, open-angle glaucoma, optic atrophy, perimeter, short wavelength automated perimetry, tonography, tonometry, tritanopia.

glaucomatous cup a large and deep excavation within the optic disc due to a raised intraocular pressure (IOP). It is characterized by overhanging walls over which the blood vessels bend sharply and reappear at the bottom of the depression. ➲ cup-disc ratio, cupped disc, glaucoma.

glaucoma valve various devices sometimes used in glaucoma to reduce raised intraocular pressure. More recent shunts incorporate a valve. The shunt is used to divert aqueous humour from the trabecular meshwork and redirect it to a subconjunctival bleb.

glazing porcelain ➲ porcelain.

Gleason grade (D Gleason, American pathologist, 20th century) a five-stage system used to assess the degree of differentiation in prostate cancer.

glenohumeral *adj* pertaining to the glenoid cavity of scapula and the humerus.

glenoid cavity *n* a cavity on the scapula into which the head of the humerus fits to form the shoulder joint.

glenoid fossa the depression in the temporal bone in which the condylar process of the mandible rests and which forms part of the temporomandibular joint

glia *n* ➲ macroglia, microglia, neuroglia—**glial** *adj.*

gliadin a protein found in the gluten present in wheat and rye. Intolerance of gliadin causes coeliac disease.

glicentin a form of enteroglucagon.

gliding joint a freely movable joint, that only allows gliding movement, such as those between the wrist and ankle bones.

glioblastoma multiforme a highly malignant brain tumour.

Table G.1 Glasgow Coma Scale

Eye opening (E)	
Spontaneous	4
To speech	3
To pain	2
Nil	1
Best motor response (M)	
Obeys	6
Localizes	5
Withdraws	4
Abnormal flexion	3
Extensor response	2
Nil	1
Verbal response (V)	
Oriented	5
Confused conversation	4
Inappropriate words	3
Incomprehensible sounds	2
Nil	1
Coma score = E + M + V	
Minimum	3
Maximum	15
Reproduced from Boon et al. (2006) with permission.	

glioma *n* a fast-growing malignant tumour that arises from neuroglial tissue, typically an astrocytoma or oligodendroglioma. Graded 1–4 based on malignancy with grade 4 being the most aggressive—**gliomata** *pl.* ⊃ astrocyte, oligodendrocyte.

gliomyoma *n* a tumour of nerve and muscle tissue—**gliomyomata** *pl.*

globin *n* the four protein molecules that join with haem to form haemoglobin.

globular grains the type of grains found in some radiographic film emulsions and have the characteristic that the light-absorbing ability of the grain depends only on its volume, they are used in blue-sensitive or monochromatic systems.

globulins *npl* a large group of proteins. Those in the plasma are classified as alpha and beta, which are concerned with substance transport, and gamma, which provides protection against infection. The gamma globulins comprise the immunoglobulins A, D, E, G and M.

globulinuria *n* the presence of globulin in the urine.

globulomaxillary cyst a developmental cyst seen in the maxillary lateral incisor tooth and canine tooth regions.

globus pallidus literally pale globe; a mass of motor grey matter situated deep within the cerebral hemispheres, lateral to the thalamus. Part of the basal nuclei.

globus pharyngis also still called globus hystericus. A subjective feeling of a lump in the throat. Can also include difficulty in swallowing and is due to tension of muscles of deglutition. It may be associated with anxiety states, dissociative disorder and depression.

glomerular filtration rate (GFR) the volume of plasma filtered by the kidneys in 1 minute. It is usually around 120 mL per min.

glomerulitis inflammation of the glomeruli.

glomerulonephritis *n* inflammation of the glomeruli (of the nephron). The term encompasses many different acute and chronic disorders of varying aetiology and prognosis—**glomerulonephritides** *pl.*

glomerulosclerosis *n* fibrosis of the glomeruli (of the nephron), often as a result of glomerulonephritis—**glomerulosclerotic** *adj.*

glomerulus *n* a coil of capillaries formed from a wide-bore afferent arteriole. It lies within the invaginated blind end of the renal tubule (Figure G.2). Together with the renal tubule it forms a nephron. Part of the filtration membrane involved in the production of urine—**glomerular** *adj*, **glomeruli** *pl.*

glomus *n* arterioles which communicate directly with veins.

glossa *n* the tongue—**glossal** *adj.*

glossectomy *n* excision of part or all of the tongue.

Glossina *n* a genus of biting flies. ⊃ tsetse

glossitis *n* inflammation of the tongue. It may be associated with infection, trauma, B vitamin deficiencies or pernicious anaemia. ⊃ median rhomboid glossitis.

glosso- a prefix that means 'tongue', e.g. *glossoplegia.*

glossodynia *n* painful tongue without visible change.

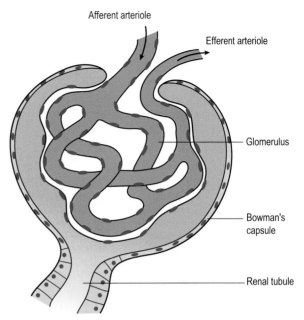

Afferent arteriole

Efferent arteriole

Glomerulus

Bowman's capsule

Renal tubule

G
H

G.2 **Glomerulus** (reproduced from Watson 2000 with permission).

glossopharyngeal *adj* pertaining to the tongue and pharynx. The ninth pair of cranial nerves, they innervate the tongue and pharynx.

glossoplegia *n* paralysis of the tongue.

glossoptosis an abnormal downward displacement of the tongue.

glossopyrosis a burning sensation felt in the tongue.

glottis *n* the opening between the abducted vocal folds in the larynx. It allows air to enter the respiratory tract and is involved in voice production—**glottic** *adj.*

glucagon *n* a catabolic polypeptide hormone secreted in the pancreatic islets by the alpha cells. It elevates blood glucose by promoting glycogenolysis (the release of glucose from liver glycogen stores) and gluconeogenesis in the liver and also mobilizes free fatty acids from adipose tissue, having opposite actions at these sites to those of insulin. Its release is stimulated by hypoglycaemia and growth hormone. The ratio of insulin to glucagon secretion appropriately decreases in exercise. Glucagon is used by injection to reverse hypoglycaemia. ⊃ gluconeogenesis, insulin.

glucagon-like peptide-1 (GLP-1) mimetics *npl* a group of hypoglycaemic drugs, e.g., exenatide. ⊃ Appendix 5.

glucagonoma a glucagon-secreting tumour of the islet cells of the pancreas. Usually malignant and often part of multiple endocrine neoplasia (MEN). It is characterized by hyperglycaemia, skin rash, cheilitis, glossitis, stomatitis, weight loss, diarrhoea and possible mental health problems, or a tendency to develop thromboembolic conditions. ⊃ islet cell tumours.

glucagon stimulation test a test of pituitary reserve, assessing the response of growth hormone and adrenocorticotrophin (ACTH) and hence cortisol to subcutaneous or intramuscular administration of glucagon.

glucans complex carbohydrates in cereals such as oats, barley and rye. They are soluble but undigested.

glucocorticoid *n* any steroid hormone which promotes gluconeogenesis and which antagonizes the action of insulin. Occurring naturally in the adrenal cortex as cortisone and cortisol (hydrocortisone), and produced synthetically as, for example, prednisolone. Produced by the adrenal cortex, under the control of adrenocorticotrophic hormone (ACTH) from the anterior pituitary. Their major actions on nutrient metabolism have the net effect of promoting glucose and free fatty acid availability as fuels. Also vital for normal cellular processes as diverse, for example, as excitation–contraction coupling and the health of connective tissues. Synthetic steroids such as prednisolone and dexamethasone have similar actions and are used in the treatment of, for example, inflammatory bowel disease, asthma, rheumatic conditions and cerebral oedema. Banned in sport due to their powerful anti-inflammatory action and effect of producing euphoria and masking pain.

glucogenesis *n* production of glucose.

gluco, glyco- a prefix that means 'sugar, glucose', e.g. *glucokinase*.

glucokinase an enzyme that catalyses the phosphorylation of glucose to glucose-6-phosphate (G6P); the initial reaction in both glycolysis and glycogenesis. It is a hexokinase and is found in the liver, intestine, pancreas and brain.

gluconeogenesis *n* the synthesis of glucose from noncarbohydrate precursors, e.g. glycerol, pyruvate, lactate, and the glucogenic amino acids derived from skeletal muscle. Gluconeogenesis occurs mainly in the liver and to a lesser extent in the renal cortex. The glucose-alanine cycle involves the conversion of alanine (an amino acid), formed in muscle, to glucose in the liver; activity of the cycle is increased during the postabsorptive state and in starvation or prolonged exercise, slowly mobilizing glycogen stores and using protein for the maintenance of normal blood glucose concentration. Gluconeogenesis and export of glucose from the liver are promoted by the hormone glucagon, and inhibited by insulin.

glucosamine an amino sugar that forms the basis of many important glycosylated lipids and proteins, such as those found in cartilage. Individuals with osteoarthritis may choose to take glucosamine supplements.

glucosan a term for the group of glucose polysaccharides that include cellulose, glycogen and starch.

glucose *n* dextrose. A hexose (a monosaccharide containing six carbon atoms). The form in which carbohydrates are absorbed through the intestinal tract and circulated in the blood. Glucose is of major importance as a source of energy in all tissues, and essential for some (brain, red blood cells, renal cortex, mammary gland and testis). Ingestion of carbohydrates provides glucose for replenishment and for accumulation of liver and muscle glycogen. When there is overconsumption of carbohydrate, excess glucose is used in the formation of triacylglycerol (triglycerides) which are stored in adipose tissue. Glucose metabolism is mainly controlled by the pancreatic hormones insulin and glucagon. The glucocorticoid hormones from the adrenal cortex and growth hormone from the anterior pituitary are also involved. ⊃ blood glucose.

glucose-electrolyte drinks ⊃ sports drinks.

glucose-6-phosphatase an enzyme that catalyses the conversion of glucose-6-phosphate to glucose.

glucose-1-phosphate a phosphorylated sugar produced at the start of glycogen breakdown (glycogenolysis) to liberate glucose for cell use. ⊃ glycogenolysis.

glucose-6-phosphate (G6P) an important phosphorylated glucose molecule in the metabolism of glucose. It is involved in glycolysis and the pentose phosphate pathway. Also concerned in glycogen production (glycogenesis) and the subsequent conversion of glycogen back to glucose (glycogenolysis). During glycogenolysis it is formed from glucose-1-phosphate. It is converted to glucose by the action of the enzyme glucose-6-phosphatase. ⊃ glycogenolysis, pentose phosphate pathway (PPP).

glucose-6-phosphate dehydrogenase (G6PD) the enzyme pivotal in the pentose phosphate pathway (hexose monophosphate shunt) and produces the reduced form of nicotinamide adenine dinucleotide phosphate (NADPH) to protect the red cell against oxidative stress. ⊃ glucose-6-phosphate (G6P), glucose-6-phosphate dehydrogenase (G6PD) deficiency, pentose phosphate pathway.

glucose-6-phosphate dehydrogenase (G6PD) deficiency deficiencies of the enzyme glucose-6-phosphate dehydrogenase are the most common human enzymopathy, affecting 10% of the world's population with a geographical distribution which parallels the malaria belt because heterozygote individuals are protected from malarial parasitization. The enzyme is a heteromeric structure made of catalytic subunits which are coded for by a gene on the X chromosome. The deficiency affects males but is carried by females, who are usually only affected in the neonatal period or in the presence of extreme lyonization or homozygosity. There are over 400 subtypes of G6PD described. The most common types associated with normal activity are the B^+ enzyme present in most Caucasians and 70% of African Caribbeans, and the A^+ variant present in 20% of African Caribbeans. The two common variants associated with reduced activity are the A^- variety in approximately 10% of African Caribbeans, and the Mediterranean or B^- variety in Caucasians. In East and West Africa up to 20% of males and 4% of females (homozygotes) are affected and have enzyme levels of approximately 15%. The deficiency in Caucasian and Oriental populations is more severe, with enzyme levels as low as 1%. Clinical features include: (a) acute drug-induced haemolysis—e.g. with aspirin, antimalarial drugs, sulphonamides, vitamin K, probenecid, etc.; (b) chronic compensated haemolysis; (c) infection or acute illness; (d) neonatal jaundice; (e) favism or acute haemolysis after ingestion of broad beans (*Vicia faba*). Management aims to stop any precipitant drugs and treat any underlying infection. Acute transfusion support may be life-saving.

glucose tolerance test (GTT) (oral glucose tolerance test) after a period of fasting, a measured quantity (75 g) of

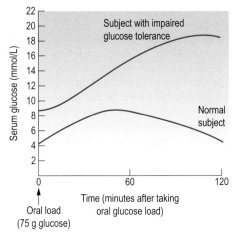

G.3 Glucose tolerance test (reproduced from Westwood 1999 with permission).

glucose is taken orally; thereafter blood samples are tested for glucose levels at intervals. A plasma glucose level ≥ 11.1 mmol/L 2 hours after the oral glucose meets the diagnostic criteria for diabetes mellitus (Figure G.3). ⟳ impaired glucose tolerance.

glucose transporters a family of membrane proteins that transport glucose across cell membranes down a concentration gradient, into most cells but out of the liver and kidney cells when gluconeogenesis occurs.

glucosinolates molecules that occur in brassicas, e.g. cabbage, broccoli, Brussels sprouts. They may have anti-cancer properties by increasing the conjugation and excretion of carcinogenic chemicals.

glucuronic acid derived from glucose. It is important in the liver and in other organs for the safe excretion of many compounds including hormones, bile pigments and drugs. For example, when drug residues are conjugated with glucuronic acid a water-soluble substance (a glucuronide) is produced, which can be safely excreted.

glue ear an accumulation of a glue-like substance in the middle ear. A cause of conductive deafness.

glue sniffing ⟳ solvent misuse.

glutamic acid (glutamate) a non-essential (dispensable) amino acid. At physiological pH glutamic acid is negatively charged and is known as glutamate. Glutamate is an important excitatory neurotransmitter in the central nervous system.

glutamic oxaloacetic transaminase ⟳ aminotransferases, AST.

glutamic pyruvic transaminase ⟳ aminotransferases, ALT.

glutamine *n* a conditionally essential (indispensable) amino acid. It is synthesized in skeletal muscle. Glutamine is one of the major fuels of the gut lining, and of the cells of the immune system. It is also a precursor for the gluconeogenesis that occurs in the kidneys after an overnight fast or in starvation. Glutamine supplementation is popular among athletes attempting to maintain a healthy immune system during training. ⟳ ergogenic aids.

glutathione *n* a tripeptide comprising three amino acids (cysteine, glutamic acid [glutamate] and glycine). It functions as a coenzyme, and as an antioxidant to protect cells against free radical damage. Required for conjugation in the liver and for red cell membrane integrity. Paracetamol overdose causes serious depletion of glutathione. In appropriate cases the administration of acetylcysteine or methionine following paracetamol overdose allows the body to replenish glutathione levels.

glutathione peroxidase an enzyme important in preventing cell damage caused by reactive oxygen species. It catalyses the reaction in which glutathione is oxidized in the presence of hydrogen peroxide. ⟳ antioxidant enzymes, reactive oxygen species.

glutathione S-transferase an enzyme important in preventing cell damage caused by reactive oxygen species. It catalyses the reaction that adds free radicals and other harmful molecules at the sulphur in the glutathione molecule. ⟳ antioxidant enzymes, reactive oxygen species.

gluteal *adj* pertaining to the buttocks.

gluten *n* a protein comprising gliadin and glutenin found in the cereals wheat and rye and products containing these cereals, e.g. bread. A gluten-free diet is used to treat coeliac disease and dermatitis herpetiformis. Such as gluten-free flour, bread, biscuits, pasta.

gluten-induced enteropathy ⟳ coeliac disease.

gluteus muscles three muscles of the buttock: gluteus maximus, g. medius, g. minimus—**gluteal**, *adj*. ⟳ Colour Section Figure 5.

gluteus maximus the largest of the three gluteal muscles, its origin is on the ilium and sacrum and the insertion on the gluteal tuberosity of the femur. It extends the thigh.

gluteus medius a gluteal muscle which has its origin on the ilium and its insertion on the greater trochanter of the femur. It abducts and medially rotates the thigh.

gluteus minimus the smallest of the three gluteal muscles, its insertion is on the ilium and the insertion on the greater trochanter of the femur. It abducts the thigh.

glycaemic index (GI) an index that ranks foods based on the extent and rate of the postprandial rise in blood glucose that they cause, compared to the response to a reference food (either glucose or white bread); the higher the glycaemic index (GI), the greater and more rapid the rise. Intake of carbohydrate (CHO)-rich foods with lower GI has been shown to be beneficial in improving glucose control, particularly in people with type 2 diabetes. Consideration of GI may also be relevant to athletic performance. High-index CHO-rich meals have been reported to enhance the storage of muscle glycogen during recovery from prolonged exercise. On the other hand, some evidence favours consumption prior to exercise of low rather than high GI CHO-rich foods, since high GI may elicit an inappropriate surge of insulin and/or attentuate fat oxidation, leading to faster depletion of glycogen and onset of fatigue. ⟳ carbohydrate intake guidelines for athletes.

glycaemic load the glycaemic index multiplied by the amount of carbohydrate present in the food.

glycated (glycosylated) haemoglobin a test used in the management of diabetes mellitus. It provides an accurate and objective measure of glycaemic control over a period of weeks to months. This can be utilized as an assessment of glycaemic control in a patient with known diabetes, but is not sufficiently sensitive to make a diagnosis of diabetes and is usually within the normal range in patients with impaired glucose tolerance. In diabetes, the slow non-enzymatic covalent attachment of glucose to haemoglobin (glycation) increases the amount in the HbA (HbA_{1c}) fraction relative to non-glycated adult haemoglobin (HbA_0). These fractions can be separated by chromatography but laboratories may report glycated haemoglobin in several ways. In many countries, however, HbA_{1c} is now the preferred measurement. The rate of formation of HbA_{1c} is directly proportional to the ambient blood glucose concentration; a rise of 1% in HbA_{1c} corresponds to an approximate average increase of 2 mmol/L in blood glucose. Although HbA_{1c} concentration reflects the integrated blood glucose control over the lifespan of the erythrocyte (120 days), half of the erythrocytes are replaced in 60 days and HbA_{1c} is weighted by changes in glycaemic control occurring in the month before measurement (representing 50% of the HbA_{1c} concentration). As HbA_{1c} is affected more by recent than by earlier events, a large shift in blood glucose control is rapidly accompanied by a change in HbA_{1c}, detectable within 2–3 weeks. Previously several methods were used to measure HbA_{1c}, precluding direct comparison of HbA_{1c} values between laboratories. HbA_{1c} testing will be standardized and reported in mmol/mol in line with the IFCC reference method. Most laboratories will give results in both mmol/mol and percentages from April 2011. HbA_{1c} estimates may be erroneously diminished in anaemia or during pregnancy, and may be difficult to interpret with some assay methods in patients who have uraemia or a haemoglobinopathy. In clinical practice, HbA_{1c} is usually measured once or twice yearly to assess glycaemic control, permitting appropriate changes in treatment and identifying inconsistency with the patient's record of home blood glucose monitoring. HbA_{1c} also provides an index of risk for developing diabetic complications.

glycated serum proteins 'fructosamine' can be measured and, because of their shorter half-life, give an indication of glycaemic control over the preceding 2 weeks. Other than in diabetic women during pregnancy, this is generally too short a period to make clinical decisions on therapeutic management.

glycation *n* the reaction between glucose and the amino groups in proteins to form a glycoprotein. Linked to the complications associated with poor glycaemic control in people with diabetes. ⊃glycated (glycosylated) haemoglobin.

glycerides *npl* the esters formed by the addition of one or more fatty acids

glycerin(e) *n* ⊃ glycerol.

glycerin thymol compound a mouthwash containing glycerol, thymol, borax, sodium carbonate, sodium benzoate, sodium salicylate, menthol, thymol, cineole, methyl salicylate and pumilio pine oil.

glycerol *n* also called glycerin(e). A three-carbon carbohydrate. It forms the 'backbone' of the triacylglycerol (triglyceride) molecule. Forms esters with three fatty acids to produce simple fats known as triacylglycerols (triglycerides). Blood glycerol concentration mainly depends on the rate of lipolysis of triacylglycerols in adipose tissue. Glycerol is an important source of glucose during periods of fasting or starvation. In sport, consumption of glycerol may be used for hyperhydration, as it reduces renal water clearance, increasing fluid retention and total body water. Glycerol is a clear, syrupy liquid, which has a hydroscopic action. It is used therapeutically as an emollient and in mouthwashes and suppositories. ⊃ gluconeogenesis, hydration status of athletes.

glycerol suppositories formally known as glycerin suppositories. They act by attracting fluid to soften hardened faeces in the rectum.

glycine *n* a conditionally essential (indispensable) amino acid. The amino acid with the simplest chemical structure. Also has neurotransmitter properties.

glycinuria *n* excretion of glycine in the urine. Associated with learning disability.

glycocholic acid a bile acid.

glycogen *n* the main carbohydrate (a branched polysaccharide) storage compound in animals. Many glucose molecules are linked together in a process called glycogenesis occurring in the liver and skeletal muscle. The conversion of liver glycogen back to glucose is called glycogenolysis. The liver normally contains ~100 g (energy value 400 kcal) and skeletal muscle ~400 g (1600 kcal) of glycogen. It is also stored in the brain. The body's upper limit for glycogen storage is ~1050 g. It is known that aerobic endurance performance is directly related to the initial muscle glycogen and that perception of fatigue during prolonged exercise parallels the decline in these stores. ⊃ carbohydrate, carbohydrate loading, glycogenesis.

glycogen loading ⊃ carbohydrate loading.

glycogenesis *n* the formation of glycogen from blood glucose by the action of the enzyme glycogen synthetase in liver and skeletal muscle. The process is very active after depletion of muscle glycogen in exercise, making rapid restoration possible, provided that there is adequate consumption of carbohydrates. Even more ample carbohydrate supply can allow glycogen supercompensation—elevation in muscle glycogen content above normal. ⊃ carbohydrate loading.

glycogenolysis *n* the breakdown of stored glycogen to glucose. It involves the removal of a glucose molecule from glycogen in a biochemical process catalysed by the action of the enzyme glycogen phosphorylase, present in liver, kidneys, muscle and brain. The products are a glycogen molecule that is one glucose residue shorter than before and glucose-1-phosphate. This in turn is converted to glucose-6-phosphate, from which free glucose can be released from the liver and kidneys (but not from skeletal muscle or brain) by the action of glucose-6-phosphatase. ⊃ glucose, glucose-6-phosphate, glycolysis.

glycogenosis ⊃ glucogen storage disease.

glycogen phosphorylase the enzyme that, with other enzymes, removes glucose molecules to form glucose-1-phosphate during glycogenolysis.

glycogen storage diseases (GSD) also known as glycogenosis. A group of inherited diseases mostly inherited as an automsomal recessive trait. The metabolic disorder is caused by a defect in one of the enzymes required for the formation (glycogenesis) or breakdown of stored glycogen (glycogenolysis). Glycogen accumulates in various organs and tissues. Hypoglycaemia occurs, and the body tends to use fat rather than glucose, leading to ketosis and acidosis. Around 11 major types of GSD are described. ⊃ Andersen's disease, Cori's disease, Hers' disease, inherited metabolic myopathies, McArdle's disease, Pompe's disease, Tarui's disease, Type VIII glycogen storage disease, Type IX glycogen storage disease, Type 0 glycogen storage disease, von Gierke's disease.

glycogen synthetase the enzyme that catalyses the reaction that adds glucose units to the glycogen molecule during glycogenesis.

glycolipid *n* a lipid and carbohydrate attached. ⊃ cerebroside, ganglioside, glycosphingolipids.

glycolysis *n* a catabolic metabolic pathway that breaks down glucose 6-phosphate (G6P), derived from glucose or glycogen, and in the process generates energy which leads to production of adenosine triphosphate (ATP). In aerobic conditions, pyruvate is the end-product. In conditions when oxygen cannot be utilized anaerobic glycolysis involves the additional step of reducing pyruvate to lactate (Figure G.4)—**glycolytic** *adj*. ⊃ aerobic exercise, anaerobic exercise, Krebs' cycle.

glyconeogenesis ⊃ gluconeogenesis.

glycopeptide antibiotics a group of antibiotics, e.g. vancomycin. ⊃ Appendix 5.

glycopeptide-resistant enterococci (GRE) *n* ⊃ vancomycin-resistant enterococci.

glycoprotein IIb/IIIa inhibitors *npl* a group of drugs that reduce blood clotting. They are used in acute coronary syndromes for high risk patients, and during percutaneous coronary interventions. Examples include abciximab, eptifibatide, tirofiban.

glycoproteins *npl* large group of proteins conjugated with one or more carbohydrate residues, e.g. collagen, mucins. The term is often used generically to include proteoglycans and mucoproteins.

glycosaminoglycan a complex macromolecule considered to be the 'glue' of the cornea. It is responsible for providing the plasticity and structural support needed for successful corneal function. Along with other molecules, it comprises the solid portion of the cornea ($\sim$22%, the remainder being water). The distribution and arrangement of glycosaminoglycans are responsible for corneal transparency and thickness.

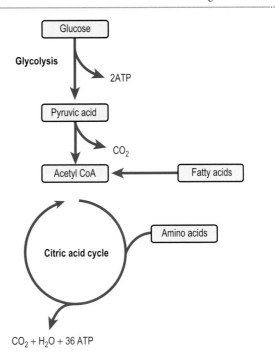

G.4 Overview of glycolysis and citric acid (Krebs') cycle (reproduced from Watson 2000 with permission).

glycosides *npl* compounds comprising a sugar joined to another molecule. If the sugar is glucose it is termed a glucoside. Many plant glycosides contain pharmacologically active substances, such as digitalis from foxgloves. *cardiac glycosides* such as digoxin increase myocardial contractility and cardiac output, and are defined as positive inotropes. ⊃ Appendix 5 (inotropes—positive).

glycosidic bond a chemical bond between a carbon of one sugar molecule and the carbon of another in a condensation reaction. For example glycogen is formed by many glucose molecules linked by glycosidic bonds.

glycosphingolipids *npl* a group of compounds that contain ceramides (lipids formed from a fatty acid and sphingosine), and a carbohydrate. They are found in the central nervous system and erythrocytes. ⊃ ganglioside.

glycosuria *n* the presence of sugar in the urine.

glycosylated haemoglobin (HbA$_{1c}$) ⊃ glycated (glycosylated) haemoglobin.

glycylcycline antibacterials a new class of antibacterial drugs. Currently tigecycline is the only example available. It is related to the tetracyclines and has demonstrated activity against several antibiotic-resistant strains of bacteria.

GM-CSF *abbr* granulocyte-macrophage colony stimulating factor.

gnathalgia *n* jaw pain.

gnathic relating to the jaw or teeth.

gnathic index a classification of skulls founded on measurements of the jaw and skull.

gnathion a craniometric point. The most anterior and inferior point of the body outline of the chin, equidistant from the pogonion and menton.

gnath/o- a prefix that means 'jaw', e.g. *gnathalgia*.

gnathodynamometer an instrument used to record and measure the forces exerted by the muscles in closing the jaws.

gnathology that branch of dental science that deals with the physiology of the masticatory mechanism.

gnathoplasty *n* plastic surgery of the jaw or cheek.

gnathosonics the study of the sounds made by the occlusion of teeth during mastication or during voluntary tooth tapping.

gnathostat a mechanical appliance used to mount and orientate plaster casts so that the Frankfort, orbital and midpalatal planes are constantly related.

GnRH *abbr* gonadotrophin-releasing hormone.

goal a clear statement of a defined outcome to be attained at a particular stage in a therapeutic intervention. A goal may be short, medium or long term. ⊃ goal setting.

goal orientation ⊃ achievement goal orientation, ego orientation, task orientation.

goal setting an essential part of any medical intervention, which occurs after identification of the client's/patient's actual and potential problems. Whenever possible, the client/patient and/or family participate in goal setting. Goals should be SMART, i.e. **S**pecific, **M**easurable, **A**chievable and **R**ealistic and **T**ime-orientated.

goblet cells mucus-secreting cells, shaped like a goblet, found in the mucosa lining the gastrointestinal and respiratory tracts. The cell has a protective mechanism since the mucus secreted acts to trap particles that have entered the respiratory tract, which are then transported via the mucociliary escalator to the mouth for clearance

Goeckerman regimen a method of treating psoriasis; exposure to ultraviolet radiation alternating with the application of a tar paste.

-gogue a suffix that means 'increasing flow', e.g. *sialagogue*.

goitre *n* struma. Thyroid gland enlargement; may be smooth (simple) or nodular, and associated with normal or abnormal thyroid function; hyperthyroid with smooth enlargement in Graves' disease, or nodular enlargement in toxic multinodular goitre; hypothyroid with glandular enlargement in Hashimoto's disease.

goitrogens *npl* agents that cause goitre. Some occur in plants, such as brassicas, e.g. cabbage.

gold (Au) *n* metallic element used in the management of rheumatoid arthritis. The radioactive isotope gold-198 (^{198}Au) is sometimes used in the treatment of some malignant diseases. Gold is heavy, soft, yellow, ductile and malleable precious metal found in its natural state and which is not dissolved by most acids. Pure gold is described as being 24 carat. Other metals may be added to it to harden it and also to change its melting point, thus reducing its carat measure of fineness. Used in dentistry, because of its favourable properties, in the construction of inlays, crowns, bridges, precision attachments and other prostheses. ⊃ carat, casting gold, fineness (of alloy), gold foil, gold solder, white gold.

gold foil a thin gold sheet historically condensed directly into cavity as a dental restorative material.

gold solder an alloy consisting of gold, silver, copper, tin and zinc, whose melting point has been adjusted to occur some 50–100°C below the melting point of the gold alloy to be soldered.

Goldenhar's syndrome (M Goldenhar, American physician, 1924–2001) a congenital condition characterized by asymmetrical facial abnormalities and associated vertebral abnormalities, low hair line, mandibular hyoplasia, low set ears, auricular appendages, sensorineural deafness, coloboma affecting the eyelids, dermoid cysts and short neck.

Goldmann applanation tonometer a contact method for measuring the intraocular pressure. ⊃ applanation, tonometry.

golfer's elbow ⊃ medial epicondylitis.

golfer's toe an inflammatory condition of the big toe, which is thought to be the result of overextension of the toe of the back foot on the follow-through. Continued overuse can lead to arthritis.

Golgi apparatus/body/complex (C Golgi, Italian histologist, 1843–1926) a cell organelle comprising a network of membranous sacs within the cytoplasm. Involved in the processing of lipids and proteins synthesized in the cell. Particularly well developed in secretory cells.

Golgi cells (C Golgi) two types of neurons; Golgi type I neurons which have a long axon and project to other parts of the nervous system, and Golgi type II neurons with short axons.

Golgi tendon organ (C Golgi) specialized proprioceptive mechanoreceptors in tendons that with skeletal muscle spindles monitor muscle stretching. Involved in proprioception. It responds to excessive muscle tension by inhibiting further muscle contraction. In so doing it protects against muscle damage. They comprise extrafusal muscle fibres that enter a funnel-like capsule that is filled with collagen fibre bundles. Nerve endings are triggered when tension in the muscle is transferred to the collagen fibres of the Golgi tendon organ. Golgi tendon organs are arranged in series with the extrafusal muscle fibres. It is designed to monitor the load or tension on a muscle, independent of its length. ⊃ extrafusal fibres.

Gompertzian growth curve a mathematical model explaining the relationship between age and the expected time of death.

gomphosis an immovable (fibrous) joint. For example, a tooth with a socket in the jaw.

gonad *n* the female or male primary reproductive structure, ovary, testis—**gonadal** *adj*.

gonadotrophic *adj* having an affinity for, or influencing, the gonads.

gonadotrophins *npl* the gonad-stimulating hormones, e.g. follicle stimulating hormone. Hormones secreted by the anterior pituitary, under the influence of the hypothalamus, which control the development and secretory function of the ovaries and testes. In pregnancy, ovarian function is under the influence of the placental secretion of human chorionic gonadotrophin (hCG), which also acts on the fetal testis. ➲ follicle stimulating hormone, human chorionic gonadotrophin, luteinizing hormone.

gonadotrophin-releasing hormone (GnRH) a hypothalamic peptide hormone that stimulates the anterior lobe of the pituitary gland to secrete the gonadotrophins.

gonad protection the use of lead rubber and/or collimation of the X-ray beam to reduce the radiation dosage to the reproductive system.

goniometer *n* protractor used to measure a joint's position when stationary, at any point over its whole range of movement; uses either a 180° or 360° system. Used in practice to assess flexibility, perhaps as part of a musculoskeletal screen—**goniometric** *adj*.

gonion a cephalometric landmark defined as the most posterior, inferior point of the angle of the mandible. It is constructed in orthodontic tracings by bisecting the angle formed by the tangents of the posterior and inferior borders of the mandible.

gonioscope an instrument used to determine how well aqueous humour is able to drain by assessing the degree to which the drainage angle of the anterior chamber of the eye is open.

gonioscopy *n* examination of the anterior chamber angle of the eye with a special lens. A routine assessment for people suspected of having glaucoma.

goniotomy *n* simple operation for congenital glaucoma. Surgical incision or use of a laser to improve the the drainage of aqueous fluid. ➲ trabeculotomy

gonococcal *adj* relating to the gonococcus or an infection caused by *Neisseria gonorrhoeae*.

Gonococcus *n* a Gram-negative diplococcus (*Neisseria gonorrhoeae*), the causative organism of gonorrhoea. It is a strict parasite—**gonococci** *pl*, **gonococcal** *adj*.

gonorrhoea *n* a sexually transmitted infection in adults. Infants can become infected during delivery, resulting in gonococcal ophthalmia neonatorum. ➲ Colour Section Figure 71. Gonococcal vulvovaginitis in girls before puberty may indicate sexual abuse. Chief manifestations of the disease in men are a purulent urethral discharge and dysuria after an average incubation period of about 6 days. The majority of women with uncomplicated infection are symptomless. Acute pelvic inflammatory disease in women, and septic arthritis with or without skin lesions, may complicate untreated gonorrhoea—**gonococcal** *adj*.

GOO *abbr* gastric outlet obstruction.

Goodell's sign softening of the cervix uteri and vagina; sign of pregnancy.

Goodpasture's disease/syndrome (E Goodpasture, American pathologist, 1886–1960) ➲ anti-GBM disease.

gooseflesh contraction of the tiny muscles attached to the hair follicles causing the hair to stand on end: it is a reaction to either cold or fear.

GORD *abbr* gastro-oesophageal reflux disease.

gothic arch tracing (arrow point tracing) ➲ tracing.

gouge *n* a chisel with a grooved blade for removing bone.

gout *n* a form of metabolic disorder in which blood levels of uric acid are raised (hyperuricaemia). It may be due to abnormal purine metabolism or increased purine intake, increased uric acid production or a reduction in the excretion of uric acid by the kidneys. Acute arthritis can result from inflammation in response to urate crystals in the joint. The big toe is characteristically involved and becomes acutely painful and swollen. Drugs that reduce uric acid levels can control the disease. If gout is untreated deposition of urate crystals can cause chronic arthritis, nodules (e.g. in the ear) and kidney damage. ➲ pseudogout, tophus.

GP *abbr* **1.** general practitioner. **2.** gas permeable (contact lens).

G6P *abbr* glucose-6-phosphate.

GPC *abbr* giant papillary conjunctivitis.

GPCL *abbr* gas permeable contact lens.

G6PD *abbr* glucose-6-phosphate dehydrogenase.

GPI *abbr* general paralysis of the insane.

GPL *abbr* gas permeable lens.

Graafian follicle a mature ovarian follicle. A minute vesicle in the ovarian stroma containing a single oocyte which is released when the vesicle ruptures at ovulation. After ovulation, the Graafian follicle forms the corpus luteum which, should fertilization occur, maintains the early pregnancy. In the absence of fertilization the corpus luteum only lasts for 12–14 days, after which it becomes the corpus albicans.

gracilis long, thin muscle of the medial thigh. The origin is on the pubis and its insertion is just below the medial condyle of the tibia. It adducts the thigh and rotates (medially) and flexes the leg. ➲ adductors of the thigh, Colour Section Figures 4, 5.

graded exercise test used to assess physiological responses to exercise, with its intensity increasing in incremental stages. ➲ exercise tolerance test (ETT).

gradient coils magnetic coils that are designed to alter the main magnetic field by a few percent. The magnetic field gradient is controlled by the electrical current passing through the coil. They are used in magnetic resonance imaging (MRI) to localize a slice and spatially encode slice information.

gradient echo (GE) a basic pulse sequence that only uses magnetic field gradient reversal to re-phase the transverse magnetization and produce echoes of the magnetic resonance signal. This allows shorter repetition times and therefore faster scanning and flip angles of less than 90°. ➲ flip angle.

gradient echo magnetic resonance imaging an advanced type of MRI scan which is more sensitive than other types of brain scan, for example computed tomography

(CT) scans. It is particularly useful in the identification of microbleeds within the brain.

gradient-index lens a lens with a refractive index (index of refraction) that changes continuously through the whole material, or part of, thus providing an area of progressive power. However, there are still problems in manufacturing these lenses reliably and without unwanted astigmatism. ⊃ progressive addition lens.

gradient test ⊃ AC/A ratio.

grading *n* **1.** in oncology, a classification of cancers based on histopathological characteristics. The level of malignancy of the tissue is determined by comparing the amount of cellular abnormality and the rate of cell division with normal cells in the same tissue. Low grade cancer generally has slow tumour growth and spread, whereas high grade cancer is aggressive with rapid spread. The grade of the disease is more important (for some types of cancer) than the stage as an indicator of prognosis and effective treatment. ⊃ differentiation, staging. **2.** in occupational therapy, the quantifiable change in activity, graded by duration, extent, level of strength or the energy needed. For example, during a therapeutic intervention aimed at increasing a client's activity or a period of time.

graft *n, v* **1.** transplanted living tissue, e.g. skin, bone and bone marrow, cornea, kidney, heart, lungs, pancreas and liver; to transplant such tissue. Grafts may involve: tissue moved from one site to another in the same individual (autograft); between genetically identical individuals (isograft); tissue obtained from a suitably matched donor (allografts or homografts); and tissue transplanted between different species (xenografts or heterografts). **2.** also includes graft material not obtained from any human or animal source, used to restore tissues or organs, e.g. acrylic, polyethylene, titanium, tantalum, chrome cobalt and stainless steel alloys.

graft versus host disease (GVHD) may follow a successful transplant, especially bone marrow, where the graft 'attacks' the tissues of the immunologically compromised host. ⊃ transplant.

grain technology the shape of the silver halide crystals in a radiographic film emulsion are referred to as grains and have two main formats, globular and tabular. ⊃ globular grains, tabular grains.

graininess random density patterns visible on a radiographic film due to the grains in the film being distributed in both area and depth and can be 'clumped' together due to the manufacturing process.

-gram a suffix that means 'a tracing', e.g. *electromyogram*.

gram (g) unit of mass. One thousand is equal to one kilogram (kg).

Gram's stain (H Gram, Danish pharmacologist and pathologist, 1853–1938) a bacteriological stain used in a basic method of identifying micro-organisms. Those staining violet are Gram-positive (+), such as *Staphylococcus aureus*, and those staining pink are Gram-negative (−), e.g. *Escherichia coli*.

grande multigravida describes a woman in her fourth or subsequent pregnancy, but who has not necessarily delivered live babies in previous pregnancies.

grande multipara describes a woman of high parity, who has delivered 4 or more babies. Increasing parity presents an increased risk of problems in pregnancy, labour and puerperium.

grand mal major epilepsy with generalized seizures. ⊃ convulsions, epilepsy, petit mal.

granular containing grains or granules.

granular cell myeloblastoma a tumour of unknown aetiology seen primarily in the tongue. Clinically, it may protrude above the surface of the tongue and histologically is made up of large cells that exhibit a granular eosinophilic cytoplasm.

granular dystrophy (*syn* corneal granular dystrophy, Groenouw's nodular type I corneal dystrophy) a hereditary condition characterized by the presence of irregularly shaped white granules of hyaline in the stroma of the cornea surrounded by clear areas. It usually develops during the first decade of life and progresses slowly throughout life. It rarely results in loss of vision although the granules are located in the centre of the cornea. If severe, though, a corneal graft/transplant is the main treatment. ⊃ corneal grafts/transplants.

granular layer of Tomes a granular layer found in the dentine immediately below the cemento-dentinal junction. It is not fully mineralized. Possibly a consequence of the unique arrangement of matrix proteins or the terminal loops of the dentinal tubules at the dentino-cementum interface.

granulation *n* **1.** the formation of new capillaries and connective tissue cells in the wound bed of an open wound, such as that occurring in a pressure ulcer that heals by secondary intention. **2.** subdivision of a solid into a small particle.

granulation tissue the new, healthy, soft tissue formed in the wound bed. Healthy granulation tissue is moist and red—**granulate** *vi*.

granulocyte *n* a cell containing granules in its cytoplasm. Describes the polymorphonuclear leucocytes—neutrophil, eosinophil and basophil.

granulocyte colony-stimulating factor (G-CSF) a growth factor that stimulates the differentiation of stem cells into granulocyte precursors.

granulocyte-macrophage colony-stimulating factor (GM-CSF) a growth factor that stimulates the differentiation of stem cells into myeloid and macrophage precursors.

granulocytopenia *n* decrease of granulocytes not sufficient to warrant the term agranulocytosis. ⊃ neutropenia

granuloma *n* a tumour formed of a mass of granulation tissue, mainly consisting of histiocytes, which occurs in reaction to chronic inflammation. ⊃ apical (dental) granuloma, eosinophilic granuloma, giant cell granuloma.

granuloma annulare a common cutaneous condition of uncertain aetiology; any association with diabetes is now thought to be spurious. Dermal nodules occur singly or in an annular configuration. They are asymptomatic but cause consternation because they commonly occur on highly visible sites such as the hands and feet. Histologically, palisading granulomas are found in the dermis. Intralesional corticosteroids can be helpful, but the natural history is spontaneous resolution after a few months to a couple of years.

granulomatosis a disorder characterized by the development of multiple granulomas. ➲ Wegener's granulomatosis.

granulomatous having the appearance of a granuloma.

granulosa cells oestradiol-secreting cells lining the Graafian follicle

granulosa lutein cells the granulosa cells remaining after ovulation which secrete oestradiol and progesterone.

granulosis the formation of a mass of granules.

graph a diagrammatical representation of two or more groups of data.

-graph a suffix that means 'instrument for writing or recording', e.g. *electrocardiograph*.

graphics computerized 'drawing', known as computer-aided drawing (CAD). The ability of the computer to produce preprogrammed graphic characters. The mode the computer has to be placed in prior to drawing graphics.

graphics interchange format (GIF) a compressed computer graphics file.

graphics tablet a piece of equipment that can digitize drawing or graphs ready for input into the computer.

graphite black lead, plumbago. One of the allotropic forms of carbon, the other being diamond. A soft, dark grey-to-black crystalline substance used as a lubricant and for the fabrication of lead pencils, furnance crucibles and as a conductor of electric currents.

grasp reflex a primitive reflex normally present in newborns; when the palm or sole is stroked the digits flex in a grasping action. If the reflex is not symmetrical or persists after 2–3 months of age it may indicate a lesion in the premotor cortex. The grasp reflex, and other primitive reflexes, may reappear in adults following a stroke or traumatic brain injury.

Graves' disease (R Graves, Irish physician, 1797–1853) hyperthyroidism due to production of stimulating thyroid-stimulating hormone (TSH) receptor antibodies; may also cause ophthalmopathy (eye disease), often evident as prominence of the eyes (exophthalmos) and pre-tibial myxoedema. ➲ hyperthyroidism.

Graves' ophthalmopathy (R Graves) a collection of eye signs associated with Graves' hyperthyroidism. These include retraction of the eyelids (Dalrymple's sign), exophthalmos, lid lag in which the upper lid follows after a latent period when the eye looks downward (von Graefe's sign), convergence weakness (Möebius' sign), raised intraocular pressure (IOP), especially on upgaze, and defective eye movements (restrictive myopathy) in addition to the signs and symptoms of hyperthypodism. If only the eye signs of the disease are present without clinical evidence of hyperthyroidism, the disease is called euthyroid or ophthalmic Graves' disease. Treatment begins with control of the hyperthyroidism (if present). Some

cases may recover spontaneously with time. Mild cases of ocular deviations and restrictions may benefit from a prismatic correction. Corticosteroids and radiotherapy may be needed and surgery is a common form of management especially when there is diplopia in the primary position of gaze. ➲ Dalrymple's sign, diagnostic positions of gaze, exophthalmos, Möebius' sign, ophthalmoplegia, thyroid ophthalmopathy, von Graefe's sign.

gravid *adj* pregnant; carrying fertilized eggs or a fetus.

gravidum gingivitis inflammation of the mucous membrane and underlying tissues of the gum. It is associated with the pregnancy hormones.

gravitation, law of relates the attraction between two bodies or objects to their masses and the distance between their centres of gravity squared. First proposed by Newton (I Newton, English scientist, 1642–1727).

gravitational *adj* being attracted by force of gravity.

gravitational acceleration acceleration caused by the gravitational attraction between two bodies or objects which depends on their masses and the distance between them squared. ➲ acceleration, angular acceleration, instantaneous acceleration, linear acceleration, tangential acceleration.

gravitational potential energy the energy due to the position of a body or object in a gravitational field. Often calculated as weight multiplied by vertical height above some base (arbitrary) datum. Also known as potential energy.

gravitational (stasis) eczema occurs on the lower legs and is often associated with signs of venous insufficiency (oedema, red or bluish discoloration, loss of hair, induration, haemosiderin pigmentation and ulceration). ➲ venous ulcers.

gravitational ulcer ➲ venous ulcer.

gravity *n* the force due to the attraction between two bodies or objects which depends on the product of their masses and inversely on the square of the distance between their centres of gravity. ➲ specific gravity.

Grawitz tumour (P Grawitz, German pathologist, 1850–1932) ➲ hypernephroma.

gray (Gy) *n* (L Gray, British medical physicist, 1905–1965) the derived Système International d'Unités (SI) unit (International System of Units) for the absorbed dose of radiation. It has replaced the rad. ➲ Appendix 2.

GRE *n* glycopeptide-resistant enterococci.

great (long) saphenous vein ➲ saphenous veins.

greater omentum ➲ omentum.

greater palatine foramen the opening that conducts the greater palatine nerve and blood vessels to and from the mucous membrane of the palate. Situated close to the posterior border of the hard palate in the region of the palatal root of the upper third molar on each side of the midline.

greater palatine nerve the nerve descending through the greater palatine foramen, running forwards in a groove in the palate to the mucous membrane of the palate. Gives rise to the lesser palatine nerve which passes through the lesser palatine foramen to supply the soft palate and its mucous membrane.

great vein of Galen a large cerebral vein passing from the midbrain and entering the junction of the inferior longitudinal and straight sinuses. The extreme, abnormal or rapid fetal skull moulding during delivery may cause the cerebral membranes, the venous sinuses and cerebral veins to be torn causing intracranial haemorrhage.

green the hue sensation evoked by stimulating the retina with rays of wavelength 490–560 nm and situated between blue and yellow. The complementary colour of green is a non-spectral colour situated in the red-purple region. ⊃ complementary colour, purple.

green blindness ⊃ deuteranopia.

green filter (*syn* red-free filter) a filter which transmits only green light. It may be used in ophthalmoscopy to increase the contrast of the blood vessels to the background facilitating the visibility of retinal circulation defects, haemorrhages and microaneurysms and the distinction between retinal and choroidal lesions. However, ophthalmoscopes actually use a filter which transmits a certain amount of red light as otherwise the observation would be so dark as to make it extremely difficult. ⊃ ophthalmoscope.

green monkey disease ⊃ Marburg disease.

green rouge a very fine polishing powder containing green chromium oxide. Used in the dental laboratory to polish chrome metal prostheses.

green stick in dentistry, a specific type of thermoplastic impression material.

greenstick fracture ⊃ fracture.

green stick impression material ⊃ impression material.

green-weakness ⊃ deuteranomaly.

gregarious *adj* showing a preference for living in a group, liking to mix and fond of company. The herd instinct is an inborn tendency of many species, including humans.

Greinacher circuit comprises two rectifiers connected in series, and two capacitors connected in series to produce a fully rectified waveform with a ripple effect on the tube voltage but a constant tube current.

grey literature reports that are unpublished or have limited distribution and are not included in the common bibliographic retrieval systems.

grey matter unmyelinated nerve fibres and nerve cell bodies situated in the central nervous system. ⊃ white matter.

grey scale display a method of showing the texture of tissue on an ultrasound display, the amplitude of each echo is represented by varying shades of grey, white outline from specular surfaces, mottled grey from various tissue areas and black from collections of fluid. The variation of shades of grey in which a computed tomography (CT) image may be represented on screen.

grey syndrome potentially fatal condition seen in preterm babies, due to reaction to the antibiotic chloramphenicol. It is characterized by an ashen grey cyanosis, vomiting, abdominal distension, hypothermia and shock.

Grey Turner's sign (G Grey Turner, British surgeon, 1877–1951) bruising around the flanks/loin. A sign of acute haemorrhagic pancreatitis. ⊃ Cullen's sign.

grid 1. a device constructed of strips of high atomic number material (e.g. lead) which absorbs the scattered radiation and low atomic number material which allows the primary beam to pass through thus improving radiographic contrast of the image. **2.** a series of horizontal and vertical lines forming squares of uniform size, used as a reference for the plotting of curves.

grid lattice the number of lines of lead per centimetre in a secondary radiation grid.

grid ratio the ratio of the height of the lead strips to the width of the spaces between them in a secondary radiation grid.

grief the emotional reaction to loss, separation or death.

grieving process describes the stages, denial, anger, bargaining, depression, acceptance and possibly fear, that an individual may experience in relation to bereavement and dying. Grieving is also associated with other situations of loss including: loss of employment or a companion animal, loss of body function, such as infertility, or of a body part, e.g. limb, breast. ⊃ bereavement.

Griffith's types subdivisions of Lancefield group A streptococci based on their antigenic structure.

grind 1. to sharpen or smooth by friction. **2.** to crush food with the posterior teeth. **3.** the elimination of high spots on tooth contours by the use of abrasive tools.

grinding-in the fine adjustment to the occlusion of artificial teeth by selective grinding.

grip dynamometer instrument for measuring the maximum isometric force with which an individual can squeeze two handles together between palm and fingers. Also known as handgrip dynamometer.

gripe *n* abdominal colic.

grocer's itch contact dermatitis, especially from flour or sugar.

Groenouw's nodular type I corneal dystrophy ⊃ granular dystrophy.

groin *n* the junction of the thigh with the abdomen.

groin pain is most common in dynamic sports where quick turns are made, such as football, martial arts and skiing. The cause can be difficult to identify. Sporting causes include strains of the muscles in the area (e.g. the adductors, gluteal muscles, iliopsoas), bursitis, osteitis pubis and hernias. Abduction of the leg against resistance is restricted by pain. Because there are more serious causes of groin pain, a full clinical examination must be carried out if the pain is persistent. Treatment can be difficult and requires a formal rehabilitation programme to prevent a chronic condition. ⊃ groin strain.

groin strain an injury which results from overstretching of the adductors in the groin, especially common in football. Requires a rehabilitation programme for both flexibility and strengthening. ⊃ groin pain.

grommet *n* ventilation tube inserted through the tympanic membrane into the middle ear. Used in the treatment of persistent otitis media with effusion ('glue ear') in children. ⊃ myringotomy, otitis media with effusion (OME).

gross motor skill ⊃ motor skill.

gross tumour volume (GTV) the total visible or palpable extent of a malignant growth.

Grotthus' law ⊃ Draper's law.

grounded theory research study where a hypothesis is elicited from the data gathered.

ground glass (*syn* depolished glass) glass which has been ground with emery, sandblasted or etched with fluoric acid to give it a matt surface. Such glass is usually translucent but not transparent. ⊃ frosted lens, translucent, transparent.

ground reaction force the force that acts on a body as a result of the body resting on or hitting the ground.

ground state when the inner orbits of an atom are filled and therefore the atom is at its lowest energy state.

group activity a structured series of actions or tasks that are carried out by a number of people acting together.

group B streptococcus (GBS) a baterial commensal found in the rectum or vagina of 20–25% pregnant women. Many infants are colonized with group B streptococci (GBS) at birth and have no ill effects, but 1 in 16 000 infants develop infection in the first week of life and it is a leading cause of neonatal bacterial sepsis, pneumonia and meningitis, with 1 in 10 affected infants dying. The maternal risk factors include preterm delivery, prolonged membrane rupture and chorioamnionitis; prophylactic intrapartum antibiotics may reduce the severity of neonatal effects. Neonatal risk factors include a previous infant with early onset GBS infection, GBS identified in maternal swabs or maternal urine, maternal pyrexia in labour >38°C, preterm labour and prolonged rupture of membranes >18 hours.

group C meningococcal disease serious disease caused by group C *Neisseria meningitidis*. It causes meningococcal meningitis and life-threatening septicaemia usually in children and young adults. Effective immunization is available and is provided as part of routine immunization programmes.

group cohesion a group's tendency to stick together in its pursuit of common goals. Also known as team cohesion.

group dynamics the social structures, relationships, behaviours, interactions and processes that occur in groups and influence how the group works.

group environment the task-related or social aspects of a group that can facilitate or undermine group cohesion.

group function the simultaneous contact of a group of mandibular and maxillary teeth in lateral movements on the working side thus distributing occlusal forces.

group integration the beliefs that individual group members hold about the cohesiveness of the group as a whole.

group psychotherapy ⊃ psychotherapy.

group therapy an approach to treatment in which clients work together with the therapist to explore feelings, learn new skills, rehearse alternative ways of interacting with others and/or complete a group task.

growth curve a graph of change-in-height against age, which shows the greatest rate of change in infancy, flattening off until the growth spurt which on average reaches a peak at about age 12 in girls and 14 in boys.

growth factor substances, usually polypeptides and proteins, that stimulate the differentiation and proliferation of new cells. Important, for example, in fetal development and wound healing. They include those that stimulate specific blood cell proliferation such as the colony-stimulating factors, platelet-derived growth factor, interleukins, nerve growth factors, insulin-like growth factor, epidermal growth factor.

growth hormone (GH) (*syn* somatotrophin). Also known as human growth hormone (HGH). A hormone secreted by the anterior pituitary gland under the influence of two hypothalamic hormones: growth hormone releasing hormone (GHRH) and growth hormone release inhibiting hormone (GHRIH) or somatostatin. As well as being vital for normal growth and development (e.g. stimulates the growth of the long bones), GH is involved throughout life in metabolism and utilization of all the macronutrients, e.g. it increases protein synthesis and raises blood glucose level. GH acts directly on some body cells e.g. on adipocytes, promoting triacylglycerol (triglyceride) breakdown but mostly indirectly, via the anabolic insulin-like growth factors (IGF) (somatomedins) which it causes the liver and other tissues to release, crucial, for example, for the muscle hypertrophy resulting from training. For this reason supplements rich in arginine, which is believed (but without conclusive evidence) to promote GH secretion, are frequently taken by body builders. Any exercise of sufficient intensity stimulates GH release; its level in the blood has been shown to rise within the first 15 minutes and it is important throughout in maintaining lipolysis and lipid metabolism. Synthetic GH is commercially available, but banned in sport. ⊃ acromegaly, dwarfism, gigantism, insulin-like growth factors.

growth hormone test a test for acromegaly. Growth hormone levels are measured during an oral glucose tolerance test. In acromegaly the level of growth hormone does not show the normal suppression with glucose.

growth scan when two or three measurements are taken of the abdomen, head and femur of a fetus in the second and third trimester using ultrasound imaging. The weight of the fetus is calculated by using charts.

grunting an abnormal breath sound heard mainly in newborns. It is a serious sign and indicates respiratory distress. It is noted on expiration indicating that the glottis has closed to the flow of air out of the lungs, usually to prevent alveolar collapse. Heard in preterm infants suffering from respiratory distress syndrome.

GSD *abbr* glycogen storage diseases.

GSL *abbr* general sales list.

GTR *abbr* guided tissue regeneration.

GTT *abbr* **1.** gestational trophoblastic tumour. **2.** glucose tolerance test.

GTV *abbr* gross tumour volume.

GU *abbr* genitourinary.

Guanarito virus a virus of the familiy *Arenaviridae*. It is the causative organism of Venezuelan haemorrhagic fever.

guanine *n* a nitrogenous base derived from purine. With other bases, one or more phosphate groups and a sugar it is

G
H

part of the nucleic acids DNA and RNA. ➲ deoxyribo-nucleic acid, ribonucleic acid.

guar *n* a soluble form of non-starch polysaccharide (NSP) fibre derived from the locust bean. Taken orally, it absorbs water from the intestine and produces a feeling of fullness and slows the rate of carbohydrate absorption. May be used in the management of some types of diabetes mellitus to reduce postprandial blood glucose levels.

guardian ad litem an individual from a social work or childcare background who is appointed to ensure that a court is fully informed of the relevant facts that relate to a child, and that the child's wishes and feelings are clearly demonstrated.

guarding intense contraction of the abdominal muscles. Occurs involuntarily in the presence of visceral pain, peritonitis, or following abdominal surgery if the abdomen is touched, such as during physical examination.

guardsman's fracture a type of jaw fracture. ➲ jaw fracture.

guard wire the baseplate of an orthodontic appliance may have a guard wire attached to its fitting surface, to limit any distortion of small springs while in use and under pressure.

gubernacular relating to a gubernaculum.

gubernacular canal a canal in the alveolar bone through which the dental follicle and unerupted teeth are connected to the oral mucosa by a cord of connective tissue known as the dental gubernaculum. ➲ dental gubernaculum.

gubernaculum *n* a guiding pathway, for example one of two strands of fibrous tissue that attach the fetal gonads within the inguinal region—**gubernacula** *pl*. ➲ dental gubernaculum.

Guedel airway (A Guedel, American anaesthetist, 1883–1956) a plastic oropharyngeal device used to maintain the airway. ➲ airway.

Guérin fracture Le Fort I fracture of the middle third of the facial skeleton. ➲ Le Fort classification.

guidance a method of controlling the direction or regulation of movements such as teeth. *anterior guidance* **1.** the moving anterior tooth contacts that guide mandibular movements. **2.** that part of an articulator on which the guide pin slides and thus mechanically reproduces mandibular movements. *canine guidance* ➲ canine protected articulation.

guided fantasy a therapeutic technique in which the therapist outlines to the client or group a theme or situation designed to stimulate their imagination. An example of this is the fantasy journey in which the therapist talks the client through the process of setting out, travelling and arriving at a destination, leaving the details to the client's imagination.

guided imagery ➲ imagery.

guided tissue regeneration (GTR) a technique used in surgical periodontics in which membranes are used to guide the path of epithelial cell regeneration and thus permit unhindered regeneration of connective tissues.

guide pin in dentistry, a metal rod attached to one part of an articulator and contacting the anterior guide table on the opposing portion of the articulator.

guide plane in dentistry, the two or more prepared parallel surfaces of abutment teeth used to limit and guide the path of insertion of a removable prosthesis.

guide table in dentistry, that part of an articulator on which the anterior guide pin rests and thus maintains the established vertical dimension. ➲ guide pin.

guidewire a device used to position an intravenous catheter, endotracheal tube, central venous line or gastric feeding tube.

Guillain–Barré syndrome (GBS) (G Guillain, French neurologist, 1876–1951; J Barré, French neurologist, 1880–1967) an acquired acute inflammatory demyelinating peripheral polyneuropathy that can occur after an infection such as campylobacter gastroenteritis. It may lead to pain, muscle weakness, sensory loss, paralysis and in some patients respiratory problems requiring support with mechanical ventilation. Management involves the prompt administration of intravenous immunoglobulins, possibly plasmapheresis and supportive measures such as respiratory support and physiotherapy.

guillotine *n* a surgical instrument for excision of the tonsils.

Guinea worm ➲ *Dracunculus medinensis*.

Gulf War syndrome/illness the set of physical and psychological effects observed in individuals who served in the Gulf War in 1991. It includes fatigue, headaches, dizziness, dyspnoea, memory problems, skin rashes, joint pains, dyspepsia.

gullet *n* the oesophagus.

GUM *abbr* genitourinary medicine. ➲ sexually transmitted infection.

gum 1. a colloquial term for gingiva. **2.** adhesive material prepared from the dried viscous sap exuded by certain trees and plants, for example gum benzoin.

gum benzoin in dentistry, balsam resin employed in Whitehead's varnish.

gumboil previously used to refer to a sinus leading from a subperiosteal abscess. ➲ dentoalveolar abscess.

gum dammar in dentistry, a natural resin used in the manufacture of waxes, baseplate materials and impression compounds.

gum scissors ➲ scissors.

gum tragacanth dried gummy exudate obtained from the incised stems of certain trees. Used in dentistry as a denture fixative.

gumma *n* a localized area of vascular granulation tissue that develops in the later stages (tertiary) of syphilis. If near the surface of the body, may form chronic ulcers—**gummata** *pl*.

gumshield ➲ protective equipment in sport.

Gunning type fixation ➲ fixation (dentistry/maxillofacial surgery).

Gunn's syndrome (R M Gunn, British ophthalmologist, 1850–1909). ➲ jaw-winking.

Gurney Mott theory theory of latent image formation stating that electrons are trapped and then escape several times before another electron is trapped forming a stable two-atom silver speck called the latent sub-image centre, this attracts further electrons causing a build up of silver atoms which eventually destroys the crystal lattice and allows development to take place. ⊃ Mitchell theory.

gustation *n* the chemical sense of taste. Closely linked to that of olfaction (smell).

gustatory *adj* relating to gustation, or to the structures involved in taste sensation. For example the gustatory pathways (via the VIIth, IXth and Xth cranial nerves) and the gustatory area of the cortex.

gustatory stimulus a substance which stimulates the taste receptor nerve endings in the mouth and causes a flow of saliva. At a basic level, the tastes are recognized as sweet, sour, salt and bitter.

gustatory sweating ⊃ Frey's syndrome.

gut *n* the intestines, large and small.

gut decontamination the use of non-absorbable antibiotics to prevent endogenous infection in patients having intestinal surgery or those who are immunocompromised because of drugs or neutropenia.

Guthrie test (R Guthrie, American physician/bacteriologist, 1916–1995) a screening test, originally for phenylketonuria, carried out within the first week of life after the infant has ingested enough phenylalanine (an amino acid) in milk feeds. Drops of blood are collected on special filter paper. Assays are performed to screen for phenylketonuria and since the development of newer analytical techniques conditions including congenital hypothyroidism, cystic fibrosis, sickle-cell diseases and, in some countries, galactosaemia. Infants with a positive test must have the diagnosis confirmed.

guttae *npl* medication in drop form, usually for use as ear or eye drops—**gutta** *sing*.

gutta percha a substance with rubber-like properties obtained from the sap of rubber trees. Available in sheets, points and sticks, it softens when warmed. Used in dentistry for a temporary dressing or in root canal treatment to obliterate the pulp canal and seal the apical foramen.

gutta percha point a slender cone of gutta percha used in endodontic treatment to obturate the entire root canal.

GVHD *abbr* graft versus host disease.

Gy *abbr* gray

gymnastic balls large air-filled balls that can be used in treatment to provide a mobile support, enabling smooth movements and stimulation of postural mechanisms. The balls need to be well inflated to withstand the weight of the person with minimum deformation.

gymnast's back injury to the back, including fractures, due to excessive hyperextension during gymnastic activity.

gynae- a prefix that means 'female', e.g. *gynaecomastia*.

gynaecoid *adj* relating to something that has female characteristics.

gynaecoid pelvis normal female pelvis, almost round at the brim, cavity and outlet, roomy, shallow and ideally shaped for childbearing.

gynaecologist *n* a surgeon who specializes in gynaecology, women's health issues and the diseases of the female reproductive system.

gynaecology *n* the science dealing with the diseases of the female reproductive system—**gynaecological** *adj*.

gynaecomastia *n* enlargement of the male mammary gland.

gynandromorphism presence of chromosomes of both sexes in different tissues of the body, producing a mosaic of male and female sexual characteristics—**gynandromorphous** *adj*.

gypsum *n* plaster of Paris (calcium sulphate).

gyromagnetic ratio (γ) is a proportionality constant and is fixed for the nucleus, for example 42.6 MHz/tesla for hydrogen.

gyrus *n* a convoluted portion of cerebral cortex.

G

H

H

[H$^+$] symbol for hydrogen ion concentration.

HAART *abbr* highly active antiretroviral therapy.

habilitation *n* the means by which a child gradually progresses towards the maximum degree of independence of which he or she is capable. ⊃ rehabilitation.

habit *n* **1.** any learnt behaviour that has a relatively high probability of occurrence in response to a situation or stimulus. Acquisition of habits may depend on both reinforcement and associative learning. **2.** in orthodontics, a persistent tendency to repeat the practice of thumb, finger, lip or tongue sucking which sometimes displaces the teeth.

habit (occupational therapy) a performance pattern in daily life, acquired by frequent repetition, that does not require attention and allows efficient function. (Reproduced with permission from the European Network of Occupational Therapy in Higher Education (ENOTHE) Terminology Project, 2008.)

habit posture instinctively and reflexively produced and maintained posture in which the muscles are in active contraction.

habitual abortion ⊃ recurrent or habitual miscarriage.

habitual posture of the mandible ⊃ rest position of the mandible.

habituation *n* describes a decreasing response to a stimulus when it becomes familiar through repeated presentation, for example becoming less aware of the feel of clothing on the skin. It is often used in a negative sense in relation to drug use or misuse, when repeated intake of the drug creates psychological dependence. ⊃ drug dependence.

HACE *abbr* high-altitude cerebral (o)edema.

haem *n* the non-protein, iron-containing pigment portion of haemoglobin. Each haemoglobin molecule contains four haem groups. A haem group is a porphyrin comprising an atom of ferrous iron (Fe^{2+}) surrounded by four pyrrole rings.

haemagglutination *n* the agglutination or clumping together of red blood cells, such as that caused by the transfusion of an incompatible blood group. ⊃ agglutination, blood groups.

haemagglutinin *n* an antibody that causes red blood cells to agglutinate. They may be autologous, homologous, or heterologous according to the source of the cells affected.

haema, haemat, haemo- a prefix that means 'blood', e.g. *haematuria*.

haemangioblastoma a tumour of vascular origin.

haemangioma *n* a malformation of blood vessels which may occur in any part of the body. When in the skin it is one form of birthmark, appearing as a red spot or a 'port wine stain'—**haemangiomata** *pl.*

Haemaphysalis a genus of ticks. Many species transmit rickettsial, bacterial and viral infections. These include some types of typhus, tularaemia and encephalitis.

haemarthrosis *n* the presence of blood in a joint cavity, such as that resulting from trauma, or those that occur spontaneously or follow minor trauma in people with haemophilia. In sport haemarthrosis is most commonly seen in the knee joint where it is always indicative of significant injury such as cruciate (70% have an anterior cruciate tear) and/or collateral ligament injury, intra-articular fractures, meniscal tears or patellar dislocation. Blood accumulates in the joint within 1–2 h in a haemarthrosis compared to the slower (24+h) accumulation in a joint effusion. Early referral to a knee specialist is recommended because of the potential for intervention to prevent chronic joint damage—**haemarthroses** *pl.* ⊃ Colour Section Figure 72.

haematemesis *n* the vomiting of blood, which may be bright red following recent bleeding. Otherwise it is of 'coffee ground' appearance due to the action of gastric juice. The bleeding is usually from the upper gastrointestinal tract and causes include: peptic ulcer, oesophageal varices, cancers, gastritis, drug erosions and coagulation defects, but blood swallowed from elsewhere, e.g. during epistaxis, or following oral trauma or dental extraction, may be vomited.

haematin *n* a ferric (Fe^{3+}) iron-containing derivative of haemoglobin formed by the oxidation of the ferrous iron molecule.

haematinuria dark urine caused by the presence of haematin or haemoglobin in the urine.

haematinic *n* a substance required for the production of red blood cells, for example iron, vitamin B$_{12}$ and folic acid.

haematocele *n* a swelling filled with blood.

haematocolpos *n* retained blood in the vagina such as caused by an imperforate hymen. ⊃ cryptomenorrhoea.

haematocrit *n* the proportion by volume of blood occupied by erythrocytes (red blood cells, RBC). Exercise-induced increase in haematocrit, together with measurement of haemoglobin concentration, allows estimation of change in plasma volume. Also known as packed cell volume (PCV). ⊃ altitude acclimatization, packed cell volume.

haematogenous *adj* relating to blood. Originating in the blood or being transported in the blood.

haematohidrosis a condition in which the sweat contains blood.

haematology *n* the science dealing with the formation, composition, functions and diseases of the blood—**haematological** *adj*, **haematologically** *adv*.

haematoma *n* a swelling composed of extravasated blood, usually traumatic in origin. One of the most common injuries in sport and one which benefits from early treatment with ice, compression and elevation—**haematomata** *pl.* ➲ extradural haematoma, subdural haematoma.

haematometra *n* an accumulation of blood (or menstrual fluid) in the uterus.

haematomyelia *n* haemorrhage in the spinal cord.

haematopoiesis *n* ➲ haemopoiesis.

haematosalpinx *n* (*syn* haemosalpinx) blood in the uterine (fallopian) tube.

haematospermia *n* the discharge of blood-stained semen. It may occur in infection of the seminal vesicles.

haematozoa *npl* parasites living in the blood—**haematozoon** *sing.*

haematuria *n* blood in the urine; may be macroscopic, i.e. visible to the naked eye, when it may be bright red, dark red or smoky in appearance; or microscopic when it is not and can only be detected by chemical tests or microscopy. Haematuria may be caused by urinary tract problems, such as glomerulonephritis, trauma to the kidney, cancers, stones, infections; or be caused by coagulation defects or anticoagulant drugs—**haematuric** *adj.*

haemoccult test a chemical test to detect minute quantities of blood in the faeces.

haemochromatosis *n* iron storage disease **1.** primary haemochromatosis (*syn* bronzed diabetes) is an inherited error in iron metabolism, usually increased iron absorption, with iron deposition in tissues, resulting in brown pigmentation of the skin, cirrhosis of the liver and iron damage to other organs such as the heart, pancreatic islet cells (causing diabetes) and endocrine glands. Management includes weekly venesection until the serum iron is normal, and thereafter at intervals that maintain iron stores at normal levels. In addition, treatment as necessary for cirrhosis and diabetes mellitus. **2.** secondary haemochromatosis may be associated with any condition requiring multiple blood transfusions, (e.g. thalassaemia and other chronic haemolytic disorders), excess intake of dietary iron and some types of porphyria. Chelating agents such as desferroxamine are used to remove the excess iron—**haemochromatotic** *adj.*

haemoconcentration *n* relative increase of volume of red blood cells to volume of plasma (i.e. an increase in packed cell volume), usually due to loss of the fluid portion of blood, but may be caused by excess red blood cell production.

haemocytometer *n* an instrument for counting the number of blood cells in a given volume of blood.

haemodiafiltration (CVVHD) *n* similar to haemofiltration, but with the addition of dialysate. Diffusion occurs and the removal of unwanted molecules is enhanced. Used as renal replacement therapy.

haemodialysis *n* dialysis involving impurity, waste or toxin removal directly from the bloodstream using a dialyser and dialysate both outside the body. Often requires the use of an arteriovenous fistula. A method of renal replacement therapy used in patients in end-stage renal disease/failure

(irreversible) or in acute renal failure (potentially reversible). The patient's blood is diverted from the body to pass through a dialyser machine for diffusion and filtration and then returned to the patient's circulation. The procedure takes from 3–8 hours and may take place daily or two or three times a week.

haemodilution *n* relative decrease of volume of red blood cells to volume of plasma, usually due to an increase in the volume of blood plasma.

haemodilution of pregnancy in spite of the normal physiological increase in red blood cell numbers during pregnancy, the concurrent increase in plasma volume leads to haemodilution. There is reduced concentration of haemoglobin, immunoglobulins and other plasma proteins.

haemodynamics the study of blood circulation.

haemofiltration (CVVH) *n* form of renal replacement therapy (artificial kidney treatment), in which the patient's blood is passed through a filter allowing separation of an ultrafiltrate containing fluid and solutes. This is discarded and replaced with an isotonic solution. Usually continuous as in continuous veno-venous haemofiltration.

haemoglobin (Hb) *n* the red, respiratory pigment in the red blood cells. A molecule comprises 4 ferrous (Fe^{2+}) iron-containing haem groups and 4 globin chains, two alpha (α) chains and two beta (β) chains (Figure H.1). It combines with oxygen and releases it to the tissues. Some carbon dioxide is carried by haemoglobin, which also acts to buffer pH changes. There is a special form of fetal haemoglobin (HbF) which has a high affinity for oxygen, and two major adult forms (HbA, HbA_2). Some adult haemoglobin is glycated or glycosylated (HbA_{1c}). HbF is normally replaced by adult forms during early childhood. However, some individuals have a genetic abnormality whereby fetal haemoglobin production continues into adulthood. There are many different haemoglobins which cause disease, e.g. Hb C, Hb E, Hb H, Hb S, etc. ➲ glycated (glycosylated)

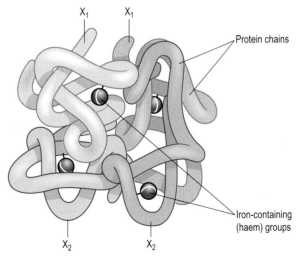

H.1 Haemoglobin (reproduced from Waugh & Grant 2006 with permission).

haemoglobin, haemoglobinopathy, oxyhaemoglobin, sickle cell disease, thalassaemia.

haemoglobinaemia *n* free haemoglobin in the blood plasma—**haemoglobinaemic** *adj*.

haemoglobinometer *n* an instrument for estimating the percentage of haemoglobin in the blood.

haemoglobinopathy *n* usually hereditary abnormality of the haemoglobin molecule. Very common genetic condition worldwide—**haemoglobinopathic** *adj*. ⊃ sickle cell disease, thalassaemia.

haemoglobinuria *n* haemoglobin in the urine. It is the result of substantial intravascular haemolysis leading to haemoglobinaemia. Also occurs as an acute transient condition in some infectious diseases—**haemoglobinuric** *adj*. ⊃ march haemoglobinuria, paroxysmal cold haemoglobinuria, paroxysmal nocturnal haemoglobinuria.

haemolysin *n* an agent capable of causing disintegration of red blood cells. Such as the substances produced by certain bacteria, e.g. streptococci.

haemolysis *n* breakdown of red blood cells, with liberation of contained haemoglobin. This happens normally at the end of the cell's lifespan and the constituent parts are dealt with by various physiological processes. Haemolysis occurs pathologically and the causes include red blood cell defects, haemoglobinopathies, transfusion of incompatible blood, infections (e.g. malaria, *Escherichia coli* type 0157), disseminated intravascular coagulation, mechanical trauma (e.g. a faulty heart valve), antibodies, hypersplenism (overactive spleen), drugs and exposure to chemicals—**haemolytic** *adj*.

haemolytic anaemia an anaemia caused by the premature destruction of red blood cells, as with some drugs and toxins, autoimmune processes, or results from an inherited red cell structural defect, red cell metabolic defects or disorders of haemoglobin. ⊃ acquired haemolytic anaemia, anaemia, congenital haemolysis, haemoglobinopathy, red cell enzymopathies, red cell membrane defects.

haemolytic disease of the newborn (*syn* erythroblastosis fetalis) a pathological condition in the newborn child due to Rhesus incompatibility between the child's blood and that of the mother. Red blood cell destruction occurs with anaemia, often jaundice and an excess of erythroblasts or primitive red blood cells in the circulating blood. Immunization of women at risk, using anti-D (Rh$_0$) immunoglobulin, can prevent haemolytic disease of the newborn. Treatment of affected infants may include: phototherapy, blood transfusion and exchange transfusion in severe cases. ⊃ anti-D (Rh$_0$) immunoglobulin, hydrops fetalis, icterus gravis neonatorum, kernicterus.

haemolytic uraemic syndrome (HUS) intravascular haemolysis and acute renal failure that occurs in association with another condition, such as food poisoning due to enterohaemorrhagic *Escherichia coli* type 0157. Those affected (mainly children) may need renal replacement therapy. The majority make a full recovery, but others will have residual renal problems.

haemopericardium *n* blood in the pericardial sac. ⊃ cardiac tamponade.

haemoperitoneum *n* blood in the peritoneal cavity.

haemophilias *npl* a group of conditions with inherited blood coagulation defects. In clinical practice the most commonly encountered defects are *haemophilia A*, factor VIII procoagulant deficiency: *haemophilia B* or Christmas disease, factor IX procoagulant deficiency. Both these conditions are X-linked recessive disorders resulting in an increased tendency to bleed, the severity of which depends on the amount of residual factor VIII or IX. Bleeding typically occurs into joints and muscles. ⊃ haemophilic arthropathy, von Willebrand's disease.

haemophilic arthropathy joint disease associated with haemophilia. The extent of joint damage has been 'staged' from radiological findings: (a) synovial thickening, (b) epiphyseal overgrowth, (c) minor joint changes and cyst formation, (d) definite joint changes with loss of joint space, (e) end-stage joint destruction and secondary changes leading to deformity.

Haemophilus *n* a genus of bacteria. Small Gram-negative rods which show much variation in shape (pleomorphism). They are strict parasites. *Haemophilus aegypticus* causes acute infectious conjunctivitis. *Haemophilus ducreyi* causes chancroid. *Haemophilus influenzae* causes acute epiglottitis, otitis media and meningitis in young children, and pneumonia in people with chronic lung disease. Effective immunization is available as part of routine programmes. ⊃ Hib vaccine. *Haemophilus pertussis* ⊃ *Bordetella pertussis*.

haemophthalmia bleeding into the vitreous body (humour) of the eye. ⊃hyphaema.

haemopneumothorax *n* the presence of blood and air in the pleural cavity.

haemopoiesis *n* (*syn* haematopoiesis) the formation of blood cells. During fetal life haemopoiesis starts in the yolk sac, liver and spleen. As fetal development progresses the active red bone marrow in all bones becomes the main site for haemopoiesis. Most of the active red marrow is replaced by yellow (fatty) marrow during childhood. In adults the red haemopoietic marrow is confined to ends of long bones, the sternum, pelvis and vertebrae. Red marrow contains pluripotent stem cells that are able to self-replicate and differentiate into any type of mature blood cell. Haemopoiesis is controlled by several growth factors, e.g. erythropoietin (EPO), granulocyte colony-stimulating factor (G-CSF), granulocyte-macrophage colony stimulating factor (GM-CSF), thrombopoietin, interleukins, etc., that cause the stem cells to differentiate into a specific blood cell type. ⊃ erythropoiesis—**haemopoietic** *adj*.

haemopoietic stem cell transplantation (HSCT) (*syn* bone marrow transplant) the infusion of stem cells into a patient's vein. The bone marrow may be obtained either on an earlier occasion from the patient (autologous transplantation) or from a suitable donor (allogeneic transplantation), or from stem cells obtained from umbilical cord blood. Usually follows myeloablative doses of chemotherapy or

G
H

radiotherapy as therapy for (most commonly) haematological cancers, other blood disorders, some genetic conditions, although also used therapeutically and experimentally for some solid tumours.

haemoptysis *n* the coughing up of blood or blood-stained mucus from the respiratory tract. The amount ranges from blood-streaked mucus up to a life-threatening haemorrhage. The blood may be bright red, frothy or rusty in appearance. Causes include chronic bronchitis, pneumonia, lung abscess, tuberculosis, bronchial cancer, pulmonary infarction, left-sided heart failure, coagulation defects and anticoagulant drugs—**haemoptyses** *pl*.

haemorrhage *n* loss of blood from a vessel—**haemorrhagic** *adj*. Usually refers to serious rapid blood loss. This may lead to hypovolaemic shock with tachycardia, hypotension, rapid breathing, pallor, sweating, oliguria, restlessness, confusion and eventually changes in conscious level. Haemorrhage can be classified in several ways. (a) according to the vessel involved, arterial, venous or capillary. (b) timing: *primary haemorrhage* that which occurs at the time of injury or operation. *reactionary haemorrhage* that which occurs within 24 hours of injury or operation. *secondary haemorrhage* that which occurs within some days of injury or operation and usually associated with sepsis. (c) whether it is internal (concealed) or external (revealed). ⊃ antepartum haemorrhage (APH), intrapartum haemorrhage (IPH), placental abruption, postpartum haemorrhage (PPH).

haemorrhagic disease of the newborn characterized by gastrointestinal, pulmonary or intracranial haemorrhage occurring from the 2nd to the 5th day of life. Caused by a physiological variation in blood clotting resulting from a transient deficiency of vitamin K which is necessary for the formation of some clotting factors. Responds to administration of vitamin K.

haemorrhagic fever a group of viral haemorrhagic diseases that include Argentine haemorrhagic fever, Bolivian haemorrhagic fever, Brazilian haemorrhagic fever, chikungunya, dengue, Ebola, Lassa fever, Marburg disease, Rift Valley fever, Venezuelan haemorrhagic fever, yellow fever. ⊃ mosquito-transmitted haemorrhagic fevers, viral haemorrhagic fevers.

haemorrhagic periostitis ⊃ periostitis.

haemorrhagic retinopathy ⊃ retinal vein occlusion.

haemorrhoidal *adj* relating to haemorrhoids or applied to nerves and vessels in the anal region.

haemorrhoidectomy *n* surgical removal of haemorrhoids.

haemorrhoids *npl* (*syn* piles) varicosity of the veins around the anus. *external haemorrhoids* those outside the anal sphincter, covered with skin. *internal haemorrhoids* those inside the anal sphincter, covered with mucous membrane.

haemosalpinx ⊃ haematosalpinx.

haemosiderin *n* an iron-protein complex related to the ferritin molecule. Some of the iron in the body is stored in this form.

haemosiderosis *n* excess iron deposition in the tissues. Especially in the monocyte-macrophage (reticuloendothelial) system, which eventually affects the liver, heart and endocrine glands. It is associated with excessive haemolysis of red blood cells. Also results from multiple blood transfusions, for example in the management of thalassaemia.

haemostasis *n* **1.** the processes that control bleeding from small vessels. Damage to the blood vessels starts a complex series of reactions between substances in the blood and others released from damaged platelets and tissue. There are four overlapping stages: vasoconstriction, platelet plug formation, coagulation and fibrinolysis. **2.** Also includes the measures used to stop bleeding during surgery or following injury.

haemostatic *adj* any agent which arrests bleeding.

haemostatic forceps artery forceps.

haemothorax *n* blood in the pleural cavity.

Hageman factor also called contact factor. Factor XII of the coagulation cascade. It is produced in the liver and is needed for the production of prothrombin activator (intrinsic system). A rare deficiency is inherited as an autosomal-recessive disorder.

HAI *abbr* hospital-acquired infection.

Haidinger's brushes an entoptic phenomenon observed when viewing a large diffusely illuminated blue field through a polarizer. It appears as a pair of yellow, brush-like shapes which seem to radiate from the point of fixation. The brushes are believed to be due to double refraction by the radially oriented fibres of Henle around the fovea. This phenomenon is used in detecting and treating eccentric fixation. ⊃ eccentric fixation, entoptic image/phenomena, Henle's fibre layer.

hair *n* thread-like appendage present on all parts of human skin except palms, soles, lips, glans penis and that surrounding the terminal phalanges. As individual hairs grow within a sheath or hair follicle, each hair grows from a bulb at the bottom of the follicle. The part of the hair within the follicle is the root and the part above the skin is the hair shaft. Types of hair are lanugo, vellus and terminal hair. ⊃ alopecia, anagen, catagen, hirsutism, hypertrichosis, telogen, Colour Section Figure 12.

hair analysis test used in preconception care to assess nutritional status and detect the concentration of up to 18 metallic elements. High levels of some metals, e.g. lead, may be associated with congenital abnormalities. Deficiencies of certain metallic elements, e.g. zinc, can be treated with dietary advice and/or supplements.

hairball ⊃ bezoar, trichbezoar.

hairy cell leukaemia a rare malignancy of haemopoietic (blood-forming) tissue—the bone and bone marrow. It is a chronic lymphoproliferative B-cell disorder. The male to female ratio is 6:1 and the median age at diagnosis is 50. Presenting symptoms are those of general ill health and recurrent infections. Splenomegaly occurs in 90% but lymph node enlargement is unusual. Severe neutropenia, monocytopenia and the characteristic hairy cells in the blood and bone marrow are typical. These cells usually type as B lymphocytes and also characteristically express CD25 and CD103. Over recent years a number of treatments have

G

H

been shown to produce long-lasting remissions. Cladribine and deoxycoformycin are effective in producing long periods of disease control.

hairy tongue (black hairy tongue) ⮑ tongue.

halal *n* the foods, including meat, permitted by Islamic dietary laws. Meat from herbivorous animals (grazing animals with cloven hooves, thus excluding pigs) slaughtered according to Islamic law. Although there are variations, fish with scales are usually permitted. ⮑ haram.

halation the reflection of light after it passes through a radiographic emulsion which may then re-expose the emulsion causing unsharpness on the film.

half-life (t$_{1/2}$) *n* amount of time taken for the radioactivity of a radioactive substance to decay by half the initial value. The half-life is a constant for each radioactive isotope, e.g. iodine-131 (^{131}I) is eight days. Or the time taken for the concentration of a drug in the plasma to fall by half the initial level. *biological half-life* time taken by the body to eliminate 50% of the dose of any substance (e.g. a drug) by normal biological processes. *effective half-life* the time taken for a combination of radioactive decay and biological processes for the activity of a radionuclide in an organ to be reduced to half its original activity.

half penetration depth (half depth) an electrotherapy term. The depth at which 50% of energy applied to an object or body remains. The preferred term now is penetration depth. The half value penetration depth of a 1 MHz beam is 4 cm whereas for a 3 MHz beam it is 2.5 cm. Therapists use this knowledge by selecting the appropriate frequency to penetrate to the desired depth. ⮑ penetration depth.

half-speed emulsion has half the speed of standard radiographic emulsions with an increase in image quality but also an increase in patient dosage. ⮑ standard contrast emulsions.

half-value thickness the thickness of a substance that will transmit exactly one-half of the intensity of radiation falling on it.

half-wave rectification ⮑ rectified.

halibut liver oil fish oil. A very rich source of vitamins A and D.

halitophobia an intense fear of having halitosis (bad breath) whether it exists or not. May be a feature of some mental health problems.

halitosis *n* bromopnoea. Foul-smelling breath. Causes include poor oral hygiene, diseased teeth, periodontal disease, a particular food item such as garlic, smoking tobacco, alcohol intake, sinusitis, suppurative respiratory conditions, gastric problems, fetor hepaticus associated with liver failure, uraemia.

Haller's layer ⮑ choroid.

Hallpike manoeuvre (C Hallpike, British otologist, 1900–1979) a diagnostic test for benign paroxysmal positional vertigo, if positive nystagmus in the eyes is seen and vertigo is provoked.

hallucination *n* a false perception occurring without any true sensory stimulus. A common psychotic symptom that can occur in schizophrenia, affective psychoses, delirium and drug intoxication. The hallcination may be auditory, gustatory, olfactory, tactile or visual.

hallucinogens *npl* (*syn* psychotomimetics) chemicals that cause hallucinations. They include cannabis, which is mildly hallucinogenic, lysergic acid diethylamide (LSD) and dimethyl-triptamine, which are potent hallucinogens, and certain fungi.

hallux *n* the great toe. ⮑ hallus rigidus, hallux valgus or hallux abducto-valgus, hallux varus.

hallux rigidus ankylosis of the metatarsophalangeal articulation due to osteoarthritis. It results in a stiff and painful toe.

hallux valgus or hallux abducto-valgus (*syn* bunion) a complex deformity of the medial column of the foot involving abduction and external rotation of the great toe and adduction and internal rotation of the first metatarsal (referenced to the midline of the body). Deformity exists when abduction of the hallux on the metatarsal is greater than 10–12°. Additional friction and pressure from poorly fitting footwear shoes cause a bursa to develop. The prominent bone, with its bursa, is known as a bunion.

hallux varus the great toe deviates toward the midline of the body and is commonly seen with metatarsus adductus.

halo *n* **1.** a coloured ring of light seen around a light source as a result of aberrations, internal reflections, diffraction or scattering. It also appears when the eye is diseased and the cornea is oedematous, as in glaucoma. ⮑ open-angle glaucoma, Sattler's veil. **2.** a titanium ring that encircles the head. ⮑ halo head frame, halopelvic traction.

halogen *n* any one of the non-metallic elements—bromine, chlorine, fluorine, iodine.

halogen lamp (*syn* tungsten-halogen lamp) a tungsten filament lamp in which the glass envelope is made of quartz and is filled with gaseous halogens. This permits a higher filament temperature and consequently provides a higher luminance and a higher colour temperature as well as a longer operating life than a conventional filament lamp of the same input power. Halogen lamps are used in some ophthalmoscopes and retinoscopes and as very bright sources for people with low vision.

halo head frame a metal band of varying design attached to the head by screws that are inserted through incisions until they contact the outside of the skull. Used for the attachment of various immobilizing devices in the treatment of fractures of the facial skeleton.

halopelvic traction a form of external fixation whereby traction can be applied to the spine between two fixed points. The device consists of three main parts: (a) a halo, (b) a pelvic loop, and (c) four extension bars.

halophiles halophilic bacteria and other micro-organisms, that are adapted to grow in high concentrations of salt (sodium chloride).

halophilic *adj* salt loving. Needing high levels of salt (sodium chloride) to grow.

hamartoma growth of new tissue which looks like tumour but results from disordered tissue development.

hamate one of the carpal bones of the wrist. It articulates with other carpal bones, the capitate, lunate and triquetral, and the fourth and fifth metacarpal bones.

hammer toe a permanent hyperextension of the first phalanx and flexion of second and third phalanges.

hamstring muscles the group of three flexor muscles that form the bulk of the posterior part of the thigh: the biceps femoris is the most lateral, the semitendinosus and medially the semimembranosus. The origins are on the ischium and they are inserted into the upper end of the fibula and tibia, or the tibia alone. Their tendons cross behind both the hip and the knee joints, so their action is to extend the hip and flex the knee. Their function is important in standing, walking and running and therefore vital in sport. Injury is common in sport, especially where sprinting or sudden acceleration is required when the muscles are under greatest tension, and is usually felt as a sudden sharp pain in the back of the thigh. ⊃ biceps femoris, hamstring strains, semimembranosus, semitendinosus.

hamstring strains are graded 1, 2 or 3 (complete rupture) depending on severity. Rehabilitation should include not only treatment of the soft tissue damage but also attempts to ascertain and where possible correct any underlying aetiological factors such as inadequate warm-up/stretching, poor low back flexibility and biomechanical abnormalities, e.g. an abnormally tilted pelvis.

hamulus a hook-like projection.

hand *n* that part of the upper limb below the wrist—a complex musculoskeletal structure, allowing the complexity of movements required. Comprises the eight carpal bones, five metacarpals and the fourteen phalanges forming the thumb and fingers. The carpal bones at the wrist articulate with the five metacarpals, and each of these in turn with the first of the phalanges of each digit. There are many small muscles attached between the various bones, which contribute to finger and thumb movements together with the long tendons of the forearm muscles which span the wrist in their tendon sheaths. ⊃ hand injury.

hand-arm vibration syndrome (HAVS) (*syn* Raynaud's phenomenon) a progressive chronic condition that arises following prolonged use of hand held vibrating equipment. Early signs are 'white finger', which is caused by constriction of and damage to the digital arteries. Other symptoms include tingling and loss of sensation caused by involvement of the digital nerves leading to loss of manual dexterity.

handedness *n* laterality. The use of the preferred hand, either right or left. The vast majority of people are right-handed and this corresponds to cerebral dominance on the left side of the brain, whereas left-handed people have cerebral dominance on the right side. Very few people are truly ambidextrous (equally skilled with either hand).

hand, foot and mouth disease a viral infection that mainly affects children. It is caused by a coxsackie virus. There are painful ulcers on the oral mucosa and vesicles on the hands and feet. Some children will feel unwell. It usually resolves after a week. ⊃ Colour Section Figure 73.

handgrip dynamometer ⊃ grip dynamometer.

handicap a term previously used to describe the individual's inability to be involved in normal life situations within society and used to be a category within the World Health Organizations model for describing Health: Impairment, Disability, Handicap. The WHO redefined these definitions in 1997, with a result that the term 'participation' replaces the term handicap, the term 'function' replaces impairment and the term 'activity' replaces disability. ⊃ impairement.

handicapped *adj* term previously applied to a person with a defect that prevents or limits the normal activities of living and achievement.

hand injury is most common in sports such as basketball, rugby, cricket, volleyball, handball, etc. Injuries include ligament sprains, fractures and dislocations.

handling a common therapeutic term used to describe assisted movement and physical contact with the patient.

hand mallet an instrument used in oral surgery. Usually metal with a cylindrical head and obtainable in various weights.

handpiece in dentistry, the hand-held connecting device placed between the driving force and rotary cutting and polishing instruments such as burs and discs. May be straight, contra-angled or miniature to hold smaller burs. Driven by the rotating shaft of an electric motor, or by compressed air. *reciprocating handpiece* a handpiece that changes the rotating movement to a reciprocating one of an alternating quarter-turn movement, e.g. the *giromatic handpiece* used in endodontic therapy. *turbine-driven handpiece* a hand-piece driven by compressed air, with friction grip chucks. The air pressure causes the small turbine or rotor in the head of the handpiece to rotate at very high speed. The rotor may be mounted on bearings or be air-borne.

hand presentation in labour with an uncorrected oblique lie, shoulder presentation and arm prolapse, or in compound presentations the fetal hand may present. If it is felt on vaginal examination it can be distinguished from a foot by the ability of the thumb to abduct, the absence of a prominent heel and fingers being longer than toes.

Hand–Schüller–Christian disease (A Hand, American paediatrician, 1868–1949; A Schüller, Austrian neurologist, 1874–1958; H Christian, American physician, 1876–1951) a rare condition usually manifesting in early childhood with histiocytic granulomatous lesions affecting many tissues. One of the diseases included in the spectrum of Langerhans' cell histiocytosis. ⊃ Letterer–Siwe disease.

handshake an electronic signal which indicates the end of the passage of data from the computer.

handwashing and hygiene a vital activity in preventing infection, both in hospital and community settings. It should include the wrists, the bulbar eminence of each thumb as well as between the fingers (Figure H.2). The hands should be washed after patient contact, and both before and after certain interventions, such as aseptic procedures, tracheal suction and emptying urine from a closed drainage system. The Infection Control Committee usually advises about the

G

H

339

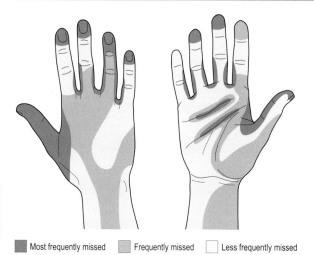

■ Most frequently missed ■ Frequently missed □ Less frequently missed

H.2 Handwashing (reproduced from Nicol et al 2004 with permission).

circumstances to be followed by handwashing, in addition to those, which have to be preceded, as well as followed, by handwashing. Local policies dictate when gloves are worn and when antiseptic hand rubs are used.

hanger a device to which radiographs are clipped in a known order during the processes of developing, fixing and drying.

hangman's fracture a type of cervical spine fracture. Bilateral fracture of pedicles of the axis (the second cervical vertebra C2).

Hannover's canal a space about the equator of the crystalline lens made up between the anterior and posterior parts of the zonule of Zinn and containing aqueous humour and zonular fibres. ⊃ zonule of Zinn.

Hansen's disease (G Hansen, Norwegian physician, 1841–1912) ⊃ leprosy.

Hantavirus a genus of viruses that cause serious haemorrhagic illnesses associated with kidney damage and failure. It is spread by the faeces of various rodents including mice and rats. Characterized by a flu-like illness that progresses to high fever, bleeding into the skin, headache, vomiting, shock and kidney failure. Cases have occurred in Korea, Russia, Japan, China and isolated cases in the United States. A *Hantavirus* also infects the respiratory system causing respiratory distress and respiratory failure.

HAPE *abbr* high-altitude pulmonary (o)edema.

haplopia single normal vision, as distinguished from diplopia. ⊃ diplopia.

hapten incomplete antigens. Low molecular weight substances such as peptides, which combine with body proteins to become antigenic. In combination with the body protein they are able to cause an immunological response, which they could not do alone. Antibiotics such as penicillin can act as haptens in susceptible individuals.

haptoglobin a plasma protein produced in several tissues that include the liver, lung and kidney. It binds to free haemoglobin in the plasma and forms a complex that can be safely removed by cells of the monocyte-macrophage system (reticuloendothelial system), such as those in the spleen and liver. The level of haptoglobin in the plasma is reduced or absent when red blood cell haemolysis occurs within the circulation, such as haemolytic anaemias. Whereas levels may be elevated in some chronic inflammatory diseases.

haplodont possessing peg-like molar teeth.

haploid *adj* refers to the chromosome complement of the mature gametes (oocytes or spermatozoa) following the reduction division of meiosis. This set represents the basic complement of 23 (n) unpaired chromosomes in humans (22 autosomes and 1 sex chromosome). The normal multiple is diploid (2n) but abnormally three or more chromosome sets can be found (triploid, tetraploid, etc.). ⊃ diploid.

haploscope an instrument used mainly in the laboratory to study various aspects of binocular vision. It presents separate fields of view to the two eyes while allowing changes in convergence or accommodation of one or both eyes, as well as providing for controls of colour, intensity or size of target and field. ⊃ amblyoscope, binocular vision.

haram foods proscribed according to Islamic dietary laws. They include alcoholic beverages, blood, meat from carnivorous or omnivorous animals, for example pork or any foods containing any product, such as lard, obtained from a pig. ⊃ halal.

hard copy the paper printout of the program or screen display.

hardener an addition to the radiographic film emulsion to make it resistant to abrasions, an addition to the developer and the fixer to reduce mechanical damage and sticking of the films to the racks.

hardiness in a psychological context, a dispositional tendency comprising a cluster of attitudes, beliefs and behavioural and mental skills that are held to promote resilience to the negative effects of stress on health and well-being.

hardness scale a scale of the ability of a material to resist indentation, scratching, abrasion or attrition. Commonly used scales in dentistry are: *Brinell hardness scale* or *number* (BHN) a scale in which a hardened steel sphere is pressed into the surface of the material being tested under a specified load. The hardness number is calculated by dividing the load by the area of indentation after removal of the load. *Knoop hardness scale* or *number* (KHN) a rhomboidal pyramid of diamond is pressed into the material being tested and the degree of hardness is calculated by measuring the length of the long axis of indentation produced. *Mohs hardness scale* or *number* (MHN) a scale for measuring the hardness of minerals by scratching one mineral against another of lower value. Diamond has an MHN of 10, quartz 7 and gypsum 2. *Rockwell hardness scale* or *number* (RHN) the hardness of the material being tested is measured by the difference in indentation produced by a hardened steel ball or diamond conical point under two different loads. *Vickers hardness scale* or *number* (VHN) the hardness is measured by indenting a material with a pyramidal diamond that has a square base.

hard palate the anterior bony part of the palate (roof of the mouth) formed by the fusion of the two maxillae in the midline, supported by the palatine processes of the maxilla and the palatine bone. Presents three foramina through which nerve and blood vessels pass carrying sensation and nutrients to and from the mucosa of the palate. ⊃ palate.

hard rollers part of the radiographic film transport system in an automatic processor made of paper wound round a stainless steel core and impregnated with epoxy resin.

hardware the mechanical and electronic part of the equipment.

hare lip obsolete term. ⊃ cleft lip.

harlequin fetus ⊃ lamellar exfoliation of newborn.

harm reduction a public health measure that seeks to reduce the harmful effects inherent in some behaviours, rather than concentrate entirely on changing the person's lifestyle. For example providing clean needle exchange for injecting drug users, or condoms to young people in high schools.

Harrington rod used in operations for scoliosis: it provides internal fixation whereby the curve is held by the rod and is usually accompanied by a spinal fusion.

Harrison's groove/sulcus (E Harrison, British physician, 1766–1838) a deformity of the lower chest caused by the pull of the diaphragm on the ribs. It may be associated with lung disease during childhood, such as, poorly controlled asthma, or rickets.

Hartmann's operation (H Hartmann, French surgeon, 1860–1952) originally a surgical procedure for colon cancer or diverticulitis in which the diseased colon was resected, the rectal stump closed and a colostomy formed. Usually a second stage operation is undertaken to restore continuity by anastomosing the distal colon to the rectum and reversing the colostomy.

Hartmann's solution (A Hartmann, American paediatrician, 1898–1964) intravenous infusion solution containing sodium lactate and chloride, potassium chloride and calcium chloride. A modified Ringer-lactate solution.

Hartnup disease named for the family in whom it was first identified. A rare recessive genetic error of neutral amino acid metabolism. It is associated with dry scaly skin, photosensitivity, hyperaminoaciduria, stomatitis, diarrhoea, ataxia and mental health problems.

Harvard step test ⊃ step test.

Harvard system of referencing a style of referencing used in an academic piece of work where strict protocols operate. The author's name takes precedence in the text, followed by the year of publication, and references are listed alphabetically in the reference list at the end of the work. ⊃ primary referencing (citation), reference, secondary referencing (citation), Vancouver system of referencing.

Hashimoto's disease (H Hasimoto, Japanese surgeon, 1881–1934) firm thyroid gland enlargement, often associated with hypothyroidism and rarely with hyperthyroidism, largely in middle-aged females, with high circulating levels of thyroid antibodies and due to autoimmune lymphocytic infiltration. The normal thyroid structures are replaced with lymphocytes and lymphoid germinal centres producing a goitre.

hashish *n* ⊃ cannabis.

Hassall-Henle bodies (A Hassall, British physician, 1817–1894; F Henle, German anatomist/pathologist, 1809–1885) ⊃ cornea guttata.

hatchet hand-held cutting chisel with bevelled blade used to trim hard tooth tissue.

haustration *n* sacculation, as of the colon—**haustrum** *sing*, **haustra** *pl*.

HAV *abbr* hepatitis A virus

haversian system/canal (C Havers, English physician, 1650–1702) the basic unit of compact bone (see Figure B.9, p. 102), an osteon. Tube-shaped structures comprising a central canal surrounded by expanding concentric rings of bone called lamellae. Spaces between the lamellae are called lacuna, these contain osteocytes. The central canal is linked, by a network of tunnels, to adjacent canals. Each central canal contains blood vessels, lymphatics and nerves.

HAVS *abbr* hand-arm vibration syndrome.

Hawley bow a variant of the short labial bow with adjustment loop in the canine region.

Hawley retainer ⊃ retainer.

Hawthorne effect an improvement in performance due to changes in environmental conditions regardless of the nature of the changes. Named after an electricity company's plant in the United States where a series of studies was conducted in the 1920s into the effects of variations in environmental conditions on workers' performance and productivity. In experimental design the term is often used to describe a threat to validity whereby participants' performance on a task improves due to them feeling that the experimenter shows concern for them. Researchers doing observation research make allowances for this reaction to their presence by not including data from the first few days in the final data analysis.

hay fever a form of allergic rhinitis in which attacks of inflammation of the conjunctiva, nose and throat are precipitated by exposure to pollen.

hazard analysis critical control process in the food industry, the identification of critical points in processing that must be controlled for food safety.

Hb *abbr* haemoglobin.

HbA *abbr* adult haemoglobin (the most abundant type).

HbA$_{1c}$ *abbr* glycated (glycosylated) haemoglobin.

HbA$_2$ *abbr* adult haemoglobin (the least abundant type).

HbA$_o$ *abbr* non-glycated (non-glycosylated) adult haemoglobin.

HbF *abbr* fetal haemoglobin.

HBIG *abbr* hepatitis B immunoglobulin.

HBV *abbr* hepatitis B virus.

HCA *abbr* healthcare assistant.

HCAI *abbr* healthcare-associated infection.

hCG *abbr* human chorionic gonadotrophin.

HCV *abbr* hepatitis C virus.

G
H

HDD *abbr* hard disk drive.

HDL *abbr* high-density lipoprotein.

HDR *abbr* high dose rate.

HDU *abbr* high dependency unit.

head a rounded portion of a bone which fits into the hollow or groove of another bone to form a movable joint. For example the hip joint formed by the head of the femur articulating within the acetabulum (a cup-like socket) on the pelvis.

headbox a perspex box placed over the infant's head into which a controlled level of additional oxygen can be administered (Figure H.3). ⊃ Gairdner headbox.

headcap in dentistry, **1.** a rigid cap made of plaster of Paris and gauze strips, incorporating anchorage wires. Used in the treatment of jaw and facial fractures. **2.** a removable head harness applied to the head and neck to provide for the transmission of extraoral forces to an orthodontic appliance.

head fitting Munro Kerr's manoeuvre. An attempt to fit a non-engaged fetal head into the maternal pelvic brim at term or in labour, to exclude cephalopelvic disproportion. If the head does not fit, ultrasound or X-ray pelvimetry provide more accurate, detailed information to assess whether vaginal delivery is possible.

headgear an apparatus applied to the head and neck for the transmission of extraoral forces to an orthodontic appliance.

head injury also know as brain injury. An injury resulting from a blow to the head causing haemorrhage or contusion. ⊃ concussion, extradural haematoma, Glasgow Coma Scale, papilloedema, subdural haematoma

head injury in sport potentially the most serious injury in sport. Injury risk is greatest in contact sports (such as boxing, rugby, football and American football) or in sports which involve a fall from height (horse riding, trampolining, gymnastics) or movement at speed (cycling, motor sports). The risk of a head injury is brain damage via either internal bleeding or a shearing force. Management of head injuries in sport requires appropriately trained personnel who adhere to the relevant guidelines especially regarding referral to hospital and advisability or otherwise of return to play. ⊃ amnesia, coma, concussion, Glasgow Coma Scale (GCS).

head lice ⊃ *Pediculosis*.

head tilt/chin lift a method of opening the airway in an unconscious casualty by placing a hand on the forehead to gently tilt the head backwards, while using the fingertips to lift the chin (Figure H.4). It is used in the adult to move the tongue forward in order to stop it from blocking the airway. In an adult head tilt/chin lift needs the neck to be hyperextended and so should not be used when a head or cervical spine injury is suspected. In infants and children head tilt/chin lift is used but without overextending the neck as this can cause the airway to close (Figure H.5). ⊃ jaw thrust.

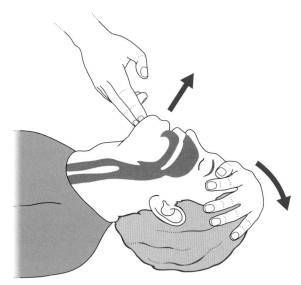

H.4 Head tilt/chin lift—adult (reproduced from Mallik et al 1998 with permission).

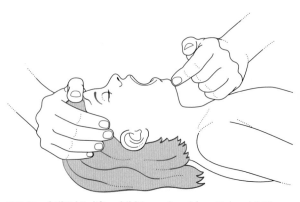

H.5 Head tilt/chin lift—child (reproduced from Huband & Trigg 2000 with permission).

Elephant tubing

Oxygen tubing

Oxygen analyser probe

Headbox comfortably positioned over head and neck

H.3 Delivery of humidified oxygen via a head box (reproduced from Huband & Trigg 2000 with permission).

Heaf test (F Heaf, British physician, 1894–1973) a tuberculin skin prick test for tuberculosis. Replaced by the Mantoux test in the UK.

healing *n* **1.** the natural process of cure or tissue repair. ➲ wound healing. **2.** in complementary or integrated medicine the term healing refers to a return to health; also the use of a therapy that may assist the healing process; a specific therapeutic form, such as spiritual healing and therapeutic touch—**heal** *vt*, *vi*.

health *n* negatively defined as a state in which no evidence of illness, disease, injury or disability is found. More positively in 1948 the World Health Organization defined health as 'a state of complete mental, physical and social well-being and not merely the absence of disease or infirmity'. The development of holistic thinking has led to the broadening of definitions of health to include social, environmental and economic influences. Health includes individuals' social and psychological resources as well as their physical capacities. A positive concept of well-being as a subjective feeling, physical fitness, normal functional capacity, resistance, resilience or hardiness. The subjective nature of what constitutes health means that individual definitions will vary from one person to another, from place to place as well as at different times.

Health and Safety legislation in the UK the statute and common law that covers health and safety duties. The Health and Safety and Welfare at Work Act 1974 sets out the responsibilities of the employer in relation to their employees, the working environment, equipment and substances, and those of individual employees to themselves and other people. The Health and Safety Commission (HSC) and the Health and Safety Executive (HSE) enforce health and safety law in the UK.

Health and Social Care Act 2008 an Act of Parliament which received Royal assent in July 2008. It has four main provisions: (a) to establish the Care Quality Commission a single regulator for health and adult social care by merging the Healthcare Commission, the Mental Health Act Commission and the Commission for Social Care Inspection. The Care Quality Commission has increased powers to make sure that services are safe and of high quality. ➲ Care Quality Commission; (b) to reform professional regulation in the wake of the Shipman Inquiry; (c) to strengthen public health protection measures in order to prevent and control the spread of specified infectious conditions and contamination caused by radioactive substances and chemicals; (d) to establish a scheme in which pregnant women are paid a 'one off' grant to assist with the expenses of healthy living, such as a healthy diet, in the later weeks of pregnancy. (Department of Health (DH) 2008 Health and Social Care Act 2008. online www.dh.gov.uk/)

health belief model the central feature of this model is that people tend not to adopt health behaviours unless they believe they are susceptible to the disease or disorder in question, that it is serious, that the recommendations will be effective and that the advantages of following the advice will outweigh the disadvantages. The individual may also require a trigger (for example the diagnosis of a friend with the disease) before any change of behaviour occurs.

health care assistant a health service employee who provides nursing support services under the direction of a qualified nurse, who remains accountable for the care given. HCAs can receive a nationally co-ordinated training, based on national vocational qualifications (NVQ/SNVQs).

healthcare-associated infection (HCAI) any infection that occurs as a result of the patient/client's care or treatment by healthcare staff, or an infection affecting healthcare staff in the course of their work. ➲ hospital-acquired (nosocomial) infection, infection.

Healthcare Commission previously established in England to encourage improvement in care (quality and effectiveness) and its provision (economy and efficiency), its remit included inspection and monitoring services, investigating serious service failures, and acting as an independent review for complaints about the NHS. As part of the provisions of the The Health and Social Care Act 2008 (which received Royal assent in July 2008) the Healthcare Commission merged with the Mental Health Act Commission and the Commission for Social Care Inspection to create a single regulator for health and adult social services—the Care Quality Commission. ➲ Care Quality Commission.

healthcare outcome the results of healthcare processes.

healthcare systems national or local organizations for providing medical/health care. The structure of the system has to accommodate progress in medical interventions, consumer demand and economic efficiency. Criteria for a successful system have been formulated: (a) adequacy and equity of access to care, (b) income protection (for patients), (c) macro-economic efficiency (national expenditure measured as a proportion of gross domestic product), (d) micro-economic efficiency (balance of services provided between improving health outcomes and satisfying consumer demand), (e) consumer choice and appropriate autonomy for care providers. There are four basic types of healthcare systems: socialized (UK NHS), social insurance (Canada, France), mandatory insurance (Germany), voluntary insurance (USA).

health centre premises from which a variety of healthcare services are provided. Includes general practice, community services such as child health, family planning and some well woman services. May be owned by local government or Primary Care Trusts, general practitioners or privately owned.

health determinant a factor that impacts on the health of individuals and populations. They include genetic inheritance, gender, age, lifestyle choices, level of education, community ties and networks, housing, working conditions,

G

H

343

unemployment, social class, accessibility of healthcare, culture, economic conditions.

Health Development Agency ⊃ National Institute for Health and Clinical Excellence

health education providing information to the public or individuals to reduce ill health and enhance positive health by influencing people's beliefs, attitudes and behaviour. The objective is to empower individuals to make appropriate choices for healthy living.

health gain an attempt at measuring the benefit of health intervention on the population. For example, health gain from a cervical cytology screening programme may be measured as the reduction in deaths from cervical cancer; coronary heart disease prevention programme measured as a reduction in deaths from coronary heart disease in men under 65 years of age, or the number of deaths avoided over a specified period of time (e.g. 5 years).

Health Improvement Programme (HImP) a focused action plan for improving health and healthcare provision at a local level. Involves a collaborative approach between Primary Care Trust(s), health professionals, local government, voluntary organizations and user groups, etc.

health level 7 the international standard for textual communication of electronic data in and between any healthcare environment.

Healthlink a centralized, data communications network for healthcare professionals which enables authorized users to exchange documents and information cheaply and efficiently.

Health Professions Council (HPC) an independent statutory body in the UK which currently regulates 13 health-related professions: art therapists, biomedical scientists, chiropodists/podiatrists, clinical scientists, dieticians, occupational therapists, operating department practitioners, orthoptists, paramedics, physiotherapists, prosthetists/orthotists, radiographers, speech and language therapists. At the time of writing there are discussions about the addition of practitioner psychologists to the list of health professions regulated by the Health Professions Council (HPC). The HPA has the responsibility for setting and maintaining standards of professional training, performance and conduct of the professions. Currently the HPA Council has 26 members, one from each of the professions and 13 lay members plus a president. Registration with the HPC means that agreed professional standards of training and proficiency have been met and that if any registrants do not uphold these standards they may be subject to having their fitness to practise investigated and dealt with by HPC.

health promotion efforts to prevent ill health and promote positive health. Five key priority areas for action formulated by the World Health Organization (1986, 1998): (a) building healthy public policy, (b) creating supportive environments for health, (c) strengthening community action for health, (d) developing personal skills for health and (e) re-orientating health services (to focus on whole populations).

Health Protection Agency (HPA) in England and Wales an agency established to protect public health and decrease the effects of chemical hazards, infectious diseases, poisons and radiation risks.

Health Service Commissioner ⊃ Parliamentary and Health Service Ombudsman.

health technology any method used by those working in health services to promote health, prevent and treat disease and improve rehabilitation and long term care.

health visitor ⊃ specialist community public health nurse.

hearing impairment impairment resulting from hearing loss. People can experience hearing loss at any stage of life. Common causes of hearing loss include glue ear, occurring most often during childhood, and presbycusis, which is a permanent sensorineural hearing loss associated with ageing. Communication with hearing impaired people can be enhanced by some simple steps including: being in front of, fairly close to, and on the same level as the affected person, reducing background noise, speaking clearly, not shouting and maintaining speech at the normal rhythm, using sentences rather than single words, not covering your face while speaking; also, avoid talking to a hearing person accompanying the patient and always make sure that you have the hearing impaired person's attention before you start to speak. ⊃ deafness.

hearing tests ⊃ acuity.

heart n the hollow muscular organ which pumps the blood around the pulmonary and general circulations. It is situated behind the sternum, lying obliquely within the mediastinum. It weighs around 300 g and is about the size of the person's fist. It is divided into a right and left side by a septum and has four chambers. There are two small upper receiving chambers, the atria, and two large lower pumping chambers, the ventricles. The wall of the heart has three layers: the outer serous pericardium, a middle of cardiac muscle (myocardium) and a lining (endocardium). Valves control blood flow between the atria and ventricles (atrioventricular valves)—tricuspid on the right and mitral (bicuspid) on the left—and the aortic and pulmonary valves (semilunar) prevent backflow from aorta and pulmonary artery. The normal heart sounds are produced when these valves close during the cardiac cycle. ⊃ cardiac nerve supply, coronary circulation, Colour Section Figures 6, 8.

heart attack a lay term for a myocardial infarction. ⊃ acute coronary syndrome, coronary heart disease, coronary thrombosis, myocardial infarction.

heart block partial or complete block to the passage of impulses through the conducting system of the atria and ventricles of the heart.

heartburn n pyrosis. Retrosternal burning due to gastro-oesophageal reflux of stomach acid.

heart failure an inability of one or both sides of the heart to pump blood effectively into the circulation. ⊃ acute heart failure, congestive heart failure.

heart-lung machine n a pump oxygenator. A machine that bypasses both the heart and lungs and is used in cardiac surgery in which the heart is stopped, or in critically ill patients to oxygenate the blood. ⊃ cardiopulmonary bypass.

heart murmur a sound additional to the normal heart sounds, heard on auscultation of the heart. Many murmurs are of no significance (innocent, physiological murmurs), particularly in young children, or due to increased blood flow through the heart during exercise, or in pregnancy. A pathological murmur may be caused by structural abnormalities of the heart or by turbulence as blood passes through a faulty heart valve (congenital or acquired: in adults most commonly following rheumatic fever). Symptoms may include breathlessness, palpitations, chest pain or fainting but many murmurs are asymptomatic and are identified, for example, during routine medical examination. All sports participants found to have a murmur should undergo full cardiovascular assessment, including echocardiography, to exclude any cause which might increase the risk of sudden death during exercise. Management is of the underlying cause and surgery may be indicated in certain conditions, especially for significantly narrowed heart valves. ⊃ heart sounds, screening in sport.

heart rate the number of heart beats per minute (bpm). The normal resting adult heart rate is 60–100 bpm and should be monitored for rate, strength and rhythm. ⊃ bradycardia, tachycardia.

heart rate reserve (HRR) maximal minus resting heart rate ($HR_{max} - HR_{rest}$): the Karvonen formula.

heart sounds the normal heart sounds correspond to the closure of the four valves of the heart. The first heart sound (S1) (heard best at the apex) is the 'LUB' sound heard on the closure of the mitral (bicuspid) and tricuspid valves (left and right atrioventricular valves) at the onset of systole. It may be abnormally soft in mitral valve regurgitation and in heart failure; the sound is louder if the circulation is hyperdynamic, such as occurs in pregnancy, hyperthyroidism and anaemia. The second heart sound (S2) (heard best at the base of the heart) is the 'DUP' sound heard on the closure of the aortic and pulmonary valves (the semilunar valves) at the end of systole. Two components of the second sound can be heard separately (split heart sound) as a normal feature. This sound may be abnormal in people with an atrial septal defect or conduction problems, for example right bundle branch block, left bundle branch block. The third heart sound (S3) heard early in diastole is normal in children and during pregnancy. S3 is present abnormally in heart failure and mitral valve regurgitation. A fourth heart (S4) heard late in diastole may be present in severe left ventricular hypertrophy. Other heart sounds include an opening snap heard early in diastole, for example in mitral valve stenosis. Systolic clicks may be heard in a variety of valve abnormalities, e.g. aortic stenosis, and from a normal replacement mechanical heart valve. ⊃ heart murmur.

heart transplant surgical transplantation of a heart from a suitable donor. May be combined with a lung transplant, for example for a person with cystic fibrosis.

heat acclimatization the process of improvement in tolerance to heat as a result of repeated sessions of exercise in a hot environment, resulting in a measurable improvement in physiological response. The body's response includes increase in the rate of sweating but decrease in sodium in the sweat, preserving salt by the action of aldosterone; increase in skin blood flow and overall control of body temperature as environmental conditions (air temperature and humidity) change. In addition, acclimatization will reduce the incidence and severity of heat illness. ⊃ acclimation.

heat and cell metabolism a great deal of what physiotherapists do is aimed at speeding up or slowing down the metabolism within a cell or group of cells. Metabolic rate increases by 13% for every 1°C rise in temperature. This means that the cells require more oxygen and nutrients and accordingly there is an increased production of metabolites or waste products. Developing a fever during an infection is one of the protective mechanisms initiated by the body in order to eliminate the microorganisms more effectively. A local infection such as a boil or spot is red and inflamed. ⊃ inflammation. Physiotherapists often use this principle. For example, a ligament that has been injured may become chronically inflamed, this means that the inflammatory response almost slows to a halt and healing ceases. By applying a treatment such as ultrasound, the metabolism in the area can be selectively increased, the inflammation changed to an acute response and the healing process recommenced. There is a limit to how far the temperature of tissues can be effectively raised. Proteins are denatured (coagulate) above a certain temperature (as happens to the white of an egg when it is fried). Generally speaking, irreversible tissue damage occurs at approximately 45°C. At normal body temperature a typical cell requires a set level of nutrients, oxygen and other essential chemicals such as hormones. The surrounding lymphatic and blood supply is responsible for clearing away waste carbon dioxide and other waste and metabolites. If a hot pack were to be placed on the area, the biochemical processes would speed up and the level of oxygen and nutrients would no longer be enough to meet demand. Much more would be needed and at a faster rate; in addition there would be increased amounts of waste products which would need to be removed, since they would be toxic if they were allowed to build up too much. As a result, the surrounding blood supply would increase. If an ice pack were to be placed on the area, as it cooled down gradually, the biochemical reactions would slow down and smaller amount of oxygen and nutrients would be needed; the cells would also produce a lower levels of waste products. The surrounding blood vessels would constrict and some local capillaries would close off. ⊃ heat therapy, ice/cold therapy.

heat cramps part of the spectrum of heat illnesses. Muscle cramps with general fatigue that occur after exercise, associated with profuse sweating and the resulting salt loss.

Treatment is removal from the hot environment, plus salt and water replacement.

heat-cured polymer used in dentistry, a mixture of powder (polymer) and liquid (monomer) which can be hardened or cured by heat.

heat exchanger in radiography, a method of maintaining the temperature of solutions in an automatic film processor with a series of separate tubes through which water, developer or fixer flows; any waste heat from the developer is absorbed and passed to the water or heat from the water can be absorbed from the fixer.

heat exhaustion part of the spectrum of heat illnesses. It is the most common heat illness in sport. Symptoms are often vague and include faintness, loss of co-ordination, profuse sweating, headache, nausea, dizziness and thirst. It is related to alterations in fluid/electrolyte balance and changes in blood volume. Treatment is removal from the hot environment, external cooling, elevation of the legs, fluid replacement and careful monitoring of airway, breathing and circulation (ABC).

heat illness the term used to describe the spectrum of conditions which result from the effects of excessive heat, whilst hyperthermia refers to any elevation of the body (core) temperature above normal. Heat problems are influenced by humidity, which reduces heat loss by evaporation. Young children have less ability to lose heat by sweating and are therefore more susceptible. ⊃ heat cramps, heat exhaustion, heat stroke, heat syncope.

heat shield a perspex shield placed over a low birth weight and/or sick infant in an incubator to prevent radiant and convective heat loss.

heat stroke part of the spectrum of heat illnesses. Heat stroke is rare but can be fatal; it is at the end of the spectrum of heat illness when the body temperature continues to rise as heat loss by sweating fails due to dehydration; the result is collapse, possible seizures, coma and death. It is a medical emergency and should be treated as such with immediate admission to hospital. ⊃ hyperthermia.

heat syncope part of the spectrum of heat illnesses. It occurs with postural pooling of blood and a decrease in venous return resulting in relative cerebral hypoperfusion. It occurs most commonly with a sudden rise in temperature or humidity. Salt and water depletion are less common than in the other types of heat illness.

heat therapy the physical effects of adding heat to an object include: (a) rise in temperature (the average kinetic energy of the molecules increases); (b) expansion of the material (molecules vibrate more and move further apart. Gases expand more than solids and liquids more than solids); (c) change in physical state; (d) acceleration of chemical reactions (Van't Hoff's law (part): any chemical reaction capable of being accelerated, is accelerated by a rise in temperature) this is of major importance to physiotherapists and (e) decrease in viscosity of fluids, e.g. synovial fluid. The distribution of heat depends on the size of heated area, the depth of absorption of specific radiation,

the duration of heating and the intensity of heating and method by which it is applied. ⊃ heat and cell metabolism, ice/cold therapy.

heat treatment in dentistry, a method of altering the physical properties of a metal by controlled temperature changes.

hebephrenia *n* a type of schizophrenia characterized by affective disturbance, thought disorder and negative symptoms. Prognosis tends to be poor—**hebephrenic** *adj*.

Heberden's nodes (W Heberden, British physician, 1710–1801) small bony swellings at terminal (distal) interphalangeal joints occurring in osteoarthritis. ⊃ Bouchard's node.

hedonism *n* excessive devotion to pleasure, so that a person's conduct is determined by an unconscious drive to seek pleasure and avoid unpleasant things.

Hedström file a tapered, flexible, endodontic file consisting of a series of sharp, milled, conical-shaped blades and used with an outward rasping motion to plane canal walls and remove materials from root canals.

heel bruise (*syn* stone bruise) contusion to the subcutaneous fat pad located over the inferior aspect of the calcaneus.

heel lock a technique of strapping, thought to ensure the stability of the subtalar joint.

heel spurs occur on the plantar surface of the calcaneus and are considered a variant of the normal point of attachment of the plantar fascia. They are insignificant when small, and may be well defined with smooth, regular cortical contours. However, when enlarged they cause pain on walking.

heel to shin test a test where the patient is asked to run their heel of one foot down the shin of the other leg. This is a test of co-ordination. Poor responses may suggest a lesion of the cerebellum and results in reduced co-ordination.

Heerfordt's syndrome ⊃ uveoparotid fever.

Hegar's sign (E Hegar, German gynaecologist, 1830–1914) extreme softening of the lower segment of the uterus at 8 weeks' gestation detected by bimanual palpation.

Heimlich's manoeuvre (H Heimlich, American surgeon, b.1920) abdominal thrusts. A first aid measure to dislodge a foreign body (e.g. food) obstructing the glottis, usually performed by holding the patient from behind and jerking the operator's clenched fists up into the victim's epigastrium (Figure H.6). In an unconscious victim it can be performed with the victim lying on the floor. ⊃ Appendix 10.

Heinz body (R Heinz, German pathologist, pharmacist, 1865–1924) refractile, irregularly shaped body composed of denatured haemoglobin present in red blood cells in some haemolytic anaemias.

helical computed tomography (CT) ⊃ spiral computed tomography (CT).

Helicobacter pylori bacterium causing a number of gastrointestinal diseases via gastric infection. These include peptic ulceration, gastric cancer and MALToma. May be diagnosed by urea breath tests, serology or gastric biopsy. Treatment with combination therapy of antibiotics (clarithromycin, with either metronidazole or amoxicillin) and a proton pump

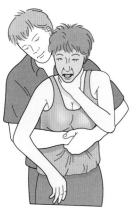

H.6 Heimlich's manoeuvre (reproduced from Peattie & Walker 1995 with permission).

inhibitor, e.g. omeprazole, is usually effective, but bacterial resistance does occur.

helium *n* an inert gas. Medical uses include pulmonary function tests and to dilute other gases.

helium–neon laser a laser which has helium–neon gas in the tube and produces red light.

helix *n* spiral. **1.** outer ridge on the auricle (pinna) of the outer/external ear. ⊃ Colour Section Figure 13. **2.** describes the structure of molecules, such as DNA.

Heller's operation ⊃ cardiomyotomy.

Hellin's law formula used to calculate the incidence of spontaneously-occurring multiple pregnancy in the UK: 1:89 pregnancies = twins; $1:89^2$, or 7921 = triplets; $1:89^3$, or 704969 = quadruplets.

HELLP *abbr* **h**aemolysis, **e**levated **l**iver enzymes and **l**ow **p**latelets.

HELLP syndrome a syndrome characterized by haemolysis, elevated liver enzymes and low platelets. It is a life-threatening condition associated with pre-eclampsia/eclampsia syndrome (pregnancy-induced hypertension). Occurring between 32 and 34 weeks' gestation it affects approximately 0.17–0.85 of all livebirths. Maternal morbidity and mortality is significant through disseminated intravacular coagulation (DIC), acute renal failure, pulmonary oedema, subcapsular liver haematoma or rupture of the liver with severe haemorrhage, or liver failure. Symptoms include malaise, epigastric or right upper quadrant pain, nausea and vomiting, as well as non-specific symptoms suggestive of viral syndrome, but blood pressure may be relatively normal; diagnosis is confirmed by blood and platelet count, liver function tests and coagulation studies. Intensive care is required to stabilize the woman's condition, expedite delivery and prevent further complications; liver transplant may be required in those with severe hepatic problems. There is also significant perinatal morbidity and mortality due to intrauterine growth retardation and birth asphyxia.

Helmholtz's law of magnification ⊃ Lagrange's law.

Helmholtz's theory of accommodation the theory that in accommodation the ciliary muscle contracts, relaxing the tension on the zonule of Zinn while the shape of the crystalline lens changes, resulting in increased convexity, especially of the anterior surface. Fincham's theory complements that of Helmholtz. ⊃ accommodation, ciliary muscle, Fincham's theory, zonule of Zinn.

Helmholtz's theory of colour vision ⊃ Young–Helmholtz theory.

helminth a worm, including cestode, nematodes, taenia, trematoda.

helminthagogue *n* an anthelmintic.

helminthiasis *n* the condition resulting from infestation with worms.

helminthology *n* the study of parasitic worms.

helper T-cells T-lymphocytes which have a key role in the immune response, both cell-mediated and antibody-mediated. Their role includes the production of cytokines and the activation of B-cells. ⊃CD4 cells.

HEMA *abbr* hydroxyethyl methacrylate.

hemeralopia (*syn* nyctalopia [this term is only synonymous with night blindness], night sight [this term is only synonymous with day blindness]) the term used to mean either night blindness in which there is a partial or total inability to see in the dark associated with a loss of rod function or vitamin A deficiency; or day blindness in which there is reduced vision in daylight while vision is normal in the dark. ⊃ dark adaptation, Oguchi's disease, retinitis pigmentosa.

hemi- a prefix that means 'half', e.g. *hemiplegia*.

hemiachromatopsia *n* a condition in which the person is colour blind in only half of the visual field.

hemianopia ⊃ hemianopsia.

hemianopsia *n* (*syn* hemianopia) loss or defect of vision in the nasal or temporal half of the visual field of one (unilateral) or both (bilateral) eyes. May be caused by brain injury. The person may bump into things on the affected side or ignore objects or people on that side of them. ⊃ altitudinal hemianopsia, binasal hemianopsia, bitemporal hemianopsia, congruous hemianopsia, heteronymous hemianopsia, homonymous hemianopsia, incongruous hemianopsia, perimeter, quadrantanopsia, scotoma, tangent screen.

hemiarthroplasty an arthroplasty procedure in which there is a partial replacement of joint structures, such as the replacement of the femoral head without replacement of the acetabulum, or a unicondylar knee placement. ⊃ arthroplasty.

hemiatrophy *n* atrophy of one half or one side. ⊃ facial hemiatrophy.

hemiballismus *n* involuntary flailing movements of limbs due in some cases to contralateral damage of the subthalamic (below the thalamus) nucleus in the basal nuclei (ganglia).

hemibody half or on one side of the body.

hemicelluloses complex carbohydrates such as mucilages and gums. Non-starch polysaccharides, which with cellulose and lignin form part of plant cell walls.

hemicephalus a condition in which a fetus has only the lower half of the brain tissue present.

hemichorea *n* choreiform movements limited to one side of the body. ⊃ chorea.

hemicolectomy *n* removal of approximately half the colon. A right hemicolectomy removes the caecum, the ascending colon and part of the transverse colon. A left hemicolectomy removes part of the transverse colon, descending colon, and possibly the sigmoid colon.

hemicrania *n* unilateral headache, as in the pain of migraine.

hemidesmosome a 'half-desmosome'. A similar structure to a desmosome but with a plate of one cell only and without a companion cell butting up against it. ⊃ cell-surface molecules, desmosomes.

hemidiaphoresis *n* unilateral sweating of the body.

hemiglossectomy *n* removal of approximately half the tongue.

hemihydrate a hydrate containing one molecule of water for every two molecules of other substance in the compound. ⊃ plaster of Paris.

hemimandibulectomy the surgical excision of one half of the mandible.

hemimaxillectomy the surgical excision of one half of the maxilla.

hemimelia a congenital developmental abnormality where the lower part of a limb is missing or shortened. It may affect either or both bones of the distal arm (radius and ulna) or leg (tibia and fibula).

hemiparesis *n* paralysis or weakness of one side of face or body. ⊃ monoparesis, paraparesis, paresis, quadriparesis.

hemiplegia *n* paralysis of one side of the body, usually resulting from a stroke (cerebrovascular accident) on the opposite side of the brain—**hemiplegic** *adj.*

hemiplegic posture the position of the head, neck, trunk and limbs after a cerebrovascular accident (stroke).

hemisection 1. the removal of one half of an organ or anatomical structure. **2.** in dentistry, the division of a tooth in half and the removal of the unwanted diseased portion together with its root or roots.

hemiseptum that portion of bone remaining between two adjacent teeth, when an infrabony lesion is present in the approximal aspect of the other tooth.

hemizygous *adj* describes an individual with a genome with only one allele for a given characteristic or trait. Having an allele present on unpaired chromosomes such as those on the X chromosome in males. The characteristic specified by the allele will be expressed whether it is dominant or recessive because there is no corresponding allele on the Y chromosome, e.g. those leading to haemophilia or Duchenne muscular dystrophy.

Henderson–Hasselbach equation a formula that explains why blood pH is dependent upon the ratio of bicarbonate (hydrogen carbonate) (HCO_3^-) and the dissolved carbon dioxide (carbonic acid H_2CO_3) which is determined by the PCO_2 The formula is:

$$\text{Blood pH} = 6.1 + \log\frac{[H_2CO_3]\text{ hydrogen carbonate}}{[CO_2]\text{ carbon dioxide in solution}}$$

A 20:1 ratio of bicarbonate (hydrogen carbonate) (base) to dissolved CO_2 (carbonic acid) is required for blood pH to remain at 7.4.

Henle's fibre layer (F Henle, German anatomist/pathologist, 1809–1885) located in the macular region, it is formed by the cone and rod fibres which run parallel to the retinal surface within the outer molecular layer of the retina. ⊃ Haidinger's brushes, macular star, retina.

Henoch–Schönlein purpura (E Henoch, German paediatrician, 1820–1910; J Schönlein German physician, 1793–1864) a small vessel vasculitis, mainly affecting children. Caused by hypersensitivity which may follow a streptococcal respiratory infection, or a drug allergy, but it may be idiopathic. Immune complexes are formed which damage capillaries in the skin, gut and elsewhere. It is characterized by purpuric bleeding into the skin, particularly shins and buttocks, and from the wall of the gut, resulting in abdominal colic and rectal bleeding; and bruising around joints with arthritis. The kidneys may be affected, leading to haematuria, proteinuria, acute glomerulonephritis, nephrotic syndrome or acute renal failure.

hepa- a prefix that means 'liver', e.g. *hepatic*.

hepar *n* the liver—**hepatic** *adj.*

heparin *n* a group of naturally occurring anticoagulant substances produced by mast cells and present in liver and lung tissue. Normally it prevents inappropriate blood coagulation in the body. Used therapeutically, heparin inhibits blood coagulation in several ways; primarily by the prevention of fibrin formation through the inhibition of thrombin activity. The two types used therapeutically are standard (unfractionated) heparin (SH) and low-molecular-weight heparin (LMWH). Heparin is used subcutaneously or intravenously for existing thromboembolic conditions, such as deep vein thrombosis, and in prophylaxis, e.g. perioperatively. Bleeding may occur as a side-effect. Its effects can be reversed with the antidote protamine sulphate. ⊃ anticoagulant, coagulation, low-molecular-weight heparin (LMWH), standard (unfractionated) heparin (SH). ⊃ Appendix 5.

heparin-induced thrombocytopenia (HIT) in a small proportion of patients treated with heparin the platelet count declines after 5–7 days due to the development of an antibody to the heparin–platelet factor 4 on the platelet surface. HIT should be considered in all patients whose platelet count falls by more than 50% after starting heparin. It is a very serious complication because it is associated with a high incidence of arterial and venous thrombosis. The diagnosis is established by detecting the antibody to PF4–heparin complex. Heparin should be discontinued as soon as HIT is diagnosed and the direct thrombin inhibitor, hirudin, given instead.

hepatalgia pain in or associated with the liver.

hepatectomy *n* excision of the liver, or more usually part of the liver.

hepat/ico, hepat/o- a prefix that means 'liver', e.g. *hepatocellular*.

hepatic *adj* pertaining to the liver.

hepatic artery the unpaired artery that branches from the coeliac artery to supply the liver with oxygenated arterial blood. It also supplies blood to the gallbladder, parts of the stomach, duodenum and pancreas.

hepatic ducts two bile ducts, right and left, that carry bile from the liver. They unite to form the common hepatic duct.

hepatic encephalopathy altered brain function associated with the wide ranging metabolic disturbances of cirrhosis and liver failure. The liver is unable to detoxify many chemicals, particularly nitrogenous substances.

hepatic flexure the right colic flexure. The 90° angle in the colon under the liver.

hepatic portal circulation venous blood rich in nutrients is carried to the liver from the small and large intestine, pancreas, spleen, distal oesophagus and stomach by the hepatic portal vein. Once in the liver the blood passes through a second capillary bed (sinusoids) so that nutrients can be modified by liver cells. The blood leaves the liver and returns to the heart via the inferior vena cava.

hepatic portal hypertension increased pressure in the hepatic portal vein. Usually caused by cirrhosis of the liver; results in splenomegaly, with hypersplenism and gastrointestinal bleeding. ⊃ oesophageal varices.

hepatic portal vein often referred to as the portal vein. A vein conveying blood into the liver; it is about 75 mm long and is formed by the union of several veins the superior mesenteric, inferior mesenteric, splenic and gastric veins.

hepatic-renal disease the presence of IgA nephropathy (kidney disease) is more common in patients with liver disease. Severe hepatic dysfunction may cause a haemodynamically mediated type of renal failure, hepatorenal syndrome. However, it also predisposes the kidney to develop acute renal failure (acute tubular necrosis) in response to relatively minor insults including bleeding and infection. Patients with such severe hepatic failure are often difficult to treat by dialysis and have a poor prognosis. Where treatment is justified—for example, if there is a good chance of recovery or of a liver transplant—very slow or continuous treatments are less likely to precipitate or exacerbate encephalopathy. ⊃ hepatorenal syndrome.

hepatic veins three large veins that carry deoxygenated blood from the liver to the inferior vena cava ⊃ hepatic portal circulation.

hepaticoduodenostomy *n* anastomosis of the hepatic duct to the duodenum.

hepaticoenteric associated with the liver and intestine.

hepaticoenterostomy *n* anastomosis of the hepatic duct to the small intestine.

hepaticojejunostomy *n* anastomosis of the hepatic duct to the jejunum.

hepatitis *n* inflammation of the liver, commonly associated with viral infection but can be due to toxic agents, such as alcohol, drugs and chemicals, or metabolic disorders, e.g. Wilson's disease. Viral hepatitis is currently a serious public health problem. It is associated with a number of different hepatitis viruses that include: hepatitis A virus (HAV), hepatitis B virus (HBV), hepatitis C virus (HCV) and hepatitis D virus (delta virus). Other types of hepatitis identified include: hepatitis E virus, hepatitis F virus and hepatitis G virus.

hepatitis A is caused by an RNA enterovirus. It is relatively common and may be epidemic, especially in institutions, e.g. schools. The virus is transmitted by the faeco-oral route, caused by poor hygiene or contaminated food.

hepatitis B is caused by a DNA virus. It is usually transmitted sexually (vaginal or anal intercourse), injection of infected blood or blood products, or via contaminated equipment, such as needles. The virus is shed in vaginal discharge, semen and saliva. Individuals at high risk include, intravenous drug users, homosexual or bisexual men, prostitutes, and healthcare professionals through needlestick injuries. Hepatitis B virus may persist, causing chronic hepatitis, or a carrier state can develop. Effective vaccine exists.

hepatitis C is caused by an RNA virus and is most common in intravenous drug users and in those who have had a transfusion of blood or blood products. The virus can remain in the blood for many years and 30 to 50% of infected people develop chronic hepatitis, cirrhosis, liver failure and possibly liver cancer. Some people become carriers of the virus.

hepatitis D (delta virus) can only replicate in the presence of hepatitis B and is therefore found infecting simultaneously with hepatitis B, or as a superinfection in chronic carriers of hepatitis B. Delta virus may increase the severity of a hepatitis B infection, increasing the risk of chronic liver disease.

hepatitis E is transmitted via the faeco-oral route and has been reported in travellers returning from the USA, Mexico, Asia and Africa.

hepatization *n* the changes that occur in the lung tissue following lobar pneumonia. The affected tissue becomes a solid mass and takes on the appearance of liver.

hepatoblastoma a rare liver cancer of infants and young children. It comprises cells that resemble primitive fetal liver cells. There is an upper abdominal mass and the alphafetoprotein level in the blood is increased.

hepatocellular *adj* pertaining to or affecting liver cells.

hepatocyte a parenchymal (functional) liver cell.

hepatoma *n* primary cancer of the liver—**hepatomata** *pl*.

hepatomegaly *n* enlargement of the liver. It is palpable below the costal margin.

hepatopancreatic ampulla *n* the enlargement formed by the union of the common bile duct with the pancreatic duct where they enter the duodenum. Previously known as the ampulla of Vater.

hepatorenal *adj* pertaining to the liver and kidneys.

G
H

hepatorenal syndrome 10% of patients with advanced cirrhosis and ascites develop the hepatorenal syndrome. There are two clinical types; both are mediated by severe renal vasoconstriction due to extreme underfilling of the arterial circulation. *Type 1 hepatorenal syndrome* is characterized by progressive oliguria, a rapid rise of the serum creatinine and a very poor prognosis (without treatment median survival is less than 1 month). There is usually no proteinuria, a urine sodium excretion below 10 mmol/day and a urine/plasma osmolarity ratio of > 1.5. Other non-functional causes of renal failure must be excluded before the diagnosis is made. Treatment consists of albumin infusions in combination with terlipressin and is effective in about two-thirds of patients. Haemodialysis should not be used routinely because it does not improve the outcome. Patients who survive should be considered for liver transplantation. *Type 2 hepatorenal syndrome* usually occurs in patients with refractory ascites, is characterized by a moderate and stable increase in serum creatinine, and has a better prognosis.

hepatosplenic *adj* pertaining to the liver and spleen.

hepatosplenomegaly *n* enlargement of the liver and the spleen, so that each is palpable below the costal margin.

hepatotoxic *adj* having an injurious effect on liver cells such as excess alcohol—**hepatotoxicity** *n*.

HER2 *abbr* human epidermal growth factor receptor 2.

herbalism *n* herbal medicine, phytotherapy. The therapeutic use of herbs or mineral remedies. The use of plant material by trained practitioners to promote health and recovery from illness.

Herbal Medicines Advisory Committee a UK committee that advises the Medicines and Healthcare Products Regulatory Agency and government ministers regarding the registration of traditional herbal medicines and on the unlicensed herbal remedies.

Herbst appliance ⊃ orthodontic appliance.

hereditary *adj* inherited; capable of being inherited.

hereditary angioedema a genetic disorder characterized by episodes of severe life-threatening angioedema and sometimes abdominal pain. It is caused by a mutation in the gene encoding C1 inhibitor, which may be absent or dysfunctional. It is treated with C1 inhibitor pooled from plasma donations.

hereditary elliptocytosis a heterogeneous group of disorders that produce an increase in elliptocytic red cells on the blood film and a variable degree of haemolysis. Hereditary elliptocytosis is due to a functional abnormality of one or more anchor proteins in the red cell membrane, e.g. alpha spectrin or protein 4.1. Inheritance may be autosomal dominant or recessive. It is less common than hereditary spherocytosis in Western countries, with an incidence of 1/10 000, but is more common in equatorial Africa and parts of Southeast Asia. The clinical course is variable and depends upon the degree of membrane dysfunction caused by the inherited molecular defect(s); most cases present as an asymptomatic blood film

abnormality but occasional cases result in neonatal haemolysis or a chronic compensated haemolytic state. Management of the latter is the same as for hereditary spherocytosis. A characteristic variant of hereditary elliptocytosis occurs in Southeast Asia, particularly Malaysia and Papua New Guinea, with stomatocytes and ovalocytes in the blood. This has a prevalence of up to 30% in some communities because it offers relative protection from malaria and thus has sustained a high gene frequency. The differential diagnosis includes iron deficiency, thalassaemia, myelofibrosis, myelodysplasia and pyruvate kinase deficiency.

hereditary gingival fibromatosis ⊃ fibromatosis gingivae, gingival fibromatosis.

hereditary haemorrhagic telangiectasia also known as Rendu–Osler–Weber disease. A hereditary disease characterized by numerous angiomatous and telangiectatic areas on the oral mucosa and the skin, that tend to undergo haemorrhage.

hereditary opalescent dentine ⊃ dentinogenesis imperfecta.

hereditary spherocytosis usually inherited as an autosomal dominant condition, although 25% of cases have no family history and represent new mutations. The incidence is approximately 1:5000 in developed countries but this may be an underestimate since the disease may present de novo in patients over 65 years and is often discovered as a chance finding on a blood count. The pathogenesis varies between families; the most common abnormalities are deficiencies of beta spectrin or ankyrin. The severity of spontaneous haemolysis varies. Most cases are associated with an asymptomatic compensated chronic haemolytic state with spherocytes present on the blood film and a reticulocytosis. Occasional cases are associated with more severe haemolysis; these may be due to co-incidental polymorphisms in alpha spectrin or co-inheritance of a second defect involving a different protein. The clinical course may be complicated by crises: (a) haemolytic crisis—occurs when the severity of haemolysis increases; this is rarely seen in association with infection; (b) megaloblastic crisis—follows the development of folate deficiency; this may occur as a first presentation of the disease in association with pregnancy; (c) aplastic crisis—occurs in association with erythrovirus infection. Patients present with severe anaemia and a low reticulocyte count. Pigment gallstones are present in up to 50% of patients and may cause symptomatic cholecystitis. The patient and other family members should be screened for features of compensated haemolysis. This may be all that is required to confirm the diagnosis. Haemoglobin levels are variable depending on the degree of compensation. The blood film will show spherocytes but the direct Coombs test is negative excluding immune haemolysis. An osmotic fragility test may show increased sensitivity to lysis in hypotonic saline solutions but is limited by lack of sensitivity and specificity. More specific flow cytometric tests detecting binding of eosin-5-maleimide to red cells are now recommended in

G
H

borderline cases. Management includes folic acid prophylaxis which should be given for life. Consideration may be given to splenectomy which improves but does not normalize red cell survival. Potential indications include moderate to severe haemolysis with complications (anaemia and gallstones), although splenectomy should be delayed until the child is over 6 years of age in view of the risk of sepsis. Acute, severe haemolytic crises require transfusion support but blood must be cross-matched carefully and transfused slowly as haemolytic transfusion reactions may occur. The typical blood film appearances are masked in the presence of iron deficiency or disorders which cause a raised mean cell volume (MCV), such as jaundice; in these situations the red cell shape is normal but spherocytes will appear when the underlying abnormality is corrected.

heredity *n* transmission from parents to children of genetic characteristics by means of the genetic material; the process by which this occurs, and the study of such processes.

Hering–Breuer reflex (K Hering, German physiologist and psychologist, 1834–1918; J Breuer, Austrian physiologist, physician and psychiatrist, 1842–1925) an inhibitory inspiratory reflex initiated by overstretching of the stretch receptors in the smooth muscle of the large and small airways. This reflex is only activated by large tidal volumes (around 900 mL) so is unimportant in quiet tidal breathing, but vital for regulation of breathing in moderate/strenuous exercise.

Hering's after-image test ⊃ after-image test.

Hering's theory of colour vision (K Hering) (*syn* opponent-process theory, tetrachromatic theory) the theory that colour vision results from the action of three independent mechanisms, each of which is made up of a mutually antagonistic pair of colour sensations: red-green, yellow-blue and white-black. The latter pair is supposed to be responsible for the brightness aspect of the sensation, whereas the former two would be responsible for the coloured aspect of the sensation. ⊃ colour vision, visual pigment, Young–Helmholtz theory.

hermaphrodite *n* individual possessing both ovarian and testicular tissue. Although they may approximate either to male or female type, they are usually sterile from imperfect development of their gonads.

hernia *n* the abnormal protrusion of an organ, or part of an organ, through an aperture in the surrounding structures: commonly the protrusion of an abdominal organ through a gap in the abdominal wall (Figure H.7). Weakness of the muscle may be due to injury or previous surgery; obesity or heavy lifting add to the risk. If the protrusion becomes stuck in the narrow gap (incarcerated hernia) the blood supply may be compromised (strangulated hernia) and surgery is required. In sport the groin is a common site of pain or discomfort, and the term sportsman's hernia is sometimes used inappropriately for a variety of other conditions that cause it (including musculotendinous injuries and osteitis of the pubic bone). It is important to diagnose accurately the cause of groin pain, as treatment options, including those

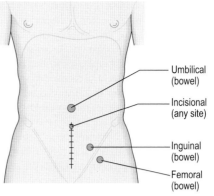

H.7 Common sites for hernias (reproduced from Waugh & Grant 2006 with permission).

involving surgery, will differ, and particularly relevant to identify a true hernia, which may be due to a tear in the external oblique muscle for which there are various methods of surgical repair. ⊃ femoral hernia, hiatus hernia, incisional hernia, inguinal hernia, irreducible hernia, strangulated hernia, umbilical hernia.

hernioplasty *n* an operation for hernia in which an attempt is made to prevent recurrence by refashioning the structures to give greater strength—**hernioplastic** *adj*.

herniorrhaphy *n* an operation for hernia in which the weak area is reinforced by some of the patient's own tissues or by some other material.

herniotomy *n* an operation to cure hernia by the return of its contents to their normal position and removal of the hernial sac.

heroin *n* diamorphine. A class A substance which is subject to considereable criminal misuse. Used medicinally as diamorphine to relieve severe pain.

herpangina *n* minute vesicles and ulcers at the back of the palate. Short, febrile illness in children caused by coxsackievirus group A.

herpes *n* a vesicular eruption caused by infection with the herpes simplex virus. *genital herpes* a sexually transmissible infection, caused by either herpes simplex virus type 1 or type 2 (HSV-1 or HSV-2), that is associated with painful, tender superficial ulcers of the genitalia or anal region. Without treatment first-episode lesions heal within about one month; antiviral therapy shortens the duration of the lesions. Recurrences are common, particularly with HSV-2, but the duration of lesions is shorter than during the initial episode. An individual can transmit the virus to a sexual partner even when there are no apparent genital or orolabial lesions.

herpes gestationis a rare immune-mediated skin disease precipitated by pregnancy. Characterized by an erythematous rash and blisters. ⊃ pemphigoid gestationis.

herpes simplex virus (HSV) there are two types of HSV—types 1 and 2 (HSV-1 and HSV-2). HSV-1 is associated with orolabial herpes (cold sores), but either type can cause genital herpes. Following infection, whether or not the individual develops symptoms, the virus becomes latent or hidden for the individual's lifetime in the trigeminal ganglion (in the case of orolabial herpes) or in the sacral ganglia (in the case of genital herpes). Reactivation of the virus can cause recurrent lesions, or the virus can be shed from the mucous membranes or skin without visible signs. ⊃ herpes, Colour Section Figure 74.

herpesviruses group of DNA viruses that include: cytomegalovirus (CMV), Epstein–Barr virus (EBV), herpes simplex virus (HSV), human herpesvirus 6 (HHV6) and varicella-zoster virus (VZV).

herpes zoster (*syn* shingles) the causative organism is the varicella-zoster virus (VZV); the same virus that causes chickenpox. Herpes zoster occurs when there is reactivation of the VZV that has remained dormant in a sensory nerve ganglion since a much earlier attack of chickenpox usually during childhood. The reactivation is associated with an event that compromises the immune system, such as stress or serious illness. It occurs in middle-aged and older people, or in individuals who are immunocompromised, especially people with HIV disease. The person with herpes zoster may infect another person with chickenpox. It is characterized by severe pain and usually, some days later, the appearance of vesicles along the distribution of a sensory nerve (usually unilateral). It is termed *herpes zoster ophthalmicus* when there is involvement of that portion of the gasserian ganglion receiving fibres from the ophthalmic division of the trigeminal nerve. Initially it leads to severe unilateral neuralgia in the region of the distribution of the nerve. This is followed by a vesicular eruption of the epithelium of the forehead, the nose, eyelids and sometimes the cornea. The vesicles rupture leaving haemorrhagic areas that heal in several weeks. Ocular complications occur in approximately 50% of all cases of herpes zoster ophthalmicus. Corneal involvement appears as acute epithelial keratitis which is characterized by small fine dendritic or stellate lesions in the peripheral cornea in association with a conjunctivitis. This keratitis usually resolves within a week. As the disease progresses it may give rise to mucous plaque keratitis which occurs usually between the third and the sixth month after the onset of the rash. It is characterized by the plaque lines on the surface of the cornea which can be easily lifted and stromal haze. Iritis also accompanies this keratitis in approximately 50% of cases. Early treatment of herpes zoster, at least 72 hours prior to the development of the rash, with an antiviral drug, such as aciclovir, famciclovir or valaciclovir, can lessen the intensity of the infection. Post-herpetic neuralgia may be particularly resistant to treatment. A live virus vaccine that reduces the risk of herpes zoster is available to people over 60 years of age in the United States. ⊃ capsaicin, iritis, keratitis, postherpetic (neuralgia), Ramsay Hunt syndrome, scleritis, Colour Section Figure 75.

herpes zoster ophthalmicus ⊃ herpes zoster.

herpetic relating to herpes.

herpetic keratitis keratitis caused by either herpes simplex (dendritic keratitis) or herpes zoster viruses. ⊃ dendritic keratitis, disciform keratitis, herpes zoster, interstitial keratitis, punctate epithelial keratitis.

herpetiform *adj* resembling herpes.

herring-bone pattern in dental radiography, the effect produced when radiographic film has been exposed with the incorrect side towards the central ray. The lead backing within the film produces the pattern on the developed film.

Hers' disease (H-G Hers, Belgian physiologist and biochemist) type VI glycogen storage disease in which there is a deficiency of liver phosphorylase enzyme. It is characterized by mild hepatomegaly.

hertz (Hz) *n* (H Hertz, German physicist, 1857–1894) derived Système International d'Unités (SI) unit (International System of Units) for wave frequency. One hertz equals one cycle per second. ⊃ Appendix 2.

Herxheimer's reaction ⊃ Jarisch–Herxheimer's reaction.

hesitancy delay in starting to void urine, even when responding to a strong desire to void. A symptom of outflow obstruction, bladder instability or hypersensitivity.

Hess test a sphygmomanometer cuff is applied to the arm and is inflated. Petechial eruption in the surrounding area after 5 min denotes weakness of the capillary walls.

HET *abbr* human enhancement technologies.

heter/o- a prefix that means 'unlikeness, dissimilarity', e.g. *heterometropia*.

heterochromia *n* (*syn* anisochromia) a difference in colour within areas in the same iris, or one iris is different in colour from the other.

heterodont possessing teeth of several shapes, such as incisors, canines, premolars and molars.

heterogametic *adj* relating to the sex which produces gametes with different sex chromosomes. Male gametes, spermatozoa have either the X or Y chromosome. They determine the sex of the offspring. ⊃ homogametic.

heterogeneity having variable qualities and characteristics.

heterogenous *adj* of unlike origin; not originating within the organism; derived from a different species. ⊃ homogenous *opp*.

heterograft ⊃ xenograft.

heterologous *adj* of different origin; from a different species. ⊃ homologous *opp*.

heterometropia a visual defect in which the refraction in one eye is slightly different from that in the other. Each eye perceives a slightly different image.

heteronymous diplopia (*syn* crossed diplopia) binocular diplopia in which the image received by the right eye appears to the left and that received by the left eye appears to the right. In this condition the images are formed on the temporal retina. ⊃ homonymous diplopia.

heteronymous hemianopsia hemianopsia involving either both nasal halves (binasal hemianopsia) or both temporal halves of the visual field (bitemporal hemianopsia). A common cause of the latter is a lesion in the optic chiasma. ⊃ circulus arteriosus, homonymous hemianopsia.

heterophile *n* a product of one species which acts against that of another, for example human antigen against sheep's red blood cells.

heterophoria (*syn* phoria) the tendency for the two visual axes of the eyes not to be directed towards the point of fixation, in the absence of an adequate stimulus to fusion. Thus, the active and passive positions do not coincide for that particular fixation distance. This tendency is characterized by a deviation which can take various forms according to its relative direction such as esophoria, exophoria, etc. ➲ associated heterophoria, compensated heterophoria, uncompensated heterophoria.

heterosexual *adj*, *n* literally, of different sexes; often used to describe an individual who is sexually attracted to members of the opposite sex. ➲ homosexual *opp*.

heterotophic ossification (HO) a condition in which bone is laid down in soft tissues. There are a number of types, neurogenic HO is found following neurological insult. Maintaining active movement and the use of medication can prevent it.

heterotopic pregnancy a pregnancy occurring in an abnormal location, such as outside the uterus.

heterotopic transplant ➲ transplant.

heterozygous *adj* having different genes or alleles at the same locus on corresponding homologous chromosomes (one of paternal origin and one maternal) ➲ homozygous *opp*.

heuristic a 'trial and error' method of trying to solve a computer problem.

Hewitt's prop ➲ mouth prop.

hex/a- a prefix that means 'six', e.g. *hexoses*.

hexachlorophene *n* a phenolic disinfectant used in preoperative skin preparation, and as a dusting powder. It should not be used on children under two years of age, during pregnancy, or on excoriated or badly burnt skin.

hexadecimal a mathematical system which employs 16 digits from 0 to 9 plus A, B, C, D, E, F.

hexokinase (HK) an enzyme that catalyzes the 'capture' of glucose after uptake from the blood, by phosphorylation of glucose to the impermanent glucose-6-phosphate. A cytoplasmic muscle enzyme present in type 1 muscle fibres, which utilize glucose directly. Important stage in glycolysis and glycogenesis. ➲ muscle enzymes.

hexosamine a hexose sugar with an amino group. For example glucosamine formed from glucose.

hexose monophosphate shunt ➲ pentose phosphate pathway.

hexoses monosaccharides containing six carbon atoms such as glucose, mannose, galactose, fructose.

HFEA *abbr* Human Fertilisation and Embryology Authority.

HFJV *abbr* high frequency jet ventilation.

HFOV *abbr* high frequency oscillation ventilation.

HFPPV *abbr* high frequency positive pressure ventilation.

HGH *abbr* human growth hormone.

HGP *abbr* hard gas permeable (contact lens).

HHNK *abbr* hyperglycaemic hyperosmolar non-ketotic (coma).

5-HIAA *abbr* 5-hydroxyindoleacetic acid.

hiatus *n* a space or opening.

hiatus hernia migration of part of the stomach through the diaphragmatic hiatus into the chest. May be asymptomatic, cause gastro-oesophageal reflux disease or strangulate. ➲ hernia—**hiatal** *adj*.

Hib vaccine *abbr* Haemophilus *influenzae* type B vaccine. An injectable vaccine that protects against the serious infections caused by *Haemophilus influenzae* is offered (in the UK) as part of the routine immunization programme at 2, 3 and 4 months of age with a booster at 12 months.

hiccough *n* (*syn* hiccup) an involuntary inspiratory spasm of the diaphragm, ending in a sudden closure of the glottis with the production of a characteristic sound.

Hick's law a law specifying the linear relationship between choice reaction time and the number of response options available, stating that choice reaction time increases as a function of the logarithm of the number of options. ➲ reaction time.

hidradenitis suppurativa a chronic suppurative condition affecting the axillae, groin and anogenital area. It is characterized by abscess formation with discharge of pus, sinuses, fibrosis and scarring.

hidrosis *n* sweat secretion.

hierarchy of evidence in evidence-based practice a ranking of types of evidence based on their ability to predict effectiveness, remove bias and control confounders. The highest level is considered to be a systematic review of several high-quality randomized controlled trials, through various levels to the lowest level of expert opinion.

HIFU *abbr* high intensity focused ultrasound.

Higginson's syringe a rubber bulb with tubes leading to and from it. Compression of the rubber bulb forces fluid forward through the nozzle for irrigation of a body cavity. Rarely used and now mostly replaced by single-use items of equipment.

high-altitude cerebral oedema (HACE) this is rare and life-threatening and is usually preceded by altitude sickness/illness. In addition to features of altitude sickness/illness, the presentation is with rapidly progressive cerebral symptoms, which may include hallucination or behavioural change, confusion, visual loss and ultimately loss of consciousness. Ataxia is usually present, papilloedema and retinal haemorrhages are common, and focal neurological signs may be found. Treatment is directed at improving oxygenation. Descent to lower altitude is the single most important intervention but, if this is impossible, nursing the patient with oxygen therapy in a portable pressurized bag may be helpful. High-dose corticosteroids, diuretics and mannitol have all been used but efficacy is difficult to assess as these treatments are usually administered in field conditions.

high-altitude pulmonary oedema (HAPE) this life-threatening condition usually occurs in the first 4 days after

G
H

ascent above 2500 m. Unlike high-altitude cerebral oedema (HACE), HAPE may occur de novo without the preceding signs of altitude sickness/illness. Presentation is with symptoms of dry cough, breathlessness and extreme fatigue. Later, the cough becomes productive of bloody sputum. It is associated with crepitations in both lung fields, profound hypoxaemia, pulmonary hypertension and radiological evidence of diffuse alveolar oedema. It is not known whether the alveolar oedema is a result of mechanical stress on the pulmonary capillaries associated with the high pulmonary arterial pressure or an effect of hypoxia on capillary permeability. It appears to occur in susceptible subjects and such individuals are at particular risk of further episodes with future ascents. Other predisposing factors include youth, rapidity of ascent, the presence of altitude sickness/illness and heavy exertion. Treatment is directed at reversal of hypoxia with immediate descent wherever possible and administration of oxygen. Reduction of pulmonary arterial pressure with nifedipine has also proved helpful and this agent has been used for prophylaxis in susceptible subjects.

high-altitude retinal haemorrhage occurs in over 30% of trekkers at 5000 m. The haemorrhages are usually asymptomatic and resolve spontaneously. Visual defects can occur with haemorrhage involving the macula, but there is no specific treatment.

high-carbohydrate diet ⊃ carbohydrate (CHO), carbohydrate intake guidelines for athletes, carbohydrate loading.

high copper amalgam alloy alloy with increased copper content to reduce corrosion. ⊃ alloy.

high-density lipoprotein (HDL) ⊃ lipoprotein.

high dependency unit (HDU) an area within a hospital with augmented levels of staff and equipment in which patients can receive levels of observation, monitoring, nursing and medical care between that available on a general ward and intensive care unit. Generally excludes those needing mechanical ventilation.

high energy bond chemical bond which is readily hydrolysed by an appropriate catalyst, and releases a large amount of energy when the hydrolysis occurs in the cytoplasm of a living cell; this energy release depends as much on the products of the hydrolysis being present at very low concentrations as it does on the properties of the bond itself. Key instances in muscle are the terminal phosphate bonds of adenosine triphosphate (ATP) and creatine phosphate (CrP) (also known as phosphocreatine).

high-fat diet one which provides more than 30% of energy as fat. Research into effects on performance indicates that 3–5 days on a high-fat diet leads to deterioration of endurance performance when compared to a carbohydrate (CHO)-rich diet. However, when adaptation to the diet is combined with training for a period of 1–4 weeks, a high-fat diet does not attenuate endurance performance compared to a high-CHO diet. When such regimens are continued and compared for longer than 4 weeks, endurance performance is markedly better on the CHO-rich diet. There is no performance benefit in switching to high-CHO after

long-term adaptation to high-fat, compared to having a high-CHO diet all along.

high frequency oscillation ventilation (HFOV) a method of mechanical ventilation used to support extremely premature infants. It is sometimes combined with nitrous oxide therapy. Pressure is used to reach optimum lung expansion and oscillation (bounce) is added to aid gas distribution. ⊃ high frequency ventilation.

high frequency ventilation a type of mechanical ventilation provided at more than four times the usual frequency, in order to reduce peak airway pressures by reducing the delivered tidal volume. Ventilation occurs through the movement of gases from a high to a low concentration gradient rather than through the exchange of gases via tidal volume changes. This type of ventilation can be delivered in three ways, classified by the method of gas delivery to the lungs: high frequency positive pressure ventilation (HFPPV), high frequency oscillation ventilation (HFOV) and high-frequency jet ventilation (HFJV). ⊃ high frequency oscillation ventilation.

high index lens a specialized lens made with higher refractive material than crown glass. Included in these are flint and titanium glasses in which the refractive index can be as high as 1.8. However, as the index increases there is usually a decrease in the constringence. For example, Zenlite (a tradename) has a refractive index of 1.805 and a constringence of 25.4. Recently, technical advances have made it possible to manufacture high index progressive lenses. High index lenses are used for high prescriptions as they can be made much thinner than crown glass lenses of equivalent power. As high index lenses have very reflective surfaces it is valuable to have them coated. ⊃ constringence.

high intensity focused ultrasound (HIFU) a type of ultrasound used to produce heat in order to destroy abnormal tissue, such as prostate cancers.

high labial bow in orthodontics, a thick stainless steel wire bent to conform to the buccal aspect of the upper dental arch above the teeth. It can carry thinner wires wound on to it in the form of T-springs or apron springs to retract the upper incisor teeth. The ends of the bow are anchored in the acrylic baseplate as a removable orthodontic appliance.

high-level fracture also known as craniofacial dysjunction fracture. A Le Fort III fracture involving the middle third of the facial skeleton. ⊃ jaw fractures, Le Fort classification.

high lip line in the upper lip, the greatest height to which the inferior border of the upper lip can be raised by muscle power. In the lower lip, the greatest height to which the superior border of the lower lip can be raised by muscle function.

highly active antiretroviral therapy (HAART) combines three different types of antiretrovial drugs that attack the human immunodeficiency virus at different stages of replication.

high-protein diet one which provides more than 15% of energy as protein. Traditionally, high-protein diets are low-carbohydrate diets. These diets are claimed to be effective for the reduction of body mass and body fat. Extremely high-protein diets are claimed to suppress appetite through reliance on fat mobilization and ketone body formation. In addition, the elevated thermic effect of dietary protein, with a relatively low coefficient of digestibility (particularly in the case of plant proteins), reduces the net calories available from ingested protein compared with a well-balanced diet of equivalent caloric value. The long-term success of high-protein diets remains questionable and they may even pose health risks, including kidney damage, increased blood lipoprotein levels and dehydration. ⊃ low-carbohydrate ketogenic diets.

high-resolution computed tomography (CT) a method of using thinner slices in computed tomography (CT) scanning in order to increase the image definition.

high risk infant an infant who is likely to suffer ill health or death.

high risk pregnancy a pregnancy which may result in injury or death to the women or the fetus.

high spatial frequency algorithm in computed tomography (CT) scanning an algorithm used to provide high spatial resolution. Frequently used to demonstrate bone, or in high resolution chest studies. ⊃ algorithm.

high temperature chemistry the chemistry used in automatic radiographic processing equipment that function in the range of 31–39°C at a pH of about 9.6, now superseded by low temperature chemistry. ⊃ low temperature chemistry.

high voltage pulsed stimulation (HVPS) an electrotherapy term. A type of pulsed current with very short monophasic pulses, shape is usually either a pulse with twin peaks or a double pulse with no interpulse interval. Duration is typically less than 50 μs, so the current is comfortable and there is little risk of skin irritation. HVPS (also known as HVPC) has a low average current, ideal for use in a battery-powered portable stimulator, charge per pulse may be too low for effective large-muscle stimulation even using multiple cathodes (option: use an alternating current or longer duration pulsed current).

hilar adenitis inflammation of the bronchial lymph nodes. ⊃ adenitis.

Hill–Sachs lesion/deformity following anterior dislocation of the shoulder, the head of the humerus can sustain a compression fracture from contact with the glenoid and its labrum. This consequent depression of the humeral head is known as a Hill–Sachs lesion.

hilot ⊃ traditional birth attendant.

hilum *n* a depression on the surface of an organ where vessels, ducts, etc. enter and leave—**hili** *pl*, **hilar** *adj*.

hindbrain the part of the brain comprising the fourth ventricle, pons, medulla oblongata and cerebellum.

hindgut the caudal or posterior part of the embryonic alimentary tract. It gives rise to the distal transverse colon, descending and sigmoid colon, rectum, part of anal canal and part of the urogenital structures. ⊃ foregut, midgut.

hindwaters the sac of amniotic fluid situated behind the fetal head and surrounding the fetus. ⊃ forewaters.

hinge angle the angle between two radiotherapy beam axes at their point of intersection.

hinge axis (dental) ⊃ transverse horizontal axis (dental).

hinge axis locating face-bow also known as hinge bow, kinematic face-bow. ⊃ adjustable axis face-bow.

hinged ankle foot orthosis (AFO) an ankle foot orthosis (AFO) with a hinge at the ankle joint so that the patient can dorsiflex their foot, but not plantarflex it further than plantargrade. It allows for a more normal gait pattern than a fixed AFO, but can be heavy and bulky for patients to wear.

hinge joint ginglymus. A synovial joint, e.g. the elbow or knee, where the bones are moulded in such a way to allow movement in one plane.

hinge movement a joint movement comparable to that of a hinge but allowing more laxity than a straight hinge. The temporomandibular joint allows forward (incisive), lateral and rotational as well as retrusive movements.

hinge or plane line articulator an articulator with a simple hinge joint preventing any lateral or sliding movement.

hip bone (innominate bone) formed by the fusion of three separate bones—the ilium, ischium and pubis.

hip injury in sport hip injury is important in sport as the initial treatment usually requires non-weight-bearing activity only and then often a prolonged rehabilitation. *acute injuries* can be the result of a fall, direct trauma or twisting; they include fractures, dislocations and soft tissue injuries to muscles and supporting ligaments. *overuse injuries* result from repetitive weight-bearing activity, such as road running, and include bursitis and tendonitis (tendinitis).

hip joint a synovial ball and socket joint formed by the cup-shaped acetabulum of the innominate (hip) bone and the almost spherical head of the femur. The capsular ligament encloses the head and most of the neck of the femur. The cavity is deepened by the acetabular labrum, a ring of fibrocartilage attached to the rim of the acetabulum, which stabilizes the joint without limiting its range of movement (Figure H.8). The hip joint is necessarily a sturdy and powerful joint, since it bears all body weight when standing upright. It is stabilized by its surrounding muscles, but its ligaments are also important. There are three main external ligaments, the iliofemoral, ischiofemoral and pubofemoral ligaments, which are localized thickenings of the joint cavity. Within the joint, the ligament of the head of femur (ligamentum teres) attaches the femoral head to the acetabulum. The lower limb movements possible at the hip are: flexion—facilitated by the psoas and iliacus (which together form the iliopsoas muscle) and satorius muscles; extension—facilitated by the gluteus maximus and the hamstring group of muscles (biceps femoris, semitendinosus, semimembranosus); abduction—facilitated by the gluteus medius, g. minimus and sartorius muscles; adduction—facilitated by the adductor longus, a. brevis and a. magnus group of muscles; medial rotation—facilitated by the gluteus medius, g. minimus and the three adductor muscles; lateral

G

H

355

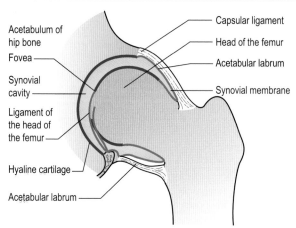

Labels (clockwise from top left): Acetabulum of hip bone, Fovea, Synovial cavity, Ligament of the head of the femur, Hyaline cartilage, Acetabular labrum; Capsular ligament, Head of the femur, Acetabular labrum, Synovial membrane.

H.8 Hip joint (reproduced from Watson 2000 with permission).

rotation—facilitated by the gluteus maximus, quadratus femoris and obturator muscles. ⊃ hip injury.

hippocampus *n* a structure located on the medial wall of each temporal lobe and which curves beneath the lateral ventricle. It is the part of the limbic system which is formed from evolutionarily older cortex. It is concerned with the initial processing of new memories and spatial orientation—**hippocampi** *pl.* ⊃ limbic system.

Hippocrates *n* Greek physician and philosopher (460–367 BC) who established a school of medicine at Cos, his birthplace. He is often termed the 'Father of Medicine'.

hip pointer a contusion of the iliac crest. Usually due to some form of trauma.

hippus the small rhythmic variations in the size of the pupils. They are present in everybody and increase slightly at high luminances. The frequency of these oscillations is about 1.4 Hz. ⊃ pupil.

hip replacement ⊃ total hip replacement procedure, arthroplasty.

Hirschsprung's disease (H Hirschsprung, Danish physician, 1830–1916) congenital intestinal aganglionosis, leading to intractable constipation or even intestinal obstruction. There is marked hypertrophy and dilation of the colon (megacolon) above the aganglionic segment. Commoner in boys and children with Down's syndrome.

hirsute *adj* hairy or shaggy.

hirsutism, hirsuties *n* any abnormal degree of coarse hairiness, (usually refers to male pattern of hair growth in a woman). ⊃ hypertrichosis.

hirudin *n* a chemical produced by the medicinal leech, which prevents the clotting of blood by acting as an anticoagulant.

hirudo *n* ⊃ leech.

HIS *acron* **H**ospital **I**nformation **S**ystem.

histamine *n* an amine released in many tissues. It causes smooth muscle contraction, gastric secretion and vasodilation depending on the type of cellular histamine receptor.

For example, constriction of bronchial muscle is mediated through (H_1) receptors, stimulation of gastric acid secretion (H_2) receptors and various actions in nervous tissue (H_3). During the inflammatory response histamine release from mast cells leads to H_1-mediated vasodilatation and increased vascular permeability, causing redness and swelling. In addition initial experiments in vivo with H_4 receptor antagonists indicate a role also for the H_4 receptor. ⊃ allergy, anaphylaxis, inflammation.

histamine receptors there are three types in the body, H_1 in the bronchial muscle, H_2 in the secreting cells in the stomach and H_3 in nerve tissue.

histamine test test previously used to determine the maximal gastric secretion of hydrochloric acid.

histidinaemia *n* an autosomal recessive metabolic condition. The lack of an enzyme needed for the metabolism of histidine leads to an increase in the amount of histidine in blood.

histidine *n* an essential (indispensable) amino acid in infants and children which is widely distributed in the proteins present in the diet.

hist/o- a prefix that means 'tissue', e.g. *histology*.

histiocytes *npl* macrophages or phagocytic tissue cells.

histiocytoma *n* benign tumour of histiocytes.

histiocytosis *n* a group of conditions in which histiocytes are abnormal in some way. Known collectively as Langerhans' cell histiocytosis. ⊃ Hand–Schüller–Christian disease, Letterer-Siwe disease.

histocompatibility the degree of similarity (compatibility) between the donor and recipient antigens in tissue or organ(s) for transplant. The closer the match the better chance of a successful transplant. ⊃ human leucocyte antigens, major histocompatibility complex.

histogram a bar graph with values for one or more variables plotted against the frequency or time. A graph displaying data in columns which are next to each other (Figure H.9).

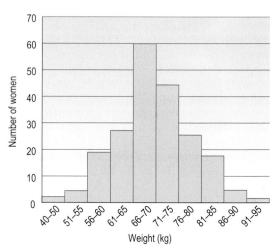

H.9 Histogram (reproduced from Gunn 2001 with permission).

histology *n* microscopic study of tissues—**histological** *adj*, **histologically** *adv*.

histolysis *n* disintegration of organic tissue—**histolytic** *adj*.

histones *npl* proteins closely associated with the chromosomal DNA of higher organisms, which coils around histone molecules.

histopathology the microscopic study of the diseases of tissues.

Histoplasma *n* a genus of fungi. *H. capsulatum* causes the condition histoplasmosis in human.

histoplasmosis *n* an infection caused by inhaling spores of the fungus *Histoplasma capsulatum*. The spores are found in the faeces of some birds including poultry and in the faeces of bats. It is endemic in parts of the United States, such as the Mississippi Valley. The primary lung lesion may be asymptomatic or be accompanied by raised temperature, malaise, cough and adenopathy. Progressive histoplasmosis can be fatal. Lung involvement increases and the infection can disseminate in the blood to affect organs that include the liver and spleen.

histotoxic hypoxia due to inability of cells to use oxygen, e.g. due to poisoning. ⊃ hypoxia.

HIT *acron* heparin-induced thrombocytopenia.

HIV *abbr* human immunodeficiency virus. ⊃ AIDS.

hives *n* nettlerash; urticaria.

HK *abbr* hexokinase.

HLA *abbr* human leucocyte antigen.

HMB *abbr* beta-hydroxy beta-methylbutyrate.

HMG-CoA reductase inhibitors (3-hydroxy-3-methyl-glutaryl-coenzyme) known colloquially as 'statins'. A group of drugs (e.g. pravastatin) that prevent the synthesis of cholesterol in the liver, thereby reducing its level in the blood. ⊃ Appendix 5.

HMM *abbr* 'heavy meromyosin'.

HNPCC *abbr* hereditary non-polyposis colorectal cancer.

HO *abbr* heterotophic ossification.

HOCM *abbr* hypertrophic obstructive cardiomyopathy.

Hodgkin's disease (T Hodgkin, British physician, 1798–1866) tumour of lymphoid tissue often originating in the mediastinum. Often occurs in young adults. A diagnostic feature is the presence of the large multinucleated Reed–Sternberg cells in the lymphatic system. The prognosis is related to the histological subtype and stage; cure rate is around 80%. Treatment may consist of radiotherapy and/or chemotherapy. ⊃ lymphoma.

hoe the chisel-like instrument used to remove hard tooth tissue by trimming and chipping. ⊃ periodontal instruments.

holandric inheritance those traits or conditions inherited through the paternal line from father to son, they are transmitted by genes on the non-homologous part of the Y chromosome.

holder a device for holding nerve canal broaches, napkins, needles, radiographic films and rubber dam.

holder method of pasteurization ⊃ pasteurization.

hole in the hand illusion ⊃ hole in the hand test.

hole in the hand test (*syn* hole in the hand illusion) a test for binocular vision in which a distant object is viewed through a tube with one eye while a hand is placed against the tube at a distance of some 20–30 cm before the other eye. Subjects who see the object through an apparent hole in the hand have binocular vision, whereas seeing either the object through the tube only or the hand only indicates an absence of binocular vision.

holes the absence of an electron in the valence band, the 'hole' has a positive charge and therefore can attract electrons.

holistic *adj* relating to the theory of holism. Describes health care that takes account of physical, psychological, emotional, social and spiritual needs and aspects of care.

Hollenhorst's plaques (R Hollenhorst, American ophthalmologist, 1913–2008) the orange-yellow spots, usually found at branching sites of retinal arterioles. They are due to necrosis and ulceration of atheromatous, cholesterol-containing emboli in the carotid arteries which discharge into the circulation. They do not usually obstruct the retinal arterioles and as such do not cause visual symptoms. However, they indicate the possible development of larger emboli (fibrinoplatelets) that may temporarily obstruct the retinal circulation and cause amaurosis fugax, and may even presage a myocardial infarction or stroke. ⊃ amaurosis fugax, corneal arcus, atheroma, xanthelasma.

holocrine gland a type of exocrine gland that disintegrates in order to discharge its secretion. For example a sebaceous gland of the skin. ⊃ apocrine gland, merocrine (eccrine) gland.

holoenzyme *n* enzyme protein combined with a prosthetic group or its coenzyme.

holography a technique for obtaining a stereoscopic image of an object without the use of lenses. It consists of recording on a photographic plate the pattern of interference between coherent light reflected from the object and light that comes directly from the same source (or is reflected from a mirror). The coherent light is usually provided by a laser. The photographic recording on the plate (called a hologram) when illuminated with coherent light yields an image which is identical in amplitude and phase distribution with the original wave from the object. It thus provides a three-dimensional image of the object in the sense that the observer's eyes must refocus to examine foreground and background and indeed 'look around' objects by simply moving the head laterally. ⊃ coherent sources, interference.

Homans' sign (J Homans, American surgeon, 1877–1954) passive dorsiflexion of foot causing pain in calf muscles. Indicative of deep vein thrombosis affecting the leg. The person lies supine or prone or sitting, the health professional passively extends the knee, then dorsiflexes the ankle. This test may give false-positive results as the movement may be painful for other reasons. Rarely used.

home assessment an evaluation of the suitability of an individual's accommodation in order to identify any adaptations, resources or services needed to enable him or her to adequately perform activities of daily living in the home environment.

G
H

357

home birth the birth of an infant at home; it may be planned or unplanned. ⊃ planned home birth, unplanned home birth.

hom/eo- a prefix that means 'like', e.g. *homeopathy*.

homeopathy *n* a method of treating disease by prescribing minute doses of drugs which, in maximum dose, would produce symptoms of the disease. The 'law of similars' or like cures like was first adopted by Hahnemann (C Hahnemann, German physician, 1755–1843)—**homeopathic** *adj.* ⊃ allopathy.

homeostasis *n* autoregulatory processes whereby functions such as body temperature, blood pressure, blood glucose and electrolyte levels are maintained within set parameters.

home visit a visit by the therapist to the client's usual living place in order to carry out assessment or treatment.

homicide *n* killing of another person: intentional killing is murder, whereas accidental (without intent) killing is manslaughter (in Scotland culpable homicide).

homo- a prefix that means 'same', e.g. *homogametic*.

homocysteine *n* an intermediate which with serine forms cysteine. It is also a precursor for methionine regeneration in reactions requiring folates and cobalamins. A deficiency in folates and other B vitamins is associated with increased amounts of homocysteine in the blood and a higher risk of coronary heart disease.

homocystinuria *n* excretion of homocystine (a sulphur-containing amino acid, homologue of cystine) in the urine. It is caused by a recessively-inherited metabolic error in which there is a deficiency of the enzyme cystathionine synthetase. The condition gives rise to slow development or learning disability of varying degree; lens of the eye may dislocate and there is overgrowth of long bones with venous and arterial thrombotic episodes which are often fatal in childhood. Osteoporosis and a Marfanoid appearance occur in homocystinuria. The diagnosis is confirmed by finding homocystine in the urine, and patients respond to treatment with pyridoxine—**homocystinuric** *adj.* ⊃ Marfan's syndrome.

homoeothermic *adj* describes an animal able to maintain a constant core body temperature despite variations in environmental temperatures.

homogametic relating to the sex which produces gametes with the same sex chromosomes. Female gametes, oocytes always have the X chromosome. ⊃ heterogametic.

homogeneous *adj* of the same type; of the same quality or consistency throughout.

homogenize *vt* to make into the same consistency throughout.

homogenous *adj* having a like nature, e.g. a bone graft from another human being. ⊃ heterogenous *opp*.

homogentisic acid an intermediate compound formed in the metabolism of the amino acids tyrosine and phenylalanine. It is responsible for the darkly-staining urine of individuals with alkaptonuria. ⊃ alkaptonuria

homograft *n* a tissue or organ which is transplanted from one individual to another of the same species. ⊃ allograft.

homolateral *adj* on the same side—**homolaterally** *adv*. ⊃ contralateral, ipsilateral.

homologous *adj* corresponding in origin and structure. ⊃ heterologous *opp*.

homologous chromosomes **1.** those that synapse (pair) during meiosis. Of the two homologues, one is paternal and the other maternal in origin. **2.** a pair of chromosomes in a diploid (2n) somatic cell which are the same in size and shape and gene loci.

homonymous *adj* consisting of corresponding halves. Pertaining to symmetrical halves of the visual fields, i.e. the nasal (inner) half of one field and the temporal (outer) half of the other. When describing a visual field defect implies loss of vision in the same side of the field in the two eyes. ⊃ homonymous diplopia, homonymous hemianopsia.

homonymous diplopia (*syn* uncrossed diplopia) binocular diplopia in which the image received by the right eye appears to the right and that received by the left eye appears to the left. In this condition, the images are formed on the nasal retina. ⊃ heteronymous diplopia.

homonymous hemianopsia hemianopsia involving the nasal half of the visual field of one eye and the temporal half of the visual field of the other eye. Common causes are occlusion of the posterior cerebral artery due to cerebrovascular accident (stroke), trauma and tumours. ⊃ heteronymous hemianopsia.

homosexual *adj*, *n* literally, of the same sex; describes an individual who is sexually attracted to members of the same sex. Individuals may prefer to be described as being gay or lesbian.

homozygous *adj* having identical genes or alleles in the same locus on both homologous chromosomes of a pair (one is paternal in origin and the other maternal). If a person has inherited a recessive allele from both parents they are homozygous for that trait or disease, e.g. cystic fibrosis; it will be expressed and their offspring will be carriers of the recessive allele. ⊃ heterozygous *opp*.

HONK *acron* **H**yper**O**smolar **N**on-**K**etotic coma.

hook a surgical instrument with a fine bent or curved tip used to retract and hold tissue at operation. ⊃ Poswillo hook.

hookworm *n* ⊃ *Ancylostoma, Necator*.

hoop traction fixed skin traction used for the treatment of fractures of the femoral shaft in children, and for the gradual abduction of the hip in children with developmental dysplasia of the hip.

hordeolum *n* ⊃ stye.

horizon a specific anatomical stage of embryonic development, of which 23 have been defined, beginning with the unicellular fertilized egg and ending 7 to 9 weeks later, with the beginning of the fetal stage.

horizontal cell a retinal cell located in the inner nuclear layer which connects several cones and rods together.

horizontal overlap ⊃ overjet.

horizontal plane ⊃ transverse plane.

hormone *n* a specific chemical messenger produced by endocrine glands and other structures. It is transported in the blood or lymph to tissues and organs elsewhere in the body where they regulate metabolic functions and cell growth. Hormones are either lipid-based, e.g. thyroid hormones, or peptides, e.g. insulin, adrenaline (epinephrine). Hormone release is regulated by negative feedback mechanisms, neurotransmitters, other hormones and releasing and inhibiting factors. Rarely regulation is through positive feedback such as the release of oxytocin during labour. Other hormones act more locally such as those secreted in the gastrointestinal tract, e.g. gastrin produced by gastric cells stimulates increased acid secretion by other gastric cells.

hormone replacement therapy (HRT) a term usually applied to oestrogen therapy (with progestogens in women who have an intact uterus) given to women to relieve menopausal symptoms and previously to prevent or minimize the development of osteoporosis. It is administered orally, by implant or transdermally with patch or gel. The term also applies to a treatment that replaces other missing or deficient hormones.

hormone-sensitive lipase enzyme responsible for hydrolysis of triacylglycerol (triglyceride) molecules and therefore release of free fatty acids and glycerol. It functions mainly in adipose tissue and muscle. Activity of the enzyme in both sites is increased during endurance-type exercise, providing free fatty acids for resynthesis of adenosine triphosphate (ATP).

Horner's syndrome (J Horner, Swiss ophthalmologist, 1831–1886) loss of sympathetic innervation to the eye and upper face causing myosis (miosis) (small pupil), ptosis (drooping of the eyelid), retraction of the eyeball (enophthalmos) and anhidrosis (loss of sweating) over the forehead on that side. It may be caused by pathology in the hypothalamus or brainstem, occur with cluster headaches when it is accompanied by unilateral lacrimation, conjunctival reddening and nasal congestion, carotid artery disease or apical bronchial cancers. ⊃ Pancoast's syndrome, Colour Section Figure 76.

horopter the locus of object points in space that stimulate corresponding retinal points of the two eyes when the eyes are fixating binocularly one of these object points. The horopter is a curve that passes through the fixation point and changes shape with fixation distance. Objects closer to the eyes than the horopter are seen double (crossed disparity) and objects further than the horopter are seen double (uncrossed disparity). There are various types of horopters depending upon the method of determination.

horseshoe kidney an anatomical variation in which the inner lower border of each kidney is joined to give a horseshoe shape. Usually symptomless, but may interfere with drainage of urine into ureters leading to hydronephrosis.

Horton's syndrome (B Horton, American physician, 1895–1980) severe headache due to the release of histamine in the body. To be differentiated from migraine.

hospice care care provided for those with chronic or terminal illnesses and their families. The care may be at home, in a day unit or in hospice premises. Individualized symptom (especially pain) control programmes are implemented which aim to minimize the physical, emotional and spiritual distress.

hospital-acquired (nosocomial) infection (HAI) one which occurs in a patient who has been in hospital for at least 72 h and did not have signs and symptoms of such infection on admission: around 8% of patients in acute hospitals develop a healthcare-associated infection. Common sites include the urinary tract, gastrointestinal tract, surgical wounds, respiratory tract and the blood stream. ⊃ healthcare-associated infection (HCAI), infection.

hospital delivery mode of delivery advised for any woman whose medical condition is unfavourable, or whose previous or current obstetric history suggests potential problems in the forthcoming labour although the mother is legally entitled to reject the advice to have her baby in hospital and to request a home birth.

hospital information system (HIS) a computerized system, the aim of which is to build a network of complementary centres, for example, hospitals, laboratories, primary care trusts and GP centres, etc. spread throughout Europe, to meet the social and healthcare needs in each area. The term can also be used to define the system used in an individual hospital or unit.

Hospital pattern (Coleman) elevator ⊃ elevator (dental).

hospital sterilization and disinfection unit (HSDU) central sterile supply units (CSSUs) that also provide disinfection of equipment.

host *n* the organic structure upon which parasites or bacteria flourish. ⊃ intermediate host.

host computer the main computer in a system containing a number of computers.

hotpacks a form of superficial heating. Types of hotpacks heated in a hydrocollator include canvas packs (moist heat) and plastic packs (dry heat). Other types of hotpacks include gelpacks and wheatpacks heated in a microwave oven and chemical packs which the user bends or breaks apart to initiate an exothermic reaction. Duration of heating depends on method and initial temperature. Dangers are mainly of burns or tissue damage if applied to an area with an insufficient blood supply.

hot spot a term used for the high uptake of a radionuclide in part of the body and thus indicating the presence of a lesion.

Hough transform a technique for electronically enhancing the edges of a feature in a digital image to improve its image quality.

Hounsfield unit/scale (G Hounsfield, British electronics engineer, 1919–2004) a standardized unit for reporting and displaying reconstructed computed tomography (CT) values. Water is given a nominal value of 0, other structures are reproduced with values relative to water. A change in one Hounsfield unit corresponds to 0.1% of the attenuation coefficient difference between water (0 Hounsfield unit) and air (–1000 Hounsfield unit).

hourglass contraction a circular constriction in the middle of a hollow organ (usually the stomach or uterus), dividing it into two portions following scar formation.

G

H

house dust mite a member of the order *Acarina* and the genus *Dermatophagoides*. They thrive in controlled environments such as those provided in houses where they are found in carpets, bedding, mattresses, pillows and furniture. They eat exfoliated skin cells, a major part of house dust. Their faecal matter, which contains partially digested food and enzymes, is a major cause of allergic conditions, including asthma.

housemaid's knee ⊃ bursitis.

Howard–Dolman test a test for measuring stereoscopic visual acuity consisting of two black vertical rods on a white background, viewed through an aperture from a distance of 6 m. By means of a double cord pulley arrangement, the subject manipulates one of the rods until it appears in the same plane as the fixed rod. The distance between the two rods is then measured, and calculations must be made to arrive at the acuity. ⊃ stereoscopic visual acuity, three-needle test, two-dimensional test.

Howe's pliers ⊃ pliers.

Howship's lacunae resorption lacunae. Depressions in the surface of mineralized tissue undergoing resorption.

HP *abbr* hypersensitivity pneumonitis.

HPA *abbr* Health Protection Agency.

HPC *abbr* **1.** Health Professions Council. **2.** history of present complaint.

HPL *abbr* human placental lactogen.

HPV *abbr* human papilloma virus.

HRCT *abbr* high-resolution computed tomography.

H_1-receptor antagonists *pl* a group of antiemetic drugs, e.g. cinnarizine, that block histamine receptors. ⊃ Appendix 5.

H_2-receptor antagonist a drug, e.g. ranitidine, which has a selective action against the H_2 histamine receptors and thereby decreases, for example, the secretion of gastric juice. ⊃ Appendix 5.

HRmax *abbr* maximal heart rate.

HRR *abbr* heart rate reserve.

HRT *abbr* hormone replacement therapy.

HSC *abbr* Health and Safety Commission

HSCT *abbr* haemopoietic stem cell transplantation.

HSDU *abbr* hospital sterilization and disinfection unit.

HSE *abbr* Health and Safety Executive.

HSSU *abbr* hospital sterile supply unit. ⊃ hospital sterilization and disinfection units.

HSV *abbr* herpes simplex virus.

5-HT *abbr* 5-hydroxytryptamine.

$5-HT_1$ agonists *npl* a group of specific antimigraine drugs such as sumatriptan, which is also used for cluster headaches. ⊃ Appendix 5.

$5-HT_3$-receptor antagonists a group of antiemetic drugs, e.g. ondansetron, that block 5-hydroxytryptamine$_3$ receptors. ⊃ Appendix 5.

HTLV *abbr* human T-cell lymphotropic viruses.

HU the measure of heat energy deposited in the anode by an exposure and is the product of the kilovoltage peak and the milliampere per second.

hub a device for connecting computers together to form a network.

Hudson–Stähli line a yellowish-brown, more or less horizontal line containing iron which runs across the cornea below the centre. It occurs in normal corneas, more frequently in older adults, or in association with corneal opacities.

Huhner's test (M Huhner, American urologist, 1873–1947) Also called Sims–Huhner test. A fertility test carried out around the time of ovulation on seminal fluid withdrawn from the vaginal fornix 1 hour after intercourse. The specimen is examined for sperm quantity, activity and survival.

human chorionic gonadotrophin (hCG) a hormone produced by the trophoblast cells and later the chorion. Also a tumour marker for testicular and choriocarcinoma.

human enhancement technologies (HET) term which may be applied widely to anything which modifies human characteristics or abilities, from antidepressant drugs to gene therapy, but mainly to those used for non-therapeutic purposes to enhance physical or mental performance. An inquiry into HET in sport, with reference chiefly to doping, was the subject of a recent UK Government Select Committee Report. ⊃ performance genes.

human epidermal growth factor receptor-2 (HER2) some breast cancers overexpress the protein HER2. Around 20% of breast cancers are HER2-positive. Breast cancers that have overexpression of HER2 receptor protein are more likely to return after treatment and have a less favourable outcome because the cancer cells are stimulated to grow by epidermal growth factors. The monoclonal antibody trastuzumab is available for the treatment of early breast cancer with HER2 overexpression with other treatment modalities. It is also used for metastatic breast cancers, which overexpress HER2.

human erythrovirus 19 previously known as parvovirus B19. The human erythrovirus 19 occurs world-wide and produces a mild or subclinical infection in normal hosts. Clinical manifestations include fifth disease (erythema infectiosum), 'gloves and socks' syndrome, arthropathies, red cell aplasia and hydrops fetalis. A biphasic illness occurs with symptoms during viraemia and at a later immune complex stage of the disease. Transmission is air-borne, although blood-borne infection has been described in people with haemophilia. A week after infection non-specific symptoms occur and a few days later the immune response commences, accompanied by bone marrow depression. Reduction of erythroid precursors progresses to thrombocytopenia, lymphopenia and neutropenia. This is transient and rarely clinically significant. The disease is relevant in individuals with a short red cell life, such as those with sickle-cell disease or spherocytosis where significant anaemia may progress to life-threatening levels. Haematopoiesis usually recovers spontaneously after 10–14 days. Two to three weeks after infection, the immune-mediated, classic red 'slapped cheek' rash with circumoral pallor and arthralgia appears. ➲ Colour Section Figure 77. A second-stage erythematous maculopapular rash may occur on the trunk and limbs. Apart from rare cases in the immunocompromised, there is spontaneous recovery. Infection during the first two trimesters of pregnancy can result in intrauterine infection and impact on fetal bone marrow; it causes 10–15% of non-immune (non-Rhesus-related) hydrops fetalis. This is rare, occurring in only 1:30 000 infected pregnancies. Erythrovirus 19 DNA may be detected in the serum and a polymerase chain reaction (PCR) test will remain positive from then until some 4 months after infection. IgM responses, although commonly used for diagnostic purposes, may persist for months. In the normal individual, this infection is self-limiting and symptomatic relief for arthritic symptoms should be given. Passive prophylaxis with normal immunoglobulin has been suggested for non-immune pregnant women exposed to infection. The pregnancy should be closely monitored by ultrasound scanning, and any suggestion of hydrops should result in consideration of fetal transfusion.

Human Fertilisation and Embryology Authority (HFEA) a UK statutory body set up in 1991. The primary purpose of the HFEA is to license and monitor clinics that provide in vitro fertilisation (IVF) and donor insemination. The HFEA also regulates the storage of sperm, eggs and embryos. They produce a Code of Practice, and information about infertility and treatments for the public. In addition, all UK-based research using human embryos must be licensed and monitored by the HFEA.

human genome project the worldwide collaboration between laboratories to decipher and document the DNA sequence of the entire human genome.

human growth hormone (HGH) ➲ growth hormone.

human immunodeficiency virus (HIV) currently designates the AIDS virus. There are two types: HIV-1 (many strains), mainly responsible for HIV disease in Western Europe, North America and Central Africa, and HIV-2, causing similar disease mainly in West Africa.

human leucocyte antigen (HLA) the major histocompatibility complexes, so called because they were first found on leucocytes. ➲ major histocompatibility complex.

human papilloma virus (HPV) there are many types of HPV, including several that are associated with anogenital warts (particularly types 6 and 11), and a few types (particularly 16 and 18) that are associated with genital tract malignancy such as cervical cancer. In the UK, a new vaccine against HPV types 6, 11, 16 and 18 has been added to the routine immunization programme for girls aged 12–13 years starting in 2008 with a catch up programme for girls aged up to 18 years. As is it does not protect against all viral types associated with cancer, normal routine cervical screening continues as before.

human parvovirus virus ➲ human erythrovirus 19.

human placental lactogen (human chorionic somato-mammotrophin) HPL a peptide hormone produced by the placenta, it is luteotrophic, lactogenic and has growth promoting activity. It is involved in the metabolism of glucose and fatty acids during pregnancy, and influences the production of hCG and prolactin. It inhibits maternal insulin activity during pregnancy. Disappears from the blood immediately after delivery. ➲ gestational diabetes.

human T-cell lymphotropic viruses (HTLV) two retroviruses, HTLV-1 and HTLV-2, both of which are linked with some forms of leukaemia.

humanism humanism is a philosophical movement which focuses on the nature and essence of the human individual. It explores and promotes the central importance of the human individual and has underpinned the reasonings behind human rights movements, patients' rights campaigns and patient-centred approaches to health care. It is one of the main philosophical movements underlying current theories of nursing practice.

humectant a substance that aids the retention of water. In the skin a humectant acts as a natural moisturizer. This is protected by lipids that control the transepidermal water loss.

humerus *n* the bone of the upper arm, between the elbow and shoulder joint—**humeri** *pl*, **humeral** *adj*. ➲ Colour Section Figure 2.

humidity *n* the amount of moisture in the atmosphere, as measured by a hygrometer.

humoral immunity immunity resulting from immunoglobulins (antibodies) produced by plasma cells derived from B lymphocytes. ➲ immunity.

humour *n* any fluid of the body. ➲ aqueous, vitreous body (humour).

Hunter's syndrome (C Hunter, Canadian physician, 1873–1955) one of the mucopolysaccharidoses. An X-linked recessive condition.

hunting reaction the phenomenon of the hunting reaction is seen in human extremities on their exposure to severe cold. On exposure to cold there is a marked increase in the affinity of the postjunctional alpha (α)-adrenoceptors for noradrenaline (norepinephrine). This results in a powerful constriction of the blood vessels and a cessation of blood flow to the distal tissue. As the temperature of the tissues rapidly falls, sympathetic nerve conduction is interrupted and vasodilatation occurs, due to the cessation of noradrenaline (norepinephrine) release and the depressor action of cold on the contractile machinery. The resultant return of blood flow rewarms the tissue, nerve conduction is re-established, and this, combined with the increased affinity of the alpha (α)-adrenoceptors for noradrenaline (norepinephrine), leads to renewed vasoconstriction. ➲ ice/cold therapy.

Huntington's disease (G Huntington, American physician, 1851–1916) rare inherited incurable neurodegenerative condition of the brain, for which the gene is known. It is transmitted as an autosomal dominant gene on chromosome 4 and affects both sexes. There is slow progressive degeneration of the nerve cells of the basal nuclei (ganglia) and

G
H

cerebral cortex. Develops in adult life (thirties and forties) or later, causing a movement disorder (usually chorea), mood changes and dementia. ⊃ chorea.

Hurler's syndrome (G Hurler, German physician, 1889–1965) one of the mucopolysaccharidoses. Inherited as an autosomal recessive trait. It is characterized by a learning disability, flattening of the nasal ridge and other skeletal abnormalities, and sometimes deafness and cardiac anomalies.

Hurter and Driffield curve (F Hurter, photographic scientist, 1844–1898; V Driffield, photographic scientist, 1848–1915) an alternative name for the characteristic curve of a radiographic film.

Hürthle cell tumour (K Hürthle, German histologist, 1860–1945) a new growth of the thyroid gland. It is characterized by large granular cells (Hürthle cells) and may be benign (adenoma) or malignant (carcinoma).

HUS *abbr* haemolytic uraemic syndrome.

Hutchinson's (notched) teeth (J Hutchinson, British surgeon/pathologist, 1828–1913) defect of the teeth which forms part of the facies of congenital syphilis. Affecting primarily the incisors, canines and first permanent molars. The teeth are hypoplastic and the incisors have a screwdriver or peg-shaped appearance.

Hutchinson's pupil a pupil which is dilated and completely inactive to all stimuli. It is associated with lesions of the central nervous system, as may occur in brain injury.

Hutchinson's sign/triad (J Hutchinson) a triad of signs present in congenital syphilis. They are interstitial keratitis, notched teeth and deafness. ⊃ interstitial keratitis.

Huygens' principle (C Huygens, Dutch physicist, 1629–1695) when an ultrasound beam generated by a single source may be considered as the sum of the beams generated by a number of point sources.

Huygens' theory ⊃ wave theory.

HVPS *abbr* high-voltage pulsed stimulation.

HVS *abbr* **1.** high vaginal swab. **2.** hyperviscosity syndrome.

HVT *abbr* half-value thickness.

hyaline *adj* like glass; transparent. ⊃ hyaline cartilage, hyaline degeneration.

hyaline bodies ⊃ drusen.

hyaline cartilage a smooth flexible tissue comprising groups of chondrocytes in a solid matrix. It provides support in the larynx, trachea and bronchi, forms the costal cartilages that join the ribs to the sternum and provides a smooth surface over the articular surfaces of long bones to allow movement at joints. ⊃ cartilage.

hyaline degeneration degeneration of connective tissue especially that of blood vessels in which tissue becomes formless in appearance.

hyaline membrane disease ⊃ neonatal respiratory distress syndrome.

hyalitis inflammation of the vitreous body (humour) of the eye.

hyaloid *adj* resembling hyaline tissue.

hyaloid artery an artery that is present during the embryological period. It arises from the ophthalmic artery, runs forward from the optic disc to the lens where it spreads over the posterior lenticular surface as a capillary net which in turn anastomoses with a capillary net located on the anterior lens surface. Thus the lens becomes enveloped by an anastomosing vascular network called the tunica vasculosa lentis. The hyaloid artery also gives rise to a large number of branches, the vasa hyaloidea propria, which at times almost fills the vitreous cavity. The hyaloid artery degenerates by the 8th month of gestation to become the central retinal artery. ⊃ hyaloid canal, hyaloid remnant, optic fissure.

hyaloid bodies ⊃ drusen.

hyaloid canal (*syn* central canal) a channel in the vitreous body (humour), running from the optic disc to the crystalline lens. In fetal life this canal contains the hyaloid artery which nourishes the lens but it usually disappears prior to birth. ⊃ hyaloid artery, vitreous body (humour).

hyaloid membrane not really a membrane, but a concentration of cells and fibres at the front surface of the vitreous body (humour). ⊃ vitreous body (humour).

hyaloid remnant (*syn* persistent hyaloid artery) a rare condition in which there remain some parts of the hyaloid artery. Posteriorly there may be a vascular loop or the thread of an obliterated vessel running forward from the optic disc and floating freely in the vitreous body (humour). Anteriorly there may be some fibrous remnants attached to the posterior lens capsule and others sometimes floating in the vitreous. The anterior attachment of the hyaloid artery to the lens may also remain throughout life as a black dot, called Mittendorf's dot, and can be seen within the pupil by direct ophthalmoscopy (it appears as a white dot with the biomicroscope). There is rarely any visual interference although patients may sometimes report seeing muscae volitantes.

hyaloideocapsular ligament (*syn* ligament of Wieger) an attachment of the anterior surface of the vitreous body (humour) to the posterior lens capsule in the shape of a ring about 8–9 mm in diameter. It forms a line called Egger's line. This adherence is strong in youth but weakens with age enabling intracapsular cataract extraction without pulling the vitreous. ⊃ cataract extraction.

hyaluronic acid mucopolysaccharide important in the extracellular matrix which holds cells together. Also present in the vitreous body (humour), and the synovial fluid, where it contributes to viscosity. It has some therapeutic uses that include intra-articular injection for osteoarthritis affecting the knee. Increasingly used in cosmetic procedures as a filler/bulking agent in the skin.

hyaluronidase *n* enzyme that breaks down hyaluronic acid. It is present in spermatozoa and its release by many spermatozoa allows one to penetrate and fertilize the oocyte. Hyaluronidase may be used therapeutically to improve the absorption of some drugs or fluids administered parenterally.

hybrid the union of two different varieties.

hybrid composite resin conventional and submicron filler particles combined. ⊃ composite resin.

hybrid denture a removable dental prosthesis which is attached to a fixed substructure (such as a Dolder bar).

G
H

hybrid layer dentine layer which has been infiltrated with resin based adhesive.

hydatid cyst the cyst formed by larvae of the tapeworm, *Echinococcus granulosa*, found in dogs and other canines. The encysted stage normally occurs in sheep but can occur in humans after eating with soiled hands from contact with dogs or infected sheep. The cysts are commonest in the liver, but can affect the brain, lungs and bone.

hydatidiform *adj* pertaining to or resembling a hydatid cyst.

hydatidiform mole a benign gestational trophoblastic tumour. Nowadays it usually known as a molar pregnancy. ➲ choriocarcinoma, gestational trophoblastic tumour, invasive mole, molar pregnancy, placental site trophoblastic tumour.

hydraemia *n* a greater plasma volume than usual compared with cellular volume of the blood; normally present in late pregnancy—**hydraemic** *adj*.

hydramnios *n* ➲ polyhydramnios.

hydrarthrosis *n* a collection of synovial fluid in a joint cavity.

hydrate *vi* combine with water—**hydration** *n*.

hydration status of athletes refers to body fluid levels. *euhydration* the normal state of body water content (typically about 40 litres in a young adult male weighing 70 kg). *hypohydration* reduced total body water which may develop by the process of dehydration due to excessive sweating under exercise heat stress. Athletes may lose 2–6% body weight during prolonged exercise. Hypohydration is detrimental to both exercise performance and health and should be prevented by provision of fluids to match water loss. In several sports (e.g. boxing, power lifting, wrestling) athletes may purposely induce dehydration to achieve weight loss prior to competition. *hyperhydration* increased total body water. It has been proposed that prior hyperhydration may improve thermoregulation during exercise heat stress, but studies have had inconsistent results. ➲ water balance.

hydro- a prefix that means 'water or hydrogen', e.g. *hydrocephalus*.

hydroa *n* a skin condition. *hydroa aestivale* a vesicular eruption that affects exposed parts and results from photosensitivity. *hydroa vacciniforme* is a more severe form of this in which scarring ensues.

hydrocele *n* a swelling due to accumulation of serous fluid between the tunica vaginalis and tunica albuginea of the testis or in the spermatic cord.

hydrocephalus *n* (*syn* 'water on the brain') an excess of cerebrospinal fluid (CSF) inside the skull due to a disruption in normal CSF circulation, impaired absorption of or excess production of CSF, or loss of brain tissue. It may be congenital when it is often associated with spina bifida, or acquired after trauma, infections, subarachnoid haemorrhage, or with tumours. A variety of shunting procedures are available to drain excess CSF and return it to the bloodstream—**hydrocephalic** *adj*. ➲ external or communicating hydrocephalus, internal or obstructive hydrocephalus

hydrochloric acid acid formed from hydrogen and chlorine; secreted by the gastric oxyntic cells and present in gastric juice.

hydrocolloid a substance which when combined with water initially forms a sol and then a gel. It may be reversible, changing its state by heat (agar), or irreversible (alginate). Used for dental impressions.

hydrocolloid dressing a type of rehydrating wound dressing. A colloid containing substances that include gelatin, cellulose, pectins and adhesives.

hydrocolloid impression material a general term to describe agar and alginate impression materials.

hydrocortisone *n* ➲ cortisol.

hydrofoil the shape of a body/object in relation to fluid (water) flow past it.

hydrogel a type of rehydrating wound dressing. Comprising a soft, water-containing gel.

hydrogen (H) *n* a colourless, odourless, combustible gas.

hydrogenase an enzyme that catalyzes the addition of molecular hydrogen in a reduction reaction.

hydrogenated oils/fats oils hardened by the addition of hydrogen, such as in food processing.

hydrogenation *n* the addition of hydrogen to a substance. ➲ reduction.

hydrogen bond a weak bond formed between polar water molecules. Or the bonds in large biological molecules such as nucleic acids and proteins. The hydrogen atoms in the bond are already bonded to other atoms such as nitrogen or oxygen. Important in maintaining the three dimensional structure of biological molecules such as enzymes.

hydrogen breath test a non-invasive test to detect disaccharide intolerance or bacterial overgrowth. ➲ lactase.

hydrogen ion concentration [H$^+$] a measure of the acidity or alkalinity of a solution. It is usually measured using a standard scale (pH), ranging from pH 0 to pH 14, 7 being approximately neutral; the lower numbers denoting acidity; the higher ones denoting alkalinity (Figure H.10). In certain situations the [H$^+$] is measured in nmol/L (see Figure P.8, p. 591). ➲ pH.

hydrogen peroxide (H$_2$O$_2$) a powerful oxidizing and deodorizing agent, used in suitable dilution in mouthwashes. Sometimes used in dentistry to irrigate root canals and as a mouthwash to destroy anaerobic micro-organisms.

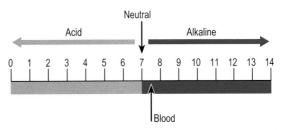

H.10 The pH scale (reproduced from Waugh & Grant 2006 with permission).

hydrolase an enzyme that catalyzes hydrolysis, the addition of water.

hydrolysis *n* the splitting into more simple substances by adding water—**hydrolytic** *adj*, **hydrolyse** *vt*.

hydrometer *n* an instrument for determining the specific gravity of fluids—**hydrometry** *n*.

hydronephrosis *n* an accumulation and distension of the renal pelvis with urine, due to an obstructed outflow. If unrelieved, pressure eventually causes atrophy of kidney tissue. It may be caused by an obstruction of the ureter by a tumour or stone, it may be congenital or caused by the constriction of the urethra by an enlarged prostate gland.

hydropericarditis *n* pericarditis with effusion.

hydropericardium *n* fluid in the pericardial sac in the absence of inflammation. Can occur in heart and kidney failure.

hydroperitoneum *n* ⊃ ascites.

hydrophilic *adj* describes an affinity for water.

hydrophobia *n* fear of water. ⊃ rabies.

hydrophobic *adj* describes an aversion to water.

hydrophthalmos ⊃ congenital glaucoma.

hydropneumopericardium *n* the presence of air and fluid in the pericardial sac surrounding the heart. It may accompany pericardiocentesis.

hydropneumoperitoneum *n* the presence of air and fluid and gas in the peritoneal cavity: it may accompany paracentesis of that cavity; it may accompany perforation of the gut; or it may be due to infection with gas-forming micro-organisms.

hydropneumothorax *n* pneumothorax further complicated by effusion of fluid into the pleural cavity.

hydrops *n* oedema—**hydropic** *adj*.

hydrops fetalis severe haemolytic disease of the newborn.

hydroquinone 1. a radiographic developer agent. **2.** in dentistry, used in minute quantities as an inhibitor to prevent premature polymerization of methylmethacrylate.

hydrosalpinx *n* distension of a uterine (fallopian) tube with watery fluid.

hydrostatic pressure that exerted by a liquid on the walls of its container, such as blood on an artery.

hydrotherapy *n* the science of therapeutic bathing, or exercise for diagnosed medical conditions. The water in hydrotherapy pools is usually warmer than in a swimming pool (allowing better muscle relaxation) and deep enough to allow the patient to exercise out of their depth for non-weight-bearing activity. Thus in sports injuries of the back, groin and lower limb, rehabilitation can begin sooner after injury and proceed at a faster rate. A water-based exercise programme will also allow maintenance and indeed improvement of fitness during the period of the injury, which results in an earlier return to sport.

hydrothorax *n* the presence of fluid in the pleural cavity. Also known as a pleural effusion.

hydroureter *n* abnormal distension of the ureter with urine.

hydrous containing water.

hydroxocobalamin *n* a commercially produced substance with vitamin B_{12} activity. Given by injection for those unable to absorb vitamin B_{12}. ⊃ cobalamin, cyanocobalamin, intrinsic factor.

hydroxyapatite *n* the calcium salts, carbonate, hydroxide and phosphate, that make bone extremely hard.

5-hydroxyindolacetic acid (5-HIAA) a breakdown product of 5-hydroxytryptamine (serotonin) metabolism. High levels in the blood or urine may confirm the presence of carcinoid syndrome.

hydroxyl (OH⁻) *n* a monovalent ion, consisting of a hydrogen atom linked to an oxygen atom. ⊃ free radical.

hydroxylysine an amino acid found only in collagen and elastin (proteins of connective tissue). Its formation requires vitamin C.

hydroxyproline an amino acid found mainly in collagen and elastin (proteins of connective tissue). Its formation requires vitamin C. Increased excretion of hydroxyproline peptides in the urine occurs during high collagen turnover.

5-hydroxytryptamine (5-HT) *n* also known as serotonin. A neurotransmitter. Also present in the gastrointestinal tract and platelets.

hygiene *n* the science dealing with the maintenance of health—**hygienic** *adj*. ⊃ communal hygiene, industrial hygiene, mental hygiene, personal hygiene, sleep hygiene.

hygienist ⊃ dental hygienist.

hygro- a prefix that means 'moisture', e.g. *hygroscopic*.

hygroma *n* a cystic swelling containing watery fluid, usually situated in the neck and present at birth, sometimes interfering with birth—**hygromata** *pl*, **hygromatous** *adj*. ⊃ cystic hygroma.

hygrometer *n* an instrument for measuring the amount of moisture in the air. ⊃ humidity.

hygroscopic *adj* describes substances that readily absorb moisture, e.g. glycerol (glycerin[e]).

hygroscopic expansion phenomenon of increased expansion, exhibited by gypsum products, after the initial set, when exposed to excess water.

hymen *n* a perforated membrane across the vaginal entrance. *imperforate hymen* a congenital condition leading to haematocolpos. ⊃ cryptomenorrhoea, imperforate hymen.

hymenectomy *n* surgical excision of the hymen.

hymenolepiasis *n* heavy infestation with *Hymenolepis nana* or *H. diminuta*. It may cause abdominal pain, anorexia and diarrhoea. Occurs in warm climates such as in the southern United States.

Hymenolepis a genus of small tapeworms that are parasitic in birds and mammals such as rats and mice. The worm eggs are eaten by insects where they mature. Humans may be infested by eating food contaminated by insects.

hymenotomy *n* surgical incision of the hymen.

hyoid *n* U-shaped.

hyoid bone the U-shaped bone situated between the thyroid cartilage and the root of the tongue. ⊃ Colour Section Figure 6.

hyper- a prefix that means 'above, excessive', e.g. *hyperemesis*.

hyperacidity *n* excessive acidity.

hyperactivity *n* excessive activity and distractibility.

hyperacuity the ability of the eye to detect the differences in the spatial locations of two or more stimuli. Hyperacuity thresholds are not based on resolution and are usually below about 15 seconds of arc. Hyperacuity tests include vernier acuity, stereoscopic acuity, orientation discrimination in which differences in the tilts of lines must be detected, the movement displacement threshold, the vertical alignment of a cluster of dots, or the ability to bisect two parallel lines. Hyperacuity is less affected by optical defocus or light scattering, as occurs for example in corneal leukoma, cataract, vitreous haemorrhage, than is Snellen acuity and can therefore be helpful in assessing macular function behind a cataract or other media opacity before surgery. ➲ cataract, clinical maxwellian view system, leukoma, movement threshold, stereoscopic visual acuity, vernier visual acuity.

hyperacusis *n* abnormally acute hearing or excessive sensitivity to sound.

hyperadrenalism ➲ Cushing's disease.

hyperaemia *n* excess of blood in an area. *active hyperaemia* caused by an increased flow of blood to a part. *passive hyperaemia* occurs when there is restricted flow of blood from a part—**hyperaemic** *adj*.

hyperaesthesia *n* excessive sensitiveness of a part—**hyperaesthetic** *adj*.

hyperaldosteronism *n* excessive production of aldosterone causing hypertension, hypokalaemic alkalosis, muscle weakness and rarely tetany. It may be primary or secondary to another condition. ➲ primary hyperaldosteronism (Conn's syndrome)**,** secondary hyperaldosteronism.

hyperalgesia *n* excessive sensibility to pain. A lowered threshold for the interpretation of pain, or hypersensitivity—**hyperalgesic** *adj*.

hyperalimentation literally large amounts of food, in excess of needs. Usually refers to the provision of parenteral nutrition (intravenous).

hyperandrogenism excess androgen hormone secretion in women. ➲ polycystic ovary syndrome.

hyperbaric *adj* term applied to gas at greater pressure than normal.

hyperbaric chamber a pressurized chamber that allows for the delivery of oxygen in high concentrations for therapeutic benefit.

hyperbaric oxygen therapy a form of treatment in which a patient is entirely enclosed in a pressure chamber breathing 100% oxygen at greater than one atmosphere pressure. Used for patients with air embolism, gas gangrene, carbon monoxide poisoning, decompression sickness, etc.

hyperbilirubinaemia *n* excessive bilirubin in the blood—**hyperbilirubinaemic** *adj*.

hypercalcaemia *n* excessive calcium in the blood usually resulting from bone resorption as occurs in hyperparathyroidism, metastatic tumours of bone, paraneoplastic syndrome associated with parathyroid hormone production in breast cancer, or Paget's disease. It results in vague symptoms of anorexia, abdominal pain, muscle pain and weakness, which can be easily missed. It is accompanied by hypercalciuria and can lead to nephrolithiasis—**hypercalcaemic** *adj*.

hypercalciuria *n* greatly increased excretion of calcium in the urine. Occurs in diseases which result in bone resorption. *idiopathic hypercalciuria* is the term used when there is no known metabolic cause. Hypercalciuria is of importance in the pathogenesis of kidney stones—**hypercalciuric** *adj*.

hypercapnia *(syn* hypercarbia) higher than normal partial pressure (tension) of carbon dioxide *(PCO$_2$)* in the lung alveoli and in arterial blood, due to hypoventilation from lung disease, or depression of breathing by drugs. Can occur with inadequate absorption of expired CO_2 in breathing apparatus, e.g. in diving. Hypercapnia may occur in more local milieu such as the tears; it is associated with the use of contact lens, especially lenses of low gas transmissibility—**hypercapnic** *adj*.

hypercarbia *n* ➲ hypercapnia.

hypercatabolism *n* excessive breakdown of body protein. Amino acids are used as a source of energy. It occurs when energy requirements are not met by dietary sources such as in situations where nutritional requirements are increased, e.g. major trauma, sepsis, surgery and burns. ➲ catabolism, nitrogen balance.

hypercementosis the excess deposition of cementum around a tooth root.

hyperchloraemia *n* excessive chloride in the blood. Occurs with hyperkalaemia and leads to metabolic acidosis as acid–base balance is disturbed—**hyperchloraemic** *adj*.

hyperchlorhydria *n* excessive hydrochloric acid in the gastric juice—**hyperchlorhydric** *adj*.

hypercholesterolaemia *n* excessive cholesterol in the blood. Predisposes to atheroma and gallstones. Also found in hypothyroidism (myxoedema)—**hypercholesterolaemic** *adj*. ➲ familial hypercholesterolaemia.

hyperchromatic lens a compound lens designed to have a large amount of chromatic aberration. It may be of use in the correction of presbyopia by extending the depth of focus of the eye; the eye receives a clear red image of distant objects and a clear blue image of near objects without having to change its focus. However, because of the reduced information in the retinal image, such a lens would be more beneficial with high contrast objects. ➲ achromatic lens, depth of focus.

hyperdontia the term used to describe greater than normal number of teeth in cases of supplemental and supernumerary teeth.

hyperemesis *n* excessive vomiting.

hyperemesis gravidarum severe nausea and vomiting that start between 4 and 10 weeks' gestation, and resolve before 20 weeks, requiring medical intervention are known as hyperemesis gravidarum. It affects 0.3–3% of all pregnant women, it is associated with fluid and electrolyte imbalance and weight loss of up to 10% of the prepregnant weight and should not be confused with the common symptoms and signs of nausea and vomiting of pregnancy that is self-limiting (Eliakim *et al* 2000). The aetiology of hyperemesis is uncertain,

G
H

with multifactorial causes such as endocrine, gastrointestinal and psychological factors proposed. Rising levels of oestrogen and human chorionic gonadotrophin (hCG) appear to be significant. Hyperemesis occurs more often where women have a multiple pregnancy, or a molar pregnancy, both of which are associated with increased hormone levels. (Eliakim R, Abulafia O, Sherer DM 2000 Hyperemesis: a current review. American Journal of Perinatology 17(4):207–218.)

hyperextension *n* overextension. Active or passive force which takes the joint into extension beyond its normal physiological range. Since human movement encompasses a wide spectrum of variations, a degree of hyperextension may be considered normal especially in the elbows or the knees.

hyperflexibility ⊃ hypermobility.

hyperflexion *n* excessive flexion.

hyperfractionation the delivery of more than one dose of radiation a day over a period of time, the dose per fraction is lower compared with conventional fractionations resulting in an increase in the overall tumour dose.

hyperglycaemia *n* increased blood glucose, usually indicative of diabetes mellitus or impaired glucose tolerance, but sometimes due to pathological stress, e.g. myocardial infarction—**hyperglycaemic** *adj*.

hyperglycinaemia *n* excess glycine in the serum. Can cause acidosis and learning disability—**hyperglycinaemic** *adj*.

hyperhidrosis *n* excessive sweating—**hyperhidrotic** *adj*.

hyperhydration a term used in sports medicine meaning increased total body water. ⊃ hydration status of athletes, water balance.

hyperinflation a state of overinflation of the lungs or chest wall, resulting in an increase in dead space, higher work of breathing and mechanical disadvantage of the respiratory muscles. Hyperinflation characteristics include an increased anteroposterior thoracic diameter, elevated horizontally positioned ribs and a flattened diaphragm.

hyperinsulinism *n* elevated circulating levels of insulin due to pancreatic tumour, insulinoma, or factitious administration of hypoglycaemic agents; resulting in hypoglycaemia, which may lead to episodic coma, confusion or even mental health disturbance.

hyperinvolution *n* reduction to below normal size, as of the uterus after parturition.

hyperkalaemia *n* excessive potassium in the blood as occurs in renal failure. An early sign may be muscle weakness. Severe hyperkalaemia causes arrhythmias and cardiac arrest—**hyperkalaemic** *adj*.

hyperkalaemic periodic paralysis brief, frequent episodes of weakness triggered by potassium ingestion. It is associated with a muscle channelopathy in which the sodium ion channels in striated muscle are abnormal. ⊃ muscle channelopathies.

hyperkeratosis *n* hypertrophy of the stratum corneum or the horny layer of the skin—**hyperkeratotic** *adj*.

hyperkinesia excessive movement. Excessive involuntary movements seen in some neurological conditions, they include such phenomena as tremor, clonus and tics—**hyperkinetic** *adj*.

hyperkinetic disorder/syndrome usually appears between the ages of 2 and 4 years. The child is slow to develop intellectually and has a marked degree of distractibility. There is an attention deficit and restlessness with uncontrolled activity. There is aggressive behaviour (especially towards siblings) even if unprovoked, and possibly antisocial behaviour. He or she is impulsive and may appear to be fearless and undeterred by threats of punishment. The parents complain of the child's cold unaffectionate character and destructive behaviour. ⊃ attention deficit hyperactivity disorder.

hyperlacrimation an overflow of tears due to excessive secretion by the lacrimal gland. It may be caused by drugs (e.g. pilocarpine), strong emotion; or as a reflex from trigeminal stimulation by an inflamed eye; or irritation of the cornea or conjunctiva by a chemical irritant in the air; cold wind; or a foreign body in the eye. The main symptoms are discomfort and blurring of vision and sometimes embarrassment. Management depends on the cause. ⊃ epiphora, lacrimal gland, tears.

hyperlipaemia *n* excessive total fat in the blood—**hyperlipaemic** *adj*.

hyperlipidaemia *n* abnormally elevated plasma lipid level. Identified as a risk factor for coronary heart disease (ischaemic heart disease), which can be familial or acquired (largely through lifestyle, especially high-saturated fat diet). The condition is asymptomatic and only diagnosed by a screening blood test or following a cardiac event. While treatment requires dietary modification, newer lipid-lowering drugs (statins) have led to much better results and a reduction in morbidity and mortality. ⊃ cholesterol, lipids, lipoproteins.

hypermagnesaemia *n* excessive magnesium in the blood; found in renal failure and in people who take excessive amounts of magnesium-containing antacids—**hypermagnesaemic** *adj*.

hypermetabolism *n* production of excessive body heat. Characteristic of hyperthyroidism—**hypermetabolic** *adj*.

hypermetria a disorder of movement where the patient tends to overshoot the intended target. ⊃ hypometria.

hypermetropia *n* longsightedness caused by low refractive power or reduced axial length of the eye, with the result that the light rays are focused beyond, instead of on, the retina—**hypermetropic** *adj*.

hypermobility *n* excessive mobility. As in a joint that has an increase in the normal range of joint movement potentially leading to instability. This is as a result of changes to connective tissue, particularly collagen, which results in laxity of the supporting structures such as ligaments and tendons. There is a spectrum from the more serious, often rare genetic, conditions to the more common, which cause fewer problems but nevertheless increase the risk of injury. Hypermobility is assessed by the Beighton Score, which measures the degree of abnormal movement at the lower back, knees, elbows and hands. The higher the score (maximum 9), indicates an increasing degree of hypermobility. However, normal joint mobility also comprises a broad spectrum and hypermobility is one end of this spectrum, as such it may not be a sign of any pathology or even produce any symptoms. ➲ flexibility.

hypermotility *n* increased movement, as peristalsis in the gastrointestinal tract.

hypernatraemia *n* increased sodium concentration in the blood most often caused by a relative loss or deficit of water. This can be due to polyuria, diarrhoea, excessive sweating or inadequate water intake. Hypernatraemia may also be caused by excessive intake of sodium—**hypernatraemic** *adj*.

hypernephroma *n* (*syn* Grawitz tumour) a malignant tumour of the kidney—**hypernephromata** *pl*, **hypernephromatous** *adj*.

hyperonychia *n* excessive growth of the nails.

hyperosmia *n* abnormally increased sense of smell.

hyperosmolar non-ketotic coma (HONK) profound dehydration due to uncontrolled type 2 diabetes leading to hyperosmolar state and ultimately coma. ➲ diabetes mellitus.

hyperosmolarity *n* (*syn* hypertonicity) a solution exerting a higher osmotic pressure than another is said to have a hyperosmolarity with reference to it. In medicine, the comparison is usually made with normal plasma.

hyperostiosis thickening of the skull vault.

hyperostosis *n* exostosis.

hyperoxaluria *n* excessive calcium oxalate in the urine—**hyperoxaluric** *adj*.

hyperparathyroidism *n* overactivity of one or more parathyroid glands, usually due to parathyroid adenoma, and resulting in elevated serum calcium levels; rarely results in parathyroid bone disease, osteitis fibrosa cystica; may be primary, or secondary/tertiary usually in response to chronic renal failure. ➲ hypercalcaemia, hypercalciuria, von Recklinghausen's disease.

hyperperistalsis *n* excessive peristalsis—**hyperperistaltic** *adj*.

hyperphagia *n* overeating. Can be caused by psychological disturbances and lesions of the hypothalamus. It is a symptom of Prader–Willi syndrome. ➲ obesity.

hyperphenylalaninaemia *n* excess of phenylalanine in the blood which results in phenylketonuria.

hyperphoria ➲ phoria.

hyperphosphataemia *n* excessive phosphates in the blood—**hyperphosphataemic** *adj*.

hyperpigmentation *n* increased or excessive pigmentation.

hyperpituitarism *n* ➲ acromegaly, Cushing's disease, gigantism, hyperprolactinaemia.

hyperplasia *n* increase in the size of an organ or other structure due to excessive formation of new cells—**hyperplastic** *adj*.

hyperpnoea *n* rapid, deep breathing; panting; gasping. Ventilation of the lungs at greater than normal resting rate, whether or not appropriate to meet the demand for increased oxygen consumption. To be distinguished from (although it includes) hyperventilation, which is defined as an increase in ventilation that reduces the carbon dioxide tension (PCO_2) in the blood—**hyperpnoeic** *adj*.

hyperpraxia restlessness, excessive activity.

hyperprolactinaemia *n* elevation in circulating prolactin levels, sometimes due to stress; if pathological results in galactorrhoea, menstrual irregularity and infertility; may be due to dopamine antagonists, such as metoclopramide or antipsychotic (neuroleptics) drugs, large, often non-functioning pituitary tumours, or prolactinomas.

hyperpyrexia *n* body temperature above 40–42°C—**hyperpyrexial** *adj*. ➲ malignant hyperthermia, neuroleptic malignant syndrome.

hyper-reactivity a state in which a reaction is greater than the normal response to a stimulus.

hyperreflexia *n* exaggerated reflexes demonstrated on electromyogram (EMG). This is part of the upper motor neuron syndrome; it may be seen following stroke or brain injury. It is thought to be related to plastic changes in the nervous system.

hypersecretion *n* excessive secretion.

hypersensitive tooth a tooth reacting more than is normal to a stimulus such as heat, cold, sweetness and pressure.

hypersensitivity *n* an abnormal or exaggerated immune response to an antigen, generally classified as type I, II, III or IV. Type I, or immediate-type, is caused by specific IgE against an allergen cross-linking Fc receptors on mast cells, causing the mast cell to degranulate and release inflammatory mediators including histamine. Type II hypersensitivity results from antibodies binding to antigens on cell surfaces. Type III reactions are due to the deposition of immune complexes in tissues. Type IV or delayed-type hypersensitivity reactions occur 24–72 hours later and are due to antigen-specific T cells and macrophages—**hypersensitive** *adj*.

hypersensitivity pneumonitis (HP) (*syn* extrinsic allergic alveolitis) results from the inhalation of certain types of organic dust which give rise to a diffuse immune complex reaction in the walls of the alveoli and bronchioles. Examples include farmer's lung, bird fancier's lung, malt worker's lung. In the UK, 50% of reported cases of hypersensitivity pneumonitis (HP) occur in farm workers; bird fanciers represent another important group. The pathology of HP suggests that both type III and type IV immunological mechanisms may be involved. Precipitating IgG antibodies may be detected in the serum and a type III Arthus reaction is believed to occur in the lung where the precipitation of immune complexes results in activation of complement and an inflammatory response in the alveolar walls characterized by the influx of mononuclear cells and foamy histiocytes. The presence of poorly formed non-caseating granulomas in the alveolar walls provides some evidence that type IV responses are also important. Chronic forms of the disease may be accompanied by a fibrotic response in the lung. For reasons that remain uncertain, there is a lower incidence of hypersensitivity

G

H

pneumonitis in smokers compared to non-smokers. The acute form of the disease should be suspected when anyone who is regularly or intermittently exposed to organic dust complains, within a few hours of re-exposure to the same dust, of influenza-like symptoms. These include headache, myalgia, malaise, pyrexia, dry cough and breathlessness. Chest auscultation reveals widespread end-inspiratory crackles and squeaks. In cases attributable to chronic low-level exposure (as may be the case with an indoor pet bird) the onset is often more insidious with progressive breathlessness, and established fibrosis may be present by the time the disease is recognized. If unchecked, the disease may progress to cause severe respiratory disability, hypoxaemia, pulmonary hypertension, cor pulmonale and eventually death. The chest X-ray shows diffuse micronodular shadowing that is classically more pronounced in the upper zones. High-resolution computed tomography (HRCT) in patients with acute disease shows bilateral areas of consolidation superimposed on small centrilobar nodular opacities and air-trapping on expiration. In more chronic disease, features of fibrosis with linear opacities and architectural distortion predominate. Pulmonary function tests show a restrictive ventilatory defect with reduced lung volumes and impaired gas transfer. The PaO_2 is reduced and in the presence of over-ventilation the $PaCO_2$ is often below normal. The diagnosis of HP is usually based on the characteristic clinical and radiological features, together with the identification of a potential source of antigen at the patient's home or place of work. Reduction in the carbon monoxide transfer factor is the most sensitive functional abnormality. The diagnosis may be supported by a positive precipitin test or by more sensitive serological tests based on the enzyme-linked immunosorbent assay (ELISA) technique. However, it is also important to recognize that the great majority of farmers with positive precipitins do not have farmer's lung, and up to 15% of pigeon breeders may have positive serum precipitins yet remain healthy. Where the diagnosis is suspected but the cause is not readily apparent, it may be helpful to visit the patient's home or workplace. Occasionally, such as when a new agent is suspected, it may be necessary to prove the diagnosis by a provocation test; if positive, inhalation of the relevant antigen is followed after 3–6 hours by pyrexia and a reduction in vital capacity (VC) and gas transfer factor. Bronchoalveolar lavage (BAL) fluid usually shows an increase in the number of CD8+ T lymphocytes. Open lung biopsy may be necessary to establish a diagnosis. Whenever possible, the patient should cease exposure to the inciting agent. However, in some cases this may be difficult to achieve, either because of implications for livelihood (e.g. farmers/farm workers) or long term hobbies (e.g. pigeon breeders). Dust masks with appropriate filters may minimize exposure and may be combined with methods of reducing levels of antigen (e.g. drying hay before storage). In acute cases prednisolone should be given for 3–4 weeks. Severely hypoxaemic patients may require high-concentration oxygen therapy initially. Most patients recover completely, but the development of interstitial fibrosis

causes permanent disability when there has been prolonged exposure to antigen.

hypersplenism *n* term used to describe depression of erythrocyte, granulocyte and platelet counts by an enlarged spleen.

hypertelorism *n* congenital defect resulting in increased interpupillary distance. May be associated with various genetic disorders.

hypertension *n* abnormally high tension, by custom abnormally high blood pressure involving systolic and/or diastolic levels. The consensus view is that hypertension is a systolic blood pressure above 140 mmHg and a diastolic blood pressure above 90 mmHg. Mild hypertension is consided to be systolic pressure between 140–159 and diastolic pressure between 90–99. Hypertension is considered to be a risk factor for the development of cardiovascular disease. No cause is found in the majority of patients and is termed *essential hypertension*. Secondary hypertension may result from coarctation of the aorta, renal artery stenosis, renal disease, phaeochromocytoma, Cushing's disease/syndrome, Conn's syndrome, various drugs, such as oral contraceptives, NSAIDs, and the pre-eclampsia of pregnancy. ➲ hepatic portal hypertension, hypertensive retinopathy, pulmonary hypertension—**hypertensive** *adj*.

hypertensive retinopathy retinal changes occurring in severe (malignant) hypertension. It is characterized by attenuation and local arteriolar constriction (grades 1 and 2). As the condition progresses, flame-shaped haemorrhages, cotton–wool exudates and oedema appear (grade 3) and at the most advanced stage (grade 4) papilloedema occurs. Arteriosclerotic retinopathy may also accompany this disease. Pregnancy-induced hypertension can lead to sudden angiospasm of retinal arterioles, later followed by the typical picture of advanced hypertensive retinopathy. In this case restitution follows rapidly after delivery of the infant. ➲ macular star.

hyperthermia *n* very high body core temperature caused by loss of thermoregulatory control. The hypothalamus in the brain malfunctions—**hyperthermic** *adj*. ➲ heat illness, hyperpyrexia, malignant hyperthermia.

hyperthyroid crisis ➲ thyroid crisis.

hyperthyroidism *n* thyrotoxicosis. A condition due to excessive production of thyroid hormones (thyroxine, triiodothyronine), usually due to Graves' disease, but also multiple or solitary toxic nodules, and resulting classically in anxiety, tachycardia, sweating, increased appetite with weight loss, and a fine tremor of the outstretched hands; much commoner in women than men.

hypertonia *n* muscle tone that is too high to permit movement; increased contractility of muscle due to excessive and inappropriate excitation of the motor neuron pools of the anterior horn of the spinal cord setting the bias on the stretch reflex too low (easily triggered), causing the muscles to be more sensitive to stretch. There are two types: spasticity and rigidity—**hypertonic** *adj*, **hypertonicity** *n*.

hypertonic *adj* **1.** pertaining to hypertonia. **2.** a fluid with a higher osmotic pressure relative to another fluid. ➲ hyperosmolarity, hypotonic, isotonic.

hypertonic saline a saline solution that has a greater osmotic pressure than physiological fluid.

hypertonic action of the uterus abnormal uterine action in which the muscle tone is excessive. The contractions are extremely painful, the intermissions brief with inadequate relaxation, labour is prolonged and exhausting to the woman and the fetus becomes hypoxic. The woman should be under medical care and may benefit from epidural analgesia, but delivery by caesarean section may be needed.

hypertonic sports drinks ➲ sports drinks.

hypertrichosis *n* excessive hairiness in a non-androgenic distribution.

hypertrophic obstructive cardiomyopathy (HOCM) one of a group of diseases of the myocardium associated with cardiac dysfunction. Hypertrophic obstructive cardiomyopathy (HOCM) is an inherited condition (the result of multiple gene defects) in which the muscle of the left ventricular wall (mainly the septum) is thickened, reducing the size of the ventricular chamber, causing possible valve dysfunction and most importantly obstruction of outflow into the aorta. Microscopically, the myocardial cells are not of normal pattern, resulting in disruption of the electrical pathways within the heart, leading potentially to fatal arrhythmias. HOCM is one of the commonest causes of sudden cardiac death in young sportspeople, when growth of the abnormal cardiac muscle is greatest. HOCM may be asymptomatic or it can cause exercise-related dizziness, breathlessness, chest pain and palpitations. Diagnosis depends on electrocardiography and echocardiography. ➲ sudden death.

hypertrophic scar an unsightly raised red scar showing continued activity and no maturation, such as may be seen with burns.

hypertrophy *n* increase in the size of tissues or structures, independent of natural growth. It may be congenital, compensatory, complementary or functional. The enlargement or overgrowth of an organ or tissue due to an increase in size of its constituent cells. For example, the increase in bulk of skeletal muscles with sports training: the individual cells (muscle fibres) become larger. Compare with hyperplasia in which bulk is increased by cell division— **hypertrophic** *adj*.

hyperuricaemia *n* excessive uric acid in the blood. Characteristic of gout. ➲ Lesch–Nyhan disease—**hyperuricaemic** *adj*.

hyperuricuria also known as hyperuricosuria, uricosuria. Excessive amounts of uric acid and urates in the urine. Causes include problems with purine metabolism (e.g. in gout), high intake of purine and renal failure.

hyperventilation *n* overbreathing. Increased ventilation of the lungs, such that in alveolar gas (and therefore also in arterial blood) the partial pressure of carbon dioxide (PCO_2) is lowered and that of oxygen (PO_2) is raised, i.e. ventilation exceeds that which would maintain the normal blood gas levels, with the rate of excretion of CO_2 exceeding that of its metabolic production until a new equilibrium is reached. Hyperventilation may accompany anxiety or be a feature of a psychological disorder, may be deliberate in order to prolong subsequent breath-holding, e.g. for diving, it may be caused by salicylate poisoning or head injury, or passively as part of a technique of general anaesthesia in intensive care. The chronic hyperventilation syndrome is a breathing pattern disorder that is often underdiagnosed, resulting in the movement of patients between departments for investigation of the many disabling physical symptoms experienced. Low PCO_2 (hypocapnia) can give rise to symptoms. Hyperventilation is associated with the development of alkalosis leading to hypocalcaemia and tetany. At sea level the raised PO_2 has no significant effect (because at normal PO_2 haemoglobin is already virtually saturated with oxygen) but in altitude acclimatization hyperventilation is a compensatory response (raising the lowered PO_2 improves oxygen saturation); also in acidaemia (decreasing PCO_2 raises pH). ➲ hypocalcaemia, tetany.

hypervitaminosis *n* any condition arising from an excessive intake of a vitamin. Can develop when large quantities of vitamin supplements are taken.

hyperviscosity an extremely viscous or thick fluid.

hyperviscosity syndrome (HVS) a condition characterized by an increase in blood viscosity; either caused by an increase in the red blood cell count or the production of excess globulins (hyperglobulinaemia) or abnormal paraproteins. It is associated with diseases that include myeloma, polycythaemia and Waldenström's macroglobulinaemia. Increased viscosity is associated with visual impairment; bleeding from the mucosae; central nervous system effects that include lethargy, seizures and altered consciousness; and cardiac and renal failure.

hypervolaemia *n* an increase in the volume of circulating blood. Can occur in athletes in association with hyponatraemia, e.g. marathon runners who drink an excess of plain water.

hyphaema *n* blood in the anterior chamber of the eye. ➲ haemophthalmia, Colour Section Figure 78.

hypno- a prefix that means 'sleep', e.g. *hypnogogic*.

hypnogogic stage the stage between being being awake and asleep. Images and hallucinations may occur.

hypnopompic stage the stage between being asleep and fully awake. Vivid images and hallucinations may occur.

hypnosis *n* a state resembling sleep, brought about by the hypnotist or the individual utilizing the mental mechanism of suggestion to produce a relaxed state and an improvement in well-being. Also used in symptom control or reduction, smoking cessation and forms of anaesthesia, as in skin suturing and pain relief such as in labour—**hypnotic** *adj*.

hypnotherapy *n* treatment that uses sleeplike state or hypnosis.

hypnotic 1. *n* a drug which produces a sleep similar to natural sleep. ➲ narcotic. ➲ Appendix 5. **2.** *adj* pertaining to hypnotism.

hypo- a prefix that means 'below, deficient', e.g. *hypocalcaemia*.

hypoaesthesia *n* also called hypaesthesia. Abnormally diminished sensitivity to stimulation—**hypoaesthetic** *adj*.

hypobaric lower pressure than normal atmopheric pressure.

hypocalcaemia *n* decreased calcium level in the blood. Causes include: disturbed kidney function, excess calcium excretion, deficiency of vitamin D, alkalosis and hypoparathyroidism. Leads to tingling in the hands and feet, and stridor and convulsions in children—**hypocalcaemic** *adj*. ⊃ carpopedal spasm, hyperventilation, tetany.

hypocalcification the lack of calcium salts in a calcified tissue. In teeth, a deficiency in the normal content of enamel due to a disturbance during the maturation period of the tooth.

hypocapnia *n* lower than normal partial pressure (tension) of carbon dioxide (PCO_2) in the lung alveoli and in the arterial blood; usually produced by hyperventilation, it can lead to respiratory alkalosis. If severe, can cause dizziness or confusion (by constrictive effect on brain blood vessels, reducing blood flow), disturbances of sensation and tetany (by reducing the amount of ionized calcium in the blood)—**hypocapnial** *adj*. ⊃ hyperventilation, tetany.

hypochloraemia *n* reduced chloride level in the blood. Leads to metabolic alkalosis as the acid–base balance is disrupted—**hypochloraemic** *adj*.

hypochlorhydria *n* decreased hydrochloric acid in the gastric juice—**hypochlorhydric** *adj*.

hypochlorite *n* salts of hypochlorous acid. They are easily decomposed to yield active chlorine, and are extensively used as disinfectants. ⊃ chlorine, sodium hypochlorite.

hypochondria *n* unnecessary anxiety about one's health—**hypochondriac, hypochondriacal** *adj*, **hypochondriasis** *n*.

hypochondriacal disorder an excessive preoccupation with the possibility of having serious health problems associated with refusal to accept professional reassurance that there is no physical illness underlying the symptoms. Symptoms are often of a bodily nature or concerned with physical appearance.

hypochondrium *n* the upper lateral region (left and right) of the abdomen—**hypochondriac** *adj*. ⊃ Colour Section Figure 18a.

hypochromic *adj* deficient in colouring or pigmentation. Of a red blood cell, having decreased haemoglobin.

hypocretins also known as orexins Two excitatory neuropeptides which, with other substances, help to regulate sleep–wake cycles and appetite. It is normally produced in the hypothalamus. Low levels have been found in the cerebrospinal fluid of people with narcolepsy. ⊃ orexins.

hypodermic *adj* below the skin; subcutaneous—**hypodermically** *adv*.

hypodermoclysis the infusion of fluids subcutaneously. Increasingly used to replace fluids and maintain adequate hydration in palliative care and older adults (Figure H.11).

hypodontia developmental absence of up to six teeth. ⊃ oligodontia.

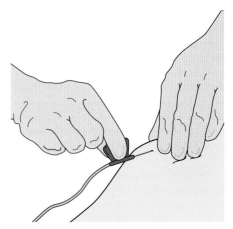

H.11 Hypodermoclysis—inserting the cannula (reproduced from Nicol et al 2004 with permission).

hypofibrinogenaemia *n* reduced amount of fibrinogen in the blood. May be hereditary or acquired and may result in an increased tendency to bleed—**hypofibrinogenaemic** *adj*.

hypofractionation the practice of giving less than the conventional fractionations for a particular treatment, is used for treating tumours which have a higher capacity for repair such as melanomas.

hypofunction *n* diminished performance.

hypogammaglobulinaemia *n* decreased gammaglobulin in the blood, occurring either congenitally or, more commonly, as a sporadic disease in adults. Lessens resistance to infection. ⊃ dysgammaglobulinaemia—**hypogammaglobulinaemic** *adj*.

hypogastric artery a branch from the internal iliac artery which in fetal life carries deoxygenated blood and communicates directly with the umbilical artery.

hypogastrium *n* that area of the anterior abdomen which lies immediately below the umbilical region—**hypogastric** *adj*. ⊃ Colour Section Figure 18a.

hypogeusia reduced sensation of taste.

hypoglossal *adj* under the tongue.

hypoglossal nerve the 12th pair of cranial nerves. They innervate tongue movements and are essential for swallowing and speech.

hypoglycaemia *n* decreased blood glucose, attended by anxiety, excitement, sweating, headache, change in personality, delirium or coma. Signs and symptoms vary markedly between individuals and can be mistakenly assumed to be due to another condition including alcohol intoxication. May be a consequence of severe fasting, but can occur in healthy well-fed people during the late stages of endurance exercise, particularly when consumption of carbohydrate drinks is neglected or, paradoxically, when a one-off intake of glucose elicits an insulin surge. Hypoglycaemia occurs most commonly in diabetes mellitus, when it is due to insulin overdosage, inadequate intake of carbohydrate or during exercise (which lowers blood glucose) unless special care is taken with blood sugar control. Blood glucose may also be low following alcohol ingestion with inadequate food intake. Acute severe hypoglycaemia can result in coma, convulsions and brain damage—**hypoglycaemic** *adj.*

hypoglycaemic drugs oral drugs that reduce blood glucose in diabetes mellitus. ⊃ alpha (α)-glucosidases inhibitor, biguanides, dipeptidyl peptidase 4 inhibitors (DPP-4 inhibitors) glitazones, glucagon-like peptide-1 (GLP-1) mimetics, prandial glucose regulators, sulphonylureas. ⊃ Appendix 5.

hypogonadism *n* a condition associated with a deficiency of ovarian or testicular secretions. Often used to mean failure of testicular function.

hypohidrosis diminished sweating. ⊃ anhidrosis.

hypohydration a term used in sports medicine meaning reduced total body water. ⊃ hydration status of athletes, water balance.

hypoinsulinism reduced production of insulin by the pancreatic cells.

hypokalaemia *n* abnormally low potassium level in the blood. Causes include: vomiting, gastrointestinal drainage, diarrhoea, starvation, excess renal loss in Cushing's syndrome or aldosteronism and with prolonged use of diuretics and other drugs. Leads to nausea, muscle weakness, arrhythmias and cardiac arrest—**hypokalaemic** *adj.*

hypokalaemic periodic paralysis episodic weakness triggered by a carbohydrate meal. It is associated with muscle channelopathies in which the sodium or calcium ion channels in striated muscle are abnormal. ⊃ muscle channelopathies.

hypokinesia *n* poverty of movement; including: inability to maintain repetitive movements or perform rapidly alternating movements (dysdiadochokinesis), lack of trunk rotation (e.g. no arm swinging), and loss of amplitude and range of movement (e.g. writing gets smaller).

hypolacrima ⊃ alacrima.

hypomagnesaemia *n* decreased magnesium level in the blood—**hypomagnesaemic** *adj.*

hypomania *n* a less intense form of mania with persistent mild elevation of mood, overactivity, increased sociability, overfamiliarity, overtalkativeness, overspending, elevated libido and decreased need for sleep. Hallucinations and delusions are usually absent—**hypomanic** *adj.*

hypomenorrhoea small amount of menstrual loss.

hypometabolism *n* decreased production of body heat. Characteristic of hypothyroidism.

hypometria a disorder of movement where the patient tends to fail to meet the intended target. ⊃ hypermetria.

hypomobility *n* decrease in the normal range of joint movement. This may include the loss of accessory movements.

hypomotility *n* decreased movement, as of the gastrointestinal tract.

hyponatraemia *n* decreased sodium concentration in the blood due to a change in the proportion of sodium and water in the blood. The causes of hyponatraemia can be categorized into (a) hypovolaemic—sodium deficit with a relatively smaller water deficit (e.g. vomiting and diarrhoea, adrenocortical failure, thiazide diuretic drugs); (b) euvolaemic—water retention only (e.g. primary polydipsia, excessive intake of plain water (such as excessive intake by athletes of water relative to sodium in their use of sports drinks) or excessive electrolyte-free water infusion, hypothyroidism, syndrome of inappropriate antidiuretic hormone secretion); (c) hypervolaemic—sodium retention with relatively greater water retention (e.g. liver cirrhosis, nephrotic syndrome, chronic renal failure during free water intake, congestive cardiac failure)—**hyponatraemic** *adj.*

hypo-osmolarity *n* (*syn* hypotonicity) a solution exerting a lower osmotic pressure than another is said to have a hypo-osmolarity with reference to it. In medicine the comparison is usually made with normal plasma.

hypoparathyroidism *n* underactivity of the parathyroid glands resulting in decreased serum calcium levels, producing tetany.

hypoperfusion inadequate blood flow in a region, organ or tissue. ⊃ ischaemia.

hypopharynx *n* that portion of the pharynx lying below and behind the larynx, correctly called the laryngopharynx.

hypophonia a weak voice with decreased phonation, which results in whispering. Also known as leptophonia.

hypophoria *n* ⊃ phoria.

hypophosphataemia *n* decreased phosphate level in the blood—**hypophosphataemic** *adj.* ⊃ phosphates.

hypophysectomy *n* surgical removal of the pituitary gland.

hypophysis cerebri ⊃ pituitary gland—**hypophyseal** *adj.*

hypopigmentation *n* decreased pigmentation. ⊃ albinism.

hypopituitarism *n* pituitary gland insufficiency, especially of the anterior lobe hormones. When the secretion of all the anterior lobe hormones is decreased it is described as panhypopituitarism or Simmonds' disease. Absence of gonadotrophins leads to failure of ovulation, uterine atrophy and amenorrhoea in women and loss of libido, pubic and axillary hair in both sexes. Lack of growth hormone in children results in short stature and a type of dwarfism. Lack of adrenocorticotrophin (ACTH) and thyrotrophin (thyroid stimulating hormone [TSH]) may result in lack of energy, pallor, fine dry skin, cold intolerance and sometimes hypoglycaemia. Usually due to tumour of or involving the pituitary gland or hypothalamus but in other cases cause is unknown. Occasionally due to postpartum infarction of the pituitary gland when it is known as Sheehan's syndrome. ⊃ Sheehan's syndrome.

hypoplasia *n* defective development of any tissue—**hypoplastic** *adj.*

hypoplastic left heart syndrome a group of congenital cardiac defects, which include defective and or underdevelopment (hypoplasia) affecting the left side of the heart including the left ventricle, the mitral (bicuspid) valve, the aortic valve and the aorta. Affected infants may, at first, appear normal, but once the ductus arteriosus closes the infant develops severe breathlessness with feeding difficulties. The infant's condition rapidly deteriorates

G

H

371

and is usually fatal in the first days or weeks of life. For some infants it may be possible to use the drug alprostadil (prostaglandin E_1) to keep the ductus arteriosus open and eventually perform a series of individualized surgical procedures, or possibly a heart transplantion.

hypopnoea abnormal slow and shallow breathing. ⊃ obstructive sleep apnoea (hypopnoea) syndrome.

hypopraxia diminished activity.

hypoproteinaemia *n* deficient protein in blood plasma, from dietary deficiency, reduced production or excessive excretion (albuminuria)—**hypoproteinaemic** *adj.*

hypopyon *n* a collection of pus in the anterior chamber of the eye (Figure H.12). It is associated with infectious diseases of the cornea (e.g. corneal ulcer), the iris or the ciliary body. The pus usually accumulates at the bottom of the chamber and may be seen through the cornea.

hyposecretion *n* deficient secretion.

hyposensitivity *n* lacking sensitivity to a stimulus.

hyposmia *n* decrease in the normal sensitivity to smell.

hypospadias *n* a congenital malformation of the male urethra. Subdivided into two types: (a) penile, when the terminal urethral orifice opens at any point along the ventral surface of the penis, and (b) perineal, when the orifice opens on the perineum and may give rise to problems of sexual differentiation. ⊃ epispadias.

hypostasis *n* **1.** congestion of blood in a part due to impaired circulation. **2.** a sediment—**hypostatic** *adj.*

hypotension *n* low blood pressure that is insufficient for adequate tissue perfusion and oxygenation; may be primary or secondary (e.g. reduced cardiac output, hypovolaemic shock, Addison's disease) or postural—**hypotensive** *adj.*

hypothalamus *n* literally, below the thalamus. It consists of an area of grey matter in the brain just above the pituitary gland. The region of the brain which links cerebral function to the endocrine system, initiates physiological responses to emotions, such as anger, and regulates eating and drinking behaviour, body temperature and circadian rhythms. Many of these actions are mediated via the autonomic nervous system. Secretes specific 'releasing' and 'inhibitory' hormones into local blood vessels that reach the anterior pituitary and influence the secretion of its hormones; also the neurohormones oxytocin and antidiuretic hormone (vasopressin or arginine vasopression [AVP]) are formed here in nerve cell bodies and travel down axons in the hypothalamohypophyseal tract to be stored in, until released from, their terminals in the posterior pituitary— **hypothalamic** *adj.* ⊃ appetite, body temperature, hormones, limbic system, thirst.

hypothenar eminence the eminence on the ulnar side of the palm below the little finger.

hypothermia *n* core body temperature below 35°C. Less severe cooling is counteracted by an increase in metabolic rate, and by shivering, stimulated by the sympathetic nervous system. Progressive cooling below 35°C leads to disturbance then loss of consciousness, and is usually fatal between 25° and 20°C, although recovery has been known from still lower temperatures. As well as extremely low ambient temperature, risks include immersion in cold water and exhaustion, e.g. on mountains, or when swimming for survival. More common in climatic conditions where low environmental temperature is combined with wet and windy conditions, adding to the rapidity and extent of the fall in body temperature. Early signs include shivering, confusion, reduced concentration and reaction time (e.g. ball skills in sport) and the inability to keep up (in outdoor sports, hill-walking, etc.). Treatment includes removal from the cold environment, removal of wet clothing and replacement with dry clothes and gradual rewarming. Further heat loss can be prevented by restriction of continued activity. Hypothermia is a particular risk at the extremes of age, in hypothyroidism and in non-sporting/recreational exposure to cold, wet and windy environmental conditions such as rough sleepers. An artificially induced hypothermia can be used in the treatment of head injuries and during cardiac surgery. It reduces the oxygen consumption of the tissues and thereby allows greater and more prolonged interference of normal blood circulation. ⊃ body temperature.

hypothermia in newborns core body temperature below 35°C. Usually occurs as a result of the infant being born in a cool room or inadequately cared for or dried at birth. There is a failure of the neonate to adjust to external cold; may be associated with infection.

hypothesis *n* a research term. A declaration that can be tested by statistical (inferential) tests. It is a prediction based on the relationship between the dependent and independent variables. The wording of a hypothesis may be a two-tailed hypothesis (no direction implied) or it may be more specific and indicate the direction of the effect, i.e. a one-tailed hypothesis. An example of a two-tailed hypothesis would be if there were a difference in intelligence between students and their lecturers. An example of a one-tailed hypothesis would be if the students were more intelligent than their lecturers.

hypothetico-deductive method theories are examined and hypotheses for testing are derived in a deductive manner. The particular research study tests the hypotheses by data analysis that either supports or repudiates the original theory.

hypothyroidism *n* conditions caused by low circulating levels of one or both thyroid hormones (thyroxine,

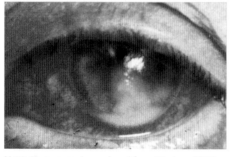

H.12 Hypopyon (reproduced from Maclean 2002).

G H

triiodothyronine). Much more common in women than men and may be: (a) associated with goitre, such as autoimmune thyroiditis, lack of iodine or as a drug side-effect, e.g. with lithium; (b) due to spontaneous atrophy; or (c) after surgical treatment for hyperthyroidism. Some individuals have a subclinical form and in others it may be transient. It results in decreased metabolic rate and may be characterized by some of the following: fatigue, bradycardia, angina, hypertension, aches and pains, carpal tunnel syndrome, low temperature and cold intolerance, weight gain, constipation, hair and skin changes (dry coarse skin), puffy face, anaemia, hoarseness, slow speech, menorrhagia and depression. Treatment is with replacement thyroxine. *congenital hypothyroidism* can be detected (by routine blood testing) soon after birth and treated successfully with thyroxine. Untreated, it leads to impaired mental and physical development. It is recognized by the presence of coarse facies and protruding tongue. The term cretinism was previously used.

hypotonia *n* muscle tone that is too low to maintain posture or permit movement against gravity; loss of contractility of muscle due to disturbance of the cerebellum or links between it and other centres in the brain causing the bias on the stretch reflex to be too high and the muscles to be less sensitive to stretch. ⇨ pendular response—**hypotonicity** *n*.

hypotonic *adj* **1.** pertaining to hypotonia. **2.** a fluid with a lower osmotic pressure relative to another fluid. ⇨ hypertonic, hypo-osmolarity, isotonic.

hypotonic saline a saline solution that has a lower osmotic pressure than normal physiological fluid.

hypotonic sports drinks ⇨ sports drinks.

hypotony decreased intraocular pressure.

hypoventilation *n* diminished breathing or alveolar hypoventilation that causes an increase in PCO_2.

hypovitaminosis *n* any condition due to lack of vitamins. For example lack of vitamin C leading to scurvy.

hypovolaemia *n* reduced volume of blood in the circulation. Under exercise conditions hypovolaemia can develop when the volume of fluid ingested is insufficient to match that lost in sweat—**hypovolaemic** *adj*. ⇨ hydration status of athletes.

hypoxaemia *n* reduced oxygen in arterial blood, shown by decreased PaO_2. Therefore lower than normal saturation of haemoglobin and oxygen content per unit volume—**hypoxaemic** *adj*. ⇨ oxygen dissociation curve.

hypoxia *n* reduced oxygen level in the tissues. If sustained, normal cellular function is disrupted and the result may be complications such as hypotension, arrhythmias and cardiac arrest. Hypoxia occurs as a result of an imbalance between the availability of oxygen in the blood and the demands of oxygen consumption, i.e. deficiency of oxygen which can be due to (a) low partial pressure of oxygen in the blood, because of (i) low oxygen in inspired air, e.g. at altitude, (ii) inadequate ventilation due to lung disease or depression of breathing by drugs (in this case accompanied by hypercapnia), (iii) defective transfer of oxygen from lung alveoli to blood; (b) low content of oxygen in the blood due to inadequate or abnormal haemoglobin; (c) failure of the heart and circulation to deliver an adequate oxygen supply to the tissues, even though the content in the blood may be normal; (d) poisoning of cells so that they cannot use the oxygen delivered to them. ⇨ anaemic hypoxia, corneal hypoxia, histotoxic hypoxia, hypoxic hypoxia, retinal hypoxia, stagnant hypoxia.

hypoxic hypoxia due to low oxygen tension in arterial blood. ⇨ hypoxia.

hysterectomy *n* surgical removal of the uterus. *abdominal hysterectomy* effected via a lower abdominal incision. *laporoscopic-assisted vaginal hysterectomy (LAVH)* a combined approach to vaginal removal of the uterus in which some of the surgical procedure is performed laparoscopically. *subtotal hysterectomy* removal of the uterine body, leaving the cervix in the vaginal vault. *total hysterectomy* complete removal of the uterine body and cervix. *vaginal hysterectomy* carried out through the vagina. *Wertheim's hysterectomy* ⇨ Wertheim's hysterectomy.

hysteresis is when a material is being magnetized the effect of magnetism lags behind the magnetizing force, the lag can be plotted to form a hysteresis loop.

hysteria *n* **1.** a state of excitement with temporary loss of emotional control. **2.** the term previously used for conversion disorder—**hysterical** *adj*.

hyster/o- a prefix that means 'uterus', e.g. *hysteroscopy*.

hysterosalpingectomy *n* excision of the uterus and uterine (fallopian) tube(s).

hysterosalpingography ⇨ uterosalpingography.

hysterosalpingo-oophorectomy surgical removal of the uterus and one or both uterine (fallopian) tubes and ovaries.

hysterosalpingosonography an examination of the uterus and uterine (fallopian) tubes using ultrasound.

hysterosalpingostomy *n* anastomosis between a uterine (fallopian) tube and the uterus.

hysteroscope an endoscope used to view the cervical canal and uterine cavity.

hysteroscopy *n* the passage of a small diameter endoscope through the cervix to visualize the uterine cavity. Used to obtain tissue for examination, remove polyps, or for treatments such as removal or transcervical resection of endometrium.

hysterotomy *n* incision of the uterus to remove a pregnancy. The word is usually reserved for a method of termination.

hysterotrachelorraphy *n* repair of a lacerated cervix uteri.

G
H

IABP *abbr* intra-aortic balloon pump.

IADL *abbr* instrumental activities of daily living.

-iasis a suffix that means 'condition of, state', e.g. *enterolithiasis*.

IAT *abbr* indirect antiglobulin test.

-iatric a suffix that means 'practice of healing', e.g. *bariatric*.

iatr/o- a prefix that means 'physician', e.g. *iatrogenic*.

iatrogenic *adj* describes a secondary condition arising from treatment of a primary condition.

I band the light area visible on electron microscopy in muscle myofibrils when the actin and myosin filaments overlap.

IBD *abbr* inflammatory bowel disease.

IBL *abbr* inquiry-based learning.

IBS *abbr* irritable bowel syndrome.

IBW *abbr* ideal body weight.

IC *abbr* inspiratory capacity.

ICCE *abbr* intracapsular cataract extraction.

ICD-10 *abbr* International Classification of Diseases.

ICE *acron* **1.** **I**ce, **C**ompress, **E**levation a first aid measure used for swelling and bruising of the limbs. An ice compress is applied to the injury and the limb is elevated to assist venous return. ➲ RICE. **2.** iridocorneal endothelial.

iceberg profile in sport psychology, a proposed ideal profile of moodstate for elite performers, characterized by low scores on negative moods (specifically tension, depression, anger, fatigue and confusion) and high scores on positive moods (specifically vigour). Known as 'iceberg' because, according to this proposition, when elite performers' moodstate scores are standardized and plotted they should show an iceberg-shaped profile with negative mood scores lying below the mean and the vigour score lying above the mean.

ice/cold therapy also known as cryotherapy. Health professionals, for example physiotherapists, use ice and cold in their practice. When an ice pack is placed on a typical blood vessel, changes will occur to minimize contact with the cold environment and the loss of any further heat, the vessel wall smooth muscle contracts, thus causing the vessel diameter to decrease (vasoconstriction). After about 5 min, the muscle in vessel wall begins to become paralysed. If this vasoconstriction were to continue, the cells and tissues that the vessel supplies would start to deteriorate and eventually die. The vessel, therefore, reopens as cold-induced vasodilatation (CIVD) occurs. However, this does not help, because as it reopens it comes into contact with more cold. For as long as the ice pack is in situ, the vessel is constantly switching between vasoconstriction and vasodilatation in an attempt to 'hunt' for the most suitable vessel diameter. This is known as Lewis' hunting reaction. Ice is best thought of as a damage limitation procedure immediately following an injury to soft tissues such as a haematoma, sprain or strain. Ice should probably be applied for little more than 2–3 min and then regularly reapplied to emphasize the vasoconstriction element of its effects. There is also little evidence about the anti-inflammatory effects of ice once the immediate acute period is over. The application of ice stimulates pain and cold sensation, but if the cold is intense enough, both of these sensations are suppressed. Some small diameter non-myelinated nerve fibres are least affected and some myelinated fibres are most affected. Muscle strength is decreased, by cooling, but increases beyond its initial value 1 hour later. Cold is useful in decreasing muscle spasm and spasticity. As skin temperature decreases, the need to produce internal heat increases, this is partly achieved by muscle contractions (shivering). Also, adopting a fetal position assists in reducing heat loss. The application of ice to some areas (e.g. hands, feet, abdomen) can be unpleasant and this should be considered when applying ice/cold therapy to patients. ➲ heat and cell metabolism, heat therapy, hunting reaction.

ICF *abbr* **1.** International Classification of Functioning, Disability and Health. **2.** intracellular fluid.

ichthyoses *npl* a group of usually congenital conditions in which the skin is scaly and feels dry. Fish skin. Xeroderma.

ICON *acron* **I**ndex of **C**omplexity of **O**rthodontic **N**eed.

icon a pictorial representation on a computer screen.

ICP *abbr* **1.** integrated care pathway. **2.** intercuspal position. **3.** intracranial pressure.

ICS *abbr* inhaled corticosteroids.

ICSH *abbr* interstitial cell stimulating hormone.

ICSI *abbr* intracytoplasmic sperm injection (transfer).

icterus *n* ➲ jaundice.

icterus gravis acute diffuse necrosis of the liver.

icterus gravis neonatorum one of the clinical forms of haemolytic disease of the newborn. ➲ haemolytic disease of the newborn.

icterus index the measurement of concentration of bilirubin in the plasma. Used in diagnosis of jaundice.

icterus neonatorum excess of the normal, or physiological, jaundice occurring in the first week of life as a result of excessive destruction of red blood cells and haemoglobin. There is yellow colouration of the skin, mucous membranes and sclera. ➲ phototherapy.

ICU *abbr* intensive care unit. ➲ intensive therapy unit.

id *n* one of the three main aspects of the personality (the others being the ego and superego); that part of the unconscious mind that comprises a system of biologically determined urges (instincts). It aspires to the immediate fulfilment of all desires and needs. According to Freud, it persists unrecognized into adult life. ⊃ ego, superego.

IDDM *abbr* insulin dependent diabetes mellitus. ⊃ diabetes mellitus type 1.

idea *n* a concept or plan of something to be aimed at, created or discovered.

idea of reference an incorrect interpretation of casual incidents and external events as having direct reference to oneself. If of a sufficient intensity may lead to the formation of delusions.

ideal occlusion based on the morphology of unworn teeth. An occlusion in which every tooth, with the exception of the lower central incisor and the upper third molar, occludes with two teeth in the opposing arch and is based on the shape of the unworn teeth.

ideal self a person's conception of how they would ideally like to be.

ideation *n* the highest function of awareness, process by which ideas are imagined, conceived and formed. It includes intellect, thought and memory.

identical twins two offspring of the same sex, derived from a single fertilized ovum. ⊃ monozygotic, uniovular.

identification *n* recognition. **1.** in psychology, the way in which personality is formed by modelling it on a chosen person, e.g. identification with the same sex parent—helping to form one's sex role; identification with a person of own sex such as a footballer or singer in the hero-worship of adolescence. **2.** a mental defence mechanism where individuals take on the characteristics of the admired role model figure.

identification dot a mark embossed on the corner of a radiographic film to indicate which side was facing the source of X-rays on exposure. Consists of a raised pimple which should face the tube head during exposure.

identity the knowledge of individuals and groups concerning who they are in relation to others in their group or society. It involves not only feelings and understandings about themselves in relation to others, but also feelings and understandings about others in relation to themselves. People may have multiple identities, for example British, health professional, author and musician.

identity bracelet currently, a plastic band attached to either a patient's wrist or ankle when they are admitted to hospital, usually giving their name and the unique patient number; it should not be removed until a patient leaves hospital. Newer technologies that include the use of bar codes are being considered as a much safer replacement.

ideomotor *adj* pertaining to the motor activity that results from an idea.

ideomotor apraxia the inability to convert an idea into the action required.

idio- a prefix that means 'private, peculiar to the individual', e.g. *idiopathic*.

idiographic relating to the study of individuals rather than groups. ⊃ nomothetic.

idiopathic *adj* of a condition, of unknown or spontaneous origin, e.g. some forms of epilepsy.

idiopathic inflammatory myopathies (IIMs) rare connective tissue disorders defined by the presence of muscle weakness and inflammation. The incidence is 2–10 per million/year with no significant world-wide variation. The aetiology is unknown and genetic associations differ amongst ethnic groups. The most common clinical forms of idiopathic inflammatory myopathies (IIMs) are polymyositis, dermatomyositis and inclusion body myositis. Other systemic autoimmune diseases such as systemic lupus erythematosus (SLE) or vasculitis can also cause myositis. Usually only skeletal muscle is affected. Occasionally, the distribution is focal (e.g. orbital myositis). There is an increased risk of malignancy in patients with dermatomyositis (about a threefold increase) and polymyositis (an increase of about 30%). Malignancy may be apparent at the time of diagnosis or manifest itself later. IIMs should be suspected in anyone who presents with proximal muscle weakness without evidence of neuropathy, particularly if there is evidence of systemic disease. Creatine kinase (CK) is usually raised and is a guide to disease activity. However, a normal CK does not exclude the diagnosis, particularly in juvenile myositis where only 70% of patients have a raised CK at the time of diagnosis. Electromyography (EMG) may confirm the presence of myopathy and exclude neuropathy. Most patients will then need a muscle biopsy to look for the typical features of fibre necrosis, regeneration and inflammatory cell infiltrate. Occasionally, a biopsy may be normal, particularly if myositis is patchy. Magnetic resonance imaging (MRI) is a useful means of identifying areas of abnormal muscle that are amenable to biopsy. When underlying malignancy is suspected screening investigations should include chest/abdomen/pelvis computed tomography (CT), gastrointestinal tract imaging and mammography. Oral corticosteroids (e.g. prednisolone) are the mainstay of initial treatment. Patients with severe weakness or evidence of respiratory or pharyngeal weakness may need methylprednisolone daily for 3 days. If there is a good response, the prednisolone dose should be reduced by approximately 25% per month to a maintenance dose. Although most patients have an initial response to corticosteroids, many will need additional immunosuppressive therapy, especially if the disease relapses. Azathioprine and methotrexate are the initial agents of choice. If these are ineffective or not tolerated, then ciclosporin, cyclophosphamide, tacrolimus and intravenous immunoglobulin are alternatives. If the patient fails to respond clinically to treatment, this may be due to steroid-induced myopathy or the development of inclusion body myositis. Further biopsy is indicated at this stage. If active necrosis and regeneration are present, then the disease is still active, whereas the presence of type 2 fibre atrophy suggests corticosteroid myopathy. ⊃ dermatomyositis, inclusion body myositis, polymyositis, systemic lupus erythematosus (SLE).

idiopathic interstitial pneumonias (IIPs) the idiopathic interstitial pneumonias (IIPs) are characterized by varying

I
J

patterns of inflammation and fibrosis in the lung parenchyma, and comprise a number of clinicopathological entities that are sufficiently different from one another to be considered as separate diseases. The most important of these is idiopathic pulmonary fibrosis (IPF). The other diseases include desquamative interstitial pneumonia (DIP), acute interstitial pneumonia (AIP), non-specific interstitial pneumonia (NSIP), respiratory bronchiolitis–interstitial lung disease (RB-ILD), cryptogenic organizing pneumonia (COP) and lymphocytic interstitial pneumonia (LIP). ⮏ acute interstitial pneumonia (AIP), cryptogenic organizing pneumonia (COP), desquamative interstitial pneumonia (DIP), lymphocytic interstitial pneumonia (LIP), non-specific interstitial pneumonia (NSIP).

idiopathic pulmonary fibrosis (IPF) the term that has replaced cryptogenic fibrosing alveolitis and refers to a specific form of diffuse parenchymal lung disease (DPLD) characterized by pathological (or radiological) evidence of usual interstitial pneumonia (UIP). The aetiology remains unknown: speculation has included exposure to infectious agents such as Epstein–Barr virus (EBV), occupational dusts such as metal or wood dusts, prior use of antidepressants, and a possible role for chronic gastro-oesophageal reflux disease (GORD). Familial cases are rare but genetic factors that control the inflammatory and fibrotic response are likely to be important. The disease displays a strong association with cigarette smoking. Idiopathic pulmonary fibrosis (IPF) is generally a disease of older adults, being uncommon before the age of 50 years. It usually presents with insidiously progressive disabling breathlessness and a non-productive cough. Constitutional symptoms are unusual but arthralgia may be reported. Finger clubbing may be observed in 25–50% of cases and late inspiratory crackles likened to the unzipping of Velcro are classically heard at the lung bases. In advanced cases central cyanosis is detectable and patients may develop features of right heart failure. Rheumatoid factor and antinuclear factor can be detected in 30–50% of patients. The erythrocyte sedimentation rate (ESR) and lactate dehydrogenase (LDH) are elevated in most cases. Pulmonary function tests show a restrictive defect with reduced lung volumes and gas transfer. However, lung volumes may be preserved in patients with concomitant emphysema. Dynamic tests are useful to demonstrate arterial hypoxaemia on exercise in patients with early disease, but as IPF advances, arterial hypoxaemia and hypocapnia are present at rest. Virtually all patients have an abnormal chest X-ray at presentation with lower zone bi-basal reticular and reticulonodular opacities. High-resolution computed tomography (HRCT) may be diagnostic, and is particularly useful in early disease when chest X-ray changes may be indistinct. Patients with typical clinical features and HRCT appearances consistent with UIP do not require lung biopsy, particularly if other known causes of interstitial lung disease have been excluded. However, bronchoalveolar lavage (BAL) and transbronchial biopsy may be used to exclude alternative diagnoses. A median survival of 3 years is typical and survival beyond 5 years unusual. However, the rate of disease progression varies considerably from death within a few months to survival with minimal symptoms for many years. The pattern of serial lung function may be helpful in predicting survival; relative preservation of lung function is a predictor of longer survival and desaturation on exercise heralds a poor prognosis. High numbers of fibroblastic foci on biopsy have been associated with a poor outcome. Treatment options remain limited. Prednisolone therapy (0.5 mg/kg) combined with azathioprine (2–3 mg/kg) is currently recommended to patients who are highly symptomatic or have rapidly progressive disease, have a predominantly 'ground-glass' appearance on computed tomography (CT) or have a sustained fall of > 15% in their forced vital capacity (FVC) or gas transfer over a 3- to 6-month period. However, response rates are notoriously poor and side-effects guaranteed. Should objective evidence of improvement be demonstrated, the prednisolone dose may be gradually reduced to a maintenance dose. New therapies are urgently required and the potential of novel therapies such as IFN-γ or acetyl-cysteine is being explored. Lung transplantation should be considered in young patients with advanced disease. Oxygen may be provided for palliation of breathlessness but opiates may be required for relief of severe dyspnoea.

idiopathic scoliosis is characterized by a lateral spinal curvature together with rotation and associated rib hump or flank recession. The treatment is by spinal brace or traction or internal fixation with accompanying spinal fusion. ⮏ halopelvic traction, Harrington rod, Milwaukee brace, scoliosis.

idiopathic thrombocytopenic purpura (ITP) a syndrome characterized by a low platelet count caused by the presence of autoantibodies. This results in purpura and intermittent bleeding from mucosal surfaces. In children it may appear following a virus infection. The onset in adults tends to be more insidious. Treatment in adults usually involves corticosteroids, with splenectomy in patients who fail to respond.

idiosyncrasy *n* a peculiar variation of constitution or temperament. It may relate to an unusual response to a particular protein, drug or food.

IE *abbr* infective endocarditis.

IEP *abbr* isoelectric point.

IFG *abbr* impaired fasting glucose/glycaemia.

IFN *abbr* interferon.

IFT *abbr* inferential therapy.

Ig *abbr* immunoglobulin.

IGF *abbr* insulin-like growth factors.

IgG *abbr* immunoglobulin G.

IGT *abbr* impaired glucose tolerance.

IHD *abbr* ischaemic heart disease.

IHE *abbr* integrated health enterprise.

IIMs *abbr* idiopathic inflammatory myopathies.

IL *abbr* interleukin.

ILD *abbr* interstitial lung disease.

ileal bladder ⮏ ileoureterostomy.

ileal conduit ⮏ ileoureterostomy.

ileal pouch ⮏ ileostomy.

ileectomy surgical procedure to remove the ileum.

I
J

ileitis *n* inflammation of the ileum, such as that caused by Crohn's disease.

ileo- a prefix that means 'ileum', e.g. *ileostomy*.

ileoanal reservoir a two-stage surgical procedure that avoids a permanent ileostomy when it is necessary to remove the colon and rectum (proctocolectomy), for instance in a person with familial polyposis coli. The colon and rectum are removed at the first operation, a temporary ileostomy is formed and a pouch or reservoir is fashioned from the distal small intestine, and this is anastomosed to the anus. Once the ileoanal anastomosis has had time to heal a second operation is performed, during which the ileostomy is reversed to re-establish bowel continuity. This allows the person to pass faeces from the anus.

ileocaecal *adj* pertaining to the ileum and the caecum.

ileocaecal valve the sphincter muscle that controls the rate at which the chyme (contents of the small intestine) enters the caecum (first part of large bowel), and prevents flow in the opposite direction. The valve opens in response to peristalsis in the small intestine and the presence of chyme. It also opens during colonic peristalsis that occurs as part of the gastrocolic reflex.

ileocolic *adj* pertaining to the ileum and the colon.

ileocolitis *n* inflammation of the ileum and the colon.

ileocolostomy *n* a surgically made fistula between the ileum and the colon, usually the transverse colon. Most often used to bypass an obstruction or inflammation in the caecum or ascending colon.

ileocystoplasty *n* operation to increase the size of the urinary bladder—**ileocystoplastic** *adj*.

ileorectal *adj* pertaining to the ileum and the rectum.

ileosigmoidostomy *n* an anastomosis between the ileum and sigmoid colon.

ileostomy *n* a surgically made fistula between the ileum and the anterior abdominal wall; a type of stoma discharging liquid faecal matter. Usually permanent when the whole of the large bowel has to be removed, e.g. in severe ulcerative colitis. ⊃ ileoanal reservoir. Special stoma bags are used to collect the liquid discharge from an ileostomy. *continent ileostomy* for some patients it may be possible to fashion an internal pouch/reservoir from the small intestine. A valve is constructed and a stoma brought out through the abdominal wall. Patients are able to use a tube to empty the pouch/reservoir at intervals instead of wearing an external stoma bag.

ileoureterostomy *n* (*syn* ureteroileostomy) transplantation of the lower ends of the ureters from the urinary bladder to an isolated loop of small bowel (ileal bladder) which, in turn, is made to open on the abdominal wall (ileal conduit).

ileum *n* the lower three-fifths of the small intestine, lying between the jejunum and the ileocaecal valve leading into the caecum. Concerned with the absorption of various nutrients such as vitamin B_{12}—**ileal** *adj*.

ileus *n* intestinal obstruction. Usually restricted to paralytic as opposed to mechanical obstruction and characterized by abdominal distension, vomiting and the absence of pain. ⊃ meconium.

iliac *adj* pertaining to the ilium.

iliac arteries *npl* two large arteries, the right and left common iliac, formed when the abdominal aorta divides. They in turn divide into external and internal iliac arteries, which carry arterial blood to the legs and pelvic organs respectively. ⊃ Colour Section Figure 9.

iliac crest the highest point of the ilium.

iliac region/fossa the abdominal region situated either side of the hypogastrium. ⊃ Colour Section Figure 18a.

iliacus ⊃ iliopsoas muscle.

iliac veins the internal iliac veins drain venous blood from the pelvic organs and the external iliac veins carry venous blood from the legs. The internal and external iliac veins unite to form the right and left common iliac veins, which unite to form the inferior vena cava. ⊃ Colour Section Figure 10.

ilio- a prefix that means 'ilium', e.g. *iliofemoral*.

iliococcygeal *adj* pertaining to the ilium and coccyx.

iliofemoral *adj* pertaining to the ilium and the femur, such as the iliofemoral ligament between the ilium and the top of the femur.

iliohypogastric nerve a nerve that arises from the lumbar plexus. It supplies the muscles and skin of the lower abdomen, upper and medial aspects of the thigh and the inguinal region. ⊃ lumbar plexus.

ilioinguinal nerve a nerve that arises from the lumbar plexus. It supplies the muscles and skin of the lower abdomen, upper and medial aspects of the thigh and the inguinal region. ⊃ lumbar plexus.

iliopectineal *adj* pertaining to the ilium and the pubis.

iliopectineal eminence small protrusion marking the fusion of ilium and os pubis.

iliopectineal line bony ridge on the internal surface of the ilium and pubic bones. It crosses the innominate bone from the sacroiliac joint to the iliopectineal eminence. Forms the dividing line between the true and false pelvis.

iliopsoas *adj* pertaining to the ilium and the loin.

iliopsoas muscle comprises two muscles—the iliacus and psoas major. The iliacus has its origin on the iliac crest and the psoas arises from the transverse processes and bodies of the lumbar vertebrae. The combined muscle inserts via a common tendon onto the lesser trochanter of the femur. Act to flex the hip and the lumbar spine.

iliotibial band a strong band of connective tissue, continuous above with the tensor fasciae latae muscle which is attached to the iliac crest, and extending down to be inserted on the outer side of the tibia below the knee. It has action over the knee (can act as a flexor at $> 30°$ of knee flexion and as an extensor at $< 30°$ of flexion) and can be affected by overuse. ⊃ iliotibial band syndrome.

iliotibial band syndrome iliotibial band syndrome is one of the commonest causes of knee pain in runners, with pain localized to the insertion on the lateral aspect of the tibia where the band rubs on the lateral tibial condyle. There may be associated crepitus or clicking. Classically caused by road running, especially on cambered surfaces, associated with excessive pronation. The key to treatment is to identify the cause and improve the flexibility and strength of the band.

ilium *n* the upper part of the innominate (hip) bone; it is a separate bone in the fetus—**iliac** *adj.*

Ilizarov frame/method (G Ilizarov, Soviet orthopaedic surgeon, 1921–1992) external fixation device used commonly in the management of fractures and for the correction of bony deformities. It incorporates an axial system of wires or pins fitted through the bone and connected to a circular ring (Figure I.1). It is sometimes used in cases of non-union. ⊃ distraction osteogenesis.

illness behaviour the ways in which people respond to illness and impairment and the type of help, if any, that they seek. Illness behaviour depends upon a multitude of factors including how symptoms are perceived and evaluated, the severity of the symptoms, past experience of illness, social support and how convenient or inconvenient it is to be ill at any given time.

illusion *n* a misidentification of a existing stimuli, e.g. of sight, a bush or tree being mistaken for a person, the bush being misrepresented in consciousness as a figure. They are a relatively 'normal' phenomenon.

IM *abbr* **1.** Index Medicus. **2.** intramedullary. **3.** intramuscular.

image *n* **1.** a revived experience of a percept recalled from memory. **2.** the optical reproduction of an object formed on the retina as light is focused through the eye. **3.** the shadow of a structure cast by X-rays on to a radiographic film.

image acquisition the collection of data in order to produce a computed tomography (CT) or magnetic resonance imaging (MRI) image.

image acquisition time the scanning time required to produce a set of images from a measurement sequence in magnetic resonance imaging (MRI). For a *two-dimensional sequence* it is the repetition time, times the number of signal excitations/averages times the number of phase encoded steps. For a *fast two-dimensional sequence* it is the two-dimensional sequence divided by the echo train length.

For *three-dimensional volume sequence* it is the two-dimensional sequence multiplied by the number of partitions.

image annotation the marking of information on a radiograph to denote the side of the body, the patient position and the exposure factors; digital systems allow preset terms, numbers and letters to be added alongside the patient image.

ImageChecker an aid to screening routine mammograms by automatically marking clusters of white areas and dense areas with radiating lines.

image distance the distance along the optical axis of a lens or optical system between the image plane and the secondary principal plane. If the system consists of a single thin lens the image distance is measured from the optical surface and the reciprocal of this quantity is called the reduced image vergence or image vergence (in air). ⊃ back vertex power, principal plane, vergence.

image format the manner in which a computed tomography (CT) image is stored or displayed such as on screen, computer disk, magnetic tape or film.

image intensifier in radiology, a means of producing a real time image of a patient. The X-ray beam passes through the patient and onto the image intensifier which converts the image to light, this image is scanned and an electrical signal is sent to a television monitor where the image is viewed.

image manipulation in computed tomography (CT) scanning the ability to digitally alter the appearance of the acquired image to enhance depiction of the required anatomy.

imaging plate a re-usable plate coated with barium phosphate that, when exposed to radiation excites the electrons, and then, when scanned by a helium-neon laser, produces an image which can be recorded.

image quality the ratio of signal over noise.

image reconstruction the process of producing an image from computer data or a set of unprocessed measurements.

imagery *n* imagination. The process of forming symbolic mental representations of objects, events or actions, which may be in any of the sensory modes. The recall of mental images of various types depending upon the specific sensory organs involved when the images were formed, e.g. smell (olfactory), sound (auditory), sight (visual), touch (tactile). *guided imagery* a technique used as part of a range of coping strategies for pain and other symptom control or anxiety in which patients are asked to imagine a particular situation, feeling or state. In *sport psychology* the effective and deliberate use of imagery is considered to be one of the fundamental mental skills for sports performers and is used for mental rehearsal, motivation, relaxation and stress management. *external imagery* is that engaged in from a third person perspective as if an external observer were watching the person doing the imaging; *internal imagery* is that engaged in from the first person perspective of the person doing the imaging. In *kinaesthetic imagery* the person images bodily movements or sensations. In *visual imagery* the person creates a mental picture of an object, event or action, also known as visualization. ⊃ psychoneuromuscular theory.

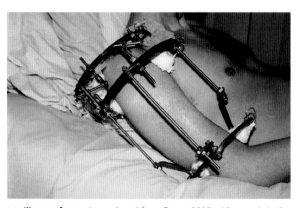

I.1 **Ilizarov frame** (reproduced from Porter 2005 with permission).

image segmentation in digital imaging, dividing an image into its various parts or taking the image from the background to increase the definition of the object.

imaging techniques diagnostic techniques used to investigate the condition and functioning of organs and structures. They include radiographic examination, radionuclide scans, ultrasonography (US), computed tomography (CT), magnetic resonance (MRI), positron emission tomography (PET), single-photon emission computed tomography (SPECT).

imago in psychoanalysis, the unconscious, often idealized image of an important/significant person, such as a parent, in the formative time during the patient's childhood.

imbalance *n* want of balance. Term refers commonly to the upset of acid–base relationship and the electrolytes in body fluids, or lack of balance in opposing muscle groups.

Imbert–Fick law applied to applanation tonometry, this law states that the intraocular pressure P (in mmHg) is equal to the tonometer weight W (in g) divided by the applanated area A (in mm^2), hence,

$$P = \frac{W}{A}$$

Strictly speaking, this law is correct only for infinitely thin, dry, elastic, spherical membranes. ⊃ applanation, intraocular pressure.

imbricated overlapped like tiles.

imbrication overlapping of adjacent incisor teeth.

immediate replacement denture a prosthesis constructed in advance of tooth extractions and fitted immediately after the removal of the teeth.

immersion foot ⊃ trench foot.

immiscible unable to be mixed, e.g. oil and water.

immobility a general term used to describe a lack of movement either locally, such as at a joint or muscle, or globally (e.g. unable to walk).

immobilization 1. a lengthy period of inactivity of a person. **2.** fixation to make a normally mobile part immobile. This includes the use of braces, splints, plaster casts, external and internal fixation of fractures or other conditions. Or surgical techniques to permanently fix a structure.

immobilization device a method of reducing movement during radiotherapy treatment or diagnostic imaging.

immune *adj* protected against infection by specific or nonspecific mechanisms of the immune system. Altered reactivity against an antigen, caused by previous exposure to that antigen. ⊃ defence mechanisms.

immune-reactive trypsin (IRT) test blood test used in newborn screening for cystic fibrosis. Deoxyribonucleic acid (DNA) analysis is undertaken if IRT results reach a certain level. ⊃ cystic fibrosis, sweat test.

immune response the specific adaptive responses of the immune system to a perceived threat, either from non-self antigens, or from self antigens during a pathological immune response. This may be against micro-organisms, malignant cells, and damaged or healthy tissues. The response may be humoral in which the B lymphocytes produce antibodies against specific antigens. Or it may be cell-mediated where T lymphocytes act in a variety of ways to counter the threat. ⊃ active immunity, cell-mediated immunity, humoral immunity, immunity, passive immunity.

immune ring of Wessley ⊃ Wessley's ring.

immune system the diverse cells, tissues and organs that protect the body from micro-organisms, foreign cells and abnormal body cells, etc. They include the lymphatic system of vessels, fluid and lymph nodes, lymphoid tissue, the spleen, the mucosal-associated lymphoid tissue, the bone marrow, thymus and the B and T lymphocytes.

immunity *n* an intrinsic or acquired state of immune responsiveness to an antigen. Immunity can be innate (from inherited qualities), or it can be acquired, actively or passively, naturally or artificially. ⊃ active immunity, cell-mediated immunity, humoral immunity, passive immunity.

immunization *n* artificial means by which immunity is initiated or augmented. Achieved by using vaccines containing attenuated micro-organisms or inactive micro-organisms or bacterial products such as toxins. Antibody production (active immunity) occurs and is generally long-lasting. In certain situations, such as during an epidemic, the injection of immunoglobulins obtained from immune humans, or very rarely sera from animals, can give temporary protection (passive immunization).

immunization programme a routine programme of immunization offered during childhood and to special groups such as healthcare workers and those travelling abroad.

immun/o- a prefix that means 'immunity', e.g. *immunoglobulin.*

immunocompromised patients (*syn* immunosuppressed patients) patients with defective immune responses, which can be inherited or acquired. Often produced by treatment with cytotoxic drugs or irradiation. Also occurs in some patients with cancer and other diseases affecting the lymphoid system. Depending on the immune defect, different patterns of infection result. Patients with cellular defects are likely to develop infections with opportunistic organisms such as *Candida*, *Pneumocystis jirovecii* (former name *Pneumocystis carinii*) and *Cryptococcus neoformans*. Patients with antibody defects are more liable to infections with encapsulated bacteria such as pneumococcus.

immunocytochemistry *n* staining cells with specific antibodies for diagnostic purposes.

immunodeficiency *n* the state of having defective immune responses, leading to increased susceptibility to infectious diseases. The problem may be with humoral immune responses where antibody production is abnormal or cell-mediated responses involving T lymphocytes are deficient.

immunodeficiency diseases inherited or acquired disorders of the immune system. They may involve B-cells or T-cells or both. ⊃ severe combined immunodeficiency.

immunofluorescence a procedure used for the identification of an antigen. The antigen is mixed with a known antibody which have been coated with fluorescein

I
J

(a fluorescent dye) and then checked for precipitation (an antigen–antibody reaction). This is confirmed by the presence of precipitate that is luminous when observed in ultraviolet light from a fluorescent microscope.

immunogenicity *n* the ability to produce immunity.

immunoglobulins (Igs) *n* (*syn* antibodies) high molecular weight glycoproteins produced by plasma cells (derived from B lymphocytes) in response to specific antigens. The basic structure of immunoglobulins is Y-shaped, consisting of two identical heavy chains, each linked to two identical light chains. Immunoglobulins are found in the blood and other body fluids where they form part of body defences. Immunoglobulins function in a variety of ways, but all involve combining with the antigen to form an immune complex. There are five classes of immunoglobulins, IgG, IgA, IgD, IgM and IgE, each with different characteristics, functions and locations. ⊃ Colour Section Figure 30.

immunohistochemistry *n* staining tissue with specific antibodies for diagnostic purposes.

immunological pregnancy test standard method to diagnose pregnancy which detects increased serum or urinary human chorionic gonadotrophin (hCG) levels by immunological methods include latex particle agglutination, or more commonly, anti-hCG antibody 'sandwich' assays which work by binding hCG with a conjugate, the mixture migrating down a test strip; when the mixture comes into contact with a line of anti-hCG antibodies a colour change occurs, indicating a positive result.

immunological response ⊃ immune response, immunity.

immunology *n* the study of the immune system of lymphocytes, inflammatory cells and associated cells and proteins, which affect an individual's response to antigens—**immunological** *adj*, **immunologically** *adv*.

immunomodulators substances which change the immune response either by augmenting or decreasing part of the response. They include both naturally occurring substances, such as cytokines, and substances used therapeutically, e.g. cytotoxic drugs, corticosteroids and drugs such as infliximab used in rheumatoid arthritis.

immunopathology *n* the study of disease involving the immune system.

immunosuppressant drugs drugs given to suppress the immune responses, e.g. azothiapine, ciclosporin, tacrolimus. ⊃ Appendix 5.

immunosuppressed patients ⊃ immunocompromised patients.

immunosuppression *n* treatment which reduces immunological responsiveness. The administration of agents to significantly interfere with the ability of the immune system to respond to antigenic stimulation by inhibiting cellular and humoral immunity. May be deliberate such as before bone marrow transplants to prevent rejection by the host or incidental such as following chemotherapy for the treatment of cancer.

immunosuppressive 1. *n* that which reduces immunological responsiveness. **2.** *adj* describes an agent such as a drug that suppresses immune system function.

immunotherapy *n* can be used to mean desensitization therapy against specific allergens, e.g. insect venom, or can refer to therapeutics which use agonists or antagonists based on immune system components, e.g. treatment based on biological modifiers such as interleukin-2 and lymphokine-activated killer cells. ⊃ immunomodulators.

impact force the force generated at the start of contact or collision. In sport this can be the impact of a jumper as they hit the ground in the long jump.

impact injury can occur in collision with another person or object when the force exceeds the strength and elasticity of the tissues. Includes both fractures and soft tissue injuries.

impact peak the high point of the sharp increase seen on a force–time trace due to impact between two bodies or objects (or one body or object and the ground).

impacted *adj* firmly wedged, abnormal immobility, as of hard constipated faeces in the colon and rectum; fracture such as some types affecting the femoral neck; a fetus in the pelvis; a tooth in its socket or a calculus in a duct. ⊃ faecal impaction.

impacted fracture ⊃ fracture.

impaction in dentistry, the state of being firmly lodged or wedged. *food impaction* the accumulation of food, generally interproximally, because of an open contact, a 'plunger' cusp or uneven marginal ridge height. *tooth impaction* a situation in which a tooth is so placed that it is unable to erupt normally. May be due to a wedging against another tooth or teeth or to the abnormal development or siting of the tooth. The impaction may be disto-angular, horizontal or mesio-angular (Figure I.2).

impaired fasting glucose/glycaemia (IFG) fasting plasma glucose levels between 6.1 and 7 mmol/L indicative of a pre-diabetic state. However, if measured, the 2-hour post-glucose load result is less than 7.8 mmol/L.

impaired glucose tolerance (IGT) fasting plasma glucose level less than 7 mmol/L. However, plasma levels between 7.8 and 11.0 mmol/L 2 hours after a glucose load is indicative of a pre-diabetic state and conferring a significantly increased risk of cardiovascular disease.

impaired glucose tolerance during pregnancy ⊃ gestational diabetes mellitus.

impairment a term used to describe the loss or abnormality of psychological, physiological or anatomical structure or function. Impairment also has a social dimension as it means different things in different societies at different times. The term was used within the World Health Organization's model for describing Health: Impairment, Disability, Handicap. The WHO redefined the definitions in 1997, with a result that the term 'function' is now used replacing the term impairment. ⊃ handicap.

impalpable *adj* not palpable; incapable of being felt by touch (palpation).

impermeable impenetrable. Refers to a substance or tissue that does not permit the passage of fluids through it.

impedance the general opposition of flow of electric current measured in ohms. In ultrasound a measure of the tissue's

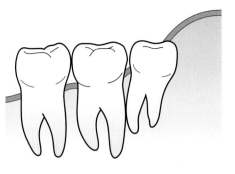

Disto-angular

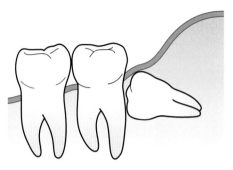

Horizontal

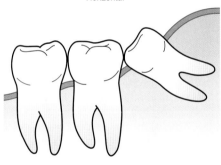

Mesio-angular

Impactions

I.2 Tooth impactions (reproduced from Heasman & McCracken 2007 with permission).

resistance to distortion by ultrasound and depends on the tissue density and the velocity of the sound.

imperforate *adj* lacking a normal opening.

imperforate anus a congenital absence of an opening into the rectum.

imperforate hymen a fold of mucous membrane at the vaginal entrance which has no natural outlet for the menstrual fluid. Rectified by a simple surgical operation. ➲ cryptomenorrhoea, haematocolpos.

impetigo *n* an inflammatory, pustular skin disease usually caused by *Staphylococcus*, occasionally by *Streptococcus*.

impetigo contagiosa a highly contagious form of impetigo, commonest on the face and scalp, characterized by vesicles which become pustules and then honey-coloured crusts. ➲ ecthyma—**impetiginous** *adj*.

impingement a term used in sports medicine when soft tissue is trapped, usually between bones, leading to pressure, inflammation, pain and loss of function. Shoulder impingement is common in repetitive overhead sports, especially swimming, where the tendons of the 'rotator cuff' are trapped between the head of the humerus and the acromion, causing pain when moving the arm forwards and upwards: the impingement sign. Treatment aims to alter poor technique and reduce inflammation (rest, ice, anti-inflammatory drugs and steroid injections). Surgery is occasionally required.

implant *n* to insert or fix. Any drug, structure or substance inserted surgically into the human body, e.g. implants of progestogens for contraception, or implants used in plastic surgery. Those used to augment tissue contour may be of two types: *alloplastic implants* synthetic foreign body implants such as those used in breast reconstruction, or *autologous implants* tissue obtained from the same patient. ➲ implant (dental).

implant (dental) can mean a tooth that has been reimplanted but usually applied to an artificial structure implanted surgically into the alveolar bone. The metal (usually titanium) screw, pin, blade or casting inserted into or placed on the alveolar bone in order to provide anchorage or stabilization either to teeth or to a prosthesis. An implant may consist of three parts: (a) the fixture (previously the body), which is placed in the bone, (b) the abutment, which connects to the fixture and is visible in the mouth and supports and/or retains the prosthesis (or superstructure) and (c) the superstructure which may be an integral part of the final restoration (a bridge) or supports the final restoration (an overdenture). *asseointegrated implant* an implant which is placed within bone; and has a direct interface between it's surface and the host's bone. ➲ diodontic implant, mandibular staple implant. *endosseous (endosteal) implant* an implant, usually of metal, introduced into bone, in dentistry this will usually be the maxilla or mandible. *subperiosteal implant* an implant that is introduced between the bone surface and overlying periosteum with a part of it protruding through the mucosa into the mouth. ➲ implant supported denture.

implant impression coping ➲ coping.

implant supported denture a prosthesis which obtains its stability and retention from a substructure lying under the soft tissues of the denture-bearing area, and which projects through the gingival tissues, e.g. asseointegrated implant fixture.

implantable defibrillator an implanted device to sense the heart rhythm. Delivers a small electric shock when ventricular tachycardia or ventricular fibrillation are detected. ➲ automatic implantable cardioverter defibrillator, sudden adult/arrhythmia death syndrome.

implantation *n* **1.** the insertion of living cells or solid materials into the tissues, e.g. accidental implantation of cancer cells in a wound. **2.** insertion of a prosthesis into

I
J

the body such as a pacemaker, breast implant or artificial replacement joint components. **3.** insertion of radioactive material such as iridium-192 (^{192}Ir) to treat cancers, or solid drugs that are released over a period of time. **4.** implantation or embedding of the fertilized ovum into the hormone-prepared endometrium or decidua. It occurs around 6–8 days following fertilization when the blastocyst becomes embedded within the decidua. The process, which is also known as nidation, is normally complete around 11 days following ovulation.

implementation in the United Kingdom, the third stage of the nursing process, when planned interventions to achieve the set goals are implemented and recorded on the patient's nursing notes, which provide cumulative information on the date set for evaluating. ⊃ assessment, evaluation, planning.

impotence *n* an outdated term, but still used by the public to describe an inability to participate in sexual intercourse, by custom referring to the male. ⊃ erectile dysfunction, premature ejaculation.

impregnate *v* fill; saturate; render pregnant.

impression an imprint, mould or negative form from which a model or positive reproduction may be obtained by casting. In dentistry or prosthetics, a negative likeness or imprint of teeth, dental arch or other body structures to use when producing a replacement part or prosthesis, such as a denture. *final, master, major, second or working impression* an impression used to make the master cast. *functional impression* an impression which, during its formation, is modified by masticatory loads and adjacent muscular activity and is mucodisplacive. *mucostatic impression* an impression made with the intention of minimizing the displacement of soft tissues. Formerly termed functional impression. *primary impression* an impression made for construction of a model or to construct a custom or special tray. *sectional impression* an impression built up in the mouth from two or more parts that are removed separately and reassembled out of the mouth for casting.

impression management the act of controlling or regulating information a person gives out in order to influence the impressions formed of them by others.

impression material material used to take an impression. *compound impression material* (compound, thermoplastic impression material, composition). Thermoplastic material consisting of natural and synthetic resins, fillers and plasticizers. Used mainly for edentulous mouth impressions. Softened by placing in hot water at 60°C or by holding over a flame. Obtainable in sticks, sheets or cones. Not sufficiently elastic to reproduce undercut areas accurately. *elastomeric impression material* very accurate impression material used in inlay, crown, bridge and precision attachment work. Especially useful for multi-unit preparations. May exhibit a rubber-like behaviour. Must be mixed and used strictly in accordance with the manufacturer's instructions. Usually presented in tubes or cartridges with mixing tips and used on preparations which must be dry. There are three main types: (a) silicone impression material—addition or condensation curing polymeric materials. Highly elastic but hydrophobic materials. Usually presented in four

viscosities (light, medium, heavy, putty) which are used in combination; (b) polyether impression material—clean to use, based on an organic polymer having an ether linkage. Marketed in tubes of pastes and accelerator; (c) polysulphide impression material—material with a characteristic odour, based on an organic polymer linked with disulphide groups. Sometimes referred to as *rubber base, thiokol* or *mercaptam.* A two-part mixture of light body, intermediate or regular, or heavy body, with a catalyst—all in tubes. *green stick impression material (tracing stick)* a thermoplastic impression material in stick form. Used to build up the margins of impression trays or in copper rings. May not be green colour. *inlay wax impression material* the wax used for obtaining patterns for castings. Blue inlay wax is harder than the green variety, the working properties being varied by their ingredients. A mixture of waxes such as paraffin wax, beeswax, ceresin, carnauba and candelilla wax. It is obtainable in sticks, sheets and prefabricated shapes used for clasps and bars. *irreversible hydrocolloid (alginate) impression material* a powder containing soluble alginates and additives mixed in correct proportion with water (at room temperature) to form a gel on setting. Cannot be re-used. Mixing instructions must be followed exactly to obtain accurate and standard results. The set material dehydrates if left exposed to air for any length of time causing shrinkage. *plaster of Paris impression material* finely ground plaster of Paris containing such substances as potassium sulphate and borax to reduce setting time and expansion. The powder is mixed with water and spatulated in a flexible bowl. Used mostly for edentulous cases but seldom as a routine. *reversible hydrocolloid (agar) impression material* an agar aqueous gel that liquefies when heated and gels on cooling. Provides very accurate impressions and is used on wet preparations. Marketed in tubes or cartridges. Heated before use in electrically controlled water baths at various temperatures. The material is contained in water-cooled impression trays held in the mouth. *zinc oxide-eugenol impression material* a paste used for rebasing or relining a complete denture, and in some cases as a wash covering an existing impression. Obtained by mixing pastes from two tubes, one containing zinc oxide, an oil and accelerator, and the other a resin dissolved in eugenol or other substance.

impression tonometer (*syn* indentation tonometer) a tonometer in which the intraocular pressure is estimated by the degree of indentation of the cornea. The excursion of the plunger of the tonometer is read from a calibrated scale and converted into values of the intraocular pressure, often using appropriate tables. The most common such instrument is that of Schiötz. ⊃ ocular rigidity.

impression tray metal or plastic tray used to carry, control and support an impression material. May be perforated to improve the adherence of the material to the tray, so reducing the possibility of distortions. *anatomical impression tray* used for edentulous cases and shaped to accommodate and follow the contours of the denture-bearing area. *box impression tray* stock impression tray of metal or plastic used for impressions of partially dentate arches. *special impression tray* tray made from an individual patient's models to control the impression material accurately. *stock impression tray* metal or plastic tray used to obtain a first impression model on which a special tray may be constructed.

imprinting *n* very early learning occurring at a critical developmental stage that results in a newborn becoming attached to a model, usually a parent, but may be a carer.

impulse *n* **1.** a sudden inclination, sometimes irresistible urge to act without deliberation. **2.** the electrochemical process involved in neurotransmission of information and stimuli throughout the body. ⊃ nerve impulse. **3.** change in momentum produced by a force. ⊃ angular impulse, linear impulse.

IMRT *abbr* intensity modulated radiotherapy.

IMTG *abbr* intramuscular triacylglycerol.

IMV *abbr* intermittent mandatory ventilation.

in- a prefix that means either 'not, lack of' e.g. *incontinence*, or 'in, on, into, within', e.g. *inborn*.

inactivated pathogen vaccines ⊃ vaccines.

inanition a state of starvation characterized by complete exhaustion with wasting. It is caused by total lack or inability to assimilate food.

inappetence usually described as having no appetite.

incarcerated *adj* imprisoned, held fast. Describes the abnormal imprisonment of a part, as in a hernia which is irreducible or a pregnant uterus held beneath the sacral promontory.

incarcerated hernia ⊃ hernia.

incentive spirometry a method of increasing lung expansion by use of a volumetric or simple flow device. Some devices provide visual feedback as to whether the desired predetermined target has been met. Incentive spirometry encourages a prolonged and maximal inspiration and increases inflation of the alveoli. There are few complications associated with their use, but these include hyperventilation, pain where pain relief is inadequate, hypoxaemia secondary to breaks in therapy and fatigue.

incest *n* sexual intercourse between close blood relatives, usually meaning those who are prohibited by law to marry. The most common type of sexual abuse occurs between father and daughter; other types of incest such as between siblings also occur. ⊃ abuse.

incidence *n* the number of times that an event happens. In epidemiology, the rate of new cases of a disease that occur in a population over a defined time period (usually a year). For example, the number of new cases of a specific cancer or an infectious disease. ⊃ prevalence.

incidental haemorrhage uncommon vaginal bleeding during pregnancy due to extraplacental causes. The causes include cervical polyps, erosions, vaginitis and more seriously cervical carcinoma. Rarely leads to dangerous haemorrhage; treatment is that of the cause.

incident beam the beam of radiation striking an object.

incident light the light travelling from the light source.

incipient *adj* initial, beginning, in its early stages.

incipient caries the very first stage of the disease process where the carious lesion is just coming into existence.

incisal angle the angle formed with the horizontal plane by drawing a line in the sagittal plane between the incisal edges of the mandibular and maxillary central incisors when the teeth are in intercuspal occlusion.

incisal edge the cutting surfaces of the incisor and canine teeth. This edge is bounded by the labial and lingual or palatal surfaces.

incisal guide or table the anterior guide of an articulator which maintains the incisal angle.

incisal guidance the guidance provided by the palatal surface of the maxillary incisors during the lateral movement of the mandible.

incisal rest ⊃ rest.

incisal surface ⊃ surface.

incised wound one which results from cutting with a sharp knife or scalpel: heals by primary intention in the absence of complications such as infection.

incision *n* the result of cutting into body tissue, using a sharp instrument—**incisional** *adj*, **incise** *vt*.

incisional biopsy the partial removal of a lesion or abnormal tissue for histological examination.

incisional hernia protrusion through the site of a previous abdominal incision. ⊃ hernia.

incisive canal the bony canal running from the incisive foramen in the anterior inferior aspect of the maxilla behind the central incisors, to the floor of the nasal cavity. Conveys the long sphenopalatine nerve, blood vessels and lymphatics.

incisive canal cyst ⊃ nasopalatine cyst.

incisive foramen (nasopalatine foramen) the opening that connects the nasal cavity to the oral mucosa. Lying in the midline internal to the upper central incisors, beneath the central papilla of the rugae. It has four openings, two for the nasopalatine nerves and two for the nasopalatine blood vessels.

incisive papilla a raised portion of soft tissue covering the incisive foramen in the hard palate.

incisor relation in orthodontics, a classification based on the anteroposterior relationship of the incisors. There are three classes with a further subdivision in one class. *class I* applies when the incisal edges of the lower incisors occlude with the central portion or cingulum of the upper central incisors. *class II* applies when the incisal edges of the lower incisors lie posteriorly to the upper central incisor cingulum— *division I* describes proclined upper central incisors with an increased overjet, and *division 2* describes retroclined upper central incisors. *class III* applies when the lower incisor edges lie anteriorly to the upper incisor edges. There is a reduced or reversed overjet.

incisor tooth a single-rooted tooth with a cutting or shearing edge (see Figure T.4b, p. 779). The four most anterior maxillary and mandibular teeth; placed first and second from the midline in both dental arches and in both the primary and secondary dentition. Classified as *central* and *lateral* incisors. The upper incisors develop and erupt in the

I
J

premaxilla and the lower incisors gain contact with them when the mouth is closed. The lateral incisors are situated on each side of the central incisors and are bounded by the canines.

inclination of pelvis the brim slopes at approximately 55° to the horizontal, and the bony outlet slopes at about 15°. ⊃ curve of Carus.

inclusion bodies microscopic particles found in the nucleus or cytoplasm of some cells of pathological and normal tissues.

inclusion body myositis a clinical form of idiopathic myopathy. The most common disease of muscle in people over the age of 50 and predominates in men. Although proximal weakness does occur, distal involvement is more common and may be asymmetrical. Creatine kinase (CK) may be marginally elevated and both myopathic and neurogenic abnormalities may be present on electromyogram (EMG). The characteristic findings on muscle biopsy are abnormal fibres containing rimmed vacuoles and filamentous inclusions in the nucleus and cytoplasm. These inclusions contain paired helical filaments that resemble those seen in the brain in Alzheimer's disease. Treatment is controversial and not as successful as in idiopathic inflammatory myopathy (IIM). Some patients do have an inflammatory component and are corticosteroid-responsive; a trial of corticosteroids is therefore warranted, and if a response occurs then immunosuppressive therapy should be substituted. ⊃ dermatomyositis, idiopathic inflammatory myopathies (IIMs), polymyositis.

inclusion conjunctivitis conjunctivitis caused by the micro-organism *Chlamydia trachomatis*. Also called trachoma inclusion conjunctivitis (TRIC). ⊃ trachoma.

inclusion criteria (in clinical study) a research term. The criteria that define who is eligible to participate in a clinical study.

inclusion cyst ⊃ fissural (inclusion) cyst.

incompatibility *n* **1.** refers to the bloods of donor and recipient in transfusion, when antigenic differences in the red cells result in reactions such as haemolysis or agglutination. Or the differences between the donor and recipient tissue types that causes transplanted tissues/organs to be rejected by the recipient's immune system. **2.** When two or more medicaments are given concurrently or consecutively they can attenuate or counteract the desired effect of each.

incompetence *n* inadequacy to perform a natural function, e.g. mitral valve regurgitation—**incompetent** *adj*.

incompetent lips a condition where the lips remain apart when the muscles of facial expression are relaxed and the mandible is in the rest position. Leads to mouth breathing and to various orthodontic and periodontal problems.

incomplete abortion ⊃ incomplete miscarriage.

incomplete fracture ⊃ fracture.

incomplete lesion a lesion in which there is a partial preservation of sensory and/or motor function found below the neurological level and includes the lowest sacral segment. With the advancement of acute intervention, more spinal injured patients are now presenting with incomplete lesions.

This is important to recognize as rehabilitation for incomplete and complete spinal injured patients takes a different approach.

incomplete lip seal ⊃ incompetent lips.

incomplete miscarriage part of the products of conception—fetus, placenta or membranes is retained in the uterus. ⊃ evacuation of retained products of conception.

incomplete overbite seen when the posterior teeth are in occlusion but the lower incisors do not occlude with the upper incisors or with the mucosa of the palate.

incongruous diplopia (*syn* paradoxical diplopia) diplopia present in individuals with abnormal retinal correspondence in which the relative positions of the two images differ from what would be expected on the basis of normal retinal correspondence. For example, a person with exotropia experiencing homonymous diplopia instead of heteronymous diplopia. ⊃ abnormal retinal correspondence, heteronymous diplopia, homonymous diplopia.

incongruous hemianopsia hemianopsia in which the defects in the two affected visual fields differ in one or more ways. A common cause of incongruous homonymous hemianopsia is a lesion of the optic tract. ⊃ congruous hemianopsia.

incontinence *n* inability to control the evacuation of urine or faeces. **1.** There are various types of urinary incontinence. *functional incontinence* with an erratic pattern of involuntary urinary incontinence. Caused by an impairment of physical or mental ability. It may be associated with cognitive problems, impaired mobility, sensory deficits and with an altered environment. *neurogenic, neurological incontinence* reflex incontinence occurs when the nerve supply to the bladder has been damaged by disease or injury, for example by multiple sclerosis, diabetes mellitus, surgery or spinal injuries. The presentation varies with the cause but may include an atonic or hypotonic bladder with overflow, reflex emptying of the full bladder or urge incontinence. ⊃ neurogenic bladder. *urge incontinence* (overactive bladder, detrusor instability) is caused by detrusor (bladder muscle) instability with unpredictable bladder contraction leading to urgency, frequency and involuntary leakage of urine on the way to the lavatory. It is the commonest cause of incontinence in older people. More common in females, because of the changes following childbirth, but also caused by having a weaker pelvic floor and a shorter urethra. May also occur in neurological conditions. *overflow incontinence* leaking or dribbling of urine from an overfull bladder. It occurs when there is an outflow obstruction such as with benign enlargement of the prostate gland in older men. *stress incontinence* occurs when the intra-abdominal pressure is raised as in coughing, giggling, laughing, sneezing and during physical exertion; there is usually some weakness of the urethral sphincter muscle coupled with anatomical stretching and displacement of the bladder neck. Stress incontinence generally affects women and is caused by bladder neck displacement due to a weakening of the pelvic floor, which follows childbirth, uterine prolapse and the climacteric. Men may have stress incontinence following prostate surgery. *mixed incontinence* a combination of urge and stress incontinence which is common in postmenopausal women. **2.** Faecal incontinence may involve involuntary defecation, lack of awareness of an urge to defecate or faecal soiling. It is commonly due to constipation with faecal impaction and leakage of liquid faeces, but may be caused by rectal prolapse, damage to the anal sphincter, neurological problems such as stroke or multiple sclerosis, episodes of infective diarrhoea, drugs causing diarrhoea and inflammatory bowel diseases. ⊃ encopresis, enuresis.

incoordinate uterine action failure of uterine polarity, resulting in weak, ineffectual contractions with delay in the first stage of labour and poor irregular cervical dilatation. Oxytocic drugs are used to coordinate rather than accelerate uterine action.

incoordination *n* inability to produce smooth, harmonious muscular movements.

increment an increase, an added amount.

incremental a variable increase in quantity. Additional small dose of a drug given at intervals.

incremental exercise exercise at gradually increasing intensity, usually achieved by stepwise increments at regular intervals, e.g. on a treadmill (incremental run) or cycle ergometer. Term may also be applied to the shuttle test, where the intervals inevitably decrease as speed increases. ⊃ Bruce protocol, shuttle test.

incremental growth lines of dentine the lines seen under the microscope to be running across the long axis of the dentinal tubules representing the rhythmic deposition of dentine matrix.

incremental growth lines of Von Ebner the microscopic lines seen in dentine, 20 μm apart, that represent 4- to 5-day increments in rhythmic growth of the tissue.

incubation *n* **1.** the period from entry of infection to the appearance of the first symptom. ⊃ latent period. **2.** the process of development, of an egg, of a bacterial culture.

incubator *n* **1.** an apparatus with controlled temperature and oxygen concentration used for preterm or sick babies. **2.** a low-temperature oven in which bacteria are cultured.

incus anvil-shaped bone of the middle ear. One of the ossicles, it transmits sound vibrations between the malleus and stapes. ⊃ malleus, stapes, Colour Section Figure 13.

incyclophoria ⊃ cyclophoria.

indentation the state of being notched. A pit or depression.

indentation tonometer ⊃ impression tonometer.

independence predominantly associated with the ability to do things for oneself, being self-supporting and self-reliant. In some cultures independence is also associated with life transitions, particularly the transition from childhood to adulthood. Independence is less valued in some cultures than others who may have a collectivist orientation. The meaning of independence in terms of 'doing things for oneself' has been increasingly challenged by people with disabilities on a number of grounds. The Disabled People's Movement views independence in terms of self-determination, control

and managing and organizing the assistance that is required. In a very real sense we are all dependent on each other for our survival so nobody is independent.

independence (occupational therapy) the condition of being able to perform everyday activities to a satisfactory level. (Reproduced with permission from the European Network of Occupational Therapy in Higher Education (ENOTHE) Terminology Project, 2008.)

independent component of nursing assessing, planning, setting goals and evaluating, in relation to problems which the patient is experiencing in everyday living activities which are amenable to nursing intervention; they may or may not be the product of the medical diagnosis.

independent living a set of ideas, sometimes referred to as a movement, developed by people with disabilities to establish their right to participate fully within society. The concept is broad and embraces the full range of human and civil rights. A key focus in the Independent Living Movement has been the availability of direct payments to buy services (Direct Payments Act 1996) and the employment of personal assistants rather than relying on statutory services. The philosophy of independent living is practised in centres of integrated (or independent) living (CILs), which are controlled by people with disabilities and which challenge the practice and philosophy of statutory services.

independent midwife self-employed midwife, either working alone or in a partnership, who contracts directly with the women for whom she cares. Practice must be contemporary, research-based and of the highest standard; the midwife is personally accountable for her practice, required to notify intention to practise to the supervisor of midwives in each of the areas in which she works, and is advised to have adequate indemnity insurance cover.

independent variable a research term. The variable which is changed (manipulated) so that its effects on the dependent variable can be seen.

index (dental) 1. method of recording the progress of a disease or condition by using established criteria. **2.** value expressing the ratio of one measurement to another. *calculus index* ⊃ oral hygiene index. *community periodontal index of treatment needs* (CPITN) World Health Organization (WHO) designated index in which a special ball ended probe is used to determine the severity of periodontal involvement and treatment need, usually in each of the sextants of the dentition. Identifies bleeding on probing, subgingival calculus, deficient restoration margins, extent of probing depth, furcation involvement and recession. Now also referred to as the basic periodontal index. *DDE index* developmental defects of enamel index. *Dean's index* used to measure dental fluorosis. *DEF index* a method of measuring caries experience. It is obtained by counting the decayed, extracted or filled teeth in the primary dentition. Missing teeth are not counted as it may be difficult to determine if they were exfoliated normally or extracted. *DEFS index* similar to DEF but filled *surfaces* rather than filled teeth are counted and added to the decayed and extracted score. *DMF index*

I
J

an index giving the total number of decayed, missing and filled permanent teeth. *DMFT/DMFS index* the decayed missing and filled components of primary teeth and primary teeth surfaces, used in dental epidemiology to measure caries prevalence and incidence. *gingival (Loe and Silness) index (GI)* the scoring depends on the severity of the condition and ranges from 0 for normal gingiva to 3 for gingiva showing severe inflammation with marked oedema, redness and ulceration. *index of tooth mobility (ITM)* tooth mobility is scored in four stages. 0—where there is no detectable mobility; 1—where there is barely discernable mobility; 2—where there is crown movement in any direction; 3—where there is crown movement in any direction including rotation and depression. *oral hygiene index (OHI)* a quantitative index for determining oral hygiene in population groups and individuals. Measurements are taken to determine the extent of debris, calculus and of plaque. *papillary bleeding index (PBI)* an index based on the bleeding resulting from the gentle probing of the interdental papilla. *periodontal disease (Ramfjord) index (PDI)* a quantitative index (now seldom used) of the periodontal state of individuals or groups. It is assessed by examining six teeth only and scoring the teeth into six grades ranging from health (0) to severe gingivitis with over 6 mm of crevice formation (6). *periodontal (Russell) index (PI)* an index (now seldom used) for assessing gingival and periodontal disease. The scoring is in six steps and ranges from 0 where there is no inflammation or loss of function and with normal radiographic appearance to 8 where there is advanced destruction of the supporting tissues, loss of masticatory function, drifting and looseness of the tooth and where there is radiographic evidence of bone loss in more than one-half of the length of the tooth root. *plaque (Silness and Loe) index* there are four criteria for scoring ranging from 0 (no plaque) to 3 where the interdental region is filled with debris and there is heavy accumulation of soft material filling the niche between the gingival margin and the tooth surface. *plaque score index* four or six surfaces of each tooth are examined for the presence or absence of plaque and the total score of surfaces expressed as a percentage. *PMA (Schour and Massler) index* this was probably the first numerical system for recording and evaluating the progress of periodontal disease. The abbreviation letters refer to the examination carried out of the Papillary, Marginal and Attached gingivae. *retention (Loe) index* this index evaluates the degree of plaque retention resulting from defective margins of restorations and from carious cavities. It is scored in four stages: 0—no caries, calculus or imperfect restorations in a gingival location, to 3—large cavity, abundant calculus and/or grossly infected margin. *Thylstrup Fejerskov index* used to measure dental fluorosis.

indexing term also called Medical Subject Headings (MESH or MeSH), thesaurus terms, subject headings or descriptors. The word assigned by a database producer to describe the content of a journal article. They are split into subject area and arranged in a hierarchy that moves from a broad subject area to increasing detail and specialism. ⊃ Allied and Complementary Medicine Database (AMED), biographical databases, Cumulative Index to Nursing and Allied Health Literature (CINHL), MEDLINE

Index Medicus (IM) a monthly bibliography of the principal worldwide biomedical literature produced by the MEDLINE system from the MEDLARS data base. It is cumulated annually into the Cumulated Index Medicus (CIM).

index myopia ⊃ lenticular myopia.

Index of Complexity of Orthodontic Need (ICON) an orthodontic index aimed to combine both treatment need and the complexity of treatment that would be required to correct a malocclusion.

Index of Orthodontic Treatment Need (IOTN) an orthodontic criteria for defining the need for treatment based on dental health and functional benefit. Categorized from 1–5 where 1 is minimum need and 5 is the greatest need.

index of refraction ⊃ refractive index.

index of tooth mobility (ITM) ⊃ index (dental).

Indian hemp ⊃ cannabis.

indican the chemical formed in the intestine from the breakdown of the amino acid tryptophan.

indicanuria *n* excess indican in the urine, associated with increased bacterial breakdown of tryptophan (an amino acid) in the bowel or with a high protein intake. ⊃ indole.

indication a substantial reason for prescribing a certain course of treatment, for instance surgery, medications or another therapy.

indicator *n* a substance used to make visible the completion of a chemical reaction or the achievement of a certain pH.

indicator lamps in radiography, situated on a control panel to give the status of equipment, for example, if the door of the treatment room is closed, or outside the room to indicate treatment is in progress.

indigenous *adj* of a disease, etc., native to a certain locality or country.

indigestion *n* (*syn* dyspepsia) a feeling of gastric discomfort, including fullness and gaseous distension, which is not necessarily a manifestation of disease.

indirect antiglobulin test (IAT) also known as indirect Coombs' test. It is used in the matching of blood products, prior to blood transfusion. ⊃ indirect Coombs' test.

indirect Coomb's test or indirect antiglobulin test (IAT). It is used to match blood products prior to transfusion in order to prevent problems with incompatibility. ⊃ indirect antiglobulin test (IAT).

indirect cost a cost that cannot be attributed to any one department and its budget. It is shared between various budgets, e.g. the cost of heating a building.

indirect ophthalmoscope an ophthalmoscope that provides an aerial image of the fundus (and not the fundus itself as with a direct ophthalmoscope) which is real, inverted, with a magnification of ×5 to ×7 and formed at approximately arm's length from the practitioner. This aerial image is usually produced by a strong positive lens ranging in power from

+13D to +30D that is held in front of the patient's eye. The practitioner views this aerial image through a sight hole with a focusing lens to compensate for ametropia and accommodation. This instrument provides a large field of view (25–40°) and allows easier examination of the periphery of the retina. This instrument has been supplanted by the binocular indirect ophthalmoscope. ⇒ binocular indirect ophthalmoscope, direct ophthalmoscope, ophthalmoscopy, scanning laser ophthalmoscope.

indirect pulp capping ⇒ pulp.

indirect retention ⇒ retention.

indirect technique in dentistry, a method of making a gold casting in which a wax pattern is obtained from a model of the tooth preparation and not directly from the preparation in the mouth.

indirect vision ⇒ peripheral vision.

individual zone of optimal functioning (IZOF) ⇒ zone of optimal functioning (ZOF).

indocyanine green angiography demonstration of the choroidal and retinal vessels using indocyanine green in the same way as with fluorescein. It provides better information about the state of the choroidal circulation, in particular the presence of abnormal new blood vessels (neovascularization).

indole *n* a product of the decomposition of the amino acid tryptophan in the intestines: it is excreted in urine as indican. ⇒ indicanuria.

indolent *adj* a term applied to a sluggish ulcer which is generally painless and slow to heal.

induced abortion ⇒ abortion.

induction *n* **1.** the act of bringing on or causing to occur, as applied to anaesthesia and labour. **2.** the derivation of rules and laws by generalizing from observations. Regarded by most 19th-century and earlier philosophers as the essence of scientific procedure, even though Hume had already, in the 18th century, pointed out that every generalization is logically liable to be invalidated by a contrary future observation. Modern thinking recognizes the subsequent development and testing of explanations for the collected observations as at least an equally crucial aspect of science. **3.** the production of an electromotive force in a conductor when it is moving relative to a magnetic field of changing intensity. ⇒ corroborating evidence, falsificationism, model.

induction of anaesthesia the initial stages in the administration of a general anaesthetic so that the patient passes smoothly from consciousness to unconsciousness.

induction of labour artificially starting labour with vaginal prostaglandins (pessaries, gels) such as dinoprostone, amniotomy or slow intravenous infusion of oxytocin (Syntocinon®). It is performed when fetal or maternal health is endangered e.g. poor fetal growth or well-being, maternal diabetes, hypertension, cardiac or renal disease, poor obstetric history, antepartum haemorrhage, breech presentation, postmaturity. If the cervix is assessed as favourable, i.e. a Bishop's score of 6 or more, induction is likely to succeed; scores of below 6 indicate caesarean section. ⇒ Bishop's score.

induration *n* the hardening of tissue, as in hyperaemia, infiltration by tumour, etc.—**indurated** *adj.*

industrial dermatitis a term used in the National Insurance (Industrial Injuries) Act to cover occupational skin conditions.

industrial disease (*syn* occupational disease) a disease contracted by reason of occupational exposure to an industrial agent known to be hazardous, e.g. dust, fumes, chemicals, irradiation, etc., the notification of, safety precautions against and compensation for which are controlled by law.

industrial hygiene (*syn* occupational health) includes all measures taken to preserve the individual's health whilst he or she is at work.

industrial therapy simulation of outside industrial working conditions within a psychiatric hospital. The main purpose is preparation for patient return to the community by occupational rehabilitation.

inelastic collisions the mutual attraction of atoms, molecules, etc. when either the energy from one particle is given to the other or only kinetic, excitation or ionization energy is transferred after the collision. ⇒ elastic collisions.

inequalities in health differences in the distribution of health associated with social class or poverty (as opposed to physiological processes: age, sex, constitution). A considerable body of evidence shows a clear relationship between poor health and deprivation (measured by income, level of education and type of employment or unemployment). Measures of inequality include differences in standardized mortality ratios, life expectancy, infant and maternal mortality rates. Low income individuals are more likely to die prematurely, suffer acute and chronic illnesses and experience long term disability.

inert lifeless. Having no chemical reactions.

inertia *n* inactivity. The reluctance of a body to start moving, or stop moving once it has started. ⇒ uterine inertia.

inertial force an imaginary force introduced to allow for analysis of the acceleration of bodies or objects from the point of view of an accelerating observer.

inertial movement motion without the need for a force. Often occurs when a body segment has been previously accelerated. Consequence of Newton's first law of motion. ⇒ ballistic movement.

inertial reference frame the use of a co-ordinate system (reference frame) that does not move (i.e. is fixed in space).

inevitable abortion ⇒ inevitable miscarriage.

inevitable miscarriage loss of the pregnancy cannot be prevented.

in extremis at the point of death.

infant *n* a child of less than 1 year old.

infanticide the killing of an infant, by its mother, in the first 12 months after the birth.

infantile cortical hyperostosis (Caffey's disease) a condition characterized by tender swellings of bone. Diagnosed radiographically.

infantile/juvenile glaucoma ⇒ congenital glaucoma.

infantile spasms a form of epilepsy that usually commences in the first year of life. It may be idiopathic or follow a variety of conditions that include hypoxia at birth, meningitis, hypoglycaemia. There is generally

I
J

a poor prognosis with learning disability, physical problems, or death.

infantilism child-like behaviour or physical characteristics that persist into adulthood.

infant mortality/death the death of an infant under the age of 12 months. The *infant mortality/death rate* is the number of deaths of infants aged under a year per 1000 live births in a specific area in a given time. Infant mortality is divided into neonatal deaths occurring in the first 28 days of life and postneonatal deaths. In developed countries most deaths occur in the first 28 days. Infant mortality rates are used as a measure of poverty and deprivation.

infarct *n* the localized area of tissue affected by anoxia caused when the end artery supplying it is occluded by atheroma, thrombosis or embolism, e.g. in myocardium or lung.

infarction *n* irreversible premature tissue death. Necrosis (death) of a section of tissue because the blood supply has been cut off. ➲ myocardial infarction, pulmonary infarction.

infection *n* the successful invasion, establishment and growth of micro-organisms on the body surfaces or in the tissues of the host, which result in a tissue reaction. It may be acute or chronic—**infectious** *adj*. ➲ autoinfection, cross infection, healthcare-associated infection, hospital-acquired (nosocomial) infection, opportunistic infection.

infection prevention and control policy the measures taken to reduce the risk of infection in all settings in which health care and social care are provided. These measures include policies that consider the level of infection risk and several specific areas. There should be policies for standard (universal) precautions, including general cleaning, handwashing and hand decontamination, use of personal protective equipment, and safe handling and disposal of sharps, such as needles. There should be policies covering the isolation of patients or residents, dealing with soiled linen and clinical waste, and the choice of cleaning agents, antiseptics and disinfectants. ➲ standard precautions.

infectious disease a disease caused by a specific, pathogenic micro-organism and capable of transmission to another individual by direct or indirect contact.

infectious mononucleosis (*syn* glandular fever) a contagious self-limiting disease caused by the Epstein–Barr virus (EBV). It mainly affects teenagers and young adults and is characterized by tiredness, headache, fever, sore throat, lymphadenopathy, splenomegaly and appearance of atypical lymphocytes resembling monocytes. Specific antibodies to EBV are present in the blood, as well as an abnormal antibody that forms the basis of the Paul–Bunnell test, which confirms a diagnosis of infectious mononucleosis.

infectious parotitis ➲ mumps.

infective *adj* infectious. Disease transmissible from one host to another. *infective hepatitis* ➲ hepatitis.

infective endocarditis (IE) previously known as acute, subacute or chronic bacterial endocarditis. Microbial infection affecting the heart lining or the heart valves. It is usually bacterial in origin, e.g. caused by *Staphylococcus aureus*, *Staphylococcus epidermidis*, *Streptococcus faecalis* and *Streptococcus viridans*. Rarely the causative organism is *Rickettsia*, *Chlamydia* or a fungus. IE may occur in people who have a diseased heart valve, after valve replacement, with congenital heart problems, patients with a central line or an intravenous cannula in place and people who inject illegal drugs. Infection from other parts of the body may also travel in the blood stream to affect the endocardium. Vegetations, comprising platelets, fibrin and micro-organisms, form on the heart valve or on the endocardium. These may break off and travel in the circulation as emboli to the brain and other sites.

infectivity the degree of infectiousness.

inferential statistics also known as inductive statistics. That which uses the observations of a sample to make a prediction about other samples, i.e. makes generalizations from the sample. ➲ descriptive statistics.

inferior *adj* lower; beneath.

inferior drawer test (sulcus test) a sulcus sign is established by pulling the patient's arm distally while relaxed. If the humeral head slides out of the glenoid an indentation will occur underneath the acromion. The sulcus sign is positive in patients with shoulder laxity (Figure I.3).

I.3 Inferior drawer test (sulcus test) (reproduced from Porter 2005 with permission).

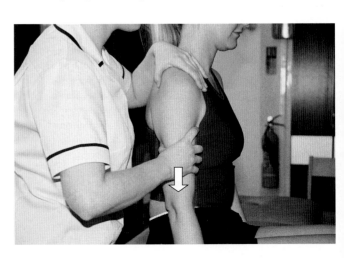

inferior colliculi (*syn* inferior corpora quadrigemina) two small rounded elevations situated on the dorsal aspect of the midbrain just below the two superior colliculi. They are relay centres for auditory fibres.

inferior corpora quadrigemina ➲ inferior colliculi.

inferiority complex feelings of being inadequate or inferior to other people. It may be unconscious but still influences behaviour. Individuals may act defensively or can compensate by displaying aggressive extrovert behaviour.

inferior longitudinal sinus a venous sinus within tentorium cerebelli which, with the superior longitudinal sinus, drains blood away from the brain; joins with great vein of Galen and straight sinus at the confluens sinuum, which tears easily if excess or rapid moulding of the fetal skull occurs, leading to tentorial tears and intracranial haemorrhage. ➲ fetal skull.

inferior nasal conchae each concha is a scroll-shaped bone, which forms part of the lateral wall of the nasal cavity and projects into it below the middle concha. ➲ ethmoid bone, nasal conchae.

inferior oblique muscle the extraocular muscle that moves the eyeball upwards and outwards; it is supplied by the oculomotor nerve (third cranial nerve). ➲ extraocular.

inferior ophthalmic vein a vein which commences as a plexus near the floor of the orbit, runs backward on the inferior rectus muscles and divides into two branches, one which runs to the pterygoid venous plexus and the other which joins the cavernous sinus, usually via the superior ophthalmic vein. The inferior ophthalmic vein receives tributaries from the lower and lateral ocular muscles, the conjunctiva, the lacrimal sac and the two inferior vortex veins.

inferior palpebral sulcus a furrow in the skin of the lower eyelid. It separates the tarsal from the orbital portion of the lid. It is often not very distinct although it becomes more so with age.

inferior rectus muscle the extraocular muscle that moves the eyeball downwards; it is supplied by the oculomotor nerve (third cranial nerve). ➲ extraocular.

inferior thyroid artery a branch from the thyrocervical trunk. It has several branches, one of which supplies blood to the posterior and inferior parts of the thyroid gland. It anastomoses with the superior thyroid artery.

inferior vena cava the major vein formed when right and left common iliac veins join at the level of the body of the 5th lumbar vertebra. This is the largest vein in the body and it conveys deoxygenated blood from all parts of the body below the diaphragm to the right atrium of the heart. It passes through the central tendon of the diaphragm at the level of the 8th thoracic vertebra.

inferosuperior radiograph a radiograph taken from below to above.

infertility *n* lack of ability to reproduce. Psychological and physical causes play their part. The problem can be with either or both partners. Specialist services exist for diagnosis, treatment and counselling. ➲ assisted conception.

infestation *n* the presence of animal parasites such as lice, threadworms or blood flukes such as *Schistosoma haematobium*—**infest** *vt*.

infibulation *n* ➲ circumcision.

infiltration *n* the entry into cells, tissues or organs of abnormal substances or cells, e.g. cancer cells, fat. Penetration of the surrounding tissues; the oozing or leaking of fluid into the tissues.

infiltration anaesthesia analgesia produced by infiltrating the tissues with a local anaesthetic.

infinity balance test ➲ Turville infinity balance test.

inflammation *n* a non-specific local defence mechanism initiated by tissue injury. The injury may be caused by trauma, micro-organisms, extremes of temperature and pH, ultraviolet (UV) radiation, or ionizing radiation. It is a process that enables the body's defensive and regenerative resources to be channelled into tissues which have suffered damage or are contaminated with abnormal material (such as invading micro-organisms). It also tends to limit the damaging effects of any contamination, to cleanse and remove foreign particles and damaged tissue debris, and allows healing processes to restore tissues towards normality. Fundamentally important for survival. It is characterized by the cardinal signs of heat (calor), redness (rubor), swelling (tumor), pain (dolor) and often with loss of function. Inflammation is one of the stages of wound healing. ➲ calor, dolor, inflammatory response, rubor, tumor.

inflammatory bowel disease (IBD) idiopathic intestinal inflammation. Commonly due to ulcerative colitis and Crohn's disease, but may also be due to lymphocytic and collagenous colitis. ➲ Crohn's disease, ulcerative colitis.

inflammatory chemical mediators chemicals released from blood cells and tissues that trigger many of the events of the inflammatory response. They include prostaglandins, histamine and kinins.

inflammatory exudate ➲ exudate.

inflammatory myopathies a disorder of muscle in which there is clinical and laboratory evidence of an inflammatory process. It is an acquired muscle disorder.

inflammatory response in acute inflammation it is the non-specific reaction of the immune system to protect the body against harmful substances or physical agents. It is one of the stages of wound healing. The inflammatory response leads to the tissue changes of inflammation, caused by inflammatory chemical mediators—vasodilatation, vascular changes whereby blood flow increases, vessel wall permeability increases with the exudation of fluid from the vessel into the tissue spaces, production of exudate, white blood cell migration (diapedesis) into the injured area for phagocytosis of micro-organisms and debris. ➲ inflammation.

influenza *n* a highly contagious acute viral infection of the nasopharynx and respiratory tract that occurs in epidemics or pandemics. The virus is spread by airbourne droplets. There are three main strains of the virus—A, B and C—which all belong to the *Orthomyxoviridae* a family of

RNA viruses. Influenza is characterized by the sudden onset of cough, headache, anorexia, myalgia and extreme lethargy and fatigue. Antiviral drugs, e.g. oseltamivir and zanamivir, are used for prophylaxis and treatment of influenza where they shorten the duration of symptoms. Complications such as pneumonia may lead to death, especially in the very young, older adults and individuals with chronic diseases including diabetes, heart and respiratory disease. An annual vaccination programme offers protection to older people (65 years and over); those with chronic conditions of the respiratory system, the heart, kidneys, diabetes and other debilitating conditions; people living in care/nursing homes; and healthcare workers and carers. Because the influenza virus changes (antigenic drift) over time a new vaccine is required each year—**influenzal** *adj*.

informal care care and assistance that is provided by unpaid carers (usually kin, but sometimes friends and neighbours) who have an emotional attachment to the person in need of assistance or a sense of obligation. Volunteers may also provide informal care.

informal patient a patient admitted to hospital without any statutory requirements. ⊃ detained patient.

informatics *n* information management and technology (IM&T). Information is needed to ensure the effective running of any organization. Data are pieces of material which, when compiled effectively, form information. Information is managed in a number of different ways but increasingly it is managed using technological means (information technology, IT). Non-technological means may be more appropriate for the target group/recipient. For example, telephone calls and notice boards are all ways in which information might be managed.

information processing in human brain function, the processes of cognition, including those to do with attention, perception, thinking, remembering, decision making and problem solving. Also parallel meanings in engineering

information theory a mathematical theory of the processing, storage and communication of information which is primarily concerned with the amount of information that needs to be conveyed in order to accurately reproduce or describe any given data.

informed choice in order to make decisions about their own care and management clients/patients need information from healthcare professionals. This means the provision of accurate, appropriate information about the person's condition, and about the treatment options available. Healthcare professionals may disagree with the patient/client's decisions, but the latter takes precedence where an adult patient is deemed to be mentally competent.

informed consent in the UK consent forms must include a signed declaration by the doctor or other healthcare professional that he or she has explained the nature and purpose of the operation or treatment to the patient or parent in non-technical terms. Any questions that the patient may have after signing the form should be referred to the doctor or other health professional who is to carry out the treatment. ⊃ consent.

infra- a prefix that means 'below', e.g. *infraorbital*.

infrabony pocket a periodontal pocket, the base of which lies below the margin of the surrounding alveolar bone. It is described according to whether it has one, two or three bony walls.

infrabulge ⊃ undercut (preferred term).

infradentale the most anterior point of the mandibular alveolar crest, situated between the lower central incisor teeth.

infra-occlusion where a tooth is below the level of the occlusal plane either due to supereruption of the adjacent teeth or due to ankylosis or other pathology preventing eruption of the tooth. ⊃ submergence.

infraorbital below the orbit.

infraorbital canal the bony canal running through the maxilla below the orbit. Conveying the infraorbital artery and the maxillary division of the trigeminal nerve carrying afferent nerve impulses from all of the upper teeth.

infraorbital foramen an opening situated on the facial aspect of the maxilla below the orbital cavity. The infraorbital artery exits from it and the afferent maxillary division of the trigeminal nerve enters it from the tissues around the nose, face and upper lip.

infraorbital pointer or indicator the part of a face-bow that records the infraorbital notch, thus aligning it with the Frankfort plane. ⊃ Frankfort plane.

infrapatellar fat pad lies deep to the patellar tendon and fills the space between the tibial condyles and the femur.

infrared optometer an optometer which uses infrared light rather than visible light. This is done so that the target used in the optometer is invisible to the patient. Otherwise when it is altered it tends to become a stimulus to accommodation. However, the instrument must be corrected for the chromatic aberration of the eye. Most modern optometers use infrared light. They are based on one of three principles: retinoscopy, Scheiner's experiment or ophthalmoscopy (indirect).

infrared radiation/rays (IRR) invisible long wavelength rays of the electromagnetic spectrum. Infrared radiation is a form of electromagnetic radiation, lying between visible light and microwaves. The wavelengths are between 760 nm and 1.0 mm and are subdivided into: near IRR (760–1500 nm) and far IRR (>1500 nm). There are both natural and artificial sources, though for therapeutic purposes, the artificial source is usual. It was previously widely used in therapy, but is much less common now. Infrared generators can be 'luminous' or 'non-luminous'. The spectral output of the non-luminous source is from 760 to 1500 nm (usually peaking at 4000 nm). The luminous generator tends to produce a shorter wavelength spectrum of IRR and also produces some visible emission. The emission spectrum is typically from 350 to 4000 nm (with a peak at 1000 nm). The red bulb (which is common) filters out short visible and any ultraviolet (UV) lights, therefore, the patient is exposed to IRR and red visible light. Near IRR (e.g. 1200 nm – luminous source) penetrates to dermis (few mm). Far IRR (>1200 nm – non-luminous source) can only penetrate superficial epidermis (1 mm or less).

The electromagnetic waves penetrate the tissues and are absorbed and as a result of the absorption, heat is generated in the tissues. The therapeutic effects of infrared include: pain relief, muscle relaxation and improved local blood flow.

infraspinatus a muscle crossing the shoulder. One of the four muscles comprising the rotator cuff. Its origin is on the scapula; it inserts on the greater tubercle of the humerus. It helps to stabilize the shoulder joint by holding the humeral head within the glenoid cavity and laterally rotates the humerus. ⊃ rotator cuff.

infravergence (*syn* deorsumvergence) the movement of one eye downward relative to the other. ⊃ supravergence, vergence.

infundibulum *n* any funnel-shaped passage, e.g. the ends of the uterine (fallopian) tubes—**infundibula** *pl*, **infundibular** *adj*.

infundibulum (uterine tube) the funnel-shaped fringed end of a uterine (fallopian) tube that is composed of many processes known as fimbrae. One fimbria is elongated to form the ovarian fimbria, which is attached to the ovary. ⊃ Colour Section Figure 17.

infusion *n* **1.** fluid flowing into the body either intravenously, or subcutaneously, or rectally. **2.** an aqueous solution containing the active principle of a drug.

infusion cholangiography the radiographic investigation of the biliary tract following the infusion of a radiographic contrast agent into the median cubital vein.

ingestion *n* **1.** taking food or drugs into the stomach. **2.** the means by which a phagocytic cell takes in material such as micro-organisms.

Ingram regimen a treatment for psoriasis using dithranol paste, tar baths and ultraviolet B radiation.

ingrowing toenail ⊃ onychocryptosis.

inguinal *adj* pertaining to the groin.

inguinal canal a tubular opening through the lower part of the anterior abdominal wall, parallel to and a little above the inguinal (Poupart's) ligament. In the male it contains the spermatic cord; in the female the uterine round ligaments.

inguinal hernia protrusion through the inguinal canal in the male. ⊃ hernia.

inguinal ligament Poupart's ligament (F Poupart, French physician, 1616–1708) a fibrous band running from the pubic bone to the anterior superior iliac spine. It is formed from the aponeurosis of the external oblique abdominal muscle.

INH *abbr* inhalation.

inhalation (INH) *n* **1.** the breathing in of air, or other vapour, etc. **2.** a medicinal substance which is inhaled, such as an inhalation anaesthetic or in the aerosols used for asthma treatment.

inhalation ('humidifier') fever characterized by self-limiting fever and breathlessness following exposure to organism-contaminated water from humidifiers or air-conditioning systems. An identical syndrome can also develop after disturbing an accumulation of mouldy hay, compost or mulch.

inhalation therapy the use of drugs administered via the respiratory tract. Commonly, bronchodilators (drugs used to open up the airways by relaxing the bronchial smooth muscle) are given via this method. In order to be taken into the lung the particle size is of extreme importance and should, ideally, be 5 μm in diameter (i.e. the thickness of a human hair) to ensure adequate pulmonary deposition. Particles larger than this will hit the upper respiratory tract while smaller particles will be exhaled.

inherent *adj* innate; inborn.

inherent filtration the filtration of the beam which is outside the operator control, for example, the target material, the glass envelope and the X-ray window of the X-ray tube.

inherent wedge a microprocessor controlled wedge used to attenuate part of the beam in radiotherapy treatment.

inherited connective tissue diseases ⊃ Ehlers–Danlos syndrome, homocystinuria, Marfan's syndrome.

inherited metabolic myopathies a large number of individually rare inherited disorders of the biochemical pathways necessary to maintain the supply of chemical energy (adenosine triphosphate, ATP) in muscles. It may present with muscle pain, weakness and fatigue. These are mostly recessively inherited deficiencies in the enzymes of the glycolytic and fatty acid metabolism pathways. Inherited disorders of the oxidative pathways of the respiratory chain in mitochondria cause a group of mitochondrial myopathies which may be associated with a range of other deficits in the nervous system, including episodic stroke-like events and myoclonic epilepsy. Many of these mitochondrial myopathies (or cytopathies) are inherited via the mitochondrial genome, down the maternal line. There is often a characteristic 'ragged-red fibre' change on muscle biopsy. ⊃ carnitine palmitoyltransferase (CPT) deficiency, chronic progressive external ophthalmoplegia (CPEO), Kearns–Sayre syndrome, McArdle's disease, mitochondrial myopathy encephalopathy lactic acidosis and stroke-like episodes (MELAS), myoclonic epilepsy with ragged red fibres (MERRF), Pompe's disease.

inhibin A a biochemical marker used in second trimester Down's syndrome screening. Affected pregnancies have increased levels, but this may be influenced by smoking. Inhibin A results are added to the three triple test biochemical markers to calculate risk of Down's syndrome, i.e. the quadruple test.

inhibins *npl* two glycoproteins—inhibin A and B. They are secreted by the ovaries and testes and inhibit the release of follicle stimulating hormone from the anterior pituitary gland. They also have a role in the production of the gametes (gametogenesis) and in the development of the embryo and fetus. Inhibin A is a biochemical marker for Down's syndrome screening. ⊃ activins.

inhibition *n* **1.** in physiology, the reduction of a physiological activity such as hormone secretion, or restraining the action of a cell, tissue or organ. **2.** in chemistry, the slowing or cessation of a chemical reaction. **3.** in psychology, the unconscious restraint of impulses or behaviour as a result of social and cultural influences. **4.** in psychology, the action of the superego to prevent the person expressing the

I
J

unconscious system of biologically determined instinctive drives and urges of the id.

inhibitor any substance that prevents or slows down the occurrence of a given process or chemical reaction, e.g. a metabolic process or the growth of bacteria.

inhibitory post synaptic potential (IPSP) a term that refers to the effect that is produced when excitatory input to a neuron causes brief hyperpolarization that spreads to the axon hillock. The balance between this and the excitatory post synaptic potential determines the final neuron output. ⊃ excitatory post synaptic potential.

inhomogeneities variations within a patient due to the different densities of bone, tissue and organs.

inhomogenicity the slight variation in uniformity of the static magnetic field in parts per million as a fractional deviation from the average value of the field.

initial assessment a process carried out at the start of an intervention of collecting and interpreting information on which to base decisions about intervention.

initial contact first touching of upper and lower teeth when the jaws are closed.

initial convergence the movement of the eyes from the physiological position of rest to the position of single binocular fixation of a distant object in the median plane and on the same level as the eyes. Initial convergence is triggered by the fixation reflex. ⊃ accommodative convergence, fusional convergence, physiological position of rest, tonic vergence.

initialize at the beginning of computation all variables are given specific values in the program.

initiator any substance that activates a given process or chemical reaction.

injected *adj* congested, with full vessels, as present in conjunctival inflammation.

injection *n* **1.** the act of introducing a fluid (under pressure) into the tissues (e.g. intradermal, intramuscularly, subcutaneously, submucosal), a vessel (e.g. intra-arterial, intravenous), cavity or hollow organ (epidural, intra-articular, intraosseous, intraperitoneal, intrapleural, intrathecal). ⊃ intraligamentary injection. **2.** the substance injected.

injection moulding a manufacturing process whereby a plastic material is forced into a mould cavity under pressure.

injection needle a hollow needle with a bevelled sharp end used to introduce fluid into the body. Produced in a variety of gauges and lengths.

injury any process causing physical damage. In sport *contact injuries* result from direct contact with another player or object (e.g. goalpost). These include fractures, ligament injuries, head and neck injuries. *overuse injuries* result from either an intrinsic cause, such as biomechanical problems, or an extrinsic cause such as the surface of the playing field. In sport, injuries to the lower limb are most common, especially to the knee. The incidence of injury in sport reflects the need for adequate, appropriately trained medical support.

injury scoring/severity scale (ISS) a system used to grade the severity of injuries sustained. Used during triage and to predict the outcomes following particular traumas.

inkjet printer a printer which sprays streams of quick-drying ink through very fine jets, building up the characters or images in very fine dots to produce an image on paper. Often a separate cartridge is used for each of the main ink colours, black, red, green and yellow.

inlay *n* in dentistry, a restoration made from composite, cast gold or porcelain to fit a prepared cavity, into which it is then cemented. Inlays can be prepared in two ways. By the *direct method* where the inlay pattern is prepared in the mouth using wax or by optical scanning of the preparation in the patient's tooth and by the *indirect technique* where an accurate impression of the prepared teeth is made, a model is poured and the resoration constructed in the laboratory on the prepared model.

inlay wax ⊃ casting wax.

inlay wax impression material ⊃ impression material.

innate *adj* inborn, dependent on genetic make-up.

inner cell mass the group of cells in the blastocyst cavity, from which the amniotic membrane and the fetus develops.

inner ear also called internal ear. The fluid-filled part of the ear that comprises the vestibule, cochlea (organ of hearing) and the semicircular canals which are concerned with balance. The cochlea and semicircular canals contain the nerve endings of the cochlear and vestibular branches of the vestibulocochlear or auditory nerve (eighth cranial).

innervation *n* the nerve supply to a part.

innervation ratio the term used to describe the ratio between the number of a motor neurons and the total number of skeletal muscle fibres. A small innervation ratio is present in muscles such as the eye muscles that need very fine control. Whereas, there is a large innervation ratio in the limb muscles. The innervation ratio increases with age as neurons die, this is one of the reasons for a loss of hand control in older people.

innocent *adj* benign; not malignant.

innominate *adj* unnamed. Applied to the hip bone formed from the ilium, ischium and pubis. Also the innominate artery and vein. ⊃ brachiocephalic (artery and vein), hip bone, innominate (hip) bone.

innominate (hip) bone each hip bone consists of three fused bones: the *ilium, ischium* and *pubis*. On its lateral surface there is a deep depression, the acetabulum, which forms the hip joint with the almost-spherical head of femur. The ilium is the upper flattened part of the bone and it presents the iliac crest, the anterior curve of which is called the anterior superior iliac spine. The ilium forms a synovial joint with the sacrum, the sacroiliac joint, a strong joint capable of absorbing the stresses of weight bearing and tends to become fibrosed in later life. The pubis is the anterior part of the bone and it articulates with the pubis of the other hip bone at a cartilaginous joint, the symphysis pubis. The ischium is the inferior and posterior part. The rough inferior projections of the ischia, the ischial tuberosities, bear the weight of the body when seated. The union of the three parts takes place in the acetabulum.

inoculation *n* **1.** the injection of substances, especially vaccine, into the body. **2.** introduction of micro-organisms into culture medium for propagation.

inorganic *adj* neither vegetable nor animal in origin. In chemistry, a compound generally containing no carbon or hydrogen.

inosine a nucleic acid derivative found naturally in brewer's yeast and organ meats. Not essential in the diet since the body can synthesize it from amino acids and glucose. Metabolically, takes part in formation of adenine, a component of adenosine triphosphate (ATP). It has been suggested that inosine supplementation might enhance exercise performance by increasing ATP supply but research studies have found no improvements. ➲ ergogenic aids

inosine monophosphate a purine nucleotide.

inositol a carbohydrate constituent of phospholipids (phosphatidyl inositols). Important in cell membrane structure and in the signalling mechanism for some hormones.

inositol triphosphate (IP$_3$) acts with other substances as a 'second messenger' molecule in cells.

inotropes *npl* substances, such as drugs, that have an effect on myocardial contractility. Those that decrease contractility are termed negative inotropes. ➲ beta (β)-adrenoceptor antagonists, calcium channel blockers (antagonists). Whereas those that increase contractility are positive inotropes. ➲ beta (β)-adrenoceptor agonists, glycosides. ➲ Appendix 5.

inotropic *adj* affecting the force of muscle contraction, applied particularly to cardiac muscle.

inquest *n* in England and Wales, a legal enquiry by a coroner into the cause of sudden or unexpected death.

inquiry-based learning (IBL) an approach to education which enables students to determine their own learning needs and seek the information they need. The approach is similar to problem-based learning (PBL), with the different term used by some educators and institutions to reflect the fact that some health professionals such as midwives mainly work with women who do not have problems.

INR *abbr* international normalized ratio.

insecticide *n* an agent which kills insects—**insecticidal** *adj*.

insemination *n* introduction of semen into the vagina, normally by sexual intercourse. *artificial insemination* instrumental injection of semen into the vagina. Using donor semen (AID), or semen from the woman's husband or partner (AIH).

insensible *adj* without sensation or consciousness. Too tiny or gradual to be noticed.

insensible perspiration ➲ perspiration.

insensible water loss the fluid lost from the body through the skin and during respiration. ➲ sensible perspiration.

insert the part of an X-ray tube which contains the anode, and cathode in a vacuum.

insertion *n* **1.** the act of setting or placing in. **2.** with reference to a skeletal muscle, the site of its attachment to bone which during its contraction is relatively mobile, compared to the site of its origin. For example, in elbow flexion contraction of the biceps moves the forearm (site of insertion) rather than the scapula (site of origin above the shoulder joint). **3.** in dentistry, the placing of an inlay into a tooth preparation or a prosthesis into the mouth.

insidious *adj* having an imperceptible commencement, as of a disease with a late manifestation of definite symptoms.

insight *n* ability to accept one's limitations while continuing to develop personally. In psychiatry means: (a) knowing that one is ill; (b) a developing knowledge of one's present attitudes and past experiences and the connection between them.

in situ in the normal position, undisturbed.

insomnia *n* sleeplessness. A chronic inability to get to sleep, or to stay asleep, or early waking.

inspiration *n* inhalation; breathing in. The phase of the breathing cycle when air is drawn into the lungs—**inspiratory** *adj*, **inspire** *vt*.

inspiratory capacity (IC) the maximum volume of air inspired following a normal expiration.

inspiratory muscles the muscles used during inspiration—the diaphragm and intercostal muscles.

inspissated *adj* thickened, as by evaporation or withdrawal of water, applied to sputum and culture media used in the laboratory.

instability term used to describe an excessive range of abnormal movements for which there is no muscular control (Maitland 2001). (Maitland GD 2001 Maitlands vertebral manipulation, 6th edn. Butterworth Heinemann, London.)

instantaneous acceleration acceleration measured over a very short (infinitesimal) period of time, effectively a continuous measurement of acceleration. ➲ acceleration, angular acceleration, gravitational acceleration, linear acceleration, tangential acceleration.

instantaneous velocity velocity of a body or object measured over a very short (infinitesimal) period of time: effectively a continuous measurement of velocity. ➲ angular velocity, linear velocity, tangential velocity, velocity.

instep *n* the arch of the foot on the dorsal surface.

instillation *n* insertion of drops into a cavity, e.g. conjunctival sac.

instinct *n* an inborn tendency to act in a certain way in a given situation, e.g. *maternal, paternal instinct* to protect children—**instinctive** *adj*, **instinctively** *adv*.

institutionalization *n* a condition of apathy resulting from lack of motivation characterizing patients, residents and staff in institutions who have been subjected to a rigid regimen with deprivation of choice and decision-making. The adverse social and psychological effects on individuals of residence in institutions, including long-stay hospitals for people with mental health problems or learning difficulties. The effects can include passivity, enforced dependency and depression. Small home settings, as well as large establishments, can create institutionalization if they are run rigidly with little regard for the needs of all those involved—patients, residents and staff.

instrument convergence ➲ proximal convergence.

instrumental activities of daily living (IADL) activities that are necessary for independent living.

insufflation *n* the blowing of air along a tube (pharyngo-tympanic, uterine) to establish patency. The blowing of powder into a body cavity.

insula *n* part of each cerebral hemisphere situated deep within the lateral sulcus.

insulator a substance which has a high resistance to the flow of electricity or heat.

insulin *n* a polypeptide hormone produced by the beta cells of the islets of Langerhans in the pancreas. Insulin secretion is regulated by the blood glucose level and it opposes the action of glucagon. Involved also in distribution, utilization and storage of protein and fat, as well as of carbohydrate, and in interconversion among them. Insulin secretion is stimulated by a rising blood glucose concentration and by the parasympathetic nervous system. It lowers blood glucose by promoting its transport into cells (notably muscle and fat cells) and diminishing its output from the liver, and it promotes formation of glycogen in liver and muscle. An absolute or relative lack of insulin results in hyperglycaemia (a high blood glucose) and glycosuria (the presence of glucose in the urine) with decreased utilization of carbohydrate and increased breakdown of fat and protein; a condition known as diabetes mellitus. Three types of insulin are available commercially: bovine insulin, porcine insulin and human insulin, produced using recombinant DNA techniques. Insulin is produced in U100 strength, i.e. 100 units per mL, a standardization that replaced the previous 20, 40 and 80 unit strengths available many years ago. Sporting activity by people with diabetics tends to reduce blood glucose, so good diabetic control with frequent blood sugar testing and adjustment of insulin dosage is important. ⊃ Appendix 5.

insulinase an enzyme that inactivates insulin.

insulin coma ⊃ hypoglycaemia.

insulin delivery devices preloaded insulin pens, reusable insulin pens and insulin dosers used by people to inject insulin as an alternative to syringe and needle (Figure I.4).

insulin dependent diabetes mellitus (IDDM) ⊃ diabetes mellitus type 1.

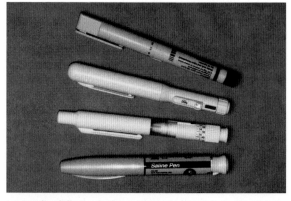

I.4 Insulin delivery devices—preloaded pens (reproduced from Brooker & Nicol 2003 with permission).

insulin-like growth factor (IGF) also called somatomedin. Two polypeptides, IGF 1 (somatomedin C) and IGF II (somatomedin A), similar in structure to insulin. They are involved in early fetal growth and later cell growth and development.

insulinoma *n* an insulin-secreting tumour of the pancreatic islet beta cells, usually benign. It causes hypoglycaemia. ⊃ islet cell tumours.

insulin resistance an alteration in the functioning of insulin-sensitive peripheral tissues. The body tissues do not respond to available insulin effectively and the pancreas produces more insulin. This results in hyperinsulinaemia (high level of insulin in the blood) and increased blood glucose, which often leads to type 2 diabetes. ⊃ metabolic syndrome.

insulin resistance syndrome ⊃ insulin resistance, metabolic syndrome.

insulin tolerance/stress test used to assess the hypothalamic-pituitary-adrenal axis and growth hormone deficiency. Intravenous soluble insulin is administered to produce hypoglycaemia (blood glucose <2.2 mmol/L) and serial blood samples are taken to measure glucose, growth hormone and cortisol levels.

Intacs the tradename of an intracorneal implant consisting of two tiny half ring segments which are inserted into the cornea to reshape its curvature and correct ametropia. The method is presently used to flatten the cornea by a given amount (the thicker the ring segments the flatter the cornea) in order to correct low myopia. It is an outpatient procedure carried out under local anaesthesia, takes less than half an hour and is reversible. The ring segments are made of clear biocompatible plastic inserted into the stroma and around the optical zone of the cornea. ⊃ LASIK.

integral dose the sum total of dose to all elements of irradiated tissue and represents the total absorbed energy.

integrated care pathway (ICP) the multidisciplinary outline of anticipated care, placed in an appropriate timeframe, designed so that patients with a specific condition, or pattern of symptoms, can move progressively through a clinical experience to a positive outcome. The pathway will include how a patient should be cared for and what should happen when and by whom. The best care pathways integrate input from all the health professionals to maximize effectiveness and are based on best available evidence and national guidelines, but applying these within the local resources and context. ICPs were initially introduced for patients having elective surgery, but now their use is widespread. Standards in the care pathways should be monitored and audited as part of a commitment to ongoing evaluation of clinical care. This is often undertaken by using a core document in which all health staff record their care.

integrated health enterprise (IHE) a consultation exercise between manufacturers and health professionals to ensure that computerization of the healthcare system achieves what the users require.

integrated medicine a term used to describe a harmonious integration of particular complementary therapies within conventional medical or other healthcare practice. Where teamwork and effective therapies (both allopathic and complementary) function together to promote health and well-being.

integrated services digital network (ISDN) a set of standards for the transfer of digital information over a telephone wire and other media.

integrated test two-stage Down's syndrome screening test. Maternal blood is assessed for pregnancy associated plasma protein-A (PAPP-A) and nuchal transparency ultrasound scan is performed. Later the triple or quadruple test is performed. The results of both stages are combined with the maternal age-related Down's syndrome risk for an overall result. The test is controversial, as parents are not informed of the results until the second stage is complete.

integration 1. in mathematics, the use of calculus to compute the cumulative addition of one variable with respect to another, displayed graphically as the area under the curve of one variable plotted against another; **2.** the summing of different types of information; **3.** in physiology, coherent function of interacting systems; **4.** in society, for example in health services or social services, the linking of different approaches or organizations.

integument *n* a covering, especially the skin.

intellect *n* the ability and power of the mind for reasoning, thinking, understanding and knowing, as contrasted with the willing and feeling faculty.

intellectualization *n* a mental defence mechanism whereby people attempt to detach themselves from painful emotions or difficult situations by dealing with the issues in an abstract, intellectual manner.

intelligence *n* inborn mental ability. Can be formally defined as that which is measured by standardized intelligence tests. Such testing, though still widely used, has been strongly criticized, in terms of objectivity, reliability and validity. There are different psychological models of intelligence, though they generally include verbal ability, problem solving and practical intelligence. More recently, the notion of emotional intelligence has emerged, which refers to the ability to interpret and use emotions in oneself and others. Intelligence, as an overall concept, has never been satisfactorily defined.

intelligence quotient (IQ) the ratio of mental age to chronological (actual) age.

intelligence tests various standardized tests designed to determine the level of intelligence. ⊃ Binet test, Stanford Binet Intelligence Scale, Wechsler Intelligence Scales.

intelligent peripheral a keypad linked to a computer that can act as a computer in its own right.

intensifying factor the ratio of the radiation exposure required to produce a density of 1.0 on a radiographic film without screens compared to the exposure required to produce a density of 1.0 with screens and using the same film.

intensifying screen a sheet of plastic coated with calcium tungstate crystals or rare earth material, positioned in contact with an unwrapped radiographic film in a cassette. X-rays striking the screen during exposure cause it to fluoresce and enhance the image on the film.

intensity the total energy of a beam of electromagnetic radiation per second at a given point. In ultrasound the intensity of the ultrasound beam is the energy flow rate per unit area in watts per square centimetre.

intensity modulated radiotherapy (IMRT) in radiotherapy, the use of a computer system to optimize the beam shape and profile to the target tissues by using multileaf, moving collimators and therefore maximizing the radiation delivery technique by evaluating millions of possible beam arrangements to create a clinically accurate treatment plan.

intensive therapy unit (ITU) a unit with augmented levels of specialist staff and equipment in which highly specialized monitoring, resuscitation and therapeutic techniques are used to support critically ill patients with actual or impending organ failure, particularly those needing mechanical ventilation. Also called intensive care unit. ⊃ high dependency unit.

intention ⊃ wound healing

intention to practice the statutory requirement of all UK registered midwives intending to practise. A designated form is completed annually or at any time when a midwife intends to provide midwifery care in a Health Authority other than her usual one.

intention-to-treat analysis ⊃ analysis by intention-to-treat.

intention tremor a tremor that occurs when the individual attempts voluntary movement, it becomes manifest as the hand approaches the target. Caused by a disorder of the nervous system, typically seen in disease affecting the cerebellum. It can be seen in patients with multiple sclerosis and this tremor is more incapacitating than a resting tremor (as seen in some patients with Parkinson's disease) as it interferes with function ⊃ tremor.

inter- a prefix that means 'between', e.g. *intercostal*.

interaction *n* when two or more things or people have a reciprocal influence on each other. ⊃ drug interaction.

interaction cross section the size of the area of the patient that lies in the field of the X-ray beam.

interactive effects an electrotherapy term. Applying two different electrophysical agents concurrently or sequentially may increase the risks to the patient. For example, applying ice or transcutaneous electrical nerve stimulation (TENS) or electrical stimulation over a region before or with ultrasound can reduce a patient's capacity to report if it becomes too hot and can lead to skin burns.

interactive sport a sport in which a player's performance or actions can directly affect the performance or actions of opposition players, such as tennis as opposed to golf.

interalveolar distance also known as interridge distance. The vertical distance between fixed points in the maxillary and the mandibular alveolar ridges at the vertical dimension of occlusion.

interarticular *adj* between joints. Within a joint, e.g. the intercondylar disc of the cartilage interposed between the

I
J

glenoid fossa and the mandibular condyle in the temporo-mandibular joint.

interatrial *adj* between the two atria of the heart.

interburst interval an electrotherapy term. The time during which no current flows following a burst or between successive bursts (continuous train of alternating pulses). ➲ alternating current, burst.

intercalated *adj* describes structures inserted between other structures. For example, the intercalated discs between the cardiac muscle cells, which link adjacent cells to form a sheet of muscle with no clear boundaries between cells. Thereby allowing the wave of contraction to pass easily across the myocardium, as it behaves like a single unit or syncytium.

intercellular *adj* between cells, such as the fluid around cells. ➲ interstitial fluid (tissue fluid).

interceptive orthodontics the method used in orthodontics to prevent malocclusion of the permanent (secondary) dentition. Generally applied during the mixed dentition period.

intercilium ➲ glabella.

intercondylar axis (dental) a hypothetical line joining the rotation centres of the condyles.

intercondylar disc an oval disc of fibrocartilage whose edges are fused with the capsular ligament of the temporo-mandibular joint, dividing the joint into an upper and a lower compartment.

intercostal *adj* between the ribs.

intercostal chest drain drains used to remove air or fluid from the pleural space enabling lung re-expansion to occur, e.g. post trauma, post operatively or after spontaneous pneumothorax. Such drains require an underwater seal drain, or in the case of a spontaneous pneumothorax a chest drain that incorporates a one way valve. The drain is used to allow restoration of the integrity of the pleural space. Suction may be applied to the drain where the air leak is brisk, but this should not be so high that it prevents the lung from sealing itself. Regular monitoring of such drains is required, with the amount, type and colour of drainage noted. Water in the tubing should fluctuate during breathing, while bubbles in the underwater seal during breathing or coughing would be indicative of an air leak (from the lung). The drains are removed when the fluid drainage and fluctuations have ceased and chest X-ray and breath sounds have returned to normal (indicating the lung is reinflated).

intercostal muscles a set of internal and external muscles. The secondary muscles of respiration situated between the ribs.

intercostal nerves the first eleven pairs of thoracic nerves (T1–11) that supply the intercostal muscles, the ribs and the overlaying skin. ➲ thoracic nerves.

intercourse *n* 1. human communication. 2. coitus.

intercurrent *adj* describes a second disease arising in a person already suffering from one disease.

intercuspal contact the contact between cusps of teeth in opposing jaws.

intercuspal occlusion also known as centric occlusion. ➲ centric occlusion, occlusion.

intercuspal position (ICP) position of the mandible when the teeth are in intercuspal occlusion.

intercuspation a condition in which the cusps of the teeth of both arches meet together.

interdental between the teeth. Situated between the approximal surfaces of adjacent teeth.

interdental brush a brush designed to remove plaque from the interdental spaces. Shaped somewhat like a small bottle brush and passed between the teeth.

interdental eyelet wiring a method of immobilizing the jaws by applying preformed eyelet wires to both the maxillary and the mandibular teeth. Intermaxillary tie wires are then passed through one eyelet in the maxilla and one in the mandible and the ends twisted tightly together, thus immobilizing the mandible against the maxilla.

interdental papilla the papilla of the gingiva situated in the interdental space.

interdental wire ➲ wiring.

interdental wood point or interdental stick hard- or softwood piece of stick used to displace food debris and plaque from the interdental spaces.

interdependence the condition of mutual dependence and influence between members of a social group. (Reproduced with permission from the European Network of Occupational Therapy in Higher Education (ENOTHE) Terminology Project, 2008.)

interdisciplinary team a type of team where health professionals and other workers meet regularly and work very closely together. There is considerable blurring of professional boundaries in order to deliver holistic and integrated care. Such teams tend to be relatively informal and are characterized by relationships of equality among members. Patients and clients should be considered central in such teams. ➲ intradisciplinary team, multidisciplinary team, teamwork.

interest the expectation that an activity will be engaging and/or pleasurable; the experience of feeling involved or committed while performing an activity.

interface the connection from the computer to other hardware, allowing free communication between the two.

interference *n* 1. in visual science, the modification of light intensity arising from the joint effects of two or more coherent trains of light waves superimposed at the same point in space and arriving at the same instant. ➲ coherent sources, holography, Young's experiment. 2. in psychology, a term that describes the contest between pieces of information that may prevent learning and retrieval from long term memory. It occurs when different pieces of information are linked to the same clue needed for retrieval.

interference filter (*syn* coloured filter) a coloured filter consisting of five layers, two outside glass, two intermediate evaporated metal films and one central evaporated layer of transparent material. These filters act not by absorption of light, but by destructive interference for all but a very narrow band of wavelengths which is transmitted.

interference fringes the alternate light and dark bands produced when two or more coherent rays of light are superimposed on a surface. ⟳ coherent sources, Fresnel's bi-prism, Young's experiment.

interferential therapy (IFT) an electrotherapy term. For 'true' or 'quadripolar' interferential therapy (IFT), two channels of alternating current are crossed, producing an amplitude modulated current in the subcutaneous area between the four electrodes. Alternatively, the current can be premodulated, so only one channel with two electrodes is required. Each burst of modulated current is called a 'beat'. While not as popular, research suggests premodulated IFT is as effective as true IFT used with large electrodes and has fewer risks and a considerably lower average current.

interferometer 1. an instrument designed to measure the wavelength of light, the refractive index of a medium, as well as the flatness, thickness, the quality of optical surfaces, etc. The interferometer is based on the phenomenon of interference between two coherent beams of light. **2.** the name given to several types of clinical maxwellian view systems used to measure visual acuity. ⟳ clinical maxwellian view system, wavelength.

interferons (IFNs) *npl* protein mediators that enhance cellular resistance to viruses. They are involved in the modulation of the immune response. Therapeutic use of interferon has caused regression of some cancers and is used in the management of some types of multiple sclerosis.

interim denture a dental prosthesis used for a short interval to check the design, the occlusion, the aesthetics or to condition the patient to accept an artificial substitute for natural teeth. The term is often used for an *immediate replacement denture*.

interlacing the construction of an image when an electron beam scans a tube phosphor, first the odd lines are scanned and then the even lines.

interleukins (ILs) *npl* large group of signalling molecules (cytokines). They are non-specific immune chemicals produced by various cells, such as macrophages. Interleukins are also involved, as growth factors, in the regulation of haemopoiesis. For example, interleukin-3 (IL-3) is a growth factor for myeloid and platelet precursors in the bone marrow.

interlobar *adj* between the lobes.

interlobular *adj* between the lobules.

interlock a safety device, for example, to protect the X-ray unit from overheating, to prevent exposure if the room door is open.

intermaxillary elastic band in orthodontics, a band applied between upper and lower dental arches to exert a pulling action when the mouth is opened.

intermaxillary fixation ⟳ fixation (dentistry/maxillofacial surgery).

intermaxillary space the space between the upper and lower jaws when the latter is in the rest position. Normally contains the teeth and the alveolar processes.

intermaxillary traction in orthodontics, treatment to produce movement of either or both dental arches, generally by means of elastic bands applied between brackets fixed to the teeth of opposing arches. Divided into three classes: *class 1* where a force is applied within the same arch to produce movement. *Class 2* where a force is applied from the posterior part of the mandibular arch to the anterior area of the maxillary arch to produce movement in one or both arches. *Class 3* where a force is applied from the anterior part of the mandibular arch to the posterior part of the maxillary arch.

intermediate care care provided after primary care and self-care, but before, instead of, or after that level of care available inside acute hospitals. Intermediate care includes preadmission assessment units, fast response specialist teams at home, multidisciplinary community assessment, rehabilitation and treatment teams, early and supported discharge schemes, intermediate care units/wards, day hospital and community hospitals. Often used for patients who are unable to manage at home and for those not quite ready to return home from acute care and require some form of rehabilitation. It is usually time limited (6 weeks). Its aim is to bridge the perceived gap between acute medical care and independence in the community.

intermediate host a host in which the parasite passes its larval or cystic stage.

intermenstrual *adj* between the menstrual periods.

intermittency during voiding the flow of urine 'stops and starts'—it is not continuous. May be associated with lower urinary tract pathology.

intermittent *adj* occurring at intervals.

intermittent claudication a condition characterized by severe pain in the legs (calves and thighs) and weakness brought on by exercise or walking. The symptoms disappear following a brief rest and the person is able to continue. Randomized clinical trials have shown that a graduated exercise programme will increase the distance walked before the symptoms are first felt. It is most often caused by atherosclerotic narrowing of the iliac and femoral arteries, often combined with lesions in distal arteries of the leg. More common in cigarette smokers and people with diabetes. ⟳ claudication, peripheral vascular disease.

intermittent peritoneal dialysis ⟳ dialysis.

intermittent pneumatic compression a stocking worn to prevent deep vein thrombosis of upper and lower limb. ⟳ phlebothrombosis.

intermittent positive pressure breathing (IPPB) a simple breathing device that responds to a spontaneous or timed trigger to deliver positive pressure to the airway throughout inspiration via a mask or mouthpiece. Its uses include delivery of bronchodilator inhaled drugs, reduction of the work of breathing and reinflation of atelectatic pulmonary areas through increases in functional residual lung capacity. The device can be used in conjunction with other therapies, such as positioning and thoracic expansion exercises.

intermittent positive pressure ventilation (IPPV) ventilation of the lungs by the intermittent application of gas under positive pressure to the airway. Used for the artificial maintenance of breathing during general anaesthesia and

I
J

397

for critically ill patients. Synonymous with artificial, assisted, controlled and mechanical ventilation.

intermittent self-catheterization (ISC) the intermittent insertion of a catheter, by the person or their carer, to drain urine from the bladder. The procedure is clean rather than one that uses aseptic technique and the catheter is removed once the bladder is empty. It is used by people who are unable to empty their bladder completely including those with spina bifida, multiple sclerosis, or following damage to the spinal cord. ⊃ self-catheterization.

internal *adj* inside.

internal conversion the transfer of energy from the nucleus of a heavy atom to an electron in the K shell.

internal ear ⊃ inner ear.

internal force force occurring inside an object or in the body, e.g. by the action of muscles.

internal haemorrhage (*syn* concealed haemorrhage) ⊃ concealed haemorrhage, haemorrhage.

internal haemorrhoids ⊃ haemorrhoids.

internal imagery ⊃ imagery.

internal jugular vein ⊃ jugular veins.

internal malleolus ⊃ malleolus.

internal market the simulation of market conditions within state services such as the NHS and social services. There is a separation between the purchaser and the provider of the services (the purchaser/provider split). Services are purchased on behalf of patients and clients by care managers and come from a variety of providers within the private, voluntary and statutory services. ⊃ mixed economy of welfare, purchaser/provider split.

internal (medial) rotation a limb or body movement where there is rotation towards the vertical axis of the body.

internal oblique muscle paired muscle of the anterior abdominal wall. ⊃ abdominal muscles.

internal (obstructive) hydrocephalus describes hydrocephalus where the excess of fluid is mainly in the ventricles of the brain. ⊃ hydrocephalus.

internal oppression oppression is internalized when those who experience it (for example, through injustice, discrimination, harassment) come to accept the views and beliefs of those who oppress them. Thus, the child with a learning disability who is treated as worthless comes to believe that he or she is worthless. Internal oppression is rarely complete and can often be dispelled if the individual is presented with alternative ideas.

internal or tissue respiration is the reverse process (to external respiration) involving gaseous exchange between the cells and blood. Oxygen moves from the blood, via the tissue fluid, to the cells, and waste cellular carbon dioxide moves into the blood for onward transport to the lungs. ⊃ external respiration.

internal os ⊃ os.

internal rotation movement at a joint which rotates the limb, or a part of a limb, inwards, e.g. rotation of the whole arm inwards at the shoulder or rotation of the forearm at the elbow, to bring the palm facing backwards; equivalent

movement possible to some extent at the hip but not at the knee. ⊃ external (lateral) rotation.

internal rotation of the fetus occurs in the second stage of labour, when the cervix is fully dilated, this is part of the mechanism performed by the fetus as it adapts to the changing shape and diameters of the birth canal.

internal scleral sulcus a slight, circular groove situated at the margin between the posterior surface of the cornea and the sclera. It contains the trabecular meshwork and the scleral venous sinus (canal of Schlemm). The posterior lip of the sulcus forms a projecting ridge called the scleral spur. ⊃ scleral spur.

internal secretions those produced by the endocrine glands; hormones.

internal skeletal fixation ⊃ fixation (dentistry/maxillofacial surgery)

internal version is turning the fetus by one hand in the uterus, and the other on the woman's abdomen. ⊃ version.

internal wire suspension a method of immobilizing the fractured facial skeleton by means of wires passing above the fractured area and threaded through the soft tissue into the mouth where they are connected to arch bars or splints.

internal work ⊃ work.

International Classification of Diseases (ICD) the 10th edition of the list of disease categories and related health problems produced by the World Health Organization.

International Classification of Functioning, Disability and Health (ICF) a classification used worldwide. It is a classification system of health and health-related domains that describe body functions and structures, activities and participation. Used for describing how people live with their health condition. The domains are classified from body, individual and societal perspectives and include a list of environmental factors. It can be used in clinical settings, health services or surveys at the individual or population level. It is the basis for defining, measuring and planning services for communities and individuals.

International Council of Nurses (ICN) at international level, the ICN, founded in 1899, represents worldwide national nurses' associations.

international normalized ratio (INR) it is the ratio of the patient's prothrombin time to an internationally recognized reference. Thus ensuring standardization of oral anticoagulation therapy. It is used only as a guide to oral anticoagulant drug dosage.

International Olympic Committee (IOC) the committee of elected representatives from member countries and sports, which oversees the running and sets the rules of the Olympic Games. The IOC has a Medical Commission, set up in 1966 to oversee doping control. This includes agreeing on the list of banned substances, administering the programme for testing athletes, and implementing appropriate sanctions.

International System of Units (SI) ⊃ Système International d'Unités, Appendix 2.

interosseous between bones.

internet a network of computers, accessible to anyone throughout the world who has access to a computer and a modem, giving access to the World Wide Web and electronic mail.

internet protocol address (IP address) a unique number given to any computer when it is connected to the Internet, it is formed by four blocks of three numbers.

internet service provider (ISP) a company that enables access to the internet.

interneuron connecting neurons in the central nervous system. For example, those in the spinal cord that connect sensory and motor neurons in a reflex arc.

interocclusal situated between opposing occlusal surfaces.

interocclusal clearance also known as freeway space. The space existing between the occlusal surfaces of the maxillary and mandibular teeth when the mandible is in the resting position.

interocclusal record record made of any occlusion position in order to transfer it to an articulator. May be retrusive, protrusive, lateral, intercuspal or initial cuspal contact. Generally obtained by using a warmed or softened occlusal wax wafer or a registration paste/material.

interosseous *adj* between bones.

interpalpebral fissure ⊃ palpebral apperture.

interpersonal skills the skills and capabilities required to engage with people in meaningful and appropriate communication.

interphalangeal *adj* between the phalanges.

interphase in cytology, the phase between two mitotic divisions during which the cell prepares for mitosis whilst performing its normal metabolic activities.

interpretive approach a research approach that incorporates the meaning and significance individuals attach to situations and behaviour. May be used in social science research.

interprofessional *adj* intense teamwork among practitioners from different healthcare professions focused on a common problem-solving purpose and requiring recognition of the core expertise and core knowledge of each profession and blending of common core skills to enable the team to act as an integrated whole. ⊃ multiprofessional.

interprofessional education (IPE) shared (or common) learning of common (or generic) core skills among students and qualified practitioners of different healthcare professions that fosters respect for each other's core knowledge and expertise, capitalizes on professional differences, and cultivates integrated teamwork to solve patients' problems.

interproximal between adjoining spaces such as those between teeth. ⊃ interproximal attrition, interproximal cavity, interproximal clearance, interproximal projection, interproximal space, interproximal stripping.

interproximal attrition the rubbing or wearing away of the proximal surfaces of adjacent teeth.

interproximal cavity (*syn* interstitial cavity) the cavity involving the mesial or distal surface of a tooth.

interproximal clearance the space between the proximal surfaces of two adjacent teeth.

interproximal projection also known as bite wing projection. A radiographic technique that demonstrates the crowns and the adjacent alveolar crests of maxillary and mandibular teeth. Primarily used in the diagnosis of interproximal caries. ⊃ bite wing (BW) radiograph.

interproximal space the triangular space between two adjacent teeth.

interproximal stripping an orthodontic technique to remove enamel from between adjacent teeth in order to provide space to allow alignment. Enamel removal is limited to the thickness of enamel and obviously limits the amount of space to be achieved using this technique.

interproximal surface ⊃ approximal surface.

interpulse interval an electrotherapy term. The time between separate pulses. A frequency of 50 Hz means there are 50 pulses/s with equal interpulse intervals between (except if catchlike current). For a pulsed current with a 50 Hz frequency and pulse duration of 300 µs, the combined interpulse intervals: $= 1\text{ s} - (50\text{ Hz} \times 300\text{ µs}) = 985\text{ ms}$. ⊃ pulsed current.

interpupillary distance (IPD, PD) (*syn* pupillary distance) the distance between the centres of the pupils of the eyes. It usually refers to the eyes fixating at distance, otherwise reference must be made to the fixation distance (e.g. near interpupillary distance). The average interpupillary distance for men is about 64 mm and for women about 62 mm (in Caucasians). The interpupillary distance is often measured from the median plane to the centre of the pupil of each eye. This is referred to as the monocular pupillary distance (MPD): it is a useful measurement, especially in dispensing progressive lenses. The interpupillary distance for near vision can be calculated using the following formula: near PD $= (\{d/d'\})$ distance PD where d is the distance between the target plane and the spectacle plane and d' the distance between the target plane and the midpoint between the centres of rotation of the eyes. ⊃ angle of convergence, metre angle, PD rule, progressive addition lens, pupillometer.

interpupillary line line joining the centre of the two orbits and is perpendicular to the median plane (midsagittal).

interpupillometer ⊃ pupillometer.

inter-radicular space the space between the roots of multi-rooted teeth.

inter-ridge distance ⊃ interalveolar distance.

interserosal *adj* between serous membrane, as in the pleural, peritoneal and pericardial cavities—**interserosally** *adv*.

intersexuality *n* the possession of both male and female characteristics.

interspinous *adj* between spinous processes, especially those of the vertebrae.

interstices *npl* small spaces.

interstitial *adj* situated in the interstices of a part; distributed through the connective structures. In anatomy, refers to the space separating the clinical crowns of adjacent and contiguous teeth.

interstitial caries ⊃ approximal caries.

interstitial cavity the cavity involving the mesial or distal surface of a tooth.

interstitial cells also called Leydig cells. Testicular cells that secrete androgen hormones, e.g. testosterone, when stimulated by interstitial cell stimulating hormone.

interstitial cell stimulating hormone (ICSH) (*syn* luteinizing hormone) a hormone released from the anterior lobe of the pituitary gland; causes production of testosterone in the male.

interstitial fluid (tissue fluid) the extracellular fluid situated in the spaces around cells.

interstitial keratitis (*syn* stromal interstitial keratitis) keratitis involving the stroma. It is characterized by deep vascularization of the cornea and is often associated with iridocyclitis. Formerly, the most common cause was congenital syphilis (syphilitic keratitis). However, nowadays it is usually the result of a herpes simplex infection, or it may be part of a syndrome (Cogan's) or other systemic diseases (e.g. leprosy, tuberculosis). Management involves cycloplegics, topical antiviral agents and in severe cases corticosteroids. ⊃ Hutchinson's sign, uveitis.

interstitial lamellae plates of bone filling the spaces between haversian systems.

interstitial lung disease (ILD) a categorization that refers to a number of lung conditions grouped together due to similarities in their clinical presentations, radiological and physiological features. The abnormalities are more consistent with changes in the interstitium rather than the airspaces. Within this category are a number of diseases with diverse causes, treatments and prognoses. Such diseases include those associated with occupational, allergic, soft tissue and idiopathic causes, e.g. asbestosis, rheumatoid lung. Sarcoidosis, drug-induced fibrosis, fibrosing alveolitis, etc. However, the usual impairment is that of a physiological restrictive deficit with reduced lung volumes (but a preserved spirometric forced expiratory ratio) and diffusing capacity for carbon monoxide. Clinical symptoms include worsening dyspnoea, cough, weight loss, lethargy, fever and arthralgia. Examination findings may include dyspnoea, digit clubbing, fine inspiratory crackles, cyanosis and rheumatoid arthritis, with death occurring as a result of a gradual deterioration terminating in respiratory failure over a 4/5 year period. However, prognosis can be varied from months to years. Management regimens (dependent upon the diagnosis of the specific interstitial lung disease) may include exposure avoidance, corticosteroids, cytotoxic agents, oxygen therapy, lung transplantation, immunization and pulmonary rehabilitation. ⊃ carbon monoxide diffusing capacity test (DLCO), spirometry.

interstitial portion (uterine tube) this portion of the uterine (fallopian) tube is 1.25 cm long and lies within the wall of the uterus. Its lumen is only 1 mm wide.

interstitial surface ⊃ approximal surface.

interstitial therapy brachytherapy where the sources are implanted directly into the affected tissue.

interstitial tubal pregnancy a pregnancy which has implanted in the narrowest part of the uterine (fallopian) tube.

intertrigo *n* superficial inflammation occurring in moist skin folds, such as under the breasts—**intertrigenous** *adj*.

intertrochanteric *adj* between trochanters such as those on the proximal femur.

interval cancer one that is discovered in the time interval between screening episodes, such as breast cancer detected between mammography examinations.

interval data measurement data with a numerical value, e.g. temperature, that has an arbitrary zero. The intervals between successive values are the same, e.g. a one degree increase from 38 to 39 is exactly the same as one from 39 to 40. ⊃ ratio data.

interval status when the numbers are ordinal and the steps between each number are of equal size.

interval training a type of training which increases aerobic endurance capacity by the use of repeating bouts of exercise with specific rest periods for recovery.

interventional radiology in radiology, the use of imaging techniques to facilitate therapeutic interventions, such as stent insertion to reopen a blood vessel or hollow structure, radiofrequency ablation, or embolization by inserting coils into an aneurysm.

interventricular *adj* between ventricles, as those of the brain or heart.

intervertebral *adj* between the vertebrae, as discs and foramina.

intervertebral disc the intervertebral disc forms a cartilaginous joint between the vertebral bodies, made up of the annulus fibrosis, nucleus pulposus and the cartilage end plates. Each disc has an inner spongy gelatinous substance (nucleus pulposus) surrounded by a protective ring of fibrocartilage (annulus fibrosus). Problems affecting the intervertebral discs are the most common cause of lumbar spine disorders. Intervertebral discs (referred to as the disc) are often described as shock absorbers, allowing load to be transmitted from one vertebra to the next, this is only part of their function. An equally important role of the disc is to permit controlled small-amplitude movements between the vertebra above and below it. Between two adjoining vertebrae, only small movements are possible (Figure I.5A). When added together, the result is a spinal column that is extremely mobile without sacrificing stability (Figure I.5B). The normal spine is self-stabilizing and for humans to stand erect takes very little muscle action, illustrated by the fact that persons who have spent prolonged periods in bed can sit upright with relative ease. ⊃ annulus fibrosus, disc herniation/protrusion, nucleus pulposus, prolapsed intervertebral disc.

intervillous between (chorionic) villi, the intervillous spaces allow maternal arterial blood to cascade round the terminal placental villi when gaseous exchange and transport of amino acids, glucose, minerals and vitamins take place.

intestinal absorption the transfer of the products of digestion, minerals and water (also drugs) from the intestine into the blood or lymph. Food products are absorbed from the small intestine, via its lining of enterocytes (where some

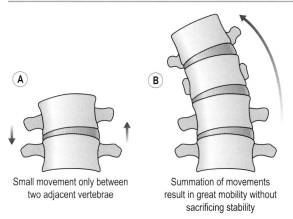

Small movement only between two adjacent vertebrae

Summation of movements result in great mobility without sacrificing stability

I.5 **Intervertebral disc movement** (A) Small movements only. (B) Summation of movements results in greater mobility (reproduced from Porter 2005 with permission).

further digestive processes take place); hexoses from carbohydrates, and amino acids and peptides from proteins, enter surrounding blood vessels, thence in the hepatic portal vein to the liver, which removes some before they reach the general circulation. Lipids enter lymph vessels and these 'lacteals' ('milky' with fat) join other lymph vessels to reach the thoracic duct, thence to the venous blood. Some water is absorbed from the small intestine, but most from the large intestine. ➲ villus.

intestinal colic abnormal peristaltic movement of an irritated gut, such as with gastroenteritis, lead poisoning (*painters' colic*) or dietary indiscretion. Colicky pain is also experienced in irritable bowel sydrome, intestinal obstruction, worm infestation, etc.

intestinal failure failure of the intestine to absorb adequate fluid and nutrients to sustain metabolic needs due to disease or resection. ➲ parenteral nutrition.

intestinal obstruction usually refers to a mechanical obstruction that prevents progress of the intestinal contents along the lumen of the intestine. The obstruction can be in the small or large intestine (colon). Causes include strangulated hernia, adhesions, intussusception, volvulus, stenosis caused by inflammatory bowel disease, foreign body, severe impaction of faeces, bowel cancers, or cancers outside the bowel. Paralytic ileus also prevents contents moving through the bowel, but in this case there is no mechanical blockage. Obstruction of the small intestine is characterized by vomiting and severe abdominal pain. Whereas obstruction in the colon tends to present with less pain, failure to pass faeces and flatus with abdominal distention, however, symptoms depend on the location of the blockage.

intestine *n* the part of the alimentary canal extending from the first part of the small intestine, the duodenum, to the anus. Consists of the small and large intestine (bowel)—**intestinal** *adj*. ➲ Colour Section Figure 18b.

intima *n* the internal coat of a blood vessel—**intimal** *adj*.

intolerance *n* the manifestation of various unusual reactions to particular substances such as nutrients or medications.

intoxication the condition of being poisoned by a toxic substance including the inebriation associated with an excess intake of alcohol.

intra- a prefix that means 'within', e.g. *intrathecal*.

intra-abdominal *adj* inside the abdomen.

intra-amniotic *adj* within or into the amniotic fluid.

intra-aortic *adj* within the aorta.

intra-aortic balloon pump (IABP) a counterpulsation device inserted into the aorta. It is used to increase cardiac output in ventricular failure that may follow myocardial infarction or shock.

intra-arterial *adj* within an artery—**intra-arterially** *adv*.

intra-articular *adj* within a joint, such as the anterior cruciate ligament of the knee.

intra-articular fractures fractures which involve the articular cartilage predispose the joint to osteoarthrosis in the future, e.g. fractures of the tibial plateau. This is due to the area of roughness that inevitably results after a fracture and also because the immobilization of the fracture results in cartilage death. Another problem with intra-articular fractures is that if callus is attempting to form within a joint cavity, it is constantly being washed away by synovial fluid, for example after a fractured neck of femur.

intrabronchial *adj* within a bronchus.

intracameral *adj* within a cavity, such as local anaesthetic drugs or antibiotics injected in the cavities of the eye.

intracanal within a canal.

intracanal medicament ➲ root canal dressing.

intracanalicular *adj* within a canaliculus.

intracapillary *adj* within a capillary.

intracapsular *adj* within a capsule, e.g. that of the lens or a joint. ➲ extracapsular *opp*.

intracapsular cataract extraction (ICCE) a surgical procedure for the removal of a crystalline lens affected by cataract. The entire lens, together with its capsule, is removed. A rarely performed procedure nowadays.

intracardiac *adj* within the heart.

intracaval *adj* within the vena cava—**intracavally** *adv*.

intracavitary therapy brachytherapy where the sources are arranged in a suitable applicator to irradiate the walls of a body cavity from the inside.

intracellular *adj* within cells.

intracellular fluid (ICF) that fluid inside the cells. In an adult with an ideal weight of 70 kg there will be around 28 L of ICF. ➲ extracellular *opp*.

intracerebral *adj* within the cerebrum, such as a haemorrhage.

intracerebral haemorrhage this usually results from rupture of a blood vessel within the brain parenchyma: a *primary intracerebral haemorrhage*. It may also occur in a patient with a subarachnoid haemorrhage if the artery ruptures into the brain substance as well as into the subarachnoid space. Haemorrhage frequently occurs into an area of brain infarction; if the volume of haemorrhage is large, this may be difficult to distinguish from primary intracerebral haemorrhage both clinically and radiologically. The risk factors and underlying causes of intracerebral haemorrhage include: (a) complex small vessel disease with disruption of vessel wall—age, high blood pressure; (b) amyloid angiopathy—familial (rare), age; (c) impaired blood coagulation—anticoagulant therapy, blood dyscrasia, thrombolytic therapy; (d) vascular anomaly—arteriovenous malformation, cavernous haemangioma; (e) substance misuse—alcohol, amphetamines, cocaine. The explosive entry of blood into the brain parenchyma causes immediate cessation of function in that area as neurons are structurally disrupted and white matter fibre tracts are split apart. The haemorrhage itself may expand over the first minutes or hours or it may be associated with a rim of cerebral oedema, which, along with the haematoma, acts like a mass lesion to cause progression of the neurological deficits. If big enough, this can cause shift of the intracranial contents, producing transtentorial coning and sometimes rapid death. If the patient survives, the haematoma is gradually absorbed, leaving a haemosiderin-lined slit in the brain parenchyma. ⇒ subarachnoid haemorrhage.

intracoronal within the crown of a tooth.

intracoronal attachment in dentistry, the precision attachment, one part of which (usually the female part) is embedded in a restoration.

intracoronal restoration a restoration lying within the confines of the crown of a restored tooth.

intracranial *adj* within the cranium (skull), such as a tumour or haemorrhage.

intracranial haemorrhage (ICH) any bleeding within the cranium (skull).

intracranial pressure (ICP) the pressure inside the rigid cranial cavity. It is maintained at a normal level by three compartments: brain tissue, blood and cerebrospinal fluid. The intracranial contents are incompressible, but they are interchangeable. While a change in any of these compartments can increase the pressure, e.g. after brain injury, the blood volume is the most rapidly and easily altered. The brain can compensate initially for a small increase in volume of one of the components but a continuing increase results in a rapid decompensation (i.e. where the brain cannot accommodate any more swelling), which untreated results in death. ⇒ cerebral perfusion pressure, coning, raised intracranial pressure.

intractable pain pain which is particulary difficult to control.

intracutaneous *adj* within the skin tissues— **intracutaneously** *adv*.

intracytoplasmic sperm injection (ICSI) a technique used in assisted conception where a single sperm is injected into an oocyte to achieve conception. ⇒ microsurgical epididymal sperm aspiration (MESA).

intradermal *adj* within the skin—**intradermally** *adv*.

intradisciplinary team a team consisting of members of the same profession who may have different levels and types of experience and expertise. Patients and clients should be considered central in such teams. ⇒ interdisciplinary team, multidisciplinary team, teamwork.

intradural *adj* inside the dura mater.

intraepidermal carcinoma (Bowen's disease) an intraepidermal carcinoma that usually presents as a slow-growing, red, scaly area with some resemblance to a plaque of psoriasis, on the lower leg of older females. Histology reveals full-thickness dysplasia. Lesions may occur at other sites, and occasionally develop into squamous cell carcinomas. They should probably be viewed as being at greater risk of transforming into squamous cell cancer than actinic keratoses. An initial incisional biopsy may be required and treatment is local destruction. Alternatively, the lesions may be managed with curettage and subsequent histology. Curettage, however, does not usually allow a squamous cell carcinoma to be positively diagnosed or excluded (because the tissue architecture is not preserved). Alternatives are cryotherapy or photodynamic therapy or imiquimod. ⇒ Colour Section Figure 79.

intrafusal fibres the bundle of fibres found within the muscle spindle; they are divided into nuclear bag and nuclear chain fibres. Invested with afferent (sensory) nerve endings and located so as to detect length changes in the main working (extrafusal) fibres of the muscle. ⇒ extrafusal fibres, gamma (γ)- motor neurons.

intragastric *adj* within the stomach.

intragluteal *adj* within the gluteal muscle of the buttock— **intragluteally** *adv*.

intrahepatic *adj* within the liver.

intrahepatic cholestasis obstruction to the flow of bile caused by blockage of the small bile ducts within the liver, such as in hepatitis or due to cirrhosis. ⇒ extrahepatic cholestasis.

intrahepatic cholestasis of pregnancy an idiopathic condition occurring in the second half of pregnancy. There is an accumulation of bile pigments and bile salts in maternal blood. It is thought to be due to changes in bile metabolism possibly due to inherited oestrogen hypersensitivity; geographical and environmental factors may also play a part. It is characterized by nocturnal pruritus without a rash, often starting in the extremities then becoming more general, insomia, fatigue, followed by mild jaundice about two weeks later persisting until delivery, dark urine, pale stools, abdominal pain, nausea and vomiting. Increased serum bile acid levels affect placental blood flow and fetal steroid metabolism; there is risk of preterm labour, fetal compromise, meconium staining and stillbirth. Treatment involves administration of antihistamines, vitamin K to prevent hypoprothrombinaemia and elective delivery after 35 weeks' gestation. Usually resolves spontaneously within 3–14 days of delivery but is likely to recur in subsequent pregnancies. ⇒ cholestasis.

intraligamentary injection in dentistry, an injection into the periodontal ligament, which produces instant analgesia.

intralobular *adj* within the lobule, e.g. vessels draining a hepatic lobule.

intraluminal *adj* within the lumen of a hollow tube-like structure—**intraluminally** *adv*.

intralymphatic *adj* within a lymphatic node or vessel.

intramaxillary elastic band in orthodontics, a band applied to orthodontic appliance in one arch only.

intramaxillary traction traction applied between groups of teeth situated in one dental arch only.

intramedullary (IM) *adj* within the bone marrow.

intramedullary fixation ⊃ fixation (dentistry/maxillofacial surgery).

intramedullary nailing intramedullary nailing has revolutionized management of long bone fractures. Here a hollow metal rod is introduced at one end of a long bone, travels down the medullary canal and may be locked with screws distally and proximally. The proximal aspect of the nail is threaded and this permits a tool to be threaded onto the nail at a later date for its removal. Intramedullary nailing for fractures of long bones has completely changed the management of many fractures, which up until a few years ago would have been managed by prolonged bed rest. The trauma is less than open techniques and results in decreased hospital in-patient stay, more rapid patient mobilization and rehabilitation with minimal risk of the complications associated with immobility. The implant rather than the bone may take stresses and strains and for this reason the surgeon may choose to remove the locking screws at a later stage. This permits the nail to move slightly and cause compaction of bone ends, this is known as dynamization. This allows the bone to once again take its normal stresses and strains and adapt in accordance with Wolff's law. Fractures of the shaft of tibia and humerus may also be nailed in this way. ⊃ Wolff's law.

intramenstrual pain uterine pain between menstrual periods; there may be an association with ovulation. ⊃ mittelschmerz.

intramural *adj* within the wall of a hollow tube or organ—**intramurally** *adv*.

intramuscular (IM) *adj* within a muscle, such a route for administration of medicines—**intramuscularly** *adv*.

intramuscular haematoma a collection of blood within a muscle. In sport this is usually the result of direct trauma, e.g. a direct blow to thigh or calf in contact sports or muscle tears in non-contact sports. Treatment is aimed at limitation of bleeding (rest, ice, compression and elevation). The collection of blood causes pain, related to either limitation of movement or the increase in pressure in the tissues. If local pressure compromises the circulation, surgery is required to relieve it and to prevent tissue necrosis by draining the haematoma. ⊃ compartment syndrome.

intranasal *adj* within the nasal cavity—**intranasally** *adv*.

intranatal *adj* ⊃ intrapartum—**intranatally** *adv*.

intranet a small local network of computers, for example, within an NHS Trust to allow limited access and enable the sharing of confidential files within the organization.

intraobserver variability a research term. The variability between the observations of the same observer on repeated occasions; for example, does the same physiotherapist give the same reading of knee flexion when goniometry is performed on more than one occasion?

intraocular *adj* within the globe of the eye.

intraocular lens (IOL) implant an artificial lens inserted into the eye following cataract surgery. There are many types including multifocal ones.

intraocular optic neuritis ⊃ optic neuritis.

intraocular pressure (IOP) the pressure within the eyeball occurring as a result of the constant formation of aqueous humour and its drainage through the trabecular meshwork and into the scleral venous sinus (canal of Schlemm) to be returned to the venous circulation. This is measured by means of a manometer. What is actually measured in the human eye is the ocular tension by means of a tonometer. This is an indirect measure of the intraocular pressure (IOP) as it depends on the thickness and rigidity of the tunics of the eye besides the IOP. Both terms, intraocular pressure and ocular pressure, are usually regarded as synonymous. Normal IOP is usually considered to be between 10 and 22 mmHg. However, there may be cases of glaucoma with lower IOP than 22 mmHg and there are also many normal cases with IOP greater than 22 mmHg. There is a slight increase in IOP with age (about 2 mmHg), in the morning as compared to the evening (about 3–4 mmHg), in the supine position as compared to the sitting position (about 3–4 mmHg), and a decrease during accommodation (about 4 mmHg). ⊃ differential intraocular pressure test, diurnal variations (intraocular pressure), glaucoma, Imbert–Fick law, iridectomy, ocular hypertension, ocular hypotonia, ocular rigidity, provocative test, scleral indentation, tonometer.

intraoperative probe a very small footprint, high-frequency ultrasound probe which is inserted into blood vessels to visualize their anatomy, for example, in cardiac procedures.

intraoperative radiotherapy radiotherapy that takes place during an operative procedure.

intraoral *adj* within the mouth, such as an intraoral appliance—**intraorally** *adv*.

intraoral anchorage the anchorage provided from within the mouth, i.e. by the teeth or other oral structures.

intraoral cassette a small cassette used with occlusal radiographic films, generally placed in the mouth. Used to reduce exposure time to X-rays by the presence of its intensifying screens.

intraoral radiograph a radiograph of a tooth, or teeth and surrounding tissues, when the film is placed inside the mouth during exposure. ⊃ periapical film.

intraoral tracing ⊃ tracing.

intraoral tube a small X-ray tube placed inside the patient's mouth when taking a panoramic dental radiograph.

intraorbital *adj* within the orbit.

intraosseous *adj* inside a bone.

intraosseous route a route for giving fluids and drugs when rapid establishment of vascular access is vital and it is not possible to gain venous access. It provides an alternative route for the administration of drugs and fluids until venous access can be achieved. The intraosseous route can safely be used to administer any intravenous drug or fluid required during a paediatric resuscitation. The onset of action and drug levels are comparable to those achieved when drugs are given

I
J

intravenously. During paediatric advanced life support it is recommended that intraosseous access should be established if reliable venous access cannot be achieved within three attempts or 90 seconds, whichever comes first. A wide-bore needle is inserted into the medullary cavity of a long bone, such as the flat anteromedial surface of the tibia in children under 6 years of age. In children under 6 years of age the marrow cavity is very large and there is less risk of injury to adjacent tissues. The main contraindication to this route is a fracture of the pelvis, or the extremity proximal to or of the chosen site.

intrapartum *adj* (*syn* intranatal) at the time of birth; during labour, as asphyxia, or infection.

intrapartum haemorrhage (IPH) excessive bleeding occurring during labour.

intraperitoneal *adj* within the peritoneal cavity—**intraperitoneally** *adv*.

intrapharyngeal *adj* within the pharynx—**intrapharyngeally** *adv*.

intraplacental *adj* within the placenta—**intraplacentally** *adv*.

intrapleural *adj* within the pleural cavity—**intrapleurally** *adv*.

intrapleural pressure (*syn* intrathoracic pressure) the negative pressure (relative to atmospheric pressure) in the intrapleural space. At the end of expiration, intrapleural pressure is about –0.5 kPa. The more the lungs are expanded, the greater their tendency to spring back to their relaxed volume. Consequently, intrapleural pressure becomes increasingly negative during inspiration. Intrapleural pressure is sometimes referred to as *intrathoracic pressure* since it is transmitted to all structures in the thorax including the heart. The negative pressure within the thorax assists venous return to the heart by exerting a slight 'sucking' force, sometimes called the *respiratory pump*. The force is increased during exercise when deeper breathing is accompanied by greater negative intrathoracic pressure.

intrapulmonary *adj* within the lungs, as intrapulmonary pressure.

intrapulmonary pressure the pressure within the lungs.

intrapulmonary receptors receptors within the lung that facilitate the regulation of breathing, e.g. juxtacapillary (J) receptors, which detect stretch.

intrapunitive *adj* self blaming.

intraretinal *adj* within the retina.

intraspinal *adj* within the spinal canal—**intraspinally** *adv*.

intrasplenic *adj* within the spleen.

intrasynovial *adj* within a synovial membrane or cavity—**intrasynovially** *adv*.

intrathecal *adj* within the meninges; into the subarachnoid space. A route used for the administration of certain drugs, such as some chemotherapy—**intrathecally** *adv*.

intrathoracic *adj* within the cavity of the thorax, such as pressures.

intrathoracic pressure ⊃ intrapleural pressure.

intratracheal *adj* within the trachea—**intratracheally** *adv*.

intratracheal intubation ⊃ endotracheal intubation.

intrauterine *adj* within the uterus.

intrauterine contraceptive device (IUCD, IUD) a device which is inserted in the cavity of the uterus to prevent conception. Its exact mode of action is not known. Some IUCDs contain a copper component, which increases their effectiveness. These can also be used for emergency contraception up to 5 days after unprotected intercourse. Other IUCDs contain the hormone progesterone and these are also used, in some cases, to manage menorrhagia or provide the progesterone component of hormone replacement therapy.

intrauterine growth restriction/retardation (IUGR) the impairment of fetal growth rate commonly arising due to placental insufficiency.

intrauterine insemination (IUI) an assisted conception technique in which prepared spermatozoa are introduced into the uterine cavity around the time of ovulation. It may be used if the man has a low sperm count. Or in cases where there is an incompatibility with the woman's cervical mucus or the presence of antibodies against sperm.

intrauterine transfer transfer of a pregnant woman to a maternity unit with facilities for neonatal intensive care, such as a woman in very preterm labour.

intrauterine transfusion ⊃ transfusion.

intravaginal *adj* within the vagina—**intravaginally** *adv*.

intravascular *adj* within the blood vessels—**intravascularly** *adv*.

intravenous (IV) *adj* within or into a vein—**intravenously** *adv*.

intravenous immunoglobulin (IVIG) immunoglobulin, mainly IgG, produced from the pooled donations of thousands of individuals, used as replacement therapy for patients with antibody deficiencies, or in higher doses as immunomodulatory therapy for a range of inflammatory and immune-mediated disorders.

intravenous infusion (IVI) commonly referred to as a 'drip': the closed administration of fluids from a containing vessel into a vein for such purposes as hydrating the body, correcting electrolyte imbalance or introducing nutrients.

intravenous injection the introduction of drugs, including anaesthetics, into a vein.

intravenous urogram (IVU) a radiographic demonstration of the urinary tract following the intravenous administration of a contrast agent. Formally known as an intravenous pyelogram. ⊃ urography.

intraventricular *adj* within a ventricle, especially a cerebral ventricle.

intraventricular haemorrhage (IVH) serious cerebral haemorrhage occurring in preterm infants below 34 weeks' gestation causing periods of apnoea and death. It is the most common lethal condition in very-low-birthweight infants. Diagnosis is by computed tomography or portable real-time ultrasound scanner.

intrinsic *adj* inherent or inside; from within; real; natural.

intrinsic detector efficiency the ability of a detector to produce a signal for each quanta of radiation falling on it.

intrinsic factor a protein released by gastric parietal cells, essential for the satisfactory absorption of vitamin B_{12} (the extrinsic factor) in the ileum.

intrinsic motivation the drive to be active for its own sake; to take pleasure in activity and in exercising one's capacities. ➲ motivation (in sport).

intrinsic motivation (in sport) ➲ motivation.

intrinsic semiconductors semiconductors that are chemically pure and have a perfect regulation of atoms in the crystal lattice. ➲ extrinsic semiconductors.

intrinsic sugars sugars found in the cell walls of foods originating from plants.

intrinsic thromboplastin ➲ thromboplastin.

intro- a prefix that means 'inward', e.g. *introversion*.

introitus *n* any opening in the body; an entrance to a cavity, particularly the vagina.

introjection *n* the unconscious incorporation of external ideas into one's mind.

intron *n* a sequence of non-coding DNA situated between the exons. ➲ exon.

introspection *n* study of one's own mental processes. May be associated in an exaggerated form in schizophrenia and other serious mental health disorders.

introversion *n* **1.** a personality trait characterized by a focus on one's own inner world rather than the outside world and a tendency to be reserved and to avoid social situations. Thoughts and interests are directed inwards to the world of ideas. **2.** a situation where a hollow structure turns in on itself (invaginates).

introvert *n* a person whose interests and behaviour patterns are directed inwards to the self. ➲ extrovert *opp*.

intubation *n* placing of a tube into a hollow organ. Commonly used in connection with tracheal intubation employed during general anaesthesia or mechanical ventilation. ➲ duodenal intubation, endotracheal tube.

intussusception *n* a condition in which one part of the bowel invaginates (telescopes) into the adjoining distal segment of bowel (Figure I.6). It causes severe colic, vomiting and the passage of blood and mucus rectally ('redcurrant jelly' stools) and intestinal obstruction. It occurs most commonly in infants around the time of weaning. It presents as an acute condition and requires emergency treatment. The intussusception is usually reduced hydrostatically

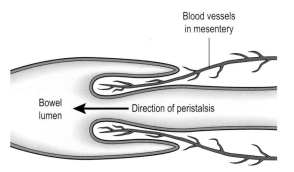

I.6 Intussusception (reproduced from Brooker 2006A with permission).

using a barium enema, but surgical intervention is sometimes required.

intussusceptum *n* the invaginated portion of an intussusception.

intussuscipiens *n* the receiving portion of an intussusception.

inulin *n* a soluble but undigested non-starch polysaccharide present in root vegetables. It is a fructose polymer. Because it is filtered by the kidney but neither reabsorbed nor secreted by the nephron it can be used in a clearance test to assess the glomerular filtration rate. ➲ clearance, creatinine.

inunction **1.** a drug in an oily base which is rubbed into the skin to be absorbed. **2.** the act of rubbing such an agent into the skin.

invagination *n* the act or condition of being ensheathed; a pushing inward, forming a pouch—**invaginate** *vt*.

invasion *n* the entry of bacteria into the body or the spread of cancer cells.

invasive having a tendency to spread and invade nearby tissues.

invasive mole a molar pregnancy that has invaded the myometrium (uterine muscle layer). Affected women will need chemotherapy and regular follow up in order to detect recurrence by monitoring the level of human chorionic gonadotrophin (hCG) in urine and blood ➲ choriocarcinoma, molar pregnancy, placental site trophoblastic tumour.

inverse bevel incision an incision made in periodontal procedures to raise a flap of gingiva from the underlying alveolus.

inverse care law states that those who are most at risk of acquiring illness and disease are least likely to receive medical and social services. This is due to a wide variety of factors relating to social inequalities and the availability of services.

inverse dynamics the calculation of forces and moments by using kinematics and data for mass and moment of inertia, effectively using Newton's second law of motion (f = ma) in reverse.

inverse square law the intensity of radiation from a small isotropic source is inversely proportional to the square of the distance from the source, used in radiography for calculating the dose rate and exposure factors when changing the focus film distance.

inverse piezoelectric effect when an electric current is applied to a material it expands and contracts producing an ultrasound pulse.

inverse treatment planning computer software to determine optimal isodose contours and maximum tumour dose for a given radiotherapy treatment, used in intensity modulated radiotherapy.

inversion *n* **1.** turning inside out, as inversion of the uterus. A rare partial or complete turning inside out of the uterus. This can occur if the third stage of labour is mismanaged. ➲ acute inversion of the uterus, procidentia. **2.** with reference to the foot: turning the sole inwards (medially).

eversion *opp*. **3.** a mutation caused by a segment of chromosome breaking off and reattaching to the chromosome in an inverted position.

inversion injury a common injury to the ankle joint in sport. Inversion of the foot usually occurs as a result of 'going over' on the ankle when the foot strikes the ground, especially if uneven or if the person is off balance. Results in damage to the lateral ligament complex, with bleeding, swelling and pain. Importantly affects proprioception and thus balance, necessitating a formal treatment and rehabilitation programme. ⊃ anterior talofibular ligament.

inversion recovery in magnetic resonance imaging (MRI) it is the basic pulse sequence which inverts the magnetization and measures the time taken for the nuclei to return to equilibrium. The rate of recovery depends on the relaxation rate (T_1).

inversion time (TI) in magnetic resonance imaging (MRI) it is the time after the middle of a 180° radiofrequency inverting pulse and the inversion recovery sequence to the middle of the 90° read pulse, and monitors the amount of longitudinal magnetization.

invert sugar glucose and fructose mixture produced by hydrolysis of sucrose. It is sweeter than sucrose. So called because the process inverts the optical rotation.

invertase sucrase the enzyme that converts sucrose to glucose and fructose.

inverted L osteotomy a surgical procedure carried out to correct prognathism or retrognathism.

inverted-U hypothesis the proposition that performance on a task progressively improves with increases in arousal up to an optimum point, beyond which further increases in arousal lead to progressive decrements in performance. For example, in sport optimal performance is held to occur at a moderate level of arousal. Also known as the Yerkes–Dodson law.

invest 1. to wrap around or envelop. **2.** in dentistry, to embed in an investment material. ⊃ investing.

investigator bias a research term. Occurs when the interviewer is aware (not blinded) of the outcome variable. An unblinded interviewer may be more vigorous in searching for the exposure of interest.

investing in dentistry, the process of investing an object such as a wax inlay pattern in a refractory investment material prior to casting. Prostheses in the wax stage are invested in plaster of Paris in metal flasks. *vacuum investing* technique in which investment material is subjected to a vacuum before, and in some cases during, the time that it is being poured into a casting ring so removing air bubbles from the mixture.

investment cast ⊃ cast.

in vitro in glass, as in a test tube.

in vitro fertilization (IVF) an assisted conception technique offered by clinics licensed to undertake the technique. Human oocytes are collected following hormone stimulation and are fertilized by spermatozoa in the laboratory. Not all oocytes will fertilize but after a period of incubation a specified number of early embryos are introduced into the uterine cavity where hopefully they will implant into the hormone-primed endometrium. The oocytes and spermatozoa may be those of the couple concerned, or either or both may come from donors. ⊃ Human Fertilisation and Embryology Authority (HFEA).

in vivo in living tissue.

involucrum *n* a sheath of new bone, which forms around necrosed bone, in such conditions as osteomyelitis. ⊃ cloaca.

involuntary *adj* independent of the will, as muscle of the thoracic and abdominal organs.

involuntary eye movements ⊃ fixation movements.

involution *n* the normal shrinkage of an organ after completing its function, e.g. uterus after labour. Or the progressive decline occurring after midlife when tissues and organs reduce in size and functional ability declines. ⊃ subinvolution—**involutional** *adj*.

IOC *abbr* International Olympic Committee.

iodine (I) *n* an element necessary in the diet (as iodides); required for the formation of thyroid hormones (T_3, T_4). Oral iodine may be prescribed preoperatively for patients with hyperthyroidism to control the release of thyroid hormones and reduce vascularity of the gland. Deficiency causes hypothyroidism. Radioactive isotopes of iodine, e.g. iodine-131 (^{131}I), are used in the diagnosis and treatment of thyroid conditions, such as cancer. Iodine is bactericidal and is used as povidone iodine for skin disinfection prior to invasive procedures. It is used within several proprietary wound dressings.

iodine seeds a source of iodine-125 (^{125}I) used to treat the pituitary gland by permanently implanting the seeds and as surface applicators to treat the cornea.

iodism *n* poisoning by iodine or iodides; presentation is similar to a common cold and the appearance of a rash.

IOFB *abbr* intraocular foreign body.

IOL *abbr* intraocular lens.

ion *n* an atom or radical with an electrical charge—**ionic** *adj*. ⊃ anion, cation.

ion channel water-filled channels in the cell membrane that allow certain ions to pass through as in the transmission of nerve impulses. Some drugs act at the level of the ion channels.

ion-exchange resins substances administered orally to reduce the level of specific ions (e.g. calcium, sodium and potassium) in the body such as may occur in renal failure. For example polystyrene suphonate resins used to reduce mild or moderate hyperkalaemia. Anion-exchange resins, such as colestyramine are used to reduce LDL-cholesterol in people with hypercholesterolaemia.

ionic bond when one or more electrons move from one atom to another and then form ions which are attracted to each other as they have an opposite charge, after the electron exchange the shells in each ion appear to be intact.

ionization *n* the dissociation of a substance in solution into ions.

ionization chamber a device, containing air for measuring the potential dosage of a beam of radiation by collecting charge on an electrode. *thimble ionization chamber* a modification to enable the device to be used practically, it is smaller in size and uses an air equivalent medium in the capsule. Used in radiotherapy planning to record the output of the X-ray tube.

ionizing radiation form of radiation that destabilizes an atom, forming an ion. Examples include gamma rays, X-rays and particle radiation. It has the ability to cause tissue damage and genetic mutations. ⊃ radiation.

ionophore *n* a molecule that facilitates the movement of ions across the lipid bilayer of the cell membrane. Some act as carrier molecules whereas others form ion channels or pores.

iontophoresis *n* an electrotherapy term. The introduction of various ions into the tissues by using a direct current. Pilocarpine is introduced into the skin by this method in order to do a sweat test for the diagnosis of cystic fibrosis. Other medications administered by this means include corticosteroids, anti-inflammatory drugs and local anaesthetics. The ionized medication is placed under the electrode (cathode or anode) with the same charge. The repulsion between like charges forces the ions through the skin directly to the area being treated.

IOP *abbr* intraocular pressure.

IORT *abbr* intraoperative radiotherapy.

IOTN *abbr* index of orthodontic treatment need.

IP₃ *abbr* inositol triphosphate.

IP address *abbr* Internet Protocol address.

IPD *abbr* interpupillary distance.

IPE *abbr* interprofessional education.

ipecacuanha *n* dried root from South America. Used in some expectorants. It is sometimes used as an emetic after poisoning but may have limited value.

IPF *abbr* idiopathic pulmonary fibrosis.

IPH *abbr* intrapartum haemorrhage.

IPPB *abbr* intermittent positive pressure breathing.

IPPV *abbr* intermittent positive pressure ventilation.

ipsilateral *adj* on the same side—**ipsilaterally** *adv*. ⊃ contralateral, homolateral.

IPSP *abbr* inhibitory post synaptic potential.

IQ *abbr* intelligence quotient.

iridectomy *n* excision of a part of the iris. The main reasons for iridectomy are to reduce the intraocular pressure in some types of glaucoma by improving drainage of aqueous humour, to enlarge an abnormally small pupil and, in cataract extraction, to prevent possible blockage of the angle of the anterior chamber. Nowadays, laser iridotomy is preferred in the treatment of angle-closure glaucoma because the incision obtained by this technique can be carried out as an outpatient procedure with only topical anaesthesia, although the cornea must not be hazy. ⊃ angle-closure glaucoma, intraocular pressure, iridotomy, iris, laser, phacoemulsification, plateau iris.

iridencleisis surgical technique previously used to reduce intraocular pressure in glaucoma.

irideremia absence of all or part of the iris. Strictly speaking a total absence of the iris is called aniridia. ⊃ aniridia.

iridiagnosis ⊃ iridodiagnosis.

iridium-192 (**¹⁹²Ir**) *n* a radioactive element used in brachytherapy to treat cancers in anus, tongue, breast as implanted wires or hair pins. Can also be used as a Selectron source.

iridium wire a source of iridium-192 used in manual afterloading systems and is purchased by specifying the activity per unit length required.

iridocele ⊃ prolapse of the iris.

iridocorneal angle ⊃ angle of the anterior chamber.

iridocorneal endothelial (ICE) syndrome a syndrome involving the proliferation of corneal endothelium, iris nodules, atrophy of the iris and synechia resulting in secondary glaucoma.

iridocyclitis *n* inflammation of the iris and ciliary body.

iridodiagnosis (*syn* iridiagnosis) the diagnosis of systemic diseases through observation of changes in form and colour of the iris. The validity of this method is questionable. ⊃ iridology.

iridodialysis *n* a separation of the iris from its ciliary body attachment.

iridodonesis *syn* tremulous iris. A tremulous condition of the iris. It usually occurs in aphakic eyes or when the lens is subluxated. ⊃ aphakia, luxation of the lens.

iridology the study of the iris (colour, shape, etc.), normal and abnormal. ⊃ iridodiagnosis.

iridoplegia paralysis of the muscle of the iris. It may be due to the instillation of drugs used to dilate the pupil, or inflammation or injury of the eye. ⊃ cycloplegia

iridoschisis a condition in which the anterior stroma of the iris atrophies and separates from the posterior layer. It mostly affects the inferior iris in older patients. In advanced cases the ruptured anterior fibres float in the aqueous humour. It often accompanies angle-closure glaucoma.

iridotomy *n* an incision into the iris; usually performed using a laser. The creation of an opening in the iris to allow aqueous humour to flow from the posterior to the anterior chamber and onward into the scleral venous sinus (canal of Schlemm). It is commonly performed with a neodymium-yag or argon laser in angle-closure glaucoma, especially that caused by pupillary block. ⊃ angle-closure glaucoma, iridectomy, pupillary block.

iris *n* part of the uveal tract. The anterior part of the vascular tunic of the eye, which is situated in front of the crystalline lens and behind the cornea. It has the shape of a circular membrane with a perforation in the centre (the pupil) and is attached peripherally to the ciliary body. The iris forms a curtain dividing the space between the cornea and the lens into the anterior and posterior chambers of the eye. The anterior surface of the iris is divided into two portions: the largest peripheral ciliary zone and the inner pupillary zone. The two zones are separated by a zigzag line, the collarette. The iris consists of four layers which are, starting in the front: (1) the layer of fibrocytes and melanocytes; (2) the stroma in which are embedded the following structures: (i) the sphincter pupillae muscle which constricts the pupil and is supplied mainly by parasympathetic fibres via the third cranial nerve, (ii) the vessels which form the bulk of the iris and, (iii) the pigment cells; (3) the posterior membrane consisting of plain muscle fibres which constitute the dilator muscle which is supplied mainly by sympathetic motor fibres, via the long ciliary nerves; (4) the posterior epithelium which is highly pigmented. Sensory fibres from the iris are contained in the nasociliary branch of the ophthalmic nerve. The blood supply is provided by the ciliary arteries. The colour of the iris is blue in Caucasian newborns and changes colour after a few months of life as pigment is deposited in the anterior limiting layer and the stroma. Iris colour is inherited; brown as a dominant trait and blue as a recessive trait. ⊃ anterior chamber, ciliary arteries, collarette, corectopia, dilator pupillae muscle, heterochromia, iridectomy, iridodialysis, iridology, iritis, melanin, posterior chamber, polycoria, pupil, pupillary membrane, sphincter pupillae muscle, Colour Section Figure 15.

iris bombe bulging forward of the iris due to pressure of the aqueous behind, when posterior synechiae are present around the pupil.

iris nodules small, solid elevations found on the iris and epithelial cells and lymphocytes. They are usually whitish or grey, depending on their location. ⊃ Busacca's nodules, Koeppe's nodules.

iritis *n syn.* anterior uveitis. Inflammation of the iris. The condition is usually characterized by ciliary injection, exudates in the anterior chamber (aqueous flare), keratitic precipitates, oedema, constricted and sluggish pupil, discoloration of the iris, posterior synechia, photophobia, lacrimation, loss of vision and pain. The chronic form exhibits most of the above signs and symptoms. In some cases the eye is not injected, in others there may be floaters and hypopyon and occasionally rubeosis iridis and an increase in intraocular pressure (IOP) due to blocking of the angle of the anterior chamber. Iritis is most often associated with choroiditis and cyclitis. Treatment includes mydriatics (to prevent synechia) and topical corticosteroid drops. It is essential to differentiate acute iritis from angle-closure glaucoma because of the possible harm of using a mydriatic in the latter. ⊃ aqueous flare, choroiditis, ciliary injection, cyclitis, floaters, Fuchs' heterochromic cyclitis, hypopyon, iridocyclitis, iridodialysis, synechia.

iron (Fe) *n* a metallic element needed in the body as a constituent of haemoglobin and several enzymes. An essential micronutrient; present in the body in the oxygen transport proteins, haemoglobin (60–70% of total iron) and myoglobin (10% of total iron). Small amounts are present in the plasma, carried by the protein transferrin, and it is stored (as ferritin) in liver, spleen and bone marrow. A small component (around 2%) is used in metabolic systems (cytochrome c, in mitochondria). Elite and recreational athletes undertaking hard training have a higher requirement and turnover of iron than less active people and quickly deplete iron stores which if untreated can lead to iron deficiency anaemia, severely impairing aerobic performance.

ironic effects in psychological terms, those that may occur when attempts to suppress a thought increase its accessibility to memory so that it is more likely to be brought to mind,

especially under conditions of stress or increased mental load. For example, in a racquet sport if a performer focuses attention on not overhitting the ball they will often do just that. Also known as ironic process.

iron-storage disease the deposition of iron in the tissues and organs, it may be primary or secondary to another disease such as thalassaemia. ⊃ haemochromatosis, haemosiderosis.

IRR *abbr* **1.** infrared radiation/rays. **2.** ionizing radiation regulations.

irradiated volume in radiotherapy, the quantity of tissue that receives a radiation dose that is considered to be significant in relation to normal tissue tolerance.

irradiation **1.** exposure to a form of radiant energy such as light, heat or X-rays. Radioactive sources of radiant heat are used in various imaging techniques and medical treatments. Gamma radiation is used to sterilize intravenous fluids, food and various items of medical equipment. Infrared is used for pain relief, muscle relaxation and to improve local blood flow. Ultraviolet light is used in the treatment of skin diseases and in the identification of some micro-organisms. **2.** the lateral scattering of light in the emulsion layer of a radiographic film causing unsharpness.

irreducible *adj* unable to be brought to desired condition.

irreducible hernia when the contents of the sac cannot be returned to the appropriate cavity, without surgical intervention. ⊃ hernia.

irregular bones cancellous bones surrounded by a thin layer of compact bone and irregular in shape, for example the vertebrae, facial bones.

irreversible unable to be reversed.

irreversible hydrocolloid (alginate) impression material ⊃ impression material.

irrigant a solution used for rinsing or washing various body sites. In endodontics, agent for flushing root canals, ideally combining antimicrobial activity and the ability to dissolve necrotic pulp tissue, for example sodium hypochlorite solution in suitable dilution.

irrigation washing out of a wound, body cavity or hollow organ, such as the bladder following prostate surgery, or a wound. In dentistry, the use of a disposable syringe with or without a curved plastic tip to irrigate sockets and cyst cavities, to wash out debris from a cavity preparation, or irrigate a pulp cavity during endodontic procedures.

irritability in the context of physiotherapy practice the amount of activity necessary to worsen the condition, the extent of the exacerbation and the duration of the response. Forms part of a patient assessment along with severity and nature. These three items are known as SIN factors, which are a valuable aid in planning frequency and duration of treatment. This has implications for the amount of assessment and treatment provided to the patient. ⊃ severity, irritability and nature factors (SIN).

irritable *adj* capable of being excited to activity; easily stimulated—**irritability** *n*.

irritable bowel syndrome (IBS) functional intestinal symptoms not explained by organic bowel disease. Symptoms include abdominal pain, bloating and change in bowel habit (alternating constipation and diarrhoea).

irritant *adj, n* describes any agent which causes irritation.

irritant eczema detergents, alkalis, acids, solvents and abrasive dusts are common causes. There is a wide range of susceptibility to weak irritants. Irritant eczema accounts for the majority of industrial cases and work loss. Older adults, those with fair and dry skin, and those with an atopic background (personal or family history of asthma, hay fever or eczema) are especially vulnerable. Napkin eczema in babies is common and due to irritant ammoniacal urine and faeces. Strong irritants elicit an acute reaction at the site of contact whereas weak irritants most often cause chronic eczema, especially of the hands, after prolonged exposure.

IRT *abbr* immune-reactive trypsin test.

Irvine–Gass syndrome ⊃ cystoid macular oedema.

ISC *abbr* intermittent self-catheterization.

ischaemia *n* also known as hypoperfusion. Deficient blood supply to any part of the body (region, organ or tissue). ⊃ angina, Volkmann's ischaemic contracture—**ischaemic** *adj*.

ischaemic heart disease (IHD) ⊃ coronary heart disease.

ischaemic optic neuropathy an obstruction of the blood supply to the optic nerve, usually to its anterior part. It causes a sudden loss of vision. It may be due to arteriosclerosis, temporal arteritis or emboli of the ciliary circulation. Treatment depends on the cause. ⊃ ciliary arteries, temporal arteritis.

ischial tuberosity avulsion detachment of a piece of bone from the tip of the ischial part of the pelvis, where the tendons of the hamstring muscles are attached, caused by their sudden strong forced contraction. This produces local pain, which can be severe. Treatment is difficult and chronic symptoms not uncommon.

ischiocavernosus muscle muscle extending from the ischium of the pelvis to the clitoris or penis, aiding in their erection.

ischiococcygeus muscle muscle extending from the ischium of the pelvis to the coccyx; the posterior portion of the levator ani muscle.

ischi/o- a prefix that means 'ischium', e.g. *ischiorectal*.

ischiorectal *adj* pertaining to the ischium and the rectum, as an ischiorectal abscess which occurs between these two structures.

ischium *n* the lower part of the innominate bone of the pelvis; the bone on which the body rests when sitting—**ischial** *adj*.

ISD *abbr* interventricular septal defect.

ISDN *abbr* integrated services digital network.

islet cell tumours uncommon hormone-secreting tumours of the islet cells of the pancreas. They include gastrinoma, glucagonoma, insulinoma and somatostatinoma.

islets of Langerhans (P Langerhans, German pathologist, 1847–1888) collections of special cells scattered throughout the pancreas, mainly concerned with endocrine function. The pancreatic islets contain four types of hormone-secreting cells: alpha cells, which secrete glucagon; beta cells, which secrete insulin and amylin; delta cells, which secrete several substances, including somatostatin or growth hormone release inhibiting hormone (GHRIH); and other cells that produce regulatory pancreatic polypeptide.

ISO *abbr* International Standards Organization.

iso- a prefix that means 'equal, alike', e.g. *isobar*.

isoantibody an antibody to isoantigens present in other individuals of the same species.

isoantigen an antigen that reacts with isoantibodies present in other individuals of the same species.

isobar **1.** any nucleus that has the same atomic mass number as another nucleus but with different atomic numbers. **2.** a line joining points of equal pressure.

isocentre the point in space at which the central beams from each beam angle intersect. In computed tomography (CT) this is the point of greatest accuracy of the reconstructed image, hence its importance when positioning a patient on the table prior to scanning. In radiotherapy, the point where the axis of rotation of the diaphragm, the horizontal axis of rotation of the gantry and the vertical axis of rotation of the couch intersect.

isocentric gantry a C-shaped structure that connects the X-ray tube to the image intensifier so that the central beam from the X-ray tube is always aligned to the centre of the image intensifier.

isocentric reference mark a point marked onto the patient to enable accuracy of repositioning, for example, in radiotherapy.

isodactylism a condition chararacterized by having digits of equal length.

isodose chart a number of isodose lines to represent the output from a specific source of radiotherapy equipment.

isodose contour a line on an isodose chart that plots doses of equal value.

isodose curve the graphical representation of the distribution of radiation dose within a uniform area.

isodose distribution lines plotting the radiation dose received by the patient throughout the radiotherapy treatment area.

isodose lines the lines that plot the areas of a patient that receive a radiation dose of equal value.

isodose surface the graphical representation of the area of skin surface receiving a radiation dose.

isoelectric point (IEP) the pH value in which a substance or system is electrically neutral. In a film emulsion it determines some characteristics of the emulsion: the minimum solubility, viscosity, conductivity and swelling and determines how easily products are removed from the emulsion.

isoenzymes *n* (*syn* isozymes) enzymes that catalyses the same reaction, but exist in several forms and at different body sites, such as lactate dehydrogenase.

isograft *n* a graft between individuals with identical genotypes, i.e. identical twins. It can also be used to describe grafts between syngeneic individuals, i.e. inbred strains of laboratory animals.

isoimmunization *n* development of anti-Rh agglutinins in the blood of a Rh-negative person who has been given a Rh-positive transfusion, or who is carrying a Rh-positive fetus.

isokinetic without change in velocity.

isokinetic activity a dynamic activity in which the velocity of the movement remains the same and the resistance varies. The movement of an object, body or body segment, by muscle action, with constant velocity. Sometimes known as isovelocity motion: rare in sport.

isokinetic dynamometer device for measuring moments at a constant velocity. The machine controls velocity (usually angular velocity) and external moment is measured. Quantitatively measures muscular strength through a preset speed of movement. Sometimes known as isovelocity dynamometer. ⊃ torque–angular velocity relation.

isolated limb perfusion a method of introducing cytotoxic drugs into an isolated arterial supply by administering a tourniquet to the limb, under general anaesthetic.

isolation *n* separation of a patient from others for a number of reasons, e.g. to prevent the spread of an infectious disease. ⊃ containment isolation, protective isolation, source isolation.

isolator *n* apparatus ranging from what is virtually a large plastic bag in which a patient can be nursed to that in which surgery can be performed. It aims to prevent pathogenic microorganisms either gaining entry or leaving the enclosed space.

isoleucine *n* an essential (indispensable) branched chain amino acid.

isomers molecules that have the same mass and formula but have different structures or functional groups. This causes them to have different properties.

isometric *adj* of equal proportions.

isometric contraction a muscle contraction where its attachments do not move and, therefore, the muscle does not shorten and joints do not move, e.g. when holding a weight steady. ⊃ force–velocity relationship.

isometric exercise (*syn* static exercise) exercise in which the muscle stays at the same length; carried out without movement. Used to maintain muscle tone.

isometric transition is the move from an excited state of a nucleus to a stable state.

isometropia both eyes having the same refractive power.

isosthenuria the kidneys are unable to produce concentrated urine; a feature of end-stage renal failure.

isotonic *adj* equal tension; applied to any solution which has the same osmotic pressure as the fluid with which it is being compared. ⊃ hypertonic, hypotonic.

isotonic exercises carried out with movement. Increases muscle strength and endurance. In practice approximated by constant angular velocity of limb movement (implying exactly isotonic muscle action only in the theoretical case of the joint concerned having constant geometry throughout the movement range, as in a simple hinge).

isotonic muscle contraction contraction in which a muscle actively shortens at constant velocity with movement of its attachments. ⊃ force–velocity relationship.

isotonic saline (*syn* normal saline, physiological saline), 0.9% solution of sodium chloride in water.

isotonic solution one that has the same osmolarity as body fluids. Most commercial sports drinks (6% carbohydrate, 20 mmol/L sodium) are isotonic. Isotonic drinks are effective in preventing exercise-induced dehydration and promoting restoration of fluid and electrolyte levels after exercise.

isotonic sports drinks ⊃ sports drinks.

isotope of an element any nucleus which contains the same number of protons as the element but has a different mass number.

isotopes *npl* two or more forms of the same element having identical chemical properties and the same atomic number but different mass numbers. Those isotopes with radioactive properties are used in medicine for research, diagnosis and treatment of disease.

isotropic to emit radiation in all directions.

ISP *abbr* internet service provider.

ispaghula husk a natural dietary fibre supplement. Used as a bulk-forming laxative. ⊃ Appendix 5.

isthmus *n* a narrowed part of an organ or tissue such as that connecting the two lobes of the thyroid gland.

isthmus of the uterine tube a narrow part of the uterine (fallopian) tube that extends for 2.5 cm from the uterus. ⊃ uterine tubes, Colour Section Figure 17.

itch *n* a sensation on the skin which makes one want to scratch. Often accompanies skin disease.

itch mite *Sarcoptes scabiei.* ⊃ scabies.

iteration to repeatedly execute an instruction in a computer program.

iterative reconstruction algorithm a mathematical method of image reconstruction which involves continually updating and adjusting the image as data are acquired.

-itis a suffix that means 'inflammation of', e.g. *iritis*.

ITM *abbr* index of tooth mobility. ⊃ index (dental).

ITP *abbr* idiopathic thrombocytopenic purpura.

ITU *abbr* intensive therapy unit.

IUCD *abbr* intrauterine contraceptive device.

IUD *abbr* **1.** intrauterine (contraceptive) device. **2.** intrauterine death (of a fetus).

IUGR *abbr* intrauterine growth restriction/retardation.

IUI *abbr* intrauterine insemination.

IV *abbr* intravenous.

IVC *abbr* inferior vena cava.

IVF *abbr* in vitro fertilization.

IVH *abbr* intraventricular haemorrhage.

IVI *abbr* intravenous infusion.

IVIG *abbr* intravenous immunoglobulin.

ivory dentine. The term is generally restricted to the teeth and tusks of elephants and other large mammals.

IVU, IVP *abbr* intravenous urogram/pyelogram ⊃ urography.

Ixodes a genus of parasitic hard-bodied ticks. Various species are associated with the spread of diseases that include Lyme disease, tularaemia, Rocky Mountain spotted fever.

IZOF *abbr* individual zone of optimal functioning.

J

J *abbr* joule.

jacket an outer covering. ⊃ jacket crown.

jacket crown a full veneer crown completely covering the prepared tooth and having a cervical shoulder. Constructed of porcelain or resin and cemented into place. ⊃ temporary crown.

Jackson cross-cylinder lens ⊃ cross-cylinder lens.

Jackson crossed cylinder test ⊃ cross-cylinder test for astigmatism.

Jacksonian epilepsy (J Jackson, British neurologist, 1835–1911) ⊃ epilepsy.

Jacobson's muscular relaxation a method for reducing physiological arousal or cognitive anxiety. *progressive muscular relaxation* a technique that involves successively tensing and relaxing different skeletal muscle groups in the body. ⊃ relaxation techniques.

Jacquemier's sign (J Jacquemier, French obstetrician, 1806–1879) darkening (blue/purple discoloration) of the vaginal mucosa; seen sometimes in early pregnancy from the fourth week. It is a possible indicator of pregnancy rather than definite evidence.

Jacquette scaler ⊃ periodontal instruments.

jactitation restlessness with muscle spasm and twitching. May accompany increase in core body temperature.

Jaeger test types test types for measuring visual acuity at near. They consist of ordinary printers' types of various sizes and are arranged as words and phrases. Depending on the size of test types read, acuity is recorded as J.1, J.2 in ascending size up to J.20 (Table J.1). The smallest Jaeger (J.1) subtends an angle of 5′ at 450 mm from the eye. ⊃ near visual acuity.

J-hook part of an external oral traction orthodontic appliance used to transmit extra-oral forces from a headgear to the appliance.

Jakob–Creutzfeldt disease ⊃ Creutzfeldt–Jakob disease.

jamais vu a sudden feeling of being a stranger in familiar places or when with people who are known to the individual. It may be associated with temporal lobe epilepsy, but also occurs infrequently as a normal phenomenon.

Janeway lesions (E Janeway, American physician, 1841–1911) haemorrhagic spots on the palm or sole. Associated with infective endocarditis.

jargon *n* technical or specialized language that is only understood by a particular group, for example health professionals, thereby excluding non-experts such as some patients and carers. Often used to describe the use of obscure and pretentious language, together with a roundabout way of expression.

Jarisch–Herxheimer's reaction (A Jarisch, Austrian dermatologist, 1850–1902; K Herxheimer, German dermatologist, 1861–1942) a reaction whereby the symptoms of a disease, such as syphilis are initially worsened when antibiotic therapy commences. Typically it is characterized by fever, chills, muscle pain, nausea and headache within a few hours of receiving the antibiotics. The reaction is not harmful and is usually short lived.

Jarman index system for weighting general practice populations according to social conditions. A composite index of social factors that general practitioners considered important in increasing workload and pressure on services. These factors were identified through a survey of one in ten general practitioners in the UK in 1981. An underprivileged area (UPA) score was then constructed based on the level of each variable in each area, weighted by the weighting assigned from the national general practitioner survey. Eight variables were used: (a) older people living alone, (b) children aged under five years, (c) unskilled, (d) unemployed (as % economically active), (e) lone parent families, (f) overcrowded accommodation (>1 person/room), (g) mobility (moved house within one year), (h) ethnic origin (new Commonwealth and Pakistan). Information on the variables were derived from the census. ⊃ Townsend index.

jaundice *n* (*syn* icterus) a condition characterized by a raised bilirubin level in the blood (hyperbilirubinaemia). Minor degrees are only detectable chemically. Major degrees are visible in the yellow discoloration of skin, sclerae and mucosae. Pruritus occurs although the mechanism is not known. Jaundice without the excretion of bilirubin in the urine is termed acholuric. Jaundice may be classified as follows: (a) *haemolytic or prehepatic jaundice* where excessive breakdown of red blood cells (erythrocytes) releases bilirubin into the blood, such as in haemolytic anaemia. ⊃ haemolysis, haemolytic disease of the newborn. (b) *hepatocellular jaundice* arises when liver cell function is impaired, such as with hepatitis or cirrhosis. (c) *obstructive or cholestatic jaundice* where the flow of bile is obstructed either within the liver (intrahepatic) or in the larger ducts of the biliary tract (extrahepatic). Causes include: cirrhosis, cancers, parasites and gallstones. ⊃ cholestasis.

java a programming language that works on all computer systems.

javelin thrower's elbow ⊃ epicondylitis, medial epicondylitis.

jaw *n* the tooth-bearing bones of the face. The upper jaw comprises the two maxillae and the premaxilla and the lower jaw, the mandible.

Table J.1 Approximate relationship between the Jaeger system, the point system (or N notation) and the Snellen equivalent

Jaeger	Point	Snellen equivalent at 40 cm	
		(m)	(ft)
1	3.5	6/7	20/23
2	4.5	6/8	20/27
3	5.5	6/11	20/37
4	6.5	6/13	20/43
5	7.5	6/14	20/47
6	8	6/15	20/50
7	9.5	6/17	20/57
8	11	6/20	20/67
9	12	6/24	20/80
10	13	6/26	20/87
11	14	6/28	20/93
12	16	6/30	20/100
13	18	6/36	20/120
14	22	6/45	20/150

Reproduced from Millodot 2004 with permission

jaw augmentation procedure a surgical technique in which various materials, usually autogenous bone or cartilage, are grafted onto the jaws.

jaw bone describes either the maxilla or, more commonly, the mandible.

jaw chattering a clonic spasm of the jaw muscles that may occur with rigor or as a habit spasm.

jaw closing reflex reflex, by mandibular elevation, following certain oral or facial stimuli.

jaw fractures jaw fractures may be *closed, comminuted, greenstick, impacted, open (compound)*, etc. ➲ fracture. Additionally, a jaw fracture may be: *indirect jaw fracture* a fracture at any distance from a point of impact or trauma, e.g. a blow on the chin may cause a fracture of one or both condyles of the mandible *(guardsman's fracture). linear jaw fracture* in which the fracture runs along the long axis of a bone. *middle third fracture* a fracture of the bony complex that comprises the middle third of the facial skeleton. Certain jaw fractures can be classified into three categories (I, II, III) using the Le Fort classification. ➲ Le Fort classification. Fractures of the jaw are treated by reducing the fracture so that the bone ends are in approximation. The fractured bone is then immobilized by means of splints, pins or wires for a period of weeks to allow the bone ends to unite, after which the splints etc. are removed.

jaw injury injury to the bones of the face which carry the teeth: the maxilla (upper jaw) and mandible (lower jaw). Jaw injuries include fractures and dislocations, and occur in road traffic accidents, violence and sport. In sport they are most common in contact sports such as boxing, rugby, lacrosse and ice hockey. These injuries require immediate assessment as they can lead to difficulty in accessing the airway or even to airway obstruction. ➲ jaw fractures.

jaw jerk reflex jaw closure occurring on stretching the jaw-closing muscles.

jaw movement profile 1. Plot of the mandibular position against time. **2.** projection of the envelope of motion on the coronal or sagittal plane.

jaw reflex reflex action produced on the muscles moving the jaws following stimulation of the oral cavity or orofacial region.

jaw relation any relationship of the mandible to the maxilla.

jaw thrust a manoeuvre used to open the airway if a head or neck injury is suspected. In adults the index and middle fingers are placed under the angle of the lower jaw and steady gentle pressure used to move the jaw upwards and forwards (Figure J.1); the mouth should then open slightly. The jaw thrust manoeuvre can be used for children and infants, but only the index finger on the lower jaw is used. ➲ head tilt/chin lift.

jaw-winking syndrome also known as Gunn's syndrome and Marcus Gunn's syndrome. Characterized by an involuntary facial movement in which the eyelid droops when the jaw closes but is raised when the jaw opens or moves from side to side. It is usually unilateral.

JCA *abbr* juvenile chronic arthritis

jejunal biopsy ➲ Crosby capsule.

jejunectomy surgical removal of all or a portion of the jejunum.

jejunileostomy a surgical anastomosis between the jejunum and the ileum.

jejun/o- a suffix that means 'jejunum', e.g. *jejunostomy.*

jejunostomy *n* a surgically made fistula between the jejunum and the anterior abdominal wall; used for feeding in cases where passage of food through the stomach is impossible or undesirable.

jejunum *n* that part of the small intestine between the duodenum and the ileum—**jejunal** *adj.*

jerk the rate of change of acceleration with respect to time.

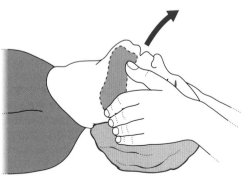

J.1 Jaw thrust—adult (reproduced from Mallik et al 1998 with permission).

Jersey finger a colloquial term used in sports medicine to describe the rupture of the flexor digitorum longus tendon from the distal phalanx of the finger due to rapid extension of the finger while being actively flexed.

jet injection a spring-loaded instrument, with no needle used to rapidly inject a small amount of a solution directly into the tissues.

jet lag disturbance to biological processes that normally have diurnal rhythms; occurs following travel through different time zones. It is characterized by changes in sleep patterns, appetite, concentration and memory, and fatigue for some days until body rhythms return to normal. People working variable shift patterns report similar effects.

jeweller's rouge ⊃ rouge.

JGA *abbr* juxtaglomerular apparatus.

Jiffy tube a small celluloid or plastic tube with an extended end of reduced dimension. Used in dentistry to introduce lubricant gels, dressings, cements and root-filling materials into a root canal.

jig a device for immobilizing patients during radiotherapy treatment.

jigger *n* a sand flea, *Tunga penetrans*, found in the tropics.

JND *abbr* just noticeable difference.

Jod-Basedow phenomenon (K von Basedow, German physician, 1799–1854) the development of hyperthyroidism following the administration of dietary iodine to a person with endemic goitre living in an iodine-deficient region. May also occur when iodine in large doses is administered to a person with a non-toxic multinodular goitre living in a region which has sufficient levels of iodine.

jogger's nipple a painful condition caused by friction of the nipple against clothing, seen particularly in both male and female distance runners. Can be reduced or prevented by the use of lubricating jelly. ⊃ cyclist's nipples

Johnstone approach a treatment approach involving a developmental progression of movement and on sensory stimulation with specific splinting techniques. It is used for patients who have had a stroke.

Johnstone splints air filled splints that envelop a limb or part of a limb. They are used in the Johnstone approach to treat patients with neurological deficit. They can also be used as a temporary measure to help with limbs that are showing signs of contractures. As with all splints they require careful monitoring.

joint *n* the articulation of two or more bones (arthrosis). There are three main classes: (a) fibrous (synarthroses), e.g. the sutures of the skull; (b) cartilaginous (amphiarthroses), e.g. between the manubrium and the body of the sternum; and (c) synovial or freely movable (diarthroses), e.g. shoulder or hip. Freely movable joints are classified by the range of movement possible. They are ball-and-socket, hinge, gliding, pivot, condyloid and saddle joints. ⊃ Charcot's joint.

joint angle angle between two body segments linked by a common joint.

joint capsule the fibrous tissue layer that covers a synovial joint, contributing to the 'hinge' of the joint. The capsule comprises two layers: a thick, tough, protective fibrous outer layer and an inner layer, which secretes synovial fluid, providing nutrition and lubrication to the joint.

joint cavity the space between the articular surfaces of bones. In the most common, synovial cavity, the ends of the bone are covered with articular hyaline cartilage and synovial fluid fills the space.

joint hypermobility syndrome a common childhood condition involving hypermobile joints (that can move beyond the normal range of motion).

joint injury damage to a joint. Joint injuries are among the most common injuries in sport and range from sprains and supporting ligament injuries to dislocations and fractures. The knee, ankle and shoulder are the most commonly injured.

joint instability during pregnancy the effects of the hormones progesterone and relaxin on the joints in pregnancy causing them to soften and have an increased range of movement, e.g. the sacroiliac joint and the symphysis pubis.

joint locking a condition, usually caused by trapping of a loose body within the joint, such as a fragment of torn meniscus at the knee. The person typically describes a history of having to push or jiggle the joint in order to unlock it.

joint mobility the ability of a joint to be moved through its range in different planes. This is dependent on the characteristics of the individual joint itself as well as the supporting muscles and ligaments, the capsule and the anatomy of the articulating surfaces. In some joints, stability is sacrificed in favour of greater mobility, e.g. the shoulder joint, where this is achieved by the shallow glenoid articulation with the humeral head. This increases the incidence of dislocation. ⊃ hypermobility.

joint picture experts group (JPEG) a compressed, computer graphics file used to store images on a computer.

joint position sense the awareness of the joints in space. Often tested by getting a patient to close their eyes and then the therapist places the impaired limb in a position and the patient tries to copy with the other. This ability is often impaired in patients with neurological problems. ⊃ kinaesthetic sense, proprioception.

joint protection techniques for managing the performance of activities to reduce or eliminate potentially damaging stresses on vulnerable joints.

joint reaction forces the forces that are transmitted through a joint's articular surfaces. The net force between the bone surfaces within a joint, not including muscle forces.

joint receptors sensory receptors in joint capsules and associated ligaments, from which information reaching the central nervous system contributes (along with other sensory inputs) to awareness of joint position and movement (proprioceptive sensation), and is necessary also for co-ordinating the action of relevant muscles. To be distinguished from the nociceptor nerve endings also present in joint tissues, which give rise to the sensation of pain resulting from overstretching, injury or inflammation.

I
J

joint replacement also known as arthroplasty. There is no typical patient who is appropriate for a joint replacement. As with all modern medicine a decision has to made that balances the risks of surgery against the potential improvements. Patient age per se is not an acceptable clinical decision making tool. Generally, the surgical team will wait until pain or disability is severe enough to cause a significant impact on the person's quality of life, where surgery would make things significantly better or prevent a major deterioration. At the time of writing, artificial joints are still not as efficient as their organic counterparts. If a synthetic joint becomes worn or damaged, it does not repair itself as a normal joint does. It will also not be as efficient at absorbing the stresses and strains of daily activity as an organic joint. The field of joint prosthetics continues to make remarkable advancements in the development of new materials and increased longevity.

joint space the space that appears on an X-ray of a joint, it is not, in fact, a space since it is occupied by articular hyaline cartilage, but this is not visible on X-ray.

joint stiffness pain and discomfort in a joint, causing difficulty in movement. Can result from medical conditions such as arthritis or from injury, especially when there is protective spasm of the surrounding muscles. Unexplained joint stiffness requires medical assessment and investigation.

joule (J) *n* the SI unit for measuring energy, work and quantity of heat. The unit (J) is the energy expended when 1 kg (kilogram) is moved 1 m (metre) by a force of 1 N (newton). The kilojoule ($kJ = 10^3$ J) and the megajoule ($MJ = 10^6$ J) are used by nutritionists for measuring large amounts of energy.

JPEG *abbr* joint picture experts group.

(J) receptors ⊃ juxtacapillary receptors.

JVP *abbr* jugular venous pressure.

judo elbow injury to the supporting ligaments around the elbow in judo. Usually the result of holding an opponent with the arms extended.

jugular *adj* pertaining to the throat.

jugular veins external and internal jugular veins pass down either side of the neck. They carry most venous blood from the head and unite with the subclavian veins to form the brachiocephalic veins, which become the superior vena cava. The *external jugular vein* begins in the neck at the level of the angle of the jaw. It passes downwards in front of the sternocleidomastoid muscle, then behind the clavicle before entering the subclavian vein. The *internal jugular veins* begin at the jugular foramina in the middle cranial fossa and each is the continuation of a sigmoid sinus (a dural venous sinus). They run downwards in the neck behind the sternocleidomastoid muscles. Behind the clavicle they unite with the subclavian veins, carrying blood from the upper limbs, to form the brachiocephalic veins ⊃ Colour Section Figure 10.

jugular venous pressure (JVP) the pressure of blood in the jugular veins; a guide to the pressure in the right side of the heart. It is estimated by assessing the blood column in the jugular veins with examination performed with the patient lying supine, with the bed head elevated to a 45° angle. When jugular venous pressure (JVP) is raised, the neck veins may be distended as high as to the angle of the jaw. In the position described above, venous distension greater than approximately 4 cm above the sternal angle is considered to be abnormal. However, examination and assessment in patients who are obese can be difficult. Raised JVP may occur with hyperinflation, right sided heart failure and hypervolaemia.

jukebox an electromechanical device for handling large numbers of optical computer disks to enable the rapid retrieval of archived data.

Julesz random-dot stereogram ⊃ random-dot stereogram (RDS).

jump test ⊃ Sargent jump test.

jumper's heel heel pain felt in jumping sports as a result of the explosive compression forces that occur on landing. The pain is usually felt on the calcaneum deep to the Achilles tendon.

jumper's knee patellar tendonitis (tendinitis). Inflammation of the patellar tendon where it attaches to the patella. An overuse injury associated with repetitive contraction of the quadriceps femoris muscle associated with the movements of athletes and dancers.

junction a joining or meeting place; an interface. ⊃ amelodentinal junction, cementoenamel junction, junctional epithelium (dentogingival junction).

junctional epithelium (dentogingival junction, epithelial cuff) epithelium at the base of the gingival sulcus which attaches the gingiva to the enamel or cementum. The term epithelial attachment is deprecated.

junctional escape rhythm a cardiac rhythm that usually arises from a focus at the junction between the atrioventricular node and the atrioventricular bundle. If the heart rate is below 50 bpm the cardiac output is reduced and the blood pressure falls leading to the person feeling dizzy and faint.

Jung, Carl Swiss psychiatrist/psychoanalyst (1875–1961).

Junin virus a virus of the family *Arenaviridae*. Discovered in 1958 it is the causative organism of Argentine haemorrhagic fever.

jurisprudence the philosophy of law.

justice *n* involves the concepts of fairness and justness. May be described as acting within a set of moral laws, respecting the views and rights of others, or equity in the distribution of resources such as health care.

just noticeable difference (JND) ⊃ difference threshold.

justominor pelvis a small gynaecoid pelvis with proportionately reduced diameters.

juvenile chronic arthritis (JCA) now more commonly termed juvenile idiopathic arthritis.

juvenile idiopathic arthritis (*syn* juvenile chronic arthritis) chronic inflammatory arthritis in children. In its systemic form (previously termed Still's disease) systemic features such as fever, rash and anaemia are prominent and may precede the arthritis.

juvenile osteochondritis a condition of the epiphyses or centres of ossification. It may be due to a poor blood supply causing the 'death of bone'.

juxtacapillary (J) receptors these are stretch receptors located in the lung parenchyma close to the pulmonary capillaries, stimulated by inflammatory processes, congestion and oedema. Tachypnoea, dyspnoea and glottic narrowing result from stimulation of these receptors. ⮥ intrapulmonary receptors.

juxtaglomerular *adj* close to the glomerulus.

juxtaglomerular apparatus (JGA) cells in the distal convoluted tubule and the afferent arteriole of the nephron. They monitor changes in pressure and sodium levels in the blood, and initiate the release of renin. ⮥ macula densa.

juxtapose *vt* to place side by side.

I

J

Kahn reaction an obsolete serological test for syphilis; used in the 20th century.

kala-azar *n* generalized leishmaniasis occurring in the tropics. Characterized by anaemia, fever, splenomegaly and wasting. It is caused by the parasite *Leishmania donovani* and is spread by sandflies.

kallidin *n* a kinin. A biologically active polypeptide that is produced in response to tissue injury. It causes vasodilation and the contraction of involuntary smooth muscle. It is similar in structure to bradykinin.

kallireins *npl* a group of enzymes involved in the release of bradykinin and kallidin.

Kallmann's syndrome (F Kallmann, German/American psychiatrist and geneticist, 1897–1965) congenital condition in which the olfactory bulbs fail to develop resulting in anosmia. There is also a deficiency of pituitary gonadotrophic hormones and hypogonadism.

Kanner's syndrome (L Kanner, Austrian/American psychiatrist, 1894–1981) autism. ➲ Asperger's syndrome.

kaolin *n* Fuller's earth. Natural aluminium silicate. Given orally it absorbs toxic substances, hence useful in diarrhoea, food poisoning and colitis. Sometimes used as a poultice.

Kaposi's disease (M Kaposi, Austrian dermatologist, 1837–1902) ➲ xeroderma pigmentosum.

Kaposi's sarcoma (M Kaposi) a cancer characterized by new blood vessel growth producing red, purple or brown lesions, often on the skin but with metastatic potential. Originally common in Africa but now often seen in immunocompromised individuals, such as those with acquired immunodeficiency syndrome (AIDS). ➲ Colour Section Figure 80.

Kaposi's varicelliform eruption widespread herpes simplex infection complicating atopic eczema. ➲ eczema herpeticum.

Kartagener's syndrome (M Kartagener, Swiss physician, 1897–1975) a rare inherited autosomal recessive condition of primary ciliary dyskinesia and transposition of the viscera, such as the heart being situated on the right side of the body. The abnormal movement of the respiratory cilia leads to chronic sinusitis and repeated respiratory tract infection, which eventually cause bronchiectasis.

karyo- a prefix that means 'nucleus', e.g. *karyotype*.

karyolysis the dissolution of the cell nucleus that occurs prior to cell division during meiosis and mitosis. It also occurs due to pathological changes to cells such as trauma or necrosis.

karyorrhexis *n* fragmentation of the cell nucleus and dissemination of nuclear chromatin within the cell cytoplasm.

karyotype *n* **1.** the number, size, structure and arrangement of chromosomes in a somatic cell of an individual. **2.** a diagrammatic representation of a set of chromosomes showing an orderly array of chromosomes the autosomes (groups A–G) and the sex chromosomes (see Figure C.9, p. 146). It is usually derived from the study of cultured cells and may be done for diagnostic purposes, or in individuals at risk of having children with chromosomal abnormalities, or for the prenatal detection of fetal abnormality.

Kawasaki disease (T Kawasaki, Japanese physician, 20th century) an inflammatory disease affecting medium size blood vessels (vasculitis). ➲ mucocutaneous lymph node syndrome.

Kayser–Fleischer ring (B Kayser, German ophthalmologist, 1869–1954; B Fleischer, German ophthalmologist, 1874–1904) a brown/green ring in the outer cornea, a sign of Wilson's disease (hepatolenticular degeneration), that results from disordered copper metabolism. ➲ Wilson's disease, Colour Section Figure 81.

KC *abbr* keratoconus.

KCS *abbr* keratoconjunctivitis sicca.

Kearns–Sayre syndrome (T Kearns, American neuro-ophthalmologist, b. 1922; G Sayre, American ophthalmologist) a mitochondrial myopathy syndrome. It has clinical features similar to chronic progressive external ophthalmoplegia (CPEO), but the onset occurs earlier (<20 years) and there is heart block and pigmentary retinopathy. ➲ chronic progressive external ophthalmoplegia (CPEO), mitochondrial myopathy syndromes.

Kegel exercises (A Kegel, American gynaecologist, 20th century) a set of pelvic floor exercises used in both women and men to minimize continence problems. Used to retrain the pelvic floor muscles after childbirth, or following prostate surgery. The person learns to identify the muscles of the pelvic floor and undertakes daily contraction of the pelvic floor to strengthen it. Thereby strengthening the muscles that surround the internal and external urinary sphincter muscles.

Kehr's sign (H Kehr, German surgeon, 1862–1913) acute referred pain felt at the top of the left shoulder caused by blood within the peritoneal cavity irritating the diaphragm. The pain impulses are transmitted by the phrenic nerve. The presence of Kehr's sign is indicative of a ruptured spleen.

Kell factor/antigen named for the person in whom the antigen was first identified. A blood group factor/antigen present in about 10% of the Caucasian population. Anti-Kell antibodies can cross the placenta. ➲ blood groups.

Keller's operation (W Keller, American surgeon, 1874–1959) arthroplasty or excision arthroplasty undertaken to correct severe hallux valgus or rigidus deformity. Excision of the proximal half of the proximal phalanx, plus any osteophytes and exostoses on the metatarsal head. The toe is fixed in the corrected position; after healing a pseudarthrosis results.

Kelly–Paterson syndrome ⊃ Plummer–Vinson syndrome.

keloid scar excessive scar production extending beyond the site of original injury. An elevated and progressive scar, which may produce contraction deformity. Keloid scarring occurs in some people who have darker skins.

Kelvin scale (K) *n* (W Thompson [Lord Kelvin], British physicist, 1824–1907) an absolute temperature scale that uses the cessation of particle vibration for determining zero degrees or absolute zero. It is calculated in degrees Celsius as $-273.15°C$. The unit the kelvin is the SI unit for temperature.

Kennedy bar also known as continuous bar connector (deprecated term). That part of a partial dental prosthesis consisting of a narrow bar lying in contact with the lingual surfaces of mandibular incisors, which connects the saddles and may provide indirect retention.

Kennedy classification a method of classifying partially edentulous mouths and the partial dentures required to restore these edentulous areas. It is based on the location of the edentulous area relative to the remaining teeth.

keratalgia pain in the cornea.

keratectomy *n* surgical excision of a portion of the cornea.

keratic precipitates (KP) clusters of inflammatory cells adherent to the posterior surface of the cornea; present following trauma or in inflammation of uvea.

keratin *n* a fibrous protein found in nails and the outer part of the skin and horns, etc.

keratinization *n* horn-like thickening of the skin. ⊃ keratosis.

keratinocytes the most numerous cells that form the epidermis. The keratinocytes produce keratin from the precursor keratohyalin. They are bound together by desmosomes which helps to prevent structural damage to the skin and maintain epidermal cohesion during renewal. Keratinocytes migrate upwards through the layers of the epidermis during epidermal renewal, eventually to be shed from the stratum corneum (surface layer).

keratitis *n* inflammation of the cornea. It can arise from various sources, the most common being: microbial infection (bacteria, fungi or viruses), hypersensitivity to staphylococcal exotoxins, nutritional deficiencies, failure of the eyelids to cover the cornea, deficiencies in the precorneal tear film, contact lens wear (especially extended wear), mechanical, radiation or chemical trauma or interruption of the ophthalmic branch of the trigeminal nerve. Keratitis is usually characterized by a dullness and loss of transparency of the cornea due to infiltrates, neovascularization, oedema and is accompanied by ciliary injection. The discomfort varies from a foreign body sensation to severe pain, with lacrimation, photophobia, blepharospasm and an impairment of vision. If the condition is severe, ulcers and pus (hypopyon) will appear and the iris and ciliary body may become involved. It is important to identify the cause and the

organism in order to treat the condition. Micro-organisms do not usually infect an intact healthy cornea so this is more likely to occur when hygiene is poor, especially if contact lenses are worn. The risk of *microbial keratitis* is increased in immunocompromised individuals, or those with existing eye disease and in eye injuries involving plant substances. It can, however, occur in people who wear soft contact lenses, especially in warmer regions. Keratitis of bacterial origin is treated with antibiotic drugs. Keratitis of viral origin (e.g. herpes) is treated with antiviral agents and that of fungal origin, such as that caused by *Fusarium* spp., are treated with antifungal drugs. Those people who do not respond to treatment and suffer corneal damage may need a corneal transplant. ⊃ ciliary injection, corneal infiltrates, corneal ulcer, disciform keratitis, hypopyon, interstitial keratitis, keratitis sicca, keratomalacia, keratomycosis, keratopathy, photokeratitis.

keratitis sicca (*syn* dry eye) keratitis due to an absence or deficiency of the lacrimal secretion. It is characterized by ciliary injection, loss of the usual glossy appearance of the cornea, mucus threads and filaments in the tear film and filamentary strands of epithelium which adhere to the cornea. The person complains of burning, itching and foreign body sensations and transient blurring of vision which are worsened by hot, dry environments. The condition is usually associated with conjunctivitis and general dryness of the skin and of the membranes of the mouth and blepharitis. Tests with fluorescein or rose bengal show tissue stains and Schirmer's test is subnormal. Keratoconjunctivitis sicca may result from: (a) a fluid deficiency of the tear film. This deficiency is also encountered in Sjögren's syndrome, for example; (b) mucin deficiency. In this case the condition is usually referred to as xerophthalmia; (c) conditions in which there is abnormal blinking; (d) lack of congruity between the cornea and the eyelids as occurs when there is a limbal lesion and dellen, for example; (e) and it follows, in some cases, juvenile idiopathic arthritis or sarcoidosis, certain medications such as antihistamines, oral contraceptives and antidepressants and living in a dry climate. Management consists mainly of artificial tears and frequent blinking. Occasionally, soft contact lenses may help although infection may be a problem. Treatment may also include moist goggles, and in severe cases, closure of the lacrimal puncta or tarsorrhaphy. ⊃ artificial tears, fluorescein, keratoconjunctivitis sicca, lacrimal apparatus, meibomian glands, Mikulicz's disease/syndrome, mucin, rose bengal, Schirmer's test, Sjögren's syndrome, tarsorrhaphy, xerophthalmia.

kerat/o- a prefix that means either 'horn, skin', e.g. *keratinocyte*, or 'cornea', e.g. *keratitis*.

keratoacanthoma a striking benign keratinocyte tumour characterized by a period of rapid growth of a lesion that may be 4 or 5 cm across or even larger, with a central keratin plug in a dome-shaped nodule. The tumour is most common on the face, back of the hands and the arms. Spontaneous resolution occurs but may take months and often results in an unsightly scar which could be improved by excision of the lesion. Clinically and histologically the lesion resembles a squamous cell carcinoma but it shows a different natural history. If there is any doubt, lesions are better managed as squamous cell carcinomas. A positive diagnosis of keratoacanthoma requires a large biopsy reflecting the architecture of the lesion is required. ⊃ squamous cell carcinoma (SCC).

keratocele (*syn* descemetocele) the herniation of Descemet's membrane through a structural defect in the cornea such as that caused by an ulcer.

keratoconjunctivitis *n* inflammation of the cornea and conjunctiva. ⊃ actinic keratoconjunctivitis, epidemic keratoconjunctivitis, keratitis sicca, keratoconjunctivitis sicca.

keratoconjunctivitis sicca (KCS) dry eye, including in Sjögren syndrome. ⊃ keratitis sicca, Sjögren syndrome.

keratoconus (KC) *n* (*syn* conical cornea) a developmental anomaly in which the central portion of the cornea becomes thinner and bulges forward in a cone-shaped fashion. Two types of cones are commonly described: a round cone and an oval (or sagging) cone. It usually appears around puberty, is bilateral, although one eye may be involved long before the other. Other corneal signs may be Vogt's striae, Fleischer's ring, scarring and fluid accumulation within the corneal stroma, as well as myopia and irregular astigmatism. The condition may be associated with osteogenesis imperfecta, ectopia lentis, aniridia, retinitis pigmentosa, Down's syndrome, Ehlers–Danlos syndrome, Marfan's syndrome. The main symptom is a loss of visual acuity due to irregular astigmatism and myopia. Correction is usually best achieved with contact lenses, especially rigid gas permeable, but if these cannot be worn or the condition is very severe, a corneal transplant is carried out. ⊃ central corneal clouding, combination lens, ectasia, Ehlers–Danlos syndrome, Fleischer's ring, keratoplasty, keratoscope, Marfan's syndrome, piggyback lens, striae, Vogt's striae, Colour Section Figure 82.

keratoderma blennorrhagica ⊃ keratosis blennorrhagica.

keratoectasia also called kerectasis. A forward bulge or protrusion affecting the cornea.

keratoglobus (*syn* macrocornea, megalocornea) a rare, bilateral corneal ectasia, especially near the limbus. The condition is usually present at birth and generally does not progress. The diameter of the cornea is normal or slightly increased and the intraocular pressure is normal as the condition is not associated with congenital glaucoma. Complications include perforation after minor trauma and corneal hydrops. It is sometimes associated with Leber's congenital amaurosis, Ehlers–Danlos syndrome and blue sclera. ⊃ Leber's congenital amaurosis, megalophthalmos.

keratolytic *adj* having the property of breaking down keratinized epidermis.

keratoma *n* ⊃ callosity—**keratomata** *pl*.

keratomalacia *n* frequently caused by lack of vitamin A, there is keratinization of corneal and conjunctival epithelia with loss of mucin-producing cells. May lead to corneal ulceration, secondary infection and corneal perforation.

keratome *n* a special knife for incising the cornea.

keratometer/ophthalmometer an optical instrument for measuring the radius of curvature of the cornea in any meridian. By measuring along the two principal meridians, corneal astigmatism can be deduced. The principle is based on the reflection by the anterior surface of a luminous pattern of mires in the centre of the cornea in an area of about 3.6 mm in diameter. Knowing the size of the pattern h and measuring that of the reflected image h' and the distance d between the two, the radius of curvature r of the cornea can be determined using the approximate formula

$$r = 2d \times \frac{h}{h'}$$

In addition, a doubling system (e.g. a bi-prism) is also integrated into the instrument in order to mitigate the effect of eye movements, as well as a microscope in order to magnify the small image reflected by the cornea. This instrument is used in the fitting of contact lenses and the monitoring of corneal changes occurring as a result of contact lens wear. The range of the instrument can be extended approximately 9D by placing a +1.25D lens in front of the objective to measure steeper corneas. The range in the other direction can be extended by approximately 6D using a −1.00D lens to measure flatter corneas. ⊃ keratoscope, liquid lens, photokeratoscopy, Topogometer, videokeratoscope.

keratomileusis (*syn* refractive keratoplasty, keratorefractive surgery) both terms also include epikeratoplasty, keratophakia and radial keratotomy. A surgical procedure on the cornea aimed at curing ametropia. An anterior layer of the cornea is sliced off with a microkeratome, frozen, ground to a new curvature and sutured back in the same location. There are many complications and technical difficulties associated with this procedure. ⊃ epikeratoplasty, keratome, keratophakia, LASIK, radial keratotomy.

keratomycosis a fungal infection of the cornea which may result in keratitis and ulceration. It is usually introduced by injury and is characterized by an ulcer which appears as a fluffy white elevated protuberance surrounded by a shallow crater on the edge of which is a sharply demarcated halo. There is ciliary and conjunctival injection. Diagnosis is best provided by laboratory analysis of a specimen of these fungal organisms which are obtained by scraping the base of the ulcer. ⊃ ciliary injection, conjunctival injection, corneal ulcer, hypopyon, keratitis.

keratophakia (*syn* refractive keratoplasty, keratorefractive surgery) both terms also include epikeratoplasty, keratomileusis and radial keratotomy. A surgical procedure on the cornea aimed at curing ametropia. A donor corneal disc (or lenticule) that was previously frozen and reshaped is inserted into the host cornea to modify the anterior corneal curvature. There are many complications and technical difficulties associated with this procedure. ⊃ epikeratoplasty, Intacs, keratomileusis, LASIK, lenticule, radial keratotomy.

keratopathy *n* any non-inflammatory disease of the cornea. ⊃ bullous keratopathy.

keratoplasty *n* ⊃ corneal graft/transplant.

keratoprosthesis *n* artificial cornea.

keratoreformation the process of improving vision following radial keratotomy by correcting a residual ametropia and an irregular corneal topography. This is usually accomplished by contact lenses. ⊃ radial keratotomy.

keratorefractive surgery ⊃ epikeratoplasty, Intacs, keratomileusis, keratophakia, keratotomy, LASIK, radial keratotomy, refractive keratoplasty.

keratoscope (*syn* Placido disc) an instrument for examining the front surface of the cornea. It consists of a pattern of alternately black and white concentric rings reflected by the cornea and seen through a convex lens mounted in an aperture at the centre of the pattern (Figure K.1). Such an instrument gives a qualitative evaluation of large corneal astigmatism, and is useful in cases of irregular astigmatism as in keratoconus, for example. ⊃ keratoconus, photokeratoscopy.

keratosis *n* thickening of the horny layer of the skin. Also referred to as hyperkeratosis. Has the appearance of warty excrescences.

keratosis blennorrhagica pustules and crusts present on the skin of the palms, soles, trunk, scrotum and scalp. It is associated with reactive arthritis and sexually acquired reactive arthritis (Reiter's syndrome).

keratosis palmaris et plantaris (*syn* tylosis) a congenital thickening of the horny layer of the palms and soles.

keratotomy an incision into the cornea.

keratouveitis *n* inflammation of the cornea and uvea (uveal tract—iris, ciliary body and choroid), often due to infection.

kerion *n* a boggy suppurative mass of the scalp associated with ringworm.

kerma kinetic energy released per unit mass of an absorber, unit joules per kilogram or grays.

kernicterus *n* staining of brain cells, especially the basal nuclei with bilirubin. It is a complication of jaundice affecting preterm babies and haemolytic disease of the newborn. It can lead to a severe encephalopathy with resultant learning disabilities.

Kernig's sign (V Kernig, Russian physician, 1840–1917) a sign of meningeal irritation such as occurs in meningitis. The patient is unable to straighten the leg at the knee when the thigh is flexed at right angles to the trunk. There is pain in the lower back and resistance to leg straightening.

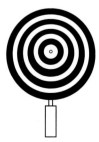

K.1 **Keratoscope** (reproduced from Millodot 2004 with permission).

Keshan's disease a condition that occurs in some areas of China where a deficiency of selenium exists. There is cardiomyopathy and hypothyroidism affecting children.

ketoacidosis *n* (*syn* ketosis) metabolic acidosis due to accumulation of ketone bodies, (β-hydroxybutyric acid, acetoacetic acid and acetone), products of the metabolism of fat. Primarily a serious complication of type 1 diabetes, but also occurs in starvation and rarely in alcohol misuse. Symptoms include drowsiness, headache and deep sighing respiration (Kussmaul's). *diabetic ketoacidosis* ketone bodies are formed as fatty acids and are incompletely oxidized when glucose is unavailable as an energy source. Acidosis and dehydration accompany hyperglycaemia. ⊃ Kussmaul's respiration.

ketogenesis the formation of ketone bodies.

ketogenic diet a high fat, low carbohydrate diet that produces ketosis (acidosis).

ketonaemia *n* ketone bodies in the blood—**ketonaemic** *adj*.

ketone bodies include acetone, acetoacetate (acetoacetic acid) and β-hydroxybutyric acid produced normally during fat oxidation. Can be used as fuel but excess production leads to ketoacidosis. This may occur when blood glucose level is high, but unavailable for metabolism, as in poorly controlled diabetes mellitus.

ketones *npl* organic compounds (e.g. ketosteroids) containing a keto group.

ketonuria *n* ketone bodies in the urine—**ketonuric** *adj*.

ketose a monosaccharide that contains a ketone group, for example the hexose fructose.

ketosis *n* ⊃ ketoacidosis.

ketosteroids *npl* adrenal corticosteroid hormones that contain a ketone group. The 17-ketosteroids are normally present in the blood and excreted in urine and are present in excess in overactivity of the adrenal glands and the gonads.

keV the energy given to an electron when passing through a potential difference of 1 kilovolt in a vacuum.

keyboard a microprocessor with a range of keys which when depressed send an electrical code to a computer which then displays the appropriate image on a monitor or carries out an appropriate action.

key hole surgery ⊃ minimally invasive surgery.

key points of control described by Bobath (1990) as areas of the body from which movement can most easily be controlled. A point in the upper thoracic region is described as the central key point, the pelvis and shoulder girdles as the proximal key points and the hands and feet as distal key points. (Bobath B 1990 Adult hemiplegia: evaluation and treatment, 3rd edn. Heinemann Medical Books, Oxford.)

keyway ⊃ dovetail (keyway).

K-file a tapered, flexible endodontic file, traditionally created by twisting lengths of square or triangular cross-section wire. Used in rotational or rasping motions to negotiate and enlarge root canals.

khat *n* also called chat, miraa, qat, etc. It is obtained from the leaves of the tree *Catha edulis* that grows in the Arabian peninsula and Africa. Khat contains psychostimulants structurally similar to amfetamine. Chewing the leaves is a widespread habit in East Africa and the Middle East. Its effects include excitement, talkativeness and feelings of euphoria. However, users may become hyperactive and serious mental health disturbances can occur. It is becoming increasingly available in the UK.

KHN *abbr* Knoop hardness scale/number.

kick chart fetal movement chart on which the woman subjectively records fetal movements over a given period of time. It is usually used in conjunction with other tests for fetal wellbeing.

kidney *n* paired retroperitoneal organs situated on the upper posterior abdominal wall in the lumbar region. ⊃ Colour Section Figures 19, 20. Vital in the maintenance of homeostasis by the production of urine in the nephrons, the microscopic functional units (comprising the glomerulus and renal tubule). This involves three processes: filtration of the blood contents, reabsorption of substances (e.g. glucose) needed by the body and secretion of unwanted substances. Urine production is vital in the excretion of nitrogenous waste products such as urea and other waste substances including drug residues, the control and maintenance of fluid balance and electrolyte balance and the maintenance of acid–base balance. The kidneys also secrete renin which is important in the control of blood pressure. In addition the kidneys produce erythropoietin, which stimulates the production of red blood cells (erythrocytes) in the bone marrow. Also involved in the metabolism of vitamin D. ⊃ horseshoe kidney.

kidney failure inability of the kidneys to maintain normal function. ⊃ renal failure.

kidney function tests a series of tests that include: routine urine testing, urine concentration/dilution tests, serum urea and electrolytes, serum creatinine and renal clearance to estimate glomerular filtration rate (GFR).

kidney machine (artificial kidney) the machine used to remove waste products from the blood in the case of renal failure and sometimes to remove poisons or toxic substances. ⊃ dialyser.

kidney transplant surgical transplantation of a kidney from a previously tested suitable live donor or a cadaveric organ. Kidneys may also be transplanted from the renal bed to other sites in the same individual in cases of ureteric disease or trauma.

Kielland's forceps (C Kielland, Norwegian obstetrician, 19th century) obstetric forceps with a sliding lock and no pelvic curve, to enable rotation of the fetal head from any position in the pelvis to an occipitoanterior position. ⊃ deep transverse arrest.

Kieselguhr ⊃ diatomaceous earth.

Kiesselbach's plexus (W Kiesselbach, German laryngologist, 1839–1902) a plexus of small blood vessels located on the anterior nasal septum. A common site of bleeding from the nose. ⊃ epistaxis, Little's area.

killers impurities added to the intensifying screen crystal to control after-glow.

kilocalorie (kcal) *n* one thousand calories. ⊃ calorie, kilojoule.

kilogram (kg) *n* one of the seven base units of the Système International d'Unités (SI) system (International System of Units). A measurement of mass. ⊃ Appendix 2.

kilojoule (kJ) *n* a unit equal to 1000 joules. It is used to measure large amounts of energy. It replaces the kilocalorie (kcal) which is still commonly used. ⊃ calorie.

kilovolt (kV) a potential difference of 1000 V. The kilovoltage determines the quality of radiation produced by the X-ray tube and thus the qualities of the final radiograph.

kilovoltage peak (kV$_p$) the maximum kilovoltage applied across an X-ray tube in a forward direction during an exposure.

kilovoltage treatment unit radiotherapy units operating in the region of either 50–150 kV for the treatment of external, superficial lesions or 150–300 kV for the treatment of metastatic bone lesions and some primary bone lesions.

kinaesthesis *n* muscle sense; perception of movement—**kinaesthetic** *adj*.

kinaesthetic imagery ⊃ imagery.

kinaesthetic sense the ability to sense body position, weight and movement. Being able to differentiate between static positions and joint action. It involves receptors in structures that include muscles, tendons and joints. ⊃ proprioception.

kinanaesthesia 1. loss of the ability to sense movement. **2.** decreased awareness of the position or movement of part of the body.

kinanthropometry *n* the utilization of a combination of anthropometry and kinesiology.

kinase *n* **1.** an enzyme activator that converts a zymogen (proenzyme) to the active form of the enzyme. **2.** enzymes that catalyze the transfer of a high-energy group of a donor, usually adenosine triphosphate (ATP), to some acceptor, usually named after the acceptor, such as fructokinase.

kin/e, kinesi/o, kin/o- a prefix that means 'motion, movement', e.g. *kinematics.*

kinematic chain exercises an engineering term that describes a system of links coupled by joints. They may be open or closed. ⊃ closed kinetic chain, open kinetic chain.

kinematic face-bow a face-bow used in conjunction with an articulator in the construction of prostheses. The ends can be adjusted to permit location of the axis of rotation of the mandible.

kinematic feedback ⊃ knowledge of performance.

kinematics the study (and measurement) of motion. ⊃ angular kinematics, linear kinematics.

kineplastic surgery operative measures, whereby certain muscle groups are isolated and used to work a modified prosthesis.

kinesiology *n* the study of muscle activity that brings together the anatomy, physiology and biomechanics of parts of the body.

-kinesis, kinetic a suffix that means 'motion', e.g. *dyskinetic.*

kinetic *adj* relating to or producing motion.

kinetic energy the energy possessed by a body or object due to movement. Can be translational or rotational (or both). ⊃ rotational kinetic energy, translational kinetic energy.

kinetics the study (and measurement) of forces and moments (torques). ⊃ angular kinetics, linear kinetics.

kinetic tremor an oscillation that occurs during movement.

kinins *npl* biologically active proteins and polypeptides such as bradykinin that cause vasodilation, increased vessel permeability, smooth muscle contraction, pain, etc.

Kirschner wire (M Kirschner, German surgeon, 1879–1942) a wire drilled into a bone to apply skeletal traction. A hand or electric drill is used, a stirrup is attached and the wire is rendered taut by means of a special wire-tightener.

kJ *abbr* kilojoule.

Klebsiella *n* (T Klebs, German bacteriologist, 1834–1913) a genus of anaerobic Gram-negative non-motile bacteria belonging to the family Enterobacteriaceae. They form part of the normal flora of the mouth and in the gut. They are opportunists and may affect immunocompromised individuals. They are commonly the cause of healthcare-associated infections of the urinary tract, respiratory tract and wounds. Some strains are resistant to many antibiotics. *Klebsiella pneumoniae* causes serious pneumonia in critically ill patients needing respiratory support.

Kleihauer test blood test used to confirm presence of fetal cells in maternal circulation following antepartum haemorrhage, placental abruption and other events. False negative results may occur if there is haemolysis of fetal cells in the maternal circulation, such as following Rhesus sensitization.

Kleine–Levin syndrome (W Kleine, German psychiatrist, 20th century; M Levin, American neurologist, 20th century) a rare episodic condition characterized by periods of extreme sleepiness and excessive eating.

kleptomania a strong impulse to steal.

Klinefelter's syndrome (H Klinefelter, American physician, b.1912) a chromosomal abnormality affecting boys. A type of genetic mosaicism, in which there is an extra X chromosome in at least one cell population. The commonest form is XXY in which the boy/man has 47 chromosomes, but some have more X chromosomes. Puberty is frequently delayed, with small firm testes, often with gynaecomastia. Associated with sterility, which may be the only symptom. The multiple X chromosome forms tend to have other abnormalities and learning disability. ⊃ mosaicism.

Klumpke's paralysis (A Déjérine-Klumpke, French neurologist, 1859–1927) paralysis and atrophy of forearm and hand muscles, caused by a birth injury. May be accompanied by Horner's syndrome with sensory and pupillary disturbances due to injury to lower roots of brachial plexus and cervical sympathetic nerves. Claw-hand results.

klystron a microwave device which amplifies the power of radiofrequency radiation. When used with a radiofrequency driver it acts as the radiofrequency power source in some linear accelerators.

knee *n* the knee is the largest and most complex joint. It is a hinge joint formed by the condyles of the femur, the condyles of the tibia and the posterior surface of the patella. The anterior part of the capsule is formed by the tendon of the quadriceps femoris muscle, which also supports the patella. Intracapsular structures include two cruciate ligaments that cross each other, extending from the intercondylar notch of the femur to the intercondylar eminence of the tibia (see Figure A.11, p. 49). They help to stabilize the joint. Semilunar cartilages or menisci are incomplete discs of white fibrocartilage lying on top of the articular condyles of the tibia. They are wedge shaped, being thicker at their outer edges, and provide stability (see Figure M.5, p. 475). They help to prevent lateral displacement of the bones, and cushion the moving joint by shifting within the joint space according to the relative positions of the articulating bones. Bursae and pads of fat are numerous. They prevent friction between a bone and a ligament or tendon and between the skin and the patella. Synovial membrane covers the cruciate ligaments and the pads of fat. The menisci are not covered with synovial membrane because they are weight bearing. External ligaments of the joint provide further support. The main ligaments are the patellar ligament, an extension of the quadriceps femoris tendon, the popliteal ligaments at the back of the knee and the collateral ligaments to each side. However, the knee is the joint most commonly injured in sport due to its relative instability and mobility. Possible movements at the knee are flexion, extension and a rotatory movement which 'locks' the joint when it is fully extended. When the joint is locked, balance is maintained with less muscular effort than when it is flexed. Thus, it is possible to stand upright for long periods without tiring the knee extensors. The main muscles extending the knee are the four muscles of the quadriceps femoris group (rectus femoris, vastus lateralis, vastus medialis and vastus intermedius). The main muscles flexing the knee are the gastrocnemius and the three muscles of the hamstring group (biceps femoris, semitendinosus, semimembranosus). ⊃ cruciate ligaments, iliotibial band, meniscus, patella, Colour Section Figure 31.

knee injury knee injuries associated with sport can be complex, involving the bones, ligaments, tendons and cartilages (menisci), and can result from both trauma and overuse.

knee jerk reflex (*syn* patellar reflex) reflex extension at the knee in response to tapping the tendon between the patella and the tibia; this stretches quadriceps muscle spindles, whence afferents to the spinal cord elicit transient reflex contraction. Elicited by a tap on the patellar tendon: usually performed with the lower femur supported behind, the knee bent and the leg limp. Tests the integrity and function of the relevant peripheral nerves and lumbar spinal segments. Persistent variation from normal usually signifies organic nervous disorder. ⊃ tendon jerk reflex.

knee presentation type of breech presentation with one or both knees below the buttocks.

knock knees ⊃ genu valgum.

Knoop hardness scale or number (KHN) ⊃ hardness scale.

knowledge classified in psychology as (a) declarative knowledge awareness of factual information; (b) procedural knowledge of how to perform a task.

knowledge of performance (KP) 1. in motor learning, feedback or information about the correct production or patterning of a movement, such as when a coach gives a gymnast feedback about the form of a movement. Also known as kinematic feedback. **2.** a term used to describe the patient's awareness of how the movement was performed. Reference to this term is made in the 'motor relearning approach' (Carr and Shepherd 1998) to the management and treatment of neurological patients. (Carr J, Shepherd R 1998 Neurological Rehabilitation: Optimizing Motor Performance. Butterworth Heinemann, Edinburgh.)

knowledge of results (KR) 1. in motor learning, feedback about the success of an action with respect to the goal of that movement, such as when an archer *sees* his or her arrow hit the target. **2.** improved information provided about success or mistakes made in achieving functional movements. It is a term used to describe the patient's awareness of the achievement, or not, or of the task. Reference to this term is made in the 'motor relearning approach' (Carr and Shepherd 1998) to the management and treatment of neurological patients. (Carr J, Shepherd R 1998 Neurological Rehabilitation: Optimizing Motor Performance. Butterworth Heinemann, Edinburgh.)

knuckles *npl* the dorsal aspect of any of the joints between the phalanges and the metacarpal bones, or between the phalanges.

Kocher's incision (E Kocher, Swiss surgeon, 1841–1917) an oblique incision in the right upper abdomen previously used for removal of the gallbladder during an open cholecystectomy. ⊃ minimally invasive surgery

Kocher's manoeuvre (E Kocher) a manoeuvre used to reduce a dislocation of the shoulder joint.

Koebner phenomenon (H Koebner, Polish dermatologist, 1838–1904) induction of a lesion of certain skin diseases, e.g. psoriasis, following non-specific trauma to the skin.

Koeppe's nodules small nodules frequently found on the iris around the pupillary margin of an eye affected by granulomatous uveitis. ⊃ Busacca's nodules, iris nodules, uveitis.

Köhler's disease (A Köhler, German physician, 1874–1947) osteochondritis of the navicular bone. Confined to children of 3–5 years.

koilonychia *n* spoon-shaped nails. The normal convex curvature of the nail is lost and it becomes slightly concave. It is more common in fingernails than toenails and is associated with iron deficiency anaemia.

Kollner's rule (*syn* Kollner's law) lesions of the outer retinal layers and changes in the ocular media produce a blue-yellow colour vision defect, whereas lesions of the inner retinal layers, the optic nerve and the visual pathway produce a red-green defect. Examples include: age-related maculopathy causes a blue-yellow defect; optic neuritis causes a red-green defect. There are exceptions to this rule, particularly during the evolution of a disease.

König bars target used to measure visual acuity consisting of two bars on a white background. The length of each bar is usually three times its width but the space between the bars is always equal to the width of one bar. The smallest pair of bars that can be perceived as separate gives a measure of the acuity. ⊃ ototype, visual acuity.

Koplik's spots (H Koplik, American paediatrician, 1858–1927) small white spots inside the mouth, during the first few days of the invasion (prodromal) stage of measles. ⊃ Colour Section Figure 83.

Korotkoff (Korotkov) sounds (N Korotkoff [Korotkov], Russian physician/surgeon, 1874–1920) the sounds audible when recording non-invasive arterial blood pressure with a sphygmomanometer and stethoscope. The phases are: (1) a sharp thud—systolic pressure, (2) a swishing/blowing sound, (3) sharper noise but softer than in phase 1, (4) a soft blowing that becomes muffled, (5) silence (Figure K.2). In the UK the diastolic pressure is normally recorded at the end of phase 4.

Korsakoff's (Korsakov's) syndrome (S Korsakoff [Korsakov], Russian psychiatrist, 1854–1900) chronic amnesia (defect of retrieval of recently acquired information) with denial, lack of insight and confabulation. ⊃ amnesic syndrome, Wernicke's encephalopathy.

kosher *n* the choice and preparation of foods which comply with the dietary laws of Judaism. Certain cuts of meat from cud-chewing animals with cloven hoofs, e.g. sheep, goats, cattle and deer are permitted. The only fish allowed are those with scales and fins. In addition animals must be slaughtered

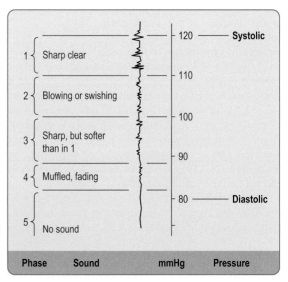

K.2 Korotkoff (Korotkov) sounds (adapted from Hinchliff et al 1996 with permission).

according to the rituals of Judaism. A food that is not kosher is termed traife. ⊃ pareve.

KP *abbr* **1.** keratic precipitates. **2.** knowledge of performance.

KR *abbr* knowledge of results.

Krabbe disease (K Krabbe, Danish neurologist, 1885–1965) genetically determined disorder of lipid metabolism that leads to degenerative changes in the central nervous system. It is associated with learning disability.

kraurosis vulvae a degenerative condition of the vaginal introitus associated with postmenopausal lack of oestrogen.

Krause's end bulbs (K Krause, German anatomist, 1797–1868) nerve endings enclosed by a capsule from 0.02 mm to 0.1 mm in length. They probably act as cold receptors. Their regular presence in the corneal limbus has been questioned. ⊃ conjunctiva, corneal limbus.

Krause's glands (K Krause) accessory lacrimal glands of the conjunctiva having the same structure as the main lacrimal gland. They are located in the subconjunctival connective tissue of the fornix, especially the superior fornix.

Krebs' cycle (*syn* citric acid cycle, tricarboxylic acid cycle) (H Krebs, British biochemist, 1900–1981) a sequence of reactions occurring within the mitochondria. It is the final common pathway for the oxidation of fuel molecules: glucose, fatty acids, glycerol and amino acids. Carbon atoms enter the cycle as acetyl-CoA and emerge as carbon dioxide, and the electrons produced are transferred to the electron transport chain. Also provides intermediates for biosynthetic processes. ⊃ electron transport chain, oxidative phosphorylation.

Kromayer's lamp (E Kromayer, German dermatologist, 1862–1933) a type of mercury vapour ultra-violet ray (UVR) lamp. The UV tube is water cooled to remove infrared radiations so applicator used in contact with skin or in cavities using special applicator.

Krukenberg tumour (F Krukenberg, German pathologist, 1871–1946) a secondary (metastatic) malignant tumour of the ovary, usually spread from primary stomach (gastric) cancer.

krypton (Kr) an inert gas. Its radioactive isotope krypton-81 m (^{81m}Kr) is used in lung ventilation scans.

krypton laser a laser with krypton gas ionized by electric current as the active medium which emits a light beam in the yellow-red region of the visible spectrum (521 nm, 568 nm or 647 nm). It may be used to perform photocoagulation or trabeculoplasty.

K-space the space that is filled with information and undergoes Fourier transformation to form a magnetic resonance image. By manipulating the K-space, faster sequences can be implemented.

KUB *abbr* kidney, ureter and bladder.

Küntscher nail (G Küntscher, German surgeon, 1902–1972) used for intramedullary fixation of fractured long bones, especially the femur. The nail has a 'clover-leaf' cross-section.

Kupffer cells (K von Kupffer, German anatomist, 1829–1902) large phagocytic macrophages lining the sinusoids of the liver. Part of the monocyte-macrophage (reticuloendothelial) system they remove micro-organisms and 'old' red blood cells from the blood and destroy them by phagocytosis.

kuru *n* a fatal prion disease (a transmissible spongiform encephalopathy, TSE) with a very long incubation period of many years. It affects the central nervous system and causes dementia, slurred speech, ataxia and paralysis. Probably transmitted by cannibalism. Rare and declining in incidence since the cessation of rituals involving cannibilism of brain tissue. Occurred exclusively among New Guinea highlanders. ⊃ Creutzfeld–Jakob disease.

Kussmaul's respiration (A Kussmaul, German physician, 1822–1902) deep sighing respiration typical of diabetic ketoacidosis.

Kveim test (M Kveim, Norwegian physician, 1892–1966) an intracutaneous test for sarcoidosis using tissue prepared from a person known to be suffering from the condition.

kV$_p$ *abbr* kilovotage peak.

kwashiorkor *n* a nutritional disorder of infants and young children associated with poverty, deprivation and infection. Develops when the diet is deficient in protein; may develop at weaning when a low protein starchy porridge is fed instead of breast milk. Characteristic features are anaemia, muscle wasting, loss of appetite, pale thin hair, oedema and a fatty liver.

Kwok's syndrome ⊃ Chinese restaurant syndrome.

Kyasanur forest disease a viral disease transmitted by ticks in parts of India. It causes headache, myalgia, fever, cough, photophobia and conjunctivitis.

kymograph *n* an apparatus for recording movements, e.g. of muscles, columns of blood. Used in physiological experiments—**kymographic** *adj*, **kymographically** *adv*.

kypho- a prefix that means 'rounded, humped', e.g. *kyphosis*.

kypholordosis *n* coexistence of kyphosis and lordosis.

kyphoscoliosis *n* coexistence of kyphosis and scoliosis. May prevent proper lung expansion and lead to respiratory problems.

kyphosis *n* as in Pott's disease, an exaggerated backward curvature of the thoracic spine in the flexion/extension axis. May be congenital or related to poor posture, especially in adolescent girls, resulting in discomfort. An exercise programme can usually correct postural kyphosis. Scheuermann's kyphosis results from a developmental defect that causes wedging of the vertebrae; it is more common in boys, is diagnosed on X-ray and requires surgical correction. In older people it is commonly associated with osteoporosis. This may result in a restrictive lung defect as detected by spirometry. If fixed as opposed to adaptive/compensatory then seating and cushions need to be adjusted to ensure appropriate support—**kyphotic** *adj*. ⊃ osteoporosis, Scheuermann's disease.

K
L

LA *abbr* left atrium.

LABAs *abbr* long-acting β₂ agonists.

labelling theory process by which socially defined labels or identities are assigned or accepted. Often linked with deviant behaviour and can make it hard for people to escape that identity. It is a long-standing and much discussed and criticized sociological theory. The central assumption is that deviance is created by society in that social groups create rules and those who infringe these rules are labelled as outsiders. Precisely who is labelled and why depends on the social context. Behaviour may, for example, be considered criminal at one time or in one culture but not at another time or in another culture. Patients and clients may be labelled 'difficult' if they do not comply with the wishes of health professionals.

labia *npl* lips—**labium** *sing*, **labial** *adj*.

labia majora ('greater lips') the two large lip-like folds of fat and areolar tissue, covered with skin and pubic hair on the outer surface. They arise in the mons veneris and merge into the perineum behind to form the vulva.

labia minora ('lesser lips') two thin folds of skin lying within the labia majora. Anteriorly they divide to enclose the clitoris; posteriorly they fuse, forming the fourchette.

labial pertaining to the labia.

labial bar a major connector of a mandibular partial denture which is placed between the reflection of the labial sulcus and the gingival margin.

labial (buccal) adjacent to the lips or cheeks.

labial frenulum ➲ frenulum or frenum.

labial surface a surface in contact with the lip. ➲ surface.

labile *adj* unstable; readily changed, as many drugs when in solution; mood in some mental health problems and blood pressure.

labile factor (proaccelerin) *n* factor V in the blood coagulation cascade. It is produced in the liver and is required for the formation of prothrombin activator. A very rare inherited (autosomal recessive) deficiency leads to a bleeding disorder

lability *n* instability. *emotional lability* rapid changes in mood.

labioglossolaryngeal *adj* relating to the lips, tongue and larynx.

labioglossolaryngeal paralysis ➲ bulbar palsy or paralysis.

labioplasty ➲ cheiloplasty.

laboratory putty a multipurpose vinyl polysiloxane material consisting of a base and a catalyst, which is mixed together by hand, used for a wide variety of applications in the dental laboratory such as matrices.

labour *n* (*syn* parturition) the act of giving birth to a child. Normal labour occurs spontaneously between 37 and 43 weeks' gestation, single fetus, vertex presentation, completed within 24 hours without maternal or fetal trauma; interaction between uterine action, maternal pelvis and fetus. In the first stage cervical effacement and dilatation occur; contractions are fundally dominant; uterine polarity facilitates contraction and retraction in upper uterine segment and contraction and dilatation in lower uterine segment. The second stage is from full dilatation of the cervix until complete delivery of the baby. The third stage involves separation and expulsion of placenta and membranes and control of haemorrhage. ➲ augmentation of labour, mechanism of labour, obstructed labour, precipitate labour, preterm labour/birth, spontaneous labour, spurious labour.

labour coach a person who assists a woman in labour and delivery by encouraging her to use previously taught techniques such as breathing patterns, concentration, positions, and the employment of massage.

labrale inferius the lowest point in the midline on the vermillion margin of the lower lip.

labrale superius the uppermost point in the midline of the vermillion margin of the upper lip.

labrum anatomical term meaning edge, rim or lip. Formed from fibrocartilage, it serves to deepen the socket and aids joint stability. For example, the labrum of the acetabulum and the one of the glenoid cavity. ➲ acetabular labrum.

labyrinth *n* the convoluted cavities of the inner ear including the cochlea and semicircular canals which form the organs concerned with hearing and balance/position sense (vestibular system which responds to changes in head position). The vestibular system conveys information about changes in head position to the muscles that move the eyes, which allows continuous visual focus when the head moves. *bony labyrinth* that part which is directly hollowed out of the temporal bone. *membranous labyrinth* the membrane lining the bony labyrinth—**labyrinthine** *adj*.

labyrinthectomy *n* surgical removal of part or the whole of the membranous labyrinth of the inner ear. Sometimes carried out for Ménière's disease.

labyrinthine righting reflexes stimulation of the labyrinth proprioceptors causes contraction of the neck muscles which bring the head back into its natural position in space.

labyrinthitis *n* inflammation of the inner ear resulting in disturbance of balance and co-ordination. Most commonly caused by viral infection but other causes include bacterial infection, side-effects of some drugs or following head injury. It causes vertigo with dizziness, loss of balance, nausea and vomiting especially on head movement. Nystagmus may be observed and hearing loss and tinnitus may also occur. Recovery may take some weeks and exercise and sport should be avoided until symptoms have resolved completely. ⊃ ear, vertigo, vestibular apparatus, vestibular rehabilitation.

laceration *n* a wound in which the tissues are torn usually by a blunt instrument or pressure: more likely to become infected and to heal by second intention. ⊃ wound healing.

Lachman's test (modified anterior drawer test) an assessment of the integrity of the anterior cruciate ligament and the diagnosis of anterior cruciate ligament injury. It is useful as it removes the limitation of the anterior drawer when the hamstrings contract, but is sometimes difficult to perform in athletes with well-developed musculature or where the examiner has small hands. The person is supine with the knee resting over the practitioner's thigh at around 20–30° of flexion. The practitioner grasps around the medial proximal aspect of the tibia with the right hand. The lateral aspect of the person's femur is stabilized by the practitioner's left hand. Anterior and posterior translation of the tibia is produced by the practitioner's right hand. The test is graded on the magnitude of movement and whether there is a firm or soft endpoint. The Lachman test has been shown to be a sensitive test for the diagnosis of anterior cruciate injury (Kim and Kim 1995). ⊃ anterior (PA) drawer test. (Kim SJ, Kim HK 1995 Reliability of the anterior drawer test, the pivot shift test, and the Lachman test. Clin Orthop 317: 237–242.)

lacrimal, lachrymal, lacrymal *adj* pertaining to tears.

lacrimal apparatus the lacrimal glands, ducts, sacs and canaliculi involved in the production and drainage of tears (Figure L.1).

lacrimal bone a tiny bone at the inner side of the orbital cavity.

lacrimal duct tiny ducts that connect the lacrimal gland to the upper conjunctival sac.

lacrimal fluid ⊃ tears.

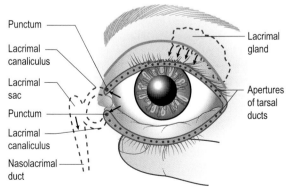

L.1 Lacrimal apparatus (reproduced from Watson 2000 with permission).

lacrimal gland situated above the upper, lateral canthus of the eye. It produces tears as a continuous process to provide a protective multilayer fluid film across the front of the eyeball. Excess production of tears occurs in response to the presence of foreign bodies, eye injury, inflammation and intense emotions. ⊃ dacryocyst.

lacrimal layer ⊃ precorneal film.

lacrimal lens ⊃ liquid lens.

lacrimal prism ⊃ tear meniscus.

lacrimation *n* a flow of tears; weeping. ⊃ alacrima, hyperlacrimation.

lacrimonasal *adj* pertaining to the lacrimal and nasal bones and ducts.

lactacid (lactic) anaerobic system a series of chemical reactions occurring within the cells whereby a very small amount of adenosine triphosphate (ATP) for energy use is produced from glucose, without oxygen. The end product being lactic acid.

lactacid oxygen debt component the amount of oxygen required to remove lactic acid from muscle tissue and blood after intense exercise; constitutes the slow phase of return to resting condition.

lactalbumin *n* one of the whey proteins found in milk. The proportion of protein as lactalbumin is higher in human milk than cows' milk.

lactase *n* (*syn* β-galactosidase) digestive enzyme present in the small intestine mucosa. It catalyses the hydrolysis of lactose to glucose and galactose.

lactase deficiency an inherited or acquired deficiency of lactase. Common in African Caribbean and Asian individuals. Consumption of lactose (milk sugar) results in colic, diarrhoea, bloating and increased flatus. May be acquired in small intestinal conditions such as coeliac disease and Crohn's disease. It may occur temporarily after a gastrointestinal tract infection. The management depends on severity and may involve the exclusion or restriction of lactose-containing foods. Various lactose-free products, such as infant formula milks, are available on prescription in the UK.

lactate the anion of lactic acid and its salts, although the term 'lactate' is commonly, but incorrectly, used interchangeably with 'lactic acid' itself. At rest and during prolonged moderate exercise, lactate level in the blood is low (0.7–1.4 mmol/L). In short-term, high-intensity exercise, lactate production in muscles, and its efflux from them, exceeds its rate of removal from the circulating blood, causing a steep increase in the concentrations of lactate and of hydrogen ions [H$^+$] both in muscle itself and in the blood. Lactate measured in blood therefore reflects the balance between release from exercising muscles and uptake (by the liver, cardiac muscle and any skeletal muscle fibres which are not themselves under anaerobic stress). Contrary to earlier assumptions, lactate is not itself deleterious to most physiological processes and can be used as fuel by well-oxygenated cells, including muscle fibres, but accumulation of [H$^+$] in muscle fibres can slow glycolysis and interfere with force generation, while in the extracellular fluid it is thought to

K
L

contribute, at extremes, to the stimulation of pain receptors. The raised [H^+] in the blood acts as an additional stimulus to ventilation, but it impairs fat oxidation by reducing release of free fatty acids from adipose tissue. ➲ anaerobic exercise, metabolic and related thresholds, monocarboxylate transporters.

lactate analyser instrument for estimating the concentration of lactate in a sample of fluid, most often blood or plasma.

lactate dehydrogenase (LDH) an enzyme, of which there are five isoenzymes, that catalyses the interconversion of lactate and pyruvate in the myocardium, skeletal muscle and the liver. The cytoplasmic muscle enzyme catalyses the reduction of pyruvate to lactate when oxygen tension is low, and the converse when it is high. The level of lactate dehydrogenase in the serum increases rapidly following necrosis of metabolically active tissue, such as after myocardial infarction. The specific isoenzyme can be distinguished in blood when either skeletal or cardiac muscle is damaged. ➲ muscle enzymes.

lactate threshold (T_{LAC}, LT) minimum work rate at which blood lactate concentration [Lac]$_b$ is found to be significantly above (sometimes defined as 1 mmol/L above) resting value. ➲ metabolic and related thresholds.

lactation *n* **1.** production and secretion of milk from the breasts. **2.** the period during which an infant receives nourishment from breast milk.

lacteals *npl* the commencing lymphatic ducts in the intestinal villi; they absorb the milky-white fluid chyle that contains digested fats and convey them to the cisterna chyli.

lactic *adj* relating to milk.

lactic acid a three carbon organic acid formed by the reduction of pyruvic acid in the last step of anaerobic glycolysis; dissociates to form lactate and hydrogen ions [H^+]. It is produced when glucose is metabolized anaerobically in vigorously contracting skeletal muscle. Also produced during the fermentation of lactose (milk sugar). ➲ monocarboxylate transporters.

lactic acid system old term for anaerobic glycolysis, referring to the production of energy by this metabolic pathway in intensive exercise of duration less than about 2 min, or in the first 40 s or so of less intensive exercise before aerobic metabolism has been fully activated. ➲ anaerobic exercise, glycolysis.

lactic acidosis results from a build-up of lactic acid in the blood and consequent reduction in pH. It is associated with conditions that cause tissue hypoxia, such as shock caused by sepsis, respiratory failure, severe anaemia and poisoning with carbon monoxide. This type of acidosis is also seen in patients with type 2 diabetes mellitus who are treated with a biguanide hypoglycaemic drug such as metformin. Other causes include liver failure, toxins (e.g. alcohol) and some drugs (e.g. salicylates).

lactiferous *adj* conveying or secreting milk.

lactiferous glands the glandular tissue of the alveoli of the breast lobules produce milk when stimulated by the hormone prolactin.

lactiferous ducts/tubules convey milk from the breast lobes to the centre of the breast where they dilate to form temporary reservoirs for milk, these are often described as the *lactiferous sinuses (ampullae)* from which milk flows to the surface of the nipple.

lactifuge an agent that decreases the production and secretion of milk.

lactitol a bulk sweetener with approximately 0.4 times the sweetness of sucrose (beet or cane sugar). Used in sugar-free foods and confectionery. ➲ sweetener.

lact/o- a prefix that means 'milk', e.g. *lactation*.

Lactobacillus *n* a genus of non-pathogenic bacteria. A large Gram-positive rod which ferments carbohydrates, producing lactic acid. They form part of the normal flora of the body, such as in the intestinal tract or the vagina during the reproductive years. The bacteria grow best in slightly acid conditions, are common in the mouth and gut and are associated with dental caries. ➲ Döderlein's bacillus.

lactoferrin an iron-binding protein with antimicrobial properties. It is a component of non-specific (innate) body defences and is found in colostrum and mature breast milk, saliva, tears and in some white blood cells.

lactogenic *adj* stimulating milk production. ➲ prolactin.

lactoglobulin globulin occurring in milk.

lacto-ovovegetarian *adj* describes a diet consisting of milk, milk products, eggs, grain, pulses, fruit and vegetables, but no meat, poultry or fish.

lactose *n* milk sugar. A disaccharide of glucose and galactose found in all types of mammalian milk. Less soluble and less sweet than ordinary sugar. Lactose can be artificially processed and is often present in carbohydrate-rich, high-calorie drinks. Broken down to glucose and galactose in the small intestine by the action of the enzyme lactase. ➲ lactase deficiency.

lactose intolerance ➲ lactase deficiency.

lactosuria the presence of lactose in the urine.

lactovegetarian *adj* describes a diet consisting of milk, milk products, grain, pulses, fruit and vegetables, but no meat, poultry, fish or eggs.

lactulose *n* a disaccharide that is not absorbed and reaches the colon unchanged. Used as an osmotic laxative. ➲ Appendix 5.

lacuna *n* a space between cells; usually used in the description of bone—**lacunae** *pl*, **lacunar** *adj*.

LAD *acron* **L**eft **A**nterior **D**escending artery.

laetrile a substance obtained from apricot stones. It is mostly amygdalin (cyanide-containing glycoside) and was thought by some to have anticancer properties. Research to date has failed to demonstrate any benefits. Also known as 'vitamin B_{17}' although it is not a vitamin.

lagophthalmos a condition whereby the eyes do not fully close. There is increased risk of corneal damage.

Lagrange's law (*syn* Helmholtz's law of magnification, Lagrange's relation, Smith–Helmholtz law) in paraxial optics, the product of the index of refraction of image space n', the image size h' and the half-angle of the refracted cone in image space u' is equal to the product of the index of refraction of object space n, the object size h and the half-angle of the incident cone in object space u, i.e. $n'h'u'=$ nhu. ⊃ sign convention.

Lagrange's relation ⊃ Lagrange's law.

LAK cells *abbr* lymphokine-activated killer cells.

lallation **1.** speech disorder characterized by problems with pronunciation in which the person uses a child-like substitution of sounds, such as using 'l' in place of 'r' sounds. **2.** unintelligible, repetitive babbling such as in an infant. It may be a feature present in some people with a learning disability or in those with serious mental health problems.

Lamaze method (F Lamaze, French obstetrician, 1890–1957) method of preparation for natural childbirth by training mind and body to modify pain perception during labour and delivery.

lambda **1.** The eleventh letter of the Greek alphabet (Λ, λ). **2.** The apex of the occipital bone of the skull where the sagittal and lamdoidal sutures unite.

lamba sign seen by ultrasound as a thickened area of placental tissue at the site of insertion of the separating membranes suggesting a dichorionic placentation and non-identical twins.

lambdoidal the suture between the occipital and parietal bones of the skull. ⊃ fontanelle

lambliasis *n* ⊃ giardiasis.

lamella *n* **1.** a thin plate-like scale or partition. **2.** a gelatin-coated disc containing a drug; it is inserted under the eyelid—**lamellae** *pl*, **lamellar** *adj*.

lamellar exfoliation of newborn congenital hereditary disorder in which the infant is completely covered with parchment-like membrane that peels off within 24 hours, after which there may be complete healing, or the scales may reform and the process repeated. In the severe form, the infant (harlequin fetus) is completely covered with thick, horny, armour-like scales, and is usually stillborn or dies shortly after birth. Also termed ichthyosis congenita, ichthyosis fetalis, lamellar ichthyosis.

lamina *n* a thin plate or layer, usually of bone. Usually describing part of a vertebra.

lamina cribrosa ⊃ cribriform plate of the sclera.

lamina dura a layer of bone forming the outer layer of the socket in which a tooth lies. It appears on a radiograph as a whitish radio-opaque line situated close to and surrounding the tooth root and its periodontal ligament image.

lamina elastica ⊃ Bruch's membrane.

lamina fusca the suprachoroid. ⊃ sclera.

lamina propria thin layer of connective tissue situated beneath the epithelium of a mucous membrane—**laminae** *pl*.

lamina vitrae ⊃ Bruch's membrane.

laminar boundary layer the layer which is next to the surface of an object, not mixing with the flow further away from the surface, and so can be considered to be a discrete layer in a plane parallel to the main flow. ⊃ boundary layer, turbulent boundary layer.

laminate veneer reconstruction conservative technique undertaken to improve the appearance of the anterior teeth. Materials that include composite resin veneers and acrylic resins are bonded onto the teeth to disguise staining/discoloration, restore malformed teeth, correct minor misalignment and deal with diastemas.

lamination layering, soft iron sheets with insulation between each sheet found in a transformer core to reduce eddy currents.

laminectomy *n* removal of part of the vertebral laminae—to expose the spinal cord nerve roots and meninges. Provides more room in the spinal (vertebral) canal and is most often performed in the lumbar region, for a herniated intervertebral disc or spinal (vertebral) canal stenosis. ⊃ spinal stenosis.

LAN *abbr* local area network.

lance to cut into, and thus obtain drainage of, a fluctuant swelling.

Lancefield's groups (R Lancefield, American bacteriologist, 1895–1981) a serological classification of the bacteria of the genus *Streptococcus* on the basis of antigenic structure. Individual species are allocated to 13 groups on the basis of their characteristic capsular polysaccharide. The streptococci that cause most infections in humans belong to Lancefield group A.

lancet *n* a device with a short pointed blade used to obtain capillary blood samples. For example to obtain blood for checking glucose levels, or for checking haemoglobin prior to the donation of blood.

lancinating *adj* describes a cutting, stabbing pain.

Landolt ring (*syn* Landolt broken ring, Landolt C, Landolt test type) a test object used for measuring visual acuity consisting of an incomplete ring resembling the letter C. The width of the break and of the ring are each one-fifth of its overall diameter. The subject must indicate where the break is located, the break being positioned in any direction. The minimum angle of resolution corresponds to the angular subtense of the just noticeable break at the eye. ⊃ visual acuity.

Lane centre prop ⊃ mouth prop.

Lang's stereotest (*syn* Lang test) a random-dot stereogram upon which is imprinted a series of parallel strips of cylindrical lenses which act to separate the views seen by each eye. There are three stereoscopic shapes which the person has to identify: a cat (inducing 1200 seconds of arc of retinal disparity), a star (600 seconds of arc) and a car (550 seconds of arc). The test is administered at 40 cm and exactly in the frontoparallel plane. As there is no need to use special spectacles it is a very useful test for young children. ⊃ random-dot stereogram.

Langer's lines (C von Langer, Austrian anatomist, 1819–1887) a pattern of cleavage lines in the skin. Surgical incisions made parallel to the cleavage lines heal with less scarring than do incisions and other wounds that cross the lines.

Langerhans' cell histiocytosis formally known as histiocytosis X. A group of disorders characterized by the proliferation of histiocytes and the presence of granulomatous changes that mainly affect the lungs and bones. ⮑ Hand–Schuller–Christian disease, histiocytosis, Letterer–Siwe disease

Langerhans' cells (P Langerhans, German pathologist, 1847–1888) dendritic cells in the epidermis that are part of the biological barrier formed by the skin. They act as antigen-presenting cells thereby protecting the body from microorganisms that breach the chemical and physical barriers.

Langhan's cell layer ⮑ cytotrophoblast.

language *n* a system of communication based on symbols or letters and gestures. The usual interpretation involves verbal language (spoken and written) that uses an 'alphabet' of letters or symbols from which many thousands of words can be formed. Particular groups of people, such as health professionals, may construct a verbal language including jargon to explain their work and inadvertently confuse and exclude clients and patients.

lanolin *n* the fat from sheep's wool. Added to ointment bases, as such bases can form water-in-oil emulsions with aqueous constituents, and are readily absorbed by the skin. Contact sensitivity to preparations containing lanolin may develop.

lantern test an occupational colour vision test used mainly to evaluate recognition of aviation and maritime signals. There are several such tests (e.g. Edridge–Green lantern, Giles–Archer lantern, Holmes–Wright lantern, Farnsworth lantern or Falant). The latter two show colours in pairs of which there are nine and the observer's task is to name the colours. ⮑ Edridge–Green lantern.

lanugo *n* the soft, downy hair sometimes present on newborn infants, especially when they are premature. Usually replaced before birth by vellus hair. ⮑ terminal hair, vellus hair.

lapar/o- a prefix that means 'flank, abdomen', e.g. *laparoscopy*.

laparoscope an endoscope used to examine the peritoneal cavity.

laparoscopy *n* (*syn* peritoneoscopy) endoscopic examination of the internal organs by the transperitoneal route. A laparoscope is introduced through the abdominal wall after induction of a pneumoperitoneum. A variety of surgical procedures are performed in this way, including biopsy, cyst aspiration, division of adhesions, tubal ligation, assisted conception techniques, appendicectomy and cholecystectomy—**laparoscopic** *adj*, **laparoscopically** *adv*.

laparotomy *n* incision of the abdominal wall. Usually the term is reserved for an exploratory operation.

large for gestational age (LGA) baby an infant whose weight is above the 90th centile. Infants who are large for gestational age are at increased risk of respiratory disease, hypoglycaemia, polycythaemia and disturbed thermoregulation. ⮑ macrosomia

large scale integration (LSI) a means of packing large numbers of electronic circuits into small chips.

Larmor equation ($\omega = \gamma B_o$) the proportional relationship between the precessional angular frequency of a nuclear magnetic moment (ω in hertz) and the main magnetic field (B_o in tesla). The gyromagnetic constant (γ) is a proportionality constant and is fixed for the nucleus, for example, 42.6 MHz/tesla for hydrogen.

Larsen's syndrome (L Larsen, American orthopaedic surgeon, b, 1914) congenital condition characterized by multiple joint dislocations, cleft palate and other skeletal abnormalities.

larva *n* an embryo that is independent before developing the characteristic features of its parents.

larva migrans itching tracks in the skin with formation of blisters; caused by the burrowing of larvae of some species of fly, and the normally animal-infesting *Ancylostoma*—**larvae** *pl*, **larval** *adj*.

larval therapy maggot therapy or biological débridement. The use of sterile blowfly (*Lucilia serricata*) larvae in the débridement of some chronic wounds. Enzymes produced by the larvae breakdown slough and necrotic tissue thus providing the conditions for the wound to heal.

larvicide *n* any agent which destroys larvae—**larvicidal** *adj*.

laryngeal *adj* pertaining to the larynx.

laryngeal mask airway (LMA) airway with inflatable cuff placed via the mouth into the oropharynx to maintain the airway during general anaesthesia (Figure L.2). It is used for spontaneously breathing patients or where help with ventilation is appropriate and can be maintained. An LMA

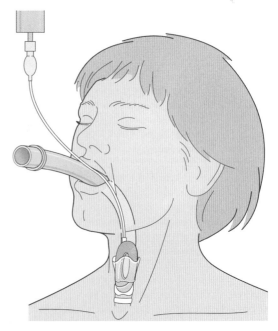

The laryngeal mask in situ

L.2 Laryngeal mask airway (reproduced from Brooker & Nicol 2003 with permission).

K
L

is not suitable in all situations, for instance when patients are repositioned during surgery, which could dislodge the mask. Furthermore, an LMA is not appropriate when there is a high risk of regurgitation and aspiration of gastric contents, such as in emergency surgery, or in obstetric emergencies.

laryngeal mirror mirror for inspecting the oral cavity and larynx.

laryngeal papilloma rare neonatal condition due to infection acquired during vaginal delivery.

laryngeal reflex a reflex cough caused by irritation of the larynx.

laryngeal spasm spasm of the larynx. ➲ laryngismus, laryngismus stridulus.

laryngectomy *n* surgical removal of the larynx. Usually for cancer.

laryngismus *n* spasm of the larynx. ➲ laryngismus stridulus.

laryngismus stridulus sudden laryngeal spasm with closure of the glottis. It is characterized by crowing sounds, respiratory distress and a period of apnoea. It is associated with the administration of an anaesthetic, inflammation, foreign bodies and hypocalcaemia of childhood rickets. ➲ croup.

laryngitis *n* inflammation of the mucosal lining of the larynx. It may be acute, which often follows an acute upper respiratory tract infection. It can be serious in small children who may develop respiratory distress. ➲ croup, laryngotracheobronchitis. Chronic laryngitis often follows a cold or influenza but precipitating factors include sudden changes in environmental temperature, chronic sinusitis, smoking, exposure to irritant fumes, drinking alcohol and over-use of the voice. It is characterized by hoarseness, dysphonia or aphonia (complete voice loss), sore throat and cough.

laryng/o- a prefix that means 'larynx', e.g. *laryngectomy*.

laryngocele *n* the presence of an air-filled sac/cavity that communicates with the larynx.

laryngologist *n* a specialist in disorders of the larynx.

laryngology *n* the study of disorders affecting the larynx.

laryngoparalysis *n* paralysis of the larynx.

laryngopharyngectomy *n* excision of the larynx and part of the pharynx. Usually performed for cancers involving the pharynx, larynx and adjacent structures in the throat.

laryngopharynx *n* the hypopharynx. The lower portion of the pharynx below the oropharynx, it gives passage to food and fluids into the oesophagus—**laryngopharyngeal** *adj.*

laryngoscope *n* instrument for visualization of the larynx, for diagnostic or therapeutic purposes or to facilitate the insertion of an endotracheal tube into the larynx under direct vision—**laryngoscopic** *adj.*

laryngoscopy *n* direct or indirect visual examination of the interior of the larynx.

laryngospasm *n* convulsive involuntary muscular contraction of the larynx, usually accompanied by spasmodic closure of the glottis, which prevents air entering the respiratory tract.

laryngostenosis *n* narrowing of the glottic aperture.

laryngotomy *n* surgical opening in the larynx.

laryngotracheal *adj* pertaining to the larynx and trachea.

laryngotracheitis *n* inflammation of the mucosal lining of the larynx and trachea.

laryngotracheobronchitis *n* inflammation (usually viral) of the mucosal lining of the larynx, trachea and bronchi. May be very serious when it occurs in small children. ➲ croup.

laryngotracheoplasty *n* surgical opening of a stenosed larynx—**laryngotracheoplastic** *adj.*

larynx *n* the organ of voice situated below and in front of the pharynx and at the upper end of the trachea. A cartilaginous box formed from nine cartilages (epiglottis, thyroid, cricoid, arytenoid [2], corniculate [2] and cuneiform [2]), ligaments (e.g. thyrohyoid) and membranes. Inspired air passes through the glottis, an opening between the vocal folds (vocal cords), before entering the trachea. During swallowing several mechanisms prevent food or fluids from entering the trachea and bronchi, for example the upward movement of the larynx which causes the epiglottis to occlude the opening into the larynx. The two vocal folds (vocal cords), which are attached at the front and the back of the larynx, produce sound—**laryngeal** *adj.* ➲ Colour Section Figure 6.

Lasègue sign/test a neurodynamic test. ➲ straight leg raise (SLR)

LASER *acron* for **L**ight **A**mplification by **S**timulated **E**mission of **R**adiation. A form of electromagnetic radiation. A tube in which stimulated emission takes place and the light produced oscillates in a regular pattern to produce a high-energy, coherent, parallel beam of light. Energy is transmitted as heat which can coagulate tissue. The penetration depth varies according to the type of laser in use. Lasers of specific type can be used in wound healing and pain control. Laser has many other therapeutic uses that include: endometrial ablation, several ocular conditions, treatment of skin lesions and cancer treatments. In ophthalmology lasers are used in the treatment of a variety of ocular conditions, especially of the cornea, the retina (e.g. detached retina, diabetic retinopathy) and glaucoma. ➲ iridectomy, photocoagulation, radial keratotomy, scanning laser ophthalmoscope. Also used in the production of modern radiographic images by exposing a film to laser light. The dangers associated with the use of lasers are primarily to eyes and, depending on class of laser, wavelength specific protecting lenses must be warn by patient and health professionals.

laser-assisted uvulopalatoplasty (LAUP) the use of lasers to modify the palate in order to relieve obstructive sleep apnoea. ➲ sleep apnoea (hypopnoea) syndrome.

laser back pointer mounted in the counterbalance of the gantry of radiotherapy equipment and projects a sheet of light in the direction of the axis of rotation of the gantry and the axis of rotation of the diaphragm system indicating the entry and exit point of the radiation beam.

laser Doppler flowmeter a device that utilizes laser technology to measure blood flow.

laser interferometry ⊃ clinical maxwellian view system.

laser iridotomy ⊃ iridectomy.

laser printer characters or images are built up by the image being scanned by a laser and then toner is fused onto the paper to produce the final print.

laser printing film in radiography, a single-sided emulsion used with imaging plates.

laser refraction a method of subjective refraction in which the person observes a slowly rotating drum on the surface of which is perceived a speckle pattern resulting from illumination by a laser. The speckle pattern appears to move only when the eye is not focused for the fixation distance. If the perceived movement of the pattern is opposite to that of the drum, the eye is myopic and if the perceived movement of the pattern is in the same direction as the drum, the eye is hyperopic. Correction can be determined by placing a lens in front of the eye which will neutralize the movement; at that point the eye is focused for the fixation distance. Astigmatism can be measured by rotating the drum in various meridians. The drum can be placed at infinity or at near (an allowance for the radius of curvature of the drum and the distance must then be made). This method can be useful for mass screening, especially children, as accommodation is not stimulated as much as with Snellen letters. It has been very useful as a research tool for accommodation studies where it is arranged as part of a Badal optometer. ⊃ Badal's optometer, refractive error.

laser trabeculoplasty a procedure aimed at improving the outflow of aqueous humour in open-angle glaucoma by producing a series of laser burns (usually with an argon laser) to the trabecular meshwork. ⊃ open-angle glaucoma, trabeculoplasty.

LASIK *abbr* **las**er **in**situ **k**eratomileusis or **l**aser **as**sisted **i**ntrastromal **k**eratoplasty. A surgical technique for correcting refractive errors—hypermetropia, myopia or astigmatism. A suction ring is applied to the globe and an increase in intraocular pressure to approximately 65 mmHg is induced for a maximum of 2 minutes. During that time an automated microkeratome advances across the cornea creating a corneal flap of about 8.5 mm in diameter. The vacuum is then switched off and the suction ring removed. The corneal flap which is hinged on one side of the cornea is turned round onto the conjunctiva and the exposed stroma is ablated with the excimer laser. On completion of the laser ablation, the corneal flap is repositioned and left to adhere without sutures. There are some complications associated with this procedure, but it gives rise to less post-operative pain and more rapid visual rehabilitation than other similar surgical procedures. Complications may include infections, problems with the flap, night glare, dry eyes and a failure to correct the refractive error (under- or overcorrection). ⊃ epikeratoplasty, excimer laser, Intacs, keratoconus, keratome, keratomileusis, keratophakia, radial keratotomy.

Lassa virus a virus of the familiy *Arenaviridae*. Discovered in 1969 it is the causative organism of Lassa fever in Africa.

Lassa fever one of the serious viral haemorrhagic fevers. Occurs as isolated cases and small outbreaks usually in West Africa. The incubation period is 3–16 days; early symptoms resemble typhoid and septicaemia. Mortality is as high as 80%. Strict isolation is required for infected people.

Lassar's paste contains zinc oxide, starch and salicylic acid in soft paraffin. Used in hyperkerototic skin conditions.

lassitude a state of weakness or weariness.

last menstrual period (LMP) determining the date of the first day of the last normal menstrual period assists in estimating the probable date of delivery. However, the woman may mistake implantation bleeding as a normal menstrual period so the midwife should check that the date refers to vaginal bleeding occurring when the woman expected a period and which lasted the normal number of days.

latent image the image produced on a film after exposure but prior to development.

latent period also known as incubation period. The period of time between exposure to a micro-organism or other agent and the develoment of symptoms. Includes the time between the exposure to a carcinogenic agent and the clinical appearance of disease.

lateral *adj* at or belonging to the side; away from the median line—**laterally** *adv*.

lateral canthus ⊃ canthus.

lateral chromatic aberration (*syn* chromatic difference of magnification, transverse chromatic aberration [TCA]) a defect of an optical system (eye, lens, prism, etc.) in which the size of the image of a point object is extended by a coloured fringe, due to the unequal refraction of different wavelengths (dispersion).

lateral compartment syndrome pain on the outer side of the leg when the plantar flexors/everters (peroneus muscles) are affected. ⊃ anterior compartment syndrome, chronic exertional compartment syndrome, compartment syndrome, posterior compartment syndrome.

lateral cutaneous nerve of the thigh a nerve arising from the lumbar plexus. It supplies the skin of the lateral aspect of the thigh including part of the front and back surfaces. ⊃ lumbar plexus.

lateral decubitus radiograph the patient lies on their side and the central ray passes from the anterior to the posterior aspect of the body. The projection is named after the side of the body that is uppermost.

lateral epicondylitis also described as 'tennis elbow', but often with no history of sport, it is associated with the origin of the common extensor tendon at the lateral humeral epicondyle.

lateral excursion the movement of the mandible in a lateral direction with the opposing teeth in contact.

lateral geniculate bodies (LGB) ovoid protuberances lateral to the thalamus in the diencephalon of the forebrain and into which the fibres of the optic tract synapse on their way to the visual cortex. However, because of the semidecussation of the optic nerve fibres in the chiasma, the lateral geniculate body in the right thalamus receives the fibres originating on the temporal retina of the right eye and the nasal fibres of the left. Each body appears, in cross-section, to consist of alternating white and grey areas. The white areas are formed by the medullated nerve fibres of the optic tract while the grey areas consist largely of the cell bodies of the optic radiations which synapse with the fibres of the optic tract. There are six grey areas or layers of cells, with layer 1 being the most ventral and layer 6 the most dorsal (or posterior). Layers 1, 4 and 6 receive the crossed or nasal fibres from the contralateral retina, while layers 2, 3 and 5 receive the uncrossed or temporal fibres of the ipsilateral retina. There are two main types of cells in the lateral geniculate bodies: in layers 1 and 2 (those most ventral) the cells are substantially larger than in the other four layers and are called *magno cells* and the layers, *magnocellular layers*. The main input to these cells are the retinal rods and the magno ganglion cells. In the other four layers (those most dorsal) the cells are smaller and are called parvo cells and the layers, *parvocellular layers*. The main input to these cells are the retinal cones and the parvo ganglion cells. The cells of the parvocellular layers seem to be mainly responsible for transmitting information about visual acuity, form vision, colour perception and low contrast targets. The cells in the magnocellular layers seem to be mainly responsible for transmitting information about motion and flicker perception, stereopsis and high contrast targets. The magnocellular and parvocellular cells project to different cells in the primary visual cortex, where they retain the same segregation as in the lateral geniculate bodies. The receptive field of the cells in the lateral geniculate body is circular with either an 'on' or 'off' centre with the opposite behaviour in the surround, but they are more sensitive to contrast than the retinal ganglion cells. ➲ ganglion, optic chiasma, optic nerve, optic radiations, optic tracts.

lateral interocclusal records ➲ interocclusal record.

lateral longitudinal arch of foot formed by the calcaneus, cuboid and two lateral metatarsals, it is supported normally by ligaments, intrinsic muscles, and the tendons of extrinsic muscles of the foot.

lateral magnification (*syn* linear magnification, transverse magnification) magnification of a lens or of an optical system, expressed as the ratio of the length of the image h' to the length of the object h. It is usually denoted by

$$M = \frac{h'}{h}$$

➲ principal plane, sine condition.

lateral periodontal cyst developmental or inflammatory cyst situated by the side of a tooth.

lateral pterygoid muscle a deep two-headed muscle of mastication; present on each side of the face. It is short and cone shaped. Its origin is on the sphenoid bone, running backwards as it diminishes in size, to insert on to the anterior aspect of the condyle of the mandible, the capsule of the temporomandibular joint and its disc. It assists in opening the jaw, protruding it and pulling it towards the opposite side to facilitate grinding action of the lower teeth.

lateral radiograph the patient is either erect or lying with the side of their body nearest the film. The projection is named after the side of the body nearest the film.

lateral rectus muscle the extraocular muscle that moves the eyeball outwards; it is supplied by the abducens (abducent) nerve (sixth cranial nerve). ➲ extraocular.

lateral release a surgical division of the lateral patellar retinaculum, from the patellar tendon to within the muscle fibres of vastus lateralis. Usually as a treatment of patellofemoral dysfunction, following the failure of conservative measures. ➲ mal tracking patella.

lateral resolution in ultrasound, the ability to see small structures that lie along the beam, this is equal to the effective beam width and is best at the focus and reduces the further away from the focus the object is.

lateral transcranial projection ➲ transcranial projection.

lateral transpharyngeal projection ➲ transpharyngeal projection.

latex allergy an allergic reaction to natural latex or one of the components used in production of latex equipment such as medical gloves and catheters. Latex allergy is increasingly common in patients having repeated invasive interventions, and in healthcare workers due to the increased use of gloves as a control of infection measure particularly following the rise in the incidence of blood-borne viruses.

lathe (dental) a machine, used in dental laboratories for holding and turning materials against a cutting tool, to shape and polish them. Dental laboratory lathes are electrically driven, double ended and have metal chucks pushed onto their rotating shafts. Chucks hold burs, stones, polishing brushes (bristle, felt and linen), felt cones and abrasive wheels. ➲ lathe cut amalgam alloy.

lathe cut amalgam alloy alloy cut on a lathe so as to produce irregular-shaped particles to be mixed with mercury. ➲ alloy.

latissimus dorsi large triangular muscle of the lower back. It attaches indirectly via the lumbodorsal fascia into the spines of the lower thoracic and lumbar vertebrae, lower ribs and iliac crest and inserts on to the humerus. It is the prime mover of arm extension. Also causes medial rotation of the arm at the shoulder and is important in arm adduction. ➲ Colour Section Figures 4, 5.

latitude the range of useful exposures a film will tolerate. ➲ useful exposure range.

latitude emulsions a film with a reduced average gradient of 2.2 to enable a large range of densities to be recorded.

lattice theory ➲ Maurice's theory.

laughing gas ➲ nitrous oxide.

LAUP *abbr* laser-assisted uvulopalatoplasty.

lavage *n* irrigation of or washing out a body cavity, for example, the stomach, colon, bladder, paranasal sinus, etc.

lavender oil *Lavandula angustifolia*. A highly concentrated essential oil used by some midwives, trained in its use, to relax, ease labour pain and aid perineal healing. It appears to facilitate uterine action and reduce blood pressure—not be used in large amounts with Syntocinon® or epidural anaesthesia, and some types may be emmenagoguic so use with caution in early pregnancy.

LAVH *abbr* laparoscopic-assisted vaginal hysterectomy. ➲ hysterectomy.

law of conservation of energy energy can neither be created nor destroyed but can be changed from one form to another. The amount of energy in a system is therefore constant.

law of conservation of matter matter is neither created nor destroyed, but it may change its chemical form as a result of chemical reaction.

law of identical visual directions (*syn* law of oculocentric visual direction) an object stimulating corresponding retinal points is localized in the same apparent monocular direction in each eye. ➲ line of direction, retinal corresponding points.

law of oculocentric visual direction ➲ law of identical visual directions.

law of refraction (*syn* Descartes' law, Snell's law) the incident and refracted rays and the normal to the surface at the point of incidence lie in the same plane and the ratio of the sine of the angle of incidence i to the sine of the angle of refraction i' is a constant for any two media, i.e.

$$\frac{\sin i}{\sin i'} = \frac{n'}{n} \text{ (or) } n \sin i = n' \sin i'$$

where n and n' are the refractive indices of the first and second medium, respectively. This constant (n'/n) is called the relative refractive index for the two media. ➲ refractive index, sign convention.

laws of motion ➲ Newton's laws of motion.

laxatives *npl* (*syn* aperients) drugs used to prevent or treat constipation. Administered orally, or rectally as suppositories or by enema. They may be: bulking agents that retain water and form a large, soft stool; faecal softeners that lubricate or soften the faeces; osmotic laxatives that increase fluid in the bowel lumen; stimulants that increase peristalsis, and combined softeners and stimulants. ➲ Appendix 5.

laxative use in sport in sports with weight categories, laxatives (sometimes in combination with food and fluid restriction, excessive exercise and use of sauna and diuretic drugs) are used to lose weight quickly prior to weigh-in; this may diminish physical performance or lead to abnormalities of bone metabolism, impairments in cognitive function and increased susceptibility to heat illness.

LBC *abbr* liquid-based cytology.

LBM *abbr* lean body mass.

LBP *abbr* low back pain.

LBW *abbr* low birthweight.

LCA *abbr* longitudinal chromatic aberration.

L-carnitine ➲ carnitine.

LCMV *abbr* lymphocytic choriomeningitis virus.

LCSS *abbr* limited cutaneous systemic sclerosis.

LD$_{50}$ *abbr* lethal dose in 50% of a population.

LDH *abbr* lactate dehydrogenase.

LDL *abbr* low-density lipoprotein.

LE *abbr* lupus erythematosus. ➲ systemic lupus erythematosus.

lead (Pb) *n* a heavy, grey, soft metal with toxic salts. It is relatively impermeable to radiation.

lead apron a protective apron used in radiography to protect the spinal column and reproductive organs from excess radiation during the taking of radiographs

lead equivalence a method of comparing protection barriers by calculating the thickness of lead required to have the same absorption to an exposure to radiation.

lead pipe rigidity increased resistance to passive stretch in any direction that is uniform throughout the whole movement, characteristic of Parkinson's disease. ➲ cogwheel rigidity.

lead poisoning (*syn* plumbism) acute poisoning is unusual, but chronic poisoning due to absorption of small amounts over time does occur. For example, young children who suck objects painted with lead paint or made from lead alloys. Lead can be ingested from drinking water contaminated from lead pipes, or from cooking utensils. Abnormally high levels of lead in the environment have been linked to the use of lead in petrol. Presentation varies and may include: colicky abdominal pain (*painters' colic*), diarrhoea and vomiting, anorexia, anaemia, and rarely the formation of a characteristic bluish-black line at the margins of the gingivae. Radiographically, dense transverse lines appear at the shafts of long bones. Neurological manifestations, including convulsions, may occur in severe poisoning.

lead professional the health professional who takes the principal responsibility for a patient's/client's care. For example, the lead professional in maternity care may be the midwife, consultant obstetrician or general practitioner obstetrician, depending on the woman's needs and wishes.

lead shielding shielding blocks of lead placed on a tray below the radiotherapy tube to shape the radiation beam so that it accurately covers the treatment area and/or shields organs at risk. Alternative products may be used, usually alloys of bismuth or cadmium. ➲ MCP block (low melting-point alloy [LMPA] block).

lead strip a contouring device formed by placing a lead strip round the patient and the skin markings are transferred to the lead using marker pen, the markings are then copied onto papers giving the patient contour.

Leadbetter–Politano operation an antireflux procedure by tunnelled reimplantation of the ureter into the urinary bladder.

leadership style the manner in which a leader typically provides direction and motivates others. *autocratic leadership style* when the leader takes a dominant, directive role; *democratic leadership style* when the leader consults with the team and involves them in the process of making decisions.

K
L

leakage radiation unwanted radiation that is emitted from an X-ray tube in directions other than the useful beam, it is reduced by the addition of lead round the X-ray tube.

lean body mass (LBM) ⊃ body composition.

learned helplessness a state of apathy and hopelessness in which the individual feels unable to affect outcomes, resulting from repeated exposure to uncontrollable situations.

learned non-use a situation that can occur when a person has some recovery in a limb affected, for example, by a stroke. They do not use the limb functionally because they have learnt not to and are not using the motor ability present in activities of daily living.

learning 1. a relatively permanent change in behaviour as a result of training, practice or experience. 2. the state of having knowledge or skills. 3. being in the process of acquiring knowledge or skills. *explicit learning* or knowledge is acquired through conscious, deliberate intention to master or understand a task; *implicit learning* or knowledge is acquired passively, without conscious awareness or deliberate effort; *incidental learning* or knowledge of a task is acquired unintentionally during the acquisition of another task.

learning disability a general term used to describe the inability to develop intellectually. The definition of and use of the term learning disability varies from country to country. In the UK the term usually refers to a variety of disorders that start before adulthood, and that have enduring effects on development. A learning disability adversely affects the acquisition, retention, understanding of new or complex information and often also the use of verbal or non-verbal communication. It has a lasting effect on development and results in a varying degree of support from others being required to cope with daily living.

learning goal a goal focused on personal improvement in performance. ⊃ performance goal, task involvement.

learning outcomes the specific quantifiable results that can be expected to follow involvement in a learning opportunity. Outcomes may focus on cognitive (knowledge), affective (attitudes) or behavioural (skills) aspects that furnish evidence that learning has been achieved.

learning strategy the manner in which people approach a learning exercise.

learning style the ways in which a person usually thinks, solves problems and remembers new knowledge.

leather bottle stomach ⊃ linitis plastica

Leber's congenital amaurosis (T Leber, German opthalmologist, 1840–1917) a rare condition causing blindness or seriously impaired vision; inherited as an autosomal recessive disorder. The eyes may appear normal at birth but results from electroretinography are abnormal.

Leber's hereditary optic neuropathy a condition inherited via mitochondrial DNA that generally affects adult males. It presents with subacute central vision loss caused by degeneration of the optic nerve and the retinal ganglion cells.

Leboyer method (F Leboyer, French obstetrician, b.1918) method of childbirth in which the infant is born gently and quietly in a darkened room, advocated by French doctor, Leboyer. The infant is born in a calm and tranquil environment, lifted on to the mother's abdomen, then put into a warm bath, so that he will cry less and be more contented since the shock of delivery is minimized.

lecithinase *n* enzyme that catalyses the decomposition of lecithin.

lecithins *npl* phosphatidylcholines. A group of phospholipids found in animal tissues. They form a vital component of cell membranes and are involved in the metabolism of fats. They are present in the liver, semen and nervous tissue. Its presence in pulmonary surfactant reduces surface tension and facilitates the exchange of gases in the alveoli.

lecithin–sphingomyelin ratio (LS) the ratio of the two substances in the amniotic fluid is used to assess the degree of fetal lung maturity. Lecithin, but not sphingomyelin, increases in amount as pregnancy progresses, so the ratio increases with fetal lung maturity. A ratio of 2 or more indicates little or no risk of neonatal respiratory distress syndrome, whereas an unfavourable ratio indicates an increased risk.

Le Cron's carver ⊃ carver.

lectins proteins from legumes such as red kidney beans, and other plants. They bind to the glycolipids and glycoproteins present on animal cell surfaces and can agglutinate red blood cells (erythrocytes) of certain blood groups. Previously known as phytoagglutinins or haemagglutinins.

lecturer practitioner a health professional, such as a nurse or midwife, who has a dual educational and clinical role. They divide their time between lecturing in the university and clinical practice.

leech *n Hirudo medicinalis*. An aquatic worm which can be applied to the human body to suck blood and thereby reduce congestion. Its saliva contains hirudin, an anticoagulant. Used after reconstructive surgery to reduce the congestion and swelling, which may compromise the blood supply.

Leeds test (*syn* triple test) a screening test similar to the Bart's test which identifies women at high risk of carrying a fetus with Down's syndrome. It measures alphafetoprotein, unconjugated oestriol, human chorionic gonadotrophin, and neutrophil alkaline phosphatase. It indicates whether a diagnostic test such as amniocentesis may be of value to an individual woman.

Leeds test objects a number of different test objects produced by the University of Leeds, used for quality control in radiology, to test, for example, film–screen combinations, television systems and computed tomography (CT) scanners, and so on.

Le Fort classification (R Le Fort, French surgeon, 1869–1951) a classification of fractures that involve the middle third of the facial skeleton. *Le Fort I fracture (Guérin type fracture)* where the maxilla is fractured transversely just above the apices of the teeth and the palatal vault thus separating this segment from the rest of the maxilla.

Le Fort II fracture (pyramidal fracture) where the fracture occurs in the central region of the middle third of the facial skeleton and passes through the bridge of the nose and backwards below the zygomatic bones. *Le Fort III fracture (high level* or *craniofacial dysjunction fracture)* where there is a transverse craniofacial bone fracture occurring above the zygomatic bones.

left anterior oblique a radiographic projection with the patient either erect or semi prone at 45° to the film with the left side of the body closest to the film and the right side away from the film.

left colic (splenic) flexure the 90° turn situated at the junction of the transverse and descending parts of the colon. It lies at a higher level than the right (hepatic) flexure.

left posterior oblique a radiographic projection with the patient either erect or semi supine at 45° to the film with the left side of the body closest to the film and the right side away from the film.

left ventricular assist device (LVAD) mechanical pump used to increase the output of blood from the left ventricle of the heart. May be used in the short term to support critically ill patients, those waiting for a heart transplant, or to give the heart muscle time to recover from disease.

leg *n* lower limb.

Leger shuttle run ⊃ shuttle test.

Legg–Calvé–Perthes disease (A Legg, American surgeon, 1874–1939; J Calvé, French orthopaedic surgeon, 1875–1954; G Perthes, German surgeon, 1869–1927) avascular necrosis affecting the upper femoral epiphysis and the head of the femur during childhood. It is usually unilateral and most common in boys from the age of 5 years up to 10 years of age. The child has pain and a limp. Revascularization occurs, but residual deformity (flattening) of the femoral head may subsequently lead to arthritic changes. Also known as Perthes' disease.

Legionella pneumophila a small Gram-negative bacillus which causes Legionnaires' disease and Pontiac fever.

Legionnaires' disease a severe and often fatal pneumonia caused by *Legionella pneumophila*; there is pneumonia, dry cough, and often non-pulmonary involvement such as gastrointestinal symptoms, renal impairment and confusion. A cause of both community- and hospital-acquired pneumonia, it is associated with an infected water supply in public buildings such as hospitals and hotels. There is no person-to-person spread.

leg length a measure from the anterior superior iliac spine (ASIS), to the tip of the medial malleolus, although this may be inaccurate in the presence of pelvic rotation or asymmetry. Leg-length discrepancies may not be significant if they are less than 6 mm, many asymptomatic individuals have a leg length difference of up to 12 mm. With the person stood or lying with their feet 18 inches apart: the true leg length is the distance from ASIS to medial malleolus, and the apparent leg length is the distance from umbilicus to medial malleolus.

leg length discrepancy difference in the true length of one leg compared to the other. It may be structural (secondary to a pre-existing condition such as Legg–Calvé–Perthes disease) or functional as a result of altered lower limb biomechanics. Differences of 0.5–1 cm are not uncommon and usually asymptomatic. Greater discrepancy will produce a compensatory pelvic tilt or secondary scoliosis (lateral curvature of the spine). This compensation, combined with repetitive exercise, can cause problems including discomfort in the back, lower limb (especially knee) pain or Achilles tendonitis (tendinitis). Treatment includes improving pelvic control and core stability and the use of orthoses. It is important to identify this problem to allow correct treatment, as treatment of the secondary effect alone will not alleviate the symptoms.

leg ulcer a wound on the leg, which can be associated with a variety of aetiologies. The vast majority of leg ulcers have a venous aetiology, less than 10% have an arterial cause, some ulcers have a mixed venous and arterial aetiology and a few are associated with other diseases. ⊃ arterial ulcer, venous ulcer.

legumen *n* the protein present in peas, beans and lentils.

legumes *npl* pulse vegetables—e.g. peas, beans, lentils. Provides valuble protein, B vitamins and iron and soluble dietary fibre. An essential component of a vegetarian and vegan diet but also very useful for people whose diet does contain meat and fish and other animal products.

Leiden abnormality ⊃ factor V Leiden, thrombophilia.

Leigh's disease (A Leigh, British neuropathologist, b. 1915) a rare inherited disorder that leads to the degeneration of the central nervous system. The disease may be the result of a deficiency of the enzyme pyruvate dehydrogenase, or because of mutations in the DNA found within the mitochondria. Signs of the disease, which progresses rapidly, are usually noticed between the ages of 3 months and 2 years. It is characterized by poor feeding, anorexia, vomiting, deteriorating motor skills, poor head control, irritability and seizures. Later there may be poor muscle tone, weakness and metabolic problems (lactic acidosis) that affect the respiratory system, kidneys and the heart. The prognosis is very poor and most children die within a few years.

leiomyoma *n* a benign tumour affecting smooth (involuntary) muscle. Very common benign tumour of the female reproductive tract where they are generally known informally as fibroids or fibromyoma, as they contain both fibrous connective tissue and muscle tissue. ⊃ fibroid. Leiomyomas also occur in the gastrointestinal tract—**leiomyomas, leiomyomata** *pl*.

leiomyosarcoma *n* a rare malignant tumour of smooth muscle tissue. They occur in the myometrium of the uterus, in the stomach and intestine.

Leishman–Donovan bodies (W Leishman, British pathologist, 1865–1926; C Donovan, Irish physician, 1863–1951) the rounded resting stage of the protozoan parasite *Leishmania* found in certain cells, e.g. macrophages, of individuals with leishmaniasis.

Leishmania *n* genus of flagellated parasitic protozoa. *Leishmania donovani* causes leishmaniasis.

leishmaniasis *n* infestation by *Leishmania*, spread by sandflies. Generalized (visceral) manifestation is kala-azar. Old World, cutaneous forms are called an *oriental sore*. New World cutaneous forms may involve the nasal and oral mucosa and the lesion is called an *espundia*. ⊃ Colour Section Figure 84.

leisure free time that is used for engaging in pleasurable activities.

leisure activities activities that are freely chosen in the expectation that they will bring pleasure and/or satisfaction.

Leksell unit a stereotactic radiotherapy unit containing a hemispherical array of 201 collimated, cobalt sources. It is usually used for the delivery of single fractions of radiation to intracranial targets.

lemniscus a band-like tract of nerve fibres in the central nervous system.

length–tension curve this relates to the relationship between a muscle's ability to contract and its length. Muscles that have been lengthened, for example by being immobilized in a plaster, generate tension more slowly than muscles that have been shortened. Short muscles are able to generate tension quickest and so tend to be recruited first. This is a fundamental principal to serial casting. Imagine an elastic band held around your index fingers, it would generate tension as you pull your fingers apart; now if you take a smaller elastic band it will generate tension quicker.

length–tension relationship the relation between a muscle's length and the isometric tension (force) which it generates when fully activated. During normal muscular activity, particularly at the longer lengths, tension partly depends on passive stretch of the connective tissue within the muscle, acting in parallel with active force generation by the muscle fibres themselves. When this contribution is subtracted, and only the actively generated force considered, the relation between force and length depends predominantly on the number of actin-myosin cross-bridges, which can be formed. Figure L.3A shows the relationship for skeletal muscle in terms of sarcomere length. Figure L.3B illustrates how this is accounted for by variations in overlap between thick and thin filaments, and therefore in the formation of cross-bridges. Over the range of decreasing sarcomere length (I–II) progressively more cross-bridges can form but when the shortest length (IV) is approached, correctly oriented cross-bridges formation diminishes as the thin filaments begin to overlap and force declines. Most muscles in the body operate only over the central, high force, part of the curve shown in Fig. L.3A. ⊃ muscle contraction, myofibrils, sliding filament hypothesis/mechanism.

lens *n* **1.** the small biconvex crystalline body which is supported by the suspensory ligament immediately behind the iris of the eye. On account of its elasticity, the lens can alter in shape, enabling light rays to focus exactly on the retina. ⊃ crystalline lens. **2.** glass or plastic used to correct refractive errors (spectacles or contact lens) or in optical

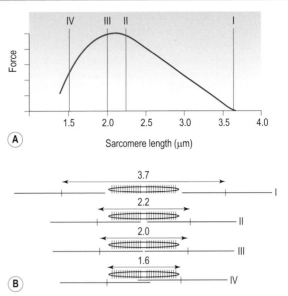

L.3 Length–tension relationship (A) Force generated at different sarcomere lengths (B) arrangement of filaments at different sarcomere lengths (reproduced from Jennett 2008 with perimission).

K
L

instruments. ⊃ bifocal lens, contact lens, Colour Section Figure 15.

lens dislocation ⊃ luxation of the lens.

lens fibres the long, six-sided bands containing few organelles and mostly lacking a nucleus, derived from epithelial cells just within the capsule of the crystalline lens and attached to an anterior and to a posterior suture. ⊃ capsule of the crystalline lens.

lens flare type of blur characterized by the presence of a secondary or ghost image. Flare may be caused by a contact lens with an optic zone diameter that is smaller than the pupil diameter or when the lens decentres so that part of the edge of the optic zone is within the pupil area. Flare is usually more apparent under conditions of reduced illumination as the pupil is larger. Management consists in refitting the patient with a lens with a larger optic zone diameter or with better centration. ⊃ ghost image.

lens flippers (*syn* flippers, flipper bar, flip lenses, flip prisms, prism flippers) two pairs of lenses mounted on a central bar, one pair on each side. One pair can be held in front of the patient's eyes and then quickly changed for the other pair by twisting the bar extension handle. The lenses may be one pair of minus lenses of equal power and the other pair of plus lenses of equal power. The most common pairs are ±2.00 D, although ±1.00 D, ±1.50 D and ±2.50 D are also available. These are used in the testing and training of accommodative facility. Prisms may also be used, as for example base-in for one pair and base-out for the other. They are used in the testing and training of vergence facility. ⊃ accommodative facility, vergence facility.

lens paradox a change of the ametropia of the eye towards hypermetropia (or less myopia) in old eyes, although the crystalline lens increases in size and the anterior and posterior surfaces become more curved. This is paradoxical since this should lead to an increase in lens power and a change towards myopia. This paradox is attributed to a reduction in the refractive index (index of refraction) occurring within the various layers of the lens, as well as to an increase in the refractive index of the vitreous body (humour) which would result in a reduction of the total lens power. ⊃ crystalline lens, refractive index.

lenticonus an abnormal protrusion on the lens of the eye. Present in Alport's syndrome.

lenticular *adj* pertaining to or resembling a lens.

lenticular myopia (*syn* index myopia) myopia attributed to an increase in the refractive index (index of refraction) of the lens. As a result there is an increase in refractive power. Such a change usually accompanies the development of some cataracts. This type of myopia may also accompany or follow an increase in blood glucose level, in which case it is usually of a transient nature, i.e. the power of the crystalline lens diminishes after the blood glucose level returns to the normal range. ⊃ cataract, diabetes mellitus.

lenticular nucleus a biconvex part of the basal nuclei (basal ganglia).

lenticule a disc-shaped piece of corneal tissue or a piece of synthetic material manufactured to produce a given curvature and thickness. It is implanted into or on top of the cornea to change its anterior curvature. ⊃ epikeratoplasty, keratophakia.

lentigo *n* a freckle with an increased number of pigment cells. ⊃ ephelides—**lentigines** *pl*.

lentulo (spiral root canal) filler ⊃ root canal (dental procedures).

Lenz's law the direction of the induced current in a conductor caused by a changing magnetic flux is such that its own magnetic field opposes the changing magnetic flux. The law only applies in closed circuits.

leontiasis *n* enlargement of the face and head giving a lion-like appearance; associated with some types of leprosy.

leprologist *n* one who specializes in the study and treatment of leprosy.

leprology *n* the study of leprosy and its treatment.

lepromata *npl* the granulomatous cutaneous eruption of leprosy—**leproma** *sing*, **lepromatous** *adj*.

leprosy (Hansen's disease) *n* a chronic and contagious disease, endemic in warmer climates and characterized by granulomatous formation in the peripheral nerves or on the skin, mucous membranes and bones with tissue destruction. Caused by *Mycobacterium leprae* (Hansen's bacillus). BCG vaccination conferred variable protection in different trials. Management includes specific care, such as that required for impaired sensation and the long term treatment with various antimicrobial drugs, including dapsone and rifampicin—**leprous** *adj*. ⊃ Colour Section Figure 85.

leptin a hormone-like peptide that is produced by adipocytes (fat cells) and plays a role in regulation of appetite and in fat storage, by acting in the hypothalamus.

It controls appetite and energy use by signalling information about the amount of body fat reserves. Normally, leptin depresses the urge to eat when food intake is maintaining ideal fat stores. With a gene defective for either adipocyte leptin production or hypothalamic leptin sensitivity, the brain cannot adequately assess adipose tissue status and the urge to eat persists, resulting in overeating. Leptin may also play a role in energy balance regulation in starvation: reduction in leptin production when food is scarce may defend against excess energy expenditure.

lepto- a prefix that means 'thin, soft', e.g. *leptomeninges*.

leptocyte ⊃ target cell.

leptomeninges the pia and arachnoid mater combined.

leptophonia ⊃ hypophonia

Leptospira *n* a genus of bacteria. Very thin, finely coiled bacteria. Common in water as saprophytes; pathogenic species are numerous in many animals. *Leptospira interrogans* serotype *icterohaemorrhagiae* causes Weil's disease in humans: *Leptospira interrogans* serotype *canicola* infects dogs and pigs, and is transmissible to humans. ⊃ leptospirosis.

leptospiral agglutination tests serological tests used to diagnose specific leptospiral infections, e.g. Weil's disease.

leptospirosis *n* infection of humans by bacteria of the *Leptospira* group found in rats and other rodents, cattle, dogs, pigs and foxes. Those at risk include abattoir and agricultural workers and water sports enthusiasts. Presentation varies according to which leptospira is responsible, but may include: high fever, headache, conjunctival congestion, rash, anorexia, jaundice, severe muscular pains, rigors and vomiting. Severe infections may cause hepatitis, myocarditis, renal tubular necrosis and less frequently meningitis with an associated mortality rate of up to 20%. ⊃ Weil's disease.

Leriche's syndrome (R Leriche, French surgeon, 1879–1955) a syndrome caused by gradual blockage of the distal aorta. It is characterized by intermittent claudication felt in the buttocks, thighs and lower legs; erectile dysfunction; absent femoral pulses; muscle wastage; cold pale legs and gangrenous toes. Management includes restoring blood flow through the aorta and iliac arteries, e.g. bypass graft, endarterectomy.

lesbianism *n* sexual attraction between women.

Lesch–Nyhan disease (M Lesch, American paediatrician, b.1939; W Nyhan, American paediatrician, b.1926) X-linked recessive genetic disorder. Overproduction of uric acid, associated with brain damage resulting in cerebral palsy and learning disability. Victims are compelled, by a self-destructive urge, to bite away the sides of their mouth, lips and fingers.

lesion *n* pathological change in a bodily tissue.

lesser omentum ⊃ omentum.

lesser palatine foramen an opening situated close and posteriorly to the greater palatine foramen at the posterior border of the hard palate. Conducts the afferent lesser palatine nerve and blood vessels from the soft palate to the sphenopalatine ganglion.

LET *acron* **L**inear **E**nergy **T**ransfer.

'let down' reflex the neurohormonal process which stimulates milk ejection from the breast (the 'let down' reflex). The release of the hormone oxytocin from the posterior pituitary gland, which is also stimulated by the infant sucking, causes contraction of myoepithelial cells which surround the glandular tissue in the breast and milk is ejected. The 'let down' reflex also stimulates the ejection of milk from the breasts, for example when the mother hears her baby crying. The release of oxytocin also causes uterine contraction, which helps the uterus to involute (return to non-pregnant state). ⊃ afterpains, milk ejection reflex, milk flow mechanism.

lethal dose 50% (LD$_{50}$) the amount of a substance, such as a drug, that produces death in 50% of the members of a species population when administered as a single dose, within a set time.

letter of referral a letter from a doctor, dentist or other health professional referring a patient to a consultant or specialist or to another health professional. The purpose of the letter being to introduce the patient, describe the clinical history and seek advice and/or treatment on behalf of the patient.

Letterer–Siwe disease (E Letterer, German pathologist, 1895–1982; S Siwe, Swedish physician, 1897–1966) a disseminated form of Langerhans' cell histiocytosis that affects young children. There is infiltration of the lungs and bones, skin lesions, hepatosplenomegaly and lymphadenopathy.

leucine *n* an essential (indispensable) branched chain amino acid.

leucocytes *npl* generic name for white blood cells (WBCs). They are nucleated, mobile and are all involved with body defences, e.g. some are phagocytic and others produce antibodies. Unlike erythrocytes (red blood cells), they are nucleated, aerobic and move freely between the blood and tissue fluids. There are two main groups: (a) polymorphonuclear cells or granulocytes (neutrophils, basophils and eosinophils); (b) monocytes and lymphocytes—these generally have no granules, but some lymphocytes are granular. Of the total white cell count, more than 50% are neutrophils, which increase in number with many common infections (leucocytosis). These together with the much smaller numbers of basophils and eosinophils have a multilobed nucleus and contain granules with different staining properties. About 35% of WBCs are lymphocytes with a major role in humoral and cell-mediated immunity. Less numerous, but largest, are the circulating monocytes equivalent to macrophages in the tissues.

leucocytolysis *n* destruction and disintegration of white blood cells—**leucocytolytic** *adj*.

leucocytosis *n* increased number of leucocytes in the blood. Often a response to infection—**leucocytotic** *adj*.

leucodepletion the removal of white blood cells from donated blood for transfusion in order to reduce the risk of transmitting variant Creutzfeld–Jakob disease.

leucoderma *n* absent skin pigmentation, especially when it occurs in patches or bands.

leuco, leuko- a prefix that means 'white, white blood cell', e.g. *leucorrhoea*.

leucoma *n* white opaque spot on the cornea—**leucomata** *pl*.

leuconychia *n* white areas on the nails. These may be dots, lines, or extend over the entire nail plate (totalis). They are usually indicative of minor trauma, e.g. resulting from too small shoes or sporting activities.

leucopenia *n* decreased number of white blood cells in the blood—**leucopenic** *adj*.

leucopheresis donated blood is separated into its components and the white cells are retained before the remaining blood is returned to the donor. The white cells so obtained are used in the treatment of severe neutropenia.

leucopoiesis *n* formation of white blood cells from stem cells. Regulated by colony stimulating factors and cytokines—**leucopoietic** *adj*.

leucorrhoea *n* a sticky, whitish vaginal discharge—**leucorrhoeal** *adj*.

leukaemia *n* a group of neoplastic diseases of the haematopoietic tissue with most commonly abnormal proliferation of immature white blood cells (leucocytes). Uncontrolled proliferation of the leukaemic cells causes secondary suppression of other blood components, and anaemia and thrombocytopenia result. The lack of mature neutrophils (polymorphonuclear white blood cells) increases the risk of infection, thrombocytopenia increases the risk of bleeding, and anaemia may be severe. Causes include ionizing radiation, previous cytotoxic chemotherapy, retroviruses (e.g. human T-cell lymphotropic virus), chemicals, such as benzene, genetic anomalies (e.g. Down's syndrome). The classification is according to cell type—lymphocytic or myelocytic, and the course acute or chronic. Acute leukaemias have a rapid onset and early immature cells are produced (blast cells), commonly of the lymphoid and myeloid series. The acute leukaemias include acute lymphoblastic leukaemia (ALL) in children and acute myeloblastic leukaemia (AML) in adults. Chronic leukaemias have an insidious onset and the cells produced are more mature, commonly lymphocytes and granulocytes. Chronic forms can become acute with blast cell proliferation. Chronic leukaemias include chronic lymphocytic leukaemia (CLL) and chronic myeloid (granulocytic) leukaemia (CML), both of which affect adults. The chronic leukaemias may enter a 'blast crisis' or acute phase. Less common leukaemias include: monocytic, eosinophilic, basophilic and hairy cell. The management of leukaemia depends upon: the cell type, whether acute or chronic and the aim of treatment: remission or palliation. Therapeutic options include chemotherapy, radiotherapy, interferon alpha, monoclonal antibodies and haemopoietic stem cell transplantation, either autologous or an allograft. Plus supportive measures that include antimicrobial drugs, blood components transfusion and protective isolation. ⊃ hairy cell leukaemia, myeloproliferative disorders, myelodysplastic syndrome (MDS), prolymphocytic leukaemia.

leukocidins exotoxins produced by streptococci and staphylococci. They cause white blood cell lysis and death. ⊃ Panton-Valentine leukocidin.

leukocoria (*syn* white pupil, white pupillary reflex) it is also spelt leucocorea, leukocorea or leukokoria. A condition characterized by a whitish reflex within the pupil. It is secondary to cataract, Coats' disease, persistent hyperplastic primary vitreous, retinoblastoma, retinopathy of prematurity, etc. ⊃ Colour Section Figure 86.

leukoma it is also spelt leucoma. Dense, white, corneal opacity caused by scar tissue. A localized leukoma appears as a whitish scar surrounded by normal cornea. A generalized leukoma involves the entire cornea which appears white, often with blood vessels coursing over its surface. Visual impairment depends on the location and extent of the leukoma. If the opacity is faint, it is called a nebula. ⊃ cornea, corneal ulcer, hyperacuity.

leukoplakia *n* white, thickened patch occurring on mucous membranes. Occurs on lips, inside mouth or on genitalia. Usually patchy and often premalignant. ⊃ kraurosis vulvae.

leukotrienes *npl* endogenous regulatory lipids derived from arachidonic acid (fatty acid). They function as signalling molecules in the inflammatory response and in some allergic responses, and are one of the triggers of asthma. ⊃ leukotriene receptor antagonists.

leukotriene receptor antagonists drugs such as montelukast and zafirlukast that block the effects of leukotrienes in the airways by blocking the leukotriene receptors. Developed as part of the treatment regimen for asthma and are particularly useful where exercise-induced symptoms are prominent or when there is associated rhinitis. ⊃ Appendix 5.

levan ⊃ extracellular polysaccharides.

levator *n* **1.** a muscle which acts by raising a part, e.g. levator scapulae. **2.** an instrument for lifting a depressed part.

lever arm distance from the fulcrum (or pivot or axis) at which a force is applied.

lever system system which has a rigid link (lever) and a fulcrum (or pivot or axis) about which the lever can turn. Can provide increases in force or in range of motion (and velocity) depending on the arrangement of the components and the forces applied. ⊃ first-class levers, lever arm, mechanical advantage, second-class levers, third-class levers.

Levin tube (A Levin, American physician, 1880–1940) a plastic catheter used for gastric intubation; it has a closed weighted tip and an opening on the side.

Lewis hunting reaction ⊃ ice/cold therapy, hunting reaction.

Lewis triple response ⊃ triple response.

Lewy bodies (F Lewy, German neurologist, 1885–1950) inclusion bodies found in damaged and dying nerve cells in the brain that is the pathological hallmark of Parkinson's disease. Also present in Lewy body dementia, Alzheimer's disease and other neurodegenerative disease.

Leydig cells (F von Leydig, German anatomist, 1821–1908) ⊃ interstitial cells.

LFA *abbr* low-friction arthroplasty.

LFTs *abbr* liver function tests.

LGB *abbr* lateral geniculate bodies.

LGVCFT *abbr* lymphogranuloma venereum complement fixation test.

LH *abbr* luteinizing hormone.

Lhermitte's sign (J Lhermitte, French neurologist, 1877–1959) sudden electric shock-like sensations moving down the body when the head is flexed. It is indicative of compression of the cervical spinal cord or multiple sclerosis.

Lhermitte–Trelles syndrome (J Lhermitte; J Trelles Montes, Peruvian neurologist, 1904–1990) flexion of the neck. It is characterized by lymphoblastic infiltrations within the peripheral nervous system—associated with paresis.

libido *n* Freud's term for the urge to obtain sensual satisfaction. Sometimes used to mean the sexual urge. Freud's meaning was satisfaction through all the senses.

lice *n* ⊃ pediculus.

lichen *n* aggregations of papular skin lesions—**lichenoid** *adj*.

lichenification *n* thickening of the skin, usually secondary to scratching. Skin markings become more prominent and the area affected appears to be composed of small, shiny rhomboids. ⊃ neurodermatitis.

lichen nitidus skin disorder characterized by minute, shiny, flat-topped, pink papules of pinhead size.

lichenoid a lesion resembling those of lichen planus.

lichen planus a rash characterized by intensely itchy polygonal papules with a violaceous hue involving the skin and less commonly the mucosae, hair and nails. The cause is unknown but an immune pathogenesis is suspected as there is an association with some autoimmune diseases such as myasthenia gravis, and with thymoma and graft-versus-host disease. Rashes with clinical and histological features of lichen planus can occur in chronic active hepatitis, in hepatitis B and C infections, and in patients taking drugs, the most common culprits being gold and other heavy metals, sulphonamides, penicillamine, antimalarials, antituberculous drugs and thiazide diuretics. They also occur in those handling colour developers. There is hyperkeratosis, a prominent granular layer, basal cell degeneration and a heavy T-lymphocyte infiltration in the upper dermis. Degenerating basal cells are seen as colloid (apoptotic) bodies. The T cell–basal cell interaction leaves a 'sawtooth' dermo-epidermal junction. The picture suggests an immune reaction to an unknown epidermal antigen. Lichen planus tends to start on the distal limbs, most commonly the volar aspects of the wrists, and the lower back. Intensely itchy, flat-topped, pink-purplish papules appear and some develop a characteristic fine white network on their surface (Wickham's striae). ⊃ Colour Section Figure 87. New lesions may appear at the site of trauma (Koebner phenomenon) and the rash may spread rapidly to become generalized. Individual lesions may last for many months and the eruption as a whole tends to last about 1 year, often leaving marked post-inflammatory pigmentation. Mucous membrane involvement, comprising an asymptomatic fine white lacy network of pinhead-sized white papules, occurs in about two-thirds of patients. The nails are usually normal but in 10% they may be affected, with changes ranging from longitudinal grooving to destruction of the nail fold and bed. Variants of the classic picture are rare; they include annular, atrophic, bullous, follicular, hypertrophic and ulcerative types. Diagnosis is usually clear-cut clinically but a skin biopsy can be helpful. Other erythematous scaly conditions should be considered in the differential diagnosis, including guttate psoriasis, pityriasis rosea, pityriasis lichenoides and drug eruptions. The condition is usually self-limiting, although rarely, particularly with oral lichen planus, it may persist for more than 10 years. Potent local corticosteroids may help with intense itch but systemic corticosteroids may be indicated, and ciclosporin, retinoids or phototherapy may be required. Topical corticosteroids applied to the buccal mucosa may also be required.

lichen sclerosis (LS) ⊃ lichen sclerosus et atrophicus (LSA).

lichen sclerosus et atrophicus (LSA) (*syn* lichen sclerosis) an uncommon autoimmune disease mainly affecting women. Ivory-white or violaceous areas occur on the perianal and vulval regions with 'cigarette paper' atrophy. There may be follicular plugging, erosions and fissuring, sclerosis and purpura. In men, the glans penis and prepuce (foreskin) may be involved, leading to phimosis or meatal stricture. Dyspareunia, soreness and pruritus often cause distress. The condition is potentially premalignant (more often in women). Potent topical corticosteroids are used initially and for phimosis or meatal strictures surgery may be necessary. ⊃ balanitis xerotica obliterans (BXO), pruritus vulvae, vulval intraepithelial neoplasia.

lichen scrofulosorum a form of tuberculide.

lichen simplex describes a plaque of lichenified eczema due to repeated rubbing or scratching, as a habit or in response to stress. Common sites include the nape of the neck, the lower legs and the anogenital area. ⊃ neurodermatitis.

lid eversion turning of the eyelid inside out so as to expose the palpebral conjunctiva. For the upper lid this is accomplished by grasping the lid by the central eyelashes, pulling it downward and forward and then folding it back over a cotton applicator (or thin plastic rod) placed at the upper margin of the tarsus, while the patient continually maintains downward fixation. Return to the normal lid position is obtained by asking the patient to look up and gently pushing the eyelashes in an outward and downward direction. Foreign bodies and even contact lenses are often lodged under the upper eyelid or in the conjunctival fornix of the upper eyelid. To inspect the superior conjunctival fornix double lid eversion is necessary. Following lid eversion (and usually with local anaesthesia of the conjunctiva), a retractor is placed between the two skin surfaces of the lid with the retractor engaging the tarsus and, after gently pulling outward and upward, the fornix will become visible. Eversion of the lower lid is performed easily by drawing the margin downward while the patient looks upward. ⊃ eyelids, subtarsal sulcus.

lie, fetal the relation of the long axis of the fetus to the long axis of the woman's uterus, normally parallel with a longitudinal lie. In an abnormal lie the fetus lies across the uterus, i.e. transverse or oblique lie, which if not corrected, causes obstructed labour.

Lieberkühn's glands (J Lieberkühn, German anatomist, 1711–1756) also called crypts of Lieberkühn. Tubular intestinal glands.

lien *n* the spleen.

lienculus *n* a small accessory spleen.

lienorenal *adj* pertaining to the spleen and kidney. ⊃ splenorenal.

lie scale in psychometrics, items included within a test or questionnaire designed to detect whether respondents have responded truthfully to the items the test is designed to tap. An example would be an item that everybody would be expected to endorse if responding truthfully (e.g. 'I sometimes get upset'). If an individual did not endorse this item it would be assumed that they are not responding truthfully.

life crisis describes an unforeseen unpleasant occurrence, such as becoming the victim of a violent crime, sudden and severe ill health or a life event, e.g. marriage or divorce, becoming unemployed, retirement.

life event in sociology a term describing the major occurrences occurring during the lifespan, such as starting school, getting married or ending a relationship, changing job, moving house, or suffering a bereavement.

life expectancy the average age at which death occurs. Influenced by health/illness and by social factors such as level of education; and environmental factors such as housing, sanitation and the supply of clean water.

lifelong learning learning throughout the person's lifespan. Particularly important for health professionals who are required to update their knowledge and skills in order to fulfil the conditions set for periodic registration and licence to practice by their statutory regulation body.

lifestyle the way that an individual organizes and balances her/his daily activities to satisfy personal needs and meet societal expectations.

lifestyle planning techniques used to enable an individual to achieve a balance between occupational roles in order to reduce stress, improve quality of life, develop potentials and attain relevant personal goals. Activity analysis is used to determine the occupational performance skills required and activities are recommended that are consistent with the individual's priorities and anticipated abilities.

life-years gained the average years of life gained per patient from a particular healthcare intervention. ⊃ quality-adjusted life years.

Li–Fraumeni syndrome (F Li, American epidemiologist, 20th century; J Fraumeni, American epidemiologist, 20th century) also known by other names, for example sarcoma, breast, leukaemia and adrenal gland (SBLA) syndrome. A very rare inherited condition that significantly increases the risk of developing several different cancers during childhood and early adulthood. These include cancers of the breast, brain, adrenal gland, osteosarcoma, soft tissue sarcoma and leukaemia. It is inherited as an autosomal dominant condition and many of those affected inherit a mutation of the TP53 gene, which normally acts as a tumour suppressor gene. Mutations of the CHEK2 gene, another tumour suppressor gene, may be associated with an increased risk of a certain cancer, such as breast cancer.

lift force force between a moving object and its surrounding medium that acts at right angles to the direction of travel of the object; may be influenced by its shape, by its angle of orientation to the direction of flow past it of fluid (liquid or gas), or by spin. ⊃ Magnus force.

ligament *n* a strong band of fibrous tissue serving to bind bones or other parts together, or to support an organ. Ligaments may form part of the capsule around a joint or be within the joint itself, such as the cruciate ligaments of the knee. Ligaments need to be flexible, to facilitate joint movement, but relatively non-elastic to provide strength and stability and to limit the range and direction of movements at a joint—**ligamentous** *adj*.

ligament of Lockwood (C Lockwood, British surgeon, 1856–1915) the lower part of the capsule of Tenon and parts of the tendons of the inferior rectus and oblique muscles which are thickened to form a hammock-like structure on which the eyeball rests. ⊃ extraocular muscles of the eye, Tenon's capsule.

ligament of Wieger ⊃ hyaloideocapsular ligament.

ligament tear disruption of a ligament, which may be partial or complete. The resultant bleeding causes pain, swelling and loss of function. Ligament tears are graded 1–3 in increasing severity: *grade* 1—microtears and stretching but ligament integrity intact; *grade* 2—partial disruption with laxity but a discernible endpoint on stressing; *grade* 3—complete rupture. Grade 3 tears, though most severe, may be relatively painless if nerve fibres are also torn. Severe or complete tears disrupt joint function and stability. Sometimes a bony fragment is torn off the bone at the ligament attachment—known as an avulsion fracture. Treatment includes RICE and anti-inflammatory medication (though 'Rest', i.e. complete immobilization, is now rare, to avoid secondary muscle wasting and loss of function). Surgery may be indicated if return to sport is important, e.g. after complete anterior cruciate ligament rupture. A graduated rehabilitation programme is required with a gradual and progressive increase in strength work, balance and flexibility, before returning to sport or exercise.

ligamentous relating to a ligament.

ligamentous position ⊃ retruded contact position.

ligamentum arteriosus vestiges of the ductus arteriosus that functioned in the fetal circulation.

ligamentum teres 1. a ligament that secures the femur in the acetabulum. **2.** the fibrous remnant of the fetal umbilical vein within the falciform ligament of the liver.

ligamentum venosum vestiges of the ductus venosus that functioned in the fetal circulation.

ligand signalling chemicals that include cytokines, hormones or neurotransmitters. They can affect cell function by binding to specific cell membrane receptors. Many drugs cause their effects by being able to imitate the natural ligand.

ligate *vt* to tie off blood vessels, etc., at operation—**ligation** *n*.

ligation *n* tying off; usually reserved for *ligation of the uterine (fallopian) tubes*, a method of sterilization.

ligature *n* the material used for tying vessels or stitching the tissues. ⊃ suture. In orthodontics, a length of soft wire or elastic material used to retain an archwire in a bracket.

ligature and pin cutting pliers ⊃ pliers.

ligature locking pliers ⊃ pliers.

ligature wire the soft, corrosion-resistant wire used in jaw fixation and splinting natural teeth. ⊃ interdental eyelet wiring.

light the electromagnetic vibration capable of stimulating the receptors of the retina and of producing a visual sensation. The radiations that give rise to the sensation of vision are comprised within the wavelength band 380–780 nm. This band is called the visible spectrum or visible light. The borders of this band are not precise but beyond these radiations the visual efficacy of any wavelength becomes very low indeed (less than 10^{-5}). For an older person, the lower boundary of the visible spectrum is closer to 420 nm than 380 nm. ⊃ absorptive lens, blue, electromagnetic spectrum, green, infrared radiations/rays (IRR), orange, quantum theory, red, spectroscope, ultraviolet (UV) rays, violet, wavelength, wave theory, yellow.

light adaptation adjustments made by the eye in bright light. The pupils constrict, rhodopsin breakdown reduces retinal sensitivity and cone activity increases. ⊃ dark adaptation.

Light Amplification by Stimulated Emission of Radiation ⊃ laser.

light beam diaphragm a light source, incorporated in the tube housing to visually indicate the area covered by the radiation emitted from the X-ray tube.

light pen a device, shaped like a pen, which interfaces with a computer screen and enables the computer to identify which part of the screen is being pointed to.

light reflex 1. (*syn* retinoscopic light) that light which appears in the pupil in retinoscopy. It is light reflected by the retina. **2.** Any reflected light. ⊃ pupillary light reflex.

light stress test ⊃ photostress test.

lightening *n* an informal term used to denote the relief of pressure on the diaphragm by the abdominal viscera, when the presenting part of the fetus descends into the pelvis in the last 3 weeks of a primigravida's pregnancy.

lightning pains symptomatic of tabes dorsalis. Occur as paroxysms of swift-cutting (lightning) stabs in the lower limbs.

lignans compounds present in various foods. They display both oestrogenic and antioestrogenic properties. ⊃ phyto-oestrogens.

ligneous conjunctivitis a rare, chronic conjunctivitis characterized by the formation of a firm, whitish membrane or pseudomembrane on the tarsal conjunctiva, usually of the upper eyelid. It is typically bilateral, begins in childhood although it may present in patients up to age 85, is more common in females than in males and may persist for months or years. Its cause is unknown but the predisposing factors include bacterial and viral infections, trauma, hypersensitivity reactions and increased vascular permeability and it is often associated with inflammations of other mucous membranes. The most effective treatment is surgical excision followed by topical ciclosporin drops, but the condition has a tendency to recur. ⊃ pseudomembranous conjunctivitis.

lignin lignocellulose. The indigestible part of the plant cell wall.

Likert scale (described by R Likert an American psychologist in 1932) a scale used in questionnaire surveys. Participants are asked to specify their degree of agreement with a particular statement, i.e. strongly agree, agree, unsure, disagree and strongly disagree. The answers may then be coded, e.g. 1–2–3–4–5, but this remains just a coding. The data collected are ordinal, i.e. they have an inherent order or sequence, but one cannot assume that the differences between each answer are equal in size, i.e. the scale is not linear.

limbal blanching a whitening of the limbal area due to pressure from the edge of a soft contact lens which fits too tightly. ⊃ corneal limbus, push-up test.

limbal conjunctiva ⊃ conjunctiva.

limb girdle muscular dystrophy a muscular dystrophy that is inherited as either an autosomal dominant condition (type 1) or as an autosomal recessive condition (type 2). It is caused by many mutations on different chromosomes. The onset is during childhood/early adulthood and the limb girdle muscles are affected. Some individuals have pseudohypertrophy of the calf muscles; some have cardiac conduction problems.

limbic system a diffuse collection of nuclei and nerve fibres in an area within the cerebral hemispheres. Its structures include the hippocampus, hypothalamus, amydala and part of the thalamus. It is part of the 'primitive' brain, formed from evolutionarily older cortex. Concerned with autonomic functions, feelings and emotions such as anger, rage, sadness, sexual arousal and pleasure. Also associated with the sense of smell and memories associated with a particular smell, motivation and memory.

limbus *n* (*syn* corneoscleral junction)—**limbal** *adj.* ⊃ corneal limbus.

lime calcium oxide (quicklime, unslaked lime). A constituent of silicate powder and some root-filling pastes.

liminal *adj* of a stimulus, of the lowest intensity that can be perceived by human sense organs. ⊃ subliminal.

liminality a transitional period between culturally defined life crises or social states.

limits of stability the range within which a person can move in any direction without a postural change or loss of balance.

limosis abnormal appetite.

linctus *n* a sweet, syrupy liquid, usually given to relieve a cough.

line 1. a thin continuous mark, ridge or strip. **2.** in anatomy and radiography, an imaginary line connecting certain landmarks on the body or passing through them. **3.** a boundary. ⊃ cervical line, finishing line, line angle, neonatal line, survey line.

linea *n* a line.

linea alba the white line visible after removal of the skin in the centre of the abdomen, stretching from the ensiform cartilage to the pubis, its position on the surface being indicated by a slight depression.

linea aspera a 'roughened' vertical ridge on the posterior surface of the femur; provides attachment for several muscles, for example the adductor brevis, adductor longus, adductor magnus.

lineae albicantes white lines which appear on the abdomen after reduction of tension as after childbirth, drainage of ascites from the abdomen, etc. ⊃ striae gravidarum.

line angle angle formed at the junction of two tooth surfaces or of two cavity walls.

linea nigra pigmented line from umbilicus to pubis which appears in pregnancy.

linear acceleration the rate of change in linear velocity with respect to time; related to force by Newton's second law of motion (often stated as force = mass × linear acceleration). Measured in metres per second squared (m/s). ⊃ acceleration, angular acceleration, gravitational acceleration, instantaneous acceleration, tangential acceleration.

linear accelerator radiotherapy equipment where electrons produced by an electron gun pass through a waveguide and are accelerated and fed into a treatment head to produce high-energy X-rays or an electron beam used in the treatment of various cancers.

linear array in ultrasound, a set of elements mounted in line and pulsed electronically in sequence to produce a rectangular field of view.

linear attenuation coefficient (μ) measures the probability of photon interaction along the path of an X-ray beam, that is the fraction of X-rays removed from a beam per unit thickness of the attenuating medium. Differences in the linear attenuation coefficient are responsible for radiographic image contrast and it is a series of these measurements which are used to produce the image in computed tomography (CT) scanning. It is dependent upon the beam energy, and the structure and density of the material traversed.

linear displacement the distance and direction between the start and end point. Contains a measure of distance (e.g. metres) and a measure of direction (e.g. an angle in degrees to the horizontal)—effectively the distance and direction 'as the crow flies'. ⊃ angular displacement, displacement.

K
L

linear energy transfer (LET) the energy that a particle dissipates, per unit length of its path, as it travels through absorbing medium.

linear expansivity is a measure of thermal expansion and is defined as the change in unit length per unit change in temperature in degrees Kelvin.

linear impulse force applied to a translating body or object multiplied by duration of the application (newtons × seconds, N/s).

linear kinematics the study of motion which takes place in straight lines (rectilinear) or curves (curvilinear). ⊃ angular kinematics, kinematics.

linear kinetics the study of forces but not torques or moments. ⊃ angular kinetics, kinetics.

linear magnification ⊃ lateral magnification.

linear measurement the measurement of a straight line between two points.

linear momentum the product of mass and velocity. The change in linear momentum is equal to the linear impulse. Conservation of linear momentum in the absence of external unbalanced forces, the total linear momentum of colliding bodies or objects will remain constant. Commonly applied to racquet/ball impacts. ⊃ angular momentum, momentum.

linear motion ⊃ motion.

linear scanner *n* radionuclide imaging in which the crystal moves backwards and forwards across an organ, the images are then recorded as a photoscan or a dot diagram. The equipment has been superseded by gamma cameras.

linear sources several collinear tubes mounted in an applicator and used in intercavitary therapy to treat line sources, for example the uterine cavity.

linear speed is usually measured in metres per second (m/s), kilometres per hour (km/h) or miles per hour (mph). ⊃ angular speed, speed, velocity.

linear velocity the linear displacement per unit time. ⊃ angular velocity, instantaneous velocity, tangential velocity, velocity.

line defects edge dislocation when an extra plane of atoms extends into the crystal lattice.

line of action direction in which a force acts upon a body or object.

line of direction the line joining an object in space with its image on the retina (allowing for the optical properties of the eye). The line joining the fixation point to the fovea is called the principal line of direction. However, the object appears to lie along a visual direction and that direction in visual space associated with the fovea is called the principal visual direction. All other visual directions associated with other retinal points are called secondary visual directions. The principal line of direction and the principal visual direction coincide, but the former indicates the direction towards the eye, while the latter indicates the direction away from the eye. ⊃ law of identical visual directions.

line of sight (*syn* principal line of vision) line joining the point of fixation to the centre of the entrance pupil. This line is more practical than the visual axis.

liner 1. a substance applied to the walls of a cavity preparation to protect the pulp from irritation by restorative materials. ⊃ cavity liner. **2.** an insulating substance placed inside a casting ring.

lingua *n* the tongue—**lingual** *adj*.

lingual pertaining to the tongue, or resembling the tongue.

lingual arch in orthodontics, the heavy-gauge archwire that is attached to bands on the posterior teeth and which lies on the palatal or lingual aspect of the standing teeth.

lingual artery a branch of the external carotid artery. It supplies the tongue, the lining membrane of the mouth, the structures in the floor of the mouth, the lingual tonsil, the sublingual salivary gland, and the epiglottis.

lingual bar major connector of a mandibular partial denture and which is normally placed between the floor of the mouth and the gingival margin.

lingual button also known as cleat or lug. An orthodontic attachment situated on the lingual aspect of a tooth and to which a wire or elastic may be secured.

lingual fraenum ⊃ frenulum or frenum.

lingual frenulum or frenum ⊃ frenulum or frenum.

lingual rest occlusal rest placed on the lingual surface of a tooth.

lingual surface any surface of an organ adjacent to the tongue. ⊃ surface.

lingual thyroid a rare developmental condition in which the thyroid tissue is found in the posterior superior surface of the tongue.

lingual tonsils ⊃ tonsils.

lingula a small, tongue-like projection of bone. The mandibular foramen is protected by a lingula of bone.

linguo-occlusion the displacement of a tooth or teeth towards the tongue.

linguoversion an unusual position of a tooth that is inclined lingually.

liniment *n* a liquid applied to the skin using gentle friction.

lining in dentistry, the covering for a surface such as the inner walls of a cavity preparation. Often contains calcium hydroxide. Applied to seal the dentinal tubules and protect the dental pulp as well as to promote the growth of reparative dentine. *resilient/soft lining* a form of relining which provides a soft or resilient tissue bearing surface for a removable prosthesis. ⊃ zinc oxide-eugenol and zinc phosphate cement.

linitis plastica also known as leather bottle stomach. A form of gastric cancer which infiltrates throughout the gastric wall. This leads to diffuse thickening and failure to inflate at endoscopy and barium examinations.

linkage in genetics, a state in which two or more genes are close together on a chromosome and so do not segregate independently during meiosis. This means that they are usually inherited together and are associated with a particular inherited characteristic. Genes located at more distant loci are more likely to cross over and become separated during meiosis.

linoleic acid an omega-6, polyunsaturated, essential fatty acid. It is found in vegetable seed oils, such as sunflower, corn and soya bean. ⊃ essential fatty acids.

linolenic acids polyunsaturated, essential fatty acids found in vegetable oils. There are two types: alpha (α)-linolenic (ALA), an omega-3 fatty acid, which is found in flax (linseed) oil and soya bean oil. ALA is used by the body to produce docosahexaenoic acid (DHA) and eicosapentaenoic acid (EPA); and gamma (γ)-linolenic (GLA), which is an omega-6 fatty acid found in evening primrose oil. GLA is important in the formation of prostaglandins. ⊃ essential fatty acids.

LIP *acron* lymphocytic interstitial pneumonia.

lip the fleshy fold bordering the external entrance to the cavity of the mouth. *Hapsburg lip* an overdeveloped thick lower lip said to be similar to that which characterized the jaws of the Hapsburg dynasty. ⊃ cleft lip, high lip line, low lip line.

lip bumper an orthodontic appliance that affects the dentition in one arch only. It is connected to the teeth and utilizes the resistance of the lips to that part of the appliance designed to displace the lips from their resting posture.

lip reading the ability of deaf and hard of hearing persons to understand the spoken word by observing the movement of the lips and associated facial muscles.

lip seal the ability of the lips to come together and thus seal the oral cavity.

lipaemia *n* increased lipids (especially cholesterol) in the blood—**lipaemic** *adj*.

lipase *n* any fat-splitting enzyme, such as pancreatic lipase. They convert fats into fatty acids and glycerol.

lipectomy surgical removal of subcutaneous fat, such as from the abdominal wall.

lipid peroxidation the oxidation of fatty acids in cell membranes by free radicals. ⊃ free radicals, reactive oxygen species.

lipids *npl* large group of fat-like organic molecules which include: neutral (true) fats (triglycerides *syn*. triacylglycerols); phospholipids in cell membranes and lung surfactant; glycolipids in the nervous system; lipoproteins; fat-soluble vitamins; steroids/sterols (including cholesterol, bile acids and steroid hormones); the regulatory prostanoids (prostaglandins, prostacyclin, leukotrienes and thromboxanes). Lipids consist of carbon, oxygen and hydrogen, and some contain phosphorus and nitrogen. They are insoluble in water, but they can be dissolved in organic solvents such as alcohol. Lipids are important in the body both structurally and functionally. Fat deposits provide an energy store, insulate and offer some physical protection. Other lipids are important constituents of cell membranes, are precursors for steroid hormones, act as regulatory molecules, e.g. prostaglandins, and transport fats around the body, and the fat-soluble vitamins are concerned with blood clotting, vision and antioxidant functions. The major lipids circulating in blood are triglycerides, cholesterol, cholesteryl esters, phospholipids and non-esterified fatty acids. ⊃ body fat, hyperlipidaemia, lipoproteins.

lipoatrophy *n* breakdown of fat cells at sites used for repeated insulin injections. There is a hollowed appearance. Compare lipohypertrophy.

lipochondrodystrophy ⊃ Hurler's syndrome.

lipodystrophy *n* a disorder of fat metabolism or the deposition of fat within the tissues. There is loss of fat tissue. It may be congenital or acquired.

lipoedema *n* the accumulation of fat in the lower extremities (hips down to ankles) with associated tenderness.

lipofuscins *npl* pigments formed mainly from the oxidation of fats that are deposited in a variety of body tissues, particularly the myocardium and liver in adults. Lipofuscins accumulate in the lysosomes during ageing.

lipogenesis *n* the formation of fatty acids from carbohydrate, mainly in the liver. It is stimulated by insulin. The fatty acids can then be combined with glycerol to form triglycerides (triacylglycerols) which are incorporated in very low-density lipoproteins (VLDL), passed into the circulation and taken up by adipose and muscle tissue; thus excess of ingested carbohydrate that is not used immediately for metabolic purposes is taken up and stored as triglyceride in adipose tissue and muscle. ⊃ free fatty acids, lipoprotein, lipase.

lipohypertrophy an increase in subcutaneous fat at sites used for repeated insulin injections. Compare lipoatrophy.

lipoid *adj*, *n* (a substance) resembling fats or oil.

lipoidosis/lipidosis *n* disease due to disorder of fat metabolism—**lipoidoses** *pl*.

lipolysis *n* the enzymatic breakdown of triglyceride molecules, in muscle and adipose tissue, catalysed by the class of enzymes known as lipases. Stimulated by glucocorticoid hormones. During endurance-type exercise, the rate of lipolysis is increased at both sites—**lipolytic** *adj*.

lipoma *n* a benign tumour of fatty tissue—**lipomata** *pl*, **lipomatous** *adj*.

lipopolysaccharide a molecule containing lipids and polysaccharides found as a component of the cell wall in some bacteria.

lipoprotein *n* lipids combined with a protein that transport triglycerides (triacylglycerols) and cholesterol around the body in the blood. They are classified into four main groups by increasing density (related inversely to the % triglyceride content): (a) chylomicrons the most rich in triglyceride, formed in intestinal cells from the absorbed breakdown products of dietary fat, carried in lymphatic vessels to reach the liver and the general circulation; (b) very low-density lipoproteins (VLDL) synthesized in and released into the blood from the liver, rich in endogenously produced triglyceride; (c) low-density lipoproteins (LDL), formed mainly from VLDL after they have lost triglyceride in the tissues. LDL have the highest cholesterol content, carrying this to all tissues. High plasma LDL is associated with increased risk of coronary heart disease, as some cells (particularly macrophages in the arterial wall) may become cholesterol-laden; (d) high-density lipoproteins (HDL), formed in liver and intestinal cells, take up cholesterol from the tissues and transport it to the liver for excretion in the bile.

High plasma HDL is associated with reduced risk of coronary heart disease. ⊃ hyperlipidaemia, lipids.

lipoprotein lipase (LPL) capillary endothelial enzyme that acts on lipoprotein particles (chylomicrons and VLDL) as they pass through capillaries in muscle, heart and adipose tissue, and hydrolyses their triglyceride (triacylglycerol) to monoglyceride and fatty acids, which then move into cells. ⊃ lipogenesis.

liposarcoma a malignant growth of fat cells—**liposarcomas, liposarcomata** *pl.*

liposome *n* a spherical body comprising a phospholipid bilayer enclosing an aqueous solution.

liposome drug delivery drug administration using drugs enclosed in vesicles. Drug release occurs when the liposome is broken down in the liver by cells of the monocyte-macrophage (reticuloendothelial) system.

liposuction *n* in cosmetic surgery a technique of vacuum extraction of subcutaneous fat using cannulae.

lipotrophic substances factors which cause the removal of fat from the liver by transmethylation.

lipotrophin hormone secreted by the anterior pituitary gland that is involved in releasing fat from the stores in adipose tissue. It has two forms: beta (β)-lipotrophin; and gamma (γ)-lipotrophin. Lipotrophins are structurally similar to adrenocorticotrophic hormone, endorphins and melanocyte stimulating hormones. ⊃ pro-opiomelanocortin.

lipping abnormal bone growth adjacent to the margin of a joint. It is demonstated radiographically and is a feature of degenerative conditions that include osteoarthritis.

lipuria *n* (*syn* adiposuria) fat in the urine—**lipuric** *adj.*

liquid-based cytology (LBC) a newer technology used in cervical screening for abnormal cells. It produces better specimens for cytological examination and early evidence suggests that sensitivity and specificity are improved. May also be used to detect infections such as the human papilloma virus.

liquid crystal display a form of flat screen imaging monitor using liquid crystals and a back light to produce the image. In colour monitors each pixel is subdivided into three colours, red, blue and green, by the use of filters, each of which can be activated independently to produce the colour image.

liquid lens (*syn* fluid lens, lacrimal lens, tear lens) the lens formed by the tear layer lying between the back surface of a contact lens and the cornea. It must be taken into account when fitting contact lenses. If the back surface of the lens is steeper than the cornea, the liquid lens is positive and the eye is made more myopic. If the back surface of the lens is flatter than the cornea, the liquid lens is negative and the eye is made more hyperopic (see Figure L.4). ⊃ contact lens, keratometer.

liquid scintillation process a method of detecting radionuclides which decay solely by beta (β) decay. The solution used contains a solvent, a scintillation solute and a secondary solute in which is dissolved a radionuclide.

liquor *n* a solution.

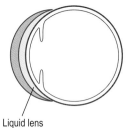

Liquid lens

L.4 **Liquid lens between a contact lens and the cornea** (it is positive in this example) (reproduced from Millodot 2004 with permission).

liquor amnii fluid surrounding the fetus. ⊃ amniotic fluid.

Lisch nodules (K Lisch, Austrian opthalmologist, 1907–1999) small circular pigmented hamartomas present in the iris in neurofibromatosis.

Lisfranc's injury (J Lisfranc, French surgeon, 1790–1847) an injury to the foot comprising a combination of dislocation of the third, fourth and fifth metatarsals with a fracture through the base of the second metatarsal.

LISP *acron* **LIS**t **P**rocessor language.

lissamine green a vital stain with dyeing quality similar to that of rose bengal, but which causes less discomfort. It stains dead or degenerated epithelial cells green and is used to facilitate the diagnosis of keratitis sicca, xerophthalmia, etc. It has a molecular weight of 577. ⊃ keratitis sicca, rose bengal, xerophthalmia.

lissencephaly a rare chromosomal disorder in which the brain is malformed. The brain surface is smooth and has no sulci or gyri. The affected infant has other brain malformations and microcephaly. It is associated with abnormalities occurring in many body systems. The effects include abnormal facial appearance, failure to thrive, feeding difficulties, dysphagia, severe developmental problems, deformity of the hands and feet, muscle hypertonia and seizures. Various types exist and it may be associated with other syndromes, such as Miller–Dieker syndrome. The prognosis for affected infants is very variable and depends on the severity of the brain malformation, but many die during the first 2 years.

listening *n* a group of complex skills used in communication; health professionals should give their whole attention to what is being said, how it is being said, and whether or not it matches the non-verbal signals.

Listeria *n* a genus of bacteria present in animal faeces and soil. *Listeria monocytogenes* causes meningitis, septicaemia, and intrauterine or perinatal infections. ⊃ listeriosis.

listeriosis *n* infection caused by *Listeria*. Transmitted via contaminated soil, contact with infected animals and by eating unpasteurized foods, such as soft cheeses, that may be infected. Infection may lead to a flu-like illness but serious consequences may occur in infants, older people, debilitated or immunocompromised individuals and pregnant women. Infection during pregnancy may lead to miscarriage, stillbirth, preterm labour and septicaemia and neonatal meningitis.

K
L

list processor language (LISP) a high-level computer language.

literature review the process of locating and appraising relevant information, usually from a range of sources. It involves a methodical and wide-ranging examination of the papers relevant to a topic. Research methods and results are analysed and presented critically. The literature review includes how the search was carried out, e.g. bibliographical databases such as Allied and Complementary Database, electronic bibliography software, MEDLINE.

-lith a suffix that means 'calculus, stone', e.g. *otolith*.

-lithiasis a suffix that means 'presence of stones', e.g. cholecystolithiasis.

lithiasis *n* any condition in which there are calculi (stones).

lithium (Li) *n* a metallic element. Lithium salts are used therapeutically in some mental health problems.

litholapaxy *n* (*syn.* lithopaxy) crushing a stone within the urinary bladder and removing the fragments by irrigation.

lithopaedion *n* a dead fetus retained in the uterus, e.g. one of a pair of twins which dies and becomes mummified and sometimes impregnated with lime salts.

lithotomy *n* general term for the surgical incision of a duct or organ for the removal of calculi, especially one from the urinary tract.

lithotomy position with the person lying down, the buttocks are drawn to the end of the table. The thighs and legs are flexed and abducted and are held in place with lithotomy poles. Each foot is placed in a sling attached to the top of the poles so that the perineum is exposed for genitourinary procedures. These include some vaginal procedures, cystoscopy and for forceps or breech delivery and perineal suturing. The person's legs must be lifted into or out of the stirrups together, preferably by two people, one on each side, to avoid possible hip dislocation. The risk of hip dislocation is increased during labour due to joint laxity resulting from relaxin and progesterone influences.

lithotripsy *n* destruction or elimination of calculi in the urinary tract or gallbladder. It may be achieved either by surgical intervention to crush the calculus, or by non-invasive means such as the use of shock waves. ⊃ extracorporeal shock wave lithotripsy.

lithotriptor *n* a machine which sends shock waves through calculi causing them to fragment. The fragments are washed out, or in the case of renal calcui they are passed naturally in the urine.

lithotrite *n* an instrument for crushing a stone in the urinary bladder.

litmus *n* a vegetable pigment used as an indicator of alkalinity (blue) or acidity (red). Often stored as paper strips: red litmus paper turns blue when exposed to an alkali; blue litmus paper turns red with an acid.

Little's area the area on the anterior nasal septum that contains Kiesselbach's plexus. A common site for epistaxis (bleeding from the nose).

Little's disease a type of cerebral palsy. There is diplegia of spastic type causing 'scissor leg' deformity. ⊃ cerebral palsy.

live attenuated vaccines ⊃ vaccines.

livedo *n* mottling and discoloration of the skin, especially in cold weather.

liver *n* the largest gland and solid organ in the body, the weight in adults is within the range 1.2–1.5 kg. The liver is situated in the right upper part of the abdominal cavity, immediately below the diaphragm and protected by the lower ribs. Functionally, it is divided into two parts (left and right) but it is frequently still described as having four lobes right, left, caudate and quadrate (Figure L.5). It receives blood from two sources—the hepatic artery carrying the oxygenated blood required by functional liver cells and the hepatic portal vein through which the liver receives all venous blood from the gut, enabling selective uptake of absorbed substances before they reach the general circulation. Deoxygenated blood leaves the liver via the hepatic vein. The liver is vital to homeostasis and its functions include: breakdown of red blood cells with the production of bile for storage and discharge into the duodenum; detoxification of drugs, chemicals and hormones; nutrient metabolism which includes protein synthesis, e.g. blood coagulation factors, the formation and storage of glycogen, and its breakdown to provide glucose to the blood as required (thus the liver is central to blood glucose homeostasis) and the regulation of cholesterol; storage of vitamins and minerals; and because of its size and level of metabolic energy it generates considerable heat.

liver function tests (LFTs) blood tests used to assess liver function including: alanine aminotransferase (ALT), alkaline phosphatase, aspartate aminotransferase (AST), coagulation tests, gamma-glutamyltransferase (GGT, gamma-GT, γ-GT), serum bilirubin and serum proteins. ⊃ aminotransferases.

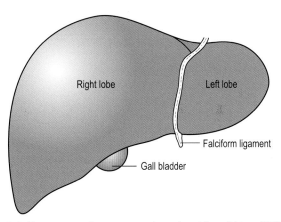

L.5 **Liver—general appearance** (reproduced from Watson 2000 with permission).

liver transplant surgical transplantation of a liver from a suitable donor or a segment from the liver of a living donor. May be used for individuals with end-stage liver failure such as that caused by congenital abnormalities of the liver and bile ducts or cirrhosis from long term alcohol misuse.

livid *adj* showing blue discoloration due to bruising, congestion or insufficient oxygenation.

living will ⮑ advance directive.

LJP *abbr* localized juvenile periodontitis.

LMA *abbr* laryngeal mask airway.

LMM *abbr* 'light meromyosin'.

LMP *abbr* last menstrual period.

LMPA *abbr* low-melting point alloy.

LMWH *abbr* low-molecular-weight heparin.

LOA *abbr* left occipitoanterior; used to describe the position of the fetal occiput in relation to the maternal pelvis.

Loa loa a parasitic nematode causing loiasis (filariasis).

lobe *n* a rounded section of an organ, separated from neighbouring sections by a fissure or septum, etc.—**lobar** *adj*.

lobectomy *n* removal of a lobe, for example lung, or liver.

lobotomy/prefrontal leucotomy a seldom performed procedure in which nerve pathways in the frontal lobe of the brain are cut.

lobule *n* a small lobe or a subdivision of a lobe—**lobular, lobulated** *adj*.

local anaesthesia administration of a drug, e.g. lidocaine, that inhibits peripheral nerve conduction so that painful stimuli fail to reach the brain. It can be achieved by injection or by topical application. ⮑ anaesthetic.

local anaesthetic a drug (e.g. lidocaine) that causes local insensibility to pain, thus facilitating a painful procedure, such as in dentistry, episiotomy, wound suturing, etc. Injected into the tissues or applied topically.

local area network (LAN) a number of computers connected together, for example in a hospital.

local authority in the UK, local government, e.g. regional councils, county councils, unitary authorities, city councils, district and town councils and parish councils. The levels of local government vary between the countries of the UK. All have powers to raise taxes and some have a statutory duty to provide services within a locality, such as environmental health, social services, education and policing.

localization the method of delineating the exact clinical target volume in a patient prior to radiotherapy treatment.

localize *vt* **1.** to limit the spread. **2.** to determine the site of a lesion—**localization** *n*.

localized alveolar osteitis also known as a dry or septic socket. Extremely painful inflammation of a tooth socket following extraction.

local muscular endurance the ability of specific muscles to maintain power output or tension, influenced by similar factors affecting whole-body endurance but with local vascularity predominating over central cardiorespiratory performance. ⮑ endurance. It is a person's ability to sustain a physical activity that relates to a particular muscle or group of muscles; for example, the number of press-ups possible in a given time gives an indication of upper arm and shoulder muscle endurance.

local rules rules outlining safe working practices of employees working with or coming into contact with radiation.

local service provider (LSP) a company that supplies computer net-working, for example, the NHS picture archieving communications system (PACS) has five LSPs to deliver the system countrywide.

local supervising authority (LSA) local organization, usually regional, which monitors midwifery practice in its area by appointing supervisors of midwifery, facilitating their education and training and enabling communication with the supervisors, developing systems to ensure eligibility to practise of each midwife working within the area and, where necessary, suspending from practice any midwife who may have acted unsafely or negligently. The local supervising authority has a nominated officer who is a practising midwife, to carry out its functions. ⮑ supervisor of midwives.

locator a device used to determine the true location of an object, such as a needle broken in the tissues.

lochia *npl* uterine discharges occurring for about 2–6 weeks after labour or miscarriage, consisting of placental site blood, shreds of decidua, vaginal epithelial cells and initially uterine debris e.g. amniotic fluid, vernix caseosa and meconium. Initially red in colour (lochia rubra), turning pinkish (lochia serosa) and finally whitish (lochia alba) as involution progresses—**lochium** *sing*, **lochial** *adj*. ⮑ lochia alba, lochia rubra, lochia serosa.

lochia alba the final whitish uterine discharges occurring after labour or miscarriage. It contains white blood cells and mucus.

lochia rubra the initial red uterine discharges occurring after labour or miscarriage. Initially contains red fresh blood that changes to browner staler blood.

lochia serosa the intermediate pinkish uterine discharges occurring after labour or miscarriage. It contains fewer red and more white cells; red, profuse lochia or sudden cessation of lochia may indicate subinvolution or, combined with offensive odour, infection.

lock in dentistry, that part of a tooth preparation used to increase the retention of a restoration.

locked-in-syndrome a paralytic condition in which there is normally critical neurological damage such that the patient is unable to move but is conscious and alert. The person has intellectual functioning but is unable to express thoughts or emotions verbally or by movement. They retain eye movement and blinking and may be able to use these in communication. It may be a transient condition.

locked twins rare cause of obstructed labour in which the bodies and heads of twins are caught together, precluding normal vaginal delivery for either infant.

locking mechanical obstruction within a joint that results in the prohibition of movement throughout its range, e.g. the inability to fully flex the knee or move from a fixed position.

In sport the knee is the most common joint to 'lock', often as a result of a loose body or meniscal tear. *false locking* may occur as a result of severe muscle spasm, e.g. of the hamstring muscle group, causing limitation of movement at the knee.

lockjaw *n* ➲ tetanus.

locomotor *adj* can be applied to any tissue or system used in movement. Most usually refers to nerves and muscles. Sometimes includes the skeletal system.

locomotor ataxia the disordered gait and loss of sense of position (proprioception) in the lower limbs, which occurs in tabes dorsalis. ➲ syphilis.

locoregional referring to a specific part of the body.

loculated *adj* divided into numerous cavities.

loculation the presence of many small spaces or cavities.

loculus in anatomy, a small space or cavity— **loculi** *pl*.

locus of causality 1. in attribution theory, a person's perception of whether the cause of their success or failure at a task is internal (due to personal factors, such as effort and ability) or external (due to external factors, such as luck or chance). 2. in self-determination theory, a person's perception of whether the origin of their reasons for engaging in a behaviour is internal (done willingly and out of free choice) or external (done because they are compelled or required to do so, either by external pressure from others or because of self-imposed pressures).

locus of control concept in health psychology. A behaviourist theory to describe individual differences in perceived control over events in people's lives. A generalized belief or expectation about whether behavioural outcomes (specifically, rewards and punishments) are within their control (the consequence of their own actions) or due to external factors (the consequence of chance, fate or the influence of powerful others). Individuals' generalized locus of control beliefs apply to most of their behaviours, especially in novel situations. Individuals also develop domain-specific control beliefs based upon personal experience, for example health locus of control beliefs: whether health outcomes are due to their own behaviour or to external, uncontrollable factors. Those people who feel that events in their lives are beyond their control, a belief in an external locus of control. This would consequently determine their response to stress and health seeking (illness) behaviour with an over-reliance on medical intervention for improving health. Others may feel that they do exercise a degree of control over events, a belief in an internal locus of control. This is more likely to lead to self-help: altered behaviour to reduce the risk of ill health, adoption of healthier lifestyles, adherence to medical advice.

Löfgren's syndrome an acute illness characterized by erythema nodosum, peripheral arthropathy, uveitis, bilateral hilar lymphadenopathy (BHL), lethargy and occasionally fever—is often seen in young women. ➲ sarcoidosis.

logarithm the logarithm of a number to a given base, is the power by which the base must be raised to give the number. For example the logarithm of 100 to the base 10 is 2 as $10^2 = 100$.

log lt curve ➲ characteristic curve.

logopaedics study of speech disorders and their treatment.

logorrhoea rapid speech that may be incoherent.

-logy a suffix that means 'science of, study of', e.g. *pathology*

loiasis *n* special form of filariasis (caused by the worm *Loa loa*) which occurs in West Africa. The vector, a large horsefly, *Chrysops*, bites in the daytime. Larvae take 2–3 years to develop and may live in humans for 15 years. There is eosinophilia. The worms move about the subcutaneous tissues causing irritation and localized swellings, and sometimes a worm crosses the eye.

loin *n* that part of the back between the lower ribs and the iliac crest; the area immediately above the buttocks.

long bones these have a shaft of compact bone with a central medullary cavity, the ends are expanded, for example, the femur, the radius.

long buccal nerve an afferent nerve running from the mucosa and outer alveolar plate, in the region of the molar and sometimes premolar teeth, obliquely across the anterior border of the ramus of the mandible between the mucous membrane and the buccinator muscle. It ascends between the two heads of the pterygoid muscle to join the mandibular nerve.

long-duration anaerobic endurance training ➲ anaerobic endurance training.

longitudinal chromatic aberration (LCA) (*syn* axial chromatic aberration) a defect of an optical system (eye, lens, prism, etc.) due to the unequal refraction of different wavelengths (dispersion) which results in an extended image along the optical axis. In the eye, blue rays are focused in front of the retina (by about 1 D) and red rays slightly behind the retina (0.25–0.5 D) when relaxed. When the eye is accommodated, blue rays tend to be focused near the retina and red rays are focused behind the retina (1 D). ➲ chromoretinoscopy, chromostereopsis.

longitudinal lie the long axis of the fetus (spine) is parallel to the long axis of the woman's uterus. The presentation can be breech or cephalic.

longitudinal magnetization (M_z) part of the macroscopic magnetization vector, parallel to the main magnetic field (B_o). Following radiofrequency excitation it returns to its equilibrium value (M_o) due to the characteristic time constant (T_1) of the tissues that have been excited.

longitudinal relaxation time (*syn* T_1, spin-lattice relaxation time, T_1 relaxation time) in magnetic resonance imaging (MRI), the time taken for the spins to give the energy obtained from the initial radiofrequency impulse, back to the surrounding environment and return to equilibrium. It represents the time required for the longitudinal magnetization (M_z) to go from 0 to 63% of its final maximum value.

longitudinal study research study where data are collected on more than one occasion, such as the study of a cohort of people over time. ➲ cohort study.

long Q-T syndrome an inherited condition with an extended Q-T interval; it predisposes to life-threatening ventricular arrhythmias leading to sudden death, often during exertion, in otherwise healthy young people.

longsighted *adj* ⊃ hypermetropia.

long slow distance training training performed at low intensity (less than 70% $\dot{V}O_{2max}$) but over time periods in excess of those during a race or other sporting competition.

long term memory (LTM) the part of memory responsible for the retention of information for longer periods. Potentially permanent and has a much greater capacity than short term memory.

long term oxygen therapy (LTOT) controlled flow rate oxygen, provided for at least 15 hours per day, usually via an oxygen concentrator. Shown to prolong survival in those with severe hypoxaemia (PaO_2 <7.3 kPa with an FEV_1 < 1.5 L) secondary to obstructive lung disease with concurrent right heart failure.

longitudinal axis (dental) ⊃ sagittal axis (dental).

longwave ultrasound (LWUS) traditionally therapeutic ultrasound employs a frequency of 1–3 MHz. Claims have been made that longwave ultrasound (LWUS), with a frequency of 45 kHz, is superior to MHz ultrasound for treating soft tissue injuries. These claims have been refuted by others, who state that the beam divergence and the energy reflection of LWUS result in a more superficial effect. By employing a lower frequency, the wavelength will be greater (assuming the velocity in tissue is approximately constant) and, hence, the theoretical penetration depth will be greater. This is estimated at around 20 times more than traditional MHz ultrasound, though it is argued that because the majority of this energy will be absorbed in the near field, the modality will actually be more effective in the superficial tissues. This can account (in part at least) for the superficial heating effect experienced by many patients. The divergent beam means that the ultrasound energy will be more diffuse at depth with LWUS. It has been estimated that the energy content of the beam has reduced to 50% at 0.5 cm and down to 10% at 2 cm from the surface. There is little clinical research evidence with regards LWUS and no substantive evidence to determine whether its physiological and cellular effects are the same as traditional MHz ultrasound. Anecdotal evidence from clinical practice is largely supportive.

loop diuretics a group of drugs, e.g. furosemide, that cause a diuretic effect by preventing the reabsorption of sodium, chloride and potassium in the thick part of the ascending limb of the loop of Henle. ⊃ Appendix 5.

loopography the radiographic investigation of an ileal conduit, a Foley catheter is inserted and dilated to block the conduit and contrast agent is injected under fluoroscopic control and plain films are taken.

loose body a fragment of loose material within a body cavity. For example a small piece of bone or cartilage within a joint, usually the result of wear and tear and/or trauma. Most common in the knee joint. Symptoms include pain, swelling and stiffness and can result in 'locking' of a joint. If symptomatic, the loose body can be surgically removed. This

can usually be achieved through minimally invasive surgical techniques. ⊃ locking.

Looser's zones pseudo (or false) fractures.

LOP *acron* **L**eft **O**ccipito **P**osterior; used to describe the position of the fetal occiput in relation to the maternal pelvis.

lordoscoliosis *n* lordosis complicated by the presence of scoliosis.

lordosis *n* an exaggerated forward, convex curve of the lumbar spine. There is a normal wide variation in spinal curvature and lordosis is common during the accelerated phases of growth. In sport it is usually the result of poor posture or unequal development of the supporting spinal musculature. Treatment is therefore targeted at correcting posture and improving muscle control, balance and strength—**lordotic** *adj*.

lordotic radiograph a chest projection where the patient is positioned for a routine PA chest and leans backwards, towards the X-ray tube by approximately 30–40°, taken to demonstrate a right middle lobe collapse or an interlobular pleural effusion.

LOS *abbr* lower oesophageal sphincter.

lost wax casting technique in dentistry, a casting process where a pattern, usually of plastic or wax, is embedded in investment material and later removed by heating in order to form a mould in which molten metal may be cast.

lotion a fluid preparation for application to the skin or a wound, for example, an antiseptic or a treatment for a skin condition.

Lou Gehrig's disease ⊃ amyotrophic lateral sclerosis.

loupe *n* a magnifying lens often attached to spectacles. ⊃ magnifier.

louse *n* ⊃ *Pediculus*—**lice** *pl*.

Løvset's manoeuvre (J Løvset, Norwegian obstetrician, 20th century) a manoeuvre used to deliver the shoulders and arms in breech presentation complicated by the arms being extended or displaced behind the neck. It involves rotating the fetus through a half circle, keeping the back uppermost, bringing the posterior arm into an anterior position below the symphysis pubis to be delivered; the fetus is then rotated a half circle in the reverse direction and the second arm is similarly delivered.

low back pain (LBP) the commonest cause seems to be posterolateral prolapse of the intervertebral disc, putting pressure on the dura and cauda equina and causing the localized pain of lumbago. It can progress to trap the spinal nerve root, causing the nerve distribution pain of sciatica.

low birthweight (LBW) defined as a weight of less than 2500 g at birth, whether or not gestation was below 37 weeks. Very low birthweight is defined as less than 1500 g at birth, and extremely low birthweight is less than 1000 g at birth. ⊃ small for gestational age. Low birthweight can result from preterm birth or from intrauterine growth restriction/retardation (IUGR).

low carbohydrate ketogenic diets emphasize carbohydrate restriction while generally ignoring total calories and the content of protein, cholesterol and saturated fat. The diet was first promoted in the 1970s by Atkins and has appeared in various forms since. These diets generate excess ketone bodies as the by-products of incomplete fat breakdown, with a high level in the plasma that supposedly suppresses appetite. Theoretically, ketones lost in the urine represent unused energy that should also facilitate weight loss. The main mechanism of action, however, may be restriction of the carbohydrate-containing foods, creating a low-calorie diet. These diets have a negative effect on ability to train and compete; they rapidly deplete glycogen stores and also induce significant loss of lean tissue.

low density lipoprotein (LDL) ⟹ lipoprotein.

low energy X-ray beam radiotherapy beam in the order of 50–160 kV, very low energy beam 8–50 kV.

low lip line the lowest position of the inferior border of the upper lip at rest. In the lower lip, the lowest position of the superior border during smiling or voluntary retraction.

lower molar forceps ⟹ forceps.

lower motor neuron the cell body is in the anterior horn of the spinal cord and the axon that passes to skeletal muscle. ⟹ neuron.

lower motor neuron (signs) signs that indicate that there may be some damage to the structures comprising the lower motor neuron. They may include diminished or loss of the reflexes, marked wasting, no muscle tone and no muscle activity.

lower oesophageal sphincter (LOS) also known as the gastro-oesophageal or cardiac sphincter. It is a physiological sphincter that prevents the reflux of acidic stomach contents into the oesophagus. Its action depends on the contribution of: (a) the mucosal folds in the lower oesophagus, which may act as a barrier; (b) the sensitivity of the involuntary, smooth muscle of the oesophageal wall to neurotransmitters and hormones; and (c) the compression of the abdominal part of the oesophagus when intra-abdominal pressure increases. ⟹ gastro-oesophageal reflux disease (GORD).

lower reference nutrient intake (LRNI) one of the UK dietary reference values. The amount of a nutrient that will be enough for that small group within a population (2.5%) who have a low requirement. ⟹ dietary reference values.

lower respiratory tract infection (LRTI) ⟹ pneumonia.

lower root forceps ⟹ forceps.

lower segment caesarean section (LSCS) involves a horizontal incision in the lower uterine segment to reduce the risks of uterine rupture during a subsequent labour.

lower urinary tract symptoms (LUTS) include - dribbling, dysuria, frequency, hesitancy, incontinence, intermittency, nocturia, poor urinary flow rate, urgency. They are indicative of pathology affecting the bladder and urethra, such as outflow obstruction due to an enlarged prostate gland, or detrusor instability.

lower uterine segment the thinner, less vascular lower part of the uterus that is formed from the isthmus and cervix during pregnancy. The uterine isthmus is a narrow area between the cavity and cervix in the non-pregnant uterus. The lower segment thins and dilates during labour as it is stretched by the powerful contrations of the upper uterine segment.

low frequency current an electrotherapy term—an alternative name for pulsed current. There is lack of agreement as to how to define low, medium and high. In clinical practice the frequency is usually from 1 Hz to approximately 200 Hz (it must be less than 1 kHz or it becomes a medium frequency current).

low-molecular-weight heparin (LMWH) a form of heparin that has fewer side effects and a longer duration of action than standard (unfractionated) heparin, examples include bemiparin, dalteparin and enoxaparin. LMWHs augment antithrombin activity preferentially against factor Xa. LMWH does not prolong the activated partial thromboplastin time (APTT), unlike standard (unfractionated) heparin and if its plasma level needs to be measured this is accomplished using a specific anti-Xa-based assay. LMWH, because of its high bioavailability after subcutaneous injection, is given as either a standard or a weight-related dose. Normally, therefore, the plasma LMWH level does not need to be measured. LMWHs are now widely used for the prophylaxis and the treatment of both deep vein thrombosis and pulmonary embolism and are replacing standard heparin as the initial treatment of choice for many patients. As injections of LMWH need only be given once daily subcutaneously and no monitoring is required, many patients can be treated at home. In older patients, those who have low body weight or renal failure, there is an increased risk of bleeding. The LMWH dose should be reduced in these groups and in those with a creatinine clearance of less than 30 ml/min. If less than 10 ml/min, the use of standard heparin should be considered, especially where reversibility may be needed. ⟹ heparin, standard (unfractionated) heparin (SH).

low spatial frequency algorithm in computed tomography (CT) scanning an algorithm used to provide high contrast resolution. Frequently used in soft-tissue studies to demonstrate inherently low contrast tissues in close proximity.

low temperature chemistry radiographic processing chemicals with a higher concentration of hydroquinone, a different restrainer and a higher concentration of preservative which have a working temperature range of 26–33°C and a pH of about 10.00. ⟹ high temperature chemistry.

low tension glaucoma (LTG) an ocular condition in which there is a glaucomatous cupping and visual field defects with an intraocular pressure of 22 mmHg or less. This glaucoma is usually associated with a cardiovascular disease or migraine.

low vision (*syn* partial sight, subnormal vision) vision below normal even after correction by conventional lenses, resulting from either congenital anomalies or ocular diseases such as cataract, glaucoma, age-related macular degeneration (maculopathy), pathological myopia, etc. The correction and rehabilitation of patients with subnormal vision is achieved by special aids called low vision aids (LVA) such as a telescopic lens, and appropriate counselling (e.g. about illumination and reading distance). The criteria which the health authorities normally use to classify a person as having partial sight take into consideration are not only the corrected visual acuity but also the extent of visual field loss, if any. ⊃ Bailey-Lovie chart, clipover, contrast sensitivity chart, cross-cylinder lens, deaf-blind, eccentric viewing, halogen lamp, low vision aids, magnifier, magnifying spectacles, pinhole spectacles, telescopic lens, typoscope.

low vision aids optical (e.g. loupe) or non-optical (e.g. large numeral telephone) appliances and devices designed to assist the partially sighted patient. ⊃ halogen lamp, loup, low vision, pinhole spectacles, telescopic lens, typoscope.

LP *abbr* lumbar puncture.

LPL *abbr* lipoprotein lipase.

LRK *abbr* laser refractive keratoplasty.

LRNI *abbr* lower reference nutrient intake.

LRTI *abbr* lower respiratory tract infection.

LS *abbr* **1.** lecithin-sphingomyelin ratio. **2.** lichen sclerosis.

LSA *abbr* **1.** lichen sclerosus et atrophicus. **2.** local supervising authority.

LSCS *abbr* lower segment caesarean section.

LSD *abbr* lysergic acid diethylamide.

LSI *abbr* large scale integration.

LSP *abbr* local service provider.

LT *abbr* lactate threshold.

LTG *abbr* low tension glaucoma.

LTM *abbr* long term memory.

LTOT *abbr* long term oxygen therapy.

lubb-dupp *n* words descriptive of the heart sounds as heard on auscultation.

lubricants *npl* **1.** substances or secretions that act as a surface-coating and reduce friction, heat or wear and tear. **2.** faecal softeners, e.g. arachis oil, that also lubricate and facilitate easy and painless defecation. ⊃ laxatives. **3.** in dentistry, a liquid or gel agent to ease the passage or use of an implement or instrument, for example the negotiation and enlargement of root canals.

lucid *adj* clear; describing mental clarity.

lucid interval a period of mental clarity which can be of variable length, occurring in people with organic mental disorder such as dementia or delirium. Importantly, a lucid interval is also a feature of extradural (epidural) haemorrhage. Bleeding is usually from the high pressure, middle meningeal artery and follows head trauma. There is initial loss of consciousness, then a variable period of lucidity, which is followed by a sudden and rapid worsening in conscious level.

Ludwig's angina ⊃ cellulitis.

lues *n* obsolete term for syphilis.

lumbago *n* incapacitating pain low down in the back.

lumbar *adj* pertaining to the loin.

lumbar nerves five pairs of spinal nerves (L1-L5).

lumbar plexus is formed by the anterior rami of the first three lumbar nerves (L1–3) and part of the fourth lumbar nerve (L4). The lumbar plexus gives rise to nerves that innervate the muscles and skin of the lower abdomen, inguinal area, thigh and lower leg and foot. The plexus is situated in front of the transverse processes of the lumbar vertebrae and behind the psoas muscle. The main branches, and their nerve roots are: iliohypogastric nerve—L1; ilioinguinal nerve—L1; genitofemoral—L1, 2; lateral cutaneous nerve of thigh—L2, 3; femoral nerve—L2, 3, 4; obturator nerve—L2, 3, 4; and the lumbosacral trunk—L4, (5). The *iliohypogastric, ilioinguinal* and *genitofemoral nerves* supply muscles and the skin in the area of the lower abdomen, upper and medial aspects of the thigh and the inguinal region. The *lateral cutaneous nerve of the thigh* supplies the skin of the lateral aspect of the thigh including part of the anterior and posterior surfaces. The *femoral nerve* is one of the larger branches. It passes behind the inguinal ligament to enter the thigh in close association with the femoral artery. It divides into cutaneous and muscular branches to supply the skin and the muscles of the front of the thigh. One branch, the *saphenous nerve*, supplies the medial aspect of the leg, ankle and foot. The *obturator nerve* supplies the adductor muscles of the thigh and skin of the medial aspect of the thigh. It ends just above the level of the knee joint. The *lumbosacral trunk* descends into the pelvis and makes a contribution to the sacral plexus. ⊃ Colour Section Figure 11.

lumbar puncture (LP) the withdrawal of cerebrospinal fluid (CSF) through a hollow needle inserted into the subarachnoid space in the lumbar region of the spine (Figure L.6). The CSF obtained is examined for its chemical (e.g. glucose)

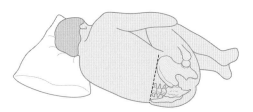

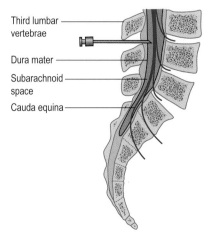

Third lumbar vertebrae

Dura mater

Subarachnoid space

Cauda equina

L.6 Lumbar puncture (reproduced from Walsh 2002 with permission).

and cellular (e.g. white blood cells) constituents and for the presence of micro-organisms; CSF pressure can be measured by the attachment of a manometer.

lumbar sympathectomy surgical removal of the sympathetic chain in the lumbar region; used to improve the blood supply to the lower limbs by allowing vasodilation.

lumbar vertebrae five bones, the largest of the vertebrae reflecting their weight-bearing function. ⇒ vertebra (typical), Colour Section Figure 3.

lumbocostal *adj* pertaining to the loin and ribs.

lumbosacral *adj* pertaining to the loin or lumbar vertebrae and the sacrum.

lumbosacral trunk a nerve trunk arising from the lumbar plexus. It comprises part of the 4th (L4) and the 5th (L5) lumbar nerve roots. It contributes to the sacral plexus. ⇒ lumbar plexus, sacral plexus.

Lumbricus *n* a genus of earthworms. ⇒ ascarides, ascariasis.

lumen *n* **1.** the space inside a tubular structure, such as an artery—**lumina** *pl*, **luminal** *adj*. **2.** the Système International d'Unités (SI) unit (International System of Units) for luminous flux and equal to 1 candela.

luminescence the emission of light by certain substances resulting from the absorption of energy (e.g. from electrical fields, chemical reaction, or other light) which is not due to a rise in temperature (unlike incandescence). The emitted radiation is characteristic of the particular substance. When the light emitted is due to exposure to a source of light the process is usually called *photoluminescence*. When the light emitted is due to either a high-frequency discharge through a gas, or to an electric field through certain solids such as phosphor which is used in fluorescent lamps, television picture tubes, etc., it is called *electroluminescence*. When luminescence persists for some time after the exciting stimulus has ceased it is termed *phosphorescence*. The term *bioluminescence* describes the luminescence produced by a living organism, such as firefly and certain fungi. ⇒ fluorescence, fluorescent lamp.

luminosity the measure of the amount of light emitted from an object.

luminous intensity (I) quotient of the luminous flux leaving the source, propagated in an element of solid angle containing the given direction, divided by the element of solid angle. It is measured in candela (cd).

lumpectomy *n* the surgical excision of a tumour with removal of minimal surrounding tissue. Increasingly used, with radiotherapy and chemotherapy, for treatment of breast cancer.

lunate one of the carpal bones of the wrist. It articulates with the radius and other carpal bones scaphoid, triquetral, hamate and capitate.

Lund and Browder's charts used to calculate more accurately a burn area and illustrate the depth of area burnt, giving a calculation of burn severity. ⇒ rule of nines, total burn surface area.

lung compliance lung compliance is the ease with which the lungs inflate and is defined as the volume change per unit of pressure change (measured in l/cm of water). Conditions resulting in poor compliance include fibrotic lung diseases, e.g. fibrosing alveolitis, tuberculosis and acute respiratory distress syndrome and chest wall abnormalities such as severe kyphoscoliosis and pectus excavatum. The lungs with low compliance are said to be 'stiff' and will yield a lower tidal volume for the same effort applied to respiration than 'normal' lungs. The lung compliance equation can be used to calculate how compliant the lungs are of a ventilated patient: $C = Vt/P$ where C = compliance; Vt = tidal volume and P is the driving pressure.

lung function a measure of how well the lungs work. Assessment includes spirometry, arterial blood gases and measures of gas transfer and lung volumes. ⇒ arterial blood gases (ABGs), respiratory function tests, spirometry.

lungs *npl* the two main organs of respiration which occupy the greater part of the thoracic cavity; they are separated from each other by the heart and other contents of the mediastinum. Arranged in lobes, they receive air during inspiration from the trachea, main bronchi and smaller airways which communicate with the alveoli, the site of gaseous exhange. The lungs are concerned with gaseous exchange—the oxygenation of blood and excretion of carbon dioxide during expiration. ⇒ Colour Section Figures 6, 7.

lung transplantation may be single, double, heart–lung transplants, or sometimes in the case of child recipients, live-related lobar transplants.

lung ventilation the passage of air in the lungs studied by the inhalation of a radioactive gas.

lung volume reduction surgery (LVRS) a procedure designed to improve respiratory function in patients with severe bullous emphysema. By excising the bullous tissue and shaping, the remaining lung expansion of the healthy lung and doming of the diaphragm can be achieved. This results in improved respiratory mechanics and symptomatic relief of dyspnoea (breathlessness).

lunula *n* the semilunar pale area at the root of the nail.

lupus *n* several destructive skin conditions, with different causes. ⇒ collagen diseases.

lupus anticoagulant ⇒ antiphospholipid antibody syndrome.

lupus erythematosus (LE) ⇒ systemic lupus erythematosus (SLE).

lupus pernio a form of sarcoidosis affecting the skin.

lupus vulgaris the commonest variety of skin tuberculosis; ulceration occurs over cartilage (nose or ear) with necrosis and facial disfigurement.

lutein *n* a naturally occurring yellow-red carotenoid pigment present in green leafy vegetables such as spinach and in some fruits. It is one of the components of macular pigment in the eye. ⇒ age-related macular degeneration, macular pigment.

luteinizing hormone (LH) a gonadotrophin secreted by the anterior pituitary gland. In females high levels in mid menstrual cycle stimulate ovulation and formation of the corpus luteum. The same hormone in males is called interstitial-cell stimulating hormone (ICSH); it stimulates the production of testosterone by the testes.

K
L

luteotrophin/luteotrophic hormone ⊃ prolactin.

luting in dentistry, the use of a cement-like substance to seal the junction of two substances such as a crown on a tooth.

luting agent fine-grained, thinly mixed cement used for the cementation of inlays, crowns, bridges and orthodontic bands.

LUTS *abbr* lower urinary tract symptoms.

lux the Système International d'Unités (SI) unit (International System of Units) of intensity of illumination.

luxation *n* partial dislocation. ⊃ subluxation.

luxation of the lens a pathological and complete dislocation of the lens relative to the pupil. If the luxation is incomplete it is called subluxation of the lens (or dislocation or ectopia lentis). Subluxation is one of the causes of monocular diplopia. If the luxation is complete the eye becomes markedly hyperopic (hypermetropia) and is unable to accommodate. Luxation occurs in contusion of the globe, in many ocular (e.g. buphthalmos) and other diseases (e.g. syphilis) or it can be inherited (e.g. the bilateral, symmetrical, superior subluxation commonly found in Marfan's syndrome). It is sometimes associated with ectopic pupils and keratoconus. Unless there are complications (e.g. secondary glaucoma) or monocular diplopia the lens is left in place and management is optical. ⊃ astigmatism, congenital glaucoma, corectopia, diplopia, Ehlers–Danlos syndrome, monocular, iridodonesis, Marfan's syndrome.

luxator in dentistry, a thin, sharpened instrument used to cut the periodontal ligament of a tooth to be extracted. Produces some luxation of the tooth but if used as an elevator is liable to fracture. Main indication for usage is preservation of bony structure for example prior to implant placement.

LV *abbr* left ventricle.

LVA *abbr* low vision aids.

LVAD *abbr* left ventricular assist device.

LVF *abbr* left ventricular failure.

LVRS *abbr* lung volume reduction surgery.

LWUS *abbr* longwave ultrasound.

Lyell's syndrome (A Lyell, British dermatologist, 20/21st century). ⊃ toxic epidermal necrolysis.

Lyme disease an infection caused by the spirochaete *Borrelia burgdorferi*. It is transmitted to humans by the bites of infected ticks of the genus *Ixodes*. It is characterized by fatigue, skin rash, lymphadenopathy, joint pains, headache, pyrexia and occasionally arthritis, meningitis and cardiac arrhythmias. First identified in Lyme, Connecticut, USA. ⊃ *Borrelia*, relapsing fever.

lymph *n* the fluid contained in the lymphatic vessels. It is formed from interstitial (tissue) fluid and is similar in composition to plasma. Unlike blood, lymph contains only one type of cell, the lymphocyte.

lymphadenectomy *n* excision of one or more lymph nodes.

lymphadenitis *n* inflammation of a lymph node.

lymphadenopathy *n* any disease of the lymph nodes—**lymphadenopathic** *adj*.

lymphangiectasis *n* dilation of the lymph vessels—**lymphangiectatic** *adj*.

lymphangiography *n* ⊃ lymphography.

lymphangioma *n* a simple tumour of lymph vessels frequently associated with similar formations of blood vessels—**lymphangiomata** *pl*, **lymphangiomatous** *adj*.

lymphangioplasty *n* any plastic surgery on lymph vessels, such as those used to improve drainage. ⊃ lymphoedema—**lymphangioplastic** *adj*.

lymphangiosarcoma rare malignancy of lymph vessels.

lymphangitis *n* inflammation of a lymph vessel.

lymphatic *adj* pertaining to, conveying or containing lymph.

lymphatic system the lymphatic system is vital in the movement of body fluids and in the functioning of the immune system. It comprises a network of lymph capillaries, vessels and the two large ducts the thoracic duct and the right lymphatic duct that empty lymph into large veins in the thorax; lymph nodes; the lymph fluid; lymph/lymphoid organs, e.g. spleen and thymus; and the diffuse lymphoid tissue or mucosa-associated lymphoid tissue (MALT), e.g. tonsils, Peyer's patches (lymphoid tissue in the small intestine), and also in the bone marrow. Networks of lymph capillaries and vessels drain extracellular fluid as lymph from all body tissues (except the central nervous system), maintaining balance with fluid that enters the tissues from blood capillary network. After passage through regional lymph nodes interpolated in the system of vessels and the two main ducts, lymph is returned to the circulating blood via the subclavian veins in the thorax. The lymph nodes 'filter' the lymph of foreign material, including bacteria, and may become inflamed if draining an area with local infection. Lymphocytes originate in the bone marrow and pass into the circulation, where they are one of the types of white blood cell (leucocytes); they also become widely distributed in lymphoid organs and tissues, notably the spleen, tonsils and gut lining, as well as in the lymph nodes. ⊃ thoracic duct.

lymph capillary begins in the tissue spaces throughout most of the body and joins others, eventually forming a lymphatic vessel.

lymph circulation that of lymph collected from the tissue spaces; it then passes via lymph capillaries, vessels, nodes and ducts to be returned to the blood.

lymph nodes accumulations of lymphatic tissue at intervals along lymphatic vessels. Sometimes erroneously referred to as lymph glands. They mainly act as filters in removing extraneous particles including micro-organisms and cancer cells, and provide a site for B and T lymphocyte/cell proliferation and the production of immunoglobulins.

lymph/o- a prefix that means 'lymph, lymphatic', e.g. *lymphocytosis*.

lymphoblast *n* an immature lymphocyte. Present in the blood and bone marrow in conditions such as acute lymphoblastic leukaemia (ALL).

lymphocele a collection of lymph in the tissues or a tumour, caused by leakage from damaged lymph vessels.

lymphocyte *n* one variety of white blood cell (leucocyte). The lymphocytic stem cells undergo transformation to T lymphocytes/cells (in the thymus), which provide cell-mediated immunity involved in destroying cancer cells, virus infected cells and transplanted cells (graft), or B-lymphocytes/cells, which form immunoglobulins (antibodies) and provide humoral immunity. The transformation is usually complete a few months after birth—**lymphocytic** *adj.* ⊃ cell-mediated immunity, humoral immunity.

lymphocytic choriomeningitis virus (LCMV) a virus of the familiy *Arenaviridae*. It is the causative organism of a type of non-bacterial meningitis.

lymphocytic interstitial pneumonia (LIP) one of the idiopathic interstitial pneumonias. It is more common in women, and is characterized by a slow onset over many years. Patients should be investigated for associations of collagen vascular disease or HIV disease.

lymphocytopenia a decrease in the number of lymphocytes in the blood.

lymphocytosis *n* an increase in lymphocytes in the blood.

lymphoedema *n* excess fluid in the tissues from abnormality or obstruction of lymph vessels that blocks or interrupts lymph drainage. There is swelling of (usually) a limb and increased risk of cellulitis. It may be primary such as with congenital abnormalities of the lymph vessels. Or secondary, for example, after lymph node resection and/or radiotherapy; most common in breast cancer, or the blockage of lymph vessels caused by filarial worms. Its effects may be minimized by careful skin care to prevent injury and infection, exercises, specific massage and containment hosiery or bandaging. ⊃ elephantiasis, filariasis.

lymphoepithelioma *n* rapidly growing malignant pharyngeal tumour. May involve the tonsil. Often has metastases in cervical lymph nodes—**lymphoepitheliomata** *pl.*

lymphogranuloma venereum a sexually transmitted infection caused by *Chlamydia trachomatis*. There are ulcers on the genitalia and local lymph node enlargement. Occurs mainly in the tropics.

lymphography *n* the radiographic examination of the lymphatic system following the direct injection of contrast agent into a lymphatic vessel of the foot. Generally replaced by computed tomography (CT) scanning—**lymphographical** *adj*, **lymphogram** *n*, **lymphograph** *n*, **lymphographically** *adv*.

lymphoid *adj* pertaining to lymph.

lymphoid tissue reticular tissue. Tissue similar to that present in lymph nodes, situated in a variety of locations, bone marrow, gut, liver, spleen, thymus and tonsils.

lymphokine-activated killer cells (LAK) cytotoxic cells that have been activated by the lymphokine interleukin-2. They do not require the presence of an antigen. LAK cells are able to destroy cancer cells that are not destroyed by natural killer cells. Used in immunotherapy for some cancers.

lymphokines *npl* a term applied to cytokines produced by stimulated T lymphocytes (e.g. interleukin-2). They function during the immune response as intercellular chemical mediators.

lymphoma *n* a group of neoplastic diseases developing in lymphoid tissue. Lymphoma is characterized by lymph node enlargement, night sweats/swinging pyrexia, pain from splenic enlargement/infarction, hepatomegaly, weight loss, malaise or recurrent infection. Causes include viral infections but most are idiopathic. Classified according to histological appearances to either Hodgkin's lymphoma or non-Hodgkin's lymphoma (NHL). Staging depends on sites involved—location and number, as well as associated 'secondary' symptoms. Therapy may be radiotherapy alone for the earliest stages, and/ or chemotherapy. Bone marrow transplantation may also be necessary. ⊃ Burkitt's lymphoma.

lymphopoiesis the production of lymphocytes in the bone marrow and other lymphoid tissues.

lymphorrhagia *n* an outpouring of lymph from a severed lymphatic vessel.

lymphosarcoma *n* obsolete term for some types of lymphoma.

lyophilization *n* freeze drying. Used to preserve biological substances such as plasma, tissue, etc.

lyophilized skin skin which has been subjected to lyophilization. It is reconstituted and used for temporary skin replacement.

lymphuria the presence of lymph in the urine.

Lyon hypothesis (M Lyon, British geneticist, b.1925) states that in females only one of the two female sex chromosomes (XX) is functional. The non-functional X chromosome becomes a Barr body. Either the paternal or maternal-derived one may be non-functioning, which explains why an X-linked characteristic is expressed in some cells but not in others. ⊃ sex chromatin.

lysergic acid diethylamide (LSD) a potent hallucinogenic agent.

lysin *n* a substance present in blood that dissolves cells. ⊃ bacteriolysin, haemolysin.

lysine *n* an essential (indispensable) amino acid necessary for growth.

lysis *n* **1.** a gradual return to normal, used especially in relation to pyrexia. ⊃ crisis *opp.* **2.** disintegration of the membrane of cells, bacteria or molecules.

-lysis a suffix that means 'breaking down, separation', e.g. *glycolysis*.

lysosome a subcellular organelle that contains lytic enzymes.

lysozyme *n* an antibacterial enzyme present in many body fluids such as tears and saliva.

lytic relating to lysis.

-lytic a suffix that means 'disintegration', e.g. *haemolytic*.

ma *abbr* ➲ metre angle.

mA the average electrical current passing through an X-ray tube during an exposure measured in milliamperes.

MAb *abbr* monoclonal antibody.

MABP *abbr* mean arterial blood pressure.

Macbeth lamp (*syn* Macbeth illuminant C) a lamp used in testing colour vision. It contains a powerful tungsten filament bulb with a blue filter of specific absorption properties such that it produces a source of a colour temperature of about 6800 K, thus approximating the spectral characteristics of natural sunlight. The lamp is also fitted with a stand to hold the colour vision booklet. ➲ CIE standard illuminants, Farnsworth test, pseudoisochromatic plates.

maceration *n* softening of the horny layer of the skin by moisture, e.g. in and below the toes (in tinea pedis), or in perianal area (in pruritus ani). Maceration reduces the protective properties of the integument and so predisposes to penetration by bacteria or fungi. Other examples include the changes that occur in a dead fetus retained in the uterus for more than 24 hours. It is characterized by discoloration, softening of tissues, peeling fetal skin and eventual disintegration. These changes indicate that a stillborn infant had been dead *in utero* before labour; may lead to disseminated intravascular coagulation.

machine code the language the computer can understand directly; all instructions are written in binary.

machine tank developer the initial developer used in an automatic processing machine and consists of developer replenisher and starter solution.

Machupo virus a virus of the familiy *Arenaviridae*. Discovered in 1963 it is the causative organism of Bolivian haemorrhagic fever in Central and South America.

Mackenrodt's ligaments also known as the transverse cervical ligaments or cardinal ligaments. ➲ uterine supports.

Macleod's syndrome (W Macleod, British physician, 1911–1977) pathological changes in one lung that resemble those in emphysema. It follows respiratory infections, e.g. bronchiolitis, in childhood and may progress to bronchiectasis.

Macmillan Cancer Support previously known as Macmillan Cancer Relief. A charity founded to improve the quality of life for people with cancer and their families. It provides nurses, cancer care units, grants, medical support and education programmes, and finances for other charities.

Macmillan nurses clinical nurse specialists experienced and skilled in symptom control and general palliative care. They provide advice and support to patients and their families in a variety of settings. They also provide specialist information, advice and support for colleagues in the multidisciplinary team.

macro- a prefix that means 'large', e.g. *macrocyte*.

macrocephaly *n* large head, not caused by hydrocephalus—**macrocephalic** *adj*.

macrocheilia *n* excessive development of the lips, usually of congenital origin.

macrocornea ➲ keratoglobus.

macrocyte *n* a large red blood cell. Occurs in megaloblastic anaemia due to lack of vitamin B_{12} and or folic acid, either because of deficient intake or poor absorption in pernicious anaemia. Macrocytes are also associated with excess alcohol intake, liver disease and hypothyroidism—**macrocytic** *adj*.

macrocytosis an increased number of macrocytes.

macrodactyly *n* excessive development of the fingers or toes.

macrodontia unusually or abnormally large teeth.

macrogenitosomia enlargement of the external genitalia in boys and pseudohermaphroditism in girls. It is congenital in origin.

macroglia a class of supporting, non-nervous tissue within the nervous system. They include astrocytes, ependymal cells, oligodendrocytes, satellite cells, Schwann cells. ➲ microglia.

macroglobulin *n* a high molecular weight globulin protein. A term used to describe monoclonal immunoglobulin (IgM) molecules when excessive amounts are present in the blood. Such as in conditions characterized by the production of abnormal IgM, for example in multiple myeloma. ➲ paraprotein.

macroglobulinaemia *n* excessive amounts of monoclonal macroglobulins (IgM) present in the blood. The IgM is overproduced by plasma cells, which is a feature of multiple myeloma and certain lymphomas such as Waldenström's macroglobulinaemia. The effects include increased blood viscosity with circulatory problems, fatigue, neurological symptoms. Moreover, normal immunoglobulin production is impaired and the person is at increased risk of serious infection. ➲ Bence Jones protein, multiple myeloma.

macroglossia *n* an abnormally large tongue.

macrognathia unusually large jaw. Overgrowth of the maxilla and/or mandible.

macrolides *npl* a group of antibiotics, (e.g. erythromycin) that may be prescribed for people with penicillin hypersensitivity. ➲ Appendix 5.

macromastia *n* an abnormally large breast.

macronutrient *n* term used to describe the energy-yielding nutrients required in large quantities; carbohydrate, fat and protein.

macrophages *npl* mononuclear cells present in the tissues. They are derived from monocytes (a type of white blood cell). Some macrophages are able to move between sites as required, whilst others, such as those in the liver, alveoli, connective tissue, spleen and neural tissue, are fixed in position. They function as part of the non-specific (innate) body defences by destroying foreign bodies and cell debris by phagocytosis. Macrocytes also have roles in specific (adaptive) defences in stimulating various immune cells, secreting regulatory chemicals (e.g. interleukin-1) and by acting as antigen-presenting cells. They form part of the monocyte-macrophage (reticuloendothelial) system. ⊃ histiocytes, Kupffer cells, microglia.

macropsia *n* (*syn* megalopsia) a visual defect in which objects are seen as much larger than they are in reality. It may occur as a result of abnormal accommodation (less than required for the fixation distance) or because of various retinal anomalies in which the visual receptors are crowded together, or because of the recent wear of either base-in prisms or a presbyopic correction, etc. ⊃ dysmegalopsia, metamorphopsia, micropsia.

macroscopic *adj* visible to the unaided eye; gross. ⊃ microscopic *opp*.

macrosomia in obstetrics, a large baby (birthweight in excess of 4000 g, some authorities define as over 4500 g). It is associated with maternal diabetes and hyperglycaemia, which leads to fetal hyperinsulinaemia and an increase in body fat and enlargement of organs. Macrosomia can be a cause of cephalopelvic disproportion and difficulties during delivery such as shoulder dystocia.

macrostomia the uni- or bilateral increase in the width of the mouth.

macrotia congenital abnormality in which the outer/external ear is enlarged.

macrotrauma *n* a single force resulting in trauma to body tissues.

macula *n* a spot—**macular** *adj*. ⊃ fovea centralis, macula lutea.

macula adherens ⊃ desmosomes.

macula densa specialized cells of the distal convoluted tubule (DCT) of the nephron. Forms part of the juxtaglomerular apparatus (JGA). The osmoreceptor/chemoreceptor cells of the macula densa monitor the level of sodium and chloride ions and fluid in the filtrate within the DCT and cause other cells of the JGA to secrete renin. ⊃ juxtaglomerular apparatus, renin, renin-angiotensin-aldosterone response.

macula lutea an oval area of the retina 3–5 mm in diameter, with the foveal depression at its centre, slightly below the level of the optic disc and temporal to it (its centre lies 3.5 mm from the edge of the disc). The side wall of the depression slopes gradually towards the centre where the fovea centralis is located and where the best photopic visual acuity is obtained. Around the fovea, the ganglion cells are much more numerous than elsewhere, being arranged in five to seven layers. The outer molecular layer is also thicker than elsewhere and there is a progressive disappearance of rods so that at the foveola only cones are found. The area responsible for sharp central vision needed for tasks such as reading and colour vision. The area of the macula lutea is impregnated by a yellow pigment (macular pigment) in the inner layers and for that reason is often called the 'yellow spot'. ⊃ age-related macular degeneration, fovea centralis.

macular degeneration *n* ⊃ age-related macular degeneration.

macular epiretinal membrane ⊃ preretinal macular fibrosis.

macular hole a condition in which there is a partial or full thickness absence of the retina in the macular area. It may occur as a result of trauma, degeneration, increasing age, preretinal macular fibrosis or pathological myopia. It appears ophthalmoscopically as a round or oval, well defined, reddish spot at the macula. There is metamorphopsia, loss of visual acuity and a central scotoma. An operculum of retinal tissue may overlie the hole. The vitreous body (humour) in front of the hole eventually condenses and separates from the retina. In partial macular hole a layer of photoreceptors may still be attached to the retinal pigment epithelium (lamellar hole), as in cystoid macular oedema. Treatment usually consists of reattaching the retina, if detached, and possibly vitrectomy. ⊃ cystoid macular oedema, metamorphopsia, pretinal macular fibrosis, retinal tear, retinopathy.

macular pigment a yellow pigment, insensitive to light and located in the inner layers of the macular area of the retina. It extends over an area of about 12° in diameter. Its density declines markedly with eccentricity. The major components of this pigment are the yellow-red carotenoid pigments—lutein and zeaxanthin. These yellow pigments absorb blue light maximally. The macular pigment has been thought to mitigate the effect of chromatic aberration and to protect the retina against short wavelength radiations. ⊃ age-related macular degeneration, macula lutea, red filter.

macular pucker ⊃ preretinal macular fibrosis.

macular star deposits of lipid material in Henle's fibre layer radiating out in a star-like pattern. It may follow retinal oedema, for example in the late stage of hypertensive retinopathy. ⊃ Henle's fibre layer.

macule *n* a non-palpable localized area of change in skin colour—**macular** *adj*.

maculopapular *adj* the presence of macules and raised palpable spots (papules) on the skin.

maculopathy a degenerative condition affecting the macula lutea.

madarosis absence or loss of the eyelashes. It may be associated with blepharitis, alopecia, or repeated trauma from rubbing.

Maddox rod not a rod but a series of cylindrical grooves ground usually into a coloured piece of glass and mounted in a rim. (Originally it consisted of a single cylindrical rod.) It is used to measure heterophoria by placing it in front of one eye of a subject viewing a spot of light binocularly.

M
N

The Maddox rod and eye together form a long streak of light perpendicular to the axis of the grooves and this retinal image is so unlike the image formed in the other eye that the fusion reflex is not stimulated. The eyes will then stay in the passive position. If there is a phoria the streak of light will not intersect the spot of light. For horizontal phorias the rod axis is placed horizontally and for vertical phorias, vertically. The amount and type of the phoria can be quantified by placing a prism of appropriate power and direction in front of either eye such that the streak appears superimposed on the spot of light. Alternatively, the angle of the phoria could be determined using a Maddox cross and placing a rod in front of one eye; the phoria can be read directly by the patient who indicates where the streak of light appears to cross the scale. The Maddox rod is also used to detect or measure cyclophoria. ⊃ cyclophoria, heterophoria, Maddox rod test, passive position, Thorington test.

Maddox rod test a test for measuring cyclophoria in which a Maddox rod is placed in front of each eye, with axes parallel, while the subject views a spot light through a 10–15 Δ prism (to displace one image relative to the other). The subject will then see two streaks. If they appear parallel there is no cyclophoria. If not, one of the Maddox rods is rotated slowly until the subject reports that the two streaks are parallel. The angle of rotation as determined with a protractor scale indicates the amount of cyclophoria.

Madura foot ⊃ mycetoma.

MAG3 *abbr* **m**ercapto**a**cetyl**tri**glycine. Used with technecium – 99m ($^{99}Tc^m$) as a tracer in radioisotope (radionuclide) imaging of the kidneys and in blood flow studies.

maggots the larvae of flies. Specific type is used in the management of some chronic wounds. ⊃ larval therapy.

magic angle artefact in magnetic resonance imaging (MRI) of a joint, if a tendon lies at an angle of 55° to the static magnetic field it appears brighter on T_1 and proton density weighted images but has a normal low signal on T_2 weighted images, and therefore can be potentially confused with pathology.

magnesium (Mg) *n* a metallic element essential to the life of all body cells, being involved in many enzyme-catalysed processes. Magnesium is mainly an intracellular positively charged ion (cation). The concentration of ionized magnesium [Mg^{2+}] in the body fluids is regulated at the correct level for normal excitability of muscle and nerve, including neuronal activity in the central nervous system. Magnesium is present in bone, and its metabolism is linked to that of calcium and phosphate. Many salts of magnesium are used therapeutically.

magnesium carbonate and trisilicate used as antacids to relieve dyspepsia and 'heartburn'. Magnesium trisilicate is also used to reduce acidity of gastric contents prior to general anaesthesia, particularly during labour to reduce risk of acid gastric contents being regurgitated into the respiratory tract. ⊃ Mendelson's syndrome.

magnesium chloride used intravenously for magnesium deficiency (hypomagnesaemia).

magnesium hydroxide an antacid and osmotic laxative.

magnesium oxide used at the back of the crystal in scintillation counters to direct light back towards the sodium iodide crystal.

magnesium sulphate (*syn* Epsom salts) an effective rapid-acting osmotic laxative. It is used topically as a paste with glycerin for the treatment of boils. Used parenterally in the treatment of eclampsia and magnesium deficiency. Magnesium sulphate is recommended by the World Health Organization (WHO) to control eclamptic convulsions (seizures), as it is more effective than diazepam or phenytoin. Administered intravenously; blood levels must be monitored regularly to ensure they remain in the range 2–4 mmol/L. Toxicity leads to loss of maternal reflexes, muscle paralysis, respiratory and cardiac arrest.

magnet a substance containing a north and a south pole.

magnetic disk an 8-inch double-sided, double-density disk for storing images of up to 1.2 Mbytes.

magnetic domain an area of a substance when all the atoms are pointing in the same direction.

magnetic field exists when a point of force is experienced by a magnetic pole placed at the point.

magnetic flux the lines of force through a magnetic field.

magnetic induction if a substance contains magnetic atoms and is placed in a magnetic field and the poles of the atoms become aligned magnetizing the substance.

magnetic moment a measure of the magnitude and direction of the magnetic properties of an object or particle that cause it to align with the static main field and form its own local magnetic field.

magnetic resonance the absorption of the emission of the electromagnetic energy by nuclei in a static magnetic field following excitation by a radiofrequency pulse. The resonant frequency of the pulse and the emitted signal are proportional to the strength of the magnetic field.

magnetic resonance angiography the use of magnetic resonance technology to demonstrate blood vessels. It may be undertaken with or without a specific contrast agent.

magnetic resonance imaging (MRI) (*syn* nuclear magnetic resonance [NMR]) a non-invasive imaging technique that does not use ionizing radiation. Instead it uses a powerful magnetic field combined with radiofrequency pulses to excite hydrogen nuclei in the body. When the hydrogen nuclei settle the signal from the body is measured and reconstructed, using computer software, into two-dimensional or three-dimensional images. MRI can demonstrate anatomy and pathology in any plane, providing superior soft-tissue contrast and functional information (some procedures require the injection of contrast media). It is an established method of imaging the central nervous and musculoskeletal systems and increasingly for investigations of the cardiovascular system, liver and breast. MRI imaging is also used to facilitate various therapeutic interventions. There are no known harmful biological effects, and MRI scanning is non-invasive, painless and safe (no ionizing radiation is used). However, there are still major safety issues to consider. Contraindications to the use of MRI include: heart pacemakers, intracerebral aneurysm clips, other metallic implants and metallic foreign objects such as coins. ➲ gradient echo magnetic resonance imaging.

magnetic resonance signal the electromagnetic signal produced by the precession of the transverse magnetism of the spins which induce a voltage in the receiver coil which is then amplified by the receiver to form the signal.

magnetic susceptibility (χ) the ability of a substance to become magnetized or to distort a magnetic field. ➲ diamagnetic, ferromagnetic, paramagnetic, superparamagnetic.

magnetic tape tape that can store 180 Mbytes of information.

magnetization transfer contrast in magnetic resonance imaging (MRI) when the image contrast is manipulated by selectively saturating a pool of protein bound water. By applying an off-resonance pulse (1000–2000 Hz) these proteins are suppressed. As the protein bound water and the bulk water protons are in rapid exchange the saturation is transferred to the bulk phase of the water protons leading to a reduction in signal from the bulk water. Used to demonstrate small peripheral vessels and aneurysms in the brain and the detection of early demyelination or protein destruction.

magneto-optical disk a disk used to store computer data by a combination of a magnetic field on the disk and the use of a laser to write or read the information thus enabling a large quantity of data to be stored on the disk.

magnetron a piece of equipment that contains an anode and a cathode in a vacuum which are placed in a uniform magnetic field which causes the electrons to travel in a spiral, curved path from the cathode to the anode to produce radiowaves. A high-power radiofrequency oscillator used to power some linear accelerators.

magnification factor ➲ cortical magnification.

magnifier (*syn* loupe) an optical device, commonly used for close viewing, which produces an apparent magnification. It can be monocular or binocular, held in the hand (hand magnifier) or mounted in front of the eye (stand magnifier). It rarely exceeds a magnification of ×10 and does not produce an inversion of the image. ➲ low vision.

magnifying spectacles spectacles containing lenses of high convex power (+10 D or higher) used for near vision. ➲ low vision.

magnitude size.

magnum *adj* large or great, such as the foramen magnum in the occipital bone through which the spinal cord passes into the cranial cavity.

Magnus force the force due to the interaction between the surface of a rotating object or body and the fluid medium (e.g. air or water) in which it is rotating. The force acts at right angles to the axis of rotation and, if the object is translating, to the path of the object. Also sometimes classified as a lift force. Examples are topspin causing downward motion of a ball (e.g. tennis) and sidespin causing sideways motion of a golf ball. (Named after the German physicist who described it in the mid-19th century.)

MAI *abbr Mycobacterium avium intercellulare.*

mainframe a large computer, usually the centre of a system. Intelligent peripherals can then be attached.

Maitland grades (G Maitland, Australian physiotherapist, 20th century) four grades proposed by Maitland for use in manual therapies aimed at relieving pain and improving joint movement. Grade I: a small-amplitude movement near the starting position of the range out of resistance and used to treat pain; Grade II: a large-amplitude movement that carries well into the range. It can occupy any part of the range that is free of muscle spasm and resistance. Used commonly to treat pain; Grade III: a large-amplitude movement, but one that does move into muscle spasm and resistance. Used commonly to treat both pain and resistance; and Grade IV: a small-amplitude movement stretching into muscle spasm and resistance. Used to treat end of range resistance.

major arterial circle of the iris a vascular circle located in the anterior part of the ciliary body near the root of the iris. It is formed by the anastomosis of the two long posterior ciliary arteries and the seven anterior ciliary arteries. It supplies the iris, the ciliary processes and the anterior choroid. ➲ ciliary arteries, minor arterial circle of the iris.

major connector ➲ connector.

major histocompatibility complex (MHC) both MHC class I and class II glycoproteins are members of the immunoglobulin superfamily, and present peptide antigens to the immune system to generate an immune response. The MHC genes are encoded on human chromosome 6. Class I MHC genes encode proteins that are expressed on all nucleated cells and present self antigens to CD8+ T cells. Class II MHC genes encode proteins that are present on antigen-presenting cells (dendritic cells, macrophages and B cells) that present antigens to CD4+ T cells. Class III MHC genes encode a variety of molecules including cytokines, complement components, and other molecules essential for antigen presentation.

major impression ➲ impression.

Makaton *n* a form of sign language. It is more basic than some other languages.

mal- a prefix that means 'abnormal, poor', e.g. *malnutrition.*

mal *n* disease.

mal de mer seasickness.

malabsorption *n* defective absorption of nutrients from the digestive tract.

malabsorption syndrome an inability to absorb nutrients in sufficient quantities for health, from the small bowel. There is loss of weight, abdominal bloating and pain and steatorrhoea, varying in severity. Caused by: (a) disease of the small intestine, such as coeliac disease, Crohn's disease; (b) lack of digestive enzymes or bile salts, e.g. cystic fibrosis, pancreatitis; (c) surgical operations, e.g. extensive small bowel resection. Leads to anaemia, fatigue, vitamin deficiencies and chronic illhealth.

malacia *n* softening of a part. ➲ keratomalacia, osteomalacia.

-malacia a suffix that means 'softening', e.g. *tracheomalacia.*

maladaptation an abnormal or maladaptive response to a situation or change. It may relate to personal relationships, or to a stress response that leads to poor health, e.g. headaches, adverse changes in body chemistry.

maladjustment *n* bad or poor adaptation to environment. It may have social, mental or physical components.

malaise *n* a feeling of illness and discomfort.

malalignment *n* faulty alignment—as of bones after a fracture. While each person has a slightly different joint configuration, malalignment is considered to be the abnormal position of a structure relative to another. In sport it can occur, for example, following incomplete treatment of a fracture and results in loss of function with secondary effects, e.g. malalignment of the tibia following a fracture can result in a variety of overuse injuries including pain in the back, lower limb and/or foot, with restriction of activity. In dentistry, the displacement of a tooth from its normal position.

malar *adj* relating to the cheek.

malar bones the cheek bones. ⟴ zygomatic bone.

malaria *n* a serious infection caused by protozoa of the genus *Plasmodium* and carried by infected mosquitoes of the genus *Anopheles*. It occurs in tropical and subtropical regions and is seen in travellers returning from malarial areas. The parasite causes haemolysis during a complex life cycle. *Plasmodium falciparum* causes the most severe disease (malignant tertian malaria). *Plasmodium malariae* causes quartan malaria. *Plasmodium ovale* and *Plasmodium vivax* cause tertian malaria. The signs and symptoms depend on the type of malaria, but include: bouts of fever, rigors, headache, cough, vomiting, anaemia, jaundice, hepatosplenomegaly. Relapses are common in malaria. Various antimalarial drugs are available for both chemoprophylaxis and treatment. Elimination of the mosquito and its habitat are important in prevention—**malarial** *adj*.

Malassezia (L Malassez, French physiologist, 1842–1909) previously known as *Pityrosporum*. A genus of fungi (yeasts) found normally on the skin suface. However, it is responsible for skin diseases including many cases of dandruff. *Malassezia furfur* is associated with tinea (pityriasis) versicolor, which in many cases represents a change in the relationship between the host and resident yeast flora. Tinea versicolor is characterized by scaly macules with changes in pigmentation, mainly on the upper trunk and arms. The altered pigmentation can persist for several months. ⟴ seborrhoeic eczema.

malathion *n* an organophosphorus insecticide, which acts by binding irreversibly to the enzyme cholinesterase. It is used in suitable dilution for the topical treatment of infestations with scabies, head lice and body lice.

malformation *n* abnormal shape or structure; deformity.

malignant *adj* virulent and dangerous—**malignancy** *n*.

malignant glaucoma ⟴ ciliary block glaucoma.

malignant growth or tumour one that demonstrates the capacity to invade adjacent tissues/organs and spread (metastasize) to distant sites; often rapidly growing and with a fatal outcome. ⟴ cancer, carcinoma, sarcoma.

malignant hyperthermia a rare inherited condition; transmitted as an autosomal dominant trait. Hyperpyrexia due to excess muscle activity, precipitated by drugs, usually volatile anaesthetic drugs, e.g. halothane, or depolarizing neuromuscular blocking muscle relaxants, e.g. suxamethonium. It is associated with a muscle channelopathy in which the calcium ion channels in striated muscle are abnormal. There is a rapid increase in body temperature, tachycardia, muscle rigidity and acidosis, which if untreated, may be fatal. Treament is with intravenous dantrolene. ⟴ muscle channelopathies, neuroleptic malignant syndrome.

malignant melanoma ⟴ melanoma.

malignant melanoma of the choroid ⟴ choroidal melanoma.

malignant pustule ⟴ anthrax.

malingering *n* the deliberate simulation of physical or psychological illness motivated by external incentives or stressors.

malleable capable of being hammered into a thin sheet, e.g. gold.

malleolus *n* a part or process of a bone shaped like a hammer. *external malleolus* at the lower end of the fibula. *internal malleolus* situated at the lower end of the tibia—**malleoli** *pl*, **malleolar** *adj*.

mallet a tool for hammering, having a head made of metal, wood, plastic, leather or horn.

Mallett fixation disparity unit an instrument used to measure the associated phoria (or compensating prism). It consists of a small central fixation letter X surrounded by two letters O, one on each side of X, the three letters being seen binocularly, and two coloured polarized vertical bars in line with the centre of the X which are seen by each eye separately. The instrument can be swung through 90° to measure any vertical fixation disparity. The associated phoria is indicated by the misalignment of the two polarized bars when the subject fixates the X through cross-polarized filters in front of the eyes. The amount of associated phoria is given by the value of the base-in or base-out prism power necessary to produce alignment. The unit can also be used to detect suppression. ⟴ associated heterophoria, compensated heterophoria, Disparometer, retinal disparity, uncompensated heterophoria.

mallet finger (*syn* hammer finger) the rupture of the extensor digitorum longus tendon from the distal phalanx as a result of a sudden forced flexion, which results in an inability to extend the joint (Figure M.1). It may even cause

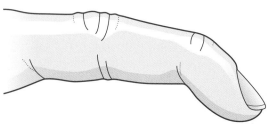

M.1 Mallet finger (reproduced from Porter 2005 with permission).

bony avulsion. Common in catching sports, especially when the ball is caught with a partially closed hand. Treatment is by splinting (Stack splint) with the finger held in full extension for about 6 weeks. Surgery is rarely required. Known as baseball finger in the USA.

malleus *n* the hammer-shaped lateral ossicle of the middle ear. It transmits sound waves from the tympanic membrane to the incus. ⮑ incus, stapes, Colour Section Figure 13.

Mallory bodies (F Mallory, American pathologist, 1862–1941) abnormal inclusions present in hepatocytes in alcohol-induced liver injury, Wilson's disease, primary biliary cirrhosis, long term cholestasis and liver cancer.

Mallory–Weiss syndrome (G Mallory, American pathologist, 20th century; S Weiss, American physician, 1898–1942) massive bleeding from a tear in the mucosa at the junction between the oesophagus and the stomach. It is caused by the straining associated with protracted vomiting. An uncommon cause of haematemesis.

malnutrition *n* the state of being poorly nourished due to the diet containing the incorrect amount of a micro- or macronutrient. Can result in disease, such as scurvy—malnutrition due to inadequate dietary intake of vitamin C, or obesity—malnutrition due to excessive energy intake. Prolonged or repeated weight-loss attempts are likely to cause nutritional deficiencies. ⮑ chronic energy deficiency, eating disorders, obesity, protein-energy malnutrition.

malocclusion *n* abnormal occlusion characterized by an incorrect relationship between the arches in any spatial plane or by abnormal anomalies in tooth position. ⮑ Angle's classification, orthodontics.

malposition *n* any abnormal position of a part. In obstetrics, a cephalic presentation other than one where the fetal head is well-flexed with the occiput in an anterior postion relative to the maternal pelvis, such as a posterior position.

malpractice *n* improper or injurious medical or nursing treatment or other healthcare intervention. Professional practice that falls below accepted standards and causes harm. It may be negligence, unethical behaviour, abuse or involve criminal activities.

malpresentation *n* any presentation in which the fetus is not in the normal vertex position before or during labour, i.e. brow, face, shoulder or breech. Failure to diagnose the condition can lead to serious complications including obstructed labour, uterine rupture, fetal or maternal death.

malrotation a congenital abnormality of the bowel when the distal limb of the midgut fails to rotate on returning to the abdomen during embryonic/fetal development. Identified on ultrasound by looking at the placement of the blood vessels supplying the bowel.

MALT *acron* mucosa-associated lymphoid tissue.

Malta fever ⮑ brucellosis.

maltase *n* (*syn* α-glucosidase) an enzyme found in intestinal juice. It converts the disaccharide maltose to glucose.

maltitol a bulk sweetener with approximately 0.8 times the sweetness of sucrose (beet or cane sugar). ⮑ sweetener.

maltodextrins water-soluble, easily digestible polymers of glucose with low sweetness produced from starch. As a convenient source of energy (4 kcal per gram) in combination with sugars added for flavour, they are used in sports drinks, energy bars and nutritional supplement beverages. The maltodextrins provide a solution of lower osmolality weight for weight than simple sugars such as dextrose, fructose and glucose and so can deliver more calories at the osmolality of body fluids.

MALToma *n* low grade B cell lymphoma of the mucosa-associated lymphoid tissue. It may be related to *Helicobacter pylori* infection which, when eradicated, may lead to disease regression.

maltose *n* malt sugar. A disaccharide composed of two molecules of glucose produced by the hydrolysis of starch by amylase during digestion. It is present in beer, cereals and germinating seeds, which makes only a small contribution to the carbohydrate content of a normal diet. Broken down by the enzyme maltase to two molecules of glucose. Also manufactured commercially.

mal tracking patella abnormal tracking of the patella (usually laterally), can be a cause of anterior knee pain and can be caused by abnormal foot or knee biomechanics or soft tissue length. Surgical management is by lateral release. As with all conditions, treatment depends on the cause but physiotherapy techniques include vastus medialis obliquus (VMO) exercises, taping, insoles if the foot is the primary cause of the problem or patellar mobilizations. ⮑ lateral release.

malunion *n* the union or healing of a fracture in a less than perfect position. For example, overlapping of the bone fragments could lead to shortening, which would affect function. Angulation or rotation of the fragments may impair function because of the resulting altered biomechanics.

mamm- a prefix that means 'breast', e.g. *mammogram*.

mamma *n* the breast—**mammae** *pl*, **mammary** *adj*.

mammaplasty, mammoplasty *n* any plastic operation on the breast—**mammaplastic** *adj*. ⮑ augmentation, implant, reduction.

mammary glands the breasts. Milk-secreting glands.

mammilla *n* **1.** the nipple. **2.** a small papilla—**mammillae** *pl*.

mammogram a radiograph of breast tissue.

mammography *n* radiographic techniques used for the demonstration of the breast, which use specially low-penetration (long wavelength) X-rays. Used in the diagnosis of or routine screening for breast conditions including cancer—**mammographic** *adj*, **mammographically** *adv*. ⮑ screening.

Manchester operation (*syn.* Fothergill's operation) anterior colporrhaphy, amputation of part of the cervix and posterior colpoperineorrhaphy, performed for genital prolapse.

Mandelbaum effect a tendency for the accommodative response to be altered when interposing a conflicting visual stimulus to the one being viewed. If the eyes are viewing a distant object through a dirty window or a wire fence the actual accommodative response will tend to be raised.

If the eyes are viewing a near object in front of a dirty window or wire fence the actual accommodative response will be less than if there were no conflicting stimulus. ⊃ accommodative response.

mandible *n* the large U-shaped bone of the lower jaw, slung below the base of the skull by two temporomandibular joints. The tooth-bearing area is known as the body and each of the two upright ends is called the ramus. The junction between the body and a ramus forms the angle of the mandible. Each ramus has an anterior process the coronoid proces and a posterior process known as the condyle. The condyle of each ramus articulates with the temporal bone at the temporomandibular joint. The alveolar process, or tooth-supporting part, lies on the superior surface of the body. The mandible forms the shape of the lower face, the floor of the mouth and supports the lower teeth and tongue. Its movement assists in mastication and speech—**mandibular** *adj.* ⊃ condyle of the mandible.

mandibular relating to the mandible.

mandibular advancement splint a splint used to correct some jaw and dental problems. It is also used to reduce snoring and to alleviate some types of sleep apnoea. A mandibular advancement splint, which is worn in the mouth, may obviate the need for therapy with a continuous positive airway pressure mask.

mandibular canal bony canal commencing at the mandibular foramen on the inner aspect of each ramus, where it is protected by the lingula. It runs through the body of the mandible, conveying the mandibular nerve, which receives afferent nerve branches from all the lower teeth.

mandibular condyle ⊃ condyle of the mandible.

mandibular displacement the deviation from a centric occlusal relationship as a result of deflection from an initial tooth contact.

mandibular foramen an opening situated on the internal aspect of the ascending ramus of the mandible, halfway between the sigmoid notch and the lower border of the body of the mandible, at the upper end of a narrow groove against which the mylohyoid nerve and blood vessels run to the floor of the mouth. The mandibular artery and vein and the afferent inferior dental nerve from all lower teeth are protected by a triangular spur of bone known as the lingula. This is the area sought when giving an inferior dental block injection.

mandibular joint ⊃ temporomandibular joint.

mandibular nerve one of the three divisions of the trigeminal nerve (fifth cranial nerve). Nerve fibres run from the skin of the lower lip and chin and the mucous membrane of the lower lip and gingivae to the mental foramen through which, as the mental nerve, it passes to join the main branch. The incisive nerve from the lower incisor teeth runs back through the body of the mandible to emerge at the mandibular foramen. It then runs deep to the ramus in front of the condyle to a foramen at the base of the skull through which it passes to the brain. The mandibular division is joined by the long buccal sensory nerve and the lingual nerve. Efferent fibres from the brain branch off the mandibular nerve to the muscles of mastication and the salivary glands.

mandibular notch also known as the sigmoid notch. Separates the condyles and coronoid process of the mandible.

mandibular or maxillary osteotomy the surgical exposure and fracturing of the mandible or of the maxilla at a predetermined plane in order to correct its position or its form.

mandibular plane in orthodontics, a line joining the gnathion and gonion and representing the lower border of the ramus of the mandible.

mandibular protrusion an abnormal protrusion of the mandible. A Class III malocclusion.

mandibular staple implant a modified endosseous implant in which the metal appliance passes through the entire height of the mandible in the anterior region where posts pierce the oral mucosa in order to give fixation points to a suitable superstructure. ⊃ implant (dental).

mandibulofacial dysostosis ⊃ Treacher–Collins syndrome.

mandrel in dentistry, a rotary metal shank to fit a mechanical handpiece having a screw (Huey's) or split stud (Moore's) at one end to secure a disc or wheel.

manganese (Mn) *n* a metallic element needed by the body for many enzyme catalysed reactions.

mania *n* a mood disorder characterized by elation, increased energy, overactivity, pressured speech, decreased need for sleep, irritability, grandiosity, distractibility, overspending. May be accompanied by psychotic symptoms, typically grandiose/religiose/persecutory delusions and hallucinations—**maniac** *adj.*

manic depressive illness ⊃ bipolar affective disorder.

manipulation *n* using the hands skilfully as in reducing a fracture or hernia, or changing an abnormal fetal position to facilitate a vaginal delivery. The technique of using the hands to move a body part, particularly to return it to its normal position after displacement, e.g. reduction of a Colles' fracture of the wrist. Manipulation implies a more powerful movement than mobilization and requires skill and experience. Indiscriminate manipulation, especially of the cervical spine, can result in further and serious damage.

manipulation time in dentistry, that part of the working time during which it is possible to manipulate a material without adversely affecting its properties. ⊃ mixing time, working time.

manipulation under anaesthesia (MUA) used for a person who has limitation of movement that is caused by adhesions or other causes that cannot be rectified by conventional physiotherapy measure. It may be appropriate for the person to be given a light anaesthetic prior to the surgeon forcefully moving the joint to regain movement, this is common following knee replacements or frozen shoulder. The role of physiotherapy is paramount after an manipulation under anaesthetic to maintain the range that the surgeon has attained.

mannitol *n* a sugar that is not metabolized in the body and acts as an osmotic diuretic. It is used to reduce cerebral oedema and raised intracranial pressure following brain injury or surgery, and to reduce intraocular pressure in the emergency treatment of glaucoma or prior to glaucoma surgery. ➲ Appendix 5. It is also used as a bulk sweetener with approximately 0.7 times the sweetness of sucrose (beet or cane sugar). ➲ sweetener.

mannose a hexose (6-carbon) sugar present in legumes.

Mann–Whitney *U* test a non-parametric statistical test comparing two sets of unmatched data using a table of values for U. If the results are less than the values in the table the results are significant. It is a substitute to Student's t test for independent groups.

manometer *n* an instrument for measuring the pressure exerted by liquids or gases. Used for example for measuring the pressure exerted by the cerebrospinal fluid during lumbar puncture, or sometimes for measuring central venous pressure.

mantle dentine the first-formed dentine layer at the periphery of the dental pulp.

mantle technique so called because the treatment area represents a cloak, the field dimensions are larger than the patient and therefore shielding of the lungs is required, used to treat Hodgkin's disease. Consists of anterior and posterior parallel pair, shielding of the spinal cord may be required from the posterior field.

Mantoux reaction (C Mantoux, French physician, 1877–1947) a skin test for tuberculosis. Tuberculin Purified Protein Derivative is injected intradermally in the forearm. After 2–4 days, if induration is greater than or equal to 5 mm, the test is positive.

manual evacuation of the bowel a rarely undertaken nursing intervention for faecal impaction. It may be required for patients who suffer chronic constipation where other measures have been unsuccessful. Apart from causing psychological distress to patients there are serious risks that include vagal nerve stimulation and rectal trauma. Manual faecal evacuation must only be undertaken by a registered practitioner who is trained and competent in the procedure. Prior to this procedure, the patient's pulse rate is recorded, noting rhythm, regularity and strength as well as rate. This will serve as a baseline, as it is important to respond to changes in the patient's condition during this procedure, as manual evacuation can cause vagal stimulation and slow the heart rate. The presence of a second person allows for constant monitoring during the procedure, and provides reassurance for the patient.

manual guidance this is where a movement or task that is performed by an individual is helped by an external force, usually by a therapist as part of a treatment intervention, i.e. if there is weakness present the patient may require assistance to fulfil the goal of movement. It is important to withdraw manual guidance as part of the re-learning process so that patients can re-educate their own movement.

manual handling the moving, lifting or supporting of a load subject to legal regulations. Back injuries are a major concern in the health and safety of health professionals, especially nursing and midwifery staff. Employers have a duty of care at common law (judge made law) and by statute (Health and Safety at Work Act 1974) to take reasonable care for the health and safety of their employees. Specific requirements have been laid down in respect of manual handling (MH). Following a Directive of the European Community, regulations were made in 1992 and brought into force in January 1993 requiring employers to implement rules relating to MH operations. MH is defined as "any transporting or supporting of a load (including the lifting, putting down, pushing, pulling, carrying or moving thereof) by hand or by bodily force." (Regulation 2(1)). The regulations require the employer: (a) so far as is reasonably practicable, to avoid the need for his employees to undertake any MH operations at work which involve a risk of their being injured; (b) where it is not reasonably practicable to avoid the need for MH, to carry out a suitable and sufficient assessment of any MH operations; (c) where it is not reasonably practicable to avoid the need for MH, to take appropriate steps to reduce the risk of injury to those employees arising out of their undertaking any such MH to the lowest level reasonably practicable; (d) to provide to the employee, where it is reasonably practicable, precise information on the weight of each load and the heaviest side of any load, whose centre of gravity is not positioned centrally; (e) to review any assessment, where there is reason to suspect that it is no longer valid or there has been a significant change in the MH operations. The MH regulations are enforced by the Health and Safety Executive, which can prosecute for any infringements in the criminal courts. In addition if any employee or other person, can show that they have suffered harm as a result of failures by the employer or other employees in following the regulations, then action can be brought in the civil courts for compensation.

manual hyperinflation a technique in which the chest is hyperinflated in order to remove pulmonary secretions and to reinflate areas of collapsed lung in patients who are intubated. Hyperinflation is usually achieved by use of a hand-bagging circuit.

manual muscle testing a specific procedure used to evaluate the functional status of a muscle's innervation and contractile tissues; uses a graded strength test performed by applying manual resistance to a body segment in order to evaluate a particular muscle or group of muscles.

manual removal of the placenta a procedure, whereby a hand inserted into the uterus is used to remove an adherant placenta from the uterine wall when other methods have failed. It is usually undertaken by a doctor using strict aseptic technique and only after vascular access has been secured by siting an intravenous infusion. Effective anaesthesia is required, either by topping-up an existing epidural anaesthetic, or by spinal or general anaesthetic.

manual rotation turning of the infant's head from a transverse position by internally applied pressure to dislodge its fixture on the ischial spines and rotating it to a more favourable position, i.e. occipitoanterior or occipitoposterior.

M
N

manual therapy encompasses many therapeutic modalities used by physiotherapists, they include manipulation, mobilization and soft-tissue techniques.

manubrium *n* a handle-shaped structure; the upper part of the sternum.

MAOI *abbr* monoamine oxidase inhibitor.

MAP *acron* **M**ean **A**rterial **P**ressure.

maple syrup urine disease an aminoacidopathy, also known as branched chain ketoaciduria. A genetic disorder transmitted as an autosomal recessive trait. The enzyme required for the metabolism of leucine, isoleucine and valine is missing. This results in high levels of the three amino acids in blood and their excretion in the urine, which has an odour similar to that of maple syrup. Symptoms vary according to the type and severity of the disease, but include poor feeding, vomiting, hypertonicity, respiratory difficulties; convulsions and severe damage to the CNS may occur leading to learning disability. A diet low in the three amino acids may be effective if started sufficiently early; without treatment the disorder is rapidly fatal. Genetic counselling may be indicated.

MAR *acron* **M**inimum **A**ngle of **R**esolution.

marasmic kwashiorkor severe form of protein-energy malnutrition in children, which is accompanied by signs and symptoms of kwashiorkor.

marasmus *n* severe protein-energy malnutrition. Wasting away of the body, especially that of a baby. ⊃ failure to thrive, kwashiorkor—**marasmic** *adj*.

marathon specifically, a footrace over a road course of 42.195 km (~26 mile 385 yd) nowadays covered by elite performers in less than 2 h 10 min (males) and 2 h 20 min (females). Named after the city of Marathon in ancient Greece, imitating the distance run by a messenger from there to Athens, with news of victory over the Persians, in 490 BC. In general, term applied to any form of very high endurance activity.

marble bones ⊃ osteopetrosis.

Marburg disease (*syn* green monkey disease) a highly infectious viral haemorrhagic fever characterized by a sudden onset of fever, severe headache and malaise, vomiting, diarrhoea, pharyngitis and mucosal bleeding. Between days 5 and 7 a rash appears. Virus can persist in the body for 2–3 months after the initial attack. Cross infection probably occurs by the aerosol route. Incubation period believed to be 4–9 days. Treatment is symptomatic only and mortality rate in previous outbreaks has been as high as 90%.

march fracture a type of stress fracture caused by an increase in physical activity which may so stress a metatarsal (usually the second) as to produce an undisplaced self-healing hair-line fracture. There is local pain, tenderness, and radiographic changes. Management usually involves moderate rest with supportive padding and strapping for a few weeks but sometimes a walking plaster is required. First described in army recruits following prolonged marching.

march haemoglobinuria redness of the urine due to presence of haemoglobin following prolonged walking/running. Occurs due to direct trauma to the blood cells in the vessels in the soles of the feet. Requires no specific treatment but can be minimized by decreasing walking/running on hard surfaces or wearing more appropriate footwear. ⊃ haemoglobinuria.

march myoglobinuria reddish-brown urine due to the breakdown of muscle myoglobin following strenuous prolonged walking or running. ⊃ myoglobinuria.

Marcus Gunn's pupil (R Marcus Gunn, British ophthalmologist, 1850–1909) (*syn* relative afferent pupillary defect [RAPD]) a defect of the pupillary reflex characterized by a smaller constriction of both pupils when the affected eye is stimulated by light as compared to that occurring when the normal eye is stimulated. It is easier, however, to observe this phenomenon when swinging a light from one eye to the other in a darkened room while the subject is fixating a distant object (this is called the *swinging flashlight test*). Stimulation of the normal eye will cause constriction of both pupils whereas rapid stimulation of the affected eye will lead to a small dilatation (a paradoxical reaction, sometimes referred to as pupillary escape). This condition is due to a lesion in one of the optic nerves which affects the afferent pupillary pathway. It is often the result of multiple sclerosis or optic neuritis or retrobulbar optic neuritis.

Marcus Gunn's syndrome (R Marcus Gunn). ⊃ jaw-winking.

Marfan's syndrome (A Marfan, French paediatrician, 1858–1942) a genetic disorder of connective tissue that mainly affects the musculoskeletal system, the cardiovascular system and the eyes. It is inherited as an autosomal dominant trait. It results from mutations of the fibrillin gene, a component of extracellular matrix. The musculoskeletal manifestations include arachnodactyly (long, thin, 'spider fingers'), skeletal disproportion with excessively long limbs that result in an arm span greater than height, excessive height (adult height usually over 1.8 metres), sternal depression, a high arched palate, poorly developed and hypotonic musculature and lax ligaments with joint hypermobility. There is dislocation of the lens of the eye and abnormalities of the iris. The most serious complications are in the cardiovascular system, with mitral valve prolapse, aortic incompetence and defective structure of the aorta, which leads to aneurysm formation and aortic dissection.

Margaria staircase test a test of short-term ('burst') anaerobic power in which, after a short run-in, the subject runs as fast as possible up a short flight of stairs of specific dimensions. In each of several versions of the test, the length of run-in, rise of each stair and the steps between which speed is measured (e.g. 8th and 12th) are all specified. Timing is by switchmats on the specified steps. Also known as Margaria–Kalamen test.

margin the edge or border of a surface—**marginal**, *adj*. ⊃ cervical margin.

marginal bone ⊃ alveolar margin.

marginal conjunctiva ⊃ conjunctiva.

marginal cost the cost of providing the extra resources required to carry out activity, such as a medical intervention, above a baseline number.

marginal placenta praevia a placenta which is low-lying, its edges located on the margin of the lower segment of the uterus, possibly reaching the internal cervical os. ⊃ placenta praevia.

marginal tear strip ⊃ tear meniscus.

marihuana, marijuana *n* (cannabis, pot, grass, hashish) one of the so-called social or recreational drugs, obtained from the hemp plant *Cannabis sativa* whose active ingredient is tetrahydrocannabinol. The use of social drugs is increasing in society and sport is no exception. UK government statistics have suggested that 40% of 16–18 year olds had taken social drugs in the 12-month period studied. Statistics of their use in sport are difficult to obtain and confirm but are likely to be significant given that the majority of sportsmen and women are young. The effects of marihuana/marijuana include relaxation, euphoria, sedation, disorientation and a lowering of aggression. It is generally accepted that regular use, and these effects, are not compatible with a training regimen required for top-level sport. The current World Anti-Doping Agency (WADA) and the International Olympic Committee (IOC) regulations ban the use of marihuana/marijuana in competition, but not out of competition. Many believe that in the absence of performance-enhancing effects, an automatic 2-year ban is not justified and that an approach based on education and rehabilitation is preferable, and will assist in maintaining the positive 'role model' example to young people. ⊃ cannabis.

Marjolin's ulcer (J Marjolin, French surgeon, 1780–1850) a squamous cell cancer that develops on damaged or chronically inflamed tissue, such as at the edge of a burn injury or a venous leg ulcer.

mark:space ratio an electrotherapy term—usually only used for pulsed ultrasound. ⊃ on:off ratio.

marrow *n* ⊃ bone marrow.

Marshall–Marchetti–Krantz operation (V Marshall, American urologist, b.1913; A Marchetti, American obstetrician, 1901–1970; K Krantz) surgical procedure for stress incontinence. A form of abdominal cystourethropexy usually undertaken in patients whose loss of continence has not been controlled by a colporrhaphy.

marsupialization *n* an operation for cystic swellings, which entails stitching the margins of an opening made into the cyst to the edges of the wound, thus forming a pouch.

Maryland bridge in dentistry, a modification of the Rochette bridge where the fitting surface of the framework is electrolytically etched in order to enhance the metal-composite-etched enamel bond. ⊃ bridge.

mAs the average electrical current passing through an X-ray tube during an exposure multiplied by the exposure time in seconds.

masculinization the development of male secondary sexual characteristics. ⊃ virilism.

masking covering up or concealing. In dentistry, the use of opaque material to cover metallic or dark areas of restorations or prostheses.

Maslow's hierarchy of needs (A Maslow, American psychologist, 1908–1970) a hierarchy of needs based on the humanistic approach. Generally shown as having five levels represented as a pyramid—commencing at the base with physiological needs required for survival; safety and security needs; love and belonging needs; self-esteem needs; and ending at the apex with self-actualization needs. A further two levels have since been added: cognitive needs and aesthetic needs, which are slotted in between self-esteem and self-actualization.

masochism *n* the deriving of pleasure from pain inflicted by others or occasionally by oneself. It may be a conscious or unconscious process and is frequently of a sexual nature. ⊃ sadism.

mass the quantity of material in an object or body. Can be measured in terms of the force needed to accelerate it. Mass is measured in kilograms (kg) and is not to be confused with weight.

mass attenuation coefficient is the linear attenuation coefficient divided by the density of the medium the beam passes through and is used to describe the probability of an interaction occurring between the X-ray beam and the tissue.

mass number the total mass of neutrons and protons within an atom.

massage *n* **1.** several different soft tissue manipulations (kneading, stroking, rubbing, tapping, etc.). They are used at different depths and rates for various purposes: to improve circulation, metabolism and muscle tone, to break down adhesions, to expel gases, and to either relax or stimulate the patient. Massage is used in sport to break down adhesions (deep friction), reduce swelling and oedema, and relax muscles. While massage will aid relaxation and reduce muscle stiffness, there is little scientific evidence of any reduction in injury rates. **2.** a complementary therapy that involves the conscious use of gentle muscle manipulation, using stroking or light kneading, to promote relaxation.

masseter the powerful, thick, square-shaped cheek muscle. One of the muscles of mastication. Its origin is on the zygomatic arch and it inserts onto the outer surface of ramus of the mandible. It closes the jaw and can be palpated when the teeth are clenched. The nerve supply is from a branch of the mandibular nerve and the blood supply from the external carotid artery.

Masson's bodies (C Masson, Canadian pathologist, 1880–1959) typical pathological changes present in lung tissue in cryptogenic organizing pneumonia.

MAST *acron* **M**ilitary **A**nti**S**hock **T**rousers.

mast cells cells produced in the bone marrow and present in connective tissues, which have similarities with basophils (a type of leucocyte). They have granules containing various chemicals that include heparin and histamine and other chemical mediators. They are generally located around small blood vessels in the skin, respiratory mucosa, gastrointestinal mucosa, the eyes, nose and mouth. They have an important role in body defences and function in the inflammatory response, allergic conditions, anaphylaxis and wound healing. Mast cells are activated to degranulate and release their chemicals in situations that include chemical or physical injury, or immunoglobulin E (IgE) binding to their receptors.

mastalgia *n* pain in the breast.

mastectomy *n* surgical removal of the breast. ⊃ lumpectomy. *simple mastectomy* removal of the breast with the overlying skin. *modified radical mastectomy* removal of the entire breast and division or excision of the pectoralis minor muscle with axillary lymph node clearance. *radical mastectomy* rarely performed operation that involves removal of the breast, pectoralis major muscle and clearance of the axillary lymph nodes.

master impression ⊃ impression.

mastication *n* chewing. When the molar teeth are used for grinding and the incisors for cutting food.

masticatory system the oral structures involved in mastication, including the muscles of mastication, the facial muscles, tongue and teeth.

mastitis *n* inflammation of the breast. *chronic mastitis* the name formerly applied to the nodular changes in the breasts now usually called fibrocystic disease.

mast/o- a prefix that means 'breast', e.g. *mastectomy*.

mastoid *adj* nipple-shaped.

mastoid air-cells extend in a backward and downward direction from the antrum.

mastoid antrum the air space within the mastoid process, lined by mucous membrane continuous with that of the tympanum and mastoid air-cells.

mastoid process the prominence of the mastoid portion of the temporal bone just behind the ear.

mastoidectomy *n* drainage of the mastoid air-cells and excision of diseased tissue. *cortical mastoidectomy* all the mastoid cells are removed making one cavity which drains through an opening (aditus) into the middle ear. The external meatus and middle ear are untouched. *radical mastoidectomy* the mastoid antrum, and middle ear are made into one continuous cavity for drainage of infection. Loss of hearing is inevitable.

mastoiditis *n* inflammation of the mastoid air-cells.

mastopexy *n* surgical fixation of a pendulous breast.

masturbation *n* non-coital sexual arousal and orgasm by stimulation of the genitalia.

mATPase *abbr* myosin ATPase.

matching hypothesis the proposition that psychological or behavioural interventions or training programmes should match the presenting problem or personal characteristics of the person being treated or trained. For example, it has been proposed that cognitive-based relaxation techniques should be used to treat cognitive anxiety whereas relaxation techniques designed to reduce physiological arousal should be used to treat somatic anxiety.

materia alba the soft, white deposit consisting of food debris, dead epithelial cells and leucocytes. Found around the necks of teeth and the gingival margin, it serves as a medium for bacterial growth and is generally associated with poor oral hygiene.

materia medica the science dealing with the origin, action and dosage of drugs.

maternal mortality death of a women due to the complications of pregnancy. In the UK the rate is calculated as the number of deaths per 100 000 births (including stillbirths) plus deaths due to abortion. The Confidential Enquiries into Maternal Deaths divides deaths into four groups: direct, i.e. due to complications of the pregnancy, most commonly thromboembolic conditions; indirect, i.e. from an existing disease that was worsened by pregnancy; coincidental, i.e. deaths unrelated to the pregnancy; and late deaths that occur between 42 days and 12 months of a miscarriage, a termination of pregnancy (abortion) or delivery.

maternity care assistant auxiliary practitioner who is not a registered midwife but specifically trained to assist mothers and midwives.

matriarchy *n* describes a situation where a female (wife, mother or daughter) inherits, dominates and controls within a social structure.

matrix *n* **1.** the foundation substance in which the tissue cells are embedded. **2.** a pattern or mould used in a casting. **3.** a thin mould, band or strip used to contain and contour filling materials in their plastic state, during insertion and setting. **4.** in dentistry, the female component of a precision attachment.

matrix band in restorative dentistry, stainless steel band or strip of polymeric material, which is wrapped around and held against multi-surface tooth preparations to provide a temporary wall against which the restorative material can be packed, and to impart a smooth surface and contour to the completed restoration. *matrix band retainer* a screw, spring or clip metal device used to retain a matrix band in position. There are two main types: those for use in cases of mesial occlusal or distal occlusal cavities in molars and premolars, and the annular type which may also be used for mesial occlusal distal cavities. (a) Ivory number 1 matrix band retainer: for use with two surfaced cavities only. The perforated ended stainless steel bands are made in various widths and thicknesses—shorter ones being available for premolar application. They are easier to remove without disturbing the completed restoration than the annular types. The perforations allow for tension adjustment. (b) Annular type matrix band retainer: for use with two or three surfaced preparations. They include: *annular ivory 8 matrix band retainer* similar to the Siqveland but the band can be released before the holder is removed separately. *Siqveland matrix band holder* a portion of ribbon band is cut and folded onto the retainer to form a ring shape which can be tightened by rotating a knurled knob. On completion of the filling the band and holder are removed together. *Tofflemire matrix band holder* one of several shaped bands is selected and placed in the holder and held by screw tension. A knurled nut is rotated to tighten the annular band round the tooth. The band can be released before the holder is removed separately.

matrix (digital imaging) the rows and columns of pixels on a display used to form a digital image.

matrix metalloproteinases a family of zinc-containing metalloendopeptidase enzymes, including collagenase, that are produced as part of the host immune and inflammatory response in a number of inflammatory, degenerative diseases and malignancies.

Matthews Duncan expulsion of placenta placental expulsion in which the maternal side appears first in third stage of labour, often due to a low-lying placenta. More severe haemorrhage is likely than with a Schultze expulsion. ⊃ Schultze expulsion of placenta.

maturation *n* 1. the process of attaining full development. 2. describes the final stage in wound healing, during which the wound is strengthened and the scar gradually fades and shrinks. 3. the process in which tooth enamel that has just been laid down becomes mineralized by the withdrawal of organic matter and water, and the deposition of apatite.

maturity onset diabetes of the young (MODY) an uncommon subtype of type 2 diabetes caused by a single gene defect. Accounts for <5% of cases of type 2 diabetes.

Matveyev's six phases system of athletic training in which the first period consists simply of general body conditioning, the second adds some sport-specific training, the third introduces competition-specific features, the fourth includes preliminary competitions, the fifth is the main competition phase and the sixth is a recuperation period before the next six-phase cycle is commenced. Normally the phase durations are of the order of months, and the complete six-phase cycle lasts a year. (Named after the Soviet scientist who established the system in the mid-20th century.)

Maurceau–Smellie–Veit manoeuvre (F Maurceau, French obstetrician, 1637–1709; W Smellie, British obstetrician, 1697–1763; A Veit, German obstetrician, 1824–1903) a manoeuvre used to deliver the aftercoming head during a breech delivery. Flexion is increased, and jaw and shoulder traction applied, which allows for better control over the delivery of the head than Burns–Marshall manoeuvre in cases where forceps delivery is not possible. ⊃ Burns–Marshall manoeuvre.

Maurice's theory (*syn* lattice theory) the theory that explains the transparency of the stroma of the cornea. It states that the stromal fibrils, which have a refractive index of about 1.55 in the dry state, are so arranged as to behave as a series of diffraction gratings permitting transmission through the liquid ground substance (refractive index 1.34). The fibrils are the grating elements that are arranged in a hexagonal lattice pattern of equal spacing and with the fibril interval being less than the wavelength of light. The diffraction gratings eliminate scattered light by destructive interference, except for the normally incident light rays. Light beams that are not normal to the cornea are also transmitted to the oblique lattice plane. However, recent work has demonstrated inconsistencies in lattice space and there is some modification to the original postulate of this theory. ⊃ diffraction.

maxilla *n* the upper jaw, consisting of two fused maxillae which support the upper teeth and are fixed to the skull. It separates the roof of the mouth from the floor of the nasal cavity and the floor of the orbit—**maxillary** *adj*.

maxillary antrum/sinus also known as the antrum of Highmore. One of two large paranasal air sinuses situated in the maxilla. It is lined with ciliated mucosa that is continuous with that lining the nasal cavity. The roots of the upper molar teeth and sometimes the premolars lie just below the floor of the antrum/sinus.

maxillary artery a terminal branch of the external carotid artery. Its many branches supply blood to the muscles of mastication, the mandible, mandibular teeth, the dura, bones of the skull, parts of the ear, etc.

maxillary disimpaction forceps ⊃ forceps.

maxillary-mandibular planes angle (MxMnPA) the cephalometric angle measured between the maxillary plane and the mandibular plane. Normal is 27 degrees plus or minus 4 degrees.

maxillary nerve a division of the trigeminal nerve (fifth cranial nerve). Afferent fibres from the eyelids, nose and upper lip pass through the infraorbital canal of the maxilla via the infraorbital foramen. Here they are joined by afferent nerve fibres from the anterior, middle and posterior superior dental nerves from all of the upper teeth. The greater palatine and nasopalatine afferent nerves from the soft palate join the maxillary nerve via the sphenopalatine ganglion as it leaves the infraorbital canal.

maxillary osteotomy the surgical repositioning of the maxilla.

maxillary plane the transverse plane through the skull represented on a lateral skull radiograph tracing by the line joining the anterior and posterior nasal spines.

maxillary resection the surgical removal of all or part of the maxilla and the related soft tissues.

maxillary tuberosity reduction the surgical removal of excess fibrous, epithelial and bone tissue which forms the tuberosity to facilitate the construction and placing of a denture.

maxillectomy the surgical resection of part (partial) or all (total) of the maxilla.

maxillofacial *adj* pertaining to the maxilla and face.

maxillofacial prosthesis a prosthesis used to restore the contour of the face and/or jaw following injury or surgery.

maxillofacial surgery branch of surgery concerned with the surgical management of developmental disorders and diseases or trauma of the facial structures.

maxillotomy cutting through the maxilla in order to move all or some parts to a better position.

maximal breathing capacity (MBC) the maximum volume of air that can be inhaled and exhaled in given time, when the person is breathing as deeply and quickly as possible.

maximal heart rate (HRmax) a term used in sports medicine. The highest heart rate that can be attained by an individual in strenuous activity, varying with fitness and, in adults, inversely with age. A 'rule of thumb' formula for the predicted maximum involves subtracting the person's age in years from 220 (HRmax = 220 − age in years), for example a person aged 60 would be expected to have a HRmax of around 160 beats per minute.

maximal intensity exercise exercise that needs the person to make a maximum effort, and where most of the energy needed for the exercise is produced from anaerobic metabolism.

maximal lactate steady state ⮎ maximum lactate steady state.

maximal oxygen consumption/uptake ($\dot{V}O_{2max}$) the rate of oxygen uptake at the highest work rate an individual can attain and sustain for some minutes, equivalent to aerobic capacity. Measured at the peak of incremental exercise or by extrapolation to predicted maximal heart rate, from successive submaximal measurements of heart rate and oxygen uptake.

maximal voluntary torque (MVT) maximal torque produced using a voluntary muscle contraction. Can be isometric (maximal voluntary isometric torque [MVIT]), isotonic or isokinetic. Used in a ratio with electrically initiated torque (EIT), but not reliable and so not recommended. ⮎ electrically initiated torque.

maximum density (D Max) in radiography, the maximum density which can be reached on a film under set exposure and processing conditions, determined using a characteristic curve. ⮎ characteristic curve.

maximum expiratory pressure (MEP) an effort-dependent measure of the maximal or peak static expiratory effort sustained for one second, measured in centimetres of water pressure using a breathing circuit with attached manometer and flanged mouthpiece. It is the highest pressure achieved during expiration after a full inspiration. This is used as an index of global muscle weakness.

maximum heart rate (HRmax) ⮎ maximal heart rate (HRmax).

maximum inspiratory pressure (MIP) this is an effort-dependent measure of the maximal or peak static inspiratory effort sustained for one second, measured in centimetres of water pressure using a breathing circuit with attached manometer and flanged mouthpiece. It is the highest pressure reached in the alveoli during a full inspiration. This is used as an index of global muscle strength.

maximum intensity projection a volume rendering technique used to visualize high-intensity structures within a data acquisition. Achieved by a step-by-step process for producing projections from a two-dimensional or three-dimensional volume data set which is processed along selected angles. The highest data value for each pixel taken from a specific viewing angle is displayed. Used to demonstrate vascular structures in computed tomography (CT) scanning and also in magnetic resonance imaging (MRI) scanning.

maximum intercuspal contacts tooth contacts in the maximum intercuspal position.

maximum intercuspation the complete intercuspation of opposing teeth independently of the position of the condyles.

maximum lactate steady state (MLSS) highest work rate which can be maintained without continuous rise in blood lactate concentration $[Lac]_b$. Functionally equivalent to critical power though this is definded in terms of $\dot{V}O_2$, not $[Lac]_b$. ⮎ metabolic and related thresholds.

maximum permitted dose the upper limit of a radiation dose received by a person during a specified period. Ionizing radiation may cause somatic or genetic injury to individuals either by a concentrated high dose or by accumulated small doses over a period of time.

maximum voluntary contraction (MVC) maximum force which a human subject can produce in a specific isometric exercise. In practice, usually taken as the best of three efforts in a single test session.

maximum voluntary ventilation (MVV) (*syn.* maximal breathing capacity [MBC]) the greatest pulmonary ventilation in L/min that a person can attain by deliberately increasing the depth and frequency of breathing.

maxwellian view system ⮎ clinical maxwellian view system.

Maxwell's spot an entopic phenomenon in which the subject can observe a dark or greyish spot in the visual field corresponding to his fovea. This is accomplished by viewing a diffusely illuminated field through a purple-blue or dark blue filter. (These are the best colours for this observation.) This phenomenon is used clinically to detect eccentric fixation by placing a fixation point in the diffusely illuminated field. The degree of eccentric fixation can thus be estimated by asking the subject to describe the position of the grey spot with respect to the fixation point. ⮎ eccentric fixation, entoptic image/phenomena.

Mayer–Rokitansky–Küster–Hauser syndrome (P Mayer, German gynaecologist, 1795–1868; C von Rokitansky, Austrian pathologist, 1804–1878; H Küster, German gynaecologist, b.1897; G Hauser, German gynaecologist, 20th century) müllerian agenesis. Congenital absence of the vagina and usually absence of the uterus and uterine (fallopian) tubes. There is normal ovarian development and function.

Mb *abbr* myoglobin.

MBC *abbr* maximal breathing capacity. ⮎ respiratory function tests.

MBP *abbr* mean (arterial) blood pressure.

MCA *abbr* **1.** Medicines Control Agency. ⮎ Medicines and Healthcare products Regulatory Agency (MHRA). **2.** middle cerebral artery.

MCADD *abbr* medium chain acyl-CoA dehydrogenase deficiency.

M
N

McArdle's disease (B McArdle, British neurologist, 1911–2002) type V glycogen storage disease in which there is a deficiency of muscle glycogen phosphorylase enzyme. It is characterized by exercise-induced fatigue and myalgia (muscle cramps), and myoglobinuria. Diagnosis is based on an elevated level of creatine kinase (CK), muscle biopsy and molecular genetic studies. ⮑ inherited metabolic myopathies.

McBurney's point (C McBurney, American surgeon, 1845–1913) a point one-third of the way between the anterior superior iliac spine and the umbilicus, the site of maximum tenderness in cases of acute appendicitis.

McCune–Albright syndrome ⮑ Albright's syndrome.

MCH *abbr* mean cell haemoglobin.

MCHC *abbr* mean cell haemoglobin concentration.

MCID *abbr* minimal clinical important difference (MCID) (of outcome scores).

McKenzie approach (R McKenzie, New Zealand physiotherapist, 20th–21st century) the approach of mechanical diagnosis and therapy developed by McKenzie that is now used worldwide by clinicians and patients for the management of spinal and non-spinal musculoskeletal problems. During the history and physical examination, the symptomatic and mechanical responses to movement and postures are determined; the analysis includes repeated movements and sustained positions. An understanding of these responses allows classification into one of the mechanical syndromes: derangement, dysfunction or postural syndrome. Direction-specific exercises are then used to treat symptoms and restore function, with the emphasis always being on patient-generated forces to maximize patient independence. Management is dependent upon good patient education. Minimal therapeutic force is always used, but force progressions are introduced if there is failure to improve. A combination of exercise and therapist intervention is used if this is necessary to produce change. There is now a wealth of research that has been done to investigate components of the approach. This research has looked at mechanical diagnosis and therapy both as an assessment tool and as a treatment approach. For instance, the symptom response of centralization has consistently been associated with a good prognosis; the assessment system is reliable when used by those who are well trained; as an intervention it is equal to chiropractic manipulation and strength-training exercises. There is an international education programme available to qualified healthcare professionals. This has five sequential courses, a credentialing examination and a diploma programme.

McKesson prop ⮑ mouth prop.

MCL *abbr* medial collateral ligament.

McMurray's osteotomy (T McMurray, British orthopaedic surgeon, 1887–1949) division of femur between lesser and greater trochanter. Shaft displaced inwards beneath the head and abducted. This position maintained by a nail plate. Restores painless weight bearing. In developmental dysplasia of the hip, deliberate pelvic osteotomy renders the outer part of the socket (acetabulum) more horizontal.

McMurray's test (T McMurray) a test of the integrity of the menisci of the knee joint. A positive test occurs if pain is elicited or a snap or click of the joint will occur if the meniscus is torn. During the test the person lies supine, with the knee flexed to 45°, hip flexed to 45°. The examiner braces the lower leg, one hand holds the ankle, other hand holds the knee. The medial meniscus assessment involves assessing for pain on palpation. The health professional palpates the medial joint line with the knee flexed; assesses for a 'click' suggesting meniscus relocation. Applies valgus stress to the flexed knee. Externally rotates the leg (toes point outward). Slowly extends the knee while still in valgus. The lateral meniscus assessment involves repeating the above with varus stress and internal rotation. The examiner may be able to detect clicking or snapping sounds when performing this test, since there are various structures in the knee joint that may produce these signs, it is easy for this test to produce a false-positive result.

MCP *abbr* multiple cosmetic phlebectomy.

MCP block (low melting-point alloy [LMPA] block) an alloy of lead, bismuth, cadmium and zinc which can be formed into individually shaped shielding blocks. These can be mounted below the head of the radiotherapy machine providing customized shielding of normal tissue.

McRoberts manoeuvre a manoeuvre used to rotate the angle of the symphysis pubis superiorly and release the impaction of the anterior shoulder in shoulder dystocia. The woman lies flat and bends her knees up to her chest with hips abducted.⮑ shoulder dystocia.

McSpadden compactor® ⮑ compactor.

MCT *abbr* medium chain triglycerides (triacylglycerols).

MCU *abbr* micturating cystourethrogram.

MCV *abbr* mean cell volume.

MDA *abbr* Medical Devices Agency. ⮑ Medicines and Healthcare products Regulatory Agency (MHRA).

MDI *abbr* metered-dose inhaler.

MDM *abbr* mental defence mechanism. ⮑ defence mechanisms.

MDR-TB *abbr* multidrug resistant tuberculosis.

MDS *abbr* myelodysplastic syndrome.

MDT *abbr* multidisciplinary team.

ME *abbr* myalgic encephalomyelitis. ⮑ chronic fatigue syndrome.

mean *n* the average. ⮑ arithmetic mean, central tendency statistic, median, mode.

mean arterial blood pressure (MABP, MAP, MBP) the arithmetic mean blood pressure in the arterial system. A mean value averaged over a cardiac cycle, derived from the arterial pulse pressure wave; typically closer to the diastolic blood pressure (DBP) than the systolic blood pressure (SBP). ⮑ pulse pressure.

mean cell (corpuscular) haemoglobin (MCH) *n* a red cell parameter estimated during a full blood count. It is the amount of haemoglobin in an average red blood cell.

mean cell (corpuscular) haemoglobin concentration (MCHC) *n* a red cell parameter measured during a full blood count. It is the weight (in grams) of haemoglobin in 100 mL of packed red blood cells.

mean cell volume (MCV) *n* a red cell parameter measured during a full blood count. It is the mean volume of red cells, which provides information about cell size. It is used to determine whether anaemia is macrocytic (MCV above normal) or microcytic (MCV below normal).

mean dose point in radiotherapy, the central dose point when all the doses are plotted by increasing or decreasing size.

mean window level the average range of pixel values in an image.

meaning the significance or importance that an object or event has for an individual or group. Meanings may be realistic or symbolic.

measles *n* (*syn* morbilli, rubeola) a paramyxovirus infection that is endemic world-wide. It is probably the most infectious of all microbial agents. Before immunization campaigns, measles occurred in almost 100% of children. Maternal antibody gives protection for the first 6 months of life. In temperate areas there is a natural epidemic cycle every 2–3 years, less obvious in the tropics. With live attenuated vaccine, the condition is potentially completely controllable by immunization and in the UK active immunization is offered as part of the routine immunization programme during childhood. The World Health Organization (WHO) has set the objective of eradicating measles by the year 2010 as part of its expanded programme of immunization. Incomplete vaccination of only 70–80% of the population may lead to outbreaks in older children and adults, in whom complications are more frequent. This necessitates repeat mass immunization campaigns or second dosing of vaccine in an older age group. At the time of writing there is a worrying increase in the number of measles cases in the UK, the increase is caused by the reduction in the uptake of the MMR vaccine. Natural illness produces lifelong immunity. Infection is by droplet spread with an incubation period of 14 days to onset of rash. A prodromal illness 1–3 days before the rash appears heralds the most infectious, 'catarrhal' stage with upper respiratory symptoms, high fever, conjunctivitis and the presence of Koplik's spots on the internal buccal mucosa. ⊃ Colour Section Figure 83. These small white spots surrounded by erythema are pathognomonic of measles. At this stage the patient is miserable, irritable and photophobic, corresponding to the peak of a second viraemia. As natural antibody develops, the rash appears, lasting 5–6 days and gradually fading with 'staining' in the pale-skinned. ⊃ Colour Section Figure 88. Generalized lymphadenopathy and diarrhoea are common, with bacterial pneumonia in approximately 4% of cases. Convulsions occur in approximately 1% and long-term damage can result in the rare occurrence of subacute sclerosing panencephalitis (SSPE) up to 7 years after infection. The typical rash may be missing in the immunocompromised and persistent infection with a giant cell pneumonitis or rapidly progressive encephalitis may occur. Complications caused by secondary bacterial infection include otitis media and corneal ulceration. As with many childhood exanthemas, disease is more severe and prolonged in adults. Measles is a serious disease in the malnourished, vitamin-deficient or immunocompromised. Mortality clustering at the extremes of age is 1:1000 in developed countries, compared to up to 1:4 in developing countries. Death usually results from bacterial superinfection such as pneumonia, diarrhoeal disease or cancrum oris. Normal immunoglobulin attenuates the disease in the immunocompromised or in non-immune pregnant women. Vaccination can be used in outbreaks and vitamin A may improve the outlook in uncomplicated disease. Antibiotic therapy is only effective where signs of superinfection already exist and should not be used empirically. ⊃ Koplik's spots.

meatotomy *n* surgery to the urinary meatus for meatal stricture in men.

meatus *n* an opening or channel—**meatal** *adj*.

mechanical advantage the difference in forces in a lever system due to the inequalities of the lever arms between the forces and the fulcrum (pivot or axis). ⊃ mechanical efficiency.

mechanical amalgamator in dentistry, the equipment, generally electrically powered, that vibrates amalgam alloy and mercury together for a controlled time to form amalgam. Other materials, such as cements and composite fillings, can also be mixed by this method.

mechanical efficiency the ratio of mechanical energy output (or work output) to the energy input.

mechanical energy may be kinetic energy (translational or rotational), gravitational potential energy (potential energy) or elastic potential energy. ⊃ conservation of mechanical energy.

mechanical stimulus any substance, such as wax, that is chewed in order to stimulate a flow of saliva.

mechanical ventilation describes various mechanical methods used to support patients where spontaneous respirations have ceased or are inadequate to maintain sufficient gas exchange of oxygen and carbon dioxide, such as respiratory failure or during general anaesthetic. Mechanical ventilation may be required to support breathing in respiratory failure. There are many causes of respiratory failure; those immediately associated with the lungs such as pneumonia, pulmonary oedema or severe acute asthma (status asthmaticus) and those that can affect the mechanics of breathing such as flail chest, Guillain–Barré syndrome or during anaesthesia. Mechanical ventilation can also be used to reduce the workload of the heart in certain conditions. A ventilator takes a mixture of oxygen and air and passes it into the lungs, commonly via an endotracheal tube or tracheostomy tube, providing inspiration. Expiration, as in normal physiology, is reliant on the natural recoil of the lungs, not the ventilator. Ventilators have controls that can alter parameters such as respiratory rate, the size of breath (tidal volume) and the percentage of inspired oxygen to suit the requirements of individual patients. Most ventilators have the capacity to provide different modes or methods of ventilation. If the patient is completely unable to breathe,

the ventilator will provide all of the breathing required. This mode (used less frequently today) is called controlled mandatory ventilation (CMV). Alternatively, if the patient can provide some of the breathing, a ventilator mode can be chosen that supplements the patient's efforts. Such modes include: pressure support ventilation (PSV) or synchronized intermittent ventilation (SIMV). Intermittent mandatory ventilation (IMV): a type of assisted ventilation where a mandatory number of respirations are mechanically imposed on spontaneous breathing. It can be used to wean patients off mechanical ventilation. ➲ intermittent positive pressure ventilation, ventilator-associated pneumonia,ventilators.

mechanics the study of forces and motion of bodies and objects.

mechanism of accommodation the process by which the eye focuses onto an object. It does so by contracting the ciliary muscle which releases the tension on the zonular fibres (zonule of Zinn) allowing the elastic lens capsule to increase its curvature, especially that of the front surface. Along with these changes are an increase in the thickness of the lens, a decrease in its equatorial diameter and a reduction in pupil size. The ciliary muscle is controlled by the parasympathetic system which is triggered by an out of focus retinal image. ➲ accommodative reflex, accommodative response, ciliary muscle, convergence accommodation, proximal accommodation.

mechanism of labour the series of passive movements of the fetus as it descends through the birth canal propelled by the uterine contractions.

mechanoreceptor sensory receptors that are responsive to mechanical forces or distortion. They include touch and pressure receptors in the skin; proprioceptors in tendons, muscles and joints; stretch receptors in the lung, bladder and gastrointestinal tract; baroreceptors in blood vessels; and receptors in the ear that respond to sound waves and changes in position.

Meckel's diverticulum (J Meckel, German anatomist, 1781–1833) a blind, pouch-like sac sometimes arising from the free border of the lower ileum. Occurs in 2% of the population: usually symptomless. May cause gastrointestinal bleeding or intussusception.

Meckel's ganglion (J Meckel) ➲ sphenopalatine ganglion.

meconium *n* the discharge from the bowel of a neonate, the first stools. It is a greenish-black, viscid substance.

meconium aspiration inhalation by the fetus of meconium-stained amniotic fluid during labour/delivery. It can cause serious respiratory distress in the newborn.

meconium ileus impaction of meconium in bowel causing bowel obstruction. It is one presentation of cystic fibrosis.

meconium plug syndrome the meconium becomes very thick and causes the large intestine to be obstructed. The newborn infant will not pass meconium, will have a distended bowel and may vomit.

medi- a prefix that means 'middle', e.g. *mediolateral*.

media 1. *n* the middle coat of a vessel. **2.** *pl* nutritive jellies used for culturing micro-organisms in the laboratory. ➲ medium.

medial *adj* pertaining to or near the midline, or to the middle layer of a structure—**medially** *adv*.

medial canthus ➲ canthus.

medial collateral ligament (MCL) usually refers to the collateral ligaments of the knee joint, but there is also a medial collateral at the ankle and the elbow joint.

medial cutaneous nerve a nerve arising from the brachial plexus, which supplies the skin of the front, medial aspect and the back of the forearm. ➲ brachial plexus.

medial epicondylitis also known as golfer's elbow or javelin thrower's elbow. An inflammatory condition affecting the common origin of the flexor tendons of the forearm which results in pain and tenderness on the inside (ulnar side) of the elbow at the medial epicondyle of the humerus. Most commonly the result of overactivity of the wrist flexors, especially with increasing intensity or duration of activity or poor technique. Treatment includes rest, anti-inflammatory medication, physiotherapy and corticosteroid injection. Prevention of recurrence depends on identifying training or technique errors which can be corrected.

medial pterygoid muscle a deep two-headed muscle of mastication; present on each side of the face. It is square shaped and thick. Its origin is on the sphenoid bone, the posterior surface of the maxilla and the palatine bone. It inserts on to the internal aspect of the ramus of the mandible, low down between the angle of the mandible and the mandibular foramen. Its action is to close the jaw, protrude it and pull the mandible to the opposite side, thus aiding grinding action.

medial rectus muscle the extraocular muscle that moves the eyeball inwards; it is supplied by the oculomotor nerve (third cranial nerve). ➲ extraocular.

medial tibial stress syndrome pain down the inner side of the shin, attributed to periostitis of the tibia. Often called shin splints, although this term is also used for pain at other sites in the leg. The most likely cause is biomechanical, related to such as poor footwear, previous injury (with altered biomechanics) or conditions of the foot such as overpronation.

median *adj* **1.** the middle. **2.** a central tendency statistic; the midway or middle value in a set of scores when placed in increasing order. ➲ arithmetic mean, central tendency statistic, mean, mode.

median cubital vein a superficial vein of the arm. A large branch of the cephalic vein; it joins the basilic vein.

median line an imaginary line passing through the centre of the body from a point between the eyes to between the closed feet.

median nerve a nerve arising from the brachial plexus. It innervates some muscles of the forearm and some skin and muscles of the thumb and fingers. Commonly entrapped in the carpal tunnel of the wrist, resulting in carpal tunnel syndrome. ➲ brachial plexus, Colour Section Figure 11.

median palatine cyst a developmental cyst arising in the median fissure of the palate.

M
N

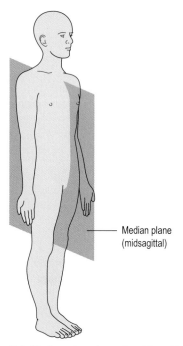

Median plane
(midsagittal)

M.2 **Median plane** (reproduced from Montague et al 2005 with permission).

M
N

median plane a vertical plane that divides the body into right and left halves (Figure M.2). Also called the midsagittal plane.

median rhomboid glossitis a condition of the tongue, in the region of a tiny pit (the foramen caecum, a remnant of the thyroglssal duct), which is reddened and lacks papillae. ⊃ glossitis.

median sternotomy a surgical incision that involves division of the sternum.

median vein a small superficial vein, which if present, carries venous blood from part of the hand and forearm to the basilic vein or the median cubital vein. ⊃ Colour Section Figure 10.

mediastinoscopy *n* a minor endoscopic surgical procedure for visual inspection of the mediastinum. May be combined with biopsy of the lymph nodes for histological examination, and diagnosis or staging in the case of cancer.

mediastinotomy *n* incision of the mediastinum.

mediastinum *n* the space between the lungs (the two pleural sacs) in the chest. Contains the heart, great vessels and the oesophagus—**mediastinal** *adj*.

mediating variable in statistics, a variable that transmits the indirect effects of an independent variable or variables on a dependent variable. For example, the relationship between social support and exercise adherence could be mediated by motivation: social support leads people to be more motivated which in turn leads them to adhere to an exercise programme. ⊃ moderating variable.

medical *adj* relating to medicine (the profession), or to conditions and treatment that are undertaken by physicians rather than surgeons.

medical audit systematic and critical review of medical care, including diagnosis and treatment, outcomes and quality of life. ⊃ quality assurance.

Medical Devices Agency (MDA) ⊃ Medicines and Healthcare Products Regulatory Agency (MHRA)

medical emergency team ⊃ critical care team.

medical ethics a set of moral values and principles of conduct for professionals working with patients. ⊃ code of ethics, ethics, ethics committees.

medicalization the predominance or orthodoxy of a set of ideas, known as the biomedical model, for conceptualizing health and illness and a whole range of social phenomena, such as disability, bereavement and homosexuality. Processes that were once considered an ordinary part of life, such as childbirth, can thus become 'medicalized' and under the control of medical professionals.

medical jurisprudence ⊃ forensic medicine.

Medical Research Council (MRC) dyspnoea scale a measurement of breathlessness useful in providing an indication of exercise limitations.

medicament *n* a medicine or remedy. ⊃ drug.

medicated *adj* impregnated with a medicine or drug.

medication *n* a therapeutic substance or drug, administered orally or by injection intra-arterially, subcutaneously, intramuscularly, intravenously, intraosseously, or into a body cavity (e.g. the bladder), or rectally, topically, transdermally, buccal or sublingual administration.

medicinal *adj* pertaining to a medicine.

medicine *n* **1.** science or art of healing, especially as distinguished from surgery and obstetrics. **2.** a therapeutic substance. ⊃ drug.

Medicines and Healthcare Products Regulatory Agency (MHRA) an agency in the UK formed from a merger between the Medicines Control Agency (MCA) and the Medical Devices Agency (MDA). Its main function is to promote and protect public health and the safety of patients by ensuring that all medicines, healthcare products and medical devices/equipment meet suitable standards of safety, quality, performance and efficacy, and are used in a safe manner. ⊃ European Medicines Agency, National Patient Safety Agency.

Medicines Commission ⊃ Commission on Human Medicines.

Medicines Control Agency (MCA) ⊃ Medicines and Healthcare Products Regulatory Agency (MHRA).

medicochirurgical *adj* pertaining to both medicine and surgery.

medicosocial *adj* pertaining to medicine and sociology.

mediolateral *adj* pertaining to the middle and one side.

meditation *n* an altered state achieved by rituals and exercises. It aims to produce relaxation (physical and mental). Various forms may be used as in relaxation as part of stress management strategies.

Mediterranean spotted fever ➲ boutonneuse fever.

medium *n* **1.** a substance used in bacteriology for the growth of micro-organisms. **2.** any substance by which something is transmitted. **3.** an environment—**media** *pl.* *separating medium* a substance used to coat surfaces to facilitate their clean separation.

medium chain acyl-CoA dehydrogenase deficiency (MCADD) a genetic metabolic disorder, which is inherited as an autosomal recessive trait. The enzyme deficiency leads to faulty nutrient metabolism. It is known to be one cause of sudden infant death syndrome (SIDS). Infants/children may have a history of altered consciousness especially if they miss a feed or meal. The previously asymptomatic disorder may become evident during an intercurrent illness such as an infection. The disorder can lead to seizures and liver failure. ➲ genetic screening, neonatal screening.

medium chain triglycerides (triacylglycerols) (MCT) triglyceride (triacylglycerol) molecules containing fatty acids with a carbon chain length of 6–10. Used in sports to provide a rapid source of fatty acid fuel. Their fatty acids are absorbed from the gut into the blood (rather than into lymphatics as are long-chain triglycerides) and thus rapidly reach the liver directly via the hepatic portal vein. Entering the general circulation, they rapidly raise the free fatty acids available to the tissues, where they readily enter cells to be used as a fuel. Being oxidized as easily as glucose, they might therefore have liver and muscle glycogen-sparing effects, delaying the onset of fatigue during endurance-type exercise. However, only a few of the numerous studies on MCT supplements have shown an increase in performance, and most reported some gastrointestinal problems. ➲ ergogenic aids.

medium frequency current (MFAC) an electrotherapy term. It is an alternative name for alternating current in the frequency range of 1 kHz to 10 kHz. Bursts of pulses with a frequency of between 1 kHz and 10 kHz. Individual pulses may be sinusoidal, rectangular or triangular. Russian current has a frequency of 2.5 kHz and interferential typically 4 kHz or between 2 kHz and 10 kHz. ➲ Russian current.

MEDLARS *abbr* medical literature analysis retrieval system. A computerized service provided by the United States National Library of Medicine. It contains references to medical journals and books published since 1966. It contains several databases including MEDLINE.

MEDLINE *n* a United States National Library of Medicine computerized database of medical science and associated literature.

medulla *n* **1.** the marrow in the centre of a long bone. **2.** the internal part of organs, e.g. kidneys, adrenals and lymph nodes, etc.

medulla oblongata the lowest part of the brainstem where it passes through the foramen magnum to become the spinal cord. It contains the nerve centres controlling various vital functions, e.g. cardiac centres. ➲ Colour Section Figure 1.

medullary *adj* pertaining to the medulla.

medullary carcinoma a malignant tumour with a soft consistency. May occur in the calcitonin-producing cells of the thyroid gland as part of some types of multiple endocrine neoplasia (MEN). ➲ Sipple's syndrome.

medullary cavity the hollow centre of a long bone, containing yellow fatty bone marrow or medulla.

medullated *adj* containing or surrounded by a medulla or marrow, particularly referring to myelinated nerve fibres.

medulloblastoma *n* malignant, rapidly growing tumour occurring in children; usually in the midline of the cerebellum. It generally occurs between 5 and 9 years of age and is more common in boys.

medulloepithelioma also called neuroepithelioma. A malignant tumour of neuroepithelial tissue, affecting the brain or the retina.

mega, megalo, mego- a prefix that means 'large', e.g. *megakaryocyte*.

megacephalic *adj* (*syn* macrocephalic, megalocephalic) large headed.

megacolon *n* dilatation of the colon. *acquired megacolon* associated with chronic constipation of any cause, or may occur in acute severe colitis of any cause (toxic megacolon). *congenital megacolon (Hirschsprung's disease)* due to absence of ganglionic cells in a distal segment of the colon with loss of relaxation resulting in dilatation of the normal proximal colon.

megakaryoblast *n* a large nucleated cell of the bone marrow. An early precursor cell in the development of megakaryocytes, which are involved in the production of platelets (thrombocytes).

megakaryocyte *n* large multinucleated cell of the bone marrow that gives rise to platelets (thrombocytes). The nonnucleated platelets form from fragments of the megakaryocytes during a process termed thrombopoiesis.

megaloblast *n* a large, nucleated, primitive red blood cell formed where there is a deficiency of vitamin B_{12}, folic acid or the intrinsic factor—**megaloblastic** *adj*.

megaloblastic anaemia an anaemia caused by a deficiency of vitamin B_{12} or folic acid. It results in the formation of large red blood cells called megaloblasts. ➲ anaemia.

megalocephalic *adj* ➲ megacephalic.

megalocornea ➲ keratoglobus.

megalomania *n* delusion of grandeur, characteristic of general paralysis of the insane.

megalophthalmos a condition in which the eye is abnormally large. It is an inherited condition and occurs mainly in males. ➲ keratoglobus.

megalopsia ➲ macropsia.

-megaly a suffix that means 'enlargement', e.g. *hepatomegaly*.

megaureter *n* dilation of one or both ureters caused by an obstruction to the flow of urine. It may be associated with vesicoureteric reflux of urine, or defective peristaltic action of the muscle layer of the ureter.

megavoltage radiotherapy units radiotherapy units operating in the range of 4–25 megavolts, for example linear accelerators, used for external beam radiotherapy treatments.

meglitinides a group of oral hypoglycaemic drugs, e.g. repaglinide, used for people with type 2 diabetes. ⊃ Appendix 5.

megophthalmia a large eyeball.

meibomian cyst ⊃ chalazion.

meibomian glands (H Meibom, German anatomist and physician, 1638–1700) (*syn* palpebral follicles, tarsal glands) sebaceous glands located in the tarsal plates of the eyelids whose ducts empty into the eyelid margin. They are arranged parallel with each other, perpendicular to the lid margin, about 25 for the upper lid and 20 for the lower. They secrete sebum. This sebaceous material provides the outermost oily (or lipid) layer of the precorneal tear film. It prevents the lacrimal fluid from overflowing onto the outer surface of the eyelid. It also makes for an airtight closure of the lids and prevents the tears from macerating the skin. The meibomian glands can be seen showing through the conjunctiva of light-skinned people as yellow streaks. ⊃ lacrimal gland, precorneal film, tarsus, tears.

meibomian gland dysfunction (MGD) (H Meibom) may be induced by blepharitis, chalazion, contact lens wear (particularly soft lenses) and ageing. The most common sign is a cloudy or absent secretion upon expression with symptoms of a mild dry eye. Hot compresses and lid massage will cure more than half of the patients; oral tetracycline will help in many of the others. ⊃ blepharitis, chalazion, hordeolum, lacrimal gland, meibomianitis, precorneal film, tarsus, tears, Tearscope plus.

meibomianitis (*syn* meibomitis) inflammation of the meibomian glands. It is believed not to be a primary bacterial disease. It is characterized by the presence of a white, frothy secretion or 'foam' on the eyelid margin. Meibomianitis is often associated with blepharitis and conjunctivitis. Symptoms include mild itching of the lids and occasionally blurred vision due to the oily secretion spreading over the cornea. This condition may also result from hard contact lens wear. Management of this disease consists of tarsal massage and removal of the secretion with a moist cotton-tipped applicator. ⊃ blepharitis, hordeolum, meibomian glands.

meibomitis ⊃ meibomianitis.

Meigs' syndrome (J Meigs, American gynaecologist and obstetrician, 1892–1963) a benign, solid ovarian fibroma associated with ascites and hydrothorax.

meiosis *n* also called a reduction division. The process which, through two successive cell divisions, results in the production of mature gametes—oocytes or spermatozoa. There is pairing of the partner chromosomes, which separate from each other at the meiotic divisions, so that the diploid (2n) chromosome number (i.e. 23 pairs) is reduced by half to 23 chromosomes, only one chromosome of each original pair: this set being the haploid (n) complement (Figure M.3). ⊃ gamete, mitosis.

Meissner's corpuscles (G Meissner, German anatomist, 1829–1905) light-pressure sensory receptors in the skin. Found in small elevations of the dermis that project up into the epidermis of glabrous skin, exclusively. These receptors

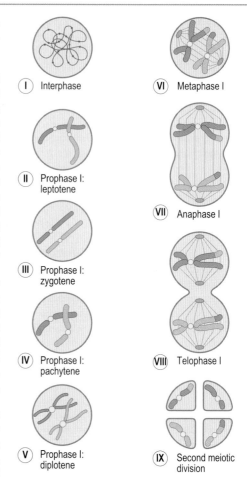

I	Interphase	VI	Metaphase I
II	Prophase I: leptotene		
III	Prophase I: zygotene	VII	Anaphase I
IV	Prophase I: pachytene	VIII	Telophase I
V	Prophase I: diplotene	IX	Second meiotic division

M.3 Meiosis (reproduced from Hinchliff et al 1996 with permission).

respond to low-frequency vibration. They lie close to the surface of the skin and have small receptive fields, but adapt rapidly to stimuli.

Meissner's plexus (G Meissner) ⊃ submucosal plexus.

melaena *n* black, tar-like stools. Contains digested blood and has a distinctive odour. Evidence of upper gastrointestinal bleeding, such as from a peptic ulcer, gastric cancer, oesophageal varices, small bowel disease, or as a drug side-effect.

melancholia *n* depression—from the Latin for black bile—**melancholic** *adj*.

melanin *n* a brown/black pigment found in hair, skin, the retinal pigment layer and the choroid of the eye.

melano melan, mel- a prefix that means 'pigment, black, dark', e.g. melanosis.

melanocytes *npl* pigment-bearing cells found in the skin, the iris, the choroid, the retina, the sclera cells that produce melanin.

melanocyte-stimulating hormones (MSH) peptide hormones produced by many species in which it is important in changing skin colour. It is produced from a large precursor molecule in the pituitary gland, and is also present in the brain where it may act as a signalling molecule.

melanoma *n* a malignant tumour arising from the pigment-producing cells (melanocytes) of the skin, or of the eye (*choroidal melanoma*). *malignant melanoma* malignant cutaneous mole or freckle (usually), it is the most dangerous of all skin cancers. Related to overexposure to ultraviolet radiation (sunburn); most common in fair skinned, blond/red haired people. It is characterized by change in colour, shape, size of mole or with bleeding or itching in a mole. ⊃ Colour Section Figure 89. The prognosis depends on Breslow's depth (thickness); staging involves lymph node status, with sentinel node biopsy (SNB) now becoming an integral part along with computed tomography (CT) scan. Surgery is the only curative treatment with chemotherapy and radiotherapy of limited effectiveness—**melanomatous** *adj.* ⊃ Breslow's depth, choroidal melanoma, Clark's level.

melanoplakia pigmented patches on the oral mucosa.

melanosis *n* dark pigmentation of surfaces as in Addison's disease, etc.

melanosis coli brown pigmentation of the colonic mucosa associated with long term misuse of stimulant laxative drugs—**melanotic** *adj.*

MELAS syndrome *abbr* **m**itochondrial **e**ncephalopathy **l**actic **a**cidosis and **s**troke-like episodes.

melasma *n* (*syn* chloasma) hypermelanosis of the face, usually in women. Known as *melasma gravidarum* when it occurs during pregnancy.

melatonin *n* a hormone produced by the pineal body (gland) in response to the amount of light entering the eye. Influences sexual development and is involved in reproductive function. Also influences mood and various circadian rhythms, such as body temperature and sleep.

Meleney's gangrene (F Meleney, American surgeon, 1889–1963) gangrene affecting the skin and subcutaneous tissues postoperatively. A synergistic bacterial gangrene that involves a non-haemolytic streptococcus and *Staphylococcus aureus*.

melioidosis *n* caused by the bacterium *Burkholderia pseudomallei* a saprophyte found in soil and water (paddy fields). It occurs in tropical areas and is endemic in Southeast Asia and northern Australia. In addition there are cases in Africa, India and the Middle East. It affects humans and many other animals including cattle, pigs, sheep, goats, dogs, cats and horses. The disease is transmitted by direct contact with contaminated water and soil. The bacterium enters the body by inhalation, ingestion or through breaks in the skin (inoculation). Patients with diabetes or severe burns are susceptible. Melioidosis may be acute when it causes pneumonia and septicaemia. Or chronic when it is characterized by abscess formation in many organs with the development of fistulas. There is high fever, prostration and sometimes diarrhoea, with signs of pneumonia and enlargement of the liver and spleen. The chest X-ray resembles that of acute caseous tuberculosis. In more chronic forms multiple abscesses recur in subcutaneous tissue and bone. Culture of blood, sputum or pus may yield *B. pseudomallei*. Except in fulminating infections, antibodies may be detected by indirect haemagglutination, direct agglutination and complement-fixation tests. In the acute illness prompt treatment, without waiting for confirmation by culture, may be life-saving. Ceftazidime 100 mg/kg, imipenem 50 mg/kg or meropenem (0.5–1 g 8-hourly) is given for about 2–3 weeks. This is followed by maintenance therapy of doxycycline 200 mg daily, plus co-trimoxazole (sulfamethoxazole 1600 mg plus trimethoprim 320 mg 12-hourly) for a minimum of 12 weeks, and chloramphenicol (500 mg 6-hourly) for the first 4 weeks. In patients with severe melioidosis in septic shock/systemic inflammatory response syndrome (SIRS), granulocyte-colony stimulating factor (G–CSF) significantly reduces mortality. Abscesses should be drained surgically. In chronic cases profound wasting is a major clinical problem. In the absence of intensive care, the disease carries a significant mortality.

melitensis *n* ⊃ brucellosis.

Melkersson–Rosenthal syndrome (E Melkersson, Swedish physician, 1898–1932; C Rosenthal, German neurologist, 1892–1937) a syndrome usually commencing during childhood or adolescence. There is chronic facial swelling, facial nerve palsy and furrowing/fissuring of the tongue. ⊃ orofacial granulomatosis.

membrane *n* a thin lining or covering substance—**membranous** *adj.* ⊃ basement membrane, hyaloid membrane, mucous membrane, plasma (cell) membrane, serous membrane, synovial membrane, tympanic membrane.

membrane attack complex a ring of complement fragments that has the ability to insert itself onto an invading cell and cause its destruction.

membrane potential electrical potential difference maintained across a cell membrane, with the inside negative to the outside: –10 mV to –30 mV in non-excitable cells, and –70 to –90 mV (the *resting potential*) in quiescent excitable cells (nerve and muscle). Due to unequal distributions mainly of potassium and sodium ions (the cell membrane being partially, but not equally, permeable to both) which in turn determines the relative movements of these ions down their respective diffusion gradients (potassium outwards and sodium inwards). The gradients are themselves maintained by the sodium–potassium (Na–K) pump which uses metabolic energy to transport the ions back 'uphill'. ⊃ action potential, depolarization, sodium-potassium (Na-K) pump.

membranes strip a procedure performed during vaginal examination, where a finger is inserted through the external cervical os and gently frees the membranes from the wall of the lower segment of the uterus. This may stimulate the release of oxytocin and commencement of labour.

membranous labyrinth ⊃ labyrinth.

memory *n* the ability to retain and recall prior learning (information and events). It is a very complex process and includes different types of memory. ⊃ episodic memory, long term memory, procedural memory, semantic memory, short term memory.

M
N

memory lapses many adults have episodes of memory loss and some time later retrieve the appropriate information. The lapses often occur when individuals are under stress and typically increase with age. ⊃ Alzheimer's disease, dementia.

MEN *acron* **M**ultiple **E**ndocrine **N**eoplasia.

menaquinones *npl* a form of vitamin K produced by bacteria in the gastrointestinal tract.

menarche *n* the first menstruation or menstrual bleed. In the vast majority of girls this usually occurs between 11 and 13 years of age but the timing depends on environment, genetics and achieving a particular body mass and percentage of body fat. The commencement of menstrual cycles is not usually accompanied by ovulation for several months.

Mendel's law (G Mendel, Austrian geneticist, 1822–1884) the fundamental theory of heredity and its laws, evolved by Mendel's work with peas. The laws determine the inheritance of different characters, and particularly the interaction of dominant and recessive traits in cross-breeding, the maintenance of the purity of such characters during hereditary transmission and the independent segregation of genetically different characteristics, such as the size of pea plants.

Mendelson syndrome (C Mendelson, American obstetrician, b.1913) the aspiration (inhalation) of regurgitated acid stomach contents, which can cause immediate death from anoxia, or it may produce extensive lung damage or pulmonary oedema with severe bronchospasm. It may happen during the administration of a general anaesthesic to women in labour, or in situations where an unconscious person vomits (e.g. inebriation caused by an excessive intake of alcohol).

Ménétrier's disease (P Ménétrier, French physician, 1859–1935) also called giant hypertrophic gastritis or hypertrophic gastropathy. A rare condition characterized by the growth of tissue within the stomach, inflammation, possible ulceration and loss of albumen. There is pain, nausea, vomiting, haematemesis, anorexia and diarrhoea. It is associated with an increased risk of stomach cancer.

Ménière's disease (P Ménière, French physician, 1799–1862) distension of membranous labyrinth of inner ear from excess fluid. Pressure causes failure of function of the cranial nerve responsible for balance and hearing (vestibulocochlear); thus there is fluctuating deafness, tinnitus and repeated attacks of vertigo.

meninges *npl* three membranes that surround the brain and spinal cord. From outside in they are the dura mater, a double layer of fibrous tissue (outer); the fibrous arachnoid membrane (middle) is separated from the dura mater by a subdural space and from the pia mater by the subarachnoid space, which contains cerebrospinal fluid; and the fragile pia mater (inner) containing many small blood vessels. The pia mater adheres to the brain and spinal cord, and follows every convolution (gyrus) and fissure (sulcus) of the brain (Figure M.4). ⊃ meningitis—**meninx** *sing*, **meningeal** *adj*. ⊃ falx cerebri, falx cerebelli, tentorium cerebelli.

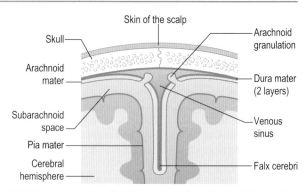

M.4 Meninges—simplified (reproduced from Brooker & Nicol 2003 with permission).

meningioma *n* a slowly growing fibrous tumour arising in the meninges—**meningiomata** *pl*, **meningiomatous** *adj*.

meningism *n* (*syn.* meningismus) a condition describing irritation and inflammation of the meninges due normally to infection or haemorrhage and consisting of neck stiffness and photophobia.

meningitis *n* inflammation of the meninges covering the brain and spinal cord usually due to infection by microorganisms. It may be viral, bacterial, fungal or caused by protozoa and parasites. Viral meningitis is the commonest cause, e.g. coxsackievirus, echovirus and mumps virus. It is usually a mild illness. Bacterial meningitis is a much more severe illness with considerable morbidity and a high mortality rate. It may be caused by *Haemophilus influenzae*, *Streptococcus pneumoniae*, *Neisseria meningitidis* (meningococcal meningitis), Group B streptococci, Gram negative bacilli and less commonly *Listeria monocytogenes*, *Cryptococcus neoformans*, *Staphylococcus aureus* and *Mycobacterium tuberculosis* (where the onset is insidious). Acute infections are characterized by a vague 'flu-like' illness, headache, cold extremities, fever, neck stiffness, photophobia, vomiting, confusion, altered consciousness, seizures, a positive Kernig's sign and changes in the CSF on lumbar puncture. In infants and small children other less specific signs may also be present. These include: irritability, abnormal high-pitched cry, poor feeding, bulging fontanelle, reduced muscle tone, mottling of the skin, reduced responses to normal stimuli. Patients with meningococcal septicaemia will also have a dark purple/red petechial rash that does not disappear when pressure is applied. Management involves the immediate administration of the appropriate antimicrobial drugs, supportive treatment, such as mechanical ventilation, and skilled nursing care and observation. ⊃ group C meningococcal disease, Colour Section Figure 90.

mening/o, mening/i- a prefix that means 'the covering membranes of the brain and spinal cord—the meninges', e.g. *meningitis*.

meningocele *n* a protrusion of the meninges through a bony defect of the skull or vertebral column. It forms a cyst filled with cerebrospinal fluid but with no neural tissue. ⊃ neural tube defect, spina bifida.

meningococcus *n* the bacterium *Neisseria meningitidis*. A Gram-negative diplococcus that causes life-threatening meningococcal meningitis and septicaemia. There are three strains - A, B and C. Group A meningococcus is a particular problem in Africa where it causes epidemics of meningitis; work to produce an effective vaccine is ongoing. An effective vaccine against the group C meningococcus has been available in the UK since 1999 and is offered as part of the routine immunization schedule. The development of a vaccine against the B strain meningococcus is in progress and (at the time of writing) it is expected that a vaccine will be available within the next few years—**meningococcal** *adj.*

meningoencephalitis *n* inflammation of the brain and the meninges—**meningoencephalitic** *adj.*

meningoencephalocele also known as encephalomeningocele. A sac containing cerebrospinal fluid, brain tissue and meninges that protrudes through a congenital defect in the skull. ⊃ neural tube defect.

meningomyelocele *n* (*syn* myelomeningocele) protrusion of a portion of the spinal cord, its enclosing meningeal membranes and cerebrospinal fluid through a bony defect in the vertebral column. It differs from a meningocele in being covered with a thin, transparent membrane which may be granular and moist. ⊃ neural tube defect.

meniscal injury meniscal injury is most common in contact sports as a result of trauma, especially with twisting or rotational stress at the joint—especially medial damage due to the attachment of the medial collateral ligament resulting in combined injury. Most tears occur in the outer border of the meniscus, which has a better blood supply and is thus more easily repaired, but cartilage repair is not favoured by professional sportsmen due to the time (and finance) lost from sport in the extended rehabilitation period. Many opt for removal of the torn fragment—partial meniscectomy—with its quicker return to action. Surgical treatment aims to minimize the amount of meniscus removed to limit the extent of later osteoarthritis. Sometimes a tear can heal spontaneously. It may result in the development of a cyst or a fragment may break off, forming a loose body inside the joint; either of these is likely to require surgical removal.

meniscectomy *n* generally refers to the removal of a meniscus (semilunar cartilage) of the knee joint, following injury and displacement. The medial cartilage is torn most commonly and occurs in excessive twisting movements of the knee. Usually a minimally invasive endoscopic removal of damaged fragments is undertaken when there is pain and in locking or instability of the knee. ⊃ arthroscopy. The term is also applied to the removal of an intra-articular disc, such as that from the temporomandibular joint.

meniscus *n* **1.** a cresent-shaped fibrocartilaginous structure that cushions the articulation of two bones (*syn* semilunar cartilages). For example the flattened crescent-shaped pieces of cartilage inside the knee joint (one medial, one lateral), wedged between the articular surfaces (condyles) of the femur and the tibia and thickest around their convexity

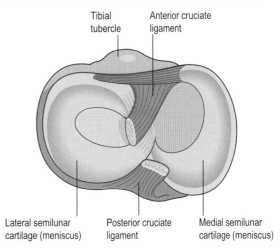

M.5 **Menisci**—upper end of the left tibia showing menisci and the cruciate ligaments (cut) (reproduced from Jennett 2008 with permission).

towards the outside of the joint (Figure M.5). They increase the joint congruency (fitting together) of joint surfaces, act as shock absorbers, assist in joint lubrication and provide joint stabilization. Often damaged, particularly in the knee, when there is a rotational force. **2.** the curved upper surface of a column of liquid and occurring because of the influence of capillarity. **3.** a concavoconvex lens, i.e. one having both concave and convex surfaces—**menisci** *pl.*

meniscus lens (*syn* bent lens, curved lens) a lens having a spherical convex surface and a spherical concave surface. Meniscus lenses often have a base of 6 D for the surface of lesser curvature. ⊃ periscopic lens, toric lens.

Menkes' disease (J Menkes, American neurologist, b.1928) an inherited disease of copper metabolism. The defective gene is transmitted on the X chromosome and mainly affects boys. The disease presents during infancy. Development may be normal or near normal for the first 3 months, after which there is marked developmental delay and loss of existing developmental skills. Affected infants fail to thrive, have seizures, low body temperature and hair that is kinky, colourless and very fragile. There is serious neurodegeneration. Although, treatment with subcutaneous or intravenous copper supplements may help, most children die before the age of 10 years.

menopause *n* the ending of menstruation. It is a single event occurring during the climacteric but is commonly used, erroneously, to describe all the changes occurring during the female climacteric. It normally occurs between the ages of 45 and 55 years. *artificial menopause* an earlier menopause caused by surgery or radiotherapy—**menopausal** *adj.* ⊃ climacteric

menorrhagia *n* an excessive regular menstrual flow. The gynaecological causes include fibroids, endometrial polyps, endometrial hyperplasia, pelvic inflammatory disease, endometriosis, cancers of the endometrium and cervix, and

M
N

intrauterine contraceptive devices. Menorrhagia may also be caused by thyroid dysfunction, coagulations disorders such as von Willebrand's disease, or with anticoagulant drugs.

menses *n* bloody fluid and tissue debris discharged from the uterus during menstruation; menstrual flow.

menstrual *adj* relating to the menses.

menstrual or uterine cycle the cyclical changes that occur as the endometrium responds to ovarian hormones. There are three phases: proliferative, secretory and menstrual in which bleeding occurs for around 5 days. The cycle is repeated approximately every 28 days (21–35), except during pregnancy, from the menarche to the menopause. ➲ Colour Section Figure 32.

menstrual cycle and sport the menstrual cycle appears to have little or no negative impact on women's athletic performance, despite the physiological changes that occur. Studies of $\dot{V}O_{2max}$ during different phases of the cycle have shown no disadvantageous effect on performance despite subjective feelings of bloating and fatigue, seen with premenstrual (cyclical) syndrome and the known effects of oestrogen and progesterone on oxygen utilization. Indeed, studies have shown that world records have been set during all phases of the menstrual cycle. ➲ amenorrhoea, female athletic triad.

menstruation *n* the flow of bloody fluid and tissue debris from the uterus once a month, or so, in the female. It usually starts at the age of 11–13 years in developed countries, and ceases around 50 years of age. ➲ menarche, menopause.

mental *adj* **1.** pertaining to the mind. **2.** pertaining to the chin

mental aberration a pathological deviation from normal thinking.

mental age the age of a person with regard to his intellectual development, which can be determined by intelligence tests.

mental defence mechanism (MDM) unconscious defence mechanism by which individuals attempt to cope with stressful, difficult or threatening emotions. ➲ defence mechanisms.

mental disorder mental illness, arrested or incomplete development of the mind, psychopathic disorder and any other disorder or disability of the mind. As defined by the relevant legislation. ➲ mental health legislation.

mental foramen an opening on the buccal aspect of the body of the mandible usually in the region below and between the premolar teeth. Afferent nerves from the lower lips and labial incisal gingivae pass through it, together with blood vessels, to join the incisive branch of the inferior dental nerve within the bone.

mental health a sense of well-being in the emotional, personal, spiritual and social domains of people's lives.

Mental Health Act 2007 recently introduced legislation (in England and Wales) that amends the Mental Health Act 1983. The changes introduce measures that include: (a) supervised community treatment (SCT)—in which suitable patients can be cared for in a community setting

following compulsory admission for treatment under the Act. Patients may be returned to hospital for treatment; (b) the introduction of a new role of approved mental health professional (AMHP)—which expands the professional groups able to deal with patients detained under the Mental Health Act 1983; (c) prescribes the classes of nurses (in England) able under the relevant section in the Mental Health Act 1983 to detain, for a maximum of 6 hours, a patient having in-patient hospital treatment for a mental disorder; (d) the introduction of a new role of approved clinician (AC)—thereby increasing the range of professional groups responsible for patients detained under the Mental Health Act. (Department of Health (DH) 2008 Mental Health Act 2007. online www.dh.gov.uk/)

Mental Health Act Commission in England and Wales the body which previously had the responsibility to review how the Mental Health (MH) Act 1983 was being applied in practice, and in particular to safeguard the interests of all patients detained under the MH Act 1983 and those patients who are liable to be detained. As part of the provisions of the The Health and Social Care Act 2008 (which received Royal assent in July 2008) the Mental Health Act Commission merged with the Healthcare Commission and the Commission for Social Care Inspection to create a single regulator for health and adult social services—the Care Quality Commission. ➲ Care Quality Commission.

Mental Health Review Tribunal in England and Wales a body with responsibility for hearing applications from or about people detained under the provisions of the Mental Health Act 1983 (amended by the Mental Health Act 2007). In Scotland the *Mental Health Tribunal* was created as part of the The Mental Health (Care and Treatment) (Scotland) Act 2003 in order to decide issues concerning the compulsory care and treatment of patients suffering from a mental disorder.

mental health legislation law pertaining to mental disorder. For example, in England & Wales the main body of mental health legislation for many years was the Mental Health Act 1983, which made provision for the compulsory detention and treatment in hospital of those with a mental disorder. The Mental Health (Patients in the Community) Act 1995 amended the 1983 Act by providing for the 'supervised discharge' of those detained patients requiring a 'high degree' of supervision on discharge from hospital. However, many people with mental health problems are in hospital as voluntary (informal) patients. The Mental Health Act 2007 (England and Wales), that introduced changes to the 1983 Act, became law in November 2008. The Mental Health (Care and Treatment) (Scotland) Act 2003 is the legal authority for mental health services in Scotland. This Act is rights-based and underpinned by a set of guiding principles. ➲ Mental Health Act 2007.

mental hygiene deals with the establishment of healthy mental attitudes and emotional reactions.

mental illness definitions predominantly characterized as a mental pathology with disturbances of mental functioning, such as delusions, hallucinations, excessive elation or low mood. The medical connotations of this term have been considered by some to be misleading or to serve the purposes of powerful groups within society. Social scientists have developed understandings of the causes of mental illnesses and of mental illness itself as social phenomena that set boundaries of what is deemed acceptable mental functioning in different cultures and societies and which regulates human conduct. People have, for example, been deemed mentally ill because of their political beliefs or because their behaviour violates a cultural norm.

mental nerve an afferent nerve arising from the skin of the lower lip and chin, and mucous membrane and gingivae between the second premolar tooth and the midline of the dental arch. It passes through the mental foramen as the incisal nerve to join the mandibular nerve.

mental practice ➲ mental rehearsal.

mental preparation the act of mentally preparing oneself for a performance.

mental rehearsal the use of imagery to practise an act mentally. An activity gaining in popularity as part of the rehabilitation process (and is also well used in the sporting arena). It is thought that if someone thinks about performing a task and mentally repeats the process in their head, it is sufficient to cause modulation of neural activity in the brain. In sport psychology, mental rehearsal is considered to be one of the fundamental mental skills for sports performers and is used for learning new skills, practising existing skills, preparing for performance and enhancing motivation. Also known as mental practice.

mental skills the set of trainable mental abilities and methods that are held to underpin successful learning and performance. The basic mental skills include concentration, goal-setting, imagery and mental rehearsal, relaxation and self-talk. Also known as cognitive skills and psychological skills.

mentoanterior *adj* forward position of the fetal chin in the maternal pelvis in a face presentation.

menton 1. the lowest point of the soft tissue of the chin. **2.** the lowest point of the bony outline of the chin.

mentoposterior *adj* backward position of the fetal chin in the maternal pelvis in a face presentation.

mentorship a system that provides support to students during their training. A mentor—a qualified and experienced practitioner—works with the student on clinical placements, ensuring he or she receives the appropriate experience. ➲ preceptorship.

mentum the chin.

menu a set of choices presented in a computer program.

MEP *abbr* **1.** maximum expiratory pressure. **2.** motor evoked potential.

meralgia paraesthetica pain, tingling and numbness felt over the lateral surface of the thigh. It is caused by the entrapment of the lateral cutaneous nerve of the thigh as it passes through the inguinal ligament.

mercurialism *n* chronic poisoning with mercury. It may occur in individuals who are exposed to mercury at work, or it may be ingested in food, such as fish in some areas of the world, which may contain high levels. There are oral manifestations such as a metallic taste, increased salivation, gingivitis and ulceration showing greyish-blue lines at the gingival margins, stomatitis, painful tongue and loosening of the teeth. Other serious effects of poisoning include gastrointestinal effects, renal failure, paraesthesia, ataxia, and visual and hearing problems.

mercury (Hg) *n* quicksilver. A highly toxic metallic element that is liquid at room temperature. Previously used in thermometers and sphygmomanometers. Toxicity means that local safety protocols should be followed in situations involving accidental spillage and contamination. Forms two series of salts: univalent mercurous salts and bivalent mercuric. ➲ mercury poisoning (acute), mercurialism.

mercury poisoning (acute) mercury, which is highly toxic, can enter the body by ingestion, inhalation and through the skin. Depending on the route and the type of mercury involved there may be dyspnoea (breathlessness), cough and haemoptysis (coughing up blood) caused by lung inflammation; gastrointestinal effects that include vomiting and abdominal pain; and renal failure and central nervous system effects. ➲ mercurialism.

meridians *npl* in complementary therapy the conceptual channels in which Qi energy flows. ➲ acupuncture, shiatsu.

Merkel cell (F Merkel, German anatomist, 1845–1919) tactile cells with granules containing neurosecretory substances. They are located in the basal/germinal layer (stratum basale) of the epidermis and are especially associated with areas where tactile sensation is enhanced. They are in contact with a sensory nerve fibre. ➲ tactile meniscus.

Merkel cell carcinoma a rare malignant tumour arising from the Merkel cells sited in the basal/germinal layer (stratum basale) of the epidermis. The tumour commonly affects the skin of the head and neck, mostly affecting older adults.

merocrine (eccrine) gland a type of exocrine gland in which the secretion is released by exocytosis into the lumen of the gland from vesicles. The gland remains intact. ➲ apocrine gland, holocrine gland.

MERRF *abbr* myoclonic epilepsy with ragged red fibres.

MESA *acron* microsurgical epididymal sperm aspiration.

mesarteritis *n* inflammation of the middle coat of an artery.

mesencephalon *n* midbrain. One of the three primary vesicles formed during embryonic delevelopment of the brain. It becomes the midbrain.

mesenchymal pertaining to mesenchyme.

mesenchyme embryonic connective tissue derived from mesoderm (one of the primary germ layers). It comprises cells embedded in a gelatinous matrix and eventually forms connective tissue including the blood and blood producing tissues. ➲ connective tissue.

mesenchymoma a new growth composed of two or more cellular elements which are not usually associated with each other and fibrous tissue.

M
N

mesentery *n* a double fan-shaped fold of peritoneum that attaches the jejunum and ileum to the posterior abdominal wall. Contains nerves, lymphatics and blood vessels—**mesenteric** *adj*.

MESH, MeSH *acron* Medical Subject Headings. ⊃ indexing term.

mesial *adj* medial. Relating to or located in the median (midsagittal) plane or line; situated in the middle. Also refers to the surfaces of the teeth in the dental arch that face towards the midline.

mesial drift the gradual movement of all teeth mesially, which occurs naturally with age. Also the movement of a tooth or teeth distal to the socket of an extracted tooth which may drift mesially in the absence of a bridge or orthodontic space maintainer.

mesial surface in anatomy, any surface of an organ situated towards the midline (or the midsagittal line). ⊃ surface.

meso- a prefix that means 'middle', e.g. *mesoderm*.

mesiodens *n* an unerupted or erupted supernumerary tooth between the central incisors of the upper jaw.

mesocolon folds of peritoneum that attach the transverse colon (transverse mesocolon) to the abdominal wall, and the sigmoid colon (sigmoid mesocolon) to the pelvic wall. Contains nerves, lymphatics and blood vessels.

mesoderm *n* middle layer of the three primary germ layers of the early embryo, between the ectoderm and endoderm. It gives rise to the cardiovascular system, lymphatic system, bone, muscles, blood, the dermis, pericardium, pleura, peritoneum, urogenital tract, gonads and the adrenal cortex. ⊃ ectoderm, endoderm, mesenchyme.

mesodermal dysgenesis of the cornea and iris ⊃ Rieger's syndrome.

mesometrium a double fold of peritoneum either side of the uterus that hangs down from the uterine (fallopian) tubes. Usually known as the broad ligaments.

mesomorph a body type (physique) characterized by a well-covered person who has a well-developed musculature—**mesomorphic** *adj*. ⊃ ectomorph, endomorph.

mesonephros the wolffian body. An excretory organ that forms in early embryonic development. It is short-lived but the duct becomes part of the structures that later develop into the male reproductive structures. ⊃ metanephros, pronephros.

mesonephric duct also known as the wolffian duct. The primitive embryonic duct that under the influence of testosterone becomes the internal genitalia (epididymis, deferent duct [vas deferens], seminal vesicles and ejaculatory ducts) in a genetically male embryo. ⊃ paramesonephric duct.

mesophile *n* a bacterium that thrives within the range 25–40°C. Most human pathogens thrive best at body temperature (37°C)—**mesophilic** *adj*.

mesopic vision (*syn* twilight vision) vision at intermediate levels between photopic and scotopic vision, and corresponding to luminances ranging from about 10^{-3} to 10 cd/m^2. ⊃ photopic vision, scotopic vision.

mesosalpinx the upper part of the broad ligament that encloses the uterine (fallopian) tubes.

mesothelioma *n* neoplasm of the pleura (commonly), pericardium or peritoneum; usually associated with asbestos exposure at least 20 years previously. Industrially related, therefore compensation usually appropriate as few are operable and the median survival post diagnosis is around 8 months. Therapy is almost universally palliative, as mesothelioma is generally chemo- and radioresistant.

mesothelium *n* a layer of flat cells that line the body cavity in the embryo. They are derived from the mesoderm layer. They continue as the layer of simple squamous epithelium that covers the serous membranes (pericardium, peritoneum, pleura) in adults.

mesovarium *n* a double fold of peritoneum that attaches the ovary to the broad ligament.

messenger RNA (mRNA) ⊃ ribonucleic acid.

meta- a prefix that means 'change, between, beyond', e.g. *metabolize*.

meta-analysis *n* a statistical summary of several research studies using complex quantitative analysis of the primary data. It involves the combining of the results from a number of studies that address the same question and report on the same outcomes to produce a summary result. The aim is to derive more precise and clear information from a large data pool. A meta-analysis is thought more likely to reliably confirm or refute a hypothesis than the individual trials.

metabolic *adj* pertaining to metabolism—**metabolically** *adv*. ⊃ basal metabolic rate (BMR).

metabolic accumulation the concentration of a substance in the body through the metabolic process, for example, iodine in the thyroid gland.

metabolic acidosis a disturbance of acid–base balance due to the generation of excess acid (including lactic acid), such as with uncontrolled diabetes mellitus (ketoacidosis), starvation, tissue hypoxia such as in severe shock (lactic acidosis), heart failure, etc., or a failure to excrete hydrogen ions [H$^+$] in renal failure. Metabolic acidosis can also occur during high-intensity exercise, due mainly to an increased rate of anaerobic glycolysis and therefore of lactic acid production. The other mechanism is through the depletion of alkali (bicarbonate), e.g. due to diarrhoea or loss from a small bowel fistula, or in renal tubular acidosis when bicarbonate ions are lost in the urine. ⊃ acid–base balance.

metabolic and related thresholds intensities of exercise (expressed as power output or as percentages of aerobic capacity, $\dot{V}O_{2max}$) at which specific metabolic and related changes are considered to take place. A plethora of thresholds has been proposed historically. These included many giving the same label to different criteria, or different labels to the same criterion; a number also embodied assumptions about bodily processes, at best unproven and sometimes now known to be false. Table M.1 lists six which appear unambiguous, the first five exactly as first described and the sixth slightly modified; however the two that are not related to observable phenomena (anaerobic and aerobic thresholds) are not recommended for further use. The [Lac]$_b$ (blood lactate concentration) values cited are representative

Table M.1 Metabolic and related thresholds

Term	Definition	[Lac]$_b$ mmol/L
Lactate threshold (LT, T$_{lact}$)	Minimum work rate at which [Lac]$_b$ is found, at least in the early minutes, to be significantly above (sometimes defined as 1 mmol/L above) resting value	2
Anaerobic threshold (AT)	Work rate at which it has been considered that shortfall in oxygen supply to working muscles causes them to begin drawing on anaerobic pathways. Previously taken as equating to LT but there is now good evidence that fully aerobic muscles release lactate	2
Ventilatory threshold (VT, T$_{vent}$)	Work rate at which the gradient of the ventilation/work rate plot increases. Attributed to rise in [Lac]$_b$ so used as non-invasive indicator of LT/AT, but precision of the agreement varies with method of determining VT	2
Aerobic threshold	Work rate considered to be minimum for achievement of aerobic training effects (not that at which aerobic metabolism starts, which is of course zero)	2
Maximum lactate steady state (MLSS)	Highest work rate which can be maintained without continuous rise in [Lac]$_b$ (see comment under OBLA). Functionally equivalent to critical power (*qv*) though this is defined in terms of $\dot{V}O_2$, not [Lac]$_b$	4
Onset of blood lactate accumulation (OBLA)	Work rate at which a *continuous* rise in [Lac]$_b$ begins. (At and a little above LT, it rises only initially, and falls gradually again after a few minutes.) OBLA is thus theoretically slightly above MLSS, but it is doubtful whether they are distinguishable in practice	4

Reproduced from Jennett (2008) with permission

approximations for a healthy but untrained young adult; they are used in some laboratories as working indices, but should *not* be taken as definitions of the term concerned. Other usages in the literature include: (a) onset of blood lactate (OBLA) as equivalent to lactate threshold (LT) or anaerobic threshold (AT)—confusions possible only if the reference to continuous rise is omitted from the OBLA definition; (b) the 4 mmol/L criterion being designated as any one of 'anaerobic', 'aerobic' or 'aerobic/anaerobic' thresholds.

metabolic alkalosis a disturbance of acid–base balance due to loss of body acids by vomiting of acidic gastric contents, excessive administration of corticosteroids and some endocrine disorders, e.g. Cushing's syndrome, primary hyperaldosteronism (Conn's syndrome), the adminstration of some diuretic drugs. Or caused by an excess of bicarbonate in the blood, such as that caused by excessive administration of alkaline antacids or infusion of intravenous fluids containing bicarbonate. ➲ acid–base balance.

metabolic equivalent (MET) expresses the approximate energy cost (in terms of oxygen consumption) of a particular activity relative to the energy expenditure at rest, i.e. at rest MET = 1, equivalent to oxygen consumption of about 3.5 mL O_2/kg/min. It is expressed as multiples of basal (resting) metabolic rate. Scores for over 500 different activities are reported in a comprehensive and well-validated list in the *Compendium of Physical Activities*, e.g. walking at 3 mph: 3.3 MET; running at 8 mph: 13.3 MET. The total daily energy expenditure can be calculated, knowing body mass, the time spent in each activity and the relevant MET scores. Used in sports medicine to estimate the intensity of exercise.

metabolic rate the rate of energy expenditure during any given state of rest or specified activity. Commonly assessed in terms of respiratory gas exchange (indirect calorimetry) by obtaining values for oxygen uptake and carbon dioxide output, and relating these to the equivalent release of energy in kJ or kcal per minute. *basal metabolic rate (BMR)* the rate of energy expenditure which is required at complete rest for all cellular function, to maintain the systems of the body and to regulate body temperature. It is measured before the person rises in the morning after fasting for at least 12 hours, requiring an overnight stay under controlled conditions in the laboratory. BMR is influenced by age, sex, body size and fat-free mass. In most sedentary healthy adults it accounts for approximately 60–80% of total daily energy expenditure, amounting to ~4000–7000 kJ per 24 hours for individuals with body mass within the normal range. In elite endurance athletes during days of competition or training, BMR may represent only 38–47% of total daily energy expenditure. *resting metabolic rate (RMR)* is more commonly measured, since it allows the person to sleep at home, to travel to the laboratory in the morning and to rest there before RMR is assessed. Values for BMR and RMR usually differ by less than 10% and sometimes are used interchangeably. RMR is typically close to 4.2 kJ per kg of body mass per hour or 3.5 mL O_2 utilized per kg of body mass per minute. ➲ Douglas bag method, oxygen consumption.

metabolic syndrome also known as metabolic syndrome X, syndrome X, insulin resistance syndrome, Reaven's syndrome. A group of risk factors for atherosclerosis manifested as macrovascular disease affecting the coronary, cerebral and peripheral arteries and type 2 diabetes. They include the degree of central (visceral) obesity— using waist circumference measurement, waist:hip ratio, waist: height ratio and body mass index; insulin resistance— hyperinsulinaemia, impaired fasting glucose/glycaemia, impaired glucose tolerance; cardiovascular risks—high blood pressure, low levels of high density (HDL) cholesterol, raised triglycerides, increased fibrinogen, increased plasminogen activator inhibitor-1, elevated plasma uric acid, the presence of microalbuminuria and increased sympathetic neural activity.

metabolic syndrome X ⊃ metabolic syndrome.

metabolic water the water produced by the cells during the oxidation of nutrients.

metabolism *n* the continuous series of biochemical processes in the living body by which life is maintained. Nutrients and tissues are broken down (catabolism), releasing energy which is utilized in the creation of new substances for growth and rebuilding (anabolism). ⊃ adenosine diphosphate, adenosine triphosphate—**metabolic** *adj. basal metabolism* the minimum energy expended in the maintenance of essential physiological processes such as respiration. ⊃ energy systems, metabolic rate.

metabolite *n* any product of or substance taking part in metabolism. An *essential metabolite* one that is necessary for normal metabolism, e.g. B vitamins needed for the synthesis of the coenzymes needed for many biochemical reactions.

metacarpal 1. *n* any one of the five slender bones forming the metacarpus. They articulate proximally with the carpal bones, and distally with the phalanges. **2.** *adj* relating to the metacarpus.

metacarpophalangeal *adj* pertaining to the metacarpus and the phalanges.

metacarpus *n* the five bones which form that part of the hand between the wrist and fingers (palm of the hand). They are numbered 1 to 5 starting at the thumb—**metacarpal** *adj*. ⊃ Colour Section Figure 2.

metachronous subsequent.

metacognition knowledge of one's own mental processes. Sometimes applied to the self-regulation of cognitive processes, such as in the application of mental skills.

Metagonimus *n* a genus of minute intestinal flukes. *Metagonimus yokogawai* may infect humans who eat undercooked fish. Infestation known as metagonimiasis causes diarrhoea and abdominal colic. It occurs in the Balkans, Far East, Siberia and Spain.

metal in dentistry, any element with the following properties: ductibility, fusibility, hardness, lustre, malleability and being a good conductor of heat and electricity. *base metal* a metal which is neither precious nor noble. *metal ceramic restoration* a restoration having a metal substructure onto which a ceramic veneer is fused. ⊃ crown (porcelain bonded). *noble metal* a metal that can not be readily dissolved by acid, nor oxidized by heat alone. *non-precious metal* ⊃ base metal. *precious metal* a metal containing primarily gold, silver and elements of the platinum group. ⊃ alloy, semiprecious metal casting alloy.

metal exchange a method of silver recovery when the fixer solution passes through a base metal which is replaced by the silver and base metal ions are released into the solution which then goes to waste.

metal gauze in dentistry, may be used as a strengthener in the construction of prostheses.

metalloenzyme *n* an enzyme that contains metal ions, such as copper or zinc as its prosthetic group. For example, carbonic anhydrase the enzyme that catalyses the rapid reversible reactions that faciltate the transport of carbon dioxide from the tissues to the lungs, contains zinc.

metalloprotein *n* a protein that contains one or more metal ions as a cofactor. For example, iron in haemoglobin.

metamorphopsia *n* an abnormality of vision in which objects appear distorted in shape or of different size or in a different location than the actual object. It may be due to a displacement of the visual receptors as a result of inflammation, tumour or retinal detachment, or it can be of central origin (e.g. migraine, drug intoxication), or it can be induced by recently prescribed myopic correction (e.g. micropsia) or presbyopic correction (e.g. macropsia) etc. Metamorphopsia can be detected with an Amsler chart. ⊃ Amsler chart/grid, dysmegalopsia, macropsia, macular hole, micropsia, pelopsia, spasm of accommodation, teleopsia.

metamyelocyte *n* an immature cell with a large kidney-shaped nucleus formed in the bone marrow during the development of the granulocyte series of white blood cells (leucocytes). Its presence in the blood is abnormal.

metanephros the final fetal excretory organ with a complex tubular structure that will develop further to become a functioning kidney. ⊃ mesonephros, pronephros.

metaphase the second stage of nuclear division in mitosis (see Figure M.7, p. 488) and both divisions in meiosis (see Figure M.3, p. 472). The chromosomes move to the middle of the cell and become arranged in the equatorial plane of the spindle. The centromeres attach to the spindle in preparation for separation. ⊃ anaphase, prophase, telophase.

metaphysis in children the area of a growing long bone situated between each epiphysis (the end) and diaphysis (shaft).

metaplasia *n* process of substituting one type of mature epithelium for a different type of mature epithelium (usually less specialized) that is better suited to cope with the adverse environment which triggered the process. For example the change from ciliated columnar epithelium to squamous epithelium in the respiratory mucosa of cigarette smokers. Metaplasia may occur in response to chronic inflammation, it is generally reversible if the cause is removed but may progress through dysplasia to malignant changes.

metastable state when an atomic nucleus is decaying and the length of time it takes can be measured.

metastasis *n* the secondary spread of malignant tumour cells from one part of the body to another. Either by the lymphatic route to the lymph nodes or to distant organs via the haematogenous (blood) route. Some cancers also spread across body cavities. Most solid tumours are not curable if metastasis has occurred—**metastases** *pl*, **metastatic** *adj*, **metastasize** *vi*.

metatarsal 1. *n* any one of the five bones forming the metatarsus. They articulate proximally with the tarsal bones, and distally with the phalanges. **2.** *adj* relating to the metatarsus.

metatarsalgia *n* pain under the metatarsal heads in the foot as a result of abnormal foot shape, intense training or overuse, altered biomechanics or poorly fitting shoes. Stress fracture should be excluded by X-ray, though this can be negative initially. Treatment initially is with rest and analgesia but aims to reverse the cause, avoid overweight and encourage good well-fitting supportive shoes. Orthoses can be helpful. ⊃ Morton's metatarsalgia.

metatarsophalangeal *adj* pertaining to the metatarsus and the phalanges.

metatarsus *n* the five bones of the foot between the ankle and the toes. They are numbered 1 to 5 from medial to lateral aspects—**metatarsal** *adj.* ⊃ Colour Section Figure 2.

metatarsus valgus a congenital deformity where the forefoot is deviated outwards away from the midline of the body in relation to the hindfoot.

metatarsus varus also known as metatarsus adductus. A congenital deformity where the forefoot is deviated inwards towards the midline of the body in relation to the hindfoot.

metencephalon *n* one of the secondary enlargements during embryonic development of the brain. It becomes part of the hindbrain—the cerebellum and the pons.

meteorism ⊃ tympanites.

meter an apparatus or instrument for measuring a physical quantity by direct reading, such as a thermometer.

metered-dose inhaler (MDI) a pressurized cannister designed to deliver an exact dose of aerosolized medication into the lungs (Figure M.6). It is frequently used by people with asthma to administer their medication. The inhaler can be used with a cone-shaped spacer device for small children and other people who are unable to coordinate the action required to use the inhaler. When used with a spacer device the lung deposition of respiratory medication is markedly improved.

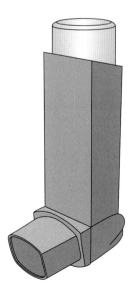

M.6 Metered dose inhaler (reproduced from Brooker & Waugh 2007 with permission).

-meter, metry a suffix that means 'measure', e.g. *tonometer*.

methadone *n* a synthetic opioid analgesic. It is used as part of a heroin withdrawal programme.

methaemalbumin *n* abnormal compound formed in blood from combination of haem with plasma albumin, under conditions of grossly accelerated red cell breakdown (haemolysis), such as the intravascular haemolysis that occurs as a complication of malaria (blackwater fever).

methaemoglobin *n* a form of haemoglobin consisting of a combination of globin with an oxidized haem, containing ferric iron. This pigment is unable to transport oxygen. Small amounts can be detected in the blood after smoking. It may be formed in babies after exposure to environmental chemicals such as the nitrates found in drinking water and some vegetables. It may form following the administration of a wide variety of drugs, including the sulphonamides. It may also be present in the blood as a result of an inherited deficiency of enzymes or in conditions where the haemoglobin is abnormal.

methaemoglobinaemia *n* methaemoglobin in the blood. If large quantities are present, individuals may show cyanosis, but otherwise no abnormality except, in severe cases, breathlessness on exertion, because the methaemoglobin cannot transport oxygen—**methaemoglobinaemic** *adj.*

methane *n* CH_4, a colourless, odourless, inflammable gas that results from the decomposition of organic matter.

methanol methyl alcohol. Also known as wood alcohol or wood spirits, it is used as a solvent, fuel and antifreeze. The ingestion, absorption or inhalation has very serious effects. It intoxicates and its breakdown product formaldehyde is toxic and causes blindness by damaging the optic nerves, depression of the nervous system, and in severe cases metabolic acidosis, respiratory failure and death.

methicillin-resistant *Staphylococcus aureus* **(MRSA)** ⊃ meticillin (methicillin)-resistant *Staphylococcus aureus* (MRSA).

methionine *n* one of the essential (indispensable) sulphur-containing amino acids. May be used in the treatment of hepatitis, paracetamol overdose and other conditions associated with liver damage.

methylcellulose *n* a bulk-forming laxative. ⊃ Appendix 5.

methylmalonic acid an intermediate formed during the metabolism of succinic acid. It tends to accumulate when there is a deficiency of vitamin B_{12}. Measuring the level in urine or serum provides information about vitamin B_{12} status.

methylmethacrylate a monomer from which polymethylmethacrylate (PMMA) is produced. ⊃ monomer.

methylxanthines a group of alkaloids that includes caffeine and related substances. Ingested caffeine is rapidly metabolized in the liver to three dimethylxanthines: paraxanthine, theophylline and theobromine; these are released in the plasma and remain in the circulation while caffeine concentration declines. As caffeine and its metabolites are often present at the same time, it is difficult

M
N

481

to resolve which tissues are directly or indirectly affected by which compound.

meticillin (methicillin)-resistant *Staphylococcus aureus* (MRSA) *n* strains of *Staphylococcus aureus* that are resistant to meticillin (not used clinically) and flucloxacillin. Causes serious and sometimes fatal infections in hospitals, and patients with MRSA are frequently encountered in community settings. Treatment depends on the sensitivity of the particular strain of MRSA to antibacterial drugs and on the site of infection. Drugs used include vancomycin, teicoplanin, combinations of rifampicin, sodium fusidate with each other or with a glycopeptide antibacterial, the streptogramin antibacterials quinupristin and dalfopristin combined, or linezolid an oxazolidinone antibacterial. Topical mupirocin is used to eliminate nasal or skin carriage. Infection prevention and control measures that include strict adherence to hand washing, proper environmental cleaning and isolation, or if single rooms are not available, patient cohorting is vital in controlling MRSA. Epidemic strains (EMRSA) have developed resistance to most antibiotics. ⮑ Panton-Valentine leukocidin, *Staphylococcus,* vancomycin-resistant *Staphylococcus aureus.*

metre (m) one of the seven base units of the Système International d'Unités (SI) (International System of Units). A measurement of length. ⮑ Appendix 2.

metre angle (ma) unit of convergence which is equal to the reciprocal of the distance (in metres) between the point of fixation assumed to lie on the median line and the base line of the eyes. Thus, if an object is located at 25 cm from the base line, each eye converges through 4 ma; at 1 metre, 1 ma, etc. Metre angles of convergence can be converted into prism dioptres of convergence by multiplying by the subject's interpupillary distance expressed in cm. *Example*: for an interpupillary distance of 6.0 cm, a convergence of 5 ma = 30Δ. ⮑ angle of convergence, base line, prism dioptre.

metritis *n* inflammation of the uterus.

metro, metra- a prefix that means 'uterus', e.g. *metrorrhagia.*

metropathia haemorrhagica a term sometimes applied to irregular, prolonged and heavy menstrual bleeding. It is associated with the persistant production of high levels of oestrogen, which causes cystic glandular hyperplasia of the endometrium. It usually occurs in women nearing the menopause.

metroplasty surgical operation to repair the uterus.

metrorrhagia *n* uterine bleeding between the menstrual periods such as after intercourse or examination.

metrostaxis persistent slight haemorrhage from the uterus.

METS *abbr* metabolic equivalents.

Meyer's loop a bundle of inferior nerve fibres that originate from the lateral portion of the lateral geniculate body, extend forward around the anterior tip of the temporal horn of the lateral ventricle and then swing backward toward the occipital lobe. A lesion in this loop may cause a superior homonymous quadrantanopsia. ⮑ optic radiations.

MFAC *abbr* medium frequency current.

mg *abbr* milligram.

MGD *abbr* meibomian gland dysfunction.

MGUS *abbr* monoclonal gammopathy of uncertain significance.

MHC *abbr* **1.** major histocompatibility complex. **2.** myosin heavy chain.

MHN *abbr* Mohs hardness scale/number.

MHRA *abbr* Medicines and Healthcare Products Regulatory Agency.

MI *abbr* myocardial infarction.

micelle tiny globules of fat and bile salts formed during fat digestion. Fatty acids and glycerol are transported into the intestinal cells (enterocytes) in this form, leaving the bile salts behind in the lumen of the bowel.

micro- a prefix that means 'small', e.g. *microalbuminuria.*

microaerophile a micro-organism that grows in an environment that contains low levels of free oxygen—**microphilic** *adj.*

microabrasion ⮑ acid-pumice microabrasion.

microalbuminuria the presence of small amounts of albumen (within a range of 20–200 μg/min) in the urine, which are not revealed using a standard routine dipstick urinalysis. There are commercial dipsticks that will detect this lower level. The presence of microalbuminuria is an indication that early nephropathy is occurring in people who have had diabetes for a number of years. It may also occur in people with hypertension and those with subclinical cardiac conditions. ⮑ diabetic nephropathy.

microaneurysm *n* tiny swelling in the wall of retinal blood vessels. May bleed or leak. It appears in the retinal capillaries as a small, round, red spot. It is commonly found in diabetic retinopathy, retinal vein occlusion or absolute glaucoma. ⮑ diabetic retinopathy.

microangiopathy *n* small vessel disease, with basement membrane thickening and endothelial dysfunction, usually in association with diabetes mellitus, but also seen in patients with connective tissue disease, infection and malignancy; results in retinopathy and nephropathy in patients with diabetes. ⮑ diabetic nephropathy, diabetic retinopathy

microbe *n* ⮑ micro-organism—**microbial, microbic** *adj.*

microbiological assay a way of measuring substances such as amino acids and vitamins, using micro-organisms. The micro-organisms are introduced into a medium containing all the nutrients needed for growth except the one being investigated. The rate of microbial growth is then proportional to the amount of the missing nutrient subsequently introduced into the medium.

microbiology *n* the science of micro-organisms—**microbiological** *adj.*

microbrush a Swedish brush, like a small bottle brush, used to remove plaque from the interproximal areas of the teeth.

microcephaly *n* an abnormally small head.

microcirculation *n* blood flow through the arterioles, capillaries and venules. Damage caused by prolonged compression to these vessels predisposes to the formation of pressure ulcers.

Micrococcus *n* a genus of Gram-positive bacteria. Found in soil and fresh water. Generally non-pathogenic, they are part of the skin flora. It can, however, cause opportunistic infections in immunocompromised individuals.

microcolon a small colon.

microcoria abnormally small pupils, usually congenital and due to an absence of the dilator pupillae muscle.

microcornea an abnormally small cornea. It may be accompanied by hypermetropia. ⊃ keratoglobus.

microcracks ⊃ crazing.

microcrystalline wax in dentistry, the synthetic wax that resembles natural wax in its physical characteristics and is used in the production of modelling waxes. Obtained by the fractional distillation of crude oil.

microcyte *n* an abnormally undersized red blood cell found for example in iron deficiency anaemia, or in anaemia caused by chronic bleeding.

microcytosis an increased number of microcytes in the circulating blood such as in iron deficiency anaemia—**microcytic** *adj*.

microdiscectomy a minimally invasive surgical procedure using an operating microscope, undertaken for some patients with back pain caused by a prolapsed intervertebral disc. It is performed through a small laminectomy (surgical procedure, which includes removal of a portion of the lamina, to provide more room in the vertebral canal). A small part of the prolapsed disc is removed to relieve the pressure on the spinal cord or the spinal nerve roots.

microdissection *n* dissection of tissue or cells under the microscope.

microdochectomy *n* a surgical procedure used in the management of intraductal papillomas of the breast, in which the affected segment of breast is excised.

microdontia *n* a condition in which the teeth are abnormally small. It my affect some or all the teeth, especially the maxillary lateral incisors and the third permanent molars.

microenvironment *n* the environment at the microscopic or cellular level immediately surrounding the body.

microepithelial cysts ⊃ epithelial microcysts.

microfilaria *n* immature filaria ⊃ filariasis.

microgenitalism abnormal smallness of the external reproductive organs.

microglia non-neural cells, a type of macrophage present in the central nervous system. They are phagocytic and are able to deal with cell debris. ⊃ macroglia.

microglossia an abnormally small tongue.

micrognathia *n* small jaw, especially the lower one. May cause problems with feeding and with the eruption of the teeth. It is a feature of the chromosomal condition Edwards' syndome, and Pierre-Robin syndrome, which is due to a developmental anomaly.

microgram (μg) *n* one millionth of a gram.

micro-leakage in dentistry, it describes the passage of liquids, micro-organisms and ions between a restoration and the walls of its cavity preparation.

micrometre (μm) *n* also still called a micron. One millionth of a metre.

micromotor in dentistry, a miniature electric motor to which a handpiece is fitted.

micron *n* ⊃ micrometre.

micronutrients *npl* nutrients needed by the body in relatively small amounts such as vitamins and minerals. They are vital for the biochemical processes of the body. With proper nutrition from a wide variety of food sources, the physically active person or competitive athlete need not consume vitamin and mineral supplements; such practices usually have no benefits and some micronutrients consumed in excess can adversely affect health and safety. ⊃ macronutrients, trace elements.

micro-organism *n* (*syn* microbe) a microscopic cell. Often synonymous with bacterium but includes virus, protozoon, rickettsia, chlamydia and fungus.

micropachometer ⊃ pachometer (pachymeter).

microphthalmia *n* (*syn* microphthalmos) a congenital condition in which one or both eyes are abnormally small.

microphthalmos ⊃ microphthalmia.

microprocessor an integrated circuit that can be pre-programmed to perform a variety of tasks.

micropsia *n* a visual defect in which objects are seen as much smaller than they are in reality. It may be due to a retinal disease in which the visual cells are spread apart, or to paresis of accommodation or to uncorrected presbyopia, or to the recent wear of either base-out prisms or a correction for myopia, etc. ⊃ dysmegalopsia, macropsia, metamorphopsia.

microscope an optical instrument used to magnify small near objects. It can consist of a single converging lens such as a loupe (*simple microscope*) or of two or more lenses or lens systems (*compound microscope*). In this latter case, one lens or lens system serves as an objective to form real and magnified images of the object while the other lens or lens system serves as an eyepiece to examine the aerial image formed by the objective. The final image is inverted with respect to the object. It can use light or a beam of electrons (*electron microscope*) which produces magnification some 50 to 100 times greater than with light. ⊃ binocular microscope, confocal microscope, electron microscope, eyepiece, slit-lamp microscope, specular microscope, Vernier (micrometer) microscope.

microscopic *adj* extremely small; visible only with the aid of a microscope. ⊃ macroscopic *opp*.

microscopic polyangiitis (MPA) an ANCA-associated vasculitis with an annual incidence of 8 per million in the UK. Classic presentation is with rapidly progressive glomerulonephritis, often associated with pulmonary alveolar haemorrhage. Cutaneous and gastrointestinal involvement is common. Other features include neuropathy and pleural

M
N

effusions. Patients are usually p-ANCA-positive. ➲ antineutrophil cytoplasmic antibodies-associated vasculitis.

microscopy the various techniques that utilize a microscope to view minute objects, such as body tissues, cells and cell organelles, or bacteria and viruses.

microsome *n* a minute fragment of endoplasmic reticulum and associated ribosomes. They result from cell breakdown during homogenization. The microsome fragments can be sorted from other subcellular organelles during centrifugation.

Microsporum n a genus of fungi. Parasitic, living in keratin-containing tissues of humans and animals. *Microsporum audouini* is the commonest cause of scalp ringworm. ➲ dermatophytes, tinea.

microstomia a condition in which the mouth is unusually small.

microstreaming (cellular streaming) the phenomenon that occurs in certain electrotherapy modalities, in particular ultrasound. It is thought to affect cell membrane permeability and, therefore, affect tissue repair.

microsurgery *n* use of the binocular operating microscope during the performance of operations that require delicate procedures involving small structures such as repairing blood vessels and nerves following a traumatic amputation. Also increases access to areas such as the brain, spinal cord and the inner ear for operative procedures—**microsurgical** *adj.*

microsurgical epididymal sperm aspiration (MESA) a technique used in assisted conception. Spermatozoa are aspirated directly from the epididymis in men who have azoospermia caused by a permanent obstruction in the duct system, such as may follow infection or vasectomy. The spermatozoa, which can be frozen and stored, are used for repeated attempts to achieve in vitro fertilization, including using intracytoplasmic sperm injection. ➲ intracytoplasmic sperm injection (ICSI).

microtia *n* a small ear. A congenital abnormality that may affect one or both ears. It is graded from a small, deformed pinna with a functional meatus/canal; through deformities that include a blocked or absent external auditory meatus/canal and absence of the tympanic membrane and conductive deafness; to complete absence of the ear (anotia).

microtome *n* an instrument used for cutting tissue sections for microscopic study, usually in the order of 4–6 micrometres in thickness.

microtrauma *n* injury to a small number of cells due to the cumulative effect of repetitive forces.

microvascular surgery surgery carried out on blood vessels using a binocular operating microscope. ➲ microsurgery.

microvilli *npl* microscopic projections from the free surface of cell membranes whose purpose is to increase the exposed surface of the cell for absorption, e.g. intestinal epithelium.

microwave electrotherapy term – electromagnetic radiation which has a frequency between 2.450 MHz and 433 MHz. Therapeutic uses include electrotherapy techniques in physiotherapy, treatment of benign prostatic enlargement, and subjecting accessible tumour cells to hyperthermia. In current physiotherapy practice the most commonly used frequency, 2.450 MHz, is the least effective for heating as electromagnetic radiation wavelength is inverse to penetration. Lower frequencies may become more commonly available leaving the higher ones for communications. It is used for deep heating, but less frequently than ultrasound or shortwave diathermy (SWD). Like SWD use, it is contraindicated within 3–5 m of a patient with an indwelling stimulator or pump and there is a risk of burns if used over indwelling metal implants. Risks common to all clinically used methods of heating are also relevant.

MICRR *abbr* multiple idiopathic cervical root resorption.

micturating cystourethrogram (MCU) radiographic examination performed during micturition, often to assess the degree of ureteric reflux, or to investigate urinary incontinence. Following intravenous injection of a contrast agent or, more commonly, after contrast is introduced into the bladder via a urinary catheter until micturating begins. A series of radiographs are taken during the act of passing urine (micturation). ➲ vesicoureteric reflux.

micturition *n* (*syn* urination) passing urine.

midbrain *n* the mesencephalon. The most anterior part of the brainstem that surrounds the cerebral aqueduct. It is situated between the cerebrum above and the pons below. It contains important nuclei and nerve tracts that connect the cerebrum with the brainstem and spinal cord. The nuclei include those of two cranial nerves (oculomotor and trochlear), the substantia nigra, the red nucleus. ➲ Colour Section Figure 1.

mid-diastolic murmur a heart murmur characteristic of mitral stenosis. ➲ heart murmur, heart sounds.

middle cerebral artery (MCA) the largest branch of the internal carotid artery. This artery is a common site for occlusion by an embolus or thrombus in cerebrovascular accident (stroke).

middle cerebral artery (MCA) flow blood flow through the middle cerebral artery, measurable with ultrasound. Increased velocities indicate severe fetal anaemia. It is a valuable test in the management and investigation of haemolytic disease from maternal red blood cell alloimmunization as it may indicate when intrauterine transfusion is required.

middle ear *n* also called the tympanum. The tympanic cavity, situated in the temporal bone. The tympanic membrane separates it from the outer ear. It is an air-filled cavity containing the three tiny bones or ossicles: malleus, incus and stapes. The ossicles transmit the sound waves to the inner ear via the oval window. The middle ear communicates with the nasopharynx via the pharyngotympanic (eustachian or auditory) tube.

middle meningeal artery a branch of the maxillary artery. It runs deeply to supply blood to the bones forming the vault of the skull.

middle superior mental nerve an afferent nerve from the first and second upper premolars and part of the first permanent upper molar. It runs upwards to the infraorbital canal, to join the maxillary division of the trigeminal nerve.

middle-third fracture ➲ jaw fracture.

midgut *n* the middle part of the embryonic alimentary tract between the foregut and the hindgut. It is endodermal tissue and will form some of the small intestine and part of the large intestine. ➲ foregut, hindgut.

midline an imaginary line that runs through the centre of the body and thus gives a reference point for assessing the anterior–posterior and rotatory alignment of individual parts of the body, i.e. head, shoulder girdle and trunk.

midline shift a term used in physiotherapy. It refers to a movement of the midline from the centre of the body. Due to tonal changes following a stroke, it is common to see a midline shift. The shift is more commonly away from the hemiplegic side, but can occur towards the hemiplegic side. ➲ pusher syndrome.

midriff *n* the diaphragm.

midsagittal plane ➲ median plane.

midstance the point of gait (walking or running) when the centre of mass of the body is above the supporting foot.

midstream specimen of urine (MSU) a specimen of urine obtained from the middle part of voiding. The first and last parts of the flow of urine are discarded. It is usually collected for microbiological examination to confirm the presence of a urinary tract infection, therefore it is collected in a sterile container and the risk of contamination is reduced by the person cleaning around the external urethral opening with the warm soapy water. Women and girls should clean from front to back. Older boys and adult males, the foreskin (if present) should be retracted, and the glans cleaned.

mid-systolic murmur a heart murmur characteristic of aortic stenosis. ➲ heart murmur, heart sounds.

mid-upper-arm-circumference (MUAC) an anthropometric test that assesses the amount of muscle tissue in the upper arm. The arm circumference is measured midway between the top of the acromion of the shoulder and the olecranon process of the elbow. Used as part of nutritional assessment. ➲ anthropometry.

midwife International Confederation of Midwives 1972 and International Federation of Gynaecologists and Obstetricians, 1973, defined a midwife as 'a person who, having been regularly admitted to a midwifery education programme, duly recognized in the country in which it is located, has successfully completed the prescribed course of studies and acquired the requisite qualifications to be registered and/or legally licensed to practise midwifery, able to give the necessary supervision, care and advice to women during pregnancy, labour and the postpartum period, conduct deliveries on her [or his] own responsibility and care for the newborn and the infant; care includes preventative measures, detection of abnormal conditions in mother and child, procurement of medical assistance and execution of emergency measures in the absence of medical help. She [or he] has an important task in health counselling and health education, ... antenatal education and preparation for parenthood and .... certain areas of gynaecology, family planning and child care. She [or he] may practise in hospitals, clinics, health units, domiciliary conditions or in any other service.'

midwifery in the UK midwives are responsible for providing care to mothers and babies in accordance with the Nursing and Midwifery Council's current *Midwives Rules and Code of Practice*. The care provided covers prenatal (antenatal), intranatal and postnatal periods. Midwives may practice in the woman's home, general practitioner's surgery, at a health centre or within a hospital. The practice of midwifery includes providing family planning advice; making a diagnosis of pregnancy; providing prenatal care and parenthood classes; care during labour and conducting deliveries; recognizing problems and abnormalities affecting mother or baby; and the care of both mother and child in the postnatal period. As midwives are members of a multiprofessional team, these activities are not pursued in isolation and midwives work with doctors, specialist community public health nurses and other professionals to provide high standards of care.

migraine *n* a condition characterized by paroxysmal headache, vomiting and focal neurological symptoms (usually visual). The presence of all three is classical migraine. Whereas, common migraine is defined as paroxysmal headache, with or without vomiting but no focal neurological symptoms. Migraine sufferers also experience photophobia and phonophobia. The aura of migraine most often takes the form of shimmering zigzag lines that move across the visual field. Migraine attacks may be triggered by certain foods and beverages such as chocolate, cheese and red wine; hormonal changes during the menstrual cycle, bright lights, and may occur during the time after stresses and strains such as weekends or holiday time—**migrainous** *adj*.

migration 1. the abnormal movement or drifting of teeth due to the inflammatory process of periodontitis. **2.** the normal physiological drift of teeth. **3.** the movement of cells, such as white blood cells, through blood vessel walls. ➲ diapedesis.

Mikulicz's disease/syndrome (J von Mikulicz-Radecki, Polish surgeon, 1850–1905) chronic hypertrophic enlargement of the lacrimal and salivary glands. It may be associated with other conditions, e.g. leukaemia, sarcoidosis.

miliaria *n* (*syn* strophulus) prickly heat common in the tropics, and affects waistline, cubital fossae and chest. Vesicular and erythematous eruption, caused by blocking of sweat ducts and their subsequent rupture, or their infection by fungi or bacteria.

miliary *adj* resembling a millet seed.

miliary tuberculosis ➲ tuberculosis.

military antishock trousers (MAST) an inflatable garment used to apply pressure to the abdomen and legs to minimize the pooling of blood in the lower body, thereby redistributing the available circulating volume to increase the perfusion of vital organs.

military attitude attitude of the fetus which is neither flexed nor extended.

milium *n* condition in which tiny, white, cystic excrescences appear on the face, especially about the eyelids; the cysts contain keratin—**milia** *pl*.

milk *n* secretion of the mammary glands. Provided that the woman is taking an adequate diet, breast milk provides the perfect nutrition for healthy infants. It contains all the essential nutrients in proportions that meet growth and development needs of infants during the first 6 months of life. Moreover, breast milk contains maternal immunoglobulins and these help to protect infants while their own immune systems develop. In addition, there are advantages to the mother that include special contact with her infant and ready availability of feeds at the correct temperature. ⊃ breast milk, colostrum.

milk flow mechanism, milk ejection reflex oxytocin released from the posterior pituitary gland in response to nervous stimulation causes contraction of myoepithelial cells. The milk is forced out of the alveoli of the breast tissue into the ducts and lacteal sinuses and is available to the baby. This occurs about 30–40 seconds after the baby takes the areola of the breast in his jaws. ⊃ 'let down' reflex.

milk sugar lactose.

milk teeth the lay term for the twenty deciduous teeth of the primary dentition.

milled bar in dentistry, a metal bar that has been milled or ground to have flat sides which serve as a means of retention for a prosthesis. Prevents rotation of the prosthesis about the bar.

Miller–Abbott tube (T Miller, American physician, 1886–1981; W Abbott, American physician, 1902–1943) double-lumen tube used for intestinal suction. The second channel leads to a balloon near the tip of the tube.

Miller–Dieker syndrome (J Miller, American physician, b.1926; H Dieker, American geneticist) ⊃ lissencephaly.

milli- a prefix that means a 'thousandth', e.g. *milligram*.

milliampere (mA) a measurement of electrical current. One thousandth part of an ampere

milligram (mg) *n* one thousandth part of a gram.

millilitre (mL) *n* one thousandth part of a litre. Equal to a cubic centimetre.

millimetre (mm) *n* one thousandth part of a metre.

millimole (mmol) *n* one thousandth part of a mole.

Milroy's disease (W Milroy, American physician, 1855–1942) a congenital condition in which there is lymphoedema caused by lymphatic obstruction. Usually affects the legs but other areas may be involved. ⊃ lymphoedema.

Milwaukee brace an orthotic device used in the corrective treatment of spinal curvature (scoliosis). It applies fixed traction between the occiput and the pelvis.

MIME *acron* **M**ultipurpose **I**nternet **M**ail **E**xtensions.

MIMS *abbr* Monthly Index of Medical Specialties.

Minamata disease a severe neurological condition caused by mercury poisoning. It is named from the place in Japan where mercury released from a factory polluted the sea and the fish, which were eaten by the inhabitants. It is characterized by ataxia, dysarthria and visual impairment.

mind–body dualism a philosophical position that takes the view that the mind and the body are essentially distinct entities with separate realms of existence. This position lies at the ideological roots of contemporary orthodox medical practice, but is increasingly being challenged by the view that the mind and body are linked and influence each other. Excessive mental stress can, for example, lead to physical ill-health.

mineralocorticoid *n* a group of corticosteroid hormones produced by the adrenal cortex. Involved in the regulation of electrolyte and water balance. ⊃ aldosterone.

mineralization the addition of mineral matter to the body tissues, such as teeth or bone.

minerals *npl* inorganic substances obtained from a varied and well-balanced diet. The substances required in the largest amounts are sodium, potassium, calcium, chloride, phosphorus and magnesium, and many others are essential in smaller amounts. They are: iron, zinc, fluoride and the trace elements cobalt, chromium, copper, iodine, manganese, molybdenum and selenium, some of which are required in extremely minute amounts. Minerals are essential in all metabolic processes, from maintenance of cell volume and structure to muscle contraction and relaxation, regulation of acid–base equilibrium, protection from oxidative stress/damage, bone metabolism, immune function and haemoglobin synthesis. No mineral supplements should be required for athletes who are consuming a well-balanced diet but they frequently take them, especially iron, magnesium and chromium. ⊃ trace elements.

mineral trioxide aggregate (MTA) the material based on building cement increasingly being used in surgical and non-surgical endodontics, especially in the treatment of open apices and repair of perforations.

miniature handpiece in dentistry, a handpiece with a small head and chuck allowing easy access into a small mouth.

mini bone plate small plates of varying thicknesses (usually <2 mm) and lengths usually used to fixate maxillofacial fractures.

Mini Mental State Examination (MMSE) a test of cognitive function used to screen for dementia or delirium. It tests five areas including orientation, recall, language, etc.

minimal carious lesion in dentistry, describes an early lesion into dentine, comprising a dark stained central pit with dark dentinal caries shining through translucent enamel with decalcification of the enamel lined walls of the pit. Usually treated using a preventive resin restoration (PRR). ⊃ preventive resin restoration.

minimal clinical important difference (MCID) (of outcome scores) a research term. The means of interpreting the score generated by an outcome measure. 'The smallest difference in score in the domain of interest which patients perceive as beneficial, and which would mandate, in the absence of troublesome side effects and excessive costs, a change in the patient's management' (Jaeschke et al 1989).

M
N

(Jaeschke R, Singer J, Guyatt G 1989 Controlled clinical trials 10: 407–415.)

minimally invasive surgery (MIS) known colloquially as 'key hole surgery'. Surgical techniques that only require minimal access; the procedure is performed through very small incisions using endoscopic instruments. An increasing variety of procedures, which cover a range of complexity, are undertaken, e.g. female sterilization, cholecystectomy, vascular surgery. ➲ laparoscopy.

minitracheostomy cricothyroidotomy. The insertion of a fine-bore minitracheostomy tube to treat or prevent the retention of sputum in a variety of conditions and situations, such as following chest surgery. ➲ tracheostomy.

minor arterial circle of the iris an incomplete vascular circle located in the region of the collarette of the iris. It is formed by arterial and venous anastomoses. It supplies the pupillary zone of the iris. ➲ major arterial circle of the iris.

minor connector ➲ connector.

minus lens method in optometry, a method of measuring the monocular amplitude of accommodation which consists in placing minus lenses in front of one eye while the subject fixates the smallest optotypes (usually subtending about one minute of arc, that is the 6/6 or 20/20 line). Progressively stronger lenses are used until the patient reports that the test appears blurred. The determination of the amplitude must take into account the vergence at the eye of the fixation point and the test must be carried out with the patient's distance correction. If the minus lens to blur is $-4D$ and the fixation distance 40 cm, the amplitude will be equal to 6.5D. ➲ amplitude of accommodation, subjective accommodation.

minute ventilation or volume also known as pulmonary ventilation. The volume of air moved into ($\dot{V}_I$) and out ($\dot{V}_E$) of the lungs in 1 minute. It is tidal volume × respiratory rate. ➲ ventilation.

mio, meio- a prefix that means 'smaller, less', e.g. *miosis*.

miosis (myosis) *n* constriction of the pupil of the eye.

miotic (myotic) *adj* an agent that causes miosis such as the drug pilocarpine. ➲ Appendix 5.

MIP *abbr* maximum inspiratory pressure.

mire a pattern used in an optical instrument to guide the observer. Examples include the luminous pattern seen in a keratometer; the two half-circles seen in an applanation tonometer. ➲ keratometer/ophthalmometer.

MIS *abbr* minimally invasive surgery.

miscarriage *n* spontaneous loss of pregnancy before 24 completed weeks of gestation (also referred to as abortion by health professionals). ➲ complete miscarriage, incomplete miscarriage, inevitable miscarriage, missed miscarriage, septic miscarriage, spontaneous miscarriage, threatened miscarriage, tubal miscarriage.

miscible able to be mixed so as to form a homogeneous substance.

missed abortion ➲ missed miscarriage.

missed miscarriage the early signs and symptoms of pregnancy disappear and the fetus dies but is not expelled for some time. ➲ carneous mole.

Misuse of Drugs Act (1971, Regulations 1985) in UK. Controls the manufacture, sale, possession, supply, storage, prescribing, dispensing and administration of certain groups of habit-forming drugs that are liable to misuse and dependence. They are called controlled drugs and are available to the public by prescription only. Drugs subject to the Act include the opioids, synthetic narcotics, cocaine, hallucinogens and barbiturates (with exceptions). The individual drugs include cocaine, diamorphine (heroin), methadone and pethidine. ➲ Appendix 5.

Mitchell's osteotomy (CL Mitchell, American orthopaedic surgeon, 20th century) a surgical procedure involving a distal osteotomy of the first metatarsal. Used for hallux valgus (bunion). It entails the lateral displacement of the distal end of the first metatarsal; slight shortening of the bone; and tightening of the medial soft tissues to correct the valgus angle at the first metatarsophalangeal joint.

Mitchell's trimmer used in dentistry. A multi-purpose hand instrument with spoonshaped end and an angled pointed blade, triangular in section.

Mitchell theory theory of latent image formation states that free silver ions come near to a shallow electron trap and deepens it, while this trap is deepened it attracts another electron and a free silver ion to form a silver atom called the pre-image centre. This then dissociates into a silver ion and an electron, the silver atom must attract a second silver ion to form a latent sub-image centre, this attracts further electrons causing a build up of silver atoms which eventually destroy the crystal lattice and allows development to take place. ➲ Gurney Mott theory.

mite a minute arachnid related to ticks and spiders. Several species are parasitic, including *Sarcoptes scabiei* which causes scabies. Some are responsible for spreading scrub typhus ➲ Trombiculidae. The house dust mite of the genus *Dermatophagoides* is an important cause of allergic asthma. ➲ house dust mite.

mitochondrial disorders result from the inheritance of faulty mitochondrial DNA. The effects of the disorders can be very variable and occur at any age. Examples include diabetes mellitus with deafness, Leber hereditary optic neuropathy, Leigh's disease and several mitochondrial myopathy syndromes.

mitochondrial genes there are a number of genes present in the mitochondria, they encode several proteins. Mitochondrial genes are inherited from the woman and mutations do occur.

mitochondrial myopathy, encephalopathy, lactic acidosis and stroke-like episodes (MELAS) a mitochondrial myopathy syndrome. It is characterized by episodic encephalopathy, stroke-like episodes often preceded by migraine-like headaches, nausea and vomiting. ➲ mitochondrial myopathy syndromes.

M
N

mitochondrial myopathy syndromes a group of inherited disorders of the oxidative pathways of the respiratory chain in mitochondria, which may be associated with a range of other deficits in the nervous system, including episodic stroke-like events and myoclonic epilepsy. Many of these mitochondrial myopathies (or cytopathies) are inherited via the mitochondrial genome, down the maternal line. There is often a characteristic 'ragged-red fibre' change on muscle biopsy. ➲ chronic progressive external ophthalmoplegia (CPEO), Kearns–Sayre syndrome, mitochondrial myopathy encephalopathy lactic acidosis and stroke-like episodes (MELAS), myoclonic epilepsy with ragged red fibres (MERRF).

mitochondrion *n* a membrane-bound subcellular organelle situated in the cytoplasm. They are the principal sites of the oxidative phosphorylation of ADP to produce ATP from the oxidation of fuel molecules. They contain nucleic acids (DNA and RNA) and ribosomes, replicate independently, and synthesize some of their own proteins. They are particularly numerous in metabolically active cells, such as skeletal muscle and liver. ➲ electron transfer/transport chain, Krebs' cycle.

mitosis *n* nuclear (and usually cell) division, in which somatic cells divide. It involves the exact replication of chromosomes, which results in two 'daughter' cells that are genetically identical to the cell of origin, i.e. they have the diploid (2n) chromosome number, 46 in humans (Figure M.7). ➲ meiosis—**mitoses** *pl*, **mitotic** *adj*.

mitotic index the ratio between the number of cells undergoing mitosis and the number of cells in total. It provides an indication of the rate of cell proliferation.

mitral *adj* mitre-shaped.

mitral (bicuspid) regurgitation (incompetence) the commonest defect associated with rheumatic heart disease. Changes in the chordae tendineae and papillary muscle of one or both cusps of the mitral valve, or dilatation of the valve ring, cause the valve to remain open during systole. The failure of the mitral valve to properly close means that blood tends to flow backwards (regurgitate) into the left atrium from the left ventricle. ➲ systolic murmur.

mitral (bicuspid) stenosis narrowing of the mitral orifice, usually due to rheumatic fever. The mitral valve is damaged and narrowed and blood flow between the left atrium and left venticle is impeded. Calcification of the valve may cause further narrowing and stiffness. ➲ mid-diastolic murmur.

mitral valve also know as the bicuspid valve (having two cusps). The atrioventricular valve between the left atrium and ventricle of the heart.

mitral valvulotomy (valvotomy) an operation to correct a stenosed mitral valve.

mittelschmerz *n* abdominal pain midway between menstrual periods, at time of ovulation.

mixed connective tissue disease an overlap connective tissue disease with features of systemic lupus erythematosus (SLE), systemic sclerosis and myositis. The usual clinical

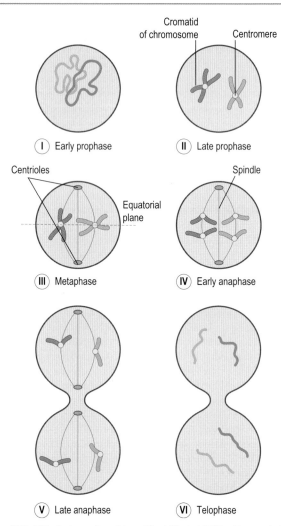

M.7 Mitosis (reproduced from Hinchliff et al 1996 with permission).

features include synovitis and oedema of the hands in combination with Raynaud's phenomenon and muscle pain/weakness. Most patients have anti-ribonucleoprotein (RNP) antibodies, although these also occur in SLE without overlap features.

mixed dentition dentition consisting of primary and permanent teeth during the period when the primary teeth are being shed.

mixed economy of welfare a means of describing the diversity of ways in which services are funded and delivered. This includes the statutory, voluntary and private sectors as well as informal care.

mixed hearing loss/deafness partial or total hearing loss due to the combined effects of an interruption of the conduction of sound waves from the atmosphere to the inner ear (conduction hearing loss/deafness) and a sensorineural defect.

mixed incontinence ⊃ incontinence.

mixed parotid tumour slow-growing adenoma of the parotid salivary gland. A benign growth of epithelial origin which may become malignant. Treatment is by excision.

mixed saliva ⊃ whole saliva.

mixed venous blood the blood flowing into the right side of the heart and thence out to the lungs in the pulmonary artery, which is a mixture of venous blood from the whole of the systemic circulation (i.e. from all parts of the body except the lungs). May be sampled by cardiac catheterization, for estimates of whole body arteriovenous difference. ⊃ arteriovenous (A-V) difference, oxygen dissociation curve.

mixed venous oxygen saturation (S$\bar{v}$O$_2$) percentage of oxygenated haemoglobin in venous blood returning to the lungs, measured in blood taken from the pulmonary artery.

mixing pad in dentistry, a pad of treated paper sheets on which powders, liquids or pastes may be mixed.

mixing slab in dentistry, a rectangular slab, usually of glass or glazed pottery, on which dental materials are mixed. One surface may be ground. When cooled the thickness of the slab retains its cool condition allowing for a slower mixing and setting time.

mixing time in dentistry, that part of the working time required to complete a satisfactory mix of the components of a material. The manufacturer's instructions for the mixing time of their products should be followed carefully. ⊃ manipulation time, working time.

mixing valve in radiography, a method of controlling the water and temperature of a unit by mixing the hot and cold water supplies together, found in automatic film processors.

mL *abbr* millilitre.

MLC *abbr* **1.** multi-leaf collimation. **2.** myosin light chains.

MLNS *abbr* mucocutaneous lymph node syndrome.

MLSO *abbr* Medical Laboratory Scientific Officer.

MLSS *abbr* maximum lactate steady state.

mm *abbr* millimetre.

MMAS *abbr* Modified Motor Assessment Scale.

mmHg *abbr* millimetres of mercury.

M mode motion modulation in ultrasound imaging when a linear scan is held while a time position graph of any motion builds up. Stationary parts are shown as straight lines and moving parts as oscillations, used in cardiac procedures to assess distances and the movement of objects.

mmol *abbr* millimole.

MMR *abbr* measles, mumps and rubella (vaccine).

MMSE *abbr* Mini Mental State Examination.

MND *abbr* motor neuron disease.

MO *abbr* medical officer.

MOA *abbr* medium opening activator.

mobile epidural low concentration of bupivacaine, sometimes with an opiate, administered into the epidural space by a 'patient-controlled epidural analgesic system' (PCEAS) pump so the woman can be mobile during labour. Pain relief may not be as complete as with conventional epidural anaesthesia. Normal labour observations should be continued and monitoring the woman's respiratory rate undertaken.

mobile unit (or cart) in dental practice, an assembly of instruments that can be moved.

mobility 1. ability to sit, stand, reach and move about. **2.** capable of movement or free flow. **3.** in dentistry, the looseness of a tooth. A numerical periodontal index of mobility may be charted according to the degree of mobility of each tooth. ⊃ mobility test.

mobility test in dentistry, a diagnostic test to determine the degree of mobility of one tooth in relation to its supporting structures.

mobilizations *npl* the manual manipulations of spinal and peripheral (limb) joints in order to free them to move more normally. Physiotherapists use several methods named for their developers, e.g. Maitland mobilizations. Whereas osteopaths and chiropractors mobilize joints with the aim of restoring function, physiotherapists also mobilize muscles, nerves and other soft tissues in order to relieve pain and restore freedom of movement. ⊃ Maitland grades.

mobilize *v* to make ready for movement. *mobilizing a patient* locomotion. *mobilize joints and soft tissues* free them to move more normally.

Mobitz type I heart block (W Mobitz, German physician, 1889–1951) a type of second degree atrioventricular (AV) block in which the P-R interval becomes progressively longer. Also known as Wenckebach heart block or phenomenon.

Mobitz type II heart block (W Mobitz) a rarer type of second degree atrioventricular (AV) block in which there is a sudden failure to conduct the atrial impulse through the atrioventricular node to the ventricle, without any lengthening of the P-R interval.

modal dose the most frequently occurring dose value in a chart.

modality 1. a sensation, such as the sense of hearing, smell, taste, touch, vision. **2.** the form or method of treatment or therapy. For example, cognitive therapies, medication, occupational therapy, physiotherapy, radiotherapy, speech and language therapy, surgery, etc.

mode *n* the most frequent (common) value in a series of scores. ⊃ central tendency statistic, mean, median.

model in the context of scientfic methodology, a simplified representation of a more complex reality. In physiology and related disciplines, the term may be applied to a physical model (e.g. an animal preparation); more widely throughout science it indicates a mental or formal (e.g. mathematical) representation. A good model of either sort enables clear and, ideally, quantitative predictions to be made; testing these predictions will thus provide evidence as to whether the simplified concepts embodied in the model sufficiently approximate the real-world system. ⊃ falsificationism, verificationism.

model A replica a three-dimensional shape representing a likeness of an existing object. In dentistry, a cast, i.e. a positive and accurate reproduction of the dentition and adjacent structures. *model A replica base former* a flexible mould used to form an acceptable base shape for plaster of Paris models, especially orthodontic models. *model A replica cement* a deprecated term for sticky wax.

model for practice a simplified representation of the components and process of intervention in a particular area of practice. A model for practice identifies the goals of intervention and suggests what actions might be taken to reach them.

modelling *n* a psychological term describing the way people learn from watching and copying the behaviour of others. Often utilized in behavioural therapies. In the context of sports training, a method whereby a person learns a skill or action by imitating another person (the model) demonstrating the skill or action. The model can be live or videotaped.

modelling wax (*syn* pink wax) a blend of waxes, usually pink, orange or red in colour, that is pliable at room temperature. Used in dentistry. The softening temperature range varies according to its intended use.

models of nursing ⊃ nursing models.

modem *abbr* **mo**dulator-**dem**odulator.

moderating variable in statistics, a variable that alters the direction or strength of the relationship between an independent or predictor variable and a dependent or criterion variable. For example, the effects of an intervention might differ depending on the gender of the participants. In this case, gender would be a moderating variable. ⊃ mediating variable.

modified Ashworth scale ⊃ Ashworth scale.

Modified Motor Assessment Scale (MMAS) ⊃ Motor Assessment Scale.

modified New York criteria criteria for the diagnosis of ankylosing spondylitis (1984), they are: (a) low-back pain for at least 3 months, improved by exercise and not relieved by rest; (b) limitation of lumbar spine movement in sagittal and frontal planes; (c) chest expansion decreased relative to normal values for age and sex; (d) bilateral sacroiliitis, grade 2–4; and (e) unilateral sacroiliitis, grade 3–4.

Modified Oxford scale (for pelvic floor contraction) a scale for describing the strength of pelvic floor contraction, it was developed by J Laycock in 1994. There are six grades: grade 0—no response, grade 1—minimal response with a flicker only, grade 2—weak contraction, grade 3—contraction moderate, with some lift, grade 4—contraction good strength, the woman can contract her pelvic floor against a degree of resistance and, 5—muscle contraction normal. The score is used to select the most suitable treatment option. ⊃ incontinence (stress incontinence). (Laycock J. (1994) *Clinical evaluation of the pelvic floor*. In: Pelvic Floor Re-education: Principles and Practice. eds. B Schussler, J Laycock, P Norton, S Stanton. Springer-Verlag, London.)

modified radical mastectomy ⊃ mastectomy.

modifier in dentistry, an agent that alters or changes a material without transforming it.

modiolus 1. the bony central pillar of the cochlea. ⊃ cochlea, ear. **2.** the point distal to the corner of the mouth where several facial muscles converge and which stabilize the cheeks and lips.

MODS *abbr* multiple organ dysfunction syndrome.

modulation an electrotherapy term. The systematic variations in one or more characteristics of a current. For example, amplitude modulation occurs with crossed sinusoidal currents with quadripolar and premodulated interferential therapy, the amplitude of successive pulses in each beat systematically increases to a peak and then decreases. The process repeats in the next beat. Some transcutaneous electrical nerve stimulation (TENS) machines offer frequency or pulse duration modulations or a combination of these to reduce adaptation to electrical stimulation.

modulation transfer function (MTF) in radiography, the assessment of an imaging system's performance at different object sizes.

modulator-demodulator (modem) a device, also known as an acoustic coupler, which allows the computer to transmit data down a conventional telephone line.

modulus of elasticity (*syn* coefficient of elasticity, Young's modulus of elasticity) the ratio of a force applied to a material to the increment of change (e.g. increase in length; angular deformation) in that material. Materials with low modulus of elasticity are less resistant to stress, while materials with high modulus of elasticity resist stress and hold their shape better. *Examples*: the modulus of elasticity of the crystalline lens capsule decreases progressively with age, being about $6 \times 10^7 \text{dyne/cm}^2$ in childhood and $1.5 \times 10^7 \text{ dyne/cm}^2$ in very old age; the modulus of elasticity of a contact lens is about $2000 \times 10^5 \text{ dyne/cm}^2$ in PMMA lenses, $500–1500 \times 10^5 \text{ dyne/cm}^2$ in siloxane acrylate gas-permeable lenses and $65–75 \times 10^5 \text{dyne/cm}^2$ in high water hydrogel lenses.

MODY *abbr* maturity onset diabetes of the young.

Möebius' sign convergence weakness; one of the eye signs occurring in Graves' hyperthyroid disease. ⊃ Graves' ophthalmopathy.

Mohs hardness scale or number (MHN) ⊃ hardness scale.

Mohs' micrographic surgery a surgical technique developed by F Mohs in the 1930s. It is a microscopically controlled excision usually of a malignant skin tumour. In particular basal cell carcinoma, squamous cell carcinoma and malignant melanoma.

moiré effect (*syn* moiré pattern) an illusory shimmering movement produced by moving one pattern superimposed on another pattern very similar to it. The phenomenon occurs because parts of the periodic patterns are in phase in some locations, and out of phase in other locations. For example: passing by a set of railings; if a transilluminated square wave grating is superimposed on an identical grating but cross each other at an angle of less than 45°, moiré fringes will appear at the intersections.

M
N

moist gangrene occurs when venous drainage is inadequate so that the tissues are swollen with fluid. ➲ gangrene.

moist wound environment débridement ➲ débridement.

moist wound healing achieved by application of an occlusive, semipermeable dressing which permits enough exudate to collect under the film to carry out its bactericidal functions and maintain wound hydration.

molality *n* the concentration of a solution expressed as the number of moles of solute (substance) per kilogram of water or other solvent.

molar *adj* describes a solution containing one mole of solute (substance) per litre of solution.

molariform having a molar shape.

molar pregnancy (previously known as a hydatidiform mole) a pregnancy in which the placental (trophoblastic) tissue shows degenerative stoma combined with neoplastic chorionic endothelium. Molar pregnancy is associated with raised levels of the hormone human chorionic gonadotrophin (hCG). It may develop as a partial (incomplete) mole or a complete mole. Molar pregnancy can be diagnosed by ultrasound examination during early pregnancy; in addition levels of hCG in the blood will be measured if a molar pregnancy is suspected. A *partial (incomplete) mole* has a chromosomally abnormal fetus (triploid chromosome complement). Whereas, a *complete mole* shows abnormal proliferation of the trophoblast and the presence of hydropic placental villi with no fetal parts. It comprises vesicles that resemble a bunch of grapes. The abnormal molar tissue is removed from the cavity of the uterus by dilatation and evacuation/curettage, but some women will also require chemotherapy. A malignant transformation to choriocarcinoma may occur, especially in pregnancies affected by a complete mole. Therefore women are followed up in a specialist unit to ensure early detection of malignant changes. Monitoring involves regular measurements of the levels of hCG in blood and urine. In the UK referral for follow up will be to one of three specialist centres (Dundee, London or Sheffield). ➲ choriocarcinoma, gestational trophoblastic tumour, invasive mole, placental site trophoblastic tumour.

molar tooth the posterior grinding teeth.They have broad multicuspal occlusal surfaces (see Figure T.4b, p. 779). There are eight primary molars, two in each quadrant, and 12 permanent molars, three in each quadrant. The upper molars normally have three roots and the lower molars have two roots. The permanent most posterior molars tend to have fused roots.

molarity *n* the concentration of a solution expressed as the number of moles of solute (substance) per litre of solution (mol/L).

mole *n* 1. one of the seven base units of the Système International d'Unités (SI) (International System of Units). The measurement of amount of substance (*abbr* mol). ➲ Appendix 2. A mole of any substance is the amount that will contain the same number of elementary particles (e.g. atoms or molecules) as there are atoms contained within 12 g of carbon-12 (6.02×10^{23}). This number is known as Avogadro's number. **2.** a pigmented area on the skin, usually brown. They may be flat, some are raised and occasionally have hairs growing from them. Alterations in shape, colour, size, or bleeding may be indicative of malignant changes.

molecular *adj* relating to molecules.

molecular distortion when the electron orbits are deformed relative to the atomic nucleus.

molecular weight the sum of the atomic weights of atoms in a molecule.

molecule *n* combination of two or more atoms to form a specific chemical substance. The smallest part of a compound that can exist on its own and retain all the properties of the compound—**molecular** *adj*.

mollities *n* softness.

mollities ossium ➲ osteomalacia.

Moll's glands (J Moll, Dutch ophthalmologist, 1832–1914) (*syn* ciliary sweat glands) sweat glands of the eyelids. They are situated in the region of the eyelashes. ➲ eyelids, hordeolum.

molluscum *n* soft swellings, masses, nodules or tumour.

molluscum contagiosum an infectious condition common in children, caused by a poxvirus. It is characterized by the formation of tiny translucent papules with a central depression.

molluscum fibrosum the superficial tumours of von Recklinghausen's disease.

molten metal sterilizer ➲ sterilizer.

MOM *abbr* multiple of the median.

moment arm the distance between an applied force and the fulcrum (pivot or axis) in a lever system.

moment of force the rotational 'turning effect' of a force. Calculated as the product of the force and the perpendicular (i.e. at 90°) distance between the point of application (and direction) of the force and the pivot; also known as torque. ➲ net moment of force.

moment of inertia a body or object's resistance to angular acceleration or deceleration. Depends on the mass of the object and the distribution of the mass in relation to the point of rotation. The summation of all the masses of the parts of the body multiplied by their distance squared from the axis of rotation ($I = \Sigma mr^2$) or the mass of the whole body multiplied by the radius of gyration squared.

momentum the 'quantity of motion' of a body or object. A vector quantity. ➲ angular momentum, linear momentum.

monarticular *adj* relating to one joint.

Mönckeberg's sclerosis (J Mönckeberg, German pathologist, 1877–1925) degenerative change resulting in calcification of the median muscular layer in arteries, especially of the limbs; leads to intermittent claudication and rarely to gangrene, if atherosclerosis coexists.

Monge's disease (C Monge-Mendrano, Peruvian pathologist, 1884–1970). ➲ chronic mountain sickness.

M
N

Mongolian blue spot a bluish-black area of skin on the sacral area of some neonates. It is commomer in infants with darker skins and usually disappears during childhood.

Monilia *n* ⊃ *Candida*.

moniliasis *n* ⊃ candidiasis.

Monitor *n* an anglicized version of the Rush Medicus quality assurance programme for use in hospitals.

monitor a device similar to a television, but which receives video signals directly from the computer, rather than RE-modulated signals, giving much more accurate resolution.

monitor photography the imaging of the video output from computed tomography (CT), magnetic resonance imaging (MRI) or ultrasound unit via a camera system.

monitoring *n* sequential recording. Term usually reserved for automatic visual display of such measurements as temperature, pulse, respiration and blood pressure.

monitoring badge ⊃ dosimeter, dosemeter.

monitrice a labour coach, usually a person with special training in the Lamaze method of childbirth. ⊃ Lamaze method.

monkey pox despite the name, the animal reservoirs for this virus are probably small squirrels and rodents. It causes a rare zoonotic infection in primitive communities in the rainforest belt of central Africa, producing a vesicular rash indistinguishable from smallpox. Little to no person-to-person transmission occurs. ⊃ smallpox.

mono- a prefix that means 'one, single', e.g. *monoclonal*.

monoamine *n* organic molecules with one amine (NH_2) group. Examples include adrenaline (epinephrine), dopamine, histamine, 5-hydroxytryptamine (serotonin), melatonin, noradrenaline (norepinephrine). ⊃ amines.

monoamine oxidase an enzyme that breaks down monoamines, such as dopamine, 5-hydroxytryptamine (serotonin) and noradrenaline (norepinephrine) in the brain.

monoamine oxidase inhibitors (MAOIs) a group of anti-depressant drugs (e.g. phenelzine, isocarboxazid) that inhibit the action of monoamine oxidase thereby preventing the breakdown of 5-hydroxytryptamine (5-HT) and other monoamines. MAOIs interact with amine-containing drugs such as decongestants which results in an increase in their pressor effect. There is a similar interaction with the tyramine present in some foods. Patients should be advised to avoid mature cheese, products made from fermented soya bean (e.g. soya sauce), meat and yeast extracts that include Bovril® and Marmite®, the pods of broad beans, pickled herring, any stale meat, offal or fish; they should also avoid game (because amines are formed when game is hung), alcoholic drinks and low-alcohol alternatives. ⊃ Appendix 5.

monoamniotic twins monozygotic twins who develop within a single amnion.

monoarthritis *n* arthritis affecting a single joint.

monoblast *n* an immature cell formed in the bone marrow during the development of the monocytes (white blood cells). Its presence in the blood is abnormal and is indicative of some types of leukaemia.

monocarboxylate transporters transmembrane carrier molecules, co-transporting monocarboxylic acid anions (typically lactate) and protons (H^+) through cell membranes, notably those of skeletal and cardiac muscle fibres. Considered to be responsible for the major part of lactate transport at low concentrations but, as saturation of the carrier approaches, simple diffusion (which is primarily of the undissociated lactic acid) becomes more important. ⊃ lactate, lactic acid.

monochorionic twins monozygotic twins who develop within a single chorion.

monochromat *n* an individual who is totally colour blind, i.e. has the condition of monochromatism. There are two types of monochromats: the *cone monochromat* whose photopic luminosity curve resembles the normal and who has normal visual acuity and dark adaptation; and the *rod monochromat* whose retina does not contain functional cones and, therefore, has poor vision, photophobia and some-times associated nystagmus and myopia. Monochromats are very rare: estimated at about three persons in 100 000. ⊃ achromatopsia, cone, defective colour vision.

monochromatic aberration (*syn* Seidel aberration) a defect of an optical system (eye, lens, prism, etc.) occurring for a single wavelength of light. There are five such aberrations: spherical aberration, coma, curvature of field, oblique astigmatism and distortion.

monochromatic emulsions in radiography, the film emulsions that are unable to detect any colours apart from the blue part of the visible spectrum, tend to be used with calcium tungstate screens. ⊃ orthochromatic emulsions, panchromatic emulsions.

monochromatic light light consisting of a single wave-length or, more usually, of a narrow band of wavelengths (a few nanometres).

monochromatism total colour blindness. ⊃ achromatopsia, defective colour vision, monochromat.

monoclonal *adj* arising from a single B lymphocyte/cell and its subsequent clones, e.g. monoclonal antibodies (MAb).

monoclonal antibodies (MAb) identical, specific anti-bodies that are increasingly used in research, and for diag-nostic assays and in treatment of cancers and other diseases. For example, bevacizumab and cetuximab for metastatic colorectal cancers; trastuzumab for some early-stage breast cancers, and metastatic breast cancer; omalizumab for asthma; and infliximab, which is used for several diseases including rheumatoid arthritis, inflammatory bowel disease and ankylosing spondylitis. Other monoclonal antibodies are currently being developed for use in the management of a wide range of disease processes.

monoclonal gammopathy of uncertain significance (MGUS) (*syn* benign monoclonal gammopathy, monoclonal gammopathy unclassified) a condition in which a paraprotein is present in the blood but with no other features of myeloma, Waldenström macroglobulinaemia, lymphoma or related disease. It is a common condition associated with increasing age; a paraprotein can be found in 1% aged over 50 years increasing to 5% over 80 years. Patients are usually asymptomatic, and the paraprotein is found on blood testing for other reasons. The routine blood count and biochemistry are normal, the paraprotein is usually present in small amounts with no associated immune paresis, and there are no lytic bone lesions. The bone marrow may have increased plasma cells but these usually constitute less than 10% of nucleated cells. After follow-up of 20 years, only one-quarter will progress to myeloma or a related disorder. There is no way of predicting progression in an individual patient and if investigations remain stable, annual monitoring is all that is required.

monoclonal gammopathy unclassified ⊃ monoclonal gammopathy of uncertain significance (MGUS).

monocular *adj* pertaining to one eye.

monocyte *n* a phagocytic white blood cell that has a kidney-shaped nucleus. Monocytes migrate to the tissues to become macrophages—**monocytic** *adj*. ⊃ macrophages.

monocyte-macrophage system (*syn.* reticuloendothelial system, mononuclear-phagocytic system) a widely disseminated system of specialized phagocytic cells in the bone marrow, alveoli, liver, lymph nodes, spleen, connective tissue, neural tissue, and other tissues. Its functions include blood cell and haemoglobin breakdown, formation of bile pigments, removal of cell breakdown products and as part of the defences against micro-organisms. ⊃ macrophages.

monocytopenia *n* a deficiency of monocytes in the peripheral blood.

monocytosis *n* an increase in the number of monocytes in the peripheral blood. The causes include some types of leukaemia and lymphomas, chronic inflammation such as with tuberculosis and autoimmune conditions.

monodactylism *n* a congenital deformity in which there is a single digit on a hand or foot.

monoenergetic single energy.

monomania *n* obsession with a single idea.

monomer **1.** a small molecule, usually organic, that bonds with other molecules (the same or different) to form polymers. Examples include: glucose bonding with other glucose molecules to form polymers of glycogen, starch and so on; and amino acids that form bonds with each other to create an enormous variety of polypeptides and proteins. ⊃ polymer. **2.** in dentistry, it refers to methylmethacrylate, a clear liquid with a characteristic smell which can be mixed with polymer powder to make a dough which polymerizes, hardens or cures, to form acrylic. Used in the construction of dental prostheses and appliances.

mononeuropathy *n* a disorder that affects a single nerve. Includes entrapment, compression from a cast or splint, the effects of radiation, or trauma.

mononuclear *adj* describes a cell with a single nucleus such as a monocyte.

monocular diplopia diplopia seen by one eye only. It is usually caused by irregular refraction in one eye (e.g. in early cataracts) or by dicoria or polycoria. It may be induced by placing a biprism in front of one eye. ⊃ cataract, dicoria, diplopia, diplopia test, ghost image, luxation of the lens, polycoria.

mononucleosis *n* an increase in the number of circulating monocytes (mononuclear cells) in the blood. ⊃ infectious mononucleosis.

monoparesis paralysis or weakness affecting a single limb or part of a limb. ⊃ hemiparesis, paraparesis, paresis, quadriparesis

monophasic an electrotherapy term. Describes a pulse with one phase. ⊃ high voltage pulsed stimulation, phases.

monoplegia *n* paralysis of only one limb—**monoplegic** *adj.*

monorchism also called monorchidism. The presence of a single testis in the scrotum. Due to the failure of the other testis to descend from the abdomen.

monosaccharide *n* a single sugar carbohydrate with the general formula $(CH_2O)_n$. They may have between 3 or 9 carbon atoms, for instance ribose is a pentose sugar with 5-carbon atoms, and glucose, fructose and galactose are hexoses with 6-carbon atoms. They are the basic unit from which other carbohydrates are formed. Monosaccharide units link together to produce disaccharides and polysaccharides.

monounsaturated fatty acid (MUFA) a fatty acid that has one double bond in its structure, such as oleic acid. They are present in olive oil, avocados, canola oil (rapeseed oil), peanuts, oil in almonds, pecans, etc. ⊃ fatty acids, oleic oil.

monosodium glutamate a sodium salt used as a flavour enhancer in savoury foods, such as soups.

monosomy *n* a type of aneuploidy. The absence of a chromosome from the normal diploid chromosome complement, resulting in 45 chromosomes rather than 46. For example, in Turner's syndrome where the female has XO instead of XX. ⊃ aneuploidy, polyploidy, trisomy.

monotrophy a woman's ability to bond with only one child of twins at a time. This may happen if one infant has remained in a special care unit after discharge of its sibling.

monovular *adj* ⊃ uniovular.

monozygotic *adj* relating to one zygote. Describes identical twins that develop from a single zygote that splits into two embryos. ⊃ dizygotic *opp*, monoamniotic twins, monochorionic twins.

Monsons' curve ⊃ curve.

mons veneris also called mons pubis. The eminence formed by the pad of fat which lies over the symphysis pubis in the female. It is covered with pubic hair from the time of puberty.

Monteggia's fracture-dislocation (G Monteggia, Italian physician, 1762–1815) an angular fracture at the junction of the proximal and middle third of ulna with associated dislocation of the head of the radius.

Montgomery's glands (W Montgomery, Irish obstetrician, 1797–1859) also known as areolar glands. Sebaceous glands in the areola surrounding the nipple.

M
N

monthly index of medical specialties (MIMS) a monthly publication containing the drugs that are currently available for prescription in the United Kingdom.

mood *n* an involuntary state of mind or feeling. It is a temporary but relatively enduring positive or negative affective state. Typically differentiated from emotion in that a mood is of longer duration and not necessarily evoked in response to a specific event. Mood variations are normal, but frequent swings from depression to over-excitement may be considered abnormal. ➲ affect, bipolar affective disorder, cyclothymia, depression, emotion, mania.

Moon's probe a dental instrument. A blunt, flat-handled probe used to explore sinuses.

Moon's teeth ➲ tooth.

Mooren's ulcer (A Mooren, German ophthalmologist, 1829–1899) peripheral ulcerative keratitis.

Moore's mandrel a split stud mandrel with latch-type end to its shank for contra-angled handpieces or smooth-end shank for straight handpieces. Used with discs and wheels.

moral development the development of a sense of right or wrong in children during the course of maturation through the influence of the social environment. Some developmentalists and educationalists claim that involvement in sport in childhood can assist in the process of moral development.

Moraxella a genus of Gram negative, non-motile bacteria. They are present as commensals and pathogens on the mucosal surfaces. *Moraxella catarrhalis* causes respiratory tract infections and otitis media. *M. lacunata* causes conjunctivitis.

morbidity *n* the state of being diseased. ➲ standardized morbidity ratio (SMBR).

morbilli *n* ➲ measles.

morbilliform *adj* describes a rash resembling that of measles.

moribund *adj* in a dying state.

Moro reflex (E Moro, German paediatrician, 1874–1951) also called the startle reflex. A normal reflex observed in infants from birth to the age of 3–4 months. Whereby, on being startled the legs are flexed and the infant throws out their arms, then brings them together in an embracing movement (Figure M.8).

-morph a suffix that means 'form', e.g. *allelomorph*.

morphoea *n* ➲ scleroderma, systemic sclerosis.

morphogenesis the formation and differentiation of the body structures and form. Especially applied to that occurring during embryonic development.

morphology *n* the study of the form and structure of living things—**morphological** *adj*, **morphologically** *adv*.

Morquio–Brailsford disease (L Morquio, Uruguayan paediatrician, 1867–1935; J Brailsford, British radiologist, 1888–1961) a mucopolysaccharidoses. An inherited disease of mucopolysaccharide storage. It is transmitted as an autosomal recessive trait. The condition is characterized by faulty musculoskeletal development leading to short stature, macrocephaly with coarse facial features and widely-spaced

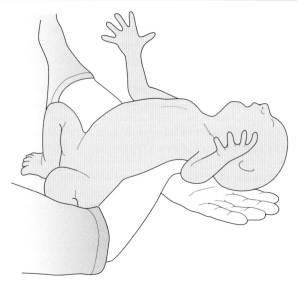

M.8 Moro or startle reflex (reproduced from Brooker 2006A with permission).

teeth, abnormal sternum, knock-knees and spinal curvature. In addition there is corneal clouding, hepatomegaly, aortic valve reguigation and neurological problems. ➲ mucopolysaccharidoses.

mortality *n* **1.** being subject to death. **2.** number or frequency of deaths.

mortality rate *n* the death rate; the ratio of the total number of deaths to the total population. There are several specialized mortality rates and ratios including: childhood mortality (children aged 1–14 years), infant mortality (first year of life), maternal mortality (deaths associated with pregnancy and childbirth), neonatal mortality (first four weeks of life), perinatal mortality (stillbirths plus deaths in the first week of life), stillbirth rate. ➲ standardized mortality rate, standardized mortality ratio.

mortar a glass receptacle with ground glass internal surface used with glass pestle to mix substances, by hand.

mortification *n* death of tissue. ➲ gangrene.

Morton's metatarsalgia (T Morton, American surgeon, 1835–1903) also called Morton's disease, Morton's neuroma. Painful neuralgia caused by a neuroma on the digital branches of the plantar nerves, most commonly that supplying the third toe cleft. Symptoms include pain and tingling in the two adjacent toes. In sport, most common in those where repetitive weight-bearing is a feature. The condition is exacerbated by ill-fitting shoes, so treatment is targeted to assess footwear and relieve pressure locally. Surgery may be required in resistant cases. ➲ metatarsalgia.

morula *n* a mass of cells formed from the cleavage (by mitosis) of the zygote prior to its implantation into the hormone-prepared uterine lining.

mosaicism *n* in genetics, a state in which an individual who develops from a single zygote has two or more cell populations that are genetically different. This may be seen

M
N

as differences in the number of chromosomes in the cells. For example, those affecting the sex chromosomes in Kleinfelter's syndrome and Turner's syndrome, or those affecting an autosomal chromosome such as in Down's syndrome.

mosquito a blood-sucking arthropod of the family *Culicidae*. They are important vectors of serious human diseases through their bite, for example malaria ⊃ *Aedes,* anopheles, filariasis, malaria, mosquito-transitted haemorrhagic fevers.

mosquito artery forceps ⊃ forceps.

mosquito-transmitted haemorrhagic fevers infections mainly occurring in tropical regions. The important ones are chikungunya, dengue, Rift Valley fever and yellow fever. ⊃ viral haemorrhagic fevers.

mossy fibre one of two fibre types (the other is a climbing fibre) carrying information to the cerebellar cortex. ⊃ climbing fibre.

mother board the main circuit board in a computer.

motile *adj* able to move spontaneously, such as certain bacteria and spermatozoa—**motility** *n*.

motilin a peptide hormone secreted by cells of the small intestine. It is concerned with gastrointestinal contraction and motility.

motion change in position of an object or body. *linear motion* motion which takes place in straight lines (rectilinear) or curves (curvilinear), but note that this does not apply to rotation. *general motion* motion which includes translation and rotation. ⊃ Newton's laws of motion.

motion sickness nausea and vomiting associated with any form of motion such as during journeys by car or plane.

motivation in psychology, the underlying causes of action. Without motivation an individual would not function. It is what impels or drives a person and is intimately related to their needs and is influenced by their emotions, values, beliefs and goals. Motivation provides people with the focus and stamina needed to undertake activities. Motivation is vitally important in the rehabilitation process and learning of skills. Motivation can be enhanced through achievement of goals and a positive learning environment. It can be adversely affected following brain injury due to factors such as poor memory, depression, cognitive and perceptual deficits.

motivation (in sport) the internal and external drives and forces that energize, direct and regulate behaviour. Motivation is often conceptualized in terms of direction (the behavioural goal) and intensity (the level of motivation from low to high). *extrinsic motivation* motivation directed towards the attainment of rewards that are separable from a behaviour or activity itself. For example, an athlete who engages in sport just to win medals would be extrinsically motivated. *intrinsic motivation* motivation driven by the pleasure and satisfaction inherent in engaging in a behaviour or activity. For example, an athlete who engages in sport purely for fun and enjoyment would be intrinsically motivated.

motivation (occupational therapy) a drive that directs a person's actions towards meeting needs. (Reproduced with permission from the European Network of Occupational Therapy in Higher Education (ENOTHE) Terminology Project, 2008.)

motivational climate the structure of the social environment with regard to the way that it influences individuals' motivation and motivational processes. In achievement goal theories it is typically described in terms of the extent to which the environment is oriented towards promoting task mastery and learning goals or social comparison and performance goals.

motivational hierarchy ⊃ need hierarchy theory.

motor *adj* pertaining to action.

motor agraphia inability to express thoughts in writing, usually due to left precentral cerebral lesions.

Motor Assessment Scale an outcome measure, used by physiotherapists, in the assessment of gross motor function. It has a modified version called the Modified Motor Assessment Scale (MMAS). It was developed by J Carr and R Shepherd and so is used by neurological physiotherapists using the motor relearning approach. ⊃ motor learning/relearning.

motor control the production and control of movement and the processes and mechanisms that underlie it. Also the study of such processes and mechanisms.

motor cortex that part of the cerebral cortex that controls voluntary skeletal muscle movement. It includes the primary motor area, motor speech area (Broca's area) and the premotor area which co-ordinates movements stimulated by the primary motor area.

motor end-plate term used variously to refer to the specialized region of skeletal muscle fibre membrane lying directly under the terminal of a motor nerve (the nerve's 'footprint' on the muscle, rich in receptors for acetylcholine, to which it responds by depolarization), or to the terminal arborization of the motor nerve. Now most frequently refers to both of these combined in the mammalian form of a neuromuscular junction. ⊃ motor unit. (Figure M.9.) ⊃ neuromuscular junction.

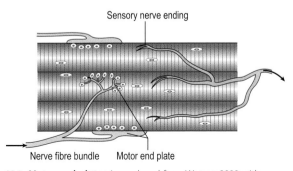

Sensory nerve ending

Nerve fibre bundle   Motor end plate

M.9 Motor end-plates (reproduced from Watson 2000 with permission).

motor evoked potentials (MEP) the stimulation of a nerve, the brain or spinal cord usually by an electrical (or magnetic) impulse and are recorded using electromyography.

motor fusion (*syn* disparity vergence, fusion reflex) one of the components of convergence in which the eyes move until the object of regard falls on corresponding retinal areas (e.g. the foveas) in response to disparate retinal stimuli. ⊃ disparate retinal points, fusional convergence, fusion field, retinal corresponding points, sensory fusion, vergence facility.

motor learning/relearning the internal processes that lead to an enduring change in a person's capacity for skilled movement. Also the study of such processes.

motor neuron(e) the nerve cell (or neuron) and its axon that supplies the electrical input to an effector structure, such as skeletal muscles. The upper motor neurons arise in the primary motor area of the cortex or the brainstem and directly or indirectly affect the functioning of the lower motor neurons. The axon runs to a synapse with another at a relay station, or directly with a lower motor neuron, the final link to muscle. The lower motor neuron directly innervates the muscle fibres or gland. The cell bodies of the lower motor neurons are in the anterior horns of grey matter in the spinal cord or in nuclei of cranial nerves. *alpha motor neurons* serve the main (extrafusal) skeletal muscle fibres; *gamma motor neurons* serve the (intrafusal) fibres of muscle spindles. ⊃ alpha(α) motor neuron, gamma (motor) system, motor unit, nerve fibre types, synapse.

motor neuron disease (MND) a group of neurodegenerative disorders affecting the nerves that supply the muscles. It is characterized by the progressive degeneration of anterior horn cells, corticospinal tracts and brainstem nuclei. Clinical features include weakness, loss of movement, pain, dyspnoea, dysarthria, dysphagia and other problems, (e.g. muscle wasting, spastic or flaccid weakness, muscle fasciculation, increased reflexes, decreased control of expression, tongue wasting and diaphragmatic paralysis) depending on the part of the nervous system affected and eventually death. Sensation and cognitive functions remains intact. ⊃ amyotrophic lateral sclerosis.

motor neuron pool all the alpha (α) motor neurons that supply the muscle fibres in an individual muscle.

motor pathways the descending pathways that arise from the brain and take movement signals primarily down to the neuronal pools in the spinal cord. The corticospinal tract is the principle route by which voluntary commands reach the motor neurones in the spinal cord.

motor pattern a co-ordinated set of movements involving both voluntary and reflex actions, such as standing, sitting, etc. Typically the initiation and cessation of such acts are voluntary but once initiated, the movements continue without conscious control.

motor point the point on a muscle or muscle belly where the supplying motor nerve enters. The small region of a skeletal muscle in which motor end-plates are aggregated; the muscle is most sensitive to electrical stimulation at this point. The usual guideline is at the junction of the upper and middle thirds of a muscle belly. The threshold for electrical stimulation at a motor point is lower than elsewhere in the muscle and is used clinically, the site of the active electrode when using unipolar stimulation technique and during strength–duration testing.

motor programme a prestructured set of commands stored in memory that, once initiated, organizes and controls a specific action or sequence of actions in an open-loop fashion without subsequent modification. *generalized motor programme* a motor programme for a class of similar actions that can be selected and modified according to the parameters (e.g. speed, direction) required for successful execution of a specific action from that class. For example, a generalized motor programme for jumping can be modified according to the distance, height, direction, etc. of a particular jump.

motor skill the ability to perform a particular task which involves significant movement of one or more joints of the body, e.g. as part of activities of daily living or a specific sports skill. A co-ordinated pattern of movements acquired through practice involving the ability to execute movements effectively to achieve intended outcomes. *gross motor skill* movement involving the co-ordinated use of large muscle groups, such as when kicking a ball. *fine motor skill* movement involving the ability to manipulate small objects.

motor unit a single motor neuron and the skeletal muscle fibres that it innervates and so controls, all of which must respond, virtually simultaneously, to an action potential in the nerve axon. The number of muscle fibres in a single motor unit ranges from about 10 to 2000: fewest in small muscles where the control is finest (e.g. for eye and finger movements) and most in large muscles (e.g. quadriceps group) designed for force rather than precision. ⊃ innervation ratio, muscle, neuromuscular junction.

motoricity index a measure of limb function with a maximum score of 100 for normal subjects. Used in neurological rehabilitation as a measure of function (impairment). Severe paralysis is defined as a score of 0–32, moderate as 33–64 and mild as 65–99.

mottle the granular appearance in areas of even density on a radiographic image. ⊃ film grain, quantum mottle, structure mottle.

mottling the surface marking of teeth caused by fluorosis or by drugs such as tetracycline.

mould *n* 1. a multicellular fungus. Often used synonymously with fungus (excluding the yeasts). It consists of filaments or hyphae, which aggregate into a mycelium. Propagates by means of spores. Occurs in infinite variety, as common saprophytes contaminating foodstuffs, and more rarely as pathogens. 2. to shape. 3. a hollow shape in which materials are cast or set.

mould chart an illustration of tooth moulds available from a particular artificial tooth manufacturer.

mould guide a mounted selection of artificial teeth available from a particular manufacturer.

moulding process of overriding of the fetal cranial bones at the sutures and fontanelles during passage through the maternal pelvis; the head is squeezed, changing shape and the length of various diameters. *normal moulding* in a vertex presentation the fetal head is well flexed; suboccipito-bregmatic and biparietal diameters present and decrease as the bones overlap, and the mentovertical diameter lengthens. (Figure M.10) *abnormal moulding* excessive or extremely rapid alterations in the diameters due to abnormal position in a cephalic presentation, such as a persistent occipitoposterior position, may cause tearing of the falx cerebri and tentorium cerebelli, leading to intracranial haemorrhage and possible death (Figure M.11).

mountain sickness ⊃ altitude sickness/illness (acute mountain sickness, AMS).

mounting 1. in dentistry, attaching a plaster case to an articulator. *mounting rings/plates* metal or plastic devices used to attach casts to an articulator. ⊃ articulator, split cast mounting. **2.** placing radiographs in a display card.

mouse a device for making the computer more 'user friendly'. Instead of accessing the computer via a keypad, the mouse is used by rolling/moving the device across a desktop, this moves a cursor to icon displays on the screen.

Mousseau-Barbin tube a plastic intubation tube which is pulled through an oesophageal tumour by the use of a string or guidewire and is attached to the stomach with a suture. Used to maintain a free passage of food and fluid.

mouth the mouth or oral cavity is bounded by muscles and bones: anteriorly—by the lips; posteriorly—it is continuous with the oropharynx; laterally—by the muscles of the cheeks; superiorly—by the bony hard palate and muscular soft palate; and inferiorly—by the muscular tongue and the soft tissues of the floor of the mouth. The oral cavity is lined throughout with mucous membrane, consisting of stratified squamous epithelium containing small mucus-secreting glands. The part of the mouth between the alveolar ridges and the cheeks is the vestibule and the remainder of the cavity is the oral cavity. The mucous membrane lining of the cheeks and the lips is reflected on to the gums or alveolar ridges and is continuous with the skin of the face. The palate forms the roof of the mouth and is divided into the anterior hard palate and the posterior soft palate. The bones forming the hard palate are the maxilla and the palatine bones. The soft palate is muscular, curves downwards from the posterior end of the hard palate and blends with the walls of the pharynx at the sides. The uvula is a curved fold of muscle covered with mucous membrane, hanging down from the middle of the free border of the soft palate. Originating from the upper end of the uvula there are four folds of mucous membrane, two passing downwards at each side to form membranous arches. The posterior folds, one on each side, are the palatopharyngeal arches and the two anterior folds are the palatoglossal arches. On each side, between the arches, is a collection of lymphoid tissue called the palatine tonsil.

mouth gag in dentistry, a two-handled instrument used to prise and hold the mouth open during an anaesthetic. It has a ratchet device to maintain the opening. The two blades are set at right angles so that they may be applied between the teeth and/or edentulous ridges. Mostly used while a mouth prop is being changed from one side to the other. Examples of mouth gags include: Mason, Ferguson, Doyen and Ackland types.

mouth guard an intraoral appliance worn during contact sports, such as boxing, rugby and hockey, to prevent or minimize damage to the teeth or other oral structures.

mouth mirror a reflecting surface designed for intraoral use and enabling the dental surgeon to see areas indirectly and to direct light into dark areas. Also used to hold the cheek and tongue away from the operating area. The mirror head unscrews from the handle. They are numbered according to size and are of three types: those reflecting from their front surfaces, those reflecting from their back surface and magnifying mirrors.

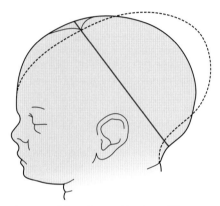

M.10 Moulding denoted by dotted line—vertex presentation, well flexed head (reproduced from Fraser & Cooper 2003 with permission).

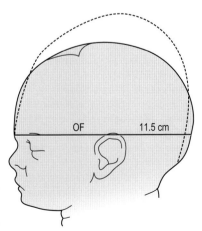

OF   11.5 cm

M.11 Upward moulding denoted by dotted line—following persistent occipitoposterior position. OF = occipitofrontal (reproduced from Fraser & Cooper 2003 with permission).

mouth prop in dentistry, a prop used during an anaesthetic to maintain the mouth in an open position. Hewitt's metal props and McKesson rubber props are in sets of three (of different sizes) joined together by a safety chain. The Lane centre prop is spring loaded and hinged so that its connecting bar may be swung from one side to the other without being removed from the mouth.

movement classification movement may be classified as passive, active assisted, active or resisted. *passive movement* a person falls asleep with their arm across a book; a friend arrives and lifts the sleeping person's arm to retrieve the book. This movement required no muscle action from the sleeping person and is, therefore, an example of passive movement. *active assisted movement* a person is helped by a friend to dress and the friend helps the person to lift their arm into a pullover. The person does some of the work, but so does their friend; the person's own muscles did some, but not all of the work. This is, therefore, an example of active assisted movement. *active movement* the person is now in the bathroom and reaches to grab the toothpaste. Their own muscles controlled the movement completely. This is, therefore, an example of active movement. *resisted movement* the person rushes down the hall; at the end of the hall a door sticks and the person needs to push it very hard. Their muscles have to work against an external force. This is, therefore, an example of resisted movement. ⊃ active movement, assisted active movement, passive movement, resisted movement.

movement diagram a concept that is useful in manipulative therapy that allows the therapist to analyse their results on examination. They have uses as self learning tools, teaching media and a means of communication.

movement science approach also known as motor relearning approach originally developed by J Carr and R Shepherd in the early 1980s. It is based on the model of motor learning and is used for the rehabilitation of patients following stroke. ⊃ motor learning/relearning.

movement threshold 1. the minimum motion of an object that can be perceived. **2.** The speed at which an object moving between two points just appears to be moving. ⊃ hyperacuity, phi movement.

movement unsharpness in radiography, blurring on an image due to movement of the equipment or the person which can be either voluntary or involuntary, for example heart beat.

moving and handling manual handling. All the activities including moving, lifting or supporting a load, which are subject to health and safety regulations.

moxibustion the use of burning mugwort (the aromatic herb *Artemisia vulgaris,* also known as moxa), to heat the needles during acupuncture. ⊃ acupuncture.

MPA *abbr* microscopic polyangiitis.

MPD *abbr* monocular pupillary distance.

MRC *abbr* Medical Research Council.

MRI *abbr* magnetic resonance imaging.

mRNA *abbr* messenger ribonucleic acid. ⊃ ribonucleic acid.

MRSA *abbr* meticillin (methicillin)-resistant *Staphylococcus aureus.*

MS *abbr* **1.** multiple sclerosis. **2.** musculoskeletal system.

MSA *abbr* multiple systems atrophy.

MSH *abbr* melanocyte stimulating hormones.

MSK *abbr* musculoskeletal.

MSP *abbr* Munchausen syndrome by proxy.

MSCC *abbr* metastatic spinal cord compression.

MSU/MSSU *abbr* midstream specimen of urine.

MSW *abbr* Medical Social Worker

MTA *abbr* mineral trioxide aggregate.

MTF *abbr* modulation transfer function.

MUA *abbr* manipulation under anaesthetic.

MUAC *abbr* mid-upper arm circumference.

mucilage *n* the solution of a gum in water—**mucilaginous** *adj.*

mucin *n* viscous, glycoprotein (mucoprotein) constituent of mucus. It is present in saliva and made up of many proteins, acting as a lubricant during swallowing. The daily output varies from person to person and from time to time. It tends to make the saliva 'ropey'—**mucinous** *adj.*

mucinase *n* a specific mucin-dissolving enzyme.

mucinolysis *n* breakdown of mucin—**mucinolytic** *adj.*

muc/o- a prefix that means 'mucus', e.g. *mucopurulent.*

mucobuccal fold the area of flexure of the mucous membrane between the maxilla or the mandible and the cheek.

mucocele, mucocoele *n* also known as a mucus retention cyst. The distension of a cavity with mucus. Such as, may be due to blockage of a salivary duct.

mucociliary escalator/transport the synchronized process occurring in the respiratory tract, whereby the mucus with any trapped foreign particles such as micro-organisms is moved upwards and out of the lungs.

mucocutaneous *adj* pertaining to mucous membrane and skin.

mucocutaneous lymph node syndrome (MLNS) a disease affecting mainly babies and children. It is an inflammatory vasculitis characterized by fever, dry lips, red mouth and strawberry-like tongue. There is a rash on the trunk, and erythema with desquamation affecting the extremities. There is cervical lymphadenopathy, polymorphonuclear leucocytosis and a raised erythrocyte sedimentation rate (ESR). Also known as Kawasaki disease.

mucodisplacement impression ⊃ impression.

mucogingival relating to gingival and alveolar mucosa.

mucogingival complex (dentogingival complex) a generic term for anything that entails both gingivae and alveolar mucosa. Includes the oral epithelium, the gingival crest and sulcus, the junctional epithelium, the complex network of collagen fibres including the periodontal ligament, the alveolar bone and the attached gingivae.

mucogingival junction an irregular line indicating the meeting of the alveolar mucosa and the attached gingiva.

mucogingival surgery the surgery conducted on the gingivae to improve or modify defects in shape, position or amount.

mucoid *adj* resembling mucus.

mucolytics *npl* drugs which reduce the viscosity of respiratory secretions, e.g. dornase alpha. ➲ Appendix 5.

mucoperiosteal flap ➲ full-thickness flap.

mucoperiosteum the periosteum with an overlying, firmly attached mucosal layer. Present in the hard palate and gingiva

mucopolysaccharide *n* complex polysaccharides containing hexosamine (amino sugar formed from hexoses). They are present as a constituent of the mucoproteins in connective tissue, e.g. chondroitin in cartilage, tendons.

mucopolysaccharidoses *npl* a group of inherited metabolic disorders in which the lack of specific enzymes causes the abnormal build-up of mucopolysaccharides. ➲ gargoylism, Hunter syndrome, Hurler syndrome, Morquio–Brailsford disease.

mucoproteins a substance containing protein and polysaccharides with several hexosamine residues. ➲ glycoproteins.

mucopurulent *adj* containing mucus and pus.

mucopus *n* mucus containing pus.

mucosa *n* a mucous membrane, such as the oral mucosa—**mucosae** *pl*, **mucosal** *adj*. ➲ mucous membrane.

mucosa-associated lymphoid tissue (MALT) collections of lymphoid tissue in the gastrointestinal tract, the respiratory tract and in the genitourinary tract. They are located in areas, which are exposed to the outside enviroment and are important in the early detection of invading pathogens. Examples include Peyer's patches and the tonsils.

mucosal pertaining to mucous membrane.

mucosal grafting vestibuloplasty (archaic) surgical deepening of the gingival sulcus by introducing a free mucous membrane graft.

mucositis *n* inflammation of a mucous membrane such as the mouth, throat or gastrointestinal tract. It occurs after cytotoxic chemotherapy, radiotherapy and immunosuppression in preparation for a haemopoietic stem cell transplant. Mucositis affecting the gastrointestinal tract compromises the integrity of the mucosa and increases the risk of micro-organisms entering the blood. This is a particular problem for neutropenic patients.

mucostatic impression ➲ impression.

mucous *adj* pertaining to or containing mucus. ➲ mucous membrane.

mucous membrane a membrane that contains glands which secrete mucus. It lines the cavities and passages that communicate with the exterior of the body, for example the respiratory tract.

mucous polyp a growth (adenoma) of mucous membrane which becomes pedunculated.

mucoviscidosis *n* cystic fibrosis.

mucus *n* viscid secretion of mucous glands. It contains water, mucin, salts and cell debris—**mucous, mucoid** *adj*.

Mueller's cell (Müller cell) a neuroglial cell in the retina with its nucleus in the inner nuclear layer and with fibres extending from the external to the internal limiting membrane. These cells support the neurons of the retina and possibly assist in their metabolism.

MUFA *abbr* monounsaturated fatty acid.

müllerian duct (J Müller, German physiologist, 1801–1858) ➲ Mayer–Rokitansky–Küster–Hauser syndrome, paramesonephric duct.

multi- a prefix that means 'many', e.g. *multicellular*.

multiagency team a team that involves practitioners from a range of different backgrounds or professions, such as health, social care and education, who work together with clients to achieve results that could not be achieved by any one agency working in isolation.

multiaxial joints a joint which has movement round more than two axes, for example, the hip joint.

multicellular *adj* having many cells.

multidisciplinary records those health records used by several groups of health and social care professionals.

multidisciplinary team (MDT) a team comprising different healthcare professionals and other workers working together to plan and deliver care for clients and may include specialist physicians and surgeons, general practitioners, nurses, midwives, specialist community public health nurses, physiotherapists, occupational therapists, speech and language therapists and dietitians. They practice relatively independently of each other with limited interaction. The team is headed by a leader and tends to be formal and hierarchical. Primary healthcare teams fall into this category where the general practitioner usually leads the team. Each team member is bound by his or her own professional education and beliefs, which may differ considerably from those of other members of the team. Patients and clients should be central in such teams. ➲ interdisciplinary team, intradisciplinary team, teamwork.

multifidus a deep lumbar spine muscle. Its primary function is to stabilize the lumbar spine.

multifocal lens a lens with various dioptric powers such as a bifocal, a trifocal, or a progressive lens.

multigravida *n* a woman who has had more than one pregnancy regardless of the outcome—**multigravidae** *pl*. ➲ multipara.

multi-infarct dementia cerebrovascular dementia. A condition arising from progressive occlusion of the blood supply to regions of the brain.

multi-leaf collimation (MLC) a method of customized beam shaping in radiotherapy without the use of lead blocks.

multilobular *adj* possessing many lobes.

multilocular *adj* possessing many small loculi or pockets, such as in a multilocular cyst.

multilocular cyst cyst with several adjoining cavities (loculi, pockets).

multinuclear *adj* possessing many nuclei, such as skeletal muscle cells—**multinucleate** *adj*.

multipara *n* a woman who has given birth to a viable infant (live or stillborn) on two or more occasions—**multiparae** *pl*. ➲ multigravida.

multiplanar reconstruction in computed tomography (CT) scanning, the formation of an image in any plane from the acquired axial data set.

M
N

multipurpose internet mail extensions (MIME) a method of sending binary objects by email.

multisection computed tomography (CT) a computed tomography (CT) scanner using multiple rows of detectors to enable several slices to be obtained at the same time thus increasing the speed of image acquisition.

multi-slice spiral computed tomography CT scanner computed tomography (CT) scanners that collect up to 64 slices (2006) of data during a spiral scan.

multiple cosmetic phlebectomy (MCP) removal of varicose veins through little stab incisions which heal without scarring.

multiple endocrine neoplasia (MEN) also known as multiple endocrine adenomas. A group of inherited autosomal dominant syndromes that are characterized by the presence of neoplasias in the endocrine glands that secrete amines or peptide hormones. Often the neoplasias are benign but some can be malignant; they may occur in the parathyroid glands, the pituitary gland, the islet cells of the pancreas (gastrinoma, insulinoma), the adrenal gland (phaeochromocytoma), gastrointestinal mucosal neuromas and the thyroid gland (medullary carcinoma). Each MEN syndrome has a typical pattern of sites of neoplasia formation. ➲ Sipple's syndrome, Werner's syndrome.

multiple idiopathic cervical root resorption (MICRR) an idiopathic condition characterized by multiple tooth root reabsorption; with reabsorption starting at the cementoenamel junction.

multiple myeloma a malignant proliferation of plasma cells. Normal plasma cells are derived from B cells and produce immunoglobulins which contain heavy and light chains. Normal immunoglobulins are polyclonal, which means that a variety of heavy chains are produced and each may be of kappa or lambda light chain type. In myeloma plasma cells produce immunoglobulin of a single heavy and light chain, a monoclonal protein commonly referred to as a paraprotein. In some cases only light chain is produced and this appears in the urine as Bence Jones proteinuria. The different paraprotein types in myeloma are: IgG, IgA, light chain only, and others (D, E, nonsectretory). Although a small number of malignant plasma cells are present in the circulation, the majority are present in the bone marrow. The malignant plasma cells produce cytokines, which stimulate osteoclasts and result in net bone absorption. The resulting lytic lesions cause bone pain, fractures and hypercalcaemia. Marrow involvement can result in anaemia or pancytopenia. The aetiology of this condition is unknown.The incidence of myeloma is 4/100 000 new cases per annum, with a male:female ratio of 2:1. The median age of diagnosis is 60–70 years and the disease is more common in African Caribbean individuals. The clinical features include: anaemia, Bence Jones proteinuria, bone pain, bruising, carpal tunnel syndrome, cerebral ischaemia, heart failure, hypercalacaemia, immune complexes, infection, lytic bone lesions, nephrotic syndrome, pancytopenia, 'panda' eyes, paraproteinaemia, raised erythrocyte sedimentation rate (ESR), retinal bleeds, spinal cord compression. The diagnosis of myeloma requires two of the following criteria: increased malignant plasma cells in the bone marrow, serum and/or urinary paraprotein and skeletal lesions. Bone marrow aspiration, plasma and urinary electrophoresis, and a skeletal survey are thus required. If patients are asymptomatic, treatment may not be required. Otherwise, treatment consists of: (a) immediate support—high fluid intake to treat renal impairment and hypercalcaemia, analgesia for bone pain, bisphosphonates for hypercalcaemia and to delay other skeletal related events, allopurinol to prevent urate nephropathy, plasmapheresis, as necessary, for hyperviscosity; (b) chemotherapy—in frail older patients, melphalan is an effective oral therapy, whilst in younger patients treatment with intravenous agents may improve response. Higher doses of intravenous melphalan appear to be well tolerated even in patients over 65 years and may produce better clinical responses; (c) radiotherapy—effective for localized bone pain not responding to simple analgesia and for pathological fractures. It is also useful for the emergency treatment of spinal cord compression complicating extradural plasmacytomas; (d) transplantation—standard treatment does not cure myeloma. Autologous stem cell transplants improve quality of life and prolong survival. All suitable patients under 65 years should be offered intravenous chemotherapy to maximum response and then an autologous stem cell transplant. Allogeneic haemopoietic stem cell transplantation (bone marrow transplantation) may cure some patients and should be considered in those under the age of 55 years with a sibling donor. Reduced-intensity allografting may improve outcomes by reducing transplant-related mortality and extending the upper age limit; (e) bisphosphonates—long-term bisphosphonate therapy reduces bone pain and skeletal events. These drugs protect bone and may cause apoptosis of malignant plasma cells; (f) thalidomide—has anti-angiogenic effects against tumour blood vessels and also immunomodulatory effects. At low doses it has been shown to be effective against refractory myeloma and when combined with dexamethasone, response rates over 50% are described. Trials are currently under way to investigate the use of thalidomide as an adjunct to other treatments earlier in the natural history of the disease. It can cause somnolence, constipation and a peripheral neuropathy. It is vital that females of childbearing age use adequate contraception as it is teratogenic. Other new agents include the proteasome inhibitor bortezomib which has also shown activity in advanced myeloma, and thalidomide derivatives which are currently being evaluated in clinical trials.The median survival of patients receiving standard treatment is approximately 40 months. Poor prognostic features include a high β_2-microglobulin, low albumin, a low haemoglobin or a high calcium at presentation. Autotransplantation improves survival and quality of life by slowing the rate of progression of bone disease. Less than 5% of patients survive longer than 10 years with standard treatment—**myelomata** *pl*, **myelomatous** *adj*. ➲ Bence Jones protein.

multiple of the median (MOM) measurement commonly used in biochemistry reports. 1 indicating the median or middle range of scores. It is considered to be more accurate than the mean as it is less likely to be skewed by extreme results. 0.5 indicates half the median and 2 indicates twice the median amount.

multiple organ dysfunction syndrome (MODS) syndrome in critically ill patients in which more than one organ system (e.g. kidneys, coagulation, gastrointestinal and respiratory) fails to function normally, may progress to multiple organ failure. It requires appropriate organ support such as mechanical ventilation and haemofiltration. ⮑ acute respiratory distress syndrome, disseminated intravascular coagulation, renal failure, systemic inflammatory response syndrome.

multiple pregnancy pregnancy with more than one fetus. Twins occur in approximately 1 in 80 pregnancies, although increasingly successful assisted conception rates have increased this number. Triplets occur in 1 in 80^2 pregnancies (i.e. 1 in 6400) and quadruplet pregnancies occur in 1 in 80^3 pregnancies (i.e. 1 in 512 000). Early ultrasound diagnosis of amnionicity and chorionicity is important, as monoamniotic (shared amniotic cavity) and monochorionic (common placenta with vascular connections) twins have a higher risk of morbidity and mortality associated with preterm labour, pregnancy induced hypertension and gestational diabetes (impaired glucose tolerance during pregnancy).

multiple sclerosis (MS) (*syn* disseminated sclerosis) a variably progressive inflammatory demyelinating disease of the central nervous system. It is possibly triggered by infection by one or more viruses and most commonly affects young adults in whom patchy, degenerative changes occur in nerve sheaths in the brain, spinal cord and optic nerves, followed by sclerosis. The presenting symptoms can vary considerably depending on the site and extent of the lesions, they include diplopia, extreme fatigue, weakness or unsteadiness of a limb, spasticity, pain; speech and swallowing difficulties; disturbances of micturition and incontinence are common. Several distinct types of multiple sclerosis are described: (a) *benign type* in which the person has minimal symptoms and long gaps between exacerbations after which they return to normal; (b) *primary progressive type* in which there is a steady, but slow progressive decline in neurological function; (c) *relapsing remitting type* in which there is a history of increasingly frequent and severe exacerbations and periods of remission without full recovery to the previous level of ability. May progress to secondary progressive type; (d) *secondary progressive type* in which the person will initially start with relapsing remitting type and then move into a stage where the disease becomes progressive. Exacerbations increase in intensity and remissions are shorter with reduced recovery until there is a constant progression of symptoms.

multiple systems atrophy (MSA) a condition characterized by rigidity and poverty of movement. It may be confused with parkinsonism or Parkinsonson's disease, but patients do not respond to the drug levodopa, whereas patients with Parkinson's disease do improve with levodopa. Usually onset is around 50–60 years with death occurring within 6 years.

multiple vision ⮑ polyopia.

multiprofessional *adj* relating to teamwork among practitioners from different healthcare professions working side by side. ⮑ interprofessional.

multivariate statistics analysis of three or more variables simultaneously. Used to clarify the association of two variables after allowing for other variables.

mumps *n* (*syn* infectious parotitis) an acute, specific inflammation of the parotid salivary glands, caused by a paramyxovirus. Spread is by droplets and the incubation period is around 18 days. There is fever, malaise, parotid salivary gland swelling and pain. Complications include pancreatitis, orchitis, oophoritis and meningitis. Active immunization is offered as part of routine programmes during childhood. ⮑ Colour Section Figure 91.

Münchausen syndrome (K von Münchhausen, German officer and story teller, 1720–1797) ⮑ factitious disorder.

Münchausen syndrome by proxy (MSP) the production of factitious disorders in a child by an adult, usually a parent or care giver.

Munro Kerr's manoeuvre ⮑ head fitting.

Munsell colour system a system of classification of colours composed of about 1000 colour samples, each designated by a letter and number system. The letter and number of each sample indicate its hue, saturation (called chroma in this system) and brightness (called value). They are represented by a three-dimensional polar coordinate system in which the hue is represented along the circumference, the value along the vertical axis and the chroma along a radius. ⮑ Farnsworth test.

mural *adj* pertaining to the wall of a structure.

murmur *n* (*syn* bruit) abnormal sound heard on auscultation of heart or great vessels. ⮑ aortic murmur, heart murmur, heart sounds, mid-diastolic murmur, mid-systolic murmur, systolic murmur.

Murphy's sign (J Murphy, American surgeon, 1857–1916) a physical sign that may be present in acute inflammation of the gallbladder. Continuous pressure over the gallbladder during a deep inspiration will cause the person to 'catch' their breath at the point of maximum inspiration.

Musca *n* genus of the common housefly, capable of transmitting many enteric infections.

muscae volitantes black dots or floaters seen before the eyes.

muscarinic *adj* a type of cholinergic receptor where muscarine would, if present, bind in place of acetylcholine. ⮑ nicotinic.

muscarinic agonists (*syn* parasympathomimetic) a group of drugs that stimulate or mimic parasympathetic activity. They have structural similarities with the neurotransmitter acetylcholine. ⮑ Appendix 5.

muscarinic antagonists (antimuscarinic drugs) (*syn.* parasympatholytic) a group of drugs that prevent the action of acetylcholine at the muscarinic receptors (ACh_m), thereby inhibiting cholinergic nerve transmission, e.g. hyoscine hydrobromide. ➲ Appendix 5.

muscle *n* one of the four basic tissues. Contractile soft tissue, responsible for all significant active movements and force-generations in an animal body. Composed of specialized contractile tissue formed from excitable cells— **muscular** *adj*. There are three types: (a) cardiac muscle— unique to the muscle layer of the heart (the myocardium); (b) skeletal muscle or voluntary muscle—the class of muscle acting, in almost all body locations, to move one bone relative to another, the more superficial skeletal muscles being visible under the skin in all but the most obese subjects; and (c) smooth muscle—the actively adjustable components of the walls of blood vessels and of the gastro-intestinal, respiratory, urinary and reproductive tracts. Skeletal and cardiac are the striated muscles; cardiac and smooth share the property of being involuntary. ➲ cardiac muscle, muscle fibres, muscle fibre types, myofibrils, red muscle, skeletal muscle, smooth muscle, white muscle, Colour Section Figures 4, 5.

muscle channelopathies inherited abnormalities of the sodium, calcium and chloride ion channels in striated muscle that produce various syndromes of familial periodic paralysis, myotonia and malignant hyperthermia which can be recognized by their clinical characteristics, provocation by exercise or eating, and associated changes in serum potassium concentration. ➲ hyperkalaemic periodic paralysis, hypokalaemic periodic paralysis, malignant hyperthermia, paramyotonia congenita, Thomsen's disease.

muscle channelopathies (calcium) inherited abnormalitities of the calcium ion channels in striated muscle. ➲ hypokalaemic periodic paralysis, malignant hyperthermia.

muscle channelopathies (sodium) inherited abnormalities of the sodium ion channels in striated muscle. ➲ hyperkalaemic periodic paralysis, hypokalaemic periodic paralysis, paramyotonia congenita.

muscle channelopathy (chloride) an inherited abnormality of the chloride ion channels in striated muscle. ➲ Thomsen's disease.

muscle conditioning training of skeletal muscles to enhance strength and/or endurance; commonly abbreviated in the sport and exercise context to 'conditioning' but note the radically different meaning of this word in behavioural work, which may be relevant to sport in attempts to modify emotions or in certain forms of skill training.

muscle contraction the process of force-generation in the fibres of any class of muscle, by the interaction of myosin head-groups in the thick filaments with actin molecules in one of the immediately neighbouring thin filaments. This is set in train ('activated') by a rise in the concentration of calcium ions [Ca^{2+}] in the muscle fibre cytoplasm in all types of muscle, but the mechanism for this rise differs in important respects between them. With reference to skeletal muscle, 'contraction', though literally implying shortening, is used to describe force-generation, whether it

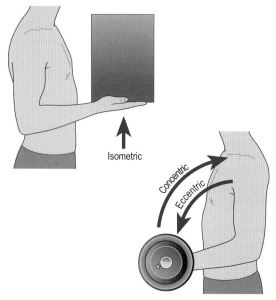

M.12 Types of skeletal muscle contraction (reproduced from Jennett 2008 with permission).

actually results in shortening (concentric action), tension without movement (isometric action) or even lengthening against the muscle's own resistance (eccentric action also known as eccentric contraction) (Figure M.12). ➲ concentric contraction, eccentric action, excitation–contraction coupling, force–velocity relationship, myofibrils.

muscle dysmorphic disorder a form of body dysmorphia that occurs almost exclusively in men, characterized by a perception that the body is too small and insufficiently muscular; also known as bigorexia. ➲ body dysmorphic disorder (BDD).

muscle enzymes the enzymes present in skeletal muscle include: actomyosin ATPase, creatine kinase, hexokinase, lactate dehydrogenase, myosin ATPase, phosphofructoki-nase, phosphorylases, pyruvate dehydrogenase, sarcoplasmic reticulum ATPase, succinate dehydrogenase. Apart from actomyosin and myosin ATPases which are associated with the contractile mechanism, they are by no means specific to muscle, being present and highly active also in other tissues. ➲ Krebs' cycle, muscle fibre types.

muscle fatigue impairment of muscle force production or of shortening speed resulting from repeated and/or prolonged activity. Causes vary greatly according to the nature and duration of the effort. In all cases they appear to consist principally in disturbances of intramuscular biochemistry, differing substantially between circumstances. However, the possibility of contributory neural factors, resulting in reduced muscle activation, should never be overlooked. Note that cytoplasmic adenosine triphosphate (ATP) concentrations never fall to less than about half resting levels in living muscle fibres (radical ATP depletion would lead to rigor, not weakness). ➲ central fatigue, fatigue, glycogen.

muscle fibre the muscle cell. Usually refers to skeletal muscle, which has greatly elongated (fibre-like) cells, up to 15–20 cm in the largest muscles of the human body. Each skeletal muscle fibre has many nuclei (more than 2000 in the largest fibres), located, after initial development, just beneath the cell membrane. These nuclei cannot divide; skeletal muscle growth and repair depend on satellite cells. The term 'muscle fibre' may also be applied to the much smaller cells of smooth and cardiac muscle, which have one central nucleus. All types of muscle fibre have longitudinally oriented contractile filaments containing actin and myosin. Each skeletal muscle fibre receives its own branch of a motor nerve, but cardiac and smooth muscle fibres are innervated in looser groupings. Skeletal muscle fibres are classified according to type of action and metabolism. ➲ muscle fibre types, myofibrils, sarcoplasmic reticulum, satellite cell.

muscle fibre types categories of muscle fibre adapted for various modes of use. Normally taken to refer to skeletal muscle unless specified otherwise. The main types found in stable human skeletal muscles after infancy are shown in Table M.2. Intermediate 'hybrid' forms also occur, commonly in non-stable states such as during intensive or recently changed training regimens, or in recovery from injury. Types termed 1, 2A and 2B, containing myosins similarly designated, have been recognized since about 1970; however, the separate existence in many mammals of type 2X (initially also known as 2D), distinguishable from 2B only by sophisticated techniques, was recognized during the 1990s and it is now accepted that most, if not all, human fibres formerly called 2B in fact have 2X myosin. The slower-contracting muscles have a majority of type 1 fibres (typically approaching 90% in the extreme instance, soleus), while the faster-contracting ones have rather more,

and often rather larger, type 2. Only some small specialist muscles (e.g. extraocular) have 80–85% fast fibres; in large limb muscles above 60% fast is reported only for sprint athletes. ➲ muscle enzymes.

muscle imbalance imbalanced muscle groups cause a wide variety of conditions, from joint wear and tear to arthritis and from tendonitis (tendinitis) to sore muscles. All joints in the body are controlled by two or more groups of muscles. Usually one set of muscles stabilizes and supports the joint, while other adjoining muscle groups create movement. However, sometimes, one group becomes unusually strong and tight, while the opposite group weakens and becomes overstretched. This imbalance leads to poor joint control and abnormal biomechanics. If these faulty movement patterns repeat many times, tissues may begin to degenerate. Muscle imbalance techniques approach patients who present with movement dysfunction and its associated problems. Several classifications of imbalance have been suggested relating to muscle structure, function and response to injury. Movement dysfunction may occur at both a segmental or local or single joint level and at a global level affecting many segments of a region. Muscles can be thought of as either stabilizers or mobilizers. Stabilizer muscles are deep, with broad attachments and their role is postural and dynamic control. Mobilizer muscles are producers of force, they are more superficially situated and have long muscle bellies. In certain pathological states these two classifications of muscles change their recruitment patterns; this typically results in an alteration in function. Mobilizer muscles that are prone to tightness include the rectus femoris, vastus lateralis, rectus abdominis, sternocleidomastoid, etc. The stabilizer muscles that are prone to weakness include the gluteus medius and minimus, serratus anterior, transversus abdominis, psoas major, etc.

M
N

Table M.2 Characteristics of the three main types of stable human skeletal muscle fibres (Reproduced from Jennett 2008 with permission)

Fibre type and myosin type	1	2A	2X (formerly '2B')
Description	Slow (-twitch) red	Fast (-twitch) red	Fast (-twitch) white
Principal energy supply system	Oxidative	Oxidative and glycolytic	Glycolytic (anaerobic)
Abbreviated description	SO	FOG	FG
Mitochondrial density	High	Medium to very high	Low
Motor neuron size	Small	Medium	Large
Contraction speed	Slow	Fairly fast	Fast
Fatigue resistance	High	Medium to high	Low
Myosin ATPase activity after pH ∼ 10.3 pre-treatment	Low	Fairly high	High
Ditto, after pH 4.6 pre-treatment	High	Low	Medium
Ditto, after pH 4.3 pre-treatment	High	Low	Low

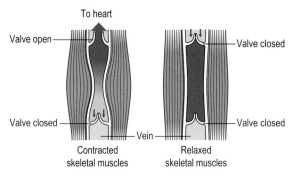

M.13 Muscle pump (reproduced from Porter 2005 with permission).

muscle pump the muscular contraction in the calf that aids venous return to the heart by squeezing the blood from one valve to the next in the leg veins (Figure M.13). Healthcare professionals, physiotherapists and nurses often encounter people who have a deficient muscle pump, for example, after joint replacement surgery or immobility. This often results in oedema in the ankles.

muscle relaxant drug used during general anaesthesia to produce muscle paralysis.

muscle reposition a surgical procedure to move a muscle attachment into a more acceptable functional position

muscles of mastication the muscles concerned with mastication are: masseter, temporalis, lateral pterygoid and medial pterygoid muscles, all innervated by the mandibular branch of the trigeminal nerve. Other muscles of mastication are: the buccinator muscle, the tongue, the anterior belly of the digastric muscle, the mylohyoid muscle and the orbicularis oris.

muscle spasm powerful involuntary muscle contraction, often of sudden onset and quite often painful, which interferes with voluntary movement; may be the consequence of neurological damage or disease. ➲ cramp, spinal injury/spinal cord injury.

muscle spindles specialized sensory structures within skeletal muscles, consisting of small intrafusal muscle fibres which do not contribute to load-bearing or power generation, but participate in control of the working (extrafusal) fibres. The intrafusal fibres are innervated towards their ends by gamma motor neurons, but are also invested more centrally by both primary and secondary sensory endings; these signal changes in length, and also rates of change in length of the muscle, to the central nervous system. The gamma motor neurons control the sensitivity of the sensory endings to stretching. They also compensate for the shortening of muscle spindles during extrafusal contraction by causing additional intrafusal contraction; this ensures that sensory feedback continues during muscle contractions. The overall system mediates both the stretch reflex and, in voluntary movement, appropriate adjustment of force-generation to load, provided the load is not varying too rapidly. ➲ gamma (motor) system, stretch reflex, tendon jerk reflex.

muscle tear rupture of the tissue of a muscle. In sport, most commonly the result of a sudden movement beyond the normal range; may reflect poor muscle strength, flexibility or preparation.

muscle tone *syn.* tonus. (a) In skeletal muscle, a state of tension that is maintained continuously—minimally even when relaxed—and which increases in resistance to passive stretch. Pathologically, loss of tone (flaccidity) can be caused, e.g. by peripheral nerve damage, and exaggerated tone (spasticity) by overstimulation, e.g. when the activity of the relevant lower motor neurons is released from higher central nervous system control in spinal injury. The term is sometimes also used, incorrectly, to indicate general muscle strength. (b) In smooth muscle, steady tension maintained in the walls of hollow vessels; regulated mainly by autonomic innervation but influenced, e.g. in the walls of arterioles, by local variables: temperature, chemical factors or intravascular pressure, contributing to autoregulation of appropriate blood flow. ➲ stretch reflex.

muscle trimming ➲ border moulding.

muscular atrophies also known as spinal muscular atrophy. The most common group of neuromuscular disease in childhood after Duchenne's muscular dystrophy. ➲ spinal muscular atrophy.

muscular dystrophies a group of inherited disorders characterized by progressive degeneration of groups of muscles, sometimes with involvement of the heart muscle or conducting tissue, and other parts of the nervous system. The onset is often in childhood, although some patients, especially those with myotonic dystrophy, may present as adults. Wasting and weakness are usually symmetrical, there is no fasciculation and no sensory loss, and tendon reflexes are preserved until a late stage, except in myotonic dystrophy. Differential diagnosis is based on the age at onset, the distribution of affected muscles and the pattern of inheritance. Myotonic dystrophy may be diagnosed clinically by the distribution of muscle weakness and other features including myotonia. Many dystrophies include cardiomyopathy amongst their clinical features. The diagnosis can be confirmed by specific molecular genetic testing, supplemented with electromyogram (EMG) and muscle biopsy if necessary. Creatine kinase is markedly elevated in Duchenne muscular dystrophy, but is normal or only moderately elevated in the other dystrophies. Screening for an associated cardiac abnormality (cardiomyopathy or arrhythmia) is important. There is no specific therapy for these conditions, but physiotherapy and occupational therapy help patients cope with their disability. Treatment of associated cardiac failure or arrhythmia (with pacemaker insertion if necessary) may be required; similarly, management of respiratory complications (including nocturnal hypoventilation) can improve quality of life. Genetic counselling is important. Patients with Duchenne dystrophy used to die within 10 years of diagnosis, but with improved general care they are now living into the third decade. The lifespan in limb girdle and facioscapulohumeral dystrophies is normal. In myotonic dystrophy, there is considerable phenotypic variation and the prognosis is very variable, limited by cardiac and respiratory complications. ➲ Becker muscular dystrophy, Duchenne muscular dystrophy, Emery–Dreifuss muscular dystrophy, facioscapulohumeral muscular dystrophy (FSH), limb girdle muscular dystrophy, myotonic dystrophy, oculopharyngeal muscular dystrophy, proximal myotonic myopathy (PROMM, DM2).

muscular endurance the ability of a muscle or group of muscles to produce force over an extended period of time, i.e. to perform repeated contractions against a sub-maximal load.

muscular power the ability of a muscle(s) to produce a force at a given time.

muscular strength the amount of force a muscle or group of muscles can exert. The ability to resist or produce a force.

musculature *n* the muscular system, or any part of it.

musculocutaneous *adj* pertaining to muscle and skin.

musculocutaneous nerve a nerve arising from the brachial plexus, which innervates the muscles of the upper arm and the skin of the forearm. ➲ brachial plexus.

musculoskeletal *adj* pertaining to the muscular and skeletal systems.

musculoskeletal system the body system consisting of the bones, their joints and skeletal (voluntary) muscles. ➲ skeletal system.

mutagen *n* any agent that causes a gene or chromosome mutation.

mutagenesis *n* the creation of mutations—**mutagenic, mutagenetic** *adj*, **mutagenetically** *adv*.

mutagenicity *n* the capacity to produce gene mutations or chromosome aberrations.

mutans streptococci a collective term used to describe a group of bacteria with characteristics similar to *Streptococcus mutans*. It comprises two human species, *S. mutans* and *S. sobrinus*, found in the oral cavity, and a variety of animal species including *S. rattus, S. downei, S. cricetus, S. ferus* and *S. macacae*. Also referred to as the *Streptococcus mutans* group.

mutant *n* a cell (or organism) that has a genetic change or mutation.

mutation *n* a gene or chromosome alteration that results in genetic changes that alter the characteristics of the affected cell. The change is transmitted through succeeding generations. Mutations may be spontaneous, or induced by agents such as ionizing radiation that alter the chromosomal DNA.

mute 1. *adj* unable to speak. **2.** *n* a person who is unable to speak.

mutilation *n* the condition resulting from the removal of a limb or other part of the body. It results in a change of body image, to which there has to be considerable physical, psychological and social adjustment for a successful outcome.

mutism *n* (*syn.* dumbness) inability or refusal to speak. It may be due to congenital causes, the most common being deafness; it may be the result of physical disease, such as a stroke, and it can be a manifestation of mental health problems.

mutual induction when a changing current is passed through one conductor and produces a changing magnetic field, if another conductor is placed in the field an electromotive force will be formed in the second conductor.

mutually protected occlusion an occlusal arrangement in which the posterior teeth prevent excessive contact of the anterior teeth in maximum intercuspation and the anterior teeth disengage the posterior teeth in all mandibular movements.

MVC *abbr* maximum voluntary contraction.

MVIT *abbr* maximal voluntary isometric torque.

MVT *abbr* maximal voluntary torque.

MVV *abbr* maximum voluntary ventilation.

MxMnPA *abbr* maxillary-mandibular planes angle.

myalgia *n* pain or ache in a muscle which may be the result of injury, inflammation, overuse or inappropriate activity. Normally settles with rest and anti-inflammatory medication. Also unexplained and persistent as part of the chronic fatigue syndrome—**myalgic** *adj. epidemic myalgia* ➲ Bornholm disease.

myalgic encephalomyelitis (ME) ➲ chronic fatigue syndrome/ME

myasthenia *n* muscular weakness—**myasthenic** *adj*.

myasthenia gravis an autoimmune disorder in which an antibody reduces the efficiency of transmission between the motor neuron and muscle. The antibody blocks receptor sites at the neuromuscular junctions and prevents the normal action of acetylcholine and nerve impulse transmission. In many cases there is a disorder of the thymus gland. It is characterized by marked fatigue affecting the voluntary muscles, especially following exercise. Other muscles involved include those of the eye, shoulder girdle and those required for speaking, swallowing, chewing and breathing.

myasthenic crisis a sudden deterioration with weakness of respiratory muscles due to an increase in severity of myasthenia. It is distinguished from cholinergic crisis by giving edrophonium chloride intravenously. Marked improvement confirms myasthenic crisis. ➲ edrophonium test.

myc, myco, myceto- a prefix that means 'fungus', e.g. *mycology*.

mycelium *n* a mass of branching filaments (hyphae) of moulds or fungi—**mycelial** *adj*.

mycetoma *n* (*syn.* Madura foot) chronic fungal disease affecting soft tissues and bones of the limbs (usually the foot), but it may occur in other sites. It causes swelling, nodules and sinus formation.

Mycobacterium *n* a genus of Gram-positive acid-fast bacteria. *Mycobacterium avium intracellulare (MAI)* atypical mycobacterium that causes infection in humans.

M
N

Mycobacterium bovis causes tuberculosis in cattle. It can be transmitted to humans. *Mycobacterium leprae* causes leprosy and *Mycobacterium tuberculosis* causes tuberculosis.

mycologist *n* an expert in mycology.

mycology *n* the study of fungi—**mycological** *adj*, **mycologically** *adv*.

Mycoplasma *n* a genus of very small micro-organisms. They have features in common with bacteria, but lack a cell wall. Some are parasites, some are saprophytes and others are pathogens; for example *Mycoplasma pneumoniae* causes primary atypical pneumonia.

mycosis *n* disease caused by any fungus—**mycotic** *adj*.

mycosis fungoides a T-cell lymphomatous condition that initially may present as scaly patches on the skin. In later stages, large tumours may develop. ⊃ Sézary's syndrome.

mycotoxins *npl* the secondary metabolites of moulds or microfungi. Many chemical substances have been identified as mycotoxins, some of which are carcinogenic as well as causing other diseases—**mycotoxic** *adj*.

mydriasis *n* dilatation of the pupil of the eye.

mydriatics *npl* drugs which dilate the pupil (mydriasis), e.g. tropicamide. ⊃ Appendix 5.

myelencephalon one of the secondary enlargements occurring during embryonic development of the brain. Part of the embryonic hindbrain, which becomes the medulla oblongata.

myelin *n* the white, fatty substance that covers and insulates some nerve fibres. An intact myelin sheath is required for smooth nerve conduction. ⊃ white matter.

myelination the process by which myelin is produced and forms the insulation around the axons of certain nerves.

myelitis *n* inflammation of the spinal cord.

myeloablative *adj* describes the therapy (e.g. radiotherapy, chemotherapy) given intentionally to completely 'knock out' the bone marrow. Used in leukaemia and often precedes a haemopoietic stem cell transplant.

myeloblasts *npl* the early precursor cells of the polymorphonuclear granulocytic white blood cells. The presence of myeloblasts in the blood is abnormal and occurs in acute myeloblastic leukaemia—**myeloblastic** *adj*.

myelocele *n* a neural tube defect. Occurs with spina bifida wherein development of the spinal cord itself has been arrested, and the central canal of the cord opens on the skin surface discharging cerebrospinal fluid.

myelocytes *npl* precursor cells of polymorphonuclear granulocytic white blood cells. The presence of myelocytes in the blood is abnormal and occurs in some leukaemias—**myelocytic** *adj*.

myelodysplastic syndrome (MDS) a group of clonal haematopoietic disorders which represent steps in the progression to the development of leukaemia. It affects predominantly older people (median age 69 years); the overall incidence is 4/100 000 rising to more than 30/100 000 in the over-70s. It is characterized by blood cytopenias and abnormal-looking (dysplastic) blood cells, including macrocytic red cells and hypogranular neutrophils with nuclear hyper- or hyposegmentation. The marrow is hypercellular with dysplastic changes in all three cell lines. Inevitably it progresses to acute myeloid leukaemia (AML), although the time to progression varies with the subtype of MDS, being slowest in refractory anaemia and most rapid in refractory anaemia with excess of blasts. The World Health Organization (WHO) classification of MDS includes the following diseases: (a) refractory anaemia (RA); (b) refractory anaemia with sideroblasts (RARS); (c) refractory cytopenias with multilineage dysplasia (RCMD); (d) refractory anaemia with excess blasts (RAEB); (e) myelodyplastic syndrome with 5q; (f) myelodysplastic syndrome unclassified. The most common presentation is due to the consequences of bone marrow failure: symptoms of anaemia, recurrent infections or bleeding. The blood film shows cytopenias and the dysplastic features indicated above. A bone marrow aspiration should be performed, which is usually hypercellular with evidence of dysplasia. Blast cells may be increased but do not reach the 20% level which indicates acute leukaemia. Chromosome analysis frequently reveals abnormalities, particularly of chromosomes 5 or 7. For the majority of patients the disease is incurable and supportive care with red-cell and platelet transfusions to maintain quality of life is the mainstay of treatment. A trial of erythropoietin and granulocyte–colony stimulating factor (G–CSF) is recommended in some patients with early disease to improve haemoglobin and white cell counts. Allogeneic haemopoietic stem cell transplantation (bone marrow transplantation) may afford a cure in younger patients. Transplantation should be preceded by intensive chemotherapy in those with more advanced disease.The survival in MDS can vary from years in patients with RA and RARS to months in those with RAEB, who rapidly transform to acute myeloid leukaemia. Poor prognostic factors include blasts > 10% in the marrow, certain cytogeneic abnormalities and more than one cytopenia in the blood.

myelodysplastic syndrome unclassified ⊃ myelodysplastic syndrome (MDS).

myelodysplastic syndrome with 5q- ⊃ myelodysplastic syndrome (MDS).

myelofibrosis a myeloproliferative disorder characterized by bone marrow fibrosis, extramedullary haematopoiesis (blood cell formation outside the bone marrow) and a leucoerythroblastic blood picture. The marrow is initially hypercellular, with an excess of abnormal megakaryocytes which release growth factors, e.g. platelet-derived growth factor (PDGF), to the marrow microenvironment, resulting in a reactive proliferation of fibroblasts. As the disease progresses, the marrow becomes fibrosed. Most patients present over the age of 50 years with lassitude, weight loss and night sweats. The spleen can be massively enlarged due to extramedullary haematopoiesis, and painful splenic infarcts may occur. The characteristic blood picture is a leucoerythroblastic anaemia, with circulating immature red blood cells (increased reticulocytes and nucleated red blood cells) and granulocyte precursors (myelocytes). The red cells are shaped like teardrops (teardrop poikilocytes) and giant platelets may be seen in the blood. The white count varies from low to moderately high and the platelet count may be high, normal or low. Urate levels may be high due to increased cell breakdown, and folate deficiency is common. The marrow is often difficult to aspirate and a trephine biopsy shows an excess of megakaryocytes, increased reticulin and fibrous tissue replacement. Median survival is 4 years from diagnosis but ranges from 1 year to over 20 years. Treatment is directed at control of symptoms, e.g. red cell transfusions for anaemia. Folic acid should be given to prevent deficiency. Cytotoxic therapy with hydroxycarbamide may help control spleen size, the white cell count or systemic symptoms. Splenectomy may be required for a grossly enlarged spleen or symptomatic pancytopenia secondary to splenic pooling of cells and hypersplenism. Haemopoietic stem cell transplantation (bone marrow transplantation) may be considered for younger patients.

myelogenous *adj* produced in or by the bone marrow.

myelography *n* radiographic examination of the spinal canal by injection of a contrast agent into the subarachnoid space. Superseded by computed tomography (CT) and magnetic resonance imaging (MRI)—**myelographic** *adj*, **myelogram** *n*, **myelograph** *n*, **myelographically** *adv*.

myeloid *adj* **1.** pertaining to the bone marrow. **2.** pertaining to the granulocyte precursor cells in the bone marrow. **3.** pertaining to the spinal cord.

myeloma ⊃ multiple myeloma.

myelomatosis *n* ⊃ multiple myeloma, Bence Jones protein.

myelomeningocele *n* ⊃ meningomyelocele.

myelo, myel- a prefix that means either 'spinal cord', e.g. *myelitis*, or 'bone marrow', e.g. *myeloblasts*.

myelopathy *n* disease of the spinal cord. Can be a serious complication of cervical spondylosis—**myelopathic** *adj*.

myeloproliferative disorders a group of chronic conditions characterized by clonal proliferation of bone marrow cellular components: erythroid precursors (primary proliferative polycythaemia/polycythaemia rubra vera, PRV), megakaryocytes (primary thrombocythaemia and myelofibrosis) or myeloid cells (chronic myeloid leukaemia, CML). Although the majority of patients are classifiable as having one of these disorders, some have overlapping features. Furthermore, there is often progression from one to another, e.g. PRV to myelofibrosis. ⊃ leukaemia, myelofibrosis, polycythaemia, primary proliferative polycythaemia, primary thrombocythaemia.

myelosclerosis a generalized increase in bone density.

myenteric plexus Auerbach's plexus. A plexus of autonomic (sympathetic and parasympathetic) nerves that innervate the smooth muscle layer and the associated blood vessels in the gastrointestinal tract.

myiasis infestation of tissues or organs with fly larvae (maggots).

mylohyoid muscle a thin sheet of muscle running the whole length of the mylohyoid ridge on the lingual surface of the body of the mandible. The two mylohyoid muscles from each side of the mandible join to form the floor of the anterior part of the mouth. Supplied by the mylohyoid branch of the inferior alveolar nerve.

mylohyoid ridge the bony ridge running along the internal surface of the body of the mandible providing attachment for the mylohyoid muscle. The ridge separates two hollows: the upper and more anterior depression against which the sublingual salivary gland lies, and the lower and more posterior depression that accommodates the submandibular salivary gland. When the alveolar bone becomes absorbed following dental extractions, the ridge becomes more superficial and is often a source of pain from the pressure of complete dentures.

mylohyoid ridge reduction the surgical removal of the mylohyoid ridge that may be affecting the comfortable fitting of a complete denture.

my/o- a prefix that means 'muscle', e.g. *myofibril*.

myocardial infarction (MI) part of the spectrum of acute coronary syndromes. Death of a part of the myocardium (heart muscle) from deprivation of blood following occlusion of a coronary artery, for example from thrombosis (Figure M.14). The patient experiences a 'heart attack' with sudden chest tightness and heaviness and intense chest pain which may radiate to the arms (especially the left), abdomen, back, neck and lower jaw, breathlessness, sweating, nausea, cyanosis and anxiety. Some groups including women may present atypically. Immediate hospital admission is required to initiate treatment and because of the risk of life-threatening arrhythmias leading to cardiac arrest. Increasingly, patients who suffer a myocardial infarction will be treated by primary angioplasty. Effectiveness of this treatment depends on it happening within 2 hours of the

M
N

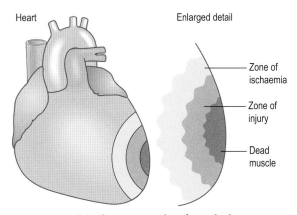

M.14 Myocardial infarction—grades of muscle damage
(reproduced from Hinchliff et al 1996 with permission).

first call for professional assistance. Where angioplasty is containdicated on health grounds or facilities are not available within the time frame patients will have thrombolytic drugs; their management includes: aspirin, early thrombolytic therapy, pain relief, antiemetics, oxygen therapy, bed rest, observations including continuous ECG and later mobilization and cardiac rehabilitation. Patients should be cared for in a coronary care unit for 12–24 hours because of the risk of life-threatening arrhythmias such as ventricular fibrillation, and the need for skilled staff to monitor the effects of thrombolytic therapy. In sport, MI is the commonest cause of sudden death in those aged over 45 years. Risk factors include cigarette smoking, high blood pressure, obesity, physical inactivity and raised cholesterol levels. Exercise programmes are recommended in the prevention of heart disease and used in the rehabilitation of patients following a heart attack. ➲ acute coronary syndromes, angina pectoris, cardiac enzymes, coronary heart disease.

myocarditis *n* inflammation of the myocardium, the muscle of the heart, usually the result of viral infection (especially *Coxsackie*), sometimes during or after bacterial and other infections. Causes enlargement of the heart, impaired function and sometimes heart failure. It can present with chest pain, breathlessness, lethargy and fatigue and arrhythmias. Diagnosis is based on history, laboratory tests (to identify infective agent and inflammatory markers), ECG and echocardiography. A rare condition, but one of the causes of sudden death during exercise, especially if a sports participant returns to activity before the infection has resolved completely.

myocardium *n* the middle layer of the heart wall. Formed from highly specialized cardiac muscle found only in the heart. It is not under voluntary control but, like skeletal muscle, striations (cross-stripes) are seen on microscopic examination. Its short branching fibres (cells) may have a single nucleus or two, and one or more branches. The ends of the cells and their branches are in very close contact with the ends and branches of adjacent cells. The boundaries between individual cells, which are not well defined, are formed by intercalated discs. Microscopically the intercalated discs, can be seen as thicker, darker lines than the ordinary striations. This arrangement gives cardiac muscle the appearance of being a sheet of muscle rather than a very large number of individual cells. Because of the end-to-end continuity of the fibres, each one does not need to have a separate nerve supply. When an impulse is initiated it spreads from cell to cell via the branches and intercalated discs over the whole 'sheet' of muscle, causing contraction. The 'sheet' arrangement of the myocardium ensures that the wave of contraction passes easily across the myocardium, which behaves as a syncitium. Thus enabling the atria and ventricles to contract in a coordinated and efficient manner. The myocardium is thickest at the apex of the heart and thins out towards the base. This reflects the amount of work each chamber contributes to the pumping of blood,

i.e. the atria receive blood whereas the ventricles pump blood out into the systemic and pulmonary circulations. It is thickest in the left ventricle. The atria and the ventricles are separated by a ring of fibrous tissue that does not conduct electrical impulses. Consequently, when a wave of electrical activity passes over the atrial muscle, it can only spread to the ventricles through the conducting system which bridges the fibrous ring from atria to ventricles. ➲ cardiac muscle, muscle, syncitium—**myocardial** *adj*.

myocele *n* protrusion of a muscle through its ruptured sheath.

myoclonic epilepsy with ragged red fibres (MERRF) a mitochondrial myopathy syndrome. It is characterized by myotonic epilepsy, cerebellar ataxia, dementia, sensorineural deafness ± peripheral neuropathy and optic atrophy. ➲ mitochondrial myopathy syndromes.

myoclonus *n* clonic contractions of individual or groups of muscles. Normal individuals occasionally experience an isolated myoclonic jerk or two during drowsiness or light sleep. ➲ clonus, dyskinetic movements.

myodioptre the contractile power of the ciliary muscle such that it induces an increase in the accommodation of the eye of 1D. ➲ dioptre.

myoelectric *adj* relating to the electrical properties of muscle.

myoepithelial cells specialized contractile cells present in myoepithelium.

myoepithelium a type of specialized epithelium that contains myoepitheial cells with contractile properties. Located around the secretory system of certain glands, e.g. mammary glands, sweat glands, it assists with secretion discharge.

myofascial pain dysfunction syndrome persistent pain of soft tissue, characterized by taut fibrous bands and focal areas of hypersensitivity known as trigger points.

myofascial trigger point trigger points are localized hyperirritable areas of hypersensitivity located within skeletal muscle. They produce localized pain, referred pain and often accompany chronic musculoskeletal disorders. Repeated microtrauma may lead to the development of stress on muscle fibres and the formation of trigger points. Patients often have persistent pain that results in a decreased range of motion in the affected muscles. These include muscles used to maintain body posture, such as those in the neck, shoulders and pelvic girdle. Trigger points may also manifest as tension headache, tinnitus, temporomandibular joint pain, decreased range of motion in the legs and low back pain. On palpation of a trigger point, a nodule of muscle fibre of harder than normal consistency is often found (Alvarez and Rockwell 2000). (Alvarez DJ, Rockwell PG 2002 Trigger points: diagnosis and management. Am Fam Physician 65(4): 653–660.)

myofibril *n* longitudinally oriented cytoplasmic components of skeletal and cardiac muscle fibres, which are the loci of force-generation when the muscle is activated. Each myofibril extends the whole length of the fibre though it is typically only ~1 μm diameter; thus a fibre of 100 μm diameter has several thousand fibrils in its cross-section. In turn, each fibril is composed of numerous parallel filaments of contractile myofibrillar proteins, chiefly myosin in thick filaments and chiefly actin in thin filaments, alternating and partially overlapping along the length of each myofibril, and so giving rise to the cross-banding pattern of the lengthwise repeating sarcomeres; these are aligned side by side across the fibre, giving it (under appropriate histological stains or optical imaging techniques) the striated appearance characteristic of these two classes of muscle. Interaction between the two proteins, myosin and actin, at the cross-bridges results in the generation of active force during muscle contraction. ➲ actin, cross-bridge, myosin, sarcoplasmic reticulum, tropomyosin, troponin.

myofibrosis *n* excessive connective tissue in muscle. Leads to inadequate functioning of part—**myofibroses** *pl*.

myofunctional appliance an orthodontic appliance, can be removable or fixed, that attempts to influence the growth of the maxilla and mandible in order to correct a malocclusion. ➲ orthodontic appliance.

myogenic *adj* originating in or starting from muscle.

myoglobin (Mb) *n* (*syn*. myohaemoglobin) iron-containing haem protein present at high density in the cytoplasm of oxidative muscle fibres (skeletal and cardiac) and substantially contributing to their redness. Related to haemoglobin (Hb), with which it shares affinity for oxygen. In diving mammals (whose tissues it makes almost black) Mb serves as a significant oxygen store but in terrestrial ones, including humans, its predominant function is considered to be facilitation of diffusion of oxygen from the blood through the cytoplasm, by the transfer of oxygen from haemoglobin (Hb) which has a lower oxygen affinity than Mb at the oxygen tension PO_2 encountered in the muscle vascular bed. Myoglobin escapes from damaged muscle and appears in the urine in 'crush syndrome'. ➲ muscle fibre types.

myoglobinuria *n* (*syn*. myohaemoglobinuria) excretion of myoglobin in the urine as in crush syndrome. ➲ march myoglobinuria.

myohaemoglobin *n* ➲ myoglobin.

myohaemoglobinuria *n* ➲ myoglobinuria.

myokymia *n* muscle twitching. In the lower eyelid it is benign. ➲ facial myokymia.

myoma *n* a tumour of muscle tissue—**myomata** *pl*, **myomatous** *adj*.

myomectomy *n* enucleation of uterine fibroid(s).

myometrium *n* the specialized muscular wall of the uterus.

myoneural *adj* pertaining to muscle and nerve.

myopathy *n* disease of muscle (usually applied to non-inflammatory conditions)—**myopathic** *adj*. ➲ acquired myopathies, congenital myopathy, inherited metabolic myopathy, muscular dystrophies, polymyositis.

myope *n* a shortsighted person—**myopic** *adj*.

myopia *n* shortsightedness caused by high refractive power or increased axial length of the eye, with the result that the light rays are focused in front of, instead of on, the retina—**myopic** *adj*.

myoplasty *n* plastic surgery of muscles—**myoplastic** *adj*.

myosarcoma *n* a malignant tumour derived from muscle—**myosarcomata** *pl*, **myosarcomatous** *adj*.

myosin *n* one of the two main myofibrillar proteins in the myofibrils of a muscle fibre. A dimeric molecule comprising two identical monomers. Each monomer consists of a long chain ('light meromyosin, LMM') which readily associates with the chains of other myosin molecules to form the thick filaments, and a more globular component ('heavy meromyosin, HMM'), itself further divisible into two subunits, S2 and S1. The latter are the myosin head-groups, embodying an ATPase and an actin-binding site; it is these that interact with actin in the thin filaments when the muscle is activated, to form the force-generating (actin-myosin) cross-bridges. This whole monomer constitutes one myosin heavy chain (MHC). However, associated with the head-groups are two myosin light chains (MLC), of uncertain function. (Since myosin is not the only constituent of thick filaments, the term 'myosin filament' is a misnomer and better avoided.) ➲ muscle contraction, sliding filament hypothesis/mechanism.

myosin ATPase (mATPase) an enzyme present in skeletal muscle. It is associated with the contractile mechanism. It is located in the myosin head groups. Catalyses the hydrolysis (calcium [Ca^{2+}]dependent, magnesium [Mg^{2+}] independent) of terminal phosphate group of adenosine triphosphate (ATP) by head group alone, not interacting with actin (so not contraction-producing: compare actomyosin ATPase). Basic histochemical marker for fast vs. slow fibres. ➲ muscle enzymes.

myosis (miosis) *n* constriction of the pupil of the eye—**myotic** *adj*.

myositis *n* inflammation of a muscle or its connective tissue. ➲ connective tissue diseases.

myositis ossificans deposition of active bone cells in muscle, resulting in hard swellings. Ossification of a haematoma, secondary to trauma. If a haematoma does not fully resolve, calcification and subsequent ossification can occur after approximately 3 weeks. Surgical intervention may then be necessary.

myotatic on-stretch reflex a reflex that involves the lengthening of a muscle followed by sudden shortening to generate power. ➲ plyometric exercise.

myotome *n* the muscles supplied by a single spinal nerve (Table M.3).

myotomy *n* cutting or dissection of muscle tissue.

myotonia *n* an increase in muscle tone at rest—**myotonic** *adj*.

myotonia congenita a genetically determined form of congenital muscular spasticity, usually presenting in infancy and due to degeneration of anterior horn cells in the spinal cord. Fibrillation of affected muscles is characteristic. It is inherited either as an autosomal dominant or autosomal recessive trait.

M
N

Table M.3 Myotomes

Myotome	Function
C1	Upper cervical flexion
C2	Upper cervical extension
C3	Cervical side flexion
C4	Shoulder shrug
C5	Shoulder abduction, external rotation
C6	Elbow flexion, wrist extension
C7	Elbow extension, wrist flexion
C8	Thumb extension, finger flexion
T1	Finger ab/adduction
L2	Hip flexion
L3	Knee extension
L4	Ankle dorsiflexion
L5	Great toe dorsiflexion (extension)
S1–2	Ankle plantar flexion, knee flexion
S3–4	Rectal sphincter

C, cervical; T, thoracic; L, lumbar; S, sacral. Reproduced from Porter (2005) with permission.

M
N

myotonic dystrophy (DM1) a multisystem autosomal dominant condition that presents with myotonia, slow relaxation of voluntary muscle after contraction, and progressive weakness and wasting of the facial, sternomastoid and distal muscles. The disorder is due to an expansion of the myotonic dystrophy gene located on the long arm of chromosome 19q. The size of the expansion correlates broadly with the severity of the disease in the individual. The age of onset is variable but the majority of those who have the expanded myotonic dystrophy gene show some symptoms by the time they reach adult life. There is great variation in severity: some people with the expanded myotonic dystrophy gene can be so mildly affected that they are unaware of it, while others can have major problems. The genetic abnormality is unstable and tends to increase in size as it is passed from one generation to the next. This explains the progressively earlier age of onset and greater severity of the disease as it is passed from generation to generation. Affected females are at risk of having a child with the severe congenital form of the disorder, as the expanded gene is thought to be more unstable when maternally inherited. Infants affected by congenital myotonic dystrophy present with respiratory failure, feeding difficulties and ongoing developmental problems requiring specialist multidisciplinary support. New mutations are thought to be rare and it should be assumed that all cases have been inherited unless there is positive evidence to the contrary. Myotonic dystrophy is no longer thought to be a rare disorder and is regarded as the most frequently occurring muscular dystrophy of adult life. The main muscle groups commonly involved are facial, sternomastoid and the distal limb muscles.

Other systems and associated problems may include: (a) eye—cataracts, ptosis; (b) endocrine—diabetes mellitus; (c) cardiac—mainly conduction defects; (d) gastrointestinal tract—dysphagia, constipation, diarrhoea and abdominal cramps; (e) central nervous system—variable cognitive impairment, specific personality changes in adults, somnolence; (f) respiratory—muscle weakness, hypoventilation, anaesthesia risks; (g) frontal balding; (h) hypogonadism. It is important that medical problems, if they occur, are diagnosed early and treated appropriately to prevent exacerbation and avoid complications. This should be stressed, both to those at risk and to those already affected. The severe degree of apathy characteristic of myotonic dystrophy can be a major obstacle to overcome and can be responsible for low attendance rates at clinics and lack of motivation in treatment regimens. Myotonic dystrophy affects a number of body systems and thus requires careful management both in daily living and when particular medical problems arise. The multidisciplinary team should be aware of the following: (a) problems with anaesthesia may arise because health professions are unaware that the patient has such a neuromuscular disorder. Individuals should be encouraged to wear a MedicAlert bracelet or to carry an alert card in case of accidents requiring surgery; (b) hypoventilation (especially nocturnal hypoventilation) can lead to recurrent chest infections, morning headaches and increased daytime sleepiness. The patient should be referred to the physiotherapist and others in the multidisciplinary respiratory team; (c) oesophageal/pharyngeal muscle weakness causing swallowing difficulty, it may be necessary to adjust the diet and to refer to the speech and language therapist; (d) the need to prevent constipation with sufficient fibre in the diet and fluids; (e) the physiotherapist will advise on preventing foot drop or will provide below-knee calipers or plastic moulded splints to help to control foot drop should it occur; (f) regular electrocardiograms (ECGs) to detect arrhythmias caused by conduction defects; (g) regular ophthalmic checks to detect the development of cataracts. Sternomastoid muscle weakness makes the use of headrests in cars imperative. Specialist obstetric/paediatric care is necessary during pregnancy and delivery due to uterine muscle involvement, the increased risk of miscarriage and the risk of the infant being affected by myotonic dystropy. The diagnosis of a hereditary, slowly progressive muscle disorder of varying severity with associated multisystem involvement can have a profound psychological effect upon the individual and the family. Living with myotonic dystrophy is not easy either for those affected, who have little energy or motivation, or for their partners or offspring. ⊃ Duchenne muscular dystrophy, muscular dystrophies.

myotonic pupil ⊃ Adie's pupil.

myringitis *n* inflammation of the eardrum (tympanic membrane).

myringoplasty *n* operation designed to close a defect in the tympanic membrane with a graft—**myringoplastic** *adj*.

myringotome *n* a delicate instrument for incising the eardrum (tympanic membrane).

myringotomy *n* incision into the eardrum (tympanic membrane). Performed for the drainage of pus or fluid from the middle ear. Middle ear ventilation is maintained by insertion of a grommet or tube.

myxoedema *n* ➲ hypothyroidism.

myxoedema coma rare but serious event characterized by alterations in consciousness and hypothermia, usually in an older person with hypothyroidism. There is a high mortality, and treatment involves parenteral thyroid hormone and supportive measures.

myxoma *n* a connective tissue tumour composed largely of mucoid material—**myxomata** *pl*, **myxomatous** *adj*.

myxosarcoma *n* a malignant tumour of connective tissue with a soft, mucoid consistency—**myxosarcomata** *pl*, **myxosarcomatous** *adj*.

myxoviruses *npl* ➲ orthomyxoviruses and paramyxoviruses.

M
N

nabothian cyst/follicle (M Naboth, German physician, anatomist and chemist, 1675–1721) cystic distension of chronically inflamed Naboth's glands (mucus-secreting glands of the uterine cervix), where the duct of the gland has become obliterated by a healing epithelial covering and the normal mucus cannot escape.

NAD *abbr* **1.** nicotinamide adenine dinucleotide. **2.** nothing abnormal detected.

NAD/NADH *abbr* nicotinamide adenine dinucleotide (oxidized and reduced forms respectively).

NADPH oxidase an enzyme complex present in neutrophils. Involved in the oxidative killing (respiratory burst) of micro-organisms phagocytosed by the neutrophils. This is achieved by the conversion of oxygen into reactive oxygen species such as hydrogen peroxide and superoxide that are lethel to micro-organisms.

NADP/NADPH *abbr* nicotinamide adenine dinucleotide phosphate (oxidized and reduced forms respectively).

Näegele's obliquity (F Näegele, German obstetrician, 1777–1851) tilting of the fetal head to one or other side to decrease the transverse diameter presented to the pelvic brim. ⊃ asynclitism.

Näegele's pelvis an asymmetrical pelvic deformity, in which one sacral alae has failed to develop.

Näegele's rule (F Näegele) a method of calculating the expected date of delivery—three calender months is subtracted from the date of the first day of the woman's last menstrual period and seven days are added. It is based on a standard gestation period of 280 days and takes no account of variation in the length of calender months. Accuracy is affected by the length of a woman's menstrual cycle and whether or not the bleeding was true menstrual bleeding.

naevoid amentia ⊃ Sturge–Weber syndrome.

naevus *n* a general term for a congenital or acquired skin lesion, including a variety of pigmented birthmarks. There is a circumscribed lesion of the skin arising from pigment-producing naevus cells or due to a developmental abnormality of blood vessels (angioma). Naevi are usually benign and only rarely undergo malignant changes —**naevi** *pl*, **naevoid** *adj*.

Nagel anomaloscope ⊃ anomaloscope.

NAI *abbr* non-accidental injury.

nail *n* unguis. The keratinized plates of stratified squamous epithelial tissue covering and protecting the ends of the digits. Similar to the claws and hooves of other species. The exposed portion of a nail (nail plate) grows out from a germinative zone of epithelial cells known as the nail bed.

A nail comprises a root, nail body/plate and a free edge. At its proximal edge the nail is thickened to form the white lunula, which is covered by eponychium (cuticle). ⊃ nail involution, nail pits, pincer nail.

nail blanch test a test of capillary refill time used to assess the amount of blood passing through the skin (skin perfusion). Light pressure is applied to the nail bed for 5 seconds so that it turns white (blanched), when the pressure is released the normal pink nail colour should return within 2 seconds.

nail involution a nail condition in which the transverse curvature increases along its longitudinal axis, reaching its maximum at the distal part. Often causes onychophosis.

nail pits describes tiny depressions on the surface of the fingernails caused by defective nail formation seen commonly in people with psoriasis.

named midwife the midwife who is primarily working with a woman; ideally in such a way that a therapeutic relationship develops. The midwife may offer continuity of carer to the woman or coordinate care from other professionals if required.

named nurse a system whereby one qualified nurse, midwife or specialist community public health nurse is accountable for the care of each patient or client and, wherever possible, the same nurse should care for, or supervise care for, the same patient during the time that person needs care. The named nurse concept can be operated within primary nursing, team nursing, or patient allocation model. ⊃ patient allocation, primary nursing, task allocation, team nursing.

nanogram (ng) *n* one thousandth part of a microgram. 10^{-9} of a gram.

nanometre (nm) *n* one thousandth part of a micrometre. 10^{-9} of a metre.

nanophthalmos congenital disorder in which the eyes are small but without other defects.

nanotechnology the technology at the atomic or molecular scale. Nanotechnological advances in dentistry have exploited the atomic or molecular properties of materials and led to the development of newer materials with better properties.

nape *n* the nucha; back of the neck.

napkin rash erythema of the napkin area. Causes include contact with ammonia formed from the decomposition of urine, candidiasis, infantile psoriasis, allergy to detergents, excoriation from diarrhoea.

narc a prefix that means 'stupor', e.g. *narcolepsy.*

narcissism *n* self-love. In psychoanalysis the narcissistic type of personality is one where the love object is the self.

narcoanalysis *n* controversial method of analysing mental content using medication—**narcoanalytic** *adj*, **narcoanalytically** *adv*.

narcolepsy *n* excessive somnolence. A condition occurring in around 0.05% of the population, commonly presenting in teenagers and young adults. Characterized by an irresistible urge to sleep, excessive daytime sleepiness, sleep paralysis and hallucinations at the onset of sleep (hypnogogic stage) or during the stage between sleep and waking (hypnopompic stage) and cataplexy (loss of muscle tone)—**narcoleptic** *adj*.

narcosis *n* drug-induced unconsciousness. ⊃ carbon dioxide narcosis, narcotic.

narcosynthesis *n* the building up of a clearer mental picture of an incident involving the client by reviving memories of it, using medication, so that both the client and the therapist can examine the incident in clearer perspective.

narcotic *n, adj* (describes) a drug causing abnormally deep sleep. Strong analgesic narcotics, such as the opioids that include morphine, may cause respiratory depression which is reversible by the use of narcotic antagonists.

nares *n* (*syn.* choanae) the nostrils—**naris** *sing*. ⊃ anterior nares, posterior nares.

narrow-angle glaucoma ⊃ angle-closure glaucoma (ACG).

nasal *adj* pertaining to the nose.

nasal bone *n* one of two facial bones that form the superior and lateral surfaces of the nasal bridge.

nasal canthus ⊃ canthus.

nasal cavity *n* an irregular cavity divided by the nasal septum and bounded by the orbit above, the hard palate below and the inner walls of the maxillary sinuses. It is lined with ciliated epithelium containing numerous mucus-producing glands. This lining is continuous with that of the paranasal sinuses. The nasal cavity is the main entry for air during inspiration. Air enters via the anterior nares and passes through the posterior nares to the nasopharynx. Nerve endings in the roof of the nose are concerned with the sense of smell (olfaction).

nasal conchae *npl* also called the turbninate bones. Three thin bones (superior, middle, inferior) that project into the nasal cavity increasing the mucosal surface area and causing air turbulence. The superior and middle conchae are parts of the ethmoid bone. The conchae collectively increase the surface area in the nasal cavity, allowing inspired air to be warmed and humidified more effectively. ⊃ ethmoid bone, inferior nasal conchae, Colour Section Figure 14.

nasal flaring enlargement of the anterior nares (nostrils) during inspiration. It is usually observed in infants and young children and can be a sign that breathing is difficult and needs more effort. Nasal flaring can be indicative of respiratory distress caused by a variety of conditions including croup, bronchiolitis, pneumonia, asthma. It may be accompanied by head bobbing as the infant or child breathes in.

nasal septum *n* a partition that divides the nasal cavity into two. The posterior bony part is formed by the ethmoid bone and the anterior part is formed from hyaline cartilage.

nasal speculum used for examination of the nose and for treatments, such as nasal cautery and packing to stop bleeding.

nasal tube a catheter inserted into the nasal passages to permit the administration of oxygen therapy.

nas a prefix that means 'nose', e.g. *nasolacrimal*.

nasion both a hard and soft tissue anatomical landmark. ⊃ bony nasion, soft tissue nasion.

nasoduodenal *adj* pertaining to the nose and duodenum, as passing a *nasoduodenal tube* via this route, for feeding. ⊃ enteral.

nasogastric (NG) *adj* pertaining to the nose and stomach, as passing a *nasogastric tube* via this route, usually for aspiration, or feeding.

nasojejunal *adj* pertaining to the nose and jejunum, usually referring to a tube passed via the nose into the jejunum for feeding.

nasolabial relating to the nose and lip, such as the area between the nose and the top lip.

nasolabial cyst developmental cyst arising in the soft tissues beneath the nasolabial fold.

nasolacrimal *adj* pertaining to the nose and lacrimal apparatus.

naso-oesophageal *adj* pertaining to the nose and the oesophagus.

nasopalatine pertaining to the nose and palate.

nasopalatine canal the canal leading from the nasopalatine or incisive foramen. The nasopalatine afferent nerve from the mucosa and gingivae of the anterior part of the hard palate runs through the incisive foramen and the canal, later to join the maxillary branch of the trigeminal nerve.

nasopalatine cyst also known as the incisive canal cyst. A developmental cyst arising from the nasopalatine duct epithelium.

nasopalatine foramen ⊃ incisive foramen.

nasopalatine nerve an afferent nerve arising from the mucous membrane of the anterior part of the hard palate and gingivae of the adjacent teeth. It ascends through the anterior palatine foramen running back to join the sphenopalatine ganglion and through this to the maxillary division of the trigeminal nerve.

nasopharyngeal pertaining to the nose and the pharynx, or to the nasopharynx. ⊃ airway.

nasopharyngeal airway ⊃ airway.

nasopharyngeal intubation the technique of passing a flexible tube into the nasopharynx through the nose.

nasopharyngeal tonsils ⊃ tonsils.

nasopharyngitis *n* inflammation of the nasopharynx.

nasopharyngoscope *n* an endoscope for viewing the nasal passages and postnasal space—**nasopharyngoscopic** *adj*.

nasopharynx *n* the portion of the pharynx behind the nose and above the soft palate. The posterior nares open into the nasopharynx. The nasopharynx communicates with

M
N

the middle ear via the pharyngotympanic (eustachian or auditory) tube. The nasopharyngeal tonsils are present on the posterior wall, these are known as adenoids when enlarged. Air passes through the nasopharaynx making it exclusively respiratory in function unlike the oral and laryngeal parts of the pharynx—**nasopharyngeal** *adj.* ⊃ Waldeyer's ring.

nasotracheal pertaining to the nose and trachea, such as passing an endotracheal tube through the nose and into trachea in order to administer a general anaesthetic.

natal teeth teeth present at birth. They may be extra teeth or may be due to the early eruption of primary teeth.

nates *npl* the buttocks. Formed from the bulk of the gluteal muscles and fatty tissue—**natis** *sing*.

National Childbirth Trust (NCT) a charitable organization offering education for pregnancy, birth and parenthood, with over 300 UK branches and groups providing antenatal classes, breastfeeding counselling and postnatal support.

National Confidential Enquiries four national enquiries that investigate clinical practice in specific areas: Confidential Enquiry into Maternal Deaths (CEMD); National Confidential Enquiry into Perioperative Deaths (NCEPOD); Confidential Enquiries into Stillbirths and Deaths in Infancy (CESDI); and Confidential Inquiry into Suicide and Homicide by People with Mental Illness (CISH).

National Health Service (NHS) a state-funded and managed system of health care established in 1948. It aims to provide universal and comprehensive health care that is financed by central government through money raised by general taxation and was intended to be free at the point of delivery. A system of charges were, however, introduced before 1950 and have gradually increased. It is a three layer system of preventive and therapeutic healthcare services and facilities available within the UK. Care and treatment is delivered by primary (e.g. general practitioners), secondary (e.g. local hospitals) and tertiary (regional and supra-regional specialist hospitals) providers. The structure and management of the NHS and the delivery of care have undergone frequent and comprehensive change in the last 60 years.

National Institute for Health and Clinical Excellence (NICE) an independent body that generates and distributes clinical guidance based on evidence of clinical and cost-effectiveness for England and Wales. For example, the cost-effectiveness of new drugs and treatments or the management of a particular condition. It merged with the Health Development Agency in 2005.

National Patient Safety Agency (NPSA) an agency set up to improve patient safety within the NHS. All NHS staff are encouraged to report patient safety incidents without fear of blame, and for colleagues to learn from such incidents (actual and near misses). The NPSA assesses reports from all areas and introduces preventative measures as necessary. For example, increased safety measures to ensure that patients receive the correct blood for transfusion; the use of the standard internal telephone number (2222), in NHS

Trusts in England and Wales, to summon the 'crash' team to an in-hospital cardiac arrest.

National Service Frameworks (NSFs) evidence-based frameworks for major care areas and particular groups of disease, e.g. Diabetes, Older People, Mental Health, Cancer, Renal Services, etc., that state what patients/clients can presume to receive from the NHS. Forthcoming NSFs include one for Chronic Obstructive Pulmonary Disease.

natriuresis the excretion of larger amounts than normal of sodium in the urine.

natural childbirth, active birth approach to labour and delivery advocating avoidance of medical interference and technology and analgesia in labour, encouraging both parents to participate in and share the experience of childbirth.

natural dentition ⊃ dentition.

natural family planning methods that do not make use of appliances or drugs. Family planning that is based on an awareness of the naturally occurring fertile and non-fertile phases of the female's menstrual cycle. Couples may use one or a combination of: a commercially-produced system for measuring urinary hormone levels to predict the fertile phase; basal body temperature recorded daily may give an indication of progesterone secretion from the ovary and thus, by observing when the basal body temperature rises, gives an approximate guide to the timing of ovulation; menstrual cycle calendar (rhythm method); or changes in the amount and consistency of cervical mucus. ⊃ Billing's method, coitus interruptus.

natural killer (NK) cells non-phagocytic, cytotoxic cells belonging to a group of large granular lymphocytes. They function as part of the non-specific (innate) body defences. NK cells kill virus-infected cells and cancer cells. They become active in response to various substances that include interferons and other cytokines. They may have a surveillance role in detecting cells with malignant changes. ⊃ interferons.

natural killer cytotoxic activity the ability of natural killer cells to kill virus-infected cells and cancer cells.

nature ⊃ severity, irritability and nature factors (SIN).

naturopathy *n* a multidisciplinary approach to health care that includes all aspects of one's lifestyle, e.g. natural foods grown without chemicals and medicines based on plants. It is founded upon the belief of the body's power to heal itself given an optimal environment for healing—**naturopathic** *adj*.

nausea *n* a feeling of impending vomiting. May be accompanied by an unpleasant feeling in the abdomen and throat with a gagging sensation, the production of excessive watery saliva, increased swallowing, sweating and pallor. Vomiting does not always occur—**nauseate** *vt*.

navel *n* ⊃ umbilicus.

navicular 1. *adj* shaped like a boat, such as the bone in the ankle. **2.** *n* one of the tarsal bones of the ankle (also known as the scaphoid bone). Situated on the medial side of the foot in front of the talus (ankle bone), with which its concave posterior surface articulates. Stress fractures of the navicular are seen in runners and should be considered if localized pain and discomfort fail to settle.

NBAS *abbr* Neonatal Behavioural Assessment Scale.

NBI *abbr* no bony injury.

NBM *abbr* nil (nothing) by mouth.

NBT *abbr* nitroblue tetrazolium reduction test.

NCT *abbr* National Childbirth Trust.

NCVQ *abbr* National Council for Vocational Qualifications.

NDT *abbr* neurodevelopmental therapy.

Nd-Yag laser *abbr* ➲ neodymium-yag (Nd-Yag) laser.

near addition (*syn* reading addition) the difference in spherical power between the distance and near corrections. A common method of arriving at the power of the addition is to measure the patient's working distance and the amplitude of accommodation. The add is obtained as follows: add = (1 metre/working distance in metre) − *x* (amplitude) where *x* is the percentage of the total amplitude of accommodation which is to be used: two-thirds is usually more appropriate for younger people with presbyopia (below about 52 years of age), while one-half is more appropriate for older people. Thus, this formula allows for a certain amount of the amplitude of accommodation to be left in reserve (usually one-third or one-half). ➲ presbyopia, reading distance.

near parallelism in dentistry, a feature of inlay and crown preparations in which the opposing surfaces or walls are only very slightly tapered (i.e. very nearly parallel to each other), thus allowing the insertion of the restoration and also providing maximum retention.

near point of accommodation (*syn* punctum proximum) the nearest point in space which is conjugate with the foveola when exerting the maximum accommodative effort. ➲ push-up method.

near point of convergence (NPC) the nearest point where the lines of sight intersect when the eyes converge to the maximum. This point is normally about 8–10 cm from the spectacle plane. If further away, the patient may have convergence insufficiency. ➲ convergence insufficiency, metre angle.

near point rule a device for measuring the near points of accommodation and convergence. The rule consists of a graduated four-sided bar on which is mounted a movable target holder which can be moved in the median plane of the head. The bar is calibrated in centimetres and dioptres. ➲ near point of accommodation, push-up method.

near point stress ➲ asthenopia.

near reflex ➲ accommodative reflex.

near-triad reflex ➲ accommodative reflex.

near visual acuity the capacity for seeing distinctly the details of an object at near. It is specified in various ways: (a) as the angle of resolution of the smallest resolvable print (in minutes of arc) at a given near distance; (b) as a Snellen fraction, either as one which is equivalent to the distance visual acuity (*Snellen equivalent*) or more correctly as one which indicates the actual distance (e.g. 16/32 if the distance is 16 inches); (c) as an arbitrary Jaeger notation (e.g. J6);

(d) as *N notation* (using Times Roman typeface) or *Points* (using any typeface), such as N8 at 40 cm (or simply 8-point), where N refers to near and the number to the amount of points (a point is a unit used by printers to specify print size and is equal to 1/72 of an inch). Thus N8 indicates that the overall height is 8/72 inch (or 2.82 mm) or about 4/72 inch (or 1.41 mm) for lower-case letters; (e) as *M Units*. For the usual font styles (e.g. Times Roman, Century) used in newsprint, 8-point print is usually considered to be approximately equal to 1 M Unit, so M units = points/8 or 1 M = N8, 2 M = N16, etc. ➲ Bailey-Lovie chart, Jaeger test types, visual acuity.

nebula *n* a cloud-like corneal opacity.

nebulizer *n* an apparatus for converting a liquid into a fine spray. It is used to deliver medicaments for application to the respiratory tract or the skin. A very common method of drug delivery used in the management of asthma (Figure N.1).

NEC *abbr* necrotizing enterocolitis.

Necator *n* a genus of parasitic nematode hookworms that includes *Necator americanus*. ➲ *Ancylostoma*.

necatoriasis infestation with the hookworm *Necator americanus*, which is found in the New World and tropical Africa. The larvae are present in the soil and gain access to the body through the skin of the lower limbs and feet, or contaminated water or food. Many infestations are asymptomatic but can cause abdominal pain, diarrhoea and iron deficiency anaemia. Infestation is prevented by wearing

M
N

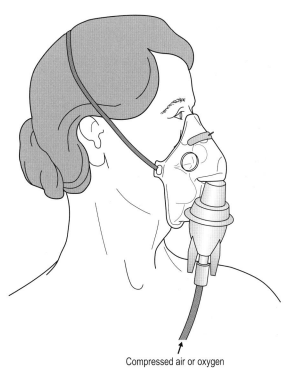

Compressed air or oxygen

N.1 Nebulizer (adapted from Nicol et al 2004 with permission).

shoes and effective sanitation to prevent contamination of soil with human faeces.

neck 1. the narrow, constricted part of an organ or other structure. For example, the neck of the femur and the humerus, the thinner area below the condylar process of the ramus of the mandible, and the neck (cervix) of the uterus. **2.** the narrow area between the head and the body. **3.** that part of the tooth where the crown joins the root.

neck injury damage to the structure of the neck including soft tissue, bones, spinal column, spinal cord and nerves. In sport, most commonly injured by direct trauma with compression (rugby) or a fall from height (trampolining, horse riding). Appropriate first aid care is vital to prevent spinal cord damage and possible paralysis. It is essential to stabilize the neck and not to move the casualty until experienced, qualified help arrives, especially if the airway is compromised. Symptoms range from pain and stiffness to numbness, paraesthesia and paralysis, but the commonest neck injuries are muscle spasm and strains, which settle with rest and physiotherapy. ➲ spinal injury/spinal cord injury.

neck strap or cervical strap a form of orthodontic headgear designed to fit around the neck only.

necr a prefix that means 'corpse, dead', e.g. *necrophilia*.

necrobiosis tissue changes characterized by swelling, the presence of basophils and the deformation of collagen in the dermis. There may be loss of normal tissue structure but with cell necrosis. ➲ necrobiosis lipoidica.

necrobiosis lipoidica a form of necrobiosis that is important to recognize because of its association with diabetes mellitus. Less than 1% of people with diabetes have necrobiosis, but more than 85% of patients with necrobiosis will have or will develop diabetes. Typically, the lesions appear as shiny, atrophic and slightly yellow plaques on the shins and arms. Underlying telangiectasia is easily seen. Minor knocks may precipitate slow-healing ulcers. No treatment is very effective. Topical and intralesional corticosteroids are used, as is long term treatment with PUVA (psoralen with ultraviolet A). ➲ Colour Section Figure 92.

necrophilia 1. an abnormal liking for dead bodies. **2.** the perversion of being sexually attracted to dead bodies. It may involve sexual gratification in the presence of a dead body, or sexual contact with the dead body, usually a man having sexual intercourse with a dead woman.

necropsy *n* the examination of a dead body.

necrosectomy *n* removal of necrotic tissue, e.g. necrotic pancreas as a consequence of severe acute pancreatitis.

necrosis *n* localized death of tissue—**necrotic** *adj*.

necrotizing enterocolitis (NEC) a condition occurring primarily in preterm or low birthweight neonates. Parts of the gut wall become necrotic, leading to intestinal obstruction and peritonitis. Probably caused by a combination of ischaemia, hypoxia and bacterial infection.

necrotizing fasciitis rare infection caused either by some strains of group A *Streptococcus pyogenes*, or a polymicrobial infection with Enterobacteriaceae and anaerobes.

There is very severe inflammation of the muscle sheath and massive soft tissue destruction. There is toxaemia and multiple-organ dysfunction syndrome leading to a mortality rate between 30–80%. ➲ Colour Section Figure 93.

necrotizing scleritis the most severe form of scleritis, much less common than the other types. About half the patients have one of the following diseases: rheumatoid arthritis, Wegener's granulomatosis, polyarteritis nodosa, systemic lupus erythematosus or herpes zoster. It is characterized by pain, and white, avascular areas next to damaged areas through which one can see the brown colour of the underlying uveal tissue, and to congested areas of the sclera. In most cases visual acuity is decreased. The necrosis gradually spreads around the globe. Treatment typically consists of topical corticosteroids, immunosuppressive agents and occasionally surgery to repair scleral or corneal perforation. ➲ scleromalacia.

necrotizing scleritis without inflammation ➲ sclerokeratitis.

necrotizing ulcerative gingivitis (NUG) previously called Vincent's angina, trench mouth, acute ulcerative necrotizing gingivitis (AUNG) and acute ulcerative gingivitis (AUG). Acute inflammation of the gingivae associated with spontaneous bleeding, pain, the presence of a grey slough called a pseudomembrane, and a characteristic halitosis. Usually occurs in young adults. Of unknown cause but associated with poor oral hygiene and the presence of a fusiform bacillus/spirochaete bacterial complex. Treatment is by prophylactic measures and, in severe cases, administration of metronidazole.

necrotizing ulcerative periodontitis acute periodontal disease in which there is redness of the gingival and alveolar mucosa. There is interdental ulceration and loss of interdental soft tissue and bone, leading to loss of periodontal attachments. ➲ periodontitis.

need for achievement ➲ achievement motivation.

need hierarchy theory the theory proposed by American psychologist Abraham Maslow (1908–1970) that human needs are hierarchically ordered such that the gratification of a need lower in the hierarchy leads to the emergence of the next higher need in the hierarchy. From lower to higher, the needs are: basic physiological needs (food, water, etc.); safety and security needs; love and belonging needs; self-esteem needs; and self-actualization needs (achieving one's true potential).

needle biopsy the removal of tissue from a lesion, for analysis by using a needle; the needle is rotated and the tissue remains in the lumen.

needle holder a hinged metal instrument with scissor handles, ratchets and serrated blades to grip suture needles without allowing any rotation. ➲ forceps.

needle phobia many children and young people who require medical intervention are most concerned about needles. Some of these children will develop an extreme fear or phobia. These children can develop manifestations of neurogenic shock when exposed to needles and this reaction can spread so that the child also fears objects or situations associated with needles. All children should be prepared effectively for any procedure involving needles to prevent the development of the phobia. Preparation involves physical and psychological interventions that include: (a) topical anaesthetic cream can be used to numb the site for most needle procedures. It is most effective when used in conjunction with psychological preparation, as the frightened child's fear will not be allayed merely by numbness of this site; (b) giving information to the child and family about the procedure. The child should be told honestly about the physical and sensory effects of the procedure in an appropriate age-related way; (c) providing a supportive environment by allowing parental presence in child-friendly surroundings with staff who are empathetic; (d) helping the child to cope by using distraction, play therapy, relaxation or guided imagery techniques during the procedure; (e) providing positive reinforcement to the child after the procedure with the use of bravery certificates or stickers, as well as verbal encouragement of their coping skills.

needle point tracing arrow point tracing produced extraorally. ⊃ tracing.

needlestick injury a particular hazard for healthcare workers and other groups, where accidental injury is sustained when skin or mucosa is penetrated by contaminated needles or other items. There is a risk of infection with various hepatitis viruses (e.g. hepatitis B or C) or, more rarely, the human immunodeficiency virus (HIV). All healthcare facilities or services should have a risk assessment, staff training, and policies and procedures in place for protective clothing, safer needles, proper disposal of equipment and action to be taken should injury occur. Post-exposure prophylaxis with antiretroviral drugs may be indicated. The person should obtain immediate expert advice.

needling *n* procedure for removal of congenital cataract, now superseded.

needs assessment estimating the need (quantifying) for services in a population. *normative,* or *assessed,* need defined by the expert or professional in any given situation; *felt need,* or *want,* perceived by the individual; *expressed need,* or *operationalized felt need*; *comparative need,* using the characteristics of a population receiving a service to define those with similar characteristics as in need. Needs assessment uses broad, non-specific indicators of need obtained through repeated health surveys of the general population (e.g. General Household Survey, Health Survey for England) and more specific indicators based on surveys of particular groups (e.g. survey of people with disabilities, loss of urinary continence). The weighted capitation formula for resource allocation uses the characteristics of populations using hospital services as indicators of need.

Neer arthroplasty a type of arthroplasty used for patients with shoulder (glenohumeral) arthritis. It takes two forms, a hemiarthroplasty may be performed or a total shoulder replacement.

Neer classification a classification used for fractures affecting the proximal humerus. There are six groups of increasing severity: group 1—minimal displacement; Group 2—anatomical neck fracture with less than 1 cm displacement; Group 3—displaced or angulated surgical neck; Group 4—displaced fracture of greater tuberosity; Group 5—fractures of the lesser tuberosity; and Group 6—fracture and dislocations.

NEFA *abbr* non-esterified free fatty acid.

negative affect a general dimension of affect reflecting a state of distress, subsuming various negative mood states including fear, anger, shame and guilt. ⊃ affect.

negative convergence ⊃ divergence.

negative correlation in statistics, when information is linked and an increase in one item will result in a decrease in the other and a decrease in one item will result in a increase in the other.

negative feedback in physiology, a homeostatic mechanism, whereby high levels, for example, of a particular hormone in the blood, 'turns off' or negates the stimulus that causes the hormone secretion (see Figure F.1, p. 284). Once hormone levels fall below the normal range, the stimulus is activated and again causes the hormone to be secreted. ⊃ feedback, homeostasis, positive feedback.

negative nitrogen balance ⊃ nitrogen balance.

negative number a number with a value of less than zero.

negative reinforcement ⊃ reinforcement.

negative transfer a degradation in performance because of practice or experience of another skill, typically where the new skill has similar characteristics and gaining familiarity with these interferes with prior learning of the similar but specific aspects of the prior skill. For example, some tennis players believe that practising other racquet sports such as badminton or squash degrades their tennis performance. ⊃ positive transfer, transfer of learning.

negative work ⊃ work.

negativism *n* active refusal by the patient to cooperate, usually shown by the patient consistently doing the exact opposite of what is asked. Seen in catatonic schizophrenia.

negatron a negative beta particle.

negligence *n* a form of professional malpractice which includes the omission of acts that a prudent health professional would have done or the commission of acts that a prudent health professional would not do. It is a professional duty to avoid patient/client injury or suffering caused in this way. It can become the basis of litigation for damages. ⊃ Bolam test, duty of care.

Neisseria *n* (A Neisser, German dermatologist, bacteriologist, 1855–1916) a genus of aerobic and facultatively anaerobic, Gram-negative bacteria. They belong to the family *Neisseriaceae.* Some are commensals found in the pharynx, genitourinary tract and on the skin in humans, but others are pathogens. *Neisseria gonorrhoeae* causes gonorrhoea and *Neisseria meningitidis* causes life-threatening meningitis and meningococcal septicaemia.

M

N

Nélaton's line (A Nélaton, French physician and surgeon, 1807–1873) an imaginary line joining the anterior superior iliac spine to the ischial tuberosity. The greater trochanter of the femur normally lies on or below this line, but in cases of the hip or femoral neck fracture, the trochanter lies above the line.

Nelson syndrome (D Nelson, American physician, b.1925) hyperpigmentation, including marked darkening of fair skin, as a result of uncontrolled adrenocorticotrophin (ACTH) secretion from a pituitary adenoma, usually after treatment of the associated Cushing's disease by bilateral adrenalectomy.

nem unit of nutrition equivalent to the nutritive value of 1 g of breast milk.

nematodes *npl* parasitic worms that can be divided into three groups: (a) those that mainly live in the intestine, e.g. *Ancylostoma duodenale* (hookworm), *Ascaris lumbricoides* (roundworm), *Enterobius vermicularis* (threadworm), *Necator americanus, Strongyloides stercoralis* and *Trichuris trichiura* (whipworm); (b) those that are mainly in the tissues, e.g. *Dracunculus medinensis* (guinea worm) and the filarial worms that include *Loa loa*; (c) those from other species (zoonotic), e.g. *Toxocara canis, Trichinella spiralis*.

neo- a prefix that means 'new', e.g. *neoplasia*.

neoadjuvant therapy in cancer treatment the use of preliminary chemotherapy or radiotherapy to reduce tumour size before further treatment such as surgery. Aims to improve the outcome of surgery and to reduce the risk of metastatic spread.

neodymium-yag (Nd-Yag) laser a solid-state laser whose active medium is a crystal of yttrium, aluminium and garnet doped with neodymium ions. It emits an infrared light beam with a wavelength of 1064 nm. It is typically used with a slit-lamp and in conjunction with a helium-neon laser which produces a red beam of light (633 nm) to allow focusing. It may be used to perform capsulotomy, iridotomy or trabecular surgery. ⊃ laser refraction.

neohesperidine DC an intense sweetener, approximately 1500–1800 times sweeter than sucrose (beet or cane sugar). ⊃ sweetener.

neologism *n* the creation of a new word. A type of thought disorder seen in schizophrenia, mania and other psychotic illnesses.

neonatal *adj* relating to the first 28 days of life.

Neonatal Behavioural Assessment Scale (NBAS) a means of assessing an infant's condition, alertness, motor function, irritability, consolability and interaction with people.

neonatal hearing screening hearing screening can be performed in young infants by use of computer-linked otoacoustic emission testing (OAE) or automated auditory brainstem response (AABR) testing. Where the two screening tests are unavailable, a less reliable distraction test using simple sounds can be performed in infants.

neonatal herpes acquired during vaginal delivery from a mother actively shedding herpes simplex virus. It is a devastating illness with a 75% mortality rate and a high incidence of severe neurological sequelae among survivors.

neonatal hypocalcaemia low level of calcium in the blood can occur within 48 hours of delivery or between the 5th and 8th days of life. Convulsions may occur, especially in infants fed on unmodified cows' milk formula as high phosphorus content contributes to the condition. It is also a very rare complication of exchange transfusion.

neonatal hypothermia the neonate may lose heat rapidly due to the body's large surface area, especially if not dried well at delivery. There is an increased risk in preterm infants who lack brown fat to help them maintain core body temperature. Extreme chilling causes the infant to use up energy and oxygen, and if the core temperature falls below 35°C, neonatal cold injury develops which may lead to death.

neonatal line a line seen under the microscope as an exaggerated incremental line in the enamel and dentine of the primary teeth and the first permanent molar. It is a sign of metabolic upset at or about the time of birth.

neonatal mortality the death rate of babies in the first 28 days of life.

neonatal respiratory distress syndrome (NRDS) respiratory failure due to surfactant deficiency in the newborn. Most commonly affects premature infants.

neonatal screening screening tests undertaken soon after birth to detect diseases and abnormalities. Screening includes a thorough physical (head-to-toe) examination, which includes checking for congenital cataracts, developmental hip dysplasia, congenital heart defects and undescended testes; a blood-spot test for various conditions including phenylketonuria, cystic fibrosis, hypothyroidism, galactosaemia (in some countries), sickle-cell diseases and thalassaemia and medium chain acyl-CoA dehydrogenase deficiency (MCADD); and a hearing test.

neonatal thermoregulation neonates are incapable of achieving a balance of heat loss and heat retention. They lose heat through conduction, radiation, evaporation and convection. Care is required to minimize heat loss by quickly drying and covering the infant (especially the head) after birth.

neonatal unit (NNU/NICU/SCBU) usually reserved for preterm and small-for-dates babies between 700 and 2000 g in weight, mostly requiring the use of high technology which is available in these units.

neonate *n* a newborn baby up to 28 days old.

neonatology *n* the scientific study of the newborn.

neonatorum *adj* pertaining to the newborn.

neoplasia *n* literally, the formation of new tissue. Customarily refers to the pathological process in the growth of a benign or malignant tumour—**neoplastic** *adj*.

neoplasm *n* a new growth; a tumour that is either cancerous or non-cancerous.

neoplastic relating to a neoplasm.

neovascular glaucoma a secondary glaucoma due to new vessel formation on the anterior surface of the iris blocking the exit of the aqueous humour through the angle of filtration. It may occur as a result of central retinal vein occlusion (this type typically develops within 3 months and is sometimes called 'ninety-day glaucoma'), or diabetes mellitus. Other causes include carotid artery occlusion, central retinal artery occlusion, retinal and choroidal tumours. The condition may initially be open-angle but eventually becomes angle-closure with severe loss of visual acuity, pain, congestion, high intraocular pressure, corneal oedema, aqueous flare, synechia and severe rubeosis iridis. The presence of new blood vessels on the iris and drainage angle distinguishes this condition from primary angle-closure glaucoma. Treatment includes topical corticosteroids to decrease the inflammation, beta (β)-adrenoceptor antagonists and carbonic anhydrase inhibitors to lower the intraocular pressure and laser treatment of the iris neovascularization and sometimes ciliodestructive procedures. ⏎ angle-closure glaucoma, ectropion uvea, rubeosis iridis.

neovascularization *n* the formation of new abnormal blood vessels. A feature of the proliferative stage of diabetic retinopathy.

nephr/o- a prefix that means 'kidney', e.g. *nephrotoxic*.

nephralgia *n* pain in the kidney.

nephrectomy *n* surgical removal of a kidney.

nephritis *n* non-specific term for inflammation within the kidney—**nephritic** *adj*.

nephroblastoma *n* the most common solid tumour of the kidney. Usually presents as an abdominal mass. Also known as Wilms' tumour. ⏎ Wilms' tumour.

nephrocalcinosis *n* the deposition of calcium salts within the renal tubules (the substance of the kidneys). It results from hyperparathyroidism and high levels of calcium in the blood, or disorders of the kidney, such as some types of renal tubular acidosis. It may lead to nephrolithiasis (the formation of renal calculi) and possible renal failure.

nephrogenic *adj* coming from or produced by the kidney.

nephrolithiasis *n* **1.** the formation of calculi in the kidney (kidney stones or renal calculi). **2.** the presence of calculi in the kidney(s).

nephrolithotomy *n* removal of a stone from the kidney by an incision through the kidney substance. ⏎ percutaneous nephrolithotomy.

nephrology *n* study of diseases of the kidney.

nephron *n* the functional unit of the kidney, comprising a glomerulus (a knot of capillaries) and a renal tubule with the associated peritubular capillary network. The tubule has a Bowman's capsule, proximal and distal convoluted tubules, loop of Henle and a collecting tubule that drains urine from many nephrons to the renal pelvis (Figure N.2).

nephronophthisis *n* rare disorder involving the growth of many small cysts in the medulla of the kidney; often leads to renal failure.

nephropathy *n* any disease of the kidney in which inflammation is not a major component. ⏎ diabetic nephropathy—**nephropathic** *adj*.

nephropexy *n* surgical fixation of a floating kidney.

nephroptosis *n* downward displacement of the kidney. The word is sometimes used for a floating kidney.

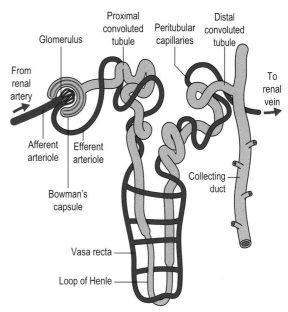

N.2 Nephron—simplified (reproduced from Brooker & Waugh 2007 with permission).

nephrosclerosis a hardening or sclerosis of the kidney. There are changes in the renal arterioles leading to ischaemia. Commonly caused by hypertension, or associated with general arteriosclerosis in older people.

nephroscope *n* an endoscope for viewing kidney tissue. It can be designed to create a continuous flow of irrigating fluid and provide an exit for the fluid and accompanying debris—**nephroscopic** *adj*.

nephrosis nephropathy. Any degenerative disease of the renal tubules. ⏎ nephrotic syndrome.

nephrostomy *n* a surgically established fistula from the pelvis of the kidney to the body surface.

nephrotic syndrome disease characterized by heavy proteinuria, low serum albumin (hypoalbuminaemia) and oedema formation; there are a wide range of causes.

nephrotoxic *adj* describes any substance or process that is injurious to renal tissue or function. For example the aminoglycoside antibiotics, (e.g. gentamicin)—**nephrotoxin** *n*.

nephroureterectomy *n* removal of the kidney along with a part or the whole of the ureter. Also known as ureteronephrectomy.

NEQ *abbr* noise equivalent quanta.

nerve block anaesthesia regional anaesthesia. The injection of a local anaesthetic, (e.g. lidocaine) into an area close to a nerve. Thus blocking the conduction in the nerve and producing anaesthesia in the structures supplied by that nerve.

nerve cell a neuron; the structural unit of the nervous system. Each consists of a cell body with a great many fine short extensions from its surface (dendrites) and a long thin extension, the nerve fibre with an axon at its core.

Other neurons which influence the activity of the cell (by excitation or inhibition) form synapses on the cell body or dendrites, and the axon terminates at a synapse on another neuron or on the effector which it innervates. ⊃ motor neuron, neuron, neurotransmitter.

nerve conduction test an electrical test used to ascertain whether nerve impulse transmission is occurring in the peripheral nerves. The nerve is electrically stimulated and a distal electrode records the impulse. Used in the diagnosis of polyneuropathies and in nerve entrapment.

nerve deafness ⊃ sensorineural hearing loss (SNHL)/ deafness.

nerve entrapment syndrome a type of mononeuropathy in which a nerve is trapped and compressed, for example as it passes through a bony canal or through fascia, such as carpal tunnel syndrome or meralgia paraesthetica. It is characterized by abnormal sensation, pain, muscle weakness and muscle wastage.

nerve fibre *n* an elongated bundle of fibres which serves for the transmission of impulses between the periphery and the nerve centres. A component of all nerves and their branches in the peripheral nervous system (PNS), and of the tracts in the central nervous system (CNS). The central axon transmits nerve impulses (action potentials) to the nerve terminal in motor (efferent) nerves, or from a receptor to a nerve cell body in sensory (afferent) nerves. Also common to all nerve fibres are an outermost covering (neurilemma) and within that the Schwann cells which are crucial to the regeneration process if a fibre is damaged. In myelinated nerve fibres (including motor nerves to skeletal muscle) there is a fatty myelin sheath between the axon and the neurilemma, interrupted at intervals by the 'nodes of Ranvier'; action potentials 'jump' between these, enabling faster conduction. Each efferent nerve fibre runs from a nerve cell body to terminal branches at a nerve-to-nerve synapse or at an effector organ; each afferent fibre runs from a sensory receptor to a relay site in the CNS.

nerve fibre types nerve fibres are classified according to how quickly they conduct impulses (conduction velocity in m/s), the diameter of the fibres (in μm), the presence or not of myelination and by function (Table N.1). Much of the confusion in fibre classification arises because there are two systems (I, II, III, IV and A, B, C) describing the same thing—the diameter and conduction velocity of the population of nerve fibres which extend from thick myelinated fibres at one extreme (group I or Aα or even simply α) to thin unmyelinated at the other extreme (group IV or C fibres). The major difference is that one focuses, but not exclusively, on afferent and the other on efferent fibres. It should be remembered that, although the group I, II, III, IV system is usually used for muscle afferents and the Aα–δ, C system for motor nerves and skin afferents, both systems are based on fibre diameter and conduction velocity and are as equivalent as measuring length in millimetres or inches.

nerve growth factor (NGF) *n* protein growth factor required for nerve differentiation and growth during embryonic development and for later nerve maintenance.

nerve impulse the transmission of electrochemical energy occurring along a nerve fibre as electrical and concentration gradients across the excitable cell membrane are caused by ion (sodium and potassium) movement (Figure N.3). ⊃ action potential, depolarization, polarized, repolarization.

nerve–muscle interaction a term relating to the functional inter-relationship of the components of movement: muscles and nerves.

nerve stimulator apparatus used to electronically stimulate peripheral nerves to locate them and test nerve blockade. ⊃ nerve conduction test.

nerve trunk a cord-like arrangement of nerve fibres from which many branches take origin.

nervous *adj* **1.** relating to nerves or nerve tissue. **2.** referring to a state of restlessness or timidity.

nervous system the structures controlling the actions and functions of the body; it comprises the brain and spinal cord

Table N.1 Nerve fibre types

Class	Myelination	Conduction velocity (m/s)	Diameter (μm)	Function
I (a & b)	+	70–120	12–20	Afferent from muscle spindles and tendon organs
II	+	25–70	4–12	Afferent from muscle spindles, touch and pressure
III	+	3–30	1–4	Afferent from cold and pain receptors
Aα	+	50–120	8–20	Efferent to extrafusal muscle fibres
Aβ	+	30–70	5–12	Efferent to intra- and extra- fusal fibres, skin afferents
Aγ	+	10–50	2–8	Efferent to intrafusal muscle fibres
Aδ	+	3–30	1–5	Afferent pain, cold
B	+	5–15	1–3	Preganglionic autonomic
C (sometimes called IV)	–	<2	<1	Postganglionic autonomic, visceral and somatic afferents for pain and temperature sensation
Reproduced from Porter (2005) with permission

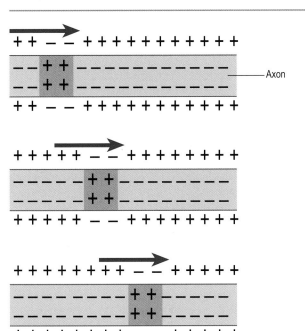

Axon

N.3 Propagation of a nerve impulse—simplified (reproduced from Waugh & Grant 2006 with permission).

(central nervous system [CNS]), and all the peripheral nerve fibres and ganglia that are outside the brain and spinal cord. The peripheral nervous system can be further subdivided into the sensory division and the motor division. The latter is in turn divided into the voluntary somatic nervous system and the involuntary autonomic system, which is divided into the sympathetic and parasympathetic nervous systems. ➲ autonomic nervous system, parasympathetic nervous system, peripheral nervous system, sympathetic nervous system, Colour Section Figures 1, 11.

Nesbit's operation (R Nesbit, American surgeon, 20th century) an operative procedure undertaken to relieve the curvature of the penis, such as that occurring in Peyronie's disease.

net force ➲ force.

net moment of force the mathematical result of all the moments applied to an object or body, taking into account the size and direction of the moments. ➲ moment of force.

net oxygen cost the oxygen used during physical activity in excess of that required at rest.

nettlerash *n* ➲ urticaria.

network a system, usually connected by telephone line, which interconnects a number of computers so that they can share information and hardware, for example, printers.

neur/o- a prefix that means 'nerve', e.g. *neuropathy*.

neural *adj* pertaining to nerves.

neural arch ➲ vertebral arch.

neural canal ➲ vertebral canal.

neural crest *n* the ectodermal cells present on the outer aspects of both sides of the neural tube during early embryonic development. The ectodermal cells migrate through the developing embryo where they will eventually form cells of the peripheral nervous system both neurons and supporting neuroglia, pigment cells, hormone-producing cells (e.g. in adrenal gland) and other cell types. ➲ neural tube.

neural fold *n* one of two folds that form during invagination of the neural plate. They come together to form the neural tube.

neuralgia *n* pain in the distribution of a sensory nerve. Neuralgia is not an illness in itself but a symptom of injury or an underlying condition. In sport usually the result of pressure from equipment (e.g. protective helmet)—**neuralgic** *adj.* ➲ trigeminal neuralgia.

neural mobilization techniques by which neural tissues are 'moved', either by movement relative to their surroundings or by tension development.

neural plate *n* the plate of ectodermal cells that forms in week 2 of embryonic development. It grows and folds in on itself (invaginates) to form the neural folds and then the neural tube, the structure which, after many changes in shape, forms the structures of the central nervous system. ➲ neural tube.

neural tension a term interchangeably used when performing assessment of neural extensibility and mobility, but should be more aptly titled neural mobility.

neural tube *n* the longtitudinal ectodermal structure formed from the fusion of the neural folds. It gives rise to the brain and spinal cord.

neural tube defect (NTD) any of a group of congenital abnormalities where there are defects in the skull and/or the vertebral column. It is caused by the failure of the neural tube to close during the first 30 days of embryonic development. NTDs include anencephaly, encephalocele, hydrocephalus, meningocele, meningoencephalocele, meningomyelocele, myelocele and spina bifida. The developing nervous system is particularly susceptible to maternal deficiency of folate (folic acid) during early pregnancy. Adequate intake of folate before conception and for the first few weeks of pregnancy is important in reducing the incidence of NTDs. ➲ alphafetoprotein, folate.

neurapraxia (neuropraxia) *n.* a measure of the extent of peripheral nerve damage (Seddon's category; Type 1 Sunderland). A transient loss of nerve function following damage. The usual mechanism is prolonged compression, direct trauma or inflammation. There is localized conduction block, but no permanent damage to the myelin sheath or axonal degeneration. The prognosis is good and recovery complete and usually takes 6–8 weeks. An example is cyclist's palsy, caused by compression of motor and sensory branches of ulnar nerve in Guyton's tunnel in the hand. ➲ axonotmesis, neurotmesis

neurasthenia *n* historically described as a form of 'nervous exhaustion'. Now regarded as an anxiety disorder characterized by persistent fatigue together with poor appetite, irritability, insomnia, headache and poor concentration—**neurasthenic** *adj.*

neurectasis *n* ➲ neurotony.

M
N

neurectomy *n* excision of part of a nerve.

neurilemma (neurolemma) *n* the thin membranous covering of a nerve fibre surrounding the myelin sheath.

neurilemmoma *n* also known as Schwann cell tumour or schwannoma. A benign tumour growing on the neurilemma of peripheral nerves.

neuritis *n* inflammation of a nerve—**neuritic** *adj*.

neuroblast *n* a primitive embryonic nerve cell.

neuroblastoma *n* a rare malignant tumour of primitive ectodermal cells arising in the adrenal medulla or any tissue of the sympathetic nervous system. Neuroblastomas metatasize to bone, liver, lungs or lymph nodes. It occurs in infants and children—**neuroblastomata** *pl*, **neuroblastomatous** *adj*.

neurodermatitis *n* (*syn* lichen simplex) leathery, thickened patches of skin secondary to pruritus and scratching. As the skin thickens, irritation increases, scratching causes further thickening and so a vicious circle is set up.

neurodevelopmental therapy (NDT) in physiotherapy practice, a common term used to describe an approach to the rehabilitation of people with neurological problems. The approach is based on principles derived from research into motor development and neurophysiology.

neurodynamic testing the mobility of the nervous system is examined by procedures known as neurodynamic tests. These tests evaluate the mechanical responses for example neural movement such as gliding and physiological responses including blood flow within the nerve (intraneural), nerve impulses and axonal transport (Shacklock 1995). ◗ passive neck flexion (PNF), prone knee bend (PKB), slump test, straight leg raise (SLR) or Lasègue sign/test. There are four upper limb neurodynamic tests, each biased towards a particular nerve. ◗ upper limb neurodynamic test 1-median nerve bias, upper limb neurodynamic test 2a-median nerve bias, upper limb neurodynamic test 2b-radial nerve bias, upper limb neurodynamic test 3-ulnar nerve bias. (Shacklock M 1995 Neurodynamics. Physiotherapy 81(1): 9–16.)

neuroendocrine relating to the close relationship between the nervous system and endocrine structures. For example, *neuroendocrine cells* (specialized neurons), which secrete neurohormones including some types of gastrin and vasopressin (or arginine vasopression [AVP]).

neuroepithelioma ◗ medulloepithelioma.

neuroepithelium specialized epithelial tissue present as sensory cells, for example, of the tongue, the olfactory epithelium of the nose and the vestibule and cochlea of the inner ear.

neurofibril microscopic threads found in the cytoplasm of neurons, they may extend into the axon.

neurofibrillary tangles a pathological change occurring in the brain of people with Alzheimer's disease. There are tangled clumps of neurofibrils within the neurons. ◗ Alzheimer's disease.

neurofibroma *n* a tumour arising from the connective tissue of peripheral nerves. A proliferation of Schwann cells—**neurofibromata** *pl*, **neurofibromatous** *adj*.

neurofibromatosis *n* a genetically determined condition in which there are many fibromata. ◗ von Recklinghausen's disease.

neurogenesis *n* the development of nervous tissue.

neurogenic *adj* originating within or forming nervous tissue.

neurogenic bladder interference with the nerve control of the urinary bladder causing either retention of urine, which presents as incontinence, or continuous dribbling without retention. When necessary the bladder is emptied by exerting manual pressure on the anterior abdominal wall. ◗ incontinence.

neurogenic, neurological incontinence ◗ incontinence.

neuroglia *n* (*syn* glia) the non-excitable supporting tissue of the central nervous system (brain and spinal cord). ◗ astrocytes, ependymal cells, macroglia, microglia, oligodendrocytes—**neuroglial** *adj*.

neurohormonal reflex the physiology of lactation involves a process in which nerves and hormones work in harmony to control the milk 'let down' reflex. ◗ 'let down' reflex.

neurohormone hormones and related chemicals produced by specialized neuron cell bodies (neurosecretory neuroendocrine cells) present in areas that include the hypothalamus, adrenal medulla and some nerve fibres. The hormones, which include vasopressin (or arginine vasopression [AVP]) and gastrin, are released into the blood, cerebrospinal fluid or directly into the spaces between cells. ◗ neuromodulators, neuropeptides, neurotransmitters.

neurohypophysis the posterior lobe of the pituitary gland. The neural part of the gland that develops from a portion of diencephalon. It stores two hormones oxytocin and antidiuretic hormone (vasopressin, or arginine vasopression [AVP]). ◗ pituitary gland.

neurokinin receptor antagonist a class of antiemetic drug, e.g. aprepitant. It is used with other drugs to control the nausea and vomiting associated with cisplatin chemotherapy.

neuroleptic malignant syndrome a rare but potentially life-threatening side-effect of neuroleptics (antipsychotic drugs) ◗ Appendix 5. It is characterized by increased temperature (hyperthermia), tachycardia, hypotension, confusion and delerium, urinary incontinence, altered consciousness, muscle tremors and rigidity, and metabolic acidosis. There is no specific treatment but the antipsychotic drug should be discontinued and appropriate supportive treatment provided.

neuroleptics *npl* usually known as antipsychotics. Drugs acting on the nervous system. ◗ antipsychotic drugs, Appendix 5.

neurolinguistic programming (NLP) communication-based techniques that seek to improve a person's awareness of their experiences and levels of 'self'. It incorporates the use of verbal and non-verbal communication, sensory events and particular patterns of behaviour.

neurological assessment of newborn an assessment performed shortly after birth with the infant awake and alert

M
N

but not crying. The infant is assessed for neck retraction, limb posture, limb hyperextension or hyperflexion, jittery or abnormal involuntary movements, high-pitched or weak cry, any of which may indicate possible antenatally-acquired or perinatal neurological disorder.

neurologist *n* a specialist in neurology. Or a medically qualified person who specializes in diagnosing and treating diseases of the nervous system.

neurology *n* **1.** the science and study of nerves—their structure, function and pathology. **2.** the branch of medicine dealing with diseases of the nervous system—**neurological** *adj*.

neurolysis the release of a nerve from adhesions. Usually refers to a surgical procedure.

neuroma a tumour of nervous tissue.

neuromodulator a chemical mediator released by neurons or from non-neuronal cells, that alters the activities of other neurons. They include glutamate (an amino acid), nitric oxide, etc.

neuromuscular *adj* pertaining to nerves and muscles.

neuromuscular disorders inherited or acquired disorders of muscle due to neuromuscular disease. They are characterized according to age of onset and site of defect.

neuromuscular electrical stimulation (NMES) various clinical devices are used to administer electrical stimulation to nerves and muscle. There is a degree of confusion in the terminology used, though neuromuscular electrical stimulation (NMES) is probably the preferred generic term. Alternatives such as chronic NMES (CNMES) imply that the stimulation is not a short-duration treatment rather than implying that it should be only employed for chronic lesions. NMES has been applied in many different clinical circumstances ranging from the reduction in spasticity in children with central nervous system lesions through to muscle strengthening in elite athletes, from electrically enhanced wound healing through to re-education of the skeletal muscles. It is probably most appropriate to describe the form of stimulation by virtue of the current being utilized (rather than using the name of a particular machine)—i.e. alternating, direct or pulsed. NMES can be used to achieve increases in muscle function for patients with significant atrophy, to prevent atrophy during immobilization, as part of a neuromuscular re-education programme, to facilitate muscle balance, as part of a programme to strengthen the pelvic floor muscles as a treatment for loss of urinary continence. It has been used for patients with scoliosis as a means to facilitate correction. In neurology, NMES can be used to facilitate motor recovery and increase strength, to reduce the impact of shoulder subluxation after stroke and to help in spasticity management programmes.

neuromuscular harmony relationship between upper and lower segments of the uterus in labour, i.e. efficient uterine action occurs when the upper uterine segment contracts and retracts and the lower segment and cervix contracts and dilates.

neuromuscular junction the communication between the axon of a myelinated nerve and the muscle fibre. The site where a motor nerve axon terminal makes close contact with the skeletal muscle fibre which it supplies. An action potential arriving at the terminal causes release of the neurotransmitter acetylcholine (ACh), which crosses the very narrow synaptic cleft to binding sites on the muscle membrane and initiates its depolarization; this triggers an action potential in the adjacent muscle fibre membrane and so sets in train the process of excitation–contraction coupling. In almost all mammalian/human extrafusal muscle fibres, the junction takes the form of a motor end-plate but less extensive structures occur in some other locations. ⊃ motor end-plate, neurotransmitters, synapse.

neuronal sprouting the process of nerve regrowth in response to injury or damage.

neuron(e) *n* a nerve cell. The basic unit of the nervous system comprising fibres (dendrites) which convey impulses to the nerve cell; the nerve cell body itself, and the fibres (axons) which convey impulses from the nerve cell body (Figure N.4). They are specialized excitable cells that are able to transmit an action potential—**neuronal, neural** *adj*. ⊃ lower motor neuron, motor neuron disease, upper motor neuron.

neuronoplasty any restorative operation to repair a nerve.

neuropathic *adj* relating to disease of the nervous system.

neuropathic pain pain experienced without any identifiable tissue damage. It is caused by faulty processing of sensory inputs by the nervous system and is associated with chronic non-malignant pain. Examples include neuralgia following an attack of herpes zoster (shingles) and phantom limb pain/syndrome.

M
N

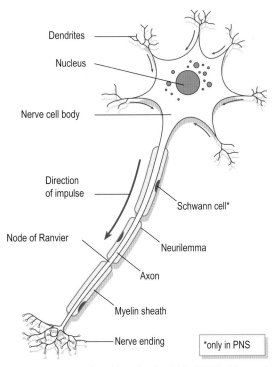

Dendrites
Nucleus
Nerve cell body
Direction of impulse
Schwann cell*
Node of Ranvier
Neurilemma
Axon
Myelin sheath
Nerve ending
*only in PNS

N.4 Neuron (reproduced from Brooker & Nicol 2003 with permission).

neuropathology *n* a branch of medicine dealing with diseases of the nervous system—**neuropathological** *adj.*

neuropathy *n* inflammation or degeneration leading to loss of function of peripheral nerves. It may be focal (e.g. carpal tunnel syndrome) known as a mononeuropathy, or generalized, as in polyneuropathy. Characterized by neuralgia, paraesthesia and loss of sensory and/or motor function. Causes include trauma, diabetes, drugs, etc. Treatment is of the cause, but it is often irreversible.

neuropeptides *npl* peptides formed and released by groups of neurons within the central nervous system, that act on other neuron populations. Comparable to neurotransmitters, often made within the same cells, but acting via different types of specific receptors. Many have been recognized, of which better known examples are enkephalins, 5-hydroxytryptamine (serotonin) and neuropeptide Y; the latter is believed to be involved in appetite control and feeding in conjunction with leptin. Neuropeptides have extensive influences, for example on mood and behaviour, pain and analgesia, appetite and the immune system. ⊃ endorphins, leptin, neurohormones, neurotransmitters.

neuropharmacology *n* the branch of pharmacology dealing with drugs that act on the nervous system—**neuropharmacological** *adj.*

neurophysiology the study of the functioning of nervous tissue and the nervous system.

neuroplasticity *n* the ability of nerve cells to change and regenerate. The functional changes in the central nervous system in response to demands from the internal or external environment. The evidence of neuroplastic changes occurring on magnetic resonance imaging scans has helped to show the benefit of therapy in the re-education of movement following brain injury.

neuroplasty *n* surgical repair of nerves—**neuroplastic** *adj.*

neuropraxia ⊃ neurapraxia.

neuroprotection a therapeutic strategy aimed at preventing the ultimate result of a neurodegenerative disease process. For example, in current glaucoma therapy, the principal objective is to lower the intraocular pressure (IOP), but that appears to be only one of the risk factors that lead ultimately to death of retinal ganglion cells and visual field loss. Neuroprotection is aimed at preventing that secondary ganglion cell degeneration in glaucomatous eyes, which may have been caused as a result of inflammatory or toxic mediators released by the primary degenerative event. Neuroprotective strategies presently being evaluated include glutamate antagonists, calcium channel blockers (antagonists), nitric oxide synthase inhibitors and various nerve growth factors (neurotrophins).

neuropsychiatry *n* a subspecialty of psychiatry dealing with mental disorder and its relationship to brain/central nervous system (dys) function—**neuropsychiatric** *adj.*

neuroretinitis inflammation affecting the optic nerve and the retina.

neurorrhaphy *n* suturing the ends of a divided nerve.

neurosensory retina this is composed of all the layers of the retina, except the outer pigmented layer (called retinal pigment epithelium). It comprises three main groups of neurons: (a) the photoreceptors, (b) the bipolar cells, and (c) the ganglion cells. In addition, there are other connecting neurons: the horizontal and amacrine cells. The neurosensory layer is derived embryologically from the inner layer of the optic cup whereas the pigmented layer is derived from the outer layer of the optic cup and they are separated by a potential space which facilitates their separation, as occurs in detached retina. ⊃ optic cup, retinal detachment, retinal pigment epithelium.

neurosis *n* an outdated term. The traditional division between psychosis and neurosis has fallen out of favour. However, the term neurotic disorders is a grouping term for anxiety disorders, phobias and obsessive-compulsive disorder—**neurotic** *adj.*

neurosurgery *n* surgery of the nervous system—**neurosurgical** *adj.*

neurosyphilis *n* infection of brain or spinal cord, or both, by *Treponema pallidum*. The variety of clinical pictures produced is large, but the two common syndromes encountered are tabes dorsalis and general paralysis of the insane (GPI). Very often symptoms of the disease do not arise until 20 years or more after the date of primary infection—**neurosyphilitic** *adj.*

neurothekeoma a soft-tissue tumour of the nerve sheath cells.

neuroticism one of the big five personality factors, characterized by a tendency to be tense, anxious and moody.

neurotmesis *n* a measure of the extent of peripheral nerve damage (Seddon's category, Types 3, 4 and 5 Sunderland). There is axonal disruption and damage to one or more layers of connective tissue in peripheral nerve. The usual mechanism is transection. Followed by Wallerian degeneration of myelin sheath by day 7. The outcome is poor, but function may be improved with microsurgical techniques. ⊃ neurapraxia (neuropraxia).

neurotomy *n* surgical cutting of a nerve.

neurotony *n* also called neurectasis. The stretching of a nerve or nerve trunk.

neurotoxic *adj* poisonous or destructive to nervous tissue—**neurotoxin** *n.*

neurotransmitters *npl* a large group of chemicals secreted by neuronal tissue. They are formed in neuron cell bodies and pass down the axon to be stored in vesicles in the axon terminals. They are released in response to action potentials, to act at a synapse with another neuron or at an effector site: skeletal muscle, smooth muscle or gland. They modify or facilitate the passage of a nerve impulse across a synapse. Examples include, acetylcholine, adrenaline (epinephrine), dopamine, endorphins, enkephalins, gamma-aminobutyrate (GABA), glutamic acid, glycine, 5-hydroxytryptamine (serotonin), noradrenaline (norepinephrine) and substance P. ⊃ acetylcholine, neuromuscular junction, noradrenaline.

neurotrophic the nutrition and maintenance of tissues as regulated by nervous influence.

neurotropic *adj* with predilection for the nervous system. *Treponema pallidum* produces neurosyphilitic complications. Neurotropic viruses (e.g. rabies, poliomyelitis) attack nerve cells.

neutral neither acid nor alkaline—pH 7.

neutral point 1. in retinoscopy, it is the point at which the sight hole of the retinoscope is conjugate with the patient's retina. At this point no reflex motion can be seen by the examiner and the entire pupil is illuminated completely, or is completely dark. This is obtained in a myopic eye when the retinoscope is placed at the far point of accommodation. When testing emmetropes and hyperopes this neutral point is reached when sufficient converging lens power has been added in order to displace the far point (artificially) to the sight hole of the retinoscope. **2.** in dichromats, it is a region of the spectrum which appears colourless. ➲ deuteranopia; protanopia; tritanopia.

neutral zone the area within the mouth in which the opposing forces of the cheeks, lips and tongue are said to be in equilibrium.

neutron *n* the subatomic particle that has no electrical charge.

neutron number (N) the number of neutrons within the nucleus of an atom.

neutropenia *n* reduction in the number of circulating neutrophils to less than $1.0 \times 10^9/L$, but not sufficiently reduced to warrant the description of agranulocytosis. It may occur as a side effect of cancer treatment with chemotherapy and or radiotherapy, which cause depression of the haemopoietic bone marrow. Because neutrophils are responsible for phagocytosis, patients with neutropenia are at high risk of serious and potentially fatal infection. Potential sites of infection include the blood, respiratory system, urinary tract and the skin, especially when vascular access devices are in situ, such as an intravenous cannula, or a central line for the administration of drugs, or nutrition—**neutropenic** *adj*.

neutrophil *n* the most numerous white blood cell (leucocyte). It is a phagocytic polymorphonuclear cell with granules (Figure N.5). A vital component of non-specific (innate) defence mechanisms.

Neville Barnes forceps obstetric forceps for operative vaginal delivery with rarely used axis traction handle attachments to allow downward traction of a high head into the pelvis.

New Ballard Score (J Ballard, American paediatrician, 20th–21st century) a system of assessing gestational age in preterm neonates. It has twelve criteria in two categories: neuromuscular, e.g. posture, popliteal angle, arm recoil; physical, e.g. skin, lanugo, eye and ear development and genitalia. ➲ Dubowitz score.

newborn bloodspot screening programme a programme to screen neonates for disorders benefiting from early diagnosis. A bloodspot sample taken on about the 6th day of life is screened for a range of disorders including phenylketonuria, congenital hypothyroidism, sickle-cell

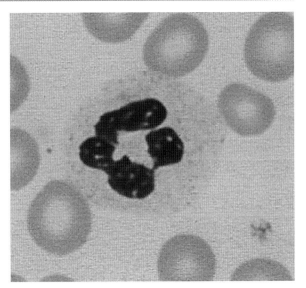

N.5 Neutrophil (reproduced from Boon et al 2006 with permission).

disease and thalassaemia, cystic fibrosis and medium chain acyl-CoA dehydrogenase deficiency (MCADD). In some countries the bloodspot is also screened for galactosaemia. ➲ neonatal screening.

newborn life support the basic life support measures used immediately after birth. Some infants, who breathe spontaneously, may only require drying and warmth. Whereas other infants will need airway clearance, oxygen therapy or even cardiopulmonary resuscitation. ➲ Appendix 10.

newton (N) *n* (I Newton, English scientist, 1642–1727) a unit of force. A derived Système International d'Unités (SI) unit (International System of Units). ➲ Appendix 2.

Newton's formula (*syn* Newton's equation, Newton's relation) an expression relating the focal lengths of an optical system (f and f') and the object x and image x' distances measured from the respective focal points. Thus, $ff' = xx$ If the optical system is a lens in air $-f = f'$ and the formula becomes $-f^2 = xx$. ➲ paraxial equation (fundamental), sign convention, gaussian theory.

Newton's laws of motion (I Newton) three laws that relate the forces and motions of bodies or objects (from the viewpoint of a fixed observer), first proposed by Isaac Newton. *Newton's first law* an object will remain at rest or continue with constant velocity unless acted on by an unbalanced force. *Newton's second law* the rate of change of momentum (or acceleration for a body/object of constant mass) is proportional to, and in the same direction as, the force applied to it (force = mass × acceleration). *Newton's third law* when two objects are in contact, the force applied by one object on the other is equal and opposite to that of the second object on the first (for every action, there is an equal and opposite reaction).

NEX in magnetic resonance imaging (MRI) the number of signal excitations repeated in a given acquisition. This is a way of increasing signal to noise ratio by increasing the time.

ng *abbr* nanogram.

NG *abbr* nasogastric.

NGF *abbr* nerve growth factor.

NGU *abbr* non-gonococcal urethritis.

NHL *abbr* non-Hodgkin's lymphoma.

NHS *abbr* National Health Service.

NHS Care Record Service (CRS) provides computerized patient records and will be linked with picture archiving communication system (PACS) to provide full clinical information on patients. ⊃ picture archiving communication system.

NHS Direct/NHS 24 telephone services—NHS Direct in England and NHS 24 in Scotland, which offer 24 hour nurse-led health information and advice services. These organizations are increasingly people's first contact with the NHS, especially out-of-hours. They also provide a comprehensive online health information service.

NHSLA *abbr* NHS Litigation Authority.

NHS Litigation Authority (NHSLA) a special health authority in England, which deals with claims of negligence against NHS bodies. The NHSLA remit also extends to risk management directed at raising standards of care and reducing claims of negligence.

NHS Trusts public accountable bodies that provide NHS health care to the population in England, either in hospital or the community.

niacin *n* one of the vitamin B complex. A generic term that includes nicotinamide and nicotinic acid.

NIBUT *abbr* non-invasive break-up time (NIBUT) test.

NICE *acron* **N**ational **I**nstitute for **H**ealth and **C**linical **E**xcellence.

nickel-titanium also known as NiTi. A highly flexible alloy of nickel and titanium with shape memory and resistance to cyclic fatigue fracture. Applications include flexible orthodontic archwires and endodontic instruments.

nicotinamide *n* the amide of nicotinic acid, a member of the vitamin B complex. It is part of the coenzymes *nicotinamide adenine dinucleotide (NAD/NADH)* and *nicotinamide adenine dinucleotide phosphate (NADP/NADPH)*, essential in metabolism. It is obtained from the meat, pulses and wholegrain cereals in the diet, and it is formed from nicotinic acid or synthesized in the liver from the amino acid tryptophan. ⊃ niacin, pellagra.

nicotinamide adenine dinucleotide (NAD/NADH) a coenzyme synthesized from nicotinamide. It is a major electron carrier in the oxidation of fuel molecules.

nicotinamide adenine dinucleotide phosphate (NADP/NADPH) a coenzyme synthesized from nicotinamide. It is an important electron carrier in the synthesis of molecules that include fatty acids.

nicotine a poisonous alkaloid present in tobacco.

nicotinic *adj* a type of cholinergic receptor where nicotine would, if present, bind in place of acetylcholine. ⊃ muscarinic.

nicotinic acid a member of the vitamin B complex, which has anti-pellagra properties and occurs in the diet. Has a direct vasodilatory action and is used in the management of peripheral vascular disease. ⊃ niacin, nicotinamide, pellagra.

nictitation *n* rapid and involuntary blinking of the eyelids.

NICU *abbr* neonatal intensive care unit.

nidation *n* implantation of the early embryo in the decidua.

NIDDM *abbr* non-insulin dependent diabetes mellitus. ⊃ diabetes mellitus type 2.

nidus *n* any structure resembling a nest in appearance or function.

nidus of infection a breeding place where bacteria and other pathological agents lodge and form a focus.

Niemann–Pick disease (A Niemann, German paediatrician, 1880–1921; L Pick, German pathologist, 1868–1944) an inherited lipid metabolic disturbance, chiefly in female Jewish infants. There are several types which are classified by age of onset and the effects on the central nervous system. Now thought to be due to absence or inadequacy of the enzyme sphingomyelinase. There is enlargement of the liver, spleen and lymph nodes caused by fat accumulation, and learning disability. Now classified as a lipid reticulosis. ⊃ cherry-red spot.

night blindness (*syn* nyctalopia) maladaptation of vision to darkness; may occur in vitamin A deficiency or genetic disorders of the retina.

night cry a shrill noise, made during sleep. May be of significance in hip disease when pain occurs in the relaxed joint.

night myopia an increase in ocular refraction (essentially accommodation) occurring at low levels of illumination. ⊃ resting state of accommodation.

night sight ⊃ hemeralopia.

night splinting the passive night time use of orthoses such as splints to maintain corrected deformities produced dynamically during walking. This may be an additional silicone digital device to maintain correction in bed, or a night splint to maintain ankle extension at 90° where there is tightening of the Achilles tendon. Night splints for the management of hallux valgus are often used as the only corrective measure.

night sweat profuse sweating, usually during sleep; typical of tuberculosis or lymphoma.

night terror ⊃ sleep terror.

night vision ⊃ scotopic vision.

nihilistic *adj* the belief that nothing is real. Nihilistic delusions.

NIHL *abbr* noise induced hearing loss.

Nikolsky's sign (P Nikolsky, Russian dermatologist, 1858–1940) slight pressure on the skin causes 'slipping' of apparently normal skin typically adjacent to a blister. Characteristic of pemphigus and other bullous conditions.

nine-hole peg test a test of manual dexterity and hand and arm speed, whereby a person is timed whilst placing nine pegs in holes on a base. The equipment comprises a wooden base with nine holes and nine wooden pegs; a stopwatch is used to measure the time taken to place the pegs in the hole.

M
N

ninety-day glaucoma ⊃ neovascular glaucoma.

Nipah virus in 1999 a newly discovered paramyxovirus in the Hendra group, the Nipah virus, caused an epidemic of encephalitis amongst Malaysian pig farmers. Infection is through direct contact with pig secretions. Mortality is around 30%. Antibodies to the Hendra virus are present in 76% of cases. ⊃ bioterrorism.

nipple *n* the conical eminence in the centre of each breast, containing the outlets of the milk ducts.

NIPPV *abbr* non-invasive intermittent positive pressure ventilation. ⊃ non-invasive ventilation.

Nissl body/granule (F Nissl, German neurologist, 1860–1919) one of the basic-staining granular structures formed from rough endoplasmic reticulum and ribosomes, present in the cytoplasm of neurons.

nit *n* the egg of the head louse (*Pediculus capitis*). It is firmly attached to the hair.

nitrates *npl* a group of drugs that act as coronary vasodilators, e.g. glyceryl trinitrate. There is a reduction in venous return to the heart and the work of the left ventricle. ⊃ Appendix 5.

nitric oxide (NO) an endogenous neuromodulator. It is involved with processes that include neurotransmission, memory, learning, gastric emptying, smooth muscle relaxation, nociception and penile erection. May be used therapeutically for patients with acute respiratory distress syndrome.

nitrogen (N) *n* **1.** an almost inert gaseous element; the chief constituent of the atmosphere (78–79%), but it cannot be utilized directly by humans. However, certain organisms in the soil and roots of legumes are capable of nitrogen fixation. It is a vital constituent of many components of living cells, e.g. proteins. **2.** the essential constituent of protein foods—**nitrogenous** *adj*.

nitrogen balance exists when nitrogen intake (in protein) equals nitrogen excretion. Nitrogen is excreted mainly as urea in the urine: ammonia, creatinine and uric acid account for a further small amount. Less than 10% total nitrogen is excreted in faeces. In *positive nitrogen balance* intake exceeds excretion, with the additional protein used to synthesize new tissues. This is required in growing children, during pregnancy, in recovery from illness and during resistance exercise training when overloading of muscle cells promotes protein synthesis. In *negative nitrogen balance* output is greater than intake, indicating that protein (primarily from skeletal muscle) is being used for energy needs. This occurs on starvation diets, those with low protein and carbohydrate intake, and in a debilitating illness (e.g. cancer), with glucocorticoid therapy, and after major surgery, trauma and sepsis when protein utilization increases; it reduces the lean tissue mass and is detrimental to exercise performance.

nitrogen narcosis a disturbance of mental function caused by an increase in the nitrogen dissolved in body fluids at high ambient pressure, e.g. diving at more than 2 atmospheres or 60 ft of water, if breathing air. Known as

the rapture of the deep. Avoided by breathing mixtures containing oxygen and helium. ⊃ diving hazards.

nitrous oxide (N_2O) gas used widely as an adjuvant for general anaesthesia and combined with oxygen for analgesia. Known colloquially as 'laughing gas'. ⊃ Entonox®

NIV *abbr* non-invasive ventilation.

NK cell *abbr* natural killer cell.

NLH *abbr* National Library for Health.

NLP *abbr* neurolinguistic programming.

nm *abbr* nanometre.

NMC *abbr* Nursing and Midwifery Council.

NMES *abbr* neuromuscular electrical stimulation.

NMR *abbr* nuclear magnetic resonance.

NNT *abbr* numbers needed to treat.

NNU *abbr* neonatal unit.

noci- a prefix that means 'pain, injury', e.g. *nociceptors*.

nociceptors *npl* receptors that respond to harmful stimuli that cause pain, such as trauma and inflammation.

nociceptive *adj* relating to nerve endings that respond to harmful stimuli.

nociceptive pain acute pain. It is associated with tissue injury, such as a cut or burn. Usually of brief duration and subsides as healing occurs.

noct- a prefix that means 'night', e.g. *nocturia*.

nocturia *n* passing urine at night.

nocturnal *adj* nightly; during the night.

nocturnal cramp occasionally disturbing sleep, particularly in older people; remains unexplained. ⊃ cramp.

nocturnal enuresis bed wetting during sleep.

nocturnal vision ⊃ scotopic vision.

nodal points in a centred optical system they are a pair of conjugate points on the axis which have the property that any incident ray which passes through the first nodal point leaves the system as though from the second nodal point and parallel to the incident ray. Thus the refracted ray is unchanged in direction, although displaced. The distance between the two nodal points is equal to the distance between the two principal points. When the refractive indices on each side of the system are equal, as in the case of a thick lens in air, the principal and nodal points coincide. They are then called *equivalent points*. In a single refracting surface, the nodal points coincide with the centre of curvature, while the principal points coincide with the vertex of the surface. ⊃ optical centre, principal plane, vertex.

node *n* **1.** a protuberance or swelling. **2.** a constriction. **3.** any computer equipment that communicates on a network.

node of Ranvier (L Ranvier, French pathologist, 1835–1922) the regular gaps in the myelin sheaf of a myelinated nerve axon. There is a concentration of voltage-gated sodium/potassium ion channels at the gap where the action potential is regenerated. Thus facilitating the transmission of the nerve impulse from node to node. ⊃ saltatory conduction.

M
N

nodule *n* a small node—**nodular** *adj*.

NOF *abbr* neck of femur.

n-of-1 trials a research methodology in which a patient undergoes pairs of treatment periods organized so that one period involves the use of the experimental treatment and one period involves the use of an alternate or placebo therapy. If possible, blinding occurs and outcomes are monitored. Treatment periods are replicated until the clinician and patient are convinced that the treatments are definitely different or definitely not different.

no fault liability acknowledgement that compensation is payable without the requirement to prove a failure in fulfilling the duty of care.

noise equivalent quanta (NEQ) in a system is the square of the signal to noise ratio and indicates the flux density of X-ray quanta that forms the image.

noise induced hearing loss (NIHL)/deafness partial or total hearing loss caused by exposure to excessive noise levels, either prolonged exposure to noise at work or during recreational activities, or a single exposure to an extremely loud noise such as an explosion. Hearing loss as a result of excess noise is an increasingly important problem. It has now become a compensatable condition if incurred in the workplace, when an employer has not taken sufficient care to protect the hearing of employees. In the past, noise-induced hearing loss was seen as a condition that affected people working in heavy industry—hence the name 'boiler-maker's disease', as it affected riveters working inside ships' boilers who were continuously exposed to loud noise. In recent years, people have become increasingly aware of the complications of loudness levels in both occupational and recreational situations: (a) occupational exposure occurs in people who work with heavy machinery or with aircraft, etc., where noise exposure is continuous; (b) recreational exposure occurs during leisure activities such as shooting, listening to music at high volume via earpieces/headphones and discos. It is postulated that the hair cells in the inner ear suffer metabolic exhaustion because of an overload of work; then, with further exposure, they are thought to become permanently non-functional. Patients usually complain of tinnitus and a decrease in the hearing in one or both ears depending on the type of exposure. A full otological history is essential to exclude other causes of hearing loss. A pure tone audiogram often shows a classical sensorineural hearing loss that is centred at the 4 kHz level and which may be unilateral or bilateral depending on the exposure. Medical management tends to involve compensation claims. Compensation may be possible for those who have worked in a noise-filled environment and amounts can be calculated according to the degree of hearing loss, the amount of noise above the acceptable limits in the working environment and the percentage disability.

noma also called cancrum oris and gangrenous stomatitis. An acute necrotizing ulceration with gangrene affecting cheek mucosa. Various micro-organisms may be involved, for example *Treponema vincentii*. It can, in severe cases, also involve the gingiva and jaw bone. In some forms the genitalia are also affected. It usually occurs in malnourished or debilitated children.

nominal data categorical data where the classes have no particular value or order, such as road names or colours. ⮌ ordinal data.

nominal power (*syn* approximate power) an estimate of the power of a lens, calculated as the sum of the front and back surface powers, i.e. $F = F_1 + F_2$. ⮌ equivalent power, surface power.

nominal scale a number given to objects that are similar to each other, a method of classification.

nominal standard dose the tolerance of normal tissues (D) can be related to the overall treatment time (T) and the number of fractions (N) by the formula: $D_N = (NSD)T^{0.11} \times N^{0.24}$.

nomogram *n* graph with several variables used to determine another related variable, such as body surface area from weight and height.

nomothetic relating to the study of groups and generalizations rather than individuals and individual differences. ⮌ idiographic.

non-accidental injury (NAI) physical maltreatment, usually of children by their parents, carers, other adults, or even other children. The injuries cannot be attributed to natural disease processes or simple accident. The injuries are often multiple and typically include bruising with finger marks, shaking injuries, fractures and burns, and involve the head, soft tissues, long bones and the thoracic cage. There may be evidence of neglect and usually there is associated psychological harm. ⮌ abuse.

non-anatomic teeth ⮌ tooth.

non-compliance *n* a term used when patients who understand their drug regimen do not comply with it.

non compos mentis not mentally competent.

non-coplanar treatment a treatment that is given in one or more planes. The rationale for this type of treatment is to avoid overlap of beam entrance and exit points.

non-disjunction the failure of homologous chromosomes to separate during the first meiotic division, or the chromatids of a chromosome do not separate during mitosis or the second meiotic division. It results in 'daughter' cells with too many or too few chromosomes. ⮌ monosomy, trisomy.

non-esterified fatty acids ⮌ fatty acids, lipids.

non-glycated haemoglobin (HbA₀) ⮌ glycated (glycosylated) haemoglobin.

non-gonococcal urethritis (NGU) (*syn.* non-specific urethritis—NSU) a common sexually transmitted disease in men. At least half of cases are caused by *Chlamydia trachomatis*. Uncommonly caused by *Trichomonas vaginalis* or herpes simplex virus. Aetiology in remaining cases uncertain, but the bacteria *Ureaplasma urealyticum* and *Mycoplasma genitalium* may be causes.

non-Hodgkin's lymphoma (NHL) tumour of lymphoid tissue. More common in older people. The cure rate is less good than Hodgkin's disease. ⊃ lymphoma.

non-immune haemolytic anaemia causes include physical trauma, infection, or chemicals or drugs. Physical trauma causing disruption of red cells may occur in a number of conditions and is characterized by the presence of red cell fragments on the blood film and markers of intravascular haemolysis: (a) mechanical heart valves—high flow through incompetent valves or periprosthetic leaks through the suture ring holding a valve in place result in shear stress damage; (b) march haemoglobinuria—vigorous exercise such as prolonged marching or marathon running can cause red cell damage in the capillaries in the feet; (c) thermal injury—severe burns cause thermal damage to red cells characterized by fragmentation and the presence of microspherocytes in the blood; (d) microangiopathic haemolytic anaemia. Fibrin deposition in capillaries can cause severe red cell disruption. It may occur in a wide variety of conditions, such as disseminated carcinomatosis, malignant or pregnancy-induced hypertension, haemolytic uraemic syndrome, thrombotic thrombocytopenic purpura and disseminated intravascular coagulation (DIC). Infections causing red cell damage include: *Plasmodium falciparum* malaria may be associated with intravascular haemolysis; when severe this is termed blackwater fever due to the associated haemoglobinuria. *Clostridium perfringens* septicaemia, usually in the context of an ascending cholangitis, may cause severe intravascular haemolysis with marked spherocytosis due to bacterial production of a lecithinase which destroys the red cell's membrane. Chemical agents or drugs may cause haemolysis by oxidant denaturation of haemoglobin. Dapsone and sulfasalazine can produce haemolysis. Arsenic gas, copper, chlorates, nitrites and nitrobenzene derivatives may all cause haemolysis. ⊃ autoimmune haemolytic anaemia.

non-insulin dependent diabetes mellitus (NIDDM) ⊃ diabetes mellitus type 2.

non-invasive *adj* describes any diagnostic or therapeutic technique that does not require penetration of the skin or of any cavity or organ.

non-invasive break-up time (NIBUT) test a test which does not require any interference with the eye used for assessing the stability of the precorneal tear film. The person's head rests on a chin rest at the centre of a hemispherical bowl of 20 cm radius which is attached at the apex to a binocular microscope. A grid of white lines on a matt black background is inscribed on the inner surface of the bowl and the image of this grid pattern projected onto the open eye is observed. The subject fixates a hole in the centre of the grid pattern and refrains from blinking. The time taken for the appearance of the first randomly distributed distortion or discontinuity of some of the reflected grid lines is a measure of the precorneal tear film break-up. The values for normal subjects vary between 5 and 200 seconds with a mean of around 40 seconds. The instrument used to measure NIBUT is often referred to as a toposcope. ⊃ break-up time test, Tearscope plus.

non-invasive ventilation (NIV) often still called non-invasive intermittent positive pressure ventilation (NIPPV). Since negative pressure devices, volume ventilators and full-face masks are all used, this phrase is now considered ambiguous and inaccurate. Non-invasive ventilation is used to provide respiratory support without the need for an endotracheal tube or a tracheostomy. Can be used in many situations including: weaning patients from invasive ventilation, acute exacerbations of chronic obstructive pulmonary disease, some obstructive sleep apnoea (hypopnoea) syndromes, etc. ⊃ biphasic positive airways pressure, continuous positive airways pressure.

non-maleficence *n* ethical principle of doing no harm. ⊃ beneficence.

non-medical prescribing in the United Kingdom, the prescribing of drugs by specially trained and qualified registered health professionals other than registered doctors and dentists. The health professionals include nurses, pharmacists, optometrists.

non-milk extrinsic sugars extrinsic sugars except that found in milk (lactose).

non-nucleated without a nucleus, such as a mature red blood cells.

non-nucleoside reverse transcriptase inhibitor a class of antiviral drugs, e.g. efavirenz, used for HIV and AIDS.

non-nursing duties duties, such as serving meals or doing clerical, administrative and domestic work, which, it may be argued, are not direct clinical care and could equally well be done by others. However, there are implications for nursing care with activities perceived to be non-nursing, such as whether the nutritional needs of patients are being met and the adequacy of domestic work in the prevention and control of infection.

nonocclusion the tooth/teeth in one arch do not make contact with those in the other arch.

non-parametric test statistical test that makes no presupposition about the distribution of data. When data are not normally distributed a non-parametric test, such as the Mann–Whitney *U* test, which does not assume a normal distribution, is the preferred option. Non-parametric tests are less powerful than the equivalent parametric test. ⊃ parametric tests.

non-proliferative diabetic retinopathy (NPDR) ⊃ background diabetic retinopathy.

non-protein nitrogen (NPN) nitrogen from nitrogenous substances other than protein, i.e. urea, uric acid, creatinine, creatine and ammonia.

non-rapid eye movement sleep (NREM) ⊃ sleep.

non-secretor a person who does not secrete their ABO blood antigens in saliva or gastric juice. ⊃ secretor.

non-shivering thermogenesis neonatal use of brown adipose tissue, stored in the mediastinum, around the nape of the neck, between the scapulae and around the kidneys and adrenal glands, to produce heat in times of cold stress.

non-small cell lung carcinoma (NSCLC) commonest type of lung cancer accounting for approximately 80% of tumours. The histological subtypes include squamous, adenocarcinoma and large cell. The doubling time is approximately 130 days. Clinical presentation may be with cough, haemoptysis, recurrent pneumonia, increasing breathlessness, weight loss or may be an incidental finding on chest X-ray. Therapy may include surgery (in approximately 20%), chemotherapy and/or radiotherapy.

non-specific interstitial pneumonia (NSIP) one of the idiopathic interstitial pneumonias. The median age of presentation is 40–50 years. There is no association with smoking and the prognosis is variable. Patients should be investigated for collagen vascular disease, hypersensitivity pneumonitis, drug-induced pneumonitis, infection or HIV disease.

non-specific urethritis (NSU) ⊃ non-gonococcal urethritis.

non-spectral colour ⊃ purple.

non-spectral purple ⊃ purple.

non-staphylococcal scalded skin syndrome ⊃ toxic epidermal necrolysis.

non-starch polysaccharides (NSP) (*syn.* dietary fibre) a form of carbohydrate (polysaccharides) other than starch that occurs in plant material that is not digested in the human gastrointestinal tract. It is found in foods such as wholegrain cereals, fruits and vegetables, and because it is not digested in the small intestine it provides no source of calories. NSP can be divided into two types: non-soluble, e.g. cellulose, and soluble, e.g. pectins and mucilages. They provide most dietary fibre in the diet. As well as providing 'bulk' and assisting weight maintenance or loss, fibre is important for preventing constipation, maintaining the health of the colon (reducing the risk of diverticular disease and colorectal cancer), reducing the risk of coronary heart disease (by combining with and preventing reabsorption of cholesterol from the gut) and assisting blood sugar regulation in diabetes mellitus (by slowing the digestion of carbohydrates).

non-steroidal anti-inflammatory drugs (NSAIDs) a large group of drugs with varying degrees of anti-inflammatory, antipyretic and analgesic action, e.g. diclofenac. Related in their action to aspirin (acetylsalicylic acid), the earliest of the group to be in common use. They act by inhibiting enzymes needed for the synthesis of prostaglandins and thromboxanes. Used in sport as an anti-inflammatory agent to treat pain and reduce swelling. Commonest used is ibuprofen, which can be bought over the counter without a prescription. Sportsmen and women can be advised to take these drugs to facilitate healing, but not to continue with sport due to the risk of masking the signs of further, potentially serious, tissue damage. ⊃ fenamates, oxicams, propionic acids, pyrazolones, salicylates. ⊃ Appendix 5.

non-union a complication of fractures in which there are distinct pathological changes and radiological evidence of non-union. There appears to be no callus formation and the fractured ends of bone become dense and the outline clearcut. The gap between the bone fragments may be filled with fibrous tissue and form a pseudoarthrosis. The lower third of the tibia has notoriously poor healing capabilities, even occasionally in young and healthy individuals.

non-vital pulp therapy strictly, any endodontic treatment that leads to successful retention of a tooth with a non-vital pulp. Generally restricted to the treatment of primary teeth with non-vital pulps in which disease is managed by chemical agents rather than shaping, cleaning and filling of the pulp space.

Noonan's syndrome (J Noonan, American paediatric cardiologist, b.1921) occurs in either males or females, with eyes set apart (hypertelorism) and other ocular and facial abnormalities; cardiac abnormalities, short stature, cryptorchidism, sometimes with neck webbing (and other Turner-like features). Generally not chromosomal; most cases sporadic; a few either dominantly or recessively inherited. ⊃ Turner's syndrome.

non-working side contacts (balancing contacts) the contacts between the mandibular and maxillary teeth or of the denture bases on the non-working side, or posteriorly in a protrusive position.

noradrenaline (norepinephrine) *n* a catecholamine neurohumoral transmitter released from adrenergic nerve endings. Also secreted into the blood stream from the adrenal medulla in response to activation of the sympathetic nervous system. It is the best known neurotransmitter at postganglionic sympathetic nerve endings (ATP and neuropeptide Y are also released). Acts on all types of adrenoceptors but is less potent than adrenaline at the β_2 adrenoceptors that dilate skeletal muscle arteries and airways. Actions include vasoconstriction, relaxation of gut musculature, dilatation of the pupils. Both noradrenaline and adrenaline (to a much lesser extent) are neurotransmitters in the central nervous system. ⊃ adrenaline (epinephrine).

norm *n* a measure of a phenomenon generally accepted as an ideal against which all other measures of the phenomenon can be measured, i.e. a standard against which values are measured.

normal distribution curve in statistics, when scores are plotted they form a symmetrical bell-shaped curve that has the mean, median and mode in the centre (Figure N.6). ⊃ skewed distribution.

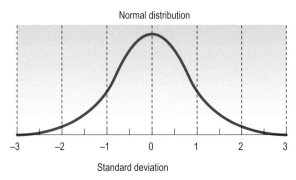

N.6 Normal distribution curve (reproduced from Gunn 2001 with permission).

normal flora ⊃ flora.

normal force force acting at right angles to the surface of a body or object. *normal reaction* the force acting at right angles on the surface of a body or object due to opposition to another force, often coming from the ground or from another body or object.

normalization a philosophy underpinning learning disability service provision. Individualized programmes of learning and goal setting are provided, which will facilitate the acquisition of the skills of daily living and maximum levels of independence. The principle of normalization has played a major role in the move from institutional to community living for people with a learning disability. When originally conceived, the prime focus was the right of people with learning disabilities to live and to be assisted to live socially valued lives of their own choosing within the community. As it has developed, the principle has been subject to much criticism, particularly as an attempt to 'normalize' people by imposing traditional, middle-class standards of behaviour. ⊃ social role valorization.

normal moulding ⊃ moulding.

normal movement the coordinated, smooth, effective, efficient, effortless and appropriate response of the nervous system for achieving the sensori-motor goal.

normal movement analysis normal movement is a learned attribute through experience and practice based on a background of activity that arises from the integration of sensori-motor skills for the execution of efficient function. Analysis of normal movement is based upon in-depth knowledge of how people move, and thus enables deviations from the norm to be recognized. It is important to acknowledge that there is a wide variation in the range of how people move and normal varies with the individual.

normal movement approach relates to the adoption of the analysis of normal movement as a basis to recognize deviations from the norm on which to formulate a plan for treatment intervention. This term is sometimes associated with the Bobath Concept.

normal occlusion an occlusion that satisfies the requirements of function and aesthetics but in which there may be minor irregularities of individual teeth. Present when the upper and lower teeth are well aligned and the cusps of the posterior teeth slot in between the opposing lower teeth. The upper and lower incisors just touch each other with a minimum of overlap, on closure.

normal population a normal distribution curve is produced when the data are plotted.

normal retinal correspondence ⊃ retinal corresponding points.

normal tissue tolerance the dose of radiation given to a specific organ or tissue that gives a certain probability of a particular complication.

normative play child-led play that aims to set up rules and norms. It is the type of play most often used and includes others and toys. It can assist in bringing normality to very strange and unfamiliar situations, such as when a child or a sibling is hospitalized. It is spontaneous and pleasurable compared with therapeutic play, which is professional led with specific goals to achieve. ⊃ therapeutic play.

normo- a prefix that means 'normal', e.g. *normocyte*.

normoblast *n* a normal-sized nucleated red blood cell, the precursor of the mature erythrocyte—**normoblastic** *adj*.

normocyte *n* a red blood cell of normal size—**normocytic** *adj*.

normoglycaemic *adj* a normal concentration of glucose in the blood—**normoglycaemia** *n*.

normotension *n* normal tension, by custom alluding to blood pressure—**normotensive** *adj*.

normothermia *n* core body temperature within the normal range, as opposed to hyperthermia or hypothermia—**normothermic** *adj*. ⊃ heat illness, hyperpyrexia, hyperthermia, hypothermia.

normotonic *adj* normal strength, tension, tone, by convention referring to muscle tissue. Spasmolytic (antispasmodic) drugs induce normotonicity in muscle, and can be used before radiography—**normotonicity** *n*.

Norn's test (*syn* tear dilution test) a test for assessing tear secretion. It consists of instilling one drop of a mixture of 1% fluorescein and 1% rose bengal into the lower conjunctival sac. After 5 minutes a slit-lamp examination is made of the colour of the stain in the central portion of the tear meniscus along the lower lid. The colour may be compared either with known dilutions of the mixture in capillary tubes or simply classified into five colours: intense red, pale red, intense orange, weak orange and yellow. In normal eyes the colour is yellow or weak orange whereas in a dry eye it is red. ⊃ dry eye, keratitis sicca, phenol red cotton thread test, Schirmer's test.

Noroviruses (Norwalk-like viruses) a group of viruses that cause outbreaks of winter gastroenteritis 'winter vomiting disease'. Transmission is via the faecal–oral route, by aerosols from vomit, enviromental contamination and contaminated food and water. It spreads rapidly in semi-closed institutions such as care homes, hospitals and schools.

Northern blot technique an electrophoretic technique used to identify the presence or not of specific messenger ribonucleic acid (mRNA). ⊃ Southern blot technique.

Norton scale a numerical scale devised by Norton, McLaren and Exton-Smith for assessing the risk of developing pressure ulcers. The risk factors used are physical condition, mental state, activity, mobility and incontinence. The total possible score is 20 and people scoring 14 or less are considered to be at risk.

nose the organ of smell. It is part of the respiratory tract and the nasal mucosa warms, moistens and filters inspired air. ⊃ nares, nasal cavity, nasal conchae, nasal septum.

nosocomial *adj* pertaining to a hospital. ⊃ infection.

nosology the science concerned with the classification of disease.

Nosopsyllus genus of fleas. *Nosopsylla fasiatus* is the common rat flea in Europe and North America. Transmits murine typhus and probably the plague bacteria.

nostalgia *n* homesickness; a longing to return to a 'place' to which, and where, one may have emotional bonds—**nostalgic** *adj*.

nostrils *npl* the anterior openings into the nose; the anterior nares; choanae.

notation a system of signs, notes, figures and symbols that convey information in abbreviated form to others who understand them. In dentistry, a charting system using a dental formula and recognized abbreviations, signs and symbols.

notifiable *adj* describes incidents or occurrences and diseases that must by law be made known to the appropriate agency. For example diseases such as tuberculosis, food poisoning and measles must be reported to the relevant department.

notochord the body of tissue comprising mesodermal cells, which forms the primitive axis in the early embryo.

NPC *abbr* near point of convergence.

NPDR *abbr* non-proliferative diabetic retinopathy.

NPF *abbr* Nurse Prescribers' Formulary.

NPN *abbr* non-protein nitrogen.

NPSA *abbr* National Patient Safety Agency.

NRDS *abbr* neonatal respiratory distress syndrome.

NREM *abbr* non-rapid eye movement (sleep). ⊃ sleep.

NSAIDs *abbr* non-steroidal anti-inflammatory drugs.

NSCLC *abbr* non-small cell lung carcinoma.

NSFs *abbr* National Service Frameworks.

NSIP *abbr* non-specific interstitial pneumonia.

NSP *abbr* non-starch polysaccharide.

NSU *abbr* non-specific urethritis. ⊃ non-gonococcal urethritis.

NT *abbr* nuchal translucency.

NTD *abbr* neural tube defect.

N-type semiconductor a device where the majority of carriers are the electrons in the conduction band and the minority of carriers are the holes in the valence band. ⊃ P-type semiconductors.

nucha *n* the nape of the neck—**nuchal** *adj*.

nuchal *adj* pertaining to the back of the neck.

nuchal displacement complication of breech labour, when a fetal arm is displaced behind the neck.

nuchal fold fat pad at the back of the fetal neck. It is measured on ultrasound scan after 14 weeks' gestation and at the 18–20 week fetal anomaly scan. Measurements of ≥ 6 mm increase chances of Down's syndrome but may be associated with other disorders, e.g. Turner's syndrome.

nuchal translucency (NT) subdermal collection of lymphatic fluid at the back of the fetal neck, best visualized between 11 and 14 weeks' gestation. Increased levels are associated with chromosomal abnormalities, structural abnormalities (e.g. cardiac), neuromuscular problems and various syndromes. ⊃ pregnancy associated plasma protein-A, combined test and integrated test.

nuchal translucency scan an ultrasound scan done to measure from the cervical vertebrae to the posterior skin surface of the fetus. A measurement of greater than 3 mm at 11–14 weeks means that there could be an increased risk of aneuploidy (a variation in the number of chromosomes).

nuclear relating to a nucleus.

nuclear energy levels the discrete energy levels occupied by nucleons in the nucleus of an atom.

nuclear family in western societies the conventional family group of two married parents and their dependent children.

nuclear force the force present in the nucleus of an atom which contains the particles inside the nucleus. The nuclear binding energy is different in different elements but is about 8 MeV per nucleon.

nuclear magnetic resonance (NMR) ⊃ magnetic resonance imaging.

nuclear medicine the use of radionuclide techniques for the diagnosis, treatment and study of disease.

nuclear reactor a method of producing electricity through controlled nuclear fusion which produces heat which turns water to steam which drives electric generators.

nuclear spin a property of nuclei which have an odd number of neutrons and/or protons which gives them angular and magnetic momentum. The spins of the nuclei have characteristic fixed values. Nuclei of paired neutrons and protons align to cancel out their spins and therefore do not resonate.

nuclease *n* an enzyme that breaks the bonds between nucleotides in nucleic acids.

nucleated *adj* possessing one or more nuclei.

nucleic acids biological macromolecules comprising many subunits called nucleotides. ⊃ deoxyribonucleic acid, ribonucleic acid.

nucleic acid synthesis inhibitor antiviral drugs, such as aciclovir, that are used for herpes simplex and varicella zoster infections.

nucle/o- a prefix that means 'nucleus', e.g. *nucleoside*.

nucleolus structures (usually two) involved in nuclear division. They are within the nuclear membrane and contain both DNA and RNA.

nucleon the protons and neutrons within the nucleus of an atom.

nucleoplasm the protoplasm within the nuclear envelope.

nucleoproteins *npl* proteins conjugated with nucleic acids found in the cell nucleus. Uric acid is an end product of nucleoprotein metabolism, which is normally excreted in the urine. ⊃ gout.

nucleoside a compound of a sugar and a nitrogenous base, either a pyrimidine or a purine.

nucleoside reverse transcriptase inhibitor a class of antiviral drugs, e.g. zidovudine, used for HIV disease. ⊃ Appendix 5.

nucleotides *npl* the subunits from which nucleic acids are formed. Consist of sugars and nitrogenous bases (nucleosides) and phosphate groups.

nucleotoxic *adj* toxic to the cell nucleus, e.g. some chemicals and viruses—**nucleotoxin** *n*.

nucleus *n* **1.** the membrane-bound cellular structure which contains the genetic material (chromosomes). **2.** a confined accumulation of nerve cells in the central nervous system associated with a particular function, **3.** the central part of an atom that contains neutrons and protons—**nuclei** *pl*, **nuclear** *adj*.

nucleus pulposus *n* the semi-gelatinous substance contained within the annulus fibrosus of the intervertebral disc. It is made up from mainly type 11 collagen, it is hydrophilic (water loving) and is kept in check by the annulus. It does not possess any nerve endings. It forms the soft, elastic core of an intervertebral disc which can prolapse into the spinal cord and cause back pain or sciatica. Internal derangement of the disc may result in leakage of the nucleus pulposus through the breached annular fibres. ⊃ annulus fibrosus (Figure N.7).

nuclide an individual atom of given atomic number and mass number.

NUG *abbr* necrotizing ulcerative gingivitis.

null hypothesis a statement that asserts there to be no relationship between the dependent and independent variables.

nullipara *n* a woman who has not borne a viable infant—**nulliparous** *adj*, **nulliparity** *n*.

numbers needed to treat (NNT) a method of stating the benefits of a therapeutic intervention. The number of subjects who need to receive treatment before one subject has a positive outcome. It is the inverse of the absolute risk reduction.

nummular *adj* coin shaped; resembling rolls of coins, as the sputum in tuberculosis.

nurse anaesthetist a nurse trained to administer general anaesthesia.

nurse consultant *n* a role for experienced clinical practitioners who have the necessary level of expertise in an area of practice; professional leadership and consultancy; education, training and development; and practice and service development, research and evaluation. Those appointed

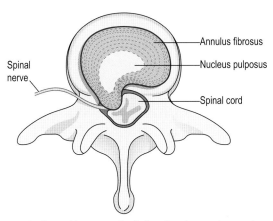

N.7 Prolapsed intervertebral disc showing nucleus pulposus (reproduced from Waugh & Grant 2006 with permission).

have considerable patient/client contact and work in diverse areas that include: critical care, mental health, continence care, dermatology, stroke services, accident and emergency, etc.

nurse practitioner a nurse who has undergone specific role preparation to enable him or her to function at an advanced level within a particular working environment. This may be within primary health care, in an accident and emergency setting, or working with certain client groups, such as homeless people. Nurse practitioners can offer a nurse-led service and invariably have highly developed skills in client assessment.

Nursing and Midwifery Council (NMC) established in 2001 to replace the United Kingdom Central Council for Nursing, Midwifery and Health Visiting (UKCC), for the statutory regulation of nursing, midwifery and specialist community public health nursing in the United Kingdom. The NMC oversees professional quality and continuing professional development standards for professional practice, discipline and conduct. It is responsible for the establishment and maintenance of a professional register for all nurses, midwives and specialist community public health nurses working in the UK, and currently has the power to remove individuals from the register in cases involving fitness to practice and professional misconduct, or in some cases to restrict practice or order specific training or conditions.

nursing bottle caries older term for dental caries during early childhood. ⊃ baby bottle tooth decay, dental caries.

nursing diagnosis a statement of actual or potential health problems requiring nurse-initiated interventions that the registered nurse is qualified and compentent to deliver. Used in North America where the North American Nursing Diagnosis Association (NANDA) has developed a series of diagnoses each of which is accompanied by a list of recommended nursing interventions. It is the second stage of the nursing process. NANDA diagnoses are not widely used in the United Kingdom.

nursing home an institution where nursing care is delivered by the independent sector, charitable organizations, social services or, rarely, the NHS.

Nursing models frameworks that identify, describe and explain a range of nursing concepts; traditionally named after the nurse theorists who first propounded them, e.g. Roy's model, Rogers' model, Roper, Logan, Tierney model, etc.

nursing process a systematic approach to nursing care. It comprises four phases (in the United Kingdom): assessment, planning, implementation and evaluation. Only for purposes of description can they be sequential; in reality, they overlap and occur and recur throughout the period a person is receiving nursing care.

nursing theory theory that explains, illuminates, or offers practical guidance about the field of nursing; generated by nursing research or, rationally, through the development of nursing ideas.

M

N

nutation *n* **1.** nodding; applied to uncontrollable head shaking. **2.** the result of the angular momentum and angular velocity vectors of a body or object being in different directions, leading to a rotation about a third axis.

nutraceuticals non-nutrient substances present in some foods, which may have potential benefits.

nutrient *n, adj* a chemical substance (e.g. protein, fats, carbohydrates, iron, calcium, vitamin C, vitamin A) found as a component of food that can be digested (as necessary) and absorbed and used to promote body function. Nutrients are used to provide energy and/or in the synthesis of substances necessary for metabolism, growth and repair, and for all physiological functions (e.g. coenzymes, hormones, haemoglobin). ⊃ macronutrient, micronutrients.

nutrient artery *n* one which enters a long bone.

nutrient foramen *n* hole in a long bone which admits the nutrient artery.

nutrition *n* the sum total of the processes by which cellular organelles, cells, tissues, organs, systems and the body as a whole obtain necessary substances from foods and use them as sources of energy and to maintain structural and functional integrity.

nutrition surveillance the process of monitoring health status, nutrition, eating behaviour, and the nutritional knowledge of the public in order to plan and evaluate nutritional policy. Particulary important in developing countries where monitoring can provide an early warning of emergencies, such as impending famine.

nutritional *adj* pertaining to nutrition.

nutritional assessment the assessment of an individual's nutritional status used to identify those who are malnourished and those who are at risk of becoming malnourished. Factors included in the assessment are dietary intake, nutritional requirements, clinical condition, physical appearance, anthropometric and biochemical measurements. ⊃ anthropometry, dietary reference values, malnutrition.

nutritional support intervention to improve nutrient intake. Interventions include increasing the number of meals and amounts of food provided, fortifying food with additional nutrients, sip-feeds, enteral and parenteral nutrition.

NVQ *abbr* National Vocational Qualification.

NWB *abbr* non-weight bearing.

nyctalgia *n* pain occurring during the night.

nyctalopia *n* night blindness. ⊃ hemeralopia.

nyct/o, nyctal/o- a prefix that means 'night', e.g. *nyctophobia*.

nyctophobia *n* abnormal fear of the night and darkness.

nymphae *npl* the labia minora.

nymphomania *n* excessive sexual desire in women— **nymphomaniac** *adj*. compare ⊃ satyriasis.

Nyquist frequency the frequency equal to or greater than twice the highest frequency in an analogue signal.

Nyquist limit the maximum frequency that can be handled to enable an accurate reconstruction to take place, for example, in pulsed wave Doppler imaging, above this level aliasing occurs. ⊃ aliasing.

Nyquist theorem states that an analogue signal waveform may be reconstructed without error from a sample which is equal to, or greater than, twice the highest frequency in the analogue signal, for example, to digitally convert a 2 MHz signal a sample must be taken at 4 MHz.

nystagmus *n* jerky, involuntary and repetitive movement of the eyeball(s). It can occur under physiological situations but can also indicate diseases, especially of the cerebellum or the inner ear.

M
N

OA *abbr* osteoarthritis.

OAE *abbr* otoacoustic emission.

oat cell carcinoma histological subtype of small cell cancer most commonly of bronchogenic epithelium. It accounts for approximately 20% of all lung cancers and is characterized by rapid growth (doubling time approximately 29 days). The highest incidence is in smokers. The lung primary may present with cough, haemoptysis, recurrent pneumonia, increasing breathlessness and weight loss or may be an incidental finding on chest X-ray. Therapy generally does not include surgery, but 90% are sensitive to chemotherapy, which is usually the treatment of choice.

Ober's test a test that determines the extensibility of the iliotibial band. It is performed with the person in side lying with the hip fully laterally rotated and the knee joint in unlocked extension. A normal finding is that the uppermost leg should be able to drop (adduct) to the plinth. An abnormal finding is that the leg cannot drop to the plinth.

obesity *n* a condition in which body fat stores are enlarged to an extent which impairs health. There is deposition of excessive fat around the body, particularly in the subcutaneous tissue, internal organs and within the abdominal cavity. Develops when the intake of food is in excess of the body's energy requirements, the most common nutritional disorder worldwide, the incidence is increasing. Defined in terms of body mass index and circumference at the waist. Obesity is linked with a variety of conditions that include: hypertension, cardiovascular disease (coronary heart disease and strokes), type 2 diabetes, sleep apnoea syndromes, osteoarthritis and some cancers. The degree of obesity is categorized by body mass index (BMI). Most authorities define obesity in adults as a BMI 30–34.9; morbid obesity as a BMI 35–39.9; and extreme obesity as BMI greater than 40. Waist circumferece, waist to height ratio, and waist to hip ratio are also used as indicators of the amount of fat present in the abdomen. ⊃ body composition, body mass index, body weight, waist circumference:height ratio, waist circumference:hip ratio.

object distance the distance along the optical axis of a lens or optical system between the object plane and the primary principal plane. If the system consists of a single thin lens the object distance is measured from the optical surface and the reciprocal of this quantity is called the reduced object vergence or object vergence (in air). ⊃ front vertex power, principal plane, vergence.

objective *adj* pertaining to things external to oneself. ⊃ subjective *opp*.

objective accommodation accommodation of the eye measured without the subject's judgement. This is accomplished by dynamic retinoscopy, by autorefractors or by visually evoked cortical potentials. The term is sometimes used incorrectly to refer to the amplitude of accommodation without the influence of the depth of focus (e.g. as measured by stigmatoscopy). ⊃ visually evoked cortical potentials, optometer, retinoscopy, stigmatoscopy, subjective accommodation.

objective optometers ⊃ optometer.

objective signs those which the observer notes, as distinct from the symptoms of which the patient complains.

objectivity a state of mind that is not influenced by personal feelings, opinions or prejudices. The notion of objectivity has been contested on the grounds that all human activity is dependent on subjective processes. For example, 'objective' research is influenced by factors relating to culture and history including what is considered worth researching.

object-to-film distance (OFD) in radiography the distance from the object being radiographed to the film.

OBLA *abbr* onset of blood lactate accumulation.

obligate *adj* distinguished by the ability to survive only in a particular set of environmental conditions, such as a micro-organism.

obligatory aerobes are micro-organisms that are unable to grow in the absence of oxygen, e.g. *Mycobacterium tuberculosis, Pseudomonas aeruginosa*.

obligatory anaerobe a micro-organism that cannot grow or survive in the presence of molecular oxygen. Examples include *Clostridium* spp., *Bacteroides* spp., ⊃ anaerobe.

oblique a slanting direction.

oblique aberration an aberration induced by a point object off the optical axis of the system. These comprise coma, curvature of field, distortion and oblique astigmatism.

oblique astigmatism 1. astigmatism in which the two principal meridians are neither approximately horizontal nor approximately vertical. **2.** an aberration of an optical system which occurs when the incident light rays form an angle with the optical axis which exceeds the conditions of gaussian optics. It gives rise to separate tangential and sagittal line foci instead of a single image point.

oblique fracture a break in bone continuity that is at an angle to the main shaft of the bone.

oblique illumination shadow test ⊃ shadow test.

oblique incidence when a radiotherapy beam enters the patient at an angle other than 90° due to the curvature of the skin surface.

oblique lateral projection an extra-oral radiographic projection that demonstrates the mandibular and maxillary teeth with minimal superimposition of the contralateral side.

oblique line the thickened line where the horizontal body of the mandible and the alveolar process merge into the ascending ramus.

oblique occlusal projection an occlusal radiographic projection in which the central ray is directed obliquely to the teeth.

oblique presentation where the long axis of the fetus (spine) is lying oblique or slanted in relation to the long axis of the woman's uterus.

oblique ridge the ridge of enamel, joining the antero-internal or mesiolingual cusp on the occlusal surfaces of all upper molar teeth to the posterobuccal cusp.

OBS *abbr* organic brain syndrome. ⊃ dementia.

observational study research in which the researcher observes, listens and records the events of concern. Where the researcher participates and has a role it is termed a *participant observational study*. May be used in qualitative social science research.

obsessive compulsive disorder (OCD) recurrent obsessional thoughts and/or compulsive acts occurring on most days for at least 2 weeks. The thoughts are usually distressing and are therefore (often unsuccessfully) resisted by the sufferer.

obstetrical conjugate ⊃ conjugate.

obstetrician *n* a qualified doctor who practises the science and art of obstetrics.

obstetrics *n* the science dealing with the care of the pregnant woman during the antenatal, parturient and puerperal stages; midwifery.

obstipation intractable constipation.

obstructed labour a situation in which there is no advance of the presenting part despite strong uterine contractions. Obstruction most commonly occurs at the pelvic brim but may occur at the outlet, e.g. deep transverse arrest in an android pelvis. The situation is avoidable with diligent midwifery care. Maternal causes of obstructed labour are a contracted bony pelvis, soft pelvic mass, such as fibroids or tumour; the fetal causes are malpresentation, malposition or abnormality, e.g. hydrocephalus. When advanced, the woman is distressed, anxious and has tachycardia, pyrexia, ketonuria and oliguria, vomiting and persistent abdominal pain. The uterus appears 'moulded' around the fetus, on palpation it is continuously hard, fetal parts cannot be felt and fetal heart sounds are absent and fetal death from anoxia occurs. Bandl's ring can be seen as a ridge running obliquely around the abdomen marking the junction between the thickened upper segment and the dangerously thinned and overdistended lower uterine segment. On examination the vagina is hot and dry with oedematous vaginal walls, a high presenting part with excessive caput succedaneum and a thick 'curtain' of cervix hanging around and below it. A multipara is in imminent danger of death from uterine

rupture and exhaustion; a primigravida may develop secondary uterine inertia. Medical aid should be summoned urgently, intramuscular pethidine is administered to relieve pain, intravenous fluids are commenced to combat shock and dehydration and a blood sample is taken for cross-matching. Caesarean section should be performed immediately wherever possible whether the fetus is alive or dead; in isolated areas it may be necessary to undertake a fetal destructive operation as the only means of emptying the uterus and saving the woman's life, although this also carries risk of rupturing the thinned overstretched lower uterine segment.

obstructive pulmonary disease a term that includes several conditions: asthma; the chronic obstructive pulmonary diseases (chronic bronchitis, emphysema, chronic bronchiolitis); and cystic fibrosis.

obstructive sleep apnoea (hypopnoea) syndrome (OSAS; OSAHS) sometimes referred to as sleep apnoea syndrome. A condition characterized by irregular breathing during sleep, episodes of apnoea/hypopnoea during sleep, snoring, choking episodes witnessed by partners and feeling tired and sleepy during the day, with poor concentration and irritability. As the person falls asleep the muscles in the pharynx relax causing the airway to narrow or close, thus reducing the airflow. The reduction in airflow and apnoea/hypopnoea means that inspiratory effort is increased and the person moves to a lighter level of sleep or to full wakefulness. The pattern is repeated throughout the night with poor quality sleep. Diagnostic procedures include full polysomnography, overnight pulse oximetry and electroencephalography, with severity calculated using the apnoea hypopnoea index. Disease management includes behavioural interventions, e.g. sleep hygiene, smoking cessation, weight control, non-surgical interventions, such as continuous positive airways pressure, intraoral devices and pharmacological interventions. Or surgical intervention, e.g. uvulopalatopharyngoplasty. ⊃ apnoea hypopnoea index (AHI), continuous positive airways pressure (CPAP), laser-assisted uvulopalatoplasty, polysomnography, uvulopalatopharyngoplasty.

obtund to dull or blunt pain or touch sensations.

obtundent pain-relieving agent, e.g. oil of cloves.

obturate to obliterate or close an opening. In endodontics, to fill a root canal.

obturator *n* that which closes an aperture. Also a device for closing any abnormal opening or cleft such as a cleft palate or a fistula between the oral and nasal cavity.

obturator externus a triangular muscle. Its origin is on the outer part of the obturator membrane and foramen, the ischium and pubis, and it inserts on the back of the femur. It facilitates lateral rotation at the hip and helps to stabilize the hip.

obturator foramen the opening in the innominate bone which is closed by muscles and fascia.

obturator internus a pelvic muscle that encloses the obturator foramen. Its origin is on the internal part of the obturator membrane and the rim of the obturator foramen, and it leaves the pelvis to insert on the greater trochanter of the femur. It facilitates lateral rotation at the hip and helps to stabilize the hip.

obturator nerve a nerve arising from the lumbar plexus. It supplies the skin of the medial aspect of the thigh and the adductor muscles of the thigh, ➲ lumbar plexus.

obturators two deep muscles of the upper thigh/ buttock. ➲ obturator externus, obturator internus.

occipital *adj* pertaining to the back of the head.

occipital artery a large branch of the external carotid artery. It supplies the posterior part of the scalp. There are two smaller branches to the sternocleidomastoid muscle.

occipital bone the occiput. The cranial bone forming the back and part of the base of the skull. It has immovable fibrous joints with the parietal, temporal and sphenoid bones. Its inner surface is deeply concave and this concavity is occupied by the occipital lobes of the cerebrum and by the cerebellum. The occiput has two articular condyles that form condyloid joints with the first bone of the vertebral (spinal) column, the atlas. This joint permits nodding movements of the head. Between the condyles is a large opening, the foramen magnum, through which the spinal cord passes into cranial cavity.

occipital cortex the superficial grey matter on the posterior part of each hemisphere of the occipital lobe of the cerebrum. ➲ visual area.

occipital lobe a small lobe of the cerebrum lying beneath the occipital bone. It has the primary visual cortex and the visual association area.

occipitoanterior *adj* describes a presentation when the fetal occiput lies in the anterior half of the maternal pelvis.

occipit/o- a prefix that means 'back of the head', e.g. *occipitoanterior*.

occipitobregmatic diameter of the fetal skull taken from below the occipital protrusion to the anterior fontanelle. In the average term infant it is approximately 10.5 cm. When measured from below the occiput it is the suboccipito-bregmatic diameter and is slightly shorter at 9.5 cm.

occipitofrontal *adj* pertaining to the occiput and the frontal bone (forehead).

occipitofrontal diameter a diameter of the partially deflexed fetal skull measured from the occipital protrusion to the forehead. It is 11.5 cm in the average term fetus.

occipitofrontal projection a radiographic technique for demonstrating the skull and jaws in the coronal plane.

occipitolateral, occipitotransverse the fetal occiput is to the side of the woman's pelvis as it enters the brim, either on the right or the left side. If the uterine contractions are efficient it will usually turn to occipitoanterior position as it reaches the resistance of the pelvic floor.

occipitomental projection (standard) a radiographic technique for demonstrating the facial bones and the maxillary sinuses. The orbitomeatal line is tilted at 45° to the plane of the film and the central ray is projected through the occipital bone perpendicular to the film.

occipitoposterior describes a presentation in which the fetal occiput is directed towards the right or left sacroiliac joint of the woman's pelvis. It is the commonest of all mechanical difficulties in labour; caused by an abnormal maternal pelvic shape, e.g. android or anthropoid. The fetal attitude is often a military (erect) one or deflexed; occurs in about 10% of all pregnancies. On examination the abdomen appears flattened below the umbilicus and a high deflexed fetal head is palpated with limbs felt over a large area on both sides of the midline. The fetal heart sounds are heard in the middle and over the flank. Vaginal examination reveals a high head with the bregma lying anteriorly or centrally. In many cases the fetal head will flex as it meets the pelvic floor, to make a long rotation to occipitoanterior position and delivery follows normally. Risks include prolonged labour, difficult delivery, cord prolapse, infection, fetal hypoxia and intracranial haemorrhage from the upwards moulding of the fetal skull. In the second stage deep transverse arrest may occur, requiring Kielland's forceps delivery or the head is born face to pubes. ➲ deep transverse arrest, face to pubes, Kielland's forceps.

occiput *n* the posterior region of the skull.

occlude to close or shut, as when the occlusal surfaces of the mandibular teeth are closed on the maxillary teeth.

occluded gas a gas dissolved in molten metal and which, when released on cooling and solidification of the metal, causes porosity.

occluding surfaces those surfaces of the natural or artificial teeth that make contact with those of the opposing jaw.

occlusal *adj* in dentistry, refers to the surfaces of teeth or their replacements that make contact with those of the opposing jaw.

occlusal adjustment, correction or equilibration the adjustment to the occlusal anatomy of the teeth, usually by grinding, in order to restore a normal occlusion and thus harmonizing cuspal relations in function. It seeks to remove premature contacts and occlusal interferences and to establish a stable occlusion.

occlusal analysis the study made of the occlusal contacts of opposing teeth.

occlusal clearance ➲ interocclusal clearance.

occlusal contact contact of the upper and lower teeth when the jaws are closed normally.

occlusal face height ➲ occlusal vertical dimension.

occlusal film a radiographic film in a waterproof envelope which the patient bites on, used to demonstrate either upper or lower 321123 on a single film.

occlusal indicator wax the wax used to register the occlusal relationship between mandibular and maxillary teeth.

occlusal overlay appliance an appliance having a component covering the occlusal or incisal surfaces of the teeth or both.

occlusal path the path of movement of one occluding surface, relative to another.

occlusal plane (plane of occlusion) an imaginary line touching the incisal surfaces of the upper incisors and the tips of the cusps of the posterior teeth. 'Plane' is a misnomer as the 'line' is usually curved.

O
P

occlusal plane guide a device used to determine the occlusal plane during denture construction.

occlusal prematurity a contact between opposing teeth occurring before the planned intercuspation.

occlusal radiograph or projection a radiograph obtained by placing the film along the occlusal plane.

occlusal registration the recording of jaw relationships, usually by means of heat-softened wax occlusal rims attached to temporary or permanent denture bases.

occlusal rehabilitation the modification of the occlusal relationships by grinding the crowns of teeth and fitting inlays, crowns and bridges. The aim is to improve the functional harmony of the dentition and the associated musculature.

occlusal reshaping ⊃ selective grinding.

occlusal rest a rest, usually of metal, that is placed on the occlusal surfaces of certain teeth to maintain the occlusal level of a prosthesis.

occlusal rim previously called a bite block or bite rim. An occluding surface formed of a mouldable material such as wax, which is attached to a temporary or permanent denture base. Intended to record jaw relationships and indicate tooth positions.

occlusal splint ⊃ occlusal overlay appliance.

occlusal surfaces those surfaces of molars which, in normal occlusion, meet the corresponding surfaces of the opposing teeth.

occlusal table the total amount of surface provided for occlusion by natural or artificial teeth.

occlusal trauma trauma to the teeth or their supporting structures caused by the opposing teeth.

occlusal vertical dimension (OVD) any vertical dimension when the teeth or occlusal rims are in contact. The Willis gauge may be used to record this measurement but is subject to inaccuracies as it has to be placed on soft tissues.

occlusally approaching clasp clasp originating on the occlusal side of a survey line and ending in the infrabulge area.

occlusion *n* **1.** the closure of an opening, especially of ducts or blood vessels. **2.** any contact between teeth of opposing arches and usually referring to their occlusal surfaces. **3.** static relationship between maxillary and mandibular teeth during maximal intercuspation—**occlusal** *adj.* ⊃ balanced occlusion, centric occlusion, edge-to-edge occlusion, ideal occlusion, mutually protected occlusion, normal occlusion, occlusion wear, traumatic occlusion.

occlusion test ⊃ cover test (CT).

occlusion treatment a method of treating amblyopia or strabismus by covering the good eye or preferred eye. Such a method is most effective below the age of 4 years and with little effect after the age of 9 years. However, this technique must be used with caution as prolonged occlusion in very young children can lead to a reversal of eye dominance in which the previously good eye becomes amblyopic (called occlusion amblyopia). Alternate occlusion is preferred as both eyes are thus stimulated. ⊃ amblyopia, penalization, pleoptics, strabismus.

occlusion wear the loss of tooth substance on opposing occlusal surfaces as a result of abrasion or attrition.

occult *adj* concealed.

occult blood minute amount of blood present in, for example, faeces, that is not visible and can only be detected by chemical tests, or microscopic or spectroscopic examination. ⊃ faecal occult blood.

occupation a group of activities that has personal and sociocultural meaning, is named within a culture and supports participation in society. Occupations can be categorized as self-care, productivity and/or leisure. (Reproduced with permission from the European Network of Occupational Therapy in Higher Education (ENOTHE) Terminology Project, 2008.)

occupational alienation a sense that one or more of the individual's occupations is meaningless and unsatisfying. This is typically accompanied by a feeling of powerlessness to change the situation.

occupational apartheid restriction or denial of access to participation in occupations for a group of people on the basis of race, disability, gender, age or other characteristic.

occupational asthma asthma caused by inhalation of specific agents in the workplace that leads to sensitization of the individual following an immune response. Symptoms do not occur on first exposure but a pattern emerges as symptoms are provoked by work exposure and relieved when away from work. Treatment is by prevention and control of exposure. Untreated the condition can become persistent and chronic.

occupational balance a condition in which the individual is able to engage in a range of occupations sufficiently varied to maintain health, wellbeing and social participation.

occupational behaviour the developmental continuum of play and work that evolves throughout an individual's life.

occupational choice the process by which a person chooses a major occupation, such as a career.

occupational deprivation the condition of being unable to access a satisfying and healthy range of occupations due to external circumstances.

occupational disease ⊃ industrial disease.

occupational disruption a transient condition of being unable to participate in a satisfying and healthy range of occupations due to temporary circumstances, such as illness.

occupational exposure job-related risk of exposure to carcinogens.

occupational form the socially accepted rules, procedures, equipment and environment that support and shape occupational performance.

occupational genesis the process by which people's daily activities evolve as they adapt to changes in the world and in their lives.

occupational health the active and proactive management of health in the workplace. Achieved through an occupational health department and the employment of occupational health doctors and or nurses, and other health professionals as appropriate.

O
P

occupational identity how a person perceives him- or herself in terms of the names of occupations which he or she feels apply to them. Having occupational identity is part of personal identity, sense of self and gives meaning to daily-living.

occupational imbalance a condition of disequilibrium in which the individual spends too much time in some occupations to the neglect of others or does not have enough to do, sufficient to pose a threat to health and wellbeing.

occupational injustice misuse of power leading to unnecessary and unfair restriction of access to participation in occupations for individuals or groups of people.

occupational justice fair and equal access to a range of occupations sufficient to maintain health, wellbeing and social participation.

occupational mapping the process of working with a client to identify his current and past occupations, the meanings that they have for him and any difficulties he has with occupational performance.

occupation performance choosing, organizing and carrying out occupations in interaction with the environment. (Reproduced with permission from the European Network of Occupational Therapy in Higher Education (ENOTHE) Terminology Project, 2008.)

occupational performance areas categories of tasks, activities and occupations that are typically part of daily life. They are usually called self-care, productivity and leisure. (Reproduced with permission from the European Network of Occupational Therapy in Higher Education (ENOTHE) Terminology Project, 2008.)

occupation performance components abilities and skills that enable and affect engagement in tasks, activities and occupations. These can be categorized, for example, as physical, cognitive, psychosocial and affective. (Reproduced with permission from the European Network of Occupational Therapy in Higher Education (ENOTHE) Terminology Project, 2008.)

occupational role the expression of an individual's occupational behaviour through various activities of daily living that identifies his or her place in society.

occupational science an academic discipline concerned with increasing understanding of the phylogenesis, ontogenesis, form and functions of occupation through research and theory generation.

occupational therapy (OT) a profession that promotes health and wellbeing in people of all ages by assisting them to carry out the occupations and activities that enable participation in everyday life.

occupational therapy assessment the use of both formal and informal screening and evaluation methods, including medical records, interview, observation, standardized and non-standardized tests, to assess occupational performance areas, performance components and occupational role performance. This provides the occupational therapist with the means to develop treatment objectives and methods to remediate, or compensate for, any problems identified.

Assessment can also be used to determine the effectiveness of treatment and any modifications that might be needed.

occupational therapy outcome the planned result of occupational therapy intervention.

occupational therapy process the flexible sequence of actions taken by the therapist, and the thinking that underpins those actions, that are used to structure intervention with a client.

OCD *abbr* obsessive compulsive disorder.

ochronosis *n* greyish discoloration of connective tissue as occurs in alkaptonuria.

OCR *abbr* optical character recognition.

octigravida a woman who is into her eighth pregnancy.

ocular *adj* pertaining to the eye. ➔ eyepiece.

ocular headache headache believed to result from excessive use of the eyes, uncorrected refractive error, especially hypermetropia and low grades of astigmatism, binocular vision anomaly or eye diseases. This headache typically occurs in the brow region but also in the occipital or neck regions. ➔ accommodative insufficiency, asthenopia, astigmatism, hypermetropia.

ocular hypertension a condition in which the intraocular pressure (IOP) is above normal but in which there are neither visual field defects nor optic disc changes. Open-angle glaucoma may or may not develop later.

ocular hypotonia abnormally low intraocular pressure.

ocular pemphigoid ➔ cicatricial pemphigoid.

ocular rigidity the resistance of the coats of the eye to indentation. This factor is taken into account in the tables used when determining the intraocular pressure (IOP) by means of an indentation tonometer such as that of Schiötz. The tables are based on an eye of average ocular rigidity but, if the eye has high or low rigidity, an error is introduced into the readings: means of minimizing this effect have been devised. ➔ impression tonometer.

oculo- a prefix that means 'eye', e.g. *oculomotor*.

oculogyric *adj* referring to movements of the eyeball.

oculogyric crisis an attack in which the eyes stay in a fixed position for minutes or even hours. Usually the eyes are positioned up and to the side, but in some cases they are fixed to the side or down.

oculomotor nerves *n* the third pair of cranial nerves. They arise from nuclei near the cerebral aqueduct and are motor only. They innervate: (a) four of the extraocular/extrinsic muscles that move the eyeball, i.e. the superior, medial and inferior recti and the inferior oblique muscle; (b) the intrinsic (intraocular)—ciliary muscles which alter the shape of the lens, changing its refractive power and the circular muscles of the iris which constrict the pupil; and (c) the levator palpebrae muscle which raises the upper eyelid.

oculopharyngeal muscular dystropy a muscular dystrophy with both autosomal dominant and autosomal recessive inheritance; there is triplet repeat expansion in *PABP2* gene chromosome 14q. The onset occurs between the ages of 30 and 50 years. The muscles affected lead to ptosis,

O
P

external ophthalmoplegia, dysphagia and weakness of the tongue. There is mild lower limb weakness.

ODA *abbr* operating department assistant.

ODD *acron* **O**ppositional **D**efiant **D**isorder.

odds ratio in statistics, the odds of a disease occurring in a person exposed to the risk factor divided by the odds of a disease occurring in a person who has not been exposed to the risk factor.

odontalgia *n* toothache.

odontoblast process protoplasmic process of the odontoblast present in the dentinal tubules and responsible for the formation of dentine.

odontoblasts the specialized cells lying on the periphery of the dental pulp that are primarily responsible for dentine formation in the teeth.

odontoclasts cells in the teeth that are responsible for the resorption of dentine and cementum.

odontodysplasia abnormal development of the teeth, with deficient formation of enamel and dentine. The teeth have a characteristic radiographic appearance and are known as *ghost teeth*.

odontogenesis the formation of the teeth.

odontogenesis imperfecta a general term that includes defects in both the epithelial and mesenchymal tissue components needed for tooth formation.

odontogenic relating to the origin and development of the teeth.

odontogenic keratocyst a developmental cyst arising from odontogenic epithelium.

odontogenic tumours several types of neoplasms arising in tooth-forming tissues, they may be benign, (e.g. odontogenic fibroma), or malignant, (e.g. odontogenic fibrosarcoma).

odontogeny the origin and formative development of the teeth.

odontoid *adj* resembling a tooth.

odontoid process also known as the dens. A peg-like projection of the axis (second cervical vertebra) that fits into the posterior part of the vertebral foramen of the atlas (first cervical vertebra). The atlas rotates around the odontoid process, which acts as a pivot during movement of the head.

odontology the scientific study of the development, structure and function of the teeth and associated oral structures.

odontolysis resorption of a tooth root.

odontoma a tumour-like anomaly of the hard tissue of teeth (e.g. dens in dente). It comprises cementum, dentine, enamel and pulp that may be ordered in the form of teeth.

odontome abnormal mass of calcified dental tissue, e.g. new growths and malformation arising from dental tissues, such as ameloblastoma (adamantinoma).

odont/o, odontia, odontic- a prefix that means 'tooth', e.g. *odontalgia*.

odontoplasty a procedure to reshape the contour of the crown or root (or both) of a tooth or the anatomy of the fissure of a tooth in order to provide a contour that allows improved plaque control and oral hygiene. The term may also be used when modifying sharp edges on teeth which may cause soft tissue and tongue lesions.

-odynia a suffix that means 'pain', e.g. *pleurodynia*.

ODP *abbr* operating department practioner.

odynophagia intense pain and burning sensation during swallowing. It results from irritation of the oesophageal mucosa caused by certain foods, gastro-oesophageal reflux disease, infection, cancer, or from muscular problems such as achalasia.

oedema *n* abnormal collection of fluid in the tissues such as around the ankles, lower leg or sacral area. Fluid may also collect in the pleural cavity, pericardial sac and within the abdominal cavity. The formation of oedema can be caused by: reduced blood albumin, such as may occur in some kidney diseases, liver disease or when protein intake is insufficient; increased hydrostatic pressure leading to venous congestion, as in chronic heart failure; 'leaky' capillaries during the inflammatory response; and when lymphatic drainage is impaired, e.g. cancer affecting the lymph nodes. ⮑ angio-oedema, ascites, pleural effusion, pulmonary oedema—**oedematous** *adj*.

oedema during pregnancy oedema is often first recognized by excess weight gain (occult oedema), then by pitting on pressure (pressure leaves a persistent depression in the tissues). Approximately 50% of pregnant women develop mild physiological ankle oedema towards term, which is normal unless accompanied by other signs and symptoms, e.g. hypertension. In the puerperium, ankle oedema often worsens temporarily, as the kidneys are unable to cope immediately with excretion of the excess fluid as a result of the autolytic process of involution. Pathological oedema occurs with chronic renal disease, pre-eclampsia, eclampsia, severe heart disease, severe anaemia and protein malnutrition.

Oedipus complex an unconscious attachment of a son to his mother resulting in a feeling of jealousy towards the father and then guilt, producing emotional conflict.

oesophageal *adj* pertaining to the oesophagus.

oesophageal atresia a congenital anomaly charaterized by the absence of the oesophageal opening. It is often suspected by the presence of maternal polyhydramnios because the fetus is unable to swallow saliva. In the neonate saliva comes out of the mouth continuously as clear mucus; a stiff tube should be passed immediately after birth via the mouth to ensure patency of the oesophagus. Oesophageal atresia is often accompanied by tracheo-oesophageal fistula. ⮑ tracheo-oesophageal fistula.

oesophageal ulcer ulceration of the oesophagus due to gastro-oesophageal reflux disease caused by hiatus hernia.

oesophageal varices varicosity of the veins at the gastro-oesophageal junction due to hepatic portal hypertension, often caused by alcohol-related cirrhosis or chronic hepatitis. These varices can bleed and may cause a massive haematemesis. Management of bleeding includes endoscopic banding, sclerotherapy or use of tissue adhesives, which are often combined with a vasoactive drug such as octreotide. Use of temporary tamponade with a Sengstaken–Blakemore tube; transjugular intrahepatic portasystemic stent shunting (TIPSS); surgery including ligation of the varices, transection of the oesophagus and various portasystemic shunts to divert blood away from the hepatic portal circulation. ⊃ Sengstaken–Blakemore tube, transjugular intrahepatic portasystemic stent shunting.

oesophagectomy *n* excision of part or the whole of the oesophagus.

oesophagitis *n* inflammation of the oesophagus.

oesophag/o- a prefix that means 'oesophagus', e.g. *oesophagotomy*.

oesophagogastroduodenoscopy (OGD) fibreoptic endoscopic examination of the oesophagus, stomach and duodenum. Used to obtain tissue samples and for treatments, which include banding of varices, coagulation of bleeding ulcers, dilation of the stomach prior to the insertion of a percutaneous gastrostomy tube.

oesophagoscope *n* an endoscope for passage into the oesophagus—**oesophagoscopy** *n*, **oesophagoscopic** *adj*.

oesophagostomy *n* a surgically established fistula between the oesophagus and the skin in the root of the neck. May be used temporarily for feeding after excision of the pharynx for malignant disease.

oesophagotomy *n* an incision into the oesophagus.

oesophagus *n* the musculomembranous canal, around 23 cm in length in adults, extending from the pharynx to the stomach—**oesophageal** *adj*. ⊃ Colour Section Figure 18b.

oestradiol (estradiol) *n* an endogenous oestrogen secreted by the corpus luteum.

oestriol (estriol) *n* an endogenous oestrogen. Produced by the fetus and placenta. Oestriol levels in maternal blood or urine can be used to assess fetal wellbeing and placental function.

oestrogen receptor surface receptors expressed in some cells. The receptors are ligand-activated and regulate the cellular response to oestrogens in both sexes. ⊃ antioestrogens, selective (o)estrogen receptor modulators (SERMS).

oestrogens (estrogens) *npl* a generic term referring to a group of steroid hormones, oestradiol, oestriol and oestrone, which have oestrogenic activity. Produced mainly by the ovaries (predominantly in the first half of the menstrual cycle) and the fetoplacental unit during pregnancy; also in small amounts by the testes, and by the adrenal cortex in both sexes. Oestrogens are responsible for female secondary sexual characteristics and the development and proper functioning of the female genital organs. Their effects produce an environment suitable for fertilization, implantation and nutrition of the early embryo. During pregnancy oestrogens stimulate growth of the uterus and duct system of the breasts. Oestrogens also influence water and electrolyte retention. Used in the combined oral contraceptive to suppress ovulation, and as hormone replacement—**oestrogenic** *adj*. ⊃ menstrual cycle.

oestrone (estrone) *n* an endogenous oestrogen.

OFD *abbr* object-to-film distance.

off-centre field of view in magnetic resonance imaging (MRI) a field of view that is not centred at the isocentre of the magnet.

OFG *abbr* orofacial granulomatosis.

OGD *abbr* oesophagogastroduodenoscopy.

-ogen a suffix that means 'precursor', e.g. *angiotensinogen*.

Oguchi's disease (C Oguchi, Japanese ophthalmologist, 1875–1945) rare congenital hereditary night blindness occurring mainly in Japan. It is inherited as an autosomal recessive trait. All other visual capabilities are usually unimpaired. It is presumed to be due to an abnormality in the neural network of the retina. ⊃ hemeralopia.

OHI *abbr* oral hygiene index.

ohm (G Ohm, German physicist, 1789–1854) the unit of electrical resistance equal to the resistance between two points on a conductor when a potential difference of one volt between the points produces a current of one ampere.

Ohm's law (G Ohm) the current flowing through a conductor is proportional to the potential difference which exists across it, providing other physical conditions remain constant. $V = I \times R$, where V is the voltage (volts) in the circuit, I is the current (amps) and R is the resistance (ohms). Used to calculate changes in circuits with direct current.

OHSS *abbr* ovarian hyperstimulation syndrome.

OID *abbr* object-to-image distance.

-oid a suffix that means 'likeness, resemblance', e.g. *android*.

oil a liquid not miscible in water and generally combustible. Oils are classified as animal or vegetable, volatile and mineral.

oil of cloves clove oil. An oil consisting of 85–90% eugenol distilled from cloves. It is obtundent, antiseptic and deodorant.

oil of eucalyptus an oil from the Australian gum or eucalyptus tree.

ointment *n* a semisolid preparation, usually greasy, for application to the skin.

-ol a suffix that means 'alcohol', e.g. *sterol*.

olecranon bursitis (*syn* student's elbow) inflammation of the bursa over the point of the elbow.

olecranon process the large process at the upper end of the ulna; it forms the point of the elbow when the arm is flexed. ⊃ olecranon bursitis.

oleic acid an omega-9 monunsaturated fatty acid, an abundant fatty acid in olive oil.

olfactory *adj* pertaining to the sense of smell—**olfaction** *n* the sense of smell.

olfactory nerve the first pair of cranial nerves, they are the nerves of the sense of smell. Their nerve endings and fibres originate in the olfactory epithelium of the upper part of the nasal cavity. They carry sensory impulses from the olfactory epithelium, upwards through the cribriform plate of the ethmoid bone and then to the olfactory bulb. The nerves then proceed backwards as the olfactory tract, to the area for the perception of smell in the temporal lobe of the cerebrum.

O
P

olfactory organ the nose. ⇒ Colour Section Figure 14.

oligaemia *n* ⇒ hypovolaemia.

oligo- a prefix that means 'few, deficiency, diminution', e.g. *oliguria*.

oligoclonal bands a marker of inflammation that is found on electrophoresis of cerebrospinal fluid (CSF) in some conditions such as multiple sclerosis.

oligodactyly *n* a developmental absence of one or more digits (fingers or toes). There is total absence of all parts of the digit, e.g. metatarsal parts and all phalanges.

oligodendrocyte *n* part of the macroglia. A neuroglial cell of the central nervous system.

oligodendroglioma *n* a tumour of glial cells (neuroglial tissue) of the brain.

oligodipsia *n* dimished sense of thirst.

oligodontia *n* a condition in which some teeth develop but not all.

oligohydramnios *n* lack of amniotic fluid. The volume, which is normally around 1 L at 38 weeks' gestation, may be between 300–500 mL but can be less. Oligohydramnios is associated with fetal urinary tract abnormalities such as absence of the kidneys (renal agenesis). There is less room for fetal movement and the cramped position can lead to talipes and other defects that include facial abnormalities, and dry leathery skin. Oligohydramnios may also occur in post-term pregnancies. ⇒ amniotic fluid, polyhydramnios, Potter's sydrome.

oligomenorrhoea *n* infrequent menstruation; the normal cycle is prolonged beyond 35 days.

oligopeptides *npl* peptides containing 4 or more amino acids, but not as many as 20.

oligosaccharides *npl* carbohydrates containing between 3 and 9 monosaccharide units. The main dietary sources are vegetables, particularly seed legumes.

oligospermia *n* reduction in number of spermatozoa in the semen. ⇒ azoospermia.

oliguria *n* reduced urine output. Usually considered to be a volume of less than 0.5 mL per kilogram body weight per hour (mL/kg/h)—**oliguric** *adj*.

Ollier's dyschondrosis (L Ollier, French surgeon, 1830–1900) a rare disorder of bone in which deposits of cartilage occur in the metaphysis (area of growing long bone between each epiphysis and the diaphysis). The cartilage remains unossified and affects the epiphyseal plate, which results in abnormal bone growth and deformity.

-ology a suffix that means 'the study of', e.g. *biology*.

-oma a suffix that means 'tumour', e.g. *adenoma*.

OME *abbr* otitis media with effusion.

omega-3 fatty acids *npl* essential polyunsaturated fatty acids which have one of their carbon–carbon (C=C) double bonds at the third carbon atom from the omega end of the molecule. The three major types contained in foods and used by the body are alpha (α)-linolenic acid (ALA), eicosapentaenoic acid (EPA) and docosahexaenoic acid (DHA). Fish oil contains EPA and DHA, while some nuts (English walnuts) and vegetable oils (canola, soybean, flaxseed/

linseed and olive oil) contain ALA. Supplements are also widely available. Research indicates that omega-3 fatty acids reduce inflammation, improve plasma lipid profile and help to prevent certain chronic conditions such as coronary artery disease and arthritis; they are highly concentrated in the brain and have been reported to be important for cognitive and behavioural function. ⇒ essential fatty acids.

omega-6 fatty acids *npl* essential polyunsaturated fatty acids which have one of their carbon–carbon (C=C) double bonds at the sixth carbon atom from the omega end of the molecule. They include linoleic acid and γ-linolenic acid. Present in most vegetable and seed oils, e.g. corn oil, sunflower oil, and also present in evening primrose.

omega-9 fatty acids *npl* monounsaturated fatty acids which have a single carbon–carbon (C=C) double bond. They include oleic oil and erucic oil. Present in avocados, nuts, olives, olive oil, sesame oil, canola (rapeseed) oil.

omentectomy the excision of all or part of the omentum.

omentum *n* a sling-like fold of peritoneum—**omental** *adj*. The functions of the omentum are support and protection, limiting infection and fat storage. *greater omentum* the fold which hangs from the lower border of the stomach and covers the front of the intestines. *lesser omentum* a smaller fold, passing between the transverse fissure of the liver and the lesser curvature of the stomach.

Ommaya reservoir a special reservoir implanted under the scalp used in specialist centres to administer drugs, e.g. anti-cancer chemotherapy, into the cerebrospinal fluid (CSF), and to obtain samples of CSF for testing. It is used in the management of some types of leukaemia, for example acute lymphoblastic. One advantage is that it avoids the need for repeated lumbar puncture.

omophagia the consumption of uncooked or raw food.

omphalitis *n* inflammation of the umbilicus.

omphalocele *n* a congenital defect in the abdominal wall resulting from abnormal development of the abdominal muscles in the fetus. Normally the developing intestine protrude into the umbilical cord until week 10 of gestation when it returns to the abdominal cavity. In omphalocele this fails to happen and loops of intestine, the liver and sometimes other structures are outside the abdomen at birth. The defect is closed surgically very soon after birth. ⇒ exomphalos, hernia.

omphalus the umbilicus.

Onchocerca *n* a genus of filarial worms such as *Onchocerca volvulus*.

onchocerciasis *n* infestation of the soft tissues, skin and eye with *Onchocerca volvulus*. Adult worms encapsulated in subcutaneous connective tissue. Larval migration to the eyes leads to partial or total visual impairment 'river blindness'.

onc/o- a prefix that means 'mass, tumour, swelling', e.g. *oncogene*.

oncofetal antigens *npl* proteins normally produced during fetal development. They include alphafetoprotein (AFP), carcinoembryonic antigen (CEA) and pancreatic oncofetal antigen (POA). The gene that produces the antigen is normally non-active in adults, but may be expressed in certain cancers, such as AFP in liver cancer, or in non-malignant diseases, e.g. CEA in pancreatitis.

oncogene *n* a gene that may be activated by physical factors, carcinogenic chemicals, radiation, or oncogenic viruses to induce cancer in the host cell.

oncogenesis *n* the cause and process that produces tumours, either benign or malignant.

oncogenic *adj* capable of tumour production.

oncogenic viruses viruses that activate an oncogene to cause tumour formation. Examples include Epstein–Barr virus (EBV) and the human papilloma virus (HPV).

oncology *n* the scientific study and therapy of neoplastic growths—**oncological** *adj*, **oncologically** *adv*.

oncolysis *n* **1.** the destruction of cancer cells and tumours. **2.** the reduction in size of a mass or swelling.

oncotic *adj* relating to or caused by swelling.

oncotic pressure also called colloid osmotic pressure. The osmotic pressure exerted by the colloids in the blood. It is vital in maintaining the fluid balance between the blood and the interstitial spaces.

one-tailed hypothesis a research term. It implies a direction to a predicted change, e.g. first year students in group A will score higher than first year students in group B. Whereas a two-tailed hypothesis implies a difference, but no direction to the change, e.g. first year students in group A will have a different score than first year students in group B. ⊃ two-tailed hypthesis.

ongoing assessment the process of collecting information about the client's performance and progress or lack of progress during an intervention. This information is used to monitor the effects of intervention, assist the therapist's clinical reasoning process and inform clinical decision making.

onlay graft a graft applied directly onto the surface of a bone.

onlay (overlay) metal, ceramic or composite restorations designed to cover the occlusal and/or incisal surfaces of teeth. ⊃ onlay graft.

on:off ratio an electrotherapy term. It is the time for which current (or another pulsed output such as ultrasound or shortwave diathermy) flows and is off in a complete cycle, measured in s or ms usually. Can be used as a ratio or to calculate duty cycle.

onomatomania an obsession with particular names or words.

onset of blood lactate accumulation (OBLA) work rate at which *continuous* rise in blood lactate concentration $[Lac]_b$ begins. (At and a little above lactate threshold, it rises only initially, and falls gradually again after a few minutes). OBLA is thus theoretically slightly above maximum lactate steady state (MLSS), but it is doubtful whether they are distinguishable in practice. ⊃ metabolic and related thresholds.

ontology a research term. The study of the fundamental categories of what sorts or kinds of things may exist. For example, propositions, facts, numbers, causal connections, ethical values, forces, substances, spiritual beings and purposes. It is

also the branch of metaphysics concerned with the fundamental categories of things.

onychatrophia *n* (*syn.* anonychia) a nail that has reached mature size and then undergoes partial or total regression.

onychauxis *n* uniform thickening of the nail. It increases from the nail base to the free edge, and is often brownish in colour.

onychia *n* acute inflammation of the matrix and nail bed; suppuration may spread beneath the nail, causing it to become detached and fall off. Frequently originates from paronychia.

onych/o- a prefix that means 'nail', e.g. *onychomycosis*.

onychocryptosis *n* (*syn.* ingrowing nail) occurs when a spike, shoulder or serrated edge of the nail pierces the epidermis of the sulcus and penetrates the dermal tissues, most frequently in the hallux of male adolescents. The portion of nail penetrates further into the tissues producing acute inflammation in the surrounding soft tissues, often becoming infected (paronychia) and resulting in excess granulation tissue.

onychogryphosis, oncogryposis *n* (*syn.* ostler's toe, ram's horn) a ridged, thickened deformity of the nails, common in older people. There is hypertrophy, and gross deformity of the nail which develops into a curved or 'ram's horn' shape. The nail is usually dark brown or yellowish in colour, with both longitudinal and transverse ridges on its surface.

onycholysis *n* separation of the nail from the bed at the distal end and/or the lateral margins—**onycholytic** *adj*. It may be idiopathic or secondary to systemic and cutaneous diseases, or may result from local causes such as harsh manicuring. It is more common in fingernails than toenails and affects women more frequently than men.

onychomadesis *n* (*syn.* onychoptosis, aplastic anonychia) the spontaneous separation of the nail, beginning at the matrix area and quickly reaching the free edge. It is often accompanied by a transient arrest of nail growth, which is characterized by a Beau's line.

onychomycosis *n* (*syn.* tinea unguium) a fungal infection of the nail bed and plate. The nail plate becomes thickened, brittle and becomes yellowish-brown in colour. Eventually it develops a porous appearance.

onychophosis *n* a condition where a callus and/or a corn forms in the nail sulcus. It causes pain and inflammation.

onychorrhexis *n* (*syn.* reed nail) a brittle nail with a series of narrow, parallel longitudinal superficial ridges.

O'nyong-nyong fever (*syn.* joint-breaker fever) caused by a togavirus transmitted primarily by infected anopheline mosquitoes in East Africa. It is characterized by high temperature, arthritis affecting several joints with effusion, a maculopapular rash, lymphadenitis, painful red eyes and chest pain.

oo- a prefix that means 'egg, oocyte, ovum', e.g. *oogonium*.

oocyte *n* an immature ovum.

oocyte donation 'egg' donation. Part of some assisted conception techniques in which a woman donates oocytes to another woman who cannot produce her own, such as following cytotoxic drugs for cancer, early ovarian failure, or

O
P

because her oocytes have a genetic defect. The donated ooytes are fertilized in the laboratory using her partner's sperm. Some couples who are undergoing an IVF fertility cycle agree to donate surplus oocytes to another infertile couple who cannot produce their own.

oogenesis *n* the formation of oocytes ('eggs') in the ovary (Figure O.1). During fetal life primordial germ cells

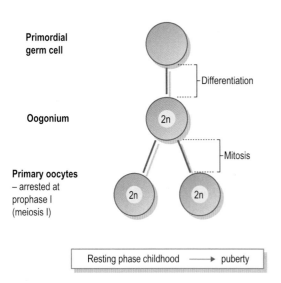

Primordial germ cell

Differentiation

Oogonium — 2n

Mitosis

Primary oocytes – arrested at prophase I (meiosis I) — 2n   2n

Resting phase childhood ⟶ puberty

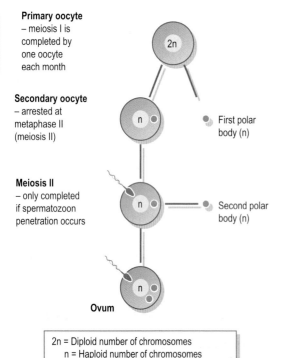

Primary oocyte – meiosis I is completed by one oocyte each month — 2n

Secondary oocyte – arrested at metaphase II (meiosis II) — n — First polar body (n)

Meiosis II – only completed if spermatozoon penetration occurs — n — Second polar body (n)

Ovum — n

2n = Diploid number of chromosomes
n = Haploid number of chromosomes

NB Polar bodies eventually degenerate within the ovum

O.1 Oogenesis (reproduced from Brooker & Nicol 2003 with permission).

differentiate to become diploid stem cells called oogonia (2n). The oogonia multiply by mitotic division to form many thousands of primary oocytes (2n). Mitosis is followed by growth and the formation of primordial follicles which surround the primary oocytes. At this stage the first meiotic division commences in the primary oocyte, but is arrested at prophase I. The primary oocyte now commences a variable-length resting stage before meiosis is completed, in a few hundred cells, some time during the woman's life. At puberty several primary oocytes are activated during each ovarian cycle. The arrested meiosis I (started during fetal life) is restarted in several primary oocytes but usually only one completes the process. During meiosis I the diploid primary oocyte produces two very dissimilar haploid cells: the secondary oocyte (n) and a polar body (n). The secondary oocyte is released from the surface of the ovary at ovulation. Meiosis II starts in the secondary oocyte, only to be arrested, this time in metaphase II, and will only be completed if it is penetrated by a spermatozoon. If this occurs the secondary oocyte completes meiosis II with the production of two haploid cells, a viable ovum (n) and a second polar body (n). The first and second polar bodies will eventually degenerate—**oogenetic** *adj.* ⊃ gametogenesis, spermatogenesis.

oogonium *n* one of the diploid precursor cells that form in the ovary during fetal development. They are derived from primordial germ cells and eventually give rise to oocytes—**oogonia** *pl.* ⊃ oogenesis.

oophorectomy *n* (*syn.* ovariectomy, ovariotomy) excision of an ovary, such as for a cyst or cancer.

oophoritis *n* (*syn.* ovaritis) inflammation of an ovary. It may occur with salpingitis, generalized pelvic inflammatory disease, or secondary to infections such as mumps.

oophor/o, - a prefix that means 'ovary', e.g. *oophoritis*.

oophoron *n* an ovary.

oophoropexy the surgical fixation of a displaced ovary to the abdominal wall or the inferior body of the uterus. It can also be done prior to radiotherapy treatment so that the ovary can be protected from receiving a large dose of radiation.

oophorosalpingectomy *n* ⊃ salpingo-oophorectomy.

opacifier a substance used in dentistry to reduce the translucency or transparency of a material and make it more opaque. Metal oxides are used to opacify dental porcelains.

opacity *n* non-transparency; cloudiness; an opaque spot, as on the cornea or lens. ⊃ dental opacity.

opacity (in radiography) the incident light over the transmitted light and is a measure of the effect the radiograph has on the original light shining on it.

opalescent having a milky appearance like an opal.

open-angle glaucoma glaucoma in which the angle of the anterior chamber is open and provides the aqueous humour free access to the drainage apparatus. It can occur: (a) as a *primary open-angle glaucoma* (POAG) (also called simple glaucoma, compensated glaucoma, chronic glaucoma). The increased intraocular pressure leads to atrophy and excavation of the optic disc and typical defects of the visual field. It is the most common type of glaucoma (opinions of incidence vary between 0.5% and 3% of the Caucasian population over 40) and because of its insidious nature is difficult to detect. It tends to occur more often after the age of 35, in people who have a family history of the disease, in African Caribbean individuals, people who have high myopia and those with diabetes mellitus. It is characterized by an almost complete absence of symptoms. Haloes around lights and blurring of vision occur in some patients when there has been a sudden increase in intraocular pressure or when the disease is very advanced. The diagnosis of this disease is made by demonstrating that the eye has a characteristic visual field loss. There may also be a raised intraocular pressure, although this is not always the case. (b) the other form is *secondary open-angle glaucoma* in which the intraocular pressure is elevated as a result of ocular trauma or iridocyclitis, crystalline lens abnormalities, etc. Management of open-angle glaucoma is usually by medication, unless this proves ineffective and surgery may be necessary. Nowadays, beta (β)-adrenoceptor antagonists such as timolol maleate or betaxolol, which act by reducing aqueous humour formation and do not affect pupil size or accommodation, are employed as the initial treatment. Also used are the carbonic anhydrase inhibitors (e.g. acetazolamide) the alpha (α)-adrenoceptor agonist (e.g. brimonidine), and the prostaglandin derivatives (e.g. latanoprost) which enhance the uveoscleral outflow. ⮑ frequency doubling perimetry, glaucomatous cup, gonioscope, laser trabeculoplasty, ocular hypertension, optic atrophy, plateau iris, provocative test, pseudoexfoliation, shadow test, tunnel vision.

open bite (open occlusal relationship, apertognathia) failure of some opposing teeth to occlude when other teeth are in maximum intercuspation. May be due to a congenital, developmental or acquired deformity; to dislocation of the temporomandibular articulation; to fracture and/or malunion of a fracture. ⮑ bite.

open chain exercise ⮑ open kinetic chain.

open fracture also known as compound fracture. There is a wound permitting communication of broken bone end with air. ⮑ fracture.

open kinetic chain in sports medicine or physiotherapy describes a motion during which the distal segment of an extremity moves freely in space, i.e. is non-weight-bearing (Figure O.2). ⮑ closed kinetic chain, kinematic chain exercises.

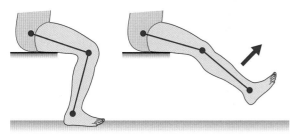

O.2 Open kinetic chain (reproduced from Porter 2005 with permission).

open loop control in motor control, movement that is executed without regard to sensory feedback. ⮑ closed loop control.

openness to experience one of the big five personality factors characterized by a tendency to be imaginative, curious, insightful and creative.

open reduction the realigning of fractures using a surgical procedure. ⮑ fracture reduction.

open reduction internal fixation (ORIF) a surgical intervention that involves the application of a plate and screws to the fracture is known as open reduction and internal fixation. It has the advantages of permitting a detailed inspection and accurate surgical assessment of the site of injury and procedure to be undertaken. The disadvantages include: (a) surgery inevitably causes additional trauma and potential exposure to micro-organisms and infection; (b) can convert a closed fracture into an open fracture; (c) requires surgery with all its sequelae and potential complications. Ironically, rigid fixation may remove the stimulus for callus formation. The implants may be removed 12–18 months in the future or if they start to become a problem, e.g. the screws may become an irritant. They will be removed in the young, as whilst they are in place bone will not grow and respond to stress normally, because some of the stresses are taken by the implants themselves. ORIF in dentistry. ⮑ fixation (dentistry/maxillofacial surgery).

open skill ⮑ skill.

operant conditioning ⮑ conditioning.

operating microscope an illuminated binocular microscope enabling surgery to be carried out on delicate tissues such as nerves and blood vessels, the brain and ear. Some models incorporate a beam splitter and a second set of eyepieces to enable a second person to view the operation site.

operating system a program that a computer loads automatically before it can run any other programs, e.g. Microsoft® Windows®, Mac® OS X®, UNIX.

operation *n* surgical procedure upon a part of the body.

operational management the management of the day-to-day activities (operations) of an organization such as a general hospital. ⮑ strategic management.

operative delivery forceps delivery of the infant, ventouse or vacuum extraction, or caesarean section.

operculum *n* **1.** the plug of mucus that occludes the cervical canal during pregnancy. It protects against ascending infection. The operculum is discharged from the vagina as the 'show' of blood-stained mucus that may precede the onset of labour or once labour commences—**opercula** *pl.* **2.** any structure resembling a lid or cover. **3.** a hood or flap of gingival tissue overlying the crown of a partially erupted tooth.

operculum opercula three areas of cerebral cortex (pars orbitalis, pars triangularis and pars basilaris), which are known collectively as the opercula of the frontal and parietal lobes. With the operculum of the temporal lobe they overlie the insula.

OPG® *abbr* orthopantomograph.

O
P

ophthalmia *n* (*syn.* ophthalmitis) inflammation of the eye. ⊃ sympathetic ophthalmia.

ophthalmia neonatorum defined as a purulent discharge from the eyes of an infant commencing within 21 days of birth. A notifiable condition.

ophthalmic *adj* pertaining to the eye.

ophthalmic applicator equipment which is sutured to the eye to hold the radioactive source, iodine-125 (^{125}I), when treating the eye. The applicator should be handled with rubber-tipped forceps to prevent damage to the thin, active window, other radiation sources can be used.

ophthalmic artery an artery arising from the internal carotid artery and which enters the orbit through the optic canal. It gives rise to numerous branches: (a) the central retinal artery; (b) the posterior ciliary arteries; (c) the lacrimal artery (and lateral palpebral and zygomatic branches); (d) muscular branches; (e) the supraorbital artery; (f) the anterior and posterior ethmoidal arteries; (g) the recurrent meningeal artery; (h) the supratrochlear artery; (i) the medial palpebral arteries; and (j) the dorsal nasal artery. Thus, the ophthalmic artery supplies all the tunics of the eyeball, most of the structures in the orbit, the lacrimal sac, the paranasal air sinuses, and the nose.

ophthalmic nerve the first division of the trigeminal nerve. It innervates the skin of the forehead, eyelids, nose and scalp, the conjunctiva, the eyeball, the lacrimal glands, nasal septum and part of the nasal mucosa, the paranasal air sinuses and part of the dura mater (outer meningeal membrane).

ophthalmic optician a term used principally in the UK and the Republic of Ireland. ⊃ optometrist.

ophthalmic prism a prism used in the correction or in the measurement of a deviation of the eyes. The power of such a prism is usually only a few prism dioptres. The power of a thin prism in air, represented by the angle of deviation *d*, is given by the approximate formula $d = (n - 1)a$ where *n* is the refractive index (index of refraction) of the prism and *a* the prism angle. ⊃ prism, prism dioptre, prism power.

ophthalmitis *n* ⊃ ophthalmia.

ophthalm/o- a prefix that means 'eye', e.g. *ophthalmoscope*.

ophthalmodynamometry an investigation used to determine the pressure of the blood in the vessels supplying the retina.

ophthalmologist *n* a medically qualified specialist in ophthalmology.

ophthalmology *n* the science that deals with the structure, function, diseases and treatment of the eye—**ophthalmological** *adj*.

ophthalmoplegia *n* paralysis of one or more extraocular/extrinsic muscles of the eye leading to an inability to move the eyes normally, or the internal muscles that control pupil size. Various causes include stroke, diabetes, brain tumours, trauma, multiple sclerosis, polyneuropathy, myasthenia gravis, exophthalmos associated with Graves' disease—**ophthalmoplegic** *adj*.

ophthalmorrhoea a discharge of mucus, pus or blood from the eye.

ophthalmoscope *n* an instrument used for viewing the media and fundus of the eye. It consists essentially of: (a) a light source (a halogen or tungsten bulb), a condenser system, a lens and a reflector (a prism, mirror or metallic plate) to illuminate the interior of the eye, and (b) a viewing system comprising a sight hole and focusing system (usually a rack of lenses of different powers) to compensate for the combined errors of refraction of the patient and the practitioner—**ophthalmoscopic** *adj*. ⊃ binocular indirect ophthalmoscope, direct ophthalmoscope, indirect ophthalmoscope, ophthalmoscopy, scanning laser ophthalmoscope.

ophthalmoscopy a method of examination of the interior of the eye with an ophthalmoscope. *red-free ophthalmoscopy* a method of ophthalmoscopy using a blue-green filter in the illumination system. This gives a better contrast between the retinal vessels and the background and helps to differentiate more easily between retinal and choroidal lesions: retinal lesions appear black while choroidal ones appear grey. However, in most ophthalmoscopes which use tungsten filament bulbs, the amount of light of short wavelength is so small that the observation is difficult and a filter which lets more long wavelengths pass is used, such as a yellow-green one. As a result of this compromise there is only a slight increase in contrast between the retinal vessels and the background.

ophthalmotomy an incision into the eyeball.

-opia a suffix that means 'eye', e.g. *myopia*.

opiate *n* strictly speaking a drug derived from the opium poppy (*Papaver somniferum*), which have analgesic and narcotic properties. Important alkaloids obtained from the poppy include codeine, morphine and papaverine. ⊃ opioids.

opioids *npl* **1.** endogenous chemicals with morphine-like effects, e.g. endorphins, enkephalins. **2.** a large group of exogenous substances that have morphine-like effects, which can be reversed by opioid receptor antagonists such as naloxone. Side-effects include constipation, dry mouth, nausea and vomiting, drowiness and respiratory depression. They include the opiates, semisynthetic morphine analogues and synthetic analogues. This list includes alfentanil, buprenorphine (agonist and antagonist actions), codeine, dextropropoxyphene, diamorphine (heroin), dihydrocodeine, fentanyl, methadone, morphine sulphate, naloxone (an antagonist), pentazocine, pethidine. ⊃ opiate, Appendix 5.

opisth/o- a prefix that means 'backward', e.g. *opisthotonos*.

opisthorchiasis *n* infestation with one of the species of *Opisthorchis* trematode liver flukes. It infests the liver and biliary tract and can lead to inflammation and cholangiocarcinoma (cancer of the gallbladder and or bile ducts), which is an usual cancer. The fluke, which is common in Southeast Asia, is associated with eating raw or inadequately cooked fish.

Opisthorchis a genus of trematode liver flukes; it includes the species *Opisthorchis felineus* and *O. viverrini*.

opisthotonic posture a posture characterized by the arched position of complete extension of the head, spine and limbs typically in severe meningeal irritation and other serious neurological conditions. ➲ opisthotonos.

opisthotonos *n* extreme extension of the body occurring in tetanic spasm. In extreme cases the patient may be resting on heels and head alone—**opisthotonic** *adj*.

opium *n* the dried juice of the opium poppy (*Papaver somniferum*). It contains morphine and other related alkaloids. ➲ opiate, opioids.

opponent-process theory ➲ Hering's theory of colour vision.

opportunistic infection a serious infection caused by a micro-organism which normally has little or no pathogenic activity but causes disease where host resistance is reduced by the effects of serious disease, invasive treatments or drugs on the ability of the immune system to resist infection. ➲ infection.

opportunity cost when a resource is used in a particular way, the opportunity to use it for another purpose is lost. This includes money, time and the activities which cannot be undertaken. An example in health care would be the decision to use money for an expensive cancer drug that prolongs life for a few months leading to a lost opportunity to spend the money for another service such as cataract surgery.

opposition *n* describes the position of the thumb and fingers when objects are picked up or grasped between thumb and fingers.

oppositional defiant disorder (ODD) a pattern of behaviour lasting longer than 6 months in which the child is abnormally defiant, hostile and disobedient to parents and other people in authority. The features include temper tantrums, argumentative behaviour, negativism, spiteful behaviour, anger, blaming others, vindictiveness, difficulty in making or keeping friends.

opsins *npl* protein part of visual pigments, which combine with retinal in the cones and rods of the retina. Found in the cones as iodopsins and in the rods as rhodopsin (visual purple). There are three iodopsins in different types of cones; they form the pigments known as chlorolabe, cyanolabe and erythrolabe.

opsoclonus rapid, erratic movements of the eyeballs in several different directions. It may occur with neurological disorders.

opsomania intense desire to consume special foodstuffs.

opsonic index a measurement that indicates the ability of phagocytes to ingest foreign bodies such as bacteria.

opsonin *n* complement protein or an antibody which coats an antigen. ➲ opsonization—**opsonic** *adj*.

opsonization *n* a process where antigens are coated with opsonins thereby increasing their susceptibility to phagocytosis.

-opsy a suffix that means 'looking', e.g. *colonoscopy*.

optic *adj* pertaining to sight.

optic atrophy pathological whitening of the optic nerve head with loss of nerve axons.

optic chiasma the meeting of the two optic nerves; where the fibres from the medial or nasal half of each retina

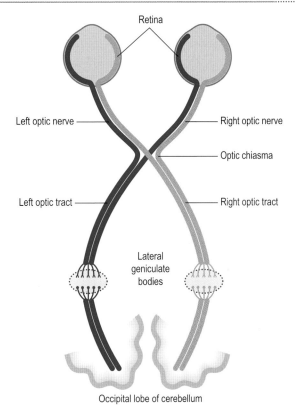

Retina

Left optic nerve

Right optic nerve

Optic chiasma

Left optic tract

Right optic tract

Lateral geniculate bodies

Occipital lobe of cerebellum

O.3 Optic chiasma (reproduced from Brooker 2006A with permission).

(supplying half the visual field in either eye) cross the middle line to join the optic tract of the opposite side (Figure O.3). ➲ chiasma.

optic cup (*syn* secondary optic vesicle) a double layered cup-shaped structure attached to the forebrain of the embryo by means of a hollow stalk. It develops into the retina and inner layers of the ciliary body and iris. It is formed by the invagination of the outer wall of the optic vesicle. Subsequently, nerve cells develop in its invaginated layer and some of these send their axons back along the hollow stalk (or optic stalk or lens stalk) to form the optic nerve. ➲ anophthalmia, optic fissure, optic vesicle.

optic disc (*syn* optic nerve head, optic papilla [this is not strictly correct because the disc is not elevated above the surrounding retina]). The region of the fundus of the eye corresponding to the optic nerve head. It can be seen with the ophthalmoscope as a pinkish-yellow area with usually a whitish depression called the physiological cup. The optic disc has an area of about 2.7 mm^2, a horizontal width of about 1.75 mm and a vertical height of about 1.9 mm. The optic disc is the anatomical correlate of the physiological blind spot. ➲ blind spot, papilloedema, retina, Colour Section Figure 15.

optic fissure (*syn* choroidal fissure, embryonic fissure) an invagination of the inferior portion of the optic stalk of the embryo. The hyaloid vessels pass through that fissure to supply the developing crystalline lens. In cases in which the invagination (or fissure) fails to fully close, colobomas will be formed. ⊃ coloboma, hyaloid artery, optic cup.

optic foramen one of two openings in the sphenoid bone that give passage to the optic nerve and the ophthalmic artery.

optic nerve head ⊃ optic disc.

optic nerves second pair of cranial nerves, they are the nerves of the sense of sight. The fibres originate in the retinae of the eyes and they combine to form the optic nerves. They convey impulses from the rods and cones in the retina to the visual area of the cerebral cortex. They are directed backwards and medially through the posterior part of the orbital cavity.They then pass through the optic foramina of the sphenoid bone into the cranial cavity and join at the optic chiasma (see Figure O.3, p. 547). The nerves proceed backwards as the optic tracts to the lateral geniculate bodies of the thalamus. Impulses pass from these to the visual area in the occipital lobes of the cerebrum and to the cerebellum. In the occipital lobe sight is perceived, and in the cerebellum the impulses from the eyes contribute to the maintenance of balance, posture and orientation of the head in space. The central retinal artery and vein enter the eye enveloped by the fibres of the optic nerve. ⊃ Colour Section Figure 15.

optic neuritis inflammation, swelling and or demyelination affecting an optic nerve. It can occur anywhere along its course from the ganglion cells in the retina to the synapse of these cell fibres in the lateral geniculate body. If the inflammation is restricted to the optic nerve head the condition is called *papillitis* (or *intraocular optic neuritis*) and if it is located in the orbital portion of the nerve it is called *retrobulbar optic neuritis* (or *orbital optic neuritis*). In papillitis the optic nerve head is hyperaemic with blurred margins and slightly oedematous. Haemorrhages and exudates may also appear. In retrobulbar optic neuritis, there are usually no visible signs in the fundus of the eye until the disease has advanced and optic atrophy may appear. However, both types are accompanied by a loss of visual acuity along with a central scotoma and impairment of colour vision. The loss of vision may occur abruptly over a few hours and recovery may be equally rapid but in other patients the loss may be slow. In retrobulbar optic neuritis, there is also pain on movement of the eyes and sometimes tenderness on palpation. The disease is usually unilateral although the second eye may become involved later. The disease is usually transient and full or partial recovery takes place within weeks. The primary cause of optic neuritis is multiple sclerosis where it may be an early and sometimes the single sign of disease, but it may also be associated with severe inflammation of the retina or choroid, vitamin B deficiency, diabetes mellitus, thyroid disease, vasculitis, autoimmune disorders, lactation, infection and toxicity. ⊃ Kollner's rule, Marcus Gunn pupil, optic nerve, papilloedema, photostress test.

optic neuropathy a non-inflammatory or degenerative disease of the optic nerve resulting in destruction of the nerve or loss of function. Causes include lack of blood supply caused by compression or an aneurysm; toxic chemicals such as methanol; and brain/head injury.

optic papilla ⊃ optic disc.

optic pit (*syn* optic sulcus) a depression on each side of the end of the neural ectoderm (or neural tube) of the embryo. The pit deepens to form the optic vesicle. ⊃ optic vesicle.

optic radiations (*syn* optic radiations of Gratiolet, geniculocalcarine tract) that part of the visual pathway which consists of axons arising in the lateral geniculate body and terminating in a fan-shaped manner in the visual area of the occipital lobe. As they emerge from the lateral geniculate body the inferior fibres loop forward in the temporal lobe before swinging back toward the occipital cortex. These fibres form what is called Meyer's loop (or Archambault's loop). They receive impulses from the inferior retinal quadrants (corresponding to the superior aspect of the contralateral visual field). They terminate on the inferior lip of the calcarine fissure. ⊃ visual area, visual pathway.

optic sulcus ⊃ optic pit.

optic tectum ⊃ tectum of mesencephalon.

optic tracts two cylindrical bands of nerve fibres carrying visual impulses. They run outward and backward from the posterolateral angle of the optic chiasma, then sweep laterally encircling the hypothalamus posteriorly on their way to the lateral geniculate bodies. ⊃ optic chiasma, hemianopsia (incongruous), visual pathway.

optic vesicle (*syn* primary optic vesicle) a hollow, spherical outgrowth from the lateral aspect of the forebrain, derived from the optic pit after closure of the embryonic neural groove. It subsequently invaginates to form the optic cup. ⊃ optic cup, optic pit.

optical *adj* relating to sight.

optical aberration an optical defect in which the rays from a point object do not form a perfect point after passing through an optical system. ⊃ oblique astigmatiam, coma, curvature of field, distortion, monochromatic aberration.

optical centre that point (real or virtual) on the optical axis of a lens which is, or appears to be, traversed by rays emerging parallel to their original direction. Applied to an ophthalmic lens, it is commonly regarded as coinciding with the vertex of either surface (British Standard). ⊃ nodal points, vertex.

optical character recognition (OCR) a means of the computer directly reading printed or written characters.

optical density 1. the light absorbed by a solution. Can be used to determine substance concentration. **2.** (*syn* absorbance [not strictly correct]). A term applied to optical filters. It is equal to the logarithm to the base 10 of the reciprocal of the transmission factor (transmittance) T thus

$$D = \log_{10} \frac{1}{T}$$

where D is the symbol for optical density. ⊃ absorption, filter, spectrophotometer.

optical disk a disk, usually a DVD or a CD that uses light in the form of a laser to burn data onto the disk and also to read information from the disk.

optical sensitizing in radiography. Increasing the spectral sensitivity of the film by adding impurities to the film emulsion, because it is done by adding coloured dyes and therefore can be called dye sensitizing, colour sensitizing or spectral sensitizing.

optical zone of cornea (*syn* corneal cap) a theoretical zone of about 4 mm in diameter in the centre of the cornea. It is assumed to be spherical for clinical purposes. ⊃ corneal apex.

optician *n* a person qualified and registered to make and fit spectacles/contact lenses (dispensing optician), or test visual acuity, prescribe and dispense spectacles or contact lenses to correct refractive errors. *ophthalmic optician*, now known as optometrist. ⊃ optometrist.

optician-optometrist a term used in some European countries. ⊃ optometrist.

opticokinetic *adj* also called optokinetic. Relating to the movement of the eyes in response to objects moving in the visual field.

optics *n* the scientific study of the properties of light.

optimum *adj* most favourable.

optimum position that which will be most useful and cause the least problems should a limb remain permanently paralysed such as following a stroke.

opto-electronic motion analysis equipment used to measure the motion of a body or object, using light (often infra-red) reflected from markers attached to its surface.

optometer (*syn* refractometer) an instrument for measuring the refractive state of the eye. There are two main types of optometers: subjective and objective. *subjective optometers* rely upon the subject's judgement of sharpness or blurredness of a test object. *objective optometers* contain an optical system which determines the vergence of light reflected from the subject's retina. Electronic optometers in which all data appear digitally within a brief period of time after the operator has activated a signal can be of either type. Objective types (also called ractors or ractometers) have become very popular and many of these ractors are now providing both objective and subjective systems within the same instrument. ⊃ autorefraction, infrared optometer, objective accommodation, photorefraction, refractive error.

optometric physician a term used in some US states, especially where therapeutic drugs are used. ⊃ optometrist.

optometrist (*syn* ophthalmic optician [term used principally in the UK and the Republic of Ireland], optician-optometrist [term used in some European countries], optometric physician [term used in some US states, especially where therapeutic drugs are used]). A person trained, qualified in the practice of optometry and registered to practice. The World Council of Optometry defines optometrists as 'the primary healthcare practitioners of the eye and visual system who provide comprehensive eye and vision care, which includes refraction and dispensing, the detection/ diagnosis and management of diseases in the eye, and the rehabilitation of conditions of the visual system'.

optometry the study of visual sciences and the management of human eye optics. An autonomous, healthcare profession involved in the services and care of the eye and visual system, and the enhancement of visual performance. ⊃ optometrist, primary care optometry.

optotype the test type used for measuring visual acuity. ⊃ Jaeger test types, König bars, Landolt ring, Snellen test type chart.

oral *adj* pertaining to the mouth—**orally** *adv*.

oral cavity that part of the mouth containing the tongue; bounded by the teeth and alveolar ridges. ⊃ mouth.

oral cholecystography the radiographic investigation of the biliary tract following the ingestion of a contrast agent, now superseded by ultrasound techniques.

oral contraceptive commonly referred to as 'the pill'. *combined oral contraceptive* contain varying amounts of the two hormones—oestrogen and progestogen. ⊃ combined oral contraceptive (COC) pill, contraceptive, progestogen-only contraceptive.

oral flora the micro-organisms normally residing in the mouth.

oral fluid ⊃ whole saliva.

oral high frequency oscillation the application of high frequency vibrations (applied either externally via a high frequency chest wall compressor or internally via devices such as the flutter) to the airways to facilitate sputum clearance. The rapid vibratory movements of small volumes of air within the airways results in the enhancement of cough and mucus clearance.

oral hygiene the maintenance of oral cleanliness by removing bacterial plaque with brushes, dental floss and other special instruments.

oral hygiene index (OHI) ⊃ index (dental).

oral medicine branch of dentistry concerned with the management of diseases of the oral mucosa and related structures, including oral manifestations of systemic diseases.

oral mucosa the layer of epithelium and subjacent connective tissue lining the oral cavity.

oral rehabilitation the restoration of the form and function of the masticatory arrangements to as nearly normal as possible.

oral rehydration solution (ORS) an oral solution for the replacement of fluids and electrolytes lost in diarrhoea. The WHO advocate a single solution, which is used flexibly depending on the specific situation. The WHO solution contains more sodium than the one used in the UK, but both provide sodium, potassium, chloride, citrate and glucose. ⊃ hydration status of athletes, sports drinks, water balance.

oral rehydration therapy (ORT) administration of oral rehydration solution by mouth to correct dehydration.

oral screen a myofunctional appliance used to exert pressure in the upper labial segment by displacing the lips from their resting position.

oral seal the seal of the oral cavity effected by the soft tissues without any conscious effort. May be at the anterior end (anterior oral seal) or the posterior end (posterior oral seal) or both. ⊃ seal.

oral stereognosis the ability to recognize the shape of an object placed in the mouth purely by intra-oral tactile information.

oral surgery branch of dental surgery concerned with minor surgery to the teeth and jaws. It includes the diagnosis and surgical treatment of the diseases, injuries and defects of the jaws and associated structures.

orange a hue corresponding to wavelengths between 590 and 630 nm. ⊃ colour, light.

ora serrata the serrated anterior boundary of the retina located some 8 mm from the corneal limbus. At the ora serrata, the retina is firmly adherent to the choroid which is the reason why a retinal detachment ends here. ⊃ ciliary body, retina, retinal dialysis, striae.

orbicular *adj* resembling a globe; spherical or circular.

orbicularis *n* a muscle that encircles an orifice.

orbicularis oculi the muscle around the eyeball, eyelid and the orbit. It contracts to close the eye and when necessary contracts strongly to 'screw' the eyes shut, such as in very bright sunlight.

orbicularis oris the unpaired muscle that encircles the mouth and blends with the buccinator muscle of the cheek. Contraction of the orbicularis oris shuts the lips and allows activities that include whistling.

orbit *n* the bony socket containing the eyeball and its appendages. It is formed from parts of the sphenoid, frontal, zygomatic, maxilla, orbital plate of the ethmoid, lacrimal and palatine bones—**orbital** *adj*.

orbital relating to the orbit.

orbital blow-out fracture a fracture of the orbital floor, possibly with the displacement of orbital tissue into the maxillary sinus.

orbital conjunctiva ⊃ conjunctiva.

orbital optic neuritis ⊃ optic neuritis.

orbitale the lowest point on the infraorbital region. ⊃ Frankfort plane.

orbitomeatal baseline a line joining the lateral canthus of the eye to the mid point of the external auditory meatus.

orchidalgia *n* pain felt in a testis. The pain may arise from testicular problems such as inflammation (orchitis) or torsion, but may be caused by a hernia or associated with renal colic.

orchidectomy *n* excision of a testis, such as following injury or to remove a cancer.

orchidometer an instrument for assessing the volume of a testis. *Prader orchidometer* (A Prader, Swiss paediatrician/endocrinologist, 1919–2001) a series of beads of different volumes (1 to 25mL) used as a comparison for assessing the volume of the patient's testes. Provides information about testicular growth and development, onset of puberty, reasons for early puberty, hypogonadism, or abnormally large testes.

orchidopexy *n* surgical procedure of bringing an undescended testis into its correct location in the scrotum, and fixing it in this position.

orchi/o, orchid/o- a prefix that means 'testis', e.g. *orchidopexy*.

orchiotomy an incision into a testis.

orchis *n* the testis.

orchitis *n* inflammation of a testis usually caused by a viral infection, particularly mumps. The testes are swollen and painful and the patient has a fever. Orchitis may occur with inflammation of the epididymis (epididymo-orchitis).

ordinal data categorical data that can be ordered or ranked, e.g. general condition—good, fair or bad, or size in general terms, as in 'smaller than'. ⊃ nominal data.

ordinal scale the numbers allotted to the ranking or ordering data in a rough sequence.

orexigenic stimulating or increasing appetite.

orexins *npl* also known as hypocretin. Two excitatory neuropeptides produced by nerve cells in the hypothalamus. With other substances, they function in the regulation of wakefulness and appetite. ⊃ hypocretin.

orf *n* purulent skin lesions caused by a type of poxvirus normally affecting sheep and goats. ⊃ Colour Section Figure 94.

organ *n* an assembly of different tissues to form a distinct functional unit, e.g. liver, uterus, able to perform specialized functions. Organs may be hollow as the stomach or compact, e.g. liver.

organelle subcellular structures, such as mitochondria, the endoplasmic reticulum and the Golgi apparatus, which perform specialized functions in the cell.

organic *adj* pertaining to an organ. Associated with life.

organic brain syndrome ⊃ dementia.

organic compounds chemical compounds containing carbon and hydrogen in their structure, e.g. glucose. They include the large biological molecules (macromolecules), such as lipids and proteins.

organic disease one in which there is structural change.

organism *n* a living cell or group of cells differentiated into functionally distinct parts which are interdependent.

organ of Corti (A Corti, Italian anatomist, 1822–1888) the spiral organ sited in the cochlea of the inner ear, it contains the auditory receptors (hair cells) which convert sound vibrations to nerve impulses. The nerve impulses are transmitted to the brain via the cochlear branch of the vestibulocochlear nerve.

organogenesis *n* the process whereby the body organs develop from embryonic tissue. It commences at about 2 weeks' gestation and is complete by week 8. The developing embryo is particularly vulnerable during this period to factors such as micro-organisms, e.g. rubella virus, that can seriously disrupt organ development.

organophosphorus compounds several highly toxic anticholinesterase compounds usually used as commercial insecticides. They cause irreversible inhibition of cholinesterase.

organs at risk the organs of the body that are more sensitive to radiation and therefore may influence treatment planning or prescribed dose, for example eyes, spinal cord and gonads.

orgasm *n* the climax of sexual excitement.

oriental sore (*syn.* Delhi boil) a form of cutaneous leishmaniasis producing papular, crusted, granulomatous skin eruptions. Occurs in tropical and subtropical regions (Old World).

orientation *n* clear awareness of one's position relative to the environment. In mental conditions orientation 'to people, space and time' means that the patient knows who people are, where he or she is and is aware of the passage of time, i.e. can give the correct date. Disorientation means the reverse. ⊃ delerium, dementia, reality orientation.

ORIF *abbr* open reduction internal fixation.

orifice *n* a mouth or opening.

orifice enlarger also called orifice opener. A endodontic instrument used to enlarge the openings of root canals to improve access.

origin *n* the commencement or source of anything.

origin of a muscle with reference to a skeletal muscle, the site of its attachment to bone which remains relatively fixed during its contraction compared to the site of its insertion. For example, in elbow extension, contraction of the triceps moves the forearm (site of insertion) while the upper arm and scapula (sites of origin) may remain still.

orlistat a drug which in conjunction with dieting has been proven to produce weight loss. It is a pancreatic lipase inhibitor which prevents fat breakdown in the intestine and therefore its absorption. About a third of ingested fat is passed through the bowel undigested when on a course of orlistat, reducing energy intake. Other beneficial effects include a lowering of serum cholesterol, reduction in blood pressure and better control of diabetes. Undesirable effects are abdominal discomfort, diarrhoea and anal leakage, and potential loss of fat-soluble vitamins. ⊃ lipolysis.

ornithine *n* an amino acid, produced from arginine during the urea cycle. Used in sport as a dietary supplement which in combination with other amino acids arginine and lysine is claimed to increase muscle growth/lean body mass to a greater extent than strength training alone, but this has not been supported by properly designed trials. ⊃ ergogenic aids.

ornithine cycle ⊃ urea cycle.

Ornithodoros a genus of ticks, some act as vectors for the bacteria causing relapsing fevers.

ornithosis *n* human illness resulting from disease of birds. ⊃ *Chlamydia*, psittacosis.

or/o- a prefix that means 'mouth', e.g. oropharynx.

oroantral pertaining to the mouth and maxillary antrum/sinus.

oroantral fistula an abnormal epithelialized connection between the oral cavity and the maxillary sinus.

orofacial pertaining to the mouth and face.

orofacial granulomatosis (OFG) a chronic granulomatous inflammatory condition of the lips and oral mucosa which may be of hypersensitivity origin ⊃ Melkersson–Rosenthal syndrome.

orofacial movements the movements of the face and mouth required for speech, eating and swallowing and non-verbal communication. Problems can occur in this area following brain injury or after Bell's palsy. The restoration of orofacial function should be of paramount importance for the physiotherapist and speech and language therapist. Problems in this area can lead to an inability to close the lips, drooling, move food around in the mouth and thus eating can become embarrassing for the patient. If eye closure is a problem then eye care is crucial to prevent drying and corneal damage. The eye is cleaned to remove debris and secretions, the eye may be protected from drying by the use of artificial tears, a hydrogel pad may be placed over the eye once closed, the eyelids may need be taped shut using hypoallogenic tape, or occasionally the eyelids may be closed with a suture (stitch).

orogenital *adj* pertaining to the mouth and the external genital area.

oropharyngeal *adj* pertaining to the mouth and pharynx, or to the oropharynx.

oropharyngeal airway ⊃ airway.

oropharynx *n* that portion of the pharynx which is below the level of the soft palate and above the level of the hyoid bone. The palatine tonsils are present in folds on the lateral walls. Air, food and fluid passes through the oropharaynx. ⊃ fauces, Waldeyer's ring.

orotic acid intermediate substance formed during the synthesis of pyrimidines.

Oroya fever ⊃ bartonellosis.

ORS *abbr* oral rehydration solution.

ORT *abbr* oral rehydration therapy.

ortho- a prefix that means 'straight', e.g. *orthodontics*.

orthochromatic emulsions in radiography, the film emulsions that have a spectral sensitivity up to and including the green part of the visible spectrum tend to be used with rare earth intensifying screens. ⊃ monochromatic emulsions, panchromatic emulsions.

orthodontic refers to the correction of irregularities in teeth. ⊃ orthodontic adhesive, orthodontic anchorage, orthodontic appliance, orthodontic band, orthodontic clasp, orthodontic elastic band, orthodontic face-bow, orthodontic ligature, orthodontic screw, orthodontic separator, orthodontic welder, orthodontic wire, orthodontics.

orthodontic adhesive used to bond orthodontic brackets to enamel.

orthodontic anchorage resistance to unwanted tooth movement during orthodontic treatment.

orthodontic appliance a device bonded or attached to the teeth used to effect or prevent movement of the teeth and associated structures. *Andresen appliance* acrylic myofunctional device to produce tooth movement and influence growth. Also known as a *monobloc activator*. A variation is the *medium opening activator* (MOA). *Bass appliance* a myofunctional appliance. *Begg appliance* a fixed, multibracket appliance ⊃ Begg technique. *Bimler appliance* a myofunctional appliance. *bionator appliance* a myofunctional appliance. *craniofacial appliance* a device used to immobilize jaw fractures. *edgewise appliance* fixed, multi-banded appliance which uses a rectangular arch wire ligated to brackets in order to achieve orthodontic tooth movement. *extra-oral appliance* apparatus using the top or back of the head or neck for anchorage—a headgear, cervical gear or halo. *fixed appliance* orthodontic device cemented or attached to the teeth. *Fraenkel appliance* an orthodontic myofunctional appliance ➲ Fraenkel. *Herbst appliance* a fixed myofunctional appliance. *Johnson twin wire appliance* an orthodontic fixed appliance using twin arch wires. *myofunctional appliance* a removable orthodontic appliance that functions by muscular action in order to try and influence growth of the jaws, e.g. Andresen, Fraenkel. *orthodontic appliance* device used to apply forces to the teeth and their supporting structures to produce changes in the relationship of the teeth and their positions. Used to carry out active or passive phases of orthodontic treatment. *pre-adjusted appliance* when the fixed appliance bracket slot is machined to incorporate the tip, torque and 'in-out' that was conventionally bent into the arch wire, so simplifying fixed orthodontic technique. *Rickett's appliance* a pre-adjusted edgewise appliance. *twin block appliance* a two-piece myofunctional appliance.

orthodontic band a retaining device for fixed orthodontic appliances. Made of stainless steel strip, which is adapted to fit individual teeth. ➲ orthodontic band tape

orthodontic band tape a stainless steel or precious metal tape, obtainable in various sizes and grades, used in the construction of fixed orthodontic appliances.

orthodontic clasp a component, made of non-staining, springy metal, of orthodontic appliances which contacts and partially surrounds a tooth to provide retention and stability.

orthodontic device *n* device used to move teeth by the controlled application of force. May be removable, myofunctional (functional) or fixed. ➲ orthodontic appliance.

orthodontic elastic band a rubber or latex elastic band used to apply forces to the teeth through appliances attached to the teeth.

orthodontic face-bow that part of extraoral traction appliance placed between the head-gear or cervical strap and the intraoral orthodontic appliance.

orthodontic ligature a soft stainless steel wire used to connect the arch or bow of a fixed orthodontic appliance to brackets either fixed onto bands or cemented to the teeth.

orthodontic scissors ➲ scissors.

orthodontic screw a device with a screw thread which is inserted into an orthodontic appliance. When turned it may bring together or separate portions of the appliance.

orthodontic separator a wire, spring or rubber band used to separate teeth prior to orthodontic band placement.

orthodontic tape ➲ orthodontic band tape.

orthodontic therapist a member of the dental team who is able to undertake orthodontic procedures under the prescription of a dentist or orthodontist.

orthodontic welder a specialized electric spot welder used with orthodontic materials.

orthodontic wire the corrosion-resistant wire used in the construction of orthodontic appliances. It may be round, square or oval in cross-section, usually constructed from stainless steel or a nickel titanium alloy.

orthodontics *n* the branch of dental science concerned with the study of the growth, development and infinite variations of the face, jaws and teeth, including dentofacial abnormalities and their corrective treatment. ➲ malocclusion.

orthodontist a dentist with specialist qualifications who diagnoses, prevents and treats malocclusion and other dental irregularities.

orthodox sleep *n* (*syn.* NREM sleep) ➲ sleep.

ortho-ethoxybenzoic acid (EBA) cement ➲ cement, ethoxybenzoic acid (EBA) cement.

orthognathic pertaining to the malposition of the bones of the jaw.

orthognathic surgery *n* surgical correction of craniofacial disharmonies by repositioning either segments of the mandible or maxilla or the entire jaws, in order to achieve a more acceptable function and appearance.

orthogonal radiographs radiographs taken at 90 degrees to one another to localize the treatment area or to verify the relative positions of radioactive sources with reference to the associated anatomy.

orthograde root filling a tooth root filling normally carried out in a root canal through the coronal access cavity. ➲ retrograde (root-end) filling.

orthomyxovirus a family of RNA viruses that cause influenza in humans.

orthopaedics *n* formerly a specialty devoted to the correction of deformities in children. It is now a branch of surgery dealing with all conditions affecting the locomotor system.

orthopantomograph (OPG®) specialist dental, tomographic equipment for imaging the upper and lower teeth on one projection. ➲ panoramic radiograph.

orthophosphoric acid ➲ phosphoric acid.

orthopic fusion fusion obtained by voluntary convergence on two targets separated in space and such that the right eye fixates the right target and the left eye the left target. This is often facilitated by looking beyond the targets and then slowly shifting one's gaze to the targets through double apertures placed in front of them. This procedure is aimed at improving negative fusional convergence. ➲ chiastopic fusion, fusional convergence.

orthopnoea *n* breathlessness that occurs when the person lies flat; often a feature of chronic cardiac failure. It occurs because this position results in the redistribution of blood, leading to an increased central and pulmonary blood volume, which gives rise to pulmonary vascular congestion and fluid accumulation in the lungs. Another cause of orthopnoea is diaphragmatic weakness or paralysis—**orthopnoeic** *adj*.

orthoptics *n* the study and treatment of eye movement disorders.

orthoptist *n* one who specializes in the assessment and treatment of eye movement disorders.

orthoptoscope ➲ amblyoscope.

orthoscopic eyepiece an eyepiece corrected for distortion, and which provides a wide field of view and high magnification. It consists of a triplet field lens and a single eye lens. It is used in high-power telescopes and range finders. ➲ triplet.

orthosis *n* from Greek *ortho*, to straighten. A custom-designed external device used to control or counteract the effect of an actual or developing deformity. Types include braces, splints, etc. In sport the term is most commonly used to describe foot-supporting insoles used to correct structural imbalance which may result in discomfort in the back, hips, knees or feet. Orthoses decrease the risk of further injury and make movement of the foot more efficient. ➲ night splint, prosthesis—**orthoses** *pl*, **orthotic** *adj*.

orthostatic *adj* caused by the upright stance.

orthostatic albuminuria the presence of albumin in the urine occurs in some healthy subjects only when they stand upright.

orthotics *n* the scientific study and manufacture of devices which can be applied to or around the body in the care of physical impairment or disability. ➲ prosthesis.

orthotist *n* a person who practises orthotics.

orthotopic transplant ➲ transplant.

orthotopic bladder substitution surgical technique of bladder reconstruction using the site of the excised native bladder with an anastomosis to the native urethra.

Ortolani's sign/test (M Ortolanli, Italian surgeon, 20th century) a test performed shortly after birth for the diagnosis of developmental dysplasia of the hip (congenital dislocation of the hip). It should always be undertaken by an experienced clinician. Often used in conjunction with Barlow's sign/test. ➲ developmental dysplasia of the hip.

os *n* a mouth. *external os* the opening of the cervix into the vagina. ➲ Colour Section Figure 17. *internal os* the opening of the cervix into the uterine cavity—**ora** *pl*.

OSAS *abbr* obstructive sleep apnoea (hypopnoea) syndrome.

OSAHS *abbr* obstructive sleep apnoea hypopnoea syndrome.

os calcis ➲ calcaneus.

oscillometry *n* measurement of vibration, using a special device (oscillometer).

oscilloscope *n* an instrument with a cathode ray tube, which displays a visual representation of electrical variations produced by a beam of electrons hitting the screen. Used to display various electrical waveforms such as that produced by the heart.

-ose a suffix that means 'sugar', e.g. *ribose*.

Osgood–Schlatter disease (R Osgood, American surgeon, 1873–1956; C Schlatter, Swiss surgeon, 1864–1934) osteochondritis/apophysitis of the tibial tubercle (tuberosity). An 'overuse' injury, which produces pain (due to inflammation) at the attachment of the patellar tendon to the tibial tubercle at an age when this is not fully developed. Most common around puberty/adolescence (rapid skeletal growth), in boys more than girls, who take part in repeated or multiple sports, especially those with repetitive running (football, athletics) or with repeated knee bending and jumping (athletics, gymnastics). Some authors suggest up to 50% are precipitated by trauma. Symptoms include swelling, pain and tenderness on direct pressure, and pain (felt precisely on the tibial tubercle) during exercise and contraction of the quadriceps muscle group. Heals spontaneously, with no individual treatment shown to be particularly helpful, except reduction in activity to levels where symptoms are acceptable. Rarely leads to problems in later life. ➲ Schlatter's disease.

Osiander's sign pulsation of the uterine arteries through the lateral fornices which can be felt on examination *per vaginam* in early pregnancy; may assist in the diagnosis of pregnancy.

os innominatum (innominate bone) the three fused bones on either side of the pelvis which form the girdle.

-osis a suffix that means 'condition, disease, excess', e.g. *osteoporosis*.

Osler's nodes (W Osler, Canadian/British physician, 1849–1919) small painful areas in pulp of fingers or toes, or palms and soles, caused by emboli. Occurs in infective endocarditis.

osmolality *n* the concentration of osmotically active particles in a solution, expressed as the number of osmoles per kilogram (Osm/kg) of solution. In blood plasma, osmolality (280–300 Osm/kg) is very slightly less than osmolarity (in Osm/L) because the presence of large molecules (e.g. lipids) adds to the volume that contains 1 kg of water (plasma is about 94% water). The two terms are often incorrectly used interchangeably; osmolality applies appropriately to body fluids. Measurement allows assessment of dehydration/overhydration.

osmolarity *n* the concentration of osmotically active particles in a solution expressed in osmoles per litre (Osm/L) of the solution. Values for human body fluids (e.g. blood plasma) are usually expressed in milliosmoles per litre (Osm/L). Compare osmolality.

osmole *n* the amount of a substance in a solution that forms 1 mole of osmotically active particles, irrespective of their size, e.g. a single sodium ion contributes as much to the osmolality as a large protein molecule; and 1 mole of glucose, which does not ionize, provides 1 osmole, while 1 mole of sodium chloride provides 2 osmoles—one of Na^+ and one of Cl^-.

osmophiles *npl* microorganisms that can thrive in a high osmotic pressure environment, e.g. in jam, honey, or pickles; the mould (yeasts) found on the surface of homemade jam.

osmoreceptors specialized cells located in the hypothalamus, sensitive to a change in the osmolality of their surroundings, which will reflect any such change in the plasma and body fluids as a whole. A rise in osmolality (tending towards dehydration) triggers thirst mechanisms and increased production and release of antidiuretic hormone (ADH) (vasopressin, or arginine vasopressin [AVP]) from the posterior pituitary (a neuroendocrine secretion), causing the renal tubules in the kidneys to retain more water. Conversely, a decrease in body fluid osmolality (due to high water intake) reduces ADH release, leading to increased and less concentrated urine output (diuresis).

O
P

osmosis *n* the passage of pure solvent across a semipermeable membrane under the influence of osmotic pressure. It is the movement of a dilute solution into a more concentrated solution. ⊃ active transport, diffusion, filtration.

osmotic diuretics inert substances such as mannitol that exert a diuretic effect. They cause an osmotic 'pull' as they are excreted by the kidney where they are filtered but not reabsorbed. ⊃ Appendix 5.

osmotic laxatives ⊃ laxatives. ⊃ Appendix 5.

osmotic pressure the 'suction' exerted by a solution of higher, upon one of lower, osmolar concentration, which moves water by osmosis in the direction that will equalize concentrations if the solutions are separated by a semipermeable membrane; this allows the passage of water but not of the solute particles. Applies to movements of water across cell membranes, maintaining osmotic equilibrium between extra- and intracellular fluids.

osseointegration the growth in bone, as it integrates with biocompatible materials, such as titanium, to form a strong and secure anchor for a dental implant or a prosthesis such as a bone-anchored hearing aid.

oss/eo, oss/i- a prefix that means 'bone', e.g. *ossicles*.

osseous *adj* relating to or resembling bone.

osseous graft in dentistry, a portion of bone taken from the patient, or a synthetic bone substitute, and used to repair or replace alveolar bone.

ossicles *npl* small bones, particularly those within the tympanic cavity of the middle ear; the malleus, incus and stapes. ⊃ Colour Section Figure 13.

ossification *n* the conversion of cartilage, etc. into bone. Also known as osteogenesis—**ossify** *vt, vi*.

ossification centres seen on X-ray at the distal end of the fetal femoral epiphysis between 35 and 40 weeks' gestation, and the proximal tibial epiphysis at 37–42 weeks; may help to determine fetal maturity. *centres of ossification* on the fetal head include frontal bosses, occipital protuberance and parietal eminences.

ostectomy the division of a bone at two lines and removal of the intervening segment.

osteitis *n* inflammation of bone.

osteitis deformans ⊃ Paget's disease.

osteitis fibrosa cavities form in the interior of bone. The cysts may be solitary or the disease may be generalized. This second condition may be the result of excessive parathyroid gland secretion and absorption of calcium from bone.

osteitis pubis an inflammatory condition causing persistent discomfort especially in the midline with tenderness on pressure over the symphysis. Most common in kicking or running sports and in gymnastics and swimming (especially breast stroke). Treatment is often difficult and sometimes requires prolonged rest.

oste/o- a prefix that means 'bone', e.g. *osteoporosis*.

osteoarthritis (OA) *n* sometimes termed degenerative joint disease (DJD) or degenerative arthritis, although the disease process is much more than simply 'wear and tear'; may be primary, or may be secondary to injury or disease involving the articular surfaces of synovial joints. It is an evolving process with much research aimed at slowing its advance. Known aetiological factors include increasing age, female sex, manual occupations, obesity, malalignment and injury in sport. Genetic factors have been implicated, though not yet identified. There is little evidence that exercise *per se* produces OA. The articular cartilage becomes worn, osteophytes form at the periphery of the joint surface and loose bodies may result. Signs and symptoms include pain, stiffness, deformity and the presence of Heberden's and Bouchard's nodes. ⊃ arthropathy, arthroplasty, Colour Section Figure 95—**osteoarthritic** *adj. primary osteoarthritis* (OA) there is no obvious cause, it is due to an intrinsic alteration of the articular tissues themselves. It affects joints in a classical pattern; intervertebral and facet joints of the cervical and lumbar vertebrae, distal interphalangeal joints of the fingers, metatarsophalangeal joint of big toes, first carpometacarpal joint, temporomandibular joint, sternoclavicular joint, acromioclavicular joint, hip and the knee joint including the patello-femoral joint. Primary OA is common in post-menopausal women who typically exhibit Heberden's and Bouchard's nodes. *secondary osteoarthritis* arises as a consequence of another condition. The causes of secondary OA can be divided into one of the following four categories: metabolic, anatomic, traumatic or inflammatory. OA appears to be more common in people with a previous injury or fracture to a particular joint (Coggon et al. 2001). Repeated minor trauma may lead to micro fractures and subsequent OA. Occupational factors are thought to be important in the development of secondary OA. For example, the first carpometacarpal and metacarpophalangeal joints may be affected in tailors, as are the elbows and shoulders of pneumatic drill operators. Joint infection puts a joint at risk of OA, as does deformity, for example, following fractures that cause biomechanical anomalies or direct cartilage damage if the fracture included the articular surface. The relationship between obesity and OA is complex and still not fully understood. Being overweight is linked to development of OA in some joints but not in others. There is a correlation between high body mass index and knee OA, which may be due to varus deformities in obese persons (Sharma et al. 2000), but the correlation is less strong between obesity and OA of the hip and with generalized OA (Sturmer et al. 2000). Being overweight may result in premature muscle fatigue, which in turn leads to abnormal kinematics and the subsequent development of OA. The relationship seems to be much stronger in women. Increased load across the joints clearly plays a role, but hormonal abnormalities associated with obesity may also be to blame, as suggested by an increase, albeit modest, in hand OA in obese women. (Coggon D, Reading I, Barret D, McLaren M, Cooper C 2001 Knee osteoarthritis and obesity. Int J Obes Relat Metab Disord 25(5): 622–627. Sharma LC, Lou C, Cahue S, Dunlop DD 2000 The mechanism of the effect of obesity in knee osteoarthritis: the mediating role of malalignment. Arthritis Rheum 43(3): 568–575. Sturmer T, Gunther KP,

O
P

Brenner H et al. 2000 Obesity, overweight and patterns of osteoarthritis: the Ulm Osteoarthritis Study. J Clin Epidemiol 53(3): 307–313.)

osteoarthrosis ⊃ osteoarthritis.

osteoblast *n* a bone-forming cell derived from embryonic mesenchyme. It produces the materials required for the osteoid matrix—**osteoblastic** *adj.*

osteocalcin a protein required for the mineralization of bone.

osteochondritis *n* originally an inflammation of bone cartilage. Usually applied to non-septic conditions, especially avascular necrosis involving joint surfaces. ⊃ osteochondritis dissecans.

osteochondritis dissecans a disease in which a portion of joint surface becomes detached from the underlying bone. A fragment of cartilage and subchondral bone may separate partially or completely to form a loose body in the joint. It is common in the knee joint. ⊃ Legg—Calvé–Perthes disease, Köhler's disease, Scheuermann's disease, Schlatter's disease, Sever's disease.

osteochondroma *n* a benign bony and cartilaginous tumour.

osteochondrosis *n* an idiopathic disease characterized by a disorder of the ossification of hyaline cartilage (endochondral). It encompasses a group of syndromes classified on the basis of their anatomical location. **1.** primary articular epiphysis—Freiberg's disease and Köhler's disease. **2.** secondary articular epiphysis—osteochondritis dissecans of the talus. **3.** non-articular epiphysis (apophyseal injury)—Sever's disease. The osteochondroses occur during the years of rapid growth. Aetiology has been linked to hereditary factors, trauma, nutritional factors and ischaemia. The articular osteochondroses such as Freiberg's, Köhler's and osteochondritis dissecans are characterized by fragmentation with a centre of ossification.

osteoclasis *n* the therapeutic fracture of a bone.

osteoclast *n* **1.** a large multinucleated bone cell that resorbs bone. **2.** an instrument used for osteoclasis (therapeutic fracture).

osteoclastoma *n* a tumour of the osteoclasts. May be benign, locally recurrent, or frankly malignant. The usual site is near the end of a long bone.

osteocyte *n* a bone cell, a mature osteoblast.

osteodystrophy *n* any generalized faulty growth of bone, usually caused by abnormal metabolism of calcium and phosphorus. It occurs in chronic renal failure—renal osteodystrophy.

osteoectomy in dentistry, an outdated procedure that involved the removal of some of the supporting alveolar bone from around the root of a tooth in order to correct an imperfect bone contour around the root.

osteogenesis *n* bone formation. ⊃ ossification.

osteogenesis imperfecta a hereditary disorder usually caused by an autosomal dominant gene. It may be present at birth or develop during childhood. The congenital form is much more severe and may lead to early death. The bones are extremely fragile and may fracture following minimal trauma.

osteogenic *adj* bone-producing.

osteogenic sarcoma *n* malignant tumour that originates from bone-producing cells.

osteology *n* the scientific study of the development, structure and function of bones and associated structures.

osteolysis *n* pathological dissolution of bone, such as following infection or where the blood supply is impaired.

osteolytic *adj* destructive of bone, e.g. osteolytic malignant deposits in bone.

osteoma *n* a benign tumour of bone which may arise in the compact tissue (*ivory osteoma*) or in the cancellous tissue. May be single or multiple.

osteomalacia *n* demineralization of the mature skeleton, with softening and bone pain. It is commonly caused by insufficient dietary intake of vitamin D or lack of sunshine, or both.

osteomyelitis *n* inflammation commencing in the marrow of bone—**osteomyelitic** *adj.*

osteon *n* a haversian system, the basic structural unit of bone (see Figure B.9 p. 102).

osteonecrosis the death of bone due to an impaired blood supply.

osteopath *n* a person qualified and registered to practise osteopathy.

osteopathy *n* an established clinical discipline. The practice of osteopathy in the UK is subject to statutory self-regulation and registration on a par with more established healthcare professions such as medicine. It is concerned with the inter-relationship between structure and function of the body. Osteopaths have a holistic approach, treating the whole person in the prevention, diagnosis and treatment of illness, injury or disease. Osteopathy may be effective for the relief or improvement of a wide variety of conditions, e.g. digestive disorders, as well as mechanical problems. Osteopaths in sport mainly treat mechanical musculoskeletal problems—**osteopathic** *adj.*

osteopenia a decrease in bone mineral density (BMD) but not as severe as that in osteoporosis. ⊃ osteoporosis.

osteopetrosis (*syn.* Albers–Schönberg disease, marble bones) a congenital abnormality giving rise to very dense bones which fracture easily.

osteophyte *n* a bony outgrowth or spur, usually at the margins of joint surfaces, e.g. in osteoarthritis—**osteophytic** *adj.*

osteoplasty *n* reconstructive operation on bone. In dentistry, it refers to an outdated procedure that involved surgical reshaping of the alveolar process to achieve as closely as possible the ideal architectural design of a healthy periodontium—**osteoplastic** *adj.*

osteoporosis *n* loss of bone density caused by excessive absorption of calcium and phosphorus from the bone, due to progressive loss of the protein matrix of bone which normally carries the calcium deposits. The WHO definition of osteoporosis is based on a woman's bone mineral density

O
P

(BMD) score and the number of standard deviations (SD) the score is from the BMD score for an average woman aged 25 years. Osteopenia an intermediate condition is defined as −1 to −2.5 SD, and osteoporosis is defined as below −2.5 SD. Osteoporosis is associated with ageing in both men and women. Common cause of fractures, particularly fractures of the wrist, crush fractures of the spine and neck of femur fractures. Changes in hormonal status influence the development of osteoporosis in both women (lack of oestrogen) and men (lack of testosterone). *osteoporosis risk factors for women* a lack of oestrogen, caused by: an early menopause (before the age of 45); an early hysterectomy (before the age of 45), particularly when both ovaries are removed by oophrectomy; amenorrhoea for 6 months or more (excluding pregnancy) as a result of excessive exercise and/or an eating disorder. *osteoporosis risk factors for men* low levels of testosterone (hypogonadism). *osteoporosis risk factors for men and women* long-term use of high dose corticosteroid drugs (e.g. prednisolone for conditions such as rheumatoid arthritis and asthma); close family history of osteoporosis (maternal or paternal), particularly with history of a maternal hip fracture before the age of 75 years; medical conditions such as Cushing's syndrome, hyperthyroidism and liver problems; malabsorption syndromes (e.g. coeliac disease, inflammatory bowel disease or extensive bowel resection); long-term immobility; smoking: excessive alcohol intake; poor diet deficient in nutrients such as calcium; and low body weight in proportion to height (Carne 2003). Prevention is through adequate diet, weight-bearing exercise, ensuring sufficient vitamin D with sensible exposure to sunlight and reducing the effects of known risk factors. Management may involve supplementation with calcium and vitamin D, bisphosphonates, parathyroid hormone, selective o(e)strogen receptor modulators (SERMS), or oestrogen hormone replacement for women who cannot tolerate other treatment modalities—**osteoporotic** *adj*. (Carne K 2003 Osteoporosis. In: Porter S (ed.) Tidy's Physiotherapy, 13th edn. Butterworth Heinemann, Oxford).

osteoradionecrosis necrosis of bone, following radiation therapy, due to a reduction in blood supply and infection.

osteosarcoma/osteogenic sarcoma *n* a malignant tumour growing from bone cells (osteoblasts)—**osteosarcomata** *pl*, **osteosarcomatous** *adj*.

osteosclerosis *n* increased density or hardness of bone— **osteosclerotic** *adj*.

osteotome *n* an instrument for cutting bone; it is similar to a chisel, but it is bevelled on both sides of its cutting edge.

osteotomy *n* division of bone followed by realignment of the ends to encourage union by healing. ⊃ mandibular or maxillary osteotomy, McMurray's osteotomy.

os tibial externum ⊃ supernumerary bones.

ostium *n* the opening or mouth of any tubular structure— **ostia** *pl*, **ostial** *adj*.

-ostomy a suffix that means 'to form an opening or outlet', e.g. *colostomy*.

os trigonum ⊃ supernumerary bones.

os vesalii ⊃ supernumerary bones.

Oswestry standing frame a standing frame, originally designed to help people with spinal injury independently stand. They are now widely used in neurological rehabilitation, but due to manual handling regulations, unless the patient is able to assist with the manoeuvre from sit to stand, they have limited use. Many standing frames are now being fitted or designed with motors to gradually move the patient from sitting to standing.

OT *abbr* occupational therapy/therapist.

otalgia *n* earache.

otalgia dentalis *n* pain felt in the ear that is caused by dental disease.

OTC *abbr* over-the-counter (medicines).

otic *adj* relating to the ear.

otic ganglion a parasympathetic ganglion arising on the glossopharyngeal nerve (ninth cranial nerve). Its nerve fibres supply the parotid salivary gland, its sensory and sympathetic fibres passing through the gland.

otitis *n* inflammation of the ear.

otitis externa inflammation of the skin of the external auditory meatus/canal.

otitis media inflammation of the middle ear cavity. The effusion can be serous, mucoid or purulent. Non-purulent effusions in children are often called 'glue ear'. ⊃ acute otitis media (AOM), acute (suppurative) otitis media (ASOM), chronic suppurative otitis media (CSOM), grommet, otitis media with effusion (OME).

otitis media with effusion (OME) (*syn* glue ear) a type of otitis media, generally occurring in children. There is a collection of viscous fluid within the middle ear as well as inflammation. Antibiotics are not generally recommended, but some children develop hearing impairment that can lead to developmental and behavioural problems, and speech and language difficulties. Treatment in this situation may involve the aspiration of the middle ear effusion and the insertion of grommets through the ear drum (tympanic membrane) into the middle ear. ⊃ grommet.

ot/o- a prefix that means 'ear', e.g. *otorrhoea*.

otoacoustic emission (OAE) testing a computer-linked hearing test used for screening babies soon after birth. It depends on the sound normally emitted by the outer hair cells of the inner ear. A microphone placed in the external auditory meatus/canal picks up the emissions. Used to determine whether the inner ear is functioning. ⊃ neonatal hearing screening.

otolaryngology *n* ⊃ otorhinolaryngology.

otoliths *npl* tiny calcareous (calcium) deposits within the utricle and saccule of the inner ear.

otologist *n* a person who specializes in otology.

otology *n* the science which deals with structure, function and disorders of the ear.

-otomy a suffix that means 'incision of', e.g. *myotomy*.

otomycosis *n* a fungal (e.g. *Aspergillus*, *Candida*) infection of the external auditory meatus/canal—**otomycotic** *adj*.

O
P

otoplasty *n* plastic operation to correct ear deformities.

otorhinolaryngology *n* the science that deals with the structure, function and disorders of the ear, nose and throat; each of these three may be considered a specialty. ➲ laryngology, otology, rhinology.

otorrhoea *n* a discharge from the ear. It may be serous, sanguineous (bloody) or purulent. The discharge may be crystal clear cerebrospinal fluid, this can occur in fractures of the base of skull.

otosclerosis *n* abnormal bone formation affecting primarily the footplate of the stapes. A common cause of progressive conductive deafness—**otosclerotic** *adj*.

otoscope *n* an instrument for examining the ear, usually incorporating both magnification and illumination. Also called an auriscope.

ototoxic *adj* having a toxic action on the ear. For example, the aminoglycoside antibiotics, (e.g. gentamicin), platinum-based chemotherapy (e.g. cisplatin) and aspirin.

-ous a suffix that means 'like, having the nature of', e.g. *delirious*.

outcome the result of an intervention, which may be planned or unexpected.

outcome expectancy in social cognitive theory, a person's expectations about the consequences of an action.

outcome goal the clearly articulated and desired result of a therapeutic or other intervention.

outcome goal (in sport) a goal that specifies the outcome of a performance, usually involving a comparison with others such as winning a race. ➲ performance goal, process goal.

outcome measurement a method for evaluating the nature and degree of change resulting from an intervention or the extent to which a therapeutic goal has been reached. ➲ outcome measures.

outcome measures tests or scales developed to measure health outcome from clinical interventions: generic measures encompassing dimensions of physical, mental and social health; disease specific scales detecting the effects of treatment of specific conditions. Prior to use, the outcome measure should be evaluated to appraise the extent to which it is valid for the intended use, can be reliably used, is sufficiently responsive, acceptable to the intended users, feasible for use in the intended setting, the results interpretable and sufficiently user-friendly. The use of outcome measures promotes the standardization of objective measurement and evaluation of practice. Outcome measures should have the key qualities of reliability, validity and responsiveness. ➲ Ashworth Scale, Motor Assessment Scale, quality-adjusted life years, Rivermead motor assessment.

outer ear also known as external ear. Comprises the auricle and the external auditory meatus/canal. ➲ ear.

outline outline form, cavosurface margin or line angle. The boundary of a restoration or preparation at its junction with the tooth surface.

output data and information leaving a computer, which can then be sent to a display screen, printer or another computer.

outreach clinic clinic, such as an antenatal clinic, situated some distance from the main maternity department, perhaps in a smaller hospital, general practitioner's surgery or public building such as a village hall. Thus enabling women to access consultant care without having to make a long or inconvenient journey to the hospital.

outrigger a type of splint used commonly after tendon or joint replacement in the hand and wrist.

ova *npl* the female gametes (reproductive cells). More correctly known as a secondary oocyte until penetration by a spermatozoon—**ovum** *sing*.

oval window fenestra ovalis. The oval opening between the middle and inner ear. The stapes vibrates in it to transmit sound waves to the inner ear.

ovarian *adj* relating to the ovaries.

ovarian cancer a common gynaecological cancer and many women present with advanced disease. Predominantly occurs in older postmenopausal women, the risk factors include childlessness, genetic factors and late menopause. Carcinomas are the most common type and FIGO has provided a classification of the stages of ovarian cancer linked to the locality and extent of the disease. Symptoms are often vague, but can include abnormal vaginal bleeding, gastrointestinal symptoms, distended abdomen, pressure symptoms, such as urinary frequency and ascites in advanced disease. Surgery involves removal of the uterus, both tubes and ovaries, part of the omentum and biopsies to ascertain the degree of spread. Chemotherapy is used after surgery, e.g. platinum-based carboplatin alone or with paclitaxel.

ovarian cycle the changes occurring in the ovary during the development of the follicle and oogenesis. It has two phases: follicular (days 1–14) when ovulation occurs, and luteal (days 15–28) when the corpus luteum develops. The cycle is controlled by follicle stimulating hormone and luteinizing hormone.

ovarian cyst a tumour of the ovary, usually containing fluid—may be benign or malignant.

ovarian hyperstimulation syndrome (OHSS) a side-effect associated with the use of gonadotrophins during an IVF cycle. Milder cases are characterized by enlargement of the ovaries, gastrointestinal symptoms, abdominal pain and weight gain. In more severe cases it is associated with fluid and electrolyte imbalance, ascites, pleural effusion, hypovolaemia, coagulation disorders and impaired renal function.

ovarian pregnancy a pregnancy which becomes implanted on the wall of or within the ovary. It does not usually survive.

ovarian vein syndrome obstruction of a ureter, most commonly the right, due to compression by an enlarged or varicosed ovarian vein. Typically the vein becomes enlarged during pregnancy, symptoms being those of obstruction or infection of the upper urinary tract.

ovariectomy *n* ➲ oophorectomy.

ovari/o- a prefix that means 'ovary', e.g. *ovariotomy*.

O
P

557

ovariotomy *n* ⊃ oophorectomy.

ovaritis *n* ⊃ oophoritis.

ovary *n* a female gonad. One of two small oval bodies situated close to the open end of each uterine (fallopian) tube on either side of the uterus on the posterior surface of the broad ligament. ⊃ Colour Section Figure 17. Controlled by pituitary hormones they produce oocytes and oestrogen and progestogen. During the fertile years, except in pregnancy, an oocyte is discharged into one of the uterine (fallopian) tubes en route for the uterus at ovulation in each menstrual cycle. The ovaries are also endocrine glands (under the influence in turn of anterior pituitary gonadotrophic hormones; follicle stimulating hormone [FSH] and luteinizing hormone [LH]), secreting the female hormones oestrogen and progestogen. These have actions both widely in the body and on the reproductive organs at specific times in the menstrual cycle and during pregnancy—**ovarian** *adj*. *polycystic ovaries* ⊃ oestrogens, polycystic ovary syndrome (PCOS).

OVD *abbr* occlusal vertical dimension.

over active bladder (*syn* urge incontinence). ⊃ incontinence.

overbite a bite in which the upper incisor teeth vertically overlap the lower incisor teeth.

overclosure reduced distance between the upper and lower teeth or occlusal rims.

overcompensation *n* a term that describes any type of behaviour which a person adopts in order to disguise a deficiency. Thus a person who is afraid may react by becoming arrogant or boastful or aggressive.

over-denture denture completely covering at least one tooth root or prepared tooth or asseo-integrated implant abutment.

over-eruption vertical migration of a tooth beyond its proper position in normal dental arches. Generally caused by absence of an opposing occlusal force because of the loss of a contacting tooth from the opposite arch.

overflow incontinence ⊃ incontinence.

overgrowth an overall increase in the size of a tissue either by an increase in the size of its cells, or in their number. ⊃ hyperplasia, hypertrophy.

overhang excess restorative material projecting beyond the preparation or cavity margin thus causing a shoulder beneath which plaque may accumulate or food may lodge.

overheads *npl* the cost of services that contribute to the general upkeep and running of the organization, e.g. grounds maintenance, that cannot be linked directly to the core activity of a department.

overjet horizontal overlap. The projection, in a horizontal plane, of teeth, usually the incisors, in one arch beyond the teeth of the opposing arch.

overjustification effect an explanation for the observation that if individuals are rewarded for engaging in an inherently enjoyable or satisfying activity, they are subsequently less likely to engage in the activity when given the opportunity to do so in the absence of a reward. It is proposed that the reward comes to justify engagement in the activity instead of the initial inherent enjoyment and when removed, there no longer remains a reason for taking part. For example, rewarding children for engaging in sport could undermine their inherent interest in sport.

overlapping 1. imbricated, like tiles on a roof. **2.** in dental radiography, a distortion of a radiological tooth image in which the structures of one tooth are superimposed on those of another.

overlay ⊃ onlay.

overlearning the learning of a task or action beyond the point of mastery so that it becomes automated. Typically acquired through repetitive drills.

overload principle a term used less now than previously, indicating the need to place increased demand upon a tissue (e.g. connective), organ (e.g. specific muscle) or system (e.g. cardiovascular) if its performance is to improve. The demand concerned may be for strength, endurance or (less commonly) speed. Must be distinguished from 'overload' in engineering, which is a load greater than a structure can bear.

over pressure a passive pressure applied to the end of a joint's active range when pain free. A movement cannot be classed as normal unless the range is pain free actively and passively and with the addition of passive overpressure at the limit of the active range.

over-the-counter (OTC) medicines describes those medicines on sale to the public without a prescription. ⊃ general sales list, pharmacy only medicine.

overtraining training exceeding the body's recovery capacity, indicated by excessive fatigue both physical and mental, and resulting in impaired performance. Also called staleness. Short-term overtraining is usually adequately countered by a period of reduced intensity or a few days' total rest but if extended, it leads to the overtraining syndrome—a set of symptoms and signs, probably of neuroendocrine origin. The psychological aspect of fatigue now usually predominates, while physical symptoms often include increased basal metabolic rate, protracted elevation of pulse rate after exercise, and negative nitrogen balance leading to weight loss. Recovery may take months or never be fully achieved. Compare the unexplained under performance syndrome (UPS) which may apply in some instances previously classed as overtraining. ⊃ burnout, under performance syndrome (UPS).

overuse injury an injury that is caused by excessive repetitive movement of a body part. Often occurs following periods of inadequate rest or recovery, over-activity, or repetitive overloading of part or structure.

overuse syndrome injury caused by accumulated microtraumatic stress placed on a structure or body area.

overwear syndrome ocular pain which may be very intense, accompanied by corneal epithelium damage, conjunctival injection, lacrimation, blepharospasm, photophobia, and hazy vision following corneal hypoxia caused by overwear of contact lenses, principally the PMMA type. The symptoms usually begin to appear 2–3 hours after the

O
P

lenses are removed and recovery usually occurs within 24 hours, although an antibiotic may be needed. ⊃ corneal abrasion, corneal exhaustion syndrome, corneal hypoxia.

overweight ⊃ body weight, body mass index, obesity.

ovi, ovo- a prefix that means 'egg, oocyte, ovum', e.g. *oviduct*.

oviduct *n* uterine or fallopian tubes.

ovulation *n* the maturation and rupture of a Graafian follicle with the discharge of an oocyte.

ovum *n* **1.** an egg. **2.** a female gamete. ⊃ ova.

oxalic acid toxic organic acid found in plants, e.g. rhubarb leaves.

oxalosis a condition in which crystals of calcium oxalates are deposited in the kidney and in other organs.

oxaluria *n* excretion of oxalates (salts of oxalic acid) in the urine.

oxazolidones *npl* a class of antibacterial drugs, e.g linezolid, which can be used to treat infections caused by meticillin (methicillin)-resistant *Staphylococcus aureus* (MRSA) and vancomycin-resistant enterococci (VRE).

Oxford scale (for movement) a relatively quick and easy-to-use scale of movement that is used widely in clinical practice. However, it is not very objective, functional or sensitive to change since the movements resisted are concentric contractions and the spaces between the grades are not linear. The scale is: 0—no contraction, 1—flicker of contraction only, movement of the joint does not occur, 2—movement is only possible with gravity counterbalanced, 3—movement against gravity is possible, 4—movement against resistance is possible, and 5—normal functional movement is possible.

Oxford scale (for pelvic floor strength) ⊃ modified Oxford scale.

oxicams a group of non-steroidal anti-inflammatory drugs. ⊃ Appendix 5.

oxidase (oxygenases) *n* any enzyme that catalyses biological oxidation reactions.

oxidation *n* the act of oxidizing or state of being oxidized. It involves the addition of oxygen, e.g. formation of oxides, or the loss of electrons or the removal of hydrogen. A part of metabolism, whereby energy is released from fuel molecules. ⊃ reduction.

oxidative phosphorylation the oxidation of products of carbohydrate, fat, protein and alcohol metabolism to carbon dioxide and water with formation of adenosine triphosphate (ATP) from adenosine diphosphate (ADP) and inorganic phosphate (P_i), associated with the transfer of electrons from substrate via coenzymes to oxygen, taking place in mitochondria. ⊃ adenosine diphosphate, adenosine monophosphate, adenosine triphosphate.

oxidative stress/damage a general term used to describe imbalance between reactive oxygen species and antioxidants. Oxidative stress/damage can damage a specific molecule or the entire organism and is known to be implicated in the pathogenesis of a wide variety of disorders, including coronary heart disease, cerebrovascular disease, chronic obstructive lung disease, some forms of cancer, diabetes, skeletal muscular dystrophy and others. Oxidative stress-induced damage in muscle could be one of the factors that terminate muscular effort, but consecutive exercise bouts seem to induce antioxidant adaptations.

oxidized cellulose prepared, haemostatic cellulose used to pack a tooth socket in the event of severe or persistent haemorrhage.

oxidoreductase an enzyme that catalyses a reaction in which one substance is oxidized and another is reduced, (e.g. dehydrogenases).

oximeter an instrument for determining, photoelectrically, the oxygen content of blood. ⊃ pulse oximetry.

oximetry ⊃ pulse oximetry.

oxyblepsia ⊃ oxyopia.

oxygen (O) *n* a colourless, odourless, gaseous element; necessary for life and combustion. Constitutes 20% of atmospheric air. Used therapeutically as an inhalation to increase blood oxygenation. Delivered as part of a general anaesthetic to maintain life. ⊃ oxygen therapy.

oxygenation *n* the saturation of a substance (particularly blood) with oxygen. Arterial oxygen tension (PaO_2) indicates degree of oxygenation (normally more than 97% saturated)—**oxygenated** *adj*. ⊃ pulse oximetry.

oxygenator *n* apparatus used to oxygenate the patient's blood during open heart surgery, or to support critically ill patients. ⊃ cardiopulmonary bypass, extracorporeal membrane oxygenator.

oxygen concentrator a device for removing nitrogen from the room air to provide a high concentration of oxygen for use by patients with chronic respiratory diseases requiring at least 15 hours of oxygen therapy each day at home. ⊃ long term oxygen therapy.

oxygen consumption/uptake ($\dot{V}O_2$) the rate of uptake of oxygen in the lungs, usually expressed in litres per minute. Measured in indirect calorimetry as an estimate of metabolic rate, taking the 'calorific value' of 1 litre of oxygen as 4.8 kcal (for an average ratio of carbohydrate to lipid oxidation), therefore 1 L/min as equivalent to 4.8 kcal/min, 20 kJ/min or 333 watts. ⊃ peak oxygen consumption/uptake.

oxygen cost the rate of oxygen usage for a particular task or work rate.

oxygen debt the amount by which oxygen consumption during recovery from exercise exceeds resting level. Consists of an initial rapid phase lasting ~1–2 min (formerly called the 'alactic' phase), in which muscle creatine phosphate (CrP) and adenosine triphosphate (ATP) stores are replenished, and a subsequent slow phase (~1 h) in which lactic acid is oxidized (hence the former term 'lactacid' phase), temperature falls toward resting level and blood hormonal concentrations are normalized. Also known as elevated post-exercise oxygen consumption (EPOC) or recovery oxygen consumption. ⊃ alactacid oxygen debt component, elevated post-exercise oxygen consumption, lactacid oxygen debt component.

oxygen deficit shortfall of oxygen consumed during activity below that required to supply all necessary energy aerobically. Post-exercise restoration of this deficit constitutes part, but not all, of the oxygen debt.

oxygen delivery (DO$_2$) amount of oxygen delivered to the tissues per minute, product of cardiac output and arterial oxygen content, typically 1000 mL/min. The rate of supply of oxygen by the arterial blood to body organs and tissues, expressed as cardiac output (L/min) × oxygen content of the blood (L/L), e.g. typical resting value would be $5 \times 0.2 = 1$ L/min. This is four times the typical oxygen usage at rest, since only a quarter of the oxygen in the arterial blood is removed by the tissues, reducing haemoglobin saturation from 100% to 75%. ⊃ oxygen dissociation curve.

oxygen dissociation curve a curve showing the different affinity each haem group of the haemoglobin molecule has for oxygen. It indicates the ease with which the oxygen dissociates and the haem groups give up the oxygen to the tissues. This is also influenced by carbon dioxide tension, temperature and pH (Figure O.4). The graph describes the relationship in the blood between partial pressure of oxygen (PO_2) and the percentage saturation of haemoglobin; it can also show the equivalent oxygen content of the blood when haemoglobin is in normal concentration. With normal lungs, saturation in arterial blood is determined by the PO_2 in the alveolar gas with which pulmonary capillary blood equilibrates. The sigmoid-shaped (S-shape) of the curve has important physiological advantages, e.g. a relatively small decrease in PO_2 encountered where blood flows through tissues causes a 'steep' removal of oxygen from the blood; but there needs to be a relatively large decrease in PO_2 in the inspired air (and therefore in the alveoli, e.g. at altitude or in a confined space) before there is a serious decline in haemoglobin saturation. ⊃ Bohr effect.

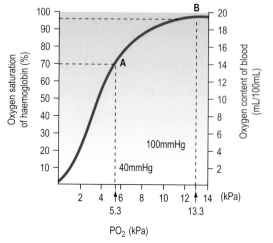

A = venous blood (at the tissues)
B = arterial blood (at the lungs)

O.4 **Oxygen dissociation curve** (at 37°C, pH 7.4, Hb 15g/dL) (reproduced from Brooker 2006A with permission).

oxygen enhancement ratio the ratio of radiation doses needed to produce a given biological effect in the presence or absence of oxygen.

oxygen permeability (Dk) the degree to which a polymer allows the passage of a gas or fluid. The oxygen permeability (*Dk*) of a material is a function of the diffusivity (*D*) (that is the speed at which oxygen molecules traverse the material) and the solubility (*k*) (or the amount of oxygen molecules absorbed, per volume, in the material). Values of oxygen permeability (*Dk*) typically fall within the range $10 - 100 \times 10^{-11}$ (cm^2/mLO$_2$)/(s/mL/mmHg). A semi-logarithmic relationship has been demonstrated between hydrogel water content and oxygen permeability. ⊃ barrier, cellulose acetate butyrate, critical oxygen requirement, equivalent oxygen pressure, refractometer, siloxane.

oxygen plateau the flattening out of oxygen consumption after the maximal value is attained in incremental exercise.

oxygen poisoning a hazard of exposure to high ambient pressure (typically in diving) when breathing high percentage oxygen. With 100% oxygen inspired oxygen pressure is ~100 kPa on the surface at 1 atmosphere, and increases by 100 kPa for every 10 m depth under water. Susceptibility varies between individuals and with the level of physical work, but limits typically advised are ~150–170 kPa, equivalent to breathing 100% oxygen at depths of 5–7 metres (or proportionately <100% mixed with nitrogen at greater depths). Toxic effects are mainly on the brain (causing epileptic-type seizures) and on the lungs (cough, pulmonary oedema, impairment of oxygen diffusion). Seizures under water can be fatal and the more slowly developing pulmonary toxicity can be irreversible if severe. (Higher pressures than those advised above are safely used to treat decompression illness by 100% oxygen at rest.)

oxygen saturation (SaO$_2$) percentage of haemoglobin saturated with oxygen present in the blood. ⊃ pulse oximetry.

oxygen tent a large plastic canopy that encloses the patient in a controlled environment used for oxygen therapy.

oxygen therapy oxygen therapy plays a vital role in the management of hypoxaemia and respiratory failure. It is a potent drug with associated potential hazards of use, e.g. fire, oxygen toxicity (which can occur if breathing >60% O$_2$ for >48 h), progression to acute/adult respiratory distress syndrome carries a high mortality and absorption atelectasis while patients' responses to its administration are varied. One hospital survey found 21% of O$_2$ prescriptions were inappropriate and 85% of patients were inadequately supervised. Similar studies in GP surgeries show inadequate prescribing of the drug. Safety and effectiveness may be achieved with prescription of flow rate, delivery system, duration and monitoring of such treatment (Bateman & Leach 1998). The amount of oxygen in the arterial blood (i.e. the oxygen content) is the vital factor for patient well-being, since this, in conjunction with cardiac output, determines oxygen delivery (i.e. the amount of oxygen delivered to the tissues per unit time). This in turn, is dependent upon blood flow to the tissues (i.e. the cardiac output) and the amount of oxygen contained in that blood (i.e. the arterial oxygen content). Oxygen is carried in combination with haemoglobin (Hb) and dissolved in plasma. Its oxygen capacity and its percent saturation with oxygen determine the amount carried by Hb, while the volume in solution depends on the partial pressure of oxygen. Normally oxygen consumption is around 250 mL/min (utilizing only one-quarter of the oxygen available), so providing a safety margin should oxygen consumption increase or delivery falls, e.g. during exercise. The normal partial pressure of oxygen in arterial blood (PaO_2) is 11–15 kPa in adults, but this value falls steadily with age (probably due to increasing ventilation–perfusion [V/Q] inequalities). Oxygen therapy should be aimed at correcting arterial hypoxaemia. When tissue hypoxia occurs without arterial hypoxaemia, treatment should address the underlying cause (e.g. cardiac failure). Treatment should be administration of a high enough concentration of oxygen to establish a PaO_2 greater than 8 kPa. Accuracy of delivery is vitally important when managing patients with chronic lung diseases (North-West Oxygen Group 2001). A fixed performance device (such as a Venturi mask) assures delivery of a stated concentration, while normal variables, such as rate and depth of breathing, equipment and peak inspiratory flow demands, will affect the concentrations delivered by the low flow devices (such as MC masks and nasal cannulae) resulting in delivery of anything between 24% and 90% oxygen concentrations. Acutely, oxygen dosages may be critical. Inadequate oxygenation results in more deaths and disability than can be justified by the relatively small risks associated with higher doses (Bateman & Leach 1998). Extra vigilance should be used when administering oxygen to the patient with a high partial pressure of carbon dioxide in arterial blood ($PaCO_2$) and hypoxia. ⊃ hyperbaric oxygen therapy, long term oxygen therapy, Venturi effect, Venturi mask. (Bateman NT, Leach RM 1998 ABC of oxygen. Acute oxygen therapy. BMJ 317: 798–801, North West Oxygen Group 2001 Emergency oxygen therapy for the breathless patient—guidelines. Emergency Med J 18(6): 421–423).

oxygen toxicity ⊃ retinopathy of prematurity.

oxygen transmissibility the degree to which oxygen may pass through a particular material of a given thickness. It is equal to the oxygen permeability divided by the thickness of the measured sample under specific conditions. Symbol: *Dk/t*; *Dk/L* The unit is Barrer/cm. ⊃ corneal exhaustion syndrome, hypercapnia, oxygen permeability.

oxygen transport ⊃ oxygen delivery, oxygen dissociation curve, partial pressure.

oxygen uptake ⊃ oxygen consumption.

oxyhaemoglobin *n* oxygenated haemoglobin, an unstable compound formed from haemoglobin on contact with air in the alveoli.

oxyhaemoglobin dissociation curve ⊃ oxygen dissociation curve.

oxyntic *adj* producing acid.

oxyntic cells the cells in the gastric mucosa which produce hydrochloric acid. Also known as parietal cells.

oxyntomodulin a form of enteroglucagon.

oxyopia (*syn* oxyblepsia) extreme acuteness of vision.

oxyphosphate cement ⊃ zinc phosphate cement.

oxytocic *adj*, *n* hastening parturition; an agent that stimulates uterine contractions. ⊃ Appendix 5.

oxytocin *n* a hormone released from the posterior pituitary. It contracts the uterine muscle and milk ducts and is involved in reflex milk ejection.

oxyuriasis ⊃ enterobiasis.

Oxyuris *n* ⊃ *Enterobius*.

ozaena *n* atrophic rhinitis.

ozone *n* a form of oxygen. O_3. Has powerful oxidizing properties and is therefore antiseptic and disinfectant. It is both irritating and toxic to the pulmonary system.

O
P

P

³²**P** *abbr* radioactive isotope of phosphorus.

P₄₅₀ enzymes *npl* the cytochrome P₄₅₀ proteins that include an important group of drug-metabolizing enzymes and those that metabolize some endogenous substances, for example thromboxanes, prostacyclins, cholesterol and vitamins A and D. ⊃ cytochromes

PA *abbr* **1.** pantoscopic angle. **2.** pernicious anaemia. **3.** posteroanterior.

pacchionian granulations/bodies (A Pacchioni, Italian anatomist, 1665–1720) the arachnoid villi/granulations through which cerebrospinal fluid returns to the blood. ⊃ cerebrospinal fluid.

pacemaker *n* the region of the heart that initiates atrial contraction and thus controls heart rate. The natural pacemaker is the sinus node (sinoatrial node) which is situated at the junction of the superior vena cava and the right atrium; the wave of contraction begins here, then spreads over the heart. The sinus node rhythmically initiates the cardiac action potential and hence the whole electrical and mechanical cardiac cycle, varying the heart rate under the influence of the sympathetic and parasympathetic nerve supply. ⊃ cardiac pacemaker.

PACG *abbr* primary angle-closure glaucoma.

pachometer (pachymeter) a device that, mounted on a slit-lamp, is used for measuring corneal thickness (or the depth of the anterior chamber). It consists of an optical system which provides two half-fields by means of two glass plates with parallel sides placed in front of one objective of the microscope, the other being occluded. These plates rest one on top of the other with the junction between them situated so as to horizontally bisect the objective. The top plate can be rotated while the bottom one is fixed. The observer viewing through the microscope sees two corneal optical sections and adjusts the top plate until the outer surface of the epithelium appears aligned with the inner surface of the endothelium. The corneal thickness is then read directly from a scale attached to the pachometer and calibrated in millimetres. To increase the accuracy of the measurement a special eyepiece is used with the microscope. It has a magnification of ×10 and has two additional components: a horizontal slit and a biprism. The role of the eyepiece is to remove from the field of view half of the two optical sections. The measurement of the depth of the anterior chamber is made with a similar device but with a different scale. An instrument with greater magnification (called a micropachometer) has been devised, principally for research purposes, using a projection system which incorporates variable doubling plates and forms two slit

images on the cornea in conjunction with the viewing system of a slit-lamp and a magnification of up to ×100, mounted on another arm. This instrument allows the measurement of the thickness of the corneal epithelium alone with a precision which can reach ±1 mm. The above pachometers are referred to as optical pachometers to differentiate them from ultrasonic pachometers which use high-frequency ultrasound waves which are reflected from the anterior and posterior corneal surfaces. ⊃ corneal epithelium, ultrasonography in ophthalmology.

pachy- a prefix that means 'thick', e.g. *pachyglossia*.

pachycheilia *n* abnormally thick or swollen lips.

pachydactyly *n* abnormally thickened fingers and toes.

pachyderma *n* thick skin. ⊃ elephantiasis.

pachyglossia *n* abnormally thickened tongue.

pachymeningitis *n* inflammation of the dura mater, the outer meningeal membrane.

pachymeninx *n* dura mater.

pachymeter ⊃ pachometer (pachymeter).

pachyonychia congenita a congenital ectodermal defect characterized by thickening of the nails, hard skin on the palms and soles, abnormality of the hair follicles and overgrowth and thickening of the skin of the knees and elbows.

pachyvaginitis an inflammation and thickening of the walls of the vagina.

pacing *n* compensatory techniques used by occupational therapists that enable an individual to perform activities of daily living in a planned, balanced, continuous manner by strictly adhering to measurable, personal goals. It involves the use of activity analysis, timing, resting, and alternating movements in order to maximize optimal performance and minimize pain, stress and fatigue by expending effort consistently over a period of time.

pacinian corpuscles (F Pacini, Italian anatomist, 1812–1883) rapidly adapting mechanoreceptors. Pacinian corpuscles contain an afferent nerve fibre surrounded by a capsule. They are sensitive to high-frequency stimuli, such as vibration.

pack 1. to fill or press into a cavity. **2.** a dressing inserted into a wound to reduce or arrest haemorrhage. *periodontal pack* a dressing designed to protect a wound created by periodontal surgery, to encourage healing. *pressure pack* sterile folded gauze pressed into a wound to arrest haemorrhage. ⊃ cyst pack.

packed cell volume (PCV) the proportion by volume of blood occupied by erythrocytes (red blood cells, RBC), expressed as a percentage of the total blood volume: on average 45%, i.e. 45 mL of red blood cells in 100 mL of whole blood. Also called the haematocrit.

packing in dentistry, filling a plaster mould in a metal flask with a plastic material which is then processed to make a prosthesis.

PaCO₂ *abbr* the partial pressure or tension of carbon dioxide in arterial blood.

PACO₂ *abbr* the partial pressure or tension of carbon dioxide in alveolar air.

PACS *abbr* picture archiving communication system.

PACS broker enables two computer systems to talk to each other by changing (translating) information into a common language.

PADL *abbr* personal activities of daily living.

paed- a prefix that means 'child', e.g. *paedophilia*.

paediatrician *n* a doctor who is a specialist in children's health and diseases.

paediatrics *n* the branch of medicine dealing with children and their diseases—**paediatric** *adj*.

paediatric advanced life support (PALS) the special techniques, drug doses and equipment appropriate to the body weight and surface area of the child being resuscitated. ⮑ advanced life support (ALS), Broselow™ paediatric resuscitation system.

paediatric basic life support the basic life support measures used for children from 1 year of age until puberty. Artificial respiration, usually by rescue breaths (mouth-to-mouth/nose breathing) and chest compressions (external cardiac massage) to save life without the use of artificial aids or equipment in the case of cardiac or respiratory arrest. ⮑ Appendix 10.

paediatric dentistry the diagnosis, prevention and treatment of dental and related diseases in children.

paediatric optometry a branch of optometry concerned with the prevention, development, diagnosis and treatment of visual problems in children.

paedodontics also known as children's dentistry. The branch of dental science concerned with the oral health of children.

paedophilia the sexual attraction to children.

PAFC *abbr* pulmonary artery flotation catheter.

Paget's disease of bone (PDB) (J Paget, British surgeon, 1814–1899) (*syn.* osteitis deformans) a common condition characterized by focal areas of increased and disorganized bone remodelling, most commonly affecting sites such as the pelvis, femur, tibia, lumbar spine, skull and scapula. Paget's disease is seldom diagnosed before the age of 40 but gradually increases in prevalence thereafter to affect up to 10% of the UK population by the age of 85. The disease is common in Caucasians from north-west and southern Europe but is rare in Scandinavians, Asians, Chinese and Japanese. These racial differences in susceptibility persist after migration, illustrating the importance of genetic factors in aetiology, but the incidence of PDB has also been found to be decreasing in some countries over the past 25 years, suggesting that environmental factors also play a role. The primary abnormality in PDB is increased osteoclastic bone resorption, which is accompanied by marrow fibrosis, increased vascularity of bone and increased osteoblast activity. The bone in PDB is architecturally abnormal and has reduced mechanical strength. Osteoclasts in PDB are increased in number, are unusually large, and contain characteristic inclusion bodies. Inclusion bodies in osteoclast nuclei have led to speculation that PDB might be caused by a slow virus infection with measles or distemper but the evidence is conflicting. Biomechanical factors may be important in determining the pattern of involvement, since PDB tends to start at the site of muscle insertions to bone and, in some cases, localizes to bones or limbs that have been subjected to repetitive trauma or overuse. Genetic factors are important in PDB. Between 15% and 40% of patients have a positive family history with autosomal dominant inheritance and a high degree of penetrance by the age of 65. Several rare inherited syndromes have also been described which are similar to PDB but have an earlier age of onset. These include the dominantly inherited conditions familial expansile osteolysis, expansile skeletal hyperphosphatasia and early-onset PDB, and the recessively inherited idiopathic hyperphosphatasia. The classic presentation of PDB is with bone pain, deformity, deafness and pathological fractures, but many patients are discovered to have asymptomatic disease as the result of an incidental finding on biochemical testing or X-ray examination. Clinical signs of PDB include bone deformity and expansion, increased warmth over affected bones and pathological fracture. Bone deformity is most evident in weight-bearing bones such as the femur and tibia, but when the skull is affected the patient may complain that hats no longer fit properly due to cranial enlargement. Neurological problems such as deafness, cranial nerve defects, nerve root pain, spinal cord compression (SCC) and spinal stenosis are recognized complications due to enlargement of the affected bones and encroachment upon the spinal cord and nerve foraminae. Surprisingly, deafness in PDB is seldom due to compression of the auditory nerve, but rather appears to be conductive in nature due to osteosclerosis of the temporal bone. The increased vascularity of Pagetic bone makes operative procedures difficult and, in extreme cases, the high bone blood flow can precipitate cardiac failure in older adults with limited cardiac reserve. Osteosarcoma is a rare but serious complication of Paget's disease that has a poor prognosis. It should be suspected in a patient with Paget's who suffers a sudden increase in pain or swelling of an affected bone. A routine biochemistry screen is helpful in diagnosis, giving the characteristic picture of an 'isolated' elevation in alkaline phosphatase in over 90% of cases. However, the alkaline phosphatase can be normal in PDB, especially when only a single bone is affected. A radionuclide bone scan is a useful way of screening for the presence of PDB and documenting its extent. If the bone scan is positive, X-rays should be taken of an affected bone to confirm the diagnosis. Typical features on X-ray are osteosclerosis alternating with osteolysis, bone expansion and bone deformity. Bone biopsy is not usually required to make the diagnosis of PDB, but it can be helpful in differentiation from osteosclerotic metastases (for example, from cancer of breast

O
P

or prostate). The treatment of PDB is primarily indicated for the control of bone pain. In many cases, pain can be adequately controlled by administration of painkillers such as paracetamol or non-steroidal anti-inflammatory drugs (NSAIDs), but if these measures are ineffective, then bisphosphonates should be tried. Aminobisphosphonates such as pamidronate, risedronate and zoledronate are more effective than older bisphosphonates such as etidronate and tiludronate at suppressing biochemical markers of bone turnover in PDB, but they have not, as yet, been shown to offer any significant advantage in terms of pain control. Calcitonin can be used as an alternative to bisphosphonate therapy in PDB, but is less convenient to administer and significantly more expensive. Repeated courses of bisphosphonates or calcitonin can be given to patients whose symptoms recur. The long-term effects of antiresorptive therapy with bisphosphonates and calcitonin on complications such as deafness, bone deformity and fracture are unknown. Currently, there is no evidence to show that prophylactic therapy with bisphosphonates in asymptomatic patients is effective in preventing complications.

Paget's disease (of the nipple) (J Paget) a manifestation of a type of breast cancer. Malignant cells are found in epidermis of the nipple and are usually associated with small multifocal areas of ductal cancer behind the nipple and deep in the breast. There is erosion and crusting of the nipple.

Paget–Schröetter syndrome (J Paget; L von Schröetter, Austrian laryngologist and physician, 1837–1908) axillary or subclavian vein thrombosis, often associated with effort in fit young persons.

PAI *abbr* plasminogen activator inhibitor.

pain *n* unpleasant sensation experienced when specialized sensory receptors known as nociceptors (from the *adj* noxious meaning harmful) are stimulated. Afferent nerve impulses reach the central nervous system (CNS), where different influences can diminish or enhance them, acting where they are relayed and transmitted to the cerebral cortex and conscious perception. The pain pathways are separate from those serving other sensations, and even vigorous stimulation of other sensory receptors does not, by itself, cause pain. Pain is individual and subjective with a physiological, emotional and social component. Pain ranges from mild to agonizing, but individual responses are influenced by factors which include: information about cause, age, whether acute or chronic and pain tolerance. ⊃ acute pain, chronic pain, neuropathic pain, nociceptive pain, phantom limb pain, referred pain.

pain assessment an important function of the nurse's role, and may be especially difficult with some adults, children and infants who are unable to articulate their pain experience. Nurses should take account of the biological, psychological and social dimensions of pain. There are several pain assessment tools. Many of them include a longitudinal scale, at one end of which is 0 for 'no pain', and at the other 10 for 'the pain is as bad as it could possibly be' (see Figure V.5, p. 826). The patient points to the number or the intensity of pain, which equates with the current experience of pain. Several pain assessment tools have been developed for use with children of varying ages, e.g. 'faces scale', in which the child points to the facial expression corresponding to his or her pain experience (Figure P.1).

pain gate theory a pain-gate theory was initially proposed in 1965 by Melzack and Wall based on the fact that small-diameter nerve fibres carry pain stimuli through a 'gate mechanism', but larger-diameter nerve fibres going through the same gate can inhibit the transmission of the smaller nerves carrying the pain signal. It is this interruption of C-fibre-mediated pain pathways by Aβ fibres that is now

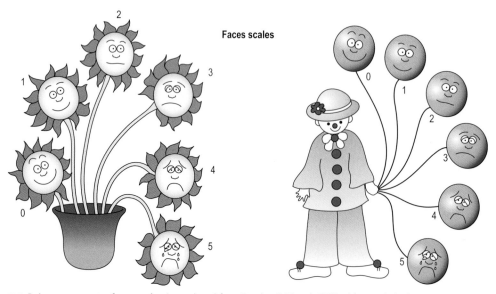

P.1 Pain assessment—faces scales (reproduced from Brooker & Waugh 2007 with permission).

known as the pain-gate theory. Chemicals released as a response to the pain stimuli also influence whether the gate is open or closed for the brain to receive the pain signal. This led to the theory that the pain signals can be interfered with by stimulating the periphery of the pain site, the appropriate signal-carrying nerves at the spinal cord, or particular corresponding areas in the brainstem or cerebral cortex. This concept is of great importance to health professionals who exert so much effort in trying to relieve pain. The 'pain-gate' may be closed by stimulating mechano-receptors, which enables the relief of pain through massage, ice packs and deep transverse frictions. Acupuncture and transcutaneous electrical nerve stimulation may also stimulate release of endogenous opioids, thereby inhibiting the transmission of pain signals. (Melzack R, Wall P 1965 Pain mechanisms: a new theory. Science 150 (699):971–979.)

pain killer colloquial term for an analgesic drug, such as paracetamol or morphine sulphate.

pain management involves a holistic multidisciplinary approach, and in many healthcare settings there is a designated pain team or nurse specialist.

pain threshold the lowest intensity at which a stimulus is felt as pain. There is very little difference between people.

pain tolerance the greatest intensity of pain that the individual is prepared to endure or put up with. There is substantial variation between people.

painful arc term that describes pain in a certain part of a movement, it usually refers to shoulder abduction, typically pain occurs in the middle of the range but inner and outer ranges are pain free. Pain is usually caused by impingement of the supraspinatus tendon under the acromion process.

paint in pharmacology, a liquid preparation that is applied to the skin or mucous membrane and contains antiseptic, analgesic or other drugs.

painter's colic the colicky abdominal pain associated with exposure to lead. For example, in people who produced or used lead-containing paint. Others affected included miners working in lead mines. ⊃ lead poisoning.

pair production when a photon with energy greater than 1.02 MeV collides with the nucleus of an atom sometimes giving up all its energy in the production of an electron and a positron.

PAIVMs *abbr* passive accessory intervertebral movements.

pakoemulsification ⊃ phacoemulsification.

PAL *abbr* **1.** physical activity level. **2.** progressive addition lens.

palatal *adj* pertaining to the palate or palatine bone.

palatal arch in orthodontics, a heavy-gauge wire between bands on posterior teeth and used to reinforce orthodontic anchorage.

palatal bar a major connector of a maxillary partial denture that crosses the palate and unites the bilateral parts of the prosthesis.

palatal foramen ⊃ incisive foramen.

palatal retractor ⊃ finger spring.

palatal spring ⊃ finger spring.

palatal surface that surface of all upper teeth which faces the tongue. ⊃ surface.

palate *n* the roof of the mouth, separating the mouth from the nasal cavity and consisting of the hard and soft palate at its posterior border. *hard palate* formed by the processes of the maxillae and palatine bones, fused in the midline during development, and covered by mucous membrane, the mucosa being exceptionally tough and having rugae on its external surface. *soft palate* movable fold of mucous membrane that tapers towards the back of the mouth to form the uvula—**palatal, palatine** *adj*. ⊃ cleft palate, hard palate, soft palate, Colour Section Figure 18B.

palatine *adj* pertaining to the palate.

palatine arches *npl* the bilateral double pillars or arch-like folds formed by the descent of the soft palate as it meets the pharynx. The two posterior palatine folds, one on each side, are the *palatopharyngeal arches* and the two anterior folds are the *palatoglossal arches*. On each side, between the arches, is a collection of lymphoid tissue called the palatine tonsil.

palatine bones *npl* two small L-shaped bones of the face. They form part of the hard palate, the orbital cavities and the lateral part of the nasal cavities.

palatine tonsils ⊃ tonsils.

palatoglossal arch ⊃ palatine arches.

palatopharyngeal arches ⊃ palatine arches.

palatopharyngoplasty ⊃ uvulopalatopharyngoplasty.

palatoplasty *n* plastic surgery to repair defects in the palate.

palatoplegia *n* paralysis of the soft palate—**palatoplegic** *adj*.

palatorrhaphy *n* also called staphylorrhaphy. An operation to repair a cleft palate.

palilalia *n* a speech disorder characterized by rapid repetition of words or phrases.

palindromic *adj* relating to symptoms or disease that worsens or recurs.

palisades of Vogt the crests of epithelium folds that run radially towards the cornea, at the limbus, from the bulbar conjunctiva. They are often seen in slit-lamp examination, especially in pigmented individuals and clearly in fluorescein angiography. They may contain stem cells that play a role in the regeneration of corneal epithelium cells. ⊃ corneal epithelium.

palladium a rare metal in the platinum group which is white, ductile and malleable. Its chief dental use is as a constituent of casting gold alloys.

palliate *v* relieve symptoms. Often refers to the option where a patient's condition is no longer curable and can only benefit from treatment to prevent or reduce distress from symptoms. It may involve surgery (e.g. stent insertion into a bile duct, stoma formation to relieve obstruction), chemotherapy, radiotherapy (e.g. to relieve pain), nerve block and drugs (typically opioids) to relieve pain, or other symptoms.

palliative *adj, n* (describes) anything that serves to alleviate but cannot cure a disease. ⊃ treatment.

O
P

palliative care the multidisciplinary specialty of symptom relief, and the care and support of the patient, their family and friends—**palliation** *n*.

palliative treatment ⊃ treatment.

pallidectomy *n* destruction of a predetermined section of globus pallidus. ⊃ chemopallidectomy, stereotactic surgery.

pallidotomy *n* surgical severance of the fibres from the cerebral cortex to the corpus striatum. Previously used for relief of tremor in Parkinson's disease.

pallor extreme paleness of the skin, such as in anaemia, or after blood loss. It may also be due to lack of natural skin pigment, for instance in individuals who are not exposed to sunlight, or those with conditions that include albinism and phenylketonuria.

palm *n* the anterior or flexor surface of the hand.

palmar *adj* pertaining to the palm of the hand.

palmar crease the tiny grooves found running across the inside of the clenched hand.

palmar arches superficial and deep, are formed by the anastomosis of the radial and ulnar arteries. Smaller arteries arise from the arches to supply blood to the fingers. ⊃ Colour Section Figure 9.

palmar grasp reflex a primitive reflex present in newborns whereby they will flex their fingers to grasp a finger placed on the palm. ⊃ grasp reflex.

palmar venous arch deep veins of the hand.

palpable *adj* capable of being palpated (felt).

palpation *n* the act of manual examination—**palpate** *vt*.

palpebra *n* an eyelid—**palpebrae** *pl*, **palpebral** *adj*.

palpebral aperture (*syn* interpalpebral fissure [this term is more accurate although used infrequently], palpebral fissure) the gap between the margins of the eyelids when the eye is open. An abnormal increase in the aperture occurs in some conditions, including Graves' disease, buphthalmos, Parinaud's syndrome and retrobulbar tumour. An abnormal decrease in the aperture occurs in some conditions, including ptosis, microphthalmia (microphthalmos) and ophthalmoplegia. ⊃ exophthalmos, eyelids.

palpebral conjunctiva ⊃ conjunctiva.

palpebral fissure the opening between the eyelids. ⊃ palprebral aperture.

palpebral follicles ⊃ meibomian glands.

palpebral ligament the connective tissue attaching the extremities of the tarsal plates of the upper and lower eyelids to the orbital margin. There are two sets: (a) the *lateral palpebral ligament* (or lateral canthal tendon) about 7 mm long and 2.5 mm wide which constitutes the deeper portion of the lateral palpebral raphe of the orbicularis muscle and attaches the tarsal plates to the lateral orbital tubercle (or Whitnall's tubercle) on the zygomatic bone; and (b) the *medial palpebral ligament* (or medial canthal tendon) which attaches the medial ends of the tarsal plates to the frontal process of the maxilla and another insertion into the posterior lacrimal crest. It lies anterior to the canaliculi and the lacrimal sac. ⊃ eyelids, tarsus.

palpebral vein one of the veins of the upper or lower eyelid which empties for the most part into the anterior facial vein as well as into the angular, supraorbital, superior and inferior ophthalmic, the lacrimal and the superficial temporal veins.

palpitation *n* beating of the heart of which the person is strongly aware, as being rapid and/or forceful or sometimes irregular. May be both unpleasant and worrying but most will experience palpitation on occasion. Physiological causes include exercise, excitement, caffeine intake, smoking and alcohol. May also be a symptom of underlying disease, e.g. anaemia, hyperthyroidism, cardiac disease (especially if linked with other symptoms such as faintness, sweating, chest pain). Investigations (ECG, ambulatory monitoring, echocardiography, exercise test) are used to identify the nature of the condition and possible underlying causes.

PALS *abbr* **1.** paediatric advanced life support. **2.** patient advocacy liaison service.

palsy *n* paralysis. An obsolete word that is only retained in compound forms—Bell's palsy, cerebral palsy and Erb's palsy.

PAM *abbr* potential acuity meter.

PAN *acron* polyarteritis nodosa.

pan- a prefix that means 'all', e.g. *pandemic*.

panacea a medicine, remedy or treatment that claims to cure all diseases.

panarthritis *n* inflammation involving all of the structures of a joint.

pancarditis *n* inflammation involving all of the structures of the heart.

panchromatic emulsions in radiography, the film emulsions that are sensitive to all wavelengths of the visible spectrum. ⊃ monochromatic emulsions, orthochromatic emulsions.

Pancoast's syndrome (H Pancoast, American radiologist, 1875–1939) shoulder pain and pain down the inner aspect of the arm caused by pressure on the lower brachial plexus. It is associated with bronchial cancer situated in the apex of the lung (superior sulcus tumour) and may be accompanied by Horner's syndrome.

pancreas *n* a tongue-shaped, mixed endocrine and exocrine gland lying below and behind the stomach. Its head is encircled by the duodenum and its tail touches the spleen. It is about 20 cm long and weighs about 100 g. The endocrine islet cells secrete hormones that include insulin and glucagon. Exocrine glands in lobules secrete alkaline pancreatic juice which contains digestive enzymes involved in the digestion of fats, carbohydrates and proteins in the small intestine. The pancreatic juice leaves the pancreas through the pancreatic duct, which unites with the common bile duct before entering the duodeum at the hepatopancreatic ampulla. ⊃ pancreatic hormones, pancreatic juice, Colour Section Figure 18b.

pancreas divisum a developmental anomaly in which parts of the pancreas fail to fuse during embryonic development. Most people are asymptomatic, but it may be associated with abdominal pain, acute pancreatitis or chronic pancreatitis in some cases.

pancreatectomy *n* excision of part or the whole of the pancreas. It may be undertaken for cancer, cysts, or sometimes for pancreatitis. Patients in whom a large amount of pancreas has been resected will need insulin therapy, oral replacement of digestive enzymes and nutritional advice and support as necessary. ⊃ Whipple's operation.

pancreatic function tests indirect tests involve measurement of pancreatic enzyme metabolites in faeces, urine, plasma or breath. Estimation of serum amylase is undertaken when acute pancreatitis is suspected. Less often pancreatic function tests involve intubation tests, in which pancreatic juice is collected from the duodeum and measured for enzyme activity and bicarbonate after endocrine or meal stimulation.

pancreatic hormones the islet cells secrete several hormones: the alpha (α) cells produce glucagon; insulin and amylin are secreted from the beta (β) cells; the delta (δ) cells secrete somatostatin (growth hormone release inhibiting hormone); and other cells produce pancreatic polypeptide which inhibits exocrine pancreatic function.

pancreatic juice the secretion from the exocrine cells of the pancreas is stimulated by the hormones secretin and cholecystokinin (CCK) produced by duodenal cells. The juice contains water, electrolytes including bicarbonate ions, enzymes and inactive enzymes. The bicarbonate ions ensure an alkaline (pH 8) environment in the duodeum by neutralizing the acidic chyme from the stomach. The enzymes are: amylase (carbohydrate digestion) and lipase (fat digestion); and the inactive proteolytic enzyme precursors chymotrypsinogen, trypsinogen, and procarboxypeptidase. Trypsinogen is converted to active trypsin by the enzyme enterokinase in the duodenum, and it in turn produces active chymotrypsin and carboxypeptidase. They are not activated until they reach the duodenum so as to avoid damage to the pancreas by autodigestion.

pancreatic oncofetal antigen (POA) an oncofetal antigen. Its presence in the serum of adults can be a tumour marker for pancreatic cancer. Lower levels may be indicative of other cancers elsewhere. ⊃ oncofetal antigens

pancreaticoduodenectomy *n* surgical excision of the duodenum and head of the pancreas, carried out in cases of cancer arising in the region of the head of the pancreas.

pancreaticojejunostomy *n* surgical procedure to establish an anastomosis between the pancreatic duct and the jejunum.

pancreatic polypeptide a polypeptide secreted by the islet cells of the pancreas, exocrine cells of the pancreas and intestinal cells. It inhibits the production of pancreatic enzymes.

pancreatin an oral supplement of digestive enzymes obtained from animal sources. They are used for people with cystic fibrosis, after pancreatectomy, or in chronic pancreatitis. In order to reduce the effects of stomach acid on the enzymes they are taken just before food, with food, or immediately after eating. Capsules are swallowed whole or the contents mixed with fluid or food and taken at once. Some preparations are enteric-coated these too are swallowed whole.

pancreatitis *n* inflammation of the pancreas which may be acute or chronic. *acute pancreatitis* usually associated with gallstones or alcohol misuse. It is a serious condition and can be life-threatening with enzyme autodigestion of the pancreas leading to peritonitis, hypovolaemia, shock and multiple organ dysfunction syndrome (MODS). Depending on severity it is characterized by severe abdominal and back pain, abdominal/flank skin discoloration, nausea and vomiting, jaundice, tachycardia, hypotension, tachypnoea, hypoxia, oliguria, an elevated serum amylase, hypocalcaemia and hyperglycaemia. Management is supportive with pain relief (not morphine), intravenous fluid replacement, antibiotics and organ support as required. Longer term complications, which include the formation of pseudocysts, pancreatic abscess and pancreatic necrosis, may require surgical intervention. ⊃ Cullen's sign, Grey Turner's sign. *chronic pancreatitis* is most often caused by alcohol misuse and may occur after acute pancreatitis. There is permanent pancreatic damage and both endocrine and exocrine functions are affected. Pancreatic failure leads to diabetes mellitus and pancreatic enzyme insufficiency. It is characterized by abdominal pain, anorexia, malabsorption and steatorrhoea, weight loss, obstructive jaundice, hypocalcaemia and impaired glucose tolerance. Management includes pain relief, pancreatic enzyme replacement, low fat diet and insulin therapy for diabetes.

pancreatography radiographic investigation, in which contrast agent is introduced into the pancreatic duct during endoscopic retrograde cholangiopancreatography, or directly at operation in order to obtain an image of the pancreas and the ducts.

pancreozymin *n* intestinal hormone chemically identical to cholecystokinin (CCK). Previously both names were used.

pancytopenia *n* describes a peripheral blood picture when red cells, granular white cells and platelets are reduced as occurs when bone marrow function is suppressed. Causes include aplastic anaemia, drug side-effects, following chemotherapy or radiotherapy.

pandemic *n* an infection spreading over a whole country or the world. For example the influenza pandemic between 1917 and 1928, or the plague (Black Death) during the 14th century.

panhypopituitarism Simmonds' disease. Deficient secretion of the hormones from the anterior lobe of the pituitary gland. ⊃ hypopituitarism.

panic attack ⊃ anxiety.

panniculitis *n* also known as Weber–Christian disease. An inflammation of the subcutaneous fat with tender nodules.

panniculus a sheet of membranous tissue, layers of fascia.

pannus *n* **1.** fibrovascular membrane usually within the anterior stroma of the cornea. Associated with trachoma or following iridocyclitis, detached retina and glaucoma. **2.** the granulation tissue derived from synovial tissue that overgrows the articular surface of the joint in rheumatoid arthritis and is associated with its subsequent breakdown.

panophthalmitis *n* a serious condition involving inflammation of all the tissues of the eyeball. ⊃ endophthalmitis.

O

P

panoramic a complete view. *panoramic film* in radiography, a type of extra-oral radiographic film used to provide a radiograph of the dental structures. *panoramic radiography* a radiographic technique where the X-ray source is placed inside the mouth in order to obtain a radiographic image of the mandibular and/or the maxillary dental arches. *panoramic(rotational) tomography* a technique of obtaining a radiograph which incorporates an image of the mandibular and maxillary dental arches. It is obtained by moving the X-ray source simultaneously and in the opposite direction to the film whilst the patient remains stationary. A panoramic radiograph is sometimes referred to as an orthopantomograph (OPG®) or a 'panorex', after the trade name of the machine used to obtain the radiograph.

panosteitis *n* inflammation of all constituents of a bone—medulla, bony tissue and periosteum.

panretinal photocoagulation (PRP) treatment of the mid-peripheral retina with laser burns to reduce proliferative retinopathy, for example in diabetes.

panting rapid shallow breathing; a mechanism in furry animals for losing heat. In humans, not a normal physiological pattern of breathing. ➲ hyperventilation, tachypnoea.

pantogram a pantographic tracing.

pantograph a complex of tracing devices attached to the mandible and the maxilla in order to obtain a record of mandibular movements in three planes.

pantographic tracing a three dimensional graphic record of mandibular movements as registered by the stylii on the recording tables of a pantograph.

pantomography a panoramic radiographic technique that produces simultaneous images of the maxillary and mandibular dental arches.

Panton-Valentine leukocidin (PVL) a toxin produced by certain strains of the bacterium *Staphylococcus aureus*. The toxin affects white blood cells. Although PVL has been detected in meticillin (methicillin)-susceptible *S. aureus* the majority of strains are meticillin (methicillin)-resistant *S. aureus*. The PVL-producing strains of *S. aureus* have a different epidemiology and pathogenesis with increased virulence. It causes a variety of infections including boils and cellulitis, septicaemia and a community-acquired necrotizing pneumonia with a high mortality, which affects previously healthy young people.

pantoscopic angle (PA) (*syn* pantoscopic tilt) the angle between the spectacle plane and the frontal plane of the face when the superior edge of the lens is farther away from the face than the inferior edge (Figure P.2). ➲ frontal plane, retroscopic plane, spectacle plane.

pantoscopic tilt ➲ pantoscopic angle.

pantothenic acid a member of the vitamin B complex. It is part of acetyl coenzyme A (acetyl-CoA) and is involved in the metabolism of macronutrients and alcohol. It is so widely distributed in food that dietary deficiency is very rare; if it develops it will be in association with other deficiency disorders.

Panum's area (*syn* fusion area) an area in the retina of one eye, any point of which, when stimulated simultaneously

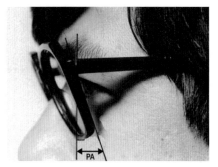

P.2 Pantoscopic angle (reproduced from Millodot 2004 with permission).

with a single point in the retina of the other eye, will give rise to a single percept. Its diameter in the fovea is about 5 minutes of arc and increases towards the periphery. ➲ horopter, retinal corresponding points, retinal disparity.

PAO *abbr* peak acid output. ➲ pentagastrin.

PaO₂ *abbr* partial pressure or tension of oxygen in arterial blood.

PAO₂ *abbr* the partial pressure or tension of oxygen in alveolar air.

PAOP *abbr* pulmonary artery occlusion pressure.

papain a proteolyic enzyme (proteose) obtained from the papaya tree (*Carica papaya*). It is prescribed in some countries for enzymatic wound débridement.

Papanicolaou test (G Papanicolaou, Greek/American cytologist and pathologist, 1883–1962) also known as a Pap smear. A smear of epithelial cells taken from the cervix using a special brush or spatula is stained and examined under the microscope for detection of the early stages of cancer. ➲ cervical intraepithelial neoplasia.

paper points absorbent, tapered cones of paper for drying root canals in endodontic treatment.

papilla *n* a minute nipple-shaped eminence, such as the gingival papilla, or those on the tongue—**papillae** *pl*, **papillary** *adj*. ➲ dental papilla, gingival papilla, incisive papilla, mammilla, renal papilla.

papillary pertaining to a papilla.

papillary bleeding index (PBI) ➲ index (dental).

papillary carcinoma a malignant tumour of the thyroid caused by irradiating the neck in childhood, it is characterized microscopically by having delicate finger-like cores of stroma lined by tumour cells.

papillary hyperplasia of the palate chronic inflammatory hyperplasia of the palate seen as closely grouped papillary projections.

papillary muscle the small muscles, which help to stabilize the atrioventricular valves of the heart. They are attached to the chordae tendineae in the cardiac ventricles. ➲ Colour Section Figure 8.

papillary necrosis infarction and necrosis of the renal papillae.

papillectomy *n* excision of a papilla.

papillitis *n* **1.** inflammation of the optic nerve head (disc). ➲ optic neuritis. **2.** inflammation of a renal papilla.

papilloedema *n* swelling of the optic nerve head (disc), seen during examination of the fundus of the eye using an ophthalmoscope. It is usually bilateral, caused by raised intracranial pressure, such as that present in cerebral oedema, expanding lesions in the skull (e.g. bleeding, tumours), hydrocephalus. ➲ Glasgow Coma Scale, head injury.

papilloma *n* a simple tumour arising from a non-glandular epithelial surface—**papillomata** *pl*, **papillomatous** *adj*.

papillomatosis *n* the growth of benign papillomata on the skin or a mucous membrane. Removal by laser means fewer recurrences.

papillomavirus a DNA-containing virus that causes warts. Many papilloma viruses are oncogenic and initiate malignant changes in cells. ➲ human papillomavirus.

Papillon–Lefèvre syndrome (M Papillon, French dermatologist; P Lefèvre, French dermatologist) a syndrome characterized by alveolar bone destruction in both the primary and the permanent (secondary) dentitions, by inflammatory gingival enlargement and by deep pocket formation and various skin lesions.

papillotomy *n* incision of a papilla, e.g. duodenal papilla for endoscopic extraction of ductal calculi.

PAPP-A *abbr* pregnancy associated plasma protein-A.

Pappataci fever also called sandfly fever. ➲ phlebotomus fever.

papule (*syn.* pimple) a small circumscribed elevation of the skin—**papular** *adj*.

papulopustular *adj* pertaining to a skin eruption with both papules and pustules.

papulosquamous *adj* pertaining to a skin eruption with both papules and scales.

PAR *acron* **1. P**eer **A**ssessment **R**eview. **2. P**hysical **A**ctivity **R**atio.

para a woman who has produced one or more viable offspring, i.e. all infants delivered over 24 weeks' gestation and all stillbirths. It is designated by numbers. *para 0* (nullipara), describes a woman who has not delivered a viable infant. *para 1* (primipara), describes a woman who has delivered one viable infant. *para 2* or more (multipara), describes a woman who has delivered two or more viable infants. Miscarriages and terminations of pregnancy are not counted but usually identified by adding [+1] after the number designating viable deliveries, e.g. para 3[+1]—**parous** *adj*.

para- a prefix that means 'beside, beyond', e.g. *parametrium*.

para-aortic *adj* near the aorta.

paracentesis *n* usually applied to the surgical puncture of the peritoneal cavity (paracentesis abdominis or abdominocentesis) for the aspiration of fluid. Either a catheter is inserted into the abdominal cavity through a small incision or a trocar and cannula is used to drain ascitic fluid—**paracenteses** *pl*.

paracentesis thoracis (thoracentesis) draining fluid from the pleural cavity. ➲ aspiration.

paracervical block infiltration of Lee-Frankenhauser nerve plexus with local anaesthetic through the lateral fornices to relieve cervical dilatation pain in labour, effective for up to 3 hours. Great care is needed because the uterine artery is in close proximity to the plexus and inadvertent injection may cause fetal bradycardia and intrauterine fetal death.

paracetamol *n* known as acetaminophen in North America. A non-opioid analgesic drug which has antipyretic properties. It is effective in mild to moderate pain, and having no anti-inflammatory action it is less likely to irritate the stomach. It is present in many over-the-counter medicines and in combination with other analgesic drugs. *paracetamol poisoning* paracetamol is toxic at relatively low levels, for example the ingestion of 10–15 g can damage liver cells (hepatocellular necrosis), and less often damage the kidneys (tubular necrosis). Paracetamol depletes the amount of glutathione in the liver and in appropriate cases the administration of acetylcysteine or methionine following paracetamol overdose helps to replenish glutathione levels and protect the liver. The decision to administer acetylcysteine or methionine depends on factors that include the time since ingestion and the concentration of paracetamol in the plasma. ➲ Appendix 5.

parachute reflex a reflex that appears between 7 and 9 months of age (i.e. before walking) in which the infant will, if held upright and suddenly moved to a horizonal prone position, extend the arms as if trying to break a fall. Persists into adulthood.

paracrine *adj* denoting a hormone, which has a localized action. Its effects are confined to adjacent cells or those in the immediate vicinity. ➲ autocrine, endocrine.

paracusis a disorder of hearing.

paradental cyst a deprecated term for lateral periodontal cyst.

paradigm *n* term introduced in 1960 by the science-historian Kuhn; a widely followed way of approaching an area of research, deriving from a notable early achievement in the field and carrying forward both its experimental methodology and its theoretical outlook. An example, model, or set of ideas or assumptions.

paradigm shift the changes that occur as the build-up of evidence causes a paradigm to be questioned and eventually replaced by a new set of ideas.

paradontal sited near or close to a tooth.

paradoxical diplopia ➲ incongruous diplopia.

paradoxical respiration abnormal breathing pattern associated with loss of chest wall integrity, such as following injuries that result in the ribs on one side being fractured in two places, such as in flail chest. The injured side of the chest moves in (deflates) on inspiration and vice versa. It may also occur in severe muscle weakness or failure. ➲ flail chest.

paradoxical sleep (*syn.* rapid eye movement [REM] sleep) ➲ sleep.

paraesthesia *n* any subjective abnormality of sensation such as tingling, 'pins and needles', a feeling of tightness or swelling, or numbness. A feature of many neurological disorders including polyneuropathy and some spinal cord lesions. Also occurs in electrolyte and pH disturbances, such as with hypocalcaemia, or in the respiratory alkalosis caused by hyperventilation. ⊃ tetany.

paraffin *n* medicinal paraffins are: *hard paraffin*, used in wax baths for rheumatic conditions; *liquid paraffin*, previously used as a lubricant/softener laxative; and *soft paraffin*, used as an ointment base.

paraffin wax wax derived from crude oil. Used as the major constituent in many dental waxes; also used for wax bath therapy to relieve pain.

parafunctional a movement that is distorted or beyond normal function, e.g. bruxism or jaw clenching. ⊃ bruxism.

paraganglioma *n* phaeochromocytoma occurring outside the adrenal medulla.

paraganglion *n* any one of the small collections of chromaffin cells around the sympathetic ganglia. The paraganglia secrete the catecholamine hormones adrenaline (epinephrine) and noradrenaline (norepinephrine).

parageusia an abnormality of the sense of taste (gustation).

paragonimiasis endemic haemoptysis. Infestation with the lung fluke *Paragonimus westermani*. It occurs mainly in the Far East but is also present in other areas that include South America and India. It is acquired by eating raw or inadequately cooked shellfish, such as fresh-water crabs and crayfish. Symptoms are similar to chronic bronchitis, including cough, haemoptysis and breathlessness. Can also cause diarrhoea and abdominal pain, or problems in the central nervous system such as encephalitis.

Paragonimus a genus of trematode flukes. For example *Paragonimus westermani*.

parainfluenza virus a paramyxovirus causing acute upper respiratory infection mainly in infants and children. Its various serotypes may cause croup, bronchiolitis, laryngotracheobronchitis, bronchopneumonia and tracheobronchitis.

parallax an apparent alteration in the relative positions of two objects when viewed from different positions. The technique is used in radiography to assess the buccolingual relationship of roots and unerupted teeth.

parallel axis theorem mathematical method of relating the moment of inertia of a body or object around one axis to the moment of inertia of the same body or object around a parallel axis. Calculated as $I_2 = I_1 + md^2$ where I_1 and I_2 are the moments of inertia, m is the mass of the object and d is the distance between the two parallel axes.

parallel-hole collimator gamma camera collimator made of a thick lead plate with several thousand parallel sided holes perpendicular to the plane of the plate, gives a 1:1 relationship between the object being recorded and the image produced.

parallel pair used in radiotherapy to describe two directly opposing treatment fields.

paralleling technique a periapical radiographic technique in which a film holder is used to align the film parallel to the long axis of the tooth and also to allow the central ray to pass perpendicular to the plane of the film.

parallelometer in dentistry, an instrument designed to ensure that preparation surfaces or prosthetic structures are parallel to one another.

paralympics the competitive events regularly held 'parallel to the Olympics' for disabled sportspeople. In the late 1940s Ludwig Guttmann, medical director of the Stoke Mandeville Spinal Injuries Unit, who had made wheelchair games a feature of rehabilitation, initiated competitive events in archery, netball and table tennis for his paraplegic patients. In 1952 he invited a small Dutch team to join in the local games, and this first international event led to his inauguration of the paralympics in Rome in 1960, with 400 wheelchair athletes. By 2004 successive occasions had extended the range of disabilities included, and there were 19 events for 4000 participants from 136 countries. ⊃ spinal injury/spinal cord injury.

paralysis *n* complete or incomplete loss of nervous function to a part of the body. This may be sensory or motor or both. Paralysis may be flaccid or spastic. ⊃ hemiplegia, monoplegia, paraplegia, quadriplegia, tetraplegia. *paralysis agitans* ⊃ parkinsonism.

paralytic *adj* pertaining to paralysis.

paralytic ileus paralysis of the intestinal muscle leading to a decrease or complete cessaion of peristalsis. Thus the bowel content cannot pass onwards even though there is no mechanical obstruction. It may occur after abdominal surgery especially gastrointestinal surgery; in peritonitis; ischaemic bowel; injury; drugs such as opiates; hypokalaemia; spinal cord injury; and hypothyroidism. ⊃ aperistalsis, ileus, intestinal obstruction, meconium ileus.

paramagnetic a substance that increases the strength of a magnetic field in which it is placed by aligning with the static magnetic field and therefore affecting the relaxation times of the tissues containing them. ⊃ diamagnetic, ferromagnetic, superparamagnetic.

paramagnetism the influence of an applied magnetic field on the electrons orbiting the nuclei within the substance which results in the formation of an elementary bar magnet.

paramedian *adj* near the middle, such as the position of an abdominal incision.

paramedical *adj* allied to medicine. Relating to the health professions closely linked to the medical profession, e.g. physiotherapy, occupational therapy, emergency paramedic, speech and language therapist. ⊃ professions allied to medicine.

paramesonephric duct also known as müllerian duct. One of the paired primitive embryonic ducts that become the internal genitalia (uterine tubes, uterus) in a genetically female embryo. ⊃ mesonephric duct, müllerian duct.

parameter 1. a numerically measured property such as blood pressure. A constant or value used in the measurement of data relating to a physiological function, for example blood chemistry, haematological indices, which are used in the assessment of health status. 2. in statistics, a measurement or value of a population characteristic, such as mean or standard deviation. 3. general term meaning boundaries or limits.

parameters (therapy) the variables that describe precisely the settings used in various therapy modalities. Ultrasound parameters include: frequency, beam non-uniformity ratio

(BNR), size and effective radiating area (ERA) of applicator, intensity (spatial average temporal average—SATA, spatial average temporal peak—SATP), duration and frequency of treatments, continuous or pulsed, location and size of area treated, brand and model of machine. Electrical stimulation parameters depend on if the current is pulsed, alternating or direct, generally they include: frequency, pulse duration and shape, intensity, duration and frequency of treatments, electrode size and location. Laser parameters include: frequency, type of laser, J/cm^2 applied, size and location of treatment area, which applicator and method, duration and frequency of treatments, etc. Shortwave diathermy (SWD) parameters include: if capacitive or magnetic field method, pulsed SWD (PSWD) or continuous SWD (CSWD), duration and frequency of treatments, size and location of electrodes or coil. Ultraviolet radiation (UVR) parameters include: which lamp, distance from skin, duration and date of treatment, etc. Ice/cold and superficial heating parameters include: method used and duration and frequency of treatments.

parametric tests statistical tests that presuppose the data are from a sample from a population that has a normal distribution curve, i.e. a histogram of values shows a bell-shaped curve, with most values lying close to the middle of the distribution, and increasingly extreme values seen with increasingly lower frequency. Parametric tests, which include Student's t test for independent groups, are more powerful than the equivalent non-parametric tests. ⊃ non-parametric tests.

parametritis *n* inflammation of the structures around the uterus, the parametrium. Pelvic cellulitis. ⊃ cellulitis, pelvic inflammatory disease.

parametrium *n* the connective tissues immediately surrounding the uterus—**parametrial** *adj*.

paramnesia 1. a distortion of memory whereby the person believes that they remember a set of circumstances that did not occur. They are unable to differentiate between reality and fantasy. **2.** the use of remembered words without having any understanding of what they mean. ⊃ confabulation, déjà vu phenomenon.

paramyotonia a condition characterized by muscle spasms resulting from an abnormality of muscle tone.

paramyotonia congenita cold-evoked myotonia with episodic weakness provoked by exercise and cold. It is associated with a muscle channelopathy in which the sodium ion channels in striated muscle are abnormal. ⊃ muscle channelopathies.

paramyxovirus a family of RNA viruses that include the measles virus, mumps virus, parainfluenza virus and the respiratory syncytial virus.

paranasal *adj* near the nasal cavities, as the various sinuses.

paranasal sinuses the air-filled sinuses in the bones around the nasal cavity. There are ethmoidal air cells and frontal, maxillary (maxillary antrum) and sphenoidal sinuses (Figure P.3). They are lined with ciliated mucous membrane,

O
P

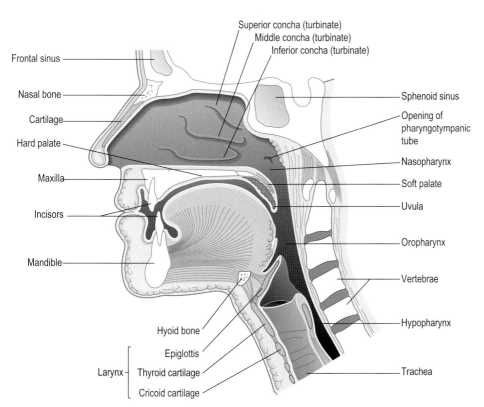

P.3 Paranasal air sinuses (frontal and sphenoid sinuses shown). (reproduced from Brooker & Nicol 2003 with permission).

which is continuous with that lining the nasal cavity. The sinuses lighten the skull and give the voice resonance.

paraneoplastic syndromes *npl* the indirect symptoms or signs associated with the presence of a cancer, but which occurs away from the primary cancer or any metastatic sites. They are caused by the production of hormones, other chemicals and immune responses. They may be haematological, endocrine, neurological or affect the skin and muscles. Examples include dermatomyositis; hypercalcaemia caused by production of parathyroid homone (PTH) in breast cancer; ectopic production of adrenocorticotrophic hormone (ACTH) in some lung cancers; myasthenia gravis associated with thymic cancers; and cerebellar degeneration associated with cancers of the ovary, breast, lung, etc.

paranoia *n* an abnormal tendency to mistrust or suspect others—**paranoid** *adj*.

paranoid behaviour acts denoting suspicion of others.

paranoid schizophrenia a form of schizophrenia characterized by (often persecutory) delusions and hallucinations.

paraoesophageal *adj* near the oesophagus.

paraparesis *n* loss of power, weakness or partial loss of movement and or sensation in the lower half of the body following damage to the spinal cord in the thoracic, lumbar or sacral regions. ➲ hemiparesis, monoparesis, paresis, quadriparesis.

paraphasia a disorder of language in which the person uses meaningless words or uses words in the wrong sense, speech is unintelligible and incoherent.

paraphimosis *n* retraction of the prepuce (foreskin) behind the glans penis so that a tight ring of skin produces oedema of the preputial skin. Thus the prepuce cannot be returned to its normal position. ➲ circumcision, phimosis.

paraphrenia *n* a persistent delusional disorder with onset in later life—**paraphrenic** *adj*.

paraplegia *n* paralysis of the lower limbs, usually affecting the nerves that control bowel and bladder function. Often the result of traumatic spinal cord damage, but also caused by multiple sclerosis or tumours—**paraplegic** *adj*. ➲ hemiplegia, monoplegia, spinal cord compression (SCC), tetraplegia.

paraprax *n* known as a 'Freudian slip'. A verbal error caused by unconscious conflicts.

paraprotein an abnormal protein including the abnormal monoclonal immunoglobulins produced in plasma cell disorders.

paraproteinaemias the over-production of one or more classes of immunoglobulin is referred to as a gammopathy. It may be polyclonal in association with acute or chronic inflammation such as infection, sarcoidosis, autoimmune disorders or some malignancies. Alternatively, a monoclonal increase in a single immunoglobulin class may occur in association with normal or reduced levels of the other immunoglobulins. Gammopathies are detected by plasma immunoelectrophoresis. Such monoclonal proteins, also called M-proteins, paraproteins or monoclonal gammopathies, occur as a feature of myeloma, lymphoma and amyloidosis, in connective tissue disease such as rheumatoid arthritis or polymyalgia rheumatica, in infection such as HIV disease and in solid tumours. In addition, they may be present with no underlying disease. ➲ monoclonal gammopathy of uncertain significance (MGUS).

parapsychology *n* the study of extrasensory perception, telepathy and other psychic phenomena.

paraquat dichloride widely used as a herbicide. Exposure leads to local effects depending on the route, but include: oral/oesophageal damage, skin blisters, epistaxis, or severe inflammation of the conjunctiva or cornea. Systemic effects that may be delayed are usually associated with ingestion and include damage to the myocardium, lungs, liver and kidneys.

pararectal *adj* near the rectum.

parasitaemia *n* parasites in the blood—**parasitaemic** *adj*.

parasite *n* an organism that obtains nutrients or shelter from another organism, the 'host'—**parasitic** *adj*.

parasiticide *n* an agent that will kill parasites.

parasitic light ➲ stray light.

parasomnias *npl* a broad class of sleep-associated disturbances; it includes sleepwalking, nightmares and bruxism.

parasternal *adj* near the sternum.

parasuicide *n* a suicidal gesture: drugs overdose or a self-mutilating act which may or may not be provoked by a real wish to die. Commonly seen in young people who are distressed but not mentally ill. May be linked to low self-esteem. ➲ deliberate self-harm, Samaritans.

parasympathetic nervous system *n* one of the two components of the autonomic nervous system. Preganglionic nerve fibres come from the brainstem and from the sacral segments of the spinal cord (craniosacral outflow), i.e. from the central nervous system above and below the sympathetic outflow. These nerves relay in ganglia close to the organs where they act (including heart, lungs, gastrointestinal tract). Most of the cranial components travel in the vagus nerves (Xth cranial nerve). In general, parasympathetic nerves stimulate the functions of the alimentary and genitourinary systems, whereas effects on the cardiorespiratory system are appropriate to relative inactivity, e.g. slowing the heart rate. Thus it is generally concerned with the normal 'at rest' body processes, such as digestion, and opposes the action of the sympathetic nervous system. ➲ acetylcholine, atropine, sympathetic nervous system, Colour Section Figure 22.

parasympatholytic *adj* usually describes a drug, that reduces or eradicates the effects of parasympathetic stimulation. ➲ muscarinic antagonist.

parasympathomimetic *adj* describes an agent, usually a drug, that causes similar effects as or stimulates parasympathetic activity. ➲ muscarinic agonist.

paratendon the fibrous sheath around a tendon, with a thin synovial lining. ➲ tendon.

parathormone *n* parathyroid hormone. ➲ parathyroid hormone.

parathyroid glands small clumps of endocrine tissue (usually four) and usually lying close to or embedded in the

O
P

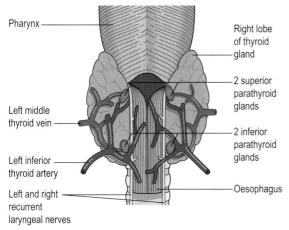

Pharynx

Right lobe of thyroid gland

2 superior parathyroid glands

Left middle thyroid vein

2 inferior parathyroid glands

Left inferior thyroid artery

Left and right recurrent laryngeal nerves

Oesophagus

P.4 Position of parathyroid glands and related structures (reproduced from Waugh & Grant 2006 with permission).

posterior surface of the thyroid gland (Figure P.4). They may, however, be located at other sites in the neck, thorax and mediastinum. They secrete parathyroid hormone. ⊃ parathyroid hormone.

parathyroid hormone (PTH) parathormone. A polypeptide hormone secreted by the parathyroid glands. Parathyroid hormone (PTH) acts to increase calcium ion concentration in the extracellular fluid, counterbalanced by the hormone calcitonin from the thyroid gland which has the opposite effects. PTH regulates calcium and phosphate homeostasis and is released when calcium concentration in serum is decreased. PTH indirectly regulates ionized calcium [Ca^{2+}] and phosphate levels by exerting an effect at three main sites in the body: (a) bone—the effects of PTH, result in the release of calcium and phosphate from the bone into the blood; (b) small intestine—this is the primary site of calcium absorption from the diet. Calcium absorption by active transport needs physiologically active vitamin D (1,25 dihydroxycholecalciferol); (c) kidney—cells in the kidney contain an enzyme that converts inactive vitamin D to the active form in the kidneys. PTH stimulates active renal tubular reabsorption of [Ca^{2+}], while simultaneously inhibiting phosphate retention. ⊃ calcitonin.

parathyroidectomy *n* excision of one or more parathyroid glands.

paratope the antigen-binding site of an antibody molecule. ⊃ epitope.

paratyphoid fever a variety of enteric fever, less severe and prolonged than typhoid fever. Caused by *Salmonella enterica* serovar Paratyphi A and B, and more rarely C.

paraurethral *adj* near the urethra.

paravaginal *adj* near the vagina.

paravertebral *adj* near the spinal column.

paravertebral block anaesthesia (more correctly, analgesia) is induced by infiltration of local anaesthetic around the spinal nerve roots as they emerge from the intervertebral foramina.

paravertebral injection of local anaesthetic into sympathetic chain can be used as a test in ischaemic limbs to see if sympathectomy is indicated.

paraxial equation (fundamental) (*syn* general refraction formula) an equation based on gaussian theory and dealing with refraction at a spherical surface:

$$\frac{n'}{l'} - \frac{n}{l} = \frac{n' - n}{r} \quad \text{(or)} \quad L' - L = \frac{n' - n}{r}$$

where n and n' are the refractive indices of the media on each side of the spherical surface, r is the radius of curvature of the surface and l and l' the distances of the object and the image from the surface, respectively. n/l and n'/l' are the vergences (or reduced vergences) of the incident and refracted light rays respectively. $L' - L$ corresponds to the change produced by the surface in the vergence of the light and is called the focal power (or vergence power, or refractive power) F of the surface. Thus

$$L' - L = F$$

Focal power is usually expressed in dioptres and can be either positive or negative. At a reflecting surface or a mirror the equation becomes

$$L' - L = \frac{2}{r}$$

where r is the radius of curvature of the surface or mirror. ⊃ dioptre, gaussian theory, image distance, object distance, refractive power, sign convention, vergence.

paraxial optics (*syn* first order optics, gaussian optics) a simplified representation of geometrical optics which deals only with paraxial rays and in which the law of refraction and the fundamental paraxial equation are applicable. ⊃ Lagrange's law, law of refraction, paraxial equation (fundamental), paraxial ray.

paraxial ray a light ray which forms an angle of incidence so small that its value in radians is almost equal to its sine or its tangent. (i.e. $\sin\theta = \theta$ or $\tan\theta = \theta$). These are approximate expressions referred to as the paraxial approximation (or the gaussian approximation.) ⊃ angle of incidence, gaussian theory, paraxial optics, paraxial region.

paraxial region (*syn* gaussian space) the hypothetical cylindrical narrow space surrounding the optical axis within which rays of light are still considered paraxial. ⊃ gaussian theory, paraxial ray.

paraxial theory ⊃ gaussian theory.

pareidolic image a sensory deception. A vivid perception of visual images in response to an indistinct stimulus. The image and the percept coexist, and the image is normally accepted as being 'unreal'. For instance faces or objects seen in a cloud formation. An example of an illusion. ⊃ eidetic, illusion.

parenchyma *n* the tissues and cells of an organ which, in contradistinction to its supporting interstitial tissue, are concerned with its function—**parenchymal, parenchymatous** *adj*.

parenchymatous salpingitis inflammation of the functional layer of the uterine (fallopian) tube.

O
P

parent radionuclide a nucleus before it has decayed. ⟂ radioactive decay.

parenteral *adj* not via the alimentary tract. Therapy such as fluid, drugs, or nutrition administered by a route other than the alimentary tract.

parenteral nutrition a method of providing nutrition by administering nutrients directly into the circulatory system via a venous catheter. It can be given temporarily in hospital, or permanently at home (home parenteral nutrition) in the treatment of intestinal failure. A special intravenous catheter is used to infuse various nutrient solutions into a central vein. Usually the catheter is sited centrally, through the subclavian vein into the superior vena cava. Sometimes it is possible to use peripherally inserted central catheters (PICC) which are inserted through the basilic vein (of the arm) to the superior vena cava via the right subclavian vein. Parenteral nutrition is used for patients whose gastrointestinal tract is not functioning. It should only be used if nutritional needs cannot be met via the enteral route. The term total parenteral nutrition is used in some countries—**parenterally** *adv*.

parenthood education health education to help parents prepare for labour and parenthood and provide a social environment for couple approaching parenthood, usually offered as a series of classes.

paresis *n* partial or slight paralysis; weakness of a limb—**paretic** *adj*. ⟂ hemiparesis, monoparesis, paraparesis, quadriparesis.

pareunia *n* coitus.

pareve (parve) a Jewish word for dishes that do not contain meat or milk. Orthodox Jews are prohibited from combining meat or milk foods, or eating or drinking milk products for 3 hours following a meal with meat. ⟂ kosher, traife.

paries a wall, such as that of a body cavity or a hollow organ—**parietes** *pl*.

parietal *adj* 1. pertaining to an outer wall, such as the parietal pleura or parietal peritoneum. 2. pertaining to the parietal lobes of the cerebrum and the parietal bones of the skull.

parietal bones the two bones which form the sides and vault of the skull. They are joined to each other at the sagittal suture, with the frontal bone at the coronal suture, with the occipital bone at the lambdoidal suture and with the temporal bones at the squamous suture. The inner surface is concave and is grooved by the brain and blood vessels

parietal cells ⟂ oxyntic.

parietal lobe the part of each cerebral hemisphere underlying the parietal bone. The parietal lobe contains the somatosensory area of the cerebral cortex and the large parieto-occipitotemporal area, which are concerned with the integration of incoming sensory impulses from receptors in the skin, those in skeleletal muscle and joints. The areas in the parietal lobe are concerned with the perception of sensations of pain, pressure, touch, temperature and the awareness of muscle and joint action; and functions that include the manipulation and identification of objects, remembering the names of objects and spatial awareness.

Parinaud's oculoglandular syndrome (H Parinaud, French ophthalmologist, 1844–1905) follicular conjunctivitis that usually affects one eye. It is accompanied by enlarged and tender preauricular lymph nodes.

Parinaud's syndrome (H Parinaud) (*syn* dorsal midbrain syndrome, tectal midbrain syndrome) paralysis of the conjugate movements of the eyes either for elevation or depression, or both, and sometimes with paralysis of convergence, fixed pupils and lid retraction. This condition is due to a lesion at the level of the superior colliculi or in the subthalamic region. ⟂ Collier's sign, convergence-retraction nystagmus, superior colliculi.

Paris system a method of introducing radioactive sources during brachytherapy using iridium-192 (^{92}I).

parity *n* status of a woman with regard to the number of children she has borne.

Parkinson facies (J Parkinson) a mask-like appearance; saliva may trickle from the corners of the mouth.

Parkinson's disease (J Parkinson, British physician, 1755–1824) an idiopathic incurable neurodegenerative condition in which there are changes in the substantia nigra and a relatively selective loss of dopamine nerve cells in the brain causing a resting tremor, bradykinesia (slowness of movement), facial musculature immobility, postural instability and rigidity in the limbs. Parkinson's disease is always progressive, although the rate of deterioration varies. It is important to try to maintain movements of extension and rotation, as posture generally becomes dominated by flexion, there is a tendency to stoop and gait becomes festinating (short shuffling steps). Some people differentiate between idiopathic Parkinson's disease and parkinsonism, the causes of which are multiple and include repeated brain trauma (as in boxing), stroke, atherosclerosis, brain cancers, Wilson's disease, various toxic agents, viral encephalitis, carbon monoxide poisoning and as a side effect of typical antipsychotic drugs (neuroleptics). ⟂ tardive dyskinesia.

parkinsonism *n* a condition resembling Parkinson's disease clinically.

Parliamentary and Health Service Ombudsman an organization that independently investigates complaints from the public about the actions of the NHS in England, government departments and many public bodies in the UK, and the service they received from them.

PARNUTS *abbr* foods for particular nutritional purposes. The term used by the European Union for the dietetic foods for people with metabolic disorders (e.g. phenylketonuria), or certain physiological conditions (e.g. coeliac disease), or for infants and young children.

paronychia *n* (*syn*. whitlow) inflammation of the tissue around a nail plate, which may be bacterial or fungal. It frequently occurs with onychia.

paroophoron *n* vestigial remains of the embryonic mesonephros located in the broad ligament between the epoophoron and the uterus. ⟂ epoophoron.

parosmia *n* altered, dysfunctional sense of smell, usually of unpleasant hallucinatory nature.

parotid salivary gland one of a pair of large salivary glands situated in front of and below the ear on either side, and wrapped round the posterior border of the ramus of the mandible (see Figure S.1, p. 688). The parotid duct (Stenson's duct) runs forward from the gland, across the masseter muscle to pass through the buccinator muscle and open into the mouth opposite the second upper molar tooth. The parotid gland secretes watery saliva containing the enzyme amylase; the volume is considerably increased during eating. It is innervated by fibres from the otic ganglion and receives arterial blood from a branch of the external carotid artery, venous blood drains via the retromandibular vein. ➲ sublingual salivary gland, submandibular salivary gland.

parotidectomy *n* excision of a parotid salivary gland, such as for removal of a tumour.

parotitis *n* inflammation of a parotid salivary gland. ➲ sialoadenitis. *infectious parotitis* ➲ mumps. *septic parotitis* refers to ascending infection from the mouth via the parotid duct, when a parotid abscess may result.

parous *adj* having borne one or more viable infants. ➲ multipara, nullipara, para, primipara.

paroxysm *n* a sudden, temporary attack.

paroxysmal *adj* coming on in attacks or paroxysms.

paroxysmal cold haemoglobinuria a condition where exposure to cold leads to intravascular haemolysis.

paroxysmal fibrillation occurs in the atrium of the heart and is associated with a ventricular tachycardia and total irregularity of the pulse rhythm.

paroxysmal nocturnal dyspnoea (PND) sudden bouts of dyspnoea occurring mostly at night in patients with cardiac disease, usually left ventricular failure. It awakens the person, following some hours of sleep. It is often accompanied by feelings of panic, respiratory distress, sweating, tachycardia and coughing up frothy sputum.

paroxysmal nocturnal haemoglobinuria (PNH) an inherited condition caused be a faulty gene on the X chromosome that results in defective blood cells including red cells. There is haemolysis, haemoglobinuria, anaemia and venous thromboses, and a decrease in the number of neutrophils and platelets in the blood.

paroxysmal tachycardia a temporary but sudden marked increase in frequency of heart beats, because the conducting stimulus is originating in an abnormal focus. It may result from ectopic impulses arising in the atrium or in the ventricle itself.

parrot disease ➲ psittacosis.

Parrot's nodes (J Parrot, French physician, 1829–1883) bossing of frontal bones and parietal bones of the skull in congenital syphilis.

pars flaccida *n* the upper part of the tympanic membrane.

pars interarticularis the segment of bone between the superior and inferior articular facets, especially in the lumbar spine.

pars tensa *n* the lower four-fifths of the tympanic membrane.

partial agonist a drug that only has a partial physiological effect, having reduced efficacy compared with a full agonist.

partial anodontia a deprecated term for hypodontia or oligodontia.

partial denture a removable dental appliance which restores one or more—but less than all—of the natural teeth and associated parts, and is supported by the teeth and/or mucosa.

partial (incomplete) mole ➲ molar pregnancy.

partial pressure the component of the total gas pressure accounted for by one gas in a mixture of gases, e.g. in air at 1 standard atmosphere (1 bar, ~101 kPa, 760 mmHg or torr), 21% is oxygen and the partial pressure of oxygen (PO_2) is ~21 kPa or 160 mmHg (torr). Partial pressure (*syn.* tension) of a gas dissolved in a liquid is defined as the partial pressure of that gas in the gaseous phase with which the liquid is, has been or would be, in equilibrium. So, given near-perfect diffusion equilibrium across the alveolar-capillary membranes, blood leaves the lungs with virtually the same PO_2 and PCO_2 as in alveolar gas (normally close to 100 mmHg PO_2 and 40 mmHg PCO_2). When blood reaches capillaries in active tissues, the lower PO_2 and higher PCO_2 in tissue fluids cause net molecular movement towards equilibrium, so that O_2 is removed from the blood and CO_2 taken up. ➲ carbon dioxide, diffusing capacity, gas exchange, nitrogen, oxygen, oxygen dissociation curve.

partial seizure ➲ epilepsy.

partial sight ➲ low vision.

partial thickness flap a surgical flap consisting of epithelium and connective tissue but not the periosteum, which is left undisturbed on the bone.

partial veneer crown (*syn* three-quarter crown) a cast-metal extracoronal restoration covering most of the surfaces of the clinical crown of a tooth.

participation involvement in life situations through activity within a social context. (Reproduced with permission from the European Network of Occupational Therapy in Higher Education (ENOTHE) Terminology Project, 2008.)

participation motive an individual's reason for engaging in activity. Often applied to reasons for engaging in exercise or sport, such as to manage weight, for enjoyment or for social reasons.

particle range the distance from its point of origin that a charged particle no longer reacts with the material it is travelling through.

particle theory the basic concept of quantum physics and considers that electromagnetic radiation of short wavelength and high velocity consists of particles or quanta or photons each having a discrete amount of energy.

partnership working in the UK a working relationship between central government, local NHS services, local government authorities, and local communities. It should enable greater coordination and cooperative multiagency/multiprofessional working that aims to improve health and well-being.

O
P

partogram/partograph *n* a chart that provides a graphic record of progress during labour. Information recorded includes fetal heart, maternal vital signs, contraction frequency and strengths, cervical dilatation and descent of presenting part, drugs administered, etc. and allows for the prompt identification of departures from normal.

parturient *adj* pertaining to childbirth.

parturition *n* ⊃ labour.

parvovirus B19 (human parvovirus B19, fifth disease, slapped cheek syndrome, erythema infectiosum) ⊃ human erythrovirus 19.

PAS *abbr* periodic acid–Schiff (reagent).

pascal (Pa) *n* derived Système International d'Unités (SI) unit (International System of Units) for pressure. The kilopascal (kPa) is now frequently used for measuring blood gases. It would be used for measuring blood pressure instead of millimetres of mercury pressure (mmHg) if the change was ever made. ⊃ Appendix 2.

PASCAL a high-level language for computers.

passive *adj* inactive. In orthodontics or prosthetics, refers to a spring or clasp which exerts no tension.⊃ active *opp.*

passive accessory intervertebral movements (PAIVMs) these are passive physiological intervertebral movements and are oscillatory physiological movements graded I–IV. They are used to assess and treat vertebral symptoms, such as pain, resistance and spasm.

passive eruption apical migration of the gingiva thus increasing the clinical crown without there being an active eruption of the tooth.

passive hyperaemia ⊃ hyperaemia.

passive immunity acquired, naturally when maternal antibodies pass to the fetus via the placenta or after birth in colostrum and breast milk, or artificially by administering immunoglobulins (usually human in origin). This type of immunity tends to be short-lived because the immune response is not stimulated to produce specific antibodies, i.e. it is passive. ⊃ immunity.

passive insufficiency the inability of a two joint muscle to fully stretch simultaneously across two joints, e.g. the hamstrings cannot stretch across hip and knee joints at the same time or the gastrocnemius cannot permit full dorsiflexion if the knee is fully extended. ⊃ active insufficiency.

passive movement a movement performed by a force, which can be another person or a machine, i.e. continuous passive motion (movement) (CPM) machine, but does not require voluntary activity of the patient's own muscles. The uses for passive movements include: (a) maintain integrity of joint and soft tissues; (b) promotion of synovial sweep over articular cartilage, thus nutrition; (c) maintain existing range of movement; (d) minimize risk of joint contractures (full range needed); (e) maintain elasticity of soft tissues; (f) assist circulation if performed quickly (stimulation of the muscle pump); (g) pain inhibition (movement can act as an analgesic); (h) relaxation; (i) promote circulation, therefore, healing: (j) preserve memory of normal movement patterns; and (k) psychological. ⊃ active assisted movement, active movement, continuous passive motion, movement classification, resisted movement.

passive neck flexion (PNF) a neurodynamic test that tests the spinal cord, meninges of the lumbar spine and sciatic nerve. The test is performed supine and the patient's head is flexed passively by the clinician. A normal response would be a full, pain-free movement. Sensitizing tests include straight leg raise and upper limb neurodynamic tests. The test evaluates all levels of the spine and should be incorporated in all cervical, thoracic and lumbar spine examinations. The test is performed in the sitting position and incorporates cervical, thoracic and lumbar flexion. Sensitized by, for example, knee extension and ankle dorsiflexion. ⊃ neurodynamic testing.

passive position the position of the eyes when they are only under the control of the postural and fixation reflexes, but not the fusion reflex, as, for example, when one eye is covered and the other is fixating an object. ⊃ heterophoria.

passive stretching stretching of a body part by use of a force other than tension in the antagonist muscles, e.g. by an examiner without assistance from the athlete.

passwords entry is forbidden into many computer-controlled systems unless a particular password has been entered. Passwords are frequently graded, so that limited access to the system is allowed by some passwords but unlimited access is provided by other passwords.

paste in pharmacy, a semi-solid preparation that is applied externally.

Paterson-Parker system a method of introducing radioactive sources during brachytherapy for gynaecological applications using caesium-137 (^{137}Cs) needles and tubes.

Pasteurella *n* (L Pasteur, French chemist, pathologist, 1822–1895) a genus of Gram negative, facultative anaerobic bacteria that causes infection in humans and domestic animals. Humans may be infected through animal bites and scratches. ⊃ *Francisella, Yersinia.*

pasteurization *n* a process whereby pathogenic organisms in fluid (especially milk) are killed by heat. *flash method of pasteurization* (HT, ST—high temperature short time), the fluid is heated to 72°C, maintained at this temperature for 15 s, then rapidly cooled, *holder method of pasteurization* the fluid is heated to 63–65.5°C, maintained at this temperature for 30 min then rapidly cooled.

Patau's syndrome (K Patau, German/American geneticist, 20th century) trisomy 13. An autosomal trisomy of chromosomes in group D (13–15) but usually chromosome 13. Closely associated with severe learning disability. Numerous physical defects include microcephaly, neural tube defect, coloboma, cleft lip and palate, polydactaly, cardiac defects and abnormalities of the genitalia. Most infants die during the first few months of life.

patch test a skin test for type IV (delayed-type) hypersensitivity to allergens, which are incorporated into an adhesive patch applied to the skin. Forty-eight hours after application the skin under the patch is examined for signs of redness and swelling. Comparison is made against a negative control containing a neutral non-allergenic compound.

patella *n* a triangular, sesamoid bone present in the patellar tendon of the quadriceps femoris muscle; the kneecap—**patellae** *pl*, **patellar** *adj*. ⊃ Colour Section Figure 2.

patella tendon (*syn.* patellar ligament) the strong flat fibrous band that runs from the lower margin of the patella to the tibial tubercle (tuberosity). The more superficial fibres are in fact continuous over the front of the patella with the quadriceps tendon, effectively providing insertion of the quadriceps onto the tibia. Injury is seen in jumping sports.

patella alta an abnormally high patella in relation to the femur; it may result in subluxation and dislocation of patella.

patella baja an abnormally low patella.

patellar dislocation/subluxation instability of the patello-femoral joint, whereby the patella usually dislocates laterally.

patellar reflex a deep tendon reflex. Also called the knee jerk reflex. ⊃ knee jerk.

patellar tap test a test to determine the presence of an effusion at the knee joint. It is performed with the patient in the supine position. Any excess fluid is squeezed out of the suprapatellar pouch by sliding the index finger and thumb from 15 cm above the knee to the level of the upper border of the patella. Then place the tips of the thumb and three fingers of the free hand squarely on the patella and jerk it quickly downwards. The abnormal finding of a 'click' sound indicates the presence of effusion. The test will be negative if the effusion is gross and tense, e.g. a haemarthrosis of the knee (blood within the joint) following an anterior cruciate rupture.

patellar tendonitis (tendinitis) inflammation of the patellar tendon. Causes include a change in training (intensity, frequency or type, e.g. more repetitive running on a hard surface), poor muscle strength and altered biomechanics at the knee. This results in pain and swelling over the tendon, especially after activity. Common in jumping sports such as basketball and athletics (jumper's knee). Treatment is as for any soft tissue injury. Rehabilitation includes changing technique, altering training load, biomechanical assessment and muscle strengthening. ⊃ knee.

patellectomy *n* excision of the patella.

patello-femoral joint (PFJ) the joint between the posterior of the patella and the femur, the patella should track up and down in the channel between the condyles, if it does not it is known as a mal tracking patella. ⊃ mal tracking patella.

patent *adj* open; not closed or occluded—**patency** *n*.

patent or persistent ductus arteriosus failure of the ductus arteriosus to close soon after birth, so that an abnormal shunt between the pulmonary artery and the aorta is preserved. If spontaneous closure does not occur, surgical correction is undertaken. Minimally invasive surgical techniques are increasingly used to close the defect. ⊃ Colour Section Figure 33.

patent interventricular communication a congenital defect in the dividing wall between the right and left ventricle of the heart. ⊃ venticular septal defect.

paternalism *n* over-protective or restricting, such as withholding information about potential risks of healthcare interventions, or well-meaning rules and regulations that reduce individual autonomy.

PATF *abbr* professionally applied topical fluoride.

path/o- a prefix that means 'disease', e.g. *pathophysiology*.

path of insertion and withdrawal in dentistry, the path along which a prefabricated restoration (e.g. crown) may be inserted into, and withdrawn from, a preparation.

path of insertion (path of placement) in dentistry, the direction followed by a prosthesis on insertion. The path is from the first contact of a removable prosthesis with the supporting tissues until it is completely seated.

pathogen *n* a disease-producing agent, usually applied to a living agent, such as a bacterium—**pathogenic** *adj*, **pathogenicity** *n*.

pathogenesis *n* the origin and development of disease—**pathogenetic** *adj*.

pathogenicity *n* the capacity to cause disease.

pathognomonic *adj* characteristic of or peculiar to a disease.

pathological fracture ⊃ fracture.

pathology *n* the science which deals with the cause and nature of disease—**pathological** *adj*, **pathologically** *adv*.

pathophobia *n* a morbid dread of disease—**pathophobic** *adj*.

pathophysiology *n* the science that deals with abnormal functioning of the human being—**pathophysiological** *adj*, **pathophysiologically** *adv*.

-pathy a suffix that means 'disease', e.g. *neuropathy*.

patient advocacy liaison service (PALS) an advocacy service to patients in NHS and Primary Care Trusts, representing their concerns and complaints to the relevant department within the trust.

patient allocation an approach to organizing nursing care introduced in the 1970s to enable nurses to focus on caring for individual patients/clients rather than a range of tasks. Nurses were allocated specific patients/clients to care for. The aim was to provide continuity of care; however, both the nursing hierarchy and relationships between charge nurses/ward sisters and other nurses remained the same and essentially task allocation continued but for smaller groups of patients/clients. ⊃ named nurse, primary nursing, task allocation, team nursing.

patient-centred medicine an approach to medicine where the views, opinions and values of patients and clients are central. The professional relinquishes control so that power within the relationship can be shared. ⊃ professional–patient relationship.

patient/client records a general term for all the health-related records held for a particular person, e.g. nursing care plan, primary care records, hospital notes. ⊃ patient held records, multidisciplinary records.

patient compliance a term used when a patient takes the prescribed drug, in the prescribed dose, at the prescribed time and by the prescribed route. ⊃ concordance, non-compliance *opp*.

O

P

patient contour the shape of a cross-section of a patient when they are initially positioned prior to radiotherapy treatment. ◌ contouring device.

patient controlled analgesia (PCA) equipment that enables patients to control the delivery of analgesic drugs, (within prescribed limits). Usually via an intravenous line, but patient controlled epidural analgesia (PCEA) may be suitable in some situations. ◌ analgesia, epidural.

patient dosimetry the measure of dose delivered to the clinical target volume.

patient held records those health records held by individual patients.

patient immobilization equipment to enable a patient to remain still during treatment or examination including, patient shells, effervescent materials, vacuum bags, bite blocks, breast boards, foam pads, sandbags.

patient participation nurses are encouraged to interact with patients, especially in the initial assessment interview, to support, prompt, reflect and help them to give their perception of their current health problem. Identification of problems with everyday living, actual and anticipated, goal setting and interventions to achieve the goal, all require patient participation, which is a criterion of good nursing practice.

patients' forum a statutory and independent body comprising patients who will represent the views of patients about how their local NHS services are run.

patient shell a clear plastic structure which is worn by the patient to enable accurate localization, patient position, patient contour, beam exit and entry points and a base for additional build-up material and shielding.

patriarchy *n* a community or family where the oldest male (father) dominates, controls and is the highest authority.

patrix in dentistry, the 'male' portion of a precision attachment that interlocks with the matrix.

pattern a form, generally in wax, that is made to be invested and so produce a mould for the 'lost wax' casting technique.

pattern, A (*syn* A syndrome) a neuromuscular anomaly of the eyes characterized by an increase in exotropia when the eyes fixate downward, or increase in esotropia when the eyes fixate upward. Upgaze and downgaze are usually measured at 25 degrees from the horizontal. ◌ strabismus (convergent strabismus, divergent strabismus).

pattern, checkerboard a square set of equal size black and white squares placed adjacent to one another. It is used to test visual acuity. The common way of using this pattern is to present it in the form of a square diamond made up of four smaller diamonds. Three of these are composed of a pattern of much smaller squares than the fourth. Resolution of the pattern with larger squares consists in indicating where it is located (top, bottom, right or left) while the other three squares appear as a uniform grey. This acuity test is less dependent on cognitive factors than letters. ◌ Snellen test type, test type, visual acuity.

pattern of distribution in statistics looks at the frequency that a qualitative result occurs.

pattern, V (*syn* V syndrome) a neuromuscular anomaly of the eyes characterized by an increase in exotropia when the eyes rotate upward, or increase in esotropia when the eyes rotate downward. ◌ strabismus (convergent strabismus, divergent strabismus).

pattern, X a neuromuscular anomaly in which the visual axes are more divergent when the eyes fixate upward and downward, as compared to the primary position of gaze.

patulous *adj* opened out; expanded.

Paul–Bunnell test (J Paul, American physician, 1893–1971; W Bunnell, American pathologist, 1895–1979) a serological test used in the diagnosis of infectious mononucleosis.

pavement epithelium ◌ squamous (pavement) epithelium.

pavementation the process in which white blood cells (leucocytes) adhere to the endothelial lining of blood vessels when blood flow slows during the inflammatory response.

Pawlik's manoeuvre a rarely used single-hand palpation method that determines the size of the fetal head, the degree of flexion and mobility.

PBD *abbr* peak bone density.

PBI *abbr* papillary bleeding index.

PBL *abbr* problem-based learning.

PBM *abbr* peak bone mass.

PBMC *abbr* peripheral blood mononuclear cells.

PCA(S) *abbr* **1.** patient controlled analgesia (system). **2.** posterior communicating artery.

PCEA *abbr* patient controlled epidural analgesia.

PCI *abbr* percutaneous coronary intervention.

PCL *abbr* posterior cruciate ligament.

PCM *abbr* protein calorie malnutrition.

PCO_2 *abbr* the partial pressure of carbon dioxide, for example in atmospheric or expired air.

PCOS *abbr* polycystic ovary syndrome.

PCP *abbr* *Pneumocystis* pneumonia.

PCr *abbr* phosphocreatine. ◌ creatine phosphate.

PCR *abbr* **1.** plaque control record. **2.** polymerase chain reaction.

PCT *abbr* Primary Care Trust.

PCV *abbr* packed cell volume.

PD *abbr* interpupillary distance.

PDA *abbr* patent ductus arteriosus.

PDB *abbr* Paget's disease of bone.

PD gauge/meter ◌ pupillometer.

PDGF *abbr* platelet-derived growth factor.

PDH *abbr* pyruvate dehydrogenase.

PDI *abbr* periodontal disease index.

PDP *abbr* personal development plan.

PDR *abbr* proliferative diabetic retinopathy.

PD rule (*syn* pupillometer [although it is an incorrect use of this term, it is frequently used as a synonym]) a ruler calibrated in millimetres used for measuring the interpupillary distance. Some have the zero point in the middle and the gradations on each side to measure two half-distances thus taking into account facial asymmetry. Many PD rules also have facilities for measuring frames. ◌ interpupillary distance, pupillometer.

O
P

PDT *abbr* photodynamic therapy.

PE *abbr* pulmonary embolism.

PEA *acron* **P**ulseless **E**lectrical **A**ctivity.

peak bone density (PBD) or mass (PBM) the greatest bone density achieved by an individual, usually achieved in their late 20s or early 30s. ⟳ bone mineral density (BMD).

peak expiratory flow rate (PEFR) often referred to as peak flow. The greatest flow of air during a forced expiration (starting with the lungs at full capacity), measured with a peak flow meter (Figure P.5). The peak expiratory flow rate is a measure of how quickly a person can exhale the air in the lungs. Peak occurs almost immediately after the start of exhalation. Usually three measurements are taken and the best of these is recorded. It is a useful test of airway function and is used to monitor various respiratory diseases, particularly asthma and chronic obstructive pulmonary disease, and to assess the effects of drug therapy.

peak force the greatest recorded instantaneous force on an object or body (e.g. during gait analysis).

peak mucus day during the menstrual cycle the last day when the cervical mucus is clear, thin, slippery and elastic. This is characteristic of the time around ovulation and can be used retrospectively in some natural family planning methods to identify the period of peak fertility. ⟳ Billings' method, spinnbarkeit.

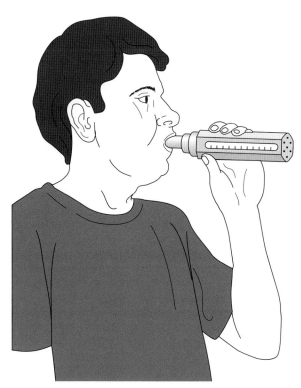

P.5 Peak flow meter (reproduced from Nicol et al 2004 with permission).

peak oxygen consumption/uptake (peak $\dot{V}O_2$) the highest oxygen consumption/uptake measured during a test of physical activity to the point of exhaustion.

peak performance a state in which the person performs to the maximum of their ability, characterized by subjective feelings of confidence, effortlessness and total concentration on the task.

peak post-exercise lactate the highest concentration of lactate in the blood reached during or just after a period of exercise.

peak sensitivity in radiography, the range of wavelengths that a film emulsion is the most sensitive to.

peak torque a measure of isokinetic performance, whereby the maximum 'torque' is achieved.

peak value the maximum value of either positive or negative current or voltage that occurs on an alternating current waveform.

peau d'orange appearance of (usually) the breast when a cancer results in lymphatic obstruction and dimpling at the hair follicles causing the breast to look (literally) like orange skin; usually a sign of locally advanced disease.

pectineus a flat muscle of the medial compartment of the thigh. Its origin is the pectineal line of the pubis and a narrow area of bone below (the superior ramus) and it inserts into the femur below the lesser trochanter. It contracts to adduct, laterally rotate and flex the thigh. ⟳ adductors of the thigh, Colour Section Figure 4.

pectoral *adj* pertaining to the chest.

pectoral girdle the shoulder girdle.

pectoral muscles two muscles of the upper anterior chest. ⟳ pectoralis major, pectoralis minor, Colour Section Figure 4.

pectoralis major a large fan-shaped muscle, its origin is on the clavicle, sternum, costal cartilages (1–6) and the aponeurosis of the abdominal external oblique muscle and it inserts onto the greater tubercle of the humerus. It is a prime mover of arm flexion, medial rotation of the arm and arm adduction.

pectoralis minor a thin, flat muscle under the *p. major*, its origin is on the ribs (3–5) and it inserts onto the coracoid process of the scapula. Contraction draws the scapula down and forwards, and rib cage upwards during a forced inspiration.

pectus *n* the chest.

pectus carinatum (*syn.* pigeon chest) a narrow chest, bulging anteriorly of the sternum (breast bone). May be seen in children with asthma.

pectus excavatum (*syn.* funnel chest) a congenital deformity in which the sternum (breast bone) is depressed towards the spine.

ped- a prefix that means 'foot', e.g. *pedometer*.

pedal *adj* pertaining to the foot.

pedal pulse the dorsalis pedis artery palpated on the dorsum of the foot. Used to check circulation to the foot in peripheral vascular disease, leg trauma and following vascular surgery.

pedicle *n* a stalk, e.g. the narrow part by which a tumour is attached to the surrounding structures.

O
P

pediculosis *n* infestation with lice (pediculi).

Pediculus *n* a genus of parasitic insects (lice) important as vectors of disease. *Pediculus humanus capitis* the head louse. ➲ Colour Section Figure 96. *Pediculus corporis* the body louse. *Pediculus* (more correctly, *Phthirus*) *pubis* the crab or pubic louse. In some regions of the world body lice are responsible for the transmission of typhus and other diseases.

pedometer a small device for counting the number of strides taken in a given period or event. Almost all modern pedometers also provide estimates of distance covered and average speed, based upon a user-entered mean value of stride length.

pedopompholyx *n* ➲ cheiropompholyx.

peduncle *n* a stalk-like structure, such as the *cerebral peduncles* and *cerebellar peduncles*, which are bands of nerves fibres that connect different parts of the brain— **peduncular, pedunculated** *adj*.

pedunculated having a peduncle or stalk.

peeling *n* desquamation.

PEEP *acron* Positive End Expiratory Pressure.

peer a person of equal rank, ability, experience and qualifications.

Peer Assessment Review (PAR) an orthodontic index for measuring the occlusion before and after treatment in order to ascertain the improvement resulting from treatment.

peer group a social group composed of people of a similar age or status.

peer review the process whereby clinicians of equal status review the practice and actions of each other. Also part of the academic process in which research and other material for publication is scrutinized by a group of eminent members of the same profession who judge whether the material is worthy of publication.

peer support support from other members of a group to which one belongs. For example, new patients perceive established patients as providing support. Likewise, health professionals use their peer groups to gain and provide support, particularly in stressful circumstances.

PEFR *abbr* peak expiratory flow rate.

PEG *acron* Percutaneous Endoscopic Gastrostomy.

peg lateral a conical tooth. ➲ tooth.

PEK *abbr* punctate epithelial keratitis.

Pel–Ebstein fever (P Pel, Dutch physician, 1852–1919; W Ebstein, German physician, 1836–1912) recurring bouts of pyrexia in regular sequence found in Hodgkin's disease. A less frequent manifestation with improving treatment.

pellagra *n* a deficiency disease caused by lack of the B vitamin niacin and or the amino acid tryptophan. Syndrome includes: glossitis; dermatitis, especially in skin exposed to sunlight; diarrhoea; mental confusion, depression and eventually dementia; and peripheral neuritis and spinal cord changes (even producing ataxia).

pellet *n* a small pill. ➲ implant.

pellicle 1. a thin layer of membrane, skin or any other substance. **2.** in dentistry, a thin film or 'membrane' of salivary proteins deposited on teeth shortly after cleaning, and which cannot be completely removed by tooth-brushing. It contains no organisms at this stage and covers most of the crown of the tooth. When it has been invaded by microorganisms it is then called plaque.

pelopsia an anomaly of visual perception in which objects appear to be much nearer than they actually are. It may be due to vision in a very clear atmosphere, recent wear of an optical correction, certain mental health disorders, etc. ➲ metamorphopsia, teleopsia.

pelvic *adj* relating to the pelvis.

pelvic bone the hip bone, comprising the ilium, ischium and pubis.

pelvic cavity the cavity formed by the pelvic bones, more particularly the part below the iliopectineal line. The pelvic cavity is roughly funnel shaped and extends from the lower end of the abdominal cavity. The boundaries are: superiorly—it is continuous with the abdominal cavity; anteriorly—the pubic bones; posteriorly—the sacrum and coccyx; laterally—the innominate bones; and inferiorly—the muscles of the pelvic floor. The pelvic cavity contains the following structures: sigmoid colon, rectum and anal canal, some loops of the small intestine, the urinary bladder, lower parts of the ureters and the urethra in the female, the female organs of the reproductive system (uterus, uterine tubes, ovaries and vagina) and in the male, some of the organs of the reproductive system (the prostate gland, seminal vesicles, spermatic cords, deferent ducts (vas deferens), ejaculatory ducts and part of the urethra (common to the reproductive and urinary systems).

pelvic cellulitis ➲ parametritis.

pelvic congestion increase in blood volume supplying the organs in the pelvis; found normally in early pregnancy and just before a woman's period is due. It also occurs in association with pelvic pathology.

pelvic diameter any diameter of the bony pelvis.

pelvic floor a mainly muscular partition with some fascia situated between the pelvic cavity above and the perineum below. The pelvic floor comprises two halves that unite along the midline, it is perforated by the urethra, vagina and anus in female, and the urethra and anus in males. The two muscles are the levator ani and the coccygeus. It supports the pelvic structures and maintains continence. In the female, weakening of the pelvic floor during childbirth, can contribute to urinary incontinence and uterine prolapse.

pelvic floor exercises ➲ Kegel exercises.

pelvic floor repair operation performed to correct genital prolapse. ➲ Manchester repair.

pelvic girdle the bony pelvis comprising two innominate bones, the sacrum and coccyx.

pelvic inflammatory disease (PID) acute or chronic inflammation of the ovaries, uterine (fallopian) tube and uterus. Infection may spread from adjacent pelvic structures including the bowel or appendix or through the cervix from the vagina and may be sexually transmitted. It is characterized by lower abdominal pain, and urgent antibiotic

O
P

treatment is essential if tubal occlusion and infertility are to be prevented.

pelvic inlet brim or entrance to the true pelvis.

pelvic outlet inferior opening of the pelvis bounded by the ischial spines, lower border of the symphysis pubis and sacrococcygeal joint.

pelvic pain syndrome (PPS) pelvic pain which occurs in women but for which no pathological cause is evident.

pelvimeter *n* an instrument especially devised to measure the pelvic diameters for obstetric purposes.

pelvimetry *n* the measurement of the dimensions of the pelvis—**pelvimetric** *adj*.

pelvis *n* (from Latin meaning 'basin') **1.** a basin-shaped cavity, e.g. pelvis of the kidney. ⊃ Colour Section Figure 20. **2.** the bony framework of the lowest part of the trunk. The large bony basin-shaped cavity formed by the innominate bones (hip bones) together with the sacrum and coccyx, containing and protecting the bladder, rectum and, in the female, the organs of generation. It is continuous above with the abdominal cavity. Each innominate bone has three fused components: the ilium with a flared upper rim, the iliac crest, and linked to the sacrum at the sacroiliac joint; the ischium with the socket for the head of the femur (the acetabulum) at the hip joint; and the pubis which is attached to its partner at the pubic symphysis, centre front—**pelvic** *adj*. ⊃ android pelvis, anthropoid pelvis, assessment of pelvis, contracted pelvis, false pelvis, gynaecoid pelvis, inclination of pelvis, Naegele pelvis, platypelloid pelvis, rachitic pelvis, Robert's pelvis, spondylolisthetic pelvis, true pelvis.

pelviureteric junction (PUJ) obstruction a condition, often congenital, resulting in obstruction at the junction of the renal pelvis and proximal ureter.

PEM *abbr* protein-energy malnutrition.

pemphigoid *n* a blistering (bullous) skin eruption, usually in the latter half of life, which is of immune-mediated cause. Histological examination of a blister differentiates it from pemphigus. Treated by systemic corticosteroids. ⊃ bullous pemphigoid.

pemphigoid gestationis (*syn* herpes gestationis) a rare immune-mediated blistering skin condition. It usually occurs in the second trimester and persists into the post natal period, but may develop after the birth. The blisters, which are tense, occur on the periumbilical area and the limbs. Only rarely involves the mucous membranes. Treatment involves systemic corticosteroids. The condition may occur in subsequent pregnancies.

pemphigus *n* a group of rare but serious blistering (bullous) skin conditions with an immune-mediated aetiology. The disease process also affects the mucous membranes, e.g pemphigus vulgaris.

pemphigus vulgaris a blistering (bullous) disease mostly of middle age, of immune-mediated aetiology. The blisters, which are flaccid and fragile, occur on the head and torso with resulting secondary infection and rupture, so that large raw areas develop. Bullae develop also on mucous membranes. The condition is treated by systemic corticosteroids and immunosuppressive drugs such as cyclophosphamide.

penalization a clinical method of treating amblyopia and eccentric fixation in which vision by the fixating eye is decreased by various means (optical overcorrection, atropinization for near vision especially, and neutral density filters) in order to compel the amblyopic eye to fixate. Sometimes the treatment consists of using the amblyopic eye for near vision and the fixating eye for distance vision. ⊃ amblyopia, eccentric fixation, occlusion treatment, pleoptics.

Pendred's syndrome (V Pendred, British physician, 1869–1946) congenital bilateral sensorineural deafness associated with the later development of goitre. There is defective synthesis of thyroxine due to deficiency of an enzyme. Inherited as an autosomal recessive trait.

pendular response a pathological response to the stretch reflex commonly seen in cerebellar disease. When a muscle is stretched by distortion of its tendon, the stretch reflex response is sluggish and is not checked by a reciprocal response in the antagonist muscle; e.g. if the knee jerk is invoked, there will not be one sharp jerk but the leg will swing like a pendulum.

pendulous *adj* hanging down.

pendulous abdomen a relaxed condition of the anterior wall, allowing it to hang down over the pubis. It is often associated with substantial weight loss, following repeated or multiple pregnancies, and other causes of abdominal distension (e.g. severe ascites). May require plastic surgery to improve the person's self-esteem and to prevent excoriation between the skin surfaces.

penetrance in genetics, the frequency in which an allele is expressed in the indiviual who has it. If the trait is expressed in the phenotype in 100% of cases it is termed fully penetrant. When expression of the trait is less than 100% it is termed reduced or incomplete penetrance. This can lead to inherited disorders missing or 'skipping' a generation. When a person who has the allele, which generally leads to an abnormal phenotype, has a normal phenotype the allele is described as nonpenetrant.

penetrating ulcer an ulcer that is locally invasive.

penetrating wound (*syn.* puncture wound) caused by a sharp, usually slim object, or a missile, which passes through the skin into the tissues beneath.

penetration depth an electrotherapy term. The depth at which 37% of energy applied to an object or body remains (i.e. 63% of applied energy has been absorbed). The extent of absorption of energy by successively deeper levels of body tissue is an exponential function. The actual value will depend on the type and intensity of the energy (e.g. if ultrasound, cold, laser or infrared) and on the type and arrangement of tissue and other structures through which it passes. For example, ultrasound at a frequency of 1 MHz has a greater penetration depth than 3 MHz ultrasound. This is why 3 MHz frequency ultrasound is often chosen to treat superficial tissues and 1 MHz frequency if deeper. To ensure energy reaches deeper tissues the general principles are to

O

P

use a lower frequency ultrasound (e.g. 0.8–1 MHz) and a higher intensity so sufficient energy is available at depth.

-penia a suffix that means 'lack of', e.g. *neutropenia*.

penicillinase ◗ beta (β)-lactamase.

penicillins *npl* a large group of β-lactam antibiotics. Many have activity against a broad range of bacteria (known as broad spectrum antibiotics) but they produce hypersensitivity reactions and many micro-organisms have developed resistance. Some penicillins are β-lactamase resistant. ◗ Appendix 5.

Penicillium *n* a genus of moulds. The hyphae bear spores characteristically arranged like a brush. A common contaminant of food. The species *Penicillium notatum* was shown by Fleming (in 1928) to produce penicillin.

penis *n* the male organ of copulation, it is homologous with the female clitoris. The urethra runs through the penis to the outside and provides passage for both urine and semen. The penis has a root embedded in the perineum and a shaft which terminates at the expanded glans penis. The glans is normally covered with the prepuce (foreskin), a loose double fold of skin. The penis comprises three columns of erectile tissue containing vascular spaces, connective tissue and involuntary muscle. There are two lateral columns, the corpora cavernosa (*sing* corpus cavernosum) and the ventral corpus spongiosum surrounding the urethra. Normally the penis is flaccid but during sexual arousal the vascular spaces fill with blood which causes it to become erect—**penile** *adj*. ◗ Colour Section Figure 16.

pentagastrin *n* a synthetic pentapeptide hormone used in gastric function tests to produce maximal gastric acid secretion. *pentagastrin test* measures gastric acid secretion by oxyntic (parietal) cells in the stomach.

pent/a, pent/o- a prefix that means 'five', e.g. *pentose*.

pentose *n* a five carbon monosaccharide (sugar) such as ribose.

pentose phosphate pathway (PPP) also called the pentose shunt or hexose monophosphate shunt/pathway. A metabolic pathway in which glucose-6-phosphate is oxidized to ribose-5-phosphate (a five-carbon sugar, a pentose) with the generation of nicotinamide adenine dinucleotide phosphate (reduced form) (NADPH), which is required in reductive biosyntheses. Ribose-5-phosphate and related molecules are constituents of many important biological molecules, including coenzyme A, adenosine triphosphate (ATP) and the nucleic acids. ◗ nicotinamide adenine dinucleotide phosphate (NADP/NADPH).

pentosuria excretion of pentose sugars in the urine. It may occur after consuming fruits such as pears. Pentosuria also occurs in an inherited metabolic disorder seen in Ashkenazi Jews; it causes no ill effects.

penumbra the area at the edge of a beam of radiation that receives some but not all of the main beam because it is not practically possible to produce an X-ray beam from a point source. ◗ geometric unsharpness.

pepsin *n* a proteolytic enzyme secreted by the stomach, as the precursor pepsinogen, which hydrolyses proteins to polypeptides. Pepsin activity has an optimum pH of 1.5–2.0.

pepsinogen *n* an inactive proenzyme secreted mainly by the chief cells in the gastric mucosa and converted to pepsin in the acidic environment created by hydrochloric acid secretion in the stomach, or existing pepsin.

peptic *adj* pertaining to pepsin or to digestion generally.

peptic ulcer a non-malignant ulcer in those parts of the digestive tract that are exposed to the gastric secretions; hence usually in the stomach or duodenum but sometimes in the lower oesophagus, in the jejunum following surgical anastomosis to the stomach, or with a Meckel's diverticulum. ◗ duodenal ulcer, gastric ulcer.

peptidase *n* an enzyme that breaks down proteins by splitting peptides into amino acids. ◗ aminopeptidases, carboxypeptidases, dipeptidases.

peptide bond a chemical bond formed during a dehydration synthesis reaction when two amino acids form peptides.

peptides *npl* organic compounds that yield two or more amino acids on hydrolysis; e.g. dipeptides and polypeptides.

peptone a mixture of protein fragments produced by the partial breakdown of a native protein by acid or enzyme.

per- a prefix that means 'by, through', e.g. *percutaneous*.

peralveolar wiring an archaic method of immobilizing a fractured maxilla by the use of stainless steel wire which traverses the alveolar process. The projecting ends are then passed over a splint and tightened. The technique is useful in the treatment of fractured edentulous jaws.

perceived ability a person's perception of their specific abilities within a given domain, such as in football versus another sport.

percentage depth dose in radiotherapy, the ratio of the absorbed dose at any given point to the absorbed dose on the beam axis at the depth of maximum dose expressed as a percentage.

percentage regulation a calculation to determine the efficiency of a transformer, the lower the percentage the more efficient is the transformer. ◗ regulation in a transformer.

percept *n* the mental product of a sensation; a sensation plus memories of similar sensations and their relationships.

perceptibility the point at which an image can be clearly seen, when contrast is equal to, or greater than the contrast threshold.

perceptibility curve a curve produced from measurable data after a phantom has been radiographed and a number of people have recorded the contrast observed at various exposure levels.

perception *n* the act or process of becoming aware of internal or external sensory stimuli or events, involving the meaningful organization and interpretation of those stimuli. In psychology, perception also applies to evaluations of one's own and others' internal states and beliefs as well as sensory stimuli and a person's perceptions are not necessarily identical to the stimulus object or event being perceived. For example, a person's perceptions of their ability might not match their actual ability. Perception is to be distinguished from sensation which refers to the subjective experience that results from excitation of the sensory apparatus without any interpretation or imposition of meaning.

perceptive hearing loss/deafness ⟳ sensorineural hearing loss (SNHL)/deafness.

perceptual motor skill any skill involving the interaction and integration of perceptual processes and voluntary physical movement, such as the ability to perform a gymnastic routine.

perch sitting sitting, with feet flat on the floor, on the edge of a high stool (called a perching stool) that has a slightly downward angulated seat that helps to attain/maintain the pelvis in a position of anterior tilt and thus encourages extensor activity in the upper body. Patients can be sat on a perching stool whilst carrying out activities of daily living and thus maximize the therapeutic effect.

percolation in dentistry, a deprecated term for microleakage.

percussion *n* tapping to determine the resonance or dullness of the area examined. Normally a finger of the left hand is laid on the patient's skin and the middle finger of the right hand (plexor) is used to strike the left finger. Used in dentistry, as a method of diagnosis by tapping a tooth, teeth or an implant to elicit the degree of sensitivity of supporting tissues (periodontal or bone) or any change from normal in the sound produced.

percutaneous *adj* through the skin.

percutaneous coronary interventions (PCI) interventions used to reopen coronary arteries stenosed by the build up of atheromatous plaques. It is used in the treatment of patients with stable angina and unstable angina and recent myocardial infarction. The term generally refers to balloon angioplasty, which is often combined with stent insertion, but other interventions include the use of lasers and other treatments to reduce risk of vessel restenosis. ⟳ percutaneous transluminal coronary angioplasty.

percutaneous endoscopic gastrostomy (PEG) gastrostomy tube inserted through the abdominal wall after the stomach has been distended endoscopically (Figure P.6). Used for long term enteral feeding.

percutaneous epididymal sperm aspiration (PESA) technique used in assisted conception. ⟳ microsurgical epididymal sperm aspiration (MESA).

percutaneous myocardial revascularization a treatment for angina. A catheter with laser energy source is introduced into the heart via the femoral artery. The laser is used to produce channels through to the myocardium, thus allowing more oxygenated blood to reach the myocardium.

percutaneous nephrolithotomy a minimally invasive technique where the kidney pelvis is punctured using X-ray control. A guide wire is inserted through which the stone is removed using a nephroscope (endoscope). ⟳ nephrolithotomy.

percutaneous transhepatic cholangiography (PTC) a radiographic image of the biliary tree achieved by injecting contrast agent though the abdominal wall directly into a small hepatic bile duct. ⟳ cholangiography.

percutaneous transluminal angioplasty (PTA) a balloon is passed into a stenosed artery and inflated with contrast agent; it presses the atheroma against the vessel wall, thereby increasing the diameter of the lumen. The technique is commonly used to reopen coronary arteries, renal arteries,

O
P

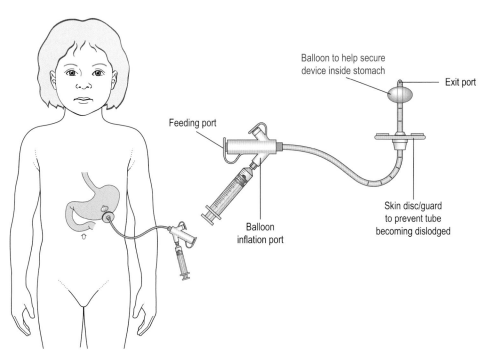

P.6 Percutaneous endoscopic gastrostomy (adapted from Huband & Trigg 2000 with permission).

Balloon to help secure device inside stomach

Exit port

Feeding port

Balloon inflation port

Skin disc/guard to prevent tube becoming dislodged

those in the leg and the carotid artery. A stent is often inserted at the same time in order to prevent the artery becoming occluded again.

percutaneous transluminal coronary angioplasty (PTCA) a procedure used in the treatment of coronary artery disease. A balloon tipped catheter is used to dilate a stenosed coronary artery. The balloon is inflated several times to compress atheromatous plaques against the walls of the vessel. Stent insertion to prevent restenosis is normally performed but not in all cases.

percutaneous umbilical cord blood sampling (PUBS) ➲ cordocentesis.

perforation *n* **1.** a hole in a previously intact sheet of tissue. Used in reference to perforation of the tympanic membrane, or the wall of the stomach or gut, constituting a surgical emergency. **2.** in endodontics, a procedural error in which a hole is created in a tooth or root during root canal treatment. *lateral perforation* a puncture hole created in the side of a root. *furcal perforation* a hole created in the floor of a pulp chamber. *strip perforation* a long, narrow hole created in the wall of a root by over enlargement of the root canal.

perforin a protein produced by cytotoxic T cells (CD8 cells) and natural killer (NK) cells. It forms a pore in the membrane of targeted cells leading to lysis and apoptosis (cell death).

performance the act of producing a co-ordinated sequence of behaviours. ➲ ability, skill.

performance profiling a method for helping athletes to identify their strengths and weaknesses in order to encourage them to be fully involved in decisions about developing appropriate training programmes to enhance their performance. It typically involves asking athletes to identify what they think are the major characteristics of an elite performer in their sport and then to rate themselves on those characteristics.

performance appraisal or review a formal procedure whereby an appraiser (manager) systematically reviews the role performance of the appraisee against a set of competencies and they jointly set goals for the future.

performance components the basic skills required to perform activities of daily living, including sensorimotor, cognitive, psychosocial, psychological and spiritual skills.

performance genes the potential uses of genetic profiling and gene therapy within sport remain experimental and controversial. Suggested applications include: (a) identification of potential athletes by the presence of the so-called performance genes, which may enable an athlete to perform at a higher level by their influence on muscle metabolism and endurance; (b) use as a screening tool to identify athletes with particular body shape, e.g. tall athletes for basketball. This could result in discrimination and have implications for the funding for young athletes, should funding be withheld from those who 'fail' to have the ideal body habitus; (c) identification of those athletes who have a genetic predisposition to sports-related injury. Other moral dilemmas exist in this area. Should the limited funding for

genetic research be used to enhance sports performance at the expense of research into disease prevention? Should there be a limit on opportunities within sport and exercise because the young person does not have the ideal 'genetic makeup'? The World Anti-Doping Agency (WADA) and the International Olympic Committee (IOC) have recently included the non-therapeutic use of genes, genetic elements and/or cells that have the capacity to enhance athletic performance in their list of proscribed substances and methods. They will continue to monitor the use of genetic testing and genetic information for identifying or selecting athletes, with a view to developing policies and guidelines for sports organizations and athletes. ➲ human enhancement technologies (HET).

performance goal 1. a goal focused on gaining favourable judgements or avoiding unfavourable judgements by others. **2.** a goal that specifies the achievement of an endproduct of performance that is relatively independent of the performance of other people, such as running a race in a certain time rather than beating others. ➲ ego involvement, learning goal, process goal, outcome goal.

performance indicators (PIs) quantitative measures of the activities and resources used in healthcare delivery.

perfusion 1. the flow of blood through tissues and organs, such as the skin, kidney or lung. ➲ blood flow. **2.** fluid and or drugs intended for a specific organ are injected into the bloodstream.

perfusionist a health professional qualified and registered to assist in procedures that involve extracorporeal circulation techniques, such as during cardiac bypass surgery, or extracorporeal membrane oxygenation in critically ill patients.

perfusion scan a radiographic technique used to assess the blood flow (perfusion) through an organ. It involves the injection of radioactive tracers. It is commonly performed to detect areas in the lung with reduced perfusion, such as caused by pulmonary emboli. A perfusion scan may be combined with a ventilation scan in which the radioactive tracer is inhaled to identify areas of the lung that are not inflated, and to calculate the ventilation perfusion ratio. ➲ ventilation–perfusion (V/Q) ratio, ventilation–perfusion scanning.

peri- a prefix that means 'around', e.g. *pericolic*.

perialveolar wire ➲ wiring.

perianal *adj* surrounding the anus.

perianal abscess also known as anorectal abscess. A cavity containing pus, which may be caused when micro-organisms infect the anal gland or enter a tear in the anal mucosa. Abscess formation may also be associated with Crohn's disease. The abscess can track further into the perianal region or into the ischiorectal fossae. It may be associated with fistulae formation. Patients report extreme pain in the perianal region, especially on sitting and during defecation.

periapical *adj* surrounding an apex. Relating to the tissues and structures around the apex of a tooth root, including the connective tissue and alveolar bone.

periapical abscess acute or chronic infection of the periapical tissues. There is pus formation at the tooth apex, and it generally results from death of the pulp tissue. The abscess may discharge into the mouth or into a maxillary air-sinus; cause cellulitis of the face; or spread to alveolar bone.

periapical curettage ⮑ apical curettage.

periapical film a small radiographic film in a waterproof envelope that is placed inside the mouth to radiograph individual teeth.

periapical projection in dental radiography, an intraoral technique for demonstrating the anatomy of the tooth and the adjacent supporting bone.

periapical radiograph ⮑ periapical projection.

periarterial *adj* surrounding an artery.

periarteritis *n* inflammation of the outer sheath of an artery and the periarterial tissue.

periarteritis nodosa ⮑ polyarteritis nodosa (PAN).

periarthritis *n* inflammation of the tissues and structures surrounding a joint. Sometimes applied to frozen shoulder.

periarticular *adj* surrounding a joint.

peribulbar *adj* around the eyeball inside the orbit.

pericardectomy *n* surgical removal of the pericardium, thickened from chronic inflammation (pericarditis) and restricting the pumping action of the heart.

pericardiocentesis *n* aspiration of fluid from the pericardial sac.

pericardiorrhaphy surgical repair of the pericardium, includes traumatic wounds and incisions made during planned surgery.

pericardiotomy an incision into the pericardium.

pericarditis *n* inflammation of the pericardial covering of the heart, it may be acute or chronic. It may or may not be accompanied by an effusion, which in extreme cases can cause tamponade, a pericardial friction rub, or the formation of adhesions between the two layers. Causes of acute pericarditis include injury, viral infection, myocardial infarction, uraemia, malignant disease and connective tissue diseases, (e.g. systemic lupus erythematosus). Chronic pericarditis is associated with bacterial infections, including tuberculosis, with rheumatoid arthritis, or may follow viral pericarditis ⮑ pericardectomy.

pericardium *n* comprises two sacs—the outer fibrous sac and an inner double serous membranous sac which envelops the heart. The fibrous sac is formed from the same tissue as the tunica adventitia of the great vessels and it is attached to the diaphragm. The fibrous sac stops overdistention as the heart fills with blood. The inner layer of the serous membrane in contact with the heart is called visceral pericardium (or epicardium); that reflected to form the outer serous membrane, which lines the fibrous sac, is called the parietal pericardium. Between the two serous membranes is a potential space, the pericardial cavity, which normally contains a thin film of serous fluid, which allows the two membranes to move easily when the heart beats—**pericardial** *adj*.

perichondritis inflammation of the fibrous connective tissue surrounding cartilage (the perichondrium). It usually refers to that affecting the outer/external ear. Trauma to the ear leading to haematoma formation can cause perichondritis and this can result in a 'cauliflower ear' deformity.

perichondrium *n* the fibrous tissue covering of cartilage (except articular cartilage in synovial joints). It has two layers, an outer layer of dense connective tissue and an inner layer from which new cartilage is produced—**perichondrial** *adj*.

pericision in dentistry, the sectioning of fibres of the periodontal ligament as an adjunct to the orthodontic movement of teeth.

pericolic *adj* around the colon, such as a *pericolic abscess* that can occur in diverticulitis.

pericorneal plexus a network of vessels situated around the corneal limbus of the eye and formed by the anastomosing of the episcleral arteries (branches of the anterior ciliary arteries) and the conjunctival arteries. It forms a series of arcades parallel to the corneal margin. This plexus is arranged in two layers: a superficial conjunctival pericorneal plexus liable to injection in inflammation of the superficial cornea or conjunctiva (conjunctival injection) and a deep episcleral plexus liable to injection in diseases of the iris, ciliary body or deep portion of the cornea, or angle-closure glaucoma (ciliary injection). ⮑ anterior ciliary vein, ciliary arteries, ciliary injection, conjunctival injection.

pericoronitis an acute inflammation of the soft tissue surrounding the crown of a partially erupted tooth.

pericranium *n* the periosteal covering of the cranium—**pericranial** *adj*.

pericystitis inflammation involving the tissues surrounding the bladder. ⮑ pelvic inflammatory disease.

perifollicular *adj* around a follicle.

perihepatitis inflammation involving the capsule of the liver and surrounding tissues.

peri-implantitis in dentistry, the inflammatory reactions with loss of supporting bone in the tissues surrounding a functioning implant.

perikymata the grooves on the surface of enamel running at right angles to the long axis of the tooth where the enamel striae of Retzius reach the surface.

perilymph *n* the fluid contained in the inner ear, between the membranous and bony labyrinth. ⮑ endolymph.

perimenopause the period of time characterized by increasing irregularity of the menstrual cycle and menopausal symptoms such as hot flushes that occurs before the menopause (the last menstrual period), and the year following the last menstrual period.

perimeter an instrument for measuring the angular extent and the characteristics (e.g. presence of scotoma) of the visual field. ⮑ campimeter, visual field.

perimetritis inflammation of the outer layer of the uterus the perimetrium

perimetrium *n* the peritoneal covering of the uterus—**perimetrial** *adj*.

perimetry *n* measurement and documentation of the field of vision, usually for the purpose of detecting anomalies in the visual pathway. ➲ glaucoma, perimeter, visual field, visual pathway.

perimolysis the mechanical wearing down of tooth enamel, or the damage caused by chemicals. For instance the frequent vomiting and exposure to acid vomit in eating disorders.

perimysium the fibrous connective tissue that covers a bundle of muscle fibres. ➲ endomysium, epimysium.

perinatal *adj* pertaining to the period around birth. The weeks before a birth, the birth and the week following. ➲ mortality.

perineal body the wedge-shaped mass of muscle and fascia situated between the scrotum and rectum in males and between the vagina and rectum in females. ➲ perineum.

perineal repair suturing of perineal lacerations or episiotomy by midwives trained and assessed as competent, or by the doctor. It involves inserting a tampon to ensure a clear visual field, followed by suturing of the vagina, commencing just above the apex of the incision or tear, with interrupted sutures; deep and superficial muscle layers, by starting in the centre of the incision to give good approximation; and perineal skin; the tampon is removed and a gloved finger is passed into the rectum to ensure no sutures encroach into it.

perineal tear a spontaneous tear occurring in the perineum during childbirth. They are classified in degrees. *first degree tear* a tear that only affects the fourchette; *second degree tear* one that involves the fourchette and the superficial muscles of the perineum (e.g. transverse perineal muscles); *third degree tear* more extensive with damage as before plus damage to the anal sphincter; and *fourth degree tear* one in which the tear involves all the structures as before but extends to involve the rectal mucosa.

perineo- a prefix/combining that means 'perineum', e.g. *perineorrhaphy*.

perineometer *n* a pressure gauge inserted into the vagina to register the strength of contraction in the pelvic floor muscles.

perineoplasty a plastic operation to enlarge the vaginal introitus.

perineorrhaphy *n* a surgical procedure for the suture of a perineal tear, an incision or defect.

perineotomy *n* episiotomy.

perinephric *adj* surrounding the kidney.

perinephric abscess an abscess in the fat around the kidney, it is usually secondary to an abscess within the kidney tissue.

perineum *n* the area of the body, which extends backwards from the pubic arch to the end of the coccyx and is bounded laterally by the ischial tuberosities. It is formed from the muscles and fascia situated at the pelvic outlet, and can be divided into the anterior urogenital triangle and the posterior anal triangle. It overlies the levator ani and coccygenus muscles of the pelvic floor and helps to support the pelvic structures—**perineal** *adj*. ➲ perineal body.

perineurium *n* connective tissue enclosing a bundle of nerve fibres. ➲ endoneurium, epineurium.

period 1. the number of seconds taken to complete one cycle of alternating current. **2.** in ultrasound the length of time required for one oscillation to occur.

periodic apnoea of the newborn, periodic breathing a period of apnoea in a newborn full term infant of 5–10 seconds followed by a period of hyperventilation at a rate of 50–60 breaths a minute, for a period of 10–15 seconds. The overall respiratory rate remains between 30 and 40 breaths per minute.

periodic table a list of the 103 elements with the number of electron shells shown horizontally and the chemical properties, that is the number of electrons in the outer shell grouped vertically.

periodization a planned variation to a training programme over a period of time, so that the athlete/sportsperson achieves optimal adaptive potential just before the race, game or other event.

periodontal 1. relating to the supporting structures of a tooth. **2.** pertaining to the periodontium.

periodontal abscess an abscess in the periodontal tissues which occurs when there is an increase in the concentration or virulence of plaque micro-organisms. ➲ phoenix abscess.

periodontal curette ➲ periodontal instruments.

periodontal cyst a cyst of inflammatory origin around the root (usually the root apex) of a pulpless tooth.

periodontal disease an inflammatory disease of the supporting tissues of the teeth. One of the most common diseases of modern civilization. In advanced cases, the patient complains of mobile teeth, teeth drifting apart, spontaneous gingival bleeding, recurrent abscess formation, difficulty in eating due to pain and mobility of teeth, sensitive teeth when being cleaned and halitosis. ➲ periodontitis.

periodontal disease (Ramfjord) index (PDI) ➲ index (dental).

periodontal dressing (or pack) a dressing designed to protect a wound following periodontal operations and to promote healing.

periodontal–endodontic procedures treatment involving both the periodontal and pulpal tissue, necessary because of a combined lesion.

periodontal fibres ➲ fibre, Sharpey's fibres.

periodontal flap operation lifting of a gingival flap to gain access for thorough instrumentation of the root surfaces to remove tooth deposits and infected cementum from the tooth surface.

periodontal hoe ➲ periodontal instruments.

periodontal (Russell) index ➲ index (dental).

periodontal instruments the instruments used to remove plaque, calculus, debris and stains from teeth, and in the treatment of periodontal disease. *electrosurgery unit* diathermy apparatus using high-frequency electric currents. May be bipolar, when the current passes between the tips of two electrodes, or unipolar, when the patient holds one electrode and the current passes from another electrode to the gingivae. *gingivectomy knife* a knife designed for gingivectomy procedures. Examples include: (a) Blake's universal gingivectomy knife—a hand instrument with a thin handle ending in a screw device to hold the tip portion of a scalpel blade at an angle to the handle. A small hexagonal spanner or key operates the screw when changing the blades. The projecting, non-cutting part of the blade is snapped off by pliers. Used in sets of four to cover all angles of approach to the gingivae. (b) Fish gingivectomy knife—a single-ended hand instrument with a fixed, double-edged sharp blade set at an angle to the handle. *Jacquette hand scaler* a sickle-shaped end with sharp edges on both sides of its cutting blade. Usually in sets of three and used to remove calculus from a tooth surface. *periodontal curette* may be universal or area specific. Hand instruments with hollow ground blade like a spoon-shaped excavator. Used to plane root surfaces. *periodontal file* an instrument with multiple, straight cutting edges used either for crushing calculus (to make removal with other instruments easier) or for removing over-burnished calculus. *periodontal hoe* a hand instrument with small blade at right angles to the shank; usually in sets of four. Used with a pulling motion. *periodontal probe* (*pocket measuring probe*) a blunt-ended graduated probe used to measure the depth of a periodontal pocket. *pocket marking forceps* left and right forceps with a pin on one blade to perforate the side of a pocket and thus mark its depth. ⊃ scaler.

periodontal ligament previously known as periodontal membrane. The system of connective tissue fibres that attach the cementum of a tooth root to the alveolar bone. It contains blood vessels, nerves and fibres that support the tooth in its socket so allowing slight mobility. The main groups of bundles of collagen fibres forming the ligament are the oblique, apical, cervical, transeptal, inter-radicular and circular. Chronic periodontitis causes destruction of the ligament, loss of bone and hence increased mobility of the tooth.

periodontal membrane ⊃ periodontal ligament.

periodontal pocket an abnormal deepening of the gingival sulcus as supporting tissues are lost. ⊃ periodontal instruments.

periodontal space in radiology, the space seen on a radiograph between the cementum on the tooth root and alveolar bone.

periodontics *n* branch of dental science concerned with the study, prevention and treatment of diseases and conditions of tissues surrounding and supporting the teeth and gingivae.

periodontitis *n* inflammation of the periodontal ligament and supporting teeth tissues with ensuing loss of bone and the periodontal ligament. Caused by bacteria. It is the main cause of loss of teeth in adults. *aggressive periodontitis* juvenile periodontitis or early-onset periodontitis. A relatively uncommon disease having an onset, classically, around adolescence. Maybe localized, usually affecting incisors and molars or more generalized. Progression of the disease is usually rapid. *necrotizing ulcerative periodontitis* possible sequela of longstanding necrotizing ulcerative gingivitis (NUG) but with involvement and necrosis of the alveolar bone as well as the overlying gingiva. Has been associated with specific microorganisms such as *Porphyromonas gingivalis* and *Prevotella intermedius* and systemic medical conditions such as HIV disease. *prepubertal periodontitis* a form of periodontitis which affects the primary dentition and is often associated with syndromes such as Papillon-Lefèvre or leucocyte deficiency syndrome.

periodontium *n* collective name given to the tissues supporting a tooth and comprising the gingivae, periodontal ligament, cementum and surrounding alveolar bone.

periodontology the study of the healthy and diseased periodontium.

periodontometer an instrument used to measure the degree of movement in a tooth.

perioperative *adj* refers to the period during which a surgical operation is carried out, as well as to the pre- and postoperative periods.

perioral *adj* around the mouth.

periosteal pertaining to or composed of periosteum.

periosteal elevator in dentistry, a hand instrument, usually double ended, used to separate the periosteum from the underlying bone.

periosteum *n* the membrane which covers a bone. In long bones only the shaft as far as the epiphysis is covered. It protects and allows regeneration—**periosteal** *adj*. ⊃ endosteum.

periostitis *n* inflammation of the periosteum. *diffuse periostitis* that involving the periosteum of long bones. *haemorrhagic periostitis* inflammation of the periosteum accompanied by bleeding between the periosteum and the bone.

peripartum *n* at the time of delivery. A precise word for what is more commonly called perinatal.

peripheral *adj* relating to the outer parts of any structure.

peripheral blood mononuclear cells (PBMC) the group of leucocytes that includes all the monocytes and lymphocytes, but excludes granulocytes.

peripheral cyanosis ⊃ cyanosis.

peripheral nervous system (PNS) that part of the nervous system outside the central nervous system. It includes all the motor and sensory peripheral nerve fibres and ganglia that are outside the brain and spinal cord. The PNS comprises 12 pairs of cranial nerves and 33 pairs of spinal nerves. The peripheral nervous system can be further subdivided into the sensory division and the motor division. The latter is in turn divided into the voluntary somatic nervous system and the involuntary autonomic system, which is divided into the sympathetic and parasympathetic nervous systems. Sometimes the term PNS is applied to those nerves which supply the musculoskeletal system and surrounding tissues to differentiate it from the autonomic nervous system.

peripheral neuropathy a disease affecting the peripheral nerves. Also called polyneuropathy or multiple neuropathy. ⊃ neuropathy, polyneuropathy.

peripheral resistance (PR) the sum total of resistance to blood flow in the systemic circulation, mostly located in the arterioles, dependent on the constriction/relaxation of the smooth muscle in their walls. The balance between

O
P

cardiac output and total peripheral resistance determines the arterial blood pressure (BP), and physiological adjustments of either or both are the means of maintaining BP despite variations in local vasodilation/vasoconstriction in different organs and tissues.

peripheral vascular disease (PVD) any abnormal condition arising in the blood vessels outside the heart, the main one being atherosclerosis. Associated with smoking, diabetes and hypertension. It is characterized by aching in the calf or buttock during exercise, eventual rest pain, numbness, diminished or absent pulses distal to the diseased area, pallor and cooling of the skin and areas with no hair growth. It can lead to thrombosis and occlusion of the vessel that can result in gangrene and the need for amputation. ⊃ intermittent claudication.

peripheral venography the radiographic investigation of the venous system of a limb following the direct injection of contrast agent into a vein.

peripheral vision (*syn* eccentric vision, extrafoveal vision, indirect vision) being able to see objects at the outer edge of the visual field, that area surrounding the central field of vision. Vision resulting from stimulation of the retina outside the fovea or macula. ⊃ central vision, sensory fusion.

periphlebitis inflammation around a vein.

periphoria ⊃ cyclophoria.

periportal *adj* surrounding the hepatic portal vein.

perirenal *adj* around the kidney.

periscopic lens a spherical lens in which the minus lenses have base curves of ±1.25 D and the plus lenses have base curves of −1.25 D. Meniscus lenses are more curved. ⊃ meniscus lens.

perisplenitis *n* inflammation of the peritoneal coat of the spleen and of the adjacent structures.

peristalsis *n* a rhythmic wave-like contraction and dilatation occurring in the smooth (involuntary) muscle of a hollow structure, e.g. ureter, gastrointestinal tract. In the intestine it is the movement by which the contents (food and waste) are propelled along the lumen. It consists of a wave of contraction preceded by a wave of relaxation—**peristaltic** *adj*.

peritomy *n* incision of the conjunctiva around the corneal limbus.

peritoneal cavity a potential space between the parietal and visceral layers of the peritoneum.

peritoneal dialysis a form of dialysis in which the peritoneum is the diffusible semipermeable membrane, and synthetic fluid is inserted into, and removed along with toxins, nitrogenous waste, excess fluid and electrolytes from the peritoneal cavity via a catheter. Different techniques exist, such as automated peritoneal dialysis and continuous ambulatory peritoneal dialysis.

peritoneal effusion (*syn.* ascites, hydroperitoneum) a collection of serous fluid in the peritoneal cavity.

peritoneal lavage irrigation of the perioneal cavity for diagnosis, such as obtaining cells for examination; or as treatment for infection.

peritoneoscopy ⊃ laparoscopy.

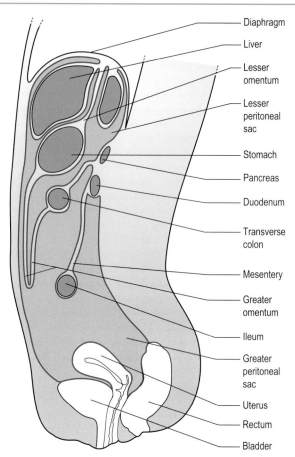

P.7 Peritoneum (female) (reproduced from Watson 2000 with permission).

peritoneum *n* the delicate serous membrane which lines the abdominal and pelvic cavities (parietal layer) and also covers some of the organs (visceral layer) contained in them (Figure P.7)—**peritoneal** *adj*. ⊃ mesentery, omentum.

peritonitis *n* inflammation of the peritoneum, usually secondary to disease of one of the abdominal or pelvic organs but it may be caused by blood borne micro-organisms, such as tubercular peritonitis. It may be bacterial (e.g. following perforation of the bowel), or chemical (e.g. in pancreatitis or a perforated peptic ulcer) in nature.

peritonsillar abscess (quinsy) abscess formation in the loose tissue around the palatine tonsil, it may occur as a complication of tonsillitis. It is characterized by a very sore throat, high temperature, dysphagia, otalgia, voice changes and sometimes trismus (unable to open the mouth). Management includes incision and drainage or aspiration of the abscess, which will relieve the pressure and pain but vitally reduces the risk that the airway will become blocked, and intravenous antibiotics. It may also involve the immediate removal of the acutely infected tonsils, but usually tonsillectomy is undertaken when the infection has subsided.

peritrichous *adj* applied to a bacterium that has flagella on all sides of the cell. ⊃ *Bacillus*.

periumbilical *adj* surrounding the umbilicus.

periurethral *adj* surrounding the urethra, as a periurethral abscess.

perivascular *adj* around a blood vessel.

periventricular haemorrhage (PVH) serious complication of preterm infants, notably under 34 weeks' gestation. The haemorrhage is graded from 0 to 3, with 3 being the most extensive.

periventricular leukomalacia cystic, ischaemic lesions in the periventricular region, diagnosed on ultrasound scan; associated with periventricular haemorrhage and a high incidence of spastic cerebral palsy.

PERLA *abbr* pupils equal reacting to light, accommodation.

perlèche *n* lip licking. An intertrigo at the angles of the mouth with maceration, fissuring, or crust formation. May result from use of poorly fitting dentures, bacterial and fungal infection, vitamin deficiency, drooling or thumb sucking.

permanent (secondary) dentition the 32 teeth present in an adult mouth and consisting of four incisors, two canines, four premolars and six molars in each jaw. ⊃ teeth.

permeability *n* **1.** in physiology, the extent to which substances dissolved in the body fluids are able to move through cell membranes or layers of cells (e.g. the walls of capillaries or absorptive tissues). **2.** the measure of the response of a material to a magnetic field. It is the ratio of the magnetic flux induced in the material to the strength of the applied magnetic field.

permittivity absolute permittivity is the ratio of the electrical displacement to the electrical field at the same point. ⊃ relative permittivity.

pernicious highly destructive, tending to a fatal outcome without effective treatment.

pernicious anaemia (PA) (Addisonian) a type of megaloblastic, macrocytic anaemia. It results from the inability of the bone marrow to produce normal red blood cells because of a deficiency of a protein released by gastric cells, called the intrinsic factor, which is necessary for the absorption of vitamin B_{12} from food in the ileum. An autoimmune mechanism may be responsible. It is characterized by the general signs and symptoms of anaemia, mild jaundice, glossitis, paraesthesia, weakness and in severe cases the development of subacute combined degeneration of the (spinal) cord. ⊃ anaemia.

perniosis *n* chronic chilblains.

perodactyly congenital deformity of the fingers or toes including absence of some digits.

peromelia *n* a teratogenic malformation of a limb.

peroneal nerve the common peroneal nerve is a branch of the sciatic nerve. It divides into the superficial peroneal (musculocutaneous) and the deep peroneal (anterior tibial) nerves, which innervate the muscles and skin of the front of the leg and dorsum of the foot and toes. ⊃ Colour Section Figure 11.

peroneal tendon subluxation occurs commonly after an inversion injury, whereby there may be a shallow peroneal groove that predisposes to the subluxation or dislocation. The patient will often complain of a 'popping' sound or a 'snapping' sensation behind the lateral malleolus.

peroneus muscles of the lateral compartment of the leg. ⊃ peroneus brevis, peroneus longus.

peroneus brevis a muscle situated under the p. longus. Its origin is on the shaft of the fibula and it inserts with a tendon on to the fifth metatarsal bone. Contraction of the muscle plantar flexes and everts the foot. ⊃ Colour Section Figure 4.

peroneus longus superficial lateral muscle of the leg. Its origin is on the upper fibula and it inserts with a long tendon on to the first metasarsal and the medial cuneiform bones. Contraction of the muscle plantar flexes and everts the foot. ⊃ Colour Section Figures 4, 5.

peropus congenital deformity of the feet.

peroral *adj* through the mouth.

peroxisome *n* minute bodies present in kidney and liver cells. They contain several enzymes including peroxidase, catalase and oxidases. They may be involved in oxidation reactions involving hydrogen peroxide, and in gluconeogenesis and in lipid and purine metabolism.

PERRLA *abbr* pupils equal, round, react to light, accommodation.

perseveration *n* constant repetition of words or phrases. Seen in organic brain disease (OBS). ⊃ delirium, dementia.

persistent ductus arteriosus ⊃ patent/persistent ductus arteriosus.

persistent hyaloid artery ⊃ hyaloid remnant.

persistent hyperplastic primary vitreous (PHPV) a congenital, abnormal vitreous development characterized by a retrolental mass formed by remnants of the hyaloid system and tunica vasculosa lentis. The eye presents with leukocoria and there may also be cataract and congenital glaucoma. Treatment should begin as early in life as possible to avoid the risk of damage to the globe and amblyopia. ⊃ hyaloid artery, hyaloid remnant.

persistent mentoposterior face presentation in which the sinciput rotates forwards and the chin rotates backwards to the sacral hollow. It is a rare cause of obstructed labour, when the thorax must present at the pelvic brim with the head.

persistent occipitoposterior deflexed vertex presentation with the sinciput rotated forwards and the occiput rotated backwards to the hollow of the sacrum. A common cause of delay in the second stage of labour; spontaneous face to pubes delivery is possible. ⊃ face to pubes delivery.

persistent trophoblastic disease ⊃ choriocarcinoma.

persistent vegetative state (PVS) a completely dependent state caused by irreparable damage to the cerebral cortex, but in which the vital functions of the brainstem continue. The person, who appears to be awake, neither responds nor is able to initiate any voluntary action. ⊃ vegetative state.

O

P

person-centred practice the process of collaboration between the therapist, the individual and relevant others, in which therapeutic goals and interventions are negotiated and agreed.

personal activities of daily living (PADL) include activities such as washing and dressing.

personal care the activities that a person does every day to maintain personal health and wellbeing, such as washing, eating and dressing.

personal construct theory a theory of personality first described by American psychologist George Kelly in 1955 that views the person as actively constructing their view of reality and acting as an incipient scientist, constantly formulating and testing hypotheses about their world in order to bring sense and meaning to their lives.

personal development plan plan developed by nurses and other health professionals as a part of their lifelong learning commitment.

personal hygiene includes all those activities which have as their objective body cleanliness; they include washing, bathing, care of hair including facial shaving for men, nails, teeth and gums, as well as changes of clothing and bedding.

personal identity each person's awareness of her/himself as an individual, separate from other people; an evolving state that unfolds and develops throughout the lifespan. Identity derives from interactions with other people and with the non-human environment.

personal protective equipment (PPE) equipment, such as eye protection, masks, gloves and aprons, used in standard precautions. ⊃ standard precautions.

personality *n* the various mental attitudes, traits and characteristics which distinguish a person. The sum total of the mental make-up—the behavioural, psychological and emotional characteristics that make a person an individual. ⊃ big five (personality factors), personality disorder, psychopathic personality, trait.

personality disorder a disturbance of personality together with deeply ingrained maladaptive behavioural patterns established by late adolescence/early adulthood resulting in personal and social difficulties.

perspiration *n* the excretion from the sweat glands through the skin pores. *insensible perspiration* the water lost by evaporation through the skin surface other than by sweating. It is significantly increased in inflamed skin. *sensible perspiration* the term used when there are visible drops of sweat on the skin.

Perthes' disease (*syn.* pseudocoxalgia) ⊃ Legg–Calvé–Perthes disease.

pertussis *n* (*syn.* whooping cough) a serious infectious respiratory disease caused by the bacterium *Bordetella pertussis*. It is spread by droplets and has an incubation period of 7–14 days. It is characterized by conjunctivitis, rhinitis, dry cough and later bouts of paroxysmal coughing with a 'whoop' and vomiting. Complications may include pneumonia, bronchiectasis and convulsions. Active immunization is available as part of the routine programme in infancy.

pes *n* a foot or foot-like structure.

PESA *abbr* percutaneous epididymal sperm aspiration.

pes anserinus bursitis inflammation of the bursa between the medial collateral ligament insertion and the 'pes' muscle group consisting of sartorius, gracilis and semitendinosus.

pes cavus (high arched foot) (*syn.* claw-foot) a pathological elevation of the longitudinal arch caused by plantar flexion of the forefoot relative to the rearfoot. The medial longitudinal arch is most affected but the lateral longitudinal arch can also be elevated. There is dorsal humping of the midfoot and associated forefoot and rearfoot deformities. These may include clawing or retraction of the lesser toes, a trigger first toe, and a depressed first metatarsal with either heel varus or equinus. It may be congenital or acquired. May be the result of underlying neuromuscular disease. Can present with pain, difficulty in getting suitable shoes or obvious foot deformity. In sport, good podiatry input and correctly fitted shoes will minimize secondary effects, which are seen primarily in weight-bearing sports.

pes planus (*syn.* flat-foot) also known as 'pronated feet'. A generic term for a foot with an abnormally low arch. The medial longitudinal arch is depressed or absent, and the foot has an increased contact area with the ground. During weightbearing the foot appears to have no longitudinal arch. It may be congenital or acquired. When young children first stand the feet appear to be flat, as adipose tissue under the medial longitudinal arch is pressed close to the ground. Older children very frequently have flattening of the medial longitudinal arch on standing but the arch reappears on standing on tiptoe (a mobile flat foot). *flexible pes planus* is generally asymptomatic in children but may become a semi-rigid condition in adulthood. It has been linked with excess laxity of the joint capsule and the ligaments supporting the arch, which allows it to collapse when weight is applied. *rigid pes planus* in adults may be a progression from flexible to semi-rigid to rigid as part of the ageing process. Structural changes due to the existing abnormal position become fixed, as soft and osseous tissues adapt. Rigidity is increased where there are significant osteoarthritic changes or inflammatory arthritic destruction.

pessary *n* **1.** a device inserted into the vagina to correct uterine displacements. A *ring* or *shelf pessary* is used to support a prolapse. A *Hodge pessary* is used to correct a retroverted uterus. **2.** a suppository containing a medication inserted into the vagina.

pestle a glass rod with ground surface used in a mortar to provide a homogeneous mixture of solids.

PET *acron* **P**ositron **E**mission **T**omography.

petechia *n* a small, haemorrhagic spot—**petechiae** *pl*, **petechial** *adj*.

Peters' anomaly (A Peters, German ophthalmologist, 1862–1938) (*syn* anterior chamber cleavage syndrome) a rare, congenital anomaly of the anterior segment of the eye. It is characterized by a central corneal opacity, usually accompanied by the adhesion of strands of iris tissue to the margins of the corneal opacity. It is frequently associated with glaucoma. ⊃ Axenfeld's syndrome, Rieger's syndrome.

petit mal minor epilepsy. ⊃ epilepsy, grand mal.

pétrissage *n* rhythmical massage manipulations of muscle and other soft tissues where pressure is used to help venous and lymphatic drainage and to mobilize skin and connective tissue. It may be slow and deep to produce relaxation and reduce spasm, or brisk to invigorate. The manipulation may be performed with one hand alone, or with both hands working alternately.

petrositis inflammation involving the petrous portion of the temporal bone.

petrous *adj* resembling stone.

Petzval surface (J Petzval, Hungarian mathematician/physicist, 1807–1891) the imaginary curved surface upon which images would be formed if curvature of field were the only aberration present. It is the curved surface in which the tangential and sagittal image shells of a point-focal lens coincide. ⊃ anastigmatic lens, curvature of field, oblique astigmatism.

Peutz–Jeghers syndrome (J Peutz, Dutch physician, 1886–1957; H Jeghers, American physician, 1904–1990) a type of familial adenomatous polyposis inherited as an autosomal dominant trait. It is characterized by excessive melanin production and pigmentation in the skin and mucosa (typically in the mouth), and the presence of many hamartomas usually in the small bowel but they also occur in the colon. ⊃ Colour Section Figure 97. It is associated with intussusception and bleeding into the bowel. People with the syndrome may have gastrointestinal cancers, and also have a tendency to develop cancers elsewhere, such as the pancreas, lung, testes, ovaries and breast.

-pexy a suffix that means 'fixation', e.g. *aortopexy*.

Peyer's patches (J Peyer, Swiss anatomist, 1653–1712) part of mucosa-associated lymphoid tissue. Aggregates of lymphatic tissue situated in the ileum. Function to prevent micro-organisms entering the blood. Site of infection in typhoid fever.

Peyronie's disease (F de la Peyronie, French surgeon, 1678–1747) deformity and painful erection of penis due to fibrous tissue formation from unknown cause. Can be associated with Dupuytren's contracture. ⊃ Nesbit's operation.

PFI *abbr* private finance initiative.

PFJ *abbr* patello-femoral joint.

PFK *abbr* phosphofructokinase.

PFM *abbr* porcelain fused to metal.

PFMC *abbr* preformed metal crown.

PGD *abbr* pre-implantation genetic diagnosis.

PGDRS *abbr* psychogeriatric dependency rating scale.

PGH *abbr* pre-implantation genetic halotyping.

pH *abbr* the negative logarithm of the hydrogen ion concentration [H^+], so a change by one pH unit means a tenfold change in [H^+]. pH 7 represents neutrality in water at 25°C, when [H^+] = 10^{-7} molar = 100 nmol/L. In the body, at 37°C, 'neutral' would be ~pH 6.8 but the extracellular pH

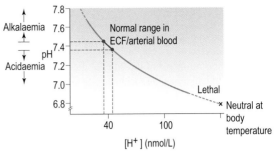

P.8 pH and hydrogen ion concentration in extracellular fluids (reproduced from Jennett 2008 with permission).

of body fluids is more alkaline than this. Arterial blood pH (the most readily measured) varies in health within the range of 7.36–7.44 or [H^+] = 40 nmol/L ± about 12%—a tiny amount compared to other ions in the blood (Figure P.8). Intracellular pH is more acidic (e.g. 6.8–7.1 in skeletal muscle fibres), so there is a gradient promoting exit of metabolically generated H^+ from cells. Regulation, vital for normal metabolic processes, depends on this gradient, on intracellular buffers (predominantly proteins and phosphates) and on variations in PCO_2. The whole-body turnover of H^+ (by ingestion, metabolic production and excretion) is of vastly greater magnitude than the body fluid concentrations. ⊃ acid–base balance.

pH meter a calibrated, electric meter used to take accurate pH readings. In radiography it is used to check the pH of processor chemicals.

phacoemulsification *n* (*syn.* pakoemulsification) procedure for removal of the crystalline lens in cataract surgery which consists of emulsifying and aspirating the contents of the lens with the use of a low frequency ultrasonic needle inserted into the eye near the limbus. This technique usually produces more rapid wound healing and early stabilization of refractive error with less astigmatism, due to the small incision. However, this technique may damage the corneal endothelium if excessive ultrasound is used. Following removal of the lens cortex and nucleus, an intraocular lens may be implanted within the remaining lens capsule. The lens is folded and inserted through a small incision (e.g. 3.2 mm) using a special injector. This procedure is preferred over other cataract extraction techniques due to both the rapid wound healing and the lower incidence of potentially vision threatening side effects (e.g. retinal detachment). ⊃ cataract extraction, intraocular lens implant, iridectomy.

phacolytic glaucoma an open-angle glaucoma secondary to a hypermature or mature cataract. It is due to a leakage of lens proteins into the anterior chamber which blocks the outflow of aqueous humour through the trabecular meshwork. It is characterized by an acute onset of pain and redness with high intraocular pressure. ⊃ cataract, open-angle glaucoma, trabecular meshwork.

phacomorphic glaucoma a form of secondary angle-closure glaucoma in which the angle of the anterior chamber

0
P

591

is closed due to swelling of the lens. Angle closure may be due to pupillary block or in some cases due to anterior pressure on the iris. ⊃ pupillary block.

phaeochromocytoma *n* (*syn.* paraganglioma) a condition in which there is a tumour of the adrenal medulla, or of the structurally similar tissues associated with the sympathetic chain. It secretes adrenaline (epinephrine) and allied hormones and the symptoms are due to the excess of these substances. Results in hypertensive crises, with associated headache, flushing and tachycardia.

-phage a suffix that means 'ingesting', e.g. *macrophage.*

phage typing identifying bacterial strains by their bacteriophages.

-phagia, phagy a suffix that means 'swallowing', e.g. *aerophagia.*

phagocyte *n* a cell capable of engulfing bacteria and other particulate material such as cell debris. Examples of phagocytic cells include neutrophils and macrophages—**phagocytic** *adj.*

phagocytosis *n* the process by which phagocytic cells engulf particles such as bacteria (Figure P.9). ⊃ bulk transport.

phagomania also called sitomania. An abnormal obsession with food.

phagophobia also called sitophobia. An abnormal fear of food.

phakic refers to an eye possessing its crystalline lens or an intraocular lens implant. ⊃ aphakia, crystalline lens, intraocular lens implant.

phalanges *n* the 14 small bones that form the fingers on each hand or the toes on each foot—**phalanx** *sing*, **phalangeal** *adj.* ⊃ Colour Section Figures 2, 3.

Phalen's test a test for carpal tunnel syndrome, whereby the wrists are held in a flexed position for one minute. If

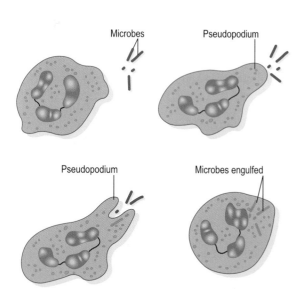

P.9 Phagocytosis (reproduced from Waugh & Grant 2006 with permission).

symptoms of paraesthesia are reproduced in the fingers, the test is positive.

phalloplasty plastic operation on the penis. Undertaken to correct congenital defects, such as hypospadias, or after injury.

phallus *n* the penis—**phallic** *adj.*

phantasy *n* ⊃ fantasy.

phantom head a manikin or simulator. Model of the head on which either artificial or extracted teeth are set up in order to allow dental students or clinicians to experience dental operative procedures.

phantom limb pain/syndrome the sensation that a limb is still attached to the body after it has been amputated. Pain may seem to come from the amputated limb. It is neuropathic pain, a type of chronic non-malignant pain. The pain is experienced because of altered pain processing by the nervous system, possibly caused by previous tissue or nerve damage. Effective pain relief before amputation is important in minimizing the risk of developing phantom limb pain. ⊃ chronic pain, neuropathic pain.

phantom pregnancy (*syn.* pseudocyesis) signs and symptoms simulating those of early pregnancy; it may occur in a childless woman who has an overwhelming desire to have a child.

pharmaceutical *adj* relating to drugs.

pharmacist *n* a person who is qualified and registered to dispense drugs. They also provide advice and information for other health professionals and the public.

pharmacodynamics *n* the study of how a drug acts in a living system and how it alters cell metabolism to exert its effects. This includes how the drug binds to cell receptor proteins: the specificity of the receptor for the drug; and its affinity for the drug, which influences the dose required to have an effect.

pharmacokinetics *n* the study of the way the body deals with a drug over time. It considers drug absorption, distribution around the body, metabolism and excretion. Each of these processes occurs at a specific rate characteristic for that drug, and the overall action of the drug (be it therapeutic or toxic), will be dependent on these processes. A number of factors can influence the pharmacokinetics of a drug and so alter its effect on the body. For example, drug absorption is affected by the formulation of the drug, the gastrointestinal contents and motility. Drug distribution depends on blood flow to the tissues, obstacles such as the blood–brain barrier that make it difficult for drugs to enter the central nervous system, and plasma protein binding. Enzymes within the liver carry out drug metabolism, and as there is considerable genetic variation in liver enzymes, the ability to metabolize drugs can vary significantly from one person to another. The presence of other drugs can also affect the rate of metabolism, either speeding it up or slowing it down. Drugs are mainly eliminated by the kidneys and are particularly affected by glomerular filtration rate, which decreases with age and disease.

pharmacology *n* the science dealing with drugs, their properties, uses and effects at their cell receptor proteins—**pharmacological** *adj*, **pharmacologically** *adv.*

pharmacopoeia *n* an authorized book detailing drugs available for prescribing in a specific country, such as the British Pharmacopoeia (BP) or United States Pharmacopoeia.

pharmacy *n* **1.** the place where drugs are prepared and dispensed. **2.** the science of preparing drugs.

pharmacy only medicine (P) in the UK, medicines that may be bought by the public from a pharmacy but only when a pharmacist is in attendance.

pharma, pharmaco- a prefix that means 'drug', e.g. *pharmacokinetics*.

pharmafoods ➲ functional foods.

pharyngeal pouch pathological dilatation of the lower part of the pharynx.

pharyngeal reflex ➲ gag.

pharyngectomy *n* surgical removal of the pharynx (partial or total), such as for cancer.

pharyngismus *n* spasm of the pharynx.

pharyngitis *n* inflammation of the pharynx, which may be acute or chronic. Acute pharyngitis leads to a sore, dry throat and pain on swallowing. Causes include tonsillitis, streptococcal infections, herpes and diphtheria.

pharyng/o- a prefix that means 'pharynx', e.g. *pharyngitis*.

pharyngolaryngeal *adj* pertaining to the pharynx and larynx.

pharyngolaryngectomy *n* surgical removal of the pharynx and larynx, such as for laryngeal cancer.

pharyngoplasty *n* any plastic operation to the pharynx.

pharyngoscope an endoscope used to examine the pharynx.

pharyngotomy *n* a surgical opening into the pharnynx.

pharyngotympanic tube (*syn.* eustachian or auditory tube) a canal, partly bony, partly cartilaginous, connecting the pharynx with the tympanic cavity. It allows air to pass into the middle ear, so that the air pressure is kept even on both sides of the eardrum. ➲ Colour Section Figure 13.

pharynx *n* a tube 12 to 14 cm long that extends from the base of the skull to the level of the 6th cervical vertebra. It lies behind the nose, mouth and larynx and is wider at its upper end. For descriptive purposes the pharynx is divided into three parts: *nasopharynx, oropharynx* and *laryngopharynx*. The pharynx is cone shaped and is lined with mucous membrane; at the lower end it opens into the oesophagus. The pharyngotympanic (eustachian or auditory) tubes pierce its lateral walls and the posterior nares pierce its anterior wall. The larynx lies immediately below it and in front of the oesophagus—**pharyngeal** *adj*. ➲ laryngopharynx, nasopharynx, oropharynx, Colour Section Figure 6.

phase the state of vibration of a light wave at a particular time. Light waves vibrating with the same frequency are said to be in phase if their peaks and troughs occur at the same time; otherwise they are said to be out of phase and one wave lags or precedes another by a phase difference (e.g. a fraction of a wavelength, or one wavelength, or a number of wavelengths). For waves exactly out of phase the phase difference is half a wavelength and for waves exactly in phase it is 0. ➲ wavelength.

phase contrast angiography a two-dimensional or three-dimensional magnetic resonance imaging (MRI) technique to distinguish flowing blood from static tissue. The magnitude image shows the blood vessels and the phase image shows the direction of flow.

phase encoding a technique used to locate a magnetic resonance signal by applying a series of varying phase-encoded, gradient pulses so that the phase of spin is altered prior to the signal readout. The spins retain the memory of the separate phase-encoded pulses.

phased array in ultrasound a sector field of view with multiple transducer elements, formed in precise sequence and under electronic control. This gives a wide field of view using a small transducer, for example, cardiac or paediatric head scans.

phases an electrotherapy term. A biphasic pulse has two phases and a monophasic has one phase. Illustrations of a phase indicate the rate of application of charge (slope and shape), the amount of charge applied (area of each phase) and the duration of each phase (duration).

-phasia a suffix that means 'speech,' e.g. *dysphasia*.

PHC *abbr* primary health care.

phenidone in radiography, a developer agent.

phenol *n* (*syn.* carbolic acid) a powerful disinfectant. Phenolic disinfectants are used in suitable dilution for environmental use. They are toxic and corrosive.

phenol red cotton thread test a test for measuring tear secretion. It is accomplished by using a special cotton thread, impregnated with phenol red dye. The thread is inserted under the lower eyelid for 15 seconds, and both eyes are closed. The absorption of tears is determined by the length of thread that has turned from red to yellow (due to the pH of tears). The average length varies between 3 and 48 mm, and less than 9 mm is usually indicative of a dry eye. This test is much quicker and much less uncomfortable than Schirmer's test and has good reliability. However, questions have been raised as to whether it is the actual secretion rate which is being measured. There exist several cotton thread tests to measure tear secretion, using different cottons of different lengths and diameters, and some are used without phenol red dye. ➲ Norn's test, Schirmer's test, tear secretion.

phenothiazines *npl* a group of typical antipsychotic drugs (neuroleptics), e.g. chlorpromazine. ➲ tardive dyskinesia. ➲ Appendix 5.

phenotype *n* the observable physical characteristics of an organism that result from the interaction between its genotype (genetic makeup) and environment. ➲ genotype.

phenylalanine *n* an essential (indispensable) amino acid required for growth and development during infancy and childhood, and for cell repair and growth during adulthood. Individuals who lack the enzyme required for its metabolism develop phenylketonuria.

phenylbutazone a powerful anti-inflammatory drug first used in the 1940s in the treatment of arthritis. Limited by its potentially serious side effects (including fatalities), it is

O

P

now rarely used in humans (ankylosing spondylitis is an exception) but interestingly is widely used in veterinary medicine such as in equestrian sports to treat soft tissue injuries in horses.

phenylketonuria (PKU) *n* metabolites of phenylalanine (e.g. phenylketones) excreted in the urine. Occurs in hyperphenylalaninaemia, owing to the lack of, or inactivity of, the liver enzyme phenylalanine hydroxylase that normally converts dietary phenylalanine into tyrosine (a non-essential [dispensible] amino acid). The enzyme defect is inherited as an autosomal recessive disease. The presence of high levels of phenylalanine are especially toxic to the developing brain. In the absence of treatment the individual will have a learning disability, eczema, their urine and skin have a 'mousy' odour, and, because they lack tyrosine, which is needed for pigmentation, they will have very fair hair. Thus routine screening for phenylketonuria is undertaken in newborns, as early detection allows for the introduction of a modified formula milk that is low in phenylalanine to prevent damage to the brain. The diet, low in phenylalanine, and regular monitoring of phenylketone levels in the blood were previously continued until brain development was complete, but many physicians recommend that a low phenylalanine diet be followed for life. Whichever regimen is followed, women with phenylketonuria planning to become pregnant are advised to recommence the low phenylalanine diet prior to conception and during pregnancy to protect the developing fetus—**phenylketonuric** *adj*.

pheromones *npl* chemicals with a specific odour. They are present in the sweat produced by the apocrine sweat glands. They are involved in communication and influence sexual behaviour.

Philadelphia chromosome (Ph¹) an anomaly of chromosome number 22. It is found in the blood cells of most people with chronic myeloid leukaemia.

-philia, phily a suffix that means 'affinity for, loving', e.g. thrombophilia.

philtrum the vertical indentation present midline of the upper lip.

phimosis *n* tightness of the prepuce so that it cannot be retracted over the glans penis.

phimosis vaginalis a congenital condition in which the vagina is narrow or closed.

phi movement (*syn* phi phenomenon) an illusion of movement created when one object disappears and an identical object appears in a neighbouring region of the same plane. If the time interval between the two sources is between 0.06 s and 0.2 s, the observer will see an apparent movement of the object from the first to the second position. The illusion of movement obtained in the cinema is based on this phenomenon. The phi phenomenon has been applied to test patients with convergent and divergent strabismus. This is Verhoeff phi phenomenon test: two light sources, separated by the angle of strabismus, are placed in front of the patient, as in a major amblyoscope. The two foveas are stimulated

with a short time interval between stimulations, and patients with normal retinal correspondence do not see a movement whereas those with abnormal retinal correspondence do. ➲ abnormal retinal correspondence, cover test, movement threshold, strabismus.

phi phenomenon ➲ phi movement.

phlebo- a prefix that means 'vein', e.g. *phlebothrombosis*.

phlebectomy *n* excision of a vein. ➲ multiple cosmetic phlebectomy (MCP).

phlebitis *n* inflammation of a vein—**phlebitic** *adj*. ➲ thrombophlebitis.

phlebography radiological examination of the venous system involving injection of a contrast agent. Mostly replaced by ultrasound. ➲ venography.

phlebolith *n* a concretion that forms in a vein.

phlebothrombosis *n* a blood clot or thrombus in a vein. ➲ deep vein thrombosis, embolism, pulmonary embolus.

phlebotomist *n* a technician who is trained to take blood samples from patients.

Phlebotomus a genus of sandfly. They transmit the parasite of leishmaniasis in old world countries. Some species of *Phlebotomus* are vectors for the arboviruses that cause a variety of diseases including phlebotomus fever (sandfly fever), and the bacterium that causes bartonellosis.

phlebotomus fever also called Pappataci fever or sandfly fever. An acute viral infection caused by several arboviruses, it occurs in hot regions that include Central Asia, Central and South America and some areas around the Mediterranean. Humans become infected by a bite from an infected sandfly. It is characterized by pyrexia, headache, conjunctivitis, muscle pain and sometimes a rash. The disease is self-limiting and treatment is symptomatic only, such as fluids and mild analgesics.

phlebotomy *n* ➲ venesection, venotomy.

phlegm *n* lay term for sputum. Mucus expectorated (coughed up) from the bronchi.

phlegmasia alba dolans also known as white leg or milk leg. Phlebitis affecting the femoral vein that leads to a swollen, white and painful leg. Sometimes occurs after childbirth or an acute illness with high temperature.

phlegmatic *adj* describes a person who is emotionally stable.

phlyctenular conjunctivitis (*syn* eczematous conjunctivitis, phlyctenulosis) conjunctivitis characterized by the presence of nodules on the bulbar conjunctiva and which sometimes may spread to the cornea. It is due to an allergic reaction to an antigen such as the bacterium *Staphylococcus aureus* or the fungus *Candida albicans*. Symptoms are soreness, and photophobia when the cornea is involved. It is associated with superficial vascularization. Treatment is generally with topical corticosteroids. ➲ conjunctiva, phlyctenular keratitis.

phlyctenular keratitis inflammation of the cornea characterized by the formation of small grey nodules (phlyctens) near the limbus. As the number of phlyctens in the cornea increases a neovascularization occurs which is called phlyctenular pannus. Phlyctenular keratitis is usually associated with an inflammation of the conjunctiva and raised nodules are also present there. ➲ phlyctenular conjunctivitis.

phlyctenule *n* a small inflammatory nodule which occurs on conjunctiva or cornea close to the corneal limbus.

phlyctenulosis *n* eye disease characterized by phlyctenules. ➲ phlyctenular conjunctivitis.

phobia *n* a morbid fear. An irrational, focused fear of an object, state or event, which causes the person to feel anxious. Specific phobias include those in respect of spiders or mice, acrophobia, agorophobia, claustrophobia, dysmorphophobia, nyctophobia, etc.—**phobic** *adj*.

-phobia a suffix that means 'fear', e.g. *phagophobia*.

phocomelia *n* teratogenic malformation. Arms and feet attached directly to trunk giving a seal-like appearance. Many cases in the 1960s were associated with the use of the drug thalidomide during pregnancy.

phoenix abscess a periodontal abscess which, after a symptom-free period, becomes symptomatic with all the characteristics of an acute periodontal abscess.

phonation *n* voice production by vibration of the vocal cords.

phonetic relating to speech sounds.

phon/o- a prefix that means 'sound, voice', e.g. *phonophobia*.

phonocardiography *n* the graphic recording of heart sounds and murmurs by electric reproduction. The fetal heart rate and its relation to uterine contraction can be measured continuously. ➲ cardiotocography—**phonocardiographic** *adj*, **phonocardiogram** *n*, **phonocardiograph** *n*, **phonocardiographically** *adv*.

phonophobia *n* a dislike of noise in general such as during an attack of migraine, or a dislike or hypersensitivity to certain sounds.

phonophoresis the process by which ultrasound waves are used to introduce a topical drug through the skin (transdermal).

phoria *n* latent strabismus. May be used as a suffix. ➲ heterophoria.

phoropter (*syn* refracting unit, refractor, refractor head) an instrument for measuring the ametropias, phorias and the amplitude of accommodation of the eyes. It consists of a large unit placed in front of the patient's head in which there are three rotating discs containing convex and concave spherical and cylindrical lenses, as well as occluders, Maddox rods, pinholes, Polaroids, prisms and coloured filters. An attachment on the instrument allows sets of rotary prisms and cross-cylinders to be swung in front of each sight hole.

phosphatases *npl* enzymes needed to catalyse the reactions concerning phosphate esters, e.g. nucleotides, carbohydrate metabolism, phospholipids. Phosphatases are present in a variety of tissues including the blood, bone, liver, kidney, prostate gland and semen. ➲ acid phosphatase, alkaline phosphatase.

phosphate-bonded investment material in dentistry, high temperature investment material. Silica, magnesium oxide and ammonium phosphate react on mixing with water to form magnesium ammonium phosphate.

phosphates *npl* salts or esters of phosphoric acid. A component of food, such as some proteins. Phosphates are present in various tissues (e.g. bone). They are vital in physiological processes including: adenosine diphosphate (ADP) and adenosine triphosphate (ATP) that function in the reactions that produce and store energy; and in the nucleotides that are part of the nucleic acids. Phosphate deficiency occurs: in preterm infants fed on human milk; patients with renal tubular phosphate loss; due to prolonged high dosage of aluminium hydroxide; when people with chronic alcohol misuse are fed with high-carbohydrate foods; and in patients receiving parenteral nutrition if inadequate phosphate is provided. Deficiency causes hypophosphataemia and muscle weakness secondary to ATP deficiency.

phosphatidylcholines phospholipids, also known as lecithins.

phosphatidylserine a phospholipid found in the brain.

phosphaturia *n* excess phosphates in the urine—**phosphaturic** *adj*.

phosphene a visual sensation arising from stimulation of the retina by something other than light. The stimulation can be either electrical, mechanical (e.g. a blow to the head or pressure on the eyeball), or some electromagnetic waves such as X-rays. ➲ entoptic image/phenomena, photopsia.

phosphocreatine (PCr) ➲ creatine phosphate.

phosphofructokinase (PFK) 6-phosphofructokinase. The most important regulatory enzyme involved in the pathway of glycolysis, enabling the phosphorylation of fructose-6-phosphate to fructose-1,6-diphosphate by adenosine triphosphate (ATP). The reaction, which is irreversible, is a key stage during glycolysis. The activity level of PFK probably limits the rate of glycolysis during maximal exercise. It is sensitive to very many stimulatory and inhibitory influences. ➲ muscle enzymes.

phospholipids *npl* organic molecules comprising a lipid plus nitrogen and phosphate groups, vital in the formation of the cell (plasma) membrane. ➲ lipids.

phosphonecrosis tissue destruction, usually involving the jaw bone ('phossy jaw'). It is caused by exposure to phosphorus, such as may occur during an industrial process and is designated as an industrial disease. It was a problem for people working without proper protection in the match industry during the 19th century and early 20th century. The phosphorus toxicity eventually caused organ failure and death.

phosphoproteins proteins that contain phosphates in their structure.

phosphor a substance that has a characteristic light emission when stimulated by an electron beam.

phosphorescence ➲ after-glow, luminescence.

phosphoric acid the main constituent of the liquid component of many dental cements. ➲ acid etchant.

O
P

phosphor layer the suspension of phosphor crystals in a binder to form the layer of an intensifying screen that converts radiation to light.

phosphor storage plate ⟾ imaging plate.

phosphor type the higher the total efficiency of a phosphor the more light is produced and therefore the thinner the phosphor, rare earth phosphors are more efficient than calcium tungstate phosphors.

phosphorus (P) *n* a poisonous element. Forms an important constituent (as phosphates) of nucleic acids, bone and all cells. *phosphorus-32* (^{32}P) radioactive phosphorus used in the treatment of thrombocythaemia. ⟾ phosphates.

phosphorylase (PPL) a cytoplasmic enzyme. It catalyses the removal of hexose units, one at a time, from glycogen, to form glucose 1-phosphate: rate-limiting enzyme of, and histochemical marker for, glycolysis. ⟾ muscles enzymes.

phosphorylases *npl* a group of enzymes needed for the addition of phosphate groups to other molecules, e.g. phosphofructokinase concerned with glucose metabolism. ⟾ muscle enzymes.

phosphorylation *n* the metabolic process of introducing a phosphate group into an organic molecule.

phosphorylation potential the concentration ratio [ATP] / [ADP] [Pi] in the cytosol of a cell (where P_i is the total of inorganic phosphate ions, HPO_4^{2-} and $H_2PO_4^-$), proposed as an index of its energy status; this ratio is directly related to the free energy available from ATP. Also known as cytoplasmic energy state. ⟾ adenosine mono-, di- and triphosphates (AMP, ADP, ATP), energy charge.

photalgia pain in the eyes caused by bright light, such as the effect of sunlight on snow.

phot/o- a prefix that means 'light', e.g. *photalgia*.

photoablation the destruction of tissue achieved by the use of light including laser. It can be used in the surgical correction of refractive errors and in some corneal conditions. It is one method used for endometrial ablation in which a laser is used to destroy the basal layer of the endometrium.

photocathode a structure made of zinc cadmium which produces electrons in proportion to the amount of light falling on it. ⟾ image intensifier.

photochemical *adj* chemically reactive in the presence of light.

photochemotherapy *n* ⟾ photodynamic therapy.

photocoagulation *n* the process of changing tissues and blood from a fluid to a coagulated (clotted) state with a powerful, focused light source, such as a laser. It may be used in the treatment of retinopathies and other conditions (e.g. detached retina, haemorrhages, diabetic retinopathy) where leaky vessels can be sealed and diseased areas on the retina destroyed, and to seal a detached retina. ⟾ age-related macular degeneration, diabetic retinopathy, laser, retinal detachment.

photodermatosis a skin condition caused by exposure to light.

photodynamic therapy (PDT) sometimes called photochemotherapy. It is a treatment that utilizes a photosensitizer drug or agent, which when activated by a specific wavelength of light produces a type of oxygen that is capable of killing nearby cells. It is used to destroy cancer cells in conditions that include: basal cell carcinoma of the skin, bladder cancer, oesophageal cancer and some types of lung cancer. PDT is used in both curative and palliative treatments. The photosensitizer is injected intravenously and is taken up by cells, but remains in cancerous cells longer than normal cells. In the next step the cancer cells are exposed to the specific wavelength of light often by use of a laser. The photosensitizer produces the form of oxygen, which destroys the cancer cells. The light source may be directed at the surface of the body for some cancers, or laser light is applied using an endoscope in other cancers, such as bladder or lung cancer. The use of PDT causes photosensitivity in the skin and eyes for around six weeks after treatment and patients are advised to avoid exposure to sunlight or bright lights during this time. PDT is also used in the management of some types of age-related macular degeneration. Research continues into further applications for PDT. ⟾ age-related macular degeneration.

photoelectric absorption when a photon collides with an orbiting electron and gives all its energy to the electron, which is then ejected from the atom.

photoendoscope *n* an endoscope incorporating a camera, thus allowing a permanent record of clinical findings to be made—**photoendoscopic** *adj*, **photoendoscopy** *n*, **photoendoscopically** *adv*.

photofluorography in radiology, the recording of the image on the output phosphor of an image intensifier.

photographic dosimeter a device containing a photographic film and several different filters that is worn over a period of time. The film is processed and the density on the film is measured. The density is proportional to the amount of radiation received by the wearer.

photographic unsharpness blurring of a radiographic image due to the recording medium. ⟾ unsharpness.

photokeratitis also known as snowblindness. Occurs as a result of excessive exposure to ultraviolet light (UV) light, as when sunlight is reflected in snow and water sports. It can be very painful, may occur several hours after exposure and may last up to 2 days. ⟾ actinic keratoconjunctivitis.

photokeratoscopy the determination of corneal curvatures and topography by photographing the corneal image of a target (usually black and white concentric rings) provided with the instrument. Measuring the size of the image and knowing the size of the object, it is possible to calculate the topography of the cornea. The theory is the same as that of the keratometer. A permanent photographic record is given with this method. The area of the cornea which is evaluated is much larger than with a keratometer. ⟾ keratometer, keratoscope, stereophotography, videokeratoscope.

photoluminescence ⟾ luminescence.

photomicrograph a photographic image of an object viewed with an electron microscope.

photomultiplier tube equipment that produces an amplified current when exposed to electromagnetic radiation, photons hitting the cathode produce electrons which in turn hit other surfaces thus producing more electrons. Used in earlier computed tomography (CT) scanner units.

photon the basic unit of radiant energy defined by the equation $E = h\nu$ where h is Planck's constant (6.62×10^{-34} joule $\times$ second), ν the frequency of the light and E the energy difference carried away by the emission of a single photon of light. The term photon usually refers to visible light whereas the term quantum refers to other electromagnetic radiations. ⊃ quantum theory, wave theory.

photonics the term referring to all the methods, procedures and systems used to measure, transmit or utilize light.

photophobia *n* dislike of bright light, usually associated with eye pain, such as in migraine and meningism—**photophobic** *adj*.

photophthalmia inflammation of the eye caused by exposure to excessively bright light.

photopic vision (*syn* daylight vision, diurnal vision) vision in bright light; at high levels of luminance (above 10 cd/m^2). That occurring in daylight involving the retinal cone photoreceptor cells. ⊃ mesopic vision, scotopic vision.

photopsia *n* the perception of flashes of light. Associated with retinal tears or detachment, migraine aura and vitreous body (humour) detachment.

photorefraction a family of photographic techniques which provide a rapid, objective method of measuring the refractive error and accommodative response of the eye. Light emitted from a small flash source placed close to the camera lens is reflected from the eye and returned to the camera. Three methods have been developed: orthogonal, isotropic and eccentric (also called photoretinoscopy). The optical design of each method results in a specific photographic pattern which varies with the degree to which the eye is defocused with respect to the plane of the camera. Photorefractive methods are not as accurate as retinoscopy but as they are entirely objective, much quicker and do not require prolonged fixation on the part of the patient, they are highly suited for testing infants and young children. ⊃ optometer, refractive error, retinoscope.

photoretinitis inflammation of the retina caused by exposure to intense light, such as looking directly at the sun. It can cause permanent damage and impaired vision.

photoscan the image from a linear scanner recorded on radiographic film.

photosensitive *adj* reactive to light.

photosensitivity *n* an exaggerated inflammatory reaction of the skin in response to light.

photostress test (*syn* light stress test) a test to differentiate the cause of a reduced visual acuity in one eye, between a lesion in the optic nerve and a disease in the fundus of the eye. A bright light is directed into the eye with the best acuity, for 10 seconds, while the defective eye is covered.

The light is then removed and the patient is instructed to read the line just above the best visual acuity line for that eye. The time taken until the patient can just read that line is recorded. The same procedure is then repeated with the defective eye. If the recovery time is about the same in both eyes, the cause of the reduced visual acuity is an optic nerve lesion (e.g. retrobulbar optic neuritis); if the recovery time is much longer for the defective eye the cause is in the fundus (e.g. retinal oedema, retinopathy, age-related maculopathy). The latter is attributed to a delay in the regeneration of visual pigments after being bleached with a bright light.

phototherapy *n* literally any treatment that involves the use of light, such as exposure to white light for seasonal affective disorder, or ultraviolet light for psoriasis. Generally refers to exposure to artificial blue light, most commonly for treatment of jaundice in neonates. Used to reduce unconjugated bilirubin levels of over 340 μmol/L at term, 210 μmol/L at 34 weeks' gestation and 150 μmol/L at 28 weeks' gestation in the jaundiced skin of a neonate, through complex changes which cause excretion of non-toxic photodegradation products without the help of the enzyme system in the liver. Effectiveness most likely due to its ability to convert bilirubin to water soluble forms that are easily excreted. Side-effects include loose green stools and skin rashes. The infant's eyes and gonads are covered to protect against any harmful effects. Phototherapy is used prophylactically for preterm infants with bruising, and those infants affected by rhesus incompatibility.

photothermographic printing uses a film containing chemicals which are activated when an image is scanned by a laser onto the film, the film is then heated to produce the image, the chemicals remain in the film. ⊃ thermographic printing.

phototransduction ⊃ transduction.

PHPV *abbr* persistent hyperplastic primary vitreous.

phren *n* the diaphragm—**phrenic** *adj*.

phrenic nerve a mixed nerve that arises mainly from the cervical nerve root 4, with minor contributions from roots 3 and 5. It supplies motor fibres to the diaphragm which stimulate contraction during inspiration, and also innervates the pleura and pericardium. Where this is disrupted, diaphragmatic pacing may be indicated (i.e. the electrical stimulation of the diaphragm to illicit a contraction and sustain breathing).

phrenicotomy *n* division of the phrenic nerve to paralyse one-half of the diaphragm.

phren/i, phrenic/o, phren/o- a prefix that either means 'diaphragm', e.g. *phrenoplegia*, or 'mind', e.g. *phrenology*.

phrenoplegia *n* paralysis of the diaphragm—**phrenoplegic** *adj*.

phrynoderma 'toad-skin'. Hyperkeratosis of the hair follicles that leads to rough, raised papules on the skin. It is possible that a deficiency of vitamins and fatty acids is responsible, but it also occurs in the absence of nutritional deficiencies.

O
P

phthiriasis *n* infestation with the pubic louse, *Phthirus pubis*. Most commonly transmitted by sexual contact, but non-sexual acquisition of the insect is also possible.

Phthirus pubis the pubic louse.

phthisis bulbi the shrinkage and atrophy of the eyeball following a severe inflammation (e.g. uveitis), absolute glaucoma or trauma.

phthisis corneae the shrinkage and atrophy of the cornea following a severe inflammation of the cornea or trauma. It is associated with shrinkage of the globe.

-phylaxis a suffix that means 'protection', e.g. *anaphylaxis*.

phylloquinone *n* a member of the vitamin K family of compounds found in green vegetables.

physical abuse ➲ abuse, non-accidental injury.

physical activity level (PAL) the ratio of daily physical energy expenditure to BMR. This factor reflects the average activity both at work and at leisure and is used to estimate average energy requirement. Average energy requirement = PAL × BMR. Examples of PALs for population groups are estimated to be: 1.4 for inactive men and women, 1.6 for moderately active women, and 1.7 for moderately active men. ➲ BMR.

physical activity ratio (PAR) the ratio of the energy cost of a specific activity to the BMR. Factors range from 1 for complete rest to 9 for very vigorous sporting activities, and are used to estimate the energy requirement of a specific activity.

physical environment non-human external factors that demand and shape occupational performance, including the natural world and man-made objects.

physical half-life is the time required for the activity of a radioactive sample to decay to half its original value.

physical self-concept a person's perception or description of their physical self, including their physical appearance, typically not involving an evaluative component.

physical self-esteem a person's evaluation of their physical self, including evaluations of both physical appearance and physical competencies. Also known as physical self-worth.

physical self-perception a general term that denotes all aspects of a person's perceptions of their physical self, including evaluative and descriptive elements.

physician *n* a qualified and registered medical practitioner who practises medicine rather than surgery.

physicochemical *adj* relating to physics and chemistry, or to physical and chemical properties or characteristics.

physio- a prefix that means 'form, nature', e.g. *physiotherapy*.

physiological *adj* often used to describe a normal process or structure, to distinguish it from an abnormal or pathological feature (e.g. the physiological level of glucose in the blood).

physiological advantage a muscle's ability to shorten. Its greatest physiological advantage is when a muscle is at rest.

physiological apex (*syn.* apical constriction, cement-dentine junction). The internal narrowing of a root canal close to the root apex, to which instruments and filling materials are extended during root canal treatment.

physiological arousal ➲ arousal.

physiological cup (*syn* physiological excavation) a funnel-shaped depression at or near the centre of the optic disc through which pass the central retinal vessels. ➲ cup-disc ratio, cupped disc, optic cup, optic disc.

physiological diplopia the normal phenomenon which occurs in binocular vision for non-fixated objects whose images fall on disparate retinal points. It is easily demonstrated to persons with normal binocular vision: the person is asked to fixate binocularly a distant object and place a pencil vertically some 25 cm in front of their nose. The person should see two rather blurred pencils. The observation of physiological diplopia has been found to be useful in the management of eso or exo deviations, suppression, abnormal retinal correspondence (ARC), etc. ➲ Brock string, retinal disparity.

physiological excavation ➲ physiological cap.

physiological nystagmus ➲ fixation movements.

physiological position of rest the position of the eyes when they are only under the control of the postural reflexes, but completely free from any visual stimuli.

physiological solution a fluid isotonic with the body fluids and containing similar salts. ➲ hypertonic, hypotonic, isotonic.

physiological third stage of labour non-interventionist management of the third stage of labour in which the placenta is allowed to separate from the uterine wall without the use of oxytocic drugs to expedite the process. The signs that the placenta has separated are the uterus rising in the abdomen, feeling small, hard and mobile, lengthening of the cord and a small gush of blood from the vagina. The placenta and membranes may then be delivered with maternal effort or controlled cord traction, in which case it is imperative to await signs of separation and descent ➲ active management of the third stage of labour.

physiology *n* the branch of biological science concerned with the normal bodily function of living organisms, hence physiologist. Also those functions themselves, as for example the physiology of digestion, of vision, of locomotion, and so on—**physiological** *adj*, **physiologically** *adv*.

physiotherapy *n* a healthcare profession concerned with human function and movement and maximizing potential. It uses physical approaches to promote, maintain and restore physical, psychological and social well-being, taking account of variations in health status. It is science-based, committed to extending, applying, evaluating and reviewing the evidence that underpins and informs its practice and delivery. The exercise of clinical judgement and informed interpretation is at its core (Chartered Society of Physiotherapy 2000). Traditionally it describes treatment to improve, restore and sometimes cure, using manipulation, electrotherapy, and exercise therapy and rehabilitation following injury or disease, e.g. stroke. Contemporarily, it also includes assessment and diagnosis, health promotion and education, and prevention of disability. ➲ extended scope physiotherapy practitioners. (Chartered Society of Physiotherapy 2000 Rules of professional conduct, 3rd edn. CSP, London.)

phytase a phosphatase enzyme that catalyses the hydrolysis of phytate to inositol and phosphate.

phytate inositol polyphosphate a substance present in plants which binds some metal ions such as ferrous iron, zinc, etc., thus reducing the bioavailability of these ions for intestinal absorption from the food. This may be a problem in certain groups, such as strict vegetarians and vegans who may become deficient in minerals leading to iron deficiency anaemia and other problems.

phytates, phytic acid chemicals present in wholegrain cereals. They can decrease intestinal absorption of some minerals, e.g. calcium, zinc and iron.

phytoagglutinins ⊃ lectins.

phyto-oestrogens chemicals with oestrogen-like effects (oestrogenic) and antioestrogenic effects that originate in plants that include soya beans, soya products such as Tofu and flax seed. Phyto-oestrogens comprise mainly flavonoids, e.g. isoflavones, with some non-flavonoids such as lignans.

phytophotodermatitis a type of contact dermatitis that is caused by exposure to a phototoxin present in certain plants such as members of the *Umbelliferae* family (e.g. cow parsley and the wild parsnip). The phototoxin results from a reaction between light-sensitive chemicals, such as psoralens, in the plant and ultraviolet light. The dermatitis is characterized by burning rather than itching, redness, possible blistering and secondary areas of hyperpigmentation.

phytotherapy phytomedicine, herbal medicine. The use of plant material or plant extracts as remedies that promote health, prevent disorders and in the treatment of disorders. In addition, there are numerous examples of the use of medicines from plant sources in conventional western medical practice, such as taxanes (cytotoxic drugs derived from the yew tree), and in some countries St John's wort is prescribed by conventionally qualified doctors for depressive illness. ⊃ herbalism.

phytotoxin toxic substances present in plants including those used for food, wild plants and those cultivated in gardens. Examples include oxalic acid and oxalates in rhubarb leaves, cardiac glycosides in foxgloves, ricin in the castor oil plant and hemlock.

PI *abbr* **1.** performance indicator. **2.** peridontal (Russell) index.

pia mater the innermost of the meninges; the delicate, vascular membrane which lies in close contact with the brain and spinal cord.

pica *n* a desire for extraordinary or abnormal types of food. Seen in pregnancy. Also known as allotriophagy, cissa and cittosis.

PICC *abbr* peripherally inserted central catheter.

PICH *abbr* primary intracerebral haemorrhage.

pickling in dentistry, a process in which a hot metal is placed in acid to remove surface oxides and other impurities. ⊃ acid bath.

Pick's disease 1. (A Pick, Czech neurologist/psychiatrist, 1851–1924) a type of cerebral atrophy producing dementia during midlife (between 40 and 60 years of age). There is

degeneration in the frontal and temporal lobes of the cerebrum. It is characterized by changes in and eventual disintegration of personality and emotions, disinhibited behaviour and changes in attitudes; impaired speech and language deficits, poor concentration, loss of motivation, poor memory and deterioration in cognitive skills and intellect, There is considerable overlap with Alzheimer's disease. **2.** (F Pick, Czech physician, 1867–1926) syndrome of ascites, hepatomegaly, oedema and pleural effusion that occurs with constrictive pericarditis.

picornavirus *n* derived from pico (very small) and RNA (ribonucleic acid). Small RNA viruses. Includes the enteroviruses (polio, coxsackie, hepatitis A and echovirus) and the rhinoviruses. They cause diverse diseases that include poliomyelitis, common cold, aseptic meningitis, gastroenteritis, hepatitis A, herpangina, etc. ⊃ virus.

picture archiving communications system (PACS) in radiography, a system which enables digital images to be stored electronically and then viewed on computer screens, and therefore allowing the transfer of images and data across the intranet. A networked system of viewing monitors connected to a central image database allows integration of image and demographic information. ⊃ NHS care record service.

PID *abbr* **1.** pelvic inflammatory disease. **2.** position indicating device. ⊃ beam guiding instrument. **3.** prolapsed intervertebral disc. ⊃ prolapse of intervertebral disc.

pie chart in statistics, a circle divided into segments, each segment represents a number of results as a proportion of the whole.

pie in the sky defect ⊃ superior quadrantanopsia.

Piedellos sign a test for the amount of movement at the sacroiliac joint. The seated patient is asked to flex forwards. The health professional palpates the sacral dimples bilaterally. Normally, both of the sacral dimples should move equally towards the head. Excessive rising of one side indicates hypomobility at that sacroiliac joint.

piedra *n* a fungal disease affecting hair. It is characterized by black or white nodules on the hair. Black piedra affects the scalp hair and is caused by *Piedraia hortae* a species of the genus *Piedraia*. Species of the genus *Trichcosporon* are responsible for white piedra which involves the beard, pubic hair and axillary hair.

pie lines in radiology, the marks on a processed film which have been caused by chemicals drying on the surface of the automatic processor rollers.

Pierre Robin syndrome (Pierre Robin, French dental surgeon, 1867–1950) a syndrome of congenital anomalies inherited as an autosomal recessive disorder. Affected infants have micrognathia and a cleft palate, often associated with abnormality of the tongue and larynx. There are feeding difficulties and some infants are at risk of inhaling fluid into the respiratory tract. Management involves protecting the airway, the selection of safe and effective feeding methods, plastic surgery to repair the cleft palate and possibly surgery to enlarge the lower jaw, speech and language therapy and specialist orthodontic treatment.

O
P

piezoelectric crystal a crystal which converts electrical impulses into sound waves and vice versa by deforming when a voltage is applied across it, for example, ceramic or quartz crystals.

piezoelectric effect when an electric current is produced by certain materials when pressure is applied to their surface. ⊃ inverse piezoelectric effect.

piezograph a form moulded by the cheeks, lips and tongue in edentulous areas of the mouth during the construction of dentures.

pigeon chest ⊃ pectus carinatum.

piggyback lens (*syn* combination system) a combination of two contact lenses; usually a rigid contact lens (preferably gas-permeable) over a hydrogel lens. The soft lens is used for comfort and the rigid lens for best visual results. Piggyback lenses can be used after corneal surgery, corneal scarring and in the management of severe keratoconus or irregular astigmatism. ⊃ combination lens, therapeutic soft contact lens.

piggyback port a special coupling device in a primary intravenous administration set, which is used for the intermittent administration of a supplementary (piggyback) intravenous solution containing a drug into the primary line.

pigment *n* any colouring matter of the body. For example the visual pigment rhodopsin; melanin in hair, iris, choroid and skin; haemoglobin; stercobilin in faeces; and the bile pigments biliverdin and bilirubin.

pigmentation *n* the deposit of pigment, especially when abnormal or excessive, such as the pigmentation associated with Addison's disease, arsenic poisoning, haemochromatosis, melanoma, melanosis coli, naevus, Nelson syndrome, etc.

PIH *abbr* pregnancy induced hypertension.

Pilates method (J Pilates, German/American exercise therapist, 1880–1967) a low impact system of focused body-mind exercises. They aim to tone, stretch, strengthen, improve exercise efficiency, improve breathing and increase body awareness.

piles *npl* ⊃ haemorrhoids.

pili *npl* hair-like appendages of many bacteria, and used for the transfer of genetic material—**pilus** *sing*.

pilomotor nerves tiny nerves that innervate the arrectores pilorum muscles of the hair follicles, causing the hairs to become erect and give the appearance of 'gooseflesh'.

pilomotor reflex the erection of the hairs on the skin causing 'gooseflesh'. It is due to the contraction of the arrectores pilorum muscles in response to cold, emotional arousal and fear.

pilonidal *adj* hair-containing.

pilonidal sinus an abnormal tract or sinus containing hairs, which is usually found in hirsute people in the cleft between the buttocks most often situated close to the tip of the coccyx. There is constant irritation and in this situation it is liable to infection and abscess formation. Initial management includes pain relief and antibiotics before a wide surgical excision and drainage. The wound is not closed and is allowed to heal by secondary intention using appropriate dressing products. Thereby ensuring that the infection is eliminated and recurrence does not occur. ⊃ wound healing.

pilosebaceous *adj* pertaining to the hair follicle and the sebaceous gland opening into it. *pilosebaceous unit* comprises the hair follicle, the hair and the associated sebaceous gland.

pilot study an early smaller-scale study carried out before the main research project to evaluate viability and to identify problems with the research methodology.

pimple *n* ⊃ papule.

pin in dentistry **1.** pin-shaped projection from the fitting surface of a cast restoration to increase retention. It fits into a tapered or cylindrical pinhole in the tooth substance which is part of the preparation. **2.** metal pin or wire that is cemented into a prepared pit in the dentine of a tooth preparation or threaded and then screwed into position in the pinhole, or held in place by friction grip. Used to retain a restoration that is placed over a pin or pins while in its plastic state. **3.** long slender metal rod used to immobilize bone fragments in fracture cases. *incisal guide pin* ⊃ guide pin. *self-threading pin* a threaded pin screwed into a prepared hole in dentine to enhance retention.

pin fixation ⊃ fixation (dentistry/maxillofacial surgery).

pinhole spectacles spectacles fitted with opaque discs having one or more small apertures. They are used as an aid in certain types of low vision (e.g. corneal scar). ⊃ low vision.

pin index system designed to prevent the wrong connection of a gas cylinder to an anaesthetic machine.

Pinard's stethoscope trumpet-shaped fetal (monaural) stethoscope; placed on the woman's abdomen over the fetal chest to hear the fetal heart sounds.

pincer nail the lateral edges of the nail practically meet. Lateral compression of the nail may cause damage to the soft tissues and reduce circulation to the nail bed. Subungual ulceration can result.

pineal body (gland) also known as the epiphysis cerebri. A tiny reddish-grey conical structure situated above the third ventricle of the brain and attached to it by a stalk. It secretes various substances which include 5-hydroxytryptamine and melatonin. The release of melatonin is influenced by the amount of light entering the eye and varies with the seasons as daylight hours change. Melatonin levels fluctuate during the 24 hours, it is at its highest level during darkness and at its lowest level around midday. Melatonin appears to influence gonadotrophin secretion, diurnal rhythms such as sleep, and mood. ⊃ depression, seasonal affective disorder.

pinguecula *n* a yellowish, slightly elevated thickening of the bulbar conjunctiva between the eyelids. Associated with the ageing eye.

pin-hole collimator gamma camera collimator with a small hole, a few millimetres in diameter at the end of a lead cone which, due to the divergence of the gamma rays, give an enlarged image of a small object.

pin ledge restoration in dentistry, a cast-metal restoration covering the lingual surface of an incisor or canine and retained by pins slotting into small ledges cut in the tooth preparation.

pink disease ⊃ erythroedema polyneuropathy.

pink eye (colloquial) ⊃ contagious conjunctivitis.

pink spot in dentistry, a term used to describe the pink-hued area on a crown of a tooth that is undergoing internal resorption. The pink hue is due to the hyperplastic vascular tissue visible through the resorbed enamel and dentine.

pink wax obsolescent term for modelling wax. ⊃ wax.

pinlay in dentistry, a cast-metal inlay or onlay that has additional retention by virtue of a pin or pins on its fitting surface.

pinna *n* the auricle. That part of the ear which is external to the head. ⊃ Colour Section Figure 13.

pinnaplasty a plastic operation on the pinna, such as for the correction of bat ears.

pinocytosis *n* the process whereby the plasma membrane engulfs a minute water droplet within a vesicle or vacule, which is taken into the cell. ⊃ bulk transport.

pinta *n* a treponemal infection caused by *Treponema pallidum* (ssp. *carateum*), it is similar to bejel. It occurs following prolonged and close contact. It is characterized by the formation of scaly papules and enlarged lymph nodes, or loss of skin pigment (dyschromatic patches). The late lesions are often depigmented and disfiguring. The infection is confined to the skin. Pinta is probably the oldest of the human treponemal infections and *T. carateum* the parent of the organism that came to Europe with the return of Christopher Columbus's sailors in 1493, starting the epidemic of venereal syphilis known as the 'Great Pox'. It is found only in South and Central America, where its incidence is declining. Pinta occurs in poor rural populations with low standards of domestic hygiene. It has features in common with bejel, notably that it is transmitted by contact, usually within the family and not sexually. The diagnosis of early stage pinta involves the detection of spirochaetes in exudate of lesions by dark ground microscopy. Both latent and early stage is diagnosed by a positive serological test for syphilis. Treatment of all stages is a single intramuscular injection of 1.2 g of long-acting benzylpenicillin. ⊃ bejel, yaws.

pinworm threadworm. ⊃ enterobiasis (oxyuriasis), *Enterobius*.

pisiform pea-shaped. One of the carpal bones of the wrist. It articulates with the triquetral bone another carpal. ⊃ Colour Section Figure 2.

piriformis a pyramidal muscle on the posterior part of the hip, situated under the gluteus minimus muscle of the buttock. Its origin is on the anterolateral part of the sacrum and it inserts on the greater trochanter of the femur. Contraction of the muscle laterally rotates the thigh, it also helps to stabilize the hip joint. ⊃ Colour Section Figure 5.

piriformis syndrome the piriformis is implicated in the irritation of the sciatic nerve, as it passes through or underneath the muscle. Often accompanied by deep buttock pain.

pit 1. in anatomy, a hollow or depression in an organ. **2.** in dentistry, a small depression in the enamel of a tooth.

pit and fissure sealant in dentistry, the material, usually resin, which may or may not contain fillers and colouring matter, used to seal the developmental pits and fissures in enamel surfaces as a preservative measure.

pitch in computed tomography (CT) scanning, is the ratio of table movement, during one 360° rotation.

pitting *n* making an indentation, e.g. in the nails as in psoriasis, or in oedematous tissues.

pituicyte a type of cell of the posterior lobe of the pituitary gland.

pituitary adenoma a tumour of the pituitary gland, often arising from the anterior part of the gland. They are usually benign.

pituitary gland (*syn.* hypophysis cerebri) a small oval endocrine gland lying in the pituitary fossa of the sphenoid bone (Figure P.10). The anterior lobe (adenohypophysis) produces and secretes several hormones; growth hormone (GH), adrenocorticotrophic hormone (ACTH), thyroid-stimulating hormone (TSH), luteinizing hormone (LH), follicle stimulating hormone (FSH) and prolactin (PRL) the lactogenic hormone. The posterior lobe (neurohypophysis) stores and secretes oxytocin and antidiuretic hormone (vasopressin or arginine vasopression [AVP]). These hormones are made by nerve fibres in the hypothalamus. ⊃ anterior pituitary, posterior pituitary.

pityriasis *n* scaly (branny) eruption of the skin. *pityriasis alba* a common eruption in children characterized by scaly hypopigmented macules on the cheeks and upper arms. *pityriasis capitis* dandruff. *pityriasis rosea* a slightly scaly eruption of ovoid erythematous lesions which are widespread over the trunk and proximal parts of the limbs. It is a self-limiting condition. *pityriasis rubra pilaris* a chronic skin disease characterized by coalescing red papules of perifollicular distribution. *pityriasis versicolor* called also 'tinea versicolor', is a yeast infection which causes the appearance of buff-coloured patches on the trunk. ⊃ Colour Section Figure 98.

Pityrosporum *n* ⊃ *Malassezia*.

pivot joint also known as a trochoid joint. A type of synovial joint in which rotation is the only movement possible.

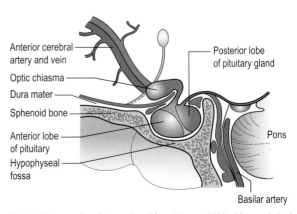

P.10 Pituitary gland (reproduced from Watson 2000 with permission).

601

The joint comprises a pivot-like bony process that fits into a ring formed from ligament and bone, and rotates within the ring. Examples include the proximal radioulnar joint, and the joint formed by the peg-like dens of the axis (second cervical vertebra) fitting into the ring formed by part of the atlas (first cervical vertebra) and the transverse ligament.

pivot shift test a test for anterolateral instability of the knee joint, with the foot in medial rotation and the knee in 30° of flexion, a valgus stress is applied to the knee whilst simultaneously extending it. A 'clunk' heard indicates a positive test and suggests anterior cruciate ligament pathology.

pixel picture cell, the dots which can be used by a character on a digital image display screen, the smaller the pixel the greater the image quality.

PJC *abbr* porcelain jacket crown.

PKB *abbr* prone knee bend.

PKU *abbr* phenylketonuria.

placebo *n* a harmless inert substance given as medicine or supplement. In a randomized placebo-controlled trial, this is identical in appearance with the material being tested. When neither the researcher nor the subjects knows which is which, the trial is said to be 'double blind'.

placebo effect a therapeutic effect which is observed after the administration of a placebo, or in the case of sport performance an enhancing effect observed after the administration of a placebo.

placenta *n* the afterbirth, a hormone-secreting vascular structure developed and functioning by about the third month of pregnancy and attached to the inner wall of the uterus. It is normally sited in the upper segment of the uterus. It is a flat structure some 17.5–20 cm in diameter and 2.5 cm thick, tapering to 1.2 cm at the periphery; weighs approximately one-sixth of the infant's birth weight at full term. It is formed by 12 weeks' gestation, developed from trophoblastic layers with a lining of mesoderm in which the blood vessels develop; composed of numerous chorionic villi grouped together in cotyledons, embedded in the uterine decidua basalis. The villi contain fetal blood vessels, ultimately joining together as the umbilical vessels, separated by intervillous spaces through which the maternal blood circulates. This structural arrangement within the placenta facilitates the exchange of substances between fetal and maternal blood thus ensuring that the fetus is supplied with nourishment and oxygen and through it the fetus gets rid of waste carbon dioxide and nitrogenous waste products. The placenta is important as a hormone-producing structure; the placental hormones include human chorionic gonadotrophin (hCG), human placental lactogen (HPL), oestrogens and progesterone. The maternal surface of the placenta is dark red in colour and lobulated (Figure P.11A). The fetal surface is covered by amnion, it is white and shiny and it is has branches of the umbilical vessels (Figure P.11B). The amnion covered umbilical vessels (two arteries and a vein) eventually leave the placenta as the umbilical cord, which links the fetus and the placenta; the chorion is continuous with the edge of the placenta. In normal labour it is

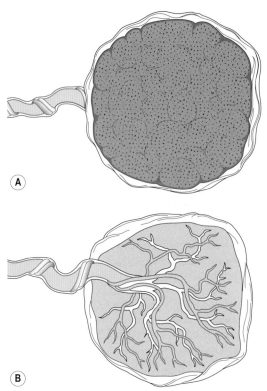

P.11 Placenta at term: A. maternal surface; B. fetal surface (reproduced from Fraser & Cooper 2003 with permission).

expelled, with the fetal membranes, during the third stage of labour. When this does not occur it is termed a retained placenta and may be an adherent placenta. Various abnormal forms of placenta include: placenta circumvallata, placenta fenestrata, placenta membranacea, succenturiate placenta— **placental** *adj.* ➲ adherent placenta, placenta accreta, placenta circumvallata, placenta fenestrata, placenta increta, placenta membranacea, placenta percreta, placenta praevia, succenturiate placenta, tripartite placenta, velamentous insertion of the umbilical cord.

placenta accreta a type of abnormally adherant placenta, which invades into the myometrium (uterine muscle layer).

placenta circumvallata (*syn.* circumvallate placenta) an abnormal placenta. It is encircled with a dense, raised, white nodular ring of attached membranes doubled back over the placental edge.

placenta fenestrata an abnormal placenta with a gap or 'window' in its structure.

placenta increta a type of abnormally adherant placenta, which invades into the perimetrium.

placenta membranacea an abnormally thin placenta, which is spread over an unusually large area of the uterus, sometimes occurring in placenta praevia.

placenta percreta a type of abnormally adherant placenta, which is through the myometrium.

O
P

placenta praevia the placenta is usually attached to the upper segment of the uterus; where part or all of it lies in the lower uterine segment it is called a *placenta praevia*. It may cause placental abruption with painless antepartum vaginal bleeding towards the end of pregnancy as the lower uterine segment stretches in preparation for labour. A placenta praevia should be considered if there is an unstable lie, non-engagement of the presenting part in a primigravida after 36 weeks' gestation or an abnormal presentation. There are four grades of placenta praevia: grade 1 where only the edge of the placenta encroaches into the lower uterine segment; grade 2 in which the whole placenta is in the lower uterine segment; grade 3 where the placenta reaches to the internal cervical os; and grade 4 where the entire placenta covers the central cervical os. Hospital admission is necessary to control bleeding, confirm the exact location of the placenta on ultrasound scan and determine the safest mode of delivery of the infant. Fetal malpresentations, e.g. oblique lie, are common and vaginal delivery is unsafe unless the degree of placenta praevia is minimal. ⊃ vasa praevia.

placental abruption premature placental separation from the uterine wall prior to the delivery of the fetus resulting in haemorrhage. ⊃ abruptio.

placental infarct death of an area of the placenta. If this is extensive it will reduce the supply of nutrients and result in fetal compromise including intrauterine growth restriction.

placental insufficiency inefficiency of the placenta. It can occur due to heavy smoking during pregnancy, diseases such as pre-eclampsia, essential hypertension, chronic renal failure or postmaturity. The fetus may be small for gestational age ('small for dates') or even die *in utero*. ⊃ intrauterine growth restriction/retardation.

placental lactogen hormone influencing breast growth and development in pregnancy. It also affects glucose metabolism in pregnancy; similar to pituitary growth hormone, but does not promote growth.

placental site trophoblastic tumour (PSTT) a rare malignant gestational trophoblastic tumour that develops in the uterine wall at the placental site. It can occur following miscarriage or a full term pregnancy. Management usually includes hysterectomy and chemotherapy if there is secondary spread outside the uterus (e.g to the lung). Radiotherapy may be required if these measures are not effective.

placentography *n* a radiographic examination of the placenta, now superseded by ultrasound.

placentophagy eating of the placenta, in the belief that its hormones prevent postnatal depression.

Placido disc ⊃ keratoscope.

plagiocephaly a congenital anomaly whereby the skull shape is distorted and asymmetrical. It is caused by abnormally early or irregular closure of the skull sutures.

plague *n* very contagious epidemic disease caused by the bacterium *Yersinia pestis*, and spread by infected rats. Transfer of infection from rat to human is through bites from rat fleas, but droplet spread may occur between humans. The main clinical types are bubonic, pneumonic or septicaemic. It is endemic in areas of Asia and Africa. There are also small scattered outbreaks in rural areas of the Western USA, where the disease is highly prevalent in wild rodents.

planar analysis motion analysis (may be kinematic or kinetic) which analyses movement in only one plane, i.e. is two-dimensional. If a body/object is moving three-dimensionally, planar analysis requires assumptions about out-of-plane movements. Kinematic planar motion analysis usually only requires one camera, so is simple.

planar implants an interstitial implant to treat a volume of tissue of the same area to a thickness of 5 mm on either side.

Planck's constant (M Planck, German physicist, 1858–1947) a constant that relates the quantum of energy (E) of a photon to the frequency (f) of the corresponding electromagnetic radiation. $E = hf$ where h is Planck's constant.

plane joint a synovial joint that allows a gliding movement only, for example, the sacroiliac joints.

plane of cut ⊃ focal plane.

plane of occlusion ⊃ occlusal plane.

planes of reference planes that locate landmarks from which anatomical and cephalometric measurements can be made.

planes *npl* in anatomy, used for reference in the description of location and movements of parts of the body, three planes perpendicular to each other, passing through the middle of the body, are defined: median (midsagittal) vertical, front-to-back; frontal (coronal) vertical, side-to-side; transverse (horizontal) horizontal. ⊃ frontal (coronal) plane, median (midsagittal) plane, principal axes, transverse (horizontal) plane.

plane warts flat small papules commonly seen on the face or hands in children.

planing in dentistry, the instrumentation of root surfaces to remove subgingival tooth deposits and necrotic cementum. ⊃ root (dental procedures).

planned home birth women can choose to deliver their infants at home and receive care from the community midwife and general practitioner, or sometimes from an independent midwife. The midwife is legally obliged to provide appropriate care for any woman within her area of practice, even if the mother's wish for a home birth is against professional advice.

planning regarded as the second stage of the nursing process. After identification of the patient's actual and potential problems with everyday living activities, the patient participates in setting appropriate goals to be achieved by the selected nursing interventions. A date is set for evaluation of whether or not the goals have been achieved. ⊃ assessment, evaluation, implementation.

planning target volume (PTV) a tissue volume used to aid the selection of the appropriate beam sizes and arrangements to ensure that the prescribed dose of radiation is delivered to the clinical target volume during radiotherapy treatment.

plantar *adj* pertaining to the sole of the foot.

O
P

plantar arch the union of the plantar and dorsalis pedis arteries in the sole of the foot.

plantar fascia the thick band of connective tissue on the sole of the foot, which runs from the calcaneus to the base of the toes.

plantar fasciitis (*syn* painful heel syndrome) inflammation (plantar fasciitis) is one of the commonest causes of heel pain, usually at the attachment to the calcaneus. Pain is felt especially first thing in the morning (overnight rest with the foot in plantar flexion allows the fascia to contract) or on weight-bearing exercise: a dull pain felt along the sole of the foot. Associated with, but not caused by, a bony spur. More common in runners, gymnasts and dancers (who use repetitive maximal plantar flexion of the foot) and in those with flat feet. The condition may be due to biomechanical abnormalities or as sequelae of other conditions such as ankylosing spondylitis. Management includes rest, anti-inflammatory medication, podiatry assessment, exercises to stretch the fascia, orthoses and, if severe, corticosteroid injection.

plantar flexion movement at the ankle joint that points the foot downwards away from the leg, or movement of the toes that curls them down towards the sole (compare dorsiflexion). ⮑ Babinski's reflex or sign.

plantar wart a wart on the sole of the foot, often painful. It is commonly caused by the human papilloma virus.

planteris a small superficial muscle of the posterior compartment of the leg. Its origin is on the posterior distal femur and its long, thin tendon inserts into the calcaneus. Contraction of the muscle assists with flexion of the knee and plantar flexion. ⮑ Colour Section Figure 5.

plaque *n* **1.** an elevated area on the skin or internal organ. **2.** a deposit of atheroma on a vessel wall. **3.** areas of demyelination (loss of myelin) and the hardening of tissue in multiple sclerosis. ⮑ dental calculus, dental plaque.

plaque score index ⮑ index (dental).

plaque (Silness and Loe) index ⮑ index (dental).

plasma *n* the pale, yellow fluid part of blood, in which the cellular components are suspended: red blood cells (erythrocytes), white blood cells (leucocytes) and blood platelets (thrombocytes). Plasma is mainly water (90–92%) and contains a variety of substances including: plasma proteins such as albumin and the clotting factors, inorganic ions (e.g. sodium, calcium, bicarbonate), amino acids, glucose, lipids, vitamins, enzymes, hormones, gases, drugs and metabolic waste. Plasma forms around 55% of blood volume.

plasma cell an immune cell that produces antibodies (immunoglobulins). It is derived from B lymphocytes/cells and is involved in humoral immunity. ⮑ humoral immunity.

plasmacytoma *n* a malignant tumour of plasma cells, it may be within the bone marrow, such as in multiple myeloma, or in other tissues—**plasmacytomas, plasmocytomata** *pl.* ⮑ multiple myeloma.

plasma membrane also known as the cell membrane. The outer membrane that encloses the cytoplasm (protoplasm) and cell organelles. The plasma membrane consists of two layers of phospholipids with some protein molecules embedded in them. Those that extend all the way through the membrane may provide channels that allow the passage of, for example, electrolytes and non-lipid-soluble substances. The phospholipid molecules have a head which is electrically charged and hydrophilic and a tail which has no charge and is hydrophobic. The phospholipid bilayer is arranged like a sandwich with the hydrophilic heads aligned on the outer surfaces of the membrane and the hydrophobic tails forming a central water-repelling layer. These differences influence the transfer of substances across the membrane. The membrane proteins perform several functions: (a) branched carbohydrate molecules attached to the outside of some membrane protein molecules give the cell its immunological identity; (b) they can act as specific receptors for hormones and other chemical messengers; (c) some are enzymes; and (d) some are involved in the transport of molecules across the membrane.

plasmapheresis *n* taking blood from a donor, removing some desired fraction, then returning the red cells and repeating the whole process. Donated plasma is used to produce fresh frozen plasma and a variety of specific components such as individual coagulation factors. Plasmapheresis is also be used in the treatment of some diseases, which are caused by antibodies or immune complexes circulating in a patient's plasma, e.g. myasthenia gravis, Guillan–Barré syndrome. Removing the plasma and replacing it with donated plasma or a plasma substitute can improve the prognosis of the disease and prevent or delay the onset of renal failure. ⮑ apheresis.

plasma thromboplastin antecedent factor XI of blood coagulation. It is produced in the liver and is required for the formation of prothrombin activator. A very rare inherited autosomal deficiency leads to a bleeding disorder.

plasmid *n* DNA present in some bacteria. The transfer of this genetic material between bacteria during sexual reproduction allows the exchange of genes for antibiotic resistance.

plasmin *n* proteolytic enzyme produced when plasminogen is activated. It breaks down fibrin clots when healing is complete. Also called fibrinolysin. ⮑ fibrinolysis.

plasminogen *n* inactive precursor of plasmin. Release of activators, e.g. tissue plasminogen activator (t-PA), from damaged tissue promotes the conversion of plasminogen into plasmin.

plasminogen activators a group of endopeptidase enzymes that convert inactive plasminogen into the active form plasmin, which is fibrinolytic. They include tissue plasminogen activator (t-PA) and urinary plasminogen activator (urokinase).

Plasmodium *n* a genus of protozoa. Parasites in the blood of warm-blooded animals which complete their sexual cycle in blood-sucking arthropods such as mosquitoes. Malaria is caused by four species of *Plasmodium*—**plasmodial** *adj*.

plaster knife in dentistry, a hand-held knife, usually with a wooden handle, used to trim plaster of Paris models.

plasterless articulator in dentistry, a fixed plate articulator that allows models to be grasped, controlling the correct occlusion without the need for plasterwork.

plaster model in dentistry, a cast of the teeth and jaw made for diagnostic purposes, such as prior to orthodontic treatment, or to produce a very precise appliance, e.g. the retainer to be bonded onto the teeth following orthodontic treatment.

plaster of Paris (POP) plaster of Paris is calcium sulphate (gypsum). It is produced as gypsum-impregnated bandage that can be moulded to the part when wet, and subsequently sets. The standard method of external splinting is still the use of plaster of Paris. Synthetic materials are now used for splinting some fractures because of their light weight and waterproof qualities. Custom-made lightweight thermoplastics can be moulded to the limb and re-moulded if swelling or atrophy cause changes in the limb contour. Some synthetic casting materials, however, are less malleable and cannot be moulded as effectively as plaster of Paris. They can occasionally cause allergies. Although plaster of Paris and synthetic material splinting has many advantages over surgery their use can lead to serious complications if swelling under the cast impedes blood supply and or causes nerve damage. Medical advice should be urgently sought if the skin of the limb becomes pale or blue, the patient complains of numbness, tingling or throbbing, excessive pain in the injured part, inability to move the fingers or toes, swelling, bulging or puffiness around the edges of the cast or a foul smell from under the cast (which may indicate the presence of an ulcer caused by pressure). It is also necessary to seek advice if the cast becomes loose and slides around. The advantages of plaster of Paris include: non-invasive thus avoiding the risk of infection; quick to apply; reduced time in hospital by avoiding surgery and its potential complications; cheap and relatively easy to apply for trained staff; can be moulded for several minutes before hardening occurs; radio translucent (bones can be X-rayed through the cast); may absorb fluids or bleeding. The extent of bleeding can be traced on the cast itself and monitored at appropriate intervals. Disadvantages of using plaster of Paris include: it may not be possible to reduce the fracture correctly or maintain reduction thus requiring surgery at a later date; the cast needs removal/or windowing (removal of a piece of the cast) to inspect the skin or a surgical site; may need removal in case of increased swelling or reapplication once swelling has subsided; smelly if it gets wet; heavy and inconvenient, may crack; the cast can rub the skin and cause pressure ulcers; inability of the patient to deal with itching under the plaster. The calcium sulphate hemihydrate powder, which when mixed with the correct proportion of water sets to a hard white solid, is used extensively in the dental laboratory for moulds and models and occasionally as an impression material.

plaster of Paris deadcap a headband of gauze and plaster of Paris into which various attachments can be incorporated. Previously used to immobilize maxillary fracture, but now largely superceded.

plaster of Paris impression material ➲ impression.

plastic *adj* **1.** capable of taking a form or mould, e.g. mixed amalgam prior to setting. Describes a body, object or substance which after deformation does not return to its initial state. Contrast elasticity. **2.** a common term for methyl methacrylate (acrylic).

plasticity the ability to change. ➲ neuroplasticity.

plasticizer 1. an addition to the radiographic film emulsion to prevent it from becoming too brittle. **2.** a substance added to plastic materials to increase their softness and flexibility.

plastic period ➲ critical period.

plastic point a tapered plastic pin of various sizes, sometimes used in conjunction with wax patterns for crown and inlay work. The pin burns out during the casting process.

plastic surgery transfer of healthy tissue to repair damaged area and the use of implants to restore form and function, or alter size or shape. Some procedures are undertaken for cosmetic reasons.

-plasty a suffix that means 'reconstructive surgery', e.g. *pharyngoplasty*.

plate ➲ bone plate, buccal plate, compression bone plate, mini bone plate.

plateau iris an anatomical anomaly in which the iris lies in a plane rather than bulging anteriorly. This is due to the fact that the root (or ciliary margin) of the iris is inserted more anteriorly into the ciliary body than usual in apposition to the trabecular meshwork. It can predispose to the development of primary closed-angle glaucoma. ➲ angle-closure glaucoma, trabecular meshwork.

platelet *n* (*syn.* thrombocyte) cellular fragments without a nucleus that are mainly concerned with blood coagulation. They are formed in the bone marrow from the megakaryocytes and released into the blood. ➲ platelet plug.

platelet-derived growth factor (PDGF) a peptide growth factor important during embryonic development; after birth it stimulates cell growth, cell differentiation, cell migration, and the development of new blood vessels (angiogenesis). It is present in granules in platelets and is released when platelets are in contact with damaged tissue. PDGF stimulates the proliferation of fibroblasts and angiogenesis during wound healing.

platelet plug one of the four overlapping stages of haemostasis. Platelets aggregate and adhere to form a temporary plug at the site of blood vessel damage (Figure P.12). ➲ coagulation, fibrinolysis, vasoconstriction.

platinum (Pt) a naturally occurring greyish-white precious metal that does not tarnish in air. In dentistry, it is used in combination with gold as an alloy for casting purposes and as platinum foil matrix in the construction of porcelain crowns.

platinum foil ➲ foil.

platinum matrix a matrix of a platinum foil that is burnished onto a crown preparation model. Wet porcelain powder is then applied to it and baked in a furnace to form a porcelain crown or inlay.

O
P

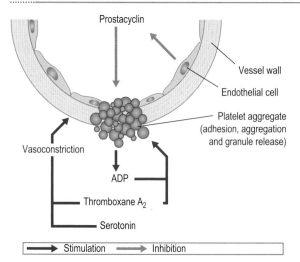

P.12 Platelet plug formation (reproduced from Hinchliff et al 1996 with permission).

platyhelminth *n* flat worm; cestodes (tapeworms) and trematodes (flukes). ⊃ *Echinococcus*, schistosomiasis, *Taenia*.

platyopnoea breathlessness experienced in an upright position.

platypelloid pelvis also known as a flat pelvis. A pelvis with oval brim, small anteroposteriorly and wide transversely.

platysma a superficial muscle of the neck. Its origin is on the fascia overlying the pectoral and deltoid muscles and it inserts into the lower edge of the mandible. It is involved in depressing the mandible and pulling the lower lip down and back. ⊃ Colour Section Figure 4.

play the natural means of self-expression for a child; the medium through which she/he learns and rehearses a wide range of life skills. ⊃ normative play, therapeutic play.

play therapist a person who uses play constructively to help children to come to terms with having to be in hospital.

PLB *abbr* pursed lip breathing.

pledget a small quantity of cotton wool, gauze or sponge compressed into a ball.

-plegia a suffix that means 'paralysis', e.g. *paraplegia*

pleiotropy the capacity of a single gene to have multiple effects on the phenotype. For example, the diverse characteristics of an inherited disease.

pleocytosis *n* the presence of an abnormal number of cells in cerebrospinal fluid.

pleomastia also known as polymastia. The presence of supernumerary breasts or nipples, usually occurring on the nipple line, i.e. on a line stretching from the midclavicular point to the pelvic girdle.

pleomorphism *n* denotes a wide range in shape and size of individuals in a bacterial population—**pleomorphic** *adj*.

pleoptics a method of treating amblyopia with eccentric fixation which consists of dazzling the eccentrically fixating retinal area with high illumination while protecting the fovea with a disc projected onto the fundus and thereby rendering the fovea more responsive to fixation stimuli. There exist several variations of this procedure, but the therapy is very fastidious. ⊃ amblyopia, occlusion treatment, orthoptics, Visuscope.

plethora *n* fullness; overloading. Previously applied to an excess of blood causing a red face—**plethoric** *adj*.

plethysmograph *n* an instrument which accurately measures blood flow. Used to measure and record changes in the volume and size of organs or an extremity—**plethysmographic** *adj*.

pleura *n* the serous membrane covering the surface of the lung including the fissures between the lobes of the lungs (visceral pleura), the diaphragm, the mediastinum and the chest wall (parietal pleura). A potential space exists between the visceral and parietal layers. A thin film of serous fluid present in the space provides the lubrication that prevents friction when the two layers glide effortlessly over each other when the volume of the lungs change during breathing. The integrity of both pleural layers is essential to keeping the underlying lung inflated—**pleural** *adj*, **pleurae** *pl*. ⊃ pneumothorax.

pleural effusion also known as hydrothorax. A collection of excess fluid in the pleural cavity, which may be an exudate or a transudate. The excess fluid may result from increased production or impaired drainage of fluid. Causes include parapneumonic, viral infection, malignancy, connective tissue diseases, lymphatic obstruction and many more. It can be associated with inflammation, pleurisy, pneumonia, tuberculosis, lung cancer, mesothelioma, other malignancies, pulmonary infarction, abdominal disorders such as pancreatitis, cardiac failure, post myocardial infarction, hypoproteinaemia, renal failure and connective tissue diseases. The clinical features vary with the size and onset, e.g. small effusions may have no symptoms while larger ones may be accompanied with dyspnoea and, if infective, cause pleuritic type pain followed by fluid accumulation. Malignant effusions are often blood stained. Turbid fluid may be present following bacterial pneumonia, this is termed empyema (pus present in the pleural fluid). Investigative procedures include chest radiology, pleural fluid aspiration and biopsy, thoracic ultrasound and video-assisted thoracoscopic biopsy. Management of effusions is determined by the cause, so may involve no intervention, analgesics, antibiotics, chest drainage or surgical interventions.

pleural pressure the negative pressure within the pleural space. It is fundamental in keeping the lung inflated and is more negative at the apex than the base (in the upright position). Disruption of the pleurae, e.g. trauma and pneumothorax, cause an increase in pleural pressure to above atmospheric pressure and will result in lung compression and collapse.

pleural rub also known as a friction rub. A grating, rubbing sound that is heard during auscultation, as the dry or roughened layers of pleura move over each other. It signifies inflammation of the pleura (pleurisy).

pleural space the potential space between the two layers of pleurae. It is filled with a thin film of serous fluid, which allows the pleural surfaces to glide easily over each other throughout the breathing cycle, while permitting chest wall forces to be transmitted to the lungs. Interruption of this space (e.g. chest trauma) can result in the separation of the two pleural surfaces when the parietal pleura will remain against the chest wall, while the visceral pleura and lung is displaced inward, away from the chest wall, e.g. pneumothorax.

pleurectomy *n* surgical stripping of the pleura to achieve a surgical pleurodesis.

pleurisy, pleuritis *n* inflammation of the pleura. It may be fibrinous (dry), be associated with an effusion (wet), or be complicated by empyema. There is pain on breathing and is usually caused by a viral infection. The pain is increased by deep breathing, coughing and chest movement. The pleural surfaces, roughened by inflammation, rub together with each breath and may produce a rough, grating sound called a friction or pleural rub. This can be heard with the stethoscope—**pleuritic** *adj*.

pleur/o- a prefix that means 'pleura', e.g. *pleurisy*.

pleurocentesis also known as paracentesis thoracis or thoracentesis. Aspiration or drainage of fluid from the pleural cavity.

pleurodesis *n* adherence of the visceral to the parietal pleura. Used therapeutically to prevent recurrence of metastatic pleural effusions, or recurrent pneumothoraces. Achieved by the use of sclerosing agents such as talc. ⊃ pleurectomy.

pleurodynia *n* intercostal myalgia or muscular rheumatism (fibrositis). ⊃ Bornholm disease.

pleurolysis *n* surgical separation of the pleura from its attachments.

pleuropneumonia-like organisms (PPLO) ⊃ Mycoplasma.

pleuropulmonary *adj* relating to the pleura and lung.

pleurotomy *n* incision of the pleura.

plexiform resembling a plexus.

plexopathy decreased movement or sensation in a joint caused by impaired function of the nerves that cause sensation and movement.

plexus *n* a network of vessels or nerves. For example, choroid plexus, cervical plexus, etc. ⊃ Colour Section Figure 11.

plica a synovial fold that is occasionally found in the knee joint, which may become pathological and painful, the most common plicae are the mediopatellar plica and the suprapatellar plica—**plicae** *pl*.

plication *n* a surgical procedure of making tucks or folds to decrease the size of an organ, such as reducing the size of the stomach in the management of morbid obesity—**plica** *sing*, **plicae** *pl*, **plicate** *adj, vt*.

pliers in dentistry, a two-handled instrument designed to grip, bend, hold or cut wires and metal strips. *Adams' pliers* pliers with solid tapered beaks that form a four-sided pyramid when closed. Used to adjust removable orthodontic appliances and to bend and form modified arrowhead (Adams') clasps. *arrowhead clasp forming pliers* used to form arrowhead wire clasps of orthodontic appliances. *band contouring pliers* used for contouring and adapting bands. There are several patterns, e.g. Adams'. Heavy pliers with tapered beaks that form a four-sided pyramid when closed. *band removing pliers* used to remove orthodontic bands from teeth. The longer beak is placed on the occlusal surface of the tooth and the shorter one levers off the band by its cervical edge. *band splitting pliers* pliers used to remove orthodontic bands by cutting them. *bird beak pliers* similar to the light wire-bending pliers but with shorter beaks. *bracket removing pliers* similar to band removing pliers. Used to remove orthodontic brackets bonded to teeth. *Howe's pliers* pliers with slender flat beaks terminating in a comma shape with serrated surfaces and meeting only at the tips. Used for tying and bending orthodontic ligature wires. *ligature and pin cutting pliers* used for cutting orthodontic ligatures and arch-retaining pins. *ligature locking pliers* used in edgewise orthodontic technique to tighten a ligature when opened. *light wire-bending pliers* pliers with short beaks, one conical and one pyramidal. Used for bending small wires and springs. *Marthew's pliers* wire-bending pliers with one conical beak closing into a hollow-ground beak. *Nance loop closing pliers* used to form parallel-sided wire loops. They have flat, thin beaks stepped down in size towards their tips. *snipe nosed pliers* pliers with square-nosed flat beaks used for wire bending. *spring-forming pliers* orthodontic wire-bending pliers with one conical and one pyramidal beak. *triple beak pliers* pliers with a single beak opposing two beaks, used to place bends in orthodontic wire. *tweed arch bending pliers* pliers with flattened blades that are parallel when gripping orthodontic wire. Used for square and rectangular wires. Another pattern forms loops or curves in such wires. *universal pliers* ⊃ Adam's pliers. *Weingart pliers* similar to How's pliers but with curved offset beaks.

plombage *n* extra-pleural compression of a tuberculous lung cavity to deprive tubercle of oxygen. Widely used surgical technique before the introduction of antibiotic therapy for tuberculosis. Now sometimes used in multidrug resistant tuberculosis.

plug a mass that closes an opening.

plugger in dentistry, 1. a hand instrument, usually double ended, with a round- or oval-shaped end, either serrated or plain. Used to plug and condense amalgam into a cavity preparation. 2. a single-ended hand instrument used to plug and condense gutta percha in a root canal.

plumbago ⊃ graphite.

plumbism *n* ⊃ lead poisoning.

Plummer's disease (H Plummer, American physician, 1874–1937) also called toxic nodular goitre. Hyperthyroidism caused by a solitary toxic adenoma in the thyroid gland. Most often affects females over the age of 40 years.

Plummer–Vinson syndrome (*syn* Kelly–Paterson, Paterson–Brown–Kelly syndrome) (H Plummer, American physician, 1874–1937; P Vinson, American surgeon, 1890–1959) sideropenic dysphagia. A combination of chronic iron deficiency anaemia, glossitis, fissuring in the corners of the mouth (angular stomatitis) and dysphagia caused by the development of a post-cricoid web. A rare condition occurring mainly in middle-aged females.

plunger cusp a cusp that forces food interproximally between teeth in the opposing arch.

pluri- a prefix that means 'many', e.g. *pluriglandular*.

pluriglandular *adj* pertaining to several glands, as in cystic fibrosis.

plyometric exercise explosive exercise that maximizes the myotatic on-stretch reflex, i.e. a lengthening of a muscle followed by a sudden shortening in order to produce power. They often involve a jumping movement. For example, skipping, bounding, lunges.

PMA *abbr* papillary, marginal and attached gingivae. The Schour and Massler index. ⊃ index (dental).

PMB *abbr* postmenopausal bleeding.

PMH *abbr* past medical history.

PMI *abbr* point of maximum impulse.

PMMA *abbr* polymethylmethacrylate.

PMR *abbr* polymyalgia rheumatica.

PMS *abbr* premenstrual syndrome.

PND *abbr* paroxysmal nocturnal dyspnoea.

pneumatocele 1. a sac or swelling that contains air. **2.** a hernia of lung tissue.

pneumaturia *n* bubbles of air or other gases in the urine. It may be the passage of flatus with urine, usually as a result of a vesicocolic (bladder–colon) fistula, such as that caused by diverticular disease when a segment of diseased bowel adheres to the bladder.

pneumococcus *n Streptococcus pneumoniae*. A Gram-positive diplococcus. Causes lobar pneumonia and other infections, e.g. meningitis—**pneumococcal** *adj*.

pneumoconiosis *n* (*syn.* dust disease) fibrosis of the lung caused by long continued inhalation of dust in industrial occupations. There is breathlessness, chronic bronchitis and a gradual decline in gaseous exchange and respiratory function with right heart failure. The most important complication is the occasional superinfection with tuberculosis—**pneumoconioses** *pl*. ⊃ anthracosis, asbestosis, byssinosis, rheumatoid pneumoconiosis, siderosis, silicosis.

Pneumocystis jirovecii formerly known as *Pneumocystis carinii*. An opportunistic micro-organism that causes pneumonia in immunocompromised individuals, such as infants, debilitated and immunosuppressed patients and those with HIV disease: mortality is high.

pneumocystis pneumonia (PCP) pneumonia caused by a fungal species of the genus *Pneumocystis*. ⊃ *Pneumocystis jirovecii*.

pneumocytes *npl* cells lining the alveolar walls in the lungs. Type I are flat cells; Type II are cuboidal and secrete surfactant.

pneumoencephalography *n* radiographic examination of the cerebral ventricles after injection of air by means of a lumbar or cisternal puncture—**pneumoencephalogram** *n*.

pneumolysis *n* separation of the two pleural layers, or the outer pleural layer from the chest wall, to collapse the lung.

pneumomediastinum the collection of air in the mediastinum and may be indicative of barotrauma or oesophageal rupture (less commonly).

pneumomycosis *n* fungal infection affecting the lung, e.g. actinomycosis, aspergillosis, candidiasis—**pneumomycotic** *adj*.

pneumonectomy *n* excision of a lung.

pneumonia *n* a lower respiratory tract infection. Acute infection of the lung by an invading organism associated with new pulmonary shadowing on a radiograph. There is inflammation of the lung parenchyma, usually as a result of bacterial or viral infection, but may occasionally be fungal or parasitic. It is now subdivided into community-acquired, hospital-acquired, and pneumonia associated with profound immunosuppression. Types include atypical pneumonia, aspiration pneumonia, bacterial pneumonia, bronchopneumonia, fungal pneumonia, lobar pneumonia, mycoplasma pneumonia, pneumocystis pneumonia, viral pneumonia. The clinical features usually present as a rapid onset of pyrexia, cough (initially unproductive) and pleuritic chest pain, with rapid shallow breathing and possibly cyanosis. The affected portion of lung will often display features of consolidation radiologically, with bronchial breath sounds and dullness to percussion being common findings. Sputum and blood cultures should be obtained as soon as possible. Close monitoring of these patients is required as severe pneumonia carries a significant risk of mortality (British Thoracic Society 2001, 2002). (British Thoracic Society 2001 Guidelines for the Management of Community Acquired Pneumonia in Adults. 56; Suppl IV. British Thoracic Society 2002 Guidelines for the Management of Community Acquired Pneumonia in Childhood. 57; Suppl I.)

pneumonic plague ⊃ plague.

pneumonitis *n* inflammation of lung tissue.

pneumoperitoneum *n* air or gas in the peritoneal cavity. It may result from the perforation of the stomach or intestine. Can be introduced for diagnostic, or therapeutic purposes such as during laparoscopic examination and operative procedures.

pneum/o, pneum/a, pneumat/o- a prefix that means 'lung', e.g. *pneumothorax*.

pneumotachograph an instrument for recording respiratory airflow in terms of the pressure drop across a low resistance in its path (flow head). Flow can be electronically integrated with respect to time, to give a continuous record of volume breathed in or out, and hence the volume per minute (ventilation).

pneumotaxic centre a respiratory control centre in the pons, which has an inhibitory effect on the nerves controlling inspiration and helps to ensure a smooth respiratory rhythm. If it is damaged the unopposed action of the apneustic centre leads to prolonged gasping inspiration with only infrequent expiration. ⊃ apneustic centre.

pneumothorax *n* air or gas in the pleural cavity separating the visceral from the parietal pleura so that underlying lung tissue collapses. Occurs spontaneously when an over-dilated pulmonary air sac ruptures, permitting communication of respiratory passages with the pleural cavity. A spontaneous pneumothorax may be treated by percutaneous needle aspiration of the air, insertion of a drain with a one way valve or an underwater seal chest drain. ⊃ underwater seal drain. Associated with many lung diseases, including asthma, bronchial cancer, chronic obstructive pulmonary disease, congenital cysts, tuberculosis. Also caused by trauma, and can occur during positive pressure ventilation. *tension pneumothorax* a valve-like wound or tear in the lung allows air to enter the pleural cavity with each inspiration, but not to escape on expiration, thus progressively increasing intrathoracic pressure and constituting an acute medical emergency. Signs are of hyperinflation, midline shift and increasing respiratory distress.

PNF *abbr* **1.** passive neck flexion. **2.** proprioceptive neuromuscular facilitation.

PNH *abbr* paroxysmal nocturnal haemoglobinuria.

PNI *abbr* psychoneuroimmunology.

PN junction is formed by fusing together a P-type semiconductor and an N-type semiconductor.

-pnoea a suffix that means 'breathing', e.g. *apnoea*.

PNS *abbr* **1.** periopheral nervous system. **2.** posterior nasal spine.

PO₂ *abbr* the partial pressure of oxygen, for example in atmospheric or expired air.

POA *abbr* pancreatic oncofetal antigen.

POAG *abbr* primary open-angle glaucoma.

pocket ⊃ periodontal instruments, periodontal pocket.

pocket marking forceps ⊃ periodontal instruments.

pockmark *n* pitted scar left on the skin at the site of a healed pustule of chickenpox or smallpox.

podalic version turning the fetus to a breech presentation. This version may be external or internal. ⊃ version.

podiatrist *n* a primary healthcare professional responsible for the assessment, diagnosis and management of conditions affecting the foot and lower limb without referral from medical practitioners. Podiatrists adopt holistic approaches to the assessment and treatment of individuals and utilize a wide range of treatment modalities many of which are performed under local anaesthesia.

podiatry *n* a term that is generally used in Western Europe and the rest of the English speaking countries to describe chiropody. Traditionally the practice of caring for the health, and treating disorders, of the feet. Now a paramedical profession responsible for the assessment, diagnosis and management of conditions of the feet and lower limbs. It recognizes the interdependence of the health of the foot with the rest of the body. The input of podiatrists in sport is increasing with the greater understanding of the role of biomechanics of the lower limb in the prevention and treatment of injury. Biomechanical assessment may, for example, suggest the benefit of custom-made insoles to partially correct an abnormality. ⊃ orthosis.

pod/o- a prefix that means 'foot', e.g. *podiatry*.

podopompholyx *n* pompholyx on the feet.

POEMS syndrome also called Crow-Fukase syndrome. A syndrome comprising **p**olyneuropathy, **o**rganomegaly, **e**ndocrinopathy, **M** protein component and **s**kin involvement. It may be associated with the presence of unusual proteins.

pogonion an orthodontic cephalometric landmark defined as the most prominent bony point of the chin. ⊃ soft tissue pogonion.

-poiesis a suffix that means 'making', e.g. *haemopoiesis*.

poikilocyte *n* red blood cell (erythrocyte) of abnormal shape, e.g. elliptical, or spherical.

poikilocytosis *n* an abnormal variation in the shape of the red blood cells (erythrocytes) in the blood, such as in elliptocytosis or spherocytosis.

poikilothermic *adj* describes an animal that is unable to maintain a constant body temperature. Their body temperture varies throughout the 24 hour period and is influenced by environmental conditions. Cold-blooded. Compare homoeothermic.

point 'A' ⊃ subspinale.

point angle the point on a tooth where three surfaces meet.

point 'B' ⊃ pogonion.

point defects the loss of an atom from a structure. *Frenkel defect* forming an interstitial ion or atom. *Schottky defect* removing the atom completely.

point of maximum impulse (PMI) the point at which the apical beat is palpated or seen at its strongest, usually just medial to the left midclavicular line, at the level of the fifth intercostal space (see Figure A.13, p. 58).

polar body one of two small haploid structures produced during the two meiotic divisions of oogenesis, in which the secondary oocyte is formed. They are non-functional and will eventually undergo disintegration. ⊃ oogenesis.

polar co-ordinates ⊃ co-ordinates.

polar graph paper in radiotherapy, the paper with a series of circular lines around a central point, intersected with radial lines from the same point forming 15° divisions, used in treatment planning.

polarity 1. gradient of strength of uterine contractions between the upper fundal pole, where the activity is strongest, and the lower segment and cervix where contractions are weak or absent, which causes cervical dilatation. **2.** the charge on a conductor, positive (anode) or negative (cathode).

polarity (in rotation) in the context of rotation, one method of signifying the direction of rotational movements. Anti-clockwise is usually positive, clockwise is negative.

polarized *adj* describes the resting state of the plasma membrane of an excitable cell where there is no impulse transmission. The inside of the membrane is electrically negative relative to the outside. ⊃ depolarization.

O
P

polar molecules when an atom contains molecules that are not coincident to the nucleus resulting in a positive and a negative end to the atom.

poles of the eyeball they are: (1) the point on the anterior surface of the cornea which constitutes the summit. It is located at the intersection of the cornea with the geometrical axis of the eye (this is the anterior pole). (2) the point of intersection of the sclera with the geometrical axis (this is the posterior pole). ⊃ anteroposterior axis of the eye, axial length of the eye.

polio- a prefix that means 'grey (as in grey matter)', e.g. *poliomyelitis.*

polioencephalitis inflammation of the grey matter of the brain. It is caused by infection with one of the polioviruses.

polioencephalomyelitis inflammation of the grey matter of the brain and that of the spinal cord. It is caused by infection with one of the polioviruses.

poliomyelitis *n* (*syn.* infantile paralysis) an epidemic infection caused by one of three polioviruses, which attack the motor neurons of the anterior horns in the brainstem (*bulbar poliomyelitis*) and spinal cord. An attack may be asymptomatic, mild without paralysis, or the paralytic form. The latter leads to paralysis of the lower motor neuron type with loss of muscular power and flaccidity. Immunization is available as part of routine programmes during infancy with booster doses before starting school, and again before leaving school.

polioviruses *npl* three enteroviruses that cause poliomyelitis. ⊃ virus.

polished surface any surface of a denture, usually polished, that is in contact with the lips, cheeks and tongue, but excluding the occlusal surfaces. The greater the polish the less the tendency for foreign bodies to stick to the surface.

polishing in dentistry, the production of a smooth glossy surface. *polishing paste* used for cleaning and polishing surfaces of teeth and restorations. A blend of fine abrasive particles containing bonding agents, flavouring and colouring matter. The term *prophylactic paste* is not recommended. *polishing strip* ⊃ abrasive strip.

pollen the airborne product of flowering plants that is capable of causing allergic reactions.

pollen count the published index of the amount of pollen in the air.

pollenosis *n* an allergic condition arising from sensitization to pollen.

pollex the thumb.

pollicization *n* a surgical procedure whereby the index finger is rotated and shortened to produce apposition as a thumb.

poly- a prefix that means 'many, much, excessive', e.g. *polycythaemia.*

polyacid-modified resin composite resin composites containing fluoroaluminosilicate glass to facilitate release of fluoride.

polyacrylic acid a polyacid formed by the polymerization of acrylic acid. In a 40% aqueous solution it is used as the liquid phase of glass ionomer and zinc polycarboxylate cements.

polyarteritis *n* inflammation of many arteries.

polyarteritis nodosa (PAN) (*syn.* periarteritis nodosa) classical polyarteritis nodosa (PAN) is a necrotizing vasculitis characterized by transmural inflammation of medium-sized to small arteries. PAN is a rare disorder with an annual incidence of 2 per million in most populations. All age groups can be affected, with a peak incidence in the fourth and fifth decades, and a male:female ratio of 2:1. Hepatitis B is a risk factor, and the incidence of PAN is 10 times higher in the Inuit population of Alaska, where hepatitis B infection is endemic. Presentation is with myalgia, arthralgia, fever and weight loss in combination with manifestations of multisystem disease. The most common skin lesions are palpable purpura, ulceration, infarction and livedo reticularis. ⊃ Colour Section Figure 99. In 70% of patients arteritis of the vasa nervorum leads to neuropathy which is typically symmetrical and affects both sensory and motor function. Severe hypertension and/or renal impairment may occur due to multiple renal infarctions; glomerulonephritis is rare. Diagnosis is confirmed by finding multiple aneurysms and smooth narrowing of either the mesenteric, hepatic or renal systems on angiography. Tissue biopsy may be definitive (muscle or sural nerve), even in the absence of angiographic abnormality. Treatment for hepatitis B-related disease is to remove the source of the antigen, i.e. antiviral therapy. Corticosteroids and cyclophosphamide are the treatment of choice for idiopathic disease. Mortality is less than 20%, although relapse occurs in up to 50% of patients. ⊃ systemic arteritis.

polyarthralgia *n* pain in several joints.

polyarthritis *n* inflammation of several joints.

polycarbonate in dentistry, a thermoplastic material derived from carbonic acid. Used to produce crown forms by injection moulding.

polycarbonate crown a preformed opaque tooth-coloured crown for temporary/provisional treatment available in a range of sizes usually for anterior teeth.

polycarboxylate cement ⊃ zinc polycarboxylate.

polychromatic multicoloured.

polycoria **1.** a rare anomaly characterized by the presence of two or more pupils in one iris. This condition may be produced by hypoplasia or hyperplasia of the iris stroma or by surgical or accidental trauma. Depending upon the location of the extra pupil, vision may be affected. ⊃ corectopia, monocular diplopia, pupil. **2.** additional reserve material within tissues, which is used for enlargement.

polycystic *adj* composed of many cysts.

polycystic kidney diseases a number of conditions which have variable effects on kidney function. *Adult polycystic kidney disease* (APKD) is a multisystem condition in which there is multiple cyst formation in the kidneys and other body sites, including the meninges and the liver. It is inherited as an autosomal dominant trait. The condition is characterized by flank or abdominal pain, bleeding into the cysts that may cause haematuria, recurrent urinary tract infection, the formation of renal calculi and hypertension. There may also be manifestions linked to cyst formation in the liver and elsewhere. Eventually there is a decline in renal function, which may lead to end-stage renal failure and the need for dialysis or renal transplantation.

polycystic ovary syndrome (PCOS) sometimes called Stein–Leventhal syndrome. A complex syndrome of amenorrhoea or oligomenorrhoea, infertility, hirsutism, acne and occasionally obesity. The ovaries contain multiple follicular cysts. In PCOS the normal feedback mechanisms do not occur, resulting in increased levels of luteinizing hormone (LH) and decreased levels of follicle-stimulating hormone (FSH). Oestrogen levels are similar to those early in the menstrual cycle and as a result women do not ovulate. There are problems associated with androgen hormone (testosterone) production. Women with PCOS also have reduced sensitivity to insulin and therefore insulin levels in the blood are raised (hyperinsulinaemia), leading to an increased risk of developing type 2 diabetes. Management includes relief of symptoms, increasing fertility if desired and preventing long term complications such as type 2 diabetes mellitus. Ovulation may be stimulated with clomiphene, and other infertility treatment offered as appropriate. Metformin may be used to increase the chances of conception. Previously, wedge resection of ovarian tissue was undertaken to induce ovulation; this has since been replaced by a laparoscopic procedure whereby laser or diathermy is used on the surface of the ovary. A reduction in weight can improve symptoms and reduce hirsutism, but cosmetic therapies such as depilatory treatments may be needed.

polycythaemia *n* increase in the number of circulating red blood cells (RBCs). This may result from dehydration or be a compensatory phenomenon to increase the oxygen carrying capacity in hypoxia, as in congenital heart disease, chronic lung disease and in healthy people living at high altitudes. This leads to stimulation of RBC production in the bone marrow. Improves oxygen transport, but at the expense of increasing blood viscosity, adding to the resistance to blood flow in the circulation. Or it may occur as an idiopathic myeloproliferative condition. ➲ primary proliferative polycythaemia (polycythaemia rubra vera).

polycythaemia rubra vera (PRV) ➲ primary proliferative polycythaemia.

polydactyly, polydactylism *n* having more than the normal number of fingers or toes. On the foot the extra digits may develop from one metatarsal or there may be duplication of metatarsal segments. Sometimes selective amputation at an early age is indicated. This ensures optimum foot function, thus facilitating shoe fitting in childhood and adult life.

polydimethylsiloxane silicone rubber. A silicone used in the manufacture of silicone impression material.

polydipsia *n* excessive thirst, such as occurs in diabetes mellitus and diabetes insipidus, or infrequently associated with a mental health problem.

polyether impression material ➲ impression material.

polygene inheritance describes physical characteristics, such as hair colour that are determined by the combined effects of several paired genes at different loci.

polygraph *n* instrument which records several variables simultaneously.

polyhydramnios *n* often referred to as hydramnios. An excessive amount of amniotic fluid, usually referring to volumes over 1.5 L. It is associated with fetal abnormality including oesophageal atresia and some neural tube defects; maternal diabetes and multiple preganancy. Polyhydramnios can lead to serious complications such as unstable fetal lie and malpresentation (e.g. shoulder, face), presentation of or prolapse of the umbilical cord, preterm labour, increased perinatal mortality and postpartum haemorrhage. ➲ amniotic fluid, oligohydramnios.

polymer *n* **1.** a molecule made up of many smaller molecules (monomers) or subunits, such as glycogen; a polymer of glucose molecules. ➲ monomer. **2.** in dentistry, powder ingredient of acrylic resin.

polymerization 1. the forming of a compound of high molecular weight by joining together similar molecules of low molecular weight. **2.** in dentistry, the curing of a mixture of polymer powder and monomer liquid to form an acrylic resin.

polymerase chain reaction (PCR) an in vitro method for the enzymic synthesis of specific DNA sequences and hence the capacity to amplify these segments of DNA. A modification of the method also allows the rapid detection and analysis of RNA.

polymethylmethacrylate (PMMA) a light transparent thermoplastic material formed by the polymerization of methylmethacrylate. It is used in the manufacture of hard contact lenses and some spectacle lenses; and also for the manufacture of acrylic resin teeth and denture bases. ➲ modulus of elasticity, refractive index, siloxane.

polymorph a shortened term for a polymorphonuclear white blood cell, includes neutrophil, eosinophil and basophil.

polymorphism existing in several different forms, for example different forms of haemoglobin.

polymorphonuclear *adj* having a many-shaped or lobulated nucleus, usually applied to the phagocytic leucocytes (granulocytes), neutrophils, basophils and eosinophils.

polymyalgia rheumatica (PMR) a syndrome of muscle pain and stiffness and, classically, an increased erythrocyte sedimentation rate (ESR). It is not a true vasculitis but there is a close association with giant cell arteritis. The prevalence is approximately 20 per 100 000 over the age of 50. The mean age of onset is 70, and diagnosis is rarely made in patients under 60. Women are affected more often than men in a ratio of 3:1. The cardinal features are muscle stiffness and pain, symmetrically affecting the proximal muscles of the neck, upper arms and, less commonly, the buttocks and thighs. There is marked early morning stiffness, often with night pain. Constitutional features of weight loss, fatigue, depression and night sweats also occur. Most patients have a rapid onset of symptoms, sometimes overnight, although occasionally the onset is more insidious. There may be stiffness and painful restriction of active shoulder movement but passive movements are preserved. Muscles may be tender to palpation but there should not be muscle-wasting; if there is, then primary muscle or neurological disease is more likely. In the majority of patients the ESR is elevated above 40 mm/hour and there may be a normochromic, normocytic anaemia. Very occasionally the ESR is low, usually in the acute situation where there has not been sufficient time for it to rise. In this situation the C-reactive protein (CRP) may be elevated prior to the ESR. The only effective treatment is corticosteroids, and prednisolone should be started. The majority of patients should have a dramatic response within 72 hours. If there is no response by 72 hours or an incomplete response by 7 days, then the diagnosis is not PMR. If there has been a good response to prednisolone, the daily dose should be reduced after 4 weeks and then by 1 mg per month, assuming that symptoms remain controlled. Most patients need corticosteroids for an average of 12–18 months and osteoporosis prophylaxis with bisphosphonates should be considered. Some patients require steroid-sparing agents such as methotrexate or azathioprine, particularly if prednisolone cannot be withdrawn at 2 years or is needed at doses greater than 7.5 mg daily. Approximately 15–20% of patients develop features of giant cell arteritis at some point in the course of their disease. All patients should therefore be instructed to seek prompt medical advice if such symptoms occur. ⊃ systemic vasculitis.

polymyositis an idiopathic inflammatory myopathy. The typical presentation is with symmetrical proximal muscle weakness, usually affecting the lower extremities first. Patients report difficulty rising from a chair, climbing stairs and lifting, sometimes in combination with muscle pain. The onset is usually between 40 and 60 years of age and is typically gradual, over a few weeks, although both more explosive and more insidious onsets may occur. Systemic features of fever, weight loss and fatigue are common. Respiratory or pharyngeal muscle involvement leading to ventilatory failure/aspiration is ominous and requires urgent treatment. Interstitial lung disease occurs in up to 30% of patients and is strongly associated with the presence of antisynthetase (e.g. Jol) antibodies. ⊃ collagen, connective tissue diseases, dermatomyositis, idiopathic inflammatory myopathies (IIMs).

polyneuritis *n* multiple neuritis, affecting many nerves—**polyneuritic** *adj*.

polyneuropathy also known as multiple neuropathy and peripheral neuropathy. It is a disorder that affects many peripheral nerves simultaneously. The types and causes are varied and include: diabetes, associated with an acute infection, Guillain–Barré syndrome, toxins and poisons such as arsenic, chronic uraemia, vitamin deficiencies and paraneoplastic syndromes.

polyol polyhydric alcohol. Many polyols have a sweet taste and low fermentability by the micro-organisms comprising

the normal flora of the mouth. They are often included in sugars-free foods, confectionery and medicines as a bulk sweetener.

polyopia *n* (*syn* multiple vision) a condition in which more than one image of a single object is perceived. It may be double vision but more commonly it is multiple vision. Irregular ocular refraction as in some cataracts may sometimes be the cause. ⊃ diplopia, triplopia.

polyp, polypus *n* a pedunculated tumour arising from any epithelial surface, e.g. cervical, uterine, nasal, intestinal. Usually benign but may be malignant. Adenomatous polyps are premalignant. ⊃ polyposis. Tissue overgrowth underlying the epithelium may also be the cause of polyp formation—**polypous** *adj*.

polypectomy *n* surgical removal of a polyp such as from the bowel or nose.

polypeptides *npl* molecules comprising several amino acids joined by peptide bonds. They are between peptides and proteins in size.

polyphagia also called hyperphagia. Excessive and abnormal eating. ⊃ Prader–Willi syndrome

polypharmacy *n* describes a situation when many drugs are prescribed for the same person, usually defined as four or more. It increases the risk of adverse drug reactions, non-compliance and readmissions to hospital. It is a particular problem in older people who are likely to be taking prescription drugs, with as many as a third of people aged 75 years or over taking more that four drugs. The problems are compounded by the use of over-the-counter medicines, or herbal medicines that the person may not mention to the prescriber.

polyphenols several groups of organic molecules, which can inhibit iron absorption from the intestine.

polyploidy *n* a multiple of the normal haploid (n) chromosome number of 23, other than the normal diploid (2n) number of 46, e.g. 69. This state is not compatible with life. ⊃ aneuploidy, monosomy, polysomy, triploid, trisomy.

polypoid *adj* resembling a polyp.

polyposis *n* a condition in which there are numerous intestinal polyps. ⊃ familial adenomatous polyposis

polyradiculitis *n* also called polyradiculopathy. Inflammation of many nerve roots. It may occur as part of a polyneuropathy.

polysaccharide *n* complex carbohydrates that contain a large number of monosaccharide units. Starch, inulin, glycogen, dextrin and cellulose are examples. Important as structural compounds and as energy storage. ⊃ non-starch polysaccharides, polymer.

polyserositis *n* inflammation of several serous membranes. A genetic type is called familial Mediterranean fever. ⊃ amyloidosis.

polysome also known as polyribosome. A structure free in the cytoplasm of the cell comprising a group of ribosomes bound to a strand of messenger ribonucleic acid (mRNA). The ribosomes 'read' the code on the mRNA and add amino acids to the growing polypeptide during the synthesis of proteins.

O
P

polysomnography a graphical recording of the changes occurring in several biophysiological parameters during sleep, such as eye movement, heart rate and rhythm, brain wave pattern, muscle contraction, oxygen saturation levels and nasal airflow. Used in the investigation of some sleep disorders.

polysomy the occurrence of more than two copies of a chromosome in a diploid cell that would otherwise be normal. An example of polysomy is a male with Klinefelter's syndrome who has three copies (trisomy) of the X chromosome (XXXY) or four copies (a tetrasomy; XXXXY); caused by non-disjunction of the chromosome during meiotic division.

polysulphide impression material ➲ impression material.

polytetrafluoroethylene (PTFE) ➲ Teflon®.

polyunsaturated fatty acid (PUFA) a fatty acid with two or more double bonds along the main carbon chain. Examples include sunflower, safflower, soybean and corn oils and fish oils. ➲ arachidonic acid, essential fatty acids, linoleic acid, linolenic acids, monounsaturated fatty acids, omega-3 fatty acids, omega-6 fatty acids.

polyuria *n* excretion of an excessive volume of urine. Causes include an abnormally large fluid intake that can occur with some mental health disorders, diabetes mellitus, diabetes insipidus, some renal diseases, with diuretic drugs and hypercalcaemia—**polyuric** *adj*.

polyvinylchloride vinyl polymer historically used for maxillofacial prostheses.

POM *abbr* prescription only medicine.

POMC *abbr* pro-opiomelanocortin.

Pompe's disease (J Pompe, Dutch physician, 20th century) type II glycogen storage disease in which there is a deficiency of α-glucosidase (acid maltase) enzyme. It classically presents during infancy and is characterized by muscle weakness, affecting promimal limb and diaphragm, which may be severe. Diagnosis is based on elevated level of creatine kinase (CK), abnormal electromyogram (EMG), lymphocyte glycogen storage, muscle biopsy and molecular genetic studies. ➲ inherited metabolic myopathies.

pompholyx recurrent vesicles and bullae occur on the palms, palmar surface of the fingers and soles, and are excruciatingly itchy. This form of eczema can occur in atopic eczema and in irritant and contact allergic dermatitis. It can be provoked by heat, stress and nickel ingestion in a nickel-sensitive patient but is often idiopathic. ➲ cheiropompholyx, podopompholyx.

POMR *abbr* problem-orientated medical record.

pons *n* a bridge; a process of tissue joining two sections of an organ. *pons varolii* part of the brainstem between the midbrain and the medulla. It comprises mainly nerve fibres (white matter), which connects the various lobes of the brain. Also contains several nuclei including those of some cranial nerves (trigeminal, abducens, facial), and the apneustic and pneumotaxic respiratory centres—**pontine** *adj*. ➲ Colour Section Figure 1.

Pontiac fever a flu-like illness with little or no pulmonary involvement and no mortality caused by *Legionella pneumophila*. ➲ legionnaires' disease.

pontic that part of a bridge which replaces the crowns of missing teeth. The suspended portion consists of one or more units made of metal, porcelain, composite or acrylic resin or a combination of metal with one of these.

PONV *abbr* postoperative nausea and vomiting.

POP *acron* **1. p**laster **of P**aris **2. p**ost **o**ffice **p**rotocol. **3. p**rogestogen-**o**nly **p**ill.

popliteal *adj* relating to the area behind the knee and associated structures; the p. fossa/space, the p. artery and p. vein.

popliteal artery formed from the femoral artery as it enters the popliteal fossa/space. The popliteal artery passes through the popliteal fossa/space behind the knee. It supplies arterial blood to the knee joint and surrounding structures. At the lower border of the popliteal fossa/space it divides into the anterior and posterior tibial arteries. ➲ Colour Section Figure 9.

popliteal fossa/space the diamond-shaped depression behind the knee, bounded by muscles and containing nerves and the popliteal vessels (artery and vein).

popliteal vein a deep vein that receives venous blood carried by the superficial saphenous veins from the lower leg. ➲ Colour Section Figure 10.

popliteus *n* a deep, triangular muscle of the posterior compartment of the leg. It is situated behind the knee in the popliteal fossa/space. Its origin is on the lateral condyle of the femur and it inserts into the proximal tibia. Contraction of the muscle flexes and rotates the leg.

population the pool of information from which statistics are drawn.

population attributable risk the rate of a condition in a population minus the rate that would occur if everyone in the population were unexposed to the risk factor. It can be expressed as the attributable risk multiplied by the prevalence of risk factor exposure in the population. Used to inform decisions about public health policies and their impact on a population. ➲ risk.

population inversion when half the atoms in a structure are in an excited state.

porcelain in dentistry, a ceramic material made of kaolin, feldspar, silica and various pigments. Used to restore the form and function of a natural tooth and to make inlays, crowns, bridge pontics and teeth for dentures. May be high, medium or low fusing according to the temperatures at which it is fired in an electrically heated furnace. *aluminous porcelain* contains a significant amount of alumina to provide increased strength. *core porcelain* contains a large proportion of alumina to provide extra strength and opacity to the core of the construction on which the covering porcelain is baked. *dentine porcelain* the translucent pigmented porcelain used to form the body of a porcelain crown and provide the overall shape and colour. *enamel porcelain* the porcelain powder applied to the outer surface of a porcelain crown during the baking process to provide translucency and pigmentation, as in natural teeth. *glazing porcelain* the clear, low-fusing porcelain used to produce

O
P

a thin glossy surface on a ceramic restoration. *stain porcelain* the low-fusing porcelain containing various metallic oxides, which is fired on to porcelain work to produce individual characteristics of colour and surface markings. *vacuum-fired porcelain* a range of ceramic materials of various types fired in a furnace under vacuum conditions in order to minimize air bubbles and produce a stronger end-product. ⊃ porcelain bonded crown, porcelain jacket crown (PJC).

porcelain bonded crown cast-metal crown to which porcelain has been bonded externally.

porcelain jacket crown (PJC) a full veneer porcelain crown possessing a shoulder at its gingival margin.

porcelain teeth artificial teeth made of porcelain, the anterior teeth being secured to the denture base by pins. Now largely superseded by acrylic teeth.

pore *n* a minute surface opening. One of the mouths of the ducts (leading from the sweat glands) on the skin surface; they are controlled by fine papillary muscles, closing in the cold and opening in the presence of heat.

pores of Kohn alveolar pores. Tiny, ventilation channels, which allow the movement of air between adjacent alveoli.

porion an orthodontic landmark defined as the most superior point of the bony external auditory meatus. ⊃ Frankfort plane.

porosity the condition of a material such as metal, porcelain or plastic having minute holes or voids on the surface or in its substance.

porous 1. having many pores. **2.** able to be permeated by fluids or air.

porphyria *n* a group of inborn errors of haem biosynthesis caused by enzyme deficiencies, usually hereditary, causing pathological changes in nervous and muscular tissue in some varieties and photosensitivity in others, depending on the level of the metabolic block involved. Excess porphyrins or precursors, produced either by the haemopoietic bone marrow or the liver, are found in the urine or stools or both. Those affected may present with bouts of abdominal pain, peripheral neuropathy, skin blistering, confusion, hypertension, tachycardia and mental health problems. ⊃ Colour Section Figure 100. In acute porphyria a porphyric crisis can be precipitated by alcohol; hormones; and certain drugs, which include some antidepressants, barbiturates, some hormones, sulphonamides, etc.

porphyrins *npl* group of organic compounds that form the basis of respiratory pigments, including the haem of haemoglobin. Naturally occurring porphyrins are uroporphyrin and coproporphyrin. ⊃ porphyria.

porphyrinuria *n* excretion of porphyrins in the urine. Such pigments are produced as a result of an inborn error of metabolism. The urine may change colour and darken on standing. ⊃ porphyria.

port a connection point on a computer for input or output hardware.

porta *n* the depression (hilum) of an organ at which the vessels enter and leave—**portal** *adj*.

porta hepatis the transverse fissure through which the hepatic portal vein, hepatic artery and bile ducts pass on the under surface of the liver.

portacaval, portocaval *adj* relating to the hepatic portal vein and inferior vena cava.

portacaval anastomosis an operation in which the hepatic portal vein is joined to the inferior vena cava with the object of reducing the pressure within the hepatic portal vein in cases of hepatic portal hypertension.

portal circulation ⊃ hepatic portal circulation.

portal hypertension ⊃ hepatic portal hypertension

portal imaging methods of verifying the radiotherapy treatment area, using either radiographic film or digital imaging methods. The portal image of the treatment area is compared to the image taken at simulation. ⊃ electronic portal imaging, therapy verification film.

portal triad (tract) comprises a branch of the hepatic artery, a branch of the hepatic portal vein and an interlobular bile duct situated at each corner of a liver lobule. Blood from the hepatic artery and the hepatic portal vein flows through the sinusoids within the lobule to drain by the central vein to eventually reach the hepatic veins and the inferior vena cava. The direction of blood flow is away from the portal triad (tract) whereas the bile secreted by the hepatocytes within the lobule flows in the opposite direction. The bile is collected in tiny bile canaliculi that unite to form the interlobular bile ducts, which eventually become the right and left hepatic ducts carrying bile away from the liver.

portal vein ⊃ hepatic portal vein.

portal venography the radiographic investigation of the (hepatic) portal venous system following a direct injection of contrast agent into the spleen.

position the location of a body or object in space that may be specified by co-ordinates (e.g. Cartesian or polar). ⊃ co-ordinates.

position indicating device (PID) ⊃ beam guiding instrument.

positioning a term used to describe the active therapeutic management of the effect of different positions on the tonal influences on the body and limbs, e.g. supine is dominated by extensor tone and thus the therapist may break up this position by the use of wedges to introduce an element of flexion. It is important to assess each individual for their optimal therapeutic positions and ensure that all members of the multidisciplinary team reinforce postures during the 24 h period.

position of the fetus eight positions relating the fetal denominator to the woman's pelvis. In a vertex presentation the denominator is the occiput, thus in the occipitoanterior position the fetal occiput is directed to the symphysis pubis, either to the right or left iliopectineal eminence, the commonest and most favourable position. In occipitolateral, occipitotransverse positions the occiput is directed to the mid-point of the left or right iliopectineal line. In occipitoposterior position the occiput is directed to the left or right sacroiliac joint; in direct or persistent occipitoposterior position the occiput is directed towards the sacrum. The breech positions are similar, but with the sacrum as the denominator.

positive affect a general dimension of affect reflecting a state of enthusiasm and alertness. ⊃ affect.

positive correlation in statistics, when information is linked and an increase in one item will result in an increase in the other and a decrease in one item will result in a decrease in the other.

positive discrimination ⊃ affirmative action.

positive energy balance ⊃ energy balance.

positive end expiratory pressure (PEEP) the maintenance of positive pressure in the airway of a ventilated patient at the end of expiration. This acts as a splinting pressure on the airways, thus holding them open. By doing so, functional residual capacity is raised and oxygenation improved.

positive expiratory pressure mask a mask device used to deliver positive expiratory pressure to facilitate the clearance of pulmonary secretions as first demonstrated by Falk et al. (1984). (Falk M, Kelstrup M, Anderson JB, Pederson SS, Rossing I, Dirksen H 1984 Improving the ketchup bottle method with positive respiratory pressure, PEP, in cystic fibrosis. Eur J Resp Dis 65: 423–432.)

positive feedback the mechanism through which a few homeostatic regulation processes work. An amplifier or cascade system in which an increase in the level of product from the process stimulates the process still further. Positive feedback usually functions in processes that occur relatively infrequently, such as parturition (labour) and normal blood clotting, which are not everyday events requiring constant regulation. For example, the events of labour are stimulated as the presenting part moves down the birth canal to exert pressure on the cervix. This pressure leads to the release of the hormone oxytocin from the pituitary gland, which in turn increases the rate and intensity of uterine muscle contractions causing the cervix to dilate and the birth of the infant. ⊃ feedback, homeostasis, negative feedback.

positive nitrogen balance ⊃ nitrogen balance.

positive pressure ventilation (PPV) positive pressure inflation of lungs to produce inspiration via endotracheal tube, tracheostomy or a nasal mask. ⊃ intermittent positive pressure ventilation.

positive regard also termed unconditional positive regard. A concept of client-centred therapy. It is the ability to hold and convey feelings for other people that are not based on negative beliefs about the person. Having positive regard for clients and patients enables the health professional to approach others with positive intentions towards them. Positive regard, along with rapport, trust, empathy, genuiness and warmth, are prerequistites for a successful therapeutic relationship.

positive signs of pregnancy audible fetal heart sounds, fetal movements and visualization of the fetus on ultrasound.

positive supporting reaction (PSR) a pattern of plantar-flexion and inversion in the foot complex is seen when the patient attempts to weight bear through the affected leg. The presence of a positive supporting reaction can lead to soft tissue shortening in the foot and affected leg and can interfere with functional activities, such as walking and sit to stand.

positive transfer an enhancement in performance because of practice or experience gained in practising another similar skill or the same skill under different conditions. For example, skill gained practising golf on a driving range should positively transfer to skill on the golf course. Similarly, practising overhand throwing of a ball should transfer positively to more complex skills such as the overhead serve in tennis. ⊃ negative transfer, transfer of learning.

positive work ⊃ work.

positivism the assertion that there is an absolute reality, which is capable of being measured, studied and understood.

positivist research paradigm a philosophy that assumes an objective measurable world. ⊃ reductionist paradigm.

positron emission tomography (PET) an imaging technique used in nuclear medicine to produce three-dimensional images showing metabolic activity in specific areas of the body. It uses cyclotron-produced isotopes of extremely short half-life that emit positrons which are introduced into the patient. When positrons react with electrons in the body gamma rays are emitted. A specialist gamma camera is used that has multiple detectors lying in a circular gantry that surrounds the patient. The detectors detect the isotopes that decay through positron emission as this produces two photons of 511 keV which are emitted at $180°$ to each other. Only if two detectors are opposite each other, each registering a photon within nanoseconds of each other, are the photons recorded. The radioactive isotopes are linked to molecules, such as glucose, that are active in metabolism (e.g. fluorodeoxyglucose) and administered to the patient, usually intravenously. The scan takes place after a suitable period to allow time for the radioactive isotope to build up in the cells. PET scanning is used in research; to evaluate the metabolic activity of organs and structures including the brain and heart; and in the detection of primary cancers and the presence of metastases.

positrons *npl* positively charged particles that combine with electrons (negative charge), causing gamma rays to be emitted.

posseting *n* regurgitation of small amounts of curdled milk in infants.

Possum derived from patient-operated selector mechanism, a device used by individuals with paralysis to achieve maximum independence by being able to operate equipment or devices that include computers, telephone and other communications systems.

post in dentistry, a tapered or cylindrical rod that is cemented into a root canal as a retention for a core or post crown.

post- a prefix that means 'after, behind', e.g. *postpartum*.

postabsorptive state the metabolic state existing between meals, such as before lunch, late afternoon and at night.

Fuel molecules for immediate energy use are in short supply and the body uses catabolic processes, e.g. glycogenolysis, lipolysis, to break down complex substances to provide energy. ⊃ absorptive state.

postanaesthetic *adj* after anaesthesia.

postanal *adj* behind the anus.

post and core in dentistry, the integral retention portion of a post crown having a post to fit the root canal and a core shaped as a crown preparation (Figure P.13).

postcibal *adj* postprandial. Relating to an event that occurs after eating, such as pain or vomiting. ⊃ 'dumping syndrome'.

postcoital *adj* after sexual intercourse.

postcoital contraception ⊃ emergency contraception.

postcoital test used during the investigation of infertility to determine spermatozoa survival in ovulatory cervical mucus. A sample of endocervical mucus is obtained around 6 hours after sexual intercourse at the likely time of ovulation. The presence of sufficient numbers of healthy motile spermatozoa indicates that there is no incompatibility between the cervical mucus and the spermatozoa.

postconcussional syndrome 1. the association of headaches, giddiness and a feeling of faintness, which may persist for a considerable time after a head injury. **2.** a term used in sports medicine to describe a progressive deterioration of cognitive function following repeated brain trauma, such as that caused during boxing.

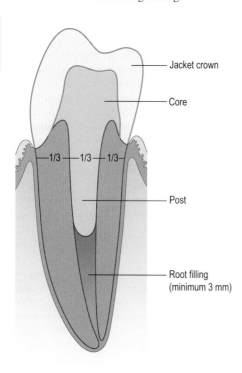

Jacket crown

Core

1/3 — 1/3 — 1/3

Post

Root filling (minimum 3 mm)

P.13 Post and core (reproduced from Heasman & McCracken 2007 with permission).

post crown a crown retained by a metal post.

post dam posterior palatal seal. ⊃ seal.

postdiphtheritic *adj* following an attack of diphtheria. Refers especially to the paralysis of limbs and palate.

postepileptic *adj* following on an epileptic seizure.

postepileptic automatism a fugue state, following on a seizure (fit), when the patient may undertake a course of action, even involving travelling long distances or violence, without having any memory of this (amnesia).

posterianterior from back to front.

posterior *adj* situated at the back. ⊃ anterior *opp*—**posteriorly** *adv.*

posterior (AP) drawer test tests the integrity of the posterior cruciate ligament. The patient is supine. The therapist sits on the patient's foot to stabilize the leg and grasps around the posterior aspect of the proximal tibia and pushes the tibia backwards. An abnormal finding is excessive translation of the tibia posteriorly. A comparison is made with the other side. Please note that a 'sag sign' is observed with the patient in crook lying whereby the tibia appears to be posteriorly displaced in relation to the femur, this may give the false impression that the patient has a rupture of the anterior cruciate ligament since when an anterior (PA) drawer test is performed a considerable amount of movement may be noted, but this is due to the tibia returning to its resting position.

posterior bite block also known as posterior bite plane and posterior capping. The platform of acrylic polymer attached to a baseplate and placed over the occlusal surface of posterior teeth.

posterior bite plane ⊃ posterior bite block.

posterior capping ⊃ posterior bite block.

posterior chamber of the eye situated between the anterior surface of the lens and the posterior surface of the iris. ⊃ aqueous.

posterior ciliary vein ⊃ vortex vein.

posterior communicating arteries two arteries branching from the basilar artery; they are part of the circulus arteriosus (circle of Willis). They supply arterial blood to the occipital cortex and the inferior part of the temporal lobe. Can be affected by a cerebrovascular accident (stroke), resulting in a homonymous hemianopia on the opposite side. ⊃ circulus arteriosus.

posterior compartment syndrome pain in the calf when the muscles in the superficial (mainly the gastrocnemius and soleus) or the deep compartment (tibialis posterior and toe flexors) are involved. ⊃ anterior compartment syndrome, chronic exertional compartment syndrome, compartment syndrome, lateral compartment syndrome, tibialis syndrome.

posterior cruciate ligament (PCL) one of two major stabilizing ligament of the knee, it limits backward movement of the tibia (Figure A.11, p. 49). Also involved in proprioception. A site of sports injury, e.g. a tear, which may occur during hockey or rugby football, or in conjunction with an anterior cruciate ligament injury. ⊃ cruciate ligaments, cruciate ligament injury, posterior (AP) drawer test.

posterior elastic lamina ⊃ Descemet's membrane.

posterior fossa lesions a term that relates to damage or injury that occurs to the brain in the region of the posterior fossa. Ataxia is commonly seen following lesions in this area.

posterior limiting layer ⊃ Descemet's membrane.

posterior nares the pair of openings from the nasal cavities into the nasopharynx.

posterior nasal spine (PNS) the tip of the posterior spine of the palatine bone.

posterior open bite condition where some of the posterior teeth do not meet on occlusion.

posterior oral seal ⊃ seal.

posterior palatal foramen ⊃ greater palatine foramen.

posterior palatal seal (post dam) ⊃ seal.

posterior pituitary not itself the site of hormone synthesis, but the site of release of two hormones formed in the hypothalamus by neurons whose axons form the hypophyseal-pituitary tract, store the hormones in their terminals, and release them into the blood stream in response to action potentials (neurohormones). Antidiuretic hormone (vasopressin or arginine vasopressin [AVP]) regulates water loss in the kidneys, by increasing water retention; oxytocin stimulates uterine contractions and the ejection of milk from the breasts. ⊃ pituitary gland.

posterior scleritis inflammation of the sclera involving the posterior segment of the eye. The condition is often associated with a systemic disease (e.g. rheumatoid arthritis). It is characterized by pain and reduced visual acuity. The severity of the visual impairment depends on the involved tissue and its location. Signs include eyelid oedema, proptosis, limitation of ocular movements and if anterior scleritis is present, redness. The ocular fundus may present disc swelling, choroidal folds, macular oedema and serous retinal detachment. Treatment mainly consists of systemic corticosteroids and immunosuppressive agents.

posterior superior dental nerve an afferent nerve running from the palatal and distobuccal roots of the first molar and all roots of the second and third molars passing backwards through the posterior aspect of the maxilla to join the maxillary division of the trigeminal nerve.

posterior teeth the premolar and molar teeth.

posteroanterior radiograph one from the back to the front of the body.

postganglionic *adj* situated distal to a collection of nerve cells (ganglion), as a postganglionic nerve fibre.

postgastrectomy syndrome covers two sets of symptoms, those of hypoglycaemia when the patient is hungry, and those of a vasovagal attack immediately after a meal.

posthepatic *adj* behind the liver.

postherpetic *adj* after herpes infection such as *postherpetic neuralgia* following an attack of herpes zoster (shingles). The pain is particularly difficult to treat. ⊃ neuropathic pain.

posthitis *adj* inflammation of the prepuce.

post hoc analysis a research term. An analysis conducted after the results are available that were not defined before the start of the trial. Such analyses have weaknesses in that they are particularly prone to false positive claims or type I error.

posthumous *adj* occurring after death.

posthumous birth 1. delivery of a baby by caesarean section after the mother's death, or 2. birth occurring after the father's death.

postmature *adj* past the expected date of delivery. An infant is postmature when labour is delayed beyond the usual 40 weeks, usually considered as being 41-42 weeks from the last menstrual period, although first trimester ultrasound scans are now considered more accurate. Expected date of delivery is used as a marker to define when induction of labour may be necessary, since placental deterioration after term may lead to fetal hypoxia—**postmaturity** *n*.

postmenopausal *adj* occurring after the menopause has been established.

postmenopausal bleeding (PMB) vaginal bleeding occurring after the menopause. Investigation is essential to exclude malignancy.

postmortem *adj* after death, usually implying dissection of the body. ⊃ antemortem *opp.*, autopsy.

postmyocardial infarction syndrome Dressler's syndrome. A late complication presenting as pericarditis developing from 2 weeks to a few months after myocardial infarction. Due to an autoimmune response to products released from dead muscle.

postnasal *adj* behind the nose and in the nasopharynx—**postnasally** *adv*.

postnatal *adj* after delivery—**postnatally** *adv*. ⊃ antenatal *opp*, postnatal depression, postnatal examination, postnatal exercises, postnatal period.

postnatal depression describes a low mood experienced by some mothers for a few days following the birth of a baby; sometimes called 'four day blues'. Less severe than puerperal psychosis.

postnatal examination 1. maternal examination undertaken frequently during the first 10 days of the puerperium to ensure that involution is taking place, lactation is becoming established and the woman is adapting physically, emotionally and psychologically to motherhood. 2. medical/midwifery examination at the end of the 6 week puerperium to ensure the woman's body has returned to the non-pregnant state without complications.

postnatal exercises exercises taught by the midwife or physiotherapist for the woman to perform regularly daily during the puerperium and, ideally, for the rest of her life. The exercises are aimed specifically at strengthening the pelvic floor and abdominal muscles, but also include deep breathing and leg exercises as a preventative measure against respiratory tract infection and thromboembolic disorders such as deep vein thrombosis.

postnatal period phase of the puerperium of between 10 and 28 days, during which the midwife practising in the UK is required by Nursing and Midwifery Council rules to attend the mother and baby regularly.

post office protocol an email system.

O
P

postoperative *adj* after surgical operation—**postoperatively** *adv.*

postpartum *adj* after a birth (parturition).

postpartum haemorrhage (PPH) excessive bleeding from the genital tract after the delivery of the infant up to 6 weeks following delivery. It may be *primary* ocurring in the first 24 hours, usually defined as blood loss in excess 500 mL. May be due to incomplete placental separation during the third stage of labour. *Secondary* postpartum haemorrhage is excessive uterine bleeding occurring more than 24 h after delivery. It is usually caused by infection associated with the retention of placental tissue.

post-patient collimation restricts scatter reaching the detectors: primarily on single slice units.

postprandial *adj* following a meal.

postprandial lipaemia the increase in blood level of triacylglycerols (triglycerides) after eating a fatty meal.

post-traumatic amnesia (PTA) the period of time between a brain injury and the point when the functions involved in memory are judged to be restored. It is a permanent memory loss and tends to reflect the severity of the damage.

post-traumatic stress disorder (PTSD) a mixed emotional disorder arising in response to an exceptional trauma, such as witnessing or being a victim of violent crime, war, natural disaster. Symptoms include autonomic arousal, intrusive images ('flashbacks' or nightmares), emotional numbness, anhedonia and avoidance of reminders of the trauma.

postural *adj* relating to posture.

postural adjustments/background movements the slight, spontaneous body adjustments occuring in response to information from proprioceptors and the vestibular apparatus, in order to maintain body alignment, centre of gravity and stability. For example, the adjustments of the trunk when reaching for a distant object.

postural albuminuria ➪ orthostatic albuminuria.

postural drainage techniques that use gravity and position to drain respiratory secretions. The airways of infected lung lobes or segments are positioned as vertically as possible. Also known as tipping because the lower lobes need to be raised higher than the mouth for secretions to drain into the trachea to stimulate the cough reflex. Apical segments of the upper lobe drain in the sitting position. The chest is percussed with clapping and vibrated, and sputum coughed into a suitable disposable container or removed by suctioning. Postural drainage may be used in conjunction with other techniques such as thoracic expansion exercises and intermittent positive pressure breathing (IPPB). Children with cystic fibrosis must have this treatment at home and family members learn the techniques required. Small children are usually tipped across an adult's thighs but bigger children and adults can be tipped by raising the foot end of the bed, or over a roll or special frame. ➪ intermittent positive pressure breathing, tapôtement.

postural hypotension orthostatic hypotension. A reduction in blood pressure when a person stands up from lying or sitting. It may occur in older people, or as a side-effect of some drugs such as alpha-adrenoceptor antagonists (alpha blockers). ➪ Appendix 5.

postural muscles those muscles, mostly extensors, which counter the downward pull of gravity to maintain the body in an upright posture, e.g. neck, back, knee and ankle extensors. They have a majority of slow (type 1, 'red') muscle fibres, e.g. the calf muscle soleus has close to 90% in most individuals and erector spinae has over 60%, although, as in all human muscles, there is substantial variation between individuals. ➪ muscle fibre types.

postural reflex describes any of the reflexes concerned with establishing or maintaining an individual's posture, particularly against the downward pull of gravity.

postural sets a term primarily used by Bobath-trained therapists to describe a patient's posture that takes into account the influence of tone on the posture, e.g. unsupported sitting is a 'mixed postural set' as it has both elements of flexion and extension, whereas the postural set of supine is dominated by extension. The term can also be found in the literature to describe adaptations of posture or adjustments that precede and accompany a movement (Bobath 1990). (Bobath B 1990 Adult hemiplegia: evaluation and treatment, 3rd edn. Heinemann Medical Books, Oxford.)

postural tremor a pathological tremor (3–5 Hz) that occurs when the body or limb is working against gravity.

posture *n* relates to the position of the body or body part in relation to space or another object or body part. The manner in which the body is held in lying, sitting, standing and walking; a particular position or attitude of the body. A good posture (Edwards 2002) is said to be the attitude of the body that facilitates maximum efficiency of a specific activity without causing damage to the body. ➪ flat back posture, hemiplegic posture, opisthotonic posture, sway back posture. (Edwards S (ed.) 2002 Neurological physiotherapy: a problem-solving approach. Churchill Livingstone, Edinburgh.)

post viral fatigue ➪ chronic fatigue syndrome/myalgic encephalomyelitis.

Poswillo hook a hook used percutaneously to elevate the zygomatic (zygoma) bone.

potash alum ➪ potassium aluminium sulphate.

potassium (K) *n* a metallic element. The major cation in intracellular fluid accounting for over 90% of the body's potassium. Its many functions include a crucial role in the generation of the membrane potential and of an action potential. The level in the blood is regulated by the kidneys, under the influence of the hormone aldosterone. Intake in food and excretion (mainly in the urine) are typically balanced at about 60 mmol/day. ➪ hyperkalaemia, hypokalaemia.

potassium aluminium sulphate (alum, potash alum, aluminium potassium bis sulphate). Chemical used in an aqueous solution to accelerate the setting reaction of gypsum products.

potassium bifluoride a deprecated term for potassium hydrogen fluoride.

potassium bromide used in radiography as a developer restrainer.

potassium-channel activator a class of drug, e.g. nicorandil. It causes vasodilation in both arteries and veins and is used in the prophylaxis and treatment of angina.

potassium chlorate a mild antiseptic used in mouthwashes and gargles.

potassium chloride used to correct hypokalaemia, and as a supplement with some diuretic drugs.

potassium citrate alkalinizes urine; still used in cystitis to minimize discomfort.

potassium deficiency ⊃ hypokalaemia.

potassium fluoride chemical constituent of fluxes used in soldering.

potassium hydrogen fluoride (potassium hydrogendifluoride) a substance used in the manufacture of silver solder fluxes.

potassium hydroxide used in radiography as a developer accelerator.

potassium metabisulphite used in radiography as a developer preservative.

potassium permanganate used in solution for some skin conditions for its cleansing and deodorizing properties.

potassium sodium tartrate ⊃ sodium potassium tartrate.

potassium sparing diuretics a group of diuretic drugs that act to retain potassium and increase loss of sodium and water, or by reducing potassium loss and sodium reabsorption. ⊃ Appendix 5.

potassium sulphate in dentistry, a chemical used to accelerate the setting time and reduce the setting expansion of gypsum plasters and investments.

potassium sulphite used in radiography as a fixing solution preservative.

potential difference also called electromotive force. A measure of electrical work on a unit positive charge in moving it from one point to another in volts (V).

potential energy the energy due to an object or body's position or form. May be elastic, gravitational or electrical.

potentiation the effect of one drug on the action of another such that their combined action, when administered together, is greater than the sum of their effects when given separately.

potter's rot one of many lay terms for silicosis arising in workers in the pottery industry.

Potter's syndrome (E Potter, American pathologist, 1901–1993) a syndrome that includes renal agenesis (absence of kidneys) and a typical flattened face associated with accompanying oligohydramnios. It is not compatible with life.

Pott's disease (P Pott, British surgeon, 1714–1788) spondylitis; spinal caries; spinal tuberculosis. The resultant necrosis of the vertebrae causes kyphosis.

Pott's fracture (P Pott) a fracture-dislocation of the ankle joint. A fracture of the lower end of the tibia and fibula, 75 mm above the ankle joint, and a fracture of the medial malleolus of the tibia.

pouch *n* a pocket or recess.

pouch of Douglas the rectouterine pouch.

poultice fomentation. Local application of heat, such as with warmed kaolin spread between two layers of gauze, used to relieve pain, act as a counter irritant or increase blood flow.

Poupart's ligament (F Poupart, French physician, 1616–1708) ⊃ inguinal ligament.

pourable denture base resin also known as pour resin, pourable resin or pour-type resin. A specially formulated denture base material that flows and fills a mould under gravity.

poverty *n* lack of material resources that is often associated with lack of social and emotional resources. It means less to spend on food, housing, clothes, transport, holidays and other human and social needs. It may be *absolute poverty* where people have insufficient resources to maintain physical health, such as not having food, shelter or the means to keep warm. Or *relative poverty* when an individual's living standards are less than those that generally exist in a particular population. They are unable to engage fully in the society of which they are a part. Poverty, in terms of lack of social and emotional resources, is not necessarily associated with wealth. Definitions of what constitutes relative poverty show considerable variation between different communities and the same community over time. There are formal government definitions of poverty (in terms of material resources) for the purposes of collecting statistics and providing financial benefits.

povidone iodine ⊃ iodine.

power **1.** In electricity, power is the rate of energy flow or dissipation, measured in watts (W). Concept applied clinically to uses of electrical stimulation and laser. For example, P (power, watts) = VI or P = I^2R where V = voltage [V], I = current [A] and R = resistance [Ω]. **2.** rate of doing work. In mechanics, over any period of constant applied force, power = force multiplied by displacement in the direction of that force, divided by the time for which it has operated, i.e. = force × velocity. ⊃ energy.

power calculation in research, a measure of statistical power. The likelihood of the research study to generate statistically significant results.

power Doppler a measure of the amplitude of the Doppler signal when scanning very slow moving structures, for example, small blood vessels in the body, it will not show the velocity or direction of flow.

power (social science context) a central concept within the social sciences, defined in different ways by different theorists. It is generally seen as a feature of all social life and interpersonal relationships and is central to understanding inequality. Those who have power have authority and influence over others. They possess and can accumulate valued resources such as wealth and property. Power is an important dimension of professional–patient/client relationships with services defined, planned and delivered by professionals.

O
P

power (ultrasound context) the power of the ultrasound beam is the energy flow rate of the whole beam which must be kept to a minimum value due to the harmful effects of ultrasound.

powerlessness *n* a feeling of being trapped and unable to control or influence the situation. People may feel powerless in their dealings with healthcare professionals and healthcare systems.

pox *n* a slang term for syphilis.

poxvirus viruses belonging to the family *Poxviridae*. Those affecting humans are the virus causing molluscum contagiosum, smallpox virus and vaccinia virus. The pox viruses are responsible for many animal diseases, e.g. orf in sheep and goats.

PPE *abbr* personal protective equipment.

PPH *abbr* post partum haemorrhage.

PPL *abbr* phosphorylase.

PPLO *abbr* pleuropneumonia-like organism. ➲ *Mycoplasma*.

ppm *abbr* parts per million.

PPP *abbr* pentose phosphate pathway.

PPS *abbr* pelvic pain syndrome.

PPV *abbr* positive pressure ventilation.

P-QRS-T complex the letters used to denote the five deflection waves of the ECG waveform (Figure P.14). The deflection waves represent the electrical activity in the heart and correspond to the events occurring during a cardiac cycle. The dome-shaped P wave represents atrial depolarization as the impulse is conducted across the atria, resulting in atrial systole (contraction). The PR interval represents the time taken for the impulse to be conducted from the sinus node, across the atria to the atrioventricular node and hence

to the ventricles. The three waves that form the large, narrow QRS complex represent depolarization of the ventricles that occurs just before contraction (ventricular systole). The gently rounded T wave represents repolarization of the ventricles (ventricular diastole). The QT interval is the time between the start of ventricular depolarization, through contraction to repolarization of the ventricles. The ST segment represents the short period of inactivity and repolarization of the ventricles that follows the QRS complex. Importantly the coronary arteries receive blood during the ST segment when the heart is relaxed.

PR *abbr* **1.** per rectum: describes the route used for examination of the rectum, or introduction of drugs or fluids into the body. **2.** peripheral resistence

P-R interval ➲ P-QRS-T complex.

practice in general, the repeated execution of an action in order to gain or improve a skill. *blocked practice* when executing a series of trials of one skill before moving on to practice another skill, typical of drills in which the same skill is repeated many times; *distributed practice* when there are periods of rest in between trials; *massed practice* when the order of executing different skills is randomized or mixed within a given session.

Prader orchidometer ➲ orchidometer.

Prader–Willi syndrome (A Prader, Swiss paediatrician/endocrinologist, 1919–2001; H Willi, Swiss paediatrician, 1900–1971) an inherited condition that arises from mutations in the paternal chromosome 15 during the formation of the gamete. There is learning disability, hypotonia, short stature, hyperphagia and morbid obesity. ➲ Angelman syndrome.

praecordial *adj* ➲ precordial.

pre- a prefix that means 'before, in front', e.g. *premenstrual*.

pre-adjusted appliance ➲ orthodontic appliance.

pre-amalgamated amalgam alloy an alloy containing a mixture of high copper amalgam, to which spherical silver copper particles and conventional lathe cut amalgam alloy are added.

preagonal *adj* pertaining to the events that may occur just before death. ➲ agonal.

preanaesthetic *adj* before an anaesthetic.

prebiotics oligosaccharides present in food that are not digested and support the growth of potentially beneficial colonic bacteria. ➲ probiotics.

precancerous outdated term. ➲ carcinoma in situ.

preceptorship *n* a system to help the newly qualified practitioner achieve confidence in the early months of registered practice, under the guidance of a preceptor.

precipitate labour a labour of very short duration perhaps as short as 1 hour but less than 2 hours. It can be due to extremely strong uterine action of which the mother may be unaware. The risks include haemorrhage, damage to the cervix and perineal tears, uterine inversion, retained placenta or postpartum haemorrhage can occur because the uterine muscle does not function normally during the third stage of labour. The fetus may be hypoxic, suffer trauma and birth injury due to rapid delivery and moulding of the head.

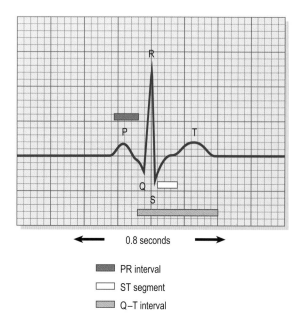

0.8 seconds

▬ PR interval
☐ ST segment
▨ Q–T interval

P.14 P-QRS-T complex (reproduced from Brooker 2006A with permission).

precipitin *n* an antibody that is capable of forming an immune complex with an antigen and becoming an insoluble precipitate, which can be detected in laboratory assays. This reaction forms the basis of many delicate diagnostic serological tests for the identification of antigens in serum and other fluids ⊃ immunoglobulins.

precision attachment in dentistry, an interlocking mechanical device, one part of which is fixed to an abutment either intra- or extracoronally, while the other is integrated into a bridge or a denture in order to provide retention and/or support to the appliance.

preclinical 1. occurring before the onset of a disease and before clinical signs or symptoms can be detected. **2.** previously described the period in the training of medical and dental students before they had contact with clients/patients.

precocious puberty the early appearance of signs of sexual development, such as breast development in girls, or the enlargement of the external genitalia in boys. It may be due to an endocrine disorder such as an ovarian tumour, or congenital adrenal hyperplasia.

preconception care refers to the medical examination and investigations, and the physical and mental preparation for childbearing of both parents before conception. Health promoting activity focuses on measures aimed at encouraging optimum health of both partners at conception and during the early weeks of pregnacy when organ development occurs (organogenesis). Thus reducing the risk of congenital abnormalities, fetal problems and maternal complications during pregnancy and labour. Preconceptual care includes a detailed history (personal, medical, family, reproductive, lifestyle history such as alcohol intake and occupational hazards). Couples are advised about the importance of measures that include the provision of sufficient folic acid in the diet of women of childbearing age, and the avoidance of alcohol, drugs (prescribed, over-the-counter and illegal) and smoking in the months before a couple decide to have a baby. Examination and investigations include a pelvic examination, cervical cytology, urinalysis and blood tests for rubella antibodies, blood count and haemoglobin, and where indicated for haemoglobinopathies. Blood tests for syphilis and human immunodeficiency virus antibodies are offered. In certain circumstances the hair and domestic water are tested for the presence of toxic metals. Referral to appropriate physician or genetic counsellor may follow.

preconceptual *adj* before conception.

preconscious *adj* information in the subconscious mind that can be evaluated and allowed to enter the conscious mind if we so wish.

precordial, praecordial *adj* relating to the area of the chest immediately over the heart.

precordial thump some authorities advocate the delivery of a sharp blow to the victim's mid-sternum during the first few seconds of ventricular fibrillation or pulseless ventricular tachycardia, i.e. a monitored or witnessed cardiac arrest, where there is no access to a defibrillator.

precorneal film (*syn* lacrimal layer, preocular tear film, tear film, tear layer) the field covering the anterior surface of the cornea which consists of lacrimal fluid and of the secretion of the meibomian and conjunctival glands. Its total thickness was thought to be about 9 μm but recent investigations have questioned that value and point to a much larger figure. It is composed of three layers: (a) the deepest and densest is the mucin layer (or mucus layer) which derives from the conjunctival goblet cells, as well as some secretion from the lacrimal gland; (b) the watery lacrimal fluid is the middle layer, called the lacrimal (or aqueous layer). It is secreted by the lacrimal gland and the accessory glands of Krause and Wolfring. It forms the bulk of the film and contains most of the bactericidal lysozyme and other proteins, inorganic salts, sugars, amino acids, urea, etc; (c) and the oily layer (or lipid layer) is the most superficial and is derived principally from the meibomian glands in the lids as well as some secretion from the glands of Zeis. It greatly slows the evaporation of the watery layer and may provide a lubrication effect between lid and cornea. Recent research is pointing to a precorneal film made up of only two layers; an innermost aqueous and mucin gel layer and an outer lipid layer. ⊃ break-up time test, conjunctival glands, goblet cell, hyperlacrimation, Krause's glands, lacrimal glands, meibomian glands, mucin, tear meniscus, tears, Tearscope plus, Wolfring's glands.

precursor *n* forerunner. For example, an inactive hormone or enzyme.

predentine the dentine that has not yet calcified and is found on the actively forming dentine surface between the calcified dentine and the odontoblast cells.

prediabetes *n* ⊃ impaired fasting glucose, impaired glucose tolerance.

predisposition *n* a natural tendency to develop or contract certain diseases.

pre-eclampsia *n* a serious hypertensive disorder of pregnancy. It is characterized by proteinuria and hypertension, with oedema, arising usually in the latter part of pregnancy. The incidence increases with maternal age. It may be suspected without proteinuria if the woman's blood pressure is raised and she complains of visual problems such as blurred vision, headache and abdominal pain. There may also be abnormal blood test results, specifically a low platelet count (thrombocytopenia) and abnormal liver enzyme levels. ⊃ eclampsia, HELLP syndrome.

pre-event fuelling ⊃ carbohydrate loading.

pre-exposed step wedges produced by film manufacturers that when processed, have a series of increased density steps which can be used to determine the consistency of the film processor.

prefabricated attachment in dentistry, a commercially manufactured precision attachment.

preformed band seamless stainless steel band manufactured in varying sizes and shapes in order to fit intimately around the crowns of teeth involved in fixed appliance orthodontic treatment.

preformed metal crown (PFMC) crown form constructed from stainless steel, but often also containing chromium, made available in a range of sizes for primary and permanent molar teeth. Used for permanent restoration of primary teeth with extensive caries or following pulp therapy and semi-permanent restoration of permanent molar teeth with hypoplasia, tooth surface loss or other dental defects (e.g. amelogenesis imperfecta).

prefrontal *adj* situated in the anterior portion of the frontal lobe of the cerebrum.

preganglionic *adj* proximal to a collection of nerve cells (ganglion), as a preganglionic nerve fibre.

pregnancy *n* being with child, i.e. gestation from the first day of the last menstrual period to parturition, normally 40 weeks or 280 days. ⊃ ectopic pregnancy, phantom pregnancy.

pregnancy and exercise ⊃ exercise during pregnancy.

pregnancy associated plasma protein-A (PAPP-A) a plasma protein originating from placental syncytiotrophoblast, levels rising as pregnancy advances. Average first trimester levels are significantly reduced in Down's syndrome pregnancies. ⊃ combined test, integrated test.

pregnancy epulis ⊃ epulis.

pregnancy gingivitis also known as gravidarum gingivitis. A transient gingivitis occurring during pregnancy and which may be avoided by strict bacterial plaque control.

pregnancy-induced hypertension (PIH) asymptomatic rise in blood pressure without proteinuria after the 20th week of pregnancy, most commonly in primigravidae and multiple pregnancy. It should be monitored closely to detect pre-eclamsia and must also be distinguished from essential hypertension. The complications include placental abruption, renal and cardiac failure, cerebral haemorrhage, placental insufficiency and intrauterine growth retardation.

pregnancy test based on the presence of beta-human chorionic gonadotrophin (hCG) in the woman's urine or serum. Commercially produced urine test kits are available for home-testing.

pregnanediol a derivative of pregnane, formed by reduction of progesterone, present in urine of pregnant women.

prehension the power of grasping or seizing.

pre-implantation genetic diagnosis (PGD) a technique used in IVF assisted conception to determine the genetic constitution of an embryo prior to implantation in the uterus.

pre-implantation genetic halotyping (PGH) a recently developed technique that can be used to check embryos produced for IVF, for several inherited conditions prior to implantation. A cell is extracted from the early embryo, the genetic material is replicated many times and the DNA is examined for the presence of chromosomes with the faulty genes that cause conditions that include cystic fibrosis and sex-linked conditions such as Duchenne muscular dystrophy. In sex-linked conditions it will be possible to distinguish between healthy male embryos and those with the faulty genes, thus allowing a male embryo to be implanted where previously only female embryos were used.

prejudice *n* literally means to pre-judge. A preconceived opinion or bias which can be negative or positive. It can be for or against members of particular groups, for example older people, migrant workers, women, people with a learning disability, and may lead to discrimination, racism, sexism or intolerance.

prelens tear film the tear film found on the front surface of a contact lens on the eye. The oily layer of the film is slightly thinner with soft lenses than in the precorneal film and almost absent with rigid lenses. The aqueous layer is thinner with rigid lenses than in the precorneal film. The exact composition of the prelens tear film varies with the characteristics of the contact lens on the eye. ⊃ precorneal film.

preload *n* the degree of stretch present in the myocardial muscle fibres at the end of diastole. It is determined by the pressure and volume of blood in the ventricles at the end of diastole (end-diastolic volume [EDV]). Thus, in situations in which venous return to the heart is decreased the preload will be reduced. ⊃ afterload, Starling's law of the heart, stroke volume.

premacular fibrosis ⊃ preretinal macular fibrosis.

premature *adj* occurring before the proper time.

premature beat ⊃ extrasystole.

premature birth ⊃ preterm birth.

premature contact initial contact of teeth which causes a deviation of the jaws on closure.

premature presbyopia ⊃ accommodative insufficiency.

premaxilla that part of the maxilla in which the incisor teeth develop and erupt. Considered as part of the maxilla in humans but a separate bone in other mammals.

premaxillary situated anteriorly to the maxilla.

premedication *n* drugs given before the administration of another drug, e.g. those given before a general anaesthesia to reduce anxiety.

premenstrual *adj* preceding menstruation.

premenstrual (cyclical) syndrome (PMS) group of physical and emotional symptoms defined as occurring in the 14 days prior to menstruation, relieved almost immediately by the onset of the period, and having at least a 7-day symptom-free break in each cycle. Women are encouraged to complete a menstrual diary to help confirm the diagnosis and rule out other gynaecological or psychological conditions. Symptoms include irritability, headache, poor concentration, mood swings, disrupted sleep pattern, headaches, breast tenderness and abdominal bloating and cramps. PMS occurs as a result of the hormonal changes, particularly the rise in progesterone, which occur at that phase of the cycle. *PMS in sport* the importance in sport is the potential effect on performance of some female athletes, though there is a huge variation among them and no attributable effect in the majority. Treatment can include lifestyle and training modification, with hormonal manipulation to alleviate the symptoms or to manipulate the cycle to avoid times of participation. ⊃ menstrual cycle.

premenstruum that part of the menstrual cycle immediately before bleeding commences.

premolar tooth one of eight permanent teeth which succeed the primary molars, two in each quadrant and lying immediately distal to the canine, i.e. placed fourth and fifth from the midline. They have two cusps (bicuspid) and are used for grinding food (see Figure T.4b, p. 779). In over 70% of cases the upper first premolar has two roots placed buccopalatally, the bifurcation of the roots occurring anywhere between the neck and the apex. The roots are usually of similar size, flattened mesiodistally. There may be three roots, the buccal one being bifurcated. The other premolars normally have one root. There are no premolars in the primary dentition.

prenatal *adj* antenatal. Pertaining to the period between the last menstrual period and birth of the child, normally 40 weeks or 280 days—**prenatally** *adv*.

Prentice's law (*syn* Prentice's rule) the prismatic effect *P* in prism dioptres at a point on a lens is equal to the product of the distance *c* in centimetres of the point from the optical centre of the lens, and the dioptric power *F* of the lens, i.e. $P = cF$. ➲ prism dioptre, prism power.

preocular tear film ➲ precorneal film.

preoperative *adj* before operation—**preoperatively** *adv*.

preoperative assessment often nurse-led clinics to assess general condition and suitability for day surgery, order appropriate investigations, and give patients information and the opportunity to ask questions and discuss worries—**preoperatively** *adv*.

preparalytic *adj* before the onset of paralysis, usually referring to the early stage of poliomyelitis.

prepatellar *adj* in front of the patella, as applied to a large bursa. ➲ prepatellar bursitis.

prepatellar bursitis (*syn.* housemaid's knee) a fluid-filled swelling of the bursa in front of the knee cap (patella). It is frequently associated with excessive kneeling. A blow can result in bleeding into the bursa and there can be infection with pyogenic pathogens.

pre-patient collimation restricts the incident beam to the required body area, determining the data set to be acquired.

prepubertal *adj* before puberty.

prepuce *n* the foreskin of the penis. The loose fold of skin that covers the glans penis, or the clitoris. In males the prepuce may be removed for cultural or religious reasons, or for the treatment of phimosis and paraphimosis—**preputial** *adj*. ➲ circumcision, Colour Section Figure 16.

prerenal *adj* literally, before or in front of the kidney, but usually refers to perfusion of the kidneys.

preretinal haemorrhage haemorrhage occurring between the retina and the vitreous body (humour). It is usually large and often shaped like a D with the straight edge at the top. It is also known as a subhyaloid haemorrhage. Others are flame shaped and occur at the level of the nerve fibre layer and tend to parallel the course of the nerve fibres (*flame haemorrhage*). Retinal haemorrhages are usually round and originate in the deep capillaries of the retina. Retinal and preretinal haemorrhages usually absorb after a period of time (except those that break into the vitreous body), but

subarachnoid haemorrhage (which is usually due to a rupture of an aneurysm in an artery of the circulus arteriosus [circle of Willis]) must be suspected as they often accompany it. ➲ circulus arteriosus, diabetic retinopathy.

preretinal macular fibrosis (*syn* epiretinal membrane, macular epiretinal membrane, macular pucker, premacular fibrosis, preretinal membrane, preretinal vitreous membrane, surface wrinkling retinopathy) the proliferation of glial cells over the surface of the internal limiting membrane of the macular region of the retina. Ophthalmoscopically the retina presents a glinting reflex. The condition may occur after trauma, eye surgery, retinal vascular disease and inflammation and with any of the causes of proliferative retinopathy (retinitis proliferans) and most commonly in older adults. Initially the patient is asymptomatic or reports some distortion of vision (metamorphopsia). This stage is often called cellophane maculopathy. As the condition develops, visual acuity diminishes, there is retinal wrinkling and the preretinal membrane becomes denser obscuring some retinal vessels in ophthalmoscopy. Some people may also develop a macular hole and posterior vitreous detachment. If vision is significantly reduced the main treatment is by vitreous surgery with removal of the layer of preretinal proliferative tissue. ➲ proliferative retinopathy.

preretinal membrane ➲ preretinal macular fibrosis.

preretinal vitreous membrane ➲ preretinal macular fibrosis.

presbycusis *n* idiopathic sensorineural hearing loss caused by or associated with age changes.

presbyopia *n* failure of accommodation in those of 45 years and onwards—**presbyopic** *adj*, **presbyope** *n*.

prescribed diseases a list of diseases which can be linked to occupation. They can be classified by the cause— physical, biological, chemical and other. Physical causes and diseases include, radiation (e.g. leukaemia and certain other cancers); vibration (e.g. blanching of fingers); noise (e.g. sensorineural deafness); and heat (e.g. cataract). Biological causes can result in a number of infections, such as tuberculosis, Weil's disease, orf, etc. Exposure to toxic chemicals cause a range of diseases that include anaemia from exposure to lead; cadmium exposure leading to the development of emphysema; a form of leukaemia following exposure to benzene; and cirrhosis of the liver after working with chlorinated naphthalenes. The last category of other causes includes the pneumoconiosis, mesothelioma, dermatitis, etc.

Prescribing Analysis and Costs the information supplied to prescribers about their prescribing.

prescription *n* a written or computer-generated formula, signed by the authorized prescriber, instructing the pharmacist to supply the required drugs.

prescription only medicine (POM) a drug that requires a written/computer-generated prescription signed by a qualified health professional who is authorized to prescribe, except in an emergency when the pharmacist may dispense the drug if certain criteria are met.

O
P

presenile dementia dementia occurring in people between 50 and 60 years of age. ⊃ dementia.

presenility *n* a condition occurring before senility is established. ⊃ dementia—**presenile** *adj*.

presentation *n* the part of the fetus which first enters the pelvic brim and will be felt by the examining finger through the cervix in labour. May be vertex, face, brow, shoulder or various types of breech.

preservative in developer, a chemical, potassium metabisulphite, that discourages oxidation and slows down the formation of discoloration products, in fixing solutions, for example, sodium sulphite or potassium sulphite is used to prevent the breakdown of the fixing agent into sulphur particles.

pressor *n* a substance which raises the blood pressure.

pressor response increase in arterial blood pressure in response to various internal or external conditions or to drugs, e.g. mental stress, sustained handgrip or other isometric exercise. A cold pressor response occurs on immersion of all or part of the body in cold water. ⊃ isometric contraction.

pressure force divided by the area over which the force acts. Measured in pascals (Pa) or newtons per square metre (N/m^2). ⊃ barometric pressure.

pressure areas any body area subjected to pressure sufficient to compress the capillaries and disrupt the microcirculation. Usually occurs where tissues are compressed between a bone and a hard surface, e.g. theatre table, trolley, bed, chair, splint, or pressure damage caused by equipment such as oxygen tubing. Areas at risk of pressure damage include: head, the ears, spine, sacral area, shoulders, elbows, hips, area over ischial tuberosities, heels and ankles. The most common site for pressure damage is the tissues over the sacral area, followed by the heels. The area over the ischial tuberosities is most at risk in people who sit for long periods. The head in infants is the most common site due to the differences in body proportions. ⊃ pressure ulcer.

pressure garment a skin-coloured, Lycra material garment used to exert firm, even pressure to a specific part of the body. Often used in the treatment of varicose veins; and burns and scalds to prevent keloid scarring.

pressure groups organizations formed to exert pressure on government (central and local) in order to further the interests of certain groups, such as older people.

pressure point a place at which an artery passes over a bone, against which it can be compressed, to stop bleeding (Figure P.15).

pressure sore ⊃ pressure ulcer.

pressure support mode of positive pressure ventilation, which augments the size of a patient's spontaneous breaths.

pressure transducer device that converts pressure into calibrated electrical signals which can be displayed on a monitor.

pressure ulcer (*syn.* decubitus ulcer, pressure sore) previously called a bedsore. Defined by the European Pressure Ulcer Advisory Panel (EPUAP) as an area of localized damage to the skin and underlying tissue caused by pressure, shear, friction, or a combination of these factors. There are

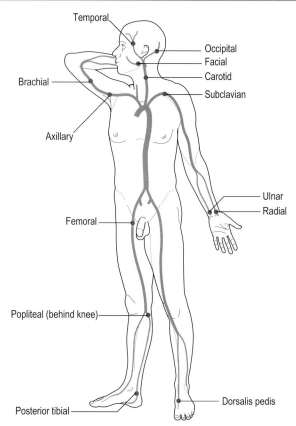

Temporal
Occipital
Facial
Carotid
Subclavian
Brachial
Axillary
Ulnar
Radial
Femoral
Popliteal (behind knee)
Posterior tibial
Dorsalis pedis

P.15 Pressure points for arresting haemorrhage (reproduced from Brooker 2006A with permission).

several grading scales, but the EPUAP advocates the use of a four point grading scale (categories of damage I-IV). Pressure ulcers develop when any area of the body is subjected to unrelieved pressure that leads to local hypoxia, ischaemia and necrosis with inflammation and ulcer formation (Figure P.16). Shearing forces also disrupt the microcirculation when they cause the skin layers to move against one another. Shearing damages the deeper tissues and can lead to an extensive pressure ulcer. Friction from continual rubbing leads to blisters, abrasions and superficial pressure ulcers, and is made worse by moisture such as urine or sweat. Factors that increase the risk of pressure ulcer formation include: poor oxygenation, incontinence, age over 65–70, immobility, altered consciousness, dehydration and malnutrition.

pressure ulcer prevention starts with assessment of skin condition and pressure areas using the most appropriate pressure ulcer risk scale on a regular basis. ⊃ Braden scale, Norton scale, Waterlow scale. Relief of pressure from the part is achieved by moving patients or encouraging them to move themselves, use of external aids such as special beds or mattresses, keeping the skin dry and clean, ensuring that fluid and nutritional needs are met, and avoiding shearing force and friction. ⊃ pressure areas, pressure ulcer, pressure ulcer risk scale, shearing force.

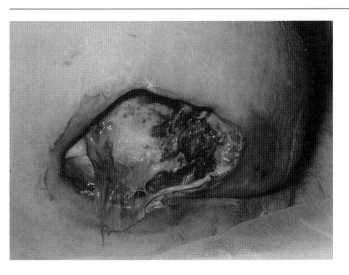

P.16 Pressure ulcer (reproduced from Brooker & Nicol 2003 with permission).

pressure ulcer risk scale various risk scales exist, they are based on a series of risk factors, each of which is given a numerical score. The patient's level of risk (low, medium or high) is ascertained by summing the scores. Individual risk scale tools differ in respect of the way the numbers relate to risk. In many risk scales, e.g. Waterlow, the higher the score, the greater the risk of pressure ulcer development; however, in other scales, such as the Braden risk scale score, the lower the total score, the greater the risk. Different risk scales with specific risk factors are intended for use in particular areas of practice, such as community settings, or with critically ill patients. ➲ Braden scale, Norton scale, Waterlow scale.

presystole *n* the period preceding the systole or contraction of the heart muscle—**presystolic** *adj.*

pretectal nucleus a complex group of nerve cells in the midbrain anterior to the superior colliculi. One of these, the pretectal olivary nucleus, receives retinal inputs via the optic tract and superior brachium and sends axons to both Edinger–Westphal nuclei. It constitutes a centre of the pupillary light reflex. Another, the nucleus of the optic tract, may be involved in the control of reflex eye movements. Other fibres from the pretectal nucleus innervate the cornea, the iris, the ciliary muscle and the extraocular mucles (except the lateral rectus and superior oblique muscles), as well as the levator palpebrae muscle. ➲ Edinger–Westphal nucleus, pupillary light reflex.

preterm infant baby born before 37 weeks' gestation, with low birth weight, and may also be small for gestational age, which is assessed using the Dubowitz score. Complications include respiratory distress syndrome, feeding difficulties due to immature sucking, swallowing and coughing reflexes, hypothermia, jaundice and infection, and poor maternal–infant relationship due to prolonged stay in the neonatal intensive care unit. ➲ Dubowitz score, low birthweight, small for gestational age, very low birthweight.

preterm labour/birth the birth of a baby before the 37th completed week of gestation, regardless of the infant's birthweight. In the UK it is a birth after 24 weeks' gestation and before 37 weeks. It may be either spontaneous due to changing hormone levels, overstretched uterus, weak cervix or infection and treated with tocolytic drugs, e.g. ritodrine hydrochloride to delay delivery; or induced due to poor maternal or fetal wellbeing, when the extrauterine environment is considered to be less hazardous and followed by controlled delivery with obstetric forceps to protect the delicate fetal head. If a fetus is delivered before 24 weeks and shows no signs of life it is termed a miscarriage. ➲ low birthweight.

pretibial laceration injury on the front of the shin especially common in older adults.

pretibial myxoedema purple/pink indurated areas of skin, usually on anterior aspect of the leg and dorsum of the foot. It is a feature of Graves' disease. The skin may be itchy and coarse hair is present.

prevalence *n* total number of cases of a disease existing in a population at a single point in time. ➲ incidence, prevalence ratio.

prevalence ratio the prevalence of a disease, expressed as a ratio of population size.

preventive dentistry the prevention of, and preventive treatment for, dental disease and the promotion of good oral health. Encompasses the community- or patient-based measures taken to prevent the incidence of dental decay or caries. Includes fissure sealing, fluoride therapy, oral hygiene instruction, dietary analysis and advice and regular review. Collectively these measures are known as the *'Pillars of Prevention'*.

preventive resin restoration (PRR) in dentistry, a restoration used to restore minimal carious lesions, usually less than 2 mm in depth using a bonded filled composite resin to replace enamel/dentine plus fissure sealant to obturate the remaining vulnerable fissure system on the tooth surface.

O
P

priapism *n* prolonged penile erection of 4–6 hours, in the absence of sexual stimulation. It is associated with spinal cord injuries and lesions, some types of leukaemia, sickle cell disease, thalassaemia and drugs, e.g. alprostadil, used to treat erectile dysfunction. It requires urgent decompression, initially by aspirating blood from one corpus cavernosum or both in order to prevent damage to penile tissues. This may include thrombosis or ischaemia and can lead to erectile dysfunction.

prickle cell a cell of the stratum spinosum layer of the epidermis.

prickly heat ⊃ miliaria.

prima facie 'at first sight', or sufficient evidence brought by one party to require the other party to provide a defence.

primary *adj* **1.** first in order. **2.** principal. **3.** in radiography, the radiation emanating directly from the focal spot.

primary amenorrhoea ⊃ amenorrhoea.

primary amyloidosis ⊃ amyloidosis.

primary antibody deficiencies are characterized by recurrent bacterial infections, particularly of the respiratory and gastrointestinal tract. The most common causative organisms are bacteria such as *Streptococcus pneumoniae* and *Haemophilus influenzae*. Severe inherited disorders of antibody production are rare and usually present at 5–6 months of age, when the protective benefit of transferred maternal immunoglobulin has waned. Three major primary antibody deficiencies present in adulthood are: (a) selective IgA deficiency—the most common primary immune deficiency, affecting 1:600 Northern Europeans. In most patients, low (<0.05 g/L) or undetectable IgA is an incidental finding with no clinical sequelae. However, 30% of individuals experience recurrent mild respiratory and gastrointestinal infections. In some patients, there is a compensatory increase in serum IgG levels; (b) common variable immune deficiency (CVID) is a heterogeneous adult-onset primary immune deficiency of unknown cause. It is characterized by low serum IgG levels and failure to make antibody responses to exogenous pathogens. Paradoxically, antibody-mediated autoimmune diseases such as idiopathic thrombocytopenic purpura and autoimmune haemolytic anaemia are common. CVID is also associated with an increased risk of malignancy, particularly lymphoproliferative disease; (c) specific antibody deficiency or functional IgG antibody deficiency—is a poorly characterized condition which causes defective antibody responses to polysaccharide antigens. Some patients are deficient in the antibody subclasses IgG2 and IgG4, and this condition was previously called IgG subclass deficiency. There is overlap between specific antibody deficiency, IgA deficiency and CVID, and some patients may progress to a more global antibody deficiency over time. Serum immunoglobulins should be measured in conjunction with protein and urine electrophoresis to exclude secondary causes of hypogammaglobulinaemia. In addition, specific antibody responses to known pathogens should be assessed by measuring IgG antibodies against tetanus, *H. influenzae* and *S. pneumoniae* (most patients will have been exposed to some of these antigens through either infection or immunization). If specific antibody levels are low, immunization with the appropriate killed vaccine should be followed by repeat antibody measurement 6–8 weeks later; failure to mount a response indicates a significant defect in antibody production. These functional tests have generally superseded IgG subclass quantitation. Quantitation of B and T lymphocytes by flow cytometry is also useful. All patients with antibody deficiencies require aggressive treatment of infections, and prophylactic antibiotics may be indicated. The mainstay of treatment is immunoglobulin replacement (intravenous immunoglobulin, IVIG), which is derived from pooled plasma and contains IgG antibodies to a wide variety of common organisms. IVIG is usually administered intravenously every 3–4 weeks with the aim of maintaining trough IgG levels within the normal range. Treatment may be self-administered, and is life-long. With the exception of selective IgA deficiency, immunization is generally not effective because of the defect in IgG antibody production. As with all primary immune deficiencies, live vaccines should be avoided.

primary care optometry a term referring to the basic field of optometry to which the public usually come directly and are not usually referred by other professionals. Primary care optometric practitioners may refer some of their patients to other practitioners such as ophthalmologists, neurologists or to other optometric specialists for specialized services such as paediatric optometry, low vision aids or highly specialized aspects of contact lens fitting.

Primary Care Trust (PCT) in England a statutory body (now rebranded, e.g. Norfolk PCT is now called NHS Norfolk) that has three core functions to: (a) work with local government departments and the voluntary sector to improve health, reduce inequalities in health and improve access to services for the local population; (b) commission appropriate health services for the local population. Including those provided by general practitioners, pharmacists, optometrists and dental surgeons in the community, secondary hospital services and services for people with mental healthcare needs; (c) directly provide community services that include district nursing, specialist community public health nursing (health visiting), rehabilitation, podiatry, dental services, children's health, etc. ⊃ Strategic Health Authority.

primary closure the immediate closure of a wound or incision by the use of sutures, staples, clips, adhesive skin tapes or tissue adhesives.

primary collimation indicates the maximum field size of an X-ray beam at a specific distance.

primary collimator defines the maximum available beam size.

primary colours (*syn* fundamental colours) any sets of three colours such as, for example, red, green and blue which, by additive colour mixture of the stimuli in varying proportions, can produce any colour sensation. ⊃ colour mixture.

primary complex (*syn*. Ghon focus) the initial tuberculous infection in a person, usually in the lung, manifesting as a small focus of infection in the lung tissue and enlarged caseous, hilar lymph nodes. It usually heals spontaneously.

primary dentine the dentine present when the tooth is fully formed.

primary dentition deciduous teeth, milk teeth. Dentition which starts to erupt about the age of 6 months and is complete at about 2½ years, after which it is gradually replaced by the permanent (secondary) dentition. When complete it consists of 20 teeth, which start to calcify before birth: one central and one lateral incisor, one canine and two molars in each quadrant. Primary teeth are usually whiter and softer, and have a relatively thin enamel covering with proportionally much larger pulp chambers than their permanent replacements. The crowns are more bulbous and the cusps are generally well worn before the teeth are shed. They are smaller than their successors except for the molars which are larger than the premolars replacing them. The first upper and lower primary molars are unlike any other teeth, each having a very bulbous crown and four cusps. The upper molar has three widely splayed roots while the lower has two widely divergent roots. ⊃ teeth.

primary disease prevention includes all activities to eradicate the cause of disease or decrease the susceptibility of the individual to the causative agent. Examples include smoking cessation advice, healthy eating, exercise, sun protection, immunization programmes. ⊃ secondary disease prevention, tertiary disease prevention.

primary glaucoma ⊃ angle-closure glaucoma, open-angle glaucoma.

primary health care (PHC) 1. the first level contact with the healthcare system. For example general practitioner or practice nurse. Health care provided in the community by general practitioners and the practice team and other health professionals. Other services include NHS and private walk-in centres; nurse-led 24 hour telephone health information and advice services. ⊃ NHS Direct/NHS 24, primary healthcare team. **2.** defined by WHO–UNICEF declaration (Alma-Ata 1978) as 'Essential health care based on practical, scientifically sound and socially acceptable methods and technology, made universally available to individuals and families in the community through their full participation and at a cost that the community and the country can afford, to maintain every stage of their development in the spirit of self-reliance and self-determination.' In its original and narrowest sense, primary health care refers to first contact care where patients contact healthcare workers directly. Principles on which effective primary health care is based are education about diseases, healthcare problems and their control; safe water and sanitation; maternal and child health, including family planning; immunization against major infectious diseases; appropriate treatment of common diseases and injuries; providing essential drugs.

primary healthcare team in the UK an interdependent multiprofessional group of individuals with a common purpose and responsibility, each member clearly understanding his or her own role, and those of other team members, in offering an equitable, efficient and effective primary healthcare service. The health professionals involved may include: community nurses, counsellors, general practitioners, specialist community public health nurses (health visitors), midwives, occupational therapists, physiotherapists, podiatrists, practice nurses, speech and language therapists, pharmacists and dental surgeons and optometrists working in the community.

primary haemorrhage ⊃ haemorrhage.

primary herpetic gingivostomatitis a common cause of severe oral ulceration in children, caused by the herpes simplex virus type 1 (HVS-1). ⊃ herpes, herpes simplex virus (HVS).

primary hyperaldosteronism (Conn's syndrome) adenoma or hyperplasia of the adrenal cortex that results in the secretion of excess aldosterone. ⊃ Conn's syndrome.

primary idiopathic acquired aplastic anaemia a rare disorder in developed countries, with 2–4 new cases per million population per annum; the disease is much more common in certain other parts of the world—for example, east Asia. The basic problem is failure of the pluripotent stem cells, producing hypoplasia of the bone marrow with a pancytopenia in the blood. Usually no cause is found but careful enquiry should be made for potential causes such as exposure to drugs, chemicals and radiation, a history taken of viral illness, particularly hepatitis, and a search undertaken to exclude rare congenital causes such as Fanconi's anaemia. Patients present with symptoms of bone marrow failure, usually anaemia or bleeding, and less commonly infections. A full blood count demonstrates pancytopenia, low reticulocytes and often macrocytosis. Bone marrow aspiration and trephine reveal hypocellularity. All patients will require blood product support and aggressive management of infection. The prognosis of severe aplastic anaemia managed with supportive therapy only is poor and more than 50% of patients die, usually in the first year. The curative treatment for patients under 30 years of age with severe idiopathic aplastic anaemia is allogeneic haemopoietic stem cell transplantation (bone marrow transplantation) if there is an available donor. Those with a compatible sibling donor should proceed to transplantation as soon as possible and have a 75–90% chance of long-term cure. In older patients, immunosuppressive therapy with ciclosporin and antithymocyte globulin gives 5-year survival rates of 75%. Such patients may relapse or evolve into other clonal disorders of haematopoiesis, such as paroxysmal nocturnal haemoglobinuria (PNH), myelodysplastic syndrome (MDS) and even acute myeloblastic/myeloid leukaemia (AML), and must be followed up long term.

primary impression ⊃ impression.

primary intention healing also known as first intention. Uncomplicated wound healing that occurs where there is little tissue loss and it is possible to draw the wound edges

O
P

together, such as in a surgical incision. ⊃ primary closure, secondary intention healing, wound healing.

primary intracerebral haemorrhage (PICH) bleeding into the cerebrum. A type of cerebrovascular accident (stroke) caused by the rupture of a small or medium-diameter artery.

primary nursing a professional model of practice, based on a belief in the therapeutic value of the nurse–patient relationship. A qualified nurse (primary nurse) is responsible and accountable for the assessment, planning and implementation of all the nursing care of a particular patient or group of patients for the entire duration of their stay in a particular care setting. The nurse is supported in this role by an associate nurse who cares for the patient while the primary nurse is absent, according to the nursing plan drawn up by the primary nurse. Other nurses, including students and healthcare assistants, may also provide care for the patient, but this is always under the supervision and co-ordination of the primary nurse. ⊃ named nurse, patient allocation, task allocation, team nursing.

primary occlusal trauma the injury caused to a tooth or teeth, with normal periodontal support, due to adverse occlusal forces.

primary optic vesicle ⊃ optic vesicle.

primary osteoarthritis ⊃ osteoarthritis (OA).

primary phagocyte deficiencies a group of conditions that usually present with recurrent bacterial and fungal infections, often affecting unusual sites. The majority present in childhood, but milder forms may present in adults. Different types include: (a) leucocyte adhesion deficiencies—disorders of phagocyte migration, where failure to express adhesion molecules results in the inability of phagocytes to exit the blood stream. These conditions are characterized by recurrent bacterial infections, and sites of infection lack pus or neutrophil infiltration. Peripheral blood neutrophil counts may be very high during acute infection because of the failure of mobilized neutrophils to exit blood vessels. Specialized tests show reduced or absent expression of adhesion molecules on neutrophils; (b) chronic granulomatous disease (CGD)—results from mutations in the genes encoding the NADPH oxidase enzyme, causing a failure of oxidative killing (respiratory burst). This may be demonstrated using the nitroblue tetrazolium reduction test (NBT), which measures the ability to reduce a colourless intracellular dye to an insoluble blue compound after neutrophil activation. The defect leads to susceptibility to catalase-positive organisms such as *Staphylococcus aureus*, *Burkholderia cenocepacia* and aspergillus. Intracellular killing of mycobacteria in macrophages is also impaired. Infections most commonly involve the lungs, lymph nodes, soft tissues, bone, skin and urinary tract and are characterized histologically by granuloma formation; (c) defects in cytokines and cytokine receptors—such as interferon (IFN-γ), interleukin (IL-12) or their receptors also result in failure of intracellular killing, and individuals are particularly susceptible to mycobacterial infections. Detailed assessment of cytokine deficiencies is currently only performed in specialized laboratories. Patients require aggressive management of existing infections, including intravenous antibiotics and surgical drainage of abscesses, and long-term prophylaxis with antifungal agents and trimethoprim-sulfamethoxazole. Specific treatment depends upon the nature of the defect, and haemopoietic stem cell transplantation (HSCT) may be considered.

primary pigmentary retinal dystrophy ⊃ retinitis pigmentosa (RP).

primary position (of the eye) the position of an eye in relation to the head, from which a pure vertical and a pure horizontal movement is not associated with any degree of torsion. The eye is usually, but not necessarily, in the straight ahead (or straightforward) position.

primary proliferative polycythaemia (*syn* polycythaemia rubra vera) also known as Vaquez–Osler disease. It is an idiopathic, myeloproliferative disorder which occurs mainly in patients over the age of 40 years and presents either as an incidental finding of a high haemoglobin, or with symptoms of hyperviscosity such as lassitude, loss of concentration, headaches, dizziness, blackouts, pruritus and epistaxis. Some present with manifestations of peripheral arterial disease or a cerebrovascular accident. Patients are often plethoric and the majority have a palpable spleen at diagnosis. Thrombotic complications may occur and peptic ulceration is common, sometimes complicated by bleeding. The diagnosis of polycythaemia requires a raised red cell mass, the absence of causes of secondary erythrocytosis, and splenomegaly. The neutrophil and platelet counts are frequently raised, an abnormal karyotype may be found in the marrow, and in vitro culture of the marrow demonstrates autonomous growth in the absence of added growth factors. Venesection gives prompt relief of hyperviscosity symptoms. Between 400 and 500 mL of blood (less in an older adult) are removed and the venesection is repeated every 5–7 days until the haematocrit is reduced to below 45%. Less frequent but regular venesection will maintain this level until the haemoglobin remains reduced because of iron deficiency. The underlying myeloproliferation can be suppressed by hydroxycarbamide or interferon. Radioactive phosphorus (5 mCi of ^{32}P intravenously) is reserved for older patients, as it increases the risk of transformation to acute leukaemia by six- to ten-fold. Treatment of marrow proliferation may reduce the risk of vascular occlusion, control spleen size and reduce transformation to myelofibrosis. Aspirin reduces the risk of thrombosis. Median survival after diagnosis in treated patients exceeds 10 years. Some patients survive more than 20 years; however, cerebrovascular or coronary events occur in up to 60% of patients. The disease may convert to another myeloproliferative disorder, with about 15% developing myelofibrosis. Acute leukaemia develops principally in those patients who have been treated with radioactive phosphorus.

primary radiation the main beam of radiation from a source which has not interacted with an object.

primary radiation barrier the floor, walls and ceiling of a room which may be exposed directly to the primary beam of radiation from X-ray equipment. ⊃ secondary radiation barrier.

primary referencing (citation) the gold standard of referencing where the source cited is the original piece of published work. ⊃ Harvard system of referencing, reference, secondary referencing (citation), Vancouver system of referencing.

primary site the initial position of tumour growth.

primary solute the main solute used in liquid scintillation counting as it fluoresces when electrons drop to their original low-energy state. ⊃ fluorescence.

primary T-lymphocyte deficiencies conditions that include autoimmune lymphoproliferative syndrome, bare lymphocyte syndromes, DiGeorge syndrome. They are characterized by recurrent viral (e.g. cytomegalovirus, Epstein–Barr virus, herpes zoster), protozoal (e.g. *Pneumocystis jirovecii, Toxoplasma gondii, Cryptosporidia*) and fungal infections (e.g. *Candida* spp., *Aspergillus* spp.). There is a pattern of infection caused by *Mycobacterium tuberculosis* and atypical mycobacteria. In addition, many T-cell deficiencies are associated with defective antibody production because of the importance of T cells in providing help for B cells. These disorders generally present in childhood. The principal tests for T-lymphocyte deficiencies are a total lymphocyte count and quantitation of lymphocyte subpopulations by flow cytometry. Serum immunoglobulins should also be quantified. Functional tests of T-cell activation and proliferation and/or an HIV test may be indicated. Patients with suspected T-cell immune deficiencies should receive anti-*Pneumocystis* and antifungal prophylaxis, and require aggressive management of specific infections. Immunoglobulin replacement may be indicated if disease is associated with defective antibody production. Haemopoietic stem cell transplantation (HSCT) may be appropriate in bare lymphocyte syndromes, and thymic transplantation has been used for DiGeorge syndrome. ⊃ autoimmune lymphoproliferative syndrome, bare lymphocyte syndromes, DiGeorge syndrome.

primary teeth ⊃ deciduous, primary dentition.

primary thrombocythaemia a myeloproliferative disorder. The malignant proliferation of megakaryocytes results in a raised level of circulating platelets that are often dysfunctional. Prior to making a diagnosis of essential thrombocythaemia it is essential to exclude reactive causes of increased platelets, e.g. chronic inflammatory disorders, malignancy, tissue damage, haemolytic anaemias, following splenectomy or haemorrhage. Patients present at a median age of 60 years with vascular occlusion or bleeding events, or without symptoms and an isolated raised platelet count. In most individuals the condition is chronic, with the platelet count gradually increasing. A very small percentage may transform to acute leukaemia and others to myelofibrosis. Low-risk patients (age less than 40 years, platelet count less than 1000×10^9/L and no bleeding or thrombosis) may require no treatment to reduce the platelet count. Aspirin therapy is often recommended. For those with a platelet count

over 1000×10^9/l or those with symptoms, treatment to control platelets should be given. Agents include oral hydroxycarbamide or anagrelide, an inhibitor of megakaryocyte maturation. Intravenous radioactive phosphorus (^{32}P) may be useful in older adults. Aspirin should be considered for all patients to reduce the risk of thrombosis and is particularly useful therapy for those with digital ischaemia.

primary tumour the neoplasm (cancer) at the site of origin.

primary visual area ⊃ visual area.

primary visual cortex ⊃ visual area.

primate spacing diastema present in some deciduous dentition between the mandibular canine and first molar and the maxillary lateral incisor and canine.

prime 1. *n* a cue given to prompt, facilitate or inhibit a particular response in experimental studies. **2.** *v* the act of presenting a prime.

primer a substance that changes the nature of the tooth surface prior to bonding.

primigravida *n* a woman who is pregnant for the first time—**primigravidae** *pl*.

primipara *n* a woman who has given birth to one viable infant—**primiparous** *adj*.

primiparous having delivered one viable child.

primitive groove the indentation at the back of the embryonic disk which will become the cephalocaudal axis (head and spine).

primitive reflexes the behaviours with which the infant is born—sucking, breathing, crying, grasping, walking and Moro reflex.

primitive streak an area at the posterior (caudal) end of the embryonic disc. It develops during the proliferation and movement of cells and produces the mesoderm layer.

primordial *adj* primitive, original; applied to the ovarian follicles present at birth.

primordial cyst ⊃ odontogenic keratocyst.

principal axes the axes of a body or object around which the moment of inertia (resistance to rotation) is greatest, least and intermediate.

principal fibre the term describing the main group of collagen fibres which make up the periodontal ligament.

principal focus (*syn* focal point) the axial image point produced by an optical system of an infinitely distant object (the second principal focus or posterior principal focus), or that axial object point for which the image will be formed at infinity (the first principal focus or anterior principal focus). A converging optical system or lens has two principal foci which are real. A diverging optical system or lens has a second principal focus which is virtual. In curved mirrors the two principal foci coincide. Depending upon whether the object is at infinity or at the principal focus, this same focal point becomes either the second principal focus or the first principal focus, respectively. ⊃ cardinal points, equivalent power, focal length, focus, sign convention.

principal line of vision ⊃ line of sight.

principal plane a plane perpendicular to the optical axis of an optical system at the point where the incident rays

O

P

parallel to the optical axis intersect the refracted rays converging to the secondary focal point (*secondary principal plane*); or in which the refracted rays parallel to the optical axis intersect the incident rays coming from the primary focal point (*primary principal plane*). Each plane is an erect image of the other, and of the same size. For this reason they are sometimes also referred to as unit planes as they are conjugate planes in which the magnification is +1. In a thin lens these planes coincide at the lens. ⮑ equivalent power, focal length, image distance, nodal points, object distance, principal points, thin lens.

principal points the points of intersection of the principal planes with the optical axis. The principal points are the usual reference points from which the focal lengths and the object and image distances are measured. ⮑ equivalent power, focal length, image distance, object distance, principal plane.

prion *n* an infectious agent consisting of protein, similar to viruses but containing no nucleic acids.

prion disease a range of disorders in which there is an abnormal deposition of prion protein in the brain of which the most common example is Creutzfeldt–Jakob disease.

prism a transparent body (e.g. plastic, glass) bounded by two inclined plane surfaces which intersect in a straight line called the apex and form an angle called the prism angle. The face opposite the apex is called the base. It is an optical element used to deviate light (towards the base of the prism). The angle of deviation d of a prism in air is given by the following formula: $d = i + i' - a$ where i is the angle of incidence, i' the angle of emergence and a the prism angle (Figure P.17). ⮑ ophthalmic prism, prism dioptre, prism power.

prism cover test ⮑ cover test.

prism dioptre **1.** a unit specifying the amount of light deviation by an ophthalmic prism. One prism dioptre (written 1Δ) represents a deviation of 1 cm on a flat surface 1 m away from the prism. The surface is perpendicular to the direction of the original light ray. Similarly, a 2Δ prism deviates light 2 cm at a distance of 1 m and so on. For small angles, conversion between prism dioptres and degrees is given by the approximate formula: 7Δ = 4° or 1Δ = 0.57° or 1° = 1.75Δ. The exact formula for any angle α less than 90° is: α in Δ = 100 tan α. Note: the current British Standard regarding ophthalmic lenses specifies a deviation (in Δ) of a ray of light of wavelength 587.6 nm incident normally at one surface. **2.** a unit of convergence of the eyes. ⮑ ophthalmic prism, Prentice's law, prism power.

prism dissociation test ⮑ diplopia test.

prism flippers ⮑ lens flippers.

prism power (*syn* prismatic power) the amount of deviation of a ray of light transmitted through a prism or lens (outside its optical centre). It is usually expressed in prism dioptres (Δ) and given by the following approximate formula for small angle prisms (in air): $P = 100(n - 1)a$ where a is the prism angle in radians and n the refractive index (index of refraction) of the prism. ⮑ Prentice's law.

prismatic power ⮑ prism power.

Private Finance Initiative (PFI) a joint venture between private and public sector to build a facility, e.g. a hospital, using private finance. The health authority then leases the building. Some non-clinical services may also be provided under the lease agreement.

PRK *abbr* photorefractive keratectomy.

PRL *abbr* prolactin.

pro- a prefix that means 'before, in front', e.g. *prodrug*.

probability the likelihood that something is going to occur. ⮑ P value.

proband *n* in the genetically inherited diseases, the first family member to present for investigation.

probe (dental) also known as an explorer. Sharp-pointed hand instrument used to explore teeth and restoration surfaces in order to detect caries, overhanging edges and other defects. May be single or double ended. *periodontal probe.* ⮑ periodontal instruments.

probe (transducer) a hand-held instrument composed of multiple elements of piezo-electric material each with its own electrodes, used in ultrasound imaging.

probiotics *npl* the addition of live micro-organisms to human food, or used as animal feed. They include species of the genera *Bifidobacterium* and *Lactobacillus*. There is increasing evidence that they may provide health benefits by re-establishing the microbial balance in the colon. ⮑ prebiotics.

problem-based learning (PBL) students are presented with a problem (trigger) and collectively discover what information they need to resolve the problem. They negotiate which member of their learning set will find which information and convey this to the group on an agreed date. This process is facilitated by an educationalist. ⮑ inquiry-based learning (IBL).

problem-orientated medical record a multiprofessional system of keeping patient records. Entries are made using

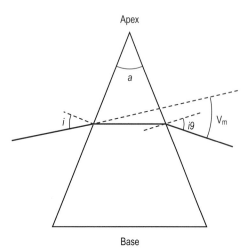

Apex

a

i $i9$ V_m

Base

P.17 Prism (*a*, prism angle; *i*, angle of incidence = *i'*, angle of emergence; *V*$_{m}$, angle of minimum deviation) (reproduced from Millodot 2004 with permission).

the SOAP formula: S = subjective, O = objective, A = assessment, P = plan.

procarcinogen *n* a substance that is not carcinogenic, but during metabolism in the body it produces a carcinogen.

procedural memory that part of memory that stores information needed to do things, e.g. take a venous blood sample or record a television programme.

process *n* 1. a prominence or outgrowth of any part. **2.** a very fine microscopic extension of a cell. **3.** in dentistry, a procedure whereby a denture base resin is polymerized (or cured) in a mould.

process goal a goal that specifies the processes a performer will engage in whilst performing. For example, a fielder in cricket might set a process goal to keep their eyes on the ball when making a catch. ⊃ outcome goal, performance goal.

procidentia *n* complete prolapse of the uterus, so that it lies within the vaginal sac but outside the contour of the body.

proclination sloping of anterior teeth in a labial direction.

proctalgia *n* pain in the anal or rectal region.

proctalgia fugax a severe, but intermittent pain in the rectum. May be caused by muscle spasm.

proctectasia abnormal dilatation of the rectum and anus.

proctectomy surgical excision of the rectum.

proctitis *n* inflammation of the rectum.

proct/o- a prefix that means 'anus', e.g. *proctology*.

proctocele ⊃ rectocele.

proctoclysis *n* introduction of fluid into the rectum for absorption. ⊃ enteroclysis.

proctocolectomy *n* surgical excision of the rectum and colon. Performed for severe ulcerative colitis or Crohn's disease and for familial polyposis coli. Requires a permanent ileostomy or some type of restorative procedure such as an ileoanal reservoir.

proctocolitis *n* inflammation of the rectum and colon.

proctodynia pain in the anal and rectal region.

proctology the branch of medicine that involves the study of diseases of the anus and rectum and their treatment.

proctorrhaphy *n* repair of a tear in the anus or rectum.

proctoscope *n* a speculum or rigid tubular instrument for examining the anal canal and rectum. ⊃ endoscope—**proctoscopic** *adj*.

proctoscopy *n* inspection of the anal canal and rectum using a rigid instrument.

proctosigmoiditis *n* inflammation of the rectum and sigmoid colon.

proctotomy surgery opening into the anus and rectum.

prodromal *adj* preceding, as the transitory rash before the true rash of an infectious disease.

prodromal labour the early stage of labour when contractions occur but are without strength and thus not felt by the woman.

prodrug *n* a drug administered as an inactive form that may be activated in a numbers of ways, e.g. by bowel bacteria, in the brain or by liver enzymes. Used for a variety of reasons such as avoiding gastrointestinal side-effects, or crossing the blood–brain barrier.

proenzyme *n* the inactive (or precursor) form of a proteolytic enzyme, such as pepsinogen or trypsinogen. Also called a zymogen.

profession a work organization with a number of characteristics, which include a central regulatory body, a code of conduct, management and control of knowledge and expertise and control of numbers, selection and training of those entering the profession. Professions can be viewed as motivated by altruism, as self-interested monopolies, or as 'agents of the state' whose function is to control 'deviant' behaviour.

professions allied to medicine ⊃ allied health professions.

professional liability the legal obligation of healthcare professionals to compensate their clients for acts of negligence in their professional practice which cause the clients suffering or damage. This is central to the concept of malpractice.

professional–patient relationship can be conceived as a power relationship through which social problems are conceived and defined, by professionals, as the needs and problems of patients and clients. The relationship also allows professionals to define solutions to these problems. The professional–patient relationship has come under considerable criticism and now a 'patient-centred' approach is advocated that allows patients and clients more power and control. ⊃ patient-centred medicine.

professional self-regulation the professional quality and continuing professional development standards set by various professional regulatory bodies for health professionals, e.g. GMC, for professional practice, discipline and conduct.

professional socialization tertiary socialization involves the acquisition of knowledge, skills and attitudes required in performing high-level occupations such as medicine, nursing and allied health professions.

profile **1.** the image captured by the detector in computed tomography (CT) scanning. **2.** a side view, especially of the face.

profiling (community) process of producing a profile of a specific community. It includes demographic information such as the age profile, social and economic make-up, existing facilities, networks and services. The profile may be produced by people living in the community with varying degrees of support from the local authority, development agencies or health services.

profunda *adj* relating to blood vessels and other structures that are deeply enclosed within the tissues.

progeria a rare congenital condition in which the person ages prematurely. It is characterized by the appearance of the signs of ageing, such as skin wrinkling and grey hair, in prepubertal children. Death frequently occurs before the teenage years from coronary artery disease.

progestational *adj* before pregnancy. Favouring pregnancy—**progestation** *n*.

progesterone *n* the 'progestation' steroid hormone secreted by the corpus luteum, ovaries, placenta and, in limited amounts, by the adrenal glands. Progesterone acts on the

O
P

endometrium, myometrium, cervical mucus and breasts. It is important in the preparation for and maintenance of pregnancy. The corpus luteum (formed in the ovary following ovulation) secretes progesterone during the second half of the menstrual cycle, with actions that prepare the lining of the uterus for a potential pregnancy. Progesterone is secreted by the ovaries in early pregnancy, and by the placenta during the later months, maintaining appropriate changes from conception onwards.

progestogen *n* any natural or synthetic progestational hormone including progesterone.

progestogen-only contraceptives available in several formulations: (a) as an oral contraceptive, the progestogen-only pill (POP) that is taken continuously and at regular time intervals to provide effective contraception; (b) for parenteral administration as an intramuscular injection, or a subdermal implant that releases hormone to provide contraception for up to 3 years; and (c) as an intrauterine device that contains progestogen. This device is also used in the management of menorrhagia and to provide progestogen where oestrogen-only hormone relacement is prescribed for a woman with an intact uterus.

proglottis a sexually mature segment of tapeworm—**proglottides** *pl*.

prognathism an anomaly in which the lower jaw bone projects forward beyond the normal distance from the cranial base.

prognosis *n* a forecast of the probable course and termination of a disease. Prognostic factors are patient or disease characteristics that influence the course. Good prognosis is associated with a low rate of undesirable outcomes; poor prognosis is associated with a high rate of undesirable outcomes—**prognostic** *adj*.

program a set of written instructions for the computer.

programmable read only memory (PROM) a specially prepared computer chip which can be programmed.

progressing stroke (*syn* stroke in evolution) describes a stroke in which the focal neurological deficit worsens after the patient first presents. Such worsening may be due to increasing volume of infarction, haemorrhage or related oedema.

progressive addition lens (PAL) (*syn* varifocal lens) a spectacle lens having a gradual and progressive change in power either over the whole lens or over a region intermediate between areas of uniform power. The progression is produced by a complex aspheric shape of one of the surfaces. This lens is used to correct presbyopia. ⟳ bifocal lens, gradient-index lens, interpupillary distance, multifocal lens.

progressive muscular atrophy ⟳ motor neuron disease.

projectile an object that moves through a resistive medium, usually the air above the surface of the earth.

projectile motion motion above the surface of the earth, under the influence of gravity and also of air resistance and lift forces, including Magnus forces.

projection *n* a defence mechanism occurring in normal people unconsciously, and in exaggerated form in some mental health problems, whereby the person fails to recognize certain motives and feelings in him or herself but attributes them to other people.

projective techniques the use of creative media to provide an external focus for the client to express feelings that they find unacceptable or difficult to voice. The therapist may invite the client to make an object onto which to project their feelings or present them with a stimulus, such as a poem or piece of music, and ask them to say what they feel about it.

prolactin (PRL) *n* a hormone secreted by the anterior pituitary, which initiates milk production. It suppresses ovulation naturally during lactation, however, this does not always happen and pregnancies may occur. Excessive secretion of prolactin can be a cause of infertility. ⟳ hyperprolactinaemia.

prolactinoma *n* prolactin secreting pituitary adenoma. ⟳ hyperprolactinaemia.

prolapse *n* descent; the falling of a structure.

prolapse of the antral mucosa the protrusion of the antral mucosa through an oroantral fistula into the oral cavity.

prolapse of the iris (*syn* iridocele) the protrusion of a portion of the iris into a corneal wound. It results from either trauma, a severe corneal ulcer or an operation. In some cases an anterior synechia may develop as the iris remains fixed in the wound by scar tissue. ⟳ corneal ulcer, synechia.

prolapse of the rectum the lower portion of the intestinal tract descends outside the external anal sphincter. The rectal mucosa may be visible outside the anus. May be associated with chronic constipation with straining.

prolapse of the uterus the uterus descends into the vagina and may be visible at the vaginal orifice. ⟳ procidentia.

prolapsed intervertebral disc (PID) (*syn.* slipped disc) disc protrusion of the nucleus pulposus through its fibrous covering into the spinal canal, due to degenerative changes, heavy lifting or injury in sport. Can press on the spinal cord or on the nerve roots, leading to pain, numbness, paraesthesia or even paralysis. Most common in the lumbar region, causing sciatica if the roots of the sciatic nerve are compressed. Diagnosis is clinical with magnetic resonance imaging (MRI) scanning to confirm. Treatment is initially rest with appropriate analgesia, then a programme of core muscle strengthening to prevent recurrence. Persistent neurological symptoms and signs require investigation and, rarely, surgical treatment with minimally invasive microdiscectomy. In sport the commonest disc injuries are in the lumbar and cervical regions, the latter typically in rugby (scrum collapse or direct injury in a tackle), in judo or in a fall from a height as in trampolining or gymnastics. These injuries highlight the need for adequately trained and experienced medical back-up.

prolapsed umbilical cord ⟳ cord prolapse.

proliferate *vi* increase by cell division—**proliferation** *n*, **proliferative** *adj*.

proliferative diabetic retinopathy (PDR) ⟳ diabetic retinopathy (DR).

proliferative retinopathy (*syn* retinitis proliferans) neovascularization of the retina extending into the vitreous body (humour) with connective tissue proliferation surrounding the vessels. The vessels usually arise from a retinal vein near an arteriovenous crossing at the posterior pole and from the surface of the optic disc. It occurs as a result of certain inflammatory conditions and in diabetes. Visual acuity may be affected. ➲ diabetic retinopathy, preretinal macular fibrosis, retinal hypoxia, vitrectomy.

prolific *adj* fruitful, multiplying abundantly.

proline *n* a conditionally essential (indispensable) amino acid.

prolonged labour labour lasting more than 24 hours due to inadequate or incoordinate uterine action, cephalopelvic disproportion or a poorly fitting presenting part as in malpresentation or malposition. The midwife must ensure that the woman receives adequate pain relief, that progress is being made and that maternal and fetal conditions are satisfactory. Fetal risks include hypoxia and trauma, excessive skull moulding causing intracranial haemorrhage; maternal risks include exhaustion, dehydration, uterine rupture, and physical trauma leading to long-term uterine, cervical or urinary tract problems.

prolonged pregnancy pregnancy lasting 42 weeks (294 days) or more from the first day of the last normal menstrual period; induction of labour is only necessary when either the maternal or fetal condition is compromised.

prolymphocytic leukaemia a variant of chronic lymphatic leukaemia found mainly in males over the age of 60; 25% of cases are of the T-cell variety. There is massive splenomegaly with little lymphadenopathy and a very high leucocyte count, often in excess of 400×10^9/L; the characteristic cell is a large lymphocyte with a prominent nucleolus. Treatment is generally unsuccessful and the prognosis very poor. Leucopheresis, splenectomy and chemotherapy may be tried.

PROM *abbr* **1.** patient reported outcome measures. **2.** programmable read only memory.

PROMM *abbr* proximal myotonic myopathy.

promontory *n* a projection; a prominent part.

promoter **1.** a sequence of deoxyribonucleic acid (DNA) that controls the start of transcription. **2.** a substance that acts with another carcinogen to stimulate cells to divide more rapidly than usual, thereby increasing the risk of malignant changes. **3.** in dentistry. ➲ accelerator (promoter).

pronate *vt* to place ventral surface downward, e.g. on the face; to turn (the palm of the hand) downwards. ➲ supinate *opp*—**pronation** *n*.

pronation *pronation of the foot* the sequence during normal gait after the heel hits the ground, the ankle tends to angle inwards, the foot is supported briefly on its inner side, the arch tends to flatten whilst weight is transferred progressively forwards towards the toes. *overpronation* flattens the arch excessively. *pronation of the forearm* the twisting movement of the forearm which brings the palm of the hand to face downwards or backwards. ➲ supination *opp*.

pronator *n* that which pronates, usually applied to a muscle, for example, the pronator teres. ➲ supinator *opp*.

pronator teres a superficial muscle of the forearm. Its origin is on the medial epicondyle of the humerus and on the coronoid process of the ulna, its common tendon inserts on to the shaft of the radius. Contraction of the muscle pronates the forearm and hand. ➲ Colour Section Figure 4.

prone *adj* **1.** lying on the anterior surface of the body with the face turned to the side. **2.** of the hand, with the palm downwards. ➲ supine *opp*.

prone knee bend (PKB) a neurodynamic test that tests the femoral nerve. Traditionally tested in prone position, however, this fails to differentiate between nervous tissue (femoral nerve) and the hip flexor muscles. Carrying out the test in side lying with the head and trunk flexed allows the cervical extension to be used as a desensitizing test. A normal response would be full range of movement so that the heel approximates the buttock and is accompanied by a strong stretch on the anterior thigh. ➲ neurodynamic testing.

prone-standing a position of half standing, where a high plinth carefully supports the trunk, head and upper limbs. The hips are generally at an angle of 90°, but this is dependent on the individual patient. This position can be used when treating people with neurological problems. It is a useful position in that the weight of the upper body is supported by the plinth and thus allowing the therapist to concentrate on the pelvis and legs.

prone test ➲ provocative test.

pronephros the earliest non-functional kidney tissue that forms in the embryo. ➲ mesonephros, metanephros.

Pronosco X-posure System™ specialist equipment for assessing bone mineral density.

pronucleus the nuclear material of the ovum and spermatozoon following the penetration of the oocyte by the spermatozoon, each contains the haploid (n) number of chromosomes, but before fusion to create the nucleus of the zygote with the diploid (2n) number of chromosomes.

pro-opiomelanocortin (POMC) a large protein prohormone which is produced in the anterior lobe of the pituitary gland and found in other tissues. It gives rise to adrenocorticotrophic hormone (ACTH), endorphins, enkephalins, lipotrophins and melanocyte-stimulating hormones.

prop a dental instrument used, generally during an anaesthetic, to maintain the mouth in an open position. ➲ mouth prop.

propagate in ultrasound to move forward through a medium, at an initial velocity and direction.

propagation speed the speed at which a wave moves through a medium in metres per second.

properdin a globulin involved in the alternative pathway of complement activation.

prophase the first stage in both mitosis (see Figure M.7, p. 488) and meiosis (see Figure M.3, p. 472). In mitosis the chromatin condenses and shortens to form a visible double set of chromosomes (from DNA replication during interphase). The double chromosomes are joined by the centromeres, each half of the chromosome is known as a chromatid. The nucleoli start to breakdown and the nuclear membrane disappears. Each pair of centrioles moves to opposite poles of the cell where they commence the formation of the mitotic spindle which eventually reaches from one pair of centrioles to the other. Prophase I in meiosis takes longer than in mitosis. Unique to meiosis there is pairing or synapsis of homologous chromosomes to form a bivalent, comprising two chromosomes, which coil around each other. The chromosome pairs undergo incomplete separation and each chromosome now has two chromatids; now each unit has four strands (quadrivalents). Several 'cross-over' points or chiasmata form between the chromatids. These facilitates the exchange of genetic material between the chromosomes of homologous pair and the production of gametes of infinite genetic variability. Separation of the two bivalents continues and the nucleolus and nuclear membrane disappear. Prophase II in the second meiotic division follows the same steps but this time with only 23 chromosomes, rather than homologus pairs. ➲ anaphase, metaphase, telophase.

prophylactic 1. pertaining to the prevention of disease. ➲ prophylaxis. **2.** an agent that prevents the development of a disease or condition, such as a vaccine.

prophylactic odontotomy a dental procedure involving the elimination of pits and fissures in tooth enamel to prevent caries.

prophylactic paste a deprecated term for polishing paste.

prophylactic (preventive) treatment ➲ treatment.

prophylaxis *n* from the Greek, to guard or prevent beforehand. The attempt to prevent a condition or disease by, for example, immunization, antibiotics for dental work in certain cardiac conditions or people exposed to an infectious disease such as meningococcal meningitis, low molecular weight heparin to prevent deep vein thrombosis for some types of surgery or prolonged immobilization, scaling, cleaning and polishing of teeth—**prophylactic** *adj*, **prophylactically** *adv*.

prophylaxis cup ➲ rubber cup (prophylaxis cup).

propionic acids a group of non-steroidal anti-inflammatory drugs, e.g. ibuprofen. ➲ Appendix 5.

proprietary name (*syn.* brand name) the name given to, for example, a drug, by the pharmaceutical company which developed it. It should always be spelt with a capital letter to distinguish it from the generic name (British Approved Name—BAN) which can be used by other companies.

proprioception *n* the process of receiving information from proprioceptors, with or without conscious awareness. The appreciation of balance and the position of the body and individual body parts in relation to each other, especially as they change during movement.

proprioceptive neuromuscular facilitation (PNF) therapeutic technique, with questionable neurophysiological basis, in which maximal static stretch is first performed, with view to enhancement of subsequent range of movement. The technique, which utilizes the properties of proprioception that respond to pressure and stretch, was developed as a therapeutic approach for the re-education of movement.

It involves the use of resistance and facilitation of movements in recognized mass patterns of spiral or diagonal movements, along with the use of stretch, repetition and verbal commands.

proprioceptor *n* sensory receptor located in muscles, joint capsules and surrounding tissues, and the vestibular apparatus of the ears whose reflex function is locomotor or postural. The receptors signal information to the central nervous system about position and movement of body parts, for example the angle at a joint or the length of a muscle. ➲ Golgi tendon organ, joint receptors, muscle spindle.

proptosis *n* forward protrusion, especially of the eyeball.

propulsive drag force the force used by sportspeople to propel themselves, usually by pushing against a fluid medium (e.g. swimmers or rowers). ➲ drag force, form drag, surface drag.

propulsive force force on a body or object used to accelerate it in a required direction (usually forward). ➲ thrust.

prosencephalon forebrain. One of the three primary vesicles formed during early embryonic development of the brain. It becomes the diencephalon and the telencephalon.

prosody *n* describes the phonological features of speech that include rate, rhythm, stress, loudness and pitch.

prospective study research that deals with future data, moving forward in time. ➲ retrospective study.

prostacyclin *n* a substance derived from prostaglandins. Produced by endothelial cells lining blood vessels. It inhibits platelet aggregation and is concerned with preventing intravascular clotting.

prostaglandins *npl* a large group of potent regulatory lipids derived from arachidonic acid. They have a short duration of action and modulate the action of several hormones. Found in most body tissues where they regulate physiological functions including: smooth muscle contraction, inflammation, gastric secretion and blood clotting. Used therapeutically to terminate pregnancy, induce labour, and for the treatment of asthma, erectile dysfunction and gastric hyperacidity. ➲ Appendix 5.

prostaglandin inhibitor an agent which prevents the production of prostaglandin and is usually a non-steroidal anti-inflammatory agent. ➲ Appendix 5.

prostate cancer common in northern Europe and the USA (particularly in the black population) but rare in China and Japan. In the UK it is the second most common malignancy in males and is increasing in frequency. It rarely occurs before the age of 50 and has a mean age at presentation of 70 years. Metastatic spread to pelvic lymph nodes occurs early and metastases to bone, mainly the lumbar spine and pelvis, are common. Prostatic specific antigen (PSA) is a good tumour marker and 40% of patients with a serum PSA > 4.0 ng/mL will have prostate cancer on biopsy. This has led to the introduction of screening programmes, principally in the USA, despite a lack of consensus about their utility. Most men present with lower urinary tract symptoms indistinguishable from benign prostatic enlargement (BPE);

dysuria, prostatis/cystitis, frequency, poor urine stream, hesitancy, dribbling, etc. Symptoms and signs due to metastases are much less common and include back pain, weight loss, anaemia and obstruction of the ureters. On rectal examination the prostate often feels nodular and stony hard. However, 10–15% of tumours are not palpable. Whenever possible, the diagnosis is confirmed by needle biopsy, usually aided by transrectal ultrasound (TRUS), or by histological examination of tissue removed by endoscopic resection if this is needed to relieve outflow obstruction. Since most men present with outflow tract obstruction, an ultrasound scan and serum creatinine determination are used to assess the urinary tract. A plain X-ray of the pelvis and lumbar spine (to investigate backache) may show bony metastases as the first evidence of prostate cancer.The patient is assessed for distant metastases by a radioisotope bone scan but high levels of serum PSA (> 100 ng/ml) almost always indicate distant bone metastases. PSA is most useful for monitoring response to treatment and disease progression. Management depends upon the stage of the cancer and whether it has spread, the treatment modalities include: (a) surgery (radical prostatectomy or transurethral resection); (b) high intensity focused ultrasound (HIFU); (c) radiotherapy (external or internal); (d) hormone manipulation (drugs or orchidectomy); (e) chemotherapy. Tumour confined to the prostate is potentially curable by either radical prostatectomy, HIFU or radical radiotherapy. A small focus of tumour found incidentally at transurethral resection of the prostate (TUR/TURP) does not significantly alter life expectancy and only requires follow-up ('watchful waiting'). Approximately half of men with prostate cancer will have metastatic disease at the time of diagnosis. Prostatic cancer is sensitive to hormonal influences; locally advanced or metastatic prostate cancer is treated by androgen depletion either by surgery (orchidectomy) or more commonly now by androgen-suppressing drugs. Anti-androgen drugs such as cyproterone acetate act by preventing the binding of dihydrotestosterone to androgen receptors in the tumour cells, so preventing cell growth. Gonadotrophin-releasing hormone (GnRH) analogues such as goserelin continuously occupy pituitary receptors, preventing them from responding to the GnRH pulses which normally stimulate luteinizing hormone (LH) and follicle stimulating hormone (FSH) release. Chemotherapy with 5-fluorouracil, cyclophosphamide or nitrogen mustard can be effective. Radiotherapy is also used as palliative treatment for generalized bone pain. ⊃ prostate specific antigen.

prostate gland *n* a small firm body at the base of the male bladder and surrounding the first part of the urethra. It is part glandular and part muscular tissue. Exocrine glands within the prostate produce fluid which comprises about 20–30% of the volume of ejaculated semen and is rich in lipids, phospholipids and enzymes including fibrinolysin, an acid phosphatase that 'activates' the sperm. Smooth muscle fibres within the prostate, under sympathetic nerve control, contract at orgasm to move seminal fluid via ejaculatory ducts into the bulbar urethra (emission)—**prostatic** *adj*. ⊃ Colour Section Figure 16.

prostate specific antigen (PSA) protein secreted by prostatic tissue. Acts as a tumour marker for prostate cancer, and its detection in the blood forms the basis for a screening test. However, conditions other than prostate cancer can cause an increase in PSA level.

prostatectomy *n* surgical removal of the prostate gland. *retropubic prostatectomy* the prostate is reached through a lower abdominal (suprapubic) incision, the bladder being retracted upwards to expose the prostate behind the pubis. *transurethral prostatectomy* ⊃ transurethral resection of prostate (TUR/TURP). *transvesical prostatectomy* the operation in which the prostate is approached through the bladder, using a lower abdominal (suprapubic) incision.

prostatic *adj* relating to the prostate. ⊃ benign prostatic enlagement (BPE).

prostatic acid phosphatase ⊃ acid phosphatase.

prostatism *n* term used to describe the symptom complex associated with bladder outflow obstruction.

prostatitis *n* inflammation of the prostate gland which may be acute or chronic. It can be caused by the same bacteria that are associated with urinary tract infection (e.g. *Escherichia coli*, *Proteus* spp., *Pseudomonas* spp., *Staphylococci epidermidis*, streptococci) or, more commonly, may be 'non-bacterial' (no organisms cultured from urine). Clinical features include frequency, dysuria, perineal or groin pain, difficulty passing urine and, in acute disease, considerable systemic disturbance. The prostate is enlarged and tender. Bacterial prostatitis is confirmed by a positive culture from urine or from urethral discharge obtained after prostatic massage, and the treatment of choice is a quinolone antibiotic such as ofloxacin. A 4- to 6-week course is required. Non-bacterial prostatitis can be treated with drugs to relax the prostate and bladder neck, such as terazosin.

prostat/o- a prefix that means 'prostate gland', e.g. *prostatism.*

prosthesis *n* artificial substitute or restoration of a part of the body that is congenitally missing, destroyed accidently or removed surgically—**prostheses** *pl*, **prosthetic** *adj*. ⊃ arthroplasty, cosmetic prothesis, dental prosthesis, dentures, implant (dental), maxillofacial prosthesis, total hip replacement, total knee replacement.

prosthetic dentistry the restoration of the function and aesthetics of missing teeth using a denture or bridge.

prosthetic group a non-protein coenzyme or metal ion which must attach to an enzyme protein in order for enzyme activity to occur. ⊃ apoenzyme.

prosthetics *n* the branch of surgery which deals with prostheses.

prosthetic surgery the surgical procedures designed to facilitate the manufacture of dentures and to improve the long term prognosis of denture wearing.

prosthion the most anterior point of the alveolar crest in the premaxilla and usually situated between the central incisors.

O
P

prosthodontics (prosthetic dentistry) branch of dental science concerned with removable dental prosthetics. This definition is applicable to the UK only. In other countries prosthodontics may refer to both removable and fixed appliances (i.e. bridge work).

prosthodontist (dental prosthetist) dental surgeon engaged in the practice of prosthodontics.

protan a person who has either protanopia or protanomaly.

protanomal a person who has protanomaly.

protanomalous trichromatism ⊃ protanomaly.

protanomalous vision ⊃ protanomaly.

protanomaly (*syn* protanomalous trichromatism, protanomalous vision, red-weakness) a type of anomalous trichromatism in which an abnormally high proportion of the red primary stimulus is needed when mixing red and green to match a given yellow. This is due to the fact that the luminosity function of a protanomal is reduced for the red radiations. The condition occurs in less than 1% of the male population. ⊃ anomaloscope, defective colour vision, pseudoisochromatic plates, trichromatism.

protanope a person who has protanopia.

protanopia (*syn* red blindness) a type of dichromatism in which only two hues are seen: below 493 nm all radiations appear bluish whereas above it they all appear yellowish. Around 493 nm is the neutral point. The luminosity function of protanopes is significantly decreased for red radiations (for which he or she is almost blind). The condition occurs in about 1% of the male population. ⊃ dichromatism, neutral pont, pseudoisochromatic plates.

protease *n* an enzyme which digests protein (proteolytic). *protease enzymes*, e.g. streptokinase, are used in the management of leg ulcers to remove slough and facilitate healing.

protease inhibitor a class of antiviral drugs, e.g. ritonavir, used in the treatment of HIV disease and AIDS.

protective barriers in radiology, the methods of protecting the patients, staff and general public from unnecessary exposure to radiation using lead panelling and/or concrete.

protective deformity the posture adopted by a person in an attempt to minimize their discomfort, pain or disability. An example may be seen in chronic back pain where a person may adopt a shifted spinal posture. This is often subconscious.

protective equipment in sport equipment which has been developed and recommended for many different sports in order to help prevent and reduce the severity of injuries where research has identified a high risk of injury in a particular sport or recreational activity. Examples include shin guards, gum shields, helmets, knee pads and fire-protection suits in motor racing.

protective isolation previously known as reverse barrier nursing. Involves separating patients who are immunocompromised and susceptible to infection, either by disease or treatment. The type of patients needing protection from infection include those with leukaemia, those having immunosuppressant treatment for organ transplantation, chemotherapy or radiation or neutropenic patients. ⊃ containment isolation, source isolation.

protective spasm muscle spasm often occurs following injury, trauma or pain. It is the body's attempt to stop movement, unfortunately the spasm is often out of all proportion to the initial injury. The intensity of the spasm is strong enough for the patient to complain that their back locked up. In some situations the spasm becomes the overriding problem rather than the initial injury. This is one reason why a hot pack or massage may be so dramatically effective in relieving pain and facilitating movement.

proteinase proteolytic enzyme that hydrolyses protein.

protein-bound iodine a former test of thyroid function superceded by tests that directly measure the thyroid hormone levels.

protein C and S deficiencies protein C is a vitamin K-dependent plasma protein. When thrombin binds to thrombomodulin on the endothelial cell surface, it becomes an anticoagulant by activating protein C. In the presence of protein S, this inactivates factors Va and VIIIa. Thus a deficiency of either protein C or S results in a prothrombotic state due to reduced inhibition of activated factor V and VIII. A deficiency of either factor is usually inherited in an autosomal fashion. ⊃ venous thromboembolism.

protein-energy malnutrition (PEM) previously known as protein-calorie malnutrition (PCM). Describes a condition in which individuals have depleted body fat and protein resulting from a diet that is deficient in both protein and energy. It develops during famine, during illness and during childhood due to inappropriate weaning. ⊃ chronic energy deficiency, kwashiorkor, marasmus.

proteins *npl* highly complex nitrogenous compounds found in all animal and vegetable tissues. They are large polymers consisting of one or more sequences of amino acid subunits joined by peptide bonds: the major functional and structural components of body cells. Essential for cell function, growth and repair of the body tissues. Those from animal sources are of high biological value since they contain the essential amino acids. Those from vegetable sources contain not all, but some of the essential amino acids. Proteins are hydrolysed in the body to produce amino acids, which are then used to build up new body proteins. The body of a 70-kg man contains about 11 kg protein. The protein mass can be influenced by nutritional status, physical activity and pathological factors. Proteins in the diet typically account for 10–15% of energy intake and the currently recommended protein requirement for sedentary individuals is 0.8 g per kilogram body mass per day. The optimal protein intake for strength athletes may be as high as 1.7–1.8 g and for endurance athletes 1.2–1.4 g per kilogram body mass per day. ⊃ nitrogen balance.

proteinuria *n* excretion of abnormally high levels of protein in the urine. ⊃ albuminuria.

proteolysis *n* the hydrolysis of the peptide bonds of proteins with the formation of smaller polypeptides. By the action of enzymes, alkalis or acids —**proteolytic** *adj*.

Proteus *n* a bacterial genus of Gram-negative motile rods of the family Enterobacteriaceae. Found in damp surroundings and is a commensal of the intestinal tract. Species including *Proteus mirabilis* and *Proteus vulgaris* cause urinary tract infections and wound infections.

prothrombin *n* inactive precursor of the enzyme thrombin produced in the liver. Factor II in blood coagulation.

prothrombin G20210A a genetic polymorphism at the non-coding $3'$ end of the prothrombin gene is associated with an increased plasma level of prothrombin and venous thrombo-embolism. It is present in about 2% of the normal population and about 6% of those with venous thrombus. ⊃ venous thromboembolism.

prothrombin time assesses the activity of the extrinsic coagulation pathway. It is the time taken for plasma to clot in vitro following the introduction of thromboplastin in the presence of calcium. It is inversely proportional to the amount of prothrombin present, a normal person's plasma being used as a standard of comparison. The prothrombin time is extended in people taking anticoagulant drugs and in some haemorrhagic conditions.

proto- a prefix that means 'first', e.g. *prototype*.

protocol written standards for a way of working or the transfer of information, for example, between different computers.

proton *n* a positively charged particle found in the nucleus of an atom.

proton density weighted image a magnetic resonance image showing contrast related to the number of mobile protons in the structure and requires scanning parameters that minimize the effects of relaxation time (T_1 and T_2) to obtain the appropriate weighting.

proton pump H^+/K^+-ATPase an enzyme concerned with the production of gastric acid. An ATP-powered pump by which hydrogen ions enter the lumen of the stomach and potassium ions move into the parietal cell in the production of hydrochloric acid.

proton pump inhibitors a group of drugs, e.g. omeprazole, that decrease gastric acid secretion by irreversibly blocking the proton pump (H^+/K^+-ATPase). ⊃ Appendix 5.

proto-oncogene *n* a gene with the potential to become a cancer-causing oncogene if stimulated by mutagenic carcinogens. ⊃ oncogene.

protopathic *adj* the term applied to the somatic sensations of fast localized pain; slow, poorly localized pain; and temperature. ⊃ epicritic *opp*.

protoplasm *n* ⊃ cytoplasm.

protoporphyrin a porphyrin produced during the synthesis of haem, it combines with ferrous iron to form haem. Excess amounts are present in the faeces in some types of porphyria. Measuring the level of protoporphyrin in the red blood cells (erythrocytes) is used as a test for iron deficiency and other states where iron is not incorporated within haem, such as in lead poisoning.

protozoa *npl* unicellular microscopic animals. Some are pathogenic. Includes the genera *Plasmodium*, *Leishmania* and *Entamoeba*—**protozoon** *sing*, **protozoal** *adj*. ⊃ amoebiasis, giardiasis, leishmaniasis, malaria, toxoplasmosis, trichomoniasis.

protraction *n* a forward movement such as thrusting out the jaw. ⊃ retraction *opp*.

protrusion 1. thrusting forward movement of the mandible. 2. the malposition of the teeth of one jaw relative to the other jaw.

protrusive interocclusal record the interocclusal record made with the mandible in a protruded position by means of thin wax films or registration pastes.

protrusive record a record of the protruded relationship of the mandible relative to the maxilla.

proud flesh excessive granulation tissue.

provisional restoration generic term for a temporary restoration, either intra- or extra-coronal, designed to provide stabilization of a tooth prior to the next stage of treatment, e.g. temporary crown or temporary filling.

provitamin *n* a vitamin precursor, e.g. β-carotene is converted into vitamin A, or 7-dehydrocholesterol in the skin that is converted into vitamin D.

provocative test a test performed to reproduce signs of a suspected disease in order to help in the diagnosis of that disease. A common provocative test for open-angle glaucoma is the water-drinking test in which a fasting person is asked to drink 1 L of water (for a 70-kg adult) within 5 minutes. The intraocular pressure (IOP) is measured before the water is taken and then at 15-minute intervals. An increase of 8 mmHg or more in 45 minutes is considered positive. Two common provocative tests for angle-closure glaucoma are: the *dark room test* in which the person is kept in a dark room for 1 hour and the IOP is measured before and after the test. An increase of 8 mmHg or more is generally considered positive; and the *prone position test* in which the person lies in the prone position for 1 hour and if the IOP increases by 8 mmHg or more, compared to the value before the test, the result is considered positive. In open-angle glaucoma provocative tests have been found to be positive in less than half of the patients but that figure is higher in angle-closure glaucoma. ⊃ angle-closure glaucoma, intraocular pressure, open-angle glaucoma.

proximal *adj* in anatomy, nearest to a reference point such as the head or source. For example, in a limb, nearer to the trunk—the forearm is proximal to the hand; in the gut, the small intestine is proximal to the large intestine. ⊃ distal *opp*—**proximally** *adv*.

proximal accommodation (*syn* psychic accommodation) that component of accommodation initiated by the awareness of a near object. ⊃ accommodation reflex, proximal convergence, resting state of accommodation.

proximal caries ⊃ approximal caries.

proximal convergence (*syn* instrument convergence, proximal vergence, psychic convergence,) that component of convergence initiated by the awareness of a near object. For example, when looking into an instrument the image may be at optical infinity yet proximal convergence may be initiated.

proximal myotonic myopathy (PROMM, DM2) a muscular dystrophy. Inheritance is autosomal dominant; quadruplet repeat expansion in Zn finger protein 9 gene chromosome 3q. The onset occurs during adulthood and it affects proximal muscles, especially those of the thigh. Sometimes there is muscle hypertrophy. There is muscle pain and other features are similar to those occurring in myotonic dystrophy, but cognition is not affected. ⊃ muscular dystrophies, myotonic dystrophy.

proximal radioulnar joint a pivot joint formed by the rim of the head of the radius rotating in the radial notch of the ulna, and is in the same capsule as the elbow joint. The annular ligament is a strong extracapsular ligament that encircles the head of the radius and keeps it in contact with the radial notch of the ulna.

proximal tibiofibular joint also called anterior or superior tibiofibular joint. A joint between the lateral condyle of the tibia and the head of the fibula.

proximal vergence ⊃ proximal convergence.

PRP *abbr* panretinal photocoagulation.

PRR *abbr* preventive resin restoration.

prune belly syndrome (Eagle–Barrett syndrome) a condition found in male infants with obstructive uropathy and atrophy of the abdominal musculature. The term is descriptive.

prurigo *n* a chronic, itching disease often associated with skin lichenification.

pruritus *n* itching. *pruritus ani* and *pruritus vulvae* may be due to a number of causes, e.g. vaginitis caused by candidiasis. Generalized pruritus may be a symptom of systemic disease, as in renal failure, Hodgkin's disease, cancer or jaundice—**pruritic** *adj*. ⊃ pruritus ani, pruritus vulvae.

pruritus ani itching of the perianal skin is common and can result from many causes, most of which result in contamination of the perianal skin with faecal contents. The causes include: (a) local anorectal conditions—anal fissure, anal fistula, haemorrhoids, inadequate personal hygiene; (b) infections/infestations—candidiasis, threadworms; (c) skin conditions—lichen planus, psoriasis, contact dermatitis; (d) other causes—diarrhoea (any cause), faecal incontinence (especially associated with chronic constipation with leakage of faecal fluid, which is a common cause of faecal incontinence in older adults), irritable bowel syndrome, anxiety. Itching may be trivial or severe and results in an itch-scratch-itch cycle which exacerbates the problem. When no underlying cause is found, all local barrier ointments and creams must be stopped. Good personal hygiene is essential, with careful washing and drying after defecation. The perineal area must be kept dry and clean. Bulk-forming laxatives may reduce faecal soiling.

pruritus vulvae (*syn* vulval itch) vulval itching is a distressing symptom that can occur at any age and its cause can be difficult to diagnose. Chronic scratching of the vulval area leads to lichenification as in other sites. In this site it can be asymmetrical and associated with quite marked oedema and swelling. The history is important to give an indication of the underlying cause. Pre-existing skin disease, such as atopic eczema, psoriasis or fungal infections, needs to be sought and an autoimmune history might be associated with lichen sclerosus et atrophicus. Also, whether there is a previous history of sexually transmitted diseases, particularly genital warts or cervical dysplasia found on colposcopy. The main dermatological causes of itch in the vulval area are candidiasis (possibly associated with diabetes), tinea cruris, eczema (including contact dermatitis), psoriasis, lichen sclerosus et atrophicus and, less commonly, lichen planus. These can usually be differentiated by careful examination, bacteriological and mycological assessment and a search for evidence of similar skin disease elsewhere on the body. A well-defined, bright red plaque on the vulva can indicate psoriasis, particularly with skin, scalp or nail signs of this condition. Oral lesions are often seen in lichen planus and this condition is often followed by marked post-inflammatory hyperpigmentation. Lichen sclerosus is characterized by ivory papules that coalesce into pale plaques with an atrophic surface. There is sometimes associated haemorrhagic blistering. Lichen sclerosus et atrophicus often forms a 'figure of eight' around the vulva and perineal area and can cause scarring of the vulva with loss of normal contours culminating in stenosis of the introitus secondary to labial fusion. Biopsy for histology is occasionally needed to differentiate these conditions and in lichen sclerosus to assess any malignant change in, for example, non-healing areas. Histology is always needed in the next group of itchy vulval lesions, neoplasia. Most tumours of the vulva can provoke the symptom of itch—in particular, vulval (squamous) intraepithelial neoplasia (VIN) and extramammary Paget's disease. Lesions of VIN can be solitary or multiple and may appear red, white, pigmented, warty, moist or eroded. As well as being itchy, VIN can be painful, particularly with superficial dyspareunia. There may be very little to see with the naked eye and then vulvoscopy is needed. In younger women there is a strong association of VIN with the human papillomavirus (HPV), immunosuppression and possibly smoking. Extramammary Paget's disease is rare, is usually asymmetrical and can be painful. It presents as a moist, red, scaly patch often mistaken for eczema; hence the importance of biopsy in 'unresponsive eczema'. Finally, vulval disease can be associated with psychological distress and careful consultation by an understanding health professional is essential to a correct diagnosis of this condition. ⊃ balanitis xerotica obliterans (BXO), lichen et atrophicus (LSA).

PRV *abbr* polycythaemia rubra vera.

PSA *abbr* prostate specific antigen.

pseud/o- a prefix that means 'false', e.g. *pseudocyst*.

pseudoangina *n* false angina. Sometimes referred to as 'left mammary pain', it occurs in anxious individuals. Usually there is no cardiac disease present. May be part of effort syndrome.

pseudoarthrosis *n* a false joint, e.g. due to ununited fracture; also congenital, e.g. in tibia.

pseudobulbar paralysis there is disturbance in the higher control of the tongue and pharynx typically with cognitive and limb abnormalities, and found most often in the context of amyotrophic lateral sclerosis (ALS) or a succession of 'strokes'. Features are due to the degeneration of corticobulbar pathways to motor nuclei of the cranial nerves V, VII, X, XI and XII. Patients present with apparent weakness when chewing and making facial expressions and can be emotionally labile.

pseudocoxalgia *n* ⊃ Legg–Calvé–Perthes disease.

pseudocrisis *n* a rapid reduction of body temperature resembling a crisis, followed by further fever.

pseudocyesis *n* ⊃ phantom pregnancy.

pseudocyst a collection of fluid or gas, which lacks a containing membrane. A feature of pancreatitis.

pseudoexfoliation (PXF) (*syn* exfoliation syndrome, pseudoexfoliation syndrome) the deposition of greyish-white, flake-like basement membrane material on the anterior lens capsule, the iris and the ciliary processes with free-floating particles in the anterior chamber. It occurs mainly in older adults. It often gives rise to open-angle glaucoma (called capsular glaucoma or pseudoexfoliation glaucoma) which is frequently resistant to medical therapy and requires laser trabeculoplasty. The origin of the pseudoexfoliative material is believed to be secondary to an abnormal basement membrane, produced by ageing epithelial cells in the eye, as well as in the skin and visceral organs. Therefore pseudoexfoliation is thought to be part of a generalized basement membrane disorder and thus also referred to as exfoliation syndrome or pseudoexfoliation syndrome (PXS).

pseudoexfoliation glaucoma ⊃ pseudoexfoliation (PXF).

pseudoexfoliation syndrome ⊃ pseudoexfoliation (PXF).

pseudofractures (Looser's zones) narrow bands of decalcification indicating osteomalacia.

pseudogout *n* an arthritis (usually monoarthritis) caused by crystals of calcium pyrophosphate dihydrate within the joint.

pseudohermaphrodite *n* a person in whom the gonads of one sex are present, whilst the external genitalia comprise those of the opposite sex.

pseudoisochromatic plates charts for testing colour vision on which are printed dots of various colours, brightness, saturation and sizes, arranged so that the dots of similar colour form a figure (a letter, a numeral, a geometrical shape or winding path) among a background of dots of another colour. The colours of the figure and the background correspond to the confusion colours of the various types of anomalous colour vision. A dichromat or an anomalous trichromat has difficulty in perceiving the pattern because it is distinguishable from the background only by its difference in hue. There are many different sets of such plates, some using figures (circles, crosses or triangles) such as the AO, HRR plates, or numbers or lines such as those of Ishihara and Dvorine, or five spots such as the City University test (CUT) in which the subject chooses the spot most closely matching the colour of the central spot, etc. ⊃ defective colour vision.

pseudologia fantastica a tendency to tell, and defend, fantastic lies plausibly.

pseudomembranous colitis inflammation of the colonic mucosa coated in pale plaques (pseudomembranes). Usually caused by superinfection with *Clostridium difficile*. Recent antibiotic usage predisposes. ⊃ antibiotic-associated colitis.

pseudomembranous conjunctivitis a non-specific inflammatory reaction characterized by the formation on the conjunctiva of a coagulated fibrinous plaque consisting of inflammatory cells and an exudate containing mucus and proteins. This plaque forms either a membrane or a pseudomembrane. The latter is loosely adherent to the conjunctival epithelium and can be peeled off without bleeding or damage to the underlying epithelium. A true membrane, on the other hand, usually occurs with intense inflammation (membranous conjunctivitis). In this case the conjunctival epithelium becomes necrotic and adheres firmly to the overlying membrane which, when peeled leaves a raw, bleeding surface. The cause of either condition may be an infection of which the common sources are herpes simplex virus, adenovirus, beta-haemolytic *Streptococcus*, *Neisseria gonorrhoeae* or as a result of the Stevens–Johnson syndrome, ligneous conjunctivitis, ocular cicatricial pemphigoid, atopic keratoconjunctivitis, chemical burns (especially alkali burns), radiation injury or post-surgical complications. ⊃ cicatricial pemphigoid, ligneous conjunctivitis, Stevens–Johnson syndrome.

Pseudomonas *n* a bacterial genus. Gram-negative motile rods. Found in water and decomposing vegetable matter. Some are pathogenic to plants and animals and *Pseudomonas aeruginosa* is a cause of urinary, wound and respiratory infection in humans. It can cause superinfection where the normal commensals have been eliminated by antibiotic usage. Produces blue-green exudate or pus with a characteristic musty odour.

pseudomucin *n* a gelatinous substance (not mucin) found in some ovarian cysts.

pseudophakia *n* presence of an artificial lens. Describes an eye after cataract surgery with intraocular lens implantation.

pseudopolyposis *n* widely scattered polypi, usually the result of previous inflammation—sometimes ulcerative colitis.

pseudoseizures *npl* attacks that can look like epileptic seizures but which have no electrical basis and are normally related to mental health problems.

PSIS *abbr* posterior superior iliac spine.

psittacosis *n* disease of parrots, pigeons and budgerigars which is occasionally responsible for atypical pneumonia in humans. Caused by *Chlamydia psittaci*.

psoas *n* two muscles of the loin, psoas major and p. minor.

psoas abscess a cold abscess in the psoas muscle, resulting from tuberculosis of the vertebrae. The abscess appears as a firm smooth swelling which does not show signs of inflammation—hence the adjective 'cold'.

psoas major ⊃ iliopsoas, Colour Section Figure 4.

O
P

psoas minor a long slender muscle, which, if present is adjacent to the psoas major.

psoralen *n* a naturally occurring photosensitive compound, used in PUVA treatment.

psoriasis *n* a genetically determined chronic inflammatory skin disease in which erythematous scaly plaques characteristically occur on the elbows, knees and scalp. Between 5% and 10% of individuals with psoriasis will also have some type of arthropathy. There are several types of psoriasis described: guttate psoriasis, erythrodermic psoriasis, pustular psoriasis. Treatment modalities include: (a) topical agents—e.g. emolients, dithranol, coal tar, calcipotriol, corticosteroids; (b) ultraviolet and PUVA treatment; (c) systemic treatments—e.g. methotrexate, hydroxycarbamide, oral retinoids, ciclosporin, and more recently cytokine modulators such as adalimumab, entanercept, infliximab. Depending upon type of psoriasis and response to treatment—**psoriatic** *adj.* ➲ Colour Section Figure 101.

psoriatic arthritis arthritis occurring in association with psoriasis.

PSR *abbr* positive supporting reaction.

PSTT *abbr* placental site trophoblastic tumour.

PSV *abbr* pressure supported ventilation.

psyche *n* Greek term for 'life force', used to describe that which makes up the mind and all its processes, and sometimes used to describe 'self'.

psychiatrist a doctor with additional qualifications in the diagnosis and treatment of mental health disorders.

psychiatry *n* the branch of medicine that addresses the diagnosis and treatment of mental health disorders—**psychiatric** *adj.*

psychic *adj* of the mind.

psychic accommodation ➲ proximal accommodation.

psychic convergence ➲ proximal convergence.

psychic stimulus any stimulus, other than the presence of food in the mouth, that results in salivation. For example, the thought of food, or the smell of cooking.

psycho- a prefix that means 'mind', e.g. *psychogenic*.

psychoactive *adj* substances and drugs that may alter mental processes.

psychoanalysis *n* a specialized branch founded by Freud. It is a method of diagnosis and treatment of some mental health problems. Briefly the method is to revive past forgotten experiences and effect a cure by helping the patient readjust his attitudes to those experiences—**psychoanalytic** *adj.*

psychodrama *n* a psychotherapy technique whereby patients act out their personal problems by adopting roles in spontaneous dramatic performances. Group discussion aims at giving the patients a greater awareness of the problems presented and possible strategies for dealing with them.

psychodynamics *n* the science of the mental processes, especially of the factors causing mental activity.

psychogenesis *n* the development of the mind.

psychogenic *adj* arising from the mind.

psychogenic symptom one that originates in the mind.

psychogeriatric *adj* outdated term, relating to the application of psychology to geriatrics. The phrase elderly mentally ill (EMI) has also been used.

psychogeriatric dependency rating scales (PGDRS) construction of these scales was based on three basic dimensions—psychological deterioration, physical infirmity and psychological agitation.

psychological skills ➲ mental skills.

psychologist a person who specializes in psychology: development, processes of the mind and behaviour. A *clinical psychologist* a suitably qualified person who provides professional services for people with emotional problems in a variety of settings.

psychology *n* the study of the behaviour and mental processes.

psychometrics the construction, validation and use of psychological tests and measurements.

psychometric properties the reliability and validity of a psychometric measurement instrument.

psychometry *n* the science involved with mental testing.

psychomotor *adj* pertaining to the motor effects of mental activity.

psychomotor epilepsy (*syn* complete partial seizure, temporal lobe epilepsy). ➲ epilepsy.

psychoneuroimmunology (PNI) *n* study of the integration of neural and immune responses in relation to psychological state. Psychological distress/stress is associated with the impairment of immune system function.

psychoneuromuscular theory the theory that mental imagery of an action provokes subliminal stimulation of the muscles that are used in the actual movement patterns being imaged. Has been used to explain why mental practice can enhance performance.

psychoneurosis *n* outdated term. ➲ neurosis.

psychopath *n* one who is morally irresponsible and intent on instant gratification—**psychopathic** *adj.*

psychopathic personality a persistent disorder of the mind (whether or not including learning disability) which results in abnormally aggressive or seriously irresponsible behaviour that requires, or is susceptible to, medical treatment. ➲ mental health legislation.

psychopathology *n* the pathology of abnormal mental states—**psychopathological** *adj*, **psychopathologically** *adv.*

psychopharmacology *n* the study and use of drugs which influence the affective and emotional state—**psychopharmacological** *adj*, **psychopharmacologically** *adv.*

psychophysics *n* the study of the relationships between the subjectively perceived magnitude of sensations and their actual magnitude, particularly with regard to the ability to detect differences between stimuli of different magnitudes—**psychophysical** *adj.*

psychoprophylactic *adj* that which aims at preventing mental health problems.

psychoprophylactic preparation for childbirth education of parents concerning the processes of birth and how to cope with/remain in control of them.

psychoprophylaxis in labour a system for coping with pain in labour based on education in the Lamaze method of relaxation.

psychosexual *adj* pertaining to the mental aspects of sexuality.

psychosexual development according to Freud's theory, development occurs through five stages (oral, anal, phallic, latent and genital). Each stage is characterized by a different area of pleasurable stimulation.

psychosexual counselling usually sought by one or both members of a partnership because one or both is unable to obtain emotional and sexual satisfaction within the relationship. Psychosexual counselling of otherwise 'healthy' people is provided by specialists and is rarely provided by the NHS in the UK. Healthcare professionals need to be aware that any health disturbance may create actual or potential psychosexual problems.

psychosis *n* the term psychotic is used as a grouping term for disorders where a lack of contact with reality occurs, e.g. by hallucinations or delusions—**psychoses** *pl*, **psychotic** *adj*.

psychosomatic *adj* pertaining to the mind and body.

psychosomatic disorder or illness a term previously used to describe physical symptoms without organic pathology. ⊃ somatization.

psychotherapy *n* treatment of emotional and psychological problems by individual or group interaction. Usually by talking but many other approaches exist—**psychotherapeutic** *adj*. *group psychotherapy or group therapy* a therapist enables and encourages people to understand and analyse their own problems and those of other group members.

psychotropic *adj* that which exerts its specific effect upon the brain cells.

psychrophiles micro-organisms that grow and divide at low temperature. Usually within a range 15–20°C, but they will grow at lower temperatures.

psych-up to mentally prepare oneself for performance.

PT *abbr* **1**. physiotherapist. **2**. prothrombin.

PTA *abbr* **1**. percutaneous transluminal angioplasty. **2**. post-traumatic amnesia.

PTC *abbr* percutaneous transhepatic cholangiography

PTCA *abbr* percutaneous transluminal coronary angioplasty.

pteroylglutamic acid ⊃ folic acid.

pterygium *n* **1**. a wing-shaped degenerative condition of the conjunctiva which encroaches on the cornea. **2**. adhesion of the eponychium (cuticle) to the nail bed. It follows destruction of the matrix due to diminished circulation or some systemic diseases. The entire nail plate is eventually shed.

pterygoid muscles two pairs of facial muscles (lateral and medial) involved in mastication. The pterygoid muscles are supplied by the mandibular branch of the trigeminal nerve and the external carotid artery. ⊃ lateral pterygoid muscle, medial pterygoid muscle.

pterygo-maxillare (PTM) the lowest point of the outline of the pterygo-maxillary fissure.

PTFE *abbr* polytetrafluoroethylene. ⊃ Teflon®.

PTH *abbr* parathyroid hormone.

PTM *abbr* pterygo-maxillare.

ptosis *n* a drooping, particularly that of the upper eyelid. Common in old age—**ptotic** *adj*.

-ptosis a suffix that means 'falling', e.g. *nephroptosis*.

PTSD *abbr* post-traumatic stress disorder.

PTV *abbr* planning target volume.

ptyalin *n* ⊃ amylase.

ptyalism a condition in which there is an excess of saliva in the mouth, due to excessive secretion or inability to swallow.

P-type semiconductor a device where the majority carriers of electrons are the positive holes in the valence band and the minority carriers are the electrons which have sufficient energy to rise to the conduction band. ⊃ N-type semiconductors.

puberty *n* the period during which the reproductive organs become functionally active and the secondary sexual characteristics develop—**pubertal** *adj*.

pubes *n* the hair-covered area over the pubic bone.

pubescent uterus the body and cervix of the uterus are the same size and length in an adult woman as in the child.

pubic symphysis the site where the two pubis bones are linked at the centre-front of the pelvis by a thick disc of fibrocartilage, allowing some flexibility, although there is no true joint cavity. Persistent pain in this area should suggest the symphysis as a possible cause but it is often misdiagnosed as arising from the groin or lower abdominal musculature. ⊃ osteitis pubis, symphysis pubis dysfunction.

pubiotomy *n* rarely performed surgery that involves cutting the pubic bone to facilitate delivery of an infant.

pubis *n* the pubic bone or os pubis. The two bones that meet at the symphysis pubis—**pubic** *adj*.

public health broadly defined as health activity for populations in small areas, regions, nations and worldwide. In the UK public health involves the following functions: Health surveillance, monitoring and analysis. Investigation of disease outbreaks, epidemics and risks to health. Establishing, designing and managing health promotion and disease prevention programmes. Enabling and empowering communities and citizens to promote health and reduce inequalities. Creating and sustaining cross-governmental and inter-sectoral partnerships to improve health and reduce inequalities. Ensuring compliance with regulations and laws to protect and promote health. Developing and maintaining a well-educated and trained, multidisciplinary public health workforce. Ensuring the effective performance of the NHS services to meet goals in improving health, preventing disease and reducing inequalities. Research, development, evaluation and innovation. Quality assuring the public health function.

pubococcygeus one part of the levator ani muscle extending from the symphysis pubis to the coccyx.

PUBS *acron* **P**ercutaneous **U**mbilical cord **B**lood **S**ampling.

pudendal block the rendering insensitive of the pudendum by the transvaginal injection of local anaesthetic. Used mainly for episiotomy and forceps delivery.

O
P

pudendum *n* the external reproductive organs, especially of the female—**pudenda** *pl*, **pudendal** *adj*.

puerperal *adj* pertaining to childbirth.

puerperal psychosis a serious mental illness (psychosis) occurring in the puerperium. ⊃ postnatal depression.

puerperal sepsis infection of the genital tract occurring within 21 days of abortion or childbirth.

puerperium *n* the period immediately following childbirth to the time when involution is completed, usually 6–8 weeks—**puerperia** *pl*.

puerper/o- a prefix that means 'childbirth', e.g. *puerperium*.

PUFA *abbr* polyunsaturated fatty acid.

PUJ *abbr* pelviureteric junction.

Pulex irritans the human flea.

pulley a hand hold placed over a bed to enable patient's, such as those in traction, to lift themselves up to relieve pressure, give themselves exercise and make bedmaking easier.

pulmonary *adj* pertaining to the lungs.

pulmonary artery the large artery that carries deoxygenated blood from the right ventricle to the lungs. It divides into two to form a right and left pulmonary artery, one to each lung. ⊃ Colour Section Figures 7, 8.

pulmonary artery flotation catheter (PAFC) specialized balloon tipped catheter which is 'floated' from the central veins, through the heart and into the pulmonary artery (Figure P.18). Allows measurement of pulmonary artery occlusion pressure. More specialized PAFCs can measure cardiac output, and from it calculate the cardiac index,

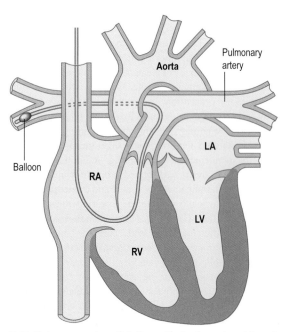

P.18 Pulmonary artery flotation catheter (reproduced from Boon et al 2006 with permission).

stroke volume, pulmonary vascular resistance and systemic vascular resistance.

pulmonary artery occlusion pressure (PAOP) pressure in the left atrium measured by inflating a balloon on the tip of a pulmonary artery catheter thereby temporarily occluding the pulmonary artery; also known as wedge pressure.

pulmonary artery pressure blood pressure in the pulmonary artery usually measured using a pulmonary artery catheter.

pulmonary circulation deoxygenated blood leaves the right ventricle in the pulmonary artery, flows through the lungs where it loses carbon dioxide, becomes oxygenated and returns to the left atrium of the heart in the pulmonary veins. ⊃ circulation of blood.

pulmonary dysmaturity syndrome also known as Wilson–Mikity syndrome. A rare respiratory insufficiency linked to poor maturation of the lungs that occurs in low birth weight infants. Pathological changes in the lungs include changes to interstitial tissues and areas of overaeration. Mortality is high.

pulmonary embolus (PE) an embolism which occurs in the pulmonary arterial system; most commonly as a result of deep vein thrombosis (DVT) in the leg or pelvic veins. Prophylaxis includes deep breathing and foot exercises, early mobilization, antithromboembolic stockings with the administration of heparin in at-risk groups. Predispositions to pulmonary embolus (PE) can include trauma, increasing age, recent surgery (certain operations), immobility, smoking, malignant disease and pregnancy, to name but a few. The size of the clot is of clinical significance since when 25% of the pulmonary circulation is obstructed, cardiac function is impaired. Clot size, patient age and existing pulmonary co-morbidities and the general health will all impact upon outcome. Clinical presentation is non-specific since signs and symptoms include dyspnoea, pain, haemoptysis, electrocardiogram (ECG) changes, peripheral oedema, tachycardia and cyanosis. Sometimes a DVT has already been diagnosed or there is a history suggestive of DVT. Investigations include ECG, chest X-ray, arterial blood gases, ventilation perfusion (V/Q) ratio scanning, angiography, spiral computerized tomography (CT) scan and D-dimer tests, though some of these are useful only in excluding the diagnosis of PE. Treatment regimens include: oxygen therapy, analgesia, anticoagulation therapy, thrombolysis and pulmonary embolectomy (though this is rarely performed and requires specialist input from a thoracic surgeon). About 10% of PEs are rapidly fatal and an additional 5% cause death later, despite diagnosis and treatment. ⊃ deep vein thrombosis, venous thromboembolism (VTE).

pulmonary emphysema a form of chronic obstructive pulmonary disease (COPD). There is overdistension and subsequent destruction of alveoli and reduced gas exchange in the lungs. It is characterized by enlargement of the terminal bronchioles and destruction of the alveolar walls without fibrosis. The total lung volume increases with added dead space due to air trapping, resulting in an increased work of breathing. Most commonly associated with tobacco smoking, but some patients may have an inherited condition called alpha$_1$ (α)-antitrypsin deficiency. Individuals with emphysema classically have a wasted general musculature, a hyperinflated chest (elevated ribs with large lung fields, a flattened diaphragm and large antero-posterior thoracic diameter and tracheal tug). They adopt a fixed posture breathing stance (i.e. fix the shoulder girdle in order to recruit the accessory respiratory muscles by leaning forward onto the arms) and automatically use pursed-lip breathing when physiologically stressed (to generate intrinsic positive end expiratory pressure, thus splinting the otherwise collapsible diseased airways open and facilitating oxygen uptake). This enables the emphysematous patient to maintain normal partial pressure levels of oxygen. ⊃ alpha$_1$ (α)-antitrypsin deficiency, bronchitis.

pulmonary fibrosis chronic inflammation and fibrosis of the alveolar walls, with steadily progressive shortness of breath resulting finally in death from oxygen lack or right-heart failure. ⊃ restrictive lung disease.

pulmonary function tests also known as respiratory function tests. Tests for assessment of the function of the lungs to aid diagnosis of respiratory disease and assess effectiveness of treatment. Includes methods for measuring lung volumes and gas transfer. In sport, primarily used in the diagnosis and monitoring of treatment of asthma, especially exercise-induced asthma; World Anti-Doping Agency (WADA) guidelines have now set criteria based on such tests, whereby an athlete may use certain inhaled medication. ⊃ arterial blood gases (ABGs), carbon monoxide diffusing capacity test (DLCO), respiratory function tests, spirometry.

pulmonary hypertension raised blood pressure within the pulmonary circulation, due to increased resistance to blood flow within the pulmonary vessels. It may be primary (genetic), or secondary due to chronic lung disease or chronic pulmonary embolism.

pulmonary infarction necrosis of lung tissue resulting from an embolus.

pulmonary oedema fluid within the alveoli. The lungs are 'waterlogged' and gas exchange is reduced such as in left ventricular failure, mitral stenosis, or fluid excess in renal failure. Hydrostatic pulmonary oedema occurs when there is a rise in the hydrostatic pressure of the lung interstitium resulting in a flooding of alveolar spaces. Non-hydrostatic pulmonary oedema involves the disruption of epithelial and endothelial barriers inducing a systemic inflammatory response associated with widespread microvascular injury including the lungs is associated with increased total lung water despite a normal hydrostatic pressure.

pulmonary rehabilitation combination of graded physical exertion, educational, psychological and behavioural interventions designed to improve symptoms in those with chronic lung disease.

pulmonary–renal disease/syndrome the pulmonary–renal disease/syndrome is a dramatic presentation with renal and respiratory failure. Anti-GBM disease (Goodpasture's disease) and small-vessel vasculitis can cause this presentation.

pulmonary tuberculosis ⊃ tuberculosis.

pulmonary valve semilunar valve situated between the pulmonary artery and right cardiac ventricle. ⊃ pulmonary valve stenosis.

pulmonary valve stenosis narrowing of the pulmonary valve. May occur in the carcinoid syndrome but is usually congenital, when it may be an isolated defect or associated with other abnormalities such as Fallot's tetralogy.

pulmonary vascular resistance (PVR) *n* the resistance in the pulmonary vascular bed which the right ventricle must overcome in order to pump blood into the pulmonary circulation.

pulmonary veins four veins, two from each lung, which convey oxygenated blood from the lungs to the left atrium of the heart. ⊃ Colour Section Figures 7, 8.

pulmonary ventilation or minute ventilation/volume. The amount of air moved in ($\dot{V}_I$) and out ($\dot{V}_E$) of the lungs in one minute.

pulp *n* **1.** the soft, interior part of some organs and structures. A soft mass of tissue. ⊃ digital pulp. **2.** in dentistry, soft tissue lying within the dentine of a tooth and containing fibres, cells and structures such as blood vessels, sensory nerves and lymphatics. These vessels pass through the apical foramen of the tooth or through accessory canals. ⊃ dental pulp. *indirect pulp capping* the technique of pulp capping when the pulp is not overtly exposed. *pulp abscess.* ⊃ pulp (or pulpal) abscess. *pulp canal* a canal running within the dentine of a tooth from the coronal portion of the tooth to the apex. *pulp cap* a wound dressing placed on the dentine floor of a deep cavity (*indirect pulp cap*) or in direct contact with pulp tissue (*direct pulp cap*) with the intention of preserving pulp vitality and promoting defensive tertiary dentine deposition. Examples include calcium hydroxide cement and mineral trioxide aggregate (MTA). *pulp capping* an application over an exposed vital pulp of one or more layers of protective and/or therapeutic material, e.g. calcium hydroxide, which promotes the production of reparative dentine. *pulp cavity* the cavity within the dentine of the tooth that contains the dental pulp. *pulp chamber* the cavity within the crown of a tooth that contains the dental pulp. *pulp cornu* (or *horn*) a horn-shaped extension of the pulp cavity extending in towards the cusp or the incisal margins. *pulp extirpation* the complete removal of the contents of the pulp chamber and root canal. *pulp horn* ⊃ pulp cornu. *pulp mummification* the application of a medicament to the pulp remnants to render them inert and preserve them in an aseptic state. *pulp stone (denticle)* a calcified area within the substance of the dental pulp. *pulp surface* that surface of the tooth cavity which overlies the pulp. *pulp sensitivity test* a diagnostic aid involving the application of an electrical, thermal or mechanical stimulus to the crown of a tooth in order to indicate the excitability of the pulp. The test is not necessarily indicative of the vitality of the pulp. *vital pulp* pulp in which the blood

O
P

supply is intact. Vitality is elicited by stimulation of the nerve endings within the pulp which are present if the blood supply is intact.

pulp (or pulpal) abscess an acute or chronic abscess in the pulp tissue of a tooth due to an irritant such as dental caries, cavity preparation, bacterial leakage around a restoration or traumatic injury.

pulpal *adj* relating to pulp.

pulpal screw ⊃ screw.

pulpectomy pulp extirpation. ⊃ pulp.

pulpitis inflammation of the dental pulp. *reversible pulpitis* a clinical diagnosis of pulp inflammation which may resolve if causative factors are eliminated. *irreversible pulpitis* a clinical diagnosis of pulp inflammation which is unlikely to resolve if causative factors are eliminated.

pulpotomy in dentistry, the removal of the coronal part of a vital pulp in order to preserve the underlying radicular portion. *partial (superficial) pulpotomy* the removal of the coronal 2–3 mm of infected pulp tissue after pulp exposure. *coronal pulpotomy* the removal of all pulp tissue from the coronal pulp chamber.

pulsatile *adj* beating, throbbing.

pulsation *n* beating or throbbing, as of the arteries or heart.

pulsativity index a method of numerically determining the low diastolic blood flow (impedance) through a vessel using the equation systolic – diastolic/mean.

pulse *n* the impulse transmitted to arteries by contraction of the left ventricle, and customarily palpated in the radial artery at the wrist. The *pulse rate* is the number of beats or impulses per minute and is about 130 in the newborn infant, 70–80 in the adult and 60–70 in old age. The *pulse rhythm* is its regularity—and can be regular or irregular; the *pulse volume* is the amplitude of expansion of the arterial wall during the passage of the wave; the *pulse force* or tension is its strength, estimated by the force needed to obliterate it by pressure of the finger.

pulsed current an electrotherapy term. One of three recognized categories of therapeutic currents (pulsed, direct and alternating currents). A series of pulses separated by interpulse intervals. The pulse duration varies, ranging from µS to ms, and the pulse may be monophasic (e.g. high-voltage pulsed stimulation—HVPS) or biphasic (typical sensory and motor stimulation currents). The distinguishing feature is that a pulsed current has an interval between successive pulses (interpulse interval). A frequency of 50 Hz, for example, means 50 separate pulses per second. ⊃ pulse (electrotherapy context).

pulsed dose-rate technique the radiotherapy method of using high-dose-rate equipment to deliver a low-dose-rate treatment by repeating a programmed cycle at predetermined intervals such as 1 hour.

pulse deficit the difference in rate of the heart (counted by stethoscope) and the pulse (counted at the wrist), as seen in atrial fibrillation.

pulse duration (width) an electrotherapy term. The time for which a pulse continues, one complete cycle of current

flow. Usually measured in µs or ms. Incorrectly referred to as 'width' as in a measure of time, not a spatial dimension. Pulse duration, together with intensity, indicates which types of nerve fibre are most likely to be stimulated and hence the probable level of comfort and type of response to stimulation.

pulsed-wave Doppler an ultrasound system which transmits bursts of ultrasound and then, after a preselected time, receives for a very short period of time, enabling a specific point within the beam to be examined.

pulse (electrotherapy context) the interrupted flow of current. The basic unit of both pulsed and alternating currents. Additional information includes: (a) type—monophasic (i.e. the pulse has one phase only, for example, high-voltage pulsed stimulation [HPVS]), interrupted galvanic or biphasic (i.e. there are two phases per pulse, for example, output of most motor stimulators); (b) symmetrical/asymmetrical—biphasic and both phases are same or different shapes; (c) shape of phase—can be rectangular, triangular, sinusoidal, sawtooth; (d) balanced/unbalanced—biphasic and balanced if the charge in each phase is equal, unbalanced if greater in one phase; (e) duration—usually measured in µs or ms; and (f) frequency: number per second (hertz, Hz).

pulse height analyser a device which can be adjusted to record input pulses within a specific range and then produce an electrical output, therefore can be used to detect different radionuclides.

pulse modulator supplies high-voltage negative pulses to the magnetron or klystron in a linear accelerator.

pulse oximetry an accurate non-invasive technique for measuring the percentage saturation of oxygen of haemoglobin in arterial blood. This is achieved by using an oximeter (a photoelectric device) with a sensor attached to a finger, an ear or the nose (Figure P.19). The oximeter device function is based on the difference in light absorbance properties of saturated and desaturated haemoglobin to provide the basis for measurement. It is used in all settings to assess oxygenation and degree of hypoxia, for example postoperatively, for patients with chronic respiratory diseases, etc. They provide constant monitoring of oxygen saturation, but there are many factors that can impair accuracy, e.g. poor peripheral tissue perfusion, optical interference and excessive patient movement. The results obtained must be considered with other criteria that include vital signs, arterial blood gases and concurrent oxygen therapy, etc. Also used to monitor oxygenation, e.g. in athletes/cyclists at high altitude or in any severely taxing exercise.

pulse pressure is the difference between the systolic and diastolic blood pressures (SBP – DBP). For example, SBP 140 – DBP 80 = pulse pressure 60. ⊃ mean arterial blood pressure.

pulser the part of an ultrasound machine that generates electrical pulses which stimulate the transducer to produce ultrasound.

pulse repetition frequency in ultrasound the number of pulses occurring in one second expressed in kilohertz (kHz).

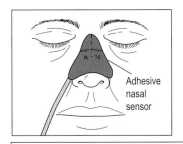

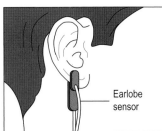

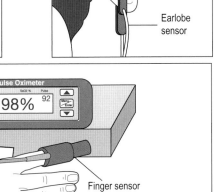

Adhesive nasal sensor

Earlobe sensor

Finger sensor

P.19 Pulse oximeter (reproduced from Nicol et al 2004 with permission).

pulseless disease progressive obliterative arteritis of the vessels arising from the aortic arch resulting in diminished or absent pulse in the neck and arms. ➲ Takayasu's disease/arteritis.

pulseless electrical activity (PEA) a type of cardiac arrest where there is a normal or nearly normal electrical activity without an effective cardiac output. Also known as electromechanical dissociation.

pulseless ventricular tachycardia a form of cardiac arrest. ➲ ventricular tachycardia.

pulsus alternans a regular pulse with alternate beats of weak and strong amplitude; associated with left ventricular heart failure.

pulsus bigeminus double pulse wave produced by interpolation of extrasystoles. A coupled beat.

pulsus paradoxus arterial pulsus paradoxus is alteration of the volume of the arterial pulse sometimes found in pericarditis. The volume becomes greater with expiration. Venous pulsus paradoxus (Kusman's sign) is an increase in the height of the venous pressure with inspiration, the reverse of normal. Sometimes found in pericardial or right ventricular disease.

pulvis *n* a powder.

pumice in dentistry, an abrasive used in polishing dentures and consisting of various silicates obtained from lava.

punch ➲ rubber dam.

punctate *adj* dotted or spotted, e.g. punctate basophilia describes red cells in which there are droplets of blue-staining material in the cytoplasm.

punctate cataract ➲ blue-dot cataract.

punctate epithelial keratitis (PEK) (*syn* superficial punctate keratitis [SPK]), although this term is more often used to describe punctate epithelial keratitis of viral origin. It is inflammation of the cornea characterized by either multiple, small, superficial, punctate lesions or minute, flat, epithelial dots resulting from bacterial infection (e.g. chlamydial, staphylococcal), vitamin B_2 deficiency, virus infection (e.g. herpes) and also from exposure to ultraviolet light, injury to the eye with aerosol products or contact lens solutions. The condition is usually associated with a conjunctivitis. Treatment depends on the causative agent (e.g. antiviral agents will be used to suppress symptoms in viral infection). ➲ herpetic keratitis, trachoma.

punctum *n* entrance to lacrimal drainage system on eyelid margin—**puncta** *pl.*

punctum proximum ➲ near point of accommodation

punctum remotum ➲ far point of accommodation.

puncture *n* a stab; a wound made with a sharp pointed hollow instrument for withdrawal or injection of fluid or other substance. ➲ cisternal puncture, lumbar puncture, penetrating wound.

punishment a stimulus that leads to a reduction in a behavioural response or, more generally, a stimulus that an organism seeks to avoid or escape. Often erroneously referred to as negative reinforcement. ➲ conditioning, reinforcement.

PUO *abbr* pyrexia of unknown origin.

pupil *n* the opening in the iris of the eye, normally circular, through which light penetrates into the eye. It is located slightly nasally to the centre of the iris. Its diameter can vary from about 2 to 8 mm. It is often slightly smaller in old age—**pupillary** *adj.* ➲ acorea, anisocoria, corectopia, dicoria, dilator pupillae muscle, dyscoria, Edinger–Westphal nucleus, hippus, iridectomy, irism, microcoria, miosis,

O
P

mydriasis, polycoria, polyopia, pupillary light reflex, sphincter pupillae muscle.

pupil block ⊃ pupillary block.

pupil light reflex ⊃ pupillary light reflex.

pupillary *adj* relating to the pupil.

pupillary block (*syn* pupil block) a blockage of the normal flow of aqueous humour from the posterior to the anterior chamber of the eye. It may be caused by a posterior annular synechia occurring during anterior uveitis, by luxation of the lens anteriorly occluding the pupil, or by adhesion of the iris to the vitreous or to the posterior capsule following extracapsular cataract extraction (called aphakic pupillary block). It may produce an attack of angle-closure glaucoma as the iris may be pushed forward blocking the drainage angle. ⊃ angle-closure glaucoma, annular synechia, iris bombé, lens luxation, seclusio pupillae.

pupillary distance ⊃ interpupillary distance (IPD, PD).

pupillary fibres axons of the optic nerve (second cranial nerve) which branch off from the visual portion of the optic tract, before the lateral geniculate body, to run in the superior brachium towards the pretectal region anterior to the superior colliculus. They mediate the pupillary reflexes. ⊃ optic nerve, optic tracts, pupillary light reflex.

pupillary light reflex (*syn* light reflex, pupil light reflex) the reflex constriction and dilatation of the pupil in response to the amount of light entering the eye. Controlled by the oculomotor nerves (third pair of cranial nerves). (a) *constriction of the pupil* in response to light stimulation of the retina. The response of an eye to light stimulation can occur either with a light shining on it directly (the direct light reflex) or when the other eye is stimulated (the consensual or indirect light reflex). The reflex arc consists of four neurons beyond the ganglion cells. The first afferent neuron transmits nervous impulses from the retina to the two pretectal nuclei, located on the lateral side of the superior colliculi, in response to light stimulation of the photoreceptors. The second neurons, called the internuncial neurons, connect each pretectal nucleus to both Edinger–Westphal nuclei which form part of the oculomotor nuclei. The third efferent neurons connect the latter nuclei, via the third nerve (oculomotor nerve) to the ciliary ganglion where there is a synapse. The fourth efferent neurons connect the latter, via the short ciliary nerves, to the sphincter pupillae muscle of each iris and constrict the pupil. The efferent path represents the parasympathetic innervation. (b) *dilatation of the pupil* in response to a reduction of the light stimulation of the retina. It is effected by cervical sympathetic innervation; the fibres pass to the superior cervical ganglion in the neck, then ascend along the internal carotid artery until they join the ophthalmic division of the trigeminal nerve. The fibres reach the dilator pupillae muscle of the iris via the nasociliary and long ciliary nerves which enter the eyeball behind the equator. ⊃ accommodative reflex, ciliary ganglion, Edinger–Westphal nucleus, oculomotor nerves, pupillary fibres, retinotectal pathway, sphincter pupillae muscle.

pupillary membrane the embryonic mesodermal tissue which is present in the centre of the iris and normally disappears by the eighth month of gestation to form the pupil. Some strands of the membrane may remain in adults; this is referred to as a persistent pupillary membrane.

pupillometer 1. (*syn* coreometer) an instrument for measuring the diameter of the pupil. There exist several types but the most common is a series of graduated filled circles whose sizes are compared with the pupil (Haab's pupillometer). It is also common to measure pupil size by photography or video after appropriate calibration of the method. **2.** (*syn* interpupillometer—the most appropriate term for this instrument, PD gauge, PD meter) although incorrectly used, it refers to an instrument for measuring the interpupillary distance (PD). These instruments are based either on using the pupil centres (e.g. Reichert PD gauge) or the corneal reflections (e.g. Essilor Corneal Reflection Pupillometer, Seiko SP-100 Pupillometer), but the latter can be used on the basis of the pupil centres as well. In the instruments using corneal reflections the subject views the image of a small illuminated target surrounding the observation aperture used by the examiner or made to appear as if it came from the observer's eye. That image is formed at infinity by a lens placed in front of the subject's eyes. The examiner moves a hair line to coincide with the centre of the corneal reflections and reads the monocular and total interpupillary distances. ⊃ interpupillary distance, PD rule.

pupillotonia ⊃ Adie's pupil.

purchaser/provider split the split between the purchasing and the provision of health and social care services. Before the NHS and Community Care Act (1990) statutory health and social care agencies typically purchased and provided services for their patients and clients. For example, social services purchased and provided residential and day-care facilities for older people. Services are now purchased from a wide variety of agencies some of which are from the private and voluntary sectors. Many hospital services, such as cleaning and laundry, are 'contracted out' to private companies and GPs may purchase services for their patients from nearby hospitals who compete for contracts. ⊃ internal market.

purgative *n* a drug that causes the evacuation of fluid faeces.

purines *npl* nitrogenous base, such as adenine and guanine, needed as constituents of nucleosides, nucleotides and nucleic acids. Uric acid is produced when purines are broken down. Increased uric acid in the blood is associated with disorders of metabolism and excretion of uric acid, and leads to the development of gout.

Purkinje cell (J Purkinje, Czech anatomist and physiologist, 1787–1869) large neurons found in the cerebellar cortex, giving rise to efferent axons and provide the only output from the cerebellar cortex.

Purkinje fibres (J Purkinje) an extensive network of branching fibres, that play an important role in the conduction of electrical impulses through the heart.

Purkinje figures/shadows/tree ➲ angioscotoma.

purple (*syn* non-spectral colour, non-spectral purple) a mixture, in suitable proportions, of short wave radiations (less than 400 nm) and long wave radiations (greater than 700 nm). It is a complementary colour to yellow-green. Purples are colour stimuli represented on the chromaticity diagram by the straight line joining the ends of the spectrum locus. ➲ chromaticity diagram, complementary colour, spectrum locus.

purposive sampling a research term. Sampling that is done with a particular group in mind, for example, if the intention was to undertake a survey of reasons of non-attendance in a specific hospital department, a purposive sample would be used, as there is no point in doing a randomized sample of attendees and non-attendees if the research question is looking at non-attendees only.

pursed lip breathing (PLB) breathing through tightly pursed lips, which results in the generation of a backpressure so avoiding compression of collapsible lung segments (i.e. the equal pressure point is moved towards the mouth). Patients with emphysema often automatically adopt this breathing in times of extreme dyspnoea.

purpura *n* superficial haemorrhage, less than 1 cm, into the skin. A disorder characterized by extravasation of blood from the capillaries into the skin, or into or from the mucous membranes. May be either small red spots (petechiae) or large bruises (ecchymoses) or by oozing from minor wounds confined to the mucous membranes. It may be due to impaired integrity of the capillary walls, or to defective quality or quantity of platelets. Purpura can be caused by many different conditions, e.g. infective, toxic, allergic, etc. ➲ Henoch–Schönlein purpura.

purulent *adj* pertaining to or resembling pus.

PUS *acron* **P**ulsed **U**ltra**S**ound.

pus *n* a liquid, usually yellowish in colour, formed in certain infections and composed of tissue fluid containing bacteria and leucocytes. Pus is a feature of infection caused by staphylococci and streptococci. Various types of bacteria are associated with pus having distinctive features, e.g. the faecal smell of pus due to *Escherichia coli*; the blue-green colour of pus due to *Pseudomonas aeruginosa*.

pusher syndrome a term used to describe the pushing behaviour present in some patients after a stroke. After a severe stroke, there is a tendency for the person to push towards their hemiplegic side and resist attempts to correct their posture towards midline. They tend to extend their unaffected arm and leg pushing them over, but their perception is that they are falling to their good side. This presentation is often accompanied by cognitive and perceptual problems.

push scaler ➲ scaler.

pustule *n* a visible collection of free pus in a blister usually indicates an infection (e.g. furuncle) but not always (e.g. pustular psoriasis)—**pustular** *adj. malignant pustule* ➲ anthrax.

push-up method (*syn* Donders' method) in optometry, a method of determining the near point of accommodation by moving a test object (made up of small optotypes subtending one minute of arc [that is the 6/6 or 20/20 line] at the eye and uniformly illuminated) closer to the patient's eye. It is usually done monocularly and then binocularly. The near point is achieved when the small test object yields a sustained blur and not just begins to blur. Alternatively, the card is moved back after appearing blurred until the small test object just appears to clear again. This is often called the push-out method. In older patients, plus lenses may be needed to carry out the test and the power of the lens is subtracted from the reading. The amplitude of accommodation is deduced by taking into account the vergence at the eye of the far point (it is at infinity in emmetropes and corrected ametropes). ➲ amplitude of accommodation, near point of accommodation, subjective accommodation.

push-up test a procedure used to ensure adequate lens movement of a soft contact lens. The lens is gently pushed upward by pressing on the patient's lower eyelid: it should move easily and return quickly to its original location. ➲ limbal blanching.

putrefaction *n* rotting; bacterial destruction of organic material.

putrescine a molecule produced when protein breaks down during the putrefaction of animal tissue. It results from the breakdown of ornithine, an amino acid, and has an extremely foul odour. ➲ cadaverine.

PUVA *abbr* psoralen with ultraviolet radiation of a long wavelength used for the treatment of skin diseases, particularly psoriasis.

PV *abbr* per vaginam: describes the route used for examination of the vagina, or the administration of drugs.

***P* value** in all inferential statistics a *P* value given. This is the probability that the results found have occurred by chance alone. The probability is measured on a scale of 0–1: a *P* value of $P = 0.05$ means 5% or a one in twenty chance, and $P = 0.01$ means a 1% or one in a hundred chance. A common error is to assume a high *P* value means the result is significant, a low value shows significance. So the probability of a test result occurring by chance is the *P* value. Lower case *p* is used for proportions.

PVD *abbr* peripheral vascular disease.

PVL *abbr* Panton–Valentine leukocidin.

PVR *abbr* pulmonary vascular resistance.

PVS *abbr* persistent vegetative state.

PWB *abbr* partial weight bearing.

PXF *abbr* pseudoexfoliation.

PXS *abbr* pseudoexfoliation syndrome.

pyaemia *n* the presence in the circulation of septic emboli. They can lodge in organs, such as the liver, brain, kidneys and lungs, to form multiple abscesses—**pyaemic** *adj*.

pyarthrosis *n* pus in a joint cavity.

pyelitis *n* obsolete term. ➲ pyelonephritis.

pyel/o- a prefix that means 'pelvis of the kidney', e.g. *pyelolithotomy*.

pyelography *n* ➲ urography.

pyelolithotomy *n* the operation for removal of a stone from the renal pelvis.

0
P

pyelonephritis *n* acute infection within the substance of the kidney, often derived either from the urine or from the blood—**pyelonephritic** *adj*.

pyeloplasty *n* a reconstructive operation on the kidney pelvis. ⊃ hydronephrosis.

pyelostomy *n* surgical formation of an opening into the kidney pelvis.

Pyemotes previously called *Pediculoides*. A genus of mites found in grain straw and hay. The species *Pyemotes ventricosus* causes an allergic dermatitis ('grain itch').

pyknosis darkening and condensation of nuclear chromatin.

pylethrombophlebitis inflammation and thrombus in the hepatic portal vein.

pyloric stenosis 1. narrowing of the pylorus due to scar tissue formed during the healing of a peptic ulcer. **2.** congenital hypertrophic pyloric stenosis due to a thickened pyloric sphincter muscle. ⊃ pyloromyotomy.

pyloroduodenal *adj* pertaining to the pylorus and the duodenum.

pyloromyotomy *n* (*syn*. Ramstedt's operation) incision of the pyloric sphincter muscle as in pyloroplasty.

pyloroplasty *n* a plastic operation on the pylorus designed to widen the passage.

pylorospasm *n* spasm of the pylorus; usually due to the presence of a duodenal ulcer.

pylorus *n* region containing the opening of the stomach into the duodenum, controlled by a sphincter muscle—**pyloric** *adj*.

py/o a prefix that means 'pus', e.g. *pyothorax*.

pyocolpos *n* pus in the vagina.

pyodermia, pyoderma *n* any purulent condition of the skin—**pyodermic** *adj*.

pyogenic *adj* relating to pus formation, such as pus-forming bacteria.

pyometra *n* pus retained in the uterus and unable to escape through the cervix—**pyometric** *adj*.

pyonephrosis *n* distension of the renal pelvis with pus—**pyonephrotic** *adj*.

pyopericarditis *n* pericarditis with purulent effusion.

pyopneumothorax *n* pus and gas or air within the pleural sac.

pyorrhoea *n* a flow of pus. Previously used term for gingivitis or chronic periodontitis.

pyosalpinx *n* a uterine (fallopian) tube containing pus.

pyothorax *n* pus in the pleural cavity.

pyramidal *adj* applied to some conical eminences in the body.

pyramidal cells (Betz cells) nerve cells in the precentral motor area of the cerebral cortex, from which originate impulses to voluntary muscles.

pyramidal fracture a fracture of middle third of the facial skeleton ⊃ Le Fort classification.

pyramidal tracts sometimes also known as the corticospinal tract. The main motor tracts in the brain and spinal cord, which transmit impulses arising from the pyramidal cells. Most decussate (cross over) in the medulla. Patients with pure pyramidal loss present with diminished fine finger control and difficulty in isolating finger movements.

pyrazolones *npl* a group of non-steroidal anti-inflammatory drugs. ⊃ Appendix 5.

pyretic relating to a fever.

pyrexia *n* core body temperature above normal, usually between 37°C and 40/41°C.

pyrexia of unknown origin (PUO) where the reason for the raised body temperature is not known. ⊃ fever, hyperpyrexia—**pyrexial** *adj*.

pyridoxal phosphate the major form of vitamin B_6 in the body.

pyridoxine *n* vitamin B_6, a mixture of the phosphates of pyridoxine, pyridoxal and pyridoxamine; important as a cofactor in glycogen and amino acid metabolism. Deficiency may lead to dermatitis and neuritic pains. Used in nausea of pregnancy and radiation sickness, muscular dystrophy, pellagra, the premenstrual syndrome, etc.

pyrimidine 5′ nucleotidase deficiency this enzyme catalyses the dephosphorylation of nucleoside monophosphates and is important during the degradation of ribonucleic acid (RNA) in reticulocytes. One of the red cell enzymopathies, the deficiency is inherited as an autosomal recessive trait and is as common as pyruvate kinase deficiency in Mediterranean, African and Jewish populations. The accumulation of excess ribonucleoprotein results in coarse basophilic stippling associated with a chronic haemolytic state. The enzyme is very sensitive to inhibition by lead and this is the reason why basophilic stippling is a feature of lead poisoning.

pyrimidines *npl* nitrogenous bases, such as cytosine, thymine and uracil, needed as constituents of nucleic acids.

pyr/o- a prefix that means 'fever', e.g. *pyrogen*.

pyrogen *n* a substance producing fever—**pyrogenic** *adj*.

pyrosis *n* (*syn*. heartburn, waterbrash) eructation of acid gastric contents into the mouth, accompanied by a burning sensation felt behind the sternum.

pyrotherapy *n* production of fever by artificial means. ⊃ hyperthermia.

pyrroles substances that form part of porphyrin and haem.

pyruvate dehydrogenase (complex) (PDH) a mitochondrial envelope enzyme present in muscle. It catalyses the oxidative decarboxylation of pyruvate (from cytoplasm) to form acetyl-CoA, which thence feeds into the Krebs'cycle. ⊃ muscle enzymes.

pyruvate kinase deficiency the second most common red cell enzyme defect and affects thousands of people worldwide. It results in deficiency of adenosine triphosphate (ATP) production and a chronic haemolytic anaemia. It is inherited as an autosomal recessive trait. The extent of anaemia is variable; the blood film shows characteristic 'prickle cells' which resemble holly leaves. Enzyme activity is only 5–20% of normal. Transfusion support may be necessary.

pyruvic acid pyruvate. An important metabolic molecule. Converted to acetyl-CoA which is used in the Krebs' cycle, or forms lactic acid during anaerobic glucose metabolism.

pyuria *n* pus in the urine (more than three leucocytes per high-power field)—**pyuric** *adj*.

QALYs *abbr* quality-adjusted life years.

Q (quadriceps)-angle the angle between the long axis of the femur (and thus the line of pull of the quadriceps muscle group) and the line of the patellar tendon (extended upwards); describes the extent to which the line of pull is not straight. In practice, it is measured as the angle between the line from the anterior superior iliac spine (ASIS) to the centre of the patella, and the line from there to the tibial tubercle. Normally less than 20° (14° in males, 17° in females) but often greater in some female runners who have a wider than average pelvis (Figure Q.1). Factors which increase the Q-angle include genu valgum (knock knees), patellar subluxation, weak quadriceps, tight hamstrings and overpronated feet. Relevant in the diagnosis of patellofemoral

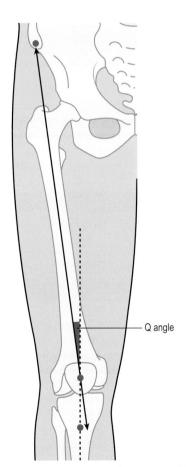

Q angle

Q.1 Q (quadriceps)-angle (reproduced from Jennett 2008 with permission).

pain and used in treatment as an indication of relative quadriceps strength, allowing appropriate strength work. Abnormal Q angles are thought to predispose to anterior knee pain and other syndromes.

Q fever a febrile disease caused by the Gram negative bacterium *Coxiella burnetii*. It is transmitted to humans from sheep, cattle or in unpasteurized milk and from domestic animals. Pasteurization of milk kills *Coxiella burnetii*.

QF-PCR *abbr* quantitative fluorescence-polymerase chain reaction.

Qi energy also known as chi, yin/yang. In complementary medicine, the person's inborn energy focused on maintaining health and well-being. The concept of Qi energy is fundamental to therapies such as acupuncture where the energy is believed to flow through meridians.

QoL *abbr* quality of life.

Q-T interval ➲ P-QRS-T complex.

quadrangular having four angles.

quadrant a fourth part. In dentistry, one half of each dental arch, the dividing line being the midpoint of the arch. There are thus four quadrants—the upper left and right and the lower left and right (Figure Q.2).

quadrantanopia ➲ quadrantanopsia.

quadrantanopsia *n* (*syn* quadrantanopia, quadrantic anopsia, quadrantic hemianopsia). Loss of vision in one quadrant of the visual field. The defect is usually bilateral as it is caused by a lesion past the optic chiasma. It may be homonymous (binasal, bitemporal, upper or lower), crossed (one upper and the other lower), congruous (equal size of the defects) or incongruous (unequal size of the defects). ➲ hemianopsia, superior quadrantanopsia.

quadrantic anopsia ➲ quadrantanopsia.

quadrantic hemianopsia ➲ quadrantanopsia.

quadrate square shaped, having four equal sides and four right angles.

quadratus having four sides.

quadratus femoris a short muscle with its origin on the ischial tuberosity and its insertion on the greater trochanter on the femur. It is a lateral rotator of the thigh and stabilizes the hip.

quadratus lumborum a muscle of the posterior abdominal wall. Its origin is on the iliac crest and it inserts onto the upper lumbar vertebrae and the last rib. If one side contracts it flexes the spine laterally, or both sides work together to maintain the upright position. ➲ abdominal muscles.

quadri- a prefix that means 'four', e.g. *quadriceps*.

quadriceps femoris *n* known colloquially as 'quads'. The large four-part extensor muscle of the anterior and lateral

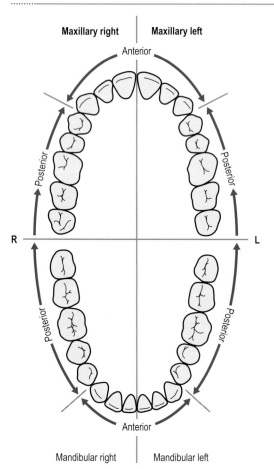

Maxillary right | Maxillary left

Anterior

R | L

Posterior | Posterior

Posterior | Posterior

Anterior

Mandibular right | Mandibular left

Q.2 Quadrants (reproduced from Heasman & McCracken 2007 with permission).

thigh, comprises the rectus femoris, vastus medialis, vastus lateralis and vastus intermedius. The lateral, intermediate and medial vasti, which all contribute to knee extension, have an origin from the shaft of the femur. The rectus femoris contributes also to hip flexion, by its origin from the ilium of the pelvis. Parts of the vasti are inserted into the top and sides of the patella, and contribute tendinous reinforcements to the joint capsule of the knee. The four muscles converge onto the single quadriceps tendon which spans the front of the knee to be inserted as the patellar tendon (ligament) into the tibial tubercle (tuberosity). ⟳ Q (quadriceps)-angle, rectus femoris, vastus, Colour Section Figure 4.

quadricusped having four cusps.

quadriparesis *n* weakness of all four limbs. ⟳ hemiparesis, monoparesis, paraparesis, paresis.

quadriplegia *n* ⟳ tetraplegia—**quadriplegic** *adj*.

quadruple test a screening test for Down's syndrome. It is the triple test with an additional serum marker, inhibin A; may be performed as part of the inregrated test.

qualitative *adj* relating to quality.

qualitative biomechanical analysis the analysis of forces and movements on (and by) the human body without regard to measurement or quantification. ⟳ biomechanical analysis, quantitative biomechanical analysis.

qualitative research research study based on observation and/or interviews to ascertain people's opinions, feelings or beliefs. Non-statistical methods often used in analysis. ⟳ quantitative research.

quality-adjusted life years (QALYs) a measurement that has been used to prioritize medical treatment. It attempts to provide an objective estimate of the costs and benefits of a medical intervention. A QALY is a measure of years of life gained through a health intervention adjusted for the quality of life (on a scale 0 to 1). For example, if an intervention prolongs life by 5 years, but at only half the quality of normal life, this produces 2.5 QALYs. Quality of Life (QoL) is a patient-centred subjective outcome measure to complement clinical outcomes. Usually measures the presence or absence of symptoms (e.g. pain), side-effects of treatment (e.g. tiredness, loss of hair), feelings of well-being, impact on income, family, work and social life. The costs per QALY can then be measured and those with the lowest costs are given priority. There are many ethical problems with this measure as it may discriminate against people needing expensive treatment and may misjudge the quality of life possible when a person is ill or has a disability. ⟳ quality of life scales.

quality assessment measures a system for evaluating patterns and programmes of clinical, administrative and consumer care.

quality assurance systematic monitoring and evaluation of agreed levels of service provision which are followed by modifications in the light of the evaluation and or audit. ⟳ benchmarking, clinical audit, performance indicators.

quality audit the review of a quality system by recording and documenting the results.

quality circles an initiative to improve the quality of care in a specific area. The health professionals in a clinical area investigate a healthcare intervention systematically and relate it to good standards of practice.

quality control the checking of performance on a regular basis to ensure consistency of results.

quality correction cycle the identification of a problem and the steps taken to rectify the fault and prevent it happening again.

quality factor factor measured in terms of linear energy transfer to express the biological effectiveness of different types of radiation. Used in the calculation of dose equivalents.

quality index an index used for comparison purposes in radiotherapy which is defined as: in a $10 \times 10 \text{ cm}^2$ field at a 100-cm source–chamber distance where the ionization measured at a depth of 20 cm is divided by the ionization measured at a depth of 10 cm at the same source–chamber distance.

quality management the steps taken to ensure constant performance; they will include protocols for safe working, monitoring and checking.

quality of life (QoL) scales quality of life is a conceptual or operational measurement that is commonly used in the oncology setting as a means to assess the impact of chemotherapy and radiotherapy treatment on the person with cancer. Conceptual measurements include well-being, quality of survival, human values and satisfaction of needs, whilst operational measures record a person's ability to independently fulfill the tasks of daily living (Montazeri et al 1996). One major critique of quality of life scales is that they seek to get quantitative (statistical) data about an aspect of life that is fundamentally subjective and qualitative and individual patients may attribute different meanings to their responses. Only the patient can make a valid assessment of their quality of life, so they are required to complete questionnaires themselves, unless they are not in a position to do so because of their physical or psychological condition. The questionnaire aims to be a broad measure usually covering domains related to physical, mental (emotional and cognitive), social and role functioning as well as the individual's perception of their own well-being. It is notable that the outcome of any assessment of the patient's quality of life is dependent upon how they feel and what life circumstances are affecting them at that time. These aspects may not be directly related to the disease and its treatment, therefore it is important to seek qualitative data to inform heathcare interventions. (Montazeri A, Gillis C R, McEwen J 1996 Measuring quality of life in oncology: is it worthwhile? European Journal of Cancer Care 5: 159–167.)

quality of radiation is dependent of the kV used, the higher the kV the more penetrating the beam, but when the kV is sufficient to penetrate the body part any further increase decreases the difference in intensity of the emerging beam and therefore decreases the subject contrast.

quality policy a set of written principles stating how people should act to provide consistent performance.

quality standard a statement or target indicating the level of performance required by teams and individuals.

quality system the management and organizational structures which underpin a high standard of working practice.

quantitative *adj* relating to quantity.

quantitative biomechanical analysis the analysis of forces and movements on (and by) the human body with emphasis on measurement and quantification. ➲ biomechanical analysis, qualitative biomechanical analysis.

quantitative fluorescence-polymerase chain reaction (QF-PCR) diagnostic chromosome test to identify trisomy and sex chromosome aneuploides. The results usually being available within 48 hours of chorionic villus sampling or amniocentesis. The polymerase chain reaction is used to multiply small samples of DNA labelled with fluorescent dyes to enable analysis; measurements of specific regions on the DNA molecule are displayed in graph form, showing the number of specific chromosomes in each cell. Heavily blood stained samples may interfere with analysis.

quantitative research research study based on the measurement and analysis of observations using statistical methods. ➲ qualitative research.

quantitative tests measure actual, numerical results.

quantitative ultrasound an ultrasound technique for measuring bone density in women at risk of osteoporosis.

quantum a unit of energy associated with electromagnetic radiation. ➲ photon.

quantum conversion efficiency in radiography, the percentage of X-rays (quanta) falling on a phosphor which are changed to light photons.

quantum detection efficiency in radiography, the percentage of X-rays (quanta) falling on a phosphor which are stopped by the phosphor.

quantum mottle in radiography, uneven density on a film due to the random distribution of image-forming X-ray quanta producing a non-uniform light emission from intensifying screens.

quantum theory (*syn* Planck's theory) the theory that radiant energy consists of intermittent and spasmodic, minute indivisible amounts called quanta (or photons). This is a somewhat modern version of the theory originally proposed by Newton. ➲ photon, wave theory.

quarantine *n* a period of isolation of infected people or those suspected of having an infectious disease with the objective of preventing spread to others. For contacts it is usually the same period as the longest incubation period for the specific disease.

quartan *adj* recurring every 72 hours (fourth day), such as the fever of quartan malaria.

quartz a crystalline substance occurring naturally as silica. Used in dentistry for investment materials as a refractory material, in some composite filling materials and in some light sources.

quasi-isometric term introduced 1997–1998 by Legg and Spurway, to indicate the condition in which muscles, though not strictly isometric, nonetheless remain for many tens of seconds under load sufficient to restrict blood flow substantially and thus produce metabolic and hence fatigue effects virtually indistinguishable from those experienced during strictly isometric contraction, sustained for similar time under equivalent load. Occurs for example in the quadriceps muscle group of a dinghy sailor in a fresh breeze or of a jockey standing in the stirrups.

Queckenstedt's test (H Queckenstedt, German physician, 1876–1918) during lumbar puncture compression on the internal jugular vein normally produces a rise in cerebrospinal fluid (CSF) pressure if there is no obstruction to circulation of fluid.

quellung reaction swelling of the capsule of a bacterium when exposed to specific antisera. It allows the identification of bacteria causing a disease.

quenching a sudden cooling of a hot metal in a cool liquid in order to temper it.

Quetelet's index (A Quetelet, Belgian mathematician/ sociologist, 1796–1874) an index of body mass. ➲ body mass index.

Q
R

quickening *n* the first perceptible fetal movements felt by the mother, usually at 16–19 weeks' gestation.

quicklime ⊃ lime.

quicksilver rarely used name for mercury.

quiescent *adj* becoming quiet or inactive.

quiet alertness the hour after an infant is born and several hours a day during which the newborn is calm and attentive, looks around and gets to know the adults around her/him and her/his environment.

quiet breathing normal resting tidal breathing.

quinine *n* an alkaloid of cinchona, previously standard treatment for malaria. Use is increasing in regions where resistance to newer antimalarials is a problem.

quininism *n* toxic effects such as headache, tinnitus and partial deafness, disturbed vision and nausea arising from an overdose or long term use of quinine.

quinsy *n* ⊃ peritonsillar abscess.

quint- a prefix that means 'five', e.g. *quintuplets*.

quotient *n* a number obtained by division. ⊃ respiratory quotient. *intelligence quotient* ⊃ intelligence.

Q
R

RA *abbr* **1.** refractory anaemia. **2.** rheumatoid arthritis. **3.** right atrium.

RA latex test used in rheumatoid arthritis. A blood test used to detect the presence of the rheumatoid factor. ⊃ sheep cell agglutination test (SCAT).

rabbit fever ⊃ tularaemia.

rabid *adj* infected with rabies.

rabies *n* (*syn*. hydrophobia) fatal infection of the central nervous system caused by a virus; infection follows the bite of a rabid animal, e.g. dog, cat, fox, vampire bat. It is distributed worldwide apart from a few areas; human and animal vaccines are available—**rabid** *adj*.

race *n* often mistakenly linked to ethnicity. However, race only applies to biological characteristics such as facial features, skin colour or hair type that distinguish a specific group. ⊃ ethnic.

racemose *adj* resembling a bunch of grapes, such as the alveoli that cluster around the terminal airways, or certain exocrine glands.

rachitic *adj* relating to rickets, or resembling or affected by rickets.

rachitic pelvis a pelvic deformity, in which the brim is flattened and kidney-shaped.

racism *n* an opinion of particular groups that is founded on race alone. It results in negative stereotyping, prejudice and discrimination. Racism may be overt, where individuals are subjected to oppressive acts, or covert, where a climate of institutional racism permits one section of society to oppress and subordinate other groups.

rad obsolete term. ⊃ gray (Gy).

radial *adj* pertaining to the radius.

radial artery the artery formed when the brachial artery divides into two below the elbow. It is the artery running down the lateral aspect of the forearm to the wrist, where it lies superficially and is easily felt in front of the radius, where the radial pulse is palpable. It is often used to count the pulse rate in adults. The artery then passes between the first and second metacarpal bones and enters the palm of the hand.

radial keratotomy (RK) (*syn* refractive keratoplasty, keratorefractive surgery—both terms also include epikeratoplasty, keratomileusis and keratophakia). A surgical procedure on the cornea aimed at curing ametropia. It consists of making incisions in the anterior part of the cornea in order to flatten it and thereby produce a reduction of its power. The incisions are usually radial, extending from the limbus to about halfway towards the centre like the spokes of a wheel, but other patterns of incision are also used. In some cases, the procedure does not produce a perfect correction

and vision is poor, especially in the dark. The use of the excimer laser provides greater accuracy and success. The technique is then called *laser refractive keratoplasty* (LRK) or *photorefractive keratectomy* (PRK). ⊃ cornea, epikeratoplasty, excimer laser, keratomileusis, keratophakia, keratoreformation, LASIK.

radial nerve the largest branch of the brachial plexus. It supplies the triceps muscle behind the humerus, crosses in front of the elbow joint then winds round to the back of the forearm to supply extensors of the wrist and finger joints. It continues into the back of the hand to supply the skin of the thumb, the first two fingers and the lateral half of the third finger. ⊃ brachial plexus.

radial nerve palsy the radial nerve can be injured, especially on the outside of the arm above the elbow, either by direct trauma, prolonged pressure, or mid-shaft humerus fractures. This commonly results in a wrist drop.

radial vein one of the deep veins of the forearm. ⊃ Colour Section Figure 10.

radiation *n* the process of heat loss from a body in the form of electromagnetic radiation; this is the only heat transfer process that can take place in a vacuum. Emanation of radiant energy in the form of electromagnetic waves including: gamma rays, infrared, ultraviolet rays, X-rays and visible light rays. Subatomic particles, such as neutrons or electrons, may also be radiated. Radiation may be non-ionizing or ionizing and has many diagnostic and therapeutic uses. ⊃ ionizing radiation.

radiation burn severe skin damage caused by exposure to ionizing radiation, either of high dosage for a short period or of small dosage over an extended period of time.

radiation caries a caries-like destruction of tooth substance following radiation therapy. The condition is associated with xerostomia.

radiation dosimetry the method of measuring the amount of radiation received by an individual. Also called radiation monitoring.

radiation hazard ionizing radiation in high doses can cause damage to the body tissues (somatic damage). Exposure (of lesser doses), especially to the gonads (ovaries, testes), can cause changes in the hereditary characteristics contained in the genes (genetic damage). In dentistry, protective measures include staying out of the surgery during radiography, and the patient wearing a rubber- or plastic-covered lead apron during exposure to X-rays.

radiation nephritis inflammation of the nephrons. It may be acute occurring 6–13 months after radiotherapy, or chronic that occurs 1.5–4 years after radiotherapy.

radiation oncologist medical specialist in the treatment of disease by X-rays and other forms of radiation.

radiation pneumonitis inflammation of the lungs caused by the radiation dosage received by the patient.

radiation protection equipment and rules to ensure that staff and patients experience safe working practices. ➲ local rules, dosimeter.

radiation protection advisor a suitably qualified and experienced person whose role is to advise staff on the safe use of ionizing radiation.

radiation protection supervisor a person directly involved with ionization who is responsible for ensuring safe working practices in a specific department and is appointed by the radiation protection advisor.

radiation safety committee a local group of radiation users, advisors and management who discuss matters related to radiation safety.

radiation sickness tissue damage from exposure to ionizing radiation leading to diarrhoea, vomiting, anorexia, and later alopecia, bleeding and bone marrow failure. Other longer term effects include fetal damage and birth defects, sterility, eye damage, leukaemia and other cancers.

radiation treatment planning the method required to graphically display the isodose distribution that results when one or more radiation beams converge on the target volume in external beam therapy.

radical *adj* pertaining to the root of a thing.

radical mastectomy ➲ mastectomy.

radical mastoidectomy ➲ mastoidectomy.

radical surgery usually extensive and aims to be curative, not palliative. Examples include Whipple's operation for cancer of the head of pancreas and radical mastectomy (rarely performed).

radical treatment ➲ treatment.

radic/o, radicul/o- a prefix that means 'nerve root', e.g. *radiculitis*.

radicular relating to nerve roots or roots of a tooth.

radicular cyst ➲ apical (radicular) cyst.

radicular fracture a fracture of the root or roots of a tooth.

radiculitis *n* inflammation affecting a nerve root.

radiculography *n* radiography of the spinal nerve roots after the introduction of a positive contrast agent via a lumbar puncture to locate the site and size of a prolapsed intervertebral disc. Superseded by computed tomography (CT) and magnetic resonance imaging (MRI)—**radiculogram** *n*.

radiculopathy *n* entrapment of the nerve as it passes out from the spinal cord to the arm or leg, and usually occurs as a result of intervertebral disc prolapse and degenerative disease in the facet joints of the spine.

radi/o- a prefix that means 'radiation', e.g. *radiotherapy*.

radioactive *adj* exhibiting radioactivity. Describes an unstable atomic nucleus which emits charged particles as it disintegrates. ➲ radioactive decay, radioisotope.

radioactive decay the process by which a nucleus of a radioactive atom spontaneously transforms by one or more discrete energy steps until a stable state is reached. ➲ half-life.

radioactive disintegration when a stable nuclide, the parent, changes to another nuclide, the daughter, which may be either stable or unstable and therefore radioactive.

radioactive equilibrium equilibrium reached, after radioactive disintegration, when the weight of each nuclide in the atom is inversely proportional to the half-life of the nuclide.

radioactive fallout release of radioactive particles into the atmosphere. Results from industrial processes or accidents, and possibly acts of terrorism and the testing or use of nuclear weapons.

radioactive source a radioactive substance sealed, in a capsule, which, when inserted into the body, delivers a predetermined dose of radiation.

radioallergosorbent test (RAST) an obsolete test for IgE antibodies against specific allergens. Now largely replaced by non-radioactive enzyme-based assays.

radiobiology *n* the study of the effects of radiation on living organisms. The use of radioactive tracers to study biological processes—**radiobiological** *adj*, **radiobiologically** *adv*.

radiocarbon *n* a radioactive form of the element carbon, such as carbon-14 (^{14}C), used for investigations, e.g. absorption tests and research.

radiodermatitis *n* the skin changes caused by exposure to ionizing radiation, such as during radiotherapy for cancer, or occupational exposure. The affected skin is red and sore with blister formation and weeping. There may be lasting effects that include fibrosis, scarring and loss of skin pigment.

radiograph *n* a photographic image formed by exposure to X-rays; the correct term for an 'X-ray'—**radiographic** *adj*.

radiographer *n* there are two distinct professional disciplines within radiography, diagnostic and therapeutic; they are registered health professionals qualified in the use of ionizing radiation and other techniques, either in diagnostic imaging or radiotherapy.

radiographic baseline also known as reference plane. In skull radiography, the orbitomeatal line. In intraoral radiography, the occusal plane of the jaw can be radiographed.

radiographic contrast the photographic differences between two adjacent areas on a film.

radiography *n* the use of X-radiation: (a) to create images of the body from which medical diagnoses can be made (diagnostic radiography). Initially referred to as 'plain' X-ray films (radiographs) but the general term has expanded to include other forms of diagnostic imaging such as ultrasound, computed tomography (CT) and magnetic resonance imaging (MRI) scanning; or (b) to treat a person suffering from a (malignant) disease, according to a medically prescribed regimen (therapeutic radiography). ➲ radiotherapy.

radioimmunoassay *n* the use of radioactive substances to measure substances such as hormones and drugs in the blood.

radioiodinated human serum albumin (RIHSA) used for detection and localization of brain lesions, determination of blood and plasma volumes, circulation time and cardiac output.

radioisotope *n* (*syn.* radionuclide) any isotope that is radioactive. Forms of an element which have the same atomic number but different mass numbers, exhibiting the property of spontaneous nuclear disintegration. Several different radioisotopes are used in diagnosis, treatment and research. Examples of radioisotopes include iodine-131 (^{131}I), strontium-90 (^{90}Sr), technecium-99 (^{99}Tc^m). When administered orally, by injection, or inhaled, they can be traced in the body by a Geiger counter. ⊃ Appendix 9.

radioisotope scan pictorial representation of the amount and distribution of radioactive isotope present in a particular organ.

radiolabel the modification of a substance to make it radioactive so that it can be used to target a particular organ or body part so that it can be detected in radionuclide imaging.

radiologist *n* a medical specialist in diagnosis by using X-rays and other allied imaging techniques.

radiology *n* the medical specialty covering the use and interpretation of X-ray images and, more recently, other imaging techniques—**radiological** *adj*, **radiologically** *adv*.

radiology information system (RIS) a computer system specifically for imaging departments which enables the booking and planning of work for inpatients and outpatients, the identification of suitable tests, the management and reporting of images and the transmission of information back to the ward, unit or individual requesting the services.

radiolucent *adj* relating to substances that permit X-rays and other types of radiant energy to pass through with minimum loss through absorption; appearing as dark images on exposed film.

radiomimetic *adj* exerting effects similar to those of ionizing radiation. For example, nitrogen mustards.

radionecrosis tissue death caused by radiation. ⊃ osteoradionecrosis.

radionuclide *n* ⊃ radioisotope.

radionuclide generator a system containing a long-lived parent radionuclide which decays to a short-lived daughter radionuclide.

radionuclide therapy the introduction of a radionuclide either orally or by injection; this is then taken up by a targeted organ which receives a calculated radiation dose to maximize the dose of radiation to the treatment area in a patient and minimize the dose to normal tissue.

radiopaque *adj* having the property of significantly absorbing X-rays, thus becoming visible on a radiograph, for example a metal tooth restoration which appears lighter than its surroundings in a dental radiograph. Barium and iodine compounds are used, as contrast agents, to produce artificial radiopacity—**radiopacity** *n*.

radiopaque denture base material denture base material to which has been added a radiopaque substance in order to facilitate the location of the appliance if swallowed, inhaled or implanted in tissues.

radioresistance the ability of tissues, both normal and some cancers, to withstand the effects of ionizing radiation.

radiosensitive *adj* applied to tissues, normal and some cancers, which are sensitive to the killing effects of ionizing radiation. The use of radiosensitizer drugs are used in some cases to increase the sensitivity of some cancers.

radiosurgery *n* (*syn.* stereotactic radiotherapy) a radiotherapy treatment based on a 3D coordinate system designed to achieve a high concentration of absorbed dose to an intracranial target.

radiotelemetry measurement based on data transmitted by radio waves from the subject to the recording apparatus; radiotelemetry of the fetal heart may be used when the woman is ambulant in labour.

radiotherapist *n* ⊃ radiation oncologist.

radiotherapy *n* the use of ionizing radiation in the treatment of proliferative disease, especially cancer, and certain non-malignant diseases, such as the use of a precisely focused radiation for the relief of pain in trigeminal neuralgia. Radiotherapy may be used alone but is more often used in combination with surgery, chemotherapy, or hormone therapy and other biological treatment modalities. It may be used as a curative treatment or as palliative treatment to reduce symptoms of advanced disease, such as pain. Total body irradiation is used to prepare patients with haemopoietic cancers for a haemopoietic stem cell transplant (bone marrow transplant). Ionizing radiation interrupts deoxyribonucleic acid (DNA) synthesis or decreases the rate of mitotic divisions. Thus cell replication is prevented, although several cell divisions may need to occur before cell death eventually occurs. The therapy may be applied by external beam methods (teletherapy) by employing a unit, which emits megavoltage radiation in order to treat cancers deep within the body, and lower energy units such as orthovoltage or kilovoltage units for more superficial cancers. A course of radiotherapy usually takes a few minutes each day, but is spread over a number of weeks. Brachytherapy describes radiotherapeutic modalities in which sealed (removed after treatment) or unsealed radiactive sources are delivered close to the cancer, such as a radioactive source placed into the body for some gynaecological cancers. In systemic therapy, radioactive isotopes (radionuclides) (e.g. yttrium-90 [^{90}Y] for neuroendocrine cancers and iodine–131 [^{131}I] for thyroid cancer) are administered orally or intravenously and are preferentially taken up by the cancerous tissue. Radiotherapy aims to deliver a homogeneous cancer-killing dose to a precisely localized area of the body, to avoid as much normal tissue as possible without compromising the treatment outcome and to avoid any critical structures such as the gonads, kidney or spinal cord, which may be particularly sensitive to radiation. Although radiation is unable to discriminate between normal and malignant tissues there is a differential effect and cancer cells are more sensitive to the effects of treatment.

radiotracer the modification of a substance to make it radioactive so that it can be used to target a particular organ or body part so that it can be detected in radionuclide imaging.

Q
R

radioulnar joint one of two joints between the radius and ulna. In addition, a fibrous membrane links the bones along their shafts, the interosseous membrane. It is an example of a fibrous joint and prevents separation of the bones when force is applied at either the elbow or the wrist. ➲ distal radioulnar joint, proximal radioulnar joint.

radium (Ra) *n* a radioactive element occurring in nature, historically a mainstay of radiotherapy. However, it has been largely replaced by radioisotopes of caesium and cobalt.

radius *n* the smaller outer bone of the forearm, it articulates with the humerus at the elbow, the carpal bones at the wrist, and with the ulna at the proximal and distal radioulnar joints. ➲ Colour Section Figures 2, 3.

radon seeds capsules containing radon—a radioactive gas produced by the disintegration of radium atoms. Historically used in radiotherapy.

RAEB *abbr* refractory anaemia with excess blasts.

raised intracranial pressure (RIP) an elevation in intracranial pressure is a serious situation. Causes include: tumours, intracranial haemorrhage, brain injury causing oedema or haematoma and obstruction to the flow of cerebrospinal fluid. The features depend on the cause, but there may be headache, vomiting, papilloedema, seizures (fits), bradycardia, arterial hypertension and changes in the level of consciousness. ➲ benign intracranial hypertension, intracranial pressure. A major consideration for health professionals, such as physiotherapists, is not to undertake treatment that might further increase intracranial pressure (ICP) in patients who already have raised intracranial pressure (RIP). So minimizing the use of suction, avoiding positioning that might raise ICP (patients should be in 30° of head and trunk elevation) and avoiding other noxious stimuli is important. However, ICP is affected by changes in respiratory blood gases so maintaining good lung function is also very important. For this reason careful clinical decision-making needs to take place for each individual patient if respiratory treatment is indicated.

râle *n* older term for the abnormal sound (crackles) heard on auscultation of lungs when fluid is present in bronchi.

RAM *acron* **R**andom **A**ccess **M**emory.

rampant caries a type of caries that may appear suddenly and become widespread rapidly.

Ramsay Hunt syndrome (J Ramsay Hunt, American neurologist, 1872–1937) herpes zoster causing vesicles on the ear lobe with pain, vertigo, impaired hearing, facial paralysis and loss of taste.

Ramstedt's operation (C Ramstedt, German surgeon, 1867–1972) ➲ pyloromyotomy.

ramus of the mandible that part of the mandible which is at an angle to its body and carries the coronoid process and the condyle (part of the temporomandibular joint). The masseter muscle is attached to its outer surface.

random access memory (RAM) the part of the memory of a computer which can be accessed by the user; the amount of random access memory available determines how much data can be stored by the user.

random-dot stereogram (RDS) (*syn* Julesz random-dot stereogram) a stereogram in which the eye sees an array of little characters or dots of a roughly uniform texture and containing no recognizable shape or contours. The only difference is that a certain region in one target has been laterally displaced with respect to the other, to produce some retinal disparity. When they are viewed in a stereoscope, that region is seen in stereoscopic relief. The shape in that region can be any pattern. The effect is remarkable as the shape usually appears to float out from the surround. The random-dot E test uses a polarized random test pattern and requires the use of Polaroid spectacles to detect whether a subject has stereopsis. The subject will see a raised letter E in the random-dot pattern of one of the test plates. At 50 cm, the retinal disparity induced by the E is 500 seconds of arc. The TNO test for stereoscopic vision also uses random-dot stereograms in which the half-images have been superimposed and printed in complementary colours, like anaglyphs. The test plates, when viewed with red and green spectacles, elicit stereopsis. There is a series of plates inducing retinal disparities ranging from 15 to 480 seconds of arc. ➲ anaglyph, Frisby stereotest, Lang stereotest, retinal disparity, stereoscopic visual acuity, two-dimensional test, vectogram.

random sampling in research. The selection process whereby every person in the population has an equal chance of being selected.

random variable background factors such as environmental conditions that may affect any conditions of the independent variables equally. ➲ independent variable, varible.

randomized controlled trial (RCT) research study using two or more randomly selected groups: experimental and control. It produces high level evidence for practice.

range *n* describes the span of values (lowest–highest) observed in a sample.

range of motion/movement (ROM) how far a joint permits rotation of the moving parts about the axis of the joint. Usually measured in degrees or radians. Depends on the articulating surfaces, the length and elasticity of ligaments and the properties of muscle, tendon and other soft tissue surrounding the joint. Used as an index of flexibility and to assess progress in rehabilitation. For example, after repair of the anterior cruciate ligament, knee movement will be restricted and as rehabilitation progresses the ROM will increase back to normal. May be assessed by direct examination and measurement or using an isokinetic dynamometer.

rank in statistics, the method of organizing data.

ranula *n* a retention cyst. A cystic swelling usually beneath the tongue due to blockage of the sublingual salivary gland duct or a mucus gland—**ranular** *adj*.

RAPD *abbr* relative afferent pupillary defect.

rape *n* unlawful sexual intercourse without consent which is achieved by force or deception. Full penetration of the vagina (or other orifice) by the penis and ejaculation of semen is not necessary to constitute rape. Many rapes include force and violence, but acquiescence because of verbal threats should not be interpreted as consent. Where women are admitted to hospital, a police surgeon will perform an examination to obtain the necessary specimens for forensic examination in the presence of specially trained female police officers who then support the victim throughout the interviews and subsequent investigation and possible prosecution of the alleged perpetrator. Male rape, the rape of a male by another male, is increasingly recognized.

raphe *n* a seam, suture, ridge or crease.

rapid eye movement sleep (REM) also known as paradoxical sleep. ⊃ sleep.

rapid plasma reagin test (RPR) a non-specific serological test for syphilis.

rare-earth metals metals having two electrons in the outer shell and either 8 or 9 electrons in the penultimate shell; they are used for the phosphors in television monitors, lasers and modern intensifying screens. Examples include lanthanum, europium, gadolinium, terbium, yttrium.

rarefaction *n* becoming less dense, as applied to diseased bone—**rarefied** *adj*.

RARS *abbr* refractory anaemia with sideroblasts.

RAS *abbr* reticular activating system.

rash *n* skin eruption, it may be described in several ways: cause, e.g. napkin rash, nettle rash; colour, e.g. rose-coloured; distribution or shape, e.g. centripetal, butterfly-shaped; and by type of lesion, e.g. macular, maculopapular, papular, papulopustular, papulosquamous, petechial, pustular. ⊃ urticaria.

Rasmussen's aneurysm (F Rasmussen, Danish physician, 1837–1877) an aneurysm of a pulmonary artery within a tuberculous cavity.

Rasmussen's encephalitis (disease or syndrome) (T Rasmussen, American neurologist, 1910–2002) a rare, progressive brain disorder, in which there is chronic inflammation of one side of the brain; possibly caused by an auto-immune process. It mainly affects children under 10 years of age and is charaterized by a deterioration in motor skills and speech, seizures, hemiparesis and a decline in mental abilities. Frequent seizures causes brain damage, which results in permanent neurological deficits.

rasp ⊃ bone file.

RAST *abbr* radioallergosorbent test.

Rastelli's operation surgical procedure to treat transposition of the great vessels in which blood circulation through the heart is diverted to effect adequate oxygenation.

raster lines the lines formed when a beam of electrons scans a phosphor to form an image. ⊃ phosphor.

rat-bite fever *n* a relapsing fever caused by the Gram-negative bacterium *Streptobacillus moniliformis* or the spirochaete *Spirillum minus*. Usually transmitted by rat bites or less often by other rodents. There is fever, joint and muscle pain and a rash; also causes local inflammation, splenomegaly and lymphadenitis.

rate-limiting enzymes ⊃ enzyme.

rating the rating of an X-ray unit is the combination of exposure settings which can occur without unacceptably damaging the unit.

rating of perceived exertion (RPE) a psychophysical measure of a person's subjective experience of the intensity of exercise based on the totality of physical sensations the person experiences during physical activity, including sensations of a racing heart, breathlessness and muscle fatigue. Often used to train people to regulate the intensity of their exercise to achieve optimal results without the need for technical equipment.

ratio data measurement data with a numerical score, e.g. height, that has a true zero of 0. It is interval data with an absolute zero. ⊃ interval data.

rationalization *n* a defence mechanism whereby a person justifies his or her actions following the event, so it looks more rational or socially acceptable.

raw data original received information.

raw data matrix in magnetic resonance imaging (MRI) it is the initial image before analysis. The points at the centre of the matrix represent areas of low spatial frequencies and the frequencies become higher the further away from the centre.

Rayleigh equation a colour equation representing a match of yellow (usually 589 nm) with a mixture of red (usually 670 nm) and green (usually 535 nm). It is used to differentiate certain types of colour deficiencies. The anomaloscope is built on this principle. ⊃ anomaloscope, defective colour vision.

Rayleigh scattering ⊃ coherent scattering.

Raynaud's disease (M Raynaud, French physician, 1834–1881) paroxysmal spasm of the digital arteries producing pallor or cyanosis of fingers or toes, and occasionally resulting in gangrene. The form of the disease most often affects young women aged 18–30 years.

Raynaud's phenomenon episodic discoloration of the fingers and sometimes the toes (classically the fingers turn white, then blue, then red), tingling, burning and pain usually in response to temperature change or stress. ⊃ CREST syndrome, hand-arm vibration syndrome.

RBC *abbr* red blood cell. ⊃ blood.

RB-ILD *abbr* respiratory bronchiolitis–interstitial lung disease.

RCA *abbr* right coronary artery.

RCMD *abbr* refractory cytopenias with multilineage dysplasia.

RCP *abbr* retruded cuspal position.

RCT *abbr* randomized controlled trial.

RD *abbr* retinal detachment.

RDA *abbr* recommended daily allowance.

RDI *abbr* recommended daily intake.

RDS *abbr* **1.** random-dot stereogram. **2.** respiratory distress syndrome.

re- a prefix that means 'again, back', e.g. *recannulation*.

reabsorb to absorb again, to resorb.

reactance the opposition to current flow and is produced by capacitors and inductors but not by resistors.

reaction *n* **1.** response to a stimulus. **2.** a chemical change. *allergic reaction* ⊃ allergy.

reationary haemorrhage ⊃ haemorrhage.

Q
R

reaction formation a defence mechanism in which attitudes completely opposite to those unconsciously held are expressed, or the person behaves in a way that is completely contary to what would normally be anticipated.

reaction time the time that elapses between the presentation of a stimulus and a response; also known as response latency. *choice reaction time* reaction time when two or more stimuli are presented and different responses are required, also known as complex reaction time. *discrimination reaction time* reaction time where a response is required to only one of two or more stimuli. *simple reaction time* reaction time when only one stimulus is presented and one response is required.

reactive arthritis (*syn.* Reiter's syndrome) arthritis that develops in response to infection, usually urogenital, gastrointestinal or throat infection. ⊃ sexually acquired reactive arthritis.

reactive oxygen species (ROS) free radicals and other highly reactive molecules formed from molecular oxygen during normal cell metabolism. From both exogenous and endogenous sources, ROS are present in all aerobic organisms, which have evolved defences against their potentially damaging effects and also ways of utilizing them (e.g. for signalling between and within cells and in the immune system, for killing invading micro-organisms). Some but not all ROS are free radicals, e.g. the superoxide anion ($^{\cdot}O_2^{-}$) and the hydroxyl radical (OH$^{\cdot}$) where an atom has one or more unpaired electrons in its outer orbital, making it particularly reactive. All the better known free radicals in the body are oxygen-based (although other atoms can also exist in this form) and are generated as by-products of oxidative metabolism. They are formed by exposure to ionizing radiation, cigarette smoke and other environmental pollutants and increased by excessive alcohol consumption and in infections. Free radicals are believed to cause cellular damage by lipid peroxidation which incorporates oxygen into membrane lipids. Protein and DNA damage are also involved. They are implicated in ageing and disease, including atherosclerosis (hence coronary heart disease and stroke), cancers and obstructive lung disease. Antioxidant enzymes protect cell membranes by reacting with the free radicals and removing them, e.g. removal of $^{\cdot}O_2^{-}$ by superoxide dismutase which produces hydrogen peroxide (H_2O_2), itself a ROS. In sport, ROS may be responsible for delayed-onset muscle soreness (DOMS). ⊃ antioxidant, antioxidant enzymes, antioxidant nutrients, oxidative stress/damage.

Read method a method of preparation for childbirth initially prepared by Dr Grantley Dick Read. It is based on the relaxation, information and pain triangle. Women are prepared for birth by being educated so that through understanding their fear may be reduced as fear is known to make pain worse. Relaxation improves the ability to cope with pain and gentle exercise promotes relaxation and fitness.

read only memory (ROM) the pre-programmed part of the computer which enables it to run programs.

reading the act of viewing and interpreting letters, words, sentences, etc. It consists of a pattern of eye movements. The eyes proceed along a line in a series of step-like saccades, separated by fixation pauses during which information from the text is acquired. The amount of reading matter correctly identified during the fixation pause is called the span of recognition or the perceptual span. Most saccadic eye movements are made from left to right but some occur in the opposite direction (called regression) to return to text recently read but not yet fully perceived. At the end of the line the eyes make a return sweep to the next line of text. ⊃ developmental eye movement test, saccadic eye movement.

reading addition ⊃ near addition.

reading distance the normal distance at which people read. It is about 33–44 cm for men and 29–40 cm for women. It is a useful measurement in determining the reading addition. ⊃ near addition.

reading slit ⊃ typoscope.

reagent *n* a substance that participates in a chemical reaction, in order to detect, measure, or produce other substances.

reagin an antibody (immunoglobulin) of the IgE class that mediates the type I hypersensitivity reactions occurring, for example in allergies to foodstuffs and atopic conditions such as asthma or hayfever.

reality orientation (RO) *n* a form of therapy useful for withdrawn, confused and depressed patients: they are frequently reminded of their name, the time, place, date and so on. Reinforcement is provided by clocks, calendars and signs prominently displayed in the environment.

real time a computer controlling, or recording, events as they are happening.

real time imaging the use of specialized recording equipment to produce images almost instantaneously, such as ultrasound scanning and other imaging techniques, particularly during interventional radiology.

real time scanning a method of producing a moving image on a screen.

real time ultrasonography an ultrasound imaging technique involving rapid pulsing to enable continuous viewing of movement to be obtained, rather than stationary images.

reamer ⊃ root canal (dental procedures).

reasonable doubt to secure a conviction in criminal proceedings, the prosecution must establish beyond reasonable doubt the guilt of the accused.

reattachment the re-establishment of attachment of the periodontal tissue to the tooth root on which viable periodontal tissue has been retained following surgery or trauma.

Reaven's syndrome (G Reaven, American endocrinologist, 20th–21st century) ⊃ metabolic syndrome.

rebase the removal and replacement of the denture base without changing the occlusal relationship.

rebore *n* ⊃ disobliteration.

recalcitrant *adj* refractory. Describes medical conditions that are resistant to treatment.

recall *n* part of the process of memory. Memory consists of memorizing, retention and recall.

recannulation *n* re-establishment of the patency of a vessel.

receiver the part of the ultrasonic transducer that detects returning sound waves and converts them to electrical signals.

receiver bandwidth the measure of a range of frequencies within which a magnetic resonance system is tuned to receive the signal. Alteration affects the signal-to-noise ratio, by narrowing the bandwidth the ratio is increased and by broadening it the ratio is decreased.

receiver operating characteristics a method of measuring the ability of an observer to make a diagnosis.

receptaculum *n* receptacle, often forms a reservoir.

receptive (sensory) aphasia a type of aphasia where there are problems of varying severity with language comprehension. Those affected may also have expressive aphasia.

receptor *n* **1.** in the nervous system, the distal ending of an afferent nerve, or specialist structure served by such a nerve, which signals the incidence of a mechanical, chemical, thermal or other stimulus (termed sensory receptor if the signal can reach consciousness). ⊃ proprioceptor. **2.** in the context of cell signalling, a molecular structure situated on the surface of the cell (membrane receptor) or inside a cell membrane, or within the cytoplasm or the nucleus. They act as binding sites for various endogenous molecules such as hormones, neurotransmitters or other signalling molecules, and exogenous drugs. Drugs exert their effects by binding to receptor proteins and interacting in one of two main ways; they may act as an agonist or an antagonist. Those that act as agonists bind to the receptor and imitate the response of the naturally occurring ligand (the endogenous chemical). Drugs can also act as antagonists and bind to receptors, preventing endogenous agonists from binding.

recession in dentistry, the migration of the gingival margin in an apical direction so exposing the root surface of a tooth.

recessive *adj* receding; having a tendency to disappear.

recessive trait a genetic character or trait that is expressed when the determining allele is present at both paired chromosomal loci (i.e. homozygous or 'in double dose'), for example in the inheritance of cystic fibrosis. When the specific allele is present in single dose the characteristic is not expressed as it is overpowered by the dominant allele at the other locus, but the person having the single allele is a carrier. However, recessive X-linked genes in males will be expressed in a single dose, such as haemophilia and red-green colour blindness. ⊃ dominant.

recipe a statement of ingredients. The heading of a prescription by the symbol R meaning 'take'.

recipient *n* the individual who receives something from a donor such as blood, an organ such as a kidney or bone marrow. ⊃ blood groups.

reciprocal anchorage a type of orthodontic anchorage in which the movement of two or more teeth is balanced against the movement of one or more opposing teeth.

reciprocal clasp a clasp arm, or other extension, of a partial denture, used to oppose the action of laterally displacing forces.

reciprocal inhibition inhibition of spinal cord motor neurons innervating muscles whose contraction would oppose an initiated movement, e.g. when flexing the elbow to lift a weight, the elbow extensors are relaxed. Term introduced in the 1890s by Charles Sherrington (British neurophysiologist and Nobel prize winner) and later known as Sherrington's law. Used as a technique in which an active contraction of the agonist muscle is used to produce a reflex relaxation of the antagonist, thereby allowing the antagonist muscle to be stretched.

reciprocal innervation the interaction between opposing muscle groups that facilitates the dynamic co-contraction for postural stability and controlled movements for function. During contraction of an agonist muscle its antagonist muscle is simultaneously inhibited to produce relaxation.

reciprocal lengthening when muscles work concentrically, the opposite muscles lengthen to permit movement. ⊃ concentric contraction.

reciprocal ponderal index a way of expressing adiposity. It is the person's height divided by the cube root of their weight.

reciprocal shortening when muscles work eccentrically, the opposite muscles have to take up the slack, but the muscle is not actively contracting, there is some cross bridge formation. ⊃ eccentric action.

reciprocating handpiece ⊃ handpiece.

reciprocity the ability to produce an accurate range of densities over a film which reflect the structure being imaged.

reciprocity failure seen with either very short exposures at high intensity or very long exposures at low intensity which do not produce the expected density on the film.

reciprocity law the amount of density produced on a film is dependent only on the total amount of light energy available.

Recklinghausen's disease ⊃ von Recklinghausen's disease.

recognition acuity the ability of an individual to recognize standard shapes.

recombinant DNA deoxyribonucleic acid produced by recombining chemically the DNA of two different organisms. Used for the study of both normal and abnormal genes and so, for example, of genetic disorders. The practical applications include diagnosis (including prenatal diagnosis) and in the manufacture of therapeutic products, e.g. human insulin, human erythropoietin.

recommended daily allowance (RDA) (*syn.* recommended daily intake—RDI) refers to national and international standards that recommend the intake level of a particular nutrient for specific groups of people. In the UK it has offically been replaced by dietary reference values (DRV) and their subcategories, but is still widely quoted on packaging with reference to vitamin content. ⊃ dietary reference values.

Q
R

Recommended International Non-proprietary Name (rINN) the system of non-proprietary drug names in use internationally.

reconstituted family a family with step-parents resulting from divorce or remarriage.

reconstruction technique a method of forming an image from a set of measurements; in computed tomography (CT) imaging this includes automatic corrections. ⊃ iterative reconstruction algorithm.

record 1. a list of facts or findings relative to a specific condition and recorded in a permanent way. **2.** in dentistry, the registration of jaw relations. *functional record* a record of the lateral and protrusive movements of the mandible on the occluding surface of the maxillary occlusal rim or other recording surface. *terminal hinge position record* a record of the relationship of the mandible relative to the maxilla at the retruded mandibular position.

recovery 1. an approach to treatment based on the belief that each person has the potential to challenge the limitations imposed by illness or disability, to make choices about occupations and activities, to participate in the life of the community and to experience a sense of wellbeing. **2.** a return to a normal state or health. It may be total or only partial.

recovery position an urgent first aid measure where a person with an altered level of consciousness is positioned so as to maintain the airway and prevent aspiration of secretions or vomit into the airway. It protects the airway of an unconscious or semi-conscious person, whatever the cause (e.g. victims of drowning, trauma or poisoning and so on) until qualified medical assistance arrives. This position prevents the tongue falling back in the mouth, obstructing the airway, or the possible aspiration of blood or vomit into the lungs. The casualty is laid on one side with the underneath leg straight while the other leg is fully flexed at the hip, with the knee bent and resting on the ground, altering the centre of gravity to prevent rolling onto the back. The head is supported by the arm, maintaining the desired position with the face tilted towards the ground (Figure R.1). It is important not to move the casualty if a spinal injury is suspected, unless for cardiopulmonary resuscitation (CPR). Also known as coma position. Figure R.2 illustrates the recovery position used for infants under one year.

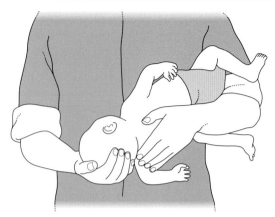

R.2 **Recovery position—infants under one year** (reproduced from Brooker & Waugh 2007 with permission).

recrudescence *n* the return of symptoms.

recruitment *n* **1.** occurs in sensorineural deafness where it describes a situation in which the person perceives a rapid increase in loudness of a sound when the increase was only very small. **2.** the activation of additional cells in response to increased stimulus strength. In skeletal muscle contraction, activation by the central nervous system of progressively more motor units, hence of more muscle fibres, as the strength of contraction increases.

rectal varices haemorrhoids.

rectified made unidirectional, when alternating current is modified so that current only flows in a positive direction. *half-wave rectification* the negative half of the cycle is suppressed. *full-wave rectification* the negative half of the cycle is made positive by the use of rectifiers.

rectifier a piece of equipment that allows current to flow in only one direction.

rect/o a prefix that means 'rectum', e.g. *rectocele*.

rectocele *n* prolapse of the rectum, so that it lies outside the anus. Usually used to describe the herniation of the anterior rectal wall into the posterior vaginal wall caused by injury to the levator ani muscles during childbirth (Figure R.3). Repaired by a posterior colporrhaphy. ⊃ cystocele, procidentia.

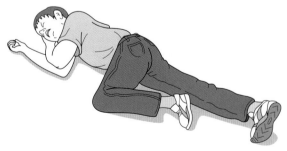

R.1 **Recovery position—adult** (reproduced from Nicol et al 2004 with permission).

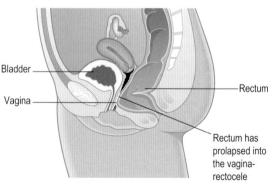

Bladder

Vagina

Rectum

Rectum has prolapsed into the vagina-rectocele

R.3 **Rectocele** (reproduced from Brooker & Nicol 2003 with permission).

rectosigmoid *adj* pertaining to the rectum and sigmoid colon.

rectouterine *adj* pertaining to the rectum and uterus, as the rectouterine pouch (pouch of Douglas).

rectovaginal *adj* pertaining to the rectum and vagina.

rectovesical *adj* pertaining to the rectum and bladder.

rectum *n* the slightly dilated, lower part of the large intestine between the sigmoid colon and anal canal. It is about 13 cm in length in adults. The rectum is normally empty until faeces moves down from the colon just before defecation—**rectal** *adj*, **rectally** *adv*. ⊃ Colour Section Figure18b.

rectus *n* a straight muscle, such as the four extraocular rectus muscles of the eye, or the rectus femoris of the thigh. ⊃ extraocular, rectus abdominis, rectus femoris.

rectus abdominis one of a pair of superficial, medial abdominal muscles. It extends from the pubis to the ribs and is covered by the aponeuroses of the other three pairs of abdominal muscles (internal and external obliques and the transversus abdominis). The two muscles are separated by the linea alba formed from the aponeuoses. Its origin is on the crest of the pubis and it inserts onto the costal cartilages of ribs 5–7 and the xiphoid process of the sternum. The rectus abdominis flexes the lower vertebral column, provides pelvic stability during movement and increases intra-abdominal pressure, such as during defecation or parturition. ⊃ abdominal muscles, Colour Section Figure 4.

rectus femoris one of the four-part quadriceps femoris muscle. A superficial muscle of the anterior aspect of the thigh. Its origin is on the pelvis and it inserts via a common tendon onto the tibial tubercle (tuberosity) and the patella. ⊃ quadriceps femoris.

recumbent *adj* lying or reclining—**recumbency** *n.*

recumbent position lying on the back with the head supported on a pillow.

recurrent caries dental caries that extends either beneath or beyond the margins of a restoration, due to the accumulation of debris resulting from inadequate cavity restoration.

recurrent (habitual) abortion ⊃ recurrent or habitual miscarriage.

recurrent or habitual miscarriage when miscarriage occurs in three successive pregnancies.

recurring costs regular and ongoing costs, such as planned maintenance and staff salaries.

red one of the hues of the visible spectrum evoked by stimulation of the retina by wavelengths beyond 630 nm. The complementary colours to red are blue-green (between 490.4 and 492.4 nm). ⊃ complementary colour.

red blindness ⊃ protanopia.

red blood cell (RBC) *n* (*syn* red cell). ⊃ erythrocytes.

red cell enzymopathies a mature red blood cell must produce energy via adenosine triphosphate (ATP) to maintain a normal internal environment and cell volume whilst protecting itself from the oxidative stress presented from oxygen carriage. Anaerobic glycolysis via the Embden–Meyerhof pathway generates ATP, and the pentose phosphate pathway (hexose monophosphate shunt/pathway) produces the reduced form of nicotinamide adenine dinucleotide phosphate (NADPH) and glutathione to protect against oxidative stress. The impact of functional or quantitative defects in the enzymes in these pathways will depend upon the importance of the steps affected and the presence of alternative pathways. In general, defects in the hexose monophosphate shunt result in periodic haemolysis induced by oxidative stress, whilst those in the Embden–Meyerhof pathway result in shortened red cell survival and chronic haemolysis. ⊃ glucose-6-phosphate dehydrogenase deficiency (G6PD), pyrimidine 5′ nucleotidase deficiency, pyruvate kinase deficiency.

red cell membrane defects the basic structure of the red cell membrane is a cytoskeleton 'stapled' on to the lipid bilayer by special protein complexes. This structure ensures great deformability and elasticity; the red cell diameter is 8 μm but the narrowest point in the circulation is 2 μm in the spleen. When this normal structure is disturbed, usually by a quantitative or functional deficiency of one or more proteins in the cytoskeleton, cells lose their normal elasticity. Each time such cells pass through the spleen they lose membrane relative to their cell volume. This results in an increase in mean cell haemoglobin concentration (MCHC), abnormal cell shape and reduced red cell survival due to extravascular haemolysis. ⊃ hereditary elliptocytosis, hereditary spherocytosis.

redistribution during fractionated radiotherapy those cells that are not killed become more resistant to radiation, they try to change to the mitotic stage of the cell cycle so that they can repopulate.

red filter a filter which transmits only red light. It may be used in ophthalmoscopy to facilitate viewing the yellow macular pigment, but other structures are seen with less contrast. It also produces a larger pupil allowing observation of a larger fundus area. ⊃ macular pigment.

red filter test ⊃ red glass test.

red-free filter ⊃ green filter.

red-free ophthalmoscopy ⊃ ophthalmoscopy.

red glass test (*syn* red filter test) a test for determining diplopia or suppression in which a bright target (e.g. a white light) is fixated while a red filter is held in front of one eye to interrupt fusion. The patient with diplopia will see a red light and a white light. The amount of deviation can be estimated by using a prism of an amount such that it eliminates the double image. The operation can be repeated in all the diagnostic positions of gaze to help identify a paretic extraocular muscle as the distance between the two images increases in the field of action of the paretic muscle. If only one light is seen it indicates suppression of one retinal image.

red muscle describes muscle consisting mainly of slow-twitch fibres. The red colour is derived from the plentiful blood supply and myoglobin. ⊃ muscle fibre types.

red-weakness ⊃ protanomaly.

reducing sugars sugars that are reducing agents, such as glucose, lactose and fructose.

reduction *n* **1.** the process of reducing or state of being reduced. It is the removal of oxygen or the addition of hydrogen or electrons to a substance. ➲ oxidation. **2.** making smaller. Commonly applied to plastic surgical procedures used to decrease the size of structures, for example the nose or breast. **3.** returning to the normal position, e.g. a hernia or after dislocation or fracture. ➲ fracture reduction.

reduction division the first division occurring during meiosis in which the chromosome numbers are halved from the diploid (2n) number to produce the haploid gametes (n). ➲ meiosis.

reductionist paradigm a research term. The belief that measurement and quantification of phenomena can be replicated by an independent observer. The fragmentation of a phenomenon into its constituent parts. ➲ positivist research paradigm.

Reed–Sternberg cell (D Reed, American pathologist, 1874–1964; K Sternberg, Austrian pathologist, 1872–1935) a large, abnormal multinucleated cell found in the lymphatic system in Hodgkin's disease.

reference the clear indication in a piece of work that a source is from another person's work. ➲ Harvard system of referencing, primary referencing (citation), secondary referencing (citation), Vancouver system of referencing.

reference nutrient intake (RNI) one of the UK dietary reference values. The amount of a nutrient required to make sure that the needs of most people in a group (97.5%) are met. Commonly used as an estimate of the micronutrient, e.g. specific vitamins, requirement of a population. ➲ dietary reference values, Appendix 4.

referred pain pain arising in the viscera but occurring at a distance from its source, e.g. pain felt in the arms, neck or jaw in angina pectoris or myocardial infarction despite there being no tissue injury at those locations. It occurs because sensory impulses from the left arm and heart enter the spinal cord at the same level and the person perceives the pain as coming from the arm. Other examples of referred pain include that from the gallbladder felt in the scapular region or the initial pain of acute appendicitis, which may be experienced in the umbilical region despite the appendix being sited in the right, lower part of the abdomen.

reference plane ➲ radiographic baseline.

refined birth rate ➲ birth rate.

reflection 1. the return or bending of light by a surface such that it continues to travel in the same medium. **2.** a mode of thinking used by the therapist (or other practitioner) to monitor their own thoughts, feelings and actions. Reflection is a tool for making sense of complex and uncertain situations and for continually improving performance. ➲ reflective practice.

reflection factor (*syn* reflectance) The ratio of the reflected luminous flux to the incident flux. There are the regular reflection factor and the diffuse reflection factor. The reflection factor is given by Fresnel's formula. ➲ diffusion, Fresnel formula, reflection.

reflective layer in radiography, the layer between the base and the phosphor layer in an intensifying screen whose function is to reflect light towards the film.

reflective practice the conscious and systematic process in which a health professional gives active and careful consideration to personal actions and feelings, aspects of practice, events that impact on the client's situation and to the process of intervention as it unfolds. The ability to review, analyse and evaluate situations, during or after events in order to develop professionally and improve practice.

reflex 1. *adj* literally, reflected or thrown back; involuntary, not controlled by will. **2.** *n* a reflex action. Examples include abdominal reflex, accommodation reflex, anal reflex, asymmetric tonic neck reflex, conditioned reflex, corneal reflex, cough reflex, doll's eye reflex, gag reflex, grasp reflex, knee jerk reflex, Moro (startle) reflex, parachute reflex, pupillary light reflex, rooting reflex, stepping reflex. ➲ deep tendon reflexes.

reflex action rapid innate response by an effector (muscle or gland) to a stimulus detected by neural receptors and signalled by afferent nerves to neurons in the central nervous system whose efferent nerves activate the effector. It results in an involuntary motor or secretory response to a sensory stimulus, e.g. tendon stretch, sneezing, blinking, coughing. Reflexes may be postural or protective. Testing reflexes provides valuable information in the localization and diagnosis of neurological diseases.

reflex arc the basic neurological components that facilitate a simple reflex action—a sensory neuron, which synapses with a motor neuron in the spinal cord or brain. In some reflexes a connector neuron(s), also known as an interneuron(s), provide the connection between sensory and motor neurons via several synapses (Figure R.4).

reflex sympathetic dystrophy (RSD) rare chronic pain syndrome. It is now more correctly termed complex regional pain syndrome as the pathophysiology is more complex and varied than first thought. ➲ complex regional pain syndrome 1.

reflexology *n* a complementary therapy based upon the assertion that the internal body structures are 'mapped out' on the soles and palms (Figure R.5). It is thought that gentle pressure upon the areas corresponding to specific structures can lead to a therapeutic response. ➲ zones.

reflux *n* backward flow. ➲ gastro-oesophageal reflux disease.

reflex nephropathy *n* previously known as chronic pyelonephritis. Caused by failure of the one-way valve system where the ureters enter the bladder. This allows urine to reflux up the ureters when pressure increases in the bladder during voiding. This urine later returns to the bladder and is not immediately voided, thus leading to urine stasis, which in turn predisposes to infection. The constant reflux of infected urine up the ureters results in damage to the renal tissue that can, without effective treatment with antibiotics and or surgical reimplanation of the ureters, lead to renal failure. ➲ vesicoureteric reflux.

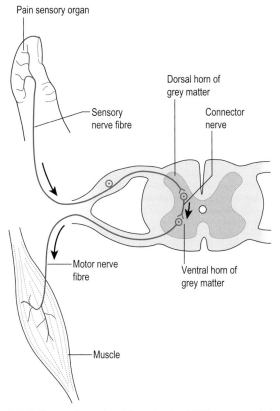

Pain sensory organ

Dorsal horn of grey matter

Sensory nerve fibre

Connector nerve

Motor nerve fibre

Ventral horn of grey matter

Muscle

R.4 Reflex arc (reproduced from Brooker 2006A with permission).

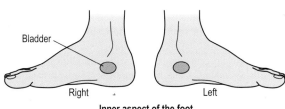

Bladder

Right   Left

Inner aspect of the foot

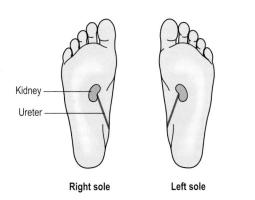

Kidney

Ureter

Right sole   **Left sole**

R.5 Reflexology pressure points on the feet (reproduced from Brooker & Waugh 2007 with permission).

refract 1. to bend a ray of light when it passes through a surface separating media of different refractive indices. **2.** to measure the refractive state of the eye.

refracting unit ⊃ phoropter.

refraction *n* the bending of light rays as they pass through media of different densities. In normal vision, this occurs so that the image is focused on the retina—**refractive** *adj*.

refractive error a condition in which the refractive power of the eye is unable to focus an image on the retina. ⊃ astigmatism, hypermetropia, myopia.

refractive index (*syn* index of refraction) the ratio of the speed of light in a vacuum or in air, *c*, to the speed of light in a given medium, *v*. *Symbol: n*. Hence,

$$n = \frac{c}{v}$$

The speed of light in a given medium depends upon its wavelength. Consequently, the refractive index (index of refraction) varies accordingly, being greater for short wavelengths (blue) than for longer wavelengths (red). The refractive index forms the basis of law of refraction (Snell's law) which quantitatively determines the deviation of light rays traversing a surface separating two media of different refractive indices. *absolute refractive index* the ratio of the speed of light in a vacuum to the speed of light in a given medium. *relative refractive index* the ratio of the speed of light in air (or other medium of reference) to the speed of light in a given medium. ⊃ dispersion, gradient-index lens, high index lens, law of refraction, refract, refractometer, speed of light, wavelength.

refractive keratoplasty ⊃ epikeratoplasty, keratomileusis.

refractive power (F) (*syn* dioptric power, focal power, vergence power) the ability of a lens or an optical system to change the direction of a pencil of rays. It is equal to

$$F = \frac{n'}{f'} = -\frac{n}{f}$$

where *n* and *n'* are the refractive indices of the object and image space, respectively, *f* and *f'* the first and second focal length, respectively, in metres, and the power *F* is expressed in dioptres. ⊃ dioptre, equivalent power, focal length, paraxial equation (fundamental), vergence.

refractometer an instrument for measuring the refractive index (index of refraction) of transparent objects. There exist several types: Abbé's refractometer which is based on the measurement of the critical angle at the interface between a sample and a prism of known index of refraction and uses white light whereas that of Pulfrich, which is based on the same principle as Abbé's, uses monochromatic light. As the refractive index of some materials is related to their water content, the hand-held Atago CL-1 Soft lens refractometer has been calibrated to provide a reading of the percentage of water content of soft contact lenses. ⊃ critical angle, optometer, oxygen permeability, water content (contact lens).

refractometry 1. the measurement of the refractive error of the eye with a refractometer or optometer. **2.** the

Q
R

measurement of the index of refraction of a medium with a refractometer (e.g. Abbé's refractometer).

refractor ⊃ phoropter.

refractor head ⊃ phoropter.

refractory *adj* **1.** resistant to treatment or unmanageable. **2.** a substance resistant to heat. **3.** in dentistry, a mineral suitable for lining furnaces and investing materials for casting moulds.

refractory anaemia (RA) ⊃ myelodysplastic syndrome (MDS).

refractory anaemia with excess blasts (RAEB) ⊃ myelodysplastic syndrome (MDS).

refractory anaemia with sideroblasts (RARS) ⊃ myelodysplastic syndrome (MDS).

refractory cytopenias with multilineage dysplasia (RCMD) ⊃ myelodysplastic syndrome (MDS).

refractory period the period of time after an action potential during which a nerve or muscle fibre is not able to respond to a stimulus. It may be an *absolute refractory period* in which the production of another action potential is impossible, regardless of the nature of the stimulus, or a *relative refractory period* when an action potential may be elicited if the stimulus is sufficiently strong.

reframing a technique for altering negative or self-defeating thought patterns by deliberately replacing them with positive, constructive self-talk. For example, athletes might reframe negative self-talk following failure in a competition by telling themselves that it was a useful learning experience. Frequently included in mental training programmes. Also known as cognitive restructuring.

refresh rate the rate at which an electron beam scans the whole of a computer screen.

regeneration *n* renewal of tissue. Some very superficial wounds may heal by regeneration to leave no visible signs. Damage to fetal tissue also heals by regeneration; healing is characterized by minimal inflammation, fibrosis or scar formation. In dentistry, regeneration techniques are used for the augmentation of alveolar ridges and in guided tissue regeneration. ⊃ guided tissue regeneration.

regional ileitis ⊃ Crohn's disease.

registered nurse, midwife, specialist community public health nurse a term protected by law in many countries including the UK. Only those, whose name appears on the Nursing and Midwifery Council register, after having successfully undergone the prescribed educational programme, can legally be called a registered nurse, midwife or specialist community public health nurse.

registrar of births, marriages and deaths official recorder of births, marriages and deaths in the UK. Part of National Statistics, which also regulates and records civil marriages/partnerships, conducts demographic research and analyses demographic material. Local registry offices are in most towns; births must be registered within 6 weeks in England (2 days in Scotland).

registration paste dental material used to physically record the occlusion of a dentate mouth, partially dentate mouth, or alternatively the occlusal surfaces of registration blocks.

Usually the material will be applied in a plastic form and will set to a rigid or semi-rigid state.

regression *n* **1.** reversion to an earlier stage of development, becoming more childish. Occurs in dementia, especially in older people, and more normally, as a defence mechanism, for instance, in a young child reacting to the birth of a sibling. **2.** in genetics, the tendency for physical characteristics in successive generations to move toward the mean for the population rather than being representative of the parents. For instance a child who has a very tall parent or very short parent is likely to be of average height for the population. **3.** describes the recovery from, or lessening of signs and symptoms of a disease, for example a patient with leukaemia following a course of treatment with cytotoxic drugs.

regression techniques in statistics, various analytical methods used in multivariate statistics. Used to predict dependent variable(s) from independent variable(s). Regression is used to answer such questions as 'how well can we predict the values of one variable, (such as survival) by knowing the value of another (such as treatment technique)'?

regular reflection (*syn* direct reflection, specular reflection) reflection from a polished surface in which there is no scattering and light travels back in a definite direction. ⊃ specular microscope.

regulation in a transformer is caused by resistance in the windings, if the electric load from the secondary winding is increased a higher current flows in the secondary winding but the potential difference across the secondary winding is decreased. ⊃ percentage regulation.

regurgitation *n* backward flow, e.g. of stomach contents into, or through, the mouth, or blood through an incompetent (regurgitant) heart valve.

rehabilitation *n* the process through which a client is helped to achieve their optimum level of functioning in order to overcome or adjust to the limitations imposed by their disability. It involves a planned, supervised and progressive programme in which convalescent or people with disabilities progress towards, or maintain, the maximum degree of physical and psychological independence of which they are capable. Planned rehabilitation programmes are provided for a variety of conditions that include acute myocardial infarction, cardiac failure, chronic respiratory diseases, musculoskeletal injuries, amputations, stroke, spinal cord injury and brain injury. ⊃ cardiac rehabilitation, Functional Independence Measure, pulmonary rehabilitation.

rehabilitation clinician in sports medicine a medical professional who is responsible for the design, progression, supervision and administration of a rehabilitation programme for an injured athlete or sports participant.

rehabilitation in sport in sports medicine, rehabilitation usually refers to the process, commencing at the time of injury or operation, which aims to return the athlete to both training and competition at their previous level, as soon as possible.

rehearsal in memory memory processing depends on two forms of rehearsal of facts: *maintenance rehearsal* where information re-enters short term memory (STM) by repetition (such as repeating the names of a new group); each time the information enters short term memory (STM) appears to enhance its chance of storage in long term memory (LTM); and *elaborative rehearsal* processing information in STM so that it can be coded for storage in LTM. It may use sensory factors, such as sound, or focus on the meaning of the information.

Reifenstein's syndrome (E Reifenstein, American physician/endocrinologist, 1908–1975) an inherited syndrome characterized by hypogonadism, gynaecomastia and azoospermia due to a partial resistance to androgen hormones.

reiki therapy a complementary therapy whereby a reiki practioner positions their hands on a part of the body or in close proximity to the part so that 'universal life force' is transferred to the client. The therapy claims to supply the necessary harmony, etc., that benefit various health problems.

reimplantation ➲ replantation.

reinforced zinc oxide-eugenol cement in dentistry, zinc oxide-eugenol cement that has been reinforced by the addition of a polymeric and/or an inorganic filler in the powder, e.g. EBA cement, or by the addition of a solution of a polymer in the eugenol liquid.

reinforcement *n* a psychological term that describes the methods employed during conditioning to increase the probability and strength of a response. **1.** In *operant conditioning*, a stimulus that, when presented following a response, leads to an increase in the frequency of emission of the response in the future. Also known as a reinforcer and more colloquially as a reward. **2.** describes the process of strengthening the frequency of a response through presenting a reinforcement. *negative reinforcement* the strengthening of the frequency of a response by removing an aversive stimulus—**reinforce** *vt*. ➲ conditioning, punishment.

Reissner's membrane (E Reissner, German anatomist, 1824–1878) the membrane separating the scala vestibuli and scala media in the cochlea of the inner ear. ➲ basilar membrane

Reiter's syndrome (H Reiter, German physician, 1881–1969) ➲ reactive arthritis, sexually acquired reactive arthritis.

reject analysis the examining of images that have been judged to be unacceptable to try to find out why the films have been rejected and whether it is due to equipment or operator problems.

rejection *n* **1.** the act of excluding or denying affection to another person. **2.** the process which leads to the destruction of grafted tissues.

relapse to drift back into a former state of ill-health. In orthodontics, to return towards the original state of malocclusion following correction.

relapsing fever louse-borne or tick-borne infection caused by spirochaetes of the genus *Borrelia*. Characterized by a febrile period of a week or so, with apparent recovery, followed by a further bout of fever.

related in statistics the data are matched—each sample has a matched sample with one or more than one variable in common.

relative afferent pupillary defect (RAPD) ➲ Marcus Gunn's pupil.

relative permittivity (or dielectric constant) of a capacitor is the ratio of its capacitance with the specific dielectric between the plates to its capacitance with air between the plates.

relative poverty ➲ poverty.

relative refractive index ➲ refractive index.

relative refractory period ➲ refractory period.

relative risk ➲ risk

relaxant *n* a drug or technique that reduces tension. ➲ muscle.

relaxation *n* a state of consciousness where individuals feel calm and peaceful. Muscle tension, anxiety and stress are all released.

relaxation techniques often used in health care and health promotion activities such as stress management. They include meditation, progressive muscle relaxation, visual guided imagery and yoga. ➲ biofeedback, hypnosis, Jacobson's progressive relaxation.

relaxin *n* polypeptide hormone secreted by the placenta and ovaries. It is considered to have a role in softening the cervix, relaxing myometrial cells and in loosening the ligaments of the pelvic girdle in preparation for labour. It modifies the collagen in target areas to increase pliability and extensibility. It also is thought to have a softening effect on connective tissue, i.e. pelvic floor and abdominal fascia, increasing their extensibility. The symphysis pubis and sacroiliac joints are particularly affected and this ligamentous laxity may continue for 6 months postpartum. Relaxin may be one of the reasons that low back pain is common during pregnancy.

relay an electrical switch in which one circuit is controlled by another ciruit.

releaser/releasing mechanism a stimulus that launches a cycle of instinctive behaviour.

reliability *n* in research, a term meaning consistency of results. The likelihood of achieving the same findings using the same research conditions over a period of time or when conducted by different researchers or observers.

relief the lessening of pain or distress. In dentistry, the reduction of pressure on a specific area below a denture base. *relief area* an area defined on a plaster model to relieve pressure on underlying tissue. Tin foil is swaged onto this area, and is removed from the processed denture before finishing, to provide a space between the mucosa and a denture. *relief chamber* a recessed area on the fitting surface of a denture obtained by the use of a tin foil spacer.

relieving prism (*syn* compensating prism) an ophthalmic prism prescribed to relieve symptoms caused by an uncompensated heterophoria. ➲ uncompensated heterophoria.

reline to add a material to the existing base of a denture in order to improve its fit.

REM sleep *abbr* rapid eye movement sleep. ⮑ sleep.

remark instruction ignored by the computer, but enables the user to add comments in plain English.

remedial *adj* describes a therapy or treatment intended to cure or improve a condition or deficit.

remineralization the restoration of mineral salts to a tissue, e.g. calcium salts to enamel or bone.

reminiscence therapy a technique, also known as nostalgia therapy, that provides older persons and others with the opportunity to reflect on, and validate, their memories of the past through the use of old pictures, music and objects. These are used to prompt shared discussion of personal experiences.

remission *n* the period of abatement of a fever or other disease. It may occur spontaneously or may result from treatment of the condition.

remittent *adj* increasing and decreasing at periodic intervals.

removable appliance an orthodontic appliance that can be removed from the mouth by the patient.

renal *adj* relating to the kidney, such as renal colic.

renal arteriography the demonstration of the renal arteries following the injection of a contrast agent into a cannula introduced via the femoral artery.

renal artery paired visceral arteries that branch from the abdominal aorta to supply around 25% of the resting cardiac output to the kidneys each minute. ⮑ Colour Section Figures 19, 20.

renal calculus stone in the kidney.

renal capsule the outer fibrous layer surrounding the kidney. ⮑ Colour Section Figure 20.

renal colic extremely severe loin pain caused by the movement of stones or debris within the ureter or kidney. Pain may also be felt in the labia or testes, or the groin. It is characterized by nausea and vomiting, tachycardia and fever if infection is present. Patients are sweaty and may thrash about in an effort to find a position that gives relief.

renal cortex a reddish-brown layer of tissue immediately below the renal capsule and outside the pyramids.

renal failure can be described as acute or chronic. Acute renal failure (ARF) occurs when previously healthy kidneys suddenly fail because of a variety of problems affecting the kidney and its perfusion with blood. This condition is potentially reversible. ARF is treated by haemofiltration or haemodiafiltration until kidney function improves. Chronic renal failure (CRF) occurs when irreversible and progressive pathological destruction of the kidney leads to end-stage renal disease/failure (ESRD). This process usually takes several years but once ESRD is reached, death will follow unless the patient is treated with some type of renal replacement therapy such as dialysis, or renal transplant. ⮑ acute tubular necrosis, crush syndrome, uraemia.

renal function tests such as glomerular filtration rate. ⮑ kidney function tests.

renal glycosuria occurs in patients with a normal blood glucose (sugar) and a lowered renal threshold for glucose.

renal medulla the innermost layer of the kidney, consisting of pale conical-shaped striations, the renal pyramids. ⮑ Colour Section Figure 20.

renal papilla the structure situated at the apex of each renal pyramid; it opens into a minor calyx.

renal pelvis the funnel-shaped structure that acts as a receptacle for urine formed in the kidney. It has a number of branches called calyces, each of which surrounds the apex of a renal pyramid. Urine formed in the nephrons passes through a papilla at the apex of the pyramid into a minor calyx, then into a major calyx before passing through the renal pelvis into the ureter. ⮑ Colour Section Figure 20.

renal rickets rickets secondary to chronic renal failure. ⮑ rickets.

renal threshold the level of a substance (e.g. glucose) in the blood at which it is excreted into the urine.

renal transplant kidney transplant. The transplantation of a single well-matched kidney from a living or cadaveric donor to a recipient with end-stage renal failure. The donated kidney is usually sited in the iliac fossa, rather than in its normal anatomical position, i.e. a heterotopic transplant.

renal tubule the tubular component of the nephron, it comprises Bowman's capsule, proximal convoluted tubule, the loop of Henle, distal convoluted tubule and the collecting tubule. ⮑ nephron.

renal vein paired veins that convey venous blood from the kidney to the inferior vena cava (IVC). The left vein is longer and receives blood from the left suprarenal and gonadal (ovarian or testicular) veins before draining into the IVC. ⮑ Colour Section Figures 19, 20.

Rendu–Osler–Weber disease (H Rendu, French physician, 1844–1902; W Osler Canadian physcian, 1849–1919; F Weber, British physician, 1863–1962) a form of hereditary haemorrhagic telangiectasia.

ren/i, ren/o- a prefix that means 'kidney', e.g. *renin*.

renin *n* a proteolytic enzyme produced and released by the kidney (juxtaglomerular apparatus) in response to low serum sodium or low blood pressure.

renin-angiotensin-aldosterone response a mechanism initiated by renin that is involved with the regulation of fluid balance, sodium level and blood pressure. A plasma protein (angiotensinogen) is activated to produce angiotensin I, which in turn is converted into the powerful vasocontrictor angiotensin II. This also causes aldosterone to be secreted, leading to sodium reabsorption with water thus further raising blood pressure. ⮑ aldosterone, angiotensin, angiotensin-coverting enzyme (ACE).

rennin *n* milk curdling enzyme found in the gastric juice of human infants and ruminants. It converts caseinogen into casein.

renogram radioisotope (radionuclide) study of the kidney.

renography *n* a method of assessing the output and function of the kidneys in radioisotope (radionuclide) imaging by producing time–activity curves.

reoxygenation the process whereby cancer cells gain access to oxygen which is released when cells are killed with

Q
R

low-energy transfer radiations—for example, between radiotherapy fractions. If the cells receive oxygen they are more likely to be killed during the next dose of treatment.

reovirus *n* a group of RNA viruses that includes the rotavirus, which causes gastroenteritis.

repair 1. a natural process to restore normal tissue function, e.g. healing of fractures, diseased and necrosed tissues. Cells injured during radiotherapy attempt to repair themselves; healthy tissue is quicker than tumour cells in achieving the repair. **2.** in dental prosthetics, a prosthesis that has been repaired.

reparative dentine similar to secondary dentine but laid down more rapidly over a period of time as a repair tissue. ➲ dentine.

repercussion ballottement, rebound of an object through a fluid.

repertory grid test an idiographic psychological test developed by American psychologist George Kelly (1905–1966) derived from his personal construct theory that elicits the ways in which an individual views their world by presenting them with a number of sets of three familiar elements (e.g. people that they know) and asking them to identify in what way any two are similar to each other but different from the third. In this way a series of bipolar constructs are elicited (e.g. friendly versus unfriendly) that are said to describe how the person construes their world. ➲ bipolar construct, personal construct theory.

repetitions repeats ('reps') of training actions at short or minimal intervals; contrast 'sets'. ➲ sets.

repetition time in magnetic resonance imaging (MRI), the time between the beginning of one radio frequency pulse sequence to the start of the next.

repetitive strain injury (RSI) a misleading term used to describe diffuse pain and inflammation randomly occurring in the hand and forearm arising from repetitive activities in the workplace, aggravated by static posture. ➲ work-related upper limb disorder.

replacement arthroplasty insertion of an inert prosthesis of similar shape into a joint, such as the hip, ankle, knee, shoulder, etc.

replantation preferred term for the replacement of a tooth in its socket following deliberate or traumatic avulsion.

replenishment in radiography, the addition of an amount of developer and fixer to the processing tank every time a film is processed to maintain the activity of the solutions.

repolarization *n* the process whereby the membrane potential of an excitable cell returns from the depolarized state to its polarized resting (negative) state.

repopulation the re-growth of tissue cells, during fractionated radiotherapy normal tissue cells can regenerate at a faster rate than the cancer cells therefore reducing the side effects of the treatment.

repression *n* a mental defence mechanism whereby painful events, unacceptable thoughts and impulses are impelled into, and remain in, the unconscious mind.

reproductive system the structures necessary for reproduction. In the male it includes the testes, deferent ducts (vas deferens), prostate gland, seminal vesicles, urethra and penis. ➲ Colour Section Figure 16. In the female it includes the ovaries, uterine (fallopian) tubes, uterus, vagina and vulva. ➲ Colour Section Figure 17.

RER or R *abbr* respiratory exchange ratio.

RES *abbr* reticuloendethelial system. ➲ monocyte-macrophage system.

rescue breaths artificial respiration used in first aid situations to oxygenate the blood when the casualty is not breathing or has suffered a cardiac arrest. Depending on the age of the casualty mouth-to-mouth or mouth-to-mouth/nose rescue breaths are used (Figure R.6). ➲ Appendix 10.

research *n* systematic investigation of data, etc., and observations to establish facts or principles, so as to produce organized scientific knowledge. Research may be quantitative or qualitative. Quantitative research defines variables to be collected and converted into numerical values. The data are analysed either to describe the data using descriptive statistics, or to test whether there are relationships between the data using inferential statistics. On the other hand, in qualitative research typically there is uncertainty about the relevance of data so predefining the data to collect is not useful. Qualitative research studies typically uses small samples, but collect more data on each subject usually by observation or interview. ➲ Appendix 14.

research design how a research study is to be undertaken such as data collection method, statistical analysis, etc.

research into practice a situation where the validated results of a piece of academic research are used to change or modify existing accepted practice (e.g. clinical or educational).

research question the question contains the population, the manoeuvre, the study population and the outcomes. The research question should specify one measurable outcome, in addition to all conditions and any other important variables.

resection *n* surgical excision.

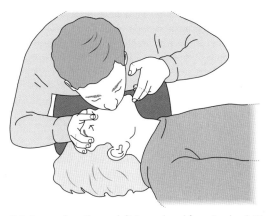

R.6 Rescue breaths—adult (reproduced from Brooker & Waugh 2007 with permission).

Q
R

resectoscope *n* an instrument passed along the urethra; it permits resection of tissue from the base of the bladder and prostate under direct vision, and for other treatments for benign enlargement of the prostate. ⮂ transurethral resection of prostate.

reservoirs of infection the skin, respiratory tract and bowel are colonized by bacteria and fungi which form the normal flora in humans. The normal flora may become pathogenic under certain circumstances.

resident flora normal flora. ⮂ transient flora.

residential home the premises where residential care is delivered by the independent sector, social services or voluntary organizations.

residual *adj* remaining.

residual air the air remaining in the lung after forced expiration.

residual caries dental caries allowed to remain on the floor of a prepared cavity, generally because its removal would lead to pulp exposure.

residual cyst cyst left behind following the removal of a pulpless tooth from which it arose.

residual ridge the bone and covering tissue that remain after the extraction of teeth.

residual thiosulphate test a method of assessing the archival permanence of a film by dropping a drop of solution on the film and comparing it with a colour chart.

residual volume (RV) the air remaining in the lungs at the end of a forced expiration. This lung volume can only be measured in the lung function laboratory by means of body box plethysmography or gas transfer tests; it cannot be measured with simple spirometry.

residual urine the volume of urine remaining in the bladder after micturition.

resin 1. Substance that is secreted naturally by certain plants and insects, e.g. rosin, or produced synthetically. **2.** Uncompounded polymeric material used in the manufacture of plastics. Many used in dentistry. *acrylic resin* general term for the resinous material of the various esters of acrylic acid. Its chief use is in the manufacture of dentures and synthetic resin teeth. *autopolymerizing resin* a resin whose polymerization is initiated by a chemical activator and without the application of heat. The preferred term is *cold curing acrylic resin*. *composite resin* hard, durable, strong filled resin used for tooth-coloured restorations. The filler may consist of finely powdered glass or quartz crystals. *epoxy resin* a synthetic resin characterized by the reactive epoxy or ethyloxyline groups. It is resistant to moderate heat and chemicals and is used as an adhesive and in the manufacture of dies. *resin bonding (bonding resin)* unfilled resin used to assist the adhesion of a resin compound to tooth structure or restorative materials. ⮂ adhesive. *resin cement* any of a group of filling or cementing materials that may be filled or unfilled and marketed in single-, dual- or multi-component systems.

resin modified glass ionomer cement ⮂ glass ionomer cement.

resistance *n* power of resisting. **1.** the impedance to the flow of electrons; it is measured in ohms. **2.** in psychology, describes the force which prevents repressed thoughts from re-entering the conscious mind from the unconscious.

resistance form a design feature of a tooth preparation that imparts strength to a restoration and the tooth when under load.

resistance to infection the capacity to withstand infection. ⮂ immunity.

resistance training strength training. In sports medicine, the training activities that increase muscle size and strength by working against resistance. ⮂ strength training.

resisted movement a movement performed that overcomes an additional resistance in addition to the weight of the body part itself, for example, an arm curl with a 5 kg weight is a resisted exercise. ⮂ active movement, assisted active movement, movement classification, passive movement.

resistivity index the ultrasonic method of numerically determining the resistance of blood flowing through a vessel by using the equation systolic – diastolic/mean.

resistor an object which opposes the flow of electrons; resistors in series are placed end to end, resistors in parallel are connected parallel to each other.

resolution *n* **1.** indicates the size of the smallest object that a system will record and the smallest distance that must exist between two objects before they are seen as two separate objects. It is expressed as line pair per millimetre. In ultrasound the ability to distinguish between two adjacent structures, the higher the frequency of the probe the better the resolution. **2.** the subsidence of inflammation; describes the earliest indications of a return to normal, as when, in lobar pneumonia, the consolidation begins to liquefy.

resolve to return to normal following an inflammatory reaction.

resonance *n* the musical quality elicited on percussing a cavity which contains air. ⮂ vocal resonance.

resonate mechanically deform, vibrate.

resorption *n* the act of absorbing again, e.g. absorption of a callus following bone fracture, the roots of the primary (deciduous teeth), or blood from a haematoma. In dentistry, the removal of the calcified parts of teeth and jaws. ⮂ alveolar resorption.

resource management a system initiated in 1986 by government aimed at increasing functional efficiency and effectiveness by devolving management to local groups. The local managers draw up business plans, are responsible and accountable for allocation of resources and are more responsive to local demands, needs and changes.

respiration *n* the gaseous exchange between a cell and its environment. (But used generally to mean breathing; hence respiratory system is the lungs and the air passages leading to them)—**respiratory** *adj*. ⮂ abdominal breathing, Cheyne–Stokes respiration, external respiration, internal or tissue respiration, Kussmaul respiration, paradoxical respiration.

respirator *n* an apparatus worn over the nose and mouth and designed to purify the air breathed through it.

respiratory acidosis a disturbance of acid–base balance due to hypoventilation and reduced alveolar ventilation with the accumulation of waste carbon dioxide. It can occur with type II respiratory failure and conditions affecting the respiratory muscles (e.g. neurological disorders). ⟶ acid–base balance.

respiratory alkalosis a disturbance of acid–base balance due to hyperventilation and lowering of carbon dioxide level. It may be due to anxiety states (panic attacks), respiratory centre stimulation following excess ingestion of salicylates and may be produced iactrogenically in patients having mechanical ventilation. ⟶ acid–base balance.

respiratory bronchiolitis–interstitial lung disease (RB-ILD) one of the idiopathic interstitial pneumonias. It is more common in men and smokers. It usually presents in the forties or fifties. The cessation of smoking may lead to an improvement. The natural history of the disease remains unclear.

respiratory centres the complex of neurons in the brainstem where the breathing rhythm is generated, and where various neural inputs influence the neural output to the respiratory muscles which in turn determines the depth and frequency of breathing. ⟶ apneustic centre, carotid bodies, chemoreceptors, Hering–Breuer reflex, pneumotaxic centre, Colour Section Figure 34.

respiratory distress syndrome (RDS) ⟶ acute/adult respiratory distress syndrome, multiple organ dysfunction syndrome, neonatal respiratory distress syndrome.

respiratory exchange ratio (RER or R) the ratio of carbon dioxide released to oxygen taken in, by exchange between the body and the atmosphere, over a period of measurement by analysis of expired gases. Used in the estimation of oxygen consumption ($\dot{V}O_2$) and from that the equivalent energy expenditure to allow calculation of the 'true' difference between inspired and expired oxygen percentage when the RER is other than 1:1. In a steady state (when carbon dioxide is neither being stored nor over-excreted by hyperventilation) RER is equal to the respiratory quotient which reflects the proportion of the different nutrients being used for energy production. ⟶ respiratory quotient.

respiratory failure failure of the lungs to oxygenate the blood adequately or remove waste carbon dioxide (CO_2). The management depends on the type, cause and severity, but includes: oxygen therapy, mechanical ventilation, tracheostomy, supportive measures and treatment of the underlying cause. It may be classified into two broad types. *type I respiratory failure* which is usually acute but may be chronic. It is characterized by hypoxia without hypercapnia. The blood gases show hypoxaemia – PaO_2 is low (<8.0 kPa) without hypercapnia and the $PaCO_2$ is normal or reduced (<6.6 kPa). It occurs in conditions that damage lung tissue. Acute causes include acute/adult respiratory distress syndrome (ARDS), asthma, pneumonia, pulmonary oedema, pulmonary embolus, pneumothorax, etc. Chronic type I failure may occur in pulmonary fibrosis, severe anaemia, etc. *type II respiratory failure* is more often chronic but can be acute when it is called asphyxia. Type II is characterized by hypoxia and hypercapnia. The blood gases show hypoxaemia – PaO_2 is low (<8.0 kPa) and hypercapnia – $PaCO_2$ is high (>6.6 kPa). It occurs in situations where alveolar ventilation is inadequate to excrete the waste carbon dioxide generated by cell metabolism. Acute causes include acute epiglottitis, foreign body in the airway, flail chest, severe acute asthma, paralysis of respiratory muscles, injury to brainstem, narcotic drugs, etc. Chronic type II failure occurs in chronic obstructive pulmonary disease.

respiratory frequency (f) number of breaths per minute; usually known as respiratory rate or breathing frequency.

respiratory function tests tests available for assessing respiratory function and aiding in diagnosis of respiratory disease. Includes spirometry to measure FEV_1 (forced expiratory volume in one second), and FVC (forced vital capacity) and in more specialized laboratories measurements of total lung volume and gas transfer factor. ⟶ arterial blood gases (ABGs), carbon monoxide diffusing capacity test (DLCO), respiratory function tests, spirometry.

'respiratory pump' ⟶ intrapleural pressure.

respiratory quotient (RQ) the ratio of carbon dioxide produced to oxygen used by the whole body, or by any of its tissues, over the period of measurement. Differs according to the metabolic substrate, ranging from 0.7 for fat alone to 1 for carbohydrate alone. Overall whole-body RQ on a typical mixed diet is about 0.8. Compare respiratory exchange ratio.

respiratory syncytial virus (RSV) a paramyxovirus that causes bronchiolitis and pneumonia in infants and small children. Infants under six months may be severely affected.

respiratory system deals with gaseous exchange. Comprises the nose, nasopharynx, larynx, trachea, bronchi and lungs. ⟶ Colour Section Figures 6, 7.

respite care short term or temporary care provided within a health or social care facility to allow relief for family and other home carers. May be residential or on a daily basis. Care may be provided within institutions or within the person's own home. It has been argued that access to respite care should be the right of all carers. Others argue that respite care demeans ill and disabled people by viewing them as a burden and by failing to resource more appropriate forms of assistance.

response latency ⟶ reaction time.

responsiveness (of a measure) the extent to which a measurement instrument detects clinically important changes over time. These changes are often defined in terms of how significant they are to patients. There is no single agreed method for expressing an instrument's responsiveness.

rest 1. natural state of relaxation. **2.** a component of a partial prosthesis resting on the occlusal, lingual, cingulum or incisal surface of a tooth to resist a vertical load.

rest face height ⟶ rest vertical dimension.

resting cell describes a cell that is between mitotic divisions. ⟶ cell cycle.

resting flow the salivary flow that occurs normally in the absence of exogenous stimulation.

Q
R

669

resting metabolic rate (RMR) ⊃ metabolic rate.

resting splint a splint that is used during night time or when a person is at rest to preserve normal joint alignments or alleviate pain/prevent deformity.

resting state of accommodation (*syn* dark accommodation, dark focus—these two terms are not strictly synonymous but as they have been found to correlate well, they have been adopted as synonyms, tonic accommodation) the passive state of accommodation of the eye in the absence of a stimulus, i.e. when the eye is either in complete darkness, or looking at a bright empty field. In this condition, the pre-presbyopic eye is usually focused at an intermediate point (about 80 cm on average, although there are large variations), that is, the emmetropic eye becomes myopic. This is presumably due to a balance between a parasympathetic innervation to the circular fibres of the ciliary muscle and a sympathetic innervation to the longitudinal fibres of the ciliary muscle. Thus, the resting state of accommodation would correspond to a position of equilibrium between the two systems. Accommodation from this state to the near point of accommodation would be the response to parasympathetic stimulation; and accommodation from this state to the far point of accommodation would be the response to sympathetic stimulation. ⊃ ciliary muscle, night myopia, vergence.

restitution restoration putting right; movement of the fetal head after delivery in the anteroposterior diameter, to correct its position in relation to the shoulders.

rest jaw relation the relationship of the mandible to the maxilla when the former is in the rest position.

restless leg syndrome restless legs characterized by paraesthesiae like creeping, crawling, itching and prickling.

restoration the end-result of dental procedures carried out to restore the form, function and appearance of teeth.

restorative dentistry a general term for the dental care provided to establish a stable and healthy functional dentition. Specializes in restoring the hard tissues of teeth that have been damaged or become diseased. Includes the use of fillings, caps, inlays, crowns, bridges, dentures and implants. Covers conservative, periodontal, prosthetic, orthodontic, endodontic and surgical procedures.

restorative material the material used to restore the form and function of a tooth.

rest pain pain in the legs and feet caused by ischaemia. The pain occurs when the patient lies down and is relieved by sitting or standing up. ⊃ peripheral vascular disease.

rest position of the mandible the natural position assumed by the mandible when the mandibular musculature is in a relaxed state and the person is in an upright position.

restrainer in radiography, a chemical to improve the selectivity of a solution; in the developer solution either benzotriazole or potassium bromide is used to ensure low fog and high image contrast.

rest re-injury cycle a pattern of injury that occurs when an athlete returns to activity after an injury and subsequently aggravates that injury due to inadequate recovery.

restrictive lung disease conditions that limit lung and chest wall expansion, thereby reducing total lung capacity. They can be caused by lung diseases such as pulmonary fibrosis; pleural disease, e.g. pneumothorax and mesothelioma; neuromuscular diseases such as muscular dystrophies and phrenic nerve palsy; bony abnormalities of the thoracic cage and spine, e.g. pectus excavatum and ankylosing spondylitis; and with subdiaphragmatic conditions, e.g. obesity and ascites. Its diagnosis is facilitated with simple spirometric measures where possible. ⊃ spirometry.

rest seat in dentistry, that part of the tooth that has been prepared to receive a rest.

rest vertical dimension the vertical dimension when the mandible is in the rest position.

resuscitation *n* restoration to life of one who is collapsed or apparently dead—**resuscitative** *adj.* ⊃ cardiopulmonary resuscitation.

retained placenta placenta which fails to be expelled within the expected time limit, dependent on whether the third stage of labour was actively or passively managed. It is caused by *placenta accreta, p. increta* or *p. percreta*, requiring manual removal under anaesthesia, or occasionally hysterectomy. Commonly the placenta is partially separated causing haemorrhage and maternal shock, as a result of poor uterine action and inadequate uterine contraction following birth of the infant; treated with manual stimulation per abdomen or administration of oxytocic drugs to encourage the uterus to contract so the placenta separates and can be delivered. ⊃ post partum haemorrhage.

retained teeth the primary teeth that are retained beyond their normal time of exfoliation.

retainer various devices used in dentistry, such as the fixed or removable retainer used to maintain the position of the teeth following orthodontic treatment. **1.** in prosthetic dentistry, an attachment such as a clasp which retains a partial denture against dislodging forces. **2.** in orthodontics, a passive removable appliance or device cemented to teeth which maintains their position following active orthodontic treatment. *bonded retainer* in orthodontics, use of a wire or other structure bonded directly to teeth in order to retain their position following orthodontic tooth movement. *Essix retainer* a clear, thin vacuum-formed retainer used in orthodontics. Can also be used to correct mild malocclusions. *Hawley retainer* an orthodontic removable appliance used to retain the tooth position achieved following orthodontic treatment. The design is a labial bow with Adams' clasps for retention. **3.** restoration cemented to an abutment tooth and serving as the retention for a bridge. *matrix band retainer* ⊃ matrix band.

retarder in dentistry, a substance that slows down a chemical reaction such as the setting of plaster of Paris or alginate impression materials.

retardation *n* **1.** the slowing of a process which has already been carried out at a quicker rate or higher level. **2.** arrested growth or function from any cause.

retching *n* straining at vomiting. The involuntary spasmodic but ineffectual attempt to vomit. May be caused by stimulation of the soft palate or the posterior third of the tongue.

rete a network, especially blood vessels.

retention *n* **1.** retaining of facts in the memory. **2.** accumulation of that which is normally excreted, such as urinary retention.

retention cyst a cyst caused by the blocking of a duct. ➲ ranula.

retention (dental) 1. in prosthetics, the resistance of a prosthesis to dislodgement along the natural path of displacement (usually vertical). *direct retention* retention obtained for a partial denture by the use of clasps or attachments to resist its dislodgement. *indirect retention* retention obtained by extending a partial denture base to provide a class II lever. **2.** in orthodontics, the use of a removable or fixed retainer. An alternative term for fixation. *acid etch retention* retention for certain filling materials provided by etching or roughening the enamel surface of a tooth by the use of dilute acids. *retention form* any design feature of a tooth preparation that prevents displacement of a restoration.

retention (Loe) index ➲ index (dental).

retention mucocoele a pathological collection of mucus within the soft tissues and arising from a salivary gland. May be due to extravasation from a gland or a duct or to retention within a duct.

retention of urine accumulation of urine within the bladder due to interference of nerve supply, outflow obstruction or psychological factors.

retentive arm the flexible component of a prosthesis that engages in an undercut of a tooth to provide retention. ➲ clasp.

reticular *adj* resembling a net.

reticular activating system (RAS) a diffuse functional area in the reticular formation of the brainstem. It has connections with other parts of the brain, including the cerebral cortex, thalamus, hypothalamus and cerebellum; it is involved in the level of consciousness, sleep–wake cycles, the state of cortical arousal and some autonomic functions.

reticular formation the collection of neurons present in the brainstem that regulate the level of consciousness and some autonomic functions. ➲ reticular activating system.

reticule a thin plastic tray holding lead markers which are positioned to delineate the geometry of the radiotherapy treatment field and a set treatment distance.

reticulin the protein found in connective reticular fibres present in lymphoid tissue.

reticulocyte *n* an immature circulating red blood cell which still contains traces of the nucleus. Accounts for up to 2% of circulating red cells.

reticulocytosis *n* an increase in the number of reticulocytes in the blood indicating active red blood cell formation in the marrow. ➲ reticulocyte.

reticuloendothelial system (RES) ➲ monocyte-macrophage system.

reticulosis abnormal proliferation of cells of the reticuloendothelial system (monocyte-macrophage system) such as occurs in lymphomas and certain leukaemias.

reticulum a network.

retina *n* the light-receptive, innermost nervous tunic of the eye. Consists of a multiple-layer complex of neurosensory retina containing nerve cells that include photoreceptors (rods and cones), and a layer of pigmented cells beyond the neurosensory retina. The retina is a thin transparent membrane (125 μm near the ora serrata and 350μm near the macula) which extends over an area of about 266 mm^2. It lies between the vitreous body (humour) and the choroid, and extends from the optic disc to the ora serrata. Near the posterior pole and temporal to the optic disc is the macula, at the centre of which is the foveola which provides the best visual acuity. The retina contains at least 10 distinct layers, of which there are two synaptic layers. They are from the outermost layer to the innermost: (1) the retinal pigment epithelium; (2) the layer of rods and cones; (3) the external limiting membrane; (4) the outer nuclear layer; (5) the outer molecular (or outer plexiform) layer; (6) the inner nuclear layer (which contains the bipolar, amacrine and horizontal cells and nuclei of the fibres of Mueller); (7) the inner molecular (or inner plexiform) layer; (8) the ganglion cell layer; (9) the nerve fibre layer (or stratum opticum); and (10) the internal limiting membrane. The two synaptic layers where visual signals must synapse as they emerge from the rods and cones on their way to the optic nerve are the two molecular layers (5 and 7) (Figure R.7)—**retinal** *adj.* ➲ amacrine cell, bipolar cell, fovea centralis, foveola, fundus, ganglion cell, horizontal cell, macula lutea, Mueller's

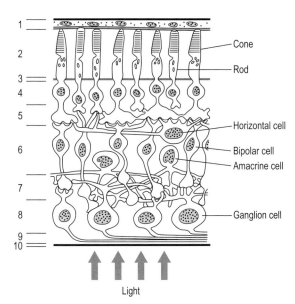

R.7 Schematic representation of the cells and layers of the central primate retina—simplified (reproduced from Millodot 2004 with permission).

cell, optic cup, optic disc, retinitis, retinopathy, rod, Colour Section Figure 15.

retinaculum tenaculum. A structure that keeps another body structure/organ in place, for example, the retinacula over the tendons of the hand—**retinacula** *pl*.

retinal 1. *adj* pertaining to the retina. **2.** *n* a light sensitive molecule present in the photoreceptors of the retina. It is derived from retinol (vitamin A) and combines with an opsin to form rhodopsin. Also known as retinene or retinaldehyde. ⮑ rhodopsin.

retinal arterial occlusion an occlusion of the central retinal artery (CRAO) is characterized by a sudden loss of vision and a defective direct pupillary light reflex. The retinal arterioles are constricted while the veins are full but a venous pulse is absent. The retina appears white and swollen, especially near the posterior pole, and the choroid is seen through it as a cherry-red spot. If the occlusion persists the cherry-red spot disappears after several weeks, the retinal arterioles remain attenuated, eventually becoming white threads, and the optic disc becomes atrophic. Occlusion is more frequently limited to one branch of the central retinal artery (BRAO). In this case, the clinical picture is limited to the area supplied by the branch and this is associated with a visual field defect in that region. Causes include retinal emboli due to a cardiovascular disease, systemic hypertension, temporal arteritis, oral contraceptives, syphilis, intravenous drug misuse or trauma. Treatment is urgent as there is an extremely serious risk of blindness. ⮑ amaurosis fugax, central retinal artery, cherry-red spot, fluorescein, pupillary light reflex, temporal arteritis, Colour Section Figure 102.

retinal corresponding points (*syn* normal retinal correspondence) two points (or small areas), one in each retina, which when simultaneously stimulated give rise to the perception of a single object. These points share a common line of direction and this explains why stimulating them is perceived as arising from the same point in space. ⮑ afterimage transfer test, horopter, law of identical visual directions, Panum's area, retinal disparity.

retinal densitometry a technique used to study visual pigments *in vivo*. It consists of measuring the small fraction of light that is reflected by the pigment epithelium of the retina before and after bleaching with a bright source of light. ⮑ visual pigment.

retinal detachment (RD) (*syn* ablatio retinae) it occurs when the neurosensory retina becomes separated from the pigmented epithelium layer. It is known as rhegmatogenous if a hole is present; detachments without a hole are sometimes described as non-rhegmatogenous. Fluid collects in that potential space (this is called serous retinal detachment). It may do so from the vitreous when there is a retinal hole or tear (a rhegmatogenous retinal detachment) or from the choroid when the retinal pigment epithelium is damaged (this is called exudative or secondary retinal detachment). Retinal detachment may also occur when the vitreoretinal membranes pull the neurosensory retina away from the

retinal pigment epithelium (this is called traction retinal detachment). It can be observed with the ophthalmoscope as it is raised above the level of the surrounding retina requiring more plus power to focus on it. The detached retina appears dark red to grey and may show some folds. Retinal detachment may be associated with degenerative myopia, ocular trauma, head trauma, age-related retinal degeneration, shrinkage of the vitreous, following cataract surgery, tumours, inflammation and diabetes. Symptoms include a loss of vision in the visual field corresponding to the detached area (a curtain or shadow in the field of vision), photopsia and a sudden shower of floaters that move with the eye. Early treatment is essential to prevent blindness in the affected eye. Retinal detachment involving the area around the macula lutea is treated as an emergency. It consists of indenting the sclera over the detached area and usually draining the subretinal fluid. The hole or detachment may be sealed using techniques that include lasers, cryotherapy, injection of a gas bubble or bands. For example, if the lesion is small, retinochoroidal adhesion may be achieved with either laser photocoagulation or cryotherapy. ⮑ central serous retinopathy, Coats' disease, Ehlers–Danlos syndrome, floaters, macular hole, metamorphopsia, photocoagulation, photopsia, retinal dialysis, retinal tear, retinopathy of prematurity, retinoschisis, vitrectomy, vitreous detachment. ⮑ Colour Section Figure 103.

retinal dialysis (*syn* retinal disinsertion) a retinal tear at the ora serrata. It usually results from trauma, although some tears occur spontaneously. If the trauma is intense there may also be a retinal tear at the optic disc but the most frequent location is in the lower temporal quadrant. The condition is most typically asymptomatic. However, as it often gives rise to retinal detachment, the patient may report some of the symptoms associated with the latter. Perimetry and binocular indirect ophthalmoscopy are essential in the examination of this condition. In some cases the tear does not progress, but because of the risk of retinal detachment, patients must be referred to a retinal specialist. ⮑ ora serrata, retinal detachment.

retinal disinsertion ⮑ retinal dialysis.

retinal disparity (*syn* binocular disparity) binocular vision in which the two retinal images of a single object do not fall on corresponding retinal points, i.e. when the object lies off the horopter. If, however, the two retinal images still fall within Panum's area the object will still be seen single. At the fixation point this may cause over or under convergence of the eyes. This particular case is called fixation disparity (or retinal slip). The presence of fixation disparity often indicates that binocular vision is under stress and the patient has an uncompensated heterophoria. Optical correction or orthoptic exercises usually eliminate the symptoms. Fixation disparity can be measured either (a) directly (e.g. Disparometer, Wesson Fixation Disparity Card, both consisting of targets with pairs of vernier lines of various angular separation, each line being seen by one eye through polarizing filters), or (b) indirectly as an associated phoria (e.g. Mallett fixation disparity unit). ⮑ depth perception, Disparometer, Mallett fixation disparity unit, Panum's area, random-dot stereogram, retinal corresponding points, stereopsis, stereoscopic visual acuity, uncompensated heterophoria.

retinal exudates exudates in the retina are opacities which result from the escape of plasma and white blood cells from defective blood vessels. They usually look greyish white or yellowish and are circular or ovoid in shape. They are sometimes classified into three groups according to size: (a) punctate hard exudates which often tend to coalesce; (b) exudates of moderate size, such as 'cotton-wool or soft exudates' as, for example, in hypertension or in diabetic retinopathy. These 'exudates' have ill-defined margins and are areas of ischaemia containing cytoid bodies, unlike hard exudates which are generally lipid deposits; (c) larger exudates, as found in the severe forms of retinopathy. ⊃ diabetic retinopathy, hypertensive retinopathy.

retinal glioma ⊃ retinoblastoma.

retinal hypoxia inadequate supply of oxygen to the retina. Retinal hypoxia leads to neovascularization.

retinal incongruity ⊃ abnormal retinal correspondence (ARC).

retinal pigment epithelium (RPE) a brown layer of the retina situated next to the choroid composed of cells filled with pigment (mainly fuscin and melanin). Depending upon the amount of pigment, the fundus will appear dark or light. It is also responsible for supplying metabolites and other needs to the photoreceptors, and helps in retinal adherence and vitamin A metabolism. A dysfunction of this tissue can be detected with the electro-oculogram. This tissue can be transplanted and this may help treat age-related maculopathy/macular degeneration. ⊃ Bruch's membrane, electro-oculogram, fuscin, melanin, Usher's syndrome.

retinal tear an opening in the retina that may be caused by trauma, degeneration or most commonly proliferative vitreoretinopathy in which the vitreous body (humour) adheres to the retina and pulls it from the point of adherence during or just after an abrupt eye movement. The tear appears horseshoe-shaped or round or occasionally slit-like. The patient often complains of photopsia and seeing floaters and they may present with a vitreous haemorrhage. Retinal tears may lead to rhegmatogenous or traction retinal detachment. Management includes laser photocoagulation or cryopexy. ⊃ retinal detachment.

retinal vasculitis ⊃ Eales' disease.

retinal vein occlusion an occlusion of the central retinal vein can be either non-ischaemic CRVO (or venous-stasis retinopathy) which is the most common type, or ischaemic CRVO (or haemorrhagic retinopathy). The non-ischaemic type is characterized by some loss of vision, slight impairment of the pupil responses to light and partial or complete central scotoma due to macular oedema. The ophthalmoscopic picture shows retinal haemorrhages, flame-shaped in appearance and distributed throughout the whole fundus, dilated and tortuous veins and a swollen optic disc. In some cases cotton-wool exudates are also noted. When the condition affects young adults it is commonly referred to as papillophlebitis (or optic disc vasculitis) in which the clinical picture is similar except that the pupillary responses to light are normal and the patient is often asymptomatic. The ischaemic type which usually affects older people is a more severe type and the signs and symptoms are much more marked than in the non-ischaemic type. Occlusion is more frequently limited to one branch of the central retinal vein (BRVO). In this case the clinical picture is limited to the retinal area drained by the occluded branch, but most patients will have some loss of vision depending on the extent of the macular oedema. Predisposing causes are cardiovascular disease, systemic hypertension, diabetes or raised intraocular pressure. Treatment depends on the primary cause. Photocoagulation is used in some cases. ⊃ central retinal vein, fluorescein, exudates, preretinal haemorrhage, Colour Section Figure 104.

retinene ⊃ retinal.

retinitis *n* inflammation of the retina. This usually follows inflammations of the vitreous body, retinal vessels and especially of the choroid. Retinitis leads to an exudation of cells into the vitreous body and, if serious, vision will be affected. If the inflammation affects the macular area there will be a loss of vision. Haemorrhages and oedema (producing a blurring of the margins of the optic disc) are also usually present.

retinitis exudativa externa ⊃ Coats' disease.

retinitis pigmentosa (RP) (*syn* primary pigmentary retinal dystrophy) a primary pigmentary dystrophy of the retina followed by migration of pigment. It is an inherited disease characterized by night blindness and constricted visual fields. Inheritance of RP is complex as many mutant genes have been identified. RP may be inherited as an autosomal dominant, autosomal recessive or as a X-linked trait. The condition is usually bilaterally symmetrical. The rod system is damaged but cones are also involved to some degree and the electroretinogram amplitude is subnormal. The disease usually begins in adolescence with night blindness, followed by a ring scotoma in the periphery that spreads until only a small contracted central field remains. Ophthalmoscopic examination reveals a yellowish atrophy of the optic nerve, severe arterial attenuation and conspicuous pigment proliferation which begins in the equatorial region. The areas of pigment have dense centres and irregular shaped processes. ⊃ electroretinogram, hemeralopia, keratoconus, tritanopia, tunnel vision.

retinitis proliferans ⊃ proliferative retinopathy.

retin/o a prefix that means 'retina', e.g. *retinopathy*.

retinoblastoma *n* (*syn* retinal glioma) a malignant tumour of the neuroglial element of the retina; occurs exclusively in children. It is usually noted in the first two years of life, although in some cases it may not be until after age 5 years. It is the most common intraocular tumour of childhood. There is a retinoblastoma gene; it was identified on chromosome 13q14. Most individuals who inherit a mutant copy of the retinoblastoma gene sustain a second hit to the remaining normal copy of the gene and develop the disease. The most

Q
R

common ocular manifestations are leukocoria and strabismus and sometimes, red eye, glaucoma and orbital cellulitis. Diagnosis is usually made by the appearance of a greyish reflex of light observed at the pupil, although often by that time the pupil is fixed and the eye is blind. Treatment includes external beam radiotherapy, photocoagulation, cryotherapy and chemotherapy, while advanced tumours are managed by enucleation. ➲ cat's eye reflex, leukocoria.

retinochoroiditis ➲ chorioretinitis.

retinoids *npl* a group of vitamin A derivatives. ➲ Appendix 5.

retinol *n* various forms of vitamin A, which can be converted to metabolically active substances, such as retinal.

retinopathy *n* disease of the retina. Includes those caused by diabetes, abnormality of the retinal vessels and hypertension, sun damage. ➲ background diabetic retinopathy, central serous retinopathy, diabetic retinopathy, hypertensive retinopathy, proliferative retinopathy, solar retinopathy.

retinopathy of prematurity previously known as retrolental fibroplasia. A bilateral retinal disease which commonly affects preterm infants exposed to high ambient oxygen concentrations. It is characterized by proliferation and tortuosity of blood vessels, usually with haemorrhages and retinal detachment accompanied by an accumulation of fibrous tissue on the surface of the retina. Some of the infants may develop cicatricial complications which may be innocuous or may progress to cover the central region of the retina and cause visual impairment. Other complications may be myopia or glaucoma. This condition is now less common, but as the concentration of oxygen which will prevent retinal damage is not known, vigilance and careful monitoring of oxygen tension level remains essential in the care of preterm babies. ➲ leukocoria.

retinoschisis a split in the layers of the retina. A vitreoretinal degeneration characterized by splitting of the retina into two layers. It occurs either as a hereditary disease or as an acquired condition (70% of these patients are hypermetropic). The X-linked hereditary condition (called juvenile retinoschisis) affects only males and usually involves the macula with loss of central vision. The congenital condition is characterized by a splitting of the nerve fibre layer from the retina whereas the acquired form, which is the most common, results in a splitting at the outer plexiform layer. The latter usually begins in the temporal periphery appearing as a coalescence of microcystoid degenerations with a smooth transparent elevation and associated with an absolute scotoma. The condition may spread to involve the entire peripheral fundus. Holes in the two layers are common and are a sign of progression. The inner layer contains blood vessels and sometimes has small whitish flakes on it which are called 'snowflakes'. ➲ retinal detachment.

retinoscope *n* (skiascope) an instrument for determining objectively the refractive state of the eye. It consists of a light source, a condensing lens and a mirror. The mirror is either semi-transparent or has a hole through which the retinoscopist can view the patient's eye along the retinoscope's beam of light. A patch of light is formed on the

patient's retina and by moving that patch in a given direction and observing the direction in which it appears to move after refraction by the patient's eye, the retinoscopist can determine whether the patient's retina is focused in front of, at, or behind the retinoscope's sight hole. If the light reflected from the patient's fundus (called the retinoscopic reflex or light reflex) and observed in the patient's pupil through the retinoscope moves in the same direction as the movement of the mirror (this is referred to as with movement), the eye is hypermetropic. If the reflex moves in the opposite direction to that of the mirror (against movement), the eye is myopic. Sometimes it is impossible to see a clear movement one way or the other but only a bipartite reflex, showing opposite movements in the two sectors of the pupils (this is called a split reflex or a scissors movement). The refractive error is determined by placing lenses of various powers in front of the patient's eye until no movement is seen, i.e. the whole pupil is either illuminated or dark and the image of the patient's retina is then conjugate with the plane of the retinoscope's sight hole. When this phenomenon occurs the neutral point has been reached. The neutral point is measured for each principal meridian of the eye if it is astigmatic. To arrive at the patient's error of refraction the dioptric power corresponding to the distance between patient and retinoscope (called the working distance) is subtracted from the total lens power used to obtain neutralization. The amount of dioptric power subtracted is called the allowance. ➲ chromoretinoscopy, neutral point, working distance.

retinoscopic reflex ➲ light reflex.

retinoscopy (*syn* skiascopy) the determination of the refractive state of the eye by means of a retinoscope. ➲ chromoretinoscopy, dynamic retinoscopy, static retinoscopy.

retinotectal pathway 1. the nervous pathway connecting the retina to the pretectal region (anterior to the superior colliculi) and from there to the Edinger–Westphal nucleus. It is involved in the pupillary light reflexes. 2. the nervous pathway between the retina and the superior colliculus. It is involved in the involuntary blink reflex to a dazzling light and in the eye movements occurring in response to the sudden appearance of a novel or a threatening stimulus. ➲ blind sight, pupillary fibres, pupillary light reflex.

retinotoxic *adj* toxic to the retina.

retractile *adj* capable of being drawn back, i.e. retracted.

retraction *n* a backward movement. ➲ protraction *opp.* A shortening of tissues. In orthodontics, the moving back of one or more teeth into a better position by the use of an appliance.

retraction cord a thin friable cord impregnated with a vasoconstrictor and placed in the gingival sulcus (previously gingival crevice) to facilitate accurate impression taking of inlay and crown preparations.

retraction ring the ridge or retraction ring that forms between the upper and lower uterine segments as the lower segment thins during labour, as the presenting part descends and the cervix dilates. ➲ Bandl's ring.

retraction syndrome ◐ Duane's syndrome.

retractor *n* a surgical instrument for holding apart the edges of a wound to reveal underlying structures. In dentistry, an instrument used to hold the cheeks, tongue or soft tissues away from the site of operation in order to improve vision and access and to protect them during surgical procedures, e.g. cheek retractor, flap retractor, lip retractor, tissue retractor, tongue retractor.

retractor spring in orthodontics, a spring used to move teeth distally. ◐ finger spring.

retro a prefix that means 'backward', e.g. *retroperitoneal*.

retrobulbar *adj* pertaining to the back of the eyeball.

retrobulbar optic neuritis inflammation of the optic nerve behind the eyeball. ◐ optic neuritis.

retrocaecal *adj* behind the caecum.

retrocalcaneal bursitis inflammation of an anatomical bursa located between the posterior angle of the calcaneus and the Achilles tendon near to its insertion. There is a fluctuant soft tissue swelling both sides of the tendon.

retroclination leaning backwards. In dentistry, lingual or palatal inclination of anterior teeth.

retroflexion *n* the state of being bent backwards, such as of the uterus. ◐ anteflexion *opp*.

retrognathia an anomaly in which there is underdevelopment of the mandible and/or the maxilla.

retrognathic *adj* pertaining to a mandible that is posterior to its normal position in relation to other facial structures.

retrograde *adj* going backward.

retrograde amnesia ◐ amnesia.

retrograde ejaculation a situation in which semen is discharged backwards into the bladder. It may follow pelvic surgery especially prostate surgery, be associated with diabetic neuropathy, spinal injuries and some drugs. ◐ ejaculation, erectile dysfunction.

retrograde filling filling placed in the apical area of a root following the surgical removal of a root apex.

retrograde menstruation the backflow of the menstrual discharge through the uterus, uterine (fallopian) tubes and into the abdominal cavity.

retrograde (reverse) root filling filling inserted into the apical end of a root during root-end surgery. ◐ apicectomy.

retrograde urography/pyelography the radiographic investigation of the renal tract when excretion urography has failed. A catheter is introduced into the renal pelvis via the urethra, bladder and ureter to enable the introduction of a contrast agent. ◐ urography.

retroillumination (*syn* transillumination) in slit-lamp examination, it is a method of illuminating a structure by using the light that is reflected by the iris or an opaque or senescent lens. This method is closely related to indirect illumination and often in corneal examination, part of the cornea will simultaneously be under retroillumination and indirect illumination. ◐ central corneal clouding.

retrolental fibroplasia ◐ retinopathy of prematurity.

retrolisthesis posterior slippage of one vertebra on another.

retromolar pad a pad of soft connective tissue found distal to the last molar in the lower jaw.

retroperitoneal *adj* behind the peritoneum, such as the kidneys and adrenal glands.

retroperitoneal abscess pus in the space behind the peritoneum of the posterior abdominal wall.

retroperitoneal fibrosis inflammation leading to the formation of fibrous tissue behind the peritoneum of the posterior abdominal wall. It may be idiopathic or associated with the use of certain drugs (e.g. methyseride used in migraine prophylaxis, pergolide used in Parkinson's disease).

retropharyngeal *adj* behind the pharynx, such as a retropharyngeal abscess.

retroplacental *adj* behind the placenta.

retroplacental clot a collection of blood behind the placenta.

retropubic *adj* behind the pubis.

retropubic prostatectomy ◐ prostatectomy.

retroscopic angle or tilt the angle between the spectacle plane and the frontal plane of the face when the superior edge of the lens is closer to the face than the inferior edge. ◐ frontal plane, pantoscopic angle, spectacle plane.

retrospection *n* morbid dwelling on the past.

retrospective study research that deals with past data, moving backwards in time. ◐ prospective study.

retrosternal *adj* behind the sternum.

retrotracheal *adj* behind the trachea.

retrusion 1. the condition of being sited behind the normal position. 2. in dentistry, the most posterior position of the mandible.

retroversion *n* turning backward—**retroverted** *adj*. ◐ anteversion *opp*.

retroversion of the uterus tilting of the whole of the uterus backward with the cervix pointing forward.

retroverted gravid uterus a pregnant uterus that is tilted backwards; a common occurrence in which the uterus usually spontaneously corrects to an anteverted position; if retroversion persists, incarceration of the retroverted gravid uterus develops, with retention of urine.

retroverted incarcerated gravid uterus retroverted pregnant uterus which does not antevert spontaneously; by 14 weeks' gestation, it is so large that it becomes trapped under the sacral promontory and cannot rise out of the pelvis. This may lead to acute retention of urine, miscarriage or, very rarely, sacculation of the uterus.

retroviruses *npl* family of ribonucleic acid (RNA) viruses that include the human immunodeficiency viruses (HIV 1 and 2) and the human T-cell lymphotropic viruses (HTLV 1 and 2).

retruded situated behind or away from.

retruded arc of closure arc formed by the movement of any joint on, or attached to, the mandible when the condyles are in their most posterior position.

retruded axis hinge axis in the retruded jaw relation.

retruded contact position position of the mandible on first tooth contact on the retruded arc of closure.

Q

R

retruded hinge axis retruded axis.

retruded jaw relation centric jaw relation. The position of the mandible on its retruded arc of closure where the condyles are in the most posterior position.

Rett's syndrome (A Rett, Austrian paediatrician, 1924–1997) a neurodegenerative disorder occurring in girls. X-linked dominant inheritance. There is progressive neurological and developmental regression from early childhood. Death occurs by the second or third decade.

revascularization *n* the regrowth of blood vessels into a tissue or organ after deprivation of its normal blood supply.

revealed haemorrhage (*syn* external haemorrhage) obvious bleeding such as from a wound, or excessive blood loss from the uterus during labour or postpartum, etc. ⊃ haemorrhage.

revenue budget the budget allocation for day to day running costs, e.g. salaries, telephone, electricity and drugs, etc. ⊃ capital budget.

reverse barrier nursing ⊃ protective isolation.

reverse bevel ⊃ bevel.

reverse bevel incision ⊃ inverse bevel incision.

reverse bias is when a battery is connected across a PN junction, the potential barrier is raised as current flow is stopped until the barrier breaks down. ⊃ forward bias *opp*.

reverse curve (anti-Monson curve) imaginary curve of the occlusal surfaces of the posterior teeth that is convex upwards and lies in a coronal plane.

reverse curve of Spee a bend commonly placed into orthodontic archwires to flatten an occlusal plane. ⊃ curve

reverse horizontal overlap (reverse overjet) a tooth relationship, in intercuspal occlusion, where the buccal maxillary cusps and/or the incisors are placed lingual to the buccal mandibular cusps and/or incisors.

reverse overjet ⊃ reverse horizontal overlap.

reversed Towne's projection a modified Towne's projection used to demonstrate the frontal bones. Used in dental radiography to demonstrate the mandibular condyles in a coronal plane. ⊃ Towne's projection.

reverse transcriptase inhibitors (nucleoside/non-nucleoside) two groups of drugs that act by inhibiting the enzyme reverse transcriptase, required for viral replication, e.g. efavirenz, zidovudine. ⊃ Appendix 5.

reversible able to change in either direction, such as some chemical reactions.

reversible hydrocolloid (agar) impression material ⊃ impression, impression material.

reversion returning to a previous position.

revert to return to a former condition or habit.

revolution one complete rotation of a body or object about an axis. Measured as 360° or 2π radians.

Reye syndrome (R Reye, Australian pathologist, 1912–1977) 'wet brain and fatty liver' as described in 1963. There is cerebral oedema without cellular infiltration, and diffuse fatty infiltration of liver and other organs, including the kidney. The age range of recorded cases is 2 months–15 years. Presents with vomiting, hypoglycaemia and disturbed consciousness, jaundice being conspicuous. There is an association with aspirin administration and infections including chickenpox and influenza. Aspirin and aspirin-containing products should not be given to children and young people under the age of 16 years, except where it is specifically indicated.

RF *abbr* rheumatoid factor.

RFLP *abbr* restriction-fragment length polymorphism.

RGB (red, green and blue) input to a computer colour monitor.

RGP *abbr* rigid gas permeable (contact lens).

Rh *abbr* Rhesus factor. ⊃ blood groups.

rhabdomyolysis *n* disease of skeletal muscle where muscle injury leads to myoglobinuria. It may also be due to crush injury or compression, which can result in acute renal failure.

rhabdomyoma *n* a benign tumour of muscle, occurring in the heart or tongue and in other sites.

rhabdomyosarcoma *n* a rare malignancy of primitive striated muscle cells.

rhagades *npl* superficial elongated scars radiating from the nostrils or angles of the mouth and which are found in congenital syphilis. One of the stigmata of the disease.

RHD *abbr* rheumatic heart disease.

rhegmatogenous *adj* pertaining to a hole or tear. ⊃ retinal detachment.

rheobase an electrotherapy term. A measure applied to a strength–duration graph to evaluate peripheral nerve function. It is defined as the intensity of current required for a minimally perceptible response (motor or sensory, depending on the test) using a monophasic pulse with a duration of 100 ms and a frequency of approximately 1 Hz. Normal values vary whether constant current or constant voltage stimulator is used (reading in current or voltage depending on the equipment).

Rhesus factor (Rh) ⊃ blood groups.

Rhesus incompatibility, isoimmunization this problem arises when a Rhesus negative woman carries a Rhesus positive fetus. During or before the birth there is mixing of fetal and maternal bloods. The woman's body then develops antibodies against the Rhesus positive blood. If a subsequent fetus is also Rhesus positive, then maternal antibodies will attack the fetal blood causing severe haemolysis. ⊃ blood groups.

rheumatic *adj* pertaining to rheumatism, a non-specific term.

rheumatic diseases a diverse group of diseases affecting connective tissue, joints and bones. They include: inflammatory joint disease, e.g. rheumatoid arthritis, septic arthritis and gout; connective tissue disease, e.g. systemic lupus erythematosus; osteoarthritis; non-articular/soft tissue rheumatism, e.g. fibromyalgia.

rheumatic fever (*syn.* acute rheumatism) a disorder, tending to recur but initially commonest in childhood, classically presenting as fleeting polyarthritis of the larger joints with swelling and pain, tachycardia, pyrexia, rash and pancarditis (inflammation involving all layers of the heart wall) of varying severity within 3 weeks following a streptococcal throat infection. Atypically, but not infrequently, the symptoms are trivial and ignored, but carditis may be severe and result in permanent cardiac damage, particularly of heart valves. It may also lead to neurological problems. ➲ chorea.

rheumatic heart disease (RHD) chronic cardiac disease with valve damage resulting from rheumatic fever.

rheumatism *n* a non-specific term embracing a diverse group of diseases and syndromes which have in common disorder or diseases of connective tissue and hence usually present with pain, or stiffness, or swelling of muscles and joints. Used colloquially to describe ill-defined aches and pains. ➲ rheumatic diseases.

rheumatoid arthritis (RA) the most common inflammatory arthritis in women. The typical clinical phenotype of RA is a symmetrical, deforming, small and large joint polyarthritis, often associated with systemic disturbance and extra-articular disease. Many rheumatologists therefore prefer the term 'rheumatoid disease'. Extra-articular manifestations of 'rheumatoid disease' include: (a) systemic—fever, extreme fatigue, weight loss, susceptibility to infection; (b) musculoskeletal—muscle wastage, tenosynovitis, osteoporosis, bursitis; (c) haematological—anaemia, thrombocytosis, eosinophilia; (d) lymphatic—splenomegaly, Felty's syndrome; (e) nodules—sinuses, fistulae; (f) ocular—episcleritis, scleritis, scleromalacia, keratoconjunctivitis sicca; (g) vasculitis—digital arteritis, ulcers, pyoderma gangrenosum, visceral arteritis; (h) cardiovascular—pericarditis, myocarditis, endocarditis, conduction defects, coronary vasculitis, granulomatous aortitis; (i) pulmonary—nodules, pleural effusion, fibrosing alveolitis, bronchiolitis, Caplan's syndrome; (k) neurological—cervical cord compression, compression neuropathies, peripheral neuropathies, mononeuritis multiplex; (l) amyloidosis. The clinical course is usually life-long, with intermittent exacerbations and remissions and highly variable severity. RA occurs throughout the world and in all racial groups. The prevalence is lowest in black Africans and Chinese, and highest in the Pima Indians of Arizona. In Caucasians it is around 1.0–1.5% with a female:male ratio of 3:1. Before the age of 45, the female:male ratio is 6:1. Prevalence increases with age, with 5% of women and 2% of men over 55 years being affected. RA is an autoimmune disease. Concordance rates are higher in monozygotic twins (12–15%) than in dizygotic twins (3%) and frequency of disease is increased in first-degree relatives of patients with RA. Up to 50% of the genetic contribution to susceptibility is due to genes in the HLA region. HLA-DR4 is the major susceptibility haplotype in most racial groups, occurring, for example, in 50–75% of Caucasian patients with RA compared to 20–25% of the normal population. However, DR1 is more important in Indians and Israelis and DW15 in Japanese. It is likely that genetic factors influence both susceptibility and severity, with DR4 positivity more common in those with severe erosive disease. Female gender is a risk factor and this susceptibility is increased post-partum and by breastfeeding. No infectious

agents have been consistently isolated and there is no evidence of disease clustering. Cigarette smoking is a risk factor for RA and for positivity for rheumatoid factor in non-RA subjects. Management depends on severity and presentation but includes: education and coping strategies; rest—both general and for specific joints with splints; maintaining joint function with local strength exercise; aerobic fitness training; good positioning and posture with expert physiotherapy; aids, appliances and enviromental modification; advice on weight loss; physical treatments (local heat, ice packs, wax baths, hydrotherapy, etc); drugs including simple analgesics, non-steroidal anti-inflammatory drugs (NSAIDs) including highly selective cyclo-oxygenase-2 inhibitors (COX-2), oral and intra-articular corticosteroids, antimalarial drugs (e.g. hydroxychloroquine), sulfasalazine, D-penicillamine, gold, cytotoxic drugs and immunosuppressants (e.g. methotrexate, azathioprine, leflunomide, cyclophosphamide, ciclosporin, etc.); biological therapies with cytokine inhibitors such as infliximab, which inhibit tumour necrosis factor α (TNF); and surgery (e.g. tendon repair, synovectomy, replacement arthroplasty, arthrodesis, etc.). ➲ connective tissue diseases, Felty's syndrome, juvenile idiopathic arthritis.

rheumatoid factors (RF) autoantibodies found in most people with rheumatoid arthritis. It is not yet known whether they are the cause of, or the result of, arthritis.

rheumatology *n* the science or the study of the rheumatic diseases.

rhinitis *n* inflammation of the nasal mucous membrane. Several types exist including allergic or atrophic. ➲ atopic syndrome, atropic rhinitis, hay fever.

rhin/o- a prefix that means 'nose', e.g. *rhinoplasty*.

rhinology *n* the study of disorders of the nose—**rhinologist** *n*.

rhinomanometry *n* a test used for assessment of the nasal airway and to measure the nasal airflow and pressure during respiration.

rhinomycosis a fungal infection affecting the nasal mucosa.

rhinophyma *n* nodular enlargement of the skin of the nose.

rhinoplasty *n* plastic surgery of the nasal framework.

rhinorrhoea *n* nasal discharge. Usually describes a thin watery fluid, but also includes the discharge of cerebrospinal fluid from the nose following a fracture of the base of the skull.

rhinoscopy *n* inspection of the nose using a nasal speculum or a flexible endoscope designed for the nasal cavity—**rhinoscopic** *adj*.

rhinoscleroma a granulomatous disease characterized by the formation of nodules in the nasal passages and nasopharynx. It may be caused by the bacterium *Klebsiella rhinoscleromatis*.

rhinosinusitis *n* inflammation of the nose and paranasal sinuses.

rhinosporidiosis *n* a fungal condition affecting the mucosa of the nose, eyes, ears, larynx and occasionally the genitalia.

Rhinosporidium *n* a genus of fungi parasitic to humans.

rhinovirus *n* a group of picornaviruses responsible for the common cold (coryza).

rhiz/o a prefix that means 'nerve root', e.g. *rhizotomy*.

Q
R

rhizotomy *n* surgical division of a root; usually the posterior root of a spinal nerve. *chemical rhizotomy* accomplished by injection of a chemical, often phenol. Generally used for the relief of persistent pain caused by trigeminal neuralgia (tic douloureux).

RHN Rockwell hardness scale/ number.

rhodopsin *n* (*syn* visual purple [no longer used], erythropsin) the visual pigment (visual purple) present in the outer segments of the rods of the retina and involved in scotopic vision. When light stimulates the retina, the chromophore of the pigment molecule '11-*cis*' retinal (which is vitamin A aldehyde) isomerizes to 'all-*trans*' retinal. This leads to other chemical transformations which carry on even in the absence of light. The first stage is *prelumirhodopsin*, then *lumirhodopsin* and finally *metarhodopsin* (of which there are two types). This last transformation may lead to the breakdown of the molecule into retinal and opsin. The molecule is regenerated by recombining retinal and opsin with some enzymes. The absorption spectrum of rhodopsin has a maximum around 498 nm. The isomerization from '11-*cis*' to 'all-*trans*' also gives rise to the process of transduction in which the membrane potential covering the pigment molecules in the outer segment changes towards a hyperpolarization of the cell. This is the first step in the nervous response to a light stimulation of the retina. ⊃ absorption spectrum, bleaching, dark adaptation, erythropsin, rod, transduction, visual pigment.

rhombencephalon hindbrain. One of the three primary vesicles formed during embryonic delevelopment of the brain. It becomes the pons, medulla oblongata and cerebellum.

rhomboid *adj* diamond shaped.

rhomboid of Michaelis diamond- or dome-shaped area at the base of the spine marked by dimpling of the skin, with the spinous process of the 5th lumbar vertebra beneath the superior angle; the posterior superior iliac spines are palpable under the lateral angles; inferiorly is the beginning of the gluteal cleft. It may be observed in the second stage of labour and represents posterior displacement of the sacrum and coccyx as the fetal occiput moves into the sacral curve. Appears to cause the woman to arch her back, push her buttocks forwards and outstretch her arms.

rhonchus *n* an adventitious whistling sound or vibration heard on auscultation of the lung. Passage of air through bronchi partially obstructed by oedema or exudate produces a musical note—**rhonchi** *pl*.

-rhythmia a suffix that means 'rhythm', e.g. *arrhythmia*.

rhythm method also known as the calendar method. ⊃ natural family planning.

RI *abbr* retention index. ⊃ index (dental).

riboflavin(e) *n* vitamin B$_2$, part of the large group of water-soluble B vitamins. Used therapeutically to treat angular stomatitis and other effects of riboflavin(e) deficiency, and for neonatal hyperbilirubinaemia. ⊃ ariboflavinosis, Appendix 4.

ribonuclease *n* an enzyme that breaks down ribonucleic acid.

ribonucleic acid (RNA) nucleic acids present in all living cells. Composed of a single chain of nucleotides formed from ribose (a 5-carbon sugar), phosphates and the nitrogenous bases: adenine (A), guanine (G), cytosine (C) and uracil (U). There are three forms: messenger (mRNA), ribosomal (rRNA) and transfer (tRNA), which have specific functions during protein synthesis. ⊃ deoxyribonucleic acid, transcription, translation.

ribose a 5-carbon (pentose) sugar; required for the formation of the nucleic acids and several coenzymes.

ribosomal RNA (rRNA) ⊃ ribonucleic acid.

ribosomes *npl* submicroscopic structures inside all cells. They are formed from ribonucleic acid and proteins. They are concerned with the synthesis of new proteins for cell use. They may be present on the rough endoplasmic reticulum, or free within the cytoplasm as single units, or in groups known as polysomes.

rib recession inwards movement of the ribs, commonly seen in the respiratory distress syndrome of neonates.

ribs *npl* the twelve pairs of bones which articulate with the twelve dorsal vertebrae posteriorly and form the walls of the thorax. The upper seven pairs are *true ribs* and are attached to the sternum anteriorly by costal cartilage. The remaining five pairs are the *false ribs*; the first three pairs of these do not have an attachment to the sternum but are bound to each other by costal cartilage. The lower two pairs are the *floating ribs* which have no anterior articulation. ⊃ Colour Section Figures 2, 3, 6.

RICE *acron* for **R**est, **I**ce, **C**ompression and **E**levation. Used in the management of acute injuries to minimize the inflammatory process and to accelerate the recovery process by eliminating swelling. ⊃ cryotherapy, ice/cold therapy.

rice-water stool the stool of cholera. The 'rice grains' are desquamated intestinal epithelium.

ricin an extremely toxic substance obtained from the castor oil plant (*Ricinus communis*).

rickets *n* bone disease caused by vitamin D deficiency during infancy and childhood (prior to ossification of the epiphyses) which results from poor dietary intake or insufficient exposure to sunlight. There is abnormal metabolism of calcium and phosphate with poor ossification and bone growth. There is muscle weakness, anaemia, respiratory infections, bone tenderness and pain, hypocalcaemia and seizures. Delays occur in motor development such as with walking, eruption of teeth and closure of the fontanelles. Later there may be bony deformities, e.g. bow legs. ⊃ rickety rosary. Rickets may be secondary to vitamin D malabsorption, or impaired metabolism, such as with chronic renal failure (*renal rickets*). The same condition in adults is known as osteomalacia.

Ricketts appliance ⊃ orthodontic appliance.

Rickettsia *n* (H Ricketts, American pathologist, 1871–1910) small pleomorphic parasitic Gram-negative micro-organisms that have similarities with both viruses and bacteria. Like viruses, they are obligate intracellular parasites. *Rickettsia* are intestinal parasites of arthropods such as fleas, lice, mites and ticks; transmission to humans is by bites from these arthropods and contact with their faeces, which may be rubbed in the eyes, or it can be airborne transmission. They cause various types of the typhus group of diseases and Rocky mountain spotted fever. ➲ rickettsial fevers, spotted fever.

rickettsial fevers a group of rickettsial diseases that include epidemic typhus caused by *Rickettsia prowazekii*; endemic typhus caused by *R. mooseri*; scrub typhus caused by *Orientia tsutsugamushi* (formally known as *R. tsutsugamushi*); and Rocky Mountain spotted fever caused by *R. rickettsii*. They are transmitted by ticks, fleas, lice and mites and are associated with overcrowding and poor hygiene (e.g. after natural disasters, during war, or in refugee camps). ➲ typhus.

rickety rosary a series of protuberances (bossing) at junction of ribs and costal cartilages in children suffering from rickets.

RIDDOR *abbr* Reporting of Injuries, Diseases and Dangerous Occurrences Regulations.

rider's bone a bony mass in the origin of the adductor muscles of the thigh, from repeated minor trauma in horse riding.

ridge a projecting structure, a crest. *alveolar ridge* that part of the alveolus and mucosa that remains following the extraction of teeth. *fibrous ridge* the excessive fibrous tissue that has replaced the bone of the crest of the ridge. *flabby ridge* the flabby tissue that has replaced the bone of the ridge crest. *marginal ridge* the ridge forming the outer margins on the occlusal surface of a premolar or molar tooth, or the lingual surface of an anterior tooth. *oblique ridge* the ridge running obliquely across the occlusal surface of a maxillary molar tooth.

Riedel's thyroiditis (B Reidel, German surgeon, 1846–1916) a chronic fibrosis of the thyroid gland; ligneous goitre.

Rieger's syndrome (H Rieger, Austrian ophthalmologist, 1898–1986) (*syn* mesodermal dysgenesis of the cornea and iris) a hereditary developmental anomaly of the cornea, iris and the angle of the anterior chamber. It is characterized by posterior embryotoxon, stromal hypoplasia of the iris, pupillary anomalies, adhesion of strands of iris tissue to the cornea at the angle of the anterior chamber and glaucoma in about half of the cases, as well as dental and skeletal abnormalities. ➲ anterior limiting ring of Schwalbe, Axenfeld's syndrome.

Rift Valley fever one of the mosquito-transmitted haemorrhagic fevers.

right anterior oblique a radiographic projection with the patient either erect or semi prone at 45° to the film with the right side of the body closest to the film and the left side away from the film.

right colic (hepatic) flexure the 90° turn between the ascending and transverse colon, beneath the liver.

right posterior oblique a radiographic projection with the patient either erect or semi supine at 45° to the film with the right side of the body closest to the film and the left side away from the film.

right hand rule 1. used to relate direction of rotation of an object to its vector representation: if the right hand is 'wrapped' from palm to tips of fingers in the direction of rotation, the vector lies in the direction of the outstretched thumb of the right hand (e.g. vector representation of angular momentum). **2.** the organization of a three-dimensional cartesian co-ordinate system. X direction can be considered as acting along the outstretched first finger of the right hand, Y direction is along the outstretched second (middle) finger of the right hand (at right angles to the first finger) and Z is along the outstretched thumb (at right angles to the other two) of the right hand.

righting reactions the automatic reactions that occur in response to alteration of body alignment, aiming to maintain and restore the head position in midline and with a normal relationship to the trunk and limbs. These can be seen in the developing infant, but are not normally able to be distinguished from equilibrium reactions in the adult.

rights *npl* an umbrella term covering entitlements and privileges enjoyed on the basis of being a human being (human rights) or a citizen (civil rights) though the two are not entirely discrete. There is the recognition in law that certain inalienable human rights should be respected, such as Article 2—'The right to life', of the Human Rights Act 1998. The articles of the Human Rights Act 1998 also include: prohibition of torture; prohibition of slavery and forced labour; right to liberty and security; right to a fair trial; no punishment without lawful authority; right to respect for private and family life; freedom of thought, conscience and religion; right to freedom of expression; freedom of assembly and association; right to marry and found a family; and prohibition of discrimination. Civil rights are recognized as belonging to all individuals within a society and can be upheld by appeal to the law. Rights play an important, though contested, role in political life, such as the conflicting claims to the right to life and the right of women to choose in relation to abortion.

rigid-body mechanics analysis of bodies or objects that do not deform due to the forces upon them. The bones of the human skeleton are often assumed to be rigid links.

rigid pes planus ➲ pes planus.

rigid splinting used in root fractured teeth where the splint usually extends to two teeth either side of damaged tooth.

rigidity *n* (*syn*. lead pipe rigidity, parkinsonian rigidity) increased tension or tone of muscle (hypertonia) with increased resistance to passive stretch in any direction that is uniform throughout the whole movement. ➲ cogwheel rigidity.

rigor *n* a sudden chill, accompanied by severe shivering. The body temperature rises rapidly and remains high until perspiration ensues and causes a gradual fall in temperature.

rigor mortis the stiffening of the body after death. It commences within a few hours of death because muscle cells have insufficient energy (ATP) and intracellular calcium levels rise causing the binding together of the muscle proteins, actin and myosin. The maximum degree of rigor will develop between 12 and 48 hours after death depending on environmental conditions. Rigor wears off as enzymic tissue decomposition begins and proteins are digested.

RIHSA *abbr* radioiodinated human serum albumin.

Riley–Day syndrome (C Riley, American paediatrician, 1913–2005; R Day, American paediatrician, 1905–1989) (*syn* familial autonomic dysfunction) a very rare inherited disorder largely confined to infants of Ashkenazic Jewish origin. It is characterized by alacrima, corneal hypoaesthesia, exotropia, myopia and excessive sweating, vomiting, attacks of high fever, incoordination and lack of pain sensitivity. Few individuals survive into adulthood ⊃ alacrima.

rim an outer border or edge of that which is roughly circular.

rima a fissure or cleft.

rima glottidis the glottis. An opening between the abducted vocal folds in the larynx.

Ringer's solution (S Ringer, British physician/physiologist, 1835–1910) an intravenous infusion solution containing sodium chloride with potassium chloride and calcium chloride. *lactated Ringer's solution (Ringer-lactate or Hartmann's solution)* one that also contains sodium lactate.

ringworm *n* (*syn.* tinea) generic term used to describe contagious fungal infection of the skin, because of the common circular (circinate) scaly patches. ⊃ dermatophytes.

rINN *abbr* Recommended International Non-proprietary Name.

Rinne's test (H Rinne, German otologist, 1819–1868) a tuning fork test used to distinguish between conductive and sensorineural deafness. ⊃ Weber's test.

RIP *abbr* raised intracranial pressure.

RIS *abbr* radiology information system.

Risdon approach a surgical technique in which the submandibular area is approached through an incision below and behind the angle of the mandible.

risk *n* a potential hazard. *attributable risk* the disease rate in people exposed to the risk factor minus the occurrence in unexposed people. *relative risk* the ratio of disease rate in people exposed to the risk factor to those not exposed. It is related to the odds ratio, which is the odds (as in betting) of disease occurring in an exposed person divided by the odds of the disease occurring in an unexposed person.

risk assessment a structured and methodical assessment of risk carried out for a particular area or activity. For example moving and handling patients in the operating theatre.

risk factors factors associated with an increase in the likelihood of ill health, disease, handicap or disability. Demonstration of the association has to fulfil Sir Austin Bradford Hill's eight criteria (e.g. smoking and lung cancer): (a) biological plausibility—tobacco tar contains known carcinogens, the stages of tumour development following exposure are clearly demonstrated; (b) reversibility—smoking cessation reduces subsequent increase in risk of lung cancer by half in the first year, to nil after ten years; (c) animal demonstration—model of beagles in laboratory experiments; (d) dose response—risk of lung cancer in smokers shown to increase progressively with the number

of cigarettes smoked per day; (e) follows exposure—temporal relationship demonstrated, lung cancer always follows exposure to cigarettes with a time lag of 20–30 years; (f) over time and overseas—relationship consistent between different case series and different places (in the world); (g) experimental design—must be reliable. Randomized controlled trials most convincing, but may be unethical. Observational studies (case control, cohort) useful if correctly carried out; (h) strength of the effect—the larger the increase in risk, the more likely the causal relationship.

risk management managing risk in healthcare settings involves: identification of the risk, analysis of the risk and controlling the risk.

risus sardonicus the spastic 'grin' of tetanus; caused by facial muscle spasm.

Ritgen manoeuvre a technique sometimes used during the second stage of labour whereby upward pressure is applied to the fetal head from the coccygeal region to extend it during actual delivery. Those who practise this manoeuvre tend to do so because they feel it will reduce the incidence of perineal tears.

Ritter's disease (G Ritter von Rittershain, German physician, 1820–1883) ⊃ staphylococcal scalded-skin syndrome.

river blindness ⊃ onchocerciasis.

Rivermead motor assessment a scale originally designed to test motor function in people who had suffered a stroke. It tests overall function and mobility by separately testing three areas: gross function, leg and trunk, and arm. It has a hierarchical structure that assumes that recovery of function has a pattern, and if a person is unable to perform a task no more tasks are attempted on that sub-area.

RK *abbr* radial keratotomy.

RMR *abbr* resting metabolic rate.

RNA *abbr* ribonucleic acid.

RNA viruses viruses that contain RNA as their nucleic acid such as picornavirus, retrovirus.

RNI *abbr* reference nutrient intake.

RNP *abbr* ribonucleoprotein.

RO *abbr* reality orientation.

ROA *abbr* right occipitoanterior; used to describe the position of the fetal occiput in relation to the maternal pelvis.

Roach clasp ⊃ gingivally approaching clasp.

Robert's pelvis an extremely rare pelvis deformity, in which both sacral alae are undeveloped with fusion to the ilium on each side. The symphysis pubis is sometimes split. The deformity prevents engagement of the fetal head.

Rochette bridge in dentistry, a type of small fixed bridge with perforated retainers at each end which are bonded by composite cements to neighbouring teeth following etching. Used to support or replace loose incisors for a limited period. ⊃ bridge.

rockerbottom feet prominent heels in infants with chromosomal disorders such as Edwards' syndrome (trisomy 18) and Patau's syndrome (trisomy 13).

Rockwell hardness scale or number (RHN) ⊃ hardness scale.

Rocky Mountain spotted fever a tick-borne rickettsial infection. Characterized by fever, myalgia, headache and petechial rash. Occurs in the USA. ➲ rickettsial fevers.

rod *n* photoreceptor cell of the retina which connects with a bipolar cell. It contains rhodopsin and is involved in scotopic vision. The molecules of rhodopsin are contained in about 1000 hollow discs (double lamellae or membranes) which are isolated from each other and from the boundary membrane of the rod cell. These discs are found in the outer segment (i.e. the part closest to the pigment epithelium) of the cell. There are about 100 million rod cells throughout the retina; only a small area, the foveola, is free of rods. ➲ cone, foveola, retina, rhodopsin, scotopic vision.

rodent ulcer ➲ basal cell carcinoma.

Rolando's fracture a fracture of the base of the first metacarpal.

role social and cultural norms and expectations of occupational performance that are associated with the individual's social and personal identity. (Reproduced with permission from the European Network of Occupational Therapy in Higher Education (ENOTHE) Terminology Project, 2008.)

role model an individual who acts as a model for another individual's behaviour in a particular role. Important for development during childhood, and also as part of professional education and development.

role play 1. the use of improvisation to act out real or imaginary social situations in order to gain insight into interpersonal difficulties, improve social skills or rehearse anticipated events. **2.** may be used during professional education when a student assumes the role of a patient/client so that other students may practise a particular skill, such as communication. Also used in therapeutic situations, e.g. patients with mental health problems.

rollator frame a mobility aid; a Zimmer-type walking frame which incorporates wheels at the front, thus allowing it to be pushed forward rather that lifted during walking.

ROM *abbr* **1.** range of motion. **2.** read only memory. **3.** resisted range of movement.

Romberg's sign (M Romberg, German neurologist, 1795–1873) a sign of impaired balance and loss of proprioception. Used to distinguish between sensory and cerebellar ataxia. The person is asked to stand with heels together, first with their eyes open and then with their eyes shut. If they show excessive sway or lose their balance only when their eyes are closed this indicates proprioceptive loss. Also called 'Rombergism'.

rongeurs (bone-nibbling forceps) ➲ forceps.

rooming-in term used when the infant remains with the mother, rather than being cared for in a nursery, which encourages development of the mother–infant relationship

root in anatomy, the origin of a structure. In dentistry, that part of the tooth, below the crown, which is normally invested in cementum. ➲ root (dental procedures). *anatomical root* that part of the tooth covered by, and including, cementum. *clinical root* that part of the anatomical root which is attached to the alveolar bone by periodontal ligament.

root canal the space within a dental root containing pulp which runs from the coronal pulp chamber to the apex of the tooth and is surrounded by dentine. Accessory or lateral canals branch off the main canal to extend to the root surface. *accessory root canal* a branch of the main canal at any point along the root.

root canal (dental procedures) in dentistry, the various therapeutic procedures undertaken on a root canal of a tooth. *root canal culturing* (clinically archaic, largely for research) a method of checking root canals for cultivable microorganisms by sampling contents. *root canal dressing* a temporary filling material placed in a root canal system to eliminate infection, reduce periapical inflammation or induce apexification. Examples include non-setting calcium hydroxide paste, corticosteroid/antibiotic pastes. *root canal file* a hand-held or engine driven tool for enlarging root canals in a rasping or planing action. *root canal filling* the material employed to fill and seal a prepared root canal. *root canal filling condenser* a thin tapered hand instrument with flat end, circular in cross-section, designed to condense materials in root canals. *root canal filling (McSpadden) compactor* a rotary instrument which softens root filling materials by frictional heat and condenses them apically into the canal by an Archimedean screw principle. *root canal preparation* the shaping and cleaning of a root canal to eliminate micro-organisms and pulp tissue in readiness for filling. *root canal filling point* (*syn* root canal filling cone) a tapered cone of material used to fill root canals. They are *master root canal filling point*—a cone of filling material used to seal the apex of the tooth, and *accessory root canal filling points*—the supplementary cones of material used to fill in canal space around the master root canal filling point. *root canal paste carrier (rotary paste filler), lentulo (spiral root canal) filler* a rotary instrument used to convey fluid materials into a root canal by Archimedean screw action. *root canal plugger* (➲ plugger) a tapered instrument with a circular cross section and flat end for vertical condensation of root filling materials. *root canal reamer* a hand held or engine driven tool for enlarging root canals in a rotational motion. *root canal sealer* the fluid cement used in root canal fillings. *root canal spreader* the tapered instrument with circular cross section and pointed tip for lateral condensation of root filling materials by a wedge-like action. *root canal treatment* (also called pulp canal treatment) a generic term to describe the processes of pulpectomy (pulp extirpation) to remove diseased pulp, root canal shaping, cleaning and filling in the preservation of pulpally compromised teeth.

root caries dental caries seen in older persons particularly where the supporting tissues have receded. The lesions occur in the cementum and are probably due to increased debris stagnation because of neglectful oral hygiene and decreased salivation.

root (dental procedures) in dentistry, the various therapeutic procedures undertaken on a tooth root. *root* *amputation* (*syn* root resection) the surgical separation and removal of one root from a multirooted tooth while retaining the remaining root or roots. *root filling* either filling and sealing of a root canal, or the material or combination of materials used to obturate root canals. *root planing* the removal of necrotic cementum and planing of root surfaces. *root splitting forceps* ➲ forceps.

root-end closure induction ➲ apexification.

root-end resection ➲ apicectomy.

rooting reflex a primitive reflex present in newborns. The infant will turn his or her head to that side when the cheek is touched. It normally disappears between 3 and 4 months of age.

ROP *abbr* right occipitoposterior; used to describe the position of the fetal occiput in relation to the maternal pelvis.

Roper, Logan and Tierney model ➲ Activities of Living (ALs).

ROS *abbr* reactive oxygen species.

rosacea *n* a skin disease which shows on flush areas of the face. In areas affected there is chronic dilatation of superficial capillaries and hypertrophy of sebaceous follicles, often complicated by a papulopustular eruption. ➲ Colour Section Figure 105.

rose bengal an iodine derivative of fluorescein having vital staining properties but unlike fluorescein it is a true histological stain which binds strongly and selectively to cellular components. The colour of this stain is red. It has the disadvantage of causing some pain in a good percentage of eyes. It stains dead or degenerated epithelial cells but not normal cells and is used to help in the detection of damaged or diseased corneal or conjunctival epithelium. ➲ fluorescein, lissamine green.

roseola *n* a rose-coloured rash.

rosin (colophony) a residue following the distillation of crude turpentine. Used in dentistry as a constituent of certain impression compounds and in varnishes.

Ross River virus disease/fever a disease caused by an alphavirus. It is transmitted by mosquitoes and is found in Australia, Papua New Guinea and other areas in the Pacific region. It is characterized by polyarthritis and a rash.

rotary instrument a hand- or power-operated instrument that is rotated in order to function, e.g. a bur.

rotary paste filler ➲ root canal (dental procedures).

rotated oblique lateral projection a modification of the oblique lateral projection in which the position of the mandible is rotated in relation to the cassette. Used to view the incisor, canine and premolar areas

rotating anode part of an X-ray tube that is made of a molybdenum disc with a tungsten/rhenium focal tract embedded in it; the positive anode rotates during exposure to enable higher intensities of X-rays than a stationary anode tube due to the larger surface allowing more heat to be deposited and then dissipated.

rotating jig in radiotherapy, a method of determining the contour of a shell. The shell is supported on four pins and the fifth pin rotates around an axis at right angles to the plane

and scaled in degrees of rotation and centimetres. The contour can then be plotted on polar graph paper.

rotation *n* movement of a body or object about an axis. The axis may be external (e.g. gymnastic high bar) or within the body (e.g. at a joint). May be combined with translation to give general motion. Turning of a body on its long axis, as in turning of the fetal head (or presenting part) for proper orientation to the pelvic axis, usually occurring naturally, but occasionally achieved through manual or instrumental manipulation. The force applied to a tooth in order to rotate it about its long axis, or the malposition of a tooth due to rotation about its long axis. Rotation also describes a specific limb movement around the axis down the centre of a long bone. ➲ translation.

rotation therapy a technique when the source of the radiation is moved through an angle of 360° during treatment.

rotational kinetic energy the mechanical energy possessed by an object due to its rotation about an axis. May be calculated as $\frac{1}{2} Iw^2$ where I is moment of inertia and w is angular velocity. Measured in joules (J). ➲ kinetic energy, translational kinetic energy

rotator *n* a muscle that acts to turn a part.

rotator cuff made up of four muscles: subscapularis, supraspinatus, infraspinatus and teres minor, which act in synergy at the shoulder joint to facilitate movement and provide stability by maintaining the head of the humerus in the glenoid cavity. Their tendons converge to form a 'cuff' over the shoulder joint, on their way to attaching from the scapula to the humerus. It runs in the subacromial space. One of its major functions is to control and produce rotation of the shoulder. They may be considered as 'dynamic ligaments', continually changing their relative tensions to maintain the stability of the humeral head. In sport, most commonly injured in throwing, swimming and racquet sports with tears, tendonitis (tedinitis) or (in young athletes) impingement. ➲ impingement.

rotaviruses *npl* viruses belonging to the reovirus group, mainly associated with gastroenteritis in children and infants. It is a very common cause worldwide of severe diarrhoeal disease in children.

Roth spots (M Roth, Swiss pathologist, 1839–1914) pale, round spots in the retina in some cases of infective endocarditis; thought to be of embolic origin.

rouge (jeweller's rouge) a finely divided ferric oxide polishing powder used mainly to polish metals.

roughage *n* an outdated term. ➲ non-starch polysaccharides.

rouleau *n* a stack of red blood cells, resembling a roll of coins.

round ligaments uterine supports that run from the uterus, through the inguinal canal, to the labia majora. ➲ Colour Section Figure 17.

round window fenestra rotunda. A round opening between the middle and inner ear. It is situated on the medial wall of the middle ear and is covered by fibrous tissue. It is in contact with the cochlea.

roundworm *n* (*Ascaris lumbricoides*) intestinal nematodes with worldwide distribution. Parasitic to humans. Eggs passed in stools; ingested; hatch in bowel; migrate through tissues, lungs and bronchi before returning to the bowel as mature worms. During migration worms can be coughed up. Heavy infections can produce pneumonia. They cause abdominal discomfort and may be vomited or passed per rectum. A tangled mass can cause intestinal obstruction or appendicitis. Adult worms can obstruct pancreatic and bile ducts. ⊃ *Toxocara*.

router computer equipment that connects computer networks together; it is more powerful than a hub, for example, used to allow access to a single internet connection (phoneline).

routine an established and predictable sequence of tasks. (Reproduced with permission from the European Network of Occupational Therapy in Higher Education (ENOTHE) Terminology Project, 2008.)

Roux-en-Y operation (C Roux, Swiss surgeon, 1857–1934) originally the distal end of divided jejunum was anastomosed to the stomach, and the proximal jejunum containing the duodenal and pancreatic digestive juices was anastomosed to the jejunum about 75 mm below the first anastomosis. The term is now used to include joining of the distal jejunum to a divided bile duct, oesophagus or pancreas, in major surgery of these structures.

Rovsing's sign (N Rovsing, Danish surgeon, 1862–1927) pressure in the left iliac fossa causes pain in the right iliac fossa in appendicitis. ⊃ Colour Section Figure 18a.

RP *abbr* retinitis pigmentosa.

RPD *abbr* removable partial denture.

RPE *abbr* **1.** rating of perceived exertion. **2.** retinal pigment epithelium.

RPP *abbr* rapidly progressive periodontitis.

RPR *abbr* rapid plasma reagin (test).

RQ *abbr* respiratory quotient.

-rrhage, rrhagia a suffix that means 'to burst forth', e.g. *haemorrhage*.

-rrhaphy a suffix that means 'suturing', e.g. *colpoperineorrhaphy*.

-rrhoea a suffix that means 'flow, excessive discharge, e.g. *diarrhoea*.

rRNA *abbr* ribosomal ribonucleic acid. ⊃ ribonucleic acid.

RS 232 a type of standard interface between computer and peripheral, defining the plug and socket sizes and how the data are transmitted between the computer and peripheral.

RSD *abbr* reflex sympathetic dystrophy.

RSI *abbr* repetitive strain injury.

RSV *abbr* respiratory syncytial virus.

RTA *abbr* **1.** renal tubular acidosis. **2.** road traffic accident.

rubber base a general term for elastic dental impression material.

rubber cup (prophylaxis cup) the flexible rubber cup used in a handpiece with polishing paste to clean and polish teeth and prostheses.

rubber dam in dentistry, a thin sheet of rubber perforated by a punch and clamped over a tooth or teeth to isolate them from the rest of the mouth. A frame keeps the rubber stretched and away from the teeth. It keeps the teeth in question dry and prevents foreign bodies, debris and strong medicaments escaping into the mouth and hence the possibility of inhaling or swallowing them. Also prevents contamination of the field of operation by saliva or microorganisms. Hypersensitivity reactions to latex has necessitated the development of latex free alternatives. *rubber dam clamp* spring clamp applied to grip the cervical area of a tooth to retain rubber dam and in some cases cotton wool rolls. There are different sizes and designs to fit molars, premolars and incisors. *rubber dam frame* flexible frame used to hold the rubber dam in a taut state, away from the field of operation. *rubber dam holder* elastic fabric band furnished with clips and placed behind the head in order to hold the rubber dam away from the field of operation. *rubber dam ligature* length of dental floss tied firmly around the neck of a tooth to retain the rubber dam. *rubber dam mask* variant of rubber dam consisting of a square of rubber dam attached to a square of tear-resistant paper with two elastic loops that may be hooked around the patient's ears. *rubber dam punch* instrument used to punch various sized holes in a sheet of rubber dam. *rubber dam weight* small metal weight clipped to the lower border of the rubber dam to control and stretch it.

rubber dam clamp forceps instrument with self-locking device used to apply and remove rubber dam clamps. ⊃ forceps.

rub, rube- a prefix that means 'red', e.g. *rubor*.

rubefacients *npl* substances which, when applied to the skin, cause redness (hyperaemia).

rubella *n* (*syn*. German measles) an acute, infectious, eruptive fever (exanthema) caused by a virus. Rubella is endemic in countries without universal vaccination policies. Outbreaks occur in spring and early summer, with epidemics every 7–10 years. The virus is transmitted by aerosol, with infectivity from up to 1 week before and 1 week after the onset of the rash. In non-immunized communities 80–85% of young adults have evidence of past infection. In childhood most cases are subclinical. In 1941 Sir Norman Gregg recognized the association between rubella infection in early pregnancy and significant congenital abnormalities. Initial infection via the upper respiratory tract and local lymph nodes is followed by viraemia to target organs such as skin, joints and placenta. If placental infection takes place in the first trimester, persistence of the virus is likely and has the potential for severe congenital disease. The severity of effects depends on the stage of pregnancy at which the woman is infected. Within the first 8 weeks of pregnancy there is considerable risk (65–85%) of multiple defects in the fetus, deafness, cataracts, brain damage or congenital heart disease, or spontaneous miscarriage; at 12 weeks' gestation there is a risk of 30–35% usually for single defect, deafness or congenital heart disease; at 16 weeks' gestation there is a 10% risk usually of deafness; and >20 weeks' gestation there is occasional deafness. Lymphadenopathy lasting several weeks occurs, usually with the involvement of post-auricular, post-cervical and suboccipital nodes and occasional splenomegaly. A maculopapular non-confluent rash starts simultaneously on the face and moves to the trunk. Petechial lesions ('Forchheimer spots') appear on the soft palate, associated with a mild coryza/conjunctivitis. Fever occurs only on the first day of the rash. Other than with congenital infection, complications are rare but are more common in adult females. An immune-mediated arthritis/arthralgia affects 30% of women and involves the fingers, wrists and knees; it takes 1–2 months to resolve. Encephalitis occurs in approximately 1 in every 5000 cases, with a 20–50% mortality. Recovery is complete in survivors. A mild hepatitis is frequently seen and haemorrhagic manifestations occur in 1:3000 cases. Laboratory confirmation of the diagnosis of rubella is required, particularly if there has been contact with a pregnant woman. Detection of rubella-specific IgG with absent IgM indicates previous infection. Specific IgM or rising IgM is indicative of recent infection. However, this may persist for 1–3 months and occur as a reaction in other common rashes such as human erythrovirus 19 (parvovirus B19) and Epstein–Barr virus (EBV) infections. The most important investigation in early pregnancy is the detection of maternal rubella-specific IgG which indicates established immunity and allows the woman and her partner to be reassured that there is no serious risk of congenital disease. Immunization is available as part of routine programmes during infancy and childhood and to non-pregnant woman of childbearing age with insufficient immunity. ◔ Colour Section Figure 106.

rubeola ◔ measles.

rubeosis iridis neovascularization of the iris characterized by numerous coarse and irregular vessels on the surface and stroma of the iris. The new blood vessels may cover the trabecular meshwork, cause peripheral anterior synechia and give rise to secondary glaucoma. The most frequent causes are diabetes mellitus and central retinal vein occlusion. ◔ iritis, neovascular glaucoma, retinal vein occlusion, secondary glaucoma, synechia.

rubidium (Rb) a metallic element. Emits some radioactivity and is used in radioisotope scanning.

Rubin's manoeuvre an invasive rotational manoeuvre used to relieve shoulder dystocia. Pressure is exerted over the fetal back to adduct and rotate the shoulders. ◔ shoulder dystocia.

Rubinstein–Taybi syndrome (J Rubinstein, American paediatrician, 1925–2006; H Taybi, Iranian/American paediatric radiologist, b.1919) includes mental and motor retardation, broad thumbs and toes, growth retardation, susceptibility to infection in the early years and characteristic facial features.

rubor *n* redness; usually used in the context of being one of the five classical signs and symptoms of inflammation—the others being calor, dolor, loss of function and tumor.

Ruffini end organs subcutaneous sensors that respond to stretching of the skin.

rugae *npl* folds present in the gastric mucosa, and the ridges present in the mucosa of the vagina. They facilitate stretching of the stomach after a meal, and of the vagina during the birth of a baby—**ruga** *sing*.

rugae palatina the ridges of mucous membrane found on the surface of the hard palate.

rule of nines a method of calculating the percentage of body surface area affected by a burn injury, using standard body maps. For example, in an adult, a burn injury affecting the front of the leg would be approximateley 9%, or a burn of the back of the head would be 4.5% (Figure R.8). Modified charts are available for infants and children because they have proportionally larger heads; a burn affecting half the head in a newborn baby would be 9.5%. ◔ total burn surface area.

Rules for Midwives rules produced by the Nursing and Midwifery Council by which all midwives practising in the UK must abide; failure to do so is likely to result in allegation of professional misconduct.

runner's haematuria ◔ march haemoglobinuria.

runner's knee a non-specific term used to describe pain felt in or around the knee in runners. Includes conditions such as patellofemoral pain and iliotibial band syndrome. ◔ chondromalacia patellae, iliotibial band, iliotibial band syndrome.

runner's nipples a colloquial expression used in sports medicine to describe the irritation of the nipples due to friction caused by the runner's shirt rubbing over their nipples; relieved by the use of lubricating jelly.

runner's toe painful, black discoloration at the base of the toe nail, usually the result of inappropriate footwear (too small or too wide) or direct trauma. A significant amount of blood gathering under the toenail may form a subungual haematoma which may require immediate release. ◔ subungual haematoma.

running economy defined as the volume of oxygen required per km, relative to body mass, to run at a submaximal speed, so expressed in mL/kg/km. Most commonly reported, however, in terms of the rate of oxygen usage relative to body mass, in mL/kg/km, in a run at a standard speed of 16 km per hour: note the lower the value, the greater the 'economy'.

rupture 1. a bursting or tearing of a body structure, e.g. uterine (fallopian) tube due to ectopic pregnancy, a ruptured uterus during pregnancy/labour. Also describes the rupture of the fetal membranes. **2.** a lay term for hernia.

Russian current an electrotherapy term, used to indicate an alternating current with a pulse frequency of 2.5 kHz (carrier frequency), sinusoidal, triangular or rectangular pulses and a burst frequency of 50 Hz, used for motor stimulation. Burst duration is typically 10 ms (interburst interval 5–10 ms), but

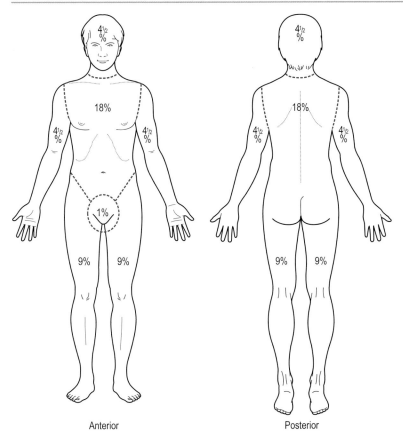

Anterior   Posterior

R.8 Rule of nines—adult (reproduced from Brooker & Waugh 2007 with permission).

can be less, especially if the aim is to reduce the rate of fatigue in the muscles being stimulated. Name of current due to use by Kots in the Soviet Union to train elite athletes prior to the Montreal Olympic games in 1976. ➲ alternating current.

ruthenium-90 an isotope contained in a silver applicator with a window thickness of 0.1 mm, attached to the sclera for 7–10 days and used to treat the eye.

RV *abbr* **1.** residual volume. **2.** right ventricle.

Ryle's tube (J Ryle, British physician, 1889–1950) a narrow-bore nasogastric tube, used mainly to aspirate gastric contents following abdominal surgery, when the bowel is obstructed or in paralytic ileus. Sometimes used for short-term enteral feeding.

Q
R

S1 *abbr* first heart sound.

S2 *abbr* second heart sound.

S3 *abbr* third heart sound.

S4 *abbr* fourth heart sound.

SA *abbr* sinoatrial.

Sabia virus a virus of the family *Arenaviridae*. It is the causative organism of Brazilian haemorrhagic fever.

Sabin vaccine (A Sabin, Polish/American physician, 1906–1993) a live attenuated poliomyelitis vaccine given orally.

sac *n* any small pouch-like structure, such as the conjunctival sac.

saccade abrupt, rapid involuntary movements, such as those of the eyes when scanning a page of print in a document—**saccades** *pl*, **saccadic** *adj*.

saccadic eye movement a short rapid and abrupt movement of the eye as occurring in reading a line of printed words or in fixating from one point to another. The peak velocity of a saccade of 10° amplitude can exceed 400°/s and be completed in 40 ms. ➲ fixation movements, reading.

sacchar/i, sacchar/o- a prefix that means 'sugar', e.g. *saccharide*.

saccharide *n* a series of carbohydrates. Includes monosaccharides, disaccharides and polysaccharides.

-saccharide a suffix that means 'basic carbohydrate molecule', e.g. *polysaccharide*.

saccharin(e) a synthetic substance with intense sweetness; used as a sweetening agent. It is approximately 500 times sweeter than sucrose (beet or cane sugar). ➲ sweetener.

saccular aneurysm a dilatation of only a part of the circumference of an artery.

sacculation *n* appearance of several saccules.

sacculation of the uterus rare complication of incarceration of a retroverted gravid uterus. The fundus remains under the sacral promontory and the anterior wall grows to accommodate the fetus.

saccule *n* a minute sac. A fluid-filled sac in the inner ear. Part of the vestibular apparatus concerned with static equilibrium; contains hair cells and otoliths—**saccular, sacculated** *adj*. ➲ utricle.

SACN *abbr* Scientific Advisory Committee on Nutrition.

sacral *adj* pertaining to the sacrum.

sacral nerves five pairs of nerves that leave the lower spinal cord.

sacral plexus a nerve plexus formed by the anterior rami of the lumbosacral trunk (the fifth lumbar nerve and part of the fourth, L4–5) and the first, second and third sacral nerves (S1–3). ➲ Colour Section Figure 11. The plexus lies in the posterior wall of the pelvic cavity. It divides into a number of branches, supplying the muscles and skin of the pelvic floor, muscles around the hip joint and the pelvic organs. In addition to these it provides the *sciatic nerve* which contains fibres from L4, 5, S1, 2, 3. The *sciatic nerve* is the largest nerve in the body. It is about 2 cm wide at its origin. It passes through the greater sciatic foramen into the buttock then descends through the posterior aspect of the thigh supplying the hamstring muscles (biceps femoris, semimembranosus, semitendinosus). At the level of the middle of the femur it divides to form the *tibial* and the *common peroneal nerves*. *The tibial nerve* descends through the popliteal fossa to the posterior aspect of the leg where it supplies muscles and skin. It passes under the medial malleolus to supply muscles and skin of the sole of the foot and toes. One of the main branches is the *sural nerve* which supplies the tissues in the area of the heel, the lateral aspect of the ankle and a part of the dorsum of the foot. The *common peroneal nerve* descends obliquely along the lateral aspect of the popliteal fossa, winds round the neck of the fibula into the front of the leg where it divides into the *deep peroneal* (anterior tibial) and the *superficial peroneal* (musculocutaneous) nerves. These nerves supply the skin and muscles of the anterior aspect of the leg and the dorsum of the foot and toes. The *pudendal nerve* (S2, 3, 4)—the perineal branch supplies the external anal sphincter, the external urethral sphincter and adjacent skin.

sacral vertebrae ➲ sacrum, vertebra (typical).

sacr/o- a prefix that means 'sacrum', e.g. *sacroiliac*.

sacroanterior *adj* describes the position of a breech presentation in the pelvis when the fetal sacrum is in the anterior part of the maternal pelvis—**sacroanteriorly** *adv*.

sacrococcygeal *adj* pertaining to the sacrum and the coccyx.

sacrocotyloid concerning the sacrum and acetabulum.

sacrocotyloid diameter the measurement from the sacral promontory and nearest point of the iliopectineal eminence; measures 9.5 cm.

sacroiliac *adj* pertaining to the sacrum and the ilium. ➲ sacroiliac joint.

sacroiliac joint (SIJ) the partly fibrous and partly a synovial joint formed between the medial surface of the ilium and the lateral aspect of the upper sacral vertebrae. Comprising and surrounded by very strong ligamentous structures. The major function is to transmit body weight, but it does have a role in movement. There is probably a small amount of rotation that occurs at this joint. It facilitates the torsional or twisting movement of the pelvis as the lower limbs move. The SIJ can be affected by various conditions including trauma, biomechanical malalignment, hormonal changes or inflammatory joint disease such as ankylosing spondylitis. Often involved in inflammatory arthritis, seen in sport in athletes with lower limb biomechanical problems.

sacroiliitis *n* inflammation of a sacroiliac joint. Involvement of both joints characterizes such conditions as ankylosing spondylitis, Reiter's syndrome and psoriatic arthritis.

sacrolumbar *adj* pertaining to the sacrum and the loins.

sacroposterior *adj* describes the position of a breech position in the pelvis when the fetal sacrum is in the posterior part of the maternal pelvis—**sacroposteriorly** *adv*.

sacrum *n* the bone lying between the 5th lumbar vertebra and the broad base of the coccyx. In adults, it comprises five vertebrae fused together to form a triangular or wedge-shaped bone with a concave anterior surface. The upper part, or base, articulates with the 5th lumbar vertebra. On each side it articulates with the ilium to form a synovial sacroiliac joint, and at its inferior tip it articulates with the coccyx. The anterior edge of the base, the promontory, protrudes into the pelvic cavity. The vertebral foramina are present, and on each side of the bone there is a series of foramina for the passage of nerves—**sacral** *adj*. ◑ vertebra (typical), Colour Section Figure 3.

SAD *acron* **S**easonal **A**ffective **D**isorder.

saddle in dentistry, that portion of a partial denture which rests on the alveolar ridge and carries the teeth. *bounded saddle* a saddle bounded at each end by a natural tooth.

saddle embolism a clot (thrombus) that straddles the bifurcation of the aorta where it divides to form the right and left common iliac arteries.

saddle joint a type of synovial joint in which bones with both concave and convex surfaces fit together. For example, the carpometacarpal joint of the thumb which allows movement in two planes; flexion and extension, and adduction and abduction.

saddle nose one with a flattened bridge; may be a sign of congenital syphilis.

sadism *n* the obtaining of pleasure from inflicting pain, violence or degradation on another person. ◑ masochism.

SADS *abbr* **S**udden **A**dult/**A**rrhythmia **D**eath **S**yndrome ◑ long Q-T syndrome.

safe-for-teeth items of food, drink or confectionery product which does not reduce plaque pH to less than 5.7 and is not dentally erosive.

safelights in radiography, lights covered with optical filters to enable staff to work in a darkened room without the film emulsion being affected by the light.

Safe Motherhood Initiative World Health Organization campaign to reduce worldwide maternal mortality and morbidity by implementation of simple, appropriate, cost-effective strategies to enable women to have access to high quality, affordable care during pregnancy and childbirth and related events such as fetal loss. It aims to improve health, nutrition and general well-being of girls and women of reproductive age before conception and into parenthood,

and to reduce long-term sequelae of childbirth which often result in lifelong disabilities.

sagittal *adj* resembling an arrow.

sagittal axis ◑ anteroposterior axis of the eye.

sagittal axis (dental) an imaginary anteroposterior line about which the mandible may rotate through a frontal plane.

sagittal plane the anteroposterior plane of the body.

sagittal sinuses two dural venous channels (sinuses) that drain blood from the brain.

sagittal split osteotomy a surgical technique to correct mandibular prognathism and anterior open bite deformity. The ramus of the mandible is split vertically between two cuts in the cortices, the first through the inner cortex horizontally above the mandibular foramen and the second through the outer cortex at various sites below the mandibular foramen.

sagittal suture the immovable joint between the two parietal bones.

sag sign the phenomenon observed in a person who has a ruptured posterior cruciate ligament, in crook lying the tibia sags posteriorly in comparison to the unaffected leg.

SAH *abbr* subarachnoid haemorrhage.

SAID *acron* **S**pecific **A**daptation to **I**mposed **D**emands.

Saint's triad (C Saint, South African radiologist, 20th century) the presence of hiatus hernia, gallstones and diverticulosis.

salbutamol short-acting beta-agonist drug, used to relieve the bronchoconstriction of asthma. ◑ Appendix 5. Use in sport is restricted due to its anabolic (and thus potentially performance-enhancing) effects. New World Anti-Doping Agency (WADA) guidelines require the degree of bronchoconstriction to be measured by formal lung function testing, with the use of salbutamol allowed only if specific criteria are reached. Requires a Therapeutic Use Exemption (TUE) form for use in sport.

salicylates *npl* a group of analgesic, antipyretic, non-steroidal anti-inflammatory drugs, such as aspirin. ◑ Appendix 5.

salicylic acid used topically, it is keratolytic and has fungicidal and bacteriostatic properties. Used in a variety of hyperkeratotic skin conditions such as corns, and combined with other substances for the treatment of scalp psoriasis.

saline *n* a solution of sodium chloride and water. Normal or physiological saline is a 0.9% solution with the same osmotic pressure as that of plasma. ◑ hypertonic, hypotonic, isotonic.

saliva *n* fluid secreted by three pairs of salivary glands—parotid, sublingual and submandibular. It contains varying amounts of water, salts, mucus and salivary amylase; the three pairs of salivary glands produce saliva of different composition. Assists in the mastication of food and its digestion by the enzyme salivary amylase. It also plays a part in speech, taste and the natural cleansing of the mouth and oral tissue and has a protective role on the teeth and the gingival and oral mucosa—**salivary** *adj*. ◑ artificial saliva, parotid salivary gland, sublingual salivary gland, submandibular salivary gland, whole saliva.

S
T

saliva ejector a tube with shaped end or tip through which saliva and other liquids are aspirated from the mouth at low velocity.

salivary *adj* pertaining to saliva.

salivary amylase previously call ptyalin. A starch-splitting enzyme present in saliva. It converts starchy foods to the disaccharide maltose. ⊃ amylase.

salivary calculus a stone formed in the salivary glands or ducts.

salivary cannula a metal or polythene cannula inserted into the duct of the gland to collect saliva.

salivary duct the duct conveying saliva from a salivary gland to the mouth. Consists of three parts: (a) the portion connecting the gland to the striated portion; (b) the striated portion that can modify the composition of saliva; and (c) the excretory duct that conveys the modified saliva into the mouth.

salivary fistula an abnormal passage conducting saliva from a salivary gland or its duct into the mouth or to the surface of the skin of the face.

salivary glands the three pairs of glands which secrete saliva, i.e. the parotid, submandibular and sublingual salivary glands (Figure S.1). ⊃ parotid salivary gland, sublingual salivary gland, submandibular salivary gland.

salivation *n* an increased secretion of saliva. The rate of salivation varies during the day; it may be increased by visual stimulation or by certain odours, such as the smell of food cooking and decreases during sleep.

Salk vaccine (J Salk, American virologist, 1914–1995) a preparation of killed poliomyelitis virus used as an antigen to produce active artificial immunity to poliomyelitis. It is given by injection.

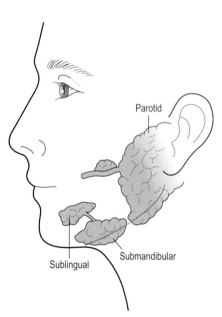

S.1 **Salivary glands** (reproduced from Brooker 2006A with permission).

Salmonella *n* (D Salmon, American veterinary pathologist, 1850–1914) a genus of bacteria of the family Enterobacteriaceae. Gram-negative rods, which are parasitic in many animals and humans in whom they are often pathogenic. Some species, such as *Salmonella enterica* serovar Typhi, are host-specific, infecting only humans, in whom they cause typhoid fever. Others, such as *Salmonella typhimurium*, may infect a wide range of host species, usually through contaminated foods. *Salmonella enteritidis* is a motile Gram-negative rod, widely distributed in domestic animals, particularly poultry, and in rodents, and sporadic in humans as a cause of food poisoning.

salmonellosis infection caused by bacterial species of the genus *Salmonella*. For example food poisoning. ⊃ food poisoning, gastroenteritis.

salpingectomy *n* excision of a uterine (fallopian) tube such as for a ruptured tubal (ectopic) pregnancy.

salpingitis *n* acute or chronic inflammation of the uterine (fallopian) tubes. ⊃ hydrosalpinx, pelvic inflammatory disease, pyosalpinx.

salping/o- a prefix that means 'uterine (fallopian) tube', e.g. *salpingitis.*

salpingography *n* radiological examination of tubal patency by retrograde introduction of contrast agent into the uterus and along the uterine (fallopian) tubes. Being superseded by ultrasound examination—**salpingographic** *adj*, **salpingographically** *adv*.

salpingolysis a procedure to divide adhesions blocking the uterine (fallopian) tubes in order to restore patency and increase the chances of conception.

salpingo-oophorectomy *n* excision of a uterine (fallopian) tube and ovary.

salpingo-oophoritis inflammation of the uterine (fallopian) tube and the ovary.

salpingostomy *n* an operation performed to restore the patency of the uterine (fallopian) tube. Or making an opening in the uterine tube.

salpinx *n* a tube, especially the uterine (fallopian) tube or the pharyngotympanic (eustachian or auditory) tube.

salt *n* a substance produced by the combination of an acid and an alkali (base), e.g. potassium chloride.

salt (sodium chloride) intake there has been controversy in the past about the potentially harmful effects of excessive salt intake (specifically the sodium component). A statement from the Faculty of Public Health of the Royal College of Physicians UK has endorsed evidence that intake above the recommended maximum of 6 g per day for adults (less for children, proportional to age group) is strongly linked to the development of hypertension, and is therefore in turn a risk factor for coronary artery disease and stroke, whereas the average intake over the population is closer to 9 g per day. More than 6 g per day is, however, likely to be appropriate for athletes whose training or competition involves excessive sweating. Salt in the diet (apart from added table salt and that used in cooking) is derived mostly from processed food and there are also other minor sources of sodium. ⊃ minerals, sodium, water balance.

salt sterilizer ⟶ sterilizer.

saltatory conduction the propagation of action potentials along a myelinated nerve in which the impulse jumps between the gaps in the myelin sheath, i.e. from one node of Ranvier to the next node. There is a concentration of voltage-gated sodium/potassium ion channels at the gap where the action potential is regenerated. Thus explaining the rapid transmission of impulses in myelinated nerves.

salvage therapy in radiotherapy, treatment given to a site where previous treatments have failed and the disease has recurred.

Samaritans *n* a voluntary befriending service available 24 hours/day to support suicidal and despairing people who make contact by telephone, electronic mail or by visiting a local centre.

sample *n* a research term. The particular subset chosen from a population. A group who meet the inclusion criteria and are entered in the research study.

sandfly *n* an insect (*Phlebotomus*) responsible for transmitting viral sandfly fever and the protozoa that causes leishmaniasis.

sandfly fever phlebotomus fever.

sandwich osteotomy a surgical technique of increasing ridge height by horizontally sectioning the mandible, above the level of the neurovascular bundle, and inserting bone or other materials.

sandwich technique an impression technique in which a light, medium and heavy impression material are used simultaneously to form layers in the set impression.

sanguineous *adj* pertaining to or containing blood.

sanitary pontic a pontic of a bridge designed to be self-cleansing.

SaO₂ *abbr* arterial oxygen saturation. ⟶ pulse oximetry.

saphenous *adj* apparent; manifest. The name given to a nerve and two superficial veins in the leg. ⟶ saphenous nerve, saphenous veins.

saphenous nerve is a branch of the femoral nerve, it innervates the medial aspects of the lower leg and the foot. ⟶ Colour Section Figure 11.

saphenous veins two superficial veins of the leg. *great (long) saphenous vein* the longest vein in the body, it carries blood from the foot, leg and thigh to the femoral vein. *small (short) saphenous vein*, which carries blood from the foot and leg to the popliteal vein. ⟶ Colour Section Figure 10.

sapro- a prefix that means 'dead, decaying', e.g. *saprophyte*.

saprophyte *n* free-living micro-organism obtaining nutrients from dead and decaying animal or plant tissue—**saprophytic** *adj*.

SARA *abbr* sexually acquired reactive arthritis.

sarc/o- a prefix that means 'flesh', e.g. *sarcoma*.

sarcoid *adj* a term applied to a group of lesions in skin, lungs or other organs, which resemble tuberculous foci in structure, but the true nature of which is still uncertain.

sarcoidosis *n* (*syn* Boeck's disease) a multisystem granulomatous disorder. The condition is more commonly seen in colder parts of Northern Europe where the incidence is approximately 40/10 000. In North America it tends to be more common, and more aggressive, in African-Caribbean populations. The aetiology remains uncertain. Links with atypical mycobacteria and viruses remain speculative; there is some evidence of familial clustering and genetic factors are undoubtedly important. Sarcoidosis appears less commonly in smokers. The mediastinal and superficial lymph nodes, lungs, liver, spleen, skin, eyes, parotid salivary glands and phalangeal bones are most frequently affected, but all tissues may be involved. The characteristic histological feature is a non-caseating epithelioid granuloma; fibrosis is seen in up to 20% of cases of pulmonary sarcoidosis. Disturbances in calcium metabolism reflect increased formation of calcitriol (1,25-dihydroxycholecalciferol vitamin D_3) by alveolar macrophages and may lead to hypercalciuria, hypercalcaemia and, rarely, nephrocalcinosis. Sarcoidosis is considered under the diagnostic term of diffuse parenchymal lung disease (DPLD) as over 90% of cases affect the lungs, but the presentation can be quite variable. Löfgren's syndrome—an acute illness characterized by erythema nodosum, peripheral arthropathy, uveitis, bilateral hilar lymphadenopathy (BHL), lethargy and occasionally fever—is often seen in young women. Alternatively, BHL may be detected in an otherwise asymptomatic individual undergoing a chest X-ray for other purposes. Pulmonary disease may also present in a more insidious manner with cough, exertional breathlessness and radiographic infiltrates; chest auscultation is often surprisingly unremarkable. Fibrosis occurs in some patients and may cause a silent loss of lung function. Pleural disease is uncommon and finger clubbing is not a feature. Complications such as bronchiectasis, aspergilloma, pneumothorax, pulmonary hypertension and cor pulmonale have been reported but are fortunately rare. The overall mortality is low (1–5%). Lymphopenia is characteristic and liver function tests may be mildly deranged. The serum calcium may be elevated and must be checked. Serum angiotensin-converting enzyme (ACE) may provide a non-specific marker of disease activity and can assist in monitoring the clinical course. Chest radiography has been used to stage sarcoid: (a) stage I—BHL usually symmetrical, paratracheal lymph nodes enlarged; (b) stage II—BHL and parenchymal infiltrates; (c) stage III—parenchymal infiltrates without BHL; (d) stage IV—pulmonary fibrosis. In patients with pulmonary infiltrates pulmonary function may show a restrictive defect accompanied by impaired gas exchange. Exercise tests may reveal oxygen desaturation. Bronchoscopy may demonstrate a 'cobblestone' appearance of the mucosa, and bronchial and transbronchial biopsy usually show non-caseating granulomas. The bronchoalveolar lavage (BAL) fluid typically contains an increased CD4:CD8 T-cell ratio. High-resolution computed tomography (HRCT) produces typical appearances. The occurrence of erythema nodosum in women in the 2nd–3rd decade with BHL on chest X-ray is often sufficient for a confident diagnosis without recourse to a tissue biopsy.

S
T

However, when there is real doubt, the diagnosis should be confirmed by histological examination of the involved organ. The majority of patients enjoy spontaneous remission and, if there is no evidence of organ damage, it is appropriate to withhold therapy for 4–6 months. Patients who present with acute illness and erythema nodosum should receive non-steroidal anti-inflammatory drugs (NSAIDs) and on occasion a short course of corticosteroids. Systemic corticosteroids are also indicated in the presence of hypercalcaemia, pulmonary impairment, and renal impairment. Topical corticosteroids may be useful in uveitis but inhaled corticosteroids have no proven benefit in lung disease. Features suggesting a less favourable outlook include: age >40, African-Caribbean origin, persistent symptoms for more than 6 months, the involvement of more than three organs, lupus pernio and a stage III/IV chest X-ray. In patients with severe disease both methotrexate and azathioprine have been used successfully and selected patients may be referred for consideration of single lung transplantation. ➲ interstitial lung disease.

sarcolemma *n* the plasma membrane that encloses the sarcoplasm (cytoplasm) of a muscle cell (fibre), plus an extracellular layer of carbohydrate and collagenous macromolecules which imparts some mechanical strength and is contiguous at fibre ends with tendons or aponeuroses of origin and insertion.

sarcoma *n* malignant tumour of connective tissue, such as bone, but the suffix is also applied to tumours of muscle, nervous or vascular tissue. Examples of sarcomas include chondrosarcoma, fibrosarcoma, myosarcoma, myxosarcoma, osteosarcoma and rhabdomyosarcoma. Treatment options include surgery, radiotherapy and chemotherapy usually in combination. ➲ Ewing's tumour—**sarcomata** *pl*, **sarcomatous** *adj*.

sarcomatosis *n* a condition in which sarcomata are widely spread throughout the body.

sarcomere *n* the segment of a myofibril that forms the smallest functional contractile unit in striated (skeletal) muscle. The length-wise repeating unit of striated muscle, from one Z line to the next; length about 2.5×10^{-6} m in fully extended muscle, less in shortened. ➲ myofibrils.

sarcopenia the atrophy of skeletal muscle and reduction in muscle mass associated with age-related changes.

sarcoplasm *n* the cytoplasm within a muscle cell (fibre).

sarcoplasmic reticulum (SR) *n* a membrane-bounded system within the cytoplasm of all muscle cells (particularly prominent in large, skeletal fibres), which on excitation releases calcium ions (thereby activating force-generation) (Figure S.2). In skeletal muscle this occurs when an action potential (AP) invades abutting t-tubes. If the AP, and thus the release process, is not repeated within a few tens of milliseconds, the active reabsorption of $[Ca^{2+}]$ into the SR by the calcium (Ca) pump leads to relaxation. ➲ t-tubes (t-tubules).

sarcoplasmic reticulum ATPase an enzyme present in the membrane of the sarcoplasmic reticulum. It catalyses the

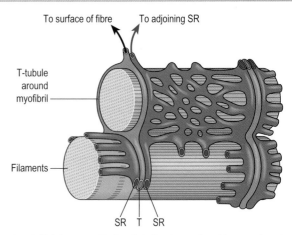

S.2 **Adjoining myofibrils of skeletal muscle**, with sarcoplasmic reticulum (SR) and t-tubes/tubules (T) (reproduced from Jennett 2008 with permission).

pumping of calcium ions $[Ca^{2+}]$ back into the sarcoplasmic reticulum after its electrically stimulated release. ➲ muscle enzymes.

Sarcoptes scabiei *n* a species of itch mite responsible for scabies.

Sargent jump test an elementary test of lower limb impulsive power, consisting of comparison between a subject's upward reach when standing and the height attained in a standing vertical jump; most simply performed against a blackboard, against which chalk is pressed by the subject's hand.

SARS *abbr* severe acute respiratory syndrome.

sartorius *n* the longest muscle in the body, it is known as the 'tailor's muscle', since it flexes one leg over the other. It is a strap-like muscle of the thigh, which crosses the hip and knee joints. Its origin is on the anterior superior iliac spine and it inserts on to the medial aspect of the tibia. It contracts to flex and laterally rotate the thigh, also a weak flexor of the knee. ➲ Colour Section Figures 4, 5.

SATA *abbr* spatial average temporal average.

satellite cell 1. cells associated with muscle cells. Important for muscle growth and repair. It is a small cell, a nucleus surrounded by minimal cytoplasm, lying outside but as close as possible to the membrane of a skeletal muscle fibre, and within the sarcolemma. When fibre enlargement (hypertrophy) or repair is required, satellite cells divide, one daughter becoming active in developing new muscle cytoplasm and the other being retained as a further-generation satellite cell. **2.** neuroglial cells that surround some neurons.

SATF *abbr* self-applied topical fluoride.

satiety with reference to food, the converse of hunger—the sensation of satisfaction or the feeling of fullness after a meal. Mediated by the hypothalamus and influenced by many complex factors, including hormone secretions from the gut in response to a full meal, vagal afferent stimulation by stomach distension, insulin and glucagon secretion and blood glucose concentration.

S
T

SATP *abbr* spatial average temporal peak.

Sattler's layer (H Sattler, Austrian ophthalmologist, 1844–1928) ⮡ choroid.

Sattler's veil (H Sattler) clouding of vision accompanied by seeing coloured haloes around lights caused by corneal oedema resulting from contact lens wear, more frequently the hard lens type (PMMA). The cause has recently been shown to be due to a circular diffraction pattern formed by the basal epithelial cells and the extracellular spaces. ⮡ central corneal clouding, halo.

saturated fatty acids (SFA) fatty acids with single bonds between carbon atoms, all the remaining bonds being attached to hydrogen. Saturated fatty acids (SFA) occur primarily in animal products such as beef, lamb, pork, chicken, cream, milk, butter. Coconut and palm oil, hydrogenated margarine, commercially prepared cakes, pies, and biscuits are also rich in SFA. High dietary intake is associated with an unfavourable (atherogenic) blood lipid profile in which low density lipoproteins (LDLs) are increased.

saturated solution one in which the maximum amount of a particular substance is dissolved.

saturation in magnetic resonance imaging (MRI), a non-equilibrium state where equal numbers of spins are aligned with and against the magnetic field. This occurs immediately following a 90° radiofrequency pulse with the longitudinal magnetization aligned in the transverse plane.

saturation analysis a technique to determine the concentration of a hormone or chemical in a small sample of blood or urine.

satyriasis *n* excessive, abnormal or uncontrolled sexual activity in males. Compare ⮡ nymphomania.

saucer a rounded, hollow depression.

saucerization in surgery, the conversion of a cyst cavity into one with a saucer-like shape.

Saving Newborn Lives global initiative lead by the Save the Children organization to ensure that safe motherhood also includes neonatal care strategies.

SBLA syndrome *abbr* sarcoma, breast, leukaemia and adrenal gland syndrome. ⮡ Li–Fraumeni syndrome.

SBP *abbr* systolic blood pressure.

SBS *abbr* short bowel syndrome.

SC *abbr* subcutaneous.

scab *n* a dried crust forming over an open wound.

scabies *n* a parasitic skin disease caused by the Acarus, *Sarcoptes scabiei* (the 'itch mite'), and is a common world-wide public health problem with an estimated global prevalence of 300 million. The infestation causes considerable discomfort and can lead to secondary infection and complications such as post-streptococcal glomerulonephritis. Highly contagious, scabies spreads in households and environments where there is a high frequency of intimate personal contact. Diagnosis is made by identifying the scabietic burrow, usually found on the edges of the fingers, toes or sides of the hands and feet. Extraction of the mite using a blunt needle can be difficult but is helpful in ensuring the correct diagnosis, appropriate treatment and compliance.

Inappropriate application of scabietic treatments can cause considerable irritation in other conditions. In small children the palms and soles can be involved with pustule formation. ⮡ Colour Section Figure 107. Involvement of the genital area in boys is pathognomonic. The main symptom is itch. The clinical features include secondary eczematization elsewhere on the body; the face and scalp are never involved except in the case of infants. Even after successful treatment the itch can continue, and occasionally nodular lesions persist. Topical treatment of scabies is usual and involves the affected individual and all asymptomatic family members/physical contacts to ensure eradication. Two applications one week apart of an aqueous solution of either permethrin or malathion to the whole body, excluding the head, are usually successful. In some clinical situations such as poor compliance, immunocompromised individuals and heavy infestations (Norwegian scabies), systemic treatment with ivermectin (200 μg/kg) as a single dose is appropriate.

scala the fluid filled structures in the cochlea; scala media (also known as the cochlear duct) containing endolymph, and the scala tympani and scala vestibuli that both contain perilymph.

scalar describes a variable, quantity or measurement that has only magnitude (size), i.e. no directional component. Can be added arithmetically. Examples are area, speed, temperature.

scald *n* an injury caused by moist heat.

scalded skin syndrome ⮡ toxic epidermal necrolysis.

scale 1. *v* in dentistry, to remove calculus and debris from the teeth. **2.** a flake of exfoliated epidermis. **3.** a sequence of numbers.

scalenus one of four paired muscles situated laterally on the neck—the scalenus anterior, medius, minimus (pleuralis) and posterior. Known collectively as the scalene muscles. The origins are on the transverse processes of the cervical vertebrae and they insert on to the first two ribs. They contract to raise the first two ribs during inspiration and may be involved in coughing; also function to flex and rotate the neck.

scalenus syndrome pain in arm and fingers, often with wasting, because of compression of the lower trunk of the brachial plexus behind scalenus anterior muscle at the thoracic outlet.

scaler in dentistry, an instrument for removing calculus and other deposits from the tooth surface. There are five main types. *curette scaler* hand instrument with a sharp, hollow, ground blade like an excavator used for debridement of periodontal pockets and tooth roots. Usually made in sets of six. *periodontal hoe scaler* hand instrument with small blade at right angles to the stem. Generally in sets of four and used with a pulling action. *push, watch-spring, Guys* or *Cushing scaler* hand scaler with thin, chisel-shaped blade, either curved or straight, in line with the handle. Used with a pushing motion. *trihedral scaler* two main types: sickle and jacquette. Instruments with two blades, one either side of the superior surface which ends in a point. Principally used for the removal of supragingival calculus or calculus located just below the gingival margin. *ultrasonic scaler* scaling instrument whose tip is activated by ultrasonic vibrations and incorporates a water spray. It has several interchangeable tips of different shapes. Theoretically, should not be used on a patient with a pacemaker as it may upset the rhythm of the heart.

scaling removal of calculus and other deposits from the crown and roots of teeth by means of scalers.

scalp *n* the hair-bearing skin which covers the cranium.

scalp cooling technique used to minimize or prevent alopecia. Associated with the administration of cytotoxic drugs such as doxorubicin.

scalp electrode small transducer applied *per vaginam* to the fetal scalp during labour to monitor fetal heart rate; the neonate may have small lesions apparent on the scalp at birth at the point where the electrode was sited.

scalpel *n* a surgeon's knife, which may or may not have detachable blades. Originally a sharp cutting blade with flat metal handle in one piece. Now consists of a metal handle with detachable, sterile-packed disposable blades of numbered assorted shapes.

scan *n* an image built up by movement along or across the object scanned, either of the detector or of the imaging agent, to achieve complete coverage, e.g. ultrasound scan.

scan delay the time between the start of the contrast agent injection and the onset of computed tomography (CT) scanning.

scan limits start and end points of data acquisition.

scanners a device which enables documents, pictures, etc. to be held as a digital image.

scanning laser ophthalmoscope (SLO) an ophthalmoscope which provides a continuous image of the ocular fundus on a television monitor. It consists of a narrow laser beam which is scanned horizontally and vertically to produce a rectangular area (called a raster) on the retina. A small beam of light is reflected back out of the eye to a light detector which monitors the brightness of each point on the raster and relays the information to the corresponding element on a monitor where the image can be viewed and/or stored. Low illumination is used to make this procedure more comfortable than conventional photography and mydriatic drugs are usually unnecessary. The field of view extends up to 40 degrees. The instrument has been especially valuable in diagnosing glaucoma and research. ⊃ binocular indirect ophthalmoscope, direct ophthalmoscope, indirect ophthalmoscope, ophthalmoscopy.

scanning speech an abnormal staccato speech pattern. The person hesitates between syllables, which are equally stressed. This produces words that sound clipped.

scan time the time taken for data acquisition.

scaphocephaly a congenital malformation that results in an abnormally long skull, it is caused by early closure of the sagittal suture.

scaphoid boat-shaped, as a bone of the carpus and the tarsus (where it is called the navicular bone).

scaphoid abdomen sunken abdomen in low birth weight babies, due to shrinkage of liver and spleen *in utero*.

scaphoid bone one of the carpal bones of the wrist. It articulates with the radius, and other carpal bones—lunate, capitate, trapezoid and trapezium. The scaphoid bone in the wrist is commonly damaged by compression, causing scaphoid fracture. The navicular bone, one of the tarsal bones of the foot, is also known as the scaphoid bone ⊃ scaphoid fracture.

scaphoid fracture a fracture of the scaphoid bone in the wrist. Commonly occurs as a result of compression of the scaphoid, when there is a fall onto the outstretched hand in hyperextension. A fracture of the scaphoid bone in the carpus of the hand is sometimes difficult to detect on the initial X-ray and it requires a repeat X-ray in around two weeks after the injury to confirm. Commonly, if the fracture involves the proximal third of the scaphoid, there is a high risk of non-union and threat of avascular necrosis, due to the poor blood supply.

scapula *n* the shoulder-blade—one of two large, flat triangular bone of the pectoral (shoulder) girdle. It is situated on the posterior thoracic wall with a layer of muscle separating it from the ribs. Each has two surfaces, three borders and three angles. The posterior surface is marked by a prominent ridge or spine which extends to the acromion process. The scapula articulates with the clavicle at the acromioclavicular joint. A shallow fossa known as the glenoid cavity, situated at the lateral angle, accommodates the head of the humerus to form the ball and socket shoulder joint. The coracoid process provides attachment for muscles that include the biceps brachii and pectoralis minor— **scapulae** *pl.* **scapular** *adj.* ⊃ Colour Section Figure 3.

scapulohumeral rhythm the movements of clavicular rotation, scapular gilding, scapular rotation and glenohumeral elevation, during movement of the shoulder complex.

scarf test a test for problems at the acromioclavicular joint (ACJ). The test is performed by forced cross body adduction in 90° flexion, pain at the extreme of motion indicates ACJ pathology.

scar *n* (*syn.* cicatrix) the dense, avascular white fibrous tissue, formed as the end result of healing, especially in the skin. ⊃ hypertrophic scar, keloid.

scarification *n* the making of a series of small, superficial incisions or punctures in the skin for the purpose of introducing a vaccine.

scarlatina scarlet fever.

scarlet fever *n* (*syn.* scarlatina) infection by β-haemolytic streptococcus (Lancefield Group A). Occurs mainly in children. Starts commonly with a throat infection, leading to fever, and a punctate erythematous rash on the skin of the trunk that is followed by desquamation. Characteristically the area around the mouth escapes (circumoral pallor).

Scarpa's triangle (A Scarpa, Italian anatomist/surgeon, 1752–1832) also known as the femoral triangle. ⊃ femoral.

SCAT *abbr* sheep cell agglutination test.

scattered when photons hit an object and are deflected from their original path, they may or may not loose energy as a result.

scattergram in statistics, where two variables are represented by a single plot against an x and y axis.

scattering cross section the area of the patient, measured in cm^2 or barns, that lies in the X-ray field, the larger the area the higher the probability that the radiation will interact with the tissue.

SCBU *abbr* special care baby unit. ⊃ neonatal unit.

SCC *abbr* **1.** spinal cord compression. **2.** squamous cell carcinoma.

Scheiner's experiment a demonstration of the refractive changes occurring in the eye when accommodating. The subject observes a target monocularly (such as a simple point of light) through a Scheiner disc (an opaque disc with two pinholes separated by a distance less than the pupil diameter). It will be seen singly at only one distance where the eye is focused, because target and retina are then conjugate. If the eye accommodates, two points of light are seen. The principle of this experiment is incorporated in several refractometers. ⊃ conjugate distances, infrared optometer, Young's optometer.

schema in psychology, an abstract mental representation or set of rules for organizing one's experience or an aspect of one's world that is based on experience and stored in memory. It is accessed either consciously or subconsciously in response to relevant environmental cues and facilitates and guides the person's perception and interpretation of events—**schemata** *pl*.

schema theory a theory of motor learning, positing that as individuals practise a motor skill, they acquire a schema for the actions involved, which generalizes and guides the execution of similar actions in the future.

Scheuermann's disease (H Scheuermann, Danish orthopaedic surgeon, 1877–1960) osteochondritis of the spine affecting the ring epiphyses of the vertebral bodies occurring during adolescence. It consists of wedging of the vertebrae, Schmorl's nodes or vertebral endplate irregularity and narrowing of the intervertebral disc spaces. Its aetiology is not clear. Scheuermann's disease commonly affects the lower thoracic and upper lumbar spine. It usually begins at puberty and males and females are equally affected. It can lead to kyphosis and half of those affected develop a scoliosis as well. ⊃ Schmorl's node.

Schick test (B Schick, American physician, 1877–1967) a skin test used to determine susceptibility or immunity to diphtheria. It consists of the intradermal injection of diphtheria toxin. A positive reaction (susceptibility to diphtheria) is indicated by the appearance of a round red area within 24–48 hours, whereas the absence of any skin reaction to the toxin indicates immunity to the disease.

Schilder's disease (P Schilder, Austrian neurologist, 1886–1940) a genetically determined degenerative disease associated with learning disability. ⊃ adrenoleucodystrophy.

Schilling test (R Schilling, American haematologist, b.1919) estimation of absorption of radioactive vitamin B_{12} for investigation of the cause of vitamin B_{12} deficiency.

Schirmer's test a test for measuring tear secretion. It is accomplished by using a 35×5 mm strip of filter paper (e.g. Whatman No. 41). The filter strip is folded so that one end, about 5 mm long, is inserted at the midportion (or lateral portion) of the lower eyelid of a patient seated in a dimly lit room. Tear secretion is considered normal if 10 mm or more of the paper from the point of the fold becomes wet in a 4-minute period. More than 25 mm of wetting would indicate excessive tear secretion. Without any additional stimulation of any kind the test, called *Schirmer's test I*, measures mainly the basal tear production, but because the filter paper tends to irritate the conjunctiva, some of the reflex tear secretion may be also be measured as well. *Schirmer's test II* is aimed at measuring mainly reflex tear secretion. It is carried out with the filter paper inserted inside the lower lid of an eye with topical anaesthesia, while the contralateral half of the nasal mucosa is irritated by rubbing it with a dry cotton-tipped applicator. The amount of tear production is measured after 2 minutes. A value of more than 15 mm is considered to be normal and less than 15 mm may indicate a deficiency of reflex tear secretion. ⊃ alacrima, keratitis sicca, Norn's test, phenol red cotton thread test, tear secretion.

Schistosoma *n* (*syn. Bilharzia*) a genus of blood flukes which require freshwater snails as an intermediate host before infesting humans. Includes: *Schistosoma haematobium* in Africa and the Middle East, *Schistosoma japonicum* in Japan, the Philippines and Eastern Asia and *Schistosoma mansoni* in the Middle East, Africa, South America and the Caribbean.

schistosomiasis *n* (*syn.* bilharziasis) infestation by *Schistosoma* that enter via the skin or mucosae. A single fluke can live in one part of the body, depositing eggs over many years. Prevention is by water chlorination, safe disposal of human waste and eradication of freshwater snails. There may be irritation at the entry site and after 3–5 weeks signs of larval migration, e.g. fever, eosinophilia, pneumonitis and hepatitis. Later, effects depend on where the eggs are deposited and the type, e.g. hepatitis, colitis, skin lesions, cystitis and haematuria. Many years later there may be organ damage due to fibrosis such as hepatic fibrosis and hepatic portal hypertension, urinary tract damage and pulmonary hypertension.

schistosomicide *n* any agent lethal to *Schistosoma*—**schistosomicidal** *adj*.

schizophrenia *n* a group of psychotic disorders characterized by disturbances of thinking, perceiving and affect. The course can be at times chronic, at times marked by acute episodes. Schizophrenia is one of the major diagnostic categories of mental illness. It may present with a variety of symptoms that include: thought echo, insertion, withdrawal, or broadcasting; delusions; hallucinations; incoherence, irrelevant speech or neologisms; catatonic behaviour; negative symptoms, including apathy, scantiness of speech and blunting of affect, usually resulting in social

S
T

withdrawal. Symptoms can be classified as positive and negative. For example, positive symptoms may be hearing voices and/or having strange thoughts, whereas negative symptoms include withdrawal from social contact and severe lack of motivation. The causes of schizophrenia are not fully understood but a genetic link is clear. Management includes medication with atypical antipsychotic (neuroleptics) drugs and other non-drug therapies that include social skills training, cognitive behavioural and psychosocial interventions—**schizophrenic** *adj.* ⊃ expressed emotion.

Schlatter's disease (*syn.* Osgood–Schlatter disease) (C Schlatter, Swiss surgeon, 1864–1934) osteochondritis of the tibial tubercle.

Schlemm's canal (F Schlemm, German anatomist, 1795–1858) ⊃ glaucoma, scleral venous sinus.

Schmidt's syndrome (M Schmidt, German pathologist, 1863–1949) also known as polyglandular autoimmune syndrome type II. An autoimmune syndrome which may affect the function of more than one endocrine gland, including the endocrine pancreas, thyroid, parathyroids, adrenals and the ovaries or testes. This is accompanied by problems caused by autoimmune processes in non-endocrine structures that include alopecia and pernicious anaemia.

Schmorl's node (C Schmorl, German pathologist, 1861–1932) the phenomenon of sequestration or breaking off of part of a disc and its herniation into the vertebral body or movement up and down the spinal canal. Sometimes described as fractured vertebral end plates, often large enough to allow the nucleus pulposus to extrude into the vertebral body. May be a feature of Scheuermann's disease of the lower thoracic and/or thoracolumbar spine. ⊃ Scheuermann's disease.

Schober's test/sign (P Schober, German physician, 1865–1943) a measure of lumbar spine flexion. May be used to assess patients with ankylosing spondylitis. Draw a line at the junction between the 4th and 5th lumbar veretbrae (L4/5), make a mark 10 cm above this line and 5 cm below it, the patient bends forwards with the knees slightly flexed. The therapist holds the end of the tape measure on the upper mark and measures between the two marks. Any increase beyond 15 cm is the lumbar flexion.

Schönlein's disease ⊃ Henoch–Schönlein purpura.

Schottky defect the result of removing an atom completely from a structure. ⊃ point defects.

Schultz–Charlton test a blanching produced in the skin of a patient showing scarlet fever rash, around an injection of serum from a convalescent case, indicating neutralization of toxin by antitoxin.

Schultze expulsion of the placenta normal expulsion of an inverted placenta with the fetal surface appearing first at the vulva. Commoner than Matthews Duncan expulsion with less bleeding. ⊃ Matthews Duncan expulsion of placenta.

Schwann cells (T Schwann, German anatomist, 1810–1882) part of macroglia. Neuroglial cells of the peripheral nervous system. They are concerned with the production of the myelin sheath that surrounds some nerve fibres.

schwannoma a benign, encapsulated tumour arising from the neurilemma of the peripheral, cranial or autonomic nerves.

sciatica *n* pain felt from the lower back to the buttock, and down the back of the leg to the outside of the foot, due to compression of the spinal nerve roots that form the sciatic nerve, aggravated by bending forwards—the 'slump test'. May cause detectable sensory loss and occasionally foot-drop. It does not include referred pain derived from spinal joints, ligaments or muscles. ⊃ disc herniation/protrusion, intervertebral disc, prolapsed intervertebral disc.

sciatic nerve the largest nerve in the body. The sciatic nerve arises from the sacral plexus and contains fibres from the 4th and 5th lumbar nerves and the first three sacral nerves. It passes into the buttock and down the posterior aspect of the thigh to supply the hamstring group of muscles. Half way down the thigh it divides into the common peroneal and tibial nerves, which innervate the muscles and skin of the lower leg, ankle and foot. ⊃ sacral plexus.

SCID *abbr* severe combined immunodeficiency.

Scientific Advisory Committee on Nutrition (SACN) provides independent expert advice to the Food Standards Agency and Government Departments including the Department of Health on matters relating to nutrients present in foods, dietary advice and the nutritional status of specific groups of the population.

scintillation counters a device used to detect small quantities of X or γ radiation from a patient using either a detector in crystalline form or as a liquid scintillation material. Gamma rays from the patient strike the detector and are converted to photons, which pass through a photomultiplier producing a pulsed voltage corresponding to the original radioactivity.

scintillation detector a device for measuring radiation emitted from a patient using a sodium iodide crystal and a photomultiplier tube.

scintillation efficiency the percentage of quantal energy stopped by a phosphor which is changed to useful light photons.

scintillography *n* (*syn.* scintiscanning) visual recording of radioactivity over selected areas after administration of suitable radioisotope (radionuclide).

scirrhous *adj* relating to something that is hard. For example, a scirrhous cancer of the breast, which contains connective tissue and feels hard and gritty.

scissor leg deformity the legs are crossed in walking—following bilateral hip-joint disease, or as a manifestation of Little's disease (spastic cerebral diplegia).

scissors cutting instrument with apposed blades and handles on a central fulcrum. *cross-beak ligature scissors* used in orthodontics for cutting ligature wires, especially against flat or tooth surfaces. *crown scissors (beebee scissors)* scissors with small stout blades, either curved or straight, used to

S
T

trim copper rings, stainless steel strips or tape and preformed metal orthodontic bands. *gum scissors (surgical scissors)* scissors with finer blades that may be curved or straight. *universal scissors* scissors with straight, broad shearing blades serrated to prevent slip when cutting metals and wires.

scissors gait one in which the legs cross each other in progressing. ⊃ gait.

SCJ *abbr* squamocolumnar junction.

SCL *abbr* soft contact lens.

sclera *n* the tough, white, opaque, fibrous outer tunic of the eyeball covering most of its surface (the cornea contributes 7% of, and completes, the outer tunic). Its anterior portion is visible and constitutes the 'white' of the eye. In childhood (or in pathological conditions) when the sclera is thin, it appears bluish, while in old age it may become yellowish, due to a deposition of fat. The sclera is thickest posteriorly (about 1 mm) and gradually becomes thinner towards the front of the eyeball. It is a sieve-like membrane at the cribriform plate of the sclera (lamina cribrosa). The sclera is pierced by three sets of apertures: (a) the posterior apertures round the optic nerve and through which pass the long and short posterior ciliary vessels and nerves; (b) the middle apertures, 4 mm behind the equator which give exit to the vortex veins; and (c) the anterior apertures through which pass the anterior ciliary vessels. The tendons of insertion of the extraocular muscles run into the sclera as parallel fibres and then spread out in a fan-shaped manner. The sclera is commonly considered to be divided into three layers from without inward: (a) the episclera; (b) the scleral stroma; and (c) the suprachoroid (or lamina fusca) which is interposed between choroid and sclera. ⊃ circle of Zinn, cribriform plate of the sclera (lamina cribrosa), episclera, optic nerve—**sclerae** *pl*, **scleral** *adj.* ⊃ Colour Section Figure 15.

scleral conjunctiva ⊃ conjunctiva.

scleral indentation a clinical procedure used in conjunction with indirect ophthalmoscopy in which some slight pressure is applied to the sclera to bring the peripheral retina into view. Pressure is usually applied with an instrument called an indentor. The technique is contraindicated in people with elevated intraocular pressure. ⊃ indirect ophthalmoscope.

scleral spur a ridge of the sclera at the level of the limbus interposed between the posterior portion of the scleral venous sinus (Schlemm's canal) and the anterior part of the ciliary body. The scleral spur is the structure from which some of the ciliary muscle fibres originate. ⊃ ciliary body, ciliary muscle, gonioscopy, internal scleral sulcus.

scleral venous sinus canal of Schlemm. A canal in the inner part of the sclera, close to its junction with the cornea, which it encircles. It drains excess aqueous humour to maintain normal intraocular pressure (IOP). Impaired drainage results in raised intraocular pressure leading to glaucoma and visual impairement in the absence of effective treatment. ⊃ glaucoma, Colour Section Figure 15.

sclerectomy *n* an operation to remove part of the sclera.

sclerema *n* a rare disease in which hardening of the skin results from the deposition of mucinous material.

sclerema neonatorum subcutaneous hardening of the tissues of the extremities, often due to hypothermia in newborn infants.

scleritis *n* inflammation of the sclera which, in its severe necrotizing or in the posterior type may cause sight-threatening complications such as keratitis, uveitis, angle-closure glaucoma or optic neuropathy. It affects females more commonly than males in the fourth to sixth decades of life. Like episcleritis it has a tendency to recur. It is characterized by pain which can be severe and redness and some people may develop nodules (nodular scleritis). It is often associated with a systemic disease. Common causes are rheumatoid arthritis, herpes zoster, ankylosing spondylitis, syphilis and lupus erythematosus. It can involve part of the sclera, e.g. anterior scleritis (that is the most common, and it is classified as diffuse, nodular and necrotizing, with or without inflammation) or posterior scleritis. Treatment includes topical and systemic corticosteroids and immunosuppressive drugs for very severe cases. ⊃ episcleritis, necrotizing scleritis, posterior scleritis.

scleritis necroticans ⊃ sclerokeratitis.

scler/o- a prefix that means 'hard', e.g. *sclerosis.*

sclerocorneal *adj* pertaining to the sclera and the cornea, as the circular junction of these two structures.

sclerodactyly *n* deformity affecting the fingers. There is fixed, partial flexion of the fingers with subcutaneous calcification. Ulceration of the finger tips may occur. Associated with systemic sclerosis. ⊃ CREST syndrome.

scleroderma *n* a connective tissue disease in which localized oedema of the skin is followed by hardening, atrophy, deformity and ulceration. It becomes generalized, producing immobility of the face, contraction of the fingers; can involve internal organs with diffuse fibrosis of the myocardium, kidneys, digestive tract and lungs. The periodontal ligament may be affected. When confined to the skin it is termed morphoea. Nowadays it is usually known as sysytemic sclerosis. ⊃ collagen, connective tissue diseases, CREST syndrome, dermatomyositis, systemic sclerosis.

sclerokeratitis (*syn* necrotizing scleritis without inflammation, scleritis necroticans) inflammation of both the sclera and the cornea.

scleromalacia *n* a bilateral and painless degenerative thinning and softening of the sclera which results in the appearance of dark bluish-grey patches, as the pigmented layer of the eye is exposed. It occurs as a systemic effect of rheumatoid arthritis; when it causes perforation it is known as *scleromalacia perforans.*

sclerose to harden.

sclerosis *n* a word used in pathology to describe abnormal hardening, induration or fibrosis of a tissue. The term is also applied to bone with an increased calcification. ⊃ amyotrophic lateral sclerosis, multiple sclerosis, tuberous sclerosis—**sclerotic** *adj.*

sclerotherapy *n* injection of a sclerosing agent for the treatment of varicose veins. When, after the injection, rubber pads are bandaged over the site to increase localized compression, the term *compression sclerotherapy* is used. Sclerotherapy is a treatment option for oesophageal varices in which the sclerosing agent is administered through an endoscope—**sclerotherapeutic** *adj*, **sclerotherapeutically** *adv*.

sclerotic *adj* relating to sclerosis. *sclerotic dentine* ⊃ dentine.

sclerotic scatter illumination in slit-lamp examination, it is a method in which the beam of light is focused on the sclera near the limbus and the cornea remains uniformly dark in the absence of an opacity. However, an opacity in the cornea becomes easily visible as it scatters light. ⊃ central corneal clouding.

sclerotome 1. parts of the embryonic mesodermal somites. It surrounds the neural tube and the notochord. During embryonic development the vertebrae and dura mater develop from the sclerotome parts of the mesodermal somites. **2.** the part of a bone that derives its nerve supply from a single spinal segment. **3.** an instrument used in surgery of the sclera.

sclerotomy *n* incision into the sclera of the eye.

scolex *n* the head of the tapeworm which it uses to attach itself to the intestine, and from which the segments (proglottides) develop.

scoliosis *n* lateral curvature of the spine, which can be congenital or acquired and is due to abnormality of the vertebrae, muscles and nerves (Figure S.3)—**scoliotic** *adj*. ⊃ halopelvic traction, Harrington rod, Milwaukee brace.

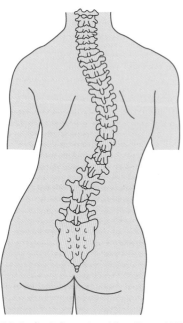

S.3 **Scoliosis** (reproduced from Porter 2005 with permission).

-scope a suffix that means 'instrument for visual examination', e.g. *endoscope*.

-scopy a suffix that means 'to examine visually', e.g. *oesophagogastroduodenoscopy*.

scorbutic *adj* relating to or affected with scurvy.

score in statistics, the total number of responses.

scoto- a prefix that means 'darkness', e.g. *scotoma*.

scotoma *n* a blind spot in the field of vision. May be normal or abnormal. *arcuate scotoma* a visual field defect in the area extending from the normal blind spot in an arc either above or below the central field. *central scotoma* a defect affecting the central field of vision. *centrocaecal scotoma* a defect extending from the normal blind spot to the central field of vision—**scotomata**.

scotopia ⊃ scotopic vision.

scotopic vision (*syn* night vision, nocturnal vision, scotopia) dark-adapted vision at low levels of luminance, below about 10^{-3} cd/m^2 and resulting from the functioning of the rod photoreceptors of the retina. ⊃ mesopic vision, photopic vision.

scrapie *n* a transmissible spongiform encephalopathy of sheep and goats caused by a prion. It is characterized by intense pruritus that leads to affected animals scraping themselves on fences (hence the name), etc., neuromuscular incoordination and eventual death. ⊃ bovine spongiform encephalopathy.

screen asymmetry the production of a pair of intensifying screens when the back screen is slightly faster than the front to compensate for any absorption that may have taken place which reduces the amount of energy reaching the screen.

screen contact test a perforated metal sheet is placed on a radiographic cassette and an exposure of 55 kV at a 2-metre focus–film distance, the film is processed and when viewed at 4 metres any dark areas indicate loss of screen film contact.

screen speed in photography, it is the ability of the phosphor to convert radiation to light, generally the faster the screen the less image detail when comparing the same phosphor, but this does not apply to comparisons between conventional and rare earth screens.

screen test ⊃ cover test (CT).

screen unsharpness blurring of an image due to the phosphor size and thickness, the presence of an absorption/ reflective layer or if a dye is used in the intensifying screen construction. It can also be influenced by poor screen/film contact.

screening *n* a preventive measure to identify potential or incipient disease at an early, asymptomatic stage when it may be more easily treated. It is carried out in a variety of settings, including primary care, hospitals, and clinics for antenatal care, and well babies, well men and well women clinics. Screening checks include: mammography; cervical cytology; blood pressure checks; urine testing for diabetes mellitus; faecal occult blood for colorectal cancer; prostatic specific antigen test for prostate cancer; ultrasound and blood tests to detect fetal abnormalities during pregnancy;

and the checks performed during neonatal screening such as tests for developmental hip dysplasia, hearing tests and blood tests. The screening process may cause anxiety even when no abnormality is found (negative result). ⊃ genetic screening, Guthrie test, neonatal screening, sensitivity, specificity.

screening assessment a process of collecting and interpreting information on which to base the decision about whether or not a person would benefit from occupational therapy intervention.

screening in sport screening can identify and stratify risk in sport, but the potential benefits must be balanced against the resultant anxiety and the fact that some conditions identified may not be treatable. Routine, organized screening in sport in the UK is uncommon: boxing is an exception with compulsory pre-fight medical examinations and annual computed tomography (CT) scanning. Screening is more common in the USA and Italy. In some sports it is compulsory when participants reach a certain level. Screening normally consists of a musculoskeletal assessment (to identify muscle imbalance, degree of flexibility, muscle strength, previous injury, biomechanical abnormalities, etc.) and testing for iron deficiency anaemia in female athletes. Cardiac screening seeks to identify abnormalities which increase the risk associated with participation in sport (especially that of sudden death); this includes a medical questionnaire (personal and family history, symptoms, etc.), clinical examination, electrocardiogram (ECG) and echocardiography. Population screening in sport is indicated and cost-effective when a condition is relatively common, easily identifiable and treatable.

screw in dentistry, a metal cylindrical object with external or internal spiral thread. *dentine screw* screw of various lengths and diameters which is inserted into a matching prepared hole in dentine to provide additional retention for a restoration. *orthodontic screw* a device used to move one or more teeth as part of a fixed or removable appliance. *pulpal screw* a tapered screw of various sizes and lengths with a square slotted head. A small finger-held box spanner or cross-sectioned screwdriver is used to insert it into a root-filled pulp canal to provide increased retention for a restoration. *screw post* a threaded post used in a root-treated tooth to provide retention for a restoration crown or precision attachment.

Scriver test biological test used for diagnosing inborn errors of metabolism, such as phenylketonuria.

scrofula *n* a form of tuberculosis that is characterized by tuberculous abscess formation affecting the lymph nodes, usually those in the cervical region. It is a rare condition but occurs in individual who are immunocompromised such as with HIV disease.

scrolling the movement of text or data on the display screen of a computer.

scrotum *n* the pouch of pigmented skin and fascia in the male, in which the testes are suspended outside the body. Each testis occupies a separate compartment within the scrotum. This arrangement helps to ensure that the testes

are kept at optimum temperature required for the production of healthy spermatozoa, i.e. 4–7°C below core body temperature. The scrotum also has numerous sweat glands, which assist in cooling the testes. In order to maintain a constant temperature the position of the scrotum can be changed by muscle contraction. This occurs in response to temperature changes: heat causes the scrotum to hang loosely away from the body, but it moves closer to the body when cold—**scrotal** *adj*. ⊃ Colour Section Figure 16.

scrub typhus a mite-borne febrile disease caused by the micro-organism *Orientia tsutsuganushi* (formerly called *Rickettia tsutsuganushi*). It occurs in the Far East, India, Pakistan, Bangladesh, parts of Australia, Indonesia and the Pacific Islands. It is characterized by sudden onset of fever, headache, enlarged lymph nodes and cough and later a maculopapular rash often appears. In severe cases it may be complicated by pneumonia and damage to other structures such as the heart.

SCT *abbr* supervised community treatment.

scurf *n* a lay term for dandruff.

scurvy a deficiency disease caused by lack of vitamin C (ascorbic acid). Clinical features include fatigue and haemorrhage. The latter may take the form of capillary bleeding from the gingivae accompanied by loose teeth and halitosis, or large ecchymoses. Tiny bleeding spots on the skin around hair follicles are characteristic. In children painful subperiosteal haemorrhage (rather than other types of bleeding) is pathognomonic.

scybala *npl* rounded, hard, faecal lumps—**scybalum** *sing*.

SD *abbr* standard deviation.

SDA *abbr* specific dynamic action.

SDH *abbr* **1.** succinate dehydrogenase. **2.** subdural haematoma.

SE *abbr* standard error.

seal a substance used to effect a closure. In dentistry, *anterior oral seal* the automatic seal of the oral cavity achieved by lip contact or contact with the lower lip and tongue and/or palatal mucosa. *border seal* the contact of a border of a denture with the soft tissues that prevents the passage of air and thus loss of retention. The term *peripheral seal* is deprecated. *posterior oral seal* the seal made by the soft palate and the dorsum of the tongue during speech and swallowing. *posterior palatal seal (post dam)* the seal at the posterior border of an upper denture.

sealant in dentistry, a substance (usually an unfilled composite resin) used to coat the pits and fissures of a tooth surface to prevent leakage.

sealer ⊃ root canal (dental procedures).

search engine a database of key words that internet users can access to find information on the web.

seasonal affective disorder (SAD) a form of mood disorder (usually depression) with a strong association with the reduced day length and longer nights of autumn and winter. The lack of exposure to light that occurs affects the secretion of melatonin by the pineal body (gland). Presentation varies but can include sleep disturbances such as early

S
T

morning awakening, sleeping longer and daytime sleepiness; poor concentration; low mood or mood swings; feeling tired and lethargic; reduced libido; increased appetite particularly for carbohydrate and sugary foods leading to weight gain; and in severe cases stress and anxiety and depression. Symptoms abate as the day length increases during spring, but it can be successfully treated with exposure to white light with the use of a light box.

seating lug a small component welded to the lingual aspect of an orthodontic band in order to provide a ledge through which pressure may be applied when seating the band onto a tooth.

sebaceous *adj* literally, pertaining to fat; usually refers to sebum.

sebaceous cyst (*syn.* wen) a benign retention cyst that actually contains keratin. Such cysts are most commonly found on the scalp, scrotum and vulva, but may occur anywhere in the body. It has a single cyst cavity.

sebaceous glands the cutaneous glands which secrete an oily substance called sebum. The ducts of these glands are short and straight and open into the hair follicles. ⊃ pilosebaceous unit, Colour Section Figure 12.

seborrhoea *n* greasy condition of the scalp, face, sternal region and elsewhere due to overactivity of sebaceous glands.

seborrhoeic eczema also known as seborrhoeic dermatitis. A condition, which is characterized by a red scaly rash, classically affects the scalp (dandruff), central face, nasolabial folds, eyebrows and central chest. It is due to a fungal infection of the skin usually *Malassezia furfur* (previously known as *Pityrosporum ovale*) but other micro-organisms may be involved. In its milder forms it is the same as dandruff, whereas when severe it may resemble psoriasis. Sebum may be permissive for the development of the rash but otherwise the name is a poor one. Treatment with anti-yeast agents improves the rash, although the course may need to be repeated. Seborrhoeic eczema is a feature of HIV/AIDS disease and can be very severe in this condition. It is very common in HIV and is present in up to 80% of patients with AIDS; severity increases as CD4 count falls. The cause is multifactorial but *Malassezia furfur* is important.

seborrhoeic warts (*syn.* basal cell papilloma) the brown, greasy warts seen in older people, commonly on the chest or back. ⊃ Colour Section Figure 108.

sebum *n* the secretion of the sebaceous glands; it contains fatty acids, cholesterol and dead cells.

seclusion used rarely for mentally ill patients who are isolated in a special room to decrease stimuli which might be causing or exacerbating their emotional distress. The use of seclusion is strictly controlled, monitored and audited.

seclusio pupillae a complete blocking of the anterior chamber from the posterior chamber by a posterior annular synechia. ⊃ annular synechia, pupillary block.

secondary *adj* second in order or importance.

secondary amenorrhoea ⊃ amenorrhoea.

secondary amyloidosis ⊃ amyloidosis.

secondary aplasia ⊃ acquired aplastic anaemia (secondary aplasia).

secondary benefits benefits resulting from a treatment in addition to the primary, intended outcome.

secondary care includes the in-patient and out-patient specialist medical and surgical services that are normally provided by district general hospitals. They include general medicine, surgery and specialist services, such as, orthopaedics, midwifery, child health, and some in-patient mental health services. Secondary care is indirectly accessed by referral from primary care practitioners, or directly as an emergency via emergency departments.

secondary collimation a method of varying the radiation fieldsize to suit individual treatment areas or diagnostic examinations. ⊃ applicator.

secondary collimators can be adjusted to restrict the field size to the treatment area in radiotherapy or the image size in diagnostic radiography. A device on a gamma camera designed to accurately project an image of radioactive distribution received from the patient on to the scintillator.

secondary dentine ⊃ dentine.

secondary dentition ⊃ permanent (secondary) dentition.

secondary disease prevention is the detection and treatment of disease before symptoms or disordered function develops, i.e. before irreversible damage occurs, generally achieved through screening. Examples include cervical cytology screening, hypertension screening. ⊃ primary disease prevention, tertiary disease prevention.

secondary epithelialization vestibuloplasty a surgical technique for the deepening of the gingival sulcus when the extended defect is allowed to epithelialize from the adjacent mucosal surfaces.

secondary generalized seizure ⊃ epilepsy.

secondary glaucoma glaucoma occurring as a result of intraocular tumour, iritis, iridocyclitis, uveitis, rubeosis iridis, traumatic cataract, tumours, etc. ⊃ angle-closure glaucoma, Graves' ophthalmopathy, hyphaemia, ICE syndrome, iritis, luxation of the lens, neovascular glaucoma, open-angle glaucoma, Rieger's syndrome, rubeosis iridis, uveitis.

secondary haemorrhage ⊃ haemorrhage.

secondary hyperaldosteronism a condition characterized by high levels of renin and aldosterone. Causes include: (a) inadequate renal perfusion—e.g. diuretic therapy, heart failure, liver failure, nephrotic syndrome, or renal artery stenosis; (b) a very rare renin-secreting renal tumour.

secondary image a phenomenon seen in panoramic dental radiography whereby the image of an object on the tube side of the patient is projected onto the opposite side.

secondary intention healing a type of wound healing that occurs when there is loss of tissue and it is neither possible nor desirable to pull the wound edges together. The healing process in wounds with considerable loss of tissue, such as traumatic wounds and pressure ulcers, usually involves granulation whereby new capillaries and healthy moist, tissue form in the wound bed, wound contraction and epithelialization where new epithelial cells migrate across the granulation tissue to cover the surface of the wound. ⊃ primary intention healing, wound healing.

secondary occlusal trauma an injury to the periodontium caused by physiologically normal occlusal forces on the tooth with a reduced periodontium.

secondary optic vesicle ⊃ optic cup.

secondary osteoarthritis the type of osteoarthritis (OA) where there is another predisposing cause rather than a problem with the cartilage itself, for example a fracture of the tibial plateau may result in secondary OA in later life. ⊃ osteoarthritis.

secondary radiation the ejection of electrons from a substance after it has been bombarded with charged particles of sufficient energy.

secondary radiation barrier a barrier that protects from the effects of scattered radiation or leakage from the X-ray tube or housing. ⊃ primary radiation barrier.

secondary referencing (citation) where the source of material is taken from a reference used in another piece of work, i.e. without accessing the original primary reference. ⊃ Harvard system of referencing, primary referencing (citation), reference, Vancouver system of referencing.

secondary solute used in liquid scintillation counting to absorb photons emitted by the primary solute and re-emit them as photons of a longer wavelength therefore increasing the efficiency of the detection by photomultiplier tubes.

secondary tumour refers to a primary cancer that has spread to other distant sites in the body, such as colorectal cancer spreading to the liver, or breast cancer spreading to the brain or bone. ⊃ metastasis.

second (s) one of the seven base units of the Système International d'Unités (SI) (International System of Units). A measurement of time and is the duration of 9 192 631 770 periods of the radiation corresponding to the transition between the two hyperfine levels of the ground state of caesium-133 (^{133}Cs) atom.

second-class levers have the resistance and force on the same side of the fulcrum with the resistance closer to the fulcrum than the force. Very rare in the human body but common in machines (e.g. wheelbarrow).

second degree tear ⊃ perineal tear.

second heart sound (S2) the 'DUP' sound heard on the closure of the aortic and pulmonary valves (the semilunar valves) at the end of systole. ⊃ heart sounds.

second impression ⊃ impression.

second messenger intracelluar signalling molecules that include cyclic adenosine monophosphate (cAMP), calcium ions [Ca^{2+}] and inositol triphosphate (IP_3), which act between the hormones and neurotransmitters that act as first messengers, and the particular cellular regulation process. Particularly important in regulatory processes where many reactions are occurring simultaneously (enzyme cascade).

second stage of labour from full dilatation of the uterine cervix to complete birth of the infant.

secretin *n* a hormone produced by cells in the duodenal mucosa, which causes the secretion of alkaline pancreatic juice that is low in enzymes, and with other regulatory peptides inhibits gastric secretion and motility.

secretion *n* a fluid or substance, formed or concentrated in a gland and passed into the gastrointestinal tract, the blood or to the exterior. ⊃ acinar secretion, apocrine gland, holocrine gland, merocrine (eccrine) gland.

secretor a person who secretes their ABO blood group antigens in saliva or gastric juice. ⊃ non-secretor.

secretory *adj* involved in the process of secretion: describes a gland which secretes.

secretory potential the electrical potential change recorded in a salivary gland during stimulation of secretion.

sectional appliance a fixed orthodontic appliance involving a number of teeth in one segment of the jaws.

sectional archwire an archwire fitted to a number of teeth and confined to one section of the dental arch.

sectional denture also known as swinglock denture, a denture made up of two or more separate parts connected with a mechanical device.

sectional impression ⊃ impression.

sectional root-filling technique a method of sealing the apical portion of a root canal with a portion of core material (e.g. gutta percha) and sealer, leaving the rest of the pulp space unfilled in order to accommodate a post.

sector probe an ultrasound probe with a small footprint used for intercostal and cardiac imaging.

secular *adj* describes the civil, state or non-religious influences on society.

secular beliefs those not overtly or specifically religious. The strong non-religious convictions/values that guide concepts of morality that affect everyday life. ⊃ spiritual beliefs.

secure socket layer (SSL) a method of verifying the identity of system users and Web sites.

sedation *n* the production of a state of lessened functional activity. In dentistry, the production of a relaxed state. *sedation technique* a method of sedating patients by the use of drugs (e.g. midazolam) to produce a state of depression of the central nervous system without complete loss of consciousness. Verbal contact with the patient is maintained and local analgesics are usually administered to produce analgesia.

sedative *n* an agent which reduces functional activity by its action on the nervous system. ⊃ anxiolytic.

sedimentation rate ⊃ erythrocyte sedimentation rate.

segment a part of an anatomical structure, such as a lung segment, or the upper and lower uterine segments.

segmental surgery the surgical mobilization and repositioning of the alveolar segments of either the maxilla or the mandible together with the teeth in that segment.

segment angle the angle of a segment of the human body (e.g. limb or trunk) to a fixed reference line (e.g. the horizontal).

segregation *n* a genetic term. The separation of the two alleles, each carried on one of a pair of chromosomes; this happens during meiosis when the haploid (n) gametes (spermatozoa, oocytes) are formed. ⊃ Mendel's law.

Seidel aberration ⊃ monochromatic aberration.

seizures *npl* result from abnormal electrical activity in the brain. They are associated with many disorders, and may take several forms some with convulsions including: absences, atonic, clonic, generalized tonic-clonic, myoclonic, partial or focal, tonic, etc. ⊃ convulsions, epilepsy, febrile seizures, pseudoseizure.

Seldinger catheter a special, small catheter and guidewire for insertion into an artery, along which it is passed to, for example, the heart. Its guidewire is used to direct large-bore cannula insertion, thereby minimizing the risk of misplacement.

selection unit remote-controlled unit for placing, for example, radioactive caesium-137 (^{137}Cs) into body cavities.

selective grinding (spot grinding) the planned adjustment of the occlusal anatomy of teeth by grinding.

selective movement in physiotherapy, a purposeful movement that is co-ordinated and precise, and is based on a suitable level of stability.

selective (o)estrogen receptor modulators (SERMs) a group of tissue specific drugs that modulate oestrogen receptors in some tissues but not others, e.g. raloxifene. They may have oestrogen-agonist or oestrogen-antagonist effects in different tissues. ⊃ Appendix 5.

selective serotonin reuptake inhibitors (SSRIs) a group of antidepressant drugs that act by preventing the reuptake of the neurotransmitter serotonin (5-hydroxytryptamine), e.g. fluoxetine. ⊃ Appendix 5.

selectivity in radiography, the ability of a developing agent to differentiate between exposed silver halide and unexposed silver halide and therefore only converting the exposed crystals to metallic silver. An agent which has no effect on either the metallic silver in the developed image or the gelatin(e) in which it is suspended.

Selectron a proprietary device which stores sealed radioactive sources of caesium, iridium or cobalt in a shielded container in readiness for intracavitary treatment in the uterus, cervix or vagina. In recent years extended to other body sites such as bronchus and oesophagus. ⊃ Colour Section Figure 109.

selenium (Se) *n* functions as an antioxidant by serving as cofactor for the enzyme glutathione peroxidase. A trace element needed in the diet to facilitate reactions that protect cells from oxidative stress/damage. Selenium deficiency causes hypothyroidism and cardiomyopathy in children and myopathy in adults. A few studies have suggested a benefit of selenium supplementation in improving antioxidant capacity and diminishing cancer occurrence. Selenium may possibly be effective in athletes who are ingesting insufficient amounts, but it is not known if marginally insufficient intake compromises efficiency of training. Excessive amounts of selenium could have toxic effects. ⊃ Keshan's disease, minerals.

self-actualization in humanistic psychology the fulfilment of one's potential. The highest level of human achievement in Maslow's hierarchy of needs. ⊃ Maslow's hierarchy.

self-advocacy most often applied to people with learning disabilities. It concerns people speaking up for themselves, defending their rights and organizing themselves to promote their interests as a group. As a political movement, it is the struggle over whose demands, concerns, choices and perspectives should prevail. ⊃ advocacy.

self-awareness the reflective ability of people to take themselves as the objects of their own thoughts. It can include self-conception and self-monitoring, which involves the observation and control of self-presentation.

self care 1. the ability to perform activities, such as, washing, dressing, eating, drinking, elimination needs, etc., without assistance. **2.** taking responsibility for one's own medical or treatment needs following suitable education. For example, self-adminstration of drug regimens, monitoring a medical condition, dialysis, or enteral or parenteral feeding.

self-catheterization *n* ⊃ intermittent self-catheterization.

self-cleansing area an area of the teeth less liable to accumulate plaque and food debris because of the action of the soft tissues and chewing.

self-concept *n* the view that the individual has of their total characteristics, ideas, feelings, qualities and negative features. A person's perceptions or description of their self, typically not involving an evaluative component. ⊃ self-esteem.

self-confidence a generalized tendency to believe that one is capable of being successful within or across behavioural domains. ⊃ self-efficacy.

self-curing acrylic ⊃ resin.

self-determination theory a theory of human personality and motivation predicated on the assumption that people have an innate tendency toward personal growth and development which is facilitated when their psychological needs to feel competent, autonomous and socially related are supported. Widely employed in the study of motivation in sport and exercise.

self-directed learning/study a student-centred learning strategy where the student determines: their learning needs, strategies to fulfil these needs, learning resources required and how to evaluate and reflect on the process.

self-efficacy in social cognitive theory, a person's belief in their ability to execute the behaviours necessary to achieve desired outcomes. In contrast to self-confidence, self-efficacy refers to beliefs about specific behaviours in specific situations. *self-efficacy level* the individual's beliefs about their expected level of performance attainment, ranging from easy to difficult, such as a tennis player's beliefs about the percentage of first serves they could successfully make in a match. *self-efficacy strength* the degree of certainty with which an individual expects to successfully execute a behaviour. ⊃ outcome expectancy.

self-esteem *n* the value or worth an individual places on themselves. Also known as self-evaluation and self-worth.

self-fulfilling prophecy a situation whereby people's expectations of another person cause them to behave in such a way as to cause the exact response that was anticipated. For example a child who is labelled 'very bright' by important people in his or her life, is likely to live up to that expectation.

self-handicapping the imposition of an impediment to successful performance by a person so that they can subsequently either attribute failure to the impediment rather than to lack of ability or effort, or gain increased credit for success. For example, an athlete might avoid training for a race in order to self-handicap.

self-help the collective activities of groups of people who are experiencing similar problems. Self-help groups may remain small but can expand into social movements, for example, the Disabled People's Movement and Gay Pride.

self-image an image of the self people suppose themselves to be. Self-image may be discrepant with what they achieve or how others see them.

self induction occurs when a current-carrying conductor induces a magnetic field in itself and the current changes.

self-infection the unwitting transfer of micro-organisms from one part of the body to another, in which it produces an infection.

self-inflating bag a bag used for ventilation of a patient during anaesthesia or resuscitation.

self-limiting relates to a disease that continues for a specific, limited period of time by reason of its own characteristics and not because of external influences.

self maintenance taking care of one's survival, health and wellbeing through personal care activities.

self-monitoring of blood glucose (SMBG) use of capillary blood, usually obtained by a finger prick, for glucose estimation by a hand-held meter allowing people to monitor and manage their diabetes.

self-serving bias the tendency to attribute successes to internal factors such as ability and effort and failures to external factors such as bad luck. ⇒ attribution.

self-straightening wire a fine stainless steel wire wound onto a labial bow orthodontic appliance as a separate fine-wire bow, to retract incisor teeth.

self-talk a person's internal dialogue, which can be positive and motivational or negative and demotivating.

sella an orthodontic landmark defined as the centre of the sella turcica.

sella turcica a fossa, in the shape of a Turkish saddle, located on sphenoid bone of the skull. It contains the pituitary gland.

Sellick's manoeuvre (B Sellick, British anaesthetist, 1918–1996) ⇒ cricoid pressure.

SEM *abbr* scanning electron microscope.

semantic differential a method for measuring affective responses or attitudes to objects or events by asking people to rate the object or event along a bipolar scale, for example ranging from good to bad.

semantic memory that part of memory that stores general information about the world, e.g. where lions and tigers are found.

semen *n* seminal fluid. Thick, white fluid ejaculated during coitus. It comprises spermatozoa from the testes and the secretions from the: seminal vesicles, which contains nutrients, prostaglandins and enzymes, and forms around 60% of semen volume; prostate gland, which contains enzymes such as acid phosphatase that activates the sperm, and forms around 30% of semen volume; and bulbourethral glands that produce a fluid which helps to maintain the slightly alkaline pH of semen. A normal ejaculate is around 5 mL in volume and contains 50–150 million sperm/mL.

semen analysis a test undertaken early during infertility investigations. A fresh sample of semen is analysed to check the number, morphology and motility of the sperm. The volume of the sample, number of sperm and their motility and the percentage of abnormal sperm are measured.

semester a period of academic time—usually 15 weeks.

semi- a prefix that means 'half', e.g. *semilunar*.

semi-adjustable articulator an articulator that allows adjustments that reproduce mandibular movements in a sagittal plane only.

semicircular canals three fluid-filled canals contained within the bony labyrinth of the inner ear. Orientated in the three planes of space they are part of the vestibular apparatus concerned with dynamic equilibrium and balance. ⇒ Colour Section Figure 13.

semicomatose *adj* describes a condition bordering on the unconscious. ⇒ Glasgow Coma Scale (GCS).

semiconductor a solid device that contains a conduction band and valence band and allows current to flow in one direction only. ⇒ diode, extrinsic semiconductors, intrinsic semiconductors, triode.

semi-finished lens (*syn* semi-finished lens blank) an ophthalmic lens of which only one surface is completely polished. The other side can be surfaced to any required curvature. If it is a bifocal lens, the side with the segment is usually the one which is completely surfaced. ⇒ blank lens, finished lens.

semi-finished lens blank ⇒ semi-finished lens.

semilunar *adj* shaped like a crescent or half moon.

semilunar cartilages the two crescentic interarticular cartilages of the knee joint (menisci) (see Figure M.5, p. 475). The are situated between the femur and the tibia, and function to stabilize the knee joint. Very commonly damaged, especially during certain sports. ⇒ meniscus.

semilunar valves valves with cusps that are half-moon shaped, such as those in the heart—the aortic valve between the aorta and the left ventricle and the pulmonary valve between the pulmonary artery and the right ventricle.

semimembranosus one of the hamstring muscles. A muscle of the posterior thigh. Its origin is on the ischial tuberosity and it inserts on to the medial condyle of the tibia. It contracts to flex the knee, medially rotate the leg and extend the thigh. ⇒ biceps femoris, semitendinosus.

seminal *adj* pertaining to semen.

seminal vesicle one of two tubular accessory glands behind the male bladder. They produce a thick alkaline fluid, which forms some 60% of semen volume. ⊃ semen, Colour Section Figure 16.

seminar a learning session where students make a presentation (usually on a something they have read) to a small group of peers and a tutor as a basis for further discussion by the group.

seminiferous *adj* carrying or producing semen.

seminiferous tubules the coiled structures present in the lobules of the testis. They are formed from sperm-producing germinal epithelium and are involved in the production of immature spermatozoa (spermatogenesis). The spermatozoa leave the seminiferous tubules to enter the epididymus where they mature during a process called spermiogenesis.

seminoma *n* a neoplasm of the testis; subtype of germ cell tumour—**seminomata** *pl*, **seminomatous** *adj*.

semipermeable *adj* selectively permeable. Describes a membrane which is permeable to some substances in solutions, but not to others.

semiprecious metal casting alloy in dentistry, an alloy with noble metal content of at least 25% but <75%. Includes low gold content and silver palladium alloys.

semiprone *adj* describes a position in which the person is partially prone, on their side with the face down, but with the knees flexed to one side. It can be used for nursing unconscious patients.

semitendinosus one of the hamstring muscles. A muscle of the posterior thigh. Its origin is on the ischial tuberosity with the long head of the biceps femoris and it inserts on to the medial aspect of the shaft of the tibia. It contracts to flex the knee, medially rotate the leg and extend the thigh. ⊃ biceps femoris, semimembranosus.

SEN *abbr* special educational needs.

senescence *n* normal physical and mental changes in increasing age—**senescent** *adj*.

Sengstaken–Blakemore tube incorporates gastric and oesophageal balloons which when inflated apply pressure to bleeding oesophageal varices (Figure S.4).

senile *adj* suffering from senescence complicated by morbid processes commonly called degeneration—**senility** *n*. *senile dementia* ⊃ dementia.

senna *n* leaves and pods of a purgative plant. Used as a stimulant laxative. ⊃ Appendix 5.

sensation *n* consciousness of a feeling that results from nerve impulses from the sensory organs reaching the brain. It describes the afferent input from the external world or from inside the body. It confers the ability to function safely and adapt in ever-changing circumstances. Sensory receptors convert information into electrical activity that is then processed by the central nervous system. Sensation requires the peripheral and central nervous system to be intact. Movement is possible without sensation but it is clumsy and slow and is heavily reliant on visual information.

sensation seeking a personality trait associated with a preference for high levels of sensory stimulation, often achieved by engaging in risk-taking behaviours and adopting non-conventional lifestyles.

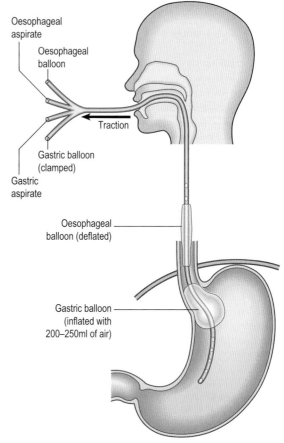

S.4 Sengstaken–Blakemore tube (reproduced from Boon et al 2006 with permission).

sensible *adj* **1.** endowed with the sense of feeling. **2.** detectable by the senses.

sensible perspiration the fluid loss through sweating which is sufficient to be observed. ⊃ insensible water loss, perspiration.

sensitive 1. capable of responding to stimuli. **2.** reacting adversely or being susceptible to an antigen, drug or other substance. **3.** describes a micro-organism that is killed or its growth is restricted by a particular antimicrobial drug. **4.** being perceptive in communication with others.

sensitive period ⊃ critical period.

sensitivity *n* **1.** high sensitivity is the ability of a screening test to accurately identify affected individuals, such as mammography screening for breast cancer. Low sensitivity can lead to false negatives, i.e. the test fails to detect all abnormal cases. ⊃ specificity. **2.** the ability of a detector, for example a film or intensifying screen, to register very small quantities of radiation, the more sensitive the detector the wider the range of intensities can be detected. The counting efficiency of a gamma camera in counts per second per megabecqueral. **3.** the extent to which a micro-organism is likely to respond to treatment with a particular antimicrobial drug. Sensitivity testing is undertaken in the microbiological laboratory. A micro-organism may be described as sensitive if the antimicrobial drug is an effective treatment, or resistant if that antimicrobial drug is not effective in inhibiting microbial growth.

sensitivity training group individuals learn about what occurs during their interactions with other people within a supportive environment. They can test and refine different behavioural responses in the light of feedback, and are encouraged to try the positively modified behaviours in situations outside the group.

sensitization *n* rendering sensitive. Persons may become sensitive to a variety of substances, which may be food (e.g. shellfish), bacteria, plants, chemical substances, drugs, sera, etc. Liability is much greater in some persons than others. ⊃ allergy, anaphylaxis.

sensitizing concept a research term. Used to describe how certain concepts may guide the researcher towards a certain behaviour.

sensitometer in radiography, an exposure device for printing a pre-determined image onto a film.

sensitometry in radiography, a method of measuring blackening on a film, plotting a characteristic curve, producing measurements from the curve and therefore comparing different films or film screen combinations. ⊃ characteristic curve.

sensorimotor feedback involves the integration and interaction of afferent (sensory) information during motor activity, which may then alter the movement or lead to adaptation of the motor response. Feedback allows errors to be corrected.

sensorimotor feed forward involves the integration and interaction of afferent (sensory) information prior to a motor activity and thus allows adaptation to be made before the execution of a movement.

sensorineural *adj* pertaining to sensory neurons.

sensorineural hearing loss (SNHL)/deafness (*syn* nerve deafness, perceptive hearing loss/deafness) is due to a lesion in the inner ear, the auditory nerve or the auditory centres in the brain. Congenital causes include maternal infections during pregnancy (e.g. rubella, cytomegalovirus, toxoplasmosis), aminoglycoside antibiotics (e.g. gentamicin) taken during pregnancy, and associated with various inherited syndromes, such as Usher's syndrome. The causes of acquired sensorineural hearing loss include: hypoxia during birth, damage caused by kernicterus, various drugs (e.g. aminoglycoside antibiotics, some antimalarial drugs, loop diuretic drugs, etc.), excessive noise, failure of the ear to develop correctly, age-related prebycusis, acoustic neuroma and some systemic conditions (e.g. underactive thyroid gland).

sensory *adj* pertaining to sensation. Strictly, applies only to the reception and processing by the nervous system of information from the outside world such that it reaches consciousness as a subjective experience (sensation); often used loosely in relation to any afferent nerve pathway or process, including those serving only reflex function.

sensory agraphia inability to interpret the written word, due to lesions in the posterior part of the left parieto-occipital region.

sensory ataxia results from lesions affecting the peripheral sensory nerves, conditions affecting the dorsal columns, such as tabes dorsalis, or lesions affecting the primary sensory cortex. Patients often have a wide based high-stepping gait pattern. ⊃ ataxia.

sensory cortex that part of the cerebral cortex that receives sensory inputs and decodes them to facilitate perception. It includes the somatosensory area, which is concerned with sensations such as pressure, touch, pain and temperature and inputs from proprioceptors in muscles and joints. It also contains specialist areas—taste, auditory, olfactory, visual and association areas that include a sensory speech area (Wernicke's area).

sensory deprivation a situation in which the usual sensory stimuli are absent, such as for patients in intensive care units, or long periods of isolation, or loss of sight. It can lead to problems that include disruption to sleep–wake patterns, tiredness, increased irritability, poor concentration, anxiety, depression, delusions or hallucinations.

sensory evoked potentials (SEP) a response that is recorded over the parietal region of the brain in response to the stimulation of a peripheral nerve. It allows the conduction time of a nerve to be calculated and so can help detect lesions in the sensory pathways.

sensory fusion (*syn* binocular fusion) the neural process by which the images in each retina are synthesized or integrated into a single percept. In normal binocular vision, this process occurs when corresponding (or nearly corresponding) regions of the retina are stimulated. This process can occur when the images are either in the central part of the retinae (*central fusion*) or in the peripheral part of the retinae (*peripheral fusion*). ⊃ amblyoscope, anaglyph, bar reading test, binocular vision, central vision, convergence insufficiency, diplopia test, fusional convergence, haploscope, peripheral vision, random-dot stereogram, retinal corresponding points, SILO response, Worth's classification of binocular vision, Worth's four dot test.

sensory integration the meaningful organization of sensory information received by the body in order to maximally function in the world at large.

sensory nerves those which transmit impulses from peripheral receptors to the brain and spinal cord.

sensory overload a situation in which the person receives more sensory inputs (usually visual or auditory but can be other stimuli) than can be meaningfully processed. It may occur in patients in hospital, particulary in critical care facilities where there is 24-hour activity involving bright light and the noise of equipment and staff talking, or in people who have difficulty processing stimuli (e.g. autistic spectrum disorders).

sentinel node biopsy (SNB) procedure used in staging (mainly) breast cancer and melanoma where (blue) dye is injected at the primary tumour site and traced to the nearest

S
T

nodal basin where the first node involved with tumour will accumulate the dye; resection of that node may improve the cure rate.

SEP *abbr* sensory evoked potentials.

separating medium a substance used to prevent one surface sticking to another, such as a plaster of Paris cast to the impression material, e.g. soap solution, glycerol, and numerous proprietary preparations.

separating strip ⊃ abrasive strip.

separating wire a soft brass wire sometimes placed between teeth to separate them prior to the placement of orthodontic bands.

separation in dentistry, the achievement of spacing between teeth in the same dental arch, usually in order to place orthodontic bands.

separation anxiety feelings of apprehension, fear and distress caused by being separated from safe and familiar situations and significant individuals, such as the mother or other main carer. For example, that occurring in preschool children separated from their mothers through admission to hospital. There are three stages: characterized first by loud protest and then despair/depression and lastly detachment or denial in which the child may appear to accept the situation. Regression to earlier behaviours may occur, such as loss of continence, clinging to parents or refusing to eat. The degree of the child's distress is influenced by factors, which include the degree of parental involvement in their care, parenting styles, parent's response, etc. ⊃ attachment.

separator an instrument using a screw force to move teeth apart. Generally, used to obtain a satisfactory contact point in dental restorations.

sepsis *n* the state of being infected with pyogenic (pus-forming) micro-organisms—**septic** *adj*.

septal defects congenital anomalies in which an opening exists between the right and left sides of the heart. The defect may be between the two atria or the two ventricles. ⊃ atrial septal defect, ventricular septal defect.

septal thickness in radiography, the thickness of the lead between the holes in a collimator of a gamma camera.

sept/i- a prefix that means 'seven', e.g. *septuagenarian*.

septic abortion ⊃ septic miscarriage.

septic miscarriage one associated with uterine infection.

septicaemia *n* the multiplication of living bacteria in the bloodstream causing infection—**septicaemic** *adj*.

septicaemic plague ⊃ plague.

septic arthritis arthritis caused by infection in the joint.

sept/o- a prefix that means 'septum', e.g. *septoplasty*.

septoplasty *n* conservative operation to straighten the nasal septum, usually undertaken for deviations and dislocations of the quadrilateral cartilage. The nasal septum is repositioned in the midline with minimal removal of nasal cartilage.

septum *n* a partition between two cavities, e.g. between the nasal cavities and the cardiac septum that separates the right and left sides of the heart. *interdental septum* the bone between the roots of teeth—**septa** *pl*, **septal, septate** *adj*.

sequela *n* pathological consequence of a disease—**sequelae** *pl*.

sequestering agent in radiography, Softens hard water, in developer EDTA sodium salt is used to prevent precipitation of calcium and magnesium salts onto the surface of the film.

sequestrated disc the complete detachment of a portion of prolapsed intervertebral disc, with migration, often into the spinal canal. ⊃ Scheuermann's disease, Schmorl's node.

sequestration the separation of a part from the whole, e.g. the rejection of necrosed bone by a pathological process.

sequestrectomy *n* excision of a sequestrum.

sequestrum *n* a piece of dead bone which separates from the healthy bone but remains within the tissues—**sequestra** *pl*.

serial extractions developed in the 1940s. Planned serial removal of primary and permanent teeth over a period of time to relieve crowding. Is no longer in common practice.

serial infra red (SIR) a wireless communication system for computers.

serial port an external socket on older computers used to plug in a mouse or a modem.

series-fibre muscle also known as short-fibre muscle. Skeletal muscle in which fibres do not extend from one end to the other, but are a fraction of muscle length and overlap their lengthwise neighbours only enough to convey force from one to another via molecular linkages between their sarcolemmae. Chief benefit is in co-ordination of contraction: in, say, the sartorius muscle, which may be 50 cm long, muscle action potential (AP) conduction over the whole length could not initiate contraction at the ends before relaxation had started under the motor endplate; 'series' construction allows motor nerve APs, propagating 10–20 times faster, to trigger contractions almost simultaneously throughout the muscle.

serine *n* a conditionally essential (indispensable) amino acid.

SERMs *abbr* selective (o)estrogen receptor modulators.

ser/o- a prefix that means 'serum', e.g. *serous*.

seroconversion a change from a negative serological test where specific antibodies are absent to a positive test in which the presence of antibodies in the serum confirms that a response to an antigen (vaccine or infection) has occurred.

serofibrinous *adj* relating to an exudate containing serum and fibrin.

serology the study of blood serum and its reactions. Important in immunological diagnostic techniques involving the detection of antigen-antibody reactions.

seropurulent *adj* relating to exudate containing serum and pus.

serosa *n* a serous membrane, e.g. the peritoneal covering of the abdominal viscera—**serosal** *adj*.

serositis *n* inflammation of a serous membrane.

serotonin *n* also called 5-hydroxytryptamine (5-HT). A monoamine formed from tryptophan (amino acid). Liberated by blood platelets after injury and found in high concentrations in the central nervous system and gastrointestinal

S
T

tract. Its widespread actions include vasoconstriction, inhibition of gastric secretion and stimulation of smooth muscle. It is also an important neurotransmitter in the central nervous system; as such it is involved in pain transmission and perception, and can influence a variety of behaviours, including tiredness, sleep–wake cycles, mood and mental fatigue. It is suggested that an increased level of serotonin makes it mentally harder to maintain a steady pace of exercise, as in running or cycling ('central fatigue'). Administration of branched-chain amino acids has been claimed to reduce uptake of tryptophan by the brain and therefore to diminish serotonin production. ⊃ ergogenic aids.

serotyping *n* classification of micro-organisms based on specific antigenic features.

serous *adj* 1. pertaining to serum. 2. describing saliva which is thin and derived from blood serum.

serous membrane a lubricating membrane lining the closed cavities of the body, and reflected over their enclosed organs. ⊃ pericardium, peritoneum, pleura.

serous secretion saliva of relatively low viscosity secreted mainly by the parotid gland at a rapid flow rate. It is rich in the enzyme amylase. ⊃ acinar secretion.

serpiginous *adj* snakelike, coiled, irregular; used to describe the margins of skin lesions, especially ulcers and ringworm.

Serratia *n* a genus of Gram-negative bacteria of the family Enterobacteriaceae. Motile bacilli capable of causing infection in humans. The species *Serratia marcescens* is an endemic hospital resident and is an opportunistic pathogen that affects immunocompromised individuals. It causes urinary tract infection, pneumonia, bacteraemia and endocarditis.

serration *n* a saw-like notch—**serrated** *adj*.

serratus anterior *n* a muscle of the anterior chest wall located over the lateral ribs. It has a serrated appearance. It arises from the first eight or nine ribs and it inserts on to the scapula. It contracts to rotate the scapula and raise the shoulder. It is important in arm abduction and in horizontal pushing or punching movements.

Sertoli cells (E Sertoli, Italian physiologist/histologist, 1842–1910) cells associated with the seminiferous tubules. They are vital in nourishing and supporting the sperm-producing germ cells of the germinal epithelium.

serum *n* the clear fluid that separates when a sample of blood coagulates after withdrawal from the body—**sera** *pl*. Has the contents that were present in plasma, except for those that have taken part in the clotting process. Used for many biochemical investigations, and in the preparation of specific immunoglobulins for short-term prevention or urgent treatment of some infections in those who are not themselves immune.

serumal calculus a deprecated term for subgingival calculus. ⊃ dental calculus.

serum sickness the allergic illness occurring 7–10 days following the injection of foreign serum for treatment or prophylaxis of infection. Rarely seen now that serum from other species has been replaced by the use of human immunoglobulins. ⊃ anaphylaxis.

server a central computer in a network that provides services and files to other computers, therefore enabling computers to communicate with each other.

service provider an organization that offers connections to the internet.

sesamoid bone a small area of bone formation (shaped like a sesame seed) in muscle tendons at points of great pressure, such as the patella (the largest sesamoid bone in the body) in the tendon of the quadriceps femoris. Some people have more sesamoid bones that others.

sesamoiditis an inflammatory condition affecting the sesamoid bones usually in the flexor tendon of the great toe. It is usually precipitated by trauma. Stress fractures of the sesamoid bone are quite common with overuse.

sessile having a broadly based attachment as distinct from a peduncle.

sessile drop test the measurement of the contact angle by observation of the formation of a drop of liquid on a solid surface. The image of the droplet may be photographed or projected. ⊃ contact angle.

setting hardening, as of plaster of Paris or dental cements. *setting time* a period of time measured from the start of a mix of a material until it has set. *setting expansion* the dimensional increase that occurs as various materials harden (or set), e.g. plaster of Paris, dental stone, casting investment.

setting (occupational therapy) the immediate surroundings that influence task, activity or occupational performance. (Reproduced with permission from the European Network of Occupational Therapy in Higher Education (ENOTHE) Terminology Project, 2008.)

sets groups of repetitions ('reps') separated by substantial recovery intervals. ⊃ repetitions.

set-up 1. the accurate positioning of a patient in preparation for the delivery of radiotherapy treatment. **2.** deprecated term for trial denture or tooth arrangement.

severe acute asthma (*syn.* status asthmaticus) severe life-threatening asthma attack. Typically there is respiratory distress, cyanosis (central), tachycardia, sweating, an unproductive cough, exhaustion and severe hypoxia. It is a medical emergency requiring immediate treatment with high concentration oxygen, intravenous access, systemic corticosteroids and inhaled β_2-adrenoceptor agonists. Respiratory support may be necessary for patients who do not improve with this treatment regimen.

severe acute respiratory syndrome (SARS) a highly infectious atypical viral pneumonia linked to the SARS coronavirus (SARS CoV) which emerged, as a new infection, in Southeast Asia in 2002 to cause a worldwide outbreak during 2003. It appears to have originated in Guangdong Province in China in November 2002, although the first reports of the disease came from Vietnam and Hong Kong in early 2003. Since then it has been reported from all parts of the world. The illness is characterized by the presence of a high fever (>38°C), malaise, headache and muscle aches and later a dry cough with shortness of breath or difficulty in breathing and typical changes indicative of pneumonia are usually present on the chest X-ray. A history of travel within 10 days of onset of symptoms to an area with documented or suspected community transmission of SARS or close contact within 10 days of onset of symptoms with a person known to be a suspect SARS case is typical. SARS has recently been attributed to the coronavirus (Urbani SARS-associated coronavirus); however, additional viruses, or other factors, may be involved. The optimum method of treating SARS remains uncertain and is largely supportive, including mechanical ventilation. In a significant proportion of infected patients, it causes severe disease and may be fatal. The role of antibacterial, antiviral and immunomodulatory therapy is still under research.

severe combined immunodeficiency (SCID) a group of immunodeficiency disorders presenting in infancy, characterized by failure of cellular and humoral immunity due to a genetic defect in a critical immune system component. There are defects in lymphoid precursors and results in the combined failure of B- and T-cell maturation. The absence of an effective adaptive immune response causes recurrent bacterial, fungal and viral infections soon after birth. SCID is generally fatal unless successfully treated by haemopoietic stem cell transplantation (HSCT) or gene therapy. Examples include adenosine deaminase (an enzyme) deficiency (ADA-SCID) and X-linked SCID caused by a defective cytokine.

severity, irritability and nature factors (SIN) three factors used by physiotherapists in the assessment of patients. They are a valuable aid in planning frequency and duration of treatment. This has implications for the amount of assessment and treatment provided to the patient. *severity* a symptom is defined as severe if the activity that causes the pain needs to be interrupted and stopped because of the intensity of the pain. In many cases this is an indication that caution is needed in examination and treatment procedures. The indicators of severity are: high number of pain killers, disturbed sleep, off work due to severity of pain and a high pain score using a visual analogue scale (VAS). *irritability* means that a little activity causes a lot of pain that takes a relatively long time to settle. In many cases this is an indication that caution is required regarding examination and treatment procedures. The indicators for irritability are: susceptibility to become painful, how painful it becomes and the length of time this pain takes to reduce. *nature of the disorder* refers to the aspects of problems that require consideration in examination and treatment procedures. It may include the pathobiological processes underlying the disorder, contributing factors such as osteoporosis, stage of healing, stage and stability of the disorder and certain personal features, such as fear of moving.

Sever's disease (J Sever, American orthopaedic surgeon, 20th century) calcaneal epiphysitis. Occurs in children and is caused by damage to the bone-cartilage layer in the heel resulting in pain. Can mimic Achilles tendonitis (tendinitis).

sex chromatin in females the chromatin in one of the sex chromosomes (pair of X chromosomes) is inactive and appears in a somatic cell nucleus as a densely staining mass called a Barr body.

sex chromosomes the two chromosomes that determine genetic sex; XX in females and XY in males.

sex hormones the steroid hormones that include the androgens, oestrogens and progesterone produced by the gonads (ovaries or testes) and to a lesser extent the adrenal glands.

sexism *n* a view that members of one sex are superior to the other. Leads to discrimination and may be a limiting influence in education, professional development, etc.

sex-limited gene *n* a gene (autosomal or sex-linked) that leads to the expression of a trait in one sex only.

sex-linked *adj* refers to genes located on the sex chromosomes or, more especially, on the X chromosome.

sex-linked gene a gene present on the X or the Y chromosome (the sex chromosomes). The genes for a number of important disorders, such as haemophilia, Duchenne muscular dystrophy and colour-blindness, are carried on the X chromosome. By convention it is usual to refer to these genes (and the characters that they determine) as X-linked. Whereas the genes on the Y chromosome are not known to cause any significant disorders.

sextuplets six infants resulting from one conception.

sexual abuse performing a sexual act with a child or with an adult against the person's wishes. The commonest type is that occurring between a father (or father figure) and daughter. ➲ abuse, incest.

sexual deviation sexual acts or behaviours that are considered to be abnormal by society. Examples include exhibitionism, fetishism, masochism, necrophilia, paedophilia, sadism, etc.

sexual diamorphism 1. physical or behavioural differences associated with sex. **2.** having some properties of both sexes, as in the early embryo and in some hermaphrodites.

sexual dysfunction a lack of desire or the ability to achieve coitus in one or both partners. ➲ dyspareunia, erectile dysfunction, frigidity, libido, vaginismus.

sexual intercourse coitus.

sexuality *n* the sum of the structural, functional and psychological characteristics as they are expressed by a person's gender-identity and sexual behaviour.

sexual orientation describes an individual's sexual attraction: towards people of the same sex (homosexuality), the opposite sex (heterosexuality) or both sexes (bisexuality). The particular preference may be transitory or life-long.

sexually acquired reactive arthritis (SARA) *n* (*syn.* Reiter's disease) often caused by infection with *Chlamydia trachomatis*, but intestinal infections can also be the triggering event. Arthritis occurs together with conjunctivitis or uveitis, urethritis (or cervicitis in women), and sometimes psoriasis and other skin lesions. ➲ reactive arthritis.

sexually transmitted disease (STD) previously called venereal disease. ⊃ sexually transmitted infection.

sexually transmitted infection (STI) the infections, including those defined legally as venereal, which are usually transmitted through sexual contact, but not exclusively so. They include: gonorrhoea, syphilis, HIV, candidiasis, chlamydial infection, genital herpes, genital warts, and trichomoniasis.

Sézary's syndrome (A Sézary, French dermatologist, 1880–1956) cutaneous T-cell lymphoma, a form of mycosis fungoides.

SF *abbr* synovial fluid.

SFA *abbr* saturated fatty acid.

SFD *abbr* **1.** small for dates. **2.** source to film distance.

SFS *abbr* Social Functioning Scale.

SGA *abbr* small for gestational age.

SGOT *abbr* serum glutamic oxaloacetic transaminase. ⊃ aminotransferase.

SGPT *abbr* serum glutamic pyruvic transaminase. ⊃ aminotransferase.

SH *abbr* standard (unfractionated) heparin.

shaded surface display algorithms in radiography, the generation of a three-dimensional outline of the surface of a patient or object from a set of stored images.

shadow mask in radiography, a thin, perforated metal plate found in colour monitors to accurately focus the electron beam onto the phosphor and therefore improve image quality.

shadow test 1. also known as oblique illumination shadow test. A test which gives an approximate evaluation of the depth of the anterior chamber. It is carried out by placing a penlight on the temporal side of the eye at the level of the pupil and directing the beam of light horizontally towards the inner side of the eye. If the iris lies in a flat plane which usually indicates a deep anterior chamber the entire iris will be illuminated. If the iris is directed anteriorly, which usually indicates a narrow anterior chamber, the iris on the temporal side of the eye will be illuminated but the iris on the nasal side will be shadowed to varying degrees depending on the narrowness of the anterior chamber. **2.** a test for the homogeneity of a lens (both material and surface quality) in which the light from a small, intense source of light passes through the lens and falls on a screen. Any defects will show as shadows. ⊃ angle-closure glaucoma, angle of the anterior chamber, open-angle glaucoma, van Herick, Shaffer and Schwartz method.

shadow tray a sheet of Perspex or perforated aluminium sheet in the form of a tray or table to hold shielding blocks during radiotherapy.

shagreen of the crystalline lens the slightly irregular or granular appearance of the surfaces of the crystalline lens when viewed with the slit-lamp with specular reflection illumination. The posterior lens shagreen has a slightly yellower tint and is less coarse than the anterior. It is believed to represent variations in the refraction of light within the lens capsule. ⊃ capsule of the crystalline lens, crystalline lens, specular reflection illumination, Vogt's sign.

shank 1. the thinner portion of a hand instrument joining the blade to the handle. **2.** the non-cutting portion of a bur.

shaping a technique used in behaviour therapy. Whereby the therapist initially reinforces behaviour that only slightly resembles the desired goal; as the programme progresses the therapist only reinforces behaviour that is increasingly close to the desired behaviour until the goal is reached.

shared care antenatal care shared between a midwife and obstetrician or general practitioner.

shared segment part of a computer network that is used by several nodes.

sharp débridement ⊃ débridement.

Sharpey's fibres (W Sharpey, British anatomist, 1802–1880) the collagen fibres that secure the periostium to the underlying bone. In dental anatomy, those portions of the principal fibres (collagen) of the periodontal ligament that are embedded in root cementum and alveolar bone proper, and which contribute to the anchorage of the tooth.

'sharps' a generic term that includes used needles, razor blades, disposable scalpels, intravenous giving sets, central venous lines and intravenous cannulae. These items should be put immediately into a rigid sharps' container of distinctive colour which is disposed of when three-quarters full. It is sealed in such a way that used needles cannot cause injury or be recovered for misuse. Arrangements have to be made for safe disposal of those used by people in their own homes, district nurses, at health centres, dental surgeries, doctors' surgeries and so on. The sharps' containers used should be manufactured to British Standard specifications in respect to aperture and closure, resistance to penetration, impact and toppling and should be coloured yellow. They should be marked with the 'sharps' biohazard symbol and marked 'Caution, biological hazard'. In the UK there is a legal responsibility to ensure that all waste is disposed of safely.

shear force force acting parallel to the surface of a material so as to tend to deform it, usually through a shear angle, the angle between a deformed body and its original position. ⊃ shearing force.

shearing force when any part of the supported body is on a gradient, the tissues nearest the bone 'slide' towards the lower gradient while the skin stays in contact with the supporting surface because of friction which is increased in the presence of moisture. The deep blood vessels are stretched and bent and the deeper tissues become ischaemic with consequent necrosis. ⊃ pressure ulcers.

sheath in anatomy, a layer of connective tissue covering structures such as muscles and nerves.

Sheehan's syndrome (H Sheehan, British pathologist, 1900–1988) hypopituitarism caused by postpartum necrosis of the pituitary gland resulting from hypovolaemia such as that occurring with severe postpartum haemorrhage. A rare condition characterized by the loss of pubic and axillary hair, possible failure of the establishment of lactation, continuing amenorrhoea as menstrual cycles do not return,

S
T

symptoms of reduced cortisol secretion and secondary hypothyroidism. ⊃ hypopituitarism, Simmonds' syndrome.

sheep cell agglutination test (SCAT) a test for the rheumatoid factor in the blood, detected by the sheep cell agglutination titre.

shelf life the length of time that a material, dressing, item of equipment or drug may be stored without deteriorating and thus remain usable.

shelf operation an operation to deepen the acetabulum in some cases of developmental dysplasia of the hip (formally known as congenital dislocation of the hip), involving the use of a bone graft. Performed at 7–8 years of age after failure of conservative treatment.

shellac a natural beetle exudate, occasionally used in the construction of temporary denture bases and impression trays. ⊃ varnish.

shell body temperature ⊃ body temperature.

shell crown a full veneer crown made from plate metal.

shells ⊃ beam direction shell, patient shell.

Shenton's line (E Shenton, British radiologist, 1872–1955) a line drawn along the medial border of the neck of femur and the superior border of the obturator foramen forming an even, continuous arc. If this arc is disrupted or displaced it indicates a fractured neck of femur or a hip dislocation.

shiatsu *n* a form of Japanese health care similar in principle to acupuncture. Specific points along the body surface are pressed using the thumbs, fingers or palms to stimulate energy flow and to start self-healing processes. The belief is that an imbalance in a person's energy may result in physical symptoms. The aims of shiatsu are to rebalance self-healing energy and so promote health and well-being.

shield the shield forms the external casing of an X-ray tube.

shielding blocks heavy metal blocks placed on a shadow tray to protect parts of the body that are in the beam of radiation but do not require treatment. They are a means of shaping the beam to individual volumes. ⊃ lead shielding, MCP block.

shift the phenomenon where a person moves a part of the body, usually the spine, in an attempt to adopt the least painful posture.

Shigella *n* (K Shiga, Japanese bacteriologist, 1870–1957) a genus of Gram-negative, non-motile bacilli of the family Enterobacteriaceae. Several species cause dysentery: *Shigella boydii*, *S. dysenteriae* and *S. flexneri* in tropical and subtropical areas. *S. sonnei* causes dysentery in temperate regions and is the most common type in the UK. Commonly affects young children and is spread by the faecal–oral route. ⊃ dysentery.

shin bone ⊃ tibia.

shin splints a collection of common problems that affect both recreational and trained athletes. Runners are often affected. Periostitis occurs further toward the front of the leg than posterior tibial shin splints and the bone itself is tender. Anterior compartment syndrome affects the outer side of the front of the leg. Stress fractures of the tibia may occur, which usually produce localized, sharp pain with tenderness below the knee. Stress fractures commonly occur several weeks into a new training programme or after commencing a more strenuous training regimen. ⊃ anterior compartment syndrome.

shingles *n* herpes zoster. A condition arising when the infecting agent (varicella-zoster virus) attacks sensory nerves causing severe pain and the appearance of vesicles along the nerve's distribution (usually unilateral). ⊃ herpes zoster, Colour Section Figure 75.

Shirodkar's operation (N Shirodkar, Indian obstetrician, 1900–1971) placing of a pursestring suture around an incompetent cervix during pregnancy around 16 weeks' gestation in an attempt to prevent miscarriage. It is removed when labour starts.

shock *n* condition in which there is inadequate flow of oxygenated blood to the tissues. There is cell hypoxia and inadequate tissue perfusion. Causes include haemorrhage, fluid deficits (hypovolaemic shock), heart failure (cardiogenic shock), infection (septic shock) and allergic reaction (anaphylactic shock). ⊃ systemic inflammatory response syndrome, toxic shock syndrome.

shock (electrical) an electrical shock: macroshock (ampere level current, person in mains to earth circuit) or microshock (issued mainly in high dependency units or intensive care units). There is a risk of a small shock with electrical stimulation. The machine should be turned on prior to testing its output and connecting the patient and turned off only after the intensity is fully down and the patient circuit disconnected. The reason for this is that a microprocessor circuit that is not fully powered is not totally predictable. ⊃ body protected areas.

short bone bones that are cuboidal in shape and are formed by cancellous bone with a thin covering of compact bone, for example the carpal bones.

short bowel syndrome (SBS) a disorder characterized by malabsorption of nutrients, which, in children, is commonly caused by congenital anomalies (e.g. small bowel atresia, gastroschisis), necrotizing enterocolitis and trauma or vascular injury, such as that caused by a volvulus. The medical management centres around maintaining nutrition through enteral feeding to ensure optimum growth and development while intestinal adaptation occurs. The initial phase of nutrition is via total parenteral nutrition (TPN), which helps to stimulate the adaptation response of the small intestine. In children, SBS results in a compensatory increase in the mucosal surface area, mostly by villus hyperplasia, and a small increase in the length and diameter of the small intestine. These changes enable a gradual increase in the absorption of nutrients.

short-cone radiography a dental radiographic technique in which the X-ray machine is fitted with a cone that is generally shorter than 20 cm.

short-duration anaerobic endurance training ⊃ anaerobic endurance training.

shortening fraction in cardiology, the difference between ventricular diameter at the end of systole and its original diameter at the end of diastole, expressed as a percentage.

Short Portable Mental State Questionnaire (SPMSQ) an assessment of cognitive function used to screen for impairment and dementia. The areas assessed are orientation, mathematical ability, practical skills, and memory (both short term and long term).

shortsightedness ⊃ myopia.

short term memory (STM) working memory. The portion of memory that is responsible for the retention of information for a few seconds only. It can only be retained if it is rehearsed or moved to long term memory (LTM). If STM is affected, for instance after stroke or brain injury, it will make the re-learning of tasks more difficult and liaison between physiotherapists, nurses, occupational therapists or psychologists is essential for compensatory strategies. ⊃ chunking, rehearsal in memory.

shortwave diathermy (SWD) an electrotherapy term. An electromagnetic radiation with a frequency of 27.12 MHz. It may be continuous SWD (CSWD) or pulsed SWD (PSWD) output. CSWD is used for deep tissue heating and PSWD to promote healing. The types used are capacitive or inductothermy. The dangers and contraindications include: indwelling pumps or stimulators within 3–5 m, indwelling metal within 30 cm and, if local circulation reduced, there is a risk of heat induced damage.

short wavelength automated perimetry (SWAP) a valuable procedure for detecting and monitoring visual defects in people with ocular hypertension and people with early glaucomatous visual field losses. It uses a blue stimulus on a yellow background, as may be arranged in an automated perimeter. It is a more sensitive and efficient method of detecting and monitoring early visual field losses than standard white-on-white automated perimetry (white stimulus on a white background). ⊃ open-angle glaucoma.

shoulder 1. describes a general area at the top of the arm or the joint. ⊃ shoulder girdle, shoulder joint. **2.** in photography the area of the characteristic curve where the film's reaction to exposure slows. ⊃ characteristic curve.

shoulder dystocia impacted shoulders. A rare complication occurring after delivery of the fetal head in which the shoulders fail to rotate, descend and deliver. It is usually due to a very large baby (over 4000 g) or a contracted pelvic outlet. The anterior shoulder is caught up behind or at the symphysis pubis. It is an obstetric emergency, which can result in perinatal morbidity or mortality, excessive blood loss and rarely, maternal death. Management may involve a change in maternal position, for example the woman should be turned into the left lateral position or asked to squat in an attempt to enlarge the outlet and deliver the baby; or an invasive manipulative procedure may be required. ⊃ macrosomia, McRoberts manoeuvre, Rubin's manoeuvre, symphysiotomy, Wood's manoeuvre, Zavanelli manoeuvre.

shoulder girdle pectoral girdle; part of the axial skeleton. The parts of the musculoskeletal system that link the upper limbs to the sternum in front and to the vertebral column behind, including sternoclavicular joint, clavicle, acromioclavicular joint, scapula and attached muscles.

shoulder-hand syndrome may also be called complex regional pain syndrome and may occur for no apparent reason or following trauma. Signs and symptoms include pain and loss of movement in the shoulder and wrist joints, with swelling of the hand and the skin may become red and shiny. It usually develops 1–6 months after a cerebrovascular accident (stroke). The syndrome is considered to develop in three consecutive phases: I—acute, II—dystrophic and III—atrophic. It is important to maintain as much range as possible in the joints but pain relief may be necessary. Sometimes a sympathetic nerve block is carried out (Zyluk & Zyluk 1999). (Zyluk A, Zyluk B, 1999 Shoulder-hand syndrome in patients after stroke. Neurol Neurochir Pol 33(1): 131–142.)

shoulder joint (*syn.* glenohumeral joint) a synovial ball- and-socket joint, the 'ball' of the head of the humerus articulating with the 'socket' of the shallow glenoid cavity of the scapula, which allows the shoulder to move around multiple axes—the greatest range of movement of any joint in the body, providing flexion, extension, abduction, adduction, circumduction, and lateral and medial rotation. These movements are facilitated by several muscles working alone or in synergy, e.g. coracobrachialis, deltoid, pectoralis major, latissimus dorsi, teres major. This flexibility sacrifices stability, which has to be maintained by the surrounding muscles and ligaments, notably the muscles of the rotator cuff (supraspinatus, infraspinatus, teres minor, subcapsularis); also the socket of the joint is deepened by the glenoid labrum, a ring of fibrocartilage attached to the rim of the glenoid cavity to which the joint capsule, ligaments and tendons are partly attached. The capsular ligament is very loose inferiorly to allow for the free movement normally possible at this joint. The tendon of the long head of the biceps brachii muscle is held in the intertubercular (bicipital) groove of the humerus by the transverse humeral ligament. It extends through the joint cavity and attaches to the upper rim of the glenoid cavity. Synovial membrane forms a sleeve round the part of the tendon of the long head of the biceps brachii muscles within the capsular ligament and covers the glenoidal labrum. The joint is stabilized partly by the glenohumeral, coracohumeral and transverse humeral ligaments but mainly by muscles (and their tendons) present in the shoulder. Labral tears are not uncommon in throwing athletes. ⊃ Bankart's lesion, dislocation, rotator cuff, superior labrum anterior-posterior (SLAP) lesions.

shoulder preparation in dentistry, a shelf or shoulder cut around, or partly around, the neck of a tooth to provide a satisfactory thickness of material (e.g. porcelain) for construction of a crown.

shoulder presentation a presentation in which the fetus lies obliquely across the uterus. It may be dorsoanterior or dorsoposterior (Figure S.5). If labour commences with the fetus in an oblique lie, one fetal shoulder is driven down into the maternal pelvis, and labour becomes obstructed. A shoulder presentation may occur in the second stage of a twin labour, after delivery of the first infant. On examination

S
T

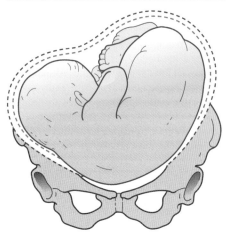

S.5 Shoulder presentation—dorsoanterior (reproduced from Fraser & Cooper 2003 with permission).

the uterus appears broad and the fundal height is less than expected for the gestation and on vaginal examination the fetal ribs may be felt and an arm may prolapse into the vagina. Caesarean section is required or, if not possible, internal podalic version and breech extraction if the fetus is alive, or possibly a destructive operation if the fetus is dead, although maternal risk of ruptured uterus is extremely high.

shoulder trimmer in dentistry, a hand instrument with a narrow serrated blade used to trim a shoulder preparation and provide a smooth surface.

'show' *n* a popular term for the bloodstained vaginal discharge that occurs at the commencement of labour.

shrinkage reduction in volume. *casting shrinkage* the contraction or volume change that occurs as a molten metal solidifies when cast in a mould. ⊃ casting.

shrinking field technique phased treatments, in radiotherapy, where a larger volume is treated first and then the volume is shrunk to allow higher doses to be delivered to the target volume while ensuring that tolerance doses to critical structures is not exceeded.

shunt *n* a term applied to the passage of fluid through other than the usual channel. This may refer to shunting of blood (e.g. some cardiac septal defects, arteriovenous shunt) or cerebrospinal fluid (e.g. ventriculoperitoneal shunt).

shuttle test test of aerobic power requiring minimal apparatus, introduced by Leger and colleagues in 1982 and also known as Leger shuttle run, multi-stage fitness test or, informally, bleep test. Starting at 8 km/h, subjects run to and fro over 20 m at a pace increased every minute until exhaustion.

SI *abbr* Système International d'Unités.

SIADH *abbr* syndrome of inappropriate antidiuretic hormone (ADH) secretion.

sialadenitis inflammation of one or more salivary glands. Causes include surgery, infection, e.g. parotitis (mumps), tumours and obstruction to salivary ducts (e.g. by calculi).

sialagogue *n* an agent which increases saliva production.

sialogram *n* a technique whereby a radiographic image of the salivary glands and ducts is produced, after injection of a contrast agent—**sialography** *n*, **sialographic** *adj*, **sialographically** *adv*.

sialograph a radiograph of the ducts and acini of the salivary glands following the introduction of contrast agent into them. Used to determine whether a gland or duct contains calculus.

sialography the radiographic examination of the salivary glands following the direct injection of a contrast agent.

sialolith *n* a calculus (stone) in a salivary gland or duct.

sialorrhoea hypersalivation. Excessive flow of saliva. It may be caused by teething, oral inflammation, poorly fitting dentures, neurological disorders and more rarely mercurialism.

Siamese twins ⊃ conjoined twins.

SIB *abbr* self-injurious behaviour.

sibilant hissing or whistling sound.

sickle cell anaemia ⊃ sickle cell disease.

sickle cell disease an inherited haemoglobinopathy; it is transmitted as an autosomal recessive condition. It is due to an abnormal haemoglobin (HbS) in which the beta-globin gene is faulty. A person who inherits one normal gene for adult haemoglobin (HbA) and one abnormal gene for sickle haemoglobin (HbS) will have sickle cell trait; they are carriers of sickle cell anaemia and can transmit the gene to their offspring, but they will not have clinical problems. The disease mainly affects people of African, African-Caribbean or African-American descent, but can also be found in those with Indian, Middle Eastern, Far Eastern and southern European ancestry. The disease is associated with regions of the world in which falciparum malaria is endemic. When HbS becomes deoxygenated, crystals form in the red cells, which become distorted and sickle-shaped. The red cells once oxygenated again can return to a normal shape, but over time the affected cells become increasingly rigid and are prematurely destroyed by the cells of the monocyte-macrophage system in the spleen and liver. The life span of these red cells is much less than the 120 days for a normal red cell. Sickle cell disease is characterized by chronic haemolytic anaemia and intermittent painful crises. Affected individuals will often have a low haemoglobin level and will usually be mildly jaundiced and have splenomegaly. At-risk populations should be screened for the abnormal HbS. Affected individuals are also offered an immunization programme that includes protection against *haemophilus influenzae* type b, influenza (annually), meningococcal C, and pneumococcal infections. Sickle cell crises occur when many red cells become sickle-shaped; the rigid cells are unable to pass through small blood vessels, the blood vessels are occluded and tissue ischaemia and infarction can result. These crises are associated with excruciating pain in the affected area of the body. Factors associated with triggering crises include: infection, reduced tissue oxygenation, general anaesthesia, dehydration, extremes of temperature, high altitude, excessive alcohol consumption, strenuous exercise, pregnancy and emotional stress. Severe crises can be life-threatening, particularly when it affects blood vessels in the brain or lungs. Management of sickle cell crises will depend on the severity; a severe crises will require admission to hospital for strong opioid analgesics, intravenous fluid replacement, oxygen therapy and close observation. Patients with chest pain, caused by a sickling crisis affecting the lungs ('chest crisis'), have a significant risk of mortality. Therefore, this may be treated by an exchange transfusion in which some of the patient's blood is removed and replaced by donated blood transfused by apheresis. At present, there is no cure for sickle cell disease apart from haemopoietic stem cell transplantation from a sibling donor. ➲ malaria, thalassaemia. ➲ Colour Section Figure 110.

sickle scaler ➲ scaler.

sick role the role a person is expected to assume when ill. This will depend on historical and cultural factors. In Britain, at the present time, the obligations of this role are to obtain competent medical help and to comply with medical treatment. In return, the individual is relieved of everyday responsibilities and is not blamed for his or her illness. The concept is more applicable to acute illness than chronic illness or impairment.

SID *abbr* source-to-image distance.

side shift ➲ Bennett movement (or shift).

side-effect *n* any physiological change other than the wanted one from a drug, e.g. oral iron causes the side-effect of black faeces. Also covers undesirable drug reactions. Some are predictable, being the result of a known metabolic action of the drug, e.g. hair loss with cytotoxic drugs. Unpredictable reactions can be: (a) immediate: anaphylaxis, angiooedema, (b) erythematous: all forms of erythema, including nodosum and multiforme and purpuric rashes, (c) cellular eczematous rashes and contact dermatitis, (d) specific, e.g. light-sensitive eruptions with griseofulvin (antifungal). ➲ adverse drug reactions.

sideroblast *n* a nucleated red blood cell precursor, a normoblast present in the bone, which contains granules of iron. The presence of *ringed sideroblasts,* which have a ring of iron granules around the cell nucleus are a feature of sideroblastic anemia.

sideroblastic anaemias *npl* a group of rare anaemias caused by defective iron metabolism; they may be inherited or acquired.

sideropenia *n* abnormally low level of iron in the serum.

siderosis *n* excess of iron in the blood or tissues. Inhalation of iron oxide into the lungs can cause one form of pneumoconiosis. ➲ haemochromatosis, haemosiderosis.

SIDS *abbr* sudden infant death syndrome.

sievert (Sv) (R Sievert, Swedish medical physicist, 1896–1966) the Système International d'Unités (SI) unit (International System of Units) for radiation dose equivalent. A measure of total biological effects of a beam of radiation. It has replaced the rem. ➲ Appendix 2.

sigmoid *adj* shaped like the letter S.

sigmoid colon the part of the descending colon after it enters the pelvis. The S-shaped bend (sigmoid flexure) at the lower end of the descending colon, which is continuous with the rectum below. ➲ Colour Section Figure 18b.

sigmoidectomy *n* excision of the sigmoid colon. Most commonly undertaken for colorectal cancer, but also may be required for other conditions, such as diverticular disease.

sigmoid notch a notch on the superior border of the ramus of the mandible lying between the condyle and the coronoid process. Also known as the mandibular notch.

sigmoidoscope *n* an instrument for visualizing the rectum and sigmoid colon. ➲ endoscope—**sigmoidoscopic** *adj*.

sigmoidoscopy *n* endoscopic examination of the rectum and distal colon (sigmoid colon). ➲ colonoscopy.

sigmoidostomy *n* the formation of a colostomy (stoma) in the sigmoid colon.

sign *n* any objective evidence of disease. For example, high temperature, a rash, swelling, abnormal breath sounds or vomiting blood.

sign convention a set of conventions regulating the direction of distances, lengths and angles measured in geometrical optics. The most common is the *New Cartesian Sign Convention*. It stipulates that: (a) all distances are measured from the lens, refracting surface or mirror. Those in the same direction as the incident light, which is drawn travelling from left to right, are positive. Those in the opposite direction are negative; (b) all distances are measured from the axis. Those above are positive. Those below are negative; (c) angles are measured from the incident ray to the axis, with anti-clockwise angles positive and clockwise angles negative; and (d) the power of a converging lens is positive and that of a diverging lens is negative. ➲ focal length, Lagrange's law, law of refraction, Newton's formula, paraxial equation (fundamental).

signal in imaging it is the information required from the system, for example a radiograph, and the minimum-sized object that can be seen by a system.

signal gain the electrical signal for a specific intensity of absorbed radiation.

signal node also known as Troisier's sign or Virchow's node. An enlarged supraclavicular lymph node, often on the left side, indicative of metastatic spread from an abdominal cancer, such as that of the stomach.

signal-to-noise ratio the ratio of the signal width to the unwanted energy (noise). In magnetic resonance imaging (MRI) it can be improved by (a) increasing the number of signal excitations, (b) increasing the field of view, or (c) increasing the strength of the main magnetic field used.

significance ➲ statistical significance.

sign language a form of non-verbal language using the hands and upper body to make signs, whereby hearing impaired people can communicate with each other and with family and friends. ➲ British sign language, finger spelling, Makaton.

sign test a statistical test used to compare two sets of results using a normal distribution table and a sign test table; the

S
T

results must be equal to or less than the results on the tables to be significant.

SIJ *abbr* sacroiliac joint.

silica (silicon dioxide) a natural substance found in three forms—quartz, cristobalite and eridymite. *fused silica* a substance used widely in dentistry in cements and as a refractory material in investment materials.

silicate cement the first direct tooth coloured filling materials and now rarely, if ever, used. Consists of a mixture of fluoride-containing aluminosilicate glass powders, and phosphoric acid causing the cement to set hard. Irritant to pulp, susceptible to erosion and must be kept moist to maintain translucency.

silicon carbide an abrasive powder incorporated in carborundum.

silicon dioxide ⇒ silica.

silicone a brittle substance occurring in amorphous and crystalline forms. It is water-repellent and is used in some types of wound dressings, as sheets, foams and gels, where it fits exactly the contours of the granulating wound to provide an ideal environment for wound healing. Also used as implants in breast reconstruction.

silicone elastomeric impression material ⇒ impression material.

silicone grease a lubricant containing silicone and used in place of a mineral or vegetable oil.

silicone hydrogel lens a contact lens made of a combination of silicone rubber and hydrogel polymer to form a co-polymer that has the properties of both. Such a lens has a high oxygen permeability, adequate wettability, good optical properties and acceptable lens movement on the eye (unlike basic silicone rubber material, which tends to adhere to the cornea). This type of lens can be used for extended wear as contact lens-induced oedema is virtually eliminated. Transmissibility (*Dk/t*) of such lenses exceeds 100.

silicone rubber (*syn* polydimethyl siloxane) a polymeric elastomeric, transparent material which is used in the manufacture of silicone rubber contact lenses. It has very high oxygen permeability but it is also very hydrophobic (wetting angle greater than 90°). The surfaces must be specially treated to render them wettable. ⇒ contact angle, refractive index, silicone hydrogel lens, siloxane.

silico-phosphate cement a silicate cement containing zinc oxide and used for temporary fillings, cementation and die making.

silicosis *n* a form of pneumoconiosis or industrial dust disease found in metal grinders, stone-workers, etc.

SILO *acron* small in large out.

siloxane a polymeric, transparent material which is used as a component in the manufacture of gas permeable contact lenses. This polymer consists of alternating silicon and oxygen atoms and two organic side groups such as methyl, propyl, phenyl, vinyl or chloropropyl attached to each silicon. Siloxane is very permeable to oxygen and carbon dioxide. Many gas permeable contact lenses are made

with a combination of siloxane and polymethylmethacrylate. ⇒ modulus of elasticity, polymethylmethacrylate, silicone rubber.

silver (Ag) a soft white, ductile and malleable metallic element.

silver bromide in radiography, a chemical used as part of a film emulsion and has a peak sensitivity of 430 nm and is not sensitive to wavelengths above 480 nm.

silver casting alloy a precious metal casting alloy composed of 95% silver and 5% copper. Used mainly in the construction of cast dental splints in surgical cases.

silver collection in radiography, used fixing solution is stored and then collected in bulk along with unwanted radiographs to enable the silver to be commercially reclaimed.

silver estimating papers in radiography, special papers used to measure the quantity of silver remaining in a solution.

silver halides silver compounds that have a natural spectral sensitivity in the blue part of the visible spectrum. ⇒ silver bromide.

Silverman–Anderson score system to evaluate breathing performance of preterm babies by assessing five categories, graded 0, 1 or 2: chest retraction compared with abdominal retraction during inspiration; retraction of the lower intercostal muscles; xiphoid retraction; flaring of the nares with inspiration; expiratory grunt. A score of 0 indicates adequate ventilation; 10 indicates severe respiratory distress.

silver nitrate used as a caustic for warts. Previously used in dentistry for its coagulant, antiseptic and caustic properties.

silver point a thin, conical metal point, mainly composed of silver, used in conjunction with a sealant to obturate the apical foramen at a root canal filling. Made in graded sizes matching reamer and file sizes. Now superseded by gutta percha.

silver recovery in radiography, the methods of recovering silver from either the fixer solution or unwanted radiographs. ⇒ electrolytic silver recovery, metal exchange, silver collection.

silver solder in dentistry, the soldering alloy composed mainly of silver, copper, zinc and tin which melts at a temperature well below that of the metals being soldered.

silver tin alloy contains silver, tin and small quantities of copper and zinc. ⇒ alloy.

SIMA *abbr* system for identifying motivated abilities.

Simmonds' disease (M Simmonds, German physician, 1855–1925) panhypopituitarism. ⇒ hypopituitarism.

simple cavity a preparation involving only one surface of the clinical crown of a tooth.

simple epithelium consists of a single layer of identical cells and is divided into four types: squamous (pavement), cuboidal, columnar or ciliated (Figure E.7, p. 264). It is usually found on absorptive or secretory surfaces, where the single layer enhances these processes, and not usually on surfaces subject to stress. The types are named according to the shape of the cells, which differs according to their

S
T

functions. The more active the tissue, the taller are the cells. ⊃ ciliatated epithelium, columnar epithelium, cuboidal epithelium, squamous (pavement) epithelium.

simple fracture ⊃ fracture.

simple glaucoma ⊃ open-angle glaucoma.

simple mastectomy ⊃ mastectomy.

simple reaction time ⊃ reaction time.

Sims' position (J Sims, American gynaecologist, 1813–1883) an exaggerated left lateral position with the right knee well flexed and the left arm drawn back over the edge of the bed.

Sims' speculum (J Sims) a type of vaginal speculum.

Sims–Huhner test (H Sims, American gynaecologist, 19th century; M Huhner, American urologist, 1873–1947) ⊃ Huhner test.

simulator used in radiotherapy treatment localization and planning. This is a specialized unit housing a diagnostic X-ray tube to identify the treatment beam–patient geometry by using an image intensifier, an isocentric therapy unit and a collimation unit.

simultaneous oppression the way in which social divisions of gender, age, class, race, sexual orientation and disability combine in important and varying ways to exacerbate the experience of oppression.

SIMV *abbr* synchronized intermittent mandatory ventilation.

SIN *acron* **S**everity, **I**rritability and **N**ature factors.

Sinding-Larsen and Johansson's disease (C Sinding-Larsen, Norwegian physician, 1866–1930; S Johansson, Swedish surgeon, 1880–1959) traction osteochondrosis affecting the inferior pole of the patella.

sine condition (*syn* Abbé's condition) the elimination of distortion and coma in an image is met when

$$M = \frac{n \sin u}{n' \sin u'}$$

where M is the lateral magnification, n and n' the refractive indices of the media in the object and image space, and u and u' are the angular apertures on the object and image sides, respectively. ⊃ angular aperture, coma (2), correction, distortion, lateral magnification.

Singer's test blood test to distinguish fetal from maternal blood.

single-cell protein a term used to describe a biomass of yeast, bacteria or algae that may be of use as human or animal food.

single-nucleotide polymorphism (SNP) a type of genetic polymorphism occurring between two genomes in which the exchange, insertion or deletion of material involves a single nucleotide.

single-photon emission computed tomography (SPECT) an imaging technique that is a variation of computed tomography. It involves the administration of radioisotopes (radionuclides) that emit gamma radiation, which is detected by several gamma cameras that are arranged to rotate around the patient. A computer constructs a three-dimensional image.

single-vision (SV) lens an ophthalmic lens having only one power.

singleton denotes the presence of a single fetus in the uterus throughout pregnancy.

sinoatrial node ⊃ sinus node.

sinus *n* **1.** a hollow or cavity, especially the paranasal air sinuses (Figure P.3, p. 571). ⊃ maxillary antrum/sinus, paranasal. **2.** a channel containing blood, especially venous blood, e.g. the dural sinuses draining venous blood from the brain. ⊃ cavernous sinus, dural sinuses. **3.** a recess or cavity within a bone. **4.** any abnormal blind tract or channel opening onto the skin or a mucous surface. ⊃ pilonidal sinus. **5.** in dentistry, the formation of a sinus is generally due to the non-vitality and periapical infection of a tooth. *sinus balloon* a rubber or plastic balloon-like device that may be expanded with either a liquid or air and is used to support depressed fractures of the zygoma and/or the maxilla.

sinus arrhythmia an increase of heart rate on inspiration, decrease on expiration.

sinusitis *n* acute or chronic inflammation of a sinus, used exclusively for the paranasal sinuses.

sinus node (sinoatrial node) the pacemaker of the heart. Part of the specialized tissue that forms the conducting system of the heart. It is situated at the junction of the superior vena cava and the right atrium. It initiates the wave of cardiac contraction. ⊃ pacemaker.

sinusoid *n* a dilated channel into which arterioles or veins open in some organs, e.g. liver, and which act in place of the usual capillaries.

sinus rhythm normal rhythm of the heart. ⊃ P-QRS-T complex.

sinuvertebral nerve a small filament of nerve that leaves from the spinal nerve, after its formation (from the joining of the ventral and dorsal nerves). The sinuvertebral nerve is joined by a branch from the sympathetic trunk.

Sipple's syndrome (J Sipple, American physician, b. 1930) a type of multiple endocrine neoplasia (MEN) in which the inheritance is usually autosomal dominant. It is characterized by medullary cancer of the thyroid, parathyroid tumours or hyperplasia leading to overactivity and the presence of phaeochromocytoma. ⊃ Wermer's syndrome.

Siqveland matrix band holder ⊃ matrix band.

SIR *acron* **S**erial **I**nfra **R**ed.

SIRS *acron* **S**ystemic **I**nflammatory **R**esponse **S**yndrome.

sitapophasis refusal to eat in people with mental health problems.

sitology the science dealing with the study of food.

sitomania also called phagomania. An abnormal obsession with food and eating.

sitophobia also called phagophobia. An abnormal fear of food.

sit-up exercise of abdominal muscles, in which the subject lying on the floor raises the upper body towards vertical before lowering again; importantly, for safety, should be performed with knees bent to approximate right angle, when

S
T

the target becomes touching of elbows to knees. Also known as the trunk curl although this term is sometimes reserved for the particular case where chin is pressed against chest during the upper-body elevation.

sitz-bath *n* a hip bath.

Sjögren–Larsson syndrome (K Sjögren, Swedish psychiatrist/physician, 1896–1974; T Larsson, Swedish statistician, 1905–1998) genetically determined congenital ectodermosis. Associated with learning disability.

Sjögren syndrome (H Sjögren, Swedish ophthalmologist, 1899–1986) an autoimmune disorder of unknown aetiology characterized by lymphocytic infiltration of salivary (leading to enlargement) and lachrimal glands, leading to glandular fibrosis and exocrine failure. The age of onset is usually in the fourth and fifth decades with a female:male ratio of 9:1. The presence of HLA-B8/DR3 is a further risk factor. The disease may be primary or secondary in association with other autoimmune disease such as rheumatoid arthritis (RA), systemic lupus erythematosus (SLE), thyroiditis, progressive systemic sclerosis, myasthenia gravis, chronic active hepatitis or primary biliary cirrhosis. The eye symptoms, termed keratoconjunctivitis sicca, are due to a lack of tears and lubrication. Conjunctivitis and blepharitis are frequent manifestations, and may lead to filamentary keratitis due to tenacious mucus filaments binding to the cornea and conjunctiva. Oral involvement typically leads to a dry mouth (xerostomia) and hoarse voice. The person needs water to swallow food, and there is a high incidence of dental caries. Other sites involved include: non-invasive arthritis, fatigue and Raynaud's phenomenon. Less common features include: low-grade fever, interstitial lung disease, anaemia, leucopenia, thrombocytopenia, cryoglobulinaemia, vasculitis, peripheral neuropathy, lymphadenopathy, lymphoreticular malignancy, glomerulonephritis and renal tubular acidosis. The disease is associated with a 40-fold increased lifetime risk of lymphoma and can be viewed as being at the crossroads between an exaggerated autoimmune response and malignancy. Most patients will have an elevated erythrocyte sedimentation rate (ESR) secondary to hypergammaglobulinaemia and one or more autoantibodies, of which antinuclear antibody (ANA) and rheumatoid factor are the most common; other antibodies include SS-A (anti-R$_0$), SS-B(anti-La), gastric parietal cell and thyroid. Keratatoconjunctivitis sicca can be established by Schirmer's tear test, which measures flow of tears over 5 minutes using absorbent paper strips placed in the lower lachrimal sac. If the diagnosis is still in doubt, it can be confirmed by finding focal lymphocytic infiltrate in the minor salivary glands on lip biopsy. Management involves artificial lubrication as the mainstay of symptomatic treatment. Lachrimal substitutes (artificial tears) containing cellulose derivatives should be used during the day in combination with more viscous lubricating ointment at night. Soft contact lenses can be useful for corneal protection in patients with filamentary keratitis, and occlusion of the lachrimal ducts is occasionally needed. Artificial saliva and oral gels can

be tried for xerostomia, but are often not effective. Stimulation of saliva flow by sugar-free chewing gum or lozenges may be helpful. Adequate post-prandial oral hygiene, prompt treatment of oral candidiasis and regular dental examination are essential. Vaginal dryness and dyspareunia can be reduced through the use of specific vaginal lubricants. Extraglandular and musculoskeletal (MSK) system manifestations may respond to corticosteroids and, if so, other immunosuppressive drugs such as azathioprine can be added for steroid-sparing effect. One of the most difficult symptoms to treat is fatigue; this is usually due to non-restorative sleep (often because of xerostomia) and is unresponsive to corticosteroids. Immunosuppression does not improve sicca symptoms. If massive lymphadenopathy or salivary gland enlargement develops during the disease course, biopsy should be performed to detect malignancy. ➲ artificial tears, connective tissue diseases, keratitis sicca, keratoconjunctivitis sicca, Schirmer's tear test.

skatole 3-methylindole. A constituent of faeces, it contributes to the characteristic odour. It is produced in the intestine from the decomposition of proteins and from the amino acid tryptophan. Its oxidation product may appear in the urine.

skeletal relating to the skeleton.

skeletal muscle striated, voluntary muscle tissue. Forms the skeletal muscles that cover the bony skeleton and allow movement. The individual cells or fibres are multinucleate and form extended cylinders. Skeletal muscle is the only muscle tissue which may be controlled consciously. However, in many cases, this control operates through reflexes. Skeletal muscle is stimulated by the voluntary motor division (somatic) of the peripheral nervous system. ➲ muscle, muscle contraction, muscle fibre, neuromuscular junction.

skeletal pattern relationships between the dental bases in the sagittal, vertical and transverse planes.

skeletal system the bones and joints of the skeleton. ➲ musculoskeletal system.

skeletal traction localized traction applied on a bone by means of a wire or pin passed through the lower fragment. ➲ traction.

skeleton *n* the bony framework of the body, supporting and protecting the soft tissues and organs and acting as attachments for muscles—**skeletal** *adj. appendicular skeleton* the bones forming the pectoral (shoulder) girdle, upper limbs, pelvic girdle and lower limbs. *axial skeleton* the bones forming the head and trunk: skull, spinal column, hyoid bone, ribs and sternum. ➲ Colour Section Figures 2, 3.

skeleton denture a prosthesis, generally of metal, designed to be as small as possible, consistent with strength, stability and retention.

Skene's glands (A Skene, American gynaecologist, 1839–1900) two small mucus-secreting glands at the entrance to the female urethra; the lesser vestibular or paraurethral glands.

skewed distribution a statistical term that describes any distribution of scores where there are a greater number of values on one side of the mean than the other, i.e. not symmetrical. ⊃ normal distribution curve.

skiascope ⊃ retinoscope.

skiascopy ⊃ retinoscopy.

skier's thumb a colloquial expression used in sports medicine to describe instability of the metacarpophalangeal joint caused by forced abduction whilst the thumb is extended (e.g. holding the ski stick in a fall); this stretches or ruptures the ulnar collateral ligament which normally limits movement of the thumb away from the hand. Also known as gamekeeper's thumb since similar damage was caused by breaking the neck of birds or rabbits held between finger and thumb.

skill *n* the learned ability to competently and consistently co-ordinate a complex pattern of behaviours in order to accomplish a task with minimum effort and maximum effect. *closed skill* a skill executed in an environment that is stable and predictable, such as a floor routine in gymnastics. *open skill* a skill executed in an environment that is variable and unpredictable, such as 'dribbling' the ball past an opponent in soccer. ⊃ ability, performance.

skill mix the level, range and variety of skills of the staff in a department, unit or team which is needed to meet the organizational outcomes.

skill (occupational therapy) an ability developed through practice which enables effective occupational performance. (Reproduced with permission from the European Network of Occupational Therapy in Higher Education (ENOTHE) Terminology Project, 2008.)

skin *n* the tissue which forms the outer covering of the body; it consists of two layers, the outer epidermis (cuticle), dermis (true skin) and the appendages; nails, hair follicles and sebaceous glands (pilosebaceous units), and sweat glands. ⊃ Colour Section Figure 12. The skin is concerned with a number of functions including: sensation, protection, thermoregulation, excretion, absorption, storage, synthesis and communication. The epidermis contains several special cell types: keratinocytes (produce keratin); corneocytes (contain water-retaining substances and moisturizing factor); immune Langerhans' cells (dendritic cells); and melanocytes (produce melanin). The epidermis has several layers of stratified epithelium through which cells progress, losing water and protein as they go. The epidermis has an outer horny zone consisting of three layers: stratum corneum (horny layer), stratum lucidum (clear layer), which is not present in all areas and stratum granulosum (granular layer)—which overlay the germinative zone. The germinative zone has two layers: stratum spinosum (prickle layer) and the stratum basale (basal layer) which contains the melanocytes responsible for melanin production and skin pigmentation. The epidermis undergoes renewal as the stratum corneum is continually shed to be replaced by new cells formed in the stratum basale which move upwards through the layers over a period of around 35 days depending on age and other factors. The continual shedding of the outer keratinized cells as flakes or scales poses a potential risk of infection in healthcare settings. The exfoliated flakes contain the micro-organisms normally resident on the skin, and these may cause infection in susceptible patients, such as those who are immunocompromised. Epidermal cohesion is maintained during the renewal by the desmosomes which bind the keratinocytes together and prevent structural disruption. As the cells migrate upwards there is nuclear disintegration, keratinization and flattening. The dermis is connective tissue containing collagen, elastin and reticular fibres, cells such as fibroblasts and macrophages, blood and lymph vessels and different types of nerve endings. ⊃ hair, nail, pilosebaceous, sebaceous glands, sweat glands.

skin cancer ⊃ basal cell carcinoma, melanoma, squamous cell carcinoma.

skin expansion a technique utilizing an inflatable prosthesis to distend and expand the skin and subcutaneous tissue.

skin flap ⊃ flap.

skin flora also called resident flora. The commensal micro-organisms normally present on the skin are part of the normal flora of the body. Micro-organisms forming the skin flora include *Candida*, corynebacteria, micrococci, *Neisseria*, staphylococci and streptococci. The type of micro-organism varies across body sites, and depends on factors that include humidity and temperature.

skinfold fold thickness an anthropometric measurement used as part of a holistic nutritional assessment. It measures subcutaneous fat in various sites, usually four, and is a guide to total body fat content. A fold of skin and subcutaneous fat is grasped between the thumb and forefinger and pulled away from the underlying muscle. The thickness of this double layer is then read, using special calipers. Measurements are taken of fat at the following sites: the middle of the posterior aspect of the upper arm (triceps), the middle of the anterior aspect of the upper arm (biceps), below the point of the scapula at an angle of 45° (subscapular) and above the iliac crest in the mid-axillary line (supra-iliac). Further measurements may be taken on the abdomen and thigh. The values are used in an equation that estimates body fat. ⊃ anthropometry, body composition.

skin graft sheet of skin containing dermis and epidermis separated from its blood supply and applied to a raw surface. *full thickness (Wolfe) graft* full thickness skin graft that requires closure of the donor site. *split thickness (Thiersch) graft* partial thickness skin graft where the donor site heals spontaneously.

skin grafting vestibuloplasty epithelial or buccal inlay. Surgical deepening of the sulcus followed by grafting a split skin thickness graft to cover the exposed portion of bone.

skin hook a surgical instrument with a fine hook at one end used to grasp tissue during dissecting or suturing.

skin shedding skin is continually shedding its outer keratinized cells as scales. As the skin has a natural bacterial flora, the scales are a potential source of infection for vulnerable patients or residents.

S
T

skin-sparing effect seen in megavoltage radiotherapy treatment machines where the maximum radiation dose is delivered below the skin surface.

skin traction or extension involves the application of weights to foam or extension plaster attached to the skin. ⊃ traction.

skull *n* the box-like bony framework of the head, the face (13 bones) and the cranium (8 bones). ⊃ calvaria. It contains and protects the brain, eyes, ears and carries the upper jaw and attached lower jaw. Its various bones are joined at their edges by bony sutures, which allow for growth. Clothed by two groups of muscles—those of expression and those concerned with mastication. ⊃ Colour Section Figures 2, 35.

skull cap a type of headgear used as an anchor for the fixation of jaw fractures and also in extraoral orthodontic therapy.

skyline X-ray a type of X-ray view that portrays the patella sitting in the groove between the femoral condyles, it is useful in highlighting mal tracking of the patella. ⊃ mal tracking patella.

SL *abbr* sublingual.

slaking in dentistry, a method of mixing zinc phosphate cement that results in a delayed setting. A small portion of the powder is allowed to remain in the liquid for up to 2 minutes before the main mix takes place.

SLAP *acron* Superior Labrum Anterior-Posterior lesion.

slap lesion a shoulder joint pathology. There is a superior glenoid labral tear in an anterior to posterior direction. ⊃ shoulder joint, superior labrum anterior-posterior (SLAP) lesion.

slapped cheek syndrome ⊃ human erythrovirus 19.

SLE *abbr* systemic lupus erythematosus.

sleep *n* a naturally altered state of consciousness occurring in humans in a 24 h biological rhythm. A *sleep cycle* consists of alternating cycles of non-rapid eye movement sleep (NREM) or orthodox sleep, which has four stages, and rapid eye movement sleep (REM) or paradoxical sleep (Figure S.6).

sleep apnoea syndrome recurrent periods of apnoea and hypopnoea while sleeping due to repeated upper airway obstruction. Associated with transient hypoxaemia, severe headaches and daytime sleepiness (somnolence). More often seen in obese individuals, or those with soft palate abnormalities. ⊃ continuous positive airway pressure, obstructive sleep apnoea (hypopnoea) syndrome (OSAS/OSAHS).

sleep deprivation a cumulative condition arising when there is interference with a person's established rhythm of paradoxical sleep. It can result in tiredness, feeling cold, headaches, reduced appetite, slurred rambling speech, irritability, disorientation, confusion, slowed reaction time, poor co-ordination, inability to perform skilled tasks, occurrence of 'microsleeps', increased risk of accidents, poor concentration, malaise, mood swings, increased aggression, progressing to illusions, delusions, hallucinations, paranoia and hyperactivity.

sleep disorder describes a change in normal sleep pattern or rhythm. They include bruxism, insomnia, narcolepsy, nightmares, sleep apnoea, sleep/night terrors and sleep walking. ⊃ parasomnias.

sleep hygiene describes the pre-sleep routines that relax, enhance settling and promote sleep. These may include going to bed and getting up at around the same time each day, and reducing activity during the evening before bedtime. Routines often include activities such as having a warm bath and changing into nightclothes, reading in bed or a bedtime story for children, a milky drink, teeth/denture cleaning and passing urine.

sleeping sickness a disease endemic in Africa; there is increasing somnolence caused by infection of the brain by trypanosomes. ⊃ trypanosomiasis.

S.6 **Sleep cycle—adults** (reproduced from Brooker & Waugh 2007 with permission).

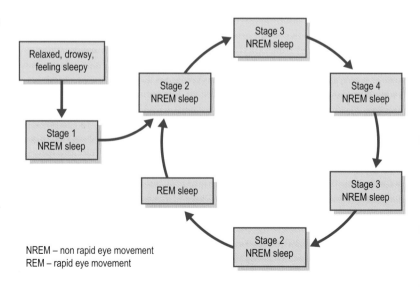

NREM – non rapid eye movement
REM – rapid eye movement

sleep study tests and observations undertaken during sleep in a specialist centre. Used in the investigation of some sleep disorders and to diagnose nocturnal hypoxaemia and apnoeic episodes. ➲ polysomnography.

sleep terror also called night terror. The person, usually a child, wakes suddenly during stage 3 or 4 of non-rapid eye movement sleep. It is characterized by episodes of sudden waking, screaming, intense fear, anxiety, agitation, confusion and disorientation. The child is sweaty and both heart rate and respiratory rate are increased.

sleep walking ➲ somnambulism.

slice a single, reconstructed computed tomography (CT) image.

slice interval in computed tomography (CT) scanning, the distance between reconstructed slices.

slice thickness in modern computed tomography (CT) scanners, reconstructed slice thickness can be selected to provide various slice thicknesses from a single data acquisition.

slide 1. in microscopy, the glass plate on which specimens are mounted for examination. **2.** a photographic slide for projection. **3.** in gnathology, the short jaw movement that occurs from the moment that the teeth first touch to the time that the jaws come to rest in centric occlusion.

sliding board a device used to move patients as part of safe-handling or no-lifting policies.

sliding filament hypothesis/mechanism an explanation of muscle contraction that proposes that the actin and myosin (contractile proteins) filaments slide against each other in the myofibrils to produce muscle shortening. The process by which striated muscles change length, the overlap of thin and thick filaments increasing as the muscle shortens and decreasing as it lengthens. Describes the manner in which these length changes occur, but is not an explanation of the mechanism of active shortening. ➲ cross-bridge, muscle fibre, myofibrils, Colour Section Figure 36.

sliding genioplasty in dentistry/maxillofacial surgery, a surgical procedure to increase the degree of mental prominence, by detaching the lower border of the mandible and repositioning it more anteriorly.

slipped disc n prolapsed intervertebral disc. ➲ prolapsed intervertebral disc.

slipped epiphysis displacement of an epiphysis, especially the upper femoral one. A condition known as slipped upper femoral (capital) epiphysis (SUF(c)E). ➲ epiphysis.

slip ring equipment to allow electrical power to be transferred from a stationary power source onto a continuously moving gantry to allow continuous motion; used in spiral or helical computed tomography (CT) scanning.

slit beam radiography a dental radiographic technique in which, by means of slit collimation of an X-ray beam that is aligned perpendicular to the dental arches during radiography, a panoramic view of the jaws is produced.

slit lamp a device used in ophthalmology to carry out a very detailed examination of the eye. It is a binocular microscope mounted on a table, with a light source that is directed through a narrow slit. It is used to provide the examiner with a three-dimensional view of the external and internal structures of the eye. The magnification and the light source can be adjusted as necessary. ➲ slit-lamp microscope.

slit-lamp microscope a compound microscope used in conjunction with a slit-lamp. It is designed to have a working distance of about 90–125 mm to allow room for the clinician or for placing certain accessories such as a tonometer or pachometer. Slit-lamp microscopes have a magnification which varies usually within the range of ×6 to ×40. ➲ slit-lamp, working distance.

SLK abbr superior limbic keratoconjunctivitis.

SLO abbr scanning laser ophthalmoscope.

SLOB acron **S**ame **L**ingual:**O**pposite **B**uccal (rule). ➲ parallax.

slough n soft, usually creamy yellow material, present at the surface of a wound. It is formed from cellular and fibrin debris, and may vary in colour as wound healing progresses.

slow release drugs drug formulations which do not dissolve until they reach the small intestine, where the drug is slowly released and absorbed. Many slow release preparations are now incorporated into transdermal patches.

slow-twitch muscle fibres skeletal muscle fibres (type 1) adapted for slow response. They contract slowly and moderately for a sustained period and are fatigue resistant. Contain abundant mitochondria, have high levels of myoglobin and are red in colour due to a good blood supply. Metabolism to produce energy is mainly aerobic (oxidative phosphorylation). ➲ fast-twitch muscle fibres, muscle fibre types.

slow virus an infective agent (prion) that only causes infection after a long latent period, perhaps many years. Many cases may never develop overt symptoms but may still be a link in the chain of infectivity. ➲ Creutzfeldt–Jakob disease.

SLR abbr straight leg raise.

SLT abbr speech and language therapist/therapy.

slump test Maitland's slump test is widely used for neurodynamic testing. It is conducted with the patient sitting on the side of a couch. In the starting position the patient sits erect with one foot on a stool and the other unsupported. A series of stages include adopting the slump position, then slump with neck flexion. The last position is further modified by adding knee extension alone and then with ankle dorsiflexion. ➲ neurodynamic testing.

SMA abbr spinal muscular atrophy.

small bowel enema the examination of the small bowel by introducing barium sulphate via a nasogastric tube, directly into the duodenum or the first part of the jejunum. ➲ barium meal, swallow.

small-cell lung carcinoma a type of lung cancer. ➲ oat cell carcinoma.

small for dates (SFD) small for gestational age.

small for gestational age (SGA) babies who weigh less than expected for a given gestational age. They are either constitutionally small or suffer from intrauterine growth restriction. ➲ low birthweight.

small in large out (SILO) response in optometry, refers to the presumed change of the perceived size of a test object that a person experiences, while maintaining fusion when convergence or divergence is varied. When convergence is increased, with base-out (BO) prisms, the object may appear to become smaller and nearer. When divergence is increased with base-in (BI) prisms the object may appear larger and further away. The SILO is not universal; children tend to respond that way, but adults commonly respond in the opposite way, that is, if the test object becomes smaller they report it as moving away from them (thus, small out large in—SOLI). The response is used in visual therapy as a feedback mechanism to patients about their performance. ➲ biofeedback, prism, sensory fusion.

small intestine that part of the alimentary tract between the pyloric sphincter and the ileocaecal valve. It has three parts duodenum, jejunum and ileum. ➲ Colour Section Figure 37.

smallpox *n* (*syn.* variola) a serious disease caused by the variola virus, which belongs to the family Poxviridae. There is a 30% mortality in the unvaccinated and no current effective therapy. The classical form is characterized by a typical deep-seated centrifugal vesicular/pustular rash, worst on the face and extremities, with no cropping (i.e. unlike chickenpox); the rash is accompanied by fever, severe myalgia and odynophagia. Smallpox was eradicated world-wide in 1980 by a successful international vaccination campaign coordinated by the World Health Organization (WHO). However, 76 laboratories world-wide retain the virus. Vaccination may be required for laboratory staff working with pox viruses and others at risk of exposure. Potential for the use of smallpox as a bioterrorist weapon is great, as deliberate release of this virus could result in major epidemics in the currently unvaccinated majority of the population. In view of this threat some developed countries have reintroduced vaccination for key health-care personnel and re-evaluated national plans for the containment of disease. ➲ bioterrorism, cowpox, vaccinia virus.

small (short) saphenous vein ➲ saphenous veins.

SMART *acron* a goal-setting acronym. **S**pecific-**M**easurable-**A**chievable-**R**ealistic-**T**ime orientated.

SMBG *abbr* self-monitoring of blood glucose.

SMBR *abbr* standardized morbidity ratio.

smear *n* a film of material spread out on a glass slide for microscopic examination. ➲ carcinoma, cervical smear, cervical intraepithelial neoplasia (CIN), colposcope, cytology.

smear layer a surface layer on prepared dentine containing cutting debris and bacteria. May interfere with bonding to dentine.

smegma *n* the sebaceous secretion which accumulates beneath the prepuce and around the clitoris.

Smith–Helmholtz law ➲ Lagrange's law.

Smith-Petersen nail (M Smith-Petersen, American orthopaedic surgeon, 1886–1953) a trifin, cannulated metal nail used to provide internal fixation for intracapsular fractures of the femoral neck.

Smith's fracture (R Smith, Irish surgeon, 1807–1873) a fracture of the distal radius with forward (volar) displacement of the distal fragment. Compare Colles' fracture.

smoking (passive) passive smoking is described as the involuntary inhalation of smoke from burning tobacco generated by another person over a period of time. It is associated with an increased risk of smoking-related illnesses such as coronary heart disease, hypertension, bronchial cancer and chronic obstructive pulmonary disease and can also trigger an asthma attack, or lead to sudden unexpected deaths in infancy. Passive smoking is an occupational hazard, for example for those working in bars and clubs, and efforts to reduce the risk include the introduction of no smoking legislation in enclosed workplaces and public places in the UK and the Republic of Ireland and encouraging employers to support smoking cessation programmes. Babies and children are especially vulnerable and have little choice about exposure to tobacco smoke. ➲ sudden unexpected deaths in infancy (sudden infant death syndrome).

smoking in pregnancy antenatal smoking is harmful as carbon monoxide reduces oxygen transport and nicotine causes vasoconstriction of arterioles leading to diminished nutrients and oxygen supplied for the fetus and resulting in poor fetal growth and development. Continued parental smoking predisposes infants to asthma and other allergenic conditions, infections and respiratory conditions.

smooth muscle unstriated, involuntary muscle tissue. Found in hollow organs, such as the gastrointestinal tract, ureter, bladder, the bronchi, blood vessels and the uterus. Spindle-shaped smooth muscle cells (fibres) have a single nucleus and form flat sheets of contractile units. Smooth muscle contraction is involuntarily; stimulation occurs through the action of autonomic nerves and various hormones and regulatory peptides. It responds slowly, and the contraction, which is less intense than that in skeletal muscle, is usually more sustained. Contractions of smooth muscle are more widespread, with all the fibres within the sheet able to contract together. In addition some smooth muscle fibres act as 'pacemakers' which are capable of initiating inherent, rhythmic contractions that may be modified by neural or hormonal influences. ➲ muscle.

SMR *abbr* **1.** standardized mortality ratio. **2.** submucous resection.

'smudge' cells cells that have been ruptured when making a blood film.

snapping hip syndrome a snapping sensation either heard or felt in the hip during movement of the joint. The nature of the signs and symptoms will indicate whether the structure at fault is more likely to be the iliotibial band or the iliopsoas tendon.

snare *n* a surgical instrument with a wire loop at the end; used for removal of polypi.

SNB *abbr* sentinel node biopsy.

Snellen test type chart (H Snellen, Dutch ophthalmologist, 1834–1908) a series of charts used for testing visual acuity. They comprise a chart of different-sized letters arranged in lines that can be read by a normal (emmetropic) eye at 60, 36, 24, 18, 12, 9, 6, 5 and 4 metres. Acuity is checked, in good light, in each eye separately and expressed as 6 over the smallest line of letters that can be read. For example, being able to read the 6-metre line at 6 metres is described as visual acuity of 6/6. Special E test-type with different orientations of the letter E can be used to test young children and other groups unable to read the letters. Charts showing objects of deceasing size can be used to test prelingual children.

Snell's law ⊃ law of refraction.

SNHL *abbr* sensorineural hearing loss.

Snoezelen *n* a controllable multisensory stimulation environment that uses light, colour, sound, tactile surfaces and scents including essential oils to stimulate the senses in a relaxing and soothing way. It has been used with people with dementia and various learning disabilities including autistic spectrum disorders.

snoring a harsh breathing sound during sleep. It is caused by vibration of the soft palate and uvula ⊃ obstructive sleep apnoea (hypopnoea) syndrome.

snowball sampling a research term. The selection of additional respondents is based on referrals from the initial respondents, continuing until no new respondents are identified.

snow blindness painful eyes and photophobia caused by overexposure to the glare from sunlight on snow. It can be accompanied by inflammation of the cornea (keratitis) and conjunctiva (conjunctivitis). ⊃ actinic keratoconjunctivitis, photokeratitis.

SNP *abbr* single-nucleotide polymorphism.

SN plane a transverse plane through the skull at a level represented by a line drawn on a lateral skull radiograph between the sella and the nasion.

snuffles *n* a snorting inspiration due to congestion of nasal mucous membrane. It is a sign of early congenital (prenatal) syphilis when the nasal discharge may be purulent or blood-stained.

Snyder's test a test used to predict a patient's susceptibility to dental caries by determining the concentration of acid producing bacteria in saliva.

SOAP *acron* **S**ubjective **O**bjective **A**ssessment **P**lan. ⊃ problem orientated medical records.

SOB *acron* **S**hortness **O**f **B**reath.

SOBOE *abbr* short of breath on exertion.

social class the classification of people into social groups. The structural position in society of an individual or a group compared to other individuals and groups. It is a central term within the social sciences and the subject of significant controversy and disagreement. In official statistics people are generally classified on the basis of occupation and income. Various classifications are used, and one such is a five category socioeconomic classification based on the householder's occupation. I, professional, e.g. lawyer; II, intermediate, e.g. nurse; III, skilled (non-manual), e.g. secretary and (manual), e.g. carpenter; IV, semi-skilled, e.g. agricultural worker; V, unskilled, e.g. cleaner.

social cognitive theory also known as social learning theory. A general theory or class of theories of human behaviour based on the assumption that thoughts, beliefs and expectations influence behaviour and that these are shaped by the person's social environment.

social deprivation measurement composite index of deprivation (poverty) in a defined population based on census-derived social and economic variables. Geographically defined populations include residents within a Strategic Health Authority (population up to several million, e.g. NHS East of England) or district (population half to one million), administrative (electoral) wards (several thousands) or enumerator districts (25 households). Deprivation indices may also be attributed to general practice populations based on the wards or enumerator districts from which the practice draws its registered patients.

social environment the people with whom the individual interacts in ways that demand and shape occupational performance.

social exclusion the lack of social connections, social support or access to social networks for particular groups in the population (community). Groups affected include rough sleepers, teenage mothers, refugees and many young people. Research has reported higher levels of ill health (illness, psychological ill health, disease, disability, mortality) in people with low levels of social support and integration, independent of physical health, socio-economic status and lifestyle. Two main theories: social support affects health directly; social support protects against life stresses. Conversely, social exclusion increases the risk of physical and psychological ill health. ⊃ underclass.

social facilitation the effects of the presence of an audience on a person's or team's performance. The term is a misnomer because the effects are not always facilitative and it has therefore been replaced with audience effects when the audience observes the activity but is not actively involved and coaction effects when the audience is concurrently engaged in the same activity.

social functioning describes the everyday activities and abilities that enable social interaction, interpersonal relationships and independent living. Social functioning ability may be severely affected by mental health problems, such as depression and schizophrenia. ⊃ Social Functioning Scale.

Social Functioning Scale (SFS) a scale used to assess aspects of everyday social functioning which are negatively affected by mental health problems. There are seven main areas, for example interpersonal behaviour, social engagement, etc.

social identity the social category of the individual and the expectations of behaviour that are attributed to them by other people.

social inclusion the full incorporation and participation of people in society as a result of fundamental changes within attitudes, behaviour and societal structures.

social isolation a term that can be applied to an individual, a family or a group of individuals. Interaction with other

S
T

people does not conform to the usual pattern, for reasons that may include immobility, poverty, etc.

socialization *n* the means by which individuals learn the social norms and the value of abiding by them. The process that facilitates the transmission of culture from one generation to another, ensuring its continuity, e.g. language, knowledge and way of life. It may occur informally in the family (primary socialization), and more formally when starting school and continuing throughout life (secondary socialization). Sometimes the term tertiary or professional socialization is applied to the acquisition of the knowledge, skills and attitude needed to perform high-level occupational roles such as medicine.

social learning theory ⊃ social cognitive theory.

social loafing a tendency for individuals to exert less effort on a task when working in groups than when they work on the same task alone.

social movement the organized efforts of significant numbers of oppressed people (including women, black people and disabled people) to change a major aspect of society. A social movement is a politically generated and committed force that is opposed to the status quo. Social movements usually operate outside regular political channels.

social norms describes socially acceptable behaviour. Norms may prescribe some forms of behaviour and prohibit others. ⊃ anomie.

social physique anxiety anxiety that individuals experience in response to a perception that others will negatively evaluate their physique.

social policy the process of developing measures to reduce social problems and implementing these measures. Social policy is also an academic field of study where these processes are analysed.

social role valorization a concept evolved from the concept of 'normalization' and was first formulated by Wolfensberger in 1998. This was partly due to mounting criticisms of the concept of 'normalization'. Social role valorization refers to the process of improving the lives and social standing of devalued groups, particularly people with a learning disability, so that their social value in the eyes of others is enhanced. Such measures include deinstitutionalization and allowing people to participate and contribute to society. ⊃ normalization.

social services personal social services that include social work and social care carried out by, or on behalf of local authority Social Services Departments, other statutory organizations, private and voluntary agencies.

social skills training a structured programme for teaching effective social skills through a combination of individual and group exercises, modelling and role play.

social stratification the means of dividing populations into unequal strata using different characteristics, for example: age, gender, income, ethnicity, etc.

socially clean a term used when articles are required to be scrupulously clean, a condition achieved without using disinfectants. To prevent nosocomial infection, it must characterize all articles which patients use, including baths, bath mats, showers, sieved water outlets, sinks and washbowls. ⊃ asepsis, disinfection, sterilization.

socio- a prefix that means 'sociology', e.g. *sociomedical*.

sociocultural *adj* pertaining to culture in its sociological context.

socio-economic status a measure for classifying individuals, families and households. Indicators include occupation, income, education and housing. ⊃ social class.

sociology *n* the scientific study of societies and groups, and interpersonal and intergroup social relationships and interactions—**sociological** *adj*.

sociology of sport area of study concerned with the social structure, social patterns and social organization of groups and subcultures in sport.

sociomedical *adj* relating to sociology and medicine. For example how social influences may predispose to diseases, e.g. sleeping rough may increase the risk for hypothermia, unemployment increasing the risk of mental health problems, such as depression, etc.

socket a hollow into which another part fits. In dentistry, the cavity in the alveolar bone of either jaw which accommodates the root of a tooth.

SOD *acron* **S**ource to **O**bject **D**istance.

sodium (Na) *n* metallic element. The main cation in the extracellular fluid (ECF). It is concerned with the composition of the fluid compartments and neuromuscular function. The concentration of ECF sodium ions, $[Na^+]$, is regulated by variations in its reabsorption and excretion in the kidneys, dependent in turn upon mechanisms within the kidneys themselves, and on the adrenal cortical hormone aldosterone (promoting renal $[Na^+]$ reabsorption), and atrial natrurietic hormone (promoting $[Na^+]$ excretion). Variations in ECF $[Na^+]$ and its renal and hormonal control are closely linked to control of blood volume and ECF fluid volume as a whole. ⊃ minerals, salt (sodium chloride) intake, water balance.

sodium bicarbonate (NaHCO₃) also known as sodium hydrogen carbonate. It functions in the body as part of a buffer system to limit pH changes in the blood. Administered intravenously to correct metabolic acidosis, such as in renal failure, or during cardiac arrest.

sodium chloride 'common salt'. Often used in intravenous fluids to replace fluids and correct electrolyte levels.

sodium citrate used as an in vitro anticoagulant, e.g. for stored blood.

sodium fluoride paste a paste containing sodium fluoride, kaolin, glycerin(e) (glycerol) and pigments. Applied to sensitive areas on teeth, such as the cervical regions, to reduce sensitivity and harden the enamel.

sodium hydroxide in radiography, used as a developer accelerator.

sodium hypochlorite a powerful disinfectant used, in suitable dilutions, in many situations, such as dealing with environmental contamination with blood and other body fluids, and disinfection of infant feeding bottles. It is effective against many micro-organisms, including the hepatitis B virus and HIV. In dentistry, used between 1% and 5.25% (free chlorine) to irrigate and disinfect root canals during root canal preparation. Dakin's Solution is a dilution (0.5% free chlorine) buffered with boric acid to pH 9.5.

sodium lactate a sodium salt present in some intravenous infusion solutions, such as compound lactate solution (Hartmann's solution, Ringer-lactate solution.)

sodium perborate a mouthwash ingredient that releases nascent oxygen, so preventing the growth of anaerobic organisms.

sodium phosphate a chemical used in alginate impression material to delay the reaction between the alginate and calcium sulphate and increase the setting time of the material.

sodium-potassium (Na-K) pump one of many similar molecular complexes embodying ion-binding sites and an ATPase, found in surface (plasma) membrane of all cells, which actively transports sodium ions [Na^+] out of the cytoplasm and potassium ions [K^+] into it (usually in the ratio $3Na^+$ out to $2K^+$ in), using energy derived from hydrolysis of adenosine triphosphate (ATP) by the action of sodium-potassium (Na-K) ATPase. All cells have at least a minimum density of these pumps but nerve and muscle cells have greater numbers to cope with the greater ion fluxes in these cells. The high intracellular [K^+] and low intracellular [Na^+] in cells (in contrast to their concentrations in extracellular fluid) are due to these pumps; the maintenance of the membrane potential and of cell volume results from this ion distribution. Formerly, on the basis of inadequate understanding, termed simply 'sodium pump'.

sodium potassium tartrate (potassium sodium tartrate) Rochelle salt. Added to dental plaster to accelerate the setting reaction.

sodium sulphite in radiography, used as a fixer preservative.

sodomy 1. anal intercourse between two men, or a man and a woman. **2.** can be used to describe intercourse between a human and an animal. This is also called beastiality or zoophilia. **3.** a more general term used to describe a sexual act or behaviour that is not acceptable to the majority in society.

soft liner a soft polymeric material processed onto the fitting surface of a prosthesis to reduce any trauma to the underlying tissues. Usually consists of a synthetic elastomer.

soft palate situated at the posterior border of the palate. A movable curtain of tissue extending downwards and backwards into the pharynx from the posterior border of the hard palate. Composed of a fold of mucous membrane whose two layers enclose muscles, glandular structures, blood vessels and nerves. During deglutition (swallowing) it is raised to assist in shutting off the nasal part of the pharynx from the portion below. The uvula hangs from its posterior free border. ⊃ palate.

soft rollers in radiography, part of the film transport system in an automatic film processor and are found where films crossover into another section and squeeze any excess liquid out of the film; they are made of a neoprene-type substance.

soft sore chancroid.

soft tissue mobilization physiotherapists and sports therapists use pétrissage or kneading techniques using the whole hand or the finger pads to stretch retracted muscles and tendons, relieve spasm and help to remove metabolic waste products from muscles. Kneading with the finger pads is also used during some natural childbirth methods. Physiotherapists use percussive manipulations, collectively called tapôtement, to move thick secretions from the respiratory tract and assist expectoration.

soft tissue nasion an anatomical landmark. The deepest point of concavity between the nose and forehead in the midline. ⊃ nasion.

soft tissue pogonion an anatomical landmark. The most anterior point on the soft tissue outline of the chin when a patient is viewed in profile. ⊃ pogonion.

software the programs run by the computer.

sol a colloidal solution in its liquid phase.

solanine *n* a very toxic compound that is naturally present in nightshade plants, such as tomatoes and potatoes. Most is ingested from eating potatoes, especially so if the potatoes have turned green and sprouted, after being exposed to light. The toxin is not completely destroyed by heat (heat stable) and if ingested, can lead to a variety of effects, mainly gastrointestinal or neurological. These include: nausea and vomiting, colicky abdominal pain and diarrhoea, low temperature, bradycardia, decreased respiratory rate, dilated pupils and visual disturbances, headache, altered sensation, delerium and hallucination. On rare occasions it results in death.

solarization when an increase in exposure results in a decrease in density on a film and therefore a reverse image can be obtained. ⊃ characteristic curve.

solar keratosis a warty skin lesion due to sun exposure which may progress to cancer.

solar plexus a large network of sympathetic (autonomic) nerve ganglia and fibres in the upper abdomen. It supplies the abdominal organs. *solar plexus punch* a blow to the abdomen that results in an immediate inability to breathe freely.

solar retinitis ⊃ solar retinopathy.

solar retinopathy macular damage caused by fixating the sun without adequate protection, usually viewing a solar eclipse, but also in people staring at the sun. The retina presents at first with retinal oedema which may develop into an atrophy of the tissue and produce a circumscribed hole or cyst in the fovea. This latter event results in a permanent central scotoma. There is no specific treament but the condition can be prevented by wearing very dense light filters or viewing through photographic film. ⊃ actinic.

solder used in dentistry. A fusible metal or metallic alloy used to join metal surfaces. When heat is applied to the joint and the solder, which has a lower melting point than the metals to be joined, it melts, runs over the join and hardens on cooling.

soldering used in dentistry. Joining of two metal parts by means of solder.

solenoid consists of several coils of wire joined together to produce magnetic lines of force. If soft iron is placed inside the loops of wire it becomes magnetized.

soleus *n* a muscle of the posterior aspect of the lower leg. It is covered by the large gastrocnemius calf muscle. Its origin is on the superior part of the tibia and fibula and it inserts on to the calcaneus (os calcis) via the calcaneal tendon (Achilles tendon) of the gastrocnemius. Contracts to plantar flex the foot; important during walking and running. ⊃ Colour Section Figure 4, 5.

SOLI *abbr* small out large in.

solid state radiation detector a silicon diode used to measure the activity of electron beams or megavoltage photon beams.

solute *n* substance dissolved in a solvent.

solution *n* a fluid that contains a dissolved substance or substances. ⊃ saturated solution.

solvent *n* an agent that is capable of dissolving other substances (solutes), e.g. in dentistry, chloroform and eucalyptus are used to dissolve gutta percha. The component of a solution that is present in excess. In photography used to dilute chemicals, for example when making up developer, developer replenisher and fixer; the solvent used is water.

solvent misuse the practice of inhaling volatile substances, such as those in some adhesives, solvents and fuels, to produce euphoria and intoxication. Characterized by odour on clothes and hair, redness and blistering around the nose and mouth, and behaviour changes. Dependence, local damage to the nasal mucosa and organ damage, e.g. the brain, may result. Death may be caused by asphyxia or toxicity. ⊃ drug misuse.

soma derived from the Greek for 'body'. **1.** the body as separate and distinct from the mind. **2.** the body excluding the gametes.

-somatia, somatic a suffix that means 'pertaining to the body', e.g. *diplosomatia*.

somatic *adj* relating to the body. **1.** the body as distinct from the mind, e.g. as in 'psychosomatic', ascribing physical symptoms to mental causes. **2.** the substance of the body, excluding the internal organs, i.e. as distinct from visceral. Hence somatic nerves, the components of the peripheral nervous system both sensory and motor, that serve the skin and musculoskeletal structures.

somatic anxiety the physiological and affective elements of anxiety including unpleasant perceptions of arousal, nervousness and tension. ⊃ anxiety.

somatic cells the body cells, as distinct from the gametes (germ cells).

somatic effect the effect of radiation on the body cells. May be produced by a high dosage of radiation or the cumulative effects of a low dosage over a period of time, e.g. radiation burn and radiation dermatitis.

somatic nerves nerves controlling the function of voluntary, skeletal muscle.

somatic/o, somat/o- a prefix that means 'body', e.g. *somatostatin*.

somatization the presence of physical symptoms without organic pathology. A number of terms have, in the past, been used to describe such events, including psychosomatic illness, functional illness, hysteria/conversion disorder, etc. Somatization is encountered in all specialisms in medicine. For example, abdominal pain with intermittent constipation and diarrhoea (irritable bowel syndrome), chest pain without cardiac pathology and atypical face pain.

somatoform disorders the *International Classification of Diseases* (ICD-10) classifies somatoform disorders in seven categories: hypochondriacal disorder, persistent somatoform pain disorder, somatoform autonomic dysfunction, somatization disorder, undiffentiated somatoform disorder, other somatoform disorders and somatoform disorder unspecified. Of these, hypochondriacal disorder and somatization disorder are the most common. The disorders have overlapping characteristics and, in practice, it is often very hard to distinguish between them. The classication in the *Diagnostic and Statistical Manual of Mental Disorders* (DSM-IV) is more specific.

somatomedin ⊃ insulin-like growth factor.

somatostatin *n* growth hormone release inhibiting hormone (GHRIH). A hormone secreted at several sites, with widespread inhibitory effects on other secretions: from the hypothalamus, as growth hormone release inhibiting hormone (GHRIH) acting in the anterior pituitary; in the pancreas, inhibits other pancreatic secretions; from the intestinal wall, inhibits many hormonal and enzyme secretions in the gut. ⊃ growth hormone.

somatostatin receptors receptors found in the pituitary gland, pancreas, upper gastrointestinal tract, small cell lung cancer, tumours of the ovary, cervix, endometrium, breast, kidney, larynx, paranasal sinus, some skin tumours and tumours in the salivary glands. They are useful in imaging a variety of tumours.

somatostatinoma *n* a rare somatostatin-secreting tumour of the islet cells of the pancreas. Causes dyspepsia, reduced secretion of gastric acid, steatorrhoea, the formation of gallstones, impaired glucose tolerance or diabetes mellitus. They also occur in the duodenum. ⊃ islet cell tumours.

somatotrophin *n* ⊃ growth hormone.

somatotyping a way of describing body type or physique using a classification that has three basic types: ectomorphic, endomorphic and mesomorphic.

somite any of the segments (somites) that form in the paired blocks of mesoderm that develop either side of the neural tube during the early days of embryonic development. The ventromedial somites will give rise to ligaments, cartilage and bone, and the dorsolateral somites will form skeletal muscle and the dermis of the skin.

somnambulism *n* (*syn.* sleepwalking) occurs during stage 4 non-rapid eye movement sleep and mostly affects children.

Following a short sleep period, the child sit ups, their eyes are open, they leave the bed and walk about. During this period they may do unusual things, such as urinating in the bedroom. Afterwards they may proceed directly to bed and will have no recall of events when they wake normally in the morning. Adults can also be affected, particularly if anxious or stressed, and may resume sleepwalking as they once did as children.

somn/i- a prefix that means 'sleep', e.g. *somnambulism*.

somnolence syndrome periods of drowsiness, lethargy, loss of appetite and irritability in children following radiotherapy treatment to the head.

Somogyi phenomenon (M Somogyi, American biochemist, 1883–1971) in diabetes mellitus, the rebound hyperglycaemia that occurs following hypoglycaemia; it is caused by the release of hormones that cause glycogenolysis, gluconeogenesis and lipolysis thus raising blood glucose.

-somy a suffix that means 'pertaining to chromosomes', e.g. *trisomy*.

-sonic a suffix that means 'sound', e.g. *gnathosonic*.

sonograph graphic record of sound waves.

sonography the means by which a sonograph is recorded and interpreted. ⊃ ultrasonography.

sonolucent without echoes.

soporific *adj, n* (describes) an agent which induces deep sleep.

sordes dried, brown crusts which form in the mouth, especially on the lips and teeth, in situations where normal oral hygiene mechanisms are impaired, such as with dehydration and pyrexia.

sorption a phenomenon of absorption and adsorption or the state in which both phenomena occur at the same time.

souffle *n* puffing or blowing sound. *funic souffle* auscultatory murmur of pregnancy. A soft whispering sound that synchronizes with the fetal heart beat and is caused by pressure on the umbilical cord. *uterine souffle* soft, blowing murmur which can be auscultated over the uterus after the fourth month of pregnancy.

sound *n* **1.** the result of mechanical energy travelling through matter as a wave, producing alternating compression and rarefaction resulting in vibration. **2.** an instrument introduced into a hollow organ or duct to detect a stone or to dilate a stricture.

source isolation is used for patients who are sources of micro-organisms that may be transmitted from them to infect others. *strict source isolation* is for highly transmissible and dangerous diseases. *standard source isolation* is for other communicable diseases/infections.

source organ an organ where radioactivity is accumulated and therefore irradiates associated organs.

source stick protocol the instructions to be followed if a machine housing a radioactive source remains in the 'beam on' position at the end of the planned exposure, i.e. the beam does not terminate.

Southern blot technique (E Southern, British biochemist, b.1938) a technique used to analyse fragments of DNA and identify the genes present. ⊃ Northern blot technique.

Souttar tube an intubation tube which comprises flexible metal coils; the tube is pushed through an oesophageal tumour to enable the free passage of food and fluid.

soya protein a protein that is extracted from soya bean, a legume used in Asiatic countries in place of meat. It is useful in dietetic preparations for those people who are allergic to cows' milk. Soya protein is a constituent of soya milk used as a substitute for cows' milk by vegans.

SP *abbr* spatial peak. ⊃ ultrasound.

space loss the loss of space in a dental arch when a tooth is lost by extraction or is developmentally absent.

space maintainer a removable or fixed appliance designed to maintain an existing space in a dental arch.

spacer the thin layer of wax or other material interposed between two structures during an impression, in order to allow for a uniform space when it is removed. Used in special trays to allow for a uniform thickness of impression material or over such retention devices as the Dolder bar. *spacer cone* ⊃ cone.

Spalding's sign gross overlapping of the fetal cranial bones, seen on abdominal radiograph, indicating that intrauterine death occurred several days previously.

spam unrequested email, usually advertising products or services.

spansule *n* a drug preparation designed to produce controlled release when given orally.

spasm *n* **1.** a sudden, involuntary contraction of a muscle. **2.** sustained contraction of a muscle or group of muscles due to pain. **3.** a seizure or convulsion of the whole body.

spasm of accommodation an involuntary contraction of the ciliary muscle producing excess accommodation. It may be constant, intermittent, unilateral or bilateral. Patients typically complain of blurred distance vision and sometimes changes in perceived size of objects, and discomfort. If the patient is a low hyperope or emmetrope, it will give rise to pseudomyopia (or false myopia or hypertonic myopia or spurious myopia). Diagnosis is facilitated by cycloplegic refraction. Management includes removal of the primary cause, if possible (e.g. uveitis, or patient taking parasympathomimetic drugs), correction of the underlying refraction, if any, changes in the visual working conditions, positive lenses, accommodative facility exercises and only rarely cycloplegics. ⊃ accommodative facility, metamorphopsia.

spasmodic dysmenorrhoea ⊃ dysmenorrhoea.

spasmolytic *adj, n* ⊃ antispasmodic.

spastic dystonia describes the sustained chronic contraction of muscle that continues in the absence of movement. It is thought to be caused by sustained efferent muscular hyperactivity, dependent upon continuous supraspinal drive to the alpha motor neurones (Burke 1988). (Burke D 1988 Spasticity as an adaptation to pyramidal tract injury. Advances in Neurology 47:401–423.)

spastic colon ⮕ irritable bowel syndrome.

spastic gait stiff, shuffling, the legs being held together. ⮕ gait.

spasticity *n* increased tension or tone of muscle (hypertonia) with increased resistance to passive movement out of the tonic posture proportional to the rate of stretch and characterized by the clasp-knife phenomenon, exaggerated deep tendon reflexes, Babinski's sign and clonus. Spasticity of one side of the body following stroke (cerebrovascular accident) is accompanied by loss of voluntary movement and postural reactions of one side of the body (spastic hemiplegia)—**spastic** *adj*.

spatial divided into partitions.

spatial awareness a knowledge of where all parts of the body are in relation to the physical characteristics of the immediate environment. Important in judging distances, such as reaching for an object, or safely going up or down steps.

spatial detail ⮕ spatial resolution.

spatial distortion when a gamma camera does not accurately distinguish between an object and its surroundings.

spatial filtering a method of improving an electronic image by modifying the pixel values that surround the area.

spatial frequency the change in brightness value of a region of an electronic image per unit distance. If an area has low spatial frequency there is little change in brightness over distance but with high spatial values there can be a large change in brightness over a small distance.

spatial neglect ⮕ unilateral neglect.

spatial relations problems a variety of problems (e.g. trips and falls, accidents involving hot liquids, etc.) caused when people are not able to work out how the position of several objects in the environment relates to them, or their own position in relation to each separate object.

spatial resolution the smallest distance between two objects that can be visually seen on an imaging system.

spatial vision ⮕ depth perception.

spatula *n* a flat flexible instrument with blunt edges for spreading creams, ointment, etc. *tongue spatula* a rigid, blade-shaped instrument for depressing the tongue during physical examination.

spatulate 1. having a flat, blunt end. **2**. to mix with a spatula.

spatulation mixing together of various materials with a spatula on a smooth flat surface to form a uniformly consistent mixture.

special educational needs (SEN) a phrase usually applied to the particular (educational) needs of a child or an adult with a learning disability. It can also apply to individuals who do not have a learning disability, e.g. the special educational needs of a child who is particularly gifted. ⮕ statement of special needs.

special needs the concept of needs is widely used in the social sciences and in service policy, practice and provision. It can denote the lack of something required by or necessary for a person, particularly for survival. Though basic human needs can be agreed, such as for food, sleep and shelter, broader social and psychological needs are contested. When applied to specific groups, particularly disabled people, the notion of needs is often qualified by the term 'special' within an individual or medical model of disability. With regard to the need for provision of services, 'special' has meant separate or segregated and is seen by many disabled people as an expression and justification of oppression. It can be argued that the needs of disabled people should be mainstream rather than 'special'.

special impression tray ⮕ impression tray.

special tray material a composite resin supplied in sheet form, which cures using a visible light source. Used for the construction of special trays and temporary bases. ⮕ tray.

specialist a health professional who, after undertaking extensive post-graduate/post-registration training and then achieving the relevant qualifications, concentrates on a special branch of medicine, dentistry, nursing, or allied health professions.

specialist community public health nurse in the UK, include health visitors, family health nurses, school nurses and occupational health nurses.

species *n* a systematic category, subdivision of genus. Individuals within a species group have common characteristics and differ, fairly obviously, from a related species.

specific *adj* special; characteristic; peculiar to.

specific action that brought about by certain remedial agents in a particular disease, e.g. antibiotics in infection.

specific activity the ratio per unit mass of radioactive to non-radioactive atoms in an element.

specific adaptation to imposed demands (SAID) principle in sports medicine the principle of specificity of training. ⮕ training.

specific disease one that is always caused by a specified organism, e.g. typhoid fever is caused by the bacterium *Salmonella enterica* serovar Typhi.

specific dynamic action (SDA) the increase in body temperature and metabolism that occurs when energy is used in the assimilation of ingested food. Protein foods in particular cause a sustained increase in basal metabolic rate that lasts for some hours.

specific gravity the relative density of one body or object compared to another. If compared to water, an object will float if its specific gravity is less than 1.0 (assuming water has a density of 1.0 kg/m^3.)

specific heat the energy in joules which is required to raise the temperature of 1 kilogram of the body by 1 kelvin unit.

specific ionization the number of ion pairs produced per millimetre by a charged particle passing through a medium.

specificity *n* **1**. high specificity is the ability of a test to accurately identify non-affected individuals, such as faecal occult blood screening for colorectal cancer. Low specificity can lead to false positives, i.e. it detects disease in cases where it is not present. ⊃ sensitivity. **2.** the ability of a detector to respond to a specific type and energy of radiation.

specific resistance of a substance is obtained when a current is measured after passing through opposing surfaces of a 1 metre cube of the material.

speckling the graininess of an ultrasound image which is caused by scatter.

SPECT *abbr* single-photon emission computed tomography.

spectacle plane a plane representing the orientation of the spectacle lenses relative to the eyes and passing through the posterior vertices of the two lenses. ⊃ pantoscopic angle, retroscopic angle, vertex, vertex distance.

spectral Doppler trace in ultrasound, a greyscale picture of a waveform showing all its components.

spectral emission the colour of light emitted by an object. In intensifying screen, lanthanum oxybromide blue, gadolinium oxysulphide green, barium fluorochloride ultraviolet and calcium tungstate blue.

spectral sensitivity the range of wavelengths of electromagnetic radiation that a film emulsion or the human eye is sensitive to.

spectral sensitizing in radiography. Increasing the spectral sensitivity of a film by adding impurities to the film emulsion, because it is achieved by adding coloured dyes and therefore can be called dye sensitizing, colour sensitizing or optical sensitizing.

spectrins a group of proteins in the red blood cell membrane that (with other proteins) controls and stabilizes red cell shape. This allows the red cell to distort to negotiate capillaries. ⊃ ankyrins, hereditary elliptocytosis, hereditary spherocytosis.

spectrophotometer *n* a spectroscope combined with a photometer for quantitatively measuring the relative intensity of different parts of a light spectrum—**spectrophotometric** *adj.*

spectroscope *n* an instrument for observing spectra of light.

spectrum locus the representation of the spectral colour stimuli on a chromaticity diagram. ⊃ chromaticity diagram.

specular microscope a light microscope utilizing specular reflection to view the component layers of the cornea and particularly to observe and photograph the endothelium. It consists of an objective which is divided longitudinally. Light in the form of a slit beam is directed down one half and is reflected from the cornea–aqueous interface to the other half of the objective to form a visible and photographic image of the endothelium. The microscope is usually fitted with a × 40 water immersion objective which has a working distance of 1.6 mm. The cornea is covered with silicone fluid into which the objective tip is immersed. Good resolution is achieved provided that the width of the slit beam is kept small, to reduce the light scatter from the overlying corneal layers. This microscope allows examination of the corneal endothelium in vitro. For clinical measurements, the specular microscope is mounted horizontally using an objective with less magnification (usually × 20). The tip of the microscope has a glass-windowed, fluid-filled, screw-on cap,

which applanates the cornea over a very small area. The field of view is usually increased by the insertion of a +10D into the incident light path before the objective. Photomicrography is accomplished with a flash unit, as otherwise eye movements make photography with long exposure impossible. However, corneal anaesthesia is necessary and clear images of the endothelium are not possible if the cornea is oedematous. For these reasons new systems have been developed which fit on a slit-lamp and facilitate photography. Their magnification is greater than other slit-lamps, being ×40 to ×70, and they do not require contact with the cornea as they have long working distances. Specular microscopy is used to monitor changes in corneal endothelium in contact lens wearers, especially those wearing extended wear lenses. ⊃ confocal microscope, corneal endothelium, endothelial polymegethism, extended wear lens, regular reflection, working distance.

specular reflection ⊃ regular reflection.

specular reflection illumination in slit-lamp examination, it is a method in which the beam of light and the microscope are placed at equal angles from the normal to the corneal or lens surface to be viewed. This is a method for examining the quality of a surface. This method is particularly useful to observe the corneal endothelium. ⊃ shagreen.

speculum *n* an instrument used to hold the walls of a cavity apart, so that the interior of the cavity can be examined or treated—**specula** *pl. nasal speculum* used for examination of the nose and for treatments, such as nasal cautery and packing to stop bleeding. *vaginal speculum* used to examine the vagina and cervix, for taking high vaginal swabs and cervical smears and for some treatments. Types include Cusco's bivalve (Figure S.7) and Sims' speculum.

speech the sound produced by the passage of air through the vocal cords and modified by the tongue, cheeks, lips and soft palate. Controlled by the speech centres of the brain.

speech and language therapist the health professional responsible for the assessment, diagnosis and treatment of speech and language disorders and disorders affecting

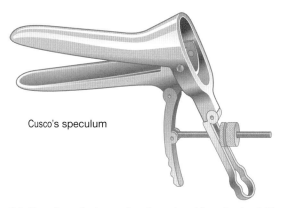

Cusco's speculum

S.7 Cusco's vaginal speculum (reproduced from Brooker & Nicol 2003 with permission).

swallowing in children and adults. In the United States and Australia they are known as speech-language pathologists.

speech and language therapy (SLT) one of the professions allied to medicine. Describes the therapy provided by a speech and language therapists to people with impaired communication, e.g. aphasia. Speech and language therapy is provided for people who are dysfluent (stammer), have impaired hearing, have language difficulties (grammar and vocabulary and the social use of language), have problems producing the correct sounds for speech so that they are difficult to understand, or have difficulties with their voice. Speech and language therapy referrals are also made for people who have dysphagia (difficulty in swallowing), particularly following a stroke or in other neurological conditions. Speech and language therapy includes assessment and treatment of these difficulties. In the UK therapy with adults is usually carried out within an NHS setting, including hospitals and nursing homes. Children may be seen in health centres but increasingly speech and language therapy services are being offered in educational settings, including mainstream schools. Speech and language therapy aims to achieve the best level of communication possible for the person concerned. As well as being provided for individuals, speech and language therapy may be provided for small groups, such as in units dedicated to stroke care, or brain injury. Programmes may also be set up for other staff (such as nurses) to carry out. Speech and language therapists are a valuable resource for other members of the multidisciplinary team and can provide advice on how to achieve optimum communication with people with difficulties in communicating.

speech mechanism normal speech involves several processes, breathing, phonation, articulation, resonance and prosody. It is disturbed in various combinations and degrees in dysarthria and dysphasia.

speech recognition software, which allows computers to be operated by human voice commands.

speech synthesis software which allows computers to 'talk' to the user.

speed the change of distance with respect to time. A scalar quantity (i.e. having no directional component). ➲ angular speed, film speed, linear speed, screen speed, velocity.

speed classification in radiography, a means of comparing different film screen combinations, it is an arbitrary scale based on 100 and combinations range between 50 and 800.

speed of light the currently accepted figure is 29 9792.5 km/s (in a vacuum). This velocity decreases, differentially with wavelength, when the radiation enters a medium. ➲ electromagnetic spectrum, refractive index, wavelength.

Spencer Wells artery forceps ➲ forceps,

sperm *n* an abbreviated form of the word spermatozoon or spermatozoa.

sperm count a test undertaken early during a series of investigations for infertility, in which semen is examined for volume, sperm numbers, morphology, motility and chemical composition. ➲ semen.

spermatic *adj* pertaining to or conveying semen.

spermatic cord suspends the testis in the scrotum and contains the testicular artery and vein and the deferent duct (vas deferens). ➲ Colour Section Figure 16.

spermatid the cells produced at the meiosis II stage of spermatocytogenesis from secondary spermatocytes. They change and mature to become functional spermatozoa during spermiogenesis. ➲ spermatogenesis.

spermatocele a swelling of the rete testis or epididymis that contains spermatozoa.

spermatocyte the primary spermatocyte is a diploid cell, derived from the spermatogonium; it undergoes meiosis I to produce two haploid secondary spermatocytes. ➲ spermatogenesis.

spermatocytogenesis the stage of spermatogenesis during which the haploid spermatids are formed.

spermatogenesis *n* the formation and development of spermatozoa. It comprises the reduction division of meiosis in which the spermatids are formed in a stage known as spermatocytogenesis, and a further maturation stage, which is called spermiogenesis. The seminiferous tubules of the adult testis contain the diploid germ cells or spermatogonia and Sertoli cells. The germ cells, which are all at different stages of development, will eventually become spermatozoa; the supporting Sertoli cells help to nourish the germ cells, secrete hormones and provide the blood–testis barrier which prevents the immune system having contact with the spermatozoa antigens, which are formed long after immuno-competence is achieved. The diploid stem cells divide by mitosis to form primary spermatocytes, which in turn enter meiosis I to produce haploid secondary spermatocytes. The secondary spermatocytes then undergo the second meiotic division which results in four haploid cells known as spermatids. Each spermatid still needs considerable modification during spermiogenesis, before it becomes a highly specialized motile spermatozoon with a head, midpiece and tail. These modifications, which occur in the epididymis, include nuclear changes, loss of excess cytoplasm and the formation of a tail (a flagellum). ➲ spermatocytogenesis, spermiogenesis.

spermatogonium the undifferentiated, diploid germ cell in the male—**spermatogonia** *pl*. ➲ spermatogenesis.

spermatorrhoea *n* involuntary discharge of semen without orgasm.

spermatozoon *n* a fully motile, mature, male gamete comprising a head, midpiece and tail (Figure S.8). The genetic material is condensed in the head, which is topped by an acrosome containing lytic enzymes. These enzymes allow the spermatozoa to pass through the cervical mucus and ultimately to penetrate the oocyte. The midpiece contains many mitochondria, arranged in a spiral, which produce the ATP required to power the movements of the tail—**spermatozoa** *pl*.

spermaturia seminuria. Spermatozoa in the urine; may be caused by retrograde ejaculation into the bladder, such as in diabetes mellitus or following prostate surgery.

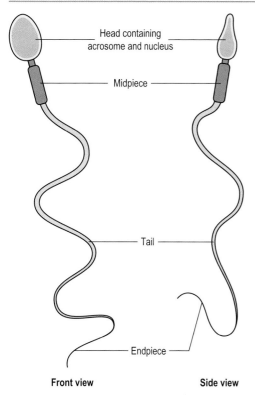

Head containing
acrosome and nucleus

Midpiece

Tail

Endpiece

Front view   Side view

S.8 Spermatozoon (reproduced from Brooker 2006A with permission).

spermicide, spermatocide *n* an agent that kills spermatozoa—**spermicidal** *adj.*

spermiogenesis the second or maturation stage of spermatogenesis. Once formed each haploid spermatid must still undergo considerable modification, before it becomes a highly specialized motile spermatozoon (or sperm cell) with the characteristic form of a head, midpiece and tail. The changes, which occur in the epididymis, include nuclear changes (condenses), with acrosome development, multiplication of mitochondria, loss of excess cytoplasm and the formation of a tail (a flagellum).

sphenoid *n* the central wedge-shaped bone at the base of the skull containing the sphenoidal sinus. It is situated beneath the brain consisting of a body, greater and lesser wings and processes. It articulates with the temporal, occipital, parietal, frontal, ethmoidal, malar, vomer and palate bones. It forms the posterior wall of each orbit. Through it pass the three nerve trunks from the trigeminal nerve (fifth cranial nerve) carrying sensations from the face and mouth and supplying the motor nerves of the muscles of mastication and salivary glands. It contains a pair of air sinuses and gives attachment to the internal and external pterygoid and the temporal muscles of mastication—**sphenoidal** *adj.*

sphenopalatine ganglion also known as Meckel's ganglion. A parasympathetic ganglion derived from the facial nerve (seventh cranial nerve). Its postganglionic fibres

supply the palatal glands, and the sensory and sympathetic fibres pass through the ganglion.

spherical aberration a defect of an optical system due to a variation in the focusing between peripheral and paraxial rays. The larger the pupil size, the greater the difference in focusing between the two rays. In the gaussian theory, the focus of the optical system is attributed to the paraxial rays. The distance, in dioptres, between the focus of the paraxial rays and the peripheral rays represents the amount of longitudinal spherical aberration of the system. When the peripheral rays are refracted more than the paraxial rays, the aberration is said to be *positive or undercorrected*. When the peripheral rays are refracted less than the paraxial rays the aberration is said to be *negative or overcorrected*. The relaxed human eye has a small amount of positive spherical aberration (up to 1 D for a pupil of 8 mm diameter).

spherical amalgam alloy alloy in the shape of spherical beads. ⟴ alloy.

spherocylindrical lens a lens with one surface spherical and the other cylindrical. It has two different refractive powers in its two principal meridians. ⟴ astigmatic lens, cylindrical lens, toric lens.

spherocyte *n* round red blood cell, as opposed to biconcave—**spherocytic** *adj.*

spherocytosis *n* an hereditary disorder transmitted as a dominant gene. It is present at birth, but symptoms may vary from non-existent to severe; thus it is sometimes discovered by a routine examination of the blood, which reveals that the red cells are predominantly spherocytic. ⟴ hereditary spherocytosis, jaundice.

sphincter *n* a circular muscle, contraction of which serves to close an orifice. For example the anal, urethral and pyloric sphincters. ⟴ Colour Section Figure 19.

sphincter pupillae muscle smooth, involuntary circular muscle about 1 mm in breadth, forming a ring all round the pupillary margin near the posterior surface of the iris. It is innervated by parasympathetic fibres of the oculomotor nerve (third cranial nerve) that synapse in the ciliary ganglion and by a few sympathetic fibres. Its contraction produces a reduction in the diameter of the pupil, i.e constriction. ⟴ dilator pupillae muscle, miosis (myosis), miotic (myotic), pupillary light reflex.

sphincterectomy surgical excision of a sphincter.

sphincteroplasty *n* plastic surgical reconstruction of a sphincter.

sphincterotomy *n* surgical incision of a sphincter.

sphingolipid *n* sphingosine combined with a lipid. A constituent of biological membranes, especially in the brain.

sphingomyelin *n* a phospholipid formed from sphingosine found as part of biological membranes.

sphingomyelinase *n* an enzyme concerned with the metabolism and storage of lipids.

sphingosine *n* an amino alcohol constituent of sphingolipids and sphingomyelin.

sphygm/o- a prefix that means 'pulse', e.g. *sphygmomanometer.*

S
T

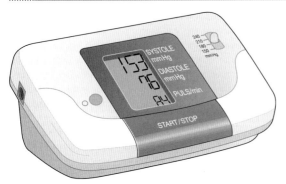

S.9 **Electronic sphygomomanometer** (reproduced from Jamieson et al 2002) with permission).

sphygmomanometer *n* an instrument used for non-invasive measurement of arterial blood pressure. Some utilize a column of mercury, but are generally being replaced with aneroid (not containing a liquid) or electronic devices that contain no mercury (Figure S.9).

spica *n* a bandage applied in a figure-of-eight pattern.

spicule *n* a small, spike-like fragment, especially of bone.

spigot *n* plastic peg used to close a tube.

spina bifida a congenital defect in which there is incomplete closure of the neural canal, usually in the lumbosacral region. *spina bifida occulta* the defect does not affect the spinal cord or meninges. It is often marked externally by pigmentation, a haemangioma, a tuft of hair or a lipoma which may extend into the spinal canal. *spina bifida cystica* an externally protruding spinal lesion. It may vary in severity from meningocele to myelomeningocele. The condition can be detected during pregnancy by an increased concentration of alphafetoprotein in the amniotic fluid or by ultrasonography. ⊃ folate, neural tube defect.

spinal *n* pertaining to the spine.

spinal accessory nerve ⊃ accessory nerve.

spinal anaesthesia 1. loss of sensation by the injection of local anaesthetic into the cerebrospinal fluid, which is accessed by introducing the needle/cannula between the vertebrae usually of the lower back, causing loss of sensation but no loss of consciousness. **2.** also used to describe the loss of feeling produced by a spinal lesion. ⊃ anaesthetic.

spinal anaesthetic a local anaesthetic solution injected into the cerebrospinal fluid within the subarachnoid space, so that it renders the area supplied by the selected spinal nerves insensitive.

spinal canal ⊃ vertebral canal.

spinal column (spine) ⊃ vertebral column.

spinal cord the part of the central nervous system (CNS) that extends, in continuity with the brain (medulla oblongata), from the base of the skull down the vertebral (spinal) canal as far as the level of the first lumbar vertebra or the top of the second lumbar vertebra in adults. It is approximately 45 cm long in an adult Caucasian male, and is about the thickness of the little finger. It is surrounded by the three meningeal membranes dura, arachnoid and pia (in continuity with the coverings of the brain) and bathed within this by cerebrospinal fluid. Consists of nerve cells (grey matter) and nerve tracts (white matter). Anterior (efferent) and posterior (afferent) spinal nerve roots leave and enter through the intervertebral foramina, linking it to the peripheral nervous system. ⊃ Colour Section Figures 1, 11. Nerves conveying impulses from the brain to the various organs and tissues descend through the spinal cord. At the appropriate level they leave the cord and pass to the structure they supply. Similarly, sensory nerves from organs and tissues enter and pass upwards in the spinal cord to the brain. Some activities of the spinal cord are independent of the brain, i.e. spinal reflexes. To facilitate these there are extensive neuron connections between sensory and motor neurons at the same or different levels in the cord. The spinal cord is incompletely divided into two equal parts, anteriorly by a short, shallow median fissure and posteriorly by a deep narrow septum, the posterior median septum. A cross-section of the spinal cord shows that it is composed of grey matter in the centre surrounded by white matter supported by neuroglia. ⊃ vertebral column.

spinal cord compression (SCC) pressure on the spinal cord. Often caused by tumour (which is commonly metastatic tumour from lung, breast or gastrointestinal cancers, when it is known as metastatic spinal cord compression [MSCC]), but other causes include spinal fractures, swelling or haemorrhage affecting the spinal cord. Early diagnosis is vital to prevent permanent effects including paralysis. Treatment usually involves corticosteroids and radiotherapy.

spinal headache a severe headache that may follow epidural anaesthesia, lumbar puncture or spinal block caused by the escape of cerebrospinal fluid during the procedure. The headache and accompanying visual disturbances may last several days.

spinal injury/spinal cord injury injury to the vertebral column (fracture-dislocation) which may or may not involve spinal cord injury and/or injury of the nerve roots within the vertebral (spinal) canal. Cord injury can occur in the cervical, thoracic and upper lumbar regions, ranging from minor damage to complete transection. Cauda equina injury occurs with damage below the first lumbar vertebra, where the 'horse's tail' of lumbar and sacral nerve roots descend to their exits from the vertebral (spinal) canal. Cord and nerve root injuries cause complete or partial paralysis of voluntary movement and sensory loss in the regions served by the nerve tracts or roots affected. ⊃ back injury, neck injury, paraplegia, tetraplegia (quadriplegia), whiplash injury.

spinal muscular atropy (SMA) also known as muscular atrophies. A group of genetic conditions, usually inherited as an autosomal recessive trait. Degeneration of nerve cells including those of anterior horn cells in the spinal cord results in muscle atrophy, weakness and death from respiratory complications during childhood. In some types of SMA individuals may survive into early adulthood. ⊃ Werdnig–Hoffmann disease.

spinal nerves 31 pairs of mixed nerves that leave the spinal cord and pass out of the spinal canal to supply the periphery. The nerves are named by the level at which they exit the spinal column; there are eight cervical nerves (C1–8), twelve thoracic nerves (T 1–12), five lumbar (L1–5), five sacral (S1–5) and a single coccygeal nerve (Co).

spinal shock the initial, temporary loss of reflexes below the level of a spinal cord injury. It can last hours, weeks or months. There is flaccid paralysis and spinal reflexes are absent. When it subsides, reflexes show a vigorous response, there is muscle hypertonia, which can lead to spasticity and deformity.

spinal stenosis also known as spinal canal stenosis. A bony narrowing of the spinal (vertebral) canal with a reduction in the anterior-posterior and lateral diameters. Although it may be congenital, it is more commonly acquired. It may occur secondary to disc degeneration and subluxation of the posterior facet joints. Symptoms include pain that ranges from a dull backache to the more severe pain and paraesthesia felt in the buttock, thighs or calves that worsens with exercise, and leg weakness.

spindle 1. the structure that forms in the nucleus during cell division; it is involved in the movement of chromosomes or chromatids during mitosis and meiosis. **2.** the end organ mechanoreceptors present in tendons and skeletal muscles. Those in skeletal muscles respond to passive stretch and are involved in the myotatic (stretch) reflex. ⊃ Golgi tendon organ. **3.** bursts of brain waves of a frequency of 14 per second that are recorded during light sleep.

spine *n* **1.** a popular term for the bony spinal or vertebral column. **2.** a sharp process of bone—**spinous, spinal** *adj*.

spin echo the reappearance of a magnetic resonance signal after the initial signal has disappeared following a 90° radiofrequency pulse followed by the application of a 180° radiofrequency pulse.

spinhaler *n* a nebulizer (atomizer) which delivers a preset drug dose.

spin-lattice relaxation time (T_1, longitudinal relaxation time, T_1 relaxation time) in magnetic resonance imaging (MRI), the time taken for the spins to give the energy obtained from the initial radiofrequency impulse back to the surrounding environment and return to equilibrium. It represents the time required for the longitudinal magnetization (M_z) to go from 0 to 63% of its final maximum value.

spinnbarkeit the cervical mucus characteristic of the time around ovulation. It is clear, thin, slippery and more elastic than usual. ⊃ Billings' method, peak mucus day.

spinocerebellar *adj* relating to the spinal cord and the cerebellum. For example the *spinocerebellar tracts* that convey touch sensation and proprioceptor information to the cerebellum.

spinocerebellar degeneration a group of inherited conditions in which degenerative changes affect the cerebellum and the tracts in the spinal cord. Resulting in ataxia.

spin-spin relaxation time (transverse or T_2 relaxation time) the time required for the transverse magnetization to decay to about 37% of its maximum value and is the characteristic time constant for loss of phase coherence among spins orientated at an angle to the static main magnetic field.

spiral computed tomography (CT) a type of computed tomography, which is capable of imaging a volume in a single breath-hold, thus reducing breathing artifacts and examination times. The patient passes through the scanner in a continuous movement thereby ensuring that the path of the beam passing through them is a continuous spiral. This is achieved by the patient table moving at a constant speed through the CT gantry while the X-ray tube rotates around the patient; the technique improves the time taken to record the scan and improves contrast and opacification.

spiral fracture a break in a bone which twists round the bone, the most common site is the shaft of the tibia.

Spirillum *n* a genus of small spiral bacteria. *Spirillum minus* is found in rodents and causes one type of rat-bite fever—**spirilla** *pl*, **spirillary** *adj*.

spiritual beliefs may be a belief system ascribed by a particular religion; a modified version of these, reached following questioning, thinking and reasoning. Other people form a strong non-religious belief system to guide their concept of morality, and to find meaning in life. ⊃ secular beliefs.

spiritual distress may occur when a person's spiritual beliefs are derived from a particular religion, which requires the person to observe certain practices in everyday living activities, e.g. the preparation of food, types of food eaten, fasting, attending public worship, prayer, personal hygiene and type of clothing. Distress is likely if they are unable to conform to the teachings of their religious faith such as might occur during illness and hospitalization.

spirochaetaemia *n* spirochaetes in the bloodstream such as occurs in the secondary stage of syphilis—**spirochaetaemic** *adj*.

spirochaete *n* a phylum of tiny spiral bacteria that includes: the genera *Borrelia*, such as *Borrelia burgdorferi*, the cause of Lyme disease; *Leptospira* such as *Leptospira interrogans* serotype *icterohaemorrhagiae*, the cause of Weil's disease; and *Treponema* such as *Treponema pallidum*, the cause of syphilis. In dentistry *Treponema denticola* is associated with the incidence and the level of severity of periodontal disease—**spirochaetal** *adj*.

spirograph *n* an apparatus which records the movement of the lungs—**spirographic** *adj*, **spirography** *n*, **spirographically** *adv*.

spirometer *n* an instrument for measuring the volume of inhaled and exhaled air. Can be used to calculate various lung capacities and changes in volume—**spirometric** *adj*, **spirometry** *n*. ⊃ respiratory function tests, spirometry.

spirometry *n* the measurement of airflow and lung volumes over time. Measurements such as the forced expiratory volume in 1 s (FEV_1), or other time specified, forced vital capacity (FVC) and forced expiratory ratio (FER), i.e. the FEV_1/FVC. Such measurements can be used for both diagnostic and monitoring purposes, but are effort dependent so correct technique is required for accurate results: (a) forced expiratory volume in 1 s (FEV_1)—the volume of air exhaled in the first second; (b) forced vital capacity (FVC)—the total volume of air exhaled from a maximal inspiration; (c) forced expiratory ratio (FER)—the ratio of FEV_1 to FVC, i.e. FEV_1/FVC × 100. This should normally be around 80%. Where the ratio is 70% airflow obstruction is detected, e.g. chronic obstructive pulmonary disease (COPD) and asthma; while a normal or raised ratio (with reduced values for both FEV_1 and FVC) is indicative of restrictive disorders such as fibrosis, oedema, chest wall deformity and neuromuscular disorders. When more detailed analysis of lung function is required, other volumes may be measured. These include: (a) functional residual capacity (FRC). This is the amount of air residual in the lungs after a normal tidal exhalation. It decreases as tidal volume increases. It is approximately 2500 mL. Plethysmography is required to measure this lung volume; (b) total lung capacity (TLC) is approximately 6 L. This is the total volume of air in the lungs after a maximal inhalation (vital capacity + residual volume); (c) residual volume (RV) is approximately 1200 mL. This is the amount of air left in the lungs after a maximal exhalation. This volume cannot be measured using normal spirometric techniques. Body plethysmography (the body box) or gas dilution techniques are required to obtain this value; (d) tidal volume (TV, V_T) is approximately 500 mL. This is the volume of air exchanged during normal resting breathing. ⊃ respiratory function tests.

Spitz–Holter valve a special valve used to drain excess cerebrospinal fluid in hydrocephalus.

SPK *abbr* superficial punctate keratitis. ⊃ punctate epithelial keratitis.

splanchnic *adj* pertaining to or supplying the viscera.

splanchnic nerves sympathetic nerve fibres that supply the viscera and other structures.

splanchnicectomy *n* surgical removal of the splanchnic nerves, whereby certain viscera are deprived of sympathetic impulses; occasionally performed in the treatment of hypertension or for the relief of certain kinds of visceral pain.

splanchnology *n* the study of the structure and function of the viscera.

spleen *n* a lymphoid, vascular organ that is part of the monocyte-macrophage (reticuloendothelial) system. It contains reticular and lymphatic tissue and is the largest lymph organ. The spleen lies in the left hypochondriac region of the abdominal cavity between the fundus of the stomach and the diaphragm. It is purplish in colour and varies in size in different individuals, but is usually about 12 cm long, 7 cm wide and 2.5 cm thick. It weighs about 200 g. The spleen is slightly oval in shape with the hilum on the lower medial border. The anterior surface is covered with peritoneum. It is enclosed in a fibroelastic capsule that dips into the organ, forming trabeculae. The cellular material, consisting of lymphocytes and macrophages, is called splenic pulp, and it lies between the trabeculae. Red pulp is the part suffused with blood and white pulp consists of areas of lymphatic tissue where there are sleeves of

lymphocytes and macrophages around blood vessels. Blood vessels, nerves and efferent lymph vessels enter and leave at the hilum. The spleen receives oxygenated blood via the splenic artery, a branch of the coeliac artery and venous blood leaves in the splenic vein, a branch of the hepatic portal vein. Blood passing through the spleen flows in sinuses which have distinct pores between the endothelial cells, allowing it to come into close association with splenic pulp. The spleen is the site of the destruction, by phagocytosis, of old or abnormal erythrocytes. The breakdown products, bilirubin and iron, are passed to the liver via the splenic and hepatic portal veins. Other cellular material, e.g. leucocytes, platelets and microbes, are phagocytosed in the spleen. Unlike lymph nodes, the spleen has no afferent lymphatics entering it, so it is not exposed to diseases spread by lymph. The spleen is able to store blood. It contains up to 350 mL of blood, and in response to sympathetic stimulation can rapidly return a large part of this volume to the circulation, e.g. in haemorrhage. The spleen is important to the immune response, it contains T- and B-lymphocytes, which are activated by the presence of antigens, e.g. in infection. Lymphocyte proliferation during serious infection can cause splenomegaly. The spleen and liver are important sites of fetal blood cell production, and the spleen can also fulfil this function in adults in times of great need—**splenic** *adj*.

splenectomy *n* surgical removal of the spleen. Loss of the spleen reduces defences against infection and patients are advised to have immunizations that offer protection against pneumococcal infections and influenza; and *Haemophilus influenzae* type b and meningococcal C, if not already protected. In elective splenectomy these should be given prior to surgery. Children up to the age of 16 years should be offered prophylactic antibiotic drugs during the 2 years following surgery.

splenic flexure the left colic flexure. The 90° angle in the colon adjacent to the spleen.

splenitis *n* inflammation of the spleen.

splen/o- a prefix that means 'spleen', e.g. *splenectomy*.

splenocaval *adj* pertaining to the spleen and inferior vena cava, usually referring to anastomosis of the splenic vein to the latter.

splenomegaly *n* enlargement of the spleen.

splenoportal *adj* pertaining to the spleen and hepatic portal vein.

splenoportogram *n* radiographic demonstration of the spleen and hepatic portal vein after injection of radiopaque contrast agent. Superseded by ultrasound examination.

splenorenal *adj* pertaining to the spleen and kidney, as anastomosis of the splenic vein to the renal vein; a procedure carried out in some cases of hepatic portal hypertension.

splenunculus an accessory spleen.

splint in dentistry, a therapeutic appliance constructed of soft plastic, hard plastic or metal covering the occlusal surfaces of one of the dental arches, such as an occlusal overlay appliance. ⊃ occlusal, orthosis.

splinter haemorrhage splinter-like haemorrhage under the finger or toe nails; may be caused by trauma or associated with infective endocarditis.

splinting used by physiotherapists and others in preventative treatment to help maintain a joint position and thus prevent loss of range of movement; corrective treatments to correct a loss of range or malalignment, e.g. serial casting; and to maximize function such as a wrist splint to maintain extension to maximize finger extension, or an ankle foot orthosis to enable safe walking. ➲ dental/maxillofacial splinting.

split cast mounting in prosthetics, a method of mounting casts on an articulator to facilitate accurate removal and replacement and as a method of checking the accuracy of jaw relations.

split course therapy radiotherapy where a gap is planned between the first and second halves of treatment to enable patients to recover from acute reactions to treatment.

split emulsion film a film having two emulsions, one on top of each other on the same side of the base, one layer providing high contrast and the other high maximum density, used for mammography.

split thickness (Thiersch) graft ➲ skin graft.

SPMSQ *abbr* Short Portable Mental State Questionnaire.

SPOD *abbr* sexual problems of the disabled.

spondyl(e) *n* a vertebra.

spondylitis *n* inflammation of the spine—**spondylitic** *adj*. ➲ ankylosing spondylitis.

spondyl/o- a prefix that means 'vertebra', e.g. *spondylolisthesis*.

spondylography *n* a method of measuring and studying the degree of kyphosis by directly tracing the line of the back.

spondylolisthesis *n* forward displacement of one vertebra on the bone below it. Most commonly seen at the 5th lumbar and 1st sacral (L5/S1). The degree of spondylolisthesis is determined by the distance the slipped vertebra travels on its lower counterpart—Grades 1–4—**spondylolisthetic** *adj*.

spondylolisthetic pelvis a pelvic deformity in which the 5th lumbar vertebra has slipped forwards on the sacrum, creating a false promontory.

spondylosis *n* a degenerative disease of the spine. It is caused by a defect in the pars interarticularis, a narrow strip of bone lying between the lamina and the inferior articular process below and the pedicle and the superior articular process above. May be congenital, traumatic or caused by overuse. The main characteristic of spondylosis is the loss of water from the disc. Tears also occur in the nucleus, annulus and vertebral endplates. The nourishment of the adult disc is more precarious than that of an immature disc and the first signs of spondylosis usually present clinically at about the age of 30 and are most common around the age of 45 years. The pathological changes that occur are the same regardless of site, but the differences in functional anatomy give rise to different clinical signs and symptoms. Pathology involves a coarsening of the annulus fibrosis, collagen fibres separate and cracks appear in the annulus.

The nucleus pulposus dehydrates and becomes more fibrous with the disc losing height overall. These changes can be present without causing any signs or symptoms. 'Lipping' of the vertebral bodies occurs, due to altered disc biomechanics, which causes traction of the periosteum by the attachments of the annulus fibrosis. There can also be decalcification within the vertebral body. The intervertebral ligaments may become contracted and thickened especially at the sites where there are gross changes. The dura mater of the spinal cord, which forms a sleeve round the nerve root, may undergo low-grade, chronic inflammatory changes. This can result in nerve-root adhesions with associated neural symptoms. Most commonly, the major change is that of osteophytosis, the formation of bony spurs along the junction of the vertebral bodies and the corresponding intervertebral discs.

spondylosyndesis spinal fusion. Usually applies to surgical procedures to immobilize unstable vertebrae. It may be performed after surgery to deal with a prolapsed intervertebral disc, or as treatment for a spinal fracture.

sponge gelatin an absorbable gelatin sponge that can be packed sterile into a tooth socket to fill a space or to control haemorrhage.

spongiform encephalopathy one of a group of degenerative neurological diseases, in humans it is a progressive dementia. ➲ bovine spongiform encephalopathy, Creutzfeldt–Jakob disease, kuru, scrapie.

spontaneous abortion ➲ spontaneous miscarriage.

spontaneous emission when an atom absorbs a photon and releases the absorbed energy as a photon of light.

spontaneous fracture ➲ fracture.

spontaneous labour labour occurring without induction or acceleration.

spontaneous miscarriage one which occurs naturally without intervention.

spontaneous vaginal delivery (SVD) delivery of an infant through the vagina without recourse to forceps or ventouse.

spoon another term for a dental excavator.

spoon denture a small, maxillary spoon-shaped prosthesis usually replacing one or two teeth. It has no clasps, fits closely to the palatal mucosa and is not extended to the palatal necks of the maxillary teeth.

sporadic *adj* scattered; occurring in isolated cases; not epidemic—**sporadically** *adv*.

spore *n* **1.** a phase in the life cycle of a limited number of bacterial genera (*Clostridium* and *Bacillus*) where the cell is encapsulated and metabolism almost ceases. Spores are highly resistant to adverse environmental conditions such as heat and desiccation. The spores are ubiquitous so that sterilization procedures must ensure their removal or death. ➲ endospore. **2.** reproductive body produced by some plants, particularly fungi, and by protozoa.

sporicidal *adj* lethal to spores—**sporicide** *n*.

sporotrichosis *n* chronic infection of a wound by the fungus *Sporotrichum schenkii*. A sore, ulcer or abscess forms with lymphangitis and subcutaneous painless granulomata. Occurs amongst agricultural workers.

sport biomechanics the study of determining optimal techniques for sport performance, the design of sports equipment and investigation of the stresses placed upon the athlete's body during performance. ⊃ biomechanics.

sport cohesion a sport team's tendency to stick together in its pursuit of common objectives.

sport competition anxiety ⊃ competitive sport anxiety.

sport psychology the application of psychological science to the study and understanding of human behaviour and mind in sport, and to the enhancement of performance in sport. Includes the areas of motor learning, sport skill acquisition, motivation and psychological skills training.

sports drinks commercially available drinks, designed for optimal delivery of water and carbohydrate during and after exercise. Water is often equally effective for hydration, but the taste of sports drinks makes them more likely to be taken in adequate quantities. The composition of commercial sports drinks is generally based on studies which have defined the content of carbohydrate (to supplement energy supply) and of electrolytes (mainly sodium salts) to promote fluid retention during and after prolonged exercise and to avoid hyponatraemia. There has, however, been some controversy about the standard recommendations, as some experts have disputed their adequacy in avoiding hyponatraemia, exemplified recently in studies of its occurrence in endurance athletes. Osmolality of these drinks varies according to the concentration of carbohydrate, most often in the form of glucose polymers. *isotonic sports drinks* contain glucose in a concentration of 6–8% and are best for events such as middle- and long-distance running and team sports, rapidly replacing fluid lost by sweating as well as supplying an energy source. *hypotonic sports drinks* are suitable, for example, for jockeys, gymnasts and dancers, who need fluid but have less need for a carbohydrate top-up. *hypertonic sports drinks* have the most carbohydrate and are taken after exercise to supplement daily intake in the replacement of muscle glycogen stores; also used during very long-distance events when high levels of energy are required. ⊃ hydration status.

sports medicine branch of medicine concerned with the diagnosis, treatment, rehabilitation and prevention of traumatic and non-traumatic injuries and disease affecting the athlete. May also be used to describe both medical and scientific aspects of sport and exercise. ⊃ sports science.

sports science a broad discipline that is mainly concerned with the processes that explain behaviour in sport and how athletic performance can be improved. Includes kinesiology, kinanthropometry, sport biomechanics, exercise physiology, sport psychology and sociology of sport.

spot grinding ⊃ selective grinding.

spotted fever ⊃ Rocky Mountain spotted fever.

spot welding the joining of metals at one point by means of pressure and heat generated by the passage of an electric current from a spot welder, without the use of filler metal.

sprain *n* injury to the soft tissues surrounding a joint, resulting in discoloration, swelling and pain. There is stretching or tearing of a ligament or capsular structure of a joint. A joint that is forced beyond its range of motion can stretch, tear and sometimes avulse the connective tissues that stabilize the joint. There are three categories: *first-degree sprain* in which a few fibres are torn; *second-degree sprain* in which approximately half of fibres are torn and: *third-degree sprain* in which there is a complete tear.

spreadsheet a program which allows forecasting and financial planning.

Sprengel's shoulder deformity (O Sprengel, German surgeon, 1852–1915) congenital high scapula, a permanent elevation of the shoulder, often associated with other congenital deformities, e.g. the presence of a cervical rib or the absence of vertebrae.

spring in dentistry, a bent or coiled metal wire, used to place a force to move teeth or to provide elasticity to a dental appliance. *spring-forming pliers.* ⊃ pliers. ⊃ auxiliary spring (finger spring), spring cantilever bridge (spring bridge).

spring cantilever bridge (spring bridge) in dentistry, a bridge in which the remote pontic is integral with one end of a bar adapted to the underlying mucosa. ⊃ bridge.

spring catarrh ⊃ vernal conjunctivitis.

sprue *n* **1.** a chronic malabsorption disorder. ⊃ coeliac, tropical sprue. **2.** in dentistry, wire (sometimes hollow), wax or plastic used during the casting process to provide an entrance for molten metal into a mould. It is attached to the wax pattern and the whole invested. When the invested material has set, the sprue is then removed or burnt out during the heating process before casting. **3.** metal that has cooled and become solid in the sprue hole. It has to be cut off from the casting. *sprue former* a conical base into which a casting sprue is fixed prior to investment.

SPSS *abbr* Statistical Package for the Social Sciences.

spur *n* **1.** a small projection of bone. **2.** a metal projection from a dental prosthesis.

spurious *adj* not genuine or what it appears to be.

spurious diarrhoea the leakage of fluid faeces past a solid impacted mass of faeces. More common in children and older people.

spurious labour contractions occuring without cervical dilatation, with no progress towards delivery; false labour.

sputum *n* the mucus and other matter expectorated (coughed up) from the lower respiratory tract.

squamocolumnar junction (SCJ) also called the transformation zone. The variable region where the columnar epithelium lining the endocervical canal meets the stratified squamous epithelium of the ectocervix (vaginal portion). It is influenced by oestrogens, particularly at puberty and during pregnancy.

squamous *adj* scaly.

squamous cell carcinoma (SCC) a carcinoma arising in squamous epithelium; epithelioma. The second most common skin cancer after basal cell carcinoma and like other forms of skin cancer is increasing in age-specific incidence. The risk factors for SCC are exposure to ultraviolet radiation

(UVR), light skin, or rarely exposure to other carcinogenic factors such as X irradiation or arsenic injection. SCC may arise in long-standing areas of inflammation such as around a chronic cutaneous ulcer, or in patients with scarring genetic syndromes of the skin such as dystrophic epidermolysis bullosa, in which up to 50% of patients may develop SCC. There is also a greatly elevated incidence in individuals who are receiving chronic immunosuppression following organ transplantation (particularly kidney and heart) and in individuals who have been treated with large amounts of psoralen with ultraviolet A (PUVA) therapy. It is a proliferative tumour that has a history of growth over a few months. Varying clinical presentations include keratotic nodules, exophytic erythematous nodules, infiltrating firm tumours and ulcers with an indurated edge. ➲ Colour Section Figure 111. Histological grade also varies from well-differentiated to anaplastic. SCCs of the lip behave more aggressively and show a greater frequency of metastasis. A number of modalities may be used, including aggressive curettage and cautery, excision or radiotherapy. In general, excision with assessment of adequacy of margins is the preferred option because of the definite risk of metastasis. Surgical excision with a 3–4 mm margin has a cure rate of 90% or more. As with basal cell carcinoma, radiotherapy can be used in selected cases.

squamous (pavement) epithelium it is composed of a single layer of flattened cells. The cells fit closely together like flat stones, forming a thin and very smooth membrane (Figure E.7, p. 264). Diffusion takes place freely through this thin, smooth, inactive lining of the following structures: the heart and blood vessels where it is also known as endothelium, the lymph vessels and the alveoli of the lungs. ➲ epithelium.

squatting a position adopted for birth in which the woman crouches close to the ground. A variation of this is the supported squat in which the woman stands with her hips and knees completely flexed supporting herself on her arms or being supported by another. The dimensions of the pelvic outlet are enlarged.

squeeze test ➲ Thompson's test.

squint *n* ➲ strabismus.

SR *abbr* sarcoplasmic reticulum.

SRBC *abbr* sheep red blood cells.

SSL *abbr* secure socket layer.

SSPE *abbr* subacute sclerosing panencephalitis.

SSRIs *abbr* selective serotonin reuptake inhibitors.

SSSS *abbr* staphylococcal scalded skin syndrome.

stability being stable. The property of an object or body that determines how difficult it is to displace it to another position. Resistance to change. In dental prosthetics, the resistance of a prosthesis to displacement by functional forces.

stabilized retinal image the image formed on the retina when neutralizing the fixation movements of the eye. The effect of these movements is thus eliminated and the image usually disappears after a few seconds. The methods used for stabilizing a retinal image are: (a) the target is placed at the end of a tube mounted on a tightly fitted contact lens. The whole device moves with every movement of the eyeball and the retinal image remains on the same retinal spot; (b) the subject is also fitted with a tight contact lens on the side of which is attached a small mirror. A test projected on the mirror is reflected onto a screen. The subject views the test through a compensating system of four mirrors and therefore as the eye moves the retinal image moves along with it and stimulates the same retinal spot; (c) presentation of a target for a length of time smaller than the time necessary for the eye to perform a small eye movement. Presentations of less than 0.01 s usually fulfil this requirement. ➲ fixation movements.

stable factor (proconvertin) *n* factor VII in the blood coagulation cascade. It is produced in the liver and requires vitamin K. It complexes with factor III (thromboplastin) to activate factor X (Stuart–Prower factor) in the extrinsic pathway. A very rare inherited (autosomal recessive) deficiency leads to a bleeding disorder.

Stafne's cavity the developmental invagination in the mandible in which lies the submandibular salivary gland.

staghorn calculus a large renal calculus that takes on the shape of the calyces and renal pelvis (Figure S.10).

staging *n* process of measuring how advanced a tumour is and to which sites it has spread; may be locally advanced or metastatic. Usually involves imaging with computed tomography, bone scan and often surgery. The TMN classification includes tumour (T) size, nodal (N) status and metastatic (M) sites present/absent.

stagnant hypoxia due to insufficient blood flow to deliver oxygen. ➲ hypoxia.

stagnant loop syndrome ➲ blind loop syndrome.

stagnation area in dentistry, the opposite of a self-cleansing area. Area where debris and plaque accumulate on a tooth and is not easily cleaned either naturally by the tongue or during mastication.

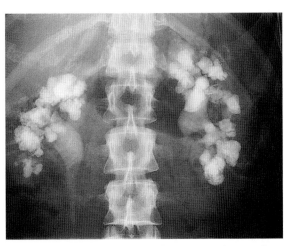

S.10 Staghorn calculi (reproduced from Boon et al 2006 with permission).

stain 1. a dye used to colour micro-organisms or tissue prior to microscopic examination, e.g. Gram stain, or to elicit a reaction. **2.** to apply a stain to tissue or micro-organisms. **3.** a mark or area of discoloration. In dentistry, tooth staining may be extrinsic or intrinsic. Extrinsic staining is caused by external agents (e.g. foods or bacteria) which can be removed with cleaning/prophylaxis. Whereas intrinsic stains occur because of changes in the structure or thickness of dental tissues, such as enamel opacities due to increased porosity of enamel, or incorporation of pigments into tooth tissues during or after tooth formation.

stain porcelain the fine pigmented porcelain used to colour a porcelain restoration.

stainless steel an alloy steel containing quantities of chromium and other elements. Very resistant to corrosion. Used extensively in orthodontic treatment in the form of wire. *stainless steel crown* ➲ preformed metal crown.

stammering stuttering. A speech disorder in which the person hesitates, repeats syllables or words and pauses.

stance way of standing or the phase of gait (walking or running) in which the body is supported, usually by one or both feet being on the ground (although can include other methods of support such as crutches).

standard a measure which forms the basis of other similar phenomena, values, substances or against which they can be compared or judged. A standard is a predetermined criterion or description of care, used to provide guidance, and can be a measure by which high quality care and professional performance are assessed.

standard contrast emulsions once the most common film emulsion types with a low base fog, an average gradient of 2.6 and a maximum density of 3.5. ➲ characteristic curve.

standard deviation (SD) in statistics, a measure of dispersion of scores around the mean value of the sample. It is the square root of variance. The standard deviation quantifies how much the values vary from each other. A normal, unskewed curve will have 34% of the cases between the mean and 1 standard deviation above or below the mean; 68% of cases between 1 standard deviation above and 1 below the mean; 95.5% of cases will be within 2 standard deviations of the mean.

standard error (SE) in statistics, a measure of variability of many mean values of different samples from a population. Used to calculate the chance of a sample mean being smaller or bigger than that for the population.

standard (unfractionated) heparin (SH) produces its anticoagulant effect by potentiating the activity of antithrombin which inhibits the procoagulant enzymic activity of factors IIa, VIIa, IXa, Xa and XIa. It is used therapeutically in the prevention and treatment of thromboembolism. Standard heparin is often reserved for treating patients with very severe, life-threatening thromboembolism, e.g. major pulmonary embolism giving rise to significant hypoxaemia or hypotension. The level of anticoagulation should be assessed by the activated partial thromboplastin time (APTT) after 6 hours and, if satisfactory, daily thereafter. It is usual to aim for a patient time which is 1.5–2.5 times the control time of the test. The half-life of intravenous heparin is about 1 hour and if a patient bleeds, it is usually sufficient just to discontinue the infusion; however, if bleeding is severe, the excess can be neutralized with intravenous protamine sulphate. The short half-life of SH makes it useful for those with a predisposition to bleeding, e.g. who have peptic ulcer, or those who may require surgery. ➲ heparin, low-molecular-weight heparin (LMWH).

standard occlusal projection mid-line, symmetrical oblique occlusal projection of the mandible or the maxilla.

standard occipital projection a radiographic technique for demonstrating the maxillary sinus (antrum) and facial bones.

standard precautions sometimes referred to as universal precautions. A set of infection control guidelines recommended by the Centers for Disease Control and Prevention (CDC) in the United States. They should be used when dealing with all hospitalized patients at all times, whatever their diagnosis or presumed infection status. They involve the universal blood and body fluids precautions and body substance isolation, which are designed to reduce the risk of transmission of pathogens present in blood, body fluids, secretions and excretions (but not sweat), non-intact skin and the mucosae. They are also required to prevent the spread of diseases that are transmitted by airborne, droplet or contact routes. These are the isolation precautions that are always used in conjunction with standard precautions. Standard precautions involve effective hand hygiene; appropriate use of personal protective equipment (PPE); safe use and disposal of sharps, such as needles or blades; effective domestic cleaning; proper decontamination, disinfection and sterilization of equipment; safe waste disposal; and safe management of used/soiled linen. ➲ containment isolation, protective isolation, source isolation.

standardized morbidity ratio (SMBR) the degree of self-reported limiting long term illness indirectly standardized for variations in age and gender.

standardized mortality rate the number of deaths per specific population standardized for age.

standardized mortality ratio (SMR) allows comparisons to be made between the death rates in populations with different demographic structures. It involves the application of national age-specific mortality rates to local populations so that a ratio of expected deaths to actual deaths can be calculated. The comparative national figure is, by convention, 100 and, for example, a local figure of 106 means that there is an increased risk of 6%, whereas a local figure of 94 indicates a risk 6% lower.

standby system a system which automatically shuts down sections of an automatic film processor when not in use to reduce running costs and conserve energy.

Stanford Binet Intelligence Scale a test adapted from Binet's test, used to test children in the USA. ➲ Binet's test.

stannic oxide ➲ tin dioxide.

stannous fluoride a form of fluoride used in toothpastes and gels to reduce the incidence of dental caries.

stanols plant substances that inhibit the absorption of cholesterol from the intestinal tract.

St Anthony's fire historical term for the mental abnormalities and painful vasoconstriction leading to gangrene of the extremities caused by ergot poisoning. Occurred through eating rye infested with a fungus containing alkaloids of ergot.

stapedectomy *n* surgical removal of stapes for otosclerosis. After stapedectomy, stapes can be replaced by a prosthesis. Normal hearing is restored in 90% of patients.

stapedial mobilization, stapediolysis release of a stapes rendered immobile by otosclerosis.

stapedius a tiny muscle of the middle ear. It contracts reflexly (sound attenuation reflex), with another muscle the tensor tympani, to protect the ear from very loud sounds by reducing conduction.

stapes *n* the stirrup-shaped medial ossicle (bone) of the middle ear. ⊃ incus, malleus, Colour Section Figure 13.

staphylectomy ⊃ uvulectomy.

staphylococcal scalded skin syndrome (SSSS) Ritter's disease. A condition mainly occurring in infants. It is caused by certain strains of *Staphylococcus aureus* that produce toxins that affect the skin. It is characterized by the presence of vesicles and bullae, erythema, peeling and necrosis of the epidermis; creating the appearance of 'scalded' skin. Compare with toxic epidermal necrolysis.

Staphylococcus *n* a genus of Gram-positive bacteria occurring in clusters. Some types are commensal on the skin and may be found in the nasopharynx, axillae, groin and perineum of some individuals. They cause infections that include: boils, impetigo, wound infection, endocarditis, pneumonia, osteomyelitis, toxic shock syndrome and septicaemia. Staphylococci cause many healthcare-associated infections. The genus includes the major pathogen *Staphylococcus aureus*, which produces the enzyme coagulase; some strains produce a powerful exotoxin, and others are meticillin (methicillin)-resistant. *Staphylococcus epidermidis* is a skin commensal (non-coagulase producer). It infects wounds and increasingly causes infection involving intravascular devices, peritoneal dialysis catheters, valves, etc. Treatment is problematic as the micro-organism has a natural resistance to many antibiotics. ⊃ meticillin (methicillin)-resistant *Staphylococcus aureus*, Panton-Valentine leukocidin, vancomycin-resistant *Staphylococcus aureus*.

staphyloma *n* a protrusion of the cornea or sclera of the eye—**staphylomata** *pl.*

staphylorrhaphy also called palatorrhaphy. Operation to repair a cleft palate.

staples pieces of wire sometimes used to close a surgical wound, or used in a special stapling device to form an anatomosis.

staple food the traditional food used as the main source of energy within a community. It varies between different communities and regions and includes maize, wheat, rice, potatoes, cassava, sago, pulses, etc.

starch *n* a polysaccharide formed from glucose molecules, the carbohydrate present in potatoes, rice and maize.

Starling's law of the heart (E Starling, British physiologist, 1866–1927) also known as Frank–Starling law of the heart (E Starling; O Frank German physiologist, 1865–1944) states that the force of myocardial contraction is proportional to the length (stretching) of the ventricular muscle fibres. Increased stretching results in the next contraction being more powerful.

starter solution in radiography, a solution containing a weak acid and bromide ions which is used with new developer in automatic processing machines to depress the activity of the developer until a number of films have been processed; the processed films produce bromide ions and therefore the solution will no longer need to be added.

startle reflex ⊃ Moro reflex.

start-up costs the costs, such as the purchase of equipment, that occur at the start of a project.

stasis *n* stagnation; cessation of motion.

-stasis a suffix that means 'stagnation, cessation of movement', e.g. *cholestasis*.

state anxiety the anxiety response to a threatening situation, such as being followed in an isolated area of town. ⊃ anxiety.

statement an instruction in a computer program.

statement of special needs a statement compiled by a local authority in England following assessment of a child. It details the child's special educational needs and sets out the help that the child should receive.

static at rest, not in motion.

static exercise ⊃ isometric contraction.

static mark in radiography, an artefact produced by static electricity during film handling.

static muscle actions actions in which muscle fibres generate force without any change in muscle.

static panoramic radiography a radiographic technique whereby the X-ray source is within the mouth and produces a single radiographic film of the teeth and surrounding structures.

static reflex a relex that maintains muscle tone and posture.

static retinoscopy retinoscopy performed with the patient fixating a target at distance or with accommodation paralysed. ⊃ dynamic retinoscopy, retinoscope.

static stretching a technique of muscle stretching used to increase range of motion; the muscle/muscle group is held at the end of its range of movement, in a static position for a period of time. It is widely suggested that an effective time to hold a static stretch for is duration of 20–30 s. By contrast with rapid ('ballistic') stretching, static stretching is considered not to elicit the stretch reflex, which would counteract the attempted muscle lengthening. Static stretching is a controlled, slow movement with emphasis on correct bodily alignment. An element of fine motor control and postural awareness is important during static stretching exercises and this can be enhanced by use of feedback and correction from the physiotherapist or trainer, as well as use of equipment such as mirrors. ⊃ dynamic stretching.

S
T

statics the study (or analysis) of systems (of bodies or objects) that are at rest or moving with constant velocity (i.e. not accelerating). Such systems are considered to be in equilibrium.

statins *npl* colloquial expression for HMG-CoA reductase inhibitors.

station location of the presenting fetal part in the birth canal, designated between −5 and −1 according to the number of centimetres above an imaginary plane passing through the ischial spines, 0 when at the plane, and +1 to +5 according to the number of centimetres the part is below the plane.

Statistical Package for the Social Sciences (SPSS) software package often used in the analysis of quantitative data.

statistical significance in research, an expression of how likely it is that a set of results happened by chance, e.g. 0.05, 0.01 and 0.001 levels. ⊃ *P* value.

statistics *n* scientific study of numerical data collection and its analysis and evaluation.

status *n* state; condition.

status asthmaticus ⊃ severe acute asthma.

status epilepticus describes epileptic seizures following each other almost continuously. It is a medical emergency and requires immediate treatment.

statutory bodies bodies such as Strategic Health Authorities, or the Health Professions Council, which are set up by legislation and provide a statutory service controlled by legislation.

STD *abbr* sexually transmitted disease.

steat/o- a prefix that means 'fat', e.g. *steatopygia*.

steatoma *n* a fatty tumour, or a sebaceous cyst.

steatopygia *n* the deposition of excessive amounts of fat in the buttocks.

steatorrhoea *n* passage of pale, frothy, foul-smelling oily stool due to fat malabsorption. It floats and is difficult to flush away.

steatosis *n* fatty infiltration of hepatocytes; occurs in alcohol misuse and protein energy malnutrition.

steering coils produce magnetic fields to ensure that an electron beam is positioned at the centre of a tube and that it is then positioned on the correct aspect of the target in a linear accelerator.

Stein–Leventhal syndrome (I Stein, American gynaecologist, 1887–1976; M Leventhal, American gynaecologist, 1901–1971) ⊃ polycystic ovary syndrome.

Steinmann's pin (F Steinmann, Swiss surgeon, 1872–1932) an alternative to the use of a Kirschner wire for applying skeletal traction to a limb. It has its own introducer and stirrup.

stellate *adj* star-shaped.

stellate fracture a star-shaped fracture with numerous cracks radiating from the point of impact.

stellate ganglion a large collection of nerve cells (ganglion) on the sympathetic chain in the root of the neck.

stellate ganglionectomy surgical removal of the stellate ganglion.

Stellwag's sign (C Stellwag, Austrian opthalmologist, 1823–1904) occurs in Graves' disease: the person blinks infrequently and the eyelids are retracted. ⊃ exophthalmos.

stem cell an undifferentiated, pluripotent cell capable of giving rise to other types of cells. For example, the stem cells normally present in the bone marrow and umbilical cord blood that are capable of developing into any of a full range of mature blood cells. They are the 'active ingredient' of haemopoietic stem cell transplants.

stenosis *n* a narrowing—**stenoses** *pl*, **stenotic** *adj*.

Stenotrophomonas maltophilia a Gram-negative bacterium. An opportunistic micro-organism that can cause infection in immunocompromised individuals including bacteraemia. It is generally sensitive to cephalosporins (third generation), co-trimoxazole and doxycycline, but is resistant to the beta-lactam antibiotic imipenem (a carbapenem) and to aminoglycoside antibiotics. ⊃ *Pseudomonas*.

Stensen's duct (N Stensen, Danish anatomist, 1638–1686) the duct of the parotid salivary gland. It runs forwards from the parotid gland to penetrate the buccinator muscle and open into the mouth opposite the upper second permanent molar tooth.

stent *n* device used to provide a shunt or keep a tube or vessel open. For example stent insertion into the bile duct to relieve obstructive jaundice, stenting the ureters to overcome urinary obstruction, and stenting the oesophagus for palliation of dysphagia caused by oesophageal cancer. ⊃ transjugular intrahepatic portasystemic stent shunting.

Stephan's curve the curve showing the change of pH of undisturbed plaque with time, originally following a rinse with a glucose solution.

step length the distance between the position (e.g. heel contact) of one foot and the next similar position of the opposite foot in gait (walking or running). May also include other support devices such as crutches. May be different for each foot. May also be positive, negative ('dragging' one foot so that it never reaches the other) or zero (when one foot is advanced only to the position beside the other foot). Usually measured in metres.

stepping reflex also called step or dance reflex. A primitive reflex normally present in newborns; when the infant is held upright over a flat surface so that their feet press on the surface they will make walking movements (reciprocal flexion and extension). The reflex normally disappears around 4–6 weeks of age.

step test test of aerobic fitness involving stepping up and down with alternate legs for a predetermined period followed by a series of measurements of post-exercise heart rate, to determine its rate of return to resting level. Variants in current use include those prescribed by the YMCA and the Association College of Sports Medicine. The original Harvard step test, devised in the 1940s, used a higher step and longer exercise period (up and down 20 inches, every 2 s, for up to 5 min) than in most recent specifications.

stepwedge a piece of equipment used in radiography. It is made up of different thicknesses of aluminium with a layer of copper on the base; wedges are calibrated so that when radiographed each step produces an exact increase or decrease in density on the film. ⊃ characteristic curves.

stercobilin *n* the brown pigment of faeces; it is formed from stercobilinogen which is derived from the bile pigments.

stercobilinogen *n* faecal urobilinogen. It is formed by bacterial action on the bile pigment bilirubin. ⊃ urobilinogen.

stercolith a hard stone-like mass of faeces.

stere/o- a prefix that means 'three dimensional, solid', e.g. *stereoisomer*.

stereognosis the faculty of recognizing the shape of objects by the sense of touch. It allows the detection of texture, weight, size and shape without the use of vision.

stereogram (*syn* stereoslide) paired similar photographs or drawings which when viewed in a stereoscope give the sensation of stereopsis. Some stereograms are used only to explore fusion. ⊃ stereoscope.

stereograph in dentistry, an instrument to record mandibular movements which allows their reproduction by a series of carved or moulded three-dimensional records.

stereoisomer chemical compounds that comprise the same atoms with the same linkages, but the atoms have a different spatial arrangement. Some of these compounds are mirror images of each other.

stereophotography photography to produce pictures which give rise to the perception of stereopsis when viewed in a stereoscope. It has been used for determining corneal and optic disc topography. ⊃ photokeratoscopy, stereoscope.

stereopsis *n* (*syn* stereoscopic vision) the ability to use both eyes together (binocular vision) for the perception of depth, distance and shape.

stereoscope an instrument which allows targets to be presented independently to the two eyes. The separation of the targets is produced either by tubes, a septum, or an arrangement of mirrors. Stereograms are the targets used with a stereoscope. Stereoscopes are used to test and train binocular fusion and stereopsis, evaluate suppression and view images in three dimensions. ⊃ stereogram.

stereoscopic visual acuity the ability to detect the smallest difference in depth between two objects. Stereoscopic visual acuity is extremely fine, varying between 5 and 15 seconds of arc. It tends to decrease with age and it is positively correlated with Snellen visual acuity. ⊃ angle of stereopsis, Howard–Dolman test, retinal disparity, three needle test, vectogram.

stereoslide ⊃ stereogram.

stereotactic radiotherapy where multiple beams of radiation are given to a tumour over a number of days to destroy the tumour.

stereotactic surgery electrodes and cannulae are passed to a predetermined point in the brain for physiological observation or destruction of tissue—**stereotaxy** *n*.

stereotype *n* a generalization about a behaviour, individual or a group; can be the basis for prejudice. Stereotypes are frequently associated with oppressed groups and provide justifications for and a means of maintaining oppression.

stereotypy inappropriate repetition of actions, postures or speech. It is a feature of some mental health disorders, autistic disorders and occurs with some types of learning disability.

sterile *adj* free from living micro-organisms including bacterial spores—**sterility** *n*.

sterility infertility. The inability to reproduce.

sterilization *n* **1.** activity that kills or removes all types of micro-organisms including spores. It is accomplished by the use of heat, radiation, chemicals or filtration. **2.** rendering incapable of reproduction, such as following vasectomy.

sterilizer in dentistry, apparatus for sterilizing precleaned objects. *autoclave sterilizer* an apparatus that sterilizes by heated water vapour under pressure. Downward displacement autoclaves rely on water vapour displacing the air from the container and any packaging whereas prevacuum autoclaves use an initial vacuum to achieve this state which effectively reduces the cycle time of the apparatus. *chemiclave sterilizer* similar in operation to an autoclave except for the use of a special solution instead of distilled water. The advantage of this method is that items liable to be damaged by either wet or dry heat can be safely sterilized in this apparatus. *dry heat sterilizer* a hot air oven that is thermostatically controlled. It is only reliable if an uninterrupted timed cycle (160°C for 1 hour) is strictly followed and no instruments are added or removed from the apparatus during the cycle time. Suitable for all metal instruments and those that should be kept dry. Not suitable for plastic and rubber articles and most turbine and mechanical slow handpieces. Cotton wool rolls and paper points may discolor slightly but their absorbency is not greatly reduced. A longer period of time is required for heat to penetrate a metal container. *ethylene oxide sterilizer* an apparatus in which objects are exposed to ethylene gas for 1 hour at 60°C. Any soft packs treated must not be used for 24 hours in order to allow the poisonous gas to dissipate. *gamma radiation sterilizer* an apparatus employed industrially to sterilize syringe needles, scalpel blades, suture materials, operating gloves, dressings and disposable syringes, by exposure to gamma-ray radiation for 24 hours. *glass bead, salt, small steel ball bearings or molten metal sterilizer* a thermostatically controlled, electrically heated small sterilizer containing beads, salt, steel balls or molten metal maintained at 250°C. Small instruments such as those used in endodontic treatment are dipped into it for 10 seconds.

sternal puncture insertion of a special guarded hollow needle with a stylet into the body of the sternum for aspiration of a bone marrow sample for examination.

Sternberg-Reed cell ⊃ Reed-Sternberg cell.

stern/o- a prefix that means 'sternum', e.g. *sternotomy*.

sternoclavicular *adj* pertaining to the sternum and the clavicle.

sternocleidomastoid muscle a strap-like, two-headed anterolateral neck muscle. Its origins are on the sternum and clavicle and it inserts onto the mastoid process of temporal bone. It contracts to flex the head. ⊃ torticollis, Colour Section Figures 4, 5.

S
T

737

sternocostal *adj* pertaining to the sternum and ribs.

sternotomy *n* surgical division of the sternum.

sternum *n* the breast bone, a flat bone felt just under the skin in the middle of the front of the chest. It has three parts, the manubrium, body and xiphoid process. The manubrium is the uppermost section and articulates with the clavicles at the sternoclavicular joints and with the first two pairs of ribs. The body or middle portion gives attachment to the ribs. The xiphoid process is the tip of the bone. It gives attachment to the diaphragm, muscles of the anterior abdominal wall and the linea alba—**sternal** *adj*. ➲ Colour Section Figure 2.

steroid hormones those secreted by the adrenal cortex, the testis and the ovary, all produced from cholesterol as precursor. A variety of synthetic steroids is used in treatment mainly of rheumatic conditions or of relevant hormonal disorders; others are marketed for body-building. ➲ aldosterone, anabolic steroids, androgens, glucocorticoid, hormones, oestrogens (estrogens), progesterone.

steroids *npl* a large group of organic compounds (lipids) that have a common basic chemical structure based on four fused carbon rings; usually three 6-carbon rings and a 5-carbon ring. They include: cholesterol, bile salts, vitamin D precursors, sex hormones and the corticosteroid hormones. ➲ steroid hormones.

sterol *n* chemicals with the basic steroid structure combined with an alcohol group such as cholesterol.

stertor *n* loud snoring; sonorous breathing—**stertorous** *adj*.

stethoscope *n* an instrument used for listening to the various body sounds, especially those of the heart and chest—**stethoscopic** *adj*, **stethoscopically** *adv*.

Stevens–Johnson syndrome (A Stevens, American paediatrician, 1884–1945; F Johnson, American physician, 1894–1934) severe variant of the allergic response—erythema multiforme. It is an acute hypersensitivity state and can follow a viral or bacterial infection, or drugs such as long-acting sulphonamides, some anticonvulsants and some antibiotics. In some cases no cause can be found. Lung complications during the acute phase can be fatal. Mostly it is a benign condition, and there is complete recovery. ➲ Colour Section Figure 112.

-sthenia a suffix that means 'strength', e.g. *neurasthenia*.

STI *abbr* sexually transmitted infection.

sticky wax blend of waxes in the form of yellow sticks which, when heated, melt and adhere to the surface to which they are applied. Used in dentistry, primarily to hold components together before they are joined permanently.

stigma *n* a defining feature or characteristic of a person, or an action usually viewed in a negative way by others. A term associated with the work of the sociologist Ervin Goffman. Its use generally denotes shame and disgrace attributed to the person (e.g. the stigma of being a prisoner), though in more formal theory it denotes a relationship of devaluation (e.g. the stigma of being disabled).

stigmata *npl* marks of disease, or congenital abnormalities, e.g. facies of congenital syphilis—**stigma** *sing*.

stigmatic lens ➲ anastigmatic lens.

stigmatoscope an instrument for observing or measuring the refractive state of the eye based on the position of best focus of a very small point source. ➲ stigmatoscopy.

stigmatoscopy A method of determining the refractive state of the eye based on the criterion of sharpness of an image. The observer determines the position at which a point source appears in the best focus, while the eye is unaccommodated: this indicates the far point of the eye. If the eye is astigmatic the point source will appear as a line or streak when at the far point of each principal meridian. The distance between the two foci corresponds to the cylinder correction and the slant of the streaks from the horizontal or vertical indicates the axis of the astigmatism. ➲ refractive error, stigmatoscope.

stilet *n* a wire or metal rod for maintaining patency of hollow instruments.

stillbirth *n* birth of a baby, after 24 weeks' gestation, that shows no sign of life.

stillbirth certificate certificate issued by a registered medical practitioner (or midwife if no medical practitioner was involved in the antenatal care) who was present at delivery of the dead infant or who examined the body; must legally be given to the qualified informant (usually the father or mother) so registration of birth can be done and a Certificate of Burial or Cremation issued to them; if there is an inquest the coroner issues the order for burial.

stillborn *n* born dead.

Stilling–Turk–Duane syndrome ➲ Duane's syndrome.

Still's disease (G Still, British physician, 1868–1941) term seldom used, having been superseded by systemic onset juvenile idiopathic arthritis. ➲ juvenile idiopathic arthritis.

stimulant *adj, n* stimulating. An agent which excites or increases function.

stimulant laxative ➲ laxatives. ➲ Appendix 5.

stimulated emission when an excited atom absorbs a photon and releases two light photons.

stimulus *n* anything which excites functional activity in an organ or part.

stippled the appearance of healthy gingival tissue whose surface is covered by minute pits. This appearance is often imitated on the buccal aspect of complete dentures.

stippling producing irregular indentations on a surface.

stirrups a technique of ankle strapping using rigid tape (usually zinc oxide). The tape is placed on the ankle, medial to lateral adhering to the undersurface of the heel, mimicking a 'stirrup'.

stitch *n* **1.** a sudden, sharp stabbing/darting pain or spasm felt in the ribcage or abdomen, usually on the right hand side during exertion. The exact cause is unknown though insufficient blood flow and thus oxygen supply to the intercostal muscles or diaphragm has been implicated. While inconvenient and painful, a stitch has no medical significance. **2.** lay term for a suture.

STM *abbr* short term memory.

S
T

stochastic effect one in which the probability of the effect occurring is governed by chance, therefore all doses of radiation carry some risk and the stochastic effects produced by radiation on an individual include radiation-induced cancer and genetic effects. ⊃ deterministic effect.

stock control the method of storing and recording purchased items, for example film in the radiography department, to ensure that the oldest is used first and all film is used before its expiry date.

stock impression tray ⊃ impression tray.

Stokes–Adams syndrome (W Stokes, Irish physician, 1804–1878; R Adams, Irish surgeon, 1791–1875) a fainting (syncopal) attack, commonly transient, which occurs in patients with heart block. If severe, may take the form of a convulsion, or patient may become unconscious.

stoma *n* the mouth; any opening. ⊃ colostomy, ileostomy, urostomy—**stomata** *pl*, **stomal** *adj*.

stomach *n* the most dilated part (J-shaped) of the digestive tube, situated between the oesophagus and the duodenum. ⊃ Colour Section Figure 18b. It lies in the epigastric, umbilical and left hypochondriac regions of the abdomen. ⊃ Colour Section Figure 18a. The stomach is continuous with the oesophagus at the region of the lower oesophageal (gastro-oesophageal [cardiac]) sphincter and with the duodenum at the pyloric sphincter. It has two curvatures. The lesser curvature is short, lies on the posterior surface of the stomach and is the downwards continuation of the posterior wall of the oesophagus. Just before the pyloric sphincter it curves upwards to complete the J shape. Where the oesophagus joins the stomach the anterior region angles acutely upwards, curves downwards forming the greater curvature then slightly upwards towards the pyloric sphincter. The stomach is divided into three regions: the fundus, the body and the antrum. At the distal end of the pyloric antrum is the pyloric sphincter, guarding the opening between the stomach and the duodenum. When the stomach is inactive the pyloric sphincter is relaxed and open and when the stomach contains food the sphincter is closed. The wall of the stomach has the same four layers of tissue that comprise the basic structure of the alimentary canal (the outer adventitia or serosa, two-layer muscle, submucosa and mucosa) but with some modifications. The stomach has three layers of smooth muscle fibres (longitudinal fibres, circular fibres and a layer of oblique fibres). This arrangement allows for the churning motion characteristic of gastric activity, as well as peristaltic movement. The mucosa of the stomach is also modified, when the stomach is empty the mucous membrane lining is thrown into longitudinal folds or rugae and there are numerous gastric glands situated below the surface in the mucous membrane, which secrete gastric juice (containing digestive enzymes, hydrochloric acid and protective mucus). The stomach receives arterial blood from branches of the coeliac artery and the venous drainage is into the hepatic portal vein. The sympathetic nerve supply to the stomach is mainly from the coeliac plexus and the parasympathetic nerve supply is from the vagus nerves (tenth cranial nerves). Sympathetic stimulation reduces the motility of the stomach and the secretion of gastric juice; vagal stimulation has the opposite effect. The function of the stomach includes: (a) temporary storage allowing time for the digestive enzymes, pepsins, to act; (b) chemical digestion—pepsins convert proteins to polypeptides; (c) mechanical breakdown—the three smooth muscle layers enable the stomach to act as a churn, gastric juice is added and the contents are liquefied to chyme; (d) limited absorption of water, alcohol and some lipid-soluble drugs; (e) non-specific defence against microbes—provided by hydrochloric acid in gastric juice. Vomiting may be a response to ingestion of gastric irritants, e.g. microbes or chemicals; (f) the preparation of inorganic iron salts for absorption further along the digestive tract—the acid environment of the stomach favours the conversion of ferric iron salts to ferrous iron salts, which are more readily absorbed; (g) the production of intrinsic factor needed for absorption of vitamin B_{12} in the terminal ileum; (h) the regulation of the passage of gastric contents into the duodenum. When the chyme is sufficiently acidified and liquefied, the pyloric antrum forces small jets of gastric contents through the pyloric sphincter into the duodenum; and (i) the secretion of the hormone gastrin. ⊃ gastric juice.

stomatitis *n* inflammation of the mouth. *angular stomatitis* fissuring in the corners of the mouth consequent upon riboflavin deficiency. Sometimes misapplied to: (a) the superficial maceration and fissuring at the labial commissures in perlèche and (b) the chronic fissuring at the site in older people with a loose lower lip or poorly fitting dentures. *aphthous stomatitis* recurring crops of small ulcers in the mouth. ⊃ aphthae. *gangrenous stomatitis* ⊃ cancrum oris—**stomal** *adj*.

stomatodynia *n* mouth soreness or pain.

stomatology *n* the study of the oral cavity; structure, function, diseases and treatment.

stomion most anterior point of the line of contact of the upper and lower lips in the midline.

stomodeum *n* in the early embryo the depression in the ectoderm of the foregut, which becomes the mouth.

-stomy a suffix that means 'to form an opening or outlet', e.g. *cholecystojejunostomy*.

stone *n* calculus; a hardened mass of mineral matter. In dentistry, **1.** rotary abrasive instrument held in a handpiece, the working end of which incorporates carborundum or similar abrasive mounted on a spindle. **2.** the second derivative of gypsum, calcium sulphate hemihydrate that has been heated to 120–150°C under steam pressure and is used extensively in dentistry to make hard models.

stone bruise ⊃ heel bruise.

stool *n* faeces.

stove-in chest there may be multiple anterior or posterior fractures of the ribs (causing paradoxical respiration) and fractures of sternum, or a mixture of such fractures.

STPD *abbr* standard temperature and pressure dry.

strabismus *n* (*syn.* squint) abnormal position of the eyes relative to each other, such that the visual axes of the two eyes fail to meet at the object of regard. *comitant (or concomitant) strabismus* consistent deviation between the eyes in all positions of gaze. *convergent strabismus* when the eyes turn inwards. *divergent strabismus* when the eyes turn outwards. *latent strabismus* deviation only present when eyes are dissociated, e.g. by converging one eye. *manifest strabismus* deviation present without dissociation.

straight leg raise (SLR) also known as Lasègue sign/test. A neurodynamic test that tests the sciatic nerve; there would be pain, strong stretching feeling or tingling in the posterior thigh, knee, calf and foot. Sensitizing tests to differentiate nervous tissue from other tissues include: ankle dorsiflexion sensitizes the tibial nerve, ankle plantarflexion and forefoot inversion sensitizes the common peroneal nerve, hip adduction sensitizes the sciatic nerve, hip medial rotation sensitizes the sciatic nerve and passive neck flexion sensitizes the meninges, spinal cord and sciatic nerve. ➲ neurodynamic testing.

straight line portion the part of the characteristic curve which is used in radiography to determine the gamma, contrast, average gradient, useful exposure range, useful density range, film latitude and film speed. ➲ sensitometry.

strain 1. a non-specific term applied to excessive or abnormal loading of tissues. Can be used interchangeably to describe the sensation felt during exercise or activity. Injury to the musculotendinous (muscle and tendon) unit resulting from excessive stretch or tension during physical activity. Strains may be classified as: *first-degree strain* in which a few fibres of muscle are stretched or torn. There is local pain, which is increased with stretch, and slight loss of strength and stability. *second-degree strain* in which approximately half of muscle and/or tendon fibres are torn. There is significant pain with muscle on stretch and moderate loss of strength and stability. *third-degree strain* in which there is complete tear of the muscle or tendon. There is sigificant loss of strength and joint stability with major loss of function (Figure S.11). **2.** a subgroup of a species, such as micro-organisms within the same species but with different characteristics. **3.** the extent to which a body or object is deformed when an external force is applied to it. Often measured as a percentage change in the object's dimensions (e.g. length) or in its position (e.g. angle moved).

strandquist isoeffect curves a series of tolerance dose curves to relate total radiotherapy dose to overall treatment time.

strangulated hernia hernia in which the blood supply to the organ involved is impaired, usually due to constriction by surrounding structures.

strangulation *n* constriction which impedes the circulation—**strangulated** *adj*.

strangury *n* a constant painful urge to micturate.

Strassman operation (P Strassman, German gynaecologist, 1866–1938) a plastic operation to make a bicornuate uterus a near normal shape.

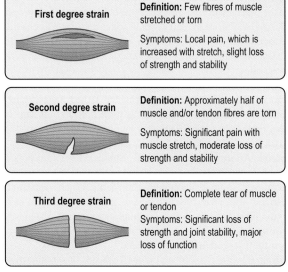

S.11 A classification of strains (reproduced from Porter 2005 with permission).

Strategic Health Authority a body responsible for strategic health planning for a geographical area with a population of many millions (e.g. NHS East of England covers the English counties of Cambridgeshire, Norfolk, Suffolk, Bedfordshire, Hertfordshire and Essex). They are also responsible for the performance management of the Primary Care Trusts (PCTs) within that area.

strategic management the management function concerned with longer-term future strategy. Financial and resource planning. ➲ operational management.

stratified *adj* arranged in layers.

stratified epithelia stratified epithelia consist of several layers of cells of various shapes. The superficial layers grow up from below. Basement membranes are usually absent. The main functions of stratified epithelium are to protect underlying structures from mechanical wear and tear and, in the urinary tract, protect against the variations in the chemical composition of urine. There are two main types: stratified squamous and transitional. ➲ stratified squamous epithelium, transitional epithelium.

stratified squamous epithelium is composed of a number of layers of cells of different shapes representing newly formed and mature cells. In the deepest layers the cells are mainly columnar (see Figure E.7, p. 264) and, as they grow towards the surface, they become flattened and are then shed. *non-keratinized stratified epithelium* is found on wet surfaces that may be subjected to wear and tear but are protected from drying, e.g. the conjunctiva of the eyes, the lining of the mouth, the pharynx, the oesophagus, the anus, the last part of the penile portion of the male urethra and the vagina. *keratinized stratified epithelium* is found on dry surfaces that are subjected to wear and tear,

S
T

i.e. skin, hair and nails. The surface layer consists of dead epithelial cells to which the protein keratin has been added. This forms a tough, relatively waterproof protective layer that prevents drying of the underlying live cells. The surface layer of skin is rubbed off and is replaced from below. ⊃ epithelium.

stratum *n* a layer or lamina, e.g. the various layers of the epithelium of the skin, i.e. stratum granulosum, stratum corneum.

strawberry naevus a red birthmark caused by a capillary haemangioma.

strawberry tongue the tongue is thickly furred with projecting red papillae. As the fur disappears the tongue is vividly red like an overripe strawberry. A characteristic of acute streptococcal disease/scarlet fever. ⊃ Colour Section Figure 113.

stray light (*syn* parasitic light) light reflected or passing through an optical system but not involved in the formation of the image such as that reflected by the surfaces of a correcting lens. ⊃ ghost image.

strength *n* the maximum force or torque that can be developed during maximal voluntary contraction of muscle(s).

strength–duration testing an electrotherapy term. A quick method (in conjunction with clinical assessment of sensory and motor deficits and functional changes) of obtaining information about a damaged peripheral nerve. Used to establish integrity and serial testing (7–14 days later) can indicate direction of change. Largely replaced by modern electrophysiological testing that is more accurate and able to provide more reliable differential diagnoses. Equipment required: monophasic pulses, frequency 1 Hz, range of 6–8 pulse durations between 10 μs and approximately 300 ms. ⊃ chronaxie, rheobase.

strength training also known as resistance training. Training achieved by working dynamically against high loads or statically against fixed resistances. In both cases the forces involved must be such that relatively few repetitions are possible without a substantial rest period. A sustained strength-training programme will progressively increase the loads and number of lifts over a period of months, the exercises being performed in several sets, each embodying a specified number of repetitions. In the first 2–3 months the main improvement in strength is attributable to increased recruitment of motor units within the pre-existing muscle mass (the 'neural phase' of strength training); thereafter, increase of muscle fibre diameters is the major factor ('hypertrophic phase'). ⊃ weight training.

Streptobacillus *n* a genus of Gram-negative bacteria. *Streptobacillus moniliformis* causes a type of rat-bite fever in humans.

Streptococcus *n* a genus of bacteria. Gram-positive cocci, often occurring in chains. They have varying haemolytic ability, α, β and non-haemolytic, and some types produce powerful toxins. Some streptococci are commensal in the intestinal tract (*Streptococcus faecalis*) and respiratory tract (*Streptococcus viridans*). The commensal streptococci, together with the pathogens *Streptococcus pyogenes* and *Streptococcus pneumoniae*, cause serious infections that include: tonsillitis, scarlet fever, otitis media, erysipelas, endocarditis, wound infections, pneumonia, meningitis, urinary infection. Glomerulonephritis and rheumatic fever may follow some streptococcal infections. Group B streptococcus, an intestinal and vaginal commensal, may cause meningitis, pneumonia and septicaemia in neonates infected by bacteria present in the maternal genital tract. ⊃ Griffith's typing, Lancefield's groups, necrotizing fasciitis.

Streptococcus mutans bacterium present in plaque and considered to be the prime causative organism of dental caries. ⊃ mutans streptococci.

streptodornase *n* a proteolytic enzyme used with streptokinase to liquefy blood clot and pus.

streptokinase *n* a streptococcal enzyme. Used with streptodornase in wound management. Plasminogen activator. Used as a fibrinolytic drug in the management of several thromboembolic conditions including acute myocardial infarction and pulmonary embolism.

streptolysins *npl* exotoxins produced by streptococci. Streptolysin antibody may be measured as an indicator of recent streptococcal infection.

Streptothrix *n* a filamentous bacterium which shows true branching. ⊃ *Streptobacillus*.

stress *n* **1.** the response of an organism to any demand made upon it by agents threatening physical or emotional well-being. Selye described such agents as stressors, which could be physical, physiological, psychological or sociocultural. Stress may be either *distress*, a negative event which has long term effects on health when it becomes chronic, or *eustress*, a more positive event that accompanies pleasurable excitement and euphoria. ⊃ anxiety, stressor. **2.** in mechanics, the force per unit area applied to a body or object. Measured in newtons per square metre (N/m^2) or pascals (Pa).

stress and tension gauge in dentistry, a gauge used to measure the force exerted by rubber bands and springs.

stress breaker in dentistry, a device intended to relieve an abutment tooth of a load.

stress fracture (*syn.* fatigue fracture) a bone fracture resulting from repeated loading with relatively low magnitude forces. Can be caused by a number of factors including overtraining, incorrect biomechanics, fatigue, hormonal imbalance, poor nutrition and osteoporosis.

stress incontinence ⊃ incontinence.

stress management a structured programme used to teach effective skills for identifying factors that create or exacerbate stress, recognizing and coping with the symptoms of stress and developing strategies to avoid or counteract stress.

stress management measures a range of measures that reduce the negative effects, such as relaxation techniques, biofeedback, etc., or reducing stress, e.g. delegation. ⊃ general adaptation syndrome.

stressors *npl* factors that cause stress responses. They may be physical, physiological, psychological and sociocultural, and include: pain, cold, trauma and blood loss, heavy workload, a life crisis such as the death of a close relative, job loss or serious illness. ⊃ burnout.

S
T

stretching exercises that may involve static or dynamic stretching. Normally used to mobilize neural and muscle tissue to the limits of the available range. Static stretching involves holding a position for a period of time; it requires the correct alignment of the body and awareness of posture and fine motor control. Dynamic stretching may be used in the management and rehabiltation of sporting injuries. ⊃ dynamic stretching, static stretching.

stretch receptor mechanoreceptors in muscle spindles and tendons that respond to stretch.

stretch reflex contraction of skeletal muscles in response to an applied stretch. Accounts for muscle tone including the continually adjusted background contraction in the postural muscles (mainly the extensors of the trunk and limbs), and for the resistance which an observer can feel in response to stretching any muscle by passive movement. Mediated by afferent impulses from the stretched intrafusal fibres in muscle spindles relayed via mono- and polysynaptic connections in the spinal cord (and also via long-loop supraspinal pathways) to the alpha (α) motor neurons that supply the extrafusal fibres of the same muscle. ⊃ tendon jerk reflex.

striae *npl* streaks; stripes; narrow bands—**stria** *sing*, **striated** *adj*. **1.** striae may occur when the abdomen enlarges such as with obesity, ascites, tumours and pregnancy, when the marks are called *striae gravidarum* they are red at first and then become silvery-white. Striae may also occur as a side-effect of corticosteroid therapy. **2.** *striae ciliares* the slight dark ridges in the pars plana of the ciliary body, which run parallel with each other from the teeth of the ora serrata to the valleys between the ciliary processes. ⊃ ciliary body, ciliary processes, ora serrata. **3.** a line in the posterior corneal stroma associated with corneal oedema and sometimes keratoconus. ⊃ keratoconus. **4.** a vein or streak seen in optical glass which has been contaminated during manufacture or in which the ingredients have been imperfectly mixed.

striae ciliares ⊃ striae.

striae retinae the concentric lines on the surface of the retina which appear after spontaneous or surgical retinal reattachment. ⊃ retinal detachment.

striate area ⊃ visual area.

striate cortex ⊃ visual area.

striated duct that part of a salivary duct that modifies the salivary composition and is so called because of the striated appearance of its lining cells.

striated muscle ⊃ skeletal muscle.

stricture *n* a narrowing, especially of a tube or canal, due to scar tissue or tumour.

strictureplasty *n* surgical reconstruction of a stricture by means of a longitudinal muscle-splitting incision and transverse suture repair, e.g. for the strictures of Crohn's disease.

stride in gait (usually walking or running): the interval between an event of one foot (e.g. heel-strike or toe-strike) and the next occurrence of the same event of the same foot.

stride length the distance between the position (e.g. heel contact) of one foot and the subsequent position of the same foot. May also include other support devices such as crutches. Should be the same for each foot as long as movement is in a straight line (i.e. not in a curve). Usually measured in metres.

stride rate the number of strides per minute.

stridor *n* a harsh breathing sound caused by turbulent airflow through constricted air passages—**stridulous** *adj*.

strip in dentistry, a long narrow piece of material used for a variety of purposes. *abrasive strip* ⊃ abrasive strip. *celluloid strip* a clear plastic strip used as a matrix during the placement of tooth coloured restorations in anterior teeth. *finishing strip* fine abrasive strip used for smoothing and polishing. *lightning strip* ⊃ separating strip. *polishing strip* ⊃ finishing strip. *separating (lightning) strip* a metal strip carrying coarse abrasives on one side and used to increase the separation between adjacent teeth.

strip crown a preformed transparent crown form used with composite resin for temporary/provisional treatment of anterior teeth and restoration of fractured incisors.

strobila the term applied to all the segments (proglottides) of a tapeworm.

stroke *n* a term for cerebrovascular accident. Sudden loss of blood supply to a part of the brain leading to a neurological defect lasting more than 24 hours. ⊃ cerebrovascular accident, completed stroke, progressing stroke, transient ischaemic attack.

stroke in evolution ⊃ progressing stroke.

stroke unit a dedicated unit for the treatment and management of stroke patients. A multidisciplinary team of specialist practitioners work collaboratively to improve patient outcomes. It is characterized by organized specialist care delivered by a multidisciplinary team, who receive ongoing training and education in stroke, meet regularly (minimum weekly) and involve the carers and relatives in the rehabilitation process. Stroke units have been found to lead to better outcome for strokes with less mortality and morbidity (Stroke Unit Trialists 2002). (Stroke Unit Trialists 2002 Organised Inpatient (Stroke Unit) Care for Stroke (Cochrane Review). In: The Cochrane Library Issue 1. Oxford: Update Software.)

stroke volume (SV) the output from each of the ventricles of the heart during a single contraction (systole). The difference between end diastolic volume (EDV) and end systolic volume (ESV). Typically ∼70 mL at rest, and rises during exercise as the venous return increases, raising the ventricular filling pressure, so that a greater volume of blood enters the relaxed ventricles during diastole, to be ejected during systole. The resting stroke volume may be doubled in exercise, exceptionally even more, but the increase is limited by the decreasing duration of diastole as heart rate increases. ⊃ cardiac output, heart rate, venous return.

stroma *n* **1.** the interstitial or foundation substance of a structure. **2.** the blood supply and supporting structures of a tumour above the size of about 2 mm.

stromal interstitial keratitis ⊃interstitial keratitis.

Strongyloides *n* a genus of small intestinal nematode worms, e.g. *Strongyloides stercoralis*. They infest humans (natural host), but can infest dogs. ⊃ strongyloidiasis.

S
T

strongyloidiasis *n* infestation with the nematode *Strongyloides stercoralis*. It commonly occurs in the tropics and subtropics, but may also infest immunocompromised people, such as those with AIDS. Infestation usually occurs through the skin from contaminated soil, but can be through the mucosae. There may be an itchy rash at the site of larval entry. The larvae migrate through the lungs and may cause respiratory symptoms as the larvae are coughed up in sputum. Some larvae are swallowed and lead to varying abdominal symptoms, e.g. pain, diarrhoea and malabsorption, as the female worm burrows into the intestinal mucosa and submucosa. Some individuals have allergic reactions such as wheezing.

strontium (Sr) *n* a metallic element present in bone. Isotopes of strontium are used in radionuclide scanning of bone.

strontium-90 (^{90}Sr) a radioisotope with a half-life of 28 years produced during atomic explosions. It is dangerous when it becomes integrated within bone tissue where turnover is slow. Used to treat the cornea by being incorporated in a rolled silver foil and bonded into a silver applicator.

Stroop effect described by American psychologist J R Stroop in 1935. A phenomenon in which individuals take longer to name the colour of words printed in a nonmatching colour, such as the word blue printed in red ink, than when the words are printed in the same colour as the word designates, such as the word blue printed in blue ink.

Stroop test a test for the Stroop effect in which individuals are presented with lists of colour words in matching and non-matching colours and the time they take to read the different words, or the number of errors they make, is recorded. Often used as a stressor in experimental studies.

structure localization a method of accurately locating small, impalpable lesions using ultrasound, computed tomography (CT) scanning or using a localizing grid and conventional radiography.

structure mottle an uneven radiographic image due to the fact that it is not possible to evenly disperse the phosphor crystals throughout the binder when manufacturing intensifying screens and therefore light from the intensifying screens is not uniformly produced.

struma a goitre.

Stryker bed/frame a proprietary bed. Designed to allow rotation of patients to the prone or supine position. Main uses include spinal injuries and burns.

S-T segment ⊃ P-QRS-T complex.

Stuart-Prower factor *n* factor X in the blood coagulation cascade. It is produced in the liver and requires vitamin K. Activation of factor X is needed for prothrombin activator through both the intrinsic and extrinsic pathways. A very rare inherited (autosomal recessive) deficiency leads to a bleeding disorder.

stud attachment in dentistry, a precision attachment having a stud-shaped patrix.

student's alloy a metal mainly consisting of brass (i.e. copper and zinc) and used in dentistry to teach casting techniques. Similar in appearance and properties to precious and semi-precious alloy.

student's elbow olecranon bursitis.

Student's paired test a parametric test for statistical significance. Used to test differences in mean values for two related measurements such as those obtained from the same subject. ⊃ Wilcoxon test.

Student's t test for independent groups a parametric test for statistical significance. Used to test differences in mean values of two groups. ⊃ Mann–Whitney *U* test.

stunting poor growth in height of children, leading to shorter stature for age, generally resulting in lifelong short stature. Especially associated with insufficient protein intake.

stupor *n* a state of marked impairment of, but not complete loss of, consciousness. The victim shows a gross lack of responsiveness, usually reacting only to noxious stimuli— **stuporous** *adj*.

Sturge–Weber syndrome (*syn.* naevoid amentia) (W Sturge, British physician, 1850–1919; F Weber, British physician, 1863–1962) a genetically determined congenital ectodermosis, i.e. a capillary haemangioma above the eye may be accompanied by similar changes in vessels inside the skull giving rise to epilepsy and other cerebral manifestations.

St Vitus' dance ⊃ chorea.

stye *n* (*syn.* external hordeolum) an abscess in the follicle of an eyelash.

stylet 1. a stout wire inserted into the lumen of a catheter or needle to stiffen it during insertion into the body. **2.** fine blunt probe.

styloid *adj* long and pointed; resembling a pen or stylus.

styloid process a projection of the temporal bone, or those on the radius and ulna.

styptic *n* an astringent applied to arrest bleeding.

sub- a prefix that means 'below, beneath', e.g. *subdural*.

subacromial *adj* under the acromion.

subacromial decompression surgical decompression of the shoulder, often with excision of the lateral portion of the clavicle, it is performed to relieve impingement.

subacromial space the region of the shoulder that is bordered by the so called subacromial joint—a joint made up by the humerus and a superior arch, consisting of the acromion process and the coracoid process of the scapula, joined by the coracoacromial ligament. This arch is lined by the synovium of the subacromial bursa. The rotator cuff runs in the subacromial space.

subacute *adj* neither acute nor chronic. Often the stage between the acute and chronic phases of disease.

subacute bacterial endocarditis ⊃ infective endocarditis.

subacute combined degeneration of the spinal cord a complication of untreated pernicious anaemia (PA) and affects the posterior and lateral columns of the spinal cord.

subacute sclerosing panencephalitis (SSPE) a rare late complication of measles with progressive and fatal loss of neurological and cognitive function due to inflammation and destruction of brain tissue.

S
T

subarachoid under the arachnoid mater (middle meningeal membrane), such as subarachnoid haemorrhage.

subarachnoid haemorrhage (SAH) the loss of blood from a vessel in the brain which leaks into the subarachnoid space. About three-quarters of those presenting with a subarachnoid haemorrhage (SAH) are under 65 years, and women are more frequently affected than men. Subarachnoid haemorrhage typically presents with a sudden, severe 'thunderclap' headache (often occipital) which lasts for hours or even days, often accompanied by vomiting. Physical exertion, straining and sexual excitement are common antecedents. There may be loss of consciousness at the onset, so subarachnoid haemorrhage should be considered if a patient is found comatose. Since subarachnoid haemorrhage is rare (incidence 6/100 000) and only 1 patient in 8 with a sudden severe headache has had a subarachnoid haemorrhage, clinical vigilance is necessary to avoid a missed diagnosis. All patients with a sudden severe headache require investigation to exclude a subarachnoid haemorrhage. On examination the patient is usually distressed and irritable, with photophobia. There may be neck stiffness due to subarachnoid blood but this may take some hours to develop. Focal hemisphere signs (hemiparesis, aphasia etc.) may be present at onset if there is an associated intracerebral haematoma. A 3rd cranial nerve palsy may be present due to local pressure from an aneurysm of the posterior communicating artery, though this is rare. Fundoscopy may reveal a subhyaloid haemorrhage, which represents blood tracking along the subarachnoid space around the optic nerve. Of all subarachnoid haemorrhages, 85% are caused by saccular ('berry') aneurysms bulging out from the bifurcations of the cerebral arteries, particularly in the region of the circulus arteriosus (circle of Willis). These rarely present before the age of 20 years. There is an increased risk in first-degree relatives of those with saccular aneurysms, and with polycystic kidney disease and congenital collagen defects, e.g. Ehlers–Danlos syndrome. Of the remainder, 10% are non-aneurysmal haemorrhages, have a very characteristic appearance on computed tomography (CT) scan and a benign outcome in terms of mortality and recurrence. Some 5% of SAHs are due to rarities including arteriovenous malformations and vertebral artery dissection. The immediate mortality of aneurysmal subarachnoid haemorrhage is about 30%. Survivors have a recurrence, or re-bleed rate of about 40% in the first 4 weeks and 3% annually thereafter. Insertion of platinum coils into an aneurysm (via an endovascular procedure) or surgical clipping of the aneurysm neck reduces the risk of both early and late recurrence. Coiling may be associated with fewer periverative complications and better outcomes. A re-bleed is not the only cause of early deterioration; it may be due to obstructive hydrocephalus, delayed cerebral ischaemia due to vasospasm, hyponatraemia and systemic complications associated with immobility, e.g. chest infection or pulmonary embolism. Nimodipine is given to prevent vasospasm in the acute phase.

subarachnoid space the space beneath the arachnoid membrane, between it and the pia mater. It contains cerebrospinal fluid.

subcarinal *adj* below a carina, usually referring to the carina tracheae.

subclavian *adj* beneath the clavicle.

subclavian artery one of two arteries with branches that supply blood to the neck, spinal cord, brain and upper limbs. ⊃ Colour Section Figure 9. The right subclavian artery branches from the brachiocephalic artery and the left subclavian artery is one of the arteries that branch directly from the aortic arch. They are slightly arched and pass behind the clavicles and over the first ribs before entering the axillae, where they continue as the axillary arteries. Before entering the axilla each subclavian artery gives off two branches: the vertebral artery, which passes upwards to supply the brain, and the internal thoracic artery, which supplies the breast and a number of structures in the thoracic cavity.

subclavian steal syndrome an occlusion of the subclavian artery (proximal to the vertebral artery) causes a reversal of blood flow in the vertebral artery on the same side from the basilar artery to the subclavian artery past the blockage. It can deprive areas of the brain of blood.

subclavian vein one of two veins that carry venous blood from the neck and upper arms to the brachiocephalic veins. ⊃ Colour Section Figure 10.

subclinical *adj* insufficient to cause the classical identifiable disease.

subcondylar osteotomy an oblique surgical section of the ramus of the mandible below the condyle to reduce mandibular prognathism.

subconjunctival *adj* deep to the conjunctiva—**subconjunctivally** *adv*.

subconscious *adj, n* that part of the mind outside the range of consciousness and full awareness, but still able to affect conscious mental or physical reactions.

subcostal *adj* beneath the rib.

subcostal nerves ⊃ thoracic nerves.

subcutaneous *adj* beneath the skin—**subcutaneously** *adv*. *subcutaneous oedema* is demonstrable by the 'pitting' produced by pressure of the finger. *subcutaneous tissue* ⊃ Colour Section Figure 12.

subdiaphragmatic *adj* underneath the diaphragm. For example the presence of air under the diaphragm following laparotomy or in the presence of a bowel perforation.

subdural *adj* beneath the dura mater; between the dura and arachnoid membranes.

subdural haematoma (SDH) the accumulation of blood beneath the dura lining the skull that can occur after head trauma. It develops slowly and may present as a space-occupying lesion with vomiting, papilloedema, fluctuating level of consciousness, weakness, usually hemiplegia on the opposite side to the clot. Finally there is a rise in blood pressure and a fall in pulse rate.

subendocardial *adj* immediately beneath the endocardium.

subgingival *adj* below the gingiva.

subgingival calculus ⊃ dental calculus.

subgingival curettage the removal of the junctional epithelium and the epithelial lining of a periodontal pocket, often accompanied by scaling and root planing.

subglossal *adj* ⊃ sublingual.

subhepatic *adj* beneath the liver.

subinvolution *n* failure of the gravid uterus to return to its normal size within a normal time after childbirth. ⊃ involution.

subject contrast the contrast seen on a radiograph varies with the body part being imaged and will change with the size of the area, the density and atomic number of the tissue, the quality of radiation and the use of contrast agents.

subjective *adj* internal; personal; arising from the senses and not perceptible to others. ⊃ objective *opp*.

subjective accommodation a measurement of the accommodation of the eye based on the subject's judgements, such as the push-up or push-out method or the minus lens method. ⊃ minus lens method, objective accommodation, push-up method.

subjective assessment the data that are gained from speaking with the patient or carer, it aims to gather all relevant information about the site, nature and behaviour of a person's symptoms and gain insight into the past behaviour and treatment. The patient's general health, previous investigations, medication and social circumstances are also recorded or reviewed.

subjective contrast the observer's opinion of the contrast seen on an image; it depends on the viewing conditions, and the observer's ability to see differences on the film.

subjective norm in the theory of reasoned action/planned behaviour, the person's perceived social pressure to engage or not engage in a behaviour.

subjective optometers ⊃ optometer.

subjectivity a state of mind which emanates from personal feelings, opinions and emotions.

sublethal damage damage caused by radiation that is insufficient to cause death of the cell.

sublimate *n* a solid deposit resulting from the condensation of a vapour.

sublimation *n* a mental defence mechanism whereby undesirable basic instinctive drives are unconsciously redirected to, and expressed through, personally approved and socially accepted behaviour, such as aggression redirected to sporting activity.

subliminal *adj* inadequate for perceptible response. Below the threshold of consciousness. ⊃ liminal.

sublingual *adj* beneath the tongue. A route used for the administration of medicines, such as glyceryl trinitrate, which are subject to first pass metabolism/effect in the liver.

sublingual bar the major connector of a mandibular partial denture that is placed on the floor of the mouth.

sublingual salivary gland the smallest of the salivary glands situated in the floor of the mouth against the deep surface of the mandible, above the mylohyoid line and close to the midline (see Figure S.1, p. 688). One of a pair of almond-shaped glands with 8–20 small ducts opening on the crest of the sublingual fold of mucous membrane beneath the tongue. It produces a viscous solution containing mucus at a fairly constant volume. The gland is innervated from the submandibular ganglion. It receives arterial blood via the lingual artery and venous blood leaves via the corresponding vein. ⊃ parotid salivary gland, submandibular salivary gland.

sublining in dentistry, the thin layer of non-irritant cement or vanish placed beneath a cement lining.

subluxation *n* incomplete dislocation of a joint. The shoulder joint is particularly vulnerable due to its inherent mobility from its anatomical structure and support given by the rotator cuff muscles. In hemiplegia or other forms of neurological damage the shoulder can sublux due to a lack of tone in the muscles surrounding the joint or in some cases the presence of increased tonal activity can cause some muscles to pull harder than others and thus cause a subluxation. Thus, great care must be taken when handling the affected shoulder in a patient with hemiplegia in order to try to prevent trauma. It is important to remember that subluxation does not necessarily lead to pain. In dentistry, minor injury to a tooth and periodontal ligament in which the tooth is mobile but not displaced.

submandibular *adj* below the mandible. ⊃ dislocation.

submandibular ganglion one of the four associated with the cranial nerves and located close to the submandibular salivary gland. Its preganglionic fibres are derived from the facial nerve (seventh cranial nerve) and its postganglionic nerve fibres supply the submandibular and sublingual salivary glands.

submandibular salivary gland one of a pair of salivary glands, about half the size of the parotid salivary gland, situated partly under cover of the mandible, below the mylohyoid line in the region of the angle (see Figure S.1, p. 688). Its duct passes forwards and upwards to open on the floor of the mouth, beneath the tongue at a small papilla on the crest of a fold of mucous membrane. The gland produces saliva containing both mucus and enzymes, the volume of which increases during talking and eating. It is innervated by nerve fibres from the submandibular ganglion. Arterial blood is supplied by branches of the facial artery, venous blood drains via corresponding veins. ⊃ parotid salivary gland, sublingual salivary gland.

submarginal calculus ⊃ dental calculus.

submaxillary *adj* below the maxilla.

submental below the chin.

submento-vertex projection a radiographic projection used to demonstrate the base of the skull and the zygomatic arches.

submergence infra-occlusion. The failure of a tooth to maintain its position relative to adjacent teeth so that its occlusal level is below that of adjacent teeth. Most often seen in the primary dentition. The mechanism appears to be related to ankylosis.

submerging teeth ⊃ infra-occlusion.

submucosa *n* the layer of connective tissue beneath a mucous membrane—**submucous, submucosal** *adj.*

submucosal plexus Meissner's plexus. A plexus of autonomic (sympathetic and parasympathetic) nerves that innervate the mucosal lining of the gastrointestinal tract.

submucosal vestibuloplasty (archaic) the surgical deepening of the gingival sulcus by freeing and displacing the tissue between the mucosa and the periosteum in order to allow the mucosa to become attached to the underlying bone.

submucous *adj* beneath a mucous membrane.

submucous resection (SMR) surgical correction of a deviated nasal septum.

subnasale the point where the lower margin columella (i.e. the terminal fleshy part of the nasal septum) meets the upper lip in the midline.

subnormal vision ⊃ low vision.

suboccipital *adj* beneath the occiput; in the nape of the neck.

suboccipitobregmatic a measurement of the fetal head taken from just above the neck posteriorly to the bregma or anterior fontanelle. It is the smallest diameter and presents when the head is well flexed.

subperiosteal *adj* beneath the periosteum of bone.

subperiosteal implant ⊃ implant (dental).

subphrenic *adj* beneath the diaphragm.

subphrenic abscess presence of pus under the diaphragm.

subpoena *n* a court order requiring a person to appear as a witness or to bring documents to court.

sub-routine a self-contained part of a computer program which can be returned to time and time again.

subscapularis a muscle crossing the shoulder, it forms part of the posterior wall of the axilla. One of the four muscles comprising the rotator cuff. Its origin is on the scapula; it inserts on the humerus (lesser tubercle). It stabilizes the shoulder joint by holding the humeral head within the glenoid cavity and medially rotates the humerus. ⊃ rotator cuff.

subspinale (point 'A') the deepest midline point between the anterior nasal spine and the prosthion.

substance misuse the misuse of alcohol, tobacco, drugs and other substances that include solvents to the point when health and or social functioning is adversely affected.

substance P a peptide neurotransmitter found in nerve cells and some endocrine cells in the gastrointestinal tract. It is a very powerful vasodilator, increases gastrointestinal smooth muscle contraction and is involved in pain transmission.

substrate *n* chemical upon which a specific enzyme is active.

substratum in radiography, an adhesive layer that attaches the emulsion to the film base, or the phosphor layer to the reflective layer of an intensifying screen.

substructure in dentistry, the metal framework, as in an implant, that is embedded beneath the tissues and in contact with the bone. Designed to support a superstructure such as an implant denture.

subsultus *n* muscular tremor.

subsultus tendinum twitching of tendons and muscles particularly around the wrist in severe fever, such as typhoid.

subtalar joint also known as talocalcaneal joint. The joint formed by the articulation of the talus with the calcaneus. This is a complex joint with a cylindrical axis.

subtarsal sulcus a groove on the inner surface of the eyelid, near the eyelid margin and parallel to it, which forms the border separating the marginal from the tarsal conjunctiva. Foreign bodies are commonly lodged in this groove. ⊃ lid eversion.

subthalamus an area below the thalamus containing many important nuclei.

subungual *adj* under a nail, such as a haematoma.

subungual exostosis a small outgrowth of bone under the nail plate near to, or immediately distal to the free edge.

subungual haematoma a collection of blood under a nail; the increased pressure causes considerable pain. The pressure and hence the pain is relieved by puncturing the nail with a sterile heated device to release the collection of blood. ⊃ Colour Section Figure 114.

subungual heloma (corn) the development of a corn or keratinized lesion under the nail plate.

succedaneous tooth a permanent tooth with a predecessor in the primary dentition, (e.g. incisors).

succenturiate placenta an abnormal placenta with a separate or accessory lobe joined to the main placenta by blood vessels running through the membranes. The lobe can become detached from the main placenta during the third stage of labour which may cause serious postpartum haemorrhage, or may possibly remain in the uterus contributing to infection.

succinate dehydrogenase (SDH) an enzyme present in the mitochondrial inner membrane of skeletal muscle. Catalyses the oxidation of succinate to fumarate, in Krebs' (tricarboxylic acid) cycle. Histochemical marker for aerobic capacity. ⊃ muscle enzymes.

succussion *n* **1.** splashing sound produced by fluid in a hollow cavity when the patient moves, e.g. liquid content of dilated stomach in pyloric stenosis. **2.** a term in homeopathy describing the vigorous shaking of natural diluted substances.

sucking blister formation of a small callous pad on the upper or lower lip of an infant which develops after sucking. It may resemble a blister.

sucrase *n* intestinal enzyme that converts sucrose to glucose and fructose.

sucrose *n* beet or cane sugar. A disaccharide that is hydrolysed into glucose and fructose during digestion. It occurs naturally in sugar and is added to many manufactured foods. Sucrose, together with plaque, produces lactic acid. Saliva makes a solution of such sugar which then bathes all the supragingival surfaces of teeth. Overconsumption of sucrose with inadequate dental hygiene can cause dental problems.

suction aspiration of fluid or gas, such as wound drainage or clearing the airway. For example, a means of removing excess bronchial secretions in a person who is unable to expectorate secretions themselves. Suction may be applied by the nasopharyngeal route where the suction catheter is inserted via the nose or oropharyngeal suction through the mouth. Suction may also be applied via an oropharyngeal airway, through an endotracheal tube in a person who is intubated, or via a tracheostomy tube. The hazards of suctioning include hypoxia as ventilation is interrupted, raised intracranial pressure, infection, trauma to the bronchial mucosa and cardiac arrhythmias (Pryor & Prasad 2002). (Pryor JA, Prasad A 2002 Physiotherapy for respiratory and cardiac problems, 3rd edn. Churchill Livingstone, Edinburgh.) In dentistry, an inaccurate term describing the process responsible for the retention of a denture that is not retained mechanically by clasps or precision attachments.

suction apparatus a vacuum pump used in many healthcare settings (e.g. operating theatres, critical care facilities, dental surgeries, by paramedics in emergency vehicles and so on) to aspirate fluid, secretions, blood and debris from the field of operation or maintain a clear airway.

suction (electrotherapy context) suction is used to hold electrodes against the skin. Can be a constant or a varying level of suction. Current passes from the stimulator output through a fine wire in each suction lead to a metal electrode in the suction cup. A damp sponge in the patient side of each suction cup completes the circuit. There is a risk of bruising if excess pressure is used or in patients with risk of bleeding, such as those taking anticoagulant medication.

sudamina *n* sweat rash.

Sudan blindness ⊃ onchocerciasis.

Sudden Adult/Arrhythmia Death Syndrome (SADS) ⊃ long Q-T syndrome.

sudden death (in sport) refers to sudden cardiovascular death, defined under the International Olympic Committee (IOC) Lausanne recommendations as death occurring without prior symptoms, or within 1 h of symptoms, in a person without a previously recognized cardiovascular condition. This specifically excludes cerebrovascular, respiratory, traumatic and drug-related causes. Ninety percent of non-traumatic sudden death in athletes is related to a pre-existing cardiac abnormality. ⊃ aortic valve stenosis, heart murmur, heart sounds, hypertrophic obstructive cardiomyopathy, long Q-T syndrome, myocardial infarction, myocarditis, Wolff–Parkinson–White syndrome.

sudden unexpected death in infancy (SUDI) (*syn.* cot death, sudden infant death syndrome [SIDS]) the unexpected sudden death of an infant, usually occurring overnight while sleeping in a cot, but may occur in other situations and under other circumstances. A common mode of death in infants between the ages of 1 month and 1 year, usually in the first 8 months of life, neither clinical nor postmortem findings being adequate to account for death. Risk factors include sleeping in the prone position, overheating, respiratory illness and infection, maternal smoking during pregnancy and being in an environment where people smoke. Parents/carers are recommended to put babies to sleep on their backs; place the baby at the foot of the cot to prevent him/her wriggling under the bedclothes; ensure that the baby's head does not become covered; that for the first six months the baby sleeps in a cot in the parents' room; not to have the baby in the parents' bed if one of the parents is very tired, is a smoker, or has consumed alcohol, medicines or drugs that may cause drowsiness; not to overheat the room; not to smoke in the same room; and seek advice from a health professional if the baby seems unwell.

Sudeck's atrophy (P Sudeck, German surgeon, 1866–1945) ⊃ complex regional pain syndrome 2.

SUDI *abbr* sudden unexpected death in infancy.

sudor *n* sweat—**sudoriferous** *adj*.

sudorific *adj*, *n* (*syn.* diaphoretic) describes an agent which induces sweating.

SUF(c)E *abbr* slipped upper femoral (capital) epiphysis.

suffocation cessation of breathing caused by an airway obstruction.

sugar the colloquial term for sucrose. Commercial sugar comes from either sugar cane or sugar beet. Chemically, the term sugars includes sucrose and other disaccharides (maltose, lactose) and also the simple sugars, the monosaccharides (pentoses, hexoses).

sugars-free the term applied to foods, drinks or medicines when they do not contain fermentable sugars and so are less likely to cause a risk to dental health.

suggestibility *n* abnormal vulnerability to suggestion. May be increased in individuals who have dependence on others such as those in hospital and some people with a learning disability.

suggestion *n* the implanting in a person's mind of an idea which he or she accepts fully. In psychology suggestion may be used as a therapeutic measure during hypnosis.

suicide *n* intentional taking of one's own life. Usually related to depression and hopelessness. Attitudes to suicide are culturally determined, and stigma may be present in some communities. ⊃ deliberate self-harm, parasuicide.

sulcus *n* 1. a furrow or groove, particularly those separating the gyri (convolutions) of the cerebral cortex. 2. space or trough, lined by mucous membrane and bounded by the cheeks on one side and the teeth and gingivae on the other—**sulci** *pl*.

sulcus deepening procedure ⊃ vestibuloplasty.

sulcus test ⊃ inferior drawer test.

sulphaemoglobin *n* (*syn.* sulphmethaemoglobin) a sulphide oxidation product of haemoglobin, produced in vivo by certain drugs. It cannot transport oxygen or carbon dioxide and, not being reversible in the body, is an indirect poison.

sulphaemoglobinaemia *n* a condition of circulating sulphaemoglobin in the blood.

sulphate salt of sulphuric acid, e.g. magnesium sulphate.

sulphonamides *npl* a group of bacteriostatic antibacterial agents, e.g. sulfadiazine. ⊃ Appendix 5.

sulphones *npl* a group of synthetic antileprotic drugs, e.g. dapsone. ⊃ Appendix 5.

sulphonylureas *npl* a group of oral hypoglycaemic drugs, e.g. glipizide. ⊃ Appendix 5.

sulphur *n* an insoluble yellow powder. Used in topical preparations and baths for acne and other skin disorders.

sulphur granules ⊃ actinomycosis.

sulphuric acid inorganic acid. Highly corrosive. In radiography, used as the acid in a fixer solution with aluminium sulphate hardener.

sunglasses spectacles which have tinted lenses. They are used to protect the eyes from bright sunlight, for special cases (e.g. fear of light) or for cosmetic reasons. ⊃ cataract, photophobia, pterygium, tinted lens, ultraviolet radiation.

sunstroke *n* ⊃ heatstroke.

superadditivity the combined activities of two chemicals is greater than the sum of their separate activities. In radiography, for example, the two chemicals phenidone and hydroquinone used in developer.

supercilium *n* the eyebrow—**superciliary** *adj*.

supercoat a thin layer of gelatin(e) that is coated on the outer surface of a film or the thin layer of cellulose acetobiturate on an intensifying screen, to protect from mechanical damage.

superego *n* one of the three main aspects of the personality (the others being the ego and id); part of the mind concerned with moral sanctions, inhibitions and self criticism; it functions at a partly conscious, but mostly unconscious level. Roughly equates to the 'conscience'. ⊃ ego, id.

superfecundation *n* the fertilization of two oocytes, released during the same menstrual cycle, by spermatozoa from sexual intercourse with different partners.

superfetation *n* the presence of two fetuses resulting from oocytes released during different menstrual cycles.

superficial *adj* near the surface such as the superficial veins of the leg.

superficial bursitis an adventitious bursa found superficial to the insertion of the Achilles tendon. It is a common condition and mainly affects adolescent females.

superficial punctate keratitis (SPK) ⊃ punctate epithelial keratitis (PEK).

superficial veins of lower limb dorsal venous arch, great (long) saphenous vein, small (short) saphenous vein. ⊃ saphenous veins.

superficial veins of upper limb basilic vein, cephalic vein, median cubital vein, median vein.

superimposition the ability to see two similar images superimposed but not mentally fused. Examples include, seeing a bird in a cage with both eyes in a Synoptophore when one eye is presented with a bird and the other with a cage; seeing the letter E in a Synoptophore when one eye is presented with the letter F and the other with the letter L. ⊃ Worth's classification of binocular vision.

superinfection *n* infection that follows the elimination of the normal flora by antibiotic usage. This permits other micro-organisms, such as *Clostridium difficile*, to thrive in the intestine without competition from micro-organisms of the normal flora. ⊃ antibiotic-associated colitis, *Clostridium,* pseudomembranous colitis, *Pseudomonas*.

superior *adj* in anatomy, the upper of two parts—**superiorly** *adj*.

superior colliculi (*syn* superior corpora quadrigemina) two small rounded elevations situated on the dorsal aspects of the midbrain, just below the thalamus. Besides receiving fibres from each other, they serve as a relay centre for movements of the eyes, head and neck in response to visual and other stimuli. ⊃ Parinaud's syndrome.

superior corpora quadrigemina ⊃ superior colliculi.

superior labrum anterior-posterior (SLAP) lesion damage to the glenoid labrum; may affect 'throwing' athletes. The lesions, which can be visualized on magnetic resonance imaging (MRI) scan, require arthroscopic surgical repair. ⊃ shoulder joint.

superior limbic keratoconjunctivitis (SLK) chronic inflammation of the superior cornea and conjunctiva. It is characterized by hyperaemia, hazy epithelium and often corneal filaments near the upper limbus and the adjacent conjunctiva, and with the sensations of burning, itching, photophobia and hazy vision. The condition is bilateral in 50% of cases. Detection of the disease in its mild form is difficult as it requires lifting the upper eyelid. The condition typically affects middle-aged women with thyroid dysfunction. It may be induced by soft contact lens wear. Smaller hard lenses, especially gas permeable, rarely cause this disease. Management involves several options: application of silver nitrate, topical medication (e.g. sodium cromoglicate), thermal cauterization of the superior bulbar conjunctiva, or occlusion of the lacrimal puncta/um to increase tear volume over the conjunctiva. ⊃ thyroid ophthalmopathy.

superior oblique muscle an extraocular muscle that moves the eyeball downwards and outwards; it is supplied by the trochlear nerve (fourth cranial nerve). ⊃ extraocular.

superior ophthalmic vein a vein which is formed near the root of the nose by a communication from the angular vein soon after it has been joined by the supraorbital vein. It passes into the orbit above the medial palpebral ligament, runs backward to the sphenoidal fissure where it usually meets the inferior ophthalmic vein, and drains into the cavernous sinus (a channel for venous blood). It has many tributaries: the inferior ophthalmic vein, the anterior and posterior ethmoidal veins, the muscular vein, the lacrimal vein, the central retinal vein, the anterior ciliary vein and two of the posterior ciliary veins (the superior ones).

superior palpebral sulcus a furrow in the skin of the upper eyelid. It separates the tarsal portion which is closest to the lid margin from the orbital portion which extends from the tarsus to the eyebrow. This furrow becomes more prominent with age. ⊃ palpebral aperture.

superior quadrantanopsia (*syn* 'pie in the sky' defect) a superior, homonymous quadrantanopsia due to a lesion of the most anterior and inferior fibres of the optic radiations

S
T

that is in Meyer's loop, on the contralateral side of the visual pathway. ➲ Meyer's loop, optic radiations.

superior rectus muscle an extraocular muscle that moves the eyeball upwards; it is supplied by the oculomotor nerve (third cranial nerve). ➲ extraocular.

superior thyroid artery a branch arising at the commencement of the external carotid artery. It slopes downwards to supply blood to the upper part of the thyroid gland and adjacent muscles. ➲ inferior thyroid artery.

superior vena cava the large vein, which drains all the venous blood from the head, neck and upper limbs, is about 7 cm long. It passes downwards along the right border of the sternum and ends in the right atrium of the heart.

supernumerary *adj* in excess of the normal number; additional. Such as with students of medicine, nursing, dentistry and allied health professions undertaking clinical practice.

supernumerary bones include os trigonum, os tibial externum and os vesalii. Such abnormalities of sesamoid bones and supernumerary bones rarely directly cause problems in the paediatric foot but may result in soft-tissue lesions. Their presence is confirmed radiographically.

supernumerary digits ➲ polydactyly.

supernumerary teeth ➲ tooth.

superovulation *n* the production of many more oocytes than normal, usually as a result of gonadotrophin administration during assisted conception techniques. ➲ ovarian hyperstimulation syndrome.

superoxide O_2^-. ➲ free radical, reactive oxygen species.

superoxide dismutases a group of enzymes that have metal ion cofactors such as copper, zinc and manganese. They clear harmful superoxide radicals from the body. ➲ free radical, reactive oxygen species.

superparamagnetic a substance which is 100–1000 times more susceptible to magnetism than a paramagnet. ➲ diamagnetic, ferromagnetic, paramagnetic.

superstructure 1. a structure that rests on another. **2.** in dentistry, the visible portion of an appliance. **3.** in dentistry, a prosthesis retained and supported by an implant substructure.

supervised area a type of designated area where a person is likely to receive a dosage of radiation in excess of one third the dose in a controlled area; access to the area is limited to those people whose presence is necessary.

supervised community treatment (SCT) ➲ Mental Health Act 2007.

supervisor of midwives a practising midwife with a minimum of 3 years' experience, at least 1 year of which must have been in the immediate past 2 years, appointed by the local supervising authority in accordance with the Nurses, Midwives and Health Visitors (Midwives Amendment) Rules and specially trained to exercise supervision over midwives in its area; responsible for receipt and monitoring of Notification of Intention to Practise forms from all midwives working in the area, submitting them to the local supervising authority; monitoring standards of midwifery practice and providing professional, clinical and educational support and guidance; issuing supply orders for controlled drugs, witnessing the destruction of controlled drugs where appropriate and ensuring that midwives are competent to administer medicines; monitoring and storing written records from all midwives in the area; investigating allegations of malpractice, negligence or misconduct; referring midwives to the Health Committee of the NMC and notifying the local supervising authority of midwives liable to be a source of infection. ➲ local supervising authority.

supinate *vt* turn or lay face or palm upward ➲ pronate *opp*—**supination** *n*.

supination *supination of the foot* during normal gait immediately before 'take-off' from the toes, the ankle tends to angle outwards and the foot is supported briefly on its outer side. *oversupination* can cause the ankle to roll over towards the outer side, with possible ligament damage. *supination of the forearm* the twisting movement which brings the palm of the hand to face upwards or forwards. ➲ pronation *opp*.

supinator *n* that which supinates, usually applied to a muscle. For example, the *supinator*, a deep muscle of the forearm. Its origin is on the lateral epicondyle of the humerus and the proximal ulna, it inserts on to the proximal radius. Assists in forearm supination. ➲ pronator *opp*.

supine *adj* **1.** lying on the back with face upwards. **2.** of the hand with palm upwards. ➲ prone *opp*.

supine hypotensive syndrome affects pregnant women during the late second and third trimesters. When lying supine the gravid uterus compresses the inferior vena cava and reduces venous return to the heart, thereby reducing cardiac output and hence blood pressure.

supplemental teeth ➲ tooth.

support a situation when an object or body has a force applied to resist the force of gravity. Often used to refer to the phase of gait when one or more feet are on the ground. ➲ stance. In dentistry. **1.** a structure resisting masticatory forces on a prosthesis. May be classified as either tooth or mucosal. **2.** an appliance that maintains a part in position.

suppository *n* medicament in a base that melts at body temperature. Administered rectally.

suppression *n* **1.** the process by which the brain inhibits the retinal image (or part of it) of one eye, when both eyes are simultaneously stimulated. This occurs to avoid diplopia as in strabismus, in uncorrected anisometropia, in retinal rivalry, etc. Also known as suspenopsia (this term actually refers to voluntary suppression as occurs, for example, when using a monocular microscope with one eye) or suspension (most often used when referring to partial suppression). **2.** in psychology, a mental defence mechanism, whereby people voluntarily force difficult or painful thoughts out of the mind; it can precipitate mental health problems. **3.** cessation of a secretion (e.g. urine) or a normal process (e.g. menstruation).

suppressor T-cell T-lymphocytes which slow or stop the activity of other T-cells and B-cells once the antigen is dealt with. ➲ CD8 cells, cytotoxic T-cell.

suppuration *n* the formation of pus—**suppurative** *adj*, **suppurate** *vi*.

suprabulge that portion of a tooth crown that converges towards the occlusal surface, i.e. is above the survey line of the crown and above the undercut (infrabulge) area of the tooth. ⊃ survey line.

suprachoroid also known as lamina fusca. ⊃ sclera.

suprachoroidal space a potential space located between the suprachoroid (or lamina fusca) layer of the sclera and the choroid. In this space are thin, pigmented strands of collagen fibres and it is traversed by the long and short posterior ciliary arteries and nerves.

supraclavicular *adj* above the clavicle.

supracondylar *adj* above a condyle.

supracondylar fracture one affecting the lower end of the femur or humerus. The latter may interfere with the blood supply to the forearm. ⊃ Volkmann's ischaemic contracture.

supragingival above the gingival margin.

supragingival calculus . ⊃ dental calculus.

supramaximal exercise ⊃ anaerobic exercise.

supramentale (bony) point 'B'. The deepest point in the bony outline between the infradentale and the pogonion.

supramentale (soft tissue) the deepest point between the nose and the forehead in the midline.

supraocclusion ⊃ over-eruption.

supraorbital *adj* above the orbits.

supraorbital artery a branch of the ophthalmic artery which supplies the upper eyelid, the scalp and also sends branches to the levator palpebrae superioris muscle and the periorbita.

supraorbital foramen a groove in the supraorbital margin of the frontal bone conducting the supraorbital nerve and vessels.

supraorbital ridge the ridge of the frontal bone covered by the eyebrows.

suprapubic *adj* above the pubis.

suprapubic catheter catheter inserted into the urinary bladder through the abdominal wall.

suprarenal *adj* above the kidney. ⊃ adrenal.

suprarenal glands ⊃ adrenal glands.

supraspinatus a muscle crossing the shoulder. One of the four muscles comprising the rotator cuff. Its origin is on the scapula; it inserts on the humerus the (greater tubercle). It helps in abduction and stabilizes the shoulder joint when heavy loads are carried, such as heavy shopping. ⊃ rotator cuff.

supraspinatus impingement if the subacromial space is narrowed, impingement of the supraspinatus tendon may occur, characterized by pain, into shoulder abduction, and positive impingement tests. The person will often attempt to deviate away from the impingement, attempting to gain the necessary movement by using a trick movement.

supraspinatus tendonitis (tendinitis) inflammation of the supraspinatus tendon. Commonly seen when there is a degree of supraspinatus tendon degeneration or degradation.

Active contraction of the supraspinatus will cause pain and there is usually an arc of pain on abduction—described as 60–120° by most authorities. ⊃ painful arc.

supraspinatus test ⊃ empty can test.

suprasternal *adj* above the sternum.

supra, super- a prefix that means 'above, excess, superior', e.g. *superfetation*.

supraventricular *adj* above the ventricles.

supraventricular tachycardia (SVT) any tachycardia originating from a focus in atrial tissue. The heart rate is greater than 100 bpm and may be as fast as 280 bpm. ⊃ Wolff–Parkinson–White syndrome.

supravergence (*syn* sursumvergence) the movement of one eye upward relative to the other. ⊃ infravergence; vergence.

surface the outermost or uppermost boundary of an object. In dental anatomy, *buccal surface* the surface of molars and premolars facing the cheeks. *distal surface* the surface of a tooth distant to the midline. *incisal surface* the cutting surface of incisors and canines. *labial surface* the surface of incisors and canines facing the lips. *lingual surface* the surface of all lower teeth facing the tongue. *mesial surface* the proximal surface of teeth facing the midline. *palatal surface* the surface of all upper teeth facing the palate.

surface applicator used in brachytherapy where the external surface of the patient is treated by locally applied sources held in shaped applicators.

surface drag the force, opposing the direction of motion, that is due to the interaction between the surface of an object and the medium through which it is passing (or that is moving past it). ⊃ drag force, form drag, propulsive drag force.

surface (or topical) analgesic/anaesthetic the jelly, spray or liquid preparations used in dentistry to provide analgesia of the mucous membrane. Contains drugs such as benzocaine or lidocaine.

surface power the dioptric power of a single refracting or reflecting surface. It is equal to

$$F = \frac{n' - n}{r}$$

where F is the power in dioptres, n and n' are the refractive indices of the media on each side of the surface and r is the radius of curvature of the lens or mirror surface, in metres. This equation forms part of the fundamental paraxial equation. For a spectacle lens in air ($n = 1$) the power of the surface becomes

$$F = \frac{n' - 1}{r}$$

⊃ paraxial equation (fundamental).

surface reflection light reflected at a surface according to Fresnel's formula. ⊃ Fresnel formula.

surface wrinkling retinopathy ⊃ preretinal macular fibrosis.

surfacing in optometry, the combined processes of roughing, smoothing and polishing of a lens surface to a given curvature. ➲ blank lens, finished lens, frosted lens, ground glass.

surfactant *n* **1.** a mixture of phospholipids secreted by type II pneumocytes. It reduces surface tension in the alveoli, allows lung inflation and prevents alveolar collapse between breaths. ➲ neonatal respiratory distress syndrome, pneumocytes. **2.** an agent which reduces the surface tension of oil or solid–water interfaces and therefore has cleaning properties. (the term is an acronym formed from; **surf**ace **act**ive **agent**). ➲ contact lens deposits, wetting solution.

surgeon a qualified doctor who specializes in surgery.

surgery *n* that branch of medicine which treats diseases, deformities and injuries, wholly or in part, by manual or operative procedures.

surgical *adj* pertaining to surgery.

surgical débridement ➲ débridement.

surgical dressings ➲ wound dressings.

surgical emphysema air in the subcutaneous tissue planes following the trauma of surgery or injury.

surgical template ➲ template.

surrogate *n* a substitute for an object or person.

surrogate motherhood where a woman agrees to have a child for an infertile couple. Surrogacy is allowed in the UK, but women may only receive reasonable financial expenses. There are, however, many informal arrangements for surrogacy.

sursumvergence ➲ supravergence.

survey *n* **1.** a data collection method. Includes: interview, postal, telephone, or via the internet. **2.** in dentistry, the procedure carried out by a surveyor (instrument) to determine the survey line and the guiding planes of a prosthetic appliance. ➲ survey line.

survey line in dentistry, a line produced on a model by a surveyor indicating the maximum convexity of a tooth or the alveolar process in relation to the planned path of insertion and natural path of displacement of a prosthesis or the optimum position for a clasp arm.

surveyor a jointed instrument holding a lead marker or a cutting blade which is used to survey models or cut parallel surfaces.

survival rate the proportion of patients who survive for a certain number of years, usually five, used for measuring the success of treatment for cancer.

susceptibility *n* the opposite of resistance. Includes a state of reduced capacity to deal with infection.

suspensory apparatus of the lens ➲ zonule of Zinn.

suspensory bandage applied so that it supports and suspends, such as the lower jaw or scrotum.

suspensory ligament a ligament whose principal function is to support another structure. Examples include: the suspensory ligament of the axilla maintaining the hollow of the axilla; the ligament of Lockwood supporting the eye ball in the orbit; the duodenum 'ligament', in fact a thin band of smooth muscle that supports the duodeno-jejunal flexure; the suspensory ligament of the penis; the zonule of Zinn. ➲ ligament of Lockwood, zonule of Zinn, Colour Section Figure 15.

sustained release device a method of administering an antimicrobial drug to a periodontal pocket. An adjunctive treatment method for periodontal disease. Designed to provide drug delivery for up to 24 hours. Examples include, minocycline gel and metronidazole gel.

sustentaculum tali the sustentaculum provides the scaffold needed by the calcaneus to sustain or hold the talus up. The scaffold is needed because although the talus sits on top of the calcaneus it does not do so completely.

suture *n*, *v* **1.** the junction of cranial bones. **2.** in surgery, a stitch or series of stitches used to appose the edges of a surgical or traumatic wound (Figure S.12). Also describes the placement of such stitches. ➲ ligature.

S$\bar{v}$O$_2$ symbol for mixed venous oxygen saturation.

Sv *abbr* sievert.

SV *abbr* **1.** single-vision (SV) lens. **2.** stroke volume.

SVD *abbr* spontaneous vaginal delivery.

SVR *abbr* systemic vascular resistence.

SVT *abbr* supraventricular tachycardia.

swab *n* **1.** a small piece of cotton wool or gauze. ➲ filamented swab. **2.** a small piece of sterile cotton wool, or similar material, on the end of a shaft of plastic, wire or wood, inside a protecting tube. It is used to collect material for microbiological examination.

swage to shape metal by hammering and adapting it to a die.

swallowing *n* deglutition. Swallowing is initiated voluntarily but completed by a reflex (involuntary) action. It occurs in three stages after mastication is complete and the food bolus has been formed. The stages are: (a) oral (buccal)—the mouth is closed and the voluntary muscles of the tongue and cheeks push the bolus backwards into the pharynx; (b) pharyngeal—the muscles of the pharynx are stimulated by a reflex action initiated in the walls of the oropharynx and coordinated in the medulla and lower pons in the brainstem. Contraction of these muscles propels the bolus down into the oesophagus. In normal swallowing, all other routes that the bolus could possibly take are closed. The soft palate rises up and closes off the nasopharynx; the tongue and the pharyngeal folds block the way back

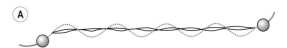

Subcuticular Prolene suture and beads

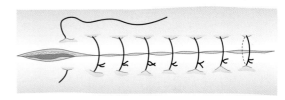

Interrupted over-and-over

S.12 Examples of skin sutures (A) continuous subcuticular prolene and beads (B) interrupted over-and-over (reproduced from Pudner 2000 with permission).

into the mouth; and the larynx is lifted up and forward so that its opening is occluded by the overhanging epiglottis preventing entry into the airway; and (c) oesophageal—the presence of the bolus in the pharynx stimulates a wave of peristalsis which propels the bolus through the oesophagus to the stomach. ➲ dysphagia.

swan-neck deformity a common finger deformity seen in rheumatoid arthritis (Figure S.13).

SWAP *acron* short wavelength automated perimetry.

sway back posture posture typified by cervical spine extension, increased upper trunk flexion, lumbar flexion, posterior pelvic tilt, hyperextended hips and knees. ➲ flat back posture.

sweat *n* the secretion from the sweat (sudoriferous) glands. Contains water, electrolytes (mainly sodium and chloride) and waste. Sweat production is primarily concerned with temperature regulation but has a small excretory role.

sweat gland two types of skin glands that produce sweat. ➲ apocrine sweat gland, eccrine, Colour Section Figure 12.

sweating secretion from the sweat glands in the skin: a major factor in the control of body temperature. Sweating is stimulated by the sympathetic nervous system and that in turn by the hypothalamus, in response to a rise in blood temperature. Corrective heat loss by evaporation of sweat is effective except in excessively humid conditions. Both sodium chloride (typically about 2.6 g/L) and water are lost in the sweat, but at a moderate sweating rate water loss is proportionately greater because sodium is reabsorbed in passage through the sweat ducts. Sweat loss can be as much as 4 litres per hour in heavy exercise in the heat, and more sodium per litre escapes reabsorption at higher flow rates: hence the need to replace both water and salt. ➲ electrolyte balance, hydration status of athletes, sodium, sports drinks.

sweat test used to measure the amount of sodium and chloride in sweat, to confirm a diagnosis of cystic fibrosis. The drug pilocarpine is introduced into the skin by iontophoresis to induce sweating. The sweat is collected and tested.

sweeteners sugar substitute, sometimes described as an alternative or artificial sweetener. Divided into two main types according to their properties and their purpose in the food and drinks in which they are used. *bulk sweeteners* (e.g. sorbitol, xylitol, maltitol, mannitol) are of low/no cariogenicity but contain calories. They are used to replace cariogenic sugars in products requiring some bulk, e.g. chocolate, baked products, and chewing gum. *intense sweeteners* (e.g. Acesulfame K, aspartame, saccharin) contain few calories and are used in small amounts to provide an intense sweet taste in diet products which do not require any bulking agent (e.g diet soft drinks).

swept gain used in ultrasound scanners to give an image of even brightness when scanning homogeneous tissue.

swimming reflex the innate ability of the infant to temporarily suspend respiration and make swimming movements when placed under water.

swing the phase of gait when one leg is being moved, to support the body when it is next placed upon the ground. Also known as swing phase.

swinglock denture ➲ sectional denture.

sycosis barbae (*syn* barber's itch) a pustular folliculitis of the beard area in men.

sycosis nuchae a folliculitis at the nape of the neck which leads to keloid thickening (acne keloid).

Sydenham's chorea (T Sydenham, English physician, 1624–1689) ➲ chorea.

sylvian aqueduct ➲ cerebral aqueduct.

symbiosis *n* a relationship between two or more organisms in which the participants are of mutual aid and benefit to one another. ➲ antibiosis *opp*—**symbiotic** *adj*.

symblepharon *n* adhesion of the lid to the eyeball.

symmelia a congenital anomaly in which the lower limbs are fused.

sympathectomy *n* surgical excision of part of the sympathetic nervous system.

sympathetic eye (*syn* sympathizing eye) the uninjured eye in sympathetic ophthalmia which becomes secondarily affected. ➲ sympathetic ophthalmia.

sympathetic nervous system part of the peripheral nervous system (PNS), it describes a division of the autonomic nervous system (ANS). Efferent fibres from nerve cells in the thoracolumbar segments (thoracolumbar outflow) of the spinal cord relay in a chain of sympathetic ganglia on each side of the spine in the thorax and abdomen; thence sympathetic postganglionic nerves reach all parts of the body except the central nervous system. They supply the heart, smooth muscle and many secretory glands. The main neurotransmitter is noradrenaline (norephinephrine) which has different actions depending on the type of receptors on the effector cells. This system is at all times active in the regulation of cardiac output, arterial blood pressure and regional blood flow (all contributing to adjustments in exercise), as well as priming the body for emergency 'fight or flight', when sympathetic nerves stimulate release of adrenaline (epinephrine) from the adrenal medulla. The outflow from the spinal cord is influenced by inputs from the hypothalamus related to body temperature control, from the cardiovascular control centres in the brainstem, and by

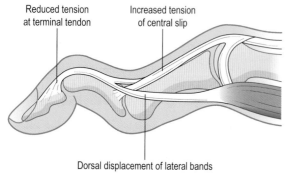

Reduced tension at terminal tendon

Increased tension of central slip

Dorsal displacement of lateral bands

S.13 **Swan-neck deformity** (reproduced from Porter 2005 with permission).

afferents from the alimentary tract and other organs. Dual sympathetic and parasympathetic innervation provides for synergistic interaction, although the effects are often opposite; most vascular smooth muscle is an exception, having only a sympathetic nerve supply. It opposes the parasympathetic nervous system and is usually involved with body stimulation. ⊃ adrenaline (epinephrine), noradrenaline (norepinephrine), parasympathetic nervous system, Colour Section Figure 22.

sympathetic ophthalmia (*syn* sympathetic ophthalmitis) a rare, bilateral inflammation of the uveal tract that usually follows perforation of one eye. The inflammation occurs first in the injured eye (called the exciting eye) and soon follows in the other eye (called the sympathetic eye). ⊃ enucleation, sympathetic eye.

sympathetic ophthalmitis ⊃ sympathetic ophthalmia.

sympathizing eye ⊃ sympathetic eye.

sympatholytic *n* an antagonist. A drug which impedes or opposes the effects of the sympathetic nervous system. ⊃ alpha (α)-adrenoceptor antagonists, beta (β)-adrenoceptor antagonists.

sympathomimetic *adj* an agonist. Producing effects similar to those produced by stimulation of the sympathetic nerves. ⊃ alpha (α)-adrenoceptor agonists, beta (β)-adrenoceptor agonists.

symphalangism the fusion of phalanges in one digit.

symphysiotomy an operation to separate the symphysis pubis and enlarge the pelvis to facilitate delivery. Rarely undertaken in developed countries. May be used for cephalopelvic disproportion or rarely for shoulder dystocia in developing countries.

symphysis *n* a fibrocartilaginous union of bones such as the symphysis pubis or symphysis menti—**symphyseal** *adj*.

symphysis–fundal height measurement taken between the upper border of the symphysis pubis and the uterine fundus, in centimetres; sequential measurements, plotted on a graph (growth chart), facilitate identification of changes in uterine or fetal growth rates.

symphysis menti the point at which the two developing bodies of the mandible join to form the chin.

symphysis pubis also called the pubic symphysis. The cartilaginous joint between the two pubis bones of the innominate bones. A limited degree of movement may take place between the two bones, as the joint is softened by circulating hormones during pregnancy.

symphysis pubis dysfunction previously known as diastasis symphysis pubis. A painful condition occurring during late pregnancy, in labour or following delivery. It is caused by the abnormal relaxation of the ligaments associated with the pubic joint. The relaxation is due to high levels of pregnancy hormones such as relaxin.

symmetrical cortical necrosis a rare complication of severe concealed abruptio placentae with destruction of large areas of the cortex of both kidneys due to internal spasm of the renal cortical arteries. Impaired renal function or death from renal failure may follow. ⊃ acute tubular necrosis.

sympodia a congenital anomaly in which the legs are fused and the feet are missing.

symptom *n* a subjective phenomenon or manifestation of disease—**symptomatic** *adj*.

symptom complex a group of symptoms which, occurring together, typify a particular disease or syndrome.

symptomatology *n* **1.** the branch of medicine concerned with symptoms. **2.** the combined symptoms typical of a particular disease.

sym, syn- a prefix that means 'together, union, with', e.g. *symphysis*.

Synacthen test ⊃ tetracosactide (Synacthen) test.

synaesthesia the occurrence of a secondary sensation accompanying another sensation, such as a particular sound producing a visual sensation.

synapse *n* the name given by Charles Sherrington in 1897 to the site of transmission of information from one neuron to another or (in current usage) to individual cells of a muscle or gland, i.e. the gap between the axon of one neuron and the dendrites of another, or the gap between the axon and a gland or muscle cell. The majority are chemical synapses involving release of a neurotransmitter, such as acetylcholine, from the presynaptic nerve ending which binds to receptors on the postsynaptic cell, opening ion channels (calcium ion release) and leading to local depolarization. At the very many fewer electrical synapses (gap junctions) the abutting cells are in tight contact and there is faster, direct electrical coupling, e.g. between neurons within the brain. ⊃ action potential, neuromuscular junction.

synapsis *n* during meiosis the pairing of homologous chromosomes.

synarthrosis an immovable fibrous joint, such as the skull sutures.

synbiotics supplements containing both prebiotics and probiotics.

synchondrosis a type of amphiarthrosis or cartilaginous joint formed by the epiphyseal plate before ossification.

synchronized intermittent mandatory ventilation (SIMV) mode of positive pressure ventilation in which the timing of the breaths is varied according to the patient's own respiratory effort.

synchysis scintillans cholesterol crystals in the vitreous body (humour) of the eye, often following vitreous haemorrhage.

synclitism state when the fetal head enters the pelvic brim with both parietal eminences at the same level. ⊃ asynclitism.

syncope *n* (*syn*. faint) literally, sudden loss of strength. Caused by reduced cerebral circulation often following a fright, when vasodilation is responsible. May be symptomatic of cardiac arrhythmia, e.g. heart block.

syncytiotrophoblast outer layer of the trophoblast which does not have cell boundaries but scattered nuclei in the protoplasm; persists throughout pregnancy covering the chorionic villi, unlike the cytotrophoblast cells. ⊃ syncytium

syncytium *n* a mass of tissue with several nuclei. Boundaries between individual cells are absent or poorly defined.

S
T

syndactyly, syndactylism, syndactylia *n* (*syn.* webbed toes, zygodactyly) a term applied to a total or partial fusion of adjacent digits. It is very common, usually bilateral and often familial. Multiple syndactyly occurs in hands and feet associated with other anomalies, as in Apert's syndrome, an autosomal dominant disorder—acrocephalosyndactyly. Treatment is not required for webbing of the toes—**syndactylous** *adj*.

syndesmophyte abnormal bony growth between vertebrae, such as in ankylosing spondylitis. It is different in appearance and direction to osteophytes. ⊃ bamboo spine.

syndesmosis a type of fibrous joint in which an interosseous ligament connects two bones, e.g. tibiofibular joint.

syndrome *n* a group of symptoms and/or signs which, occurring together, produce a pattern or symptom complex, typical of a particular disease.

syndrome of inappropriate ADH secretion (SIADH) syndrome in which excessive antidiuretic hormone leads to water retention and low serum sodium.

syndrome X ⊃ metabolic syndrome.

synechia *n* abnormal union of structures, especially adhesion of the iris to the cornea in front (anterior synechia), or to the capsule of the crystalline lens behind (posterior synechia)—**synechiae** *pl*. ⊃ cloverleaf pupil, glaucoma, iris bombé, iritis, Peter's anomaly, prolapse of the iris, Rieger's syndrome, uveitis.

synergism, synergy *n* the harmonious working together of two agents, such as drugs, micro-organisms, muscles, etc.—**synergistic** *adj*.

synergist *n* an agent cooperating with another. Commonly refers to a muscle which acts together with another muscle to produce a greater effect; may also be applied to any pair or group of biological agents of the same kind, e.g. hormones—**synergistically** *adv*.

synergistic action that brought about by the cooperation of two or more muscles, neither of which could bring about the action alone.

synkinesis *n* the ability to carry out precision movements.

synkinetic near reflex ⊃ accommodative reflex.

Synoptiscope ⊃ Worth's amblyoscope.

Synoptophore a type of major amblyoscope. ⊃ Worth's amblyoscope.

synostosis union between bones occurring by ossification.

synovectomy *n* excision of synovial membrane.

synovial *adj* relating to joints that have a cavity lined by synovial membrane which secretes synovial fluid.

synovial cavity the potential space in a synovial joint.

synovial fluid (SF) the fluid secreted by the synovial membrane lining a freely movable joint cavity. Synovial fluid is a clear or straw-coloured fluid, which is thixotropic. Thixotrophy is an unusual property, whereby the more quickly a joint moves, the less viscous its synovial fluid becomes. Synovial fluid contains nutrients and the glycoprotein hyaluronate. It bathes and nourishes the joint and it also plays an important role in absorbing joint stresses. When moving from sitting to standing, stresses on the hip joint

have been calculated to be in excess of 2610 pounds per square inch. Studies show that 90% of this load may be borne by hydrostatic pressure within the synovial fluid between the articulating surfaces. An increase in the volume of synovial fluid often occurs after trauma, presence of infection, loose bodies or as a response to other pathology. Too much synovial fluid in a joint is known as a joint effusion. ⊃ synovial fluid analysis.

synovial fluid analysis the pivotal investigation in patients suspected of having septic arthritis, crystal-associated arthritis and intra-articular bleeding, and it should be performed in all patients with acute monoarthritis, especially with overlying erythema. Synovial fluid (SF) can readily be obtained from most peripheral joints and for diagnostic purposes only a small volume is required. Normal SF is present in small volume, contains very few cells, is clear and either colourless or pale yellow, and has high viscosity. With increasing joint inflammation the volume increases, the total cell count and proportion of neutrophils rise (causing turbidity), and the viscosity lowers (due to enzymatic degradation of hyaluronan and aggrecan). However, because of considerable variation and overlap between arthropathies these features have little diagnostic value. Frank pus or 'pyarthrosis' results from very high neutrophil counts and is not specific for sepsis. High concentrations of crystals, mainly urate or cholesterol, can make SF appear white. Non-uniform blood-staining of SF is common, reflecting inconsequential needle trauma to the synovium. Uniform blood-staining—haemarthrosis—commonly accompanies florid synovitis but may also result from a bleeding diathesis, trauma or pigmented villonodular synovitis. A lipid layer floating above blood-stained fluid is diagnostic of intra-articular fracture with release of lipid from the bone marrow. If sepsis is suspected, SF should be sent for urgent microscopy, Gram stain and culture in a sterile universal container. If gonococcal sepsis or uncommon organisms are suspected, especially in immunocompromised patients, the microbiologist should be consulted to ensure that optimal cultures are established and that molecular techniques of antigen detection are used if appropriate. Identification of common SF crystals is by compensated polarized light microscopy of fresh unrefrigerated SF (to avoid problems of crystal dissolution and post-aspiration crystallization). Urate crystals are long and needle-shaped and show a strong light intensity with a negative sign of birefringence. Calcium pyrophosphate crystals are smaller, rhomboid in shape, usually less numerous than urate and have weak intensity and positive birefringence. ⊃ Colour Section Figure 115.

synovial joint diarthrosis or freely movable joint. (Figure S.14). One of the three main classes of joints.

synovial membrane the membrane lining the intra-articular parts of bones and ligaments. It does not cover the articular surfaces.

synovial sweep the phenomenon whereby articular hyaline cartilage gains its source of nutrition (from synovial fluid). The process of joint movement and compression facilitates

S
T

the spread of synovial fluid across the surface of a joint. For this reason many intra-articular fractures are now managed by early movement or continuous passive movement (CPM).

synovioma *n* a tumour of synovial membrane—benign or malignant.

synovitis *n* inflammation of a synovial membrane.

syntax error two words which are shown on the computer display when an incorrect input or statement has been made.

synthesis *n* the process of compiling complex substances from less complex ones by chemical reactions—**synthetic** *adj*.

synthetic produced artificially.

synthetic resin one of a number of synthetically produced compounds on which the manufacture of a large group of plastics is based. In dentistry, the most commonly used synthetic resin is polymethylmethacrylate.

syphilide *n* a syphilitic skin lesion.

syphilis *n* a sexually transmitted infection caused by the spirochaete *Treponema pallidum* (ssp. *pallidum*). It may be congenital or acquired. *acquired syphilis* is contracted during sexual intercourse with an infected person. There are two main stages: (a) early, characterized by a primary lesion (chancre) at the site of entry into the body that heals within about one month, and may be followed by a generalized illness (secondary syphilis) characterized by a skin rash, fever, generalized lymph node enlargement, mucosal ulcers (snail track); (b) late (occurring many years after the infection) with skin or visceral lesions (gumma), neurosyphilis (tabes dorsalis and general paralysis of the insane), or cardiovascular syphilis (including aneurysm formation in the ascending aorta). In many individuals there

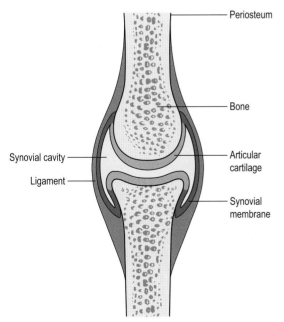

S.14 Typical synovial joint (reproduced from Waugh & Grant 2006 with permission).

may be no clinical signs of syphilis (latent syphilis), the diagnosis being made on the basis of positive serological tests for *T. pallidum*. *congenital syphilis* the spirochaete is transmitted from mother to fetus via the placenta. The affected infant may exhibit characteristic features that include a generalized rash, generalized lymphadenopathy and hepatitis. ⊃ Colour Section Figure 116.

syringe *n* a hand-held device for injecting, instilling or withdrawing fluids and pastes. Consists of a cylindrical barrel to one end of which a hollow needle may be attached, and a close-fitting plunger. *air syringe* in dentistry, an instrument conveying cold or warmed compressed air to the mouth in order to blow away debris or to dry the field of operation. *aspirating syringe* an instrument devised to inject and withdraw fluids from tissues. A dental syringe with the facility of withdrawing the plunger of a local analgesic cartridge. It enables the clinician to see whether a blood vessel has been penetrated, so reducing the possibility of the solution passing directly into the bloodstream. *cartridge syringe* injection syringe accommodating cartridges containing measured quantities of sterile drug solutions. In dentistry, such syringes have a threaded end to which is screwed the hub of an injection needle. *chip syringe* in dentistry, a syringe with metal nozzle and soft rubber bulb, used to puff away debris and to dry tooth preparations. Now superseded by the three-in-one (compressed air/water) syringe. Sometimes used to irrigate an operation site during oral surgery. *Higginson syringe* a two-way rubber bulb syringe previously used for irrigating maxillofacial wounds. *Hunt's syringe* metal syringe with spring-loaded plunger, used for irrigation. *impression material syringe* in dentistry, a syringe with detachable nozzle and plunger, used to convey mixed impression material to the site of operation. *plastic syringe* in dentistry, syringe of various sizes used to convey pastes and other materials to the mouth. *safety syringe* in dentistry, a semi-disposable syringe that allows safe disposal without the need for removal of the needle. *self-aspirating automatic syringe* cartridge syringe that allows aspiration without withdrawal of the syringe plunger rod. *three-in-one syringe* in dentistry, a combination instrument to deliver air, water or an atomized spray through a nozzle and having a variable control.

syringe driver medical device for the continuous delivery of drugs intravenously or subcutaneously. Commonly used in end-of-life care to control symptoms including vomiting and pain.

syringe shield a device made of either metal with a high atomic number or thick Perspex which is designed to protect the hands of staff when handling syringes containing radioactive material.

syringomyelia *n* an uncommon, progressive disease of the spinal cord of unknown cause, beginning mainly in early adult life. Cavitation and surrounding fibrous tissue reaction, in the upper spinal cord, interferes with sensation of pain and temperature, and sometimes with the motor pathways. There

S
T

is painless injury, particularly of the hands. Touch sensation is typically intact in the early stages. ⊃ Charcot's joint.

syringomyelocele *n* the most severe form of meningeal hernia (spina bifida). The central canal is dilated and the thinned-out posterior part of the spinal cord is in the hernia.

syrinx *n* a cyst-like cavity in the spinal cord.

systematic desensitization a technique that utilizes classical conditioning to treat anxiety disorders and phobias. ⊃ conditioning, desensitization.

systematic review a systematic approach to literature reviews of both published and unpublished material that lessens bias and random errors. A research process that summarizes the evidence on a clearly formulated question according to a pre-defined protocol and using a thorough approach. The report should make explicit the methods used to identify, select and appraise relevant studies and to extract, collate and report their findings. It may or may not use meta analysis.

Système International d'Unités (SI) (International System of Units) system of measurement used for scientific, technical and medical purposes. There are seven base units: ampere, candela, kelvin, kilogram, metre, mole and second, and various derived units, e.g. pascal, becquerel, etc. ⊃ Appendix 2.

system for identifying motivated abilities (SIMA) a self-explanatory term. The tests are especially useful in diagnosing the level of mental deterioration.

systemic 1. relating to a system as a whole, e.g. with reference to pathological conditions, affecting the whole body, as opposed to being localized. **2.** with reference to the circulation of the blood, the route from the left atrium and left ventricle of the heart through the aorta and arteries and arterioles supplying the whole body except the lungs, and returning to the right side of the heart.

systemic circulation circulation of oxygenated blood from the left ventricle to aorta, to tissues and back to right atrium of heart in the superior and inferior venae cavae. ⊃ circulation of blood.

systemic connective tissue disease the connective tissue diseases are a group of chronic inflammatory disorders that involve multiple body systems and therefore exhibit a wide spectrum of clinical manifestations. Their aetiology is multifactorial and involves genetic, immunological (especially autoantibody production) and environmental factors. Although each disease displays different clinical and pathological features, the group shares enough characteristics to be considered a family of overlapping conditions. They were initially grouped as 'collagen disease' because of common pathological changes (especially fibrinoid changes in the connective tissues) but the term connective tissue disease is now preferred as it avoids confusion with unrelated monogenic disorders of collagen such as Marfan's syndrome. ⊃ dermatomyositis, inclusion body myositis, inherited connective tissue disease, mixed connective tissue disease, polymyositis, systemic lupus erythematosus (SLE), systemic sclerosis.

systemic inflammatory response syndrome (SIRS) generalized inflammatory response, which may be triggered by a range of processes (e.g. poor perfusion). Features include: abnormal temperature, altered white cell count, increased respiratory rate and increased heart rate. SIRS and multiple organ dysfunction syndrome frequently occur together in critically ill patients.

systemic lupus erythematosus (SLE) the most common multisystem connective tissue disease. For example, it can involve sun-exposed skin, lungs, heart and blood vessels, kidneys and joints, etc. Thus, it is characterized by a wide variety of clinical features and a diverse spectrum of auto-antibody production. There may be skin changes with a typically butterfly-shaped (malar) facial rash, alopecia, pyrexia, pleurisy, pericarditis, alveolitis, arthritis, vasculitis and renal damage. The prevalence varies according to geographical and racial background, from 30/100 000 in Caucasians to 200/100 000 in African-Caribbeans. Around 90% of affected individuals are women, with peak onset in the second and third decades. None of the diverse manifestations of SLE can be attributed to a single antigenic stimulus, and it is likely that this wide spectrum of auto-antibody production results from polyclonal B- and T-cell activation. In normal health these antigens are 'hidden' from the immune system and do not provoke an immune response. Although the triggers that lead to autoantibody production in SLE are unknown, one mechanism may be exposure of intracellular antigens on the cell surface during apoptosis (cell death). This hypothesis is supported by the fact that environmental factors that associate with flares of lupus—such as sunlight and artificial ultraviolet (UV) light, pregnancy and infection—increase oxidative stress and subsequent apoptosis. Few of the autoantibodies found in SLE have been ascribed a specific pathological role. An exception is in the antiphospholipid syndrome, in which antibodies against components of the coagulation cascade are responsible for the predisposition to thromboembolic disease. ⊃ Colour Section Figure 117.

systemic sclerosis previously known as scleroderma. a generalized disorder of connective tissue affecting the skin, internal organs and vasculature. The clinical hallmark is the presence of sclerodactyly in combination with Raynaud's phenomenon or digital ischaemia. The peak age of onset is in the fourth and fifth decades, and overall prevalence is 10–20 per 100 000 with a 4:1 female:male ratio. It is subdivided into diffuse cutaneous systemic sclerosis (DCSS) and limited cutaneous systemic sclerosis (LCSS). Many patients with LCSS have features which are phenotypically grouped into the CREST syndrome (calcinosis, Raynaud's, (o)esophageal involvement, sclerodactyly, telangiectasia). The aetiology is unknown, with no consistent genetic, geographical or racial associations. Environmental factors are important in isolated cases that result from exposure to silica dust, vinyl chloride, hypoxy resins and trichloroethylene. Early in the disease there is skin infiltration by T lymphocytes and abnormal fibroblast activation

S
T

that leads to increased production of extracellular matrix in the dermis, primarily type I collagen. This results in symmetrical thickening, tightening and induration of the skin. In addition to skin changes there is arterial and arteriolar narrowing due to intimal proliferation and vessel wall inflammation. Endothelial injury causes release of vasoconstrictors and platelet activation, resulting in further ischaemia. Systemic sclerosis is predominantly a clinical diagnosis based on the presence of sclerodactyly. ⊃ Colour Section Figure 118. Most patients are antinuclear antibody (ANA) positive, and approximately 30% of patients with diffuse disease and 60% with limited disease have antibodies to topoisomerase 1 and centromere respectively. Raynaud's phenomenon is universal and may precede other clinical features. The initial phase of skin disease is characterized by non-pitting oedema of the fingers and flexor tendon sheaths. Subsequently, the skin becomes shiny and taut, and distal skin creases disappear. The face and neck are usually involved next, with thinning of the lips and radial furrowing. In some patients skin thickening stops at this stage. Skin involvement restricted to sites distal to the elbow or knee (apart from the face) is classified as *limited cutaneous disease* or CREST syndrome. ⊃ Colour Section Figure 119. Involvement proximal to the knee and elbow and on the trunk is classified as *diffuse cutaneous disease*. In the distal extremities, the combination of intimal fibrosis and vessel wall inflammation may cause critical tissue ischaemia, leading to skin ulceration over pressure areas, localized areas of infarction and pulp atrophy at the fingertips. Arthralgia, morning stiffness and flexor tenosynovitis are common. Restricted hand function is due to skin rather than joint disease and erosive arthropathy is uncommon. Muscle weakness and wasting are usually due to myositis. Gastrointestinal involvement is common. Smooth muscle atrophy and fibrosis in the lower two-thirds of the oesophagus lead to acid reflux with erosive oesophagitis. Since this may progress to further fibrosis, adequate treatment of reflux (usually with proton pump inhibitors) is important. Dysphagia and odynophagia (painful dysphagia) may also occur. Involvement of the stomach causes early satiety and occasionally outlet obstruction. Recurrent occult upper gastrointestinal bleeding may indicate a 'watermelon stomach' (antral vascular ectasia), which occurs in up to 20% of patients. Small intestine involvement may lead to malabsorption due to bacterial overgrowth and intermittent bloating, pain or constipation. Dilatation of large or small bowel due to autonomic neuropathy may cause pseudo-obstruction. Pulmonary involvement is a major cause of morbidity and mortality. Fibrosing alveolitis mainly affects patients with diffuse disease. Pulmonary hypertension is a complication of long-standing disease and is six times more prevalent in limited than in diffuse disease. The clinical features are rapidly progressive dyspnoea (more rapid than interstitial lung disease), right-sided heart failure and angina, often in association with rapidly progressing digital ischaemia. Treatment strategies include vasodilators, continuous infusions of epoprostenol, the oral endothelin 1 antagonist bosentan and heart-lung transplantation. One of the main causes of death is hypertensive renal crisis characterized by rapidly developing malignant hypertension and renal failure. Treatment is by angiotensin-converting enzyme (ACE) inhibition even if renal impairment is present. The five-year survival is approximately 70%. Self-management to maintain core body temperature and avoid peripheral cold exposure is important. Infection of ulcerated skin should be treated with prompt antibiotic therapy. Antibiotics penetrate poorly into the skin lesions and therefore need to be given at higher dose for longer periods. Calcium antagonists (e.g. amlodipine) or angiotensin II receptor antagonists (e.g. valsartan) may be effective for Raynaud's symptoms. For severe digital ischaemia, intermittent infusions of epoprostenol may be helpful. Corticosteroids and cytotoxic drugs are indicated in patients with myositis or alveolitis. No agent has been shown to arrest or improve skin changes.

systemic vascular resistence (SVR) the resistance against which the left ventricle must pump blood into the systemic circulation. It is influenced by the degree of vasoconstriction in the peripheral arterioles, i.e. peripheral resistance.

systemic vasculitis a heterogeneous group of diseases characterized by inflammation and necrosis of blood vessel walls. It can be classified by vessel size: (a) large vessel—giant cell arteritis, Takayasu's disease/arteritis; (b) medium vessel—classical polyarteritis nodosa, Kawasaki disease; (c) small vessel—Wegener's granulomatosis, Churg–Strauss syndrome, Henoch–Schönlein purpura, etc. The spectrum of disease ranges from benign and self-limiting (e.g. cutaneous leucocytoclastic vasculitis limited to skin) to life-threatening (e.g. fulminant Wegener's granulomatosis with renal failure and pulmonary haemorrhage). Vasculitis may occur in many types of inflammatory or infectious diseases, such as systemic lupus erythematosus (SLE), rheumatoid arthritis (RA), endocarditis and hepatitis B and C. Primary systemic vasculitis is less common, with an annual incidence of approximately 18–40 new cases per million, which peaks in the 65- to 74-year age group. The aetiology remains unclear, although geographic, environmental and genetic factors are important. Clinical features are due to a combination of local tissue ischaemia (caused by vessel inflammation and narrowing) and the systemic effects of widespread inflammation. Systemic vasculitis should be considered in any patient with fever, weight loss, fatigue, evidence of multisystem involvement, rashes, raised inflammatory markers and abnormal urinalysis. Early diagnosis and management are essential to prevent irreversible organ damage. Vasculitis may be difficult to distinguish from widespread malignancy, occult sepsis (particularly infective endocarditis and meningococcal septicaemia), cholesterol emboli, atrial myxoma and the antiphospholipid syndrome. If vasculitis is suspected, the diagnosis should ideally be confirmed by tissue biopsy, in order to determine the vessel size involved and guide therapy. Skin biopsies are easily obtained. Nasal septal tissue can be taken from areas of ulceration or granulation.

S
T

Muscle biopsy is positive in about 50% of patients with muscle pain. The most important near-patient test is the urine dip test for protein and blood, and subsequent microscopy, since the prognosis of vasculitis is often determined by the degree of renal involvement. In patients with abnormal renal function and active urinary sediment, renal biopsy should be considered. Visceral angiography to detect microaneurysms is most useful where involved tissue is not available to biopsy. Antineutrophil cytoplasmic antibodies (ANCA) are directed against enzymes present in neutrophil granules. However, positive ANCAs occur in many other diseases, including malignancy, infection (bacterial and HIV disease), inflammatory bowel disease, RA, lupus and pulmonary fibrosis.

systole *n* the contraction phase of the cardiac cycle, as opposed to diastole—**systolic** *adj*.

systolic blood pressure the maximum blood pressure measured during the cardiac contraction phase of the cardiac cycle, i.e. when blood is ejected from the heart into the aorta and the systemic arteries.

systolic function the measurement of the ventricular contraction of the heart.

systolic murmur a cardiac murmur occurring between the first and second heart sounds due to ventricular septal defect or valvular disease, e.g. mitral regurgitation.

S
T

T

T *abbr* tesla.

T₃ *abbr* triiodothyronine.

T₄ *abbr* thyroxine.

t₁/₂ *abbr* half-life.

T₁ relaxation time (*syn* T₁, spin-lattice relaxation time, longitudinal relaxation time) in magnetic resonance imaging (MRI) the time taken for the spins to give the energy obtained from the initial radio frequency impulse back to the surrounding environment and return to equilibrium. It represents the time required for the longitudinal magnetization (M_z) to go from 0 to 63% of its final maximum value.

T₂ relaxation time (*syn* transverse or spin-spin relaxation time) the time required for the transverse magnetization to decay to about 37% of its maximum value and is the characteristic time constant for loss of phase coherence among spins orientated at an angle to the static main magnetic field.

TA *abbr* temporal average. ⇨ ultrasound.

tabe- a prefix that means 'wasting', e.g. *tabes*.

tabes *n* wasting away—**tabetic** *adj*.

tabes dorsalis a variety of neurosyphilis characterized by a staggering gait and 'lightning' limb pains. ⇨ Charcot's joint, locomotor ataxia.

tabetic gait the foot is raised high then brought down suddenly, the whole foot striking the ground. ⇨ gait.

table in dentistry, a horizontal flat surface serving a specific purpose, such as guide table. ⇨ guide table, occlusal.

table incrementation time the time taken for the patient's couch to move from one slice location to the next in sequential (non-spiral) computed tomography (CT) scanning.

tablet a solid form of a drug. It may be designed to be swallowed whole, or chewed, or dissolved in water, or absorbed from the buccal cavity, or sublingually. It may be a slow release preparation, or enteric-coated to ensure that absorption occurs in the small intestine.

taboo *n* a behaviour forbidden by individual societies, such as incest or cannibalism.

taboparesis *n* a form of neurosyphilis in which there are clinical features of both brain and spinal cord involvement.

tabular grains are 'flattened' grains that are used only in sensitized film emulsions in screen film technology; they have a large surface area and small volume. The added dye can increase the amount of absorption resulting in a high-speed, high-resolution film with relatively low silver coating weights.

tache noir the black lesion that forms at the bite site in tick-borne boutonneuse fever.

tachy- a prefix that means 'fast', e.g. *tachycardia*.

tachycardia *n* excessively rapid action of the heart at rest (in excess of 100 beats per minute in adults). ⇨ paroxysmal tachycardia.

tachyphagia eating very rapidly.

tachyphasia *n* extreme rapidity of speech. It can be a feature of some mental health disorders.

tachyphylaxis the decreasing effectiveness of some drugs during long term administration.

tachypnoea *n* rapid breathing; abnormal frequency of respiration (in excess of 20 respirations per minute in adults at rest). In most situations when ventilation increases, there is normally an increase in both depth and frequency of breathing. Increase in frequency alone may occur in response to sudden immersion in cold water, and also can accompany anxiety. Tachypnoea with shallow breathing may increase only the dead space ventilation (as in panting) and so may not affect gas exchange—**tachypnoeic** *adj*.

TACI *abbr* total arterial cerebral infarction.

tactile *adj* relating to the sense of touch.

tactile meniscus a cup-shaped nerve ending within the epidermis and other locations; has contact with a specialized tactile receptor (Merkel cell). ⇨ Merkel cell.

taenia *n* a flat strip.

taenia coli three bands of longtitudinal muscle of the colon, because they are shorter than the colon they produce haustrations or puckering.

Taenia *n* a genus of flat, parasitic worms; cestodes or tapeworms. *Taenia saginata* larvae present in infested, undercooked beef. In the human (the definitive host) intestinal lumen they develop into the adult tapeworm, which by its four suckers attaches itself to the wall of the intestine. *Taenia solium* has hooklets as well as suckers. The larvae are ingested in infested, undercooked pork; humans can also be the intermediate host for this worm by ingesting eggs, which develop into larvae in the stomach and pass via the intestinal wall to reach organs where they develop into cysts. In the brain these may cause seizures. ⇨ cysticercosis, cysticercus, *Echinococcus*.

taeniacide *n* an agent that destroys tapeworms—**taeniacidal** *adj*.

taeniafuge *n* an agent that causes the expulsion of a tapeworm.

tagged information file format (TIFF, TIF) a graphics or picture computer file used for photographs. The file is not compressed and therefore the picture quality is good but the file size is very large.

tailor's muscle a colloquial name for the sartorius muscle, so called because tailors used to sit cross legged (the combined actions of sartorius hip flexion, abduction and lateral rotation).

Takayasu's disease/arteritis (M Takayasu, Japanese ophthalmologist, 1860–1938). (*syn* pulseless disease—colloquial term) a chronic inflammatory granulomatous panarteritis of elastic arteries. The vessels most commonly involved are the aorta and its branches, and the carotid, ulnar, brachial, radial and axillary arteries. Pulmonary arteries are occasionally affected. It is more common in women (female:male ratio 8:1) with a typical onset at the age of 25–30 years. It has a world-wide distribution but is most common in Asia. The aetiology is unknown. In contrast to other vasculitides, Takayasu's arteritis is characterized by thickened and inflamed intima without fibrinoid degeneration. The usual presentation is with claudication and systemic symptoms of fever, arthralgia and weight loss. Clinical examination may reveal loss of pulses, bruits, hypertension and aortic incompetence. Investigations are usually nonspecific, with high erythrocyte sedimentation rate (ESR) and normocytic, normochromic anaemia. Diagnosis is usually based on angiographic findings of coarctation, occlusion and aneurysmal dilatation.The 5-year survival rate is ~80%. Most patients respond to initial high-dose oral prednisolone. Additional therapy with methotrexate or cyclophosphamide is usually required. Reconstructive vascular surgery should be avoided during periods of active inflammation but may benefit selected patients, especially those with hypertension secondary to aortic or renal lesions. ⊃ systemic arteritis.

talar tilt test a musculoskeletal test used to assess the integrity of the calcaneo-fibular ligament. The person is supine or in side lying with a relaxed foot. The talus is tilted into abduction and adduction. Excessive tilting means excessive laxity or rupture of this ligament.

talipes *n* any of a number of congenital deformities of the foot and ankle. ⊃ talipes calcaneovalgus, talipes equinovarus.

talipes calcaneovalgus a congenital foot deformity usually caused by intrauterine posture. The foot having been fixed in an upturned position with the sole against the uterine wall. Improvement and usually complete recovery occurs with active movement after birth.

talipes equinovarus a common congenital foot deformity in which the heel is drawn up, the foot inverted and the hindfoot adducted—in the equinovarus position.

talipomanus clubhand.

talocalcaneal joint ⊃ subtalar joint.

talus *n* the astragalus. A tarsal bone situated between the tibia proximally and the calcaneus distally, thus directly bearing the weight of the body. It is the second largest bone of the ankle and articulates with the malleoli of the tibia and fibula at the ankle, with the calcaneus at the subtalar joint and with the navicular bone.

tapetum used as a general term for a covering of a cell layer. A mass of fibres of the corpus callosum that extend into the cerebral hemispheres. It forms part of the lateral wall of the lateral ventricle of the brain.

tapetum lucidum a reflecting pigment layer lying behind the visual receptors of the retina of certain mammals (e.g. cats, dogs), birds and fish which gives a shining appearance to the eyes when illuminated in the dark. The tapetum is located either in the pigment epithelium or in the choroid and covers either the whole fundus or more often only the upper and back portion. The role of the tapetum lucidum is to increase the probability of visual stimulation of the photoreceptors by reflecting light after having already traversed them once, thus aiding vision in dim illumination. In some species the tapetum consists of guanine crystals.

tampon *n* a plug used in the nose, vagina or other orifice to absorb blood or secretions.

tampon shock syndrome ⊃ toxic shock syndrome.

tamponade *n* **1.** insertion of a tampon to apply pressure to a structure in order to control haemorrhage. **2.** the abnormal compression of an organ, such as the heart, caused by the accumulation of blood or other fluid. ⊃ cardiac tamponade.

T_AN *abbr* anaerobic threshold.

tangential when a beam enters the body at an angle to avoid critical structures, for example, in the treatment technique for cancer of the breast.

tangential acceleration the acceleration of an object or body acting at a tangent to its direction of motion, e.g. when it is moving in a circle or around a curve. ⊃ acceleration, angular acceleration, gravitational acceleration, instantaneous acceleration, linear acceleration.

tangential velocity the velocity of an object or body acting at a tangent to its direction of motion (often when it is moving in a circle or around a curve). ⊃ angular velocity, instantaneous velocity, linear velocity, velocity.

tangent screen (*syn* Bjerrum's screen) a large plane surface for detecting and plotting the central visual field (about 50° in diameter) by moving the position of a stimulus (e.g. a white 1-mm pinhead). It consists of dull black cloth or other material perpendicular to the line of sight and placed usually 1 m away from the subject (2 m gives more accuracy). In the centre of the screen is a white spot that provides a fixation point and a series of radial and circumferential lines are sewn or drawn to facilitate the localization of the stimulus. ⊃ campimeter, perimeter.

tannins substances present in some plants. They bind to divalent metal ions such as zinc, ferrous iron, calcium, etc., present in foods, thus reducing the bioavailability of these ions for absorption from the food. Can lead to a deficiency of certain nutrients, (e.g. iron), if intake is marginal, such as can occur with a strict vegetarian diet.

tantalum (Ta) a metal used for various prostheses including plates for repairing defects in the skull.

tape a wide form of dental floss. ⊃ dental floss/tape.

taper to make or to become gradually more narrow. In endodontics. **1.** denoting the shape of root canal instruments and materials. ISO taper = 0.02 mm/mm (2%) taper. Equipment and materials may have increased tapers of 4–12%. **2.** to shape or flare a root canal so that it is narrowest apically and widest coronally.

tapeworm *n* cestodes. They include *Taenia saginata* (beef tapeworm), *Taenia solium* (pork tapeworm) and *Diphyllobothrium latum* (fish tapeworm). Dogs and cats are the definitive host for the tapeworm *Dipylidium caninum*, which may cause human disease. ⮑ *Diphyllobothrium, Taenia.*

taping the use of tape to prevent or treat injury. Taping is used to limit movements which would exacerbate the injury, whilst not inhibiting function. There is a lack of scientific evidence on its use to prevent injury, but it is widely used in the treatment of conditions such as ankle sprains and patellofemoral pain.

tapôtement *n* (*syn* tapping) massage manipulations in which the hands strike, or percuss, the body alternately and rhythmically; used to eliminate secretions, as in postural drainage, and in an invigorating massage. It may involve: beating with loosely clenched fists, clapping using clapped hands and producing a deep-toned sound, hacking using the ulnar (little finger side) borders of the hands and fingers, and pounding with the ulnar sides of loosely clenched fists.

tapping *n* 1. ⮑ aspiration. 2. ⮑ tapôtement.

TAR *acron* **T**otal **A**nkle **R**eplacement.

tardive dyskinesia abnormal movements. Repeated involuntary movements of the face, tongue, trunk and limbs. Associated with the long term use of typical antipsychotic (neuroleptics) drugs, particularly the phenothiazines, e.g. fluphenazine.

target thin tungsten plate on the anode of an X-ray tube which, when bombarded with electrons, produces X-rays.

target angle the angle between the X-ray beam and the face of the target, the target of an X-ray tube is set at an angle to maximize the target area and minimize the geometric unsharpness.

target cell 1. a leptocyte. A red blood cell that has a dark centre surrounded by a paler ring. It can occur in various blood disorders, such as haemoglobinopathies, iron deficiency anaemia, or in liver disease, or following splenectomy. 2. a general term applied to cells that have a specific receptor that is targeted by specific T-cells, antibodies, hormones, other chemicals, etc.

target heart rate heart rate (HR) range aspired to during aerobic training, with view to enhancing cardiovascular fitness. Always best set in relation to the individual's measured maximal heart rate (HR_{max}) or heart rate reserve (HRR), rather than general population figures. In exercise for health, 60–85% HR_{max} or 55–80% HRR may typically be prescribed.

target organ the organ that a dose of radiation is calculated for.

target zone (*syn* training zone) the use of heart rate ranges to indicate the intensity of effort required during exercise programmes.

tarsal 1. *adj* relating to the seven bones of the ankle or tarsus. 2. *adj* relating to the fibrous tissue of the eyelids (tarsus), or the tarsal glands. 3. *n* one of the seven bones of the ankle or tarsus.

tarsal coalition (peroneal spastic flat foot) an anomaly in which adjacent tarsal bones are fused together. Fusion may be bony or cartilaginous. The most common occurs between the calcaneus and the navicular with union across the mid-tarsal joint. Talocalcaneal coalition also occurs.

tarsal conjunctiva ⮑ conjunctiva.

tarsalgia *n* pain in the foot.

tarsal gland also called meibomian glands. Modified sebaceous glands of the eyelid. ⮑ meibomian glands.

tarsal tunnel syndrome common, painful foot condition, caused by compression of the posterior tibial nerve as it passes through the tarsal tunnel on the inner side of the ankle to the foot. Results in pain, numbness, burning and tingling along the sole of the foot towards the first three toes. Often the result of excessive pronation. Treatment aims to reverse the cause but surgery may be required.

tars/o- a prefix that either means 'foot', e.g. *tarsometatarsal*, or 'edge of eyelid', e.g. *tarsorrhaphy.*

tarsometatarsal *adj* relating to the tarsal and metatarsal region.

tarsoplasty blepharoplasty. Plastic surgery of the eyelid.

tarsorrhaphy *n* suturing of the eyelids lids together to protect the cornea.

tarsus *n* 1. the posterior half of the foot, containing the seven tarsal bones of the ankle. They are the talus, calcaneus, navicular, cuboid and three cuneiform bones. ⮑ Colour Section Figure 2. 2. the dense connective tissue found in each eyelid, contributing to its form and support—**tarsal** *adj.*

tartar *n* lay term for ⮑ dental calculus.

Tarui's disease (S Tarui, Japanese physician, 20th century) type VII glycogen storage disease in which there is a deficiency of muscle phosphofructokinase enzyme. It is characterized by exercise-induced fatigue and myalgia.

task a series of structured steps (actions and/or thoughts) intended to accomplish a specific goal. This goal could either be: 1. the performance of an activity. 2. a piece of work the individual is expected to do. (Reproduced with permission from the European Network of Occupational Therapy in Higher Education (ENOTHE) Terminology Project, 2008.)

task allocation the main approach to organizing nursing care when hospitals were established; it still persists to some extent in many areas of nursing. Where it continues, this is usually due to autocratic leadership styles and the continuing use of the biomedical model. Task allocation is based on a hierarchy of tasks where tasks are carried out according to the status of the caregiver and has much in common with an industrial production line, with each carer carrying out a limited range of care-related tasks for many patients/clients. It also reflects the hierarchical, ecclesiastical and military roots of nursing that value obedience and subservience. For example, in a hierarchy (on a surgical ward), tasks are allocated by seniority where: (a) senior nurses—administer drugs, care for wounds/dressing changes, speak to relatives, liaise with medical and other staff, serve meals; (b) junior nurses—carry out bed baths, give bedpans, complete fluid balance charts, take observations of vital signs; (c) untrained nurses/care assistants—help people to wash, serve drinks, feed patients, undertake general tidying up, arrange flowers; (d) domestic staff—undertake general cleaning, tidying, distribute water jugs and washing up. ⊃ named nurse, patient allocation, primary nursing, team nursing.

task analysis the process of identifying the sequence of structured steps that make up an activity.

task involvement a state in which the individual's goal is to demonstrate mastery of a task or personal improvement relative to self-referenced criteria, such as improving on their previous personal best. ⊃ ego involvement, learning goal.

task orientation a dispositional tendency to feel most successful in an activity when one demonstrates ability relative to one's self and personal improvement rather than in comparison to the performance of others. ⊃ achievement goal orientation, ego orientation.

task performance choosing, organizing and carrying out tasks in interaction with the environment. (Reproduced with permission from the European Network of Occupational Therapy in Higher Education (ENOTHE) Terminology Project, 2008.)

taste *n* gustation. A chemical sense closely linked with olfaction (smell) and, like smell, also involves stimulation of chemoreceptors by dissolved chemical. Taste buds contain sensory receptors (chemoreceptors) that are found in the papillae of the tongue and widely distributed in the epithelia of the tongue, soft palate, pharynx and epiglottis. They consist of small sensory nerve endings of the glossopharyngeal (ninth cranial nerves), facial (seventh cranial nerves) and vagus nerves (tenth cranial nerves). Some of the cells have hair-like microvilli on their free border, projecting towards tiny pores in the epithelium. The sensory receptors are stimulated by chemicals that enter the pores dissolved in saliva. Nerve impulses are generated and conducted along the glossopharyngeal, facial and vagus nerves before synapsing in the medulla and thalamus. Their final destination is the taste area in the parietal lobe of the cerebral cortex where taste is perceived. There are four basic tastes—sweet, sour, bitter and salt; all other tastes are combinations of these. This is probably an over-simplification because perception varies widely and many 'tastes' cannot be easily classified. However, some tastes consistently stimulate taste buds in specific parts of the tongue: sweet and salty, mainly at the tip, sour, at the sides, bitter, at the back. The sense of taste triggers salivation and the secretion of gastric juice. It also has a protective function, e.g. when foul-tasting food is eaten then reflex gagging or vomiting may be induced. The sense of taste is impaired when the mouth is dry because substances can be 'tasted' only if they are in solution.

tattoos permanent skin markings to facilitate accurate daily set up of patients during a course of radiotherapy.

taurine substance derived from the amino acid cysteine; it has a role in the conjugation of bile salts.

taurocholic acid one of the bile acids.

taurodontism a variation in tooth form in which the pulp chamber is enlarged, elongated and extends into the roots.

Taussig–Bing syndrome (H Taussig, American paediatric cardiologist, 1898–1986; R Bing, German/American surgeon, b.1909) transposition of the great vessels of the heart with ventricular septal defect straddled by a large pulmonary artery.

-taxia, taxis, taxy a suffix that means 'arrangement, coordination, order', e.g. *ataxy*.

taxis 1. movement towards or away from a stimulus. **2.** manual manipulation for restoring a structure to its normal position, such as a hernia.

taxonomy a classification system for naming organisms.

Tay–Sachs disease (*syn* gangliosidosis) (W Tay, British ophthalmologist, 1843–1927; B Sachs, American neurologist/psychiatrist, 1858–1944) an inherited lipid storage disease in which GM_2 ganglioside (carbohydrate-rich sphingolipid) accumulates within the nervous system. It is due to a deficiency of the enzyme β-N-acetylhexosaminidase and results in mental deterioration, blindness and death. The gene responsible is most commonly carried by individuals of Ashkenazic Jewish origins. ⊃ cherry-red spot.

TB *abbr* tuberculosis.

TBA *abbr* traditional birth attendant.

T-bandage used to hold a perineal dressing in position.

TBI *abbr* **1.** total body irradiation. **2.** traumatic brain injury.

TBSA *abbr* total burn surface area.

TCA *abbr* **1.** transverse chromatic aberration. ⊃ lateral chromatic aberration **2.** tricyclic antidepressant.

T-cell ⊃ lymphocyte.

T-cell receptor (TCR) receptor situated on the surface of T-cells. They recognize specific antigens presented to them by antigen presenting cells (APCs).

TCR *abbr* T-cell receptor.

TCRE *abbr* transcervical resection of endometrium.

T-cytotoxic (killer) cell ⊃ cytotoxic-T cell.

T-delayed hypersensitivity cell ⊃ delayed hypersensitivity T-cell.

TE *abbr* echo time.

TEA *acron* thermic effect of activity.

tea tree oil an aromatherapy essential oil.

team cohesion ⊃ group cohesion.

team midwifery system of midwifery management with midwives divided into teams to care for identified groups of women in order to improve communication and continuity of care by reducing the number of midwives whom an individual woman sees for maternity care. ⊃ caseload midwifery, continuity of care.

team nursing a method of care delivery designed to provide maximum continuity of patient-centred care. A small team of nurses, working together but led by one registered nurse, is responsible and accountable for the care of a particular group of patients for the length of time they require care in a particular setting. It differs from patient allocation or primary nursing in that it is based on the belief that a small group of nurses working together can give better care than if working individually, using the skills of all the team members to the benefit of each patient, but retaining continuity of care. Effective verbal and written communication between the team members is vital. ⮑ named nurse, patient allocation, primary nursing, task allocation.

teamwork working in collaboration with others. Most healthcare professionals work in teams and there is a widespread belief that they achieve more when working collaboratively than when working alone. Teams work by pooling skills, knowledge and resources. Each individual has his or her specific role but the team has common interests and objectives. Each member shares responsibility for the decisions made within the team, its overall functioning and the quality of its output. Teamwork allows for a broader base of skills, attitudes and values to be brought into practice and the decision-making process. Patients and clients should be central to any team involved in their care. ⮑ interdisciplinary team, intradisiplinary team, multidisciplinary team.

tear dilution test ⮑ Norn's test.

tear film ⮑ precorneal film.

tear layer ⮑ precorneal film.

tear lens ⮑ liquid lens.

tear meniscus (*syn* marginal tear strip, lacrimal prism, tear prism) a thin strip of tear fluid with concave outer surface at the upper and lower lid margins. It contains most of the exposed tear volume. The absence of a tear meniscus is an indication of a dry eye. ⮑ precorneal film.

tear prism ⮑ tear meniscus.

tear pumping the mechanism involving blinking which acts to bring fresh tears with oxygen and nutrients to the cornea behind a contact lens, and pumping stale tears containing carbon dioxide, lactic acid and other waste products from beneath the lens. It occurs most readily with hard contact lenses (between 14% and 20% of the tear volume is exchanged with each blink) and to a much smaller extent with soft lenses (between 1% and 5% of the tear volume is exchanged with each blink). ⮑ corneal hypoxia, oxygen transmissibility.

tear secretion there are two types of tear secretion: (a) basal tear secretion which occurs normally without any stimulation and comes mainly from the accessory glands of Krause and Wolfring. It maintains the cornea and conjunctiva continuously moist, but is reduced in dry eyes (e.g. keratitis sicca) and in older people; and (b) reflex tear secretion which is produced mainly by the lacrimal gland in response to an irritant and also depends on psychological factors. The amount of tears secreted amounts to 14–33 g per 24 hours or 0.5–2.2 µL/min, being about 2 µL/min at 15 years of age and less than 1 µL/min at 65 years of age. ⮑ basic secretion test, Schirmer's test, tearing reflex.

tearing reflex tears produced in response to irritation to the cornea or to the conjunctiva. ⮑ Schirmer's test, tears, tear secretion.

tears (*syn* lacrimal fluid) the clear watery fluid secreted by the lacrimal gland which, together with the secretions from the meibomian glands, the goblet cells, the gland of Zeis, as well as the accessory lacrimal glands of Krause and Wolfring, helps to maintain the conjunctiva and cornea moist and healthy. Periodic involuntary blinking spreads the tears over the cornea and conjunctiva and causes a pumping action of the lacrimal drainage system, through the lacrimal puncta into the nasolacrimal duct. Approximately 25% of the tears is lost by evaporation, the remaining 75% is pumped into the nasal cavity and over 60% of the tear volume is drained through the lower canaliculus. Tears contain water (98.2%), salts, lipids (e.g wax esters, sterol esters, hydrocarbons, polar lipids, triglycerides and free fatty acids), proteins (e.g. lysozyme, lactoferrin, albumin, IgA, IgE, IgG, complement proteins C3, C4, C5 and C9, and beta-lysin), magnesium, potassium, sodium, calcium, chloride, bicarbonate, urea, ammonia, nitrogen, citric acid, ascorbic acid and mucin. Tears have a pH varying between 7.3 and 7.7 (shifting to a slightly less alkaline value when the eye is closed) and the quantity secreted per hour is between 30 and 120 µL. ⮑ alacrima, blink, break-up time test, epiphora, fluorescein, hyperlacrimation, lacrimal apparatus, lacrimal gland, lysozyme, mucin, non-invasive break-up time test, precorneal film, phenol red cotton thread test, Schirmer's test, Sjögren's syndrome.

Tearscope plus the tradename of a hand-held instrument designed to view the tear film non-invasively. It uses a cold light source to minimize any drying of the tear film during the examination. It can be used directly in front of the eye or in conjunction with a slit-lamp biomicroscope to gain more magnification. Evaluation of the interference patterns of the anterior surface of the tear film lipid layer facilitates the diagnosis of the cause of dry eye symptoms, as well as screening patients for contact lens wear. The instrument also allows the measurement of the non-invasive break-up time. ⮑ meibomian glands, non-invasive break-up time test, precorneal film.

technetium (Tc) *n* a radioactive element which is produced by irradiation of molybdenum. An isotope of technetium ($^{99}Tc^m$) is used in radionuclide imaging for brain scanning.

technetium (Tc) bone scan a sensitive imaging investigation, utilizing the isotope technetium-99m ($^{99}Tc^m$). It can be used to estimate bone density as well as other bony pathology. In sport, it is used in the diagnosis of bony injury, especially for suspected stress fractures which may not show up on a conventional X-ray at an early stage. ⮑ osteoporosis.

technetium generator used to produce radionuclides artificially by bombarding the nuclei of elements with particles. Molybdenum-98 is placed in a neutron stream and neutrons are absorbed to produce molybdenum-99

S
T

which results in the emission of gamma rays; the molybdenum decays to form technetium-99m and this is removed from the generator as sodium pertechnetate which is used for radionuclide imaging.

tectal midbrain syndrome ➲ Parinaud's syndrome.

tectum of midbrain ➲ tectum of mesencephalon.

tectum of the mesencephalon (*syn* optic tectum, tectum of the midbrain) the structure comprising the plate of grey and white matter (called the tectal lamina) which forms the roof of the midbrain and from which project the inferior and superior colliculi. The area anterior to it is called the pretectal region. ➲ convergence-retraction nystagmus, inferior colliculi, pupillary fibres, retinotectal pathway, superior colliculi.

tectum of the midbrain ➲ tectum of the mesencephalon.

TEDs *acron* **T**hrombo**E**mbolic **D**eterrents.

teeth the 20 teeth of first or primary dentition ('baby teeth', deciduous, 'milk teeth') erupt between the age of 5/6 months and 2½ years (Figure T.1A). The permanent (secondary) dentition (adult teeth) of 32 teeth start to replace the deciduous teeth at about 6 years of age. The process is nearly complete by 12 years of age; the third molars or 'wisdom' teeth, if they erupt, will do so during the late teens and early 20s (Figure T.1B). ➲ Appendix 11, primary dentition, permanent (secondary) dentition, tooth.

teething *n* lay term for the discomfort during the eruption of the primary dentition in babies and young children. The process of tooth eruption, most commonly associated with the eruption of the relatively large primary molars in 1–2 year olds. May sometimes be associated with local and systemic signs of local irritation, e.g. redness and swelling of mucosa over the erupting tooth, increased salivation, irratibility and sleeplessness.

teeth whitening the application of chemical agents to the teeth in order to remove staining and improve cosmetic appearance.

TEF *abbr* thermic effect of food.

Teflon® polytetrafluoroethylene. A proprietary material used in surgery as a barrier membrane. May be used in guided bone or tissue generation procedures in surgical periodontics or prior to or during implant placement.

tegument *n* the skin or covering of the body.

teichopsia *n* also called scintillating scotoma. The appearance of shimmering zigzag lines that move across the visual field. Occurs during the aura of some types of migraine.

telangiectasis *n* dilatation of small blood vessels. Leads to small red lesions in the skin and mucosae.

telecentric pertains to an optical system in which its aperture stop is positioned so that the entrance pupil falls in the first focal plane, the exit pupil is at infinity, and the rays through the centre of the entrance pupil from all points on the object are parallel to the axis in the image space. Similarly, if the exit pupil lies in the second focal plane the entrance pupil will be at infinity, and the rays through the centre of the exit pupil will be parallel to the axis in the object space.

teleisotope unit equipment containing a radioactive source producing X or γ rays for teletherapy.

telemedicine the use of electronic technologies, such as telephone and the Internet, for consultations and diagnosis, monitoring patients with chronic diseases, for health professionals to seek advice from an expert and for patients to seek advice, etc. ➲ telemetry.

telemetry *n* literally 'measurement at a distance'. The electronic transmission of data including clinical measurement between distant sites. May be used for cardiac monitoring and monitoring fetal heart and uterine contractions, thus enabling ambulation during labour. Achieved by portable radio transmitter sending data measured from the subject to the observer's receiver. In exercise physiology, these data invariably include heart rate (HR); more sophisticated (but bulkier) equipment will also report other values, e.g. oxygen consumption.

telencephalon one of the secondary enlargements during embryonic development of the brain. It becomes the cerebrum and the basal nuclei.

teleopsia an anomaly of visual perception in which objects appear to be much further away than they actually are.

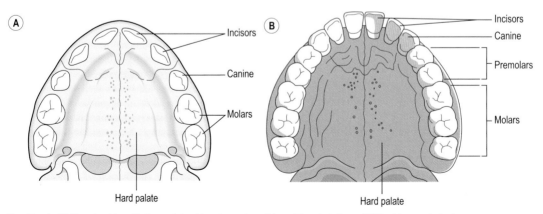

T.1 **Teeth** (A) First dentition (B) Second dentition (reproduced from Waugh & Grant 2006 with permission).

It may be due to vision in a hazy atmosphere, intoxication, certain mental health disorders, etc. ⊃ metamorphopsia, pelopsia.

teleradiology the electronic transfer of images and reports to remote centres, for example, general practitioner practices.

telescopic crown a two-part crown, the inner part being cemented to the tooth and the outer part fixed over it. Used in bridgework when there are problems concerning parallelism of the abutment teeth.

telescopic lens a thick lens system forming a galilean telescope used to magnify the image. It is mounted in some form of frame and is lighter than an actual telescope. It is used to help low vision patients for either distance or near vision, although for the latter the lens system (or sometimes a single lens) is often referred to as a microscopic lens. ⊃ low vision.

Teletex the sending of documents at high speed electronically.

Teletext the non-interactive public information service on television; BBC transmits Ceefax, the ITA transmits Oracle.

teletherapy *n* when an external source of radiation (X-rays or γ-rays) is directed to a tumour to give the maximum radiation dose to the tumour and the minimum dose to the surrounding healthy tissue—**teletherapeutic** *adj*, **teletherapeutically** *adv*.

telocentric *adj* describes a chromosome that has the centromere at one end.

telogen the resting stage in the hair growth cycle prior to shedding. ⊃ anagen, catogen.

telomeres *npl* protective regions of DNA at the ends of chromosomes that become shorter with age. Normally they stop chromosomal damage during cell division, but with increasing age the telomeres no longer function properly. Results eventually in genetic damage and cell death. ⊃ apoptosis.

telophase the last stage of nuclear division in mitosis (see Figure M.7, p. 488) and in both divisions of meiosis (see Figure M.3, p. 472). The set of chromosomes at each pole of the cell uncoil, the nuclear membrane reforms, the nucleoli reform and the mitotic spindle disappears. If the cell is to divide the cleavage furrow develops further until two cells are produced by cytokinesis. ⊃ anaphase, metaphase, prophase.

temperament *n* the usual mental attitude of the person.

template a pattern or mould. In dental prosthetics, a curved plate useful in arranging teeth along the imaginary curve of Spee during denture manufacture. ⊃ curve of Spee. *surgical template* a transparent pattern or mould used as an orientation guide for the surgical placement of osseo-integrated implants. Alternatively may aid in shaping the alveolar process prior to the insertion of immediate dentures.

temple *n* that part of the head situated between the outer angle of the eye and the top of the pinna.

temporal *adj* relating to the temple, to the side of the head, or the temporal bone, artery and so on.

temporal adaptation 1. awareness of time, the ability to remember the past, live in the present and plan for the future. **2.** the constructive use of time to achieve personal goals and maintain health and life satisfaction through daily activities.

temporal arteritis (*syn* giant cell arteritis—strictly speaking this term is usually reserved for the more generalized condition). An inflammatory disease of the wall of arteries, mainly of the extracranial vessels, which occurs in people who are over 60 years of age. The condition is characterized by headache and pain in muscles and joints, such as those of the jaws, and sometimes fever. A sudden loss of vision in one eye (amaurosis fugax) may occur in the first few weeks after the onset of the disease due to an occlusion of either the central retinal artery or of the short posterior ciliary arteries that supply the optic nerve. Prompt administration of systemic corticosteroids has been found to be of great value in the management of this condition. ⊃ Adie's pupil, amaurosis fugax, giant cell arteritis, ischaemic optic neuropathy.

temporal artery a branch of the external carotid artery, it has three branches that supply blood to the skin and muscles of the temporal, frontal and parietal scalp. The pulse may be felt in front of the upper part of the ear.

temporal bones the skull bones that lie one on each side of the head and form immovable joints with the parietal, occipital, sphenoid and zygomatic bones. Each temporal bone has several important features. The squamous part is the thin fan-shaped part that articulates with the parietal bone. The zygomatic process articulates with the zygomatic bone to form the zygomatic arch (cheekbone). The mastoid part contains the mastoid process, a thickened region behind the ear. It contains a large number of very small air sinuses which communicate with the middle ear and are lined with squamous epithelium. The petrous portion forms part of the base of the skull and contains the organs of hearing (the spiral organ) and balance. The temporal bone articulates with the mandible at the temporomandibular joint, the only movable joint of the skull. Immediately behind this articulating surface is the external auditory meatus/canal, which passes inwards towards the petrous portion of the bone.

temporal canthus ⊃ canthus.

temporalis the temporal muscle. A fan-shaped muscle of the head. Its origin is on the zygomatic arch and it inserts onto the coronoid process of the mandible. Important in mastication as its action is to close the mouth and retrude/protrude the mandible. It is innervated by the mandibular division of the trigeminal nerve (fifth cranial nerve).

temporal lobe lateral lobe of the cerebrum, beneath the temporal bone. It is concerned with audition and olfaction and also contains some association areas for learning and memory.

temporal lobe epilepsy (*syn* complete partial seizure, psychomotor epilepsy). ⊃ epilepsy.

temporary bridge in dentistry, a bridge made of temporary materials which is placed into position on bridge preparations

S
T

765

during the period in which the proper bridge is being constructed by the dental technician. ⊃ bridge.

temporary crown a full veneer crown made of aluminium, resin, stainless steel or acrylic resin to protect a tooth preparation and the soft tissues surrounding it. It is easily removed, maintains the occlusion and is placed in position while a permanent restoration is being constructed.

temporary filling in dentistry, a filling, usually of temporary cement that is intended to remain in place for a short time only. ⊃ provisional restoration.

temporary post crown a temporary crown that incorporates a post.

temporomandibular *adj* relating to the temporal region or bone, and the lower jaw.

temporomandibular joint (TMJ) one of two synovial joints (modified hinge or bicondylar joints) lying on each side of the skull, its bony components being the condyle of the mandible and the glenoid or articular fossa of the temporal bone. There are separate joints on each side of the face, but these function together as a single unit. The joint has two cavities divided by a flat fibrocartilage disc lying between the two bony surfaces. A loose fibrous capsule is arranged around the joint, attached to the temporal bone at the periphery of the articular fossa and eminence, and passing like a sleeve over the head of the condyle of the mandible, to be attached at its neck. It is strengthened by a stronger fibrous band laterally—the lateral ligament. The capsule, but not the disc of bony surface, is lined by a smooth shiny synovial membrane that secretes the lubricating synovial fluid filling both joint cavities. The articular disc is moulded to the rounded shape of the condylar head on its lower surface and the articular fossa and eminence of the temporal bone above it. The lateral pterygoid muscle of mastication is inserted into the articular disc, fibrous capsule and neck of the condyle. On contraction, the condylar head and disc move together to glide forwards onto the eminence. Dislocation of the joint occurs when they move beyond the height of the eminence.

temporomandibular joint dysfunction syndrome Costen's syndrome. Uni- or bilateral disturbance of the normal function of the temporomandibular joint. Symptoms may be clicking or grating of the joint, swelling and tenderness over the joint, and areas of pain in the face, neck, and muscles of mastication. May be associated with malocclusion of the teeth, resulting in malposition of the condylar heads in the joint and abnormal muscle activity, and by bruxism.

TEN *acron* Toxic Epidermal Necrolysis.

ten steps to successful breastfeeding ⊃ Baby Friendly Initiative (BFI).

tenaculum 1. an instrument for grasping and holding tissue. **2.** band of tissue that secures a body part in place. ⊃ retinaculum.

Tenckhoff catheter (H Tenckoff, American nephrologist, 20th century) a commonly used peritoneal dialysis catheter.

tendin/o, tend/o, ten/o- a prefix that means 'tendon', e.g. *tendinitis*.

tendon *n* a band of white, fibrous connective tissue that joins muscle to bone. Tendons consist of parallel bundles of collagen with little elastic tissue. This results in excellent mechanical strength but little elasticity. Tendons focus the strength of muscle contraction on a relatively small area of bone, maximizing pull and facilitating movement of the bone—**tendinous** *adj.* ⊃ paratendon, tendonitis (tendinitis).

tendonitis (tendinitis) *n* inflammation of a tendon. Usually the result of repetitive overuse movements, especially at high intensity. This causes micro-tears in the collagen matrix with inflammation, swelling, tenderness and pain, especially on specific movements. Pain is reproduced with resisted movements and tendon stretching, with active range of motion often normal, but with pain experienced at the end of range. More common in older athletes. Treatment aims to identify and reverse the cause, together with local anti-inflammatory measures such as RICE (rest, ice, compression and elevation), anti-inflammatory medication, electrotherapy and occasionally corticosteroid injection (into the paratendon to avoid tendon rupture). ⊃ epicondylitis, tenosynovitis.

tendon jerk reflex rapid reflex contraction of a muscle in response to a sudden stretch, elicited by tapping its tendon, and involving direct (monosynaptic) excitation of alpha (α) motor neurons in the spinal cord by afferent fibres from primary sensory endings in muscle spindles. The best known is the knee jerk: when the patellar tendon is tapped, the quadriceps muscle is caused to contract. Similar rapid monosynaptic reflexes operate, e.g. when the tendon of the biceps is tapped at the elbow or the Achilles tendon at the ankle. Also known as a phasic stretch reflex. ⊃ stretch reflex.

tendon organ ⊃ Golgi tendon organ.

tendonosis degenerative changes in tendons.

tenesmus *n* painful, ineffectual straining to empty the bowel or bladder.

tennis elbow ⊃ lateral epicondylitis.

Tenon's capsule (J Tenon, French pathologist/surgeon, 1724–1816) (*syn* Bonnet's capsule, capsule of the eyeball, fascia bulbi) the fascia around the globe of the eye in the socket. A fibrous membrane which envelops the globe from the margin of the cornea to the optic nerve. Its inner surface is in close contact with the episclera to which it is connected by fine trabeculae. These trabeculae also attach it to the extraocular muscles. The posterior surface of the capsule is in contact with the orbital fat. Anteriorly, it becomes thinner and merges gradually into the subconjunctival connective tissue. ⊃ episclera, ligament of Lockwood.

tenoplasty *n* a reconstructive operation on a tendon—**tenoplastic** *adj.*

tenorrhaphy *n* the suturing of a tendon.

tenosynovitis *n* also called tendosynovitis. Inflammation of the thin synovial lining of a tendon sheath, as distinct from

S
T

its outer fibrous sheath. It may be caused by mechanical irritation, overuse, trauma or by bacterial infection. There is pain, swelling and/or restricted movements. The swelling has a characteristically linear appearance, along the tendons.

tenotomy *n* division of a tendon.

tenovaginitis thickening of the fibrous tendon sheath.

TENS *acron* **T**ranscutaneous **E**lectrical **N**erve **S**timulation.

tensile force force applied along the fibres of a tissue. Excessive tensile forces cause a tearing of the tissues as they are stretched beyond their normal length.

tension the force with which a body or object resists extension. Also known as tension load. A measure of force developed within a muscle during contraction when it is not allowed to shorten, i.e. isometric contraction.

tension pneumothorax ⊃ pneumothorax.

tensor tympani a tiny muscle of the middle ear. It contracts reflexly (sound attenuation reflex), with another muscle the stapedius, to protect the ear from very loud sounds by reducing conduction. ⊃ stapedius.

tenth-value thickness the thickness of a substance that will transmit exactly one-tenth of the intensity of radiation falling on it.

tentorium cerebelli a fold of dura mater between the cerebellum and cerebrum. Damage during birth may result in intracranial bleeding.

TEPP *abbr* tetraethyl pyrophosphate.

teratogen *n* anything capable of disrupting embryonic/fetal growth and producing malformation. Classified as drugs, poisons, radiations, physical agents such as electroconvulsive therapy (ECT), infections, e.g. rubella and Rhesus and thyroid antibodies—**teratogenic, teratogenetic** *adj*, **teratogenicity, teratogenesis** *n*.

teratogenesis the processes by which teratogens, such as drugs, produce physical malformations, particularly during organogenesis during embryonic development.

teratology *n* the scientific study of teratogens and their mode of action—**teratological** *adj*, **teratologist** *n*, **teratologically** *adv*.

teratoma *n* commonly a tumour of the testis or ovary. It is of embryonic origin and usually malignant. Some testicular tumours have both seminoma and teratoma components. The cure rate for germ cell tumours has increased 10-fold with use of platinum-based chemotherapy—**teratomata** *pl*, **teratomatous** *adj*.

teres rounded and smooth. ⊃ ligamentum teres, teres major, teres minor.

teres major a rounded muscle crossing the shoulder. It forms part of the posterior axillary wall. Its origin is on the posterior scapula; it inserts, via a joint insertion tendon with the latissimus dorsi, on the anterior part of the humerus (lesser tubercle). It contracts to extend, adduct and medially rotate the humerus.

teres minor an elongated muscle crossing the shoulder. One of the four muscles comprising the rotator cuff. Its origin is on the scapula; it inserts on the humerus (greater tubercle). It stabilizes the shoulder joint by holding the humeral head

within the glenoid cavity and laterally rotates the humerus. ⊃ rotator cuff.

term 1. normal gestation period, a pregnancy of 40 weeks' gestation. **2.** a specific period of time, e.g a fixed term contract.

term infant a neonate born after 37 completed weeks' but before 43 weeks' gestation.

terminal hair coarse pigmented hair of the scalp and eyebrows. During puberty it replaces the vellus hair found around the external genitalia and axillae in both sexes, and forms the facial and body hair in males. ⊃ lanugo, vellus hair.

terminal hinge axis (dental) ⊃ transverse horizontal axis (dental).

terminal hinge position record ⊃ record.

termination of pregnancy (TOP) ⊃ abortion.

termination or stop codon the three-nucleotide sequence in mRNA that signals the end of a sequence of amino acids in a polypeptide chain. There are three stop codons: UAG, UGA and UAA (A = adenine, G = guanine, U = uracil).

ternary alloy a deprecated term for high copper amalgam alloy. ⊃ alloy.

terra alba ⊃ kaolin.

tertian *adj* recurring every 48 hours such as the fever in some types of malaria.

tertiary *adj* third in order.

tertiary care highly specialized healthcare services accessed through indirect referral via secondary care. Deals usually with uncommon or rare conditions. The specialized hospital care is provided by a regional or national centre, e.g. spinal injuries, certain cancers.

tertiary disease prevention is the monitoring and management of established disease in order to prevent the complications of the disease process, disability or handicap. For example monitoring of patients with diabetes in order to detect and treat early complications. ⊃ primary disease prevention, secondary disease prevention.

tesla (T) a unit for measuring the strength of a magnetic field. A magnetic flux density of 1 tesla exists if the force on a 1 metre long straight wire, carrying a current of 1 ampere, is 1 newton and the wire is placed at right angles to the direction of magnetic flux.

test cavity a dental diagnostic test used when all other vitality tests have proved inconclusive. The tooth is pulp-tested by cutting a small cavity in dentine (without a local analgesic) and observing the reaction.

testicle *n* ⊃ testis—**testicular** *adj*.

testicular artery one of two arteries that branch from the abdominal aorta to supply blood to the testes.

testicular cancer relatively rare cancers, but the most common cancer in young men under 35 years of age. Early detection is vital, as the cancer is highly curable if detected at an early stage; all men should be encouraged to examine their testes on a regular basis. Presentation is usually with a lump or painless swelling in one testis, or a dull ache or heavy feeling in the lower abdomen, anal or scrotal area.

S
T

The treatment modalities, which can be used alone or in combination, include orchidectomy, chemotherapy or radiotherapy.

testicular self-examination (TSE) regular examination undertaken by men to detect cancers or other testicular abnormalities.

testis *n* a male gonad. One of the two glandular structures contained in the scrotum of the male. The testis is the site of spermatogenesis (spermatozoa production). Immature cells the spermatids mature in a process called spermiogenesis (maturation stage of spermatogenesis); the mature spermatozoa are discharged via the vas deferens into the urethra at ejaculation. The testis secretes male sex hormones (androgens - testosterone and related hormones) and other hormones that include inhibins and activins. Spermatogenesis and testicular endocrine function are under the control of gonadotrophic hormones (follicle stimulating hormone [FSH] and interstitial cell stimulating hormone [ICSH], which is identical to luteinizing hormone in the female) from the anterior pituitary, and in turn of the hypothalamus. ⊃ spermatogenesis, spermiogenesis—**testes** *pl*. ⊃ undescended testes, Colour Section Figure 16.

testosterone *n* the major androgen, an anabolic steroid hormone produced by the testes. It is responsible for the development of the male secondary sexual characteristics and reproductive functioning.

tests (electrotherapy context) three specific tests are used on the relevant cutaneous area prior to applying a specific electrophysical agent. They are: (a) thermal discrimination if risk of thermal burns. This tests patient's ability to accurately distinguish heated from cooled objects applied cutaneously in treatment area; (b) sharp/blunt discrimination if there is risk of skin irritation, pain or electrolytic skin burns. This tests patient's ability to accurately differentiate sharp and blunt objects applied cutaneously in treatment area; (c) ice reaction test if there is risk of adverse skin reaction to ice. This tests the response of skin to local application of ice for 30 s or by checking under an icepack after 5 min. Prior to using many electrotherapeutic machines the therapist should test the output to ensure the machine is working and to obviate any risks to the patient. For example, *testing ultrasound output* by placing the applicator in a small metal bowl with face covered by water, rapidly increase and decrease output, bulk streaming visible as beam reflects from side of bowl (using other methods can damage applicator crystal); testing *electrical stimulation machine* by turning on and setting the output parameters, connecting the leads and the therapist placing damp fingers on electrodes or end of leads, gradually increasing output until they can feel it. Turn back to zero and connect to patient if operating satisfactorily; *laser* testing needs specialized equipment (photodiode) as does a pulsed shortwave diathermy machine. Other specific tests include assessing the grade of erythema (reddening of the skin) caused in response to a dose of ultraviolet rays (UVR) and the strength-duration test, which tests the normality of the

response of a nerve to electrical stimulation. ⊃ chronaxie, rheobase, strength–duration testing.

test-tube baby one produced by in vitro fertilization.

test type any letter, figure or character used for vision testing. The term test object or test target is a more general term which encompasses any pattern or object (e.g. checkerboard).

tetanus *n* **1.** (*syn* lockjaw) disease caused by the bacterium *Clostridium tetani*, an anaerobic spore-forming microorganism present in the intestine of domestic animals and humans, commonly found in soil, dust and manure. It produces a powerful exotoxin that affects the motor nerves causing muscle spasms, rigidity and convulsions. Active immunization with tetanus toxoid (TT) is available as part of routine programmes, as regular booster doses and when risk is increased. Tetanus immunoglobulin is available for passive immunization. ⊃ opisthotonos, risus sardonicus, trismus—**tetanic** *adj*. **2.** in the contraction of muscle, the summation that increases the force of contraction by increasing the frequency of stimulation to the maximum to produce a sustained contraction.

tetany *n* occurs in all syndromes or situations in which ionized calcium concentrations in the blood are low, for example as a result of alkalosis from hyperventilation (which may also be seen in sport) or alkali ingestion, or hypocalcaemia associated with hypoparathyroidism. Low ionized calcium concentrations cause increased excitability of peripheral nerves. In the absence of alkalosis, tetany usually occurs in adults only if total serum calcium is <2.0 mmol/L (8 mg/dl). Children are more sensitive than adults. In children, a characteristic triad of carpopedal spasm, stridor and seizures occurs, although one or more of these may be found independently of the others. The hands in carpal spasm adopt a characteristic position. Pedal spasm is much less frequent. Stridor is caused by spasm of the glottis. Adults complain of tingling in the hands and feet and around the mouth. Less often there is painful carpopedal spasm, while stridor and seizures are rare. Latent tetany may be present when signs of overt tetany are lacking. It is best recognized by eliciting Trousseau's sign; inflation of a sphygmomanometer cuff on the upper arm to more than the systolic blood pressure is followed by carpal spasm within 3 minutes. A less specific sign of hypocalcaemia is that described by Chvostek, in which tapping over the branches of the facial nerve as they emerge from the parotid salivary gland produces twitching of the facial muscles. ⊃ calcium, carpopedal spasm, Chvostek's sign, Trousseau's sign.

tetra- a prefix that means'four', e.g. *tetraplegia*.

tetrachromatic theory ⊃ Hering's theory of colour vision.

tetracosactide (Synacthen) test a test of adrenocortical function. Adrenocortical insufficiency is indicated if the plasma cortisol concentration fails to rise following an intramuscular injection of tetracosactide (an ATCH analogue).

tetracyclines *npl* a group of broad spectrum antibiotics, e.g. doxycycline. Problems associated with the tetracyclines include superinfection with gastrointestinal disturbances, bacterial resistance and vitamin B deficiency. They are also deposited in teeth and bone and should not be prescribed for pregnant or lactating women, or for children because they can lead to discoloration of the second dentition and bone abnormalities. ➲ Appendix 5.

tetradactylous *adj* having four digits on each limb.

tetraethyl pyrophosphate (TEPP) organophosphorous compound used as a commercial insecticide. Toxicity results from its powerful and irreversible anticholinesterase action.

tetralogy of Fallot ➲ Fallot's tetralogy.

tetraplegia *n* (*syn* quadriplegia) paralysis of all four limbs—**tetraplegic** *adj*.

tetrodotoxin the toxin present in the puffer fish.

TFR *abbr* total fertility rate.

TFT *abbr* thin film transistor.

TG *abbr* **1.** triacylglycerol. **2.** triglyceride.

TGC *abbr* time gain control.

TGF *abbr* transforming growth factor.

thalamencephalon the area of the brain containing the thalamus, epithalamus and subthalamus.

thalamic pain/syndrome pain that arises in the central nervous system. Caused by damage to the thalamus, usually caused by a stroke, leading to intractable pain and increased sensitivity affecting the contralateral (opposite) side of the body. The pain is described as intense burning pain, which is often made worse by touch.

thalamotomy *n* usually operative (stereotaxic) destruction of a portion of thalamus. Can be done for intractable pain.

thalamus *n* a collection of grey matter at the base of the cerebrum. Sensory impulses from the whole body pass through the thalamus en route to the cerebral cortex—**thalami** *pl*, **thalamic** *adj*. ➲ limbic system.

thalassaemia *n* a group of inherited haemoglobinopathies in which mutation or deletion of one or more globin genes results in an imbalance in the production of α and β globin molecules. Because it affects the deformability of the red cell, this imbalance leads to increased red cell breakdown and a failure of bone marrow red cell precursors to produce fully mature erythrocytes. This in turn leads to anaemia, the severity of which depends on the nature of the genetic defect. *beta thalassaemia* results most often from genetic mutations in the β globin genes. If both copies of the gene are affected (patient is homozygous for a mutation), a severe, transfusion-dependent anaemia, with jaundice and hepatosplenomegaly may result (beta thalassaemia major). By contrast, in the carrier (heterozygous) state where only one copy of the gene is mutated, there is often only a mild asymptomatic anaemia. The situation with *alpha thalassaemia* is more complex as there are four α globin genes, and the severity of alpha thalassaemia varies from asymptomatic, if only one gene is affected, to usually fatal in utero if four genes are affected (hydrops fetalis). Persons with three affected genes have so-called haemoglobin H disease and are often transfusion dependent.

thallium (Tl) a metallic element. Many thallium compounds are highly toxic.

thallium activator luminescent centres where about 10–15% of the energy deposited is converted to light energy. Used with sodium iodide as a scintillator crystal.

thallium-201 myocardial perfusion scintigraphy scan the radioisotope (radionuclide) thallium-201 (^{201}Tl) is administered intravenously to study myocardial perfusion. Useful in identifying myocardial ischaemia in the diagnosis of coronary artery disease when it can be combined with an exercise stress test; or a resting scan in the localization of a myocardial infarction.

thanatology *n* the scientific study of death, including its cause and diagnosis.

THC *abbr* total haemolytic complement.

theca *n* an enveloping sheath, especially of a tendon, or the dura mater—**thecal** *adj*.

thelarche *n* the commencement of female breast development; normally starts very early in puberty.

T-helper cell ➲ helper T-cells.

thematic analysis a research term. In qualitative research, the researcher attempts to categorize and analyse the themes that are produced from interviews.

thenar *adj* relating to the palm (hand) and the sole (foot).

thenar eminence the palmar eminence below the thumb.

theoretical saturation (data saturation) a research term. Used in qualitative research, the point where no new themes or concepts emerge from the data being collected.

theory of planned behaviour an extension to the theory of reasoned action which incorporates the construct of perceived behavioural control, these being a person's beliefs about whether or not they possess the necessary skills and resources to overcome any difficulties in engaging in the behaviour.

theory of reasoned action a social cognitive theory of relationships between attitudes and volitional behaviour which holds that intention is the immediate determinant of behaviour and that intentions are determined jointly by attitudes towards the behaviour and perceived social pressures to engage in the behaviour. It is underpinned by the belief that human beings usually behave in a rational way. Behavioural intentions, for example, to give up smoking, are influenced by the person's belief that a desired outcome will occur and that the outcome will be beneficial. Beliefs about what other people think the individual ought to do, the individual's motivation to comply with the wishes of others and how much control the individual believes he or she has are also important.

therapeutic abortion ➲ abortion.

therapeutic environment an environment that is arranged and designed to allow patients and clients to achieve their best performance. Environment has been shown to be a very important factor in rehabilitation, both physically and mentally.

therapeutic index an indicator of the difference between the therapeutic dose of a drug and a dose that causes toxicity. It can vary between individuals.

S
T

therapeutic play play that is structured and initiated by adults. It can be used for distraction, creating normality, helping children to express their fears and wishes, giving information, assessing developmental stages, etc. ⊃ normative play.

therapeutic soft contact lens (*syn* bandage lens) a hydrophilic contact lens used as a protective device for the cornea, as in entropion, trichiasis, or damage by application of a tonometer; as a pressure bandage to relieve pain, as in bullous keratopathy; to facilitate corneal healing, as in corneal erosion due to trauma; to improve vision during the healing process; and as a delivery mechanism for drugs, since soft contact lenses placed on the eye can slowly release a drug which was previously absorbed. Because of the risks associated with this type of lens, it is important to follow the patient very assiduously. ⊃ bullous keratopathy, Cogan's microcystic epithelial dystrophy, combination lens, entropion, piggyback lens, trichiasis.

therapeutics *n* the branch of medicine concerned with the treatment of disease states—**therapeutic** *adj*, **therapeutically** *adv*.

therapeutic use exemption (TUE) the authorization granted by the World Anti-Doping Agency for an athlete to use a drug such as salbutamol for the relief of bronchcospasm if strict criteria of therapeutic need are met.

therapy *n* treatment of a range of psychological or physical conditions. ⊃ occupational therapy, physiotherapy, speech and language therapy.

therapy verification film an X-ray film shielded by a lead sheet, which is placed behind the patient during one treatment to verify the area being treated. ⊃ portal imaging.

thermal *adj* pertaining to heat.

thermal capacity the heat energy in joules which is required to raise the temperature of the body by 1 kelvin unit.

thermal effect of ultrasound the heating of tissue by breaking down the air bubbles and cavities in the tissues.

thermal strain the physiological and psychological reaction to environmental thermal stress.

thermal stress the build-up of environmental conditions that stresses the thermoregulatory structures

thermic effect of activity (TEA) the energy expenditure of physical activity.

thermic effect of food (TEF) ⊃ diet-induced thermogenesis.

thermionic emission the process of releasing electrons from an emitter.

thermionic emitter a substance that releases electrons when heated.

thermistor *n* a device used to detect very small changes in temperature.

therm/o- a prefix that means 'heat', e.g. *thermography*.

thermoalgesia pain caused by high temperature.

thermoanaesthesia also known as thermoanalgesia. The inability to perceive the sensations of cold or heat.

thermoduric describes bacteria that are not destroyed by pasteurization.

thermogenesis *n* the production of heat by the body. It might be for maintaining temperature, or in response to food intake or drugs —**thermogenetic** *adj*. ⊃ brown adipose tissue (brown fat), diet-induced thermogenesis, non-shivering thermogenesis.

thermographic printing utilizes a film containing silver behenate that when exposed to light the resultant heat activates the silver and produces the image. ⊃ photo-thermographic printing.

thermography *n* an investigation that detects minute temperature differences over different body areas by use of an infrared thermograph that is sensitive to radiant heat. The uses include the study of blood flow and detection of cancers, such as breast cancer.

thermolabile *adj* capable of being easily changed or destroyed by heat.

thermoluminescence a property exhibited by some substances. When the substance is irradiated it stores energy, when heated photons of light are produced in proportion to the energy stored.

thermoluminescent dosimeters small disks containing lithium fluoride can be attached to a patient's body, the disks are then heated and the amount of light produced is compared to a standard to ascertain the amount of radiation received by the patient. A badge containing two lithium fluoride disks worn by radiation workers to estimate the radiation dose they have received to the skin and the whole body dose.

thermolysis *n* heat-induced chemical dissociation. Dissipation of body heat—**thermolytic** *adj*.

thermometer *n* an instrument for measuring temperature—**thermometric** *adj*. ⊃ clinical thermometer.

thermoneutral environment conditions designed so that the body temperature can be maintained with the least consumption of oxygen and energy.

thermophiles bacteria that grow best at temperatures above 55°C and can tolerate temperatures up to 80°C—**thermophilic** *adj*.

thermoplastic a substance that becomes softened on warming and then hardens on cooling. *thermoplastic impression material* (or *compound*) ⊃ impression material.

thermoreceptor a specialized nerve ending that responds to heat and cold.

thermoregulation the homeostatic mechanisms that maintain core body temperature within a normal range.

thermostable *adj* unaffected by heat. Remaining unaltered at a high temperature, which is usually specified—**thermostability** *n*.

thermostat equipment for controlling temperature.

thermotherapy *n* heat treatment, such as diathermy, warm compresses, electric pads, warm baths, etc.

thiamin(e) *n* a member of the vitamin B complex. It is concerned in carbohydrate, fat and alcohol metabolism. Deficiency causes beri-beri, mental confusion or cardiomyopathy. ⊃ Appendix 4, Korsakoff's psychosis/syndrome, Wernicke's encephalopathy.

S
T

thiazide diuretics a group of diuretics, e.g. bendro-flumethiazide (bendrofluazide), that act on the first part of the distal tubule of the nephron. They reduce sodium and chloride reabsorption, which increases the amount of water, sodium and chloride excreted. ⊃ Appendix 5.

thiazolidinediones a group of antidiabetic drugs (oral hypoglycaemics), e.g. rosiglitazone, which reduce blood glucose. ⊃ Appendix 5.

thick filaments ⊃ myofibrils, myosin.

Thiersch skin graft (K Thiersch, German surgeon, 1822–1895) ⊃ skin graft.

thimble in dentistry, a bridge retainer consisting of a thin, tube-like metal substructure to which a crown may be cemented. Has previously been used to overcome bridge insertion and retention problems. ⊃ bridge, bridge retainer.

thimble ionization chamber ⊃ ionization chamber.

thin filaments ⊃ actin, myofibrils.

thin film transistor (TFT) the technology used in laptop computer screens.

thin lens a lens or combination of lenses in which the refracting surfaces are regarded as coincident, that is in which the separation between surfaces does not appreciably alter the total power of the system. Most ophthalmic lenses are thin lenses, but the crystalline lens of the eye is considered to be a thick lens. For optical purposes contact lenses are also regarded as thick lenses. ⊃ principal plane.

third-class levers have the resistance and force on the same side of the fulcrum with the force closer to the fulcrum than the resistance; very common in the human body (e.g. biceps brachii concentric action in elbow flexion).

third degree tear ⊃ perineal tear.

third heart sound (S3) a sound heard early in diastole is normal in children and during pregnancy. ⊃ heart sounds.

third stage of labour from birth of the infant to complete expulsion of placenta and membranes, involving separation and expulsion of the placenta and membranes and control of haemorrhage. It may be managed physiologically (duration 5 minutes to 2 hours with an average of 20–30 minutes) or actively managed when an oxytocic drug is administered to expedite placental separation and to control haemorrhage. Active delivery of placenta and membranes using controlled cord traction may also be undertaken. ⊃ active management of the third stage of labour, physiological third stage.

thirst sensation arising when there is body fluid depletion, in response to increase in local osmolality in the hypothalamus and to neural and hormonal signals related to decreased blood volume and/or blood pressure; accompanied by production by cells in the hypothalamus of the water-retaining antidiuretic hormone (ADH) and its release from the posterior lobe of the pituitary gland. Normally, if fluid is lost from the body or intake is inadequate the person feels thirsty and usually remedies the situation by having a drink. However, certain groups of people are unable to respond to thirst; infants, small children, people with mobility problems, unconscious patients, people with a severe learning disability, or dementia and older adults (who may not experience thirst) are all at risk of fluid depletion.

thixotropy a term, which originates in engineering, relates to the inherent stiffness or viscosity in a muscle. It has been likened to the property of paint before and after stirring. The synovial fluid within joints has thoxotropic properties, whereby the fluid becomes less viscous as joint activity increases.

Thomas' test (H Thomas, British orthopaedic surgeon, 1834–1899) a test used to determine the presence of a fixed flexion deformity at the hip. The patient is supine, the hip is fully passively flexed and the lumbar lordosis is obliterated. If the opposite hip rises off the bed, this indicates a fixed flexion deformity of that hip. This may be due to tightness or restriction in the capsule, iliopsoas or rectus femoris muscles. To differentiate between the iliopsoas and rectus femoris as the source of restriction, the patient's knee is passively extended. If this results in the patient's hip dropping down into less flexion, then the restriction is in the rectus femoris muscle, since, by extending the knee, an element of stretch has been removed. If the hip is unaffected and remains in the same degree of flexion, independently of the knee extension, then the restriction is in the iliopsoas muscle.

Thomas' splint (H Thomas) splint used to immobolize fractures of the leg during transportation, and for use with various types of traction (Figure T.2).

Thompson's test also known as squeeze test. This tests the integrity of the gastrocnemius/soleus Achilles tendon complex. The patient lies prone. The physiotherapist or doctor squeezes the calf firmly just distal to its maximum circumference. If the tendon is intact, the foot will plantarflex. A positive test will occur if the tendon or muscle is ruptured and the ankle will not plantarflex. A palpable gap in the tendon or muscle belly may sometimes be observed if the tendon is ruptured.

Thomsen's disease (A Thomsen, Danish physician, 1815–1896) generalized myotonia with muscle hypertrophy. It is associated with a muscle channelopathy in which the

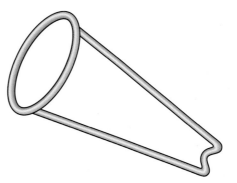

T.2 Thomas' splint (reproduced from Brooker 2006A with permission).

chloride ion channels in striated muscle are abnormal. ➲ muscle channelopathies.

thoracentesis *n* aspiration of the pleural cavity.

thoracic *adj* pertaining to the thorax.

thoracic aorta that portion of the descending aorta within the thorax. ➲ Colour Section Figure 9.

thoracic breathing inhalation by expanding the thorax, using the intercostal muscles to elevate the ribs, as compared to abdominal breathing using the diaphragm.

thoracic cage framework (ribs, costal cartilages, sternum and thoracic vertebrae), which protects the internal thoracic structures (especially lungs, heart and great vessels) and provides muscle attachments. Traumatic damage such as in road traffic accidents or in sport can range from local discomfort to fractured ribs and potential damage to the lungs and, rarely, the heart. The liver and spleen, although not in the thorax, are also protected by the lower ribs and can be damaged by their injury. ➲ pneumothorax.

thoracic cavity the chest. The cavity situated in the upper part of the trunk. Its boundaries are formed by a bony framework and supporting muscles: anteriorly—the sternum and costal cartilages of the ribs; laterally—12 pairs of ribs and the intercostal muscles; posteriorly—the thoracic vertebrae and the intervertebral discs between the bodies of the vertebrae; superiorly—the structures forming the root of the neck; and inferiorly—the diaphragm, a dome-shaped muscle, which separates it from the abdominal cavity. The main organs and structures contained in the thoracic cavity are: the trachea, two bronchi, two lungs, the heart, aorta, superior and inferior vena cava, numerous other blood vessels, the oesophagus, lymph vessels, lymph nodes and nerves.

thoracic duct the main channel commencing in the abdomen (cisterna chyli) that conveys lymph (chyle) from the legs, abdomen, left side of the chest and head and the left arm to the left subclavian vein.

thoracic nerves the thoracic nerves do not intermingle to form plexuses. There are 12 pairs and the first 11 are the *intercostal nerves*. They pass between the ribs supplying them, the intercostal muscles and overlying skin. The 12th pair are the *subcostal nerves*. The 7th to the 12th thoracic nerves also supply the muscles and the skin of the posterior and anterior abdominal walls. ➲ Colour Section Figure 11.

thoracic outlet syndrome although it involves the structures at the thoracic inlet in the neck, it is known as thoracic outlet syndrome. The cause may be structural due to the presence of a supernumerary rib (cervical rib) in the cervical region. Signs and symptoms are caused by compression of the brachial plexus (comprising the lower cervical nerves C5–C8 and the first thoracic nerve T1). Sometimes compression of the subclavian artery also gives rise to signs and symptoms. Presentation depends on the structures involved and can include shoulder and arm pain, numbness, paraesthesia, muscle wasting, muscle weakness, Raynaud's phenomenon affecting one arm, or loss of radial

pulse when the arm is abducted and externally rotated (Adson's sign). ➲ Adson's sign.

thoracic vertebrae twelve bones of the vertebral column. They have facets on their transverse processes and bodies for articulation with the ribs. ➲ vertebra (typical), Colour Section Figure 3.

thorac/o- a prefix that means 'thorax', e.g. *thoractomy*.

thoracolumbar fascia the fascia that covers the deep muscles of the back.

thoracoplasty *n* an operation on the thorax in which the ribs are resected to allow the chest wall to collapse and the lung to rest; previously used in the treatment of tuberculosis. Since the advent of antituberculous drugs it is extremely rare.

thoracoscope *n* an instrument which can be inserted into the pleural cavity through a small incision in the chest wall, to permit inspection of the pleural surfaces and division of adhesions by electric diathermy—**thoracoscopic** *adj*, **thoracoscopy** *n*.

thoracotomy *n* surgical exposure of the thoracic cavity. Usually undertaken to resect part or all of a lung. It involves rib resection and transection of major chest wall muscles.

Thoraeus filter ➲ compound filters.

thorax *n* the chest cavity—**thoracic** *adj*.

Thorington test a test for the measurement of heterophoria at near and at distance. It consists of a horizontal row of letters on one side of a light source and a horizontal row of numbers on the other side of that source. A Maddox rod, orientated horizontally, is placed in front of one eye and the patient who is fixating the light source is asked to report through which letter or number the vertical streak appears to pass, or to which it is closest. At 6 m the number of letters must be placed 6 cm apart to represent 1Δ steps. If the Maddox rod is in front of the right eye, the numbers on the right side of the source and the letters on the left, each number represents 1Δ of esophoria and each letter represents 1Δ of exophoria. The Thorington test can also be used at near. At 40 cm, for example, the separation of the letters and numbers must be 0.4 cm to represent 1Δ. It can also be placed vertically with the Maddox rod orientated vertically to measure vertical heterophoria. ➲ heterophoria, Maddox rod.

Thorn initiative training programme supported by funding from the Sir Jules Thorn Charitable Trust, the Thorn initiative training programme was established in 1991, in London, at the Institute of Psychiatry and at Manchester University. The programme provided mental health practitioners with the opportunity to develop skills in psychosocial interventions and management strategies to help reduce relapse rates. Initial evidence from the original programmes confirmed that training could enhance practitioners' knowledge and attitudes towards clients and their relatives who in turn derive significant benefits from the psychological interventions they receive.

thought stopping a technique of cognitive behaviour therapy in which individuals are trained to stop intrusive negative thoughts when they occur, either by the self-administration of a painful stimulus, such as snapping an elastic band worn around the wrist, or by bringing to mind a vivid mental image such as a stop sign. Typically, individuals are also trained to reframe the negative thoughts or replace them with positive self-talk. Sometimes known as thought stoppage.

THR *abbr* total hip replacement.

threadworm (pinworm) *n Enterobius vermicularis.* Tiny thread-like nematode worm that infests the intestine. ⊃ enterobiasis.

threatened abortion ⊃ threatened miscarriage.

threatened miscarriage characterized by slight vaginal bleeding whilst the cervix remains closed.

three-components theory ⊃ Young–Helmholtz theory.

three-dimensional reconstruction a digitally produced image that shows the depth, height and width of an object or objects.

three-dimensional ultrasound the creation of a computerized, reconstructed ultrasound image which represents the anatomical structure being investigated, for example, used to visualize the fetal face and the adult heart valves.

three-dimensional volume sequence ⊃ image acquisition time.

three-in-one syringe ⊃ syringe.

three-needle test a test for measuring stereoscopic visual acuity consisting of three fine rods placed vertically, two of them being fixed in the same plane, while the third one is movable in between. The subject views them through an aperture. The centre rod is placed in various positions backward and forward until the subject judges whether it is nearer or farther than the others. ⊃ Howard–Dolman test, stereopsis.

three phase a form of alternating current formed by three phases of current and voltage to enable more power to be supplied for static X-ray equipment. The line voltage is 398 volts in a three-phase supply.

three-quarter crown ⊃ partial veneer crown.

threonine *n* an essential (indispensable) amino acid.

threshold 1. the level at which a stimulus produces an effect or response. ⊃ pain threshold. **2.** in radiography, the point at which a film first shows a reaction to exposure. ⊃ sensitometry.

thrill *n* vibration as perceived by the sense of touch.

thrombectomy *n* surgical removal of a thrombus from within a blood vessel.

thrombin *n* the active enzyme formed from prothrombin. Thrombin is formed during both the extrinsic and intrinsic coagulation pathways; it converts fibrinogen to fibrin. ⊃ coagulation, prothrombin, thromboplastin.

thromb/o- a prefix that means 'blood clot', e.g. *thrombosis*.

thromboangiitis *n* clot formation within an inflamed vessel.

thromboangiitis obliterans ⊃ Buerger's disease.

thromboarteritis *n* inflammation of an artery with clot formation.

thromboasthenia *n* also called thrombasthenia. A decrease in platelet function. A rare inherited haemorrhagic disorder in which the platelets do not function normally in haemostasis.

thrombocyte *n* (*syn* platelet) functions in the coagulation of blood. ⊃ blood, platelet.

thrombocythaemia *n* a condition in which there is an increase in circulating blood platelets, which can encourage clotting within blood vessels. ⊃ myeloproliferative disorders, primary thrombocythaemia, thrombocytosis.

thrombocytopenia *n* a reduction in the number of platelets in the blood, which can result in spontaneous bruising and prolonged bleeding after injury—**thrombocytopenic** *adj.* ⊃ idiopathic thrombocytopenic purpura (ITP).

thrombocytosis *n* an increase in the number of platelets in the blood. It may arise in reaction to infection, bleeding, inflammation or malignancy or may indicate the presence of a bone marrow disorder.

thromboembolic *adj* describes the phenomenon whereby a thrombus or clot detaches itself and is carried to another part of the body in the bloodstream to block a blood vessel there. ⊃ deep vein thrombosis (DVT), pulmonary embolus (PE), venous thromboembolism (VTE).

thromboembolic deterrents (TEDs) ⊃ anti-embolism hoisery/stockings.

thromboendarterectomy *n* removal of a thrombus and atheromatous plaques from an artery.

thromboendarteritis *n* inflammation of the inner lining of an artery with clot formation.

thrombogenic *adj* capable of clotting blood—**thrombogenesis, thrombogenicity** *n*, **thrombogenically** *adv*.

thrombokinase *n* ⊃ thromboplastin.

thrombolytic *adj* pertaining to disintegration of a blood clot—**thrombolysis** *n*.

thrombolytic therapy the use of fibrinolytic drugs, such as alteplase, reteplase, tenecteplase and streptokinase to dissolve preformed intravascular fibrin occlusions in acute myocardial infarction, acute arterial thrombosis, deep venous thrombosis, pulmonary embolus and central retinal venous and arterial thrombosis.

thrombophilia *n* an inherited or acquired tendency to develop venous thrombosis. ⊃ factor V Leiden.

thrombophilia screen a series of tests used to identify familial or acquired disorders which increase thrombosis risk, e.g. antithrombin, protein C, protein S, activated protein C resistance, factor V Leiden and factor II variant lupus type inhibitor. Used to identify those individuals at increased risk of thrombosis. Pregnant women with a personal or family history of venous thromboembolism (VTE) (deep vein thrombosis or pulmonary embolus) should be offered the test to identify those at increased risk of intrauterine growth restriction, pre-eclampsia and fetal loss.

thrombophlebitis *n* inflammation of the wall of a vein with secondary thrombosis within the involved segment—**thrombophlebitic** *adj*.

thrombophlebitis migrans recurrent episodes of thrombophlebitis affecting short lengths of superficial veins:

S
T

deep vein thrombosis (DVT) is uncommon and pulmonary embolism (PE) rare.

thromboplastin *n* (*syn* thrombokinase) a substance released from damaged tissue to start the extrinsic coagulation pathway. *intrinsic thromboplastin* produced by the interaction of several factors during coagulation. It is more active than *tissue thromboplastin* (factor III) of blood coagulation, which interacts with other factors in the formation of a fibrin clot. ➲ activated partial thromboplastin time (APTT).

thrombopoiesis the formation of platelets from megakaryocytes in the bone marrow. The process is stimulated by cytokines, such as thrombopoietin.

thrombosis *n* the unwanted, intravascular formation of a blood clot—**thromboses** *pl*, **thrombotic** *adj*. ➲ coronary thrombosis, deep vein thrombosis.

thromboxanes *npl* regulatory lipids derived from arachidonic acid (fatty acid). They are released from platelets and cause vasospasm and platelet aggregation during platelet plug formation. ➲ haemostasis.

thrombus *n* an intravascular blood clot—**thrombi** *pl*.

thrush *n* ➲ candidiasis.

thrust force that propels a body or object in the required direction of motion. ➲ propulsive force.

Thylstrup Fejerskov index index (dental).

thymectomy *n* surgical excision of the thymus gland.

thymic-parathyroid aplasia absence of the thymus gland and parathyroid glands. ➲ DiGeorge's syndrome.

thymine *n* a nitrogenous base derived from pyrimidines. With other bases, one or more phosphate groups and a sugar it is part of the nucleic acid DNA. ➲ deoxyribonucleic acid.

thymocytes *npl* cells found in the dense lymphoid tissue of the thymus gland—**thymocytic** *adj*.

thymol a colourless crystalline substance used as an antifungal or antibacterial medicament.

thymoma *n* a tumour arising in the thymus—**thymomata** *pl*.

thymopoietin *n* peptide hormone secreted by the thymus gland.

thymosin *n* peptide hormone secreted by the thymus gland.

thymus *n* a lymphoid gland lying behind the sternum and extending upward as far as the thyroid gland. It is well developed in infancy and attains maximum size during puberty; thereafter the lymphatic tissue is replaced by fatty tissue. It produces thymic hormones (thymosins and thymopoietin) that ensure the proper development of T lymphocytes. The autoimmune condition myasthenia gravis results from pathology of the thymus gland—**thymic** *adj*.

thyratron a gas-filled device allowing current to flow in one direction only, containing an anode, a cathode and a grid. A negative potential on the grid can stop the electron flow and therefore can act as an on–off switch.

thyristor a solid-state replacement for a thyraton which can act as an electric switch.

thyrocalcitonin *n* ➲ calcitonin.

thyrocervical trunk a branch from the subclavian artery. It divides into three branches; the inferior thyroid artery, transverse cervical artery and the suprascapular artery.

thyroglobulin *n* a colloid stored in the thyroid follicles used for the production of thyroxine, one of the thyroid hormones.

thyroglossal *adj* pertaining to the thyroid gland and the tongue.

thyroglossal cyst a retention cyst caused by blockage of the thyroglossal duct: it appears on one or other side of the neck.

thyroglossal duct the embryonic passage from the thyroid gland to the back of the tongue. In this area thyroglossal cyst or fistula can occur.

thyrohyoid *n* a muscle of the throat involved in the co-ordinated events of swallowing. Its origin is on the thyroid cartilage and it inserts onto the hyoid bone.

thyroid *adj* pertaining to the thyroid gland.

thyroid acropachy periosteal hypertrophy of the digits that occurs rarely in some thyroid diseases.

thyroid antibody test the presence and severity of autoimmune thyroid disease is diagnosed by the levels of thyroid-stimulating immunoglobulins in the blood.

thyroid cartilage the main cartilage of the larynx; it has two halves, which fuse in the midline. ➲ Colour Section Figure 6.

thyroid crisis also known as hyperthyroid crisis or thyroid storm. A very rare complication of hyperthyroidism caused by a sudden release of thyroid hormones into the blood. It is associated with infection or may occur following thyroidectomy in a patient insufficiently prepared with antithyroid drugs, or treatment with radioactive iodine. It is a life-threatening medical emergency characterized by pyrexia, tachycardia, atrial fibrillation, restlessness, confusion, agitation and possibly altered consciousness.

thyroid eye disease ➲ thyroid ophthalmopathy.

thyroid gland a two-lobed endocrine gland, either side of the trachea (Figure T.3). It secretes three hormones: triiodothyronine (T_3) and thyroxine (T_4) under pituitary control, which stimulate metabolism, and calcitonin from the follicular cells, which helps to regulate calcium and phosphate homeostasis. The two iodine-containing hormones thyroxine (T_4) and triiodothyronine (T_3) are necessary for normal growth in childhood, and crucial in the control throughout life of energy metabolism. Their release is regulated by thyroid-stimulating hormone (thyrotrophin) from the anterior pituitary, and in turn by the hypothalamus. Thyroxine and triiodothyronine target most body cells (except in the central nervous system) where they modify enzyme synthesis, thereby controlling the rate of aerobic metabolism and heat production. Thus overactivity (hyperthyroidism) causes increase in basal metabolic rate (BMR) and body temperature with weight loss, and deficiency (hypothyroidism) the reverse. ➲ hyperthyroidism, hypothyroidism.

thyroid ophthalmopathy (*syn* dysthyroid eye disease, thyroid eye disease) disease of the thyroid gland which leads to

S
T

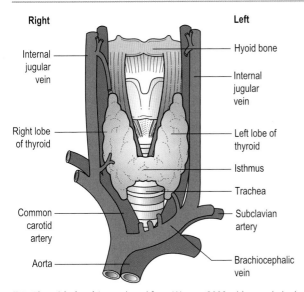

Right | Left

Internal jugular vein — Hyoid bone

— Internal jugular vein

Right lobe of thyroid — Left lobe of thyroid

— Isthmus

— Trachea

Common carotid artery — Subclavian artery

Aorta — Brachiocephalic vein

T.3 Thyroid gland (reproduced from Watson 2000 with permission).

ocular manifestations. There are two main types: mild and severe. The mild type occurs in Graves' disease in which most or some of the typical signs may be present and to a different extent. The severe type is much less common and affects the sexes equally in middle age. All the signs of Graves' disease are present but are more pronounced with the addition of oedema of the eyelids and of the conjunctiva, conjunctival injection, enlargement of the extraocular muscles and in a few cases there is also optic neuropathy due to compression of the optic nerve or its blood supply with consequent visual loss, colour vision impairment and often diplopia. ⊃ accommodative insufficiency, Graves' ophthalmopathy, optic neuropathy, superior limbic keratoconjunctivitis.

thyroid-stimulating hormone (TSH) also called thyrotrophin. Pituitary hormone that stimulates the secretion of the thyroid hormones thyroxine and triiodothyronine.

thyroid-stimulating hormone assay radioimmunoassay of the level of thyroid-stimulating hormone in the serum. Used in the diagnosis of hypothyroidism.

thyroidectomy *n* surgical removal of part or the whole of the thyroid gland.

thyroiditis *n* inflammation of the thyroid gland; can occur postpartum, following viral infection (De Quervain's), or due to autoimmune diseases. ⊃ Hashimoto's disease, Riedel's thyroiditis.

thyr/o, thyroid/o- a prefix that means 'thyroid gland', e.g. *thyroxine*.

thyrotoxicosis ⊃ hyperthyroidism.

thyrotrophic *adj* (describes) any substance that stimulates the thyroid gland, e.g. thyrotrophin (thyroid-stimulating hormone [TSH]) secreted by the anterior pituitary gland.

thyrotrophin-releasing hormone (TRH) a hypothalamic peptide which stimulates the release of thyroid-stimulating hormone by cells in the anterior pituitary gland.

thyroxine (T$_4$) *n* the principal hormone of the thyroid gland, it contains four atoms of iodine. It is essential for metabolism and development. Used in the treatment of hypothyroidism. ⊃ triiodothyronine.

TI *abbr* **1.** inversion time. **2.** treatment index.

TIA *abbr* transient ischaemic attack.

tibia *n* the shin bone; the larger of the two bones in the lower part of the leg; it articulates with the femur superiorly and the talus inferiorly, it also joins the fibula at the proximal (anterior or superior) and the distal (inferior) tibiofibular joints. ⊃ Colour Section Figures 2, 3.

tibial *adj* relating to the tibia.

tibial arteries anterior and posterior tibial arteries formed by the division of the popliteal artery, supply blood to the lower leg. The anterior tibial artery passes forwards between the tibia and fibula and supplies the structures in the front of the leg. It lies on the tibia, runs in front of the ankle joint and continues over the dorsum (top) of the foot as the *dorsalis pedis artery*. The posterior tibial artery runs downwards and medially on the back of the leg. Near its origin it gives off a large branch called the *peroneal artery*, which supplies the lateral aspect of the leg. In the lower part it becomes superficial and passes medial to the ankle joint to reach the sole of the foot where it continues as the *plantar artery*. ⊃ Colour Section Figure 9.

tibialis anterior a superficial, anterior muscle of the lower leg. The origin is on the lateral condyle of the tibia, the upper tibia and the interosseous membrane. It inserts on the medial cuneiform bone (a tarsal bone) and the first metatarsal by way of a long tendon. It contracts to facilitate dorsiflexion of the foot. ⊃ Colour Section Figure 4.

tibialis muscles muscles occupying the anterior and posterior compartments of the lower leg with tendons extending into the foot. ⊃ tibialis anterior, tibialis posterior, tibialis syndrome.

tibialis posterior a deep, posterior muscle of the lower leg. Its origin is on the top of the tibia and fibula and on the interosseous membrane. It inserts on the tarsal bones and the second to the fourth metatarsals on the underside of the foot arch. It contracts to facilitate plantarflexion and foot inversion; contributes to the stability of the medial longitudinal foot arch.

tibialis syndrome acute inflammation, usually the result of overuse, results in the so-called *tibialis syndrome* where swelling in the tight compartment causes pain and tenderness on specific movements. Treatment is of the inflammation and of any identified cause such as over-pronation. ⊃ anterior compartment syndrome, chronic exertional compartment syndrome, compartment syndrome, posterior compartment syndrome.

tibial nerve a branch of the sciatic nerve. It descends through the popliteal fossa/space to the posterior aspect of the leg where it innervates the skin and muscles. It passes under the medial malleolus to supply the muscles and skin of the sole of the foot and toes. ⊃ Colour Section Figure 11.

tibial veins anterior and posterior tibial veins form the popliteal vein. ⊃ Colour Section Figure 10.

S
T

tibi/o- a prefix that means 'tibia', e.g. *tibial*.

tibiofibular *adj* pertaining to the tibia and the fibula. ➲ distal tibiofibular joint, proximal tibiofibular joint.

tic *n* purposeless involuntary, spasmodic muscular movements and twitchings, due partly to habit, but may be associated with a psychological factor.

tic douloureux ➲ trigeminal neuralgia.

tick *n* a blood-sucking parasite, larger than a mite. Some of them are involved in the transmission of relapsing fever, typhus, etc.

tidal volume/air the volume of air that passes in and out of the lungs in normal quiet breathing.

tied numbers results of the same value.

Tietze syndrome (A Tietze, German surgeon, 1864–1927) costochondritis. A self-limiting condition of unknown aetiology. There is no specific treatment. Differential diagnosis is myocardial infarction.

TIFF (TIF) *abbr* tagged information file format.

tight junction a junction between cells where the cell membranes are tightly bound together, it limits or prevents the movement of molecules between cells. ➲ gap junction.

tilt table a standing device that can be used for patients who are unable to stand, such as those with paraplegia or quadriplegia. It can be used to position patients at any angle between horizontal and vertical.

time bomb a device used by some software suppliers to prevent piracy of programs.

time gain control (TGC) a method of compensating for the attenuation of ultrasound as it passes through the tissues so that the deep echoes appear equally as reflective as superficial echoes.

time-of-flight angiography a technique in magnetic resonance imaging (MRI) to enhance the blood flowing into a slice by ensuring that the blood does not become saturated by previous radiofrequency pulses.

timer an electronic or mechanical clock used in the processing of radiographs. *X-ray timer* an electric or mechanical switch mechanism used to complete the electrical circuit during the production of X-rays.

time scale sensitometry a method of producing a characteristic curve by keeping all exposure factors constant, covering the film with a piece of lead rubber and exposing the film a number of times, moving the rubber to reveal more film for each exposure or producing darkened strips on the film by doubling the exposure time for each subsequent step.

time-to-event paradigm in sport psychology, a research paradigm for manipulating the components of anxiety or examining their relationships with other variables based on the reliable observation that cognitive and somatic anxiety tend to dissociate during the period leading up to a competitive event. Cognitive anxiety tends to be high and stable during the days leading up to an event and then falls when the event begins, whereas somatic anxiety remains low and stable during the days leading up to an event, rises just before the start of the event, and falls once the event begins. ➲ cognitive anxiety, somatic anxiety.

tin (Sn) a white metallic element.

tin dioxide in dentistry, a white insoluble compound used as a polishing agent.

tin foil an extremely thin base metal foil used as a separating medium in denture construction.

tincture a drug or other substance prepared in an alcoholic solution.

tine a prong, such as the point of a probe.

tinea *n* (*syn* ringworm) a fungal infection of the skin, hair or nails caused by a variety of dermatophytes: *Trichophyton*, *Epidermophyton* and *Microsporum*. Usually named for the area of the body affected, i.e. *tinea barbae*, the beard area; *tinea capitis*, the head; *tinea corporis* (circinata), the body; *tinea cruris* (dhobie itch), the groin; *tinea pedis*, the foot (athlete's foot); *tinea unguium*, the nails.

Tinel's sign (J Tinel, French neurologist, 1879–1952) a test of nerve regeneration, tapping the area over the nerve causes tingling distal to the injury. It can also be used as a diagnostic sign in carpal tunnel syndrome.

tinnitus *n* an abnormal perception of buzzing, thumping or ringing sounds in the ears.

tinted lens an absorptive lens having a noticeable colour and absorbing certain radiations more than others. ➲ absorptive lens, bleaching, cosmetic contact lens, glass, photophobia, sunglasses, transmission curve.

TIPSS *abbr* transjugular intrahepatic portasystemic stent shunting.

tissue *n* a collection of cells or fibres of similar function, forming a structure, often in a background stroma. There are four main groups of tissue in the body—connective, epithelial, muscular and nervous.

tissue–air ratio the ratio of the dose rate at a point in the patient to that at the same point in air without the patient being present.

tissue compensator an attenuator placed in the primary beam during radiotherapy of irregular parts of the body, to maintain the dose distribution and the skin sparing effect.

tissue conditioner in dentistry, a type of soft liner for prostheses used for a short period and intended to improve the condition of the soft tissues lying beneath the prostheses.

tissue culture cells or tissues grown in vitro and maintained artificially.

tissue Doppler imaging the analysis of the Doppler signals from a moving structure, for example, the myocardium of the heart, exhibiting a large amplitude but low frequency.

tissue equivalent material a substance that interacts with ionizing radiation in the same way that a patient would interact with the radiation, it therefore has the same scattering and absorption properties of human tissue.

tissue forceps ➲ forceps.

tissue harmonic imaging in ultrasound, using the secondary frequencies sent back to the probe by tissue or contrast media such as air bubbles to improve contrast and spatial resolution in larger subjects as the far field is improved. ➲ contrast, spatial resolution.

tissue phantom ratio the ratio of the axis dose rate at a depth d in a phantom to the axis dose rate at a reference depth in the same phantom.

tissue plasminogen activator (t-PA) an endopeptidase enzyme that activates plasminogens. Produced naturally by endothelial cells lining blood vessels and other cells. Needed for fibrinolysis, the last stage of haemostasis, in which the fibrin clot is dissolved by plasmin when healing is complete. Also produced by recombinant DNA technology for use in thrombolytic therapy. ⊃ urokinase.

tissue respiration ⊃ respiration.

tissue surface in dentistry, that part of a denture that is in contact with the denture-bearing area.

tissue thromboplastin ⊃ thromboplastin.

tissue typing a number of tests used to determine the degree of histocompatibility between the tissue of the donor and prospective recipient. ⊃ human leucocyte antigen, major histocompatibility complex.

tissue viability primarily the management of wounds, but also involves the prevention of tissue damage, protecting vulnerable skin and maintaining the health of tissue.

titanium (Ti) a metallic element used alone or as an alloy for surgical implants.

titanium oxide in dentistry, a pigment used to provide white colour in opaque fissure sealants.

titration *n* volumetric analysis using standard solutions to determine the concentration of a substance in solution.

titre *n* a standard of concentration per volume, as determined by titration. Unit of measure used to assess antibody concentration in serum.

titubation *n* abnormal head and trunk movements when sitting, and unsteady stumbling gait.

TIVA *abbr* total intravenous anaesthesia.

TKR *abbr* total knee replacement.

T$_{LAC}$ *abbr* lactate threshold.

TLC *abbr* total lung capacity.

TLS *abbr* tumour lysis syndrome.

T-lymphocyte (T-cell) ⊃ lymphocyte.

TMJ *abbr* temporomandibular joint.

TMS *abbr* transcranial magnetic stimulation.

TNF *abbr* tumour necrosis factor.

TNM classification *abbr* tumour, node (lymph) and metastasis. ⊃ staging.

tobacco amblyopia toxic amblyopia.

toco- a combining form meaning 'childbirth'. For example *tocolytics*.

tocography *n* process of recording uterine contractions using a tocograph or a parturiometer. ⊃ cardiotocography.

tocolytics *npl* a group of drugs that relax uterine muscle. They have a restricted role in the inhibition of preterm labour. ⊃ beta (β)-adrenoceptor agonists. ⊃ Appendix 5.

tocopherols *npl* group of chemicals with vitamin E activity which includes the important α-tocopherols. They are widely distributed in many foods and function as important antioxidants in biological membranes. ⊃ alpha (α)-tocopherols.

tocotransducer a piece of electronic equipment used to measure the pressure felt over the abdomen during a uterine contraction.

tocotrienols *npl* a group of chemicals that have vitamin E activity. They have similar biological action to tocopherols but are less potent.

Todd's paralysis (R Todd, British physician, 1809–60) the short-lived paralysis that can follow some types of epileptic seizure.

togaviruses a family of RNA viruses they include the rubella virus and several spread by insects, such as those causing yellow fever, dengue and encephalitis.

token part of a computer network that indicates if a node can write to the network.

token ring the circular computer network which carries the tokens enabling them to signal to the nodes.

tokophobia morbid fear of childbirth.

tolerable upper intake level the maximum intake of a nutrient through foods with added nutrients, or nutritional supplements that is not likely to pose a risk of being harmful to health.

tolerance *n* the ability to endure the application or administration of a substance, usually a drug; or to undertake a specific activity. ⊃ drug tolerance, exercise tolerance.

Toller view ⊃ transpharyngeal projection.

-tome a suffix that means 'cutting instrument', e.g. *microtome*.

tomography *n* a radiographic technique to produce a sharp plane within the body by blurring the structures above and below the image by moving the X-ray tube and film around a fulcrum—**tomographic** *adj*, **tomogram** *n*, **tomograph** *n*, **tomographically** *adv*.

-tomy a suffix that means 'incision of', e.g. *enterotomy*.

tone *n* a quality of sound, or the normal, healthy state of tension. ⊃ muscle tone.

tongue *n* the mobile muscular organ situated in the floor of the mouth. It is attached by its base to the hyoid bone and by a fold of its mucous membrane covering, called the frenulum, to the floor of the mouth. The superior surface consists of stratified squamous epithelium, with numerous papillae (little projections), containing nerve endings of the sense of taste, sometimes called the taste buds. There are three varieties of papillae. Vallate papillae, usually between 8 and 12 altogether, are arranged in an inverted V shape towards the base of the tongue. These are the largest of the papillae and are the most easily seen. Fungiform papillae are situated mainly at the tip and the edges of the tongue and are more numerous than the vallate papillae. Filiform papillae are the smallest of the three types. They are most numerous on the surface of the anterior two-thirds of the tongue. The main arterial blood supply to the tongue is by the lingual branch of the external carotid artery. Venous drainage is by the lingual vein which joins the internal jugular vein. The nerves that innervate the tongue are: the hypoglossal nerves (twelfth cranial nerves) which supply the voluntary muscle tissue, the lingual branch of

S
T

the mandibular nerves which are the nerves of somatic (ordinary) sensation, i.e. pain, temperature and touch, the facial and glossopharyngeal nerves (seventh and ninth cranial nerves) which are the nerves of the special sensation of taste. The tongue plays an important part in: the mastication (chewing) of food, swallowing (deglutition), speech and taste (gustation). ⊃ taste. *bifid tongue* a tongue that is split in the anterior region by a longitudinal fissure. *black hairy tongue* a condition characterized by elongation of the filliform papillae on the dorsum of the tongue, without desquamation, which forms a thick matted brown or black layer. Usually due to heavy smoking or to broad spectrum antibiotic therapy. *cleft tongue* ⊃ bifid tongue. *fissured, furrowed tongue* a tongue with several longitudinal fissures or grooves. *hairy tongue* ⊃ black hairy tongue. *magenta tongue* a magenta-coloured tongue due to a deficiency of the B vitamin riboflavin. ⊃ geographic tongue, strawberry tongue, tongue tie.

tongue depressor a flat spatula used to depress the tongue during examination of the fauces.

tongue guard a metal device, usually attached to a saliva ejector, designed to protect the tongue from rotating instruments during tooth preparation.

tongue thrust thrusting of the tongue between the teeth during the act of swallowing or speech. May cause a malocclusion.

tongue tie ankyloglossia. A congenital condition in which the tongue is fixed to floor of the mouth.

tonic *adj* 1. used to describe a state of continuous muscular contraction, as opposed to intermittent contraction. 2. *n* a lay term for a medicinal product that increases general well-being.

tonic accommodation ⊃ resting state of accommodation.

tonic-clonic seizure ⊃ epilepsy.

tonic contraction of the uterus sustained abnormal uterine contraction, either generalized which may lead to fetal anoxia, or localized, i.e. a constriction ring, which forms most commonly round the fetal neck, adversely affecting the progress of labour.

tonic convergence ⊃ tonic vergence.

tonicity 1. the normal tone or tension present in muscle. 2. describes the effective osmotic pressure of a solution. ⊃ hyperosmolarity, hypo-osmolarity.

tonic pupil ⊃ Adie's pupil.

tonic vergence (*syn* dark vergence, tonic convergence) the passive state of vergence of the eyes in the absence of a stimulus, i.e. when the eyes are in total darkness or when looking at a bright empty field. This position is maintained by the tonus of the extraocular muscles. Only at death or when paralysed do the eyes return to their anatomical position of rest and tonic vergence disappears. ⊃ physiological position of rest, resting state of accommodation, tonus.

tonofibril bundles of very fine tonofilaments present in epithelial cells. They are part of the supportive cytoskeleton of cells and are involved in intercellular contact and adhesion by converging at the desmosomes.

tonography *n* continuous measurement of blood, or intraocular, pressure. *carotid compression tonography* normally occlusion of one common carotid artery causes an ipsilateral fall of intraocular pressure. Used as a screening test for carotid insufficiency.

tonometer *n* an instrument for measuring intraocular pressure. ⊃ applanation, Goldmann tonometer.

tonometry the measurement of pressure or tension. Usually applied to intraocular pressure (IOP).

tonsillectomy *n* surgical removal of the palatine tonsils.

tonsillectomy position the three-quarters prone position to prevent inhalation (aspiration) pneumonia and asphyxiation.

tonsillitis *n* inflammation of the tonsils. It is often caused by *Streptococcus pyogenes*. There is a severe sore throat, dysphagia, pyrexia, earache and enlarged lymph nodes. ⊃ Colour Section Figure 120.

tonsilloliths *npl* concretions arising in the body of the tonsil.

tonsillopharyngeal *adj* relating to the tonsils and pharynx.

tonsils *npl* small aggregations of lymphoid tissue located around the pharynx. Forming part of body defences they contain macrophages and are a site for lymphocyte proliferation. There are *lingual tonsils* under the tongue, *nasopharyngeal tonsils* located on the posterior wall of the nasopharynx (called adenoids when enlarged) and the *palatine tonsils* found in the oropharynx, one on each side in the fauces between the palatine arch—**tonsillar** *adj*. ⊃ Waldeyer's ring.

tonus muscle tone. The normal condition of partial muscle contraction controlled by reflexes.

tooth *n* hard calcified structures in the mouth used for masticating food. Composed largely of dentine with enamel covering the crown and cementum covering the root surface. The pulp occupies the central cavity at the core of the crown (pulp chamber) and the channel running along the length of the root (root canal) (Figure T.4A)—**teeth** *pl*. There are four basic types in permanent (secondary) dentition: incisor, canine, premolar, molar (Figure T.4B). The different types have specific actions, for example the incisors have a cutting or shearing edge and the molars are adapted for grinding food. ⊃ canine tooth, Hutchinson's teeth, incisor tooth, molar tooth, permanent (secondary) dentition, premolar tooth, primary dentition, teeth, wisdom tooth. *accessory tooth* ⊃ supernumerary tooth. *acrylic (resin) tooth* a tooth made of acrylic resin. *anatomic (anatomical tooth)* artificial tooth whose crown simulates the morphology of a natural tooth. *anchor tooth* ⊃ anchorage. *ankylosed tooth* ⊃ ankylosis. *artificial tooth* manufactured tooth used as a substitute for a natural tooth in a prosthesis and usually made of porcelain or acrylic resin. *avulsed tooth* tooth that has been forcibly displaced from the alveolus. *baby tooth* colloquial name for a primary tooth. *buck tooth* colloquialism for prominent projecting anterior maxillary teeth. *conical (peg-shaped) tooth* malformed teeth found in ectodermal dysplasia and other disorders and occasionally in unaffected children. *cracked tooth* ⊃ cracked tooth syndrome. *cuspless tooth* also known

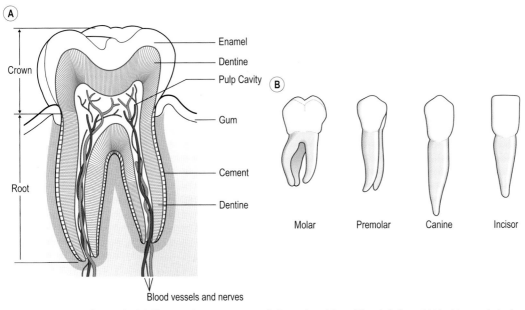

T.4 (A) Structure of a tooth. (B) Shapes of permanent teeth (reproduced from Waugh & Grant 2006 with permission).

as *flat cusp teeth*. Teeth designed without cusps and used in a prosthesis where the registration of centric occlusion presents difficulties. *dead tooth* common but erroneous term for a pulpless tooth. *diatoric tooth* artificial tooth with holes in its base into which the denture base material flows when processed and thus attaches the tooth to the base. Also called *pinless tooth. dilacerated tooth* ⊃ dilaceration. *double tooth* term used to describe either a geminated tooth, formed by the partial splitting of a tooth germ, or a fused tooth, formed by the fusion of two tooth germs. *eye tooth* ⊃ canine tooth. *embedded tooth* tooth that has not erupted because of lack of eruptive force. *flat cusp tooth* ⊃ cuspless tooth. *Fournier's tooth* ⊃ Moon's tooth. *fused tooth* teeth that have undergone partial or complete union of their tooth germs during development. *geminated tooth* ⊃ gemination. *hereditary brown opalescent tooth* ⊃ dentinogenesis imperfecta. *Hutchinson's (notched) tooth* a tooth abnormality seen in congenital syphilis and affecting primarily the incisors, canines and first permanent molars. The teeth are hypoplastic and the incisors have a screwdriver or peg-shaped appearance. *hypoplastic tooth* ⊃ hypoplasia. *impacted tooth* tooth prevented from erupting normally either by overlying bone or by an adjacent tooth. *milk tooth* ⊃ primary dentition. *missing tooth* tooth missing from the dentition because of congenital factors, exfoliation, extraction, avulsion, etc. *molar tooth* ⊃ molar tooth. *Moon's tooth* malformed, small, domed first molars seen in patients with congenital syphilis, also known as *Fournier's teeth. natal tooth* teeth present prior to birth. *neonatal tooth* teeth that erupt during the first month of life. *non-anatomic tooth* artificial tooth whose occlusal surfaces are not copies of the natural dentition, but have been given special forms designed to more nearly fulfil the requirements

of mastication and tissue tolerance. *non-functional tooth* tooth that is not in occlusion because of the absence of the opposing tooth in the other jaw. *non-vital tooth* tooth that does not respond to normal pulp testing stimuli. Term often inaccurately used to refer to a pulpless tooth. *notched tooth* ⊃ Hutchinson's tooth. *peg-shaped tooth* ⊃ conical tooth. *permanent tooth* ⊃ permanent (secondary) dentition. *pink tooth* tooth that has undergone idiopathic internal resorption which gives it a pink coloration due to the visibility of the granulation tissue within the pulp chamber. *pinless tooth* ⊃ diatoric tooth. *plastic tooth* ⊃ acrylic (resin) tooth. *posterior tooth* the premolar and molar teeth. *primary tooth* ⊃ primary dentition. *pulpless tooth* tooth from which the pulp has been extirpated. Commonly but inaccurately called a *dead* or *non-vital tooth. secondary tooth* ⊃ permanent (secondary) dentition. *Steele's interchangeable tooth* or *facing*. Artificial tooth manufactured with a standardized slot that fits in a matching metal backing, thus allowing its easy replacement should the facing fracture. *supernumerary tooth* tooth of abnormal form in excess of the usual number. *supplemental tooth* supernumerary tooth of normal appearance. *temporary tooth* ⊃ primary dentition. *tooth ache* pain in a tooth, generally due to caries or trauma producing a pulpitis. *tooth-borne* term describing a prosthesis that relies entirely on the abutment teeth for support. *tooth brush* a manual or powered brush designed to remove plaque from teeth. *tooth brush injury* an injury to a tooth or gingiva caused by incorrect or excessive tooth brushing, or by the use of a stiff textured brush. *tooth brushing* ⊃ tooth brushing technique. *tooth cleaning* or *polishing paste* a blend of fine abrasive particles, bonding agents, flavouring and colouring matter together with medicaments and other chemicals. Used to clean and polish

S
T

the surfaces of teeth and restorations. Also called toothpaste or dentifrice. *tooth depression* ⟶ extrusion. *tooth fracture* uncomplicated fracture involving enamel or enamel and dentine without involving the pulp. Complicated fracture involving enamel, dentine and pulp. *tooth fulcrum* axis about which a tooth moves when a lateral force is applied. *tooth germ* group of embryonic cells that develop to form a complete tooth. *tooth position* deprecated term for intercuspal position. *tooth preparation* ⟶ tooth or cavity preparation. *Turner's tooth* hypoplastic permanent tooth due to injury or inflammation of the preceding primary tooth. *tube tooth* artificial tooth constructed with a vertical circular hole in its base into which a pin or cast post can be inserted for attachment to a denture base. *unerupted tooth* ⟶ embedded tooth. *wisdom tooth* the lay term for a third molar.

tooth brushing technique *Bass tooth brushing technique* an effective method for the removal of dental plaque. The toothbrush filaments are placed at an angle of 45° to the long axis of the teeth, with the filament ends pointed towards the gingival margins. Slight pressure is then applied to remove the filaments into the sulcular regions where, once they are engaged, a vibratory motion is utilized, moving the brush back and forth with very short strokes, keeping the ends of the filaments in the sulcus. *Charter's tooth brushing technique* a method of cleaning utilized when the interdental papillae do not fill the embrasure spaces. The technique is contraindicated where there are full inter-dental spaces. The filaments of the brush are placed at a 45° angle, directed towards the occlusal surfaces. The sides of the filaments are then placed against the mar-ginal gingivae and the teeth, extending the filaments into the approximal spaces. A firm, rotary/vibratory movement is utilized while keeping the filaments in position. A soft multitufted brush is recommended, particularly after peri-odontal surgery. *roll tooth brushing technique* a technique in which the toothbrush is placed buccally in the first selected quadrant with its bristles resting on the gingivae, pointing away from the teeth. The filaments are then rolled across the gingiva, up the teeth towards their occlusal surfaces allowing the filaments to sweep into the inter-proximal spaces. This should be repeated about eight times before moving to another quadrant and after dealing with the lingual aspect in a similar manner.

tooth buds the embryonic teeth. The deciduous teeth by 6 weeks' gestation and those of the permanent teeth by week 10.

tooth drifting the migration of teeth from their normal position in the dental arches.

toothfriendly ⟶ safe-for-teeth.

tooth or cavity preparation the preparation of a tooth or cavity involves the removal of carious and weakened tissue from a tooth and the shaping of sound tissue to accept and retain a temporary or permanent restoration.

toothpaste a dentifrice. Powder or paste used on a toothbrush to clean accessible areas of teeth. Contains mild abrasives, flavouring, colouring, often fluoride and sometimes medicaments.

tooth surface loss the loss of surface tooth structure or toothwear due to abrasion, attrition, or erosion, or a combination of these processes.

tooth transplantation the removal of a tooth from its socket and its replacement in a new position in the alveolar bone of the maxilla or mandible.

TOP *acron* termination of pregnancy.

tophus *n* a small, hard concretion forming on the ear lobe, on the joints of the phalanges, etc. in gout—**tophi** *pl.*

topical *adj* describes the local application of drugs to skin and mucous membrane—**topically** *adv.*

topical analgesic surface (or topical) analgesic/anaesthetic.

topical fluoride the application to the surface of the teeth of a substance containing a fluoride agent, in order to render them more resistant to caries. May be in the form of a solution, gel, foam, mouthwash, varnish or paste. *professionally applied topical fluoride (PATF)* the topical fluoride gels, foams, solutions varnishes and prophylactic pastes applied in the dental surgery by dentists and dental care professionals. *self-applied topical fluoride (SATF)* the topical fluoride toothpastes and mouthrinses applied by individuals, usually at home.

Topogometer a device attached to a keratometer that allows a measurement of the curvature of the cornea off the visual axis. It consists of an illuminated fixation light that can be moved along two axes, both of which are perpendicular to the axis of the keratometer. Scales are provided with the device to indicate, in millimetres, the amount of decentration of the visual axis from the optical axis of the keratometer at the corneal surface. This device helps in the fitting of contact lenses, by providing an estimation of the flattening of the peripheral cornea and of the position of the corneal apex. This instrument has been superseded by computerized instruments. ⟶ keratometer, videokeratoscope.

topographical occlusal projection ⟶ oblique occlusal projection.

topography *n* a description of the regions of the body—**topographical** *adj*, **topographically** *adv.*

top up epidural anaesthesia repeat administration of the bupivicaine used for epidural anaesthesia following insertion of the cannula and administration of the first dose of the drug by the anaesthetist. Appropriately trained and assessed midwives are permitted by the Nursing and Midwifery Council (NMC) to perform this technique, sub-ject to cross-checking with a colleague and written instructions from the anaesthetist. Maternal blood pressure must be recorded every 5 minutes for 30 minutes and quarter hourly thereafter.

TORCH infection a group of infections (including **t**oxoplasmosis, **o**ther (syphilis), **r**ubella, **c**ytomegalovirus and **h**erpes) for which the neonate can be screened especially on admission to a special care unit.

toric lens this is usually a meniscus-type lens with a toroidal convex or concave surface. A toroidal surface is a surface with meridians of least and greatest curvature located at

S
T

right angles to each other. ⊃ astigmatic lens, meniscus lens, spherocylindrical lens.

torpor *n* **1**. decreased response to a stimulus. **2**. physical or mental inactivity.

torque ⊃ moment of force.

torque–angular velocity relation obtained from a series of measurements of the two parameters on an isokinetic dynamometer; the nearest approximation to a muscle force–velocity relationship which can be obtained from an intact limb but falling short of exact fit, both inevitably, because no anatomical joint retains constant geometry throughout its range of movement, and also often for neurophysiological reasons, as voluntary muscle activation varies with shortening velocity, a feature which is particularly marked in knee extension. ⊃ moment of force, momentum.

Torres bodies intranuclear eosinophilic inclusions found in the liver in cases of yellow fever. ⊃ yellow fever.

torsion *n* **1**. twisting, for example a torsion of a testis, or an ovarian cyst. **2**. force applied to a body or object that deforms (or tends to deform) it in a 'twisting' manner. Also known as torsion load.

torsion of the testis twisting of the structures supporting the testis. The blood supply is disrupted and can result in testicular infarction.

torticollis *n* (*syn* wryneck) a painless contraction of one sternocleidomastoid muscle. The head is slightly flexed and drawn towards the contracted side, with the face rotated over the other shoulder.

torulosis ⊃ cryptococcosis.

torus a swelling, a rounded projection. *torus mandibularis* a developmental bony protuberance sometimes found on the lingual aspect of the mandible in the premolar region. May cause difficulty in the fitting of complete dentures. *torus palatinus* a developmental bony eminence sometimes found in the midline of the hard palate.

total ankle replacement (TAR) a replacement arthroplasty in which the diseased painful ankle joint is totally removed and replaced with a prosthesis. It is usually performed to restore ankle function and relieve pain in patients who have severe arthritis (rheumatoid arthritis or osteoarthritis).

total arterial cerebral infarction a cerebrovascular accident (stroke) caused by an infarct involving the total anterior circulation supplying the brain. ⊃ circulus arteriosus.

total body imaging the radionuclide imaging of the whole of the body to detect metastatic spread from cancers.

total body irradiation (TBI) a treatment used in the management of some cancers, e.g. haemopoietic tissue. The aim of the treatment is to deliver a uniform dose to the whole body, using megavoltage photons and tissue compensation. Used prior to a haemopoietic stem cell transplantation (bone marrow transplant).

total burn surface area (TBSA) a formula for predicting outcomes after a burn injury: 100 − (age + TBSA) = percentage chance of surviving. ⊃ Lund and Browder's charts, rule of nines.

total efficiency the ability of a phosphor to produce light; it is dependent of its ability to absorb energy and convert it to light.

total fertility rate (TFR) a fertility rate expressed as the average number of children per woman. ⊃ fertility rate.

total gastrectomy ⊃ gastrectomy.

total glycated haemoglobin (GHb) ⊃ glycated (glycosylated) haemoglobin.

total hip replacement (THR) procedure the hip joint is the largest and deepest joint in the body that takes the form of a multi-axial spheroidal joint with three degrees of freedom of movement with high levels of congruency (stability and surface area for stress transmission) and extensive range of movement. In total hip replacement a metal alloy femoral head and stem (e.g. stainless steel, chromium cobalt) with high-molecular-weight (high-density) polyethylene cup are used. Where the small head of the Charnley prosthesis is used the procedure is known as the low-friction arthroplasty (LFA). Operating time is around 90 minutes and the surgical approach to the hip-joint depends on surgeon's preference and impacts upon postoperative rehabilitation. Commonly used approaches include the lateral trans-trochanteric division necessitating trochanteric rewiring at closure and posterolateral intermuscular division. The femoral neck is divided, the joint dislocated (where possible) and the head removed. The femoral canal and acetabulum are reamed down to fresh bleeding bone and prepared for component implantation. The cavity size depends on fixation technique. If the components are to be cemented *in situ*, trial components are inserted and size/fit determined. These are then removed and the quick-setting cement, available impregnated with antibiotics, is pushed into the cavities. The implants (surfaces protected) are pushed into the cement—a complete cement mantle between the implant and the bone is essential for even distribution of forces and therefore implant life/procedure success. Significant pressure is applied to ensure this. The joint is then relocated and tested for stability. Once the surgeon is satisfied, the joint is adducted, flexed and medially rotated to dislocate the joint. The surface protection is removed, the joint relocated and closure commenced. If the greater trochanter was sawn off for access then it is rewired back onto the femur with specialized wiring techniques, developed to resist breaking. The soft tissues are repaired in their layers and deep and superficial drains may or may not be used (Birch and Price 2003). (Birch A, Price A 2003 Joint arthroplasty. In: Porter S (ed.) Tidy's Physiotherapy, 13th edn. Butterworth Heinemann, Oxford.)

total intravenous anaesthesia (TIVA) general anaesthetic produced with intravenous drugs only and no gases.

total knee replacement (TKR) a replacement arthroplasty in which the diseased painful knee joint is totally removed and replaced with prostheses for the tibial and femoral parts of the joint. It is usually performed to relieve pain and minimize disability in patients who have severe arthritis (rheumatoid and osteoarthritis); it may be undertaken to

S
T

correct deformity and or instability of the knee joint. ⊃ unicondylar (unicompartment) knee replacement.

total linear attenuation coefficient (μ) the fraction of the X-rays removed from a beam per unit thickness of the attenuating material.

total lung capacity (TLC) the volume of air in the lungs after the greatest inspiratory effort.

total mass attenuation coefficient graphs the sum of the individual mass attenuation processes, that is: energy spectrum of the X-ray beam, density and atomic number of the tissue passed through and the separation of the patient, plotted as a graph of energy against incidence.

total parenteral nutrition (TPN) ⊃ parenteral nutrition.

total quality management (TQM) a whole organization approach to quality where all employees are expected to take responsibility for quality. It aims to ensure quality at every interface and improve effectiveness and flexibility throughout the organization.

total replacement arthroplasty replacement of the entire joint. For example, replacement of the head of femur and the acetabulum, both being cemented into the bone. ⊃ hemiarthroplasty, total ankle replacement (TAR), total knee replacement (TKR), total hip replacement (THR) procedure, unicondylar knee replacement.

total scanning time with multi-slice computed tomography (CT) this is commonly reduced to the time of data acquisition as large volumes can be scanned in a single breath hold.

total transmittance ⊃ transmittance.

Tourette's syndrome also known as Gilles de Tourette syndrome. A disorder characterized by involuntary grimaces, tics and arm movements and shouting, and the use of obscene language (coprolalia) and rude gestures.

tourniquet *n* an apparatus for the compression of the blood vessels of a limb. Designed for compression of a main artery to control bleeding. It is also often used to obstruct the venous return from a limb and so facilitate the withdrawal of blood from a vein. Tourniquets vary from a simple rubber band to a pneumatic cuff.

Towne's projection a radiographic technique for demonstrating the occipital region of the skull. Used to demonstrate the mandibular condyles in the coronal plane. ⊃ reversed Towne's projection.

Townsend index composite index of deprivation in the population. Sum of the standardized values of the percentages of households without cars, households not owner-occupied, overcrowded and unemployed in an electoral ward. The components (socio-economic variables) are drawn from census information. ⊃ Jarman.

toxaemia *n* a generalized poisoning of the body by the products of bacteria or damaged tissue—**toxaemic** *adj*.

tox, toxic/o- a prefix that means 'poison', e.g. toxicity.

toxic *adj* poisonous, caused by a poison.

toxic epidermal/epidermolytic necrolysis (TEN) also known as Lyell's syndrome or non-staphylococcal scalded skin syndrome. A condition that usually occurs in adults in response to an adverse drug reaction. There is erythema

and hyperpigmentation, the formation of bullae and scaling, which gives the appearance of scalded skin. ⊃ staphylococcal scalded skin syndrome, Colour Section Figure 121.

toxic shock syndrome (TSS) (*syn* tampon shock syndrome), a potential but rare complication of tampon use, but it does occur in non-menstruating women and men. It is caused by the toxins of the bacterium *Staphylococcus aureus* found at various sites including the perineal area in healthy people. Bacterial contamination of the tampon occurs and the bacteria multiply within the vagina. The bacterial toxins enter the bloodstream and cause pyrexia, headache, vomiting and diarrhoea, rash, and sometimes life-threatening hypovolaemic shock.

toxicity *n* the quality or degree of being poisonous.

toxicology *n* the science dealing with poisons, their mechanisms of action and antidotes to them—**toxicological** *adj*, **toxicologically** *adv*.

toxin *n* a poison, for example a bacterial toxin that damages or kills cells, or a chemical. Examples include poisonous substances produced by a living organism, e.g. snake venom, and a wide variety of substances produced by some fungi (mycotoxins), such as alphatoxin and plants including many alkaloids such as hemlock. Bacterial toxins are described as either endotoxin or exotoxins such as botulinum toxin which causes botulism and various enterotoxins produced by virulent strains of *Escherichia coli* (E. coli) which cause acute gastroenteritis; the effects of which may range from mild illness to life-threatening haemolytic uraemic syndrome. ⊃ endotoxin, *Escherichia*, exotoxin.

Toxocara *n* genus of nematode roundworm of the dog and cat, e.g. *Toxocara canis, Toxocari cati*. Humans can be infested. ⊃ toxocariasis.

toxocariasis *n* also known as visceral larva migrans. Infestation with *Toxocara*. Infestation occurs by eating with hands contaminated from contact with affected animals, especially puppies. The ova can exist for several months in soil contaminated by infected faeces from dogs or cats. Because the worms cannot develop properly in humans (incorrect host) the larvae move through the body before dying. This can lead to problems in the skin, liver and the eye: rashes, skin irritation, fever, hepatomegaly and possible blindness.

toxoid *n* a toxin altered in such a way that it has lost its poisonous properties but retained its antigenic properties. *toxoid antitoxin* a mixture of toxoid and homologous antitoxin in floccule form, used as a vaccine, e.g. in immunization against diphtheria.

toxoid vaccines ⊃ vaccines.

Toxoplasma a genus of protozoon, e.g. *Toxoplasma gondii*. It is an intracellular parasite and the definitive host is the domestic cat and other felines and rodents are the intermediate host. It can cause serious infections in humans and other mammals, e.g. sheep. ⊃ toxoplasmosis.

toxoplasmosis *n* infection with *Toxoplasma gondii*. Infected animals contaminate the environment with faeces containing cysts. Human infection occurs through environmental contact, such as gardening, playing and cleaning cat litter trays, or by contacting infected animals, or by eating undercooked meat. Most infections are symptomless or may cause a mild non-specific illness with tiredness and myalgia. However, it can be more serious with pyrexia and lymphadenopathy, with complications that include myocarditis. There is serious disease in immunocompromised individuals, e.g. AIDS patients, who develop encephalitis and eye involvement of variable severity. The more common lesion being a non-specific intraocular inflammation involving either the anterior or posterior segment of the eye. It is possible to be infected from a donated organ during transplant surgery. Primary toxoplasmosis during pregnancy can lead to the disease being passed to the fetus via the placenta. This is extremely serious and can lead to stillbirth or an infant with problems such as microcephaly or hydrocephaly, convulsions, or liver damage, thrombocytopenia and purpura or serious eye involvement. There is bilateral retinochoroiditis in which the fovea is frequently destroyed, resulting in loss of central vision. The infants who survive may have a learning disability and develop encephalitis, liver cirrhosis and blindness. ➲ Colour Section Figures 38, 123.

TP *abbr* temporal peak. ➲ ultrasound.

t-PA, tPA *abbr* tissue plasminogen activator.

TPHA *abbr* *Treponema pallidum* haemagglutination assay.

TPN *abbr* total parenteral nutrition.

TPR *abbr* temperature, pulse, respiration.

TQM *abbr* total quality management.

trabeculae *npl* the septa or fibrous bands projecting into the interior of an organ, e.g. the spleen—**trabecula** *sing*, **trabecular** *adj*.

trabecular meshwork the meshwork of connective tissue located at the angle of the anterior chamber of the eye and containing endothelium-lined spaces (the intertrabecular spaces) through which passes the aqueous humour to Schlemm's canal. It is usually divided into two parts: the corneoscleral meshwork which is in contact with the cornea and the sclera and opens into Schlemm's canal and the uveal meshwork which faces the anterior chamber. ➲ angle of the anterior chamber, aqueous humour, glaucoma, scleral venous sinus (Schlemm's canal).

trabeculectomy *n* operation used in glaucoma to reduce intraocular pressure by creating a drainage channel from the anterior chamber of the eye to the subconjunctival space.

trabeculoplasty *n* various laser-assisted procedures used in glaucoma to reduce intraocular pressure. It involves the modification of the trabecular meshwork in order to improve drainage of aqueous fluid.

trabeculotomy *n* operation for congenital glaucoma. Creation of a channel from the scleral venous sinus (canal of Schlemm) into the anterior chamber.

trace elements elements that are present in very small amounts in the tissues and known to be essential for normal metabolism. For example: chromium (Cr)—appears to be involved with insulin activity; cobalt—ulitized as vitamin B_{12}; copper (Cu)—needed for many enzymes, e.g. superoxide dimutase, cytochrome oxidase, and the production of neuropeptides and amines, e.g. enkephalins, catecholamines; fluorine (F)—a constituent of bone and teeth as calcium fluorapatite; iodine (I)—a constituent of the thyroid hormones thyroxine (T_4) and triiodothyronine (T_3); manganese (Mn)—a component of many enzymes, e.g. superoxide dimutase, and involved in the activation of other enzymes, e.g. kinases; molybdenum (Mo)—needed for enzymes involved in the metabolism of DNA; selenium (Se)—needed for the enzyme glutathione peroxidase.

tracer *n* a substance or instrument used to gain information. Radioactive tracers are used in the diagnosis of some cancers, e.g. brain, and thyroid disease, or in the investigation of metabolic processes. In dentistry, a device to record jaw positions and movements.

trachea *n* (*syn* windpipe) the major airway marking the commencement of the respiratory tract. It is about 115 mm long and about 25 mm wide and lies mainly in the median plane in front of the oesophagus. It is a continuation of the larynx and extends downwards to about the level of the 5th thoracic vertebra where it bifurcates (divides) at the carina into the right and left main bronchi, one bronchus going to each lung. ➲ Colour Section Figure 6. The structures associated with the trachea are: *superiorly*—the larynx; *inferiorly*—the right and left main bronchi; *anteriorly*—the upper part: the isthmus of the thyroid gland, and the lower part: the arch of the aorta and the sternum; *posteriorly*—the oesophagus separates the trachea from the vertebral column; and *laterally*—the lungs and the lobes of the thyroid gland. ➲ Colour Section Figure 39. The trachea is composed of three layers of tissue, and is held open by between 16 and 20 incomplete C-shaped rings of hyaline cartilage lying one above the other. The rings of cartilage are incomplete posteriorly. Connective tissue and involuntary muscle join the cartilages and form the posterior wall where they are incomplete. The soft tissue posterior wall is in contact with the oesophagus. Three layers of tissue 'clothe' the cartilages of the trachea: (a) the outer layer consists of fibrous and elastic tissue and encloses the cartilages; (b) the middle layer of cartilages and bands of involuntary, smooth muscle that wind round the trachea in a helical arrangement. There is some areolar tissue, containing blood and lymph vessels and autonomic nerves. The arrangement of cartilage and elastic tissue prevents kinking and obstruction of the airway as the head and neck move. The absence of cartilage posteriorly allows the trachea to dilate and constrict in response to nerve stimulation, and for indentation as the oesophagus distends during swallowing. The cartilages prevent collapse of the tube when the internal pressure is less than intrathoracic pressure, i.e. at the end of forced expiration; (c) the inner lining consists of ciliated columnar epithelium, containing mucus-secreting goblet cells. The lining membrane of the trachea functions as a mucociliary escalator in which synchronous and regular beating of the cilia of the mucous membrane lining wafts mucus with adherent

S
T

foreign particles upwards towards the larynx where it is swallowed or expectorated. The lining mucosa warms, humidifies and filters the air as in the nose, although air is normally saturated and at body temperature when it reaches the trachea. The trachea receives arterial blood from the inferior thyroid and bronchial arteries and the venous return is by the inferior thyroid veins into the brachiocephalic veins. The nerve supply is by parasympathetic and sympathetic fibres. The parasympathetic supply is by the recurrent laryngeal nerves and other branches of the vagus nerves (tenth cranial nerves). Sympathetic supply is by nerves from the sympathetic ganglia. The trachea is involved in the cough reflex. Nerve endings in the larynx, trachea and bronchi are sensitive to irritation that generates nerve impulses which are conducted by the vagus nerves to the respiratory centre in the brainstem. The reflex motor response is deep inspiration followed by closure of the glottis. The abdominal and respiratory muscles then contract and suddenly the air is released under pressure expelling mucus and/or foreign material from the mouth. Lymph from the respiratory passages passes through lymph nodes situated round the trachea and in the carina, the area where it divides into two bronchi—**tracheal** *adj*.

tracheitis *n* inflammation of the trachea; most commonly the result of a viral infection such as the common cold.

trachelorrhaphy *n* operative repair of a uterine cervical laceration.

trache/o- a prefix that means 'trachea', e.g. *tracheitis*.

tracheobronchial *adj* pertaining to the trachea and the bronchi.

tracheobronchitis *n* inflammation of the trachea and bronchi. ⮑ bronchitis.

tracheomalacia a congenital or acquired softening and weakening of the tracheal cartilages. The acquired form may follow a long period of endotracheal intubation. The structural changes allow the trachea to collapse during inspiration leading to breathing difficulties, such as wheezing, cough or stridor, or apnoea caused by compression of the trachea by other structures such as the aorta. ⮑ aortopexy.

tracheo-oesophageal *adj* pertaining to the trachea and the oesophagus.

tracheo-oesophageal fistula a congenital defect that often occurs in conjunction with oesophageal atresia. The fistula usually connects the distal oesophagus to the trachea.

tracheostomy *n* surgical opening between the front of the neck and the trachea to create an artificial airway. It is kept open with a tracheostomy tube (Figure T.5). A tracheostomy may be short or long term. It may be performed for a variety of reasons including: to bypass an obstruction in the upper airway; for long-term mechanical ventilation; to facilitate tracheobronchial suction when sputum is retained; to prevent the aspiration of secretions; following head and neck surgery; and in situations where laryngeal reflexes are absent, such as after brain injury or stroke— **tracheostome** *n*.

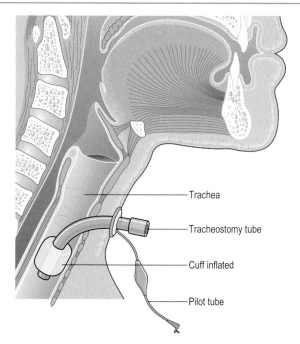

Trachea
Tracheostomy tube
Cuff inflated
Pilot tube

T.5 Cuffed tracheostomy tube (adapted from Brooker & Nicol 2003 with permission).

tracheotomy *n* vertical slit in the anterior wall of the trachea at the level of the third and fourth cartilaginous rings. Undertaken to access the airway below an obstruction caused by swelling or a foreign body. It may be performed as an emergency both in hospital or the community.

trachoma *n* a chronic, bilateral, contagious conjunctivitis caused by the serotypes A, Ba and C of *Chlamydia trachomatis* spread by flies. The conjunctivitis results in conjunctival scarring (Arlt's line) and may lead to entropion and trichiasis and dry eyes. Follicles at the limbus may leave some sharply defined depressions (Herbert's pits). There is also keratitis with corneal infiltrates, pannus and vascularization. As the disease progresses there is corneal ulceration and opacification which may result in visual impairment. Trachoma is one of the main causes of blindness in the world. It is a disease most commonly encountered in hot regions of the globe where hygienic conditions are poor, commonly encountered in communities with sparse water supplies. Treatment includes a course of tetracycline or erythromycin and surgical correction of entropion and trichiasis may be necessary—**trachomatous** *adj*. ⮑ adult inclusion conjunctivitis, alacrima, pannus.

trachoma inclusion conjunctivitis (TRIC) ⮑ adult inclusion conjunctivitis.

tracing line or pattern made on paper or a plate representing movement, such as cardiovascular activity or mandibular movement. *arrow point tracing* (gothic arch tracing). *gothic arch tracing* method of illustrating, by means of a tracing, the posterior position of the mandible in determining the normal occlusion for the construction of dentures or

S
T

rehabilitation cases. The horizontal tracing resembles an arrow head or gothic arch and is obtained by a series of mandibular movements using a tracing device on a horizontal recording plane. *tracing stick* ⊃ green stick, impression material.

traction *n* a drawing or pulling on the patient's body to overcome muscle spasm and to reduce or prevent deformity. A steady pulling exerted on some part (limb or head) by means of weights, pulleys and cords in conjunction with a variety of splints or frames. It may be skeletal or skin traction. ⊃ beam, Braun's frame, Bryant's gallows traction, halopelvic traction, hoop traction, Kirschner wire, skeletal traction, skin traction, Steinmann's pin, Thomas' splint.

tractotomy *n* incision of a nerve tract. Surgical relief of intractable pain, using stereotactic measures.

traditional birth attendant unqualified women, usually mothers themselves, who traditionally help other women to deliver their babies, found in developing countries where midwifery or obstetric help may not be available; indigenous midwife, hilot, dunken, dai.

tragacanth used in dentistry. A gum obtained from a vegetable plant. ⊃ adhesive.

tragus *n* the projection in front of the external auditory meatus/canal. Physiotherapists sometimes use this as an objective marker when measuring spinal movements against a wall for example—**tragi** *pl*.

traife items of food that do not comply with the dietary laws of Judaism. ⊃ kosher.

training *n* in sports medicine describes a deliberate scheme or programme to assist learning and/or improve fitness. The four principles of training are: specificity, individual differences, overload and reversibility. Training programmes will vary depending on the nature of the sport or activity being trained for and the goals to be achieved.

trait *n* an individual physical or mental characteristic which is inherited or develops. Describes an enduring individual behavioural characteristic or aspect of personality that is exhibited in a wide range of contexts.

trait anxiety a general disposition to respond to situations with a high level of state anxiety. ⊃ anxiety.

trajectory the plotted path of an object through space.

TRAM flap *acron* **T**ransverse **R**ectus **A**bdominis **M**yocutaneous flap.

trance *n* a term used for hypnotic sleep and for certain self-induced hysterical stuporous states.

tranexamic acid an antifibrinolytic drug that is useful in the management of patients with bleeding disorders (such as Von Willebrand's disease) who are having dental extractions or other intraoral surgery. It can be administered orally, by injection or topically as a mouthwash.

tranquillizers *npl* drugs that relieve anxiety or deal with psychotic symptoms without excessive sedation. ⊃ antipsychotic drugs (neuroleptics), anxiolytics. ⊃ Appendix 5.

trans- a prefix that means 'across, through', e.g. *transcutaneous*.

transabdominal *adj* through the abdomen—**transabdominally** *adv*.

transactional analysis a form of psychotherapy based on the theory that inter-relationships between people can be analysed in terms of transactions with each other as representing 'child', 'adult' and 'parent'. The aim is to give the adult ego decision-making power over the child and parent egos.

transaminases ⊃ aminotransferases.

transamniotic *adj* through the amniotic membrane and fluid, as a transamniotic transfusion of the fetus for haemolytic disease.

transbuccal or cheek wiring (archaic) a method of immobilizing fractures by wires from a halo head frame passed through the cheeks and fastened to a dental splint.

transcervical resection of endometrium (TCRE) a hysteroscopic procedure of removing the endometrium in cases of menorrhagia.

trans configuration means on the opposite side. In chemistry, describes an isomerism in which the two substituent groups are on the opposite side of a carbon-carbon double bond. ⊃ cis configuration, trans-fatty acids.

transcranial magnetic stimulation (TMS) a neuropsychological test whereby magnets are placed on the skull and stimulation can be applied to the brain to cause muscle movement dependent on the site of the stimulus. TMS can be more easily used in a clinical setting to provide a measurement tool of cerebral activity.

transcranial projection a radiographic technique used for demonstrating the temporomandibular joint, particularly the relationship of the condyle head to the glenoid fossa. ⊃ transpharyngeal projection.

transcription *n* first stage in protein synthesis where genetic information is transferred from DNA to mRNA. ⊃ translation.

transcutaneous *adj* through the skin, for example monitoring, e.g. oxygen saturation by pulse oximetry, or drug absorption.

transcutaneous blood gas monitor measurements of neonatal PO_2 and PCO_2 via a skin probe heated to 44°C. Accuracy depends on peripheral circulation and is usually used with intermittent arterial sampling.

transcutaneous electrical nerve stimulation (TENS) a method of non-invasive pain control using pads placed appropriately to apply a mild electric current from a battery-operated device, which can be controlled by the patient for pain relief. Used with good effect by women during labour, and in the control of chronic pain symptoms. TENS involves the delivery of short duration (50–250 µs) electrical pulses which target sensory nerves and can thereby achieve effective symptomatic pain relief. It is a widely used modality and one that is well supported by the evidence. TENS devices are usually small, battery-powered and well suited to patient self-management. Some of the larger, clinic-based electrical stimulators offer a TENS option that will achieve the same effects. TENS is a generally well tolerated form of electrical stimulation. With traditional or high TENS at (80–150 Hz) the target nerves are the sensory (Aß) fibres. Once stimulated, they will serve to close the

S
T

pain gate and thus reduce the awareness of pain. Stimulation at lower frequencies (2–5 Hz) using acupuncture like AL-TENS aims to stimulate the Aδ sensory fibres and stimulate opioid production at spinal cord level by means of descending extrasegmental modulation. Burst-mode TENS employs an interrupted output with machines commonly pre-set to burst at 2–3 times a second. Modulated output is also a standard feature and can be achieved by varying the ampli-tude, frequency or duration of the stimulating pulses. Electrodes are commonly placed either side of the painful site, providing segmental stimulation. Alternative (and evidenced) electrode placements include stimulation of spinal nerve roots, peripheral nerves, motor points, dermatome, myotome or sclerotome, acupuncture and trigger points.

transdermal *adj* through the skin. A drug administration system using patches, creams and gels. Thus drugs delivered in this way, e.g. hormone replacement, avoid first pass metabolism/first pass effect in the liver.

transducer (probe) *n* device that converts one form of energy into another to facilitate its electrical transmission. A hand-held instrument composed of multiple elements of piezoelectric material each with its own electrodes, used in ultrasound imaging.

transduction *n* **1.** generally, the conversion of one form of energy into another. For example, the transformation of light energy into receptor potentials in the photoreceptors of the retina (also called phototransduction). The absorption of light by the pigments of the photoreceptors triggers a cascade of biochemical events that leads to a change in ionic fluxes across the plasma membrane and to a change in resting potential from around –40 mV in the dark, to around –70 mV in light, that is a hyperpolarization of the cells. ⊃ rhodopsin. **2.** in microbiology, one of the sexual reproductive processes in certain bacteria whereby genetic material (DNA) is transferred from one bacterium to another. In transduction the transfer is by a bacteriophage (a parasitic virus of bacteria). It allows the genes that confer antibiotic resistance to be passed between bacteria. ⊃ conju-gation, transformation.

transection *n* the cutting across or mechanical severance of a structure.

trans-fatty acids *npl* stereoisomers of cis-fatty acids formed during food processing, such as those produced by the hydrogenation of oils during the manufacture of marga-rine and other fats. They appear to have the same adverse effects on health as saturated fats, thus food manufacturers are reducing or eliminating them from foods.

transfer coping ⊃ coping.

transfer of learning the extent to which practice or learning of one skill influences the learning or performance of a different skill, or the same skill in a different context. Also known as generalizability of learning. ⊃ negative transfer, positive transfer.

transfer RNA (tRNA) ⊃ ribonucleic acid.

transfer tubes in radiotherapy, the tubes used to connect catheters to an afterloading machine.

transferable skills particular skills: academic, problem solving, interpersonal, practical, etc. that can be transferred to new or different situations.

transferase an enzyme that catalyses the transfer of chemical radicals or groups between molecules, such as aminotransferases.

transference in psychotherapy or psychoanalysis, the unconscious transfer of a client's emotions regarding a significant person in their life, usually a person from child-hood such as a dominant parent, to the therapist. *counter transference* the unconscious or conscious emotional reaction of therapist to client.

transferrin *n* a plasma protein that has a high affinity for ferric iron. It binds the iron and transports it around the body in the blood.

transformation in microbiology, one of the sexual reproductive processes in certain bacteria whereby genetic material (DNA) is transferred from one bacterium to another. In transformation a strand of extrachromosomal DNA is transferred from one bacterium to another through the cell wall. It allows the genes that confer antibiotic resistance to be passed between bacteria. ⊃ conjugation, transduction.

transformation zone ⊃ squamocolumnar junction.

transformer a piece of equipment that either raises or lowers electric current in a circuit, a step-up transformer raises current, a step-down transformer reduces current.

transformer efficiency the ratio of output power to input power of the transformer.

transforming growth factor (TGF) a cytokine produced by some T-cells.

transfrontal *adj* through the frontal bone; an approach used for hypophysectomy.

transfusion *n* the introduction of fluid into the tissue or into a blood vessel. *blood transfusion* the intravenous replace-ment of lost or destroyed blood by compatible citrated human blood. Also used for severe anaemia with deficient blood production. Fresh blood from a donor or stored blood from a blood bank may be used. It can be given 'whole', or as plasma-depleted blood (packed-cell transfusion). If incompatible blood is given, severe reaction follows. ⊃ blood donor, blood groups. *intrauterine transfusion* can be used from about 20 weeks' gestation for a fetus endangered by Rhesus incompatibility. Red cells may be administered by intraperitoneal transfusion, but increasingly intravascular transfusion is possible with the development of more advanced ultrasound equipment. One or more transfusions may be needed. This enables the induction of labour to be postponed until a time more favourable to fetal survival.

transhiatal across the opening.

transient flora the micro-organisms that are present on a host for a short period. They colonize the superficial layers of the skin and healthcare workers acquire them during contact with patients, contaminated equipment, or the environment.

transient global amnesia ⊃ amnesia.

transient ischaemic attack (TIA) a brief loss of neurological function as a result of a disturbance of blood supply that lasts for minutes to 24 hours. The term describes cerebrovascular accidents (strokes) in which symptoms resolve within 24 hours—an arbitrary cut off which has little value in practice apart from perhaps indicating that underlying cerebral haemorrhage or extensive cerebral infarction is extremely unlikely. The term transient ischaemic attack (TIA) traditionally also includes patients with transient monocular blindness (also known as amaurosis fugax), usually due to a vascular occlusion in the retina. Transient symptoms, such as syncope, amnesia, confusion and dizziness, which do not reflect focal cerebral dysfunction, are often mistakenly attributed to TIA.

transient tachypnoea of newborn a condition affecting neonates. Common after caesarean section, it is characterized by rapid respirations up to 120 per minute for up to five days, cyanosis but with mostly normal blood gases; there is little rib recession or expiratory grunt. Oxygen therapy is administered and other causes of respiratory distress must be eliminated, e.g. infection, respiratory distress syndrome.

transillumination *n* the transmission of light through a tissue for examination, such as the sinuses for diagnostic purposes. In dentistry, projection of light rays through a crown and its associated structures in order to detect caries, calculus, debris, fractures, foreign bodies or the position of root canals. ⊃ retroillumination.

transistor a solid-state replacement of a diode which consists of an emitter, a base and a collector; it allows current to flow in one direction only.

transitional cell carcinoma a malignant tumour of the transitional epithelium of the urinary tract (urothelium) present in the urethra, bladder, ureters and the renal pelvis.

transitional epithelium a type of stratified epithelium found only in the urinary tract, where it lines the renal pelvis, the ureter, the bladder and the entire length of the female urethra and all but the last part of the penile portion of the male urethra, which is lined with stratified squamous epithelium. Structurally it is composed of cuboidal, columnar and dome-like surface cells (see Figure E.7, p. 264), which allow distension when the urinary structures fill with urine. Its surface cells are also able to withstand the normal chemical variations in the pH and composition of urine.

transjugular intrahepatic portasystemic stent shunting (TIPSS) a stent placed between the hepatic portal vein and the hepatic vein in the liver to reduce hepatic portal pressure by providing a shunt between the hepatic portal and systemic circulations. Performed to prevent further bleeding from oesophageal varices.

translation *n* **1.** movement from one position to another along a straight or curved line (rectilinear or curvilinear motion)—**translational** *adj*. **2.** the second stage of protein synthesis in which tRNA and rRNA translate the base sequences required to make a new polypeptide. ⊃ transcription.

translation table a method of modifying digital pixel values to adjust the contrast of a computed tomography (CT) image; the table is loaded into the video interface of the display system.

translational movement along a path.

translational kinetic energy the energy possessed by an object due to its movement along a straight or a curved line. May be calculated as $\frac{1}{2}\,mv^2$ where m is the mass of the object and v is linear velocity. ⊃ kinetic energy, rotational kinetic energy.

translocation *n* transfer of a chromosomal segment to a different site on the same chromosome (shift) or to a different chromosome. Can be a cause of several congenital abnormalities.

translucent *adj* in between transparent and opaque. Pertains to a medium or substance that transmits light but diffuses or scatters it on the way so that objects cannot be seen through it, e.g. paraffin wax, tracing paper, cloth, smoke, fog, opaque light shades, ground glass, etc. ⊃ ground glass, transparent.

translucent dentine ⊃ dentine.

translumbar *adj* through the lumbar region. Route used for injecting contrast agent into the aorta prior to aortography.

translumbar aortography the radiographic investigation of the aorta and its major branches by the direct injection of a contrast agent into the abdominal aorta.

transluminal angioplasty a method of dilating arterial narrowing by passing a guidewire through the lesion and then a catheter over the guidewire to dilate the artery.

transmethylation *n* a process in which methyl groups are donated by amino acids and transferred to other compounds.

transmigration *n* ⊃ diapedesis.

transmission the passage of radiations through a medium or a substance. Transmission can be either diffuse (light is scattered in all directions) or regular (i.e. without diffusion). ⊃ absorption, translucent, transmittance, transparent.

transmission curve a graph in which the transmission of an optical medium is plotted against the wavelength. ⊃ tinted lens.

transmission factor ⊃ transmittance.

transmittance (*syn* transmission factor, total transmittance) the measure of transmission expressed as the ratio of the transmitted luminous flux to the incident flux. ⊃ transmission.

transmitted when photons pass through an object without interacting with it. ⊃ transmitted beam, transmitted light.

transmitted beam the radiation leaving an object.

transmitted light the light seen by the viewer after it has passed through an X-ray film, used to calculate the opacity of the film. ⊃ opacity.

transmitter bandwidth the range of frequencies within a radiofrequency pulse delivered by the transmitter in magnetic resonance imaging.

transmural *adj* through the wall, e.g. of an organ, etc. For example, a transmural myocardial infarction that extends from the epicardium to the endocardium—**transmurally** *adv*.

S
T

transmyocardial revascularization a laser technique used to increase the blood supply to the myocardium and reduce anginal pain by creating a series of tiny channels from the subepicardial surface to the endothelium. It may be a treatment option for patients with severe angina in whom angioplasty or coronary artery bypass surgery is not appropriate.

transnasal *adj* through the nose—**transnasally** *adv*.

transoesophageal echo a tiny ultrasound probe on the end of an endoscope, used in cardiac work to examine the heart valves.

transoesophageal echocardiography ⊃ echocardiography.

transonic describes a material that allows the passage of a beam of ultrasound without any reflection back to the transducer.

transorbital (transmaxillary) projection a dental radiographic technique for demonstrating the articular eminence and the head of the condyle in cross-sectional view in an oblique coronal plane.

transparent able to see through clearly, e.g. window glass. Pertains to a medium or a substance which transmits light without scattering and with little absorption, so that objects can be seen through it. Optical lenses, prisms, etc. are made of such material. ⊃ translucent.

transparent grid a transparent material marked with a calibrated grid and used to make accurate comparisons or measurements of drawings, radiographs, models or casts.

transperitoneal *adj* across or through the peritoneal cavity. ⊃ dialysis, laparoscopy.

transpharyngeal projection also known as a lateral transpharyngeal projection or Toller view. A radiographic technique for demonstrating the temporomandibular joint, particularly the head of the condyle in lateral view. ⊃ transcranial projection.

transplacental *adj* through the placenta, such as the exchange of subtances between maternal and fetal blood—**transplacentally** *adv*.

transplant *n* customarily refers to the surgical operation of grafting an organ or tissue, which has been removed from a person who has been declared brain dead, from a living relative, or other suitable donor. If the recipient's malfunctioning organ is removed and the transplant is placed in its bed, it is referred to as an *orthotopic transplant* (e.g. liver and heart). If the transplanted organ is not placed in its normal anatomical site the term *heterotopic transplant* (e.g. a kidney) is used—**transplantation** *n*, **transplant** *vt*, **transplantation** *n* ⊃ graft, tooth transplantation.

transport system in radiography, the part of an automatic film processor that moves the film through the system and comprises a number of various diameter. ⊃ hard rollers, soft rollers.

transposition 1. the movement of genetic material from one chromosome to another. Associated with various congenital abnormalities. **2.** an embryonic developmental abnormality in which a structure is located on the right side of the body when it is normally on the left or vice versa.

⊃ transposition of the great vessels. **3.** in dentistry, the interchange of position of adjacent teeth during development and eruption.

transposition of the great vessels a congenital anomaly in which the pulmonary artery arises from the left ventricle and the aorta from the right ventricle.

transpulmonary pressure the difference between intrapleural pressure and alveolar pressure.

transrectal *adj* through the rectum.

transrectal ultrasonography (TRUS) method used to perform an ultrasound examination of the prostate gland—**transrectally** *adv*.

trans-sexualism a condition in which a person feels intensely uncomfortable with their biological gender and wishes to live as the opposite sex. They may cross-dress, but some will eventually have hormonal modification and surgery. Extensive counselling is required before any medical or surgical treatment is undertaken.

trans-sphenoidal *adj* through the sphenoid bone; an approach used for hypophysectomy.

transthoracic *adj* across or through the chest, as in transthoracic needle biopsy of a lung mass, or transthoracic echocardiography. ⊃ echocardiography.

transthoracic echo the examination of the heart through the thorax with the probe in the parasternal and apical positions.

transudate *n* a fluid that has passed out of the cells into a body cavity (e.g. ascitic fluid in the peritoneal cavity): it contains few cells and only small amounts of protein. ⊃ exudate.

transudation *n* the movement of fluid through a membrane or cell boundary.

transurethral *adj* through the urethra.

transurethral resection of prostate (TUR, TURP) the procedure whereby prostatic tissue is resected from within the urethra using an electric cautery. ⊃ prostatectomy, resectoscope.

transurethral vaporization of the prostate (TUVP) a minimally invasive technique used to reduce the effects of benign prostatic enlargement (BPE). An electric current is used to vaporize the prostate gland using an electrode passed through a resectoscope.

transvaginal *adj* through the vagina—**transvaginally** *adv*.

transvaginal probe an ultrasound probe that is inserted into the vagina to allow imaging of the cervix, uterine (fallopian) tubes, uterus, ovaries and related structures.

transvaginal ultrasound scan ultrasound examination of the pelvic structures using a transvaginal probe. It produces higher resolution images than the use of a transabdominal probe. Used in assisted conception techniques, in early pregnancy and to examine the uterus and ovaries for pathology. It is commonly performed in the first trimester of pregnancy, as intrauterine detail is often much clearer using this route. Used to confirm first trimester non-viability, and to visualize fetal parts in the pelvic cavity in late pregnancy.

S
T

transventricular *adj* through a ventricle. Term used mainly in cardiac surgery—**transventricularly** *adv*.

transverse arrest deflexed fetal head is caught above the level of the ischial spines with the sagittal suture in the transverse diameter of the pelvis; causes cephalopelvic disproportion and obstructed labour. ➲ deep transverse arrest.

transverse chromatic aberration (TCA) ➲ lateral chromatic aberration.

transverse colon the part of the colon between the right colonic (hepatic) flexure and the left colonic (splenic) flexure. ➲ Colour Section Figure 18b.

transverse condylar axis an imaginary line drawn through the condyle of the mandible about which it rotates.

transverse frictions ➲ deep transverse friction.

transverse horizontal axis (dental) (*syn* hinge axis, terminal hinge axis) an imaginary line about which the mandible rotates on its condyles during opening and closing without any sideways movement.

transverse lie the longitudinal fetal axis lies across that of the maternal uterus; if uncorrected it may cause shoulder presentation and obstructed labour. It is due to lax abdominal and uterine muscles, as in grande multiparae, multiple pregnancy, placenta praevia or contracted pelvic outlet. On examination the uterus usually appears broad, asymmetrical with a low fundus and the fetal head is felt in the flank or iliac fossa. After 30 weeks' gestation a persistent transverse lie may require external cephalic version and, towards term, controlled membrane rupture/induction of labour if appropriate, or elective caesarean section.

transverse magnification ➲ lateral magnification.

transverse myelitis a rare acute inflammatory condition that is associated with viral infections such as measles, mumps, herpes zoster/simplex. It is characterized by sensory loss, weakness or paralysis, incontinence and lower motor neuron signs, such as decreased or absent reflexes and muscle wasting. It may be preceded by fever, back and/or limb pain.

transverse plane a horizontal plane that divides the body into superior and inferior parts. Also called the horizontal plane (Figure T.6).

transverse rectus abdominis myocutaneous (TRAM) flap a flap from the abdominal wall muscle, which is used in breast reconstruction following mastectomy.

transverse relaxation time (T$_2$ or spin-spin relaxation time) the time required for the transverse magnetization to decay to about 37% of its maximum value and is the characteristic time constant for loss of phase coherence among spins orientated at an angle to the static main magnetic field.

transverse tubules ➲ sarcoplasmic reticulum, t-tubes (t-tubules).

transversus abdominis paired muscle of the anterior abdominal wall. ➲ abdominal muscles.

transvesical *adj* through the urinary bladder—**transvesically** *adv*.

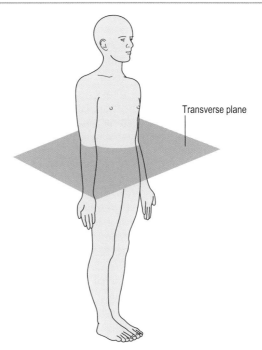

Transverse plane

T.6 Transverse plane (reproduced from Montague et al 2005 with permission).

transvesical prostatectomy ➲ prostatectomy.

transvestism cross-dressing in clothes of the opposite gender.

trapezium *n* one of the carpal bones of the wrist. It articulates with other carpal bones scaphoid and trapezoid, and the first and second metacarpal bones.

trapezius large, triangular, superficial muscle on each side of the upper back, its origin extending in the midline from the base of the skull down to the spine of the lowest thoracic vertebra. From there its fibres converge towards the shoulder, and partly over it, round the side of the lower neck, to be inserted in a continuous line into the outer end of the clavicle and the spine of the scapula. The tone of the two muscles keeps the shoulders braced and they act with the scapular spine as a lever when lifting the arms at the shoulder. ➲ Colour Section Figures 4, 5.

trapezoid *n* one of the carpal bones of the wrist. It articulates with the scaphoid bone, and the second metacarpal bone.

trauma *n* bodily injury—**traumatic** *adj*. ➲ Abbreviated Injury Scale, advanced trauma life-support, post-traumatic stress disorder.

traumatic exposure ➲ exposure.

traumatic head injury an insult to the brain from an external force, which may lead to altered consciousness and loss of movement, speech and altered cognition amongst other impairments. Head injury is a common cause of accidental death.

traumatic occlusion any occlusion of the teeth that is injurious to the oral or related structures, teeth or periodontium.

S
T

789

traumatologist *n* a doctor or nurse who specializes in traumatology.

traumatology *n* the branch of medicine dealing with injury—**traumatological** *adj*, **traumatologically** *adv*.

traveller's diarrhoea infectious illness common where hygiene conditions are poor and caused by a variety of infectious agents. Seen in sport where teams travel to countries where food and water hygiene and sanitation are poor. Can be passed from one member to another quickly, limiting numbers available to compete.

tray in dentistry, a flat shallow vessel with raised edges. ⊃ impression tray, tray adhesive, tray compound, special tray material.

tray adhesive the substance used to ensure adhesion of impression material to the impression tray containing it. It prevents impression materials lifting from impression trays, thus causing distorted models. Some adhesives are designed for use exclusively with certain materials.

tray compound a thermoplastic material used in making special impression trays on the preliminary models.

Treacher Collins syndrome (E Treacher Collins, British ophthalmologist, 1862–1932) a form of mandibulofacial dysostosis inherited as an autosomal dominant trait. It is characterized by slanting eyes, microtia, poorly developed facial bones, micrognathia, high palate, abnormal positioning of the teeth and atypical hair growth. ⊃ Colour Section Figure 122.

treadmill training a form of therapy intervention that focuses on gait retraining following a neurological insult. It usually involves a specialist treadmill with a body de-weighting support system.

treated volume the volume of tissue inside an isodose surface that is appropriate to receive a radiation dose during radiotherapy treatment.

treatment methods of curing, minimizing or controlling the effects, or preventing a disease, disorder or injury. *conservative treatment* using drugs, rest, exercise or diet rather than surgery or other drastic means. ⊃ conservative dentistry. *curative treatment* measures aimed at complete cure. *empirical treatment* treatment based on experience and observation rather than scientific knowledge. *endodontic treatment* ⊃ endodontics. *orthodontic treatment* ⊃ orthodontics. *palliative treatment* the measures taken to control symptoms such as nausea, pain, etc. without hope of cure. *periodontal treatment* ⊃ periodontics. *prophylactic (preventive) treatment* measures taken to prevent disease such as antibiotics after exposure to an infectious disease, or immunization. In dentistry, the instructions given to a patient to prevent the development of dental disease particularly as related to caries and periodontal disease. *prosthetic treatment* ⊃ prosthetics, prosthodontics (prosthetic dentistry). *radical treatment* measures aimed at complete cure, which may for example involve extensive surgery, use of radiotherapy and drugs. *root canal treatment* the technique of removing vital or non-vital pulp tissue from a root canal, its sterilization and preparation to receive a permanent root filling. ⊃ root canal (dental procedures). *treatment plan* ⊃ dental treatment plan.

treatment allocation a research term. Assigning a participant to a particular arm of the clinical trial.

treatment index (TI) in dentistry, an obsolescent term based on the DMF index and sometimes used to show the extent to which treatment has been successful. ⊃ DMF index, index (dental).

Trematoda *n* a class of parasitic flukes which include many human pathogens of the blood, hepatobiliary system, the lungs and the intestine, such as the *Schistosoma* of schistosomiasis.

tremor *n* rhythmic movement disorder that can affect any part of the body but typically the hands and which can be seen in Parkinson's disease. ⊃ dyskinetic movements, intention tremor.

trench foot (*syn* immersion foot) occurs in frostbite or other conditions of exposure when local blood supply is impaired and secondary bacterial infection is present.

trench mouth an outdated term for necrotizing ulcerative gingivitis (NUG). ⊃ necrotizing ulcerative gingivitis (NUG).

Trendelenburg gait (F Trendelenburg, German surgeon, 1844–1924) an intrinsic disorder of the abductors of the hip due to either a weakness or an inhibition to function. As a result, the hip abductors are unable to stabilize the hip, as body weight is transferred to the affected side, resulting in a pelvic drop or tilt towards the opposite side.

Trendelenburg's position (F Trendelenburg) lying on an operating or examination table, with the head lower than the pelvis with the legs raised. It is used for varicose vein surgery and pelvic surgery.

Trendelenburg's sign/test (F Trendelenburg) a test of the stability of the hip, and particularly of the ability of the hip abductors (gluteus medius and g. minimus) to steady the pelvis upon the femur. Normally, when one leg is raised from the ground the pelvis tilts upwards on that side, through the hip abductors of the standing limb. If the abductors are inefficient (e.g. in poliomyelitis, severe coxa vara and developmental dysplasia of the hip), they are unable to sustain the pelvis against the body weight and it tilts downwards instead of rising (Figure T.7).

trephine *n* an instrument with sawlike edges for removing a circular piece of tissue, such as the cornea or skull.

Treponema *n* a genus of slender spiral-shaped bacteria that are actively motile. Best visualized with dark-ground illumination. Cultivated in the laboratory with great difficulty. *Treponema carateum* causes pinta; *Treponema pallidum* causes syphilis; *Treponema pertenue* causes yaws.

***Treponema pallidum* haemagglutination assay (TPHA)** *n* a specific serological test for syphilis and other treponemal diseases.

treponematosis *n* any treponemal diseases.

treponemicide *n* lethal to *Treponema*—**treponemicidal** *adj*.

trespass against the person a general term that covers any interference with the person's bodily integrity and liberty, it includes assault and battery. ⊃ assault, battery.

Trexler isolator a flexible film, negative pressure, bed isolator for dangerous infections such as viral haemorrhagic disease.

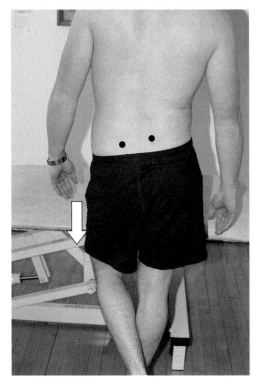

T.7 Positive Trendelenberg sign (note the different levels of the posterior superior iliac spine (PSIS) indicated by the black dots (reproduced from Porter 2005 with permission).

TRH *abbr* thyrotrophin-releasing hormone.

tri- a prefix that means 'three', e.g. *tricuspid.*

triacylglycerol (TG) *n* the officially approved term to replace the older but still widely used triglyceride. A hydrophobic compound made from the combination of glycerol and three fatty acids, which is the major energy store of the body and main component of dietary fat. Present in the body in adipose tissue, in the circulating blood and as intramuscular triacylglycerol (IMTG). ➲ lipids, lipoproteins, medium-chain triglycerides.

triad a group of three. ➲ portal triad (tract).

triage *n* **1.** a system of priority classification of casualties in any emergency situation, such as in hospital emergency departments and at accidents and disasters with several casualties. The modern use of triage has developed from its military use with injured soldiers in the Napoleonic wars. In battle, the aim was to return soldiers to the front line, so those with serious injuries were left in favour of the 'walking wounded'. There are several triage classifications ranging from a simple three category system to much more sophisticated systems based on specific criteria. At its most basic level triage is: people who need immediate treatment in order to survive, those who can wait for treatment and those people who will not survive under any circumstances. ➲ Abbreviated Injury Scale (AIS), Advanced Trauma Life-Support (ATLS). **2.** a system of sorting patients according to

their illness or severity of injury so that patients can be steered to the most appropriate health worker.

triage nurse a nursing role in emergency departments. It is not merely a means of allocating a category rating to a patient, although pressures on emergency departments to speed up the flow of patients present a difficult task. Triage encompasses assessment, prioritization of need, first aid, the initiation of relevant investigations and the provision of health promotion. Skills include effective communication, objectivity and the ability to make rapid clinical decisions, in order to achieve the best care for every patient. Many emergency departments have a designated triage area, providing some privacy from the rest of the waiting area. However, a difficult balance has to be struck between the preservation of dignity, and visibility and access to and from the triage nurse. The triage nurse is faced with the difficult task of identifying the sickest patients, whilst providing a service for the large numbers of people whose problem may not be serious, yet who suffer long waits. Triage is a dynamic process. The condition of patients may improve or deteriorate and their need for attention will alter. People in pain require special attention, as their distress can lead to dissatisfaction. Pain relief must therefore be seen as a high priororiry. Triage nurses also work in general practice where they see patients with minor illnesses to make a decision about whether the person can be treated by the nurse or needs to see a doctor.

trial denture a denture in the process of construction when the teeth are set up in wax. It is tried in the mouth for suitability, aesthetics and stability before completion. Formerly called a '*set up*' or '*try in*'.

trial labour conducted in consultant obstetric unit when the fetal head is not engaged, due to slight cephalopelvic disproportion, to ascertain whether normal vaginal delivery is possible. If good contractions occur the head may flex and descend with moulding through the pelvic brim facilitating normal delivery; if there is lack of progress in descent of the head and dilatation of the cervix despite good contractions, or signs of fetal or maternal distress caesarean section can be performed.

trial lens clip ➲ clipover.

trial of scar controlled, often induced labour in order to observe the woman's condition and progress when she has a uterine scar from a previous caesarean or other uterine surgery. The increased risk of scar dehiscence, particularly in multigravidae, requires labour to be carefully monitored in a consultant unit so that emergency measures can be implemented if necessary.

triangular bandage used for arm slings, for securing splints, in first aid and for inclusive dressings of a part, as a whole hand or foot.

triangulation a research term. The process whereby the same data are obtained from various means as an attempt to improve its validity. Determining the consistency of evidence gathered from different sources of data and/or different research methods about a particular research question

S

T

of interest. For example, it may involve a questionnaire, individual interviews and a focus group as a means of data triangulation.

Triatoma a genus of bloodsucking bug of the family Reduviidae. They act as vectors for the protozoon *Trypanosoma cruzi* which causes Chagas' disease, a form of trypanosomiasis, present in South America.

tricarboxylic cycle ⊃ Krebs' cycle.

TRIC *abbr* trachoma inclusion conjunctivitis. ⊃ adult inclusion conjunctivitis.

triceps brachii *n* the major extensor muscle of the elbow and the only muscle on the back of the upper arm. It is three-headed (long, lateral and medial heads) and arises partly from the scapula below the shoulder joint but the main bulk arises from the back of the humerus. It forms a single, broad tendon which passes behind the elbow joint (separated from it by a small bursa) to be inserted on the back of the olecranon process of the ulna. It contracts to extend the forearm and adduct the arm. ⊃ Colour Section Figures 4, 5.

trichobezoar a mass of hair present in the stomach. The person may swallow their own hair, or animal hair. ⊃ bezoar.

trichiasis *n* abnormal ingrowing eyelashes.

Trichinella a genus of parasitic nematode worms, e.g. *Trichinella spiralis* a parasite of pigs and rats that causes human disease. ⊃ trichinosis.

trichinosis *n* also called trichiniasis. Caused by eating undercooked pork infected with *Trichinella spiralis* (the trichina worm). The female worms in the small intestine produce larvae which invade the body and, in particular, form cysts in skeletal muscles; usually causes diarrhoea, nausea, colicky pain, fever, facial oedema, muscle pains and stiffness.

trich/o- a prefix that means 'hair', e.g. *trichobezoar*.

trichoglossia 'hairy tongue', associated with fungal infection.

trichology the study of hair and the scalp, and related diseases.

trichomonacide *n* an agent that is lethal to the protozoa belonging to the genus *Trichomonas*.

Trichomonas *n* a genus of motile protozoan parasites; e.g. *Trichomonas vaginalis* causes vaginitis in females and urethral infection in males. The organism is easily recognized by wet microscope preparations of the discharge. ⊃ trichomoniasis.

trichomoniasis *n* inflammation of the vagina (urethra in males) caused by the protozoan *Trichomonas vaginalis*.

trichomycosis fungal disease affecting the hair.

Trichophyton *n* a genus of fungi affecting the skin and nails. ⊃ dermatophytes, tinea.

trichophytosis *n* infection with a species of the fungus *Trichophyton*, e.g. ringworm of the hair or skin.

Trichosporon *n* a genus of fungi. ⊃ piedra.

trichotillomania an impulsive disorder in which the person pulls out their hair. It may be a feature of some learning disabilities.

trichromacy ⊃ trichromatism.

trichromatic *adj* pertaining to normal colour vision; having cones with the three visual pigments that respond to bright light of green, blue or red wavelengths.

trichromatic theory ⊃ Young–Helmholtz theory.

trichromatic vision ⊃ trichromatism.

trichromatism (*syn* trichromacy, trichromatic vision) colour vision characterized by the fact that any perceived hues can be matched by three independent primaries (e.g. red, green and blue). *anomalous trichromatism* a form of defective colour vision in which three primary colours are required for colour matching, but the proportion of each primary is not the same as those required by a normal trichromat. There are three types of anomalous trichromatism; deuteranomaly, protanomaly and tritanomaly. Also known as anomalous trichromacy, anomalous trichromatic vision. ⊃ defective colour vision.

trichuriasis *n* infestation with *Trichuris trichiura*. Infestation occurs from ingesting contaminated soil or food. Usually produces few symptoms but heavy infestation may cause blood-stained diarrhoea, abdominal pain and sometimes anaemia if blood loss is severe.

Trichuris *n* a genus of nematode worms. *Trichuris trichiura* (whipworm) common in hot, humid regions. ⊃ trichuriasis.

tricuspid *adj* having three cusps. *tricuspid valve* the right atrioventricular valve of the heart between the right atrium and ventricle.

tricyclic antidepressants (TCA) a group of antidepressant drugs, e.g. amitriptyline. They act by inhibiting the uptake of the neurotransmitters serotonin (5-hydroxytryptamine) and noradrenaline (norepinephrine). ⊃ Appendix 5.

tridactyly *n* a congenital absence of digits, there are only three on a hand or foot.

trifurcation an anatomical area where the roots divide in a three-rooted tooth.

trigeminal *adj* triple; separating into three sections, e.g. the trigeminal nerve, the fifth cranial nerve, which has three branches, ophthalmic, maxillary and mandibular.

trigeminal nerves the fifth and among the largest of the twelve pairs of cranial nerves. They are mixed nerves containing both motor and sensory fibres. They are the chief sensory nerves for the face and head (including the oral and nasal cavities and teeth), receiving impulses of pain, temperature and touch. The motor fibres stimulate the muscles of mastication. There are three main divisions or branches of the trigeminal nerve: (a) the ophthalmic nerves are sensory only and supply the lacrimal glands, conjunctiva of the eyes, forehead, eyelids, anterior aspect of the scalp and mucous membrane of the nose; (b) the maxillary nerves are sensory only and receive impulses from the cheeks, all the upper teeth and gingivae and the lower eyelids; and (c) the mandibular nerves contain both sensory and motor fibres. These are the largest of the three divisions and they receive sensory impulses from all the teeth and gingivae of the lower jaw, pinnae of the ears, lower lip and the anterior two-thirds of the tongue. They also send motor (efferent) impulses to the salivary glands and the muscles of mastication.

trigeminal neuralgia also known as tic douloureux. Spasms of sudden, excruciating pain in the distribution of the trigeminal nerve. Although the pain may soon pass off, it can be repeated rapidly over several hours. The location of pain depends on the branch of the nerve involved, but it may be the forehead, around the eye; the nose, upper lip and cheek; or the lower lip and jaw. Various activities can trigger an attack and include touching or moving the face and mouth, such as during eating and talking, or cold air blowing on the face. It usually affects people aged over 50 years and more women are affected than men.

trigeminy a group of three. Often applied to abnormal heart rhythms in which the arrhythmia occurs in groups of three, such as two ectopic beats followed by a normal beat.

trigger finger a condition in which the finger can be actively bent but cannot be straightened without help. It usually occurs secondary to tenosynovitis (usually due to overuse) or to rheumatoid arthritis. It occurs when there is thickening and nodule formation within the flexor tendon of the hand which prevents free gliding. Most commonly, the nodule is trapped under the metacarpophalangeal ligament, as the tendon flexes. Corticosteroid injection may relieve the symptoms, but sometimes surgery is indicated.

trigger point a localized hypersensitive band of tissue which, when irritated, refers pain to another part of the body. For example, shoulder trigger point resulting in headache. ⊃ myofascial trigger point.

triglyceride (TG) n triacylglycerol or neutral fat. A lipid with three fatty acids and a glycerol molecule. Forms the fat deposits of the body within the cytoplasm of the adipocytes (fat cells) in adipose tissue and is the major source of stored energy. ⊃ triacylglycerol (TG).

trigone n a triangular area, especially applied to the bladder base, bounded by the two ureteral openings at the back and the urethral opening at the front—**trigonal** *adj*.

trigonocephaly a congenital malformation that results in a skull with a sharp angulation present on the forehead; there is defective closure of the suture between the two parts of the frontal bone.

triiodothyronine (T₃) n a thyroid hormone that is involved in the regulation of growth, development and in maintaining the body's metabolic processes. It contains three iodine atoms and is more active than thyroxine from which it is formed.

tri-malleolar fracture a fracture that involves both malleoli and the posterior part of the tibial articular surface.

trimester n a period of 3 months. Applied especially to the first, second and third trimesters of pregnancy.

trimmer a machine-operated or hand instrument used to reduce the size of prostheses, models, restorations or preparations.

triode a device allowing current to flow in one direction only, containing an anode, a cathode and a grid in a vacuum,

a negative potential on the grid can stop the electron flow and therefore can act as an on–off switch.

triose n a monosaccharide containing three carbon atoms, such as glyceraldehyde.

tripartite placenta a placenta divided into three lobes, each with a cord leaving it which join to form one cord a short distance from the lobes.

triple syringe in dentistry, a three-in-one syringe. ⊃ syringe.

triple test blood test offered to some pregnant women between 15 and 20 week' gestation. It measures three biochemical markers: alphafetoprotein (AFP), unconjugated oestriol (UE₃) and total human chorionic gonadotrophin (hCG) in maternal serum. The results are used in conjunction with the mean value for gestational age to predict the estimated risk of conditions such as Down's syndrome and neural tube defects. A higher than average hCG and lower than average AFP and UE₃ levels are associated with increased risk of Down's syndrome. Maternal age, gestation and biochemical marker levels are calculated together to give a combined Down's syndrome risk; if the risk is higher than 1 in 250 at term, the woman is in the higher risk range and is offered further diagnostic tests. ⊃ amniocentesis, chorionic villus sampling, nuchal translucency.

triple response the triple response described by Lewis in 1927. A three part response to skin injury: redness caused by changes to blood vessels; increased capillary permeability caused by the release of inflammatory chemicals results in a wheal as fluid leaks from the capillaries into the tissues; and lastly a more generalized flare occurs when adjacent arterioles dilate, which is initiated by a local axon reflex. This effect can be demonstrated by drawing a blunt instrument firmly across the skin (for convenience the forearm is often used) and watching the following sequence of events, which are similar irrespective of the type of injury. Instantly, a white line forms following the 'injury'. This is due to vasoconstriction of the underlying arterioles as a direct response to the injury and is only transient. This vasoconstriction is not considered to be fully part of the inflammatory process. A flush rapidly follows, seen as a dull red line which occurs as the capillaries dilate. To the naked eye, the vasodilation can give the impression that the injured tissue contains a greater number of blood vessels. This dilation may last for as long as the inflammatory process persists. The formation of a wheal (a raised area of skin) occurs owing to the fluid passing out of the blood vessels and into the extravascular space, so leading to oedema. The flare is where an irregular red zone develops. This occurs due to the response of the surrounding arterioles, which have been affected by both nervous and chemical mediators. At the same time, the endothelial cells that form the internal wall of the blood vessels retract such that they no longer form a completely continuous lining of the vessel. Consequently, the vessels become 'leaky' to the extent that fluid, namely water and some of the salts and smaller proteins (e.g. fibrinogen), contained in plasma may pass out directly into the extracellular spaces of the damaged

S
T

area. The fluid exudate becomes transformed into a cellular exudate. This is achieved through circulating neutrophils leaving the blood vessels and entering the extracellular spaces in the area of tissue damage. In the first 6–24 h of an inflammatory response it is the neutrophils that predominate; between 24 and 48 h, however, they are superseded by monocytes and lymphocytes acting in a similar way (Court & Lea 2003). (Court E, Lea R 2003 Tissue inflammation and repair. In: Porter S (ed.) Tidy's Physiotherapy, 13th edn. Butterworth Heinemann, Oxford.)

triple vaccine contains diphtheria, tetanus and pertussis antigens (DTaP). Offered as part of a routine immunization programme.

triplet 1. one of three infants resulting from a single pregnancy. **2.** the three sequential bases in a molecule of deoxyribonucleic acid or ribonucleic acid, which code for a specific amino acid in the synthesis of a polypeptide chain. ⟳ codon. **3.** a lens system composed of three lenses as, for example, a convex crown glass lens cemented between two concave flint lenses. The aim of such a system is to minimize optical aberrations. ⟳ achromatizing lens, crown glass, doublet, flint glass, orthoscopic eyepiece.

triploid *adj* possessing three chromosomal sets (3n). ⟳ diploid, genome, haploid, polyploidy, triploidy.

triploidy (69XXX, 69XXY) a syndrome in which three haploid sets of chromosomes are present. It may occur when two sperm fertilize one oocyte. The normal human karyotype contains 46 chromosomes (23 from each parent). Many triploid pregnancies miscarry spontaneously but liveborn infants may have craniofacial abnormalities, eye defects and other anomalies and developmental delay.

triplopia a condition in which a subject sees three images of a single object. This condition may be the result of crystalline lens sclerosis, multiple pupils, etc. ⟳ diplopia, polycoria, polyopia.

triquetral *n* one of the proximal carpal bones of the wrist, it is situated between the pisiform and lunate bones.

trismus *n* spasm in the muscles of mastication such as that occurring in tetanus.

trisodium orthophosphate ⟳ sodium phosphate.

trisomy *n* a type of aneuploidy. The presence of three chromosomes where normally they would be paired. Results in an increase in the chromosome number by one (single trisomy), e.g. to 47 in humans. For example, *trisomy* 13 ⟳ Patau's syndrome. *trisomy* 18 ⟳ Edward's syndrome. *trisomy* 21 ⟳ Down's syndrome. ⟳ aneuploidy, monosomy, polyploidy.

tritan a person who has either tritanopia or tritanomaly.

tritanomal a person who has tritanomaly.

tritanomaly (*syn* tritanomalous trichromatism; tritanomalous vision) a type of anomalous trichromatism in which an abnormally high proportion of blue is needed when mixing blue and green to match a given blue-green stimulus. This condition is exceedingly rare: it is estimated at about one person in a million. ⟳ anomaloscope, defective colour vision, pseudoisochromatic plates, trichromatism.

tritanope a person who has tritanopia.

tritanopia (*syn* blue blindness, blue-yellow blindness) a rare type of dichromatism in which blue and yellow are confused. The tritanope only sees two colours: reds on the long-wave side, and greens or bluish greens on the other side of his neutral point which is situated around 570 nm. Tritanopia occurs more often as an acquired type as a result of retinal disease or detachment, glaucoma, diabetes, retinitis pigmentosa, etc. Congenital tritanopia is very rare: it is estimated at about five males and three females in 100 000. ⟳ defective colour vision, dichromatism, Farnsworth test.

tritiated water when one hydrogen atom is replaced with tritium, an isotope of hydrogen-3. It is used to study electrolyte and water absorption problems.

triton tumour a tumour affecting peripheral nerves. It is associated with neurofibromatosis.

trituration grinding, rubbing or pounding of a mixture in order to pulverize it. In dentistry describes the process of mixing amalgam alloy particle with mercury.

trizygotic formed from three separate zygotes.

tRNA *abbr* transfer ribonucleic acid. ⟳ ribonucleic acid.

trocar *n* a pointed rod which fits inside a cannula.

trochanteric bursitis often associated with tendonitis (tendinitis) of gluteus medius muscle, it is characterized by an inflammation of the bursae overlying the greater trochanter of the femur. There is pain over the greater trochanter—the bony prominence on the femur on either side of the thigh. Occurs as a result of repeated friction due to poor running gait or technique, altered biomechanics or poor muscle co-ordination. Pain is often reproduced on stretch (hip flexion to 90° with full lateral rotation of hip) or contraction of the gluteus medius as in resisted hip abduction. Management is as for bursitis elsewhere, including analgesia and identification of the underlying cause.

trochanters *npl* two processes, the larger one (*greater trochanter*) on the outer, the other (*lesser trochanter*) on the inner side of the femur between the neck and shaft; they provide attachment for muscles—**trochanteric** *adj*.

trochlea *n* any part which is like a pulley in structure or function, such as the trochlea or pulley-like end of the humerus that articulates with the ulna—**trochlear** *adj*.

trochlear nerves the fourth pair of cranial nerves. They innervate the extraocular/extrinsic muscle that moves the eyeball in an outwards and downward direction.

trochoid joint a pivot joint.

Troisier's sign (C Troisier, French pathologist, 1844–1919) ⟳ signal node.

Trombiculidae a family of mites that include harvest mites. They act as vectors for diseases including scrub typhus.

trophic *adj* pertaining to nutrition.

troph/o- a prefix that means 'nourishment', e.g. *trophoblast*.

trophoblast *n* cells covering the embedding ovum and concerned with the nutrition of the ovum, invasion of the endometrium and secretion of human chorionic gonadotrophin (hCG)—**trophoblastic** *adj*. ⟳ cytotrophoblast.

trophoblastic tissue ⤷ cytotrophoblast, syncytiotrophoblast.

-trophy a suffix that either means 'nourishment', e.g. *hypertrophy*.

tropia *n* manifest strabismus. May be used as a suffix.

tropical sprue chronic malabsorption of unknown aetiology occurring in residents or visitors to tropical regions.

-tropic, tropy a suffix that either means 'affininity for', e.g. *lymphotropic*.

tropomyosin *n* one of the control proteins present in the thin filaments of striated muscle myofibrils; works in partnership with troponin. It winds along the actin 'thin filament' and covers the myosin-binding sites in the absence of inonized calcium. ⤷ myofibril, troponin.

troponin *n* one of the control proteins present in the thin filaments of striated muscle myofibrils; works in partnership with tropomyosin. Troponin has high affinity for calcium ions, which are released into the cytoplasm from the sarcoplasmic reticulum in response to excitation. When ionized calcium [Ca^{2+}] binds to it, the troponin molecule changes shape and in so doing, is thought to move the associated tropomyosin molecule around the thin filament, making previously masked binding sites on a number of actin molecules accessible to the head-groups of myosin. The resultant myosin/actin interaction then develops force. ⤷ cardiac enzymes, myofibrils.

T-roll a T-shaped piece of equipment that is used to help position patients by breaking up established patterns of tone and distributing weight more equally in patients with soft tissue shortening.

Trousseau's sign (A Trousseau, French physician, 1801–1867) a test for latent tetany. Spasm of the forearm muscle is observed, within 3 minutes of inflating a cuff on the upper arm to a pressure above the systolic blood pressure. ⤷ carpopedal spasm, Chvostek's sign.

troy a system of weights used to assess quantities of precious metals, such as those used in dentistry.

true birth rate ⤷ birth rate.

true conjugate ⤷ conjugate.

true lateral projection a radiographic technique for demonstrating all or part of the skull by directing the central ray at right angles to the plane of the film.

true occlusal projection a dental radiographic technique in which the central ray is directed along the long axis of the teeth.

true pelvis the bony pelvis from the level of the brim and below, forming the bony canal through which the fetus must pass to be born normally. Consists of the brim or inlet, bounded by the sacral promontory and alae, upper sacroiliac joints, iliopectineal lines, upper inner borders of the upper pelvic rami and symphysis pubis; the cavity, bounded by the sacral hollow, sacrospinous ligaments, ischial and pubic bones and symphysis pubis; and the anatomical outlet, bounded by the coccyx, sacrotuberous ligaments, ischial tuberosities and pubic arch. The obstetrical outlet is bounded posteriorly by the lower aspect of the sacrum and laterally by the ischial spines and is the lowest level of bone surrounding the fetus in the birth canal.

true power ⤷ equivalent power.

truncal ataxia unco-ordinated movements of the postural muscles of the trunk.

truncus main part of an anatomical structure, such as a vessel, from which smaller branches arise.

truncus arteriosus an early embryonic structure that opens from both primitive ventricles; it will become the pulmonary artery and the aorta.

TRUS *abbr* transrectal ultrasonography.

try in a trial denture ⤷ denture.

trypanocide a drug that kills trypanosomes.

Trypanosoma *n* a genus of parasitic protozoa. Their life cycle alternates between blood-sucking arthropods and vertebrate hosts. A limited number of species are pathogenic to humans. ⤷ trypanosomiasis.

trypanosomiasis *n* disease caused by infection with *Trypanosoma*. In Africa these include: *Trypanosoma rhodesiense* or *Trypanosoma brucei gambiense*. Both are transmitted by the bite of infected tsetse flies. The disease caused by *T. brucei gambiense* is usually chronic. Central nervous system involvement causes headache, confusion, insomnia, daytime sleepiness and eventual coma and death. ⤷ sleeping sickness. Infection with *T. rhodesiense* is more acute, with myocarditis, hepatitis, pleural effusion and central nervous system involvement that leads to coma, tremors and death. In South America, trypanosomiasis is also known as Chagas' disease. It is caused by *Trypanosoma cruzi* transmitted by bugs. ⤷ *Triatoma*.

trypsin *n* active proteolytic enzyme. ⤷ trypsinogen.

trypsinogen *n* inactive precursor of trypsin secreted by the pancreas. It is activated by enterokinase (enteropeptidase) in the intestine.

tryptophan *n* one of the essential (indispensable) amino acids necessary for growth. It is a precursor of serotonin. Nicotinamide is synthesized from tryptophan.

TSE *abbr* testicular self-examination.

tsetse fly a fly of the genus *Glossina*, the vector of *Trypanosoma* in Africa. The *Trypanosoma* are transferred to new hosts, including humans, in the salivary juices when the fly bites for a blood meal.

TSF *abbr* triceps skinfold thickness.

TSH *abbr* thyroid stimulating hormone.

T-spring a removable orthodontic appliance spring, working from its palatal aspect to move a tooth or teeth buccally or labially. It is made by a double length of fine wire with a t-shaped tip.

TSS *abbr* toxic shock syndrome.

T-suppressor cell ⤷ suppressor T-cell.

Tsutsugamushi disease scrub typhus. ⤷ rickettsial fevers, typhus.

T4 syndrome the symptoms associated with a hypomobility lesion at thoracic vertebra 4 (T4) (plus or minus one or two levels). The person complains of vague arm pain or discomfort, accompanied by paraesthesia, which does not follow any dermatome patterns. Hand symptoms are also considered to be an integral part of T4 syndrome. The pathology is unknown, but autonomic nerve control may be compromised.

TT *abbr* tetanus toxoid.

TTTS *abbr* twin to twin transfusion syndrome.

T-tube a T-shaped tube that may be used to drain bile from the common bile duct following surgery.

t-tubes (t-tubules) in full transverse tubules. Tubules continuous with the surface membrane of a striated muscle fibre, which contain extracellular fluid yet penetrate in a network pattern the whole cellular cross-section, encircling every myofibril. The tubules are separated from the sarcoplasmic reticulum (SR) only by closely adjoining membranes, and are the route of excitation as an action potential spreads inward from the surface of the fibre to instigate $[Ca^{2+}]$ release from the SR. ➲ sarcoplasmic reticulum.

tubal *adj* pertaining to a tube.

tubal abortion ➲ tubal miscarriage.

tubal ligation tying of both uterine (fallopian) tubes as a means of sterilization.

tubal miscarriage an ectopic pregnancy in which the embryo dies and is expelled from the fimbriated end of the uterine (fallopian) tube.

tubal pregnancy ➲ ectopic pregnancy.

tube head the protective metal head covering containing the X-ray tube, tube housing, transformers and cooling oil. The removable cone is placed at the aperture of the head.

tube insert an evacuated tube which contains a negative cathode, which when heated produces a stream of electrons, and a positive anode or target that when bombarded by electrons produces a beam of radiation.

tube side that side of an X-ray film packet or cassette which faces the source of X-rays from an X-ray machine.

tubercle *n* **1.** a small rounded prominence, usually on bone. Often used interchangeably with tuberosity. **2.** the specific lesion produced by *Mycobacterium tuberculosis*.

tubercle of Carabelli ➲ Carabelli's cusp.

tuberculide, tuberculid *n* a small lump. Metastatic manifestation of tuberculosis, producing a skin lesion, e.g. papulonecrotic tuberculide, rosacea-like tuberculide.

tuberculin *n* a sterile extract of tuberculoprotein. Utilized in skin testing for tuberculosis or in some cases before administration of BCG immunization. ➲ Heaf test, Mantoux test.

tuberculoid *adj* resembling tuberculosis. One of the two types of leprosy.

tuberculoma *n* a caseous tubercle, usually large, its size suggesting a tumour.

tuberculosis (TB) *n* chronic granulomatous infection caused by *Mycobacterium tuberculosis* (human type). Immunization with BCG is used to protect vulnerable individuals. ➲ BCG. Tuberculosis causes systemic effects such as pyrexia, night sweats, anorexia and weight loss, plus site-dependent signs and symptoms, e.g. cough and purulent sputum in lung disease (pulmonary TB), haematuria in renal TB and infertility if the uterine (fallopian) tubes are affected.

A diagnosis of pulmonary TB is made on clinical signs, chest X-ray, biopsy, skin tests (e.g. Heaf, Mantoux) and the presence of acid-fast bacilli in cultures of sputum or gastric washings. The mycobacterial infection is usually confirmed by direct microscopy (Ziehl-Neelsen or auramine staining) and culture of samples. A stain-positive sputum sample requires confirmation by use of standard culture methods (growth characteristics, pigment production and biochemical tests) or molecular DNA technology (hybridization probes, polymerase chain reaction [PCR]). Following decontamination, samples should be cultured on a solid medium (Löwenstein-Jensen or Middlebrook). However, as the organism grows slowly, simultaneous culture in liquid culture media should be performed to expedite the testing of drug sensitivities (typically within 7–21 days). However, treatment is started ahead of culture results if clinical signs and histology are indicative of TB. In the UK treatment is with a combination of antituberculosis drugs in two distinct phases, initial and continuation. Four drugs are used in the initial phase: rifampicin, ethambutol, isoniazid and pyrazinamide for a period of two months. Rifamicin and isoniazid are used during the continuation phase for another four months. The incidence, especially of multidrug resistant tuberculosis (MDR-TB) is increasing, in Asia, Africa and Eastern Europe, in association with poverty and homelessness, in debilitated individuals and in those who are immunocompromised due to HIV disease. Where MDR-TB is suspected, molecular tools may be employed to test for the presence of the rpo gene, currently associated with around 95% of rifampicin-resistant cases. Rapid tests for other forms of drug resistance are under development. If a cluster of cases suggests a common source, fingerprinting of isolates with restriction-fragment length polymorphism (RFLP) or DNA amplification can help confirm this. In addition extensively drug-resistant TB (XDR-TB) strains have been isolated in many countries including a case in Scotland. Bovine tuberculosis (caused by *Mycobacterium bovis*) is endemic in cattle and transmitted to humans by drinking infected milk. Pasteurization of milk and monitoring of dairy herds are the mainstays of disease control. *M. avium intracellulare (MAI)* is an atypical mycobacterium, which may infect severely immunocompromised individuals (such as those with advanced AIDS). *miliary tuberculosis* so called because of the appearance of many small areas resembling millet seeds on the chest X-ray. There is widespread disease with dissemination of tubercle bacilli in the blood. It can affect bone, spleen, liver and the meninges. *primary tuberculosis* occurs during childhood and there is lung involvement, fever and skin rash. *post primary tuberculosis* the most common form of pulmonary TB but other sites may be affected—**tubercular, tuberculous** *adj*.

tuberculum a small rounded swelling or projection.

tuberosity *n* a bony prominence, such as that of the humerus. Provides for the attachment of ligaments or muscles. Often used interchangeably with tubercle.

S
T

tuberosity of fifth metatarsal a tubercle at the base of the fifth metatarsal to which the tendon of the peroneus brevis muscle attaches.

tuberous sclerosis (*syn* epiloia) also known as Bourneville's disease. An inherited autosomal dominant disorder characterized by cognitive defects, skin lesions and epilepsy. There may also be gum hyperplasia, changes in the basal nuclei, tumour formation and retinal changes.

tubo-ovarian *adj* pertaining to or involving both uterine (fallopian) tube and ovary, e.g. tubo-ovarian abscess.

tubo-ovarian gestation an ectopic pregnancy which develops between the ovary and the uterine (fallopian) tube.

tubule *n* a small tube. *collecting tubule* straight tube in the kidney medulla conveying urine to the renal pelvis. *convoluted tubule* coiled tube in the kidney cortex. *renal tubule* part of a nephron. *seminiferous tubule* coiled tube in the testis.

TUE *abbr* therapeutic use exemption.

tularaemia *n* (*syn* deer-fly fever, rabbit fever, tick fever) an infection of mammals, including wild rabbits, domestic cats and dogs, and birds caused by the Gram-negative bacterium *Francisella tularensis*; it occurs in the northern hemisphere and is transmitted by bites from ticks and flies. Humans acquire the infection either from ticks or from handling infected animal carcasses, such as rabbits. Skin ulceration at the inoculation site is followed by painful lymphadenopathy and fever with constitutional upset. It can be acquired by the inhalation of infected material that leads to pulmonary tularaemia and pneumonia. An infrequent presentation is conjunctivitis with ulceration. Rarely it causes septicaemia. Treatment is with an aminoglycoside antimicrobial drug, gentamicin or streptomycin.—**tularaemic** *adj.* ⊃ Colour Section Figure 124.

tumescence *n* a state of swelling; turgidity. Usually due to oedema, or the collection of blood in the part.

tumor *n* swelling; usually used in the context of being one of the five classical signs and symptoms of inflammation, the others being calor, dolor, loss of function and rubor.

tumour *n* a swelling. A mass of abnormal tissue which resembles the normal tissues in structure, but which fulfils no useful function and which grows at the expense of the body. Benign, simple or innocent tumours are encapsulated, do not infiltrate adjacent tissue or cause metastases and are unlikely to recur if removed—**tumorous** *adj. malignant tumour* not encapsulated, infiltrates adjacent tissue and causes metastases. ⊃ cancer.

tumour infiltrating lymphocyte lymphocytes found in solid cancers; when cultured in interleukin–2 they exhibit specific activity against the cancer from which they originated.

tumour lysis syndrome (TLS) may occur following intensive chemotherapy treatment for some haematological malignancies. As cancer cells are destroyed there is release of cellular breakdown products. This results in metabolic problems (e.g. hyperkalaemia, hypocalcaemia, hyperuricaemia, hyperphosphataemia) that may cause renal failure and possibly circulatory and respiratory failure.

tumour marker chemical detected in the serum that may be associated with a specific cancer or sometimes non-malignant diseases. They include: alphafetoprotein (AFP), cancer cell surface antigen 125 (CA-125), carcinoembryonic antigen (CEA), human chorionic gonadotrophin (hCG), pancreatic oncofetal antigen (POA) and prostate specific antigen (PSA). They may be used for monitoring disease progress and efficacy of treatment, but are of limited use for population screening.

tumour necrosis factor (TNF) a cytokine that is toxic to cancer cells and activates other leucocytes. It causes profound metabolic effects that include inflammatory responses, pyrexia and weight loss leading to cachexia.

tumourocidal dose a dose of radiation capable of destroying a tumour.

tumour-specific antigen an antigen produced by specific cancer cells, but is not present on the non-cancerous cells in the tissue from which the cancer was derived.

tungsten carbide the abrasive powder used in grinding wheels and some rotary cutting instruments used in dentistry. Also incorporated in certain steels to produce a harder, longer-lasting cutting edge.

tungsten-halogen lamp ⊃ halogen lamp.

tunica *n* a lining membrane; a coat.

tunica adventitia the outer fibrous coat of an artery, arteriole or vein.

tunica albuginea the inner fibrous tissue covering of the testis, it is beneath the tunica vaginalis. It dips down into the glandular substance of the testis to form septa that divide the substance of the testis into many wedge-shaped lobules.

tunica intima the smooth endothelial (squamous epithelium) lining of an artery, arteriole or vein. In the veins of the limbs the tunica intima is modified to form valves that prevent backflow and pooling of blood in the limbs. ⊃ muscle pump, venous return.

tunica media the middle smooth muscle and elastic tissue coat of an artery and arteriole; the tunica media of veins is thinner with less muscle and elastic tissue.

tunica vaginalis the outer, double membrane covering the testis, it is derived from the pelvic and abdominal peritoneum during embryonic development when the testes are within the abdomen.

tunica vasculosa a network of connective tissue and capillaries within the testis.

tunica vasculosa lentis an anastomosing vascular network that develops during embryonic life to envelop the lens of the eye. ⊃ hyaloid artery.

tunnel procedure ⊃ furcation.

tunnel vision the loss of the peripheral part of the visual field. It may be a symptom of the final stage of primary open-angle glaucoma (POAG) or retinitis pigmentosa. The onset of POAG is insidious and because central vision remains intact, patients may fail to discern the peripheral loss of vision. Occasionally patients suffer more bumps and scrapes because of visual field loss, which they erroneously attribute to ageing.

S
T

TUR/TURP *abbr* transurethral resection of prostate.

turbid cloudy, not clear. Normal urine containing mucus may be turbid. However, urine may be cloudy because it contains abnormal substances, e.g. protein, or pus and white blood cells if a urinary tract infection is present.

turbinate *adj* shaped like an inverted cone.

turbinate bones also known as nasal conchae. One of three structures on either side forming part of the lateral nasal walls. ⮑ concha, ethmoid bone, inferior nasal conchae, nasal conchae.

turbine-driven handpiece turbine handpiece or air rotor. In dentistry, a handpiece incorporating a rotor that is driven at high speed up to 300 000 rpm by compressed air flow. The head contains a friction grip chuck and one or more water jets acting as a coolant for the burs, etc. ⮑ handpiece.

turbinectomy *n* removal of a nasal turbinate bone.

turbulent boundary layer the layer which is next to the surface of an object, but in this case mixing with the flow further away from it. An example of a boundary layer change is that due to a dimpled golf ball in flight: the dimples make the boundary layer turbulent, which reduces drag caused by the pressure being lower behind the ball, so less energy is lost to the flow. ⮑ boundary layer, laminar boundary layer.

turbulent flow the flow of a medium (e.g. air or water) in which the molecules are moving in a random, non-ordered manner. Can be an effect of an object or body travelling through the medium.

turf toe a colloquial expression used in sports medicine to describe the sprain and subsequent inflammation of the first metatarsophalangeal joint.

turgid *adj* swollen; firmly distended, as with blood by congestion—**turgescence** *n*, **turgidity** *n*.

turgor indicates the elasticity and resilience of the skin; these are influenced by the amount of fluid in the cells and the interstitial spaces. Skin turgor decreases with age, but it can be useful as part of a holistic assessment of the state of hydration. Skin turgor is assessed by lifting a fold of skin, usually on the back of the hand. On release, it should quickly return to its original position. During normal ageing the skin loses elasticity and takes longer to return to its original position in older people. Reduced turgor may be an early sign of dehydration. Conversely the presence of oedema will increase turgor, the skin is tight and shiny and cannot be lifted.

Turk's disease ⮑ Duane's syndrome.

Turner's syndrome (H Turner, American endocrinologist, 1892–1970) a chromosomal abnormality affecting around 1 in 2500/3000 females who have a single sex chromosome, the X, and thus they have one less chromosome than normal. The karyotype is usually XO with a total of only 45 chromosomes, but there may be mosaic forms, (e.g. XO/XX). The condition is characterized by multiple abnormalities, which include webbed neck, low set ears, abnormal facial structure, short stature, cubitus valgus, shield chest, aortic coarctation and other cardiovascular abnormalities. There may be some degree of learning disability and spatial processing defects are common. There is infantile genital development and underdeveloped breasts; the ovaries are almost completely devoid of germ cells and there is failure of pubertal development. Affected women are at risk of poor bone mineral density, hypertension and type 2 diabetes.

turnkey a term used to denote a company which will provide all the necessary software and hardware and back-up support to enable the user to 'turn a key' and use the equipment.

turtle a wheeled mechanical device, used for graphics, attached to a computer via cables.

Turville infinity balance test (*syn* infinity balance test) a test for balancing the accommodative state of the eyes. It can also be used for detecting suppression, vertical and horizontal associated phorias and (with a target composed of two horizontal lines) aniseikonia in the vertical meridian. It consists of a 3 cm wide vertical septum placed in the centre of a mirror on which is reflected a reversed illuminated chart. Thus the patient can only see the right side of the chart with the right eye, and the left side with the left eye, which allows for simultaneous comparison of the chart seen by both eyes, while still retaining fusion for peripheral objects near the border of the chart. If the chart is projected onto a screen, the septum is placed halfway between patient and screen. The test is carried out after the conventional refractive procedures. ⮑ associated heterophoria, balancing test.

tussis *n* a cough.

TUVP *abbr* transurethral vaporization of the prostate.

TV *abbr* **1.** tidal volume/air. **2.** transvaginal. **3.** *Trichomonas vaginalis*.

T_vent *abbr* ventilatory threshold.

tweed arch bending pliers ⮑ pliers.

tweezer a hand instrument with two narrow and/or pointed, straight or curved beaks used to grasp small objects. May have a locking device to maintain the beaks in a closed position until released.

twilight vision ⮑ mesopic vision.

twin block appliance ⮑ orthodontic appliance.

twins one of two infants resulting from a single pregnancy. ⮑ binovular, conjoined twins, dichorionic twins, monoamniotic twins, monochorionic twins, monozygotic, uniovular.

twin to twin transfusion syndrome (TTTS) ⮑ fetofetal transfusion syndrome.

twin wire arch a part of a fixed orthodontic appliance consisting of twin, fine stainless steel archwires attached to bands cemented onto the teeth or brackets bonded to the teeth. The natural effect of the wire tending to straighten itself is the force used to align such teeth.

twitch a rapid contraction of muscle in response to single stimulus.

two-dimensional test a test for stereopsis consisting of two-dimensional objects as test material such as targets,

S
T

cards, etc. as used in a stereoscope or a major amblyoscope (e.g. random-test stereogram; Titmus stereotest). Other tests for stereopsis are three-dimensional (3-D), the Howard–Dolman test being the most well known. Two-dimensional tests (2-D) are the most commonly used in clinical practice. ⊃ Howard–Dolman test, random-dot stereogram, stereoscope, vectogram.

two-dimensional sequence ⊃ image acquisition time.

two-tailed hypothesis a research term. It implies a difference but no direction to the change, e.g. first year students in group A will have a different score than first year students in group B. Whereas a one-tailed hypothesis implies a direction to a predicted change, e.g. first year students in group A will score higher than first year students in group B. ⊃ one-tailed hypothesis.

tylosis *n* ⊃ keratosis, keratosis palmaris et plantaris.

tylosis palmaris a scaling condition of the palms of the hands.

tylosis plantaris a scaling condition of the soles of the feet.

tympanic *adj* pertaining to the tympanum.

tympanic cavity the cavity of the middle ear; contains the three ossicles.

tympanic light reflex a reflection of light shining on the tympanic membrane. Normally this is seen as a cone of bright light in the antero-inferior segment of the tympanic membrane (Figure T.8).

tympanic membrane the eardrum. It separates the outer ear from the middle ear and transmits sound vibrations to the ossicles. Most of the tympanic membrane comprises three layers: an epithelial lining continuous with the external auditory meatus/canal, a fibrous layer which provides strength and the ability to vibrate, and a mucosal layer that is continuous with that of the middle ear. The three layers are present in the lower four-fifths of the tympanic membrane, known as the pars tensa. The fibrous layer is absent in the upper tympanic membrane, known as the pars flaccida. ⊃ Colour Section Figure 13.

tympanic thermometer accurate core body temperature recorded by means of an electronic probe introduced into the external auditory meatus/canal.

tympanites, tympanism *n* (*syn* meteorism) abdominal distension due to accumulation of gas in the intestine.

tympan/o- a prefix that means 'eardrum, middle ear', e.g. *tympanoplasty.*

tympanoplasty *n* reconstructive operation on the middle ear designed to improve hearing or prevent otorrhoea in ears damaged by chronic suppurative otitis media—**tympanoplastic** *adj.*

tympanum *n* the cavity of the middle ear.

Tyndall effect (*syn* Tyndall scatter) diffusion of light by the particles present in a liquid or gas. It is because of this effect that heterogeneities (e.g. increased proteins) of the media of the eye can be seen, as occurs in iris and/or ciliary body inflammation. ⊃ aqueous flare.

Tyndall scatter ⊃ Tyndall effect.

type I error (alpha α error) in research, rejecting a null hypothesis that is true. The investigator determines that there is something going on when in fact there is not.

type II error (beta β error) in research, not rejecting a null hypothesis that is false. The investigator determines that there is nothing going on when in fact there is.

type VIII glycogen storage disease (GSD) a GSD in which there is a deficiency of liver phosphorylase kinase enzyme. It is characterized by very mild disease, hepatomegaly, growth retardation, elevated liver enzymes, hyperlipidaemia and fasting hyperketosis.

type IX glycogen storage disease (GSD) a GSD in which there is a deficiency of liver glycogen phosphorylase kinase enzyme. It is characterized by mild hepatomegaly. It can be inherited as an autosomal or X-linked recessive trait.

type 0 glycogen storage disease (GSD) a GSD in which there is a deficiency of liver glycogen synthase enzyme. It is characterized by fasting hypoglycaemia and postprandial hyperglycaemia.

S
T

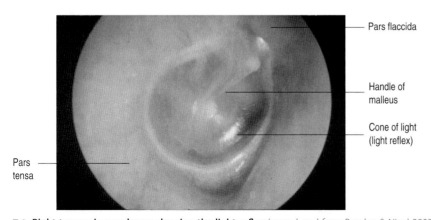

Pars flaccida

Handle of malleus

Cone of light (light reflex)

Pars tensa

T.8 Right tympanic membrane showing the light reflex (reproduced from Brooker & Nicol 2003 with permission).

type 1 hepatorenal syndrome ⊃ hepatorenal syndrome.

type 2 hepatorenal syndrome ⊃ hepatorenal syndrome.

types of nipples the nipple type influences the establishment of successful breast feeding. Types include: normal where the ducts protrude in the aerola beyond the curve of the breast tissue; flat where the ducts are flush with the soft tissue of the breast; depressed where the ducts are below the level of the skin of the breast, forming a small saucer shape; and inverted where the tiny muscles of the erectile tissue are contracted, drawing the ducts down into the soft tissue of the breast. They are likely to be kinked, obstructing the flow of milk.

typhlitis *n* inflammation of the caecum.

typhoid fever an infectious enteric fever usually spread by contamination of food, milk or water supplies with *Salmonella enterica* serovar Typhi, either directly by sewage, indirectly by flies or by poor personal hygiene. Symptomless carriers harbouring the micro-organism in the gallbladder and excreting it in faeces are the main source of outbreaks of disease in the UK. The average incubation period is 10–14 days. A progressive febrile illness with a 'stepladder' rise in temperature marks the onset of the disease, which develops as the micro-organism invades lymphoid tissue, including the spleen and that of the small intestine (Peyer's patches), to produce profuse diarrhoeal (pea soup) stools which may become frankly haemorrhagic due to bowel ulceration. The bowel can perforate. Patients may have a slow pulse, headache, drowsiness, delirium and a cough. A rose-spot rash may appear on the upper abdomen and back at the end of the first week. Ultimate recovery usually begins at the end of the third week. Immunization is available for travellers to regions where sanitation is poor and the infection is endemic, and for laboratory staff, but it is not a substitute for meticulous personal hygiene measures. ⊃ paratyphoid.

typhoid vaccine a capsular polysaccharide vaccine for intramuscular administration and a live attenuated vaccine for oral administration.

typhus *n* a group of acute infectious diseases. The presentation varies between types but generally includes sudden onset of high fever, a skin eruption (maculopapular or petechial depending on type), lymphadenopathy, severe headache, weakness, cough, bronchitis and limb pains. In severe infections there may be pneumonia, haemorrhage, renal failure and heart failure. It is a disease of war, famine or catastrophe, being spread by lice, ticks, mites or fleas. It is only sporadic in the UK. ⊃ rickettsial fevers.

typodont an articulated apparatus with hollowed-out upper and lower bases that can be filled with wax or acrylic to support metal or plastic teeth and on which students can practise dental techniques. Commonly used in orthodontics to practise tooth movement using appliances.

typoscope (*syn* reading slit) a reading shield made of black material in which there is a rectangular aperture allowing one or more lines of print to be seen (Figure T.9). It reduces

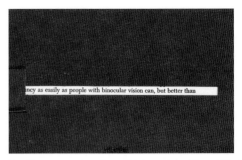

T.9 Typoscope (reading slit) (reproduced from Millodot 2004 with permission).

extraneous light reflected from the surface of the paper and assists in staying on the correct line. It can be helpful for people with low vision who have, for example, media involvement. Recent models embody built-in lighting to provide even and controlled illumination. ⊃ low vision.

tyramine *n* a monamine derived from the amino acid tyrosine that is present in several foodstuffs and beverages, especially mature cheese, red wine, ripe fruit, broad bean pods, fermented soya bean foods, e.g. tofu and soy sauce, meat and yeast extracts. It has a similar effect in the body to adrenaline (epinephrine) and causes an increase in systemic blood pressure. It is normally metabolized by the enzyme monoamine oxidase in the wall of the intestine and in the liver; consequently patients taking drugs in the monoamine oxidase inhibitor (MAOI) group (e.g. the antidepressants phenelzine, isocarboxazid) should not eat foods containing tyramine such as mature cheese, otherwise a dangerously high blood pressure may result. ⊃ monoamine oxidase inhibitor (MAOI) antidepressant drugs.

tyrosinaemia *n* an aminoacidopathy resulting from abnormal metabolism of tyrosine and the build up of toxic metabolites caused by a specific enzyme deficiency; there are several types. (a) neonatal tyrosinaemia in which there is a transitory inability to metabolize tyrosine, especially in preterm infants. It results in increased levels in the blood and increased excretion of tyrosine and its metabolites in the urine (aminoaciduria). (b) type I tyrosinaemia is inherited as an autosomal recessive trait. It is due to a deficiency of the enzyme fumarylacetoacetate hydrolase. This is the most severe type and leads to liver and kidney damage. It may be acute, with symptoms occurring soon after birth. The infant fails to thrive, there is a cabbage-like odour, diarrhoea and vomiting, jaundice, liver damage, liver failure and death without a successful liver transplant. The chronic form occurs later during childhood and is characterized by delays in achieving developmental milestones, renal tubular malfunction, chronic liver disease and polyneuropathy. (c) type II tyrosinaemia is inherited as an autosomal recessive trait in which the enzyme tyrosine aminotransferase is deficient. There are hyperkeratotic lesions on the palms and soles and affected individuals have photophobia, excessive tearing and eye pain. A learning disability is often present. (d) type III tyrosinaemia, an autosomal dominant condition, which occurs much less commonly is caused by the lack of the enzyme 4-hydroxyphenylpyruvate dioxygenase. Affected individuals have a learning disability and experience seizures and intermittent problems with co-ordination and balance.

tyrosine *n* a conditionally essential (indispensable) amino acid required for growth. Combines with iodine to form the hormone thyroxine. If phenylalanine intake is restricted, as in phenylketonuria (PKU), the diet needs to be supplemented with tyrosine.

tyrosinosis *n* abnormal metabolism of tyrosine. Usually known as tyrosinaemia.

ubiquinone *n* also known as coenzyme Q10. A quinone derivative that acts as an electron carrier in the mitochondrial respiratory chain (electron transport chain). In the body it is located primarily in the mitochondria, especially in skeletal and cardiac muscle. It is a non-essential lipid-soluble nutrient found predominantly in animal foods and at low levels in plant foods. As a component of the electron transport chain, it is important for ATP formation. It is also believed to have an antioxidant function, protecting DNA and cell membranes from oxidative stress/damage. For athletes, ubiquinone (coenzyme Q10) supplements are claimed to enhance energy production through the electron transport chain, and to reduce the oxidative stress/damage of exercise. Research does not support the claim, reporting either no effect or in some cases an ergolytic rather than ergogenic effect. ➲ ergogenic aids.

UE₃ *abbr* unconjugated oestriols.

UIP *abbr* usual interstitial pneumonia.

ulcer *n* destruction of either mucous membrane or skin from whatever cause, producing a crater or indentation. An inflammatory reaction occurs and if it penetrates a blood vessel bleeding ensues. If the ulcer is in the lining of a hollow organ it can perforate through the wall. ➲ arterial ulcer, leg ulcer, peptic ulcer, pressure ulcer, venous ulcer.

ulcerative *adj* pertaining to or of the nature of an ulcer.

ulcerative colitis superficial inflammatory condition affecting the colon. It always involves the rectum and spreads continuously for a variable distance. It is characterized by diarrhoea containing blood, passage of mucus and pus, pain, loss of weight and anaemia. Complications include severe inflammation, perforation of the bowel, haemorrhage, fistulae, fluid and electrolyte imbalance, toxic dilatation (megacolon) and colorectal cancer. Systemic complications include liver disease, iritis, arthralgia, mouth ulcers, gallstones, etc. ➲ colitis, inflammatory bowel disease, Colour Section Figure 125.

ulcerative gingivitis ➲ gingivitis, necrotizing ulcerative periodontitis.

ulcerogenic *adj* capable of producing an ulcer.

Ullrich syndrome (O Ullrich, German paediatrician, 1894–1957) ➲ Noonan's syndrome.

ulna *n* the inner (medial) bone of the forearm. The longer of the two forearm bones, it articulates with the humerus at the elbow, the carpals at the wrist and with the radius at the proximal and distal radioulnar joints. ➲ Colour Section Figure 2.

ulnar *adj* pertaining to the ulna. As in descriptions of forearm structures: on or towards the side of the ulna, i.e. the fifth finger side.

ulnar artery the artery running down the medial aspect of the forearm that carries blood to muscles of the forearm and wrist. It crosses the wrist to become the superior palmar arch of the hand. ➲ Colour Section Figure 9.

ulnar nerve a branch of the brachial plexus. It descends through the upper arm lying medial to the brachial artery. It passes behind the medial epicondyle of the humerus to supply the muscles on the ulnar aspect of the forearm. It continues downwards to supply the muscles in the palm of the hand and the skin of the whole of the little finger and the medial half of the third finger. It gives off no branches above the elbow. ➲ brachial plexus, cubital tunnel external compression syndrome, Colour Section Figure 11.

ulna vein one of the deep veins of the forearm. ➲ Colour Section Figure 10.

U-loop an orthodontic wire such as a buccal bow bent into a U-shape, to allow for adjustment by closing or opening the loop.

ultra- a prefix that means 'beyond, excess', e.g. *ultrasound*.

ultradian *adj* pertaining to a biological rhythm that has a cycle of less than 24 hours. ➲ circadian.

ultrafiltration *n* filtration under pressure; e.g. in haemofiltration where the blood is filtered under pressure.

ultrasonic *adj* relating to mechanical vibrations of very high frequency. ➲ ultrasound. Used in dentistry for various purposes—*ultrasonic cleaning bath* an electronic high frequency generator which agitates a cleaning solution in the bath thus loosening any debris adhering to dental instruments and appliances prior to sterilization. *ultrasonic endodontic instrumentation* conventional and diamond coated endodontic instruments are energized by the piezo-electric effect and used to remove pulp tissue and other debris and in enlarging and irrigating root canals. *ultrasonic instrument removal* use of ultrasonic energy to loosen and remove fractured instruments from root canals. *ultrasonic post-removal* the use of ultrasonic energy to loosen and remove root canal posts. *ultrasonic root-end preparation* cutting cavities in the root tip during endodontic surgery with ultrasonically-energized instruments. *ultrasonic scaler* a scaling instrument with interchangeable tips of several shapes. The tips vibrate at ultrasonic speeds under a water spray. Should not be used on patients with a heart pacemaker. *ultrasonic troughing* cutting dentine with ultrasonically energized tools to locate root canal entrances.

ultrasonogram picture of an internal organ or structure produced by ultrasound scanning.

ultrasonography *n* formation of a visible image from the use of ultrasound. A controlled beam of sound is directed

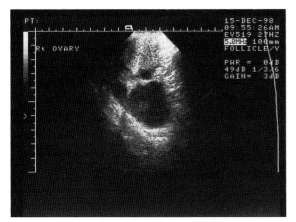

U.1 Ultrasound image showing a right-sided 6 cm cyst ovarian swelling (reproduced from Gangar 2001 with permission).

into the relevant part of the body. The reflected ultrasound is used to build up an electronic image of the various structures of the body (Figure U.1). ➲ transrectal ultrasonography, ultrasound. Routinely offered during pregnancy to monitor progress and detect fetal and placental abnormalities. *diagnostic ultrasonography* is used across all specialties. ➲ ultrasonography in ophthalmology. Information is derived from echoes which occur when a controlled beam of sound energy crosses the boundary between adjacent tissues of differing physical properties. Used in sports medicine as a diagnostic tool in both cardiovascular and musculoskeletal assessment, e.g. cardiac screening, muscle tears. Ultrasound equipment is portable and accessible, costs less than magnetic resonance imaging (MRI) scanning but requires a skilled operator. It also allows dynamic imaging, e.g. of rotator cuff during shoulder movement. *real-time ultrasonography* an ultrasound imaging technique involving rapid pulsing to enable continuous viewing of movement to be obtained, rather than stationary images—**ultrasonograph** *n*, **ultrasonographically** *adv*.

ultrasonography in ophthalmology a technique utilizing high frequency ultrasound waves (greater than 18 000 Hz) emitted by a transducer placed near the eye. The silicone probe, which rests on the eye, is separated from the transducer by a water column to segregate the noise from the transducer. The technique is used to make biometric measurements such as the axial length of the eye, the depth of the anterior chamber, the thickness of the lens, the distance between the back of the lens and the retina and the thickness of the cornea. The ultrasound wave is reflected when it encounters a change in density (or elasticity) of the medium through which it is passing. The reflected vibration is called an echo. Echoes from the interfaces between the various media of the eye are converted into an electrical potential by a piezoelectrical crystal and can be displayed as deflections or spikes on a cathode-ray oscilloscope. Two types of ultrasonographic measurements are used— the *time-amplitude or A-scan* which measures the time or

distance from the transducer to the interface and back. Thus echoes from surfaces deeper within the eye take longer to return to the transducer for conversion into electrical potential and so they appear further along the time base on the oscilloscope display. The A-scan is more useful for the study of the biometric measurements, as well as measurements of intraocular tumour size (e.g. choroidal melanoma); and the *intensity-modulated or B-scan* in which various scans are taken through the pupillary area and any change in acoustic impedance is shown as a dot on the oscilloscope screen, and these join up as the transducer moves across a meridian. The B-scan is useful to indicate the position of a retinal or vitreous detachment, or of an intraocular foreign body, and for the examination of the orbit. The B-scan is especially useful in the examination of the posterior structures of the eye when opacities prevent ophthalmoscopic examination (e.g. cataract, corneal oedema). ➲ axial length of the eye.

ultrasound (US, U/S) *n* sound waves with a frequency of over 20 kHz, not audible to the human ear. Ultrasound is used to promote healing (frequency 0.8–3 MHz), for diagnosis (frequency 1–10 MHz and applicator has receiver) and for tissue destruction (varies). Ultrasound requires 'coupling' of applicator to skin with gel or water or similar as it is not transmitted in air at MHz frequency. The penetration is inversely proportional to frequency (i.e. 3 Hz absorbed more rapidly in superficial tissue depth than 1 MHz frequency). The absorption rate is higher in collagen-based tissues than, for example, adipose tissue (fat). The properties of kHz frequency ultrasound are very different from those of MHz ultrasound. Used for teeth and jewellery cleaning and car alarms (i.e. travels in air). The beam divergence is very wide and most energy penetrates through bodies with little effective absorption. Ultrasound energy heats tissue (thermal effects) and has mechanical pressure effects (non-thermal) at the same time to different degrees depending on intensity and frequency and underlying tissue properties. The mechanical pressure effects: acoustic streaming is either bulk streaming (i.e. movement of fluid in a direction in response to the ultrasound) or microstreaming (i.e. fluid eddies adjacent to a source of ultrasound). The contribution of streaming to treatment outcomes is not clear. Cavitation, the formation of bubbles from gas previously in solution, does not occur in the human body at usual frequency or intensity range of therapeutic ultrasound, though is a risk near gas-filled body cavities such as lungs and gut. Ultrasound output can be continuous US (CUS) or pulsed US (PUS). The operator sets intensity. The average intensity in the beam at a defined point is called the spatial average (SA). The peak intensity set is the temporal peak (TP). If pulsed, the intensity is described as the temporal average (TA)—the equivalent intensity if it were continuous and not pulsed (i.e. TA = TP × pulsing rate; if 2 W/cm^2 output [TP] pulsed at 20% duty cycle the TA is 0.4 W/cm^2). The ultrasound beam is complex, changing with distance from the applicator according to the frequency of ultrasound and diameter of applicator. For 1 MHz frequency, near zone

U
V

803

(Fresnel) extends 10–15 cm from applicator, very uneven energy distribution, beam remains collimated (~4 divergence). The far zone (Fraunhofer) beam is less intense and has more even energy distribution. Variations in energy distribution is reported as beam non-uniformity ratio (BNR). BNR = spatial peak intensity (SP)/spatial average intensity (SA). The usual BNR for therapeutic equipment is 5–6, for fracture healing it is 2.16. This has practice implications as the energy distribution in higher BNR beam is very irregular and the applicator must be moved (even if pulsed output) during treatment to avoid effects of localized high-intensity beam energy. Energy is applied with applicator for therapeutic US. The applicator is the site of production of ultrasound. The applicator contains a crystal, which is stimulated by high-frequency alternating current (reverse piezoelectric effect). The applicator sizes are usually 1, 2, 5 or 10 cm^2 depending on area being treated. The actual radiating area is usually less than the applicator face size—effective radiating area (ERA). Couple energy is produced in applicator to skin with gel or water or other transmissive substance as US is not transmitted through air at MHz frequencies. The effectiveness of MHz frequency ultrasound for acute soft-tissue injuries is still debated. One reason is that it is very difficult to identify a reduction in healing time over 5–7 days healing time. Another reason is unreliable equipment output, as intensity is often not accurate. There is clear evidence of the effectiveness of MHz frequency ultrasound in fracture healing of delayed and non-uniting fractures. In chronic conditions, each application is for longer and there are more of them. Ultrasound dosage includes frequency, size of applicator and ERA, intensity (spatial average temporal average—SATA, spatial average temporal peak—SATP), location and size of area treated, duration of treatment, which machine, etc. ⊃ ultrasonography.

ultraviolet radiation (UVR) short wavelength electromagnetic radiation outside the visible spectrum. There are three types of ultraviolet radiation (UVA, UVB and UVC) divided by wavelength because of differences in effects and hence clinical uses. UVA has a wavelength between 400–315 nm and is also called long UV. It is used with sensitizers, e.g. psoralen (PUVA) method, to treat psoriasis. The main component of solar UVR. UVB has a wavelength between 315–280 nm and is also known as medium UV or erythemal UV. It is the main cause of skin damage from sun. UVC has a wavelength between 280–100 nm and is also called short UV or abiotic UV. It is used to treat wounds as it has a bactericidal effect. UVC has a zero component in solar UVR as it is absorbed in ozone layer. In dentistry UVR is used to polymerize and harden certain fissure sealants or composite filling materials.

umbilical catheterization the passing of a fine catheter into the umbilical vein of the umbilicus and to the liver for purposes of feeding and assessing the condition of a sick neonate.

umbilical cord the cord connecting the fetus to the placenta. It contains a vein and two arteries and a gelatinous embryonic connective tissue called Wharton's jelly (Figure U.2).

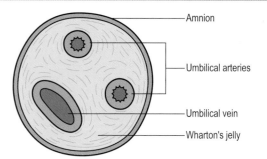

U.2 Umbilical cord (cross-section) (reproduced from Fraser & Cooper 2003 with permission).

umbilical cord blood stem cells stem cells harvested from blood taken from the umbilical cord or the placenta soon after birth. The stem cells, which will only produce blood cells, are stored and subsequently used in haemopoietic stem cell transplantation for a variety of conditions including some types of leukaemia.

umbilical hernia protrusion of a portion of intestine through the area of weakness at the umbilical scar. ⊃ hernia.

umbilicated *adj* having a central depression.

umbilicus, omphalus *n* (*syn* navel) the abdominal scar left by the separation of the remnant of umbilical cord after birth—**umbilical** *adj*.

unciform bone ⊃ hamate.

uncinate hook-shaped, or having hooks.

uncinate epilepsy a varient of temporal lobe epilepsy involving the uncinate area in which the person experiences olfactory and gustatory hallucinations.

uncompensated heterophoria (*syn* decompensated heterophoria) any heterophoria which gives rise to symptoms or to suppression. The symptoms are associated with visual tasks, especially close work, but also occasionally inadequate illumination. Resting the eyes will usually lessen the symptoms. Unbalanced spectacle correction, a deterioration in the patient's general health, worry and anxiety can also sometimes give rise to an uncompensated heterophoria. This type of heterophoria is presumed to manifest itself as fixation disparity. ⊃ compensated heterophoria, Disparometer, Mallett fixation disparity unit, relieving prism, retinal disparity.

unconditioned response in classical conditioning, a response to an unconditioned stimulus that is naturally evoked by that stimulus. For example, in Pavlov's experiments with dogs, salivation at the presentation of food is the unconditioned response. ⊃ conditioning.

unconditioned stimulus in classical conditioning, a stimulus that automatically evokes a particular reflexive response. For example, in Pavlov's experiments with dogs, the presentation of food is the unconditioned stimulus that automatically evokes the salivatory response. ⊃ conditioning.

unconscious 1. unresponsive to stimuli. **2.** that part of the mind comprising the instincts, feelings, emotions and experiences of which the person is not normally aware.

Although they are not easily recalled they may influence behaviour.

unconsciousness *n* state of being unconscious; insensible. ➲ Glasgow Coma Scale.

uncrossed diplopia ➲ homonymous diplopia.

uncut lens ➲ finished lens.

underclass *n* a group who are deprived, disenfranchised and marginalized in society, such as rough sleepers.

undercut in dentistry **1.** a design feature of a tooth preparation achieved by cutting away tooth substance from below, or occurring by chance or error. It prevents the displacement of a restoration when set. **2.** an overhung area of a tooth beneath which a clasp or band may be placed for retention of a prosthesis as may be indicated by a survey line. *under ridge* the alveolar ridge in an edentulous mouth that has resorbed leaving an undercut below its crest thus making denture construction and insertion difficult.

underperformance syndrome (UPS) an enduring deficit in performance which persists despite a period of rest or reduced training load and is not explained by any major diagnosed pathology. Characterized by a wide range of symptoms including fatigue, frequent minor infections and disturbed mood. It differs from chronic fatigue syndrome in that the symptoms do not have to last at least 6 months. ➲ chronic fatigue syndrome/myalgic encephalomyelitis, overtraining.

underwater seal drain a type of drainage whereby a tube exiting from the chest is placed under water (the seal) to prevent air entering the chest. The underwater seal drain may be used to remove air, blood or other fluids from the pleural cavity. A chest drain that incorporates a one way valve may be used for spontaneous pneumothorax. ➲ haemothorax, intercostal chest drain, pneumothorax.

underwater weighing (*syn* hydrostatic weighing) an accurate method for the measurement of body density from which the percentages of body fat and lean body mass can be determined using standard equations. Weight in air is compared with weight in water during brief immersion, holding the breath after full expiration (at residual lung volume which is separately measured). Density is calculated from the volume of water displaced according to the Archimedes principle, which states that an object submerged in water is buoyed up by the weight of water displaced. ➲ body composition, body fat.

undescended testis (*syn* cryptorchism) a testis that has failed to migrate to the correct position in the scrotum. The types of undescended testis are ectopic, where the testis may be found in the abdominal wall or near the base of the penis, and incomplete, where the testis is mobile (i.e. it can move up and down). The complications of undescended testes are: torsion of the testis leading to damage, infertility and testicular cancer. Ectopic and incomplete descent of the testes require surgical mobilization by orchiopexy, i.e. mobilization of the testes into the scrotum. Most male infants' testes will descend within 12 months of birth. If the testes have not descended after 12 months, an orchiopexy is normally required. This is usually performed before the child reaches 3 years. If an undescended testis were found in an adult male, an orchidectomy would be required, given the risk of developing cancer.

undine *n* a small glass flask with a spout that produces a fine stream of liquid; used for irrigating the eye.

undulant fever brucellosis.

unengaged head on abdominal examination the fetal head is palpated above the pelvic brim. ➲ engagement.

unerupted describes teeth not yet erupted into the mouth.

unexplained under performance syndrome (UUPS) also known as overtraining syndrome, sports fatigue syndrome, staleness, etc. In sports medicine, a decline in performance lasting for more than two weeks despite sufficient recovery.

ungual *adj* pertaining to the fingernails and toenails.

unguentum *n* ointment.

unguis *n* a nail.

uni- a prefix that means 'one', e.g. *unicellular*.

uniaxial joint a joint with movement round one axis only, for example, flexion and extension.

UNICEF *abbr* United Nations International Children's Emergency Fund.

unicellular *adj* consisting of only one cell, such as a bacterium.

unicondylar knee replacement also known as unicompartment knee replacement. A hemiarthroplasty in which either the medial or the lateral part of the tibiofemoral joint is replaced. ➲ total knee replacement.

uniformity in radiology, the variations in count rate detected by a gamma camera when it is exposed to a regular source of gamma rays emitted from a radionuclide.

uniform resource locator (URL) the address of internet files.

unilateral *adj* relating to or on one side only—**unilaterally** *adv*.

unilateral neglect also called spatial neglect and visiospatial neglect. It is recognized in patients with brain injury and is characterized as a failure to respond, report to or orientate to meaningful stimuli presented to the side contralateral to the cerebral lesion (Heilman et al. 1993). This may present as the patient ignoring their own arm, eating half their food on the plate and bumping into objects on their affected side. (Heilman KM, Watson R, Valenstein E 1993 Neglect and related disorders. In: Heilman KM, Valenstein E (eds) Clinical neuropsychology, 3rd edn. Oxford University Press, Oxford).

uniocular *adj* pertaining to, or affecting, one eye.

union healing; restoration of continuity, as in the healing of a fractured bone.

uniovular *adj* (*syn* monovular) pertaining to one ovum, as uniovular twins (identical, same sex). ➲ binovular *opp*.

unipara *n* a woman who has borne only one child. ➲ primipara—**uniparous** *adj*.

unipolar *adj* having a single pole. Also describes a neuron that has a single process.

U
V

unipolar (electrotherapy) the use of an electrode arrangement in which one electrode (indifferent electrode) is larger than the other (stimulating or active electrode). The higher current density under the active electrode means stimulation of nearby nerve or muscle is more likely than if under the larger indifferent electrode with its lower current density. The outcome depends on the relative sizes of the electrodes. In order to stimulate the quadriceps femoris muscle: unipolar—a small electrode is used over the femoral nerve, as it exits with the femoral artery under the inguinal ligament, the larger indifferent electrode is placed on the lateral aspect of the contralateral thigh or the abdomen or lower back. ⊃ bipolar.

unipolar disorder a disorder of mood that is characterized by repeated episodes of depression. ⊃ bipolar affective disorder, depression.

unit cost an average cost for a specific activity, for example a surgical procedure, an investigative procedure, or a home visit. It is calculated by dividing the total cost of the service by the number of outputs.

United Nations International Children's Emergency Fund a fund set up in 1946 by the United Nations to aid children in devastated areas of the world through the provision of food, medical treatment, vaccinations, vitamins and education.

univariate statistics descriptive statistics that analyse one variable, such as frequency distributions.

universal pliers ⊃ pliers.

universal precautions the routine infection control precautions taken during contact, or the possibility of contact, with blood and body fluids, such as wearing gloves or using eye protection. The aim being to prevent the transmission of blood-borne viruses such as hepatitis B and C. These infection prevention/control activities are now part of standard precautions. ⊃ infection, standard precautions.

universal scissors ⊃ scissors.

universal serial bus (USB) a serial port on a computer used to attach hardware such as the mouse, keyboard or a scanner.

unloading reflex reflex inhibition of the jaw closing muscles that occurs following the sudden reduction of forces between the jaws caused by the collapse of a food or other material to which a force was being applied by the muscles of mastication.

unmyelinated fibres nerve fibres that are not covered by myelin. Type C fibres are very small in diameter and carry sensory information about pain and temperature.

unplanned home birth one that occurs when an infant who is intended to be born in hospital is born unexpectedly or prematurely at home, or where the pregnancy is concealed.

unrelated in statistics, the whole groups of data are roughly matched but the individual samples are not.

unsharpness blurring on a radiograph (photographic unsharpness) which can be caused by movement unsharpness, screen unsharpness and/or geometric unsharpness.

unstable cavitation ⊃ cavitation (electrotherapy).

unstable lie in obstetrics, the lie of a fetus that changes between longtitudinal, oblique or transverse after 36 weeks' gestation. There is a risk of cord prolapse. Causes include placenta praevia, contracted pelvis, polyhydramnios.

unsupported mother a pregnant woman without a partner to provide psychological or financial support to herself and assist with caring for the infant.

upper anterior forceps (straight) ⊃ forceps.

upper limb neurodynamic test 1-median nerve bias consists of shoulder girdle depression, shoulder joint abduction, forearm supination, wrist and finger extension, shoulder joint lateral rotation and elbow extension. The sensitizing test involves cervical lateral flexion away from the symptomatic side and the desensitizing movement involves cervical lateral flexion towards the symptomatic side. ⊃ neurodynamic testing.

upper limb neurodynamic test 2a-median nerve bias consists of shoulder girdle depression, shoulder joint abduction of 10°, lateral rotation of the whole arm, elbow extension and wrist, finger and thumb extension. The sensitizing test is cervical lateral flexion away from the symptomatic side or shoulder abduction. Desensitizing movement involves cervical lateral flexion towards the affected side or release of the shoulder girdle. ⊃ neurodynamic testing.

upper limb neurodynamic test 2b-radial nerve bias consists of shoulder girdle depression, shoulder joint abduction of 10°, elbow extension, medial rotation of the whole arm, wrist, finger and thumb flexion. The sensitizing test is cervical lateral flexion away from the symptomatic side and shoulder abduction. The desensitizing movement is cervical lateral flexion towards the symptomatic side or release of the shoulder girdle. ⊃ neurodynamic testing.

upper limb neurodynamic test 3-ulnar nerve bias consists of shoulder girdle depression, wrist and finger extension, forearm pronation, elbow flexion, lateral rotation of the shoulder and shoulder abduction of 90°. The sensitizing test is cervical lateral flexion away from the symptomatic side and shoulder abduction. The desensitizing movement is cervical lateral flexion towards the symptomatic side or release of the shoulder girdle. ⊃ neurodynamic testing.

upper molar forceps ⊃ forceps.

upper motor neuron the cell body is in the motor cortex and the axon terminates in the anterior horn of the spinal cord. ⊃ neuron.

upper motor neuron syndrome a collection of positive and negative signs that are associated with cerebral lesions. The positive features include spasticity, increased tendon reflexes, clonus and resistance to passive movement. The negative features include muscle weakness, loss of dexterity and coordination and slowness of movement.

upper respiratory tract infection (URTI) the upper respiratory tract is the commonest site of infection in all age groups. The infections include rhinitis—usually viral—sinusitis, tonsillitis, adenoiditis, pharyngitis, otitis media and croup (laryngitis), often involving the tonsils and cervical lymph nodes. Such infections seldom require hospital treatment, but epiglottitis can be rapidly fatal.

upper root baynet pattern forceps ⊃ forceps.

upper root forceps ⊃ forceps.

upper uterine segment upper three-quarters of the uterus which contracts and retracts during labour.

UPPP *abbr* uvulopalatopharyngoplasty.

UPS *abbr* underperformance syndrome.

uptake count for a particular organ, is expressed as a percentage of the total radiation administered to the patient for radionuclide imaging purposes.

urachus *n* the stemlike structure connecting the bladder with the umbilicus in the fetus; after birth it becomes a fibrous cord situated between the apex of the bladder and the umbilicus, known as the median umbilical ligament—**urachal** *adj*.

uracil *n* nitrogenous base derived from pyrimidines. With other bases, one or more phosphate groups and a sugar it is part of the nucleic acid RNA. ⊃ ribonucleic acid.

uraemia *n* azotaemia. A syndrome in which endogenous waste products including urea and other nitrogenous substances accumulate in the blood, accompanied by disturbance of electrolytes and acid–base balance. It is caused by severely impaired renal function or renal failure, which may be due to renal disease, or to conditions such as systemic inflammatory response syndrome. It leads to a number of symptoms, particularly nausea, vomiting, headache, lethargy, altered taste, hiccups, anorexia, pruritus, visual problems, cardiac arrhythmias, altered consciousness and seizures. Renal replacement therapy such as haemodialysis may be required—**uraemic** *adj*.

uranoschisis cleft palate.

uranostaphyloplasty the surgical repair of a cleft palate.

urataemia *n* the presence of urates in the blood.

urate *n* any salt of uric acid.

uraturia *n* the excretion of urates in the urine.

urea *n* the main nitrogenous end-product of protein metabolism: produced mainly in the liver, it is excreted in the urine. ⊃ urea cycle.

urea breath test a non-invasive diagnostic test for the presence of *Helicobacter pylori* in the stomach.

urea cycle the biochemical reactions occurring in the liver in which the ammonia derived from the metabolism of amino acids is detoxified through conversion to urea. Amino acids not needed by the body are broken down, or deaminated. The nitrogenous part, the amino group (NH_2), is converted to ammonia (NH_3) and then combined with carbon and oxygen derived from carbon dioxide (CO_2) to form urea ($CO(NH_2)_2$), which is excreted in the urine.

Ureaplasma urealyticum *n* a bacterium of the genus *Ureaplasma*. Commonly found in the genitourinary system of women and men where it it may be asymptomatic. One of the micro-organisms responsible for non-gonococcal urethritis.

urease *n* bacterial enzyme that splits urea.

ureter *n* the tube passing from each kidney to the bladder for the conveyance of urine; its average length in an adult is 25–30 cm. It comprises an outer fibrous layer, a middle layer of smooth muscle, which contracts to produce the peristaltic movements by which urine passes down the tube and a mucosal lining called urothelium—**ureteric, ureteral** *adj*. ⊃ Colour Section Figures 19, 20.

ureterectomy *n* excision of a ureter.

ureteritis *n* inflammation of a ureter.

ureter/o- a prefix that means 'ureter', e.g. *ureterectomy*.

ureterocele *n* prolapse of the distal portion of the ureter into the bladder. It may obstruct the flow of urine and lead to ureteral dilatation and hydronephrosis.

ureterocolic *adj* pertaining to the ureter and colon, usually indicating anastomosis of the two structures.

ureteroileal *adj* pertaining to the ureters and ileum as in the anastomosis necessary in ileal conduit.

ureterolith *n* a calculus in the ureter.

ureterolithotomy *n* surgical removal of a stone from a ureter.

ureterolysis *n* surgical technique of freeing encased ureters.

ureteroneocystostomy *n* reimplantation of the ureters; usually as treatment for vesicoureteric reflux. Also known as ureterocystoneostomy, ureterocystostomy, ureterovesicostomy. ⊃ Leadbetter–Politano operation.

ureteronephrectomy *n* surgical excision of the ureter and kidney. Also called nephroureterectomy.

ureteroplasty *n* a plastic operation on the ureter, such as that to relieve a stricture.

ureteroscope *n* a fibreoptic endoscope that can be used to examine the ureters and renal pelvis, and to remove stones. ⊃ nephroscope.

ureteroscopy *n* endoscopic visualization of the ureters.

ureterostomy *n* the formation of a permanent fistula through which the ureter discharges urine. ⊃ cutaneous, ileal conduit.

ureterosigmoidostomy *n* operation to implant a ureter into the sigmoid colon.

ureterotomy *n* surgical incision into a ureter.

ureterovaginal *adj* pertaining to the ureter and vagina.

ureterovesical *adj* pertaining to the ureter and urinary bladder.

urethra *n* the passage that drains urine from the bladder to the outside at the external urinary meatus; in the vesitbule in females and the glans penis in males. ⊃ Colour Section Figure 19. The female urethra is straight and approximately 4–5 cm in length. The male urethra, which has several curves and is surrounded by the prostate gland, is around 20–25 cm in length. Additionally the male urethra transports semen during ejaculation. The urethra has two muscular sphincters; an internal and external sphincter. The urethral muscle layer is formed from smooth muscle with elastic tissue at its junction with the bladder; this forms an internal musclar sphincter under the control of autonomic nerves. Further down the urethra it changes to skeletal muscle, which forms the external sphincter and is under voluntary

U
V

control once continence is achieved during childhood. In addition there is a submucosal layer and a mucosal lining, which is continuous with the urothelium of the bladder in the upper part but changes to stratified squamous epithelium in the lower part—**urethral** *adj*.

urethral caruncle *n* prolapse of urethral mucosa at the external urinary meatus in women. It is prone to bleeding.

urethral dilatation the use of instruments to dilate the urethra narrowed by stricture.

urethral syndrome symptoms of urinary infection although the urine is sterile when withdrawn by catheter.

urethritis *n* inflammation of the urethra from any cause, but usually caused by a bacterial or a viral infection. Commonly part of infection affecting the bladder or the kidneys. It is characterized by dysuria and with some infections (e.g. gonorrhoea) a purulent discharge. *non-specific urethritis* ⊃ non-gonococcal urethritis.

urethr/o- a prefix that means 'urethra', e.g. *urethrocele*.

urethrocele *n* prolapse of the urethra, usually into the anterior vaginal wall.

urethrocystitis inflammation of the urethra and bladder.

urethrography *n* radiological examination of the urethra. Can be an inclusion with cystography either retrograde (ascending) or during micturition—**urethrographic** *adj*, **urethrogram** *n*, **urethrograph** *n*, **urethrographically** *adv*.

urethrometry *n* measurement of the urethral lumen using a urethrometer—**urethrometric** *adj*, **urethrometrically** *adv*.

urethroplasty *n* any reconstructive operation on the urethra.

urethrorrhaphy repair of the urethra, such as after an injury.

urethrorrhoea abnormal discharge from the urethra; mucus or pus.

urethroscope *n* an instrument designed to allow visualization of the interior of the urethra—**urethroscopic** *adj*, **urethroscopy** *n*, **urethroscopically** *adv*.

urethrostomy a surgical procedure in which the urethra is opened in the perineum in men.

urethrotomy *n* incision into the urethra; usually part of an operation for urethral stricture.

urethrotrigonitis *n* inflammation of the urethra and the trigone area of the urinary bladder between the ureteric openings and the urethra. ⊃ trigone.

urge incontinence ⊃ incontinence.

urgency the feeling of an immediate need to pass urine, it can lead to urge incontinence. It may be associated with a high intake of caffeine-containing drinks, diuretic drugs, detrusor muscle instability, urinary tract infection, or bladder outflow obstruction, e.g. benign prostatic enlargement.

-uria a suffix that means 'urine', e.g. *glycosuria*.

uric acid substance formed during purine metabolism, which is present in nucleic acids and some foods and beverages. Uric acid is excreted in the urine and may give rise to kidney stones. High levels of uric acid in the blood may be due to faulty excretion of uric acid, excessive cell breakdown, or associated with high purine intake. ⊃ gout.

uricosuria *n* ⊃ hyperuricuria.

uricosuric agents drugs that enhance renal excretion of uric acid, e.g. allopurinol. ⊃ Appendix 5.

uridrosis *n* excess of urea in the sweat; it may be deposited on the skin as fine white crystals (sometimes referred to as urea snow or frost).

urinalysis *n* physical, chemical or microbiological examination of the urine. Routine ward or clinic-based urinalysis involves checking the colour, clarity and odour of urine; and testing with reagent strips for pH, specific gravity, protein, blood, glucose, ketones, urobilinogen and bilirubin. Some reagent strips also test for the presence of nitrites and white blood cells, which may be indicative of bacteriuria and urinary tract infection. Microbiological examination is used to detect infection, blood cells, crystals or casts.

urinary *adj* pertaining to urine.

urinary bladder a muscular distensible bag situated in the pelvis. The bladder has an outer connective tissue layer, a middle smooth muscle layer known as the detrusor muscle and a mucosal lining of transitional epithelium (urothelium), which has folds known as rugae that allow the bladder to distend as it fills with urine. It receives urine from the kidneys via two ureters and stores it until micturition occurs. ⊃ Colour Section Figures 16, 19.

urinary incontinence ⊃ incontinence.

urinary plasminogen activator ⊃ urokinase.

urinary system comprises two kidneys, two ureters, one urinary bladder and one urethra. The kidneys produce urine of variable content; the ureters convey the urine to the bladder, which stores it until there is sufficient volume to elicit reflex emptying or the desire to pass urine and it is then conveyed to the exterior by the urethra. ⊃ Colour Section Figures 19, 20.

urinary tract infection (UTI) includes urethritis, cystitis, pyelonephritis. A common healthcare-associated infection. It occurs most frequently in the presence of an indwelling catheter. It is most commonly caused by Gram-negative bacterium, such as *Escherichia coli*, suggesting that self-infection via the periurethral route is a common pathway. ⊃ bacteriuria.

urination *n* ⊃ micturition.

urine *n* the clear straw-coloured fluid excreted by the kidneys. Urine contains water, nitrogenous waste and electrolytes. Normally adults produce about 1500 mL every 24 h, but this depends on fluid intake, activity and age. Usually slightly acidic (pH 6.0), but varies between 4.5 and 8.0. The specific gravity is usually within the range 1005–1030.

uriniferous tubule ⊃ renal tubule.

urinogenital *n* ⊃ urogenital.

urinometer *n* an instrument for estimating the specific gravity of urine.

uri, urin/o- a prefix that means 'urine', e.g. *urinometer*.

URL *abbr* uniform resource locator.

ur/o- a prefix that means 'urine, urinary organs', e.g. *urobilinuria*.

urobilin *n* a brownish pigment excreted in the faeces. Formed by the oxidation of urobilinogen.

urobilinogen *n* (*syn* stercobilinogen) a pigment formed from bilirubin in the intestine by bacterial action. It may be reabsorbed into the circulation and converted back to bilirubin in the liver and re-excreted in the bile or urine.

urobilinuria *n* the presence of increased amounts of urobilin in the urine. Evidence of increased production of bilirubin in the liver, e.g. after haemolysis.

urocele a swelling in the scrotum caused by extravasated urine.

urochezia the passage of urine in faeces.

urodynamics *n* the method used to study bladder function. ⊃ cystometry.

urogenital *adj* (*syn* urinogenital) pertaining to the urinary and the genital organs.

urography *n* radiographic visualization of the renal pelvis and ureter by injection of a contrast agent. The agent may be injected into the bloodstream whence it is excreted by the kidney (intravenous urography) or it may be injected directly into the renal pelvis or ureter by way of a fine catheter introduced through a cystoscope (retrograde or ascending urography)—**urographic** *adj*, **urogram** *n*, **urographically** *adv*. *intravenous urography (IVU)* also called intravenous pyelography although other structures are demonstrated. The demonstration of the urinary tract following an intravenous injection of an opaque agent.

urokinase *n* an endopeptidase enzyme that activates plasminogens. Produced naturally by the kidney and is excreted in the urine. It is used therapeutically in vitreous haemorrhage (eye), to clear intravenous catheters, thrombosed arteriovenous shunts and other thromboembolic conditions.

urolith *n* a stone or calculus that forms in the urinary tract.

urologist *n* a medically qualified person who specializes in disorders of the female urinary tract and the male genitourinary tract.

urology *n* that branch of biomedical science which deals with disorders of the female urinary tract and the male genitourinary tract—**urological** *adj*, **urologically** *adv*.

uropathy *n* disease in any part of the urinary system.

uroporphyrin a naturally occurring porphyrin excreted in the urine in small amounts. The excretion of excessive amounts are indicative of porphyria.

urostomy *n* the collective term for cutaneous ureterostomy, ileal conduit, ureterosigmoidostomy.

URTI *abbr* upper respiratory tract infection.

urticaria *n* (*syn* nettlerash, hives) skin eruption characterized by multiple, circumscribed, smooth, raised, pinkish, itchy weals, developing very suddenly, usually lasting a few days and leaving no visible trace. The cause is unknown in most cases. ⊃ angio-oedema, dermographia, Colour Section Figure 126.

US, U/S *abbr* ultrasound.

USB *abbr* universal serial bus.

useful density range the range of densities, between 1.36 and 2.16, that make up a radiographic image; above and

below this range it is not possible to determine differences visually between adjacent densities. ⊃ useful exposure range.

useful exposure range the range of exposures that make up a radiographic image; above and below this range it is not possible to determine differences visually between adjacent densities. To calculate the range the characteristic curve of the film is used at a particular kV, a vertical line is drawn from density 1.36 and 2.16, the antilogs of the range of values on the horizontal, log It, axis gives the useful exposure range in mAs. ⊃ characteristic curve.

Usher's syndrome (C Usher, British ophthalmologist, 1865–1942) a hereditary condition inherited as a recessive autosomal trait. It is characterized by a degeneration of the retinal pigment epithelium, and accompanied by sensorineural deafness.

uterine *adj* pertaining to the uterus.

uterine arterial embolization ⊃ embolization.

uterine bruit the sound heard with a stethoscope as blood pulsates through the arteries of the uterus.

uterine cavity that of the uterus, the base extending between the orifices of the uterine (fallopian) tubes. It opens distally at the internal os of the cervix.

uterine colic ⊃ dysmenorrhoea.

uterine inertia lack of co-ordinated contraction of parturient uterus. Hypotonic uterine action with the inability of the uterine muscle to contract efficiently. A common cause of prolonged labour, and may lead to haemorrhage from the placental site.

uterine isthmus the narrow part of the uterus between the uterine cavity and the cervix, which is 7 mm long. It enlarges during pregnancy to form the lower uterine segment.

uterine rupture bursting apart of the uterus following obstructed labour, in which the Bandl's ring, a ridge running obliquely across the abdomen, marks the junction between the grossly thickened upper uterine segment and the dangerously thinned and over-stretched lower segment; or of a uterine scar from a previous caesarean section during pregnancy or labour. Dehiscence may occur insidiously towards term or rapidly during labour due to powerful contractions. Blood loss must be replaced and shock treated before attempting to suture the rupture; occasionally hysterectomy may be required to save the life of the woman.

uterine souffle ⊃ souffle.

uterine supports muscles of the pelvic floor, the peritoneum and various ligaments; pubocervical, round, transverse cervical (Mackenrodt's or cardinal) and the uterosacral ligaments that hold the uterus in the correct anteverted and anteflexed position (Figure U.3).

uterine tetany prolonged uterine contractions.

uterine tubes (*syn* fallopian tubes, oviducts) two tubes that extend laterally from the upper part of the uterus to open into the peritoneal cavity. Each measures 10 cm in length, but the diameter varies greatly along the length. The tube is divided into four distinct parts—a funnel-like infundibulum ending in the finger-like projections known as fimbrae, which help

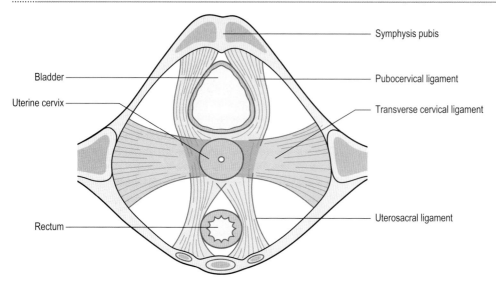

Bladder

Uterine cervix

Rectum

Symphysis pubis

Pubocervical ligament

Transverse cervical ligament

Uterosacral ligament

U.3 Uterine supports, at the level of the cervix (reproduced from Fraser & Cooper 2003 with permission).

to waft the oocyte from the ovary into the tube, a dilated ampulla where fertilization usually occurs, an isthmus and an interstitial part within the uterine wall which is extremely narrow. ⊃ Colour Section Figure 17. The wall of a tube has three layers: it is covered with and supported by part of the broad ligament known as the mesosalpinx, a middle layer of smooth muscle, which contracts to produce the peristaltic movements that assist in moving the oocyte towards the uterus, and a highly specialized, ciliated mucosal lining containing secreting cells with microvilli. Rhythmic ciliary movement move the oocyte into the uterus and the secretions help to maintain the oocyte and spermatozoa in good condition.

uter/o- a prefix that means 'uterus', e.g. *uterosacral*.

uteroplacental *adj* pertaining to the uterus and placenta. Refers to the junction where the placenta meets the inner lining of the uterus.

uterorectal *adj* pertaining to the uterus and the rectum.

uterosacral *adj* pertaining to the uterus and sacrum.

uterosalpingography *n* (*syn* hysterosalpingography) radiological examination of the uterus and uterine (fallopian) tubes involving retrograde introduction of an opaque contrast agent during fluoroscopy. Used to investigate patency of uterine (fallopian) tubes. Is being superseded by ultrasound examination.

uterovaginal *adj* pertaining to the uterus and the vagina.

uterovesical *adj* pertaining to the uterus and the urinary bladder.

uterus *n* the womb. A hollow muscular organ into which the ovum is received through the uterine (fallopian) tubes and where it is retained during development, and from which the fetus is expelled through the vagina. ⊃ Colour Section Figure 17. The uterus is divided into—the fundus (top), corpus (body) and the cervix (neck).The corpus and the cervix are divided by a narrow isthmus. The wall of the

uterus has three layers—an outer layer of peritoneum known as the perimetrium, the myometrium, a middle layer of interlocking smooth muscle fibres, which form a 'living ligature' by compressing blood vessels to prevent bleeding after childbirth, and the mucosal lining the highly vascular endometrium that contains many glands. The endometrium has two layers, the permanent stratum basalis and the stratum functionalis, which is shed each month during menstruation. ⊃ bicornuate—**uteri** *pl*, **uterine** *adj*.

uterus didelphys a double uterus. ⊃ bicornuate.

UTI *abbr* urinary tract infection.

utilitarianism *n* ethical theory that holds that an action should always produce more benefits than harm. It aims to provide the greatest good for the majority of individuals. ⊃ deontological.

utility measure a means of determining the strength of an individual's preference for a specific health state in relation to alternative health states. A utility measure assigns numerical values on a scale from 0 (death) to 1 (optimal or perfect health). As health states can be considered worse than death, negative values can be recorded.

utricle *n* a little sac or pocket. A fluid-filled sac in the membranous labyrinth of the inner ear. Part of the vestibular apparatus; contains the hair cells and otoliths that are concerned with static equilibrium. ⊃ saccule.

UUPS *abbr* unexplained under performance syndrome.

UV *abbr* ultraviolet.

uvea *n* (*syn* uveal tract, vascular tunic of the eye) the pigmented, vascular middle coat of the eye, consisting of the choroid, ciliary body and the iris. The last two structures are usually considered to form the anterior uvea. The uvea contains most of the blood supply—**uveal** *adj*. ⊃ uveitis, vortex vein.

UVPPP *abbr* uvulopalatopharyngoplasty.

UVR *abbr* ultraviolet radiation.

U
V

uveal meshwork ⊃ trabecular meshwork.

uveal tract ⊃ uvea.

uveitis *n* inflammation of the uvea of the eye. All three tissues of the uvea tend to be involved to some extent in the same inflammatory process because of their common blood supply. However, the most severe reaction may affect one tissue more than the others as in iritis, cyclitis or choroiditis or sometimes two tissues, e.g. iridocyclitis. The symptoms also vary depending upon which part of the tract is affected. Anterior uveitis will be accompanied by pain, photophobia and lacrimation and some loss of vision because of exudation of cells (aqueous flare), protein-rich fluid and fibrin into either the anterior chamber or vitreous body (humour) as well as ciliary injection, adhesion between the iris and lens (posterior synechia) and keratic precipitates. The condition is often associated with ankylosing spondylitis, rheumatoid arthritis, sarcoidosis or syphilis. Treatment includes corticosteroids (e.g. prednisolone) and mydriatics (e.g. homatropine) to reduce the risk of posterior synechia and to relieve a spasm of the ciliary muscle. ⊃ aqueous flare, choroiditis, ciliary injection, cyclitis, hypopyon, iridocyclitis, iritis, keratic precipitates, Koeppe's nodules, mydriatics, phthisis bulbi, posterior synechia, synchisis scintillans.

uveoparotid fever (Heerfordt's syndrome) a condition characterized by an intermittent pyrexia accompanied by enlargement of the salivary glands, inflammation of the uveal tracts of the eye and cranial nerve involvement. Xerostomia may also occur.

uvula *n* the central tag of muscle tissue covered with mucous membrane that hangs down from the free edge of the soft palate. It is involved in phonation. The lesser palatine nerve runs from it through the lesser palatine foramen to join the maxillary branch of the trigeminal nerve (fifth cranial nerve). ⊃ palatine arches.

uvulectomy *n* excision of the uvula. Also known as staphylectomy.

uvulitis *n* inflammation of the uvula.

uvulopalatopharyngoplasty (UPPP, UVPPP) *n* also known as palatopharyngoplasty, uvulopalatoplasty. An operation on the soft palate and pharyngeal tissue for relief of excessive snoring and obstructive sleep apnoea (hypopnoea) syndrome.

U

V

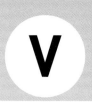

V̇ symbol for volume (of gas) per unit time.

V̇ₐ alveolar ventilation.

V1 ⊃ visual area1.

VA *abbr* visual acuity.

vaccinate *vt* to inoculate with a vaccine in order to produce immunity from a specific disease.

vaccination *n* originally described the process of inoculating persons with discharge from the lesions of cowpox to protect them from smallpox. Now applied to the inoculation of any antigenic material for the purpose of producing active artificial immunity to specific infectious diseases.

vaccines *npl* suspensions or products of infectious agents, e.g. attenuated or killed micro-organisms, used chiefly for producing active immunity. *component vaccines* are prepared using an isolated and purified component of the disease causing micro-organism, for example a mixture of capsule polysaccharides from the major disease associated strains of *Streptococcus pneumoniae*. In some cases the antigen may be isolated, cloned in another organism and harvested for vaccine preparation e.g. surface antigen from hepatitis B virus (HBV); *conjugate vaccines* are prepared using, usually, a purified carbohydrate antigen attached to an unrelated protein which serves to promote an immune response, e.g. meningococcal C-conjugate vaccine. *inactivated pathogen vaccines* are prepared using whole bacteria or viruses which have been killed by either heat or chemicals, e.g. rabies, influenza and hepatitis A; *live attenuated vaccines* are prepared using live pathogens which are subjected to processes (attenuation) that reduces pathogenicity whilst preserving antigenicity, e.g. BCG, MMR and oral poliomyelitis. *toxoid vaccines* are prepared from toxins which have been rendered harmless by some form of chemical treatment, usually formaldehyde, but which still elicit an antigenic response in the host, e.g. tetanus toxoid. ⊃ BCG, Hib vaccine, human papilloma virus, immunization, MMR, Sabin, Salk, triple vaccine, typhoid vaccine.

vaccinia virus *n* a pox virus causing disease in cattle. This poxvirus, derived in the laboratory, is the basis of the existing vaccine to prevent smallpox. Widespread vaccination is no longer recommended due to the likelihood of local spread from the vaccination site (potentially life-threatening in those with eczema [eczema vaccinatum] or immune deficiency) and of encephalitis (1:10–30 000 doses).

vacuole a small cavity or space within the cytoplasm of a cell. Some types contain water, whereas others are part of the Golgi apparatus where they contain and condense cellular secretions prior to discharging them at the cell surface. ⊃ bulk transport.

vacuum space entirely without matter.

vacuum bag a sealed plastic bag containing small expanded polystyrene spheres, the patient is positioned on the bag which has the air pressure reduced until it is hardened. This mould can be used during radiotherapy to accurately immobilize the patient and enable daily reproducibility of positioning. ⊃ patient immobilization.

vacuum extractor 1. a device used to assist delivery of the fetus. ⊃ Ventouse extraction. **2.** an aspiration device used as a method of terminating a pregnancy.

vacuum-fired porcelain ⊃ porcelain.

vacuum forming in dentistry, a method of forming flat plastic sheets into three-dimensional shapes by the use of moulds, heat and a vacuum.

vacuum investing in dentistry, the investment of a waxy pattern under vacuum conditions to reduce the possibility of small air bubbles being incorporated in the investment material itself.

VADAS *abbr* voice activated domestic appliance system.

vagal *adj* pertaining to the vagus nerve.

vagina *n* literally, a sheath; the musculomembranous passage extending from the vulva to the cervix uteri. ⊃ Colour Section Figure 17. It runs obliquely upwards and backwards at an angle of 45°. The anterior wall is about 7.5 cm in length and is close to the urethra and bladder, and the posterior wall, which is longer at 9 cm, is in front of the rectum and the rectovaginal pouch. The difference in length is due to the angle of insertion of the cervix through the anterior wall. Normally the vaginal walls are in apposition, but the presence of rugae (folds) allows the vagina to distend in order to facilitate coitus and childbirth. The projection of the cervix into the vagina forms four fornices (deep folds or gutters). The hymen, a perforated membrane, partially occludes the distal opening of the vagina. The vagina has: an outer covering of connective tissue, a middle layer of smooth muscle (a strong outer coat of longtitudinal fibres and a weaker inner coat of circular fibres) and a stratified squamous epithelial lining, which affords some protection against the trauma of childbirth. The vagina has no secretory glands but the surface is kept moist by cervical secretions and transudate that leaks out from the blood vessels in the vaginal wall. Between puberty and the menopause the vagina is acidic (pH between 4.9 and 3.5) due to the production of lactic acid by bacteria of the *Lactobacillus* spp. which form part of the normal vaginal flora. The lactic acid is produced by bacterial action on glycogen present in the stratified squamous epithelium. The acidic environment inhibits the growth of most other micro-organisms, thus helping to protect the vagina from many pathogenic micro-organisms that may enter from the perineum. The vagina receives arterial blood from an arterial plexus formed by the uterine and vaginal arteries that branch from the internal iliac arteries. The venous return is via a venous plexus that drains into the internal iliac veins. The lymphatic drainage is through the internal iliac and superficial inguinal lymph nodes. The vagina is innervated by parasympathetic fibres from the sacral outflow, sympathetic fibres from the lumbar outflow and somatic sensory fibres from the pudendal nerves—**vaginal** *adj*.

vaginal cytology antenatal examination of desquamated cells from the vaginal wall for changes which show hormone changes suggesting placental insufficiency and fetal risk.

vaginal examination (VE) examination *per vaginum*. In midwifery/obstetric practice the index and middle fingers are passed through the vagina to assess the dilatation, thickness and consistency of the cervix, the state of the membranes, the presentation, position and station of the presenting part of the fetus. ⊃ Bishop's score.

vaginal speculum ⊃ Cusco's speculum, speculum, Sims' speculum.

vaginismus *n* painful muscular spasm of the vaginal walls occurring when the external genitalia are touched, such as during medical examination or sexual contact. It results in dyspareunia or painful coitus, or indeed preventing coitus in extreme cases.

vaginitis *n* inflammation of the vagina. It is caused by a variety of micro-organisms that include: *Chlamydia trachomatis, Trichomonas vaginalis, Gardnerella vaginalis, Neisseria gonorrhoeae* and yeasts, particularly *Candida albicans*. There is discharge, intense pruritus, vulval excoriation and soreness and sometimes dysuria. *atrophic vaginitis* is characterized by thinning of the vaginal mucosa and reduced acid secretions associated with the postmeno-pausal decrease in oestrogen secretion, which make the vagina more prone to infection. Infection with *Candida albicans* is particularly common in older women. Atrophic changes affecting the vaginal mucosa may cause inflamma-tion, dryness, itching and dyspareunia even when infection is not present. Any associated postmenopausal bleeding must be fully investigated.

vaginoplasty *n* also called colpoplasty. A plastic surgical procedure undertaken on the vagina.

vaginosis *n* vaginal infection caused by a proliferation of commensal micro-organisms such as *Gardnerella vaginalis*. ⊃ bacterial vaginosis.

vagolytic *adj, n* that which neutralizes the effect of a stimulated vagus nerve.

vagotomy *n* surgical division of the branches of the vagus nerves that innervate the stomach; done in conjunction with gastroenterostomy in the treatment of peptic ulcer, or with pyloroplasty.

vagus nerves the tenth pair of cranial nerves (mixed nerves). The vagus nerves have a more extensive distribu-tion than any other cranial nerves. Originating from the brain stem they descend through the neck, thorax and abdomen, giving off branches with both afferent and efferent components to many organs and tissues. The efferent fibres are mainly part of the parasympathetic nervous system, including those that slow the heart and those that innervate smooth muscle and glands in the pharynx, larynx, trachea, heart, oesophagus, stomach, intestines, exocrine pancreas, gallbladder, bile ducts, spleen, kidneys, ureters and blood vessels in the thoracic and abdominal cavities. The main afferent fibres are visceral afferents from thoracic and abdominal organs—**vagi** *pl*, **vagal** *adj*.

valence band a band which contains the outer electrons of an atom and may be partially or completely full.

valency the ability of one atom to join another.

valency bond the electron linkage between two atoms.

valgus, valga, valgum *adj* exhibiting angulation away from the midline of the body, e.g. hallux valgus.

valgus deformity refers to a lateral inclination of a distal bone, of a joint, from the midline.

valgus stress test (medial collateral ligament of the knee) the patient lies supine. The therapist applies a valgus strain to the knee joint. An abnormal finding is excessive opening up on the medial side of the joint or pain. The test is normally performed with the knee in 20–30° of flexion. If the test is done with the knee held in full extension, a positive sign would suggest major ligamentous injury involving the medial collateral, posterior cruciate and potentially the anterior cruciate injury.

validation the process of assessing an academic course and determining whether it meets the criteria for recognition. Often this is done by the professional body, licensing agency and university at the same time.

validity a research term. The 'truth' of the research. In simple terms, does a test record accurately what it is supposed to record? A clinical example would be that asking a person to perform a straight leg raise is not a particularly reliable test of quadriceps function, since it is isometric only and mainly works the hip flexors instead. There are many types of validity: content, criterion, external, face, internal and predictive.

validity (content) similar to face validity, but this time examines the concepts and thinking behind a tool to ensure it has the potential to obtain the right information.

validity (criterion) a term that indicates the ability of a test to correlate with other tools.

validity (external) a term that indicates the degree to which research findings can be generalized to other populations and in other settings.

validity (face) in research, the subjective assessment of the measurement tool to ensure that it is relevant and clear, e.g. when designing a questionnaire, clarity is vital.

validity (internal) in research, a term that indicates the extent to which a method or test measures what it intends to measure.

validity (predictive) a term that indicates the ability to predict outcomes.

U
V

valine *n* an essential (indispensable) amino acid.

vallate having a rim, as in the vallate papilla of the tongue. ⮑ placenta circumvallata, tongue.

Valsalva manoeuvre (A Valsalva, Italian anatomist, 1666–1723) the maximum intrathoracic pressure achieved by forced expiration against a closed glottis; occurs in such activities as lifting heavy objects, changing position and during defecation: the glottis narrows simultaneously with contraction of the abdominal muscles.

value–expectancy theory ⮑ expectancy–value theory.

value for money (VFM) a means of obtaining the best quality of service within the resource allocation. It involves economy, efficiency and effectiveness.

values *npl* the individual and personal view of the worth of an idea or specific behaviour. Principles of living which are refined from life experiences that guide behaviour.

value systems an accepted set of values, conduct and way of behaving in a particular social group. ⮑ beliefs, secular beliefs.

valve *n* a fold of membrane in a passage or tube normally permitting the flow of contents in one direction only. For example, the atrioventricular valves of the heart—**valvular** *adj*.

valvoplasty *n* a plastic operation on a valve, usually reserved for the heart; to be distinguished from valve replacement or valvotomy—**valvoplastic** *adj*.

valvotomy, valvulotomy *n* incision of a stenotic valve, by custom referring to the heart, to restore normal function.

valvulitis *n* inflammation of a valve, particularly in the heart.

valvulotomy *n* ⮑ valvotomy.

vancomycin-resistant enterococci (VRE) also known as glycopeptide-resistant enterococci (GRE). Enterococci such as *Enterococcus faecium* that have developed resistance to vancomycin (a glycopeptide antibiotic). ⮑ *Enterococcus*.

vancomycin-resistant *Staphylococcus aureus* (VRSA) strains of metacillin-resistant *Staphylococcus aureus* that have developed full resistance to the antibiotic vancomycin. Although the strain is sensitive to some older antibiotics and some newer drugs, this develoment further restricts the choice of antibiotic treatment for serious infections caused by *Staphylococcus aureus*.

Vancouver system of referencing a referencing system used in academic publications which uses superscript numbers inserted into the text. For example, the first reference cited in the text is numbered [1] and the citation is listed first in the full reference list at the end and so on. This system of referencing is used in some medical journals. ⮑ Harvard system of referencing, reference, primary referencing (citation), secondary referencing (citation).

van den Bergh's test (A van den Bergh, Dutch physician, 1869–1943) estimation of serum bilirubin. Direct positive reaction (conjugated) occurs in obstructive and hepatic jaundice. Indirect positive reaction (unconjugated) occurs in haemolytic jaundice.

van Herick, Shaffer and Schwartz method a technique for estimating the angle of the anterior chamber. It is based on the fact that the width of the angle of the anterior chamber is correlated to the distance between the posterior corneal surface and the anterior iris as viewed near the corneal limbus. This is done using a slit-lamp with a narrow slit beam perpendicular to the temporal or nasal corneal surface, viewing from the straight-ahead position and comparing the depth of the anterior chamber to the thickness of the cornea. If the anterior chamber depth is equal to or greater than the corneal thickness, the angle is considered to be *grade 4* (corresponding to a wide open angle). If the anterior chamber depth is equal to one-half the corneal thickness, the angle is considered to be *grade 3* (this is the most common angle width). If the anterior chamber depth is equal to one-fourth the corneal thickness, it is considered to be *grade 2,* and if the anterior chamber depth is less than one-fourth the corneal thickness, it is considered to be *grade 1* (corresponding to a very narrow angle). *Grade 0* is considered to be a closed angle. The method is most useful for predicting the possibility of angle-closure glaucoma. ⮑ angle-closure glaucoma, angle of the anterior chamber, gonioscope, shadow test.

vanillylmandelic acid (VMA) a metabolite of adrenaline (epinephrine) which is excreted in the urine. The level in a 24-hour urine collection is used to assess adrenal medulla function and in the diagnosis of adrenal tumours.

vanishing twin syndrome a situation in which one fetus in a twin pregnancy is reabsorded, usually during the first trimester.

Van't Hoff's law part of the law states that any chemical reaction capable of being accelerated is accelerated by a rise in temperature. This concept is of key importance to physiotherapists, particularly when dealing with electrotherapy modalities. ⮑ heat therapy, heat and cell metabolism.

VAP *abbr* ventilator-associated pneumonia.

vaporize to change into a vapour by heating.

vaporizer a device that produces a vapour containing small droplets of a drug in liquid form for inhalation. ⮑ nebulizer.

Vaquez–Osler disease *n* (L Vaquez, French physician, 1860–1936; W Osler, Canadian physician, 1849–1919) primary proliferative polycythaemia. ⮑ primary proliferative polycythaemia.

variable *n* a research term that describes any factor or circumstance that is part of the study. *confounding variable* one that affects the conditions of the independent variables unequally. *dependent variable* one that depends on the experimental conditions. *independent variable* the variable conditions of an experimental situation, e.g. control or experimental. *random variable* background factors such as environmental conditions that may affect any conditions of the independent variables equally. ⮑ mediating variable, moderating variable.

variance *n* a mathematical term used in statistics. The distribution range of a set of results around the mean. ⮑ standard deviation.

varicella *n* ⊃ chickenpox—**varicelliform** *adj*.

varicella-zoster immunoglobulin (VZIG) polyclonal immunoglobulin (largely IgG) from donors exposed to varicella-zoster. Contains high concentrations of specific antibody, and used to convey passive immunity to varicella.

varicella-zoster virus (VZV) herpesvirus causing chickenpox (varicella) and shingles (herpes zoster).

varices *npl* dilated, tortuous (or varicose) veins. ⊃ oesophageal varices, varicose veins—**varix** *sing*.

varicocele *n* varicosity of the veins of the pampiniform plexus in the spermatic cord.

varicose ulcer (*syn* gravitational ulcer) ⊃ venous ulcer.

varicose veins dilated veins, the valves of which become incompetent so that blood flow may be reversed (Figure V.1) Most commonly found in the lower limbs where they can result in a gravitational ulcer; in the rectum, when the term 'rectal varices' (haemorrhoids) is used; and in the lower oesophagus, when they are called oesophageal varices.

varicotomy *n* an incision into a varix.

varifocal lens ⊃ progressive addition lens (PAL).

variola *n* ⊃ smallpox.

varioloid *n* attack of smallpox modified by previous vaccination.

varix *n* ⊃ varices.

varnish a solution of resin, shellac, copal, sandrac and other medicaments in a volatile solvent such as ether or alcohol. On evaporation it forms a thin protective adherent coating or film that may be a barrier against the deleterious effects of moisture, for example on glass ionomer cements. *fluoride varnish* an adherent varnish containing a high concentration (up to 23 000 ppm) of fluoride, designed for professionally applied topical use on teeth with early enamel caries to arrest and prevent caries.

varus, vara, varum *adj* displaying displacement or angulation towards the midline of the body, e.g. coxa vara.

varus deformity refers to medial inclination of a distal bone, of a joint, from the midline.

varus stress test (lateral collateral ligament of the knee) the patient lies supine. The therapist applies a varus force (i.e. the femur is pushed laterally and the leg pulled medially) to the knee joint. A positive sign is observed as excessive opening up or pain on the lateral side of the joint. The test is normally performed with the knee in 20–30° of flexion. With the knee held in extension a positive sign suggests major ligamentous injury involving the lateral collateral, posterior cruciate and potentially the anterior cruciate injury. The test is performed again with the knee in 20–30° of flexion.

VAS *acron* visual analogue scale.

vas *n* a vessel—**vasa** *pl*.

vasa praevia a situation in which the umbilical blood vessels run through the membranes before inserting into the placenta (a velamentous insertion). If the placenta is sited low down in the uterus the blood vessels may be across the internal os, ahead of the presenting part. In this situation there is a high risk of damage to the vessels when the membranes rupture resulting in fetal exsanguination and death.

vasa vasorum the minute nutrient vessels of the artery and vein walls.

vascular *adj* supplied with vessels, especially referring to blood vessels.

vascular endothelial growth factor inhibitors monoclonal antibodies, such as ranibizumab, that inhibit vascular endothelial growth factor. Thereby reducing the abnormal growth of new blood vessels (neovascularization). ⊃ age-related macular degeneration.

vascular tunic of the eye ⊃ uvea.

vascularization *n* the acquisition of a blood supply; the process of becoming vascular.

vasculitis *n* (*syn* angiitis) inflammation of blood vessels. May be part of a systemic disease.

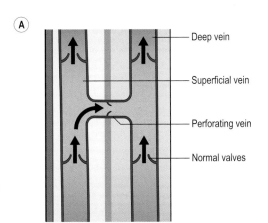
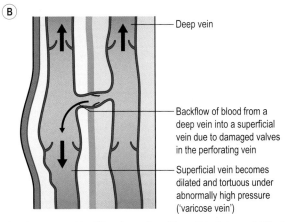

V.1 Formation of varicose veins: (A) normal veins and valves, (B) valve damage and backflow (reproduced from Bale & Jones 1997 with permission)

vasculotoxic *adj* any substance or agent that causes harmful changes in blood vessels.

vas deferens duct carrying spermatozoa from the epididymis. ⊃ deferent duct.

vasectomy *n* surgical excision of all or part of the deferent duct (vas deferens), usually for male sterilization.

vas/o- a prefix that means 'vessel, duct', e.g. *vasomotor*.

vasoactive *adj* having an effect on the diameter of blood vessels, causing vasocontriction or vasodilation.

vasoactive intestinal peptide (VIP) a regulatory peptide hormone/neurotransmitter present in the hypothalamus, other areas of the brain, the intestine and pancreas. It acts to relax smooth muscle in the intestine, increases the amount of water and electrolytes in pancreatic and intestinal juices, stimulates the release of pancreatic hormones and inhibits gastric acid secretion and motility. ⊃ VIPoma.

vasoconstriction *n* any narrowing of the lumen of a blood vessel due to contraction of the smooth muscle in its wall, mediated by neural (autonomic) control, local or blood-borne chemical factors, or fall in temperature. Part of the rationale for the use of ice in acute injury to minimize blood flow (and therefore swelling) in the damaged tissue. Also the first stage of the four overlapping stages of haemostasis. ⊃ coagulation, fibrinolysis, platelet plug.

vasoconstrictor *n* any agent causing vasoconstriction. For example, the drug adrenaline (epinephrine) that causes constriction of blood vessels, especially arterioles, and is used topically to reduce bleeding during dental procedures. When added in very small quantities to a local anaesthetic solution it delays the absorption of the solution into the circulation and hence prolongs the effect of the local anaesthetic. ⊃ adrenaline (epinephrine).

vasodilation *n* (*syn* vasodilatation) widening of the lumen of a blood vessel, due to relaxation of the smooth muscle in its wall, mediated by neural (autonomic) control, local or blood-borne chemical factors, or rise in temperature.

vasodilator *n* any agent causing vasodilation.

vasoepididymostomy *n* anastomosis of the vas deferens to the epididymis.

vasography *n* radiographic demonstration of the deferent duct (vas deferens) after the introduction of contrast agent. An investigation of male infertility.

vasomotor *adj* relating to nerves and muscles that control blood vessel lumen size.

vasomotor centre (VMC) a centre, located in the cardiovascular centre in the medulla oblongata. Concerned with controlling lumen size of peripheral arterioles and peripheral resistence and heart rate as part of the regulation of arterial blood pressure. It operates through autonomic sympathetic nerve activity in response to baroreceptor signals. The degree of VMC activity depends on the amount of inhibition by the baroreceptors, the pressure receptors located in the carotid sinus and aortic arch.

vasomotor symptoms symptoms caused by vasomotor instability experienced by many women during the climacteric; typically hot flushes (flashes) and excess sweating including night sweats.

vasopressin *n* antidiuretic hormone. The substance produced in the hypothalamus and stored in the posterior lobe of the pituitary gland. ⊃ antidiuretic hormone.

vasopressor *n* a drug which increases blood pressure. Usually by constricting arterioles but not always.

vasospasm *n* constricting spasm of blood vessel walls—**vasospastic** *adj*.

vasovagal *adj* pertaining to the effects of the vagus nerve upon the vascular system.

vasovagal reflex stimulation of the vagus nerve that results in a rapid fall in blood pressure and heart rate. Frequently associated with the transient loss of consciousness (vasovagal syncope) caused by insufficient blood reaching the brain, pallor, nausea and sweating. May be caused by stimulation of the soft palate (gag reflex), Valsalva manoeuvre, pain or emotional episodes.

vasovasostomy *n* a surgical procedure to restore the patency of the deferent ducts (vas deferens), which aims to re-establish fertility; the reversal of a previous vasectomy.

vastus *n* one of three muscles of the four-part quadriceps femoris muscle. All three extend the knee—**vasti** *pl.* ⊃ vastus intermedius, vastus lateralis, vastus medialis.

vastus intermedius the muscle of the quadriceps femoris group on the anterior aspect of the thigh beneath the rectus femoris muscle; it extends the knee. The fibres lie in a plane parallel with the anterior aspect of the shaft of the femur.

vastus lateralis the muscle of the quadriceps femoris group on the lateral aspect of the thigh; it extends the knee.

vastus medialis also known as vastus medialis obliquus (VMO). The muscle of the quadriceps femoris group on the anteromedial aspect of the thigh. Recently investigated for its role in patellar stability, with particular reference to patellofemoral pain.

VATS *acron* videoassisted thoracoscopy.

VBI *abbr* vertebrobasilar insufficiency.

VC *abbr* vital capacity.

$\dot{V}_D$ symbol for dead space ventilation.

VDT *abbr* visual display terminal.

VDU *abbr* visual display unit.

$\dot{V}_E$ symbol for the volume of air leaving the lungs in one minute.

VECP *abbr* visual-evoked cortical potential.

vectogram a polarized stereogram consisting of two polarized images at right angles to each other. When viewed through polarizing filters it presents one image to one eye and another image to the other eye. The Vectograph is a chart based on this principle in which almost one half of a chart is seen by one eye and almost the other half by the other eye while some lines, letters or numbers are seen binocularly to lock fusion. The Vectograph is useful for balancing refraction and to detect suppression and fixation disparity. Various types of vectograms are available,

U
V

including those that provide finer tests for stereoscopic acuity. ⮑ balancing test, random-dot stereogram, retinal disparity, stereoscopic visual acuity, two-dimensional test.

vector *n* **1.** a carrier of disease, e.g. ticks, fleas, mites, lice, mosquitoes, sandflies and so on. **2.** a variable, quantity or measurement that has both size and directional components. Cannot be added arithmetically due to directional component.

vegan *n* a person who excludes all foods of animal origin from their diet, so does not eat meat, fish, eggs, dairy produce, and also honey. The diet consists totally of vegetables, vegetable oils, fruit, grains and seeds. Protein is provided by nuts, grains and pulse vegetables. With careful food choices and combinations the diet can be nutritionally adequate but the vegan diet may be deficient in protein, iron and vitamin B$_{12}$.

vegetable dye a colouring matter extracted from vegetables and used in dentistry for plaque disclosing tablets and solution, e.g. erythrocin (which is not toxic).

vegetarian a person who excludes any meat, fish, seafood or animal-body by-products such as gelatin, but may include milk, cheese (made with non-animal rennet) and eggs in their diet. ⮑ lacto-ovovegetarian, lactovegetarian.

vegetations *npl* growths or accretions composed of fibrin and platelets occurring on the edge of the cardiac valves in infective endocarditis.

vegetative *adj* relating to the non-sporing stage of a bacterium.

vegetative state the vegetative state may result from severe brain injury or disease that irrevocably damages the central nervous system. The person is rendered dependent on others for all activities of daily living. There are three primary features of the vegetative state: (a) the person has sleep–wake cycles; (b) all responses can be identified as reflex patterns; and (c) the person makes no meaningful responses and has no awareness (Andrews 1999). At the recommendation of the International Working Party (1996), the terms 'persistent' or 'permanent' should no longer be used as they confuse prognosis with diagnosis. ⮑ persistant vegetative state. (Andrews K 1999 The vegetative state—clinical diagnosis. Postgraduate Medical Journal 75: 321–324. International Working Party 1996 Report on the Vegetative State. The Royal Hospital for Neurodisability, London.)

vehicle a substance with which a drug is mixed for administration, such as sterile water.

vein *n* a vessel conveying blood from the capillaries and venules back to the heart in the pulmonary and systemic circulations. It has the same basic three coats as an artery, but with some differences including an inner coat which is modified to form valves in some veins to aid venous return to the heart—**venous** *adj*. ⮑ tunica adventitia, tunica intima, tunica media.

veined denture base material denture base material treated by the addition of coloured nylon threads to give an appearance of blood vessels.

velamentous like a veil.

velamentous insertion of the umbilical cord a type of placenta in which the umbilical cord vessels divide before reaching the placenta. ⮑ vasa praevia.

vellus hair short downy hair found on most hair bearing parts of the body in children and in women except that on the scalp and the axillae and external genitalia. ⮑ lanugo, terminal hair.

velocity rate of change of position with respect to time. A vector quantity so has both magnitude (speed) and direction. ⮑ angular velocity, displacement, instantaneous velocity, linear velocity, tangential velocity.

vena cava one of two large veins emptying into the right atrium of the heart. The superior vena cava drains venous blood from the head, neck and upper limbs, and the inferior vena cava drains venous blood from structures below the diaphragm—**venae cavae** *pl*, **vena caval** *adj*. ⮑ Colour Section Figures 8, 10.

vena vorticosa ⮑ vortex vein.

veneer *n* in dentistry, a thin restoration that covers the surface of a tooth, usually made from tooth coloured composite resin or porcelain. It is bonded to the underlying tooth tissue to mask discoloured or malformed teeth.

venepuncture *n* also called venipuncture. The insertion of a needle into a vein.

venereal *adj* pertaining to or caused by sexual intercourse.

venereal disease ⮑ sexually transmitted infection.

venereal disease research laboratory (VDRL) test a non-specific serological test for syphilis.

venereology *n* the study and treatment of sexually transmitted infections.

venesection *n* (*syn* phlebotomy) a clinical procedure whereby blood is removed via venepuncture. It is used in the treatment of iron overload, e.g. haemochromatosis and occasionally acutely for congestive heart failure.

ven/e, ven/i, ven/o- a prefix that means 'vein', e.g. *venotomy*.

venography *n* (*syn* phlebography) radiological examination of the venous system involving injection of a contrast agent. Mostly replaced by ultrasound—**venographic** *adj*, **venogram** *n*, **venograph** *n*, **venographically** *adv*.

venom *n* a poisonous fluid produced by some snakes, spiders and scorpions.

venotomy *n* incision of a vein. ⮑ venesection.

venous *adj* pertaining to the veins.

venous haemorrhage bleeding from a vein; the blood is dark red (low in oxygen—deoxygenated) in colour and tends to gush or flow from the vein/ wound. ⮑ haemorrhage.

venous return the flow of blood from the whole body (except the lungs) via the great veins (superior and inferior venae cavae) to the right atrium of the heart. It is achieved by means of the respiratory pump (created by intrathoracic pressure changes during breathing), the calf muscle pump in conjunction with one way valves in the leg veins and changes in venomotor tone. Apart from minor beat-by-beat variations, this is equal at any one time to the cardiac output (from each of the ventricles), as the whole circulation, with

U
V

the systemic and pulmonary components in series, is a closed loop. When heart rate increases and muscle supply vessels dilate in exercise, stroke volume is maintained (so that cardiac output is increased) by an increase in venous return, assisted by further constriction of peripheral veins, reduction in the blood flow to the abdominal organs, and by the 'pumping' effects of increased depth of breathing (promoting flow into the thorax), and of the contracting muscles in the legs, which 'milk' blood along their local veins towards the heart.

venous sinus any one of the sinuses or channels that convey venous blood from the dura mater, or the coronary sinus which conveys venous blood from the myocardium. ⟳ coronary sinus, dural sinuses, sagittal sinuses.

venous stasis retinopathy ⟳ retinal vein occlusion.

venous thromboembolism (VTE) venous thrombosis may arise either because of damage to, or pressure on veins (e.g. varicose veins or pelvic tumour), slowing of bood flow (venous stasis) or as a result of changes in the plasma or cellular elements of the blood. Predisposing conditions for venous thrombosis and venous thromboembolism (VTE) are: (a) patient factors—age > 40 years, obesity (body mass index greater than 30 kg/m^2), varicose veins, previous deep vein thrombosis or pulmonary embolus, oral contraception, pregnancy and puerperium, dehydration, paralysis affecting lower limb, immobility; (b) surgical conditions—surgery, especially if > 30 minutes' duration, abdominal or pelvic surgery, orthopaedic surgery to lower limb; (c) medical conditions—myocardial infarction, heart failure, inflammatory diseases such as inflammatory bowel disease, malignancy, chronic respiratory disease, nephrotic syndrome, acute infection such as pneumonia, homocystinaemia; (d) haematological disorders—primary proliferative polycythaemia, essential thrombocythaemia, paroxysmal nocturnal haemoglobinuria, myelofibrosis; (e) deficiency of anticoagulants—antithrombin, protein C, prothrombin G20210A, protein S, factor V Leiden; (f) antiphospholipid antibody—lupus anticoagulant, anticardiolipin antibody. When a thrombotic event arises in an individual under the age of 40 years, particularly if there is a family history of thrombosis, investigations for a predisposing blood abnormality should be undertaken. Often several other risk factors are present when an acute deep venous thrombosis (DVT) occurs, e.g. obesity and surgery in a patient with factor V Leiden. The treatment of a venous thrombosis depends on its site and extent and on the age of the thrombus. Prior to any antithrombotic therapy it is essential to consider whether the patient has a significant contraindication to anticoagulant therapy such as thrombocytopenia, recent cerebral haemorrhage, recent surgery, especially eye or central nervous system, liver disease, renal failure, haemophilia, peptic ulcer, uncontrolled hypertension, recent falls in older adults, etc. On occasion therapy may have to be given to a patient who has a contraindication and in this instance the potential benefits have to be weighed against the risk of serious haemorrhage. ⟳ antiphospholipid antibody

syndrome, antithrombin deficiency, deep vein thrombosis, factor V Leiden, protein C and S deficiencies, prothrombin G20210A, pulmonary embolus, thrombophilia screen.

venous ulcer (*syn* gravitational ulcer) ulcer with a venous aetiology. They usually occur close to the ankle or between ankle and knee. There is often brown staining to the skin and dermatitis. Ulcers are large and shallow with large amounts of exudate. They frequently occur in people who have a history of deep vein thrombosis or varicose veins. They are chronic wounds and can be difficult to treat effectively. ⟳ ankle-brachial pressure index (ABPI), compression therapy, larval therapy, Colour Section Figure 127.

ventilation *n* the supply of fresh air. Ventilation in physiology and medicine, refers to pulmonary ventilation, the movement of air in and out of the lungs, whether during normal breathing, or by artificial means. Total ventilation or minute ventilation (volume) $\dot{V}_E$ (or $\dot{V}_I$) is the volume breathed out (or in) in litres per minute: the tidal volume multiplied by the number of breaths per minute. May be measured, e.g. by collecting the expired gas over a known time (Douglas bag method), or by integrating inspired or expired airflow with respect to time (by pneumotachograph). The effective component, alveolar ventilation $\dot{V}_A$, refers to that which reaches the regions of the lungs where gas exchange occurs, and is equal to the total ventilation minus dead space ventilation $\dot{V}_D$. Normally, at rest, $\dot{V}_A : \dot{V}_D = 2:1$ or typically, $\dot{V}_E - \dot{V}_D = \dot{V}_A$, 6 −2 = 4 L/min. When ventilation increases in exercise, the dead space is unchanged, so $\dot{V}_D$ rises only in proportion to the rise in frequency of breaths, but $\dot{V}_E$ rises relatively more as tidal volume also increases. ⟳ dead space.

ventilation–perfusion (V/Q) ratio the ratio between gases in the alveoli (alveolar ventilation) and blood flow in the pulmonary capillaries (pulmonary perfusion). Homeostatic autoregulatory mechanisms normally control the ratio to ensure that gas exchange is as efficient as possible. For example, mechanisms operate to compensate for adopting an upright posture. However, differences between the apex and the base of the lung are not fully compensated by the autoregulatory mechanisms; even in healthy lungs there will be areas of lung where ventilated alveoli are not perfused and areas where poorly ventilated alveoli are perfused, which results in less efficient gas exchange. For example if the normal V (ventilation) is 4 L air/min and the normal Q (perfusion) is 5 L blood/min, the normal V/Q ratio is 0.8. If the V/Q is higher than 0.8, it means ventilation exceeds perfusion and if the V/Q is less than 0.8, there is a VQ mismatch caused by poor ventilation. Where a substantial mismatch occurs, gas exchange is impaired and leads to the development of hypoxia and possibly hypercapnia. The mismatch may be due to alveolar underventilation (e.g. with chronic obstructive pulmonary disease), or poor blood flow in the pulmonary capillaries, (e.g. after pulmonary embolus and infarction).

ventilation–perfusion scanning an imaging technique used in nuclear medicine to investigate lung ventilation and perfusion, such as after pulmonary embolus. The investigation has two parts; a radioactive gas (e.g. krypton [Kr-81m], xenon [Xe-133]) is inhaled to investigate ventilation and radioactive albumin is administered intravenously to demonstrate perfusion.

ventilator *n* invasive type is known colloquially as a 'life support machine'. Specialized equipment for mechanically inflating a patient's lungs. Used to support or replace the patient's own breathing. These may be of invasive ventilators that require tracheal intubation or tracheostomy, or non-invasive mask system ventilators. There are now numerous applications of ventilation with many combinations of control, phase and variables. These can broadly be explained in three categories: (a) controlled mandatory ventilation (CMV) (infrequently used today), in which a precise minute ventilation can be delivered thus providing full ventilatory support; (b) intermittent mandatory ventilation (IMV), which combines both patient and machine triggered breaths; and (c) spontaneous breath modes, which are all patient initiated. Such modes include continuous positive airway pressure (CPAP), biphasic positive airway pressure (BIPAP) and pressure supported ventilation (PSV). ⊃ mechanical ventilation.

ventilator-associated pneumonia (VAP) ventilator-associated pneumonia is a common cause of hospital-acquired pneumonia. It is defined as pneumonia diagnosed in a patient more than 48 hours following the insertion of an endotracheal tube and the commencement of mechanical ventilation. The normal reflexes of cough and sneeze, and the mucus-clearing action of the mucucilliary escalator are absent, thereby allowing pathogenic micro-organisms from the upper respiratory tract to enter and contaminate the lower respiratory tract (bronchioles and alveoli). The risk of VAP in critically ill patients is increased as they are exposed to many invasive procedures and will be prescribed antibiotic therapy. ⊃ mechanical ventilation.

ventilatory equivalent describes the ratio of ventilation (minute ventilation/volume) to oxygen intake, or to carbon dioxide output. For oxygen, the volume of gas breathed out (and in) in litres per minute (ventilation, $\dot{V}_E$) divided by the oxygen consumption in litres per minute ($\dot{V}O_2$) over the same period: an index of the efficiency of oxygen uptake in the lungs. When there is significant anaerobic metabolism, decrease in blood pH is countered by stimulation of ventilation to increase CO_2 excretion, such that $\dot{V}_E$ increases at a higher rate than $\dot{V}O_2$, raising the ventilatory equivalent (CO_2 the ventilatory equivalent, $\dot{V}_E/\dot{V}CO_2$, increases in this instance less than that for O_2 because as CO_2 in the blood and lungs decreases, the same output is achieved by a smaller expired volume).

ventilatory threshold (VT, T_{vent}) work rate at which the gradient of the ventilation/work rate plot increases. Attributed to rise in blood lactate concentration $[Lac]_b$ so used as non-invasive indicator of lactate threshold (LT)/ anaerobic threshold (AT), but precision of the agreement varies with the method of determining ventilatory threshold.

Ventouse extraction use of the vacuum extractor in obstetrics to facilitate the delivery of the fetus. It is used more commonly than forceps in northern Europe and Africa. The vacuum extractor is an instrument that applies traction via a soft of rigid cup (Figure V.2). It can be used as an alternative to a forceps delivery. The cup cleaves to the fetal scalp by suction and is used to assist maternal effort during pushing. The women is usually in the lithotomy position and the same precautions are observed as for forceps delivery. Local anaesthesia or inhalational analgesia may be sufficient. Pudendal nerve block may be employed or epidural, if already in situ, may be topped up. Episiotomy is not routinely carried out. ⊃ chignon.

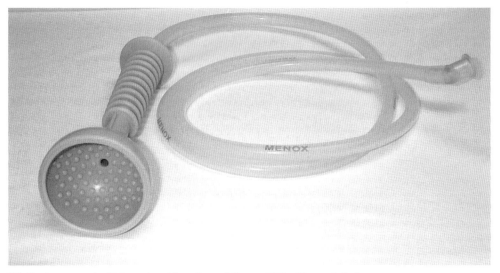

V.2 Ventouse cup (soft) (reproduced from Fraser & Cooper 2003 with permission)

ventral *adj* pertaining to the abdomen or the anterior surface of the body. Applies to the front of the hands and arms in the anatomical position when the palms face forwards—**ventrally** *adv*. ⊃ dorsal *opp*.

ventral decubitus radiograph the patient lies prone and the central ray passes through the body from side to side.

ventricle *n* a small belly-like cavity—**ventricular** *adj*.

ventricle of the brain one of four cavities filled with cerebrospinal fluid within the brain.

ventricle of the heart the two lower muscular pumping chambers of the heart. The left ventricle receives oxygenated blood from the lungs via the left atrium, and in an average-sized person at rest ejects a stroke volume of around 70 mL at each beat (contraction, systole) into the aorta, increasing during exercise by virtue of greater filling and stretching during each relaxation (diastole); the right ventricle receives venous blood from the rest of the body via the right atrium, and ejects the same volume as the left ventricle, in synchrony with it. The heart beat can normally be felt over the apex of the left ventricle. ⊃ Colour Section Figure 8.

ventricular aqueduct ⊃ cerebral aqueduct.

ventricular fibrillation (VF) a serious, life-threatening cardiac arrhythmia where uncoordinated ventricular activity, which is characterized by fast quivering rather than contraction, fails to produce any output of blood into the circulation. Thus the person will have neither a pulse nor a blood pressure. VF occurs when abnormal foci in the ventricles fire in a completely chaotic manner. The ECG shows rapid fibrillation (Figure V.3). It becomes a fatal arrhythmia in the absence of initial basic life support, successful defibrillation and advanced life support. A common cause of sudden death following myocardial infarction. ⊃ automated external defibrillator (AED), cardiac arrest, Appendix 10.

ventricular septal defect (VSD) *n* a hole or holes in the interventricular septum. Most commonly due to a congenital defect, but can also follow a myocardial infarction. VSD is the commonest congenital heart defect and accounts for 30% of defects, and can be associated with maternal rubella infection during pregnancy or Down's syndrome; it is also a feature of complex congenital heart defects, such as Fallot's tetralogy. The defect results in a left-to-right shunt of blood in the heart with a murmur, and sometimes cardiac failure in infants aged 4–6 weeks. Small defects may close spontaneously, but where surgical repair is indicated it is increasingly performed using percutaneous minimally invasive techniques.

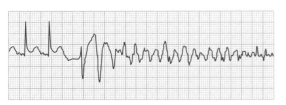

V.3 Ventricular fibrillation (reproduced from Boon et al 2006 with permission)

VSD can result in ventricular overload and hypertrophy, and changes to pulmonary vascular resistance and pulmonary hypertension that lead eventually to shunt reversal and Eisenmenger's syndrome. ⊃ Colour Section Figure 40.

ventricular tachycardia (VT) a very serious ventricular arrhythmia characterized by a rapid ventricular rate of 140–200 per minute. It may lead to cardiac arrest—ventricular fibrillation or pulseless ventricular tachycardia.

ventriculitis *n* inflammation of a ventricle. Usually refers to that affecting the cerebral ventricles in conjunction with encephalitis.

ventricul/o- a prefix that means 'ventricle', e.g. *ventriculoatrial*.

ventriculoatrial shunt *n* an artificial communication between the cerebral ventricles and the right atrium of the heart. Accomplished by the use of a plastic tube, which contains a pressure-flow regulator. Used to drain excess cerebrospinal fluid in hydrocephalus.

ventriculoatriostomy *n* ⊃ ventriculoatrial shunt.

ventriculocysternostomy *n* ventriculocisternal shunt. An artificial communication between the cerebral ventricles and the cisterna magna. Previously used as a drainage procedure for hydrocephalus.

ventriculography *n* **1.** radiographic demonstration of the cardiac ventricles following the insertion of contrast agent, or an imaging technique using a radioisotope (radionuclide). **2.** an obsolete radiographic examination of the cerebral ventricles, now replaced by CT and MRI scanning.

ventriculoperitoneal shunt *n* an artificial communication between the cerebral ventricles and the peritoneal cavity. Accomplished by the use of a plastic tube, which contains a non-return valve. A commonly used technique for draining excess cerebrospinal fluid in hydrocephalus.

ventriculopleural shunt *n* an artificial communication between the cerebral ventricles and the pleural cavity. Accomplished by the use of a plastic tube, which contains a pressure-flow regulator. Used to drain excess cerebrospinal fluid in hydrocephalus.

ventriculoscopy *n* direct visualization of the cerebral ventricles using an endoscope.

ventriculostomy *n* an artificial opening into a ventricle. Usually refers to a drainage operation for hydrocephalus.

ventriculovenous shunt *n* an artificial communication between the cerebral ventricles and the internal jugular vein. Accomplished by the use of a plastic tube, which contains a pressure-flow regulator. Used to drain excess cerebrospinal fluid in hydrocephalus.

ventrosuspension *n* fixation of a displaced uterus to the anterior abdominal wall.

Venturi effect (G Venturi, Italian physicist, 1746–1822) a principle of gas behaviour used for the mixing and delivery of gases, such as oxygen masks. ⊃ Venturi mask.

Venturi mask an oxygen therapy mask designed to direct atmospheric air to mix it with a given flow of prescribed oxygen. A variety of masks are available that allow the administration of oxygen at different concentrations.

U
V

venule *n* a small vein that connects the capillary bed to larger veins.

verbal feedback verbal or auditory feedback can be used by health professionals, such as physiotherapists, in reinforcing treatment goals in relation to performance. It is important to encourage appropriate effort, as accurate feedback is essential to the learning process. There should not be a mismatch between the action of the patient and the feedback of the therapist. However, negativity can also be non-motivational and so care should be taken to achieve a balance when treating patients.

verbigeration the stereotyped repetition of words and phrases; a feature of some types of schizophrenia.

Veress needle a sharp needle with a blunt ended trochar which has a lateral hole; it is used for a pneumoperitoneum. When the trochar projects from the needle, the gut is pushed safely away from the needle point.

vergence 1. denotes divergence of light travelling from, or convergence of light travelling from, or to an object or image. The unit of vergence is the dioptre. **2.** Disjunctive movements of the eyes such as convergence, divergence, cyclovergence, infravergence or supravergence. ⊃ convergence, disjunctive eye movements, divergence.

vergence facility the ability of the eyes to make fusional vergence movements in a given period of time. Clinically, this is measured by introducing a relatively large prism in front of one or both eyes of a patient fixating a target until it appears single. The operation is repeated many times and the results are commonly presented in cycles per minute (one cycle indicates that single vision was reported both with the prism and after removing the prism). ⊃ fusional convergence, lens flippers, motor fusion.

vergence power ⊃ refractive power (*F*).

Verhoeff's circles (F Verhoeff, American ophthalmic scientist and pathologist, 1874–1968) (*syn* Verhoeff's rings) two black concentric circles designed for use with the duochrome test and as a target for the cross-cylinder method. The thickness and overall diameter of the inner ring are equivalent to a 6/6 (or 20/20) Snellen letter while the thickness and overall diameter of the outer ring are equivalent to a 6/15 (or 20/50) Snellen letter. ⊃ cross-cylinder test for astigmatism, duochrome test, Snellen test type chart.

verification the process of confirming the accuracy of radiotherapy planning prior to treatment taking place.

vermicide *n* an agent which kills intestinal worms—**vermicidal** *adj*.

vermiform *adj* wormlike.

vermiform appendix the vestigial, hollow, wormlike structure attached to the caecum. ⊃ appendix vermiformis.

vermifuge *n* an agent that expels intestinal worms.

vermillion border the exposed red border of the lips.

vermis *n* **1.** a worm. **2.** the narrow worm-like structure situated between the two hemispheres of the cerebellum.

vernal catarrh ⊃ vernal conjunctivitis.

vernal conjunctivitis (*syn* vernal keratoconjunctivitis [VKC]—although this is not strictly speaking a synonym

since the condition often involves the cornea, spring catarrh, vernal catarrh) chronic, bilateral conjunctivitis which recurs in the spring and summer and is more often seen in boys than girls. Its origin is probably due to an allergy. It is characterized by hard flattened papillae of a bluish-white colour separated by furrows and having the appearance of 'cobblestones' located in the upper palpebral portion of the conjunctiva. A second type of vernal conjunctivitis exists which affects the limbal region of the bulbar conjunctiva, characterized by the formation of small, gelatinous white dots called Trantas' dots or Horner–Trantas' dots. The chief symptom of the disease is intense itching. Treatment consists mainly of cold compresses and limited (because of side effects) use of topical corticosteroids (e.g. dexamethasone, prednisolone). Sodium cromoglicate or lodoxamide have also been found to be very successful in treating this condition and with fewer side effects than corticosteroids. ⊃ Colour Section Figure 128.

vernal keratoconjunctivitis (VKC) ⊃ vernal conjunctivitis.

vernier an instrument used to accurately measure length.

vernier (micrometer) microscope a microscope mounted on a movable slide and used to measure accurately the dimension of small objects.

vernier visual acuity (*syn* aligning power) the ability to detect the alignment or otherwise of two lines as in the reading of a vernier scale. This is the finest acuity being of the order of 1–5 seconds of arc depending on the length of the line; the longer the line, the more acute the detection. ⊃ hyperacuity.

vernix caseosa the fatty substance which covers and protects the skin of the fetus from maceration caused by amniotic fluid and friction. It is present from 18 weeks' gestation, but increases dring the last trimester.

verocytotoxin *n* powerful enterotoxin produced by enterohaemorrhagic *Escherichia coli* such as *E. coli* 0157. It can cause haemolytic uraemic syndrome. ⊃ haemolytic uraemic syndrome.

verruca *n* ⊃ wart, condyloma—**verrucae** *pl*, **verrucous**, **verrucose** *adj*.

version *n* turning—applied to the manoeuvre to alter the position of the fetus in utero. ⊃ cephalic version, external cephalic version (ECV), internal version, podalic version.

vertebra (typical) *n* one of the irregular bones making up the vertebral column (spinal column). A typical movable vertebra has a body, which is situated anteriorly (Figure V.4). The size varies with the site. They are smallest in the cervical region and become larger towards the weight-bearing lumbar region. The vertebral (neural) arch encloses a large vertebral foramen. The ring of bone consists of two pedicles that project backwards from the body and two laminae. Where the pedicles and laminae unite, transverse processes project laterally and where the two laminae meet in the midline posteriorly they form a spinous process. The vertebral (neural) arch has four articular surfaces: two articulate with the vertebra above and two with the one below.

U
V

821

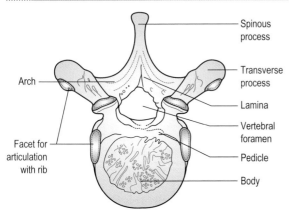

Spinous process

Transverse process

Arch

Lamina

Vertebral foramen

Facet for articulation with rib

Pedicle

Body

V.4 Typical thoracic vertebra (from above) (Reproduced from Watson 2000 with permission)

The vertebral foramina form the vertebral (neural) canal that contains the spinal cord—**vertebrae** *pl*, **vertebral** *adj*. ⊃ vertebral column.

vertebra prominens the seventh cervical vertebra.

vertebral arch (neural arch) *n* the arch formed by the pedicles and laminae at the posterior part of a vertebra; encloses the vertebral canal or foramen.

vertebral artery *n* one of two arteries. They contribute to the circulus arteriosus (circle of Willis) that supplies blood to the brain. The two vertebral arteries branch from the subclavian arteries, run upwards through foramina in the cervical vertebra and pass into the skull through the foramen magnum to form the basilar artery.

vertebral artery occlusion the vertebral arteries can be occluded by pathologies that include atherosclerosis, arthritis and deformities of the spine. The vertebral arteries can also be occluded by certain movements of the cervical spine including rotation and extension. Subjective symptoms arising from vertebral artery insufficiency are known as the five 'Ds', they are diplopia, dizziness, dysphagia, dysarthria and drop attacks. Before performing any mobilization/manipulation or traction of the cervical spine, it is essential for the therapist to ask the patient specifically if they have experienced any of the above symptoms. If the patient has positive signs on subjective examination, it is necessary to conduct vertebral artery tests to support or negate vertebral artery insufficiency. Equally, if a patient is undergoing a technique that will compromise the vertebral artery, such as grade III/IV rotation of the cervical spine, vertebral artery insufficiency needs to be cleared objectively.

vertebral canal (neural canal) also called vertebral foramen. The cavity within the vertebral column that houses and protects the spinal cord.

vertebral column (*syn* spinal column) The dorsal axis of the body in all vertebrates. A bony and ligamentous structure extending from the uppermost (the first cervical or atlas) vertebra which articulates with the base of the skull, and ending above and behind the anus. It is made up of 33/34 vertebrae, articulating with the skull above and the pelvic girdle below.

Consists of 24 separate vertebrae linked by joints and by the intervertebral discs—7 cervical,12 thoracic (which give attachment to the ribs), 5 lumbar—and 9 or 10 fused bones—5 sacral and 4 or 5 coccygeal. The fused vertebrae form the sacrum (articulating with the ilium of the pelvic bones) and four or five rudimentary 'tail' vertebrae fused in the coccyx. The vertebral column allows a limited amount of movement of the trunk. The vertebrae are so shaped that they enclose a cavity (vertebral, spinal or neural canal), which provides a protected tunnel for the spinal cord and the paired anterior and posterior spinal nerve roots, which leave through openings (intervertebral foramina) at the sides of the column, each being numbered according to that of the vertebra above the foramen. ⊃ cervical spine, intervertebral disc, spinal injury/spinal cord injury.

vertebral end plate the vertebral end plates are found above and below each intervertebral disc, they are approximately 1 mm thick and have several functions: the end plate is thought to permit osmosis of nutrients between the vertebral body and the disc, it restrains the disc and may also protect the vertebra from pressure.

vertebrate having a backbone or vertebral column.

vertebrobasilar insufficiency (VBI) a poorly understood condition in which there is thought to be transient disturbances in the blood flow to the brainstem.

vertex *n* **1.** the top of the head. **2.** the point where the optical axis intersects a reflecting or refracting surface. In a spectacle lens the back vertex is the point of intersection of the optical axis with the surface nearest to the eye, the other being the front vertex—**vertices** *pl*.

vertex distance the distance along the line of sight between the apex of the cornea and the posterior surface of a spectacle lens. This distance normally varies between 11 mm and 15 mm. ⊃ apical clearance, spectacle plane.

vertex focal length the linear distance separating the principal focal point (or focus) of an optical system or lens from the front or back vertices. They are called the front vertex focal length (f_v) and the back vertex focal length (f'_v), respectively. In the case of a biconcave or biconvex lens the front and back vertex focal lengths are equal. In the case of a positive meniscus lens, the back vertex focal length is shorter than the front vertex focal length and vice versa in the case of a negative meniscus lens. ⊃ back vertex power, front vertex power.

vertex occlusal projection axial true occlusal projection of the maxilla often used to demonstrate the buccolingual position of unerupted teeth.

vertex power ⊃ back vertex power, front vertex power.

vertical perpendicular. Positioned directly above a given place or point at right angles to the horizontal plane.

vertical angulation in radiography, the direction of the central ray in a vertical plane.

vertical axis (dental) a hypothetical line around which the mandible rotates in the horizontal plane.

vertical dimension (of the face) a measurement of the face taken by selecting two midline points above and below the mouth. A Willis facial height gauge may be used for this measurement.

vertical overlap (vertical overbite) overlap of the upper teeth over the lower teeth in a vertical direction when all teeth are in occlusion.

vertical subsigmoid osteotomy an osteotomy to correct mandibular prognathism by the vertical sectioning of the ramus commencing at the mandibular notch.

vertical transmission transmission of disease from mother to fetus, via the placenta, during delivery or via breast milk, e.g. HIV.

vertigo *n* giddiness, dizziness. It can be caused by an infection such as sinusitis, or disease of the ear (e.g. benign paroxysmal positional vertigo, Ménière's disease, labyrinthitis), or following damage to the vestibular nerve or its central connections, or as a side effect of medication. Vertigo gives the patient an illusion of rotatory movement due to disturbed orientation of the body in space, leaving the affected person with feeling that the environment around them is moving. It is often accompanied by nausea or vomiting—**vertiginous** *adj*.

very low birthweight (VLBW) very low birthweight is defined as less than 1500 g at birth, and extremely low birthweight is less than 1000 g at birth ⊃ low birthweight, small for gestational age.

very-low-density lipoprotein (VLDL) ⊃ lipoprotein.

vesical *adj* pertaining to the urinary bladder.

vesicant *n* a drug or other substance that causes blistering of the skin.

vesicle *n* **1.** a small bladder, cell or hollow structure. **2.** a fluid-filled skin blister less than 5 mm in diameter—**vesicular** *adj*, **vesiculation** *n*.

vesic/o- a prefix that means 'bladder', e.g. *vesical*.

vesicocolic *adj* pertaining to the urinary bladder and the colon. *vesicocolic fistula* an abnormal communication between the urinary bladder and the colon, for example with diverticular disease. ⊃ pneumaturia.

vesicostomy ⊃ cystostomy.

vesicoureteric *adj* pertaining to the urinary bladder and ureter.

vesicoureteric reflux (VUR)) retrograde passage of urine up the ureters following a rise of pressure within the bladder during voiding. It can lead to reflux nephropathy (chronic pyelonephritis). ⊃ reflux nephropathy.

vesicovaginal *adj* pertaining to the urinary bladder and vagina. *vesicovaginal fistula* an abnormal communication between the bladder and the vagina. Causes include advanced cancer of the cervix, radiotherapy and damage during labour.

vesiculitis *n* inflammation of a vesicle, particularly the seminal vesicles.

vesiculography radiographic demonstration of the seminal vesicles following the introduction of contrast agent.

vesiculopapular *adj* pertaining to or exhibiting both vesicles and papules.

vesiculopustular *adj* pertaining to or exhibiting both vesicles and pustules.

vessel *n* a tube, duct or canal, holding or conveying fluid, especially blood and lymph.

vestibular *adj* relating to the space of the vestibule. *vestibular aspect* or *surface* the surface of teeth or gingivae that face the vestibule.

vestibular apparatus the sensory organs of the inner ear concerned with position sense and balance—the otolith organs and the semicircular canals. They detect tilt of the head with respect to the ground, and the direction and rate of any acceleration of the head in space. This input interacts with sensory information from muscles and joints, eyes and ears to co-ordinate reflex postural adjustments.

vestibular aqueduct a minute canal of the vesibule of the inner ear. It is occluded by a tiny vein and the endolymphatic duct and conveys no fluid.

vestibular aqueduct vein a tiny vein from the inner (internal ear); it travels through the vestibular aqueduct (which it occludes) and empties blood into the superior petrosal venous sinus.

vestibular ataxia may occur with peripheral vestibular disorders or central disorders that affect the vestibular nuclei and/or their afferent/efferent connections via the vestibular branch of the vestibulocochlear nerve (VIII cranial nerve). Peripheral lesions may be either bilateral or, more commonly, unilateral. Patients with vestibular ataxia may demonstrate poor balance reactions, have a wide-based gait, those with unilateral lesions leaning towards the side of the lesion and people with bilateral lesions have a tendency to lean backwards. Patients also tend to rely heavily on visual information and so may have increased problems with movement in reduced lighting or the dark. ⊃ acoustic neuroma.

vestibular deepening ⊃ vestibuloplasty.

vestibular glands four mucus-secreting glands that open into the vestibule of the female external genitalia. The greater vestibular glands (Bartholin's glands) and the lesser vestibular or paraurethral glands (Skene's glands).

vestibular rehabilitation a type of rehabilitation for people suffering from vertigo. Physiotherapists can help with vestibular rehabilitation by assessing the problems and prescribing specific exercises such as Cawthorne Cooksey and activities to increase independence. The Cawthorne Cooksey exercises comprise a series of movement initially undertaken in bed with a gradual progression, as the condition improves and confidence increases, to performing them sitting, standing and then moving about. Physiotherapists must make a distinction when assessing individuals between positional triggers and movement triggers. Peripheral problems respond better to these habituation exercises, central vertigo often only has limited success. ⊃ benign paroxysmal positional vertigo, vertigo.

vestibule *n* a connecting passage. **1.** the middle part of the inner ear, lying between the semicircular canals and the cochlea. **2.** the triangular area between the labia minora. **3.** the area of the mouth between the buccal and labial aspect of the teeth and gingivae, and the inner aspect of the cheeks and lips—**vestibular** *adj*.

vestibulocochlear *adj* relating to the vestibule and the cochlear.

vestibulocochlear nerve auditory nerve. The eighth pair of cranial nerves. There are two branches: the vestibular, which transmits impulses from the vestibular apparatus of the ear to the cerebellum, and the cochlear, which transmits impulses from the cochlea in the ear to the auditory cortex situated in the temporal lobe of the cerebrum.

vestibulo-ocular reflex compensatory eye movement stimulated by head movement to stabilize gaze in space.

vestibuloplasty in dentistry, a surgical procedure to deepen the vestibule—often required to facilitate fitting a denture. Some techniques allow for the adjacent mucous membrane to grow together, others use skin grafts of various kinds to line the deepened area.

vestige the remaining part of a structure that formerly existed in a previous stage of development.

vestigial *adj* pertaining to a rudimentary structure, a remnant of something formerly present.

VF *abbr* ventricular fibrillation.

VFM *abbr* value for money.

VHF *abbr* **1.** very high frequency. **2.** viral haemorrhagic fever.

VHN Vickers hardness scale/number.

V̇ₗ symbol for the volume of air entering the lungs in one minute.

viable *adj* capable of living a separate existence—**viability** *n*.

vibrating line the line of junction between the movable soft palate and the static tissues anterior to the soft palate.

vibration *n* a form of massage manipulation. A fine tremor transmitted through the hands and finger tips to body cavities in order to move fluids and gases. Vibration is sometimes used as a stimulation technique and can be applied to muscle or tendon. High-frequency vibration (100–300 Hz) will elicit a reflex called the tonic vibratory response. It can be used to facilitate activity in a hypotonic muscle or inhibit hypertonicity in a muscle belly.

vibration syndrome (*syn* Raynaud's phenomenon) ⊃ hand-arm vibration syndrome.

vibration—whole body arises from use of equipment in which the worker is supported by the vibrating machinery, e.g. a vehicle seat or ship's deck. The cardiovascular system is affected, with an increase in heart rate and interference with circulation; musculoskeletal problems are common particularly involving the spine. Fatigue and poor concentration are also thought to be significant.

vibrator in dentistry, a pulsating machine for removing air bubbles from impression and investment materials during mixing.

Vibrio *n* a genus of curved, motile micro-organisms. *Vibrio cholerae* causes cholera.

vibrissae *npl* the coarse hairs growing within the nasal cavity.

vicarious *adj* substituting the function of one organ for another.

vicarious experience knowledge or information about a skill or behaviour derived from seeing the performance of others.

vicarious liability describes the liability of the employer, such as an NHS Trust, for the wrongful acts of an employee committed during the course of employment.

Vickers hardness scale or number (VHN) ⊃ hardness scale.

victim blaming a tendency to blame the person who is experiencing ill-health or other difficulties. A heavy smoker, for example, may be blamed for contracting lung cancer. Victim blaming denies the influence of wider social, economic and political factors on people's behaviour, over which they may have little control.

video analysis the use of video cameras and equipment to analyse motion, often for kinematic analysis.

videokeratoscope an electro-optical instrument for measuring the corneal topography. It produces a colour coded three-dimensional map of the shape of the cornea and of the dioptric power of the different corneal regions. These instruments are computer-assisted providing rapid, on-line analysis of the image and most of them are based on the corneal reflection of the Placido pattern. They are used to evaluate keratoconus, irregular corneal shape, contact lens fitting, monitor the cornea after keratoplasty or refractive surgery, etc. There are many commercial models (e.g. EyeSys, Tomey, Humphrey, Dicon, Orbscan II). The latter, which incorporates a scanning slit measurement system, simultaneously measures both corneal surfaces enabling a diagnosis of anterior and posterior keratoconus. ⊃ keratoconus, photokeratoscopy, Topogometer.

videokymography recording vibrations, such as those of the vocal folds of the larynx, using a high-speed camera.

videotext the interactive public information service broadcast on television, known as Prestel.

vignetting shading round an image.

villonodular synovitis a joint problem, usually affecting the hips or knees, where the lining of the joint becomes swollen and extra synovial fluid is secreted causing swelling and pain.

villus *n* a microscopic fingerlike projection; found on the mucosal surface of the small intestine, or on the outside of the chorion of the embryonic sac. Those on the intestinal mucosa increase the surface area available for the absorption of water and nutrients. The villus contains blood vessels and a central lymphatic lacteal for absorption—**villi** *pl*, **villous** *adj*. ⊃ Colour Section Figure 41.

VIN *abbr* vulval intraepithelial neoplasia.

vinca alkaloids a group of cytotoxic drugs extracted from the periwinkle plant, e.g. vincristine. They prevent mitosis and cell division by inhibiting microtubule formation. ⊃ cytotoxic. ⊃ Appendix 5.

Vincent's angina (*syn* ulcerative gingivitis) (H Vincent, French physician, 1862–1950) outdated term for necrotizing ulcerative gingivitis (NUG). ⊃ necrotizing ulcerative gingivitis (NUG).

violet one of the hues of the visible spectrum evoked by stimulation of the retina by wavelengths shorter than 450 nm and somewhat longer than 380 nm. ⊃ colour, light.

VIP *abbr* vasoactive intestinal peptide.

VIPoma a rare tumour that secretes vasoactive intestinal peptide. Usually occurs in the pancreas where it is often malignant, but it does occur elsewhere. They cause diarrhoea, hypokalaemia (reduced potassium level in the blood) and hypochlorhydria (reduced gastric acid).

viraemia *n* the presence of viruses in the blood—**viraemic** *adj*.

viral *adj* pertaining to or caused by a virus, such as viral meningitis.

viral haemorrhagic fevers fevers occurring mainly in tropical areas in both old and new world countries; they are often transmitted by mosquitoes or ticks and other animal vectors (rats, mice); they may cause a petechial skin rash. Mortality is often very high. They include: Argentine haemorrhagic fever, Bolivian haemorrhagic fever, Brazilian haemorrhagic fever, chikungunya, Ebola, dengue, Lassa fever, Marburg disease, Rift Valley fever, Venezuelan haemorrhagic fever, and yellow fever.

viral hepatitis ⊃ hepatitis.

Virchow's node (R Virchow, German pathologist, 1821–1902) ⊃ signal node.

Virchow's triad (R Virchow) three factors that predispose to the formation of deep vein thrombosis—slowing of blood flow (venous stasis), abnormal or inappropriate coagulation processes, or damage to veins. ⊃ deep vein thrombosis, venous thromboembolism (VTE).

virement *n* financial term meaning to move money from one expenditure category to another.

viricidal *adj* lethal to a virus—**viricide** *n*.

virilism *n* the appearance of secondary male characteristics in the female. It may be caused by abnormal adrenal secretion of androgenic substances, or by drugs.

virologist *n* an expert in viruses and viral diseases.

virology *n* the study of viruses and the diseases caused by them—**virological** *adj*.

virtue ethics an ethical approach that focuses on and encourages the intellectual and moral characteristics that allow individuals and groups to analyse ethical dilemmas and make sound ethical judgements. It is deemed important for people to possess the personality traits of courage, wisdom, sensitivity, compassion and empathy in order to be capable of making sound ethical judgements. This approach may lead to the erroneous assumption that ethical decision making is simply about being the 'right' sort of person rather than having the ability to analyse ethical dilemmas skilfully and thoroughly.

virulence *n* infectiousness; the disease-producing power of a micro-organism and its power to overcome host resistance—**virulent** *adj*.

viruses *npl* a diverse group of micro-organisms which are only visible using electron microscopy. They contain either deoxyribonucleic acid (DNA) or ribonucleic acid (RNA), and can only replicate within the host cell. Viruses infect humans, animals, plants and other micro-organisms (bacteriophages). Diseases caused by viruses in humans include: colds, influenza, measles, rabies, hepatitis, chickenpox, poliomyelitis, dengue and HIV disease. Viruses are widely considered not to be themselves truly 'living', and not possible to destroy directly without also destroying the host cells. Antiviral drug treatment is developing, but remains limited (antibiotics have no effect) but vaccination can provide immunity and in the second half of the 20th century this eradicated smallpox worldwide and much reduced the incidence of poliomyelitis. Some viruses are associated with cancer of the cervix, Burkitt's lymphoma and some types of leukaemia. ⊃ Epstein–Barr virus, human papilloma virus, human T-cell lymphotropic virus.

viscera *n* the internal organs—**viscus** *sing*, **visceral** *adj*.

visceral pertaining to the viscera or internal organs. Hence visceral afferents are the components of the peripheral nervous system that carry information from the organs. The outgoing nerves to the viscera are the sympathetic and parasympathetic nerves of the autonomic nervous system but are not usually known as visceral efferents.

viscid *adj* thick, sticky and glutinous, may be used to describe sputum, mucus, etc.

viscosity the property of a fluid medium that provides resistance to motion of the fluid itself or of an object moving through it. Also can be considered to be friction within fluids.

visible spectrum the small part of the electromagnetic spectrum containing the range of wavelengths that can be seen by the human eye.

vision one of the five senses. The appreciation of differences in the external world, such as form, colour, position, etc. resulting from the stimulation of the retina by light. ⊃ colour vision, visual acuity.

visiospatial neglect ⊃ unilateral neglect.

visual *adj* pertaining to vision. ⊃ colour vision, visual acuity.

visual acuity (VA) the sharpness of vision; the ability to see the difference between two points of light. Capacity for seeing distinctly the details of an object. Quantitatively, it is represented in two ways: (a) as the reciprocal of the minimum angle of resolution (in minutes of arc). This is the *resolution visual acuity*. Also known as minimum separable visual acuity. (b) as the Snellen fraction. This is measured using letters or Landolt rings or equivalent objects. Average clinical visual acuity varies between 6/4 and 6/6 (or 20/15 and 20/20 in feet). Visual acuity varies with the region of the retina (being maximum in the foveola), with general illumination, contrast, colour and type of test, time of exposure, the refractive error of the eye, etc. ⊃ contrast sensitivity, hyperacuity, optotype, photostress test, Snellen test type chart.

visual analogue scale (VAS) a self-reporting scale for pain. Uses a 10 cm horizontal line with indicators of pain severity such as 'pain free/no pain' at one end right up to 'worst pain

U
V

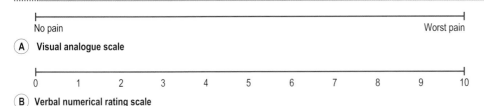

(A) **Visual analogue scale**

(B) **Verbal numerical rating scale**

V.5 **(A) Visual analogue scale. (B) Verbal numerical rating scale** (reproduced from Brooker & Waugh 2007 with permission)

possible' at the other end (Figure V.5A). Patients are asked to indicate the point on the scale that best describes their current pain. It can be modified by adding numbers (a verbal numerical rating scale), for example 0 = no pain and 10 = worst possible pain. These can be more reliable in 'measuring' pain (Figure V.5B).

visual area 1. any region of the brain in which visual information is processed. **2.** (*syn* primary visual area, primary visual cortex, striate area, striate cortex, V1, visual cortex) this is Brodmann's area 17 in each occipital lobe. It contains six layers of cells numbered 1 to 6 from top, layer 4 being subdivided into three sublayers 4A, 4B and 4C. Layer 4C receives inputs from the photoreceptors in the retina via the lateral geniculate bodies. There are also some afferents to layers 1 and 6. The primary visual area is identified by a white striation (line of Gennari) on each side of the calcarine fissure. This white line appears in the middle of the fourth layer of the visual cortex and is composed of fibres from the optic radiations. **3.** it also refers to all parts of each occipital lobe related to visual functions. ➲ cortical magnification, lateral geniculate bodies, occipital cortex, visual pathway.

visual axis (*syn* visual line) the line joining the object of regard to the foveola and passing through the nodal points which are often considered as coincident, as they are very close to each other. Strictly, this axis is not a single straight line as it consists of two parts: one line connecting the object of regard to the first nodal point and the other line parallel and connecting the second nodal point to the foveola. ➲ line of sight.

visual cortex ➲ visual area.

visual-evoked cortical potential (VECP) an electrical potential measured at the level of the occipital cortex in response to a light stimulation. Recording requires repetition of the stimulus and a computer synchronized with the onset of that stimulus, to average out the background noise produced by the spontaneous brain potentials (e.g. alpha, beta, delta, theta waves). This potential has clinical application and is used to objectively measure refraction, visual acuity, amblyopia, binocular anomalies, problems with the optic nerve and visual pathways; especially useful in the diagnosis of some demyelinating diseases such as multiple sclerosis, which have early optic nerve damage, etc. Many abbreviations are also used, although they are not strictly correct. They are EP (evoked potential), VEP (visually evoked potential), VER (visual evoked response), and

pVER (indicating that this potential is pattern-elicited). ➲ electrodiagnostic procedures, multiple sclerosis, objective accommodation.

visual fatigue a feeling of weariness resulting from a visual task. It can be of ocular, muscular or psychic origin. However, there does not seem to be objective proof of a reduction in visual aptitude (e.g. visual acuity) accompanying visual fatigue. ➲ asthenopia.

visual field also called field of vision. The area in which objects can be seen without moving the eye. In binocular vision, the overlap of the fields of both eyes across the nose allows perception of depth (stereoscopic vision).

visual imagery ➲ imagery.

visual impairment some degree of low vision, sight impairment or blindness. Common causes worldwide include: macular degeneration, diabetic and other retinopathies, glaucoma, cataracts, vitamin A deficiency, infections (e.g. trachoma) and trauma.

visual line ➲ visual axis.

visual pathway the neural path starting in the receptors of the retina and travelling through the following structures: the optic nerve (second cranial nerve), the optic chiasma, the optic tract, the lateral geniculate bodies, the optic radiations and the visual (occipital) cortex where the pathway ends. The fibres of the optic nerve of one eye meet with the fibres from the other eye at the optic chiasma, where approximately half of them (the nasal half of the retina) cross over to the other side. Thus, there is semidecussation in the visual pathway. ➲ lateral geniculate bodies, optic chiasma, optic radiations, optic tracts, Colour Section Figure 42.

visualization ➲ imagery.

visual motor coordination the ability to co-ordinate vision with movement or parts of the body.

visual pigment the photosensitive pigment contained in the outer segments of both rods and cones. The pigment in the rods is called rhodopsin. The cones contain three other types of pigments (one in each type of cone) which have spectral absorption curves with a maximum around 420, 530 and 560 nm. These three pigments form the basis of normal trichromatic colour vision. The cone visual pigments are cyanolabe, chlorolabe and erythrolabe, names sometimes used for the short-wave, middle-wave and long-wave sensitive cone pigments, respectively. Erythrolabe, meaning red pigment, has, in fact, its maximum spectral absorption around 560 nm which is in the green-yellow portion of the visible spectrum. ⊃ bleaching, cone, defective colour vision, photostress test, retinal densitometry, rhodopsin, rod, trichromatism, Young–Helmholtz theory.

visual purple rarely used term for rhodopsin. ⊃ opsins, rhodopsin, visual pigment.

Visuscope a modified ophthalmoscope containing a small graticule target for the measurement of eccentric fixation. The examiner projects a shadow of the target on the patient's retina. The patient is asked to look at the centre of the target. The position of the foveal reflex relative to the centre of the graticule target indicates whether the patient has eccentric fixation and in which direction and by how much. A modified version is the Euthyscope in which the graticule target consists of black spots rather than a star and concentric circles as in the Visuscope. The Euthyscope is used more for eccentric fixation therapy. ⊃ eccentric fixation, pleoptics.

vital necessary to life.

vital capacity (VC) the amount of air expelled from the lungs after a maximal inspiratory effort. ⊃ forced vital capacity.

vital centre specialized nerve cells usually located in the brainstem or the hypothalamus that control vital autonomic functions that include heart rate, respiration, blood pressure, etc. For example, the cardiac centre, respiratory centres and vasomotor centre.

vitality the state of being alive and capable of responding to a stimulus.

vital pulp tooth pulp that reacts positively to a pulp test or shown to have an intact blood supply.

vital pulpotomy the removal of the coronal portion of a vital tooth pulp, followed by the placement of a medicament on the remaining radicular stump, in order to retain the remaining pulp in a healthy and vital condition.

vital pulp therapy the procedures undertaken to preserve all or part of an injured dental pulp in health, such as pulp capping. ⊃ pulp, pulpotomy.

vital signs those signs that indicate life. Usually refers to the measurement of temperature, pulse and respiration. Within the context of basic monitoring of the condition of patients, it is usual to also record blood pressure.

vitallium *n* an alloy used in the manufacture of nails, plates, etc., used in orthopaedic and other surgical procedures.

vitalograph *n* apparatus for measuring the vital capacity. Tests lung function and is able to produce a trace that is very useful for diagnosis and assessment of treatment efficacy.

vitalograph trace a useful diagnostic tool to identify normal lung function and to differentiate between obstructive or restrictive airway disease states.

vital signs monitor apparatus that automatically records and displays physiological measurements such as blood pressure and electrocardiogram (ECG).

vitamin A retinol. A fat-soluble anti-infective substance present in all animal fats. In its provitamin form, β-carotene, it is present in carrots, cabbage, lettuce, tomatoes and other fruits and vegetables: in the body it is converted into retinol.

It is essential for healthy skin and mucous membranes: it aids night vision. Deficiency can result in stunted growth, night blindness and xerophthalmia and is an important cause of blindness in certain parts of the world, e.g. India.

vitamin B any one of a group of water-soluble vitamins— the vitamin B complex, all chemically related and often occurring in the same foods. ⊃ biotin, cobalamins, folate, nicotinic acid, pantothenic acid, pyridoxine, riboflavin, thiamin.

vitamin B_1 thiamin diphosphate or thiamin pyrophosphate. It occurs in wheatgerm, wheat products, yeast extracts, meat and fortified breakfast cereals. Functions as a coenzyme in carbohydrate metabolism. Deficiency results in beri-beri and Wernicke–Korsakoff syndrome. ⊃ Korsakoff's syndrome, Wernicke's encephalopathy.

vitamin B_2 riboflavin. Occurs in most foods, the best sources are milk, milk products, offal and fortified breakfast cereals. It functions as part of the coenzymes flavin mononucleotide (FMN) and flavin adenine dinucleotide (FAD), the electron carrier/transfer molecules involved in the oxidation of fuel molecules in the mitochondria. ⊃ oxidative phosphorylation. Deficiency symptoms are angular stomatitis, cheilosis and anaemia.

vitamin B_3 niacin, nicotinic acid, nicotinamide. Occurs in meat, fish, pulses, wholegrains, fortified breakfast cereals, etc. It functions as part of the coenzymes nicotinamide adenine dinucleotide (NAD) and nicotinamide adenine dinucleotide phosphate (NADP), the electron carriers in the oxidation of fuel molecules and the synthesis of molecules that include fatty acids. Deficiency leads to pellagra.

vitamin B_5 pantothenic acid. It is widespread in foods, e.g. eggs, liver, pulses, cereals, vegetables, etc., and deficiency is rare. It functions in the metabolism of protein, carbohydrate and fat.

vitamin B_6 pyridoxine. Occurs in unprocessed cereal foods, vegetables, meat and eggs. It functions as a coenzyme in protein metabolism. Deficiency symptoms include general weakness, peripheral neuropathy, dermatitis, glossitis and impaired immunity.

vitamin B_{12} cobalamins. Occurs in meat, eggs, milk and cheese. It functions as a coenzyme in protein metabolism. It is essential for the maturation of erythrocytes and nerve function, cannot be synthesized in the body and must be supplied in the diet. Its absorption in the terminal ileum requires the presence of the intrinsic factor secreted by the stomach. Deficiency may develop where absorption is impaired or with a dietary deficiency such as may occur with a vegan diet. Symptoms include megaloblastic anaemia and neurological dysfunction. Vitamin B_{12} is promoted as an ergogenic aid to enhance deoxyribonucleic acid (DNA) synthesis and increase muscle growth in strength training, but research indicates no effect. ⊃ intrinsic factor, pernicious anaemia.

vitamin C ascorbic acid. A water-soluble antioxidant vitamin, which is present in fruits (e.g. citrus, blackcurrants) and vegetables (e.g. potato, green leafy vegetables). It is destroyed by cooking in the presence of air and by plant enzymes released when chopping, cutting or grating food: it is also lost during storage. Deficiency leads to scurvy, sore gums and mouth, poor wound healing, etc. ➲ ascorbic acid.

vitamin D a fat-soluble vitamin needed for the absorption of calcium and the calcification of the skeleton. It occurs in two forms—cholecalciferol (vitamin D_3) formed by the action of ultraviolet radiation on 7-dehydrocholesterol, which occurs naturally in the skin, and ergocalciferol (vitamin D_2, calciferol) formed by the action of ultraviolet radiation on ergosterol, which occurs naturally in plants. Occurs in oily fish, eggs, fortified margarine. Deficiency leads to rickets and osteomalacia.

vitamin E a group of chemically related compounds known as tocopherols and tocotrienols. It is an intracellular fat-soluble antioxidant and maintains the stability of polyunsaturated fatty acids and other fat-like substances. It is thought that deficiency results in muscle degeneration, a haemolytic blood disease, and is associated with the ageing process.

vitamin E deficiency syndrome occurs in small infants, less than 2 kg and under 35 weeks' gestation. Diagnosis at between 6 and 11 weeks reveals low haemoglobin and reticulocytosis; there is good response to vitamin E including a rise in haemoglobin and loss of oedema. The condition is aggravated by giving iron. Deficiency in older children results in cerebellar ataxia and is associated with abetalipoproteinaemia.

vitamin K occurs in three forms—phylloquinone, menaquinones and menadione. Phylloquinone occurs in green vegetables and menaquinones are produced by bacteria in the gastrointestinal tract. It is required for the synthesis of several clotting factors. Deficiency leads to reduced blood clotting.

vitaminoids *npl* compounds that display vitamin-like activity. For example choline, flavonoids, inositol and essential fatty acids.

vitamins *npl* organic substance or group of substances that have specific biochemical functions in the body. They are required in very small quantities and most must be obtained from dietary intake. They are either fat-soluble—vitamins A, D, E and K, or water-soluble—vitamin B complex and vitamin C. They are essential for normal metabolism and are provided by the diet. Some vitamins can also be synthesized in the body, e.g. vitamin D. Their absence causes deficiency diseases. The recommended daily allowance (RDA) for any vitamin, widely quoted on food and drink labels, is less than 200 mg. Originally identified by alleviation of conditions caused by their deficiency (e.g. of scurvy in ships' crews in the 1750s by providing citrus fruit, the vital component being found later to be ascorbic acid, vitamin C). Nowadays hypovitaminosis due to lack of one or more vitamins is rare on a well-balanced diet, although occasionally an athlete may suffer from a deficiency, e.g. if dieting for weight loss or eliminating particular foods or food groups from the diet. Hypervitaminosis can occur with excessive intake of one or more vitamins. The International Olympic Committee (IOC) states that no vitamin supplements should be required if the diet is well balanced but athletes do often take them, especially vitamins C, B-complex and E, with a possible danger to their health by overconsumption. ➲ Appendix 4.

vitellin a protein containing lecithin found in egg yolk.

vitelline artery the vessels which circulate blood through the yolk sac to and from the early embryo.

vitellus the yolk of an ovum.

vitiligo *n* a skin disease of probable autoimmune origin characterized by areas of complete loss of pigment, often on the face and hands.

vitrectomy *n* surgical removal of the vitreous body (humour) from the vitreous chamber.

vitreous *adj* resembling glass.

vitreous body (humour) the clear, jelly-like substance contained by a membrane within the vitreous chamber. It is formed during embryonic life within a closed system and it lasts for life. ➲ Colour Section Figure 15.

vitreous chamber the posterior cavity inside the eyeball and behind the lens; contains the vitreous body (humour).

vitreous detachment detachment from the posterior retina can occur as the vitreous body (humour) liquefies during normal ageing. It is also associated with diabetes mellitus. Vitreous detachment can cause tears in the retina and possible retinal detachment.

vitritis inflammation within the vitreous body (humour).

VKC *abbr* vernal keratoconjunctivitis.

VLBW *abbr* very low birth weight.

VLDL *abbr* very low density lipoprotein.

VMA *abbr* vanillylmandelic acid.

VMC *abbr* vasomotor centre.

V_{max} the maximum velocity of an enzyme-catalysed reaction in which the substrate concentration is not limiting.

VMO *abbr* vastus medialis obliquus.

$\dot{V}O_2$ symbol for oxygen consumption/uptake.

$\dot{V}O_{2max}$ symbol for maximum oxygen consumption/uptake.

vocal cords ➲ vocal folds (cords).

vocal folds (cords) the vocal folds (true vocal cords) are two membranous folds stretched anteroposteriorly across the larynx. The ventricular folds (or false vocal cords) are situated lateral to the vocal folds. Sound is produced by vibration of the vocal folds as air from the lungs passes between them. Their length varies, which is why men, with longer vocal cords, have deeper voices than women. An opening (the glottis) between the true vocal cords allows air movement through the larynx.

vocal resonance is the reverberating note heard through the stethoscope when the patient is asked to say 'one, one, one' or '99'.

vocational assessment the objective evaluation of a person's ability to perform a specific job consistently and competently. This may include the identification of the need for training or the provision of compensatory techniques.

vocational rehabilitation the process of helping someone to overcome barriers to employment and to find or return to work after an episode of illness or trauma.

U
V

Vogt's line ⊃ Vogt's striae.

Vogt's sign the loss of the normal shagreen of the front surface of the crystalline lens indicating anterior capsular cataract.

Vogt's striae (*syn* Vogt's line) thin vertical streaks located in the posterior corneal stroma. These folds disappear with external pressure on the globe. They are often present in patients with keratoconus. ⊃ keratoconus.

voice activated domestic appliance system (VADAS) a microprocessor and voice input system that allows people with severe physical impairments to control their environment and live as independently as possible.

volar *adj* relating to the palm of the hand or the sole of the foot.

volatile *adj* evaporating rapidly.

volatile anaesthetic agent drug in the form of a liquid which when vaporized induces general anaesthesia.

volition *n* the will to act—**volitional** *adj*. ⊃ conation.

volition (occupational therapy) the ability to choose to do or continue to do something, together with an awareness that the performance of the activity is voluntary. (Reproduced with permission from the European Network of Occupational Therapy in Higher Education (ENOTHE) Terminology Project, 2008.)

volitional behaviour in the theory of reasoned action, behaviour that a person intentionally enacts and that has no barriers or obstacles that would impede its enactment.

Volkmann's ischaemic contracture (R von Volkmann, German surgeon, 1830–1889) a flexion deformity of the wrist and fingers from fixed contracture of the flexor muscles in the forearm. The cause is ischaemia of the muscles by injury or obstruction to the brachial artery, near the elbow. For example caused by a supracondylar fracture of the humerus.

Volkmann's spoon in dentistry, a spoon-shaped hand instrument used as a curette, usually double ended.

volt (V) *n* the derived Système International d'Unités (SI) unit (International System of Units) for electromotive force (also known as potential difference or electrical potential). It is the potential that exists at a point when 1 joule of work is done in moving coulomb of positive charge from infinity to that point; volt of potential difference exists between two points if 1 joule of work is done moving coulomb of positive charge from one point to the other. ⊃ Appendix 2.

voltage the number of volts in a circuit; in Britain the mains voltage is 240 volts for the domestic supply and 398 volts for a three-phase supply.

volume the amount of space taken up by an object or fluid. Expressed as cubic metres (m^3). The more commonly used litre (L or l) and it subdivisions are not SI units, but accepted for use with them: 1 L = 1 cubic decimetre (1 dm^3) = $10^{-3} m^3$.

volumetric reconstruction the production of a three-dimensional image in computed tomography (CT) scanning.

voluntary *adj* under the control of the will; free and unrestricted, as opposed to reflex or involuntary.

voluntary muscle ⊃ skeletal muscle.

voluntary patient informal patient. A person with a mental health problem who is an in-patient on a voluntary basis, i.e. not detained there under any provision of mental health legislation.

voluntary sector the organizations controlled and run by volunteers, e.g. Samaritans, MIND. Many have charitable status, some receive grants from government, and some employ professionals and other paid staff to facilitate their work.

volvulus *n* torsion of a loop of intestine, so as to occlude the lumen causing intestinal obstruction.

vomer the thin flat bone that extends upwards from the middle of the hard palate to form most of the inferior part of the nasal septum. Superiorly it articulates with the perpendicular plate of the ethmoid bone.

vomit *n* **1.** *v* ejection of the stomach contents through the mouth and sometimes the nose; sickness. **2.** *n* the material vomited, the vomitus.

vomiting *n* reflex expulsion of stomach contents through the mouth, it is often accompanied by feelings of nausea. It may occur effortlessly, be accompanied by abdominal pain, or be projectile, such as with pyloric stenosis. The vomiting reflex is initiated and co-ordinated by two centres in the medulla of the brain—the vomiting (emetic) centre and the chemoreceptor trigger zone (CTZ).

vomiting (emetic) centre a centre in the medulla oblongata that has overall control of vomiting. It responds to various stimuli such as those from the gastrointestinal organs. ⊃ chemical trigger zone.

vomiting of pregnancy ⊃ hyperemesis.

vomitus *n* vomited matter.

von Gierke's disease (E von Gierke, German pathologist 1877–1945) type I glycogen storage disease in which there is a deficiency of glucose-6-phosphatase enzyme. It presents during childhood and is characterized by hypoglycaemia and hepatomegaly.

von Graefe's sign (F von Graefe, German ophthalmologist, 1828–1870) immobility or lagging of the upper eyelid when looking downward; one of the eye signs occurring in Graves' hyperthyroid disease. ⊃ Graves' ophthalmopathy.

von Recklinghausen's disease (*syn* Recklinghausen's disease) (F von Recklinghausen, German pathologist, 1833–1910) describes two conditions: (a) osteitis fibrosa cystica—the result of hyperparathyroidism leading to decalcification of bones and formation of cysts; (b) multiple neurofibromatosis—the tumours can be felt beneath the skin along the course of nerves. There may be pigmented spots (café au lait) on the skin and neurofibroma in the endocrine glands and the gastrointestinal tract. Tumour growth may also occur in any of the structures of the eye or adnexa.

von Willebrand's disease (E von Willebrand, Finnish physician, 1870–1949) an inherited bleeding disease due to deficiencies relating to the von Willebrand factor in plasma. The inheritance is autosomal dominant, affecting both sexes. Essentially a disorder of the primary haemostatic

U
V

mechanism with abnormal platelet–endothelial cell interaction. In rare, severe cases von Willebrand's disease results in a clotting defect resembling haemophilia.

vortex vein (*syn* posterior ciliary vein, vena vorticosa) one of usually four (two superior and two inferior) veins which pierce the sclera obliquely on either side of the superior and inferior recti muscles, some 6 mm behind the equator of the globe. The two superior ones open into the superior ophthalmic vein and the two inferior open into the inferior ophthalmic vein. These veins drain the posterior uveal tract. ⊃ anterior ciliary vein, inferior ophthalmic vein, superior ophthamic vein.

voxel a three-dimensional pixel.

V/Q *abbr* ventilation–perfusion (ratio).

VRE *abbr* vancomycin resistant enterococci.

VRSA *abbr* vancomycin resistant *Staphylococcus aureus*.

VSD *abbr* ventricular septal defect.

VSO *abbr* Voluntary Service Overseas.

V syndrome ⊃ pattern, V.

VT *abbr* **1.** ventilatory threshold. **2.** ventricular tachycardia.

V$_T$ *abbr* tidal volume.

VTE *abbr* venous thromboembolism.

vulcanite rubber to which sulphur has been added and which hardens when heated. Previously used to construct denture bases, now superseded by acrylic resins.

vulcanization the processing of rubber to form vulcanite by the application of heat under steam pressure.

vulva *n* the external genitalia of the female—**vulval** *adj*.

vulval intraepithelial neoplasia (VIN) the staging of cellular changes occuring in the skin of the vulva. It is generally diagnosed in women over 50 years of age, but does occur in younger women. In some women the cell changes may later become more abnormal and a small percentage will become cancerous. Some authorities grade vulval intraepithelial neoplasia (VIN) in three stages: VIN I, II and III where VIN III represents carcinoma-in-situ. One type of VIN is commonly associated with infection by the human papilloma virus (HPV). Treatment depends on the grade of VIN and the degree of risk of it becoming cancerous. It may be treated by laser ablation, surgery (local excision or very rarely vulvectomy) or diathermy. Various clinical trials have involved the use of HPV vaccine, photodynamic therapy and the local application of imiquimod cream. ⊃ pruritus vulvae.

vulval itch ⊃ pruritus vulvae.

vulvectomy *n* excision of the vulva.

vulvitis *n* inflammation of the vulva.

vulv/o- a prefix that means 'vulva', e.g. *vulvovaginitis*.

vulvodynia *n* chronic painful vulval discomfort such as burning, rawness and stinging. Previously regarded by many as a psychogenic condition, vulvodynia is an organic disease that presents with surface changes or as an aberration of sensory function in which surface changes may be absent.

vulvovaginal *adj* pertaining to the vulva and the vagina.

vulvovaginitis *n* inflammation of the vulva and vagina.

vulvovaginoplasty *n* operation for congenital absence of the vagina, or acquired disabling stenosis—**vulvovaginoplastic** *adj*.

VUR *abbr* vesicoureteric reflux.

V-value ⊃ constringence.

VZIG *abbr* varicella-zoster (hyperimmune) immunoglobulin.

VZV *abbr* varicella-zoster virus.

U
V

Waardenburg's syndrome (P Waardenburg, Dutch ophthalmologist, 1886–1979) a syndrome inherited as an autosomal dominant trait. There are facial abnormalities, multicolour irises (heterochromia), a striking white forelock and white eyelashes, and sometimes hearing impairment. **2.** also known as Klein–Waardenburg syndrome. Inherited as an autosomal dominant trait. Problems include cranial and facial abnormalities, cleft palate, short digits, congenital heart defects and glaucoma.

WADA *abbr* World Anti-Doping Agency.

wafer wax thin strip of wax, in which a thin metal foil is sometimes embedded, used to make interocclusal records.

WAGR syndrome **W**ilms' tumour-**a**nhidria-**g**enitourinary abnormalities-learning disability (mental **r**etardation), caused by a deletion affecting chromosome number 11.

waist circumference:height ratio ⊃ Ashwell scale.

waist circumference:hip ratio (WHR) a way of assessing the distribution of fatty tissue; whether it is mainly subcutaneous or intra-abdominal. It is the circumference at the waist divided by that at the hips; an index of body fat distribution, said to be ideally not >0.8 in women and not >0.9 in men, i.e. a low ratio ('pear-shape') is healthier than a high ratio ('apple shape'). Some large-scale studies have found evidence that WHR is a better predictor than body mass index for coronary heart disease. ⊃ Ashwell scale.

Waldenström's macroglobulinaemia (J Waldenström, Swedish physician, 1906–1996) a low-grade lymphoma associated with an IgM paraprotein causing clinical features of hyperviscosity syndrome. It is a rare tumour occurring in older adults and affects a slight excess of males. Patients classically present with features of hyperviscosity such as nosebleeds, bruising, confusion and visual disturbance. However, presentation may be with anaemia, systemic symptoms, splenomegaly or lymphadenopathy. Patients are found on investigation to have an IgM paraprotein associated with a raised plasma viscosity. The bone marrow has a characteristic appearance, with infiltration of lymphoid cells and prominent mast cells. Severe hyperviscosity and anaemia may necessitate plasmapheresis to remove IgM and make blood transfusion possible. Treatment with oral agents such as chlorambucil is effective but rather slow and fludarabine may be more active in this disease. The median survival is 5 years.

Waldeyer's ring (H Waldeyer, German anatomist, 1836–1921) a lymphoid tissue circle surrounding the pharynx; the lingual, palatine and pharyngeal tonsils. ⊃ tonsils.

walking aids walking sticks, crutches, tripods and various types of metal frame that allow people to regain or retain independence for walking.

Wallace's rule of nines ⊃ rule of nines.

wallerian degeneration (A Waller, British physician/physiologist, 1816–1870) degeneration in a nerve fibre that is separated from its nerve cell body.

WAN *acron* **W**ide **A**rea **N**etwork.

WAP *abbr* wireless application protocol.

warm autoimmune haemolysis ⊃ autoimmune haemolytic anaemia.

warm-down period of progressively less intense dynamic activity and stretching, undertaken promptly after a competition or bout of high-intensity training with a view to preventing blood pooling (leg exercise), better clearing of lactate and other waste products and minimizing subsequent stiffness. Also known as cool-down.

warm-up techniques used to increase circulation, and local muscle and core body temperature prior to vigorous exercise. A period of dynamic activity and stretching, initially gentle and loose but increasing in intensity and focus over 5–10 min, which gradually elevates heart rate and oxygen uptake as well as raising the temperature of muscle and other soft tissues. Undertaken shortly before a competition or bout of high-intensity training (which itself may be dynamic or static), with a view to enhancing performance and reducing the likelihood of soft tissue injury or cardiovascular incident. Can be either active or passive and may be specific to the sport or exercise about to be performed. Warm-up exercise may also limit metabolite build up and subsequent acidosis during exercise. Proprioception may also be significantly more sensitive after warm-up.

wart *n* verruca. ⊃ common wart, plane wart, plantar wart, seborrhoeic warts.

Warwick James elevator ⊃ elevator (dental).

washing in film processing is to remove fixer solution and the remaining soluble silver complex salts from the film surface.

Wassermann reaction (A von Wassermann, German bacteriologist, 1866–1925) an early complement fixation test on blood or cerebrospinal fluid for syphilis. Now obsolete.

watch spring scaler ⊃ scaler.

water birth labour care in which the woman chooses to labour and may deliver in water for relaxation and pain relief; midwives should receive adequate training before taking responsibility for this type of care.

water balance the state when the amount of water consumed in food and drink plus that generated by metabolism equals the amount of water excreted. Intake is regulated by behavioural mechanisms, including thirst and salt cravings. While almost a litre of water per 24 hours is unavoidably lost via the skin, lungs and faeces, the kidneys are the site of regulated excretion of water in the urine. In a moderate climatic environment, to achieve water balance a sedentary individual should consume ~2 litres of water daily; in hot dry environments up to 4 litres may be needed. Athletes require additional intake to match the loss due to a high sweating rate, depending in turn on the type and severity of exercise, on the temperature and humidity, and on heat acclimatization. ⊃ hydration status of athletes, sports drinks, thirst.

waterbrash ⊃ pyrosis.

water coolant a water spray directed on to a tooth surface being cut by a highspeed cutting instrument, in order to reduce and prevent pulpal damage caused by friction heat.

water content (contact lens) the water in a contact lens expressed as a percentage of the total mass of the lens in its hydrated state under equilibrium conditions. The US Food and Drug Administration (FDA) has categorized hydrogel contact lenses into four groups according to their water content and their surface reactivity (referred to as ionic if it contains more than 0.2% ionic material, and non-ionic otherwise). Group 1: water content less than 50% and non-ionic. Group 2: water content greater than 50% and non-ionic. Group 3: water content less than 50% and ionic. Group 4: water content greater than 50% and ionic.

Waterhouse–Friderichsen syndrome (R Waterhouse, British physician, 1873–1958; C Friderichsen, Danish paediatrician, 1886–1979) shock with widespread skin haemorrhages occurring in meningitis, especially meningococcal. There is bleeding into the adrenal glands.

Waterlow scale a pressure ulcer risk scale developed in the UK by Judy Waterlow a nurse educator in 1985. It is more comprehensive than earlier risk scales and includes six main criteria: build/weight for height, continence, skin condition (skin type/visual risk areas), mobility, sex, age, nutrition (appetite and weight loss), and a number of special risks: tissue malnutrition, neurological deficit, major surgery/trauma and medication.

water phantom a water tank containing a small ionization chamber; the radiation beam can enter the tank either horizontally or vertically. The signal is displayed on a television monitor and the image is analysed for radiotherapy treatment planning.

water-soluble vitamins those of the B group and vitamin C. ⊃ fat-soluble vitamins.

watt (W) *n* (J Watt, British mechanical engineer, 1736–1819) derived Système International d'Unités (SI) unit (International System of Units) for electrical power, watts equal volts times amps (W = VI). ⊃ Appendix 2.

wavefront a virtual surface emanating from an object or an optical system, perpendicular throughout to a bundle of rays. ⊃ wavefront aberration.

wavefront aberration (*syn* wavefront error) the amount of deviation between an output wavefront emanating from an optical system and a conceptualized ideal (reference) wavefront. The specification of the deviation (or error) is usually fitted with a normalized Zernike expansion. The measurement of this aberration can be done subjectively or objectively (e.g. with an aberrometer based on the Hartmann–Shack principle). The method (called aberrometry) has been applied clinically to measure the aberrations displayed by optical systems, such as the eye, the eye with a correction, contact lenses (in vitro or in situ), intraocular lenses (in vitro or in situ), in corneal refractive surgery, cataract, etc.

wavefront error ⊃ wavefront aberration.

waveguide a series of chambers with small iris diaphragms between them and varying distance apart. The function is to control the velocity of the electron beam that passes through it. ⊃ klystron, magnetron.

wavelength (λ) the distance in the direction of propagation of a periodic wave between two successive points at the same position in the wave (e.g. the distance between two crests). The wavelength in a medium is equal to the wavelength in vacuum divided by the refractive index of the medium. Unless otherwise stated, values of wavelength are generally those in air. The refractive index of standard air (15°C, 101 325 N/m^2) lies between 1.000 27 and 1.000 29 for visible radiations. The reciprocal of the wavelength is called the wave number. The wavelength is longer for red light than for blue light. Wavelength λ is equal to

$$\lambda = \frac{c}{v}$$

where c is the velocity of light and v is the frequency of light. ⊃ electromagnetic spectrum, fluorescence, infrared radiations/rays, light, phase, refractive index, ultraviolet radiation, wave theory.

wave theory (*syn* Huygens' theory) the theory that light is propagated as continuous waves. This theory was quantified by the Maxwell equations. The wave theory of light can satisfactorily account for the observed facts of reflection, refraction, interference, diffraction and polarization. However, the interchange of energy between radiation and matter, absorption and the photoelectric effect are explained by the quantum theory. Both the wave and quantum theories of light were combined by the concept of quantum mechanics, and light is now considered to consist of quanta travelling in a manner that can be described by a wave form. ⊃ light, photon, quantum theory, wavelength.

wax 1. pliable substance obtained from plants and insects or synthetically produced. It has many dental applications. ⊃ baseplate wax, bite wax, bone wax, candelilla wax, carnauba wax, carving wax, casting wax, inlay wax, modelling wax, paraffin wax, sticky wax, wafer wax, wax knife, wax pattern. **2.** a mixture of paraffin wax and mineral oil usually heated to 42–52°C in a purpose-designed container (wax bath). Used to provide superficial tissue heating, especially of hands to relieve chronic pain associated with various arthritic conditions or post fracture. Particular dangers are those associated with heating.

wax bath a purpose-specific container, thermostat controlled and used to heat therapeutic wax clinically. Larger volumes usually require the container is within a surrounding water jacket to ensure even heating.

waxing up the use of wax by the dental technician in making trial dentures.

wax knife metal instrument used to melt, carve and convey molten wax during the construction of dentures. It has a pointed flat blade at one end and a hollowed blade at the other, separated by a wooden or plastic handle.

wax pattern accurate pattern of a crown or inlay preparation made in blue or green inlay wax and used in the lost wax process during the casting of gold and other casting materials.

WBC *abbr* white blood cell (leucocyte). ⊃ blood.

WD *abbr* working distance.

weal *n* a superficial swelling, characteristic of urticaria, nettle-stings, etc.

wear facet the characteristic polished surface of a tooth produced by moving contacts between occluding surfaces.

Weber–Christian disease (F Weber, British physician, 1863–1962; H Christian, American physician, 1876–1951) ⊃ panniculitis.

Weber's test a tuning fork (512 Hz) test for the interpretation of asymmetric deafness. ⊃ Rinne's test.

web server a computer which 'fetches' or stores images or web pages and makes them available over the internet or intranet on request.

Wechsler Intelligence Scales (D Wechsler, American psychologist, 1896–1981) a set of standardized tests for measuring the IQ of children and adults.

wedge 1. to force apart or fix firmly. **2.** a wooden, plastic or metal object, thick at one end and tapered to a point, used to force apart or prevent free movement. In dentistry, a small wedge-shaped piece of wood or plastic made in various sizes and thicknesses. Used to hold a matrix band tightly against the cervical margin of a prepared cavity and also to separate teeth. **3.** in radiotherapy, a wedge-shape piece of metal used to attenuate the beam over part of the field during radiotherapy treatment.

wedge angle for a particular wedge is the angle that the 50% isodose line makes with the central axis of the X-ray beam. The angle defined at a specific depth of tissue in a patient, usually 10 cm.

wedged pair dose distribution when two beams of the same wedge angle are used to produce an ideal dose distribution when used with a hinge angle of (180–200) degrees.

wedge factor the increase in set monitor units required to the same dose at D_{max} with a wedge as without the wedge present for the same field size.

wedges available in a variety of sizes and can be used to help position patients and break up patterns of muscle activity, i.e. a wedge under the knees in supine lying can introduce flexion into an otherwise dominated extensor position. Alternatively, they can also be used to support areas of low tone, i.e. under the head and upper thorax to stop a low-tone shoulder 'dropping backwards'. Wedges are a useful adjunct to treatment.

WeeFIM a paediatric version of the Functional Independence Measure (FIM). ⊃ Functional Independence Measure (FIM).

Wegener's granulomatosis (WG) (F Wegener, German pathologist, 1907–1990) a rare antineutrophil cytoplasmic antibodies (ANCA)-associated vasculitis affecting small vessels. The annual incidence is 5–10 per million. The most common presentation is with upper airway involvement (typically epistaxis, nasal crusting and sinusitis), haemoptysis, mucosal ulceration and deafness due to serous otitis media. Symptoms may have been present for several months and erroneously attributed to infection or allergy. The most common ocular abnormality is proptosis, due to inflammation of the retro-orbital tissue. This may cause diplopia due to entrapment of the extraocular muscles, or loss of vision due to optic nerve compression. Untreated nasal disease ultimately leads to destruction of bone and cartilage. Migratory pulmonary infiltrates and nodules occur in 50% of patients. A minority of patients present with glomerulonephritis. Patients are usually c-ANCA-positive. ⊃ antineutrophil cytoplasmic antibodies-associated vasculitis.

weight the force due to the effect of gravity on the mass of a body or object. Can be calculated by multiplying the mass by the acceleration due to gravity. Correctly, expressed in newtons. Commonly (usually in the public context) but incorrectly referred to in units of mass (e.g. kg).

weight-bearing exercise exercise in which the legs support the body weight.

weight distribution the distribution of body weight is a significant factor influencing postural stability. For instance, a person is more stable on a wide base of support than when standing on tiptoes on one foot. For stability the centre of gravity of a body must fall within the base of support. A common problem for patients with hemiplegia following a stroke is their difficulty in moving the centre of gravity over the hemiplegic foot and hence problems with moving the so called unaffected leg, but this is really due to their weight distribution still being proportionately more over the non-affected side.

weighted capitation the allocation of resource based on the number of people in an area but adjusted for the age profile or the relative economic and social conditions, e.g. areas with a high level of social deprivation would be allocated extra resource.

weight gain during pregnancy during pregnancy normal weight gain is usually about 10–12 kg, approximately 2.5 kg in the first 20 weeks and 0.5 kg per week thereafter. This is accounted for by: fetus at term 3.4 kg, placenta 0.7 kg, amniotic fluid 1 kg, uterus 1 kg, increase in blood volume 1.4 kg, breasts 1 kg plus tissue fluid, fat and protein deposition. Excess weight gain may be due to oedema as in pre-eclampsia, multiple pregnancy or a large fetus. Poor weight gain may indicate intrauterine growth retardation.

weight gain in neonates a neonate loses up to 10% of their birth weight in the first few days of life due to passage of

W
X

meconium. Normally this weight should have regained by 10–14 days after birth; weight gain is then approximately 200 g per week.

weight-lifting sport consisting of lifting maximum possible free weights through a variety of previously stipulated body positions.

weight training strength or resistance training using either free weights or those providing the loads in exercise machines. ⊃ strength training.

Weil–Felix test (E Weil, Austrian bacteriologist, 1879–1922; A Felix, Polish bacteriologist, 1887–1956) a non-specific agglutination reaction used in the diagnosis of rickettsial disease, e.g. typhus.

Weil's disease (A Weil, German physician, 1848–1916) serious bacterial disease caused by infection with spirochaetes of the genus *Leptospira* such as *Leptospira icterohaemorrhagica*. Transmission is via the infected urine of rats and other animals. ⊃ leptospirosis.

welding the joining together of separate metal parts by heat and/or pressure without the use of solder, such as in dentistry. ⊃ spot welding.

welfare state a system whereby government provides minimum, guaranteed services and income. In Britain the welfare state is linked to wide-ranging legislation, which was passed after the Second World War and which includes the National Health Service Act (1948) and the National Assistance Act (1948). The origins of the welfare state can, however, be traced back much further.

Welland's test ⊃ bar reading test.

well counter a scintillation counter containing a sodium iodide crystal with a depression cut out of it, a bottle containing the sample is placed in the depression and the gamma emission from the sample is measured.

wen *n* ⊃ sebaceous cyst.

Wenckebach heart block/phenomenon (K Wenckebach, Dutch/Austrian physician, 1864–1940). ⊃ Mobitz I heart block.

Werdnig–Hoffmann disease (G Werdnig, Austrian neurologist, 1844–1919; J Hoffman, German neurologist, 1857–1919) a type of spinal muscular atrophy inherited as an autosomal recessive trait. Death occurs from respiratory complications/failure during early childhood.

Wermer's syndrome (P Wermer, American physician, 1898–1975) a type of multiple endocrine neoplasia (MEN) in which the inheritance is usually autosomal dominant. It is charaterized by the presence of a pituitary adenoma causing excessive anterior lobe hormone secretion, which in turn causes over stimulation of the thyroid and adrenal glands, parathyroid tumours or hyperplasia leading to overactivity, and tumours of the pancreatic islet cells insulinomas and gastrinomas. ⊃ Sipple's syndrome, Zollinger–Ellison syndrome.

Wernicke's area (K Wernicke, Polish/German neurologist, 1848–1905) a sensory speech area located in the temporal lobe of the brain. In right-handed people it is dominant in the left cerebral hemisphere and vice versa.

Wernicke's encephalopathy (K Wernicke) a level of impaired consciousness and thinking due to thiamin(e) deficiency and which is therefore commonly seen in long term alcohol misuse.

Wertheim's hysterectomy (E Wertheim, Austrian gynaecologist, 1864–1920) a radical and extensive abdominal operation performed for cancer of the cervix, where the uterus, cervix, upper vagina, uterine (fallopian) tubes, ovaries and regional lymph nodes are removed.

Wessley's ring (*syn* immune ring of Wessley) a disc-shaped greyish opacity made up of inflammatory cells consisting of antigen-antibody complexes located in the corneal stroma. It is seen in stromal interstitial keratitis resulting from a herpes simplex virus or disciform keratitis. The ring may attract neovascularization. ⊃ disciform keratitis, interstitial keratitis.

Western blot also known as immunoblotting, a process of identifying antigens in a mixture using specific antibodies. The antigens are separated using an electrophoretic technique, transferred to a sheet of nitrocellulose, and then identified by radio- or enzyme-labelled antibodies.

West Nile fever a zoonosis. It is a sporadic disease caused by West Nile viruses (WNV), arboviruses of the genus *Flavivirus*. It is found in wild birds and transmitted to humans from a bite by an infected *Culex* mosquito. There have been reports of infection after a blood transfusion. Originally confined to Israel and the Nile region, it has recently spread, probably via infected birds, to a large area over the eastern seaboard of the USA, the Middle East and to parts of Europe (e.g. Portugal). The infection may be asymptomatic, or after 3–14 days' incubation presents with 'flu-like' symptoms—fever, headache, lymphadenopathy and vague muscle aches and pains, and with relatively mild meningitic or encephalitic symptoms. Rarely there is encephalitis or meningoencephalitis (inflammation of the brain and spinal cord). A small proportion of older or very young sufferers ($<1\%$) present with a severe encephalitic illness with cranial nerve signs, ataxia and extrapyramidal features; these may evolve to the Guillain–Barré syndrome. If there is a history of travel to relevant areas the diagnosis should be sought by IgM serology or demonstration of the virus from cerebrospinal fluid (CSF) samples. Supportive therapy is all that can be offered and the disease carries a significant mortality.

wet nurse a woman who breastfeeds infants who are not her own.

wetting agent 1. in radiography, an addition to the film emulsion to reduce the surface tension and allow the easy penetration of chemicals, an addition to developer to reduce the surface tension of the film. **2.** material that reduces the surface tension of a liquid thus aiding its spread over a solid surface.

wetting angle ⊃ contact angle.

wetting solution a solution which (a) transforms a hydrophobic surface into a hydrophilic one; (b) acts as a lubricant; (c) helps to clean the surface; (d) and helps to prevent contamination of the lens while being inserted. It is spread on both surfaces of a rigid contact lens prior to insertion. However, the effect of a wetting solution only lasts a short time because it is quickly removed by the tear layer. A common wetting agent is polyvinyl alcohol which also has viscosity building properties. ⊃ artificial tears.

WFP *abbr* World Food Programme.

WG *abbr* Wegener's granulomatosis.

Wharton's duct (T Wharton, English anatomist, 1614–1673) the duct of the submandibular salivary gland. It runs from the medial aspect of the submandibular gland to open on the ridge of mucous membrane (the sublingual fold) in the floor of the mouth beneath the tip of the tongue.

Wharton's jelly (T Wharton) embryonic connective tissue contained in the umbilical cord.

wheel a disc or circular frame that revolves around a shaft or axle passing through its centre. In dentistry, an abrasive wheel mounted on a mandrel or chuck and used to reduce or polish materials.

wheezing *n* a high-pitched whistling or rasping breathing sound. Associated with the bronchospasm of asthma and other conditions.

whiplash injury damage to the structures of the neck, particularly the cervical vertebrae, muscles, tendons and ligaments and, most importantly, the spinal cord and nerve roots. Term describes the mechanism of injury rather than a precise diagnosis. Usually caused by the sudden, uncontrolled movement of the neck forwards and backwards, like the crack of a whip. It is particularly associated with road traffic accidents in which there is sudden acceleration or deceleration, such as a vehicle being struck from behind or when a vehicle comes to a sudden stop at speed. In sport, most common in rugby and American football when a player is tackled. ⊃ spinal injury/spinal cord injury.

Whipple's disease (G Whipple, American pathologist, 1878–1976) a rare condition with steatorrhoea, malabsorption, weight loss, anaemia and joint pain. It is characterized by infiltration of small intestinal mucosa by 'foamy' macrophages which stain positive with periodic acid–Schiff (PAS) reagent. The disease is a multisystem one and almost any organ can be affected, sometimes long before gastrointestinal involvement becomes apparent. Electron microscopy reveals small Gram-positive bacilli (*Tropheryma whipplei*) within the macrophages. Villi are widened and flattened; densely packed macrophages occur in the lamina propria. These may obstruct lymphatic drainage, causing fat malabsorption. Middle-aged men are most commonly affected and the presentation depends on the pattern of organ involvement. Low-grade fever is common and most patients have joint symptoms to some degree, often as the first manifestation. Occasionally, neurological manifestations may predominate. Whipple's disease is often fatal if untreated but responds well, at least initially, to co-trimoxazole and to a lesser degree, to tetracycline. Symptoms usually resolve quickly and biopsy changes revert to normal in a few weeks. Long-term follow-up is essential, as relapse occurs in up to one-third of patients.

This often occurs within the central nervous system, in which case 2 weeks of parenteral ceftriaxone, followed by 6–12 months of oral co-trimoxazole, are necessary.

Whipple's operation (A Whipple, American surgeon, 1881–1963) radical operation sometimes performed for cancer of the head of pancreas. It involves: partial pancreatectomy, and excision of the pylorus, duodenum and bile duct with a gastrojejunostomy, choledochojejunostomy and pancreaticojejunostomy (Figure W.1).

Whipple's triad (A Whipple) three essential features of an insulinoma: spontaneous attacks of severe hypoglycaemia; symptoms including sweating and dizziness associated with the hypoglycaemia; and symptoms are reversed by the administration of glucose.

whipworm *n Trichuris trichiura.* ⊃ trichuriasis.

whistle blowing a process whereby somebody employed by an organization makes known the incompetent or unethical practices or behaviour of colleagues. People who 'blow the whistle' are frequently victimized and, therefore, in 1998 the Public Interest and Disclosure Act was passed to provide them with some protection.

white blood cell ⊃ leucocytes.

white body a sample exhibiting diffuse reflection and having a reflectance of approximately 100%. Examples include coating of magnesium oxide, sand-blasted opal glass surface, plaster of Paris. ⊃ coating, diffusion.

white finger ⊃ hand-arm-vibration sydrome (HAVS), Raynaud's phenomenon.

white gold a gold alloy with a high platinum content.

white gold casting alloy ⊃ semiprecious metal casting alloy.

Whitehead's varnish in dentistry, an antiseptic solution occasionally used as a dressing following some surgical procedures. It is manufactured by dissolving iodoform, green benzoin, storax and tolu balsam in ether.

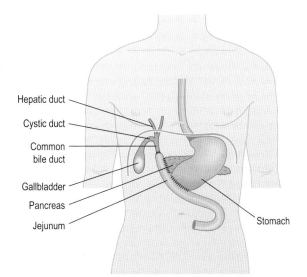

W.1 **Whipple's operation** (reproduced from Brooker & Nicol 2003 with permission)

white leg thrombophlebitis occurring in women after childbirth. ➲ phlegmasia alba dolens.

white light light perceived without any attribute of hue. Any light produced by a source having an equal energy spectrum will appear white after the eye is adapted. Some of the CIE illuminants are often used as a source of white light, e.g. B, C and D. Sunlight is a source of white light. ➲ chromaticity diagram, CIE standard illuminants, equal energy spectrum.

white matter white nerve tissue of the central nervous system, the myelinated fibres. ➲ grey matter.

white muscle a term used to describe muscle consisting mainly of fast-twitch fibres. It is white because there is very little myoglobin and a less abundant blood supply than in red muscle.

white noise sounds of different frequency within a specific band all having equal intensity. Used in noise generators worn to mask the distressing symptoms of tinnitus.

white pupil ➲ leukocoria.

white pupillary reflex ➲ leukocoria.

white spot in dentistry, a white area produced by acid attack from the prolonged presence of bacterial plaque which demineralizes the enamel. An early indication of dental caries.

whiting in dentistry, a finely ground white chalk used with water on a soft lathe brush to promote a high polish.

whitlow *n* acute paronychia or purulent infection of the finger pulp. ➲ paronychia.

WHO *abbr* World Health Organization.

wholefoods unrefined foods, those subjected to the minimum amount of processing. The food has no additions and nothing has been taken out. For example wholemeal flour made by grinding the entire cereal grain.

whole (or mixed) saliva oral fluid. The fluid present in the mouth and consisting of the combined secretions of the salivary glands, gingival fluid, cellular elements and possibly food remnants.

whooping cough ➲ pertussis.

WHR *abbr* waist–hip ratio.

Wickham's striae (L Wickham, French dermatologist/pathologist, 1861–1913) a characteristic fine white network present on the surface of the papules of lichen planus. ➲ lichen planus.

Widal reaction/test (G Widal, French physician, 1862–1929) an agglutination reaction for typhoid fever.

wide area network (WAN) the connection of a group of computer networks.

Wilcoxon test a statistical test used as a non-parametric alternative to Student's paired test.

William's pin a tapered plastic pin placed in prepared pin holes of an inlay or crown preparation and incorporated in a wax pattern. It burns out during the casting process.

Williams' syndrome (J Williams, New Zealand cardiologist, 20th century) rare genetic disorder usually caused by a deletion affecting chromosome number 7. It is characterized by a learning disability, distinctive 'elfin' facial features, short stature, cardiac problems (e.g. aortic stenosis), episodes of hypercalcaemia and an excessively friendly, outgoing personality.

Willis (facial height) gauge an adjustable, flat-handled metal instrument used to measure the distance between two points. May be used to decide whether the interalveolar distance is satisfactory when checking dentures, or to compare the length of incisor teeth. May also be modified to measure the length of orthodontic instruments.

Wilms' tumour (M Wilms, German surgeon, 1867–1918) the commonest abdominal tumour of childhood, and one which usually affects the kidneys. Usually diagnosed during the preschool period. Prognosis is uncertain and depends on the stage of the tumour and child's age at onset of diagnosis and treatment. ➲ nephroblastoma.

Wilson's disease (S Wilson, British neurologist, 1878–1937) rare inherited hepaticolenticular degeneration. Due to disturbance of copper metabolism with copper deposition in various organs, such as the liver and basal nuclei (ganglia). Associated with dementia, tremor, chorea, cirrhosis, hepatic portal hypertension and liver failure. Treatment is with penicillamine, which binds the copper. Relatives with the disease should have prophylactic penicillamine, even if they have no symptoms. ➲ Kayser–Fleischer ring.

Wilson–Mikity syndrome ➲ pulmonary dysmaturity syndrome.

winchester disk a large-capacity *hard* disk, is housed in a hermetically sealed container, as any ingress of dust or dirt, no matter how microscopic, could possibly destroy very large amounts of data.

windchill the heat loss from the body caused by exposure to cool air currents. It is directly related to wind speed.

window 1. the range of grey scale (or colour scale) values displayed in a digital image. **2.** ➲ exit port.

window centre the central point in a range of grey scale (or colour scale) values.

window level the centre of the window width, another term for window centre.

window mean the average range of pixel values in an image.

window width the range of displayed pixel values in a digital image.

windowing ➲ window.

windpipe *n* ➲ trachea.

Wingate test test of anaerobic power production, originating in the Wingate Institute, Israel, in 1974. Consists of flat-out pedalling on a cycle ergometer for 30 s against a resistance chosen to suit the subject's body weight (BW), sex and fitness, and the design of the ergometer, e.g. 7.5% BW for a normally healthy young adult male on the widely used Monark ergometer. Both peak power output and the extent to which output is maintained over the 30 s are usually reported.

winging scapula an abnormality elicited when the extended arm is pushed against resistance. The scapula 'wings' out when there is a weakening of the serratus anterior muscle, usually caused by a long thoracic nerve lesion.

W
X

Winter elevator ➲ elevator (dental).

WinZip® a computer program that is used to compress computer files prior to storage or sending to another computer thus saving on storage space or transmission time.

wire 1. a slender, pliable strand of metal used in surgery and dentistry. **2.** to join together structures by the use of wire. *ligature wire* ➲ ligature. *wire brush* a metal tube holding several strands of brass wire protruding just beyond the tube. Used to clean debris from burs and metal instruments. *wire gauge* a metal plate perforated by holes of a known diameter through which a wire may be threaded to determine its size. ➲ archwire.

wire diaphragms in radiotherapy, an additional set of wires attached to a simulator to accurately display the edges of the treatment area.

wireless application protocol a standard to allow text messages from the web to be available to mobile phones.

wiring in maxillofacial surgery/dentistry, method of immobilizing bony tissues following a fracture or surgery, in order to allow them to reunite without undue disturbance. There are several types named according to their position or the technique used. *archwire* a bent metal bar is wired bucally to the teeth by soft stainless steel wires. *bridle wire* a method of temporarily reducing a fracture in a dentate segment by passing a wire around teeth either side of the fracture line and twisting it clockwise. *cheek wire* (archaic) wires from a head halo are passed through the cheek to a splint or wires fixed to the lower teeth. *circumferential wire* stainless steel wires are passed from the mouth round the lower border of the body of the mandible and back into the mouth, the ends being tied over a splint or denture. *continuous loop wire* technique for the reduction and fixation of fractures by loop wiring the mandibular and maxillary teeth and using intermaxillary elastics. *direct bone wire* (archaic) used to immobilize bone fragments permanently or temporarily to allow open reduction internal fixation (ORIF). Holes are drilled in the bone, the fragments are repositioned and the wires passed through the holes, twisted and secured. *interdental wire* the teeth are held together by passing wires round the necks of the teeth, twisting the ends together and then twisting these ends onto similar wires from the opposing teeth. *perialveolar wire* used in the treatment of edentulous fracture cases. A wire is passed through the maxillary alveolus, buccopalatally.

wisdom tooth lay term for the third molar tooth placed eighth from the midline in the permanent (secondary) dentition. The last teeth to erupt, usually during late teens or early twenties.

Wiskott–Aldrich syndrome (A Wiskott, German paediatrician, 1898–1978; R Aldrich, American paediatrician, b. 1917) an immunodeficiency disorder resulting in increased susceptibility to viral, bacterial and fungal infections. Inheritance is X-linked recessive. Affected individuals have a reduction in platelet numbers (thrombocytopenia), reduced lymphocytes in the blood and reduced cellular immunity. It is associated with eczema and the development of lymphoma.

withdrawal bleeding blood loss from the uterus occurring after the cessation of oestrogen and progesterone preparations, as happens with each course of a combined oral contraceptive.

WNV *abbr* West Nile virus.

WOB *abbr* work of breathing.

wobble board a device used by physiotherapists and others, during rehabilitation in order to improve proprioception and balance (Figure W.2).

Wolfe graft ➲ skin graft.

wolffian body (K Wolff, German anatomist/embryologist, 1733–1794) ➲ mesonephros.

wolffian duct (K Wolff) ➲ mesonephric duct.

Wolff–Parkinson–White (WPW) syndrome (Wolff L, American cardiologist, 1898–1972; J Parkinson, British cardiologist, 1885–1976; P White, American cardiologist, 1886–1973) a cardiac arrhythmia resulting from an abnormal conduction pathway between the atria and ventricles. Usually results in a supraventricular tachycardia. The characteristic ECG pattern has a wide QRS complex with a 'delta wave' and a short PR interval. A recent study of routine ECGs in over 130 000 adults over a wide age range detected the syndrome in about 1 in 1000, with the highest incidence in the 20–40 age group, equally in men and women. Usually asymptomatic but requires further investigation (by echocardiography and exercise testing) if discovered opportunistically or by cardiac screening. ➲ sudden death (in sport).

Wolff's law (J Wolff, German anatomist, 1835–1902) as bones are subjected to stress, they will change their internal architecture accordingly. Put simply, bone is laid down when it is needed and absorbed when it is not. This is of key importance to health professionals, such as physiotherapists and nurses, since a person on prolonged bed rest will quickly start to lose bone mass, conversely a person who takes up jogging or weight lifting will begin to deposit extra bone—bone is alive.

Wolfram syndrome (D Wolfram, American physician, 20th century) also called DIDMOAD syndrome—**d**iabetes **i**nsipidus, **d**iabetes **m**ellitus, **o**ptic **a**trophy and **d**eafness. A rare syndrome inherited as an autosomal recessive trait.

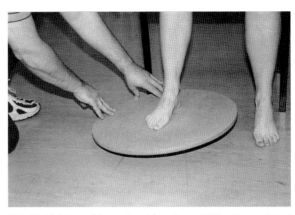

W.2 Wobble board (reproduced from Porter 2005 with permission)

W
X

Wolfring's glands (E Wolfring, Polish opthalmologist, 1832–1906) (*syn* glands of Ciaccio) accessory lacrimal glands of the upper eyelid situated in the region of the upper border of the tarsus. ⊃ Krause's glands, lacrimal gland, precorneal film.

womb *n* the uterus.

wood point a small, hard- or soft-wood stick, of many shapes, used to remove food debris from the inter-dental spaces and the approximal surfaces of the teeth. Some are medicated.

Wood's light (R Wood, American physicist, 1868–1955) special ultraviolet light used for the detection of fungal diseases such as ringworm. The infected hair or skin become fluorescent under the light.

Wood's manoeuvre an invasive rotational or screw manoeuvre to relieve shoulder dystocia. Pressure is exerted on the fetal chest to rotate and abduct the shoulders. ⊃ shoulder dystocia.

woolsorter's disease the pulmonary form of anthrax, haemorrhagic bronchopneumonia. ⊃ anthrax.

wool test (*syn* colour wool test) a test for assessing colour vision deficiencies. It consists of a set of wool strands which are to be matched with loose wool strands of the same colour. The most well known of these is the Holmgren's test.

Woolwich shell a plastic domed appliance with a flat base containing a hole. Used to encourage retraction of flat nipples. The nipple is inserted into the hole and the appliance is worn inside the brassiere.

word blindness ⊃ alexia.

work *n* the magnitude of a force applied to a body or object multiplied by the distance through which it is moved (linearly) in the direction of that force. Also the moment applied to a rotating body or object multiplied by the angular displacement through which it is moved (angularly). If there is no motion of the object there is no mechanical work done on it. A scalar quantity. Measured in joules (J). *external work* work done on an external body or object (e.g. by the human body); *internal work* work by forces inside a body or object (e.g. the human body); *negative work* the usually accepted convention for the situation of an object having work done on it by an external force, e.g. a muscle being extended by an external load during eccentric action. *positive work* the usually accepted convention for work done by an agent on surroundings, e.g. when a net muscle moment acts in the same direction as the direction of motion that it induces in the object.

work–energy theorem states that the change in the energy of a body or object is equal to the work performed.

workload in general usage, the amount of any type of work to be done, or being done, by a person or group. Used often, but inappropriately, in describing the level of various types of exercise and should be avoided since it has no precise definition or specific units, whereas each type may be properly quantified, e.g. as power output in cycling or treadmill exercise, or as force or tension during isometric contraction. The term 'intensity' has been recommended as preferable when referring to the level of activity during any exercise; it does not imply any particular units of measurement and so can be used with respect to the magnitude of force (in N), of power (in W), of speed (in km/h) or to any of these as percentage of maximal.

work (occupational therapy) productive activities that use the individual's skills, contribute to the maintenance or advancement of society and may be a means of generating income.

work of breathing (WOB) the amount of energy required to overcome the opposing forces of breathing (i.e. the elastic and resistive properties of the lung and chest wall). In order to move a given volume of air into the lung, a certain amount of effort is required.

workrate term used in exercise physiology for the power produced by a living body. May be expressed directly in units of power (joules per second [J/s] or watts [W]) or indirectly in terms of oxygen consumed per unit time.

work-related upper limb disorder (WRULD) occurs as a result of prolonged persistent repetitive overuse of the upper limb with maintenance of static postures. It is common in keyboard workers, production workers and telephonists. The soft tissues in the shoulders, arms, wrists and hands are affected, leading to various diagnoses, e.g. tendonitis (tendinitis), tenosynovitis, carpal tunnel syndrome and tennis elbow. It can be prevented by adequate ergonomic-based risk assessment of the workplace.

working distance (WD) 1. the distance at which a person reads or does close work. **2.** in retinoscopy, the distance between the plane of the sighthole and that of the patient's spectacles. **3.** in microscopy, the distance between an object and the front surface of the objective. ⊃ retinoscope.

working impression ⊃ final impression.

working side (ipsilateral side) the side to which a mandible moves during a lateral excursion.

working time in dentistry, the period of time during which a dental material can be manipulated without loss of property. Includes the mixing time, doughing time for acrylics, and the manipulation time. ⊃ doughing time, manipulation time, mixing time.

World Anti-Doping Agency (WADA) the organization that produces a list of banned doping classes and methods. The list, with some modifications, is adopted by the governing bodies of sport. ⊃ banned substance, doping (in sport).

World Food Programme (WFP) international food aid donated by countries with a surplus; organized and implemented by the United Nations.

World Health Organization (WHO) health organization that coordinates health activity and promotes public health world-wide. Established through a 'declaration' during the United Nations Conference on International Organization held in San Francisco in 1945. A number of disparate health organizations were joined together under the aegis of the United Nations with a headquarters in Geneva, Switzerland.

World Health Organization (WHO) International Code of Marketing of Breast Milk Substitutes the World Health Organization and UNICEF code to protect and promote breastfeeding and control marketing of products for artificial feeding, especially in developing countries. The code recommends prohibition of advertising and promotion direct to the public; no free breast milk substitute samples or other free gifts, no special offers and discounts for mothers; no financial or other rewards for health workers to promote breast milk substitutes; professional information on breast milk substitutes should contain only scientific factual data, in no way implying superiority over human breast milk.

World Wide Web (www) an information and resource centre for the internet.

WORM *acron* **W**rite **O**nce **R**ead **M**any.

wormian bone *n* (O Worm, Danish anatomist, 1588–1654) any of the tiny bones located within the sutures (fibrous joints) between the skull bones.

worms *npl* cestode, helminth, nematodes, taenia, trematoda.

Worth's amblyoscope a modified haploscope introduced by Worth consisting of two angled tubes held in front of the eyes which present a different image to each eye, and which can be turned to any degree of convergence or divergence. If the instrument is incorporated into a table, it is called a major amblyoscope of which there are various types called Synoptiscope or Synoptophore. ➲ haploscope.

Worth's classification of binocular vision for the purpose of visual rehabilitation, binocular vision is often classified into three grades: (a) simultaneous binocular vision (or first-degree fusion or superimposition); (b) fusion (or sensory fusion or second-degree fusion or flat fusion); (c) stereopsis (or third-degree fusion). ➲ sensory fusion, superimposition.

Worth's four dot test (*syn* four dot test) a test for determining the presence of binocular vision. It consists of four illuminated discs: two green, one red and one white on a black background. The test is viewed at any distance by a subject wearing red and green filters such that one eye sees the red and the white discs, while the other eye sees the two green discs and the white disc. Subjects are asked to report how many dots they see: four dots indicates normal binocular vision; two dots, both red, indicates suppression of the image in the eye wearing the green filter; three dots, all green, indicates suppression of the image in the eye wearing the red filter; and five dots, two red and three green, indicates diplopia. ➲ FRIEND test, suppression, Worth's classification of binocular vision.

wound *n* most commonly used when referring to injury to the skin or underlying tissues or organs by a blow, cut, missile or stab. It also includes injury to the skin caused by chemicals, cold, friction, heat, pressure and radiation. Wounds may be acute, e.g. surgical incision, or chronic such as venous leg ulcers and pressure ulcers. Surgical wounds are usually classified according to the risk of wound infection, as being: (1) clean—non-traumatic wounds, such as during planned surgery using aseptic technique, which neither involves opening an organ nor has septic focus, e.g. excision of a breast lump; (2) clean contaminated—

non-traumatic wounds, such as planned elective surgery, which involves opening an organ but without significant spillage of its contents, e.g. cholecystectomy, or with only a negligible breach in aseptic technique; (3) contaminated—traumatic wounds that are from a relatively clean source, such as a clean kitchen knife, or significant spillage of contents from an open organ, or when aseptic technique is seriously breached, or when acute non-purulent infection is present, e.g. removal of an inflamed appendix; (4) and dirty—traumatic wounds from a dirty source, such as a puncture wound from a garden fork, or a delay in treating a wound, or when there is acute bacterial contamination or release of pus, e.g. surgery following trauma sustained in a road traffic accident or where an organ, such as the bowel, is perforated and peritonitis is present. ➲ incised wound, laceration, penetrating wound, puncture, tissue viability.

wound drains most commonly used in surgical wounds. They may be inserted as treatment, e.g. to drain pus, or prophylactically, e.g. to prevent haematoma formation. Drains may be attached to a vacuum system or suction apparatus, producing a closed system of wound suction.

wound dressings a variety of proprietary materials applied to surgical or medical wounds, e.g. leg ulcers. Modern dressings should be permeable to water vapour and gases but not to bacteria or liquids, thus retaining serous exudate. They do not adhere to the wound surface and can be removed without damage to new tissue.

wound healing there are four stages/phases in normal wound healing: haemostasis, inflammation, proliferation and maturation, which may take many months. Wound healing may be delayed by local factors, e.g. mechanical stress, inadequate blood supply, or by general factors that include: malnutrition, ageing, drugs such as corticosteroids, etc. ➲ angiogenesis, débridement, epithelialization, granulation, moist wound healing. Wound healing may be by *primary (or first) intention* in a clean wound with the edges in apposition. There is minimal scarring and deformity; *secondary (or second) intention* when the wound edges are not in apposition and there is loss of tissue the gap must be filled by granulation tissue before epithelialization can take place; or by *third intention* when a wound is left open until local factors such as infection have been treated before the wound edges are brought together.

WPW *abbr* Wolff–Parkinson–White syndrome.

wrap around (aliasing, fold-over) an artefact that occurs in magnetic resonance imaging (MRI) due to the image-encoding process. It occurs when the field of view is smaller than the area being imaged.

Wrigley's forceps obstetric forceps used to grip the fetal head. Traction is applied to effect delivery of the fetus when the second stage of labour is delayed. The head needs to be low in the pelvic cavity for a 'lift out'. They are also used during caesarean section or to control the aftercoming head in a medically managed breech delivery.

wrinkle *n* furrow or skin crease, increase in number with ageing.

W
X

wrist *n* the carpus. Formed by eight carpal bones in two rows.

wrist drop paralysis of the extensor muscles of the wrist and hand which are needed to raise the wrist result in the wrist being flexed. It is due to damage to the radial nerve, such as following fractures of the shaft of the humerus (the radial nerve winds around the radial groove on the shaft of the humerus), or compression caused by sleeping with the arm in an abnormal position over the back of a chair. ⊃ radial nerve palsy

wrist joint the condyloid joint between the distal radius and three of the proximal carpals, the scaphoid, lunate and triquetral. A disc of white fibrocartilage separates the ulna from the joint cavity and articulates with the carpal bones. It also separates the distal radioulnar joint from the wrist joint. It links the forearm bones to the proximal row of the carpal bones. Thus allowing movement of the hand forward (palmar flexion), backward (dorsiflexion) and side-to-side (adduction and abduction) and combinations of these by the action of muscles (flexor carpi radialis, extensor carpi radialis [longus and brevis], flexor carpi ulnaris, extensor carpi ulnaris) that have their origins in the forearm and around the elbow, and tendons that span the wrist to be inserted beyond it. Extracapsular structures consist of medial and lateral ligaments and anterior and posterior radiocarpal ligaments. ⊃ carpus, Colour Section Figure 2.

wrist injury is most common in sports where a strong grip is required, especially with twisting, such as gymnastics, golf and tennis, or in throwing sports (causing soft tissue injuries), contact sports or where falls are likely such as boxing or horse riding (causing fractures).

Write **O**nce **R**ead **M**any **(WORM)** optical disks which are used once to receive data for archiving and can subsequently be read as often as is required.

write protect a method of protecting a computer file or disk to prevent the contents being altered or deleted.

wrought metal that has been shaped and worked on.

WRULD *abbr* work-related upper limb disorder.

wryneck *n* ⊃ torticollis.

Wuchereria *n* (O Wucherer, German physician, 1820–1873) a genus of parasitic filarial worms, such as *Wuchereria bancrofti* that causes elephantiasis. They are found in subtropical and tropical regions that are warm and humid. ⊃ elephantiasis, *Filaria,* filariasis.

www *abbr* **W**orld **W**ide **W**eb.

W
X

xanthaemia ⊃ carotenaemia, carotinaemia.

xanthelasma *n* a variety of xanthomas. *xanthelasma palpebrarum* a cutaneous deposition of lipid material which appears in the skin of the eyelids, most commonly near the inner canthi. It appears as a yellowish, slightly elevated area. It is a benign and chronic condition that occurs primarily in older people. It may be associated with an abnormal blood lipid profile, leading to heart disease or diabetes. ⊃ corneal arcus, Hollenhorst's plaque.

xanthine *n* an intermediate product formed during the breakdown of nucleic acids to uric acid. It is excreted in the urine.

xanthinuria *n* **1.** the excretion of excessive amounts of xanthine in the urine. **2.** a rare inherited disorder of purine metabolism in which the enzyme xanthine oxidase is lacking, resulting in excessive urinary xanthine and hypoxanthine instead of uric acid. It is inherited as an autosomal recessive trait and may cause the formation of renal calculi.

xanth/o- a prefix that means 'yellow', e.g. *xanthelasma.*

xanthochromia yellow discoloration of the cerebrospinal fluid due to the presence of breakdown products of haemoglobin, such as after subarachnoid haemorrhage.

xanthogranuloma a tumour of granulation tissue.

xanthogranulomatous pyelonephritis a granulomatous reaction within the kidney usually secondary to chronic infection and stone disease.

xanthoma *n* nodules showing a yellow discoloration—**xanthomata** *pl.*

xanthomatosis yellow discoloration present in many tissues, such as that occurring in various inherited disorders of fat metabolism.

xanthophylls yellow-orange derivatives of carotene.

xanthopsia 'yellow vision'. A disorder of colour vision in which all objects are seen as yellow.

X chromosome sex chromosome that is paired in genetic females. Present in every oocyte and in half of spermatozoa. It is larger than the Y chromosome and carries many major genes. ⊃ sex-linked, Y chromosome.

XCP *abbr* extension-cone paralleling technique.

XDR-TB *abbr* extensively drug-resistant tuberculosis.

xenobiotic *adj* relating to substances, such as drugs, that are foreign to the body.

xenogenesis the changing of genes as they are passed down several generations to produce different traits.

xenograft (*syn* heterograft) a graft between individuals of two different species.

xenon (Xe) *n* a rare inert gas. *xenon*-133 (^{133}Xe) radioactive isotope used in ventilation-perfusion scanning of the lungs.

xenotransplantation ⊃ xenograft.

Xenopsylla *n* a genus of fleas. *Xenopsylla cheopis* is the rat flea that transmits diseases, including bubonic plague.

xer/o- a prefix that means 'dry', e.g. *xerderma.*

xeroderma, xerodermia *n* dryness of the skin.

xeroderma pigmentosum (*syn* Kaposi's disease) a rare inherited skin condition where there is severe photosensitivity to ultraviolet radiation. It is characterized by the formation of freckles, keratoses, telangiectases and malignant skin tumours. Those affected must avoid exposure to ultraviolet radiation.

xerophthalmia *n* (*syn* xeroma, xerosis of the conjunctiva if the cornea is not involved) extreme dryness of the conjunctiva and cornea due to a failure of the secretory activity of the mucin-secreting goblet cells of the conjunctiva. The conjunctiva and cornea lose their lustre and become skin-like in appearance. The condition may even propagate to the cornea and give rise to keratoconjunctivitis sicca and, if severe, keratomalacia. It can cause ulceration of the cornea which may lead to blindness. Xerophthalmia may be due to trauma, exposure or systematic deficiency of vitamin A, etc. ⊃ Bitot's spots, keratitis sicca, keratomalacia, mucin.

xeroradiography a method of image recording using a re-usable, electrically charged selenium plate which is sprayed with blue powder and the image is transferred to paper; was used for soft tissue imaging, including mammography. Now obsolete.

xeroma ⊃ xerophthalmia.

xerosis *n* dryness. ⊃ xerophthalmia.

xerosis conjunctivae ⊃ xerophthalmia.

xerosis of the conjunctiva ⊃ xerophthalmia.

xerostomia *n* dryness of the mouth due to lack of saliva. May be due to lack of proper function of the salivary glands, blockage of the salivary ducts or the action of certain drugs (e.g. tricyclic antidepressants, diuretics, etc.), or the effects of head and neck radiotherapy. ⊃ artificial saliva.

xiph/i, xiph/o- a prefix that means 'ensiform cartilage of sternum', e.g. *xiphoid process.*

xiphoid process also called ensiform process, xiphoid, xiphisternum. The sword-shaped cartilage at the lower end of the sternum.

X-linked agammaglobulinaemia (XLA) a primary (inherited) immunodeficiency affecting boys. A gene mutation results in absent B cells and hence absent immunoglobulin production.

X-linked hyper-IgM syndrome (XHIM) a primary (inherited) immunodeficiency affecting boys. There is defective antibody production, particularly very high IgM levels, and impaired cellular immunity.

X-linked lymphoproliferative syndrome (XLP) Duncan disease/syndrome. A rare X-linked immunodeficiency disorder. Affected individuals have abnormal immune responses to the Epstein–Barr virus (EBV). There is lymphoproliferation, B-cell lymphomas, severe infectious mononucleosis with hepatitis, or hypogammaglobulinaemia.

XO the anomaly in which cells have a single sex chromosome. All those with XO are female and have Turner's syndrome. Although the karyotype is usually XO with only 45 chromosomes, there may be mosaic forms.

X-ray digitizer a computer linked to an electronic palate in order to allow the input of cephalometric orthodontic points digitally to calculate cephalometric landmarks, angles and measurements.

X-rays *npl* short-wavelength electromagnetic ionizing radiation, which can penetrate the body structures to varying degrees. Produced by electrical equipment. Discovered in 1895 by Wilmhelm Röntgen, a German physicist (the very first X-ray photograph showed the bones of his wife's hand, with her wedding ring). Used in general, and in sport, to produce photographic images of body structures, notably bones (to detect fractures), also heart and lungs. The word is popularly used to mean radiographs, radiography, radiology.

X-ray tracing table an illuminated table used when tracing cephalometric radiographs.

X-ray tube equipment formed by either a stationary or rotating anode and a cathode assembly in an evacuated glass envelope which is contained in an oil-filled, lead-lined housing.

XX sex chromosomes of normal females.

XXY syndrome Klinefelter syndrome.

XY sex chromosomes of normal males.

xylitol bulk sweetener, with the same intensity of sweetness as sucrose (beet or cane sugar). ⊃ sweetener.

xylose *n* a five-carbon sugar (a pentose) present in plant material.

xylose absorption test a test for malabsorption. Xylose is given orally and its urinary excretion is measured. Less than 16% excretion indicates malabsorption.

XYY syndrome males with an extra Y chromosome thus having 47 chromosomes in total. Occasionally there are two extra Y chromosomes (XYYY). The extra Y chromosome may be associated with tallness, learning disability and behavioural problems. However, it does occur in normal men.

W
X

-y a suffix that means 'condition, process, state', e.g. *neuropathy*.

YAG *abbr* yttrium aluminium garnet. A crystal used in certain lasers (YAG-laser).

y-axis ⊃ anteroposterior axis of the eye.

Y axis (of growth) a line joining the sella to the gnathion.

yawning *n* an involuntary action whereby the person takes a deep breath in through an open mouth and exhales slowly. Often occurs with stretching and moving the upper body. It is associated with boredom, tiredness and drowsiness.

yaws *n* a granulomatous disease, mainly involving the skin and bones, which is caused by *Treponema pertenue*, morphologically indistinguishable from the causative organisms of syphilis and pinta. The three infections induce similar serological changes and possibly some degree of cross-immunity. Organisms are transmitted by bodily contact from a patient with infectious yaws through minor abrasions of the skin of another patient, usually a child. The mass World Health Organization (WHO) campaigns between 1950 and 1960 treated over 60 million people and eradicated yaws from many areas, but the disease has persisted patchily throughout the tropics; there was a resurgence in the 1980s and 1990s in West and Central Africa and the South Pacific. A proliferative granuloma containing numerous treponemes develops at the site of the inoculation. This primary lesion is followed by secondary eruptions. In addition, there may be hypertrophic periosteal lesions of many bones, with underlying cortical rarefaction. Lesions of late yaws are characterized by destructive changes which closely resemble the osteitis and gummas of tertiary syphilis and which heal with much scarring and deformity. The incubation period is 3–4 weeks. In early yaws the primary lesion or 'mother yaw' is usually on the leg or buttocks. The secondary eruption usually follows a few weeks or months later, as crops of papillomas covered with a whitish-yellow exudate, especially in the flexures and around the mouth. Sometimes a lesion erupts through the palm or sole, and walking becomes painful ('wet crab yaws'). Phalanges, nasal bones and tibiae swell and become distorted. Most of the lesions of early yaws will eventually subside, even if untreated. In the 'latent yaws' stage, following the spontaneous resolution of 'early yaws', serological changes may persist, to be followed by further manifestations of 'early yaws' or, after an interval of as much as 5–10 years, by the tertiary lesions of 'late yaws'. In late yaws, solitary or multiple lesions appear as nodules or ulcers in the skin, hyperkeratotic lesions of palms or soles ('dry crab yaws') and gummatous lesions of bone. They heal with scarring. Lesions of the facial and palatal bones cause terrible disfigurement (gangosa). The diagnosis of early stage yaws involves the detection of spirochaetes in exudate of lesions by dark ground microscopy. Both latent and early stage is diagnosed by a positive serological test for syphilis. Treatment of all stages is a single intramuscular injection of 1.2 g of long-acting benzylpenicillin. Prevention involves improving hygiene and housing; the disease disappears with improved housing and cleanliness. In few fields of medicine have chemotherapy and improved hygiene achieved such dramatic success as in the control of yaws ⊃ bejel, pinta.

Y chromosome the sex chromosome found singly in the genetic male. Present in half of spermatozoa and none of the oocytes. It is shorter than the X chromosome and has fewer major genes, but carries the genes that stimulate the development of male characteristics.

yeast *n* a general term for fungi from various taxonomic families which are unicellular some of which are opportunistic human pathogens, e.g. *Candida albicans*, *Cryptococcus neoformans*, *Malassezia furfur*. For example, candidiasis or cryptococcosis can be particular problems for immunocompromised individuals.

yellow one of the hues of the visible spectrum evoked by stimulation of the retina by wavelengths situated in a narrow region between about 560 and 590 nm, i.e. between red and green. The complementary colours to yellow are blues. ⊃ complementary colour, light.

yellow card reporting in the UK a system for reporting suspected adverse drug reactions (ADRs), this includes prescription medicines, over-the-counter drugs and herbal remedies. It is administered by the Medicines and Healthcare products Regulatory Agency (MHRA) and the Commission on Human Medicines (CHM). All health professionals (both prescribers and non-prescribers) and patients or their families are encouraged to report ADRs. Online reporting, using an electronic yellow card accessed on the MHRA website, is encouraged, but yellow cards are available from various sources including from the MHRA, regional offices, in the British National Formulary, or as a download from the MHRA.

yellow fever caused by a flavivirus, is normally a zoonosis of monkeys that inhabit tropical rainforests in West and Central Africa and South and Central America, where it may cause devastating epidemics. It is transmitted by mosquitoes living in tree-tops. *Aedes africanus* in Africa and the *Haemagogus* species in America are the vectors. The infection is brought down to humans either by infected mosquitoes when trees are felled, or by monkeys raiding human settlements. In towns

843

yellow fever may be transmitted between humans by *Aedes aegypti*, which breeds efficiently in small collections of water. The distribution of this mosquito is far wider than that of yellow fever and poses a continual risk of spread. It is surprising that there is no yellow fever in Asia; this may be because there are strain differences between the Asian and African *Aedes* mosquitoes or there may be unrecognized demographic obstacles to transmission. The number of cases of yellow fever is estimated to be around 200 000 with 30 000 deaths each year, mainly in sub-Saharan Africa, where it remains a major public health problem. Humans are infectious during the viraemic phase, which starts 3–6 days after the bite of the infected mosquito and lasts for 4–5 days. The incubation period is 3–6 days. In the liver, acute mid-zonal necrosis leads to deposits of hyalin called Councilman bodies, and intranuclear eosinophilic inclusions called Torres bodies. Another characteristic feature is the absence of inflammatory infiltrate. The kidneys show tubular degeneration, which may partly be due to reduced blood flow. Widespread petechial haemorrhages are most marked in the stomach and duodenum. Haemorrhage is due to liver damage and disseminated intravascular coagulation (DIC). Yellow fever is often a mild febrile illness lasting less than 1 week. In severe cases the disease starts suddenly with rigors and high fever. Backache, headache and bone pains are severe. Nausea and vomiting then develop. The face is flushed and the conjunctivae are injected. Bradycardia and leucopenia are characteristic of this phase of the illness, which lasts 3 days and is followed by a period of remission lasting a few hours or days. The fever then returns with acute hepatic and renal failure. There is jaundice and a haemorrhagic diathesis with petechiae, haemorrhages into the mucosa and gastrointestinal bleeding plus oliguria. Patients commonly die in the third stage, often after a period of coma. A diagnosis of yellow fever is made on the following: clinical features in endemic area; virus isolation from the blood in the first 24 hours; a fourfold rise in antibody titre; a post-mortem liver biopsy; differentiation from malaria, typhoid, viral hepatitis, leptospirosis, haemorrhagic fevers, alphatoxin poisoning. Treatment is supportive, with meticulous attention to fluid and electrolyte balance, urine output and blood pressure. Blood transfusions, plasma expanders and peritoneal dialysis may be necessary. Patients should be isolated as their blood and body products may contain viral particles. A single vaccination with the 17D non-pathogenic strain of virus gives full protection against yellow fever for at least 10 years. The vaccine does not produce appreciable side-effects, unless there is allergy to egg protein. Vaccination is not recommended in people who are immunosuppressed, whether this is the result of immunosuppressive therapy or of underlying disease.

yellow spot *n* ⮑ macula lutea.

yellow vision ⮑ xanthopsia.

Yergason's test (R Yergason, American surgeon, 20th century) a test for subluxation of the biceps tendon, at the shoulder. The physiotherapist resists shoulder flexion, elbow flexion and forearm supination. The biceps tendon is palpated to feel for any subluxation.

Yerkes–Dodson law ⮑ inverted-U hypothesis.

Yersinia *n* (A Yersin, French bacteriologist, 1862–1943) a genus of Gram-negative bacilli of the family Enterobacteriaceae. For example, the species *Yersinia pestis*, the cause of plague; and *Yersinia enterocolitica* is a cause of gastroenteritis and mesenteric lymphadenitis.

yin and yang the philosophy of complementary therapies, such as acupuncture and shiatsu. They describe a dynamic, symbiotic relationship between active and passive energy forces believed to be present in the universe (true Qi) and the human body (Qi). Keeping equilibrium between the two aspects is important in maintaining health and well-being.

yips a movement disorder that can affect sports performers, seen particularly in golfers but also in cricketers and darts players, involving uncontrollable movements of the hand or wrist or an inability to release the ball or dart, making effective performance impossible. Its causes are unknown but both neurological deficits due to long-term overuse and psychological factors such as performance anxiety have been implicated.

yoga *n* complementary therapy that utilizes breathing techniques, postures and exercises to relax, reduce stress and generally enhance well-being.

yolk *n* nutrient of the ovum.

yolk sac an early embryonic structure, it provides nutrients until the early placenta takes over, and is a site for very early blood cell formation. The blood formed from yolk sac mesoderm provides the embryo with blood until the liver commences haemopoiesis around week 5. Part of the yolk sac is eventually incorporated into the embryo to form the lining epithelium of the gut tube.

Young–Helmholtz theory (*syn* Helmholtz's theory of colour vision, three-components theory, trichromatic theory) the theory that colour vision is due to a combination of the responses of three independent types of retinal receptors whose maximum sensitivities are situated in the blue, green and red regions of the visible spectrum. This theory has been shown to be correct, except that the pigment in the third receptor has a maximum sensitivity in the yellow and not in the red region of the spectrum. Hering's theory of colour vision, which explains phenomena at a level higher than that of the cone receptors, complements this theory. ⮑ colour vision, Hering's theory of colour vision, visual pigment.

Young's experiment a method of producing interference of light which was shown by Young in 1801. He used two coherent beams of light that were produced by passing light through a very small circular aperture in one screen, then through two small circular apertures very close together in a second screen. On a third screen, behind the second screen, there will be two overlapping sets of waves and, if the original source is emitting monochromatic light, interference fringes will appear on the third screen. ⮑ coherent sources, interference fringes.

Young's modulus of elasticity ⮑ modulus of elasticity.

Young's optometer a simple optometer consisting of a single positive lens and using the Scheiner's disc principle.

The target is either a single point of light or a thread which is moved back and forth until it is seen singly by the observer. When the target is out of focus, it is seen double and slightly blurred. ⊃ Scheiner's experiment.

Young's syndrome a rare condition in which there is obstructive azoospermia, and primary ciliary dyskinesia that leads to rhinosinusitis, recurrent respiratory tract infection and bronchiectasis.

Y-plasty in plastic surgery, the use of a Y-shaped incision to relieve scar tissue or contractures.

yttrium 90 (^{90}Y) a substance emitting beta particles with a half-life of 64 h. Implantations of ^{90}Y in bone wax are left in the pituitary fossa after hypophysectomy for breast cancer. Also used in a number of interstitial cancer treatments.

Y
Z

Z *abbr* **1.** acoustic impedance. **2.** atomic number.

zap a small alteration to a computer program.

Zavanelli manoeuvre an invasive manipulation for shoulder dystocia when all other manoeuvres have been unsuccessful. It is performed by an obstetrican; the fetal head is returned to the vagina, in order to facilitate delivery of a live infant by caesarean section.

zeaxanthin a yellow-red carotenoid pigment; one of the components of macular pigment in the eye. ⊃ age-related macular degeneration, macular pigment.

Zeis' glands (E Zeis, German opthalmologist, 1807–1868) (*syn* ciliary sebaceous glands) the sebaceous glands of the eyelids which are attached directly to the follicles of the eyelashes. Their secretion contributes to the oily layer of the precorneal film. ⊃ blepharitis, hordeolum, precorneal film.

zeitgeber 'time-givers'. The external cues that act as signals to influence the circadian rhythms. They may be natural events that fluctuate, such as the light–dark cycle, or be socially constructed, e.g. work shift times, set meal times, alarm clocks, etc.

Ziehl–Neelsen stain (ZN) (F Ziehl, German bacteriologist, 1857–1926; F Neelsen, German pathologist, 1854–1894) a microbiological staining technique used in the identification of acid-fast bacilli, e.g. *Mycobacterium tuberculosis*.

Zieve's syndrome (L Zieve, American physician, b.1915) a syndrome associated with an excessive intake of alcohol. It is characterized by mild anaemia, high levels of cholesterol and triglyceride in the blood, hepatosplenomegaly and a fatty liver.

ZIFT *abbr* zygote intrafallopian tube transfer.

Zimmer frame a four-point walking aid used in rehabilitation and to enhance independence in people with enduring mobility problems. Whilst assisting independence, the health professional must be careful that the frame is at the right height so as to reduce the flexion influence, which may compound a balance problem. In some cases, wheels may be used to replace the solid struts at the front of the frame in order to encourage a more-fluid pattern of walking. As with all walking aids, the Zimmer frame relies on upper-limb support and this needs to be taken into account when assessing the suitability of the patient.

Z–line the point of insertion of thin filaments of a myofibril. The region between two Z-lines constitutes one sacromere (the smallest contractile unit of skeletal muscle).

zinc (Zn) *n* a metallic element needed by the body in small amounts as a cofactor for certain enzyme reactions (including carbonic anhydrase, alcohol dehydrogenase and alkaline phosphatase), insulin storage, cell multiplication and wound healing. Zinc is present in most foods of vegetable and animal origin but phytates in the diet can reduce absorption. Acute zinc deficiency has been reported in patients receiving prolonged zinc-free parenteral nutrition and causes diarrhoea, apathy, a moist eczematoid dermatitis especially around the mouth, and loss of hair. Zinc deficiency is responsible for the clinical features seen in the very rare congenital disorder known as acrodermatitis enteropathica (growth retardation, hair loss and chronic diarrhoea). In the Middle East chronic deficiency has been described in association with dwarfism and hypogonadism. Zinc deficiency has also been observed secondary to protein-energy malnutrition (PEM), malabsorption syndromes, and chronic alcohol misuse and associated hepatic cirrhosis. In PEM, associated zinc deficiency causes thymic atrophy, and zinc supplements may accelerate the healing of skin lesions, promote general well-being, improve appetite and reduce the morbidity associated with the malnourished state. Also a metal used in alloys such as brass in some dental amalgams and in galvanizing iron. Several of its salts are used in dentistry.

zinc acetate (or diacetate) in dentistry, used in small quantities to accelerate the setting of zinc oxides and eugenol cements.

zinc chloride astringent, antiseptic, styptic, caustic and obtundent. Used as an astringent with gingival retraction cord to control bleeding and temporarily displace the gingival tissues. May be used as a 40–50% solution in water and applied to desensitize a sensitive tooth area. Zinc chloride has been incorporated into toothpaste as a desensitizing agent. Has also been used diluted as a daily mouthwash. Continued use changes the composition of the saliva.

zinc free amalgam alloy absence of zinc minimizes the adverse effects of contamination by moisture and saliva. ⊃ alloy.

zinc oxide a white, amorphous, odourless and tasteless powder with mild astringent properties usually mixed with other medicaments to form creams, powders or pastes. It is a widely used mild astringent, present in calamine lotion and cream and several other dermatological applications. In dentistry, widely used as a solid component in filling materials, impression materials, periodontal packs and in some polishing agents.

zinc oxide/EBA cement ⊃ EBA cement.

zinc oxide-eugenol cement cement formed by mixing zinc oxide and eugenol—the principal constituent of oil of cloves. Modifiers may be added to speed up the setting reaction. Used as an obtundent, antiseptic temporary dressing in a cavity, or as a means of temporarily cementing crowns, bridges and splints into place. May also be used as a root canal filling material in combination with gutta percha.

zinc oxide–eugenol impression paste ⊃ impression material.

zinc phosphate cement (*syn* zinc oxyphosphate cement is deprecated). Hard cement made of a mixture of powder containing deactivated zinc oxide and colouring matter and of a solution of phosphoric acid in water. It should not be used too thin as its acidity may damage the tooth pulp. May be slaked to provide a longer working time.

zinc polycarboxylate cement (*syn* zinc polyacrylate cement). Deactivated zinc oxide powder mixed with a viscous 40% aqueous solution of polyacrylic acid to provide a non-irritant, adhesive cement. It should not be used after the cobweb stage has been reached.

zinc sulphate used as a supplement in zinc deficiency, such as that caused by deficient intake, malabsorption, or loss of zinc (e.g. with extensive burns).

zirconium oxide a finely ground powder used as a polishing agent in dentifrices.

ZN *abbr* Ziehl–Neelsen stain.

Zn symbol for zinc.

ZOF *abbr* zone of optimal functioning.

Zollinger–Ellison syndrome (R Zollinger, American surgeon, 1903–1992; E Ellison, American physician, 1918–1970) gastrin-secreting tumour (gastrinoma) of the pancreatic islets resulting in hypersecretion of gastric acid, fulminating ulceration of the oesophagus, stomach and duodenum and jejunum. Diagnosed by high basal gastric acid secretion and elevated fasting serum gastrin levels. ⊃ multiple endocrine neoplasia, Wermer's syndrome.

zona *n* a zone; a girdle; a term applied to shingles.

zona fasciculata the middle layer of the adrenal cortex, secretes glucocorticoid hormones such as cortisol.

zona glomerulosa outer layer of the adrenal cortex, secretes mineralocorticoid hormones such as aldosterone.

zona orbicularis fibres of the articular capsule of the hip joint that encircle the neck of the femur.

zona pellucida membrane around the oocyte.

zona reticularis inner layer of the adrenal cortex, secretes some glucocorticoids and sex hormones (androgens and oestrogens).

zone *n* a term used in reflexology. The suggestion is that inborn Qi energy flows through different zones (reflexes) that end in the feet or hands.

zone of optimal functioning (ZOF) in sport psychology, a model of optimal performance, proposed in 1980 by Russian psychologist Yuri L Hanin, that hypothesizes a bandwidth of arousal within which an athlete will perform at their optimal level. This bandwidth is held to be different for different individuals with some performing better within higher bandwidths and others within lower bandwidths. In acknowledgement of these individual differences, the model was later renamed the individual zone of optimal functioning model (IZOF). The more recent conceptualization also extends the model to include optimal patterns of positive and negative affect, taking account of particular emotions that might influence different performers differently and the optimal intensity of those emotions.

zonula *n* also called zonule. A small zone, belt or girdle.

zonula ciliaris *n* ⊃ zonule of Zinn.

zonule of Zinn (J Zinn, German anatomist/botanist, 1727–1759) (*syn* suspensory apparatus of the lens, suspensory ligament, zonular fibres) a suspensory ligament attaching the periphery of the lens of the eye to the ciliary body. It comprises a series of fibres passing from the ciliary body to the capsule of the lens at or near its equator, holding the lens in position and enabling the ciliary muscles to act upon it. The lens and zonule form a diaphragm that divides the eye into a small anterior area (the anterior and posterior chambers) which contains aqueous humour, and a larger posterior cavity which contains the vitreous body (humour). The zonule forms a ring that is roughly triangular in a meridional section. It is made up of fibres that are transparent and straight for the most part. The tension of these fibres varies with the state of contraction of the ciliary muscle and thus affects the convexity of the lens. The zonule of Zinn is made up of many noncellular fibres, the fibrils of which consist of a cysteine-rich microfibrillar component of the elastic system, fibrillin. The fibres have been classified as follows: (a) the hyaloid zonule (or orbiculoposterior capsular fibres) which originate from the pars plana of the ciliary body and insert into the capsule just posterior to the equator at the edge of the patellar fossa. (b) the anterior zonule (or orbiculoanterior capsular fibres or anterior zonular sheet), which originate from the pars plana of the ciliary body and insert into the capsule just anterior to the equator. These are the strongest and thickest of the zonular fibres. (c) the posterior zonule (or cilioposterior capsular fibres or posterior zonular sheet), which originate from the pars plicata of the ciliary body and insert into the lens capsule posterior to the equator. These are the most numerous. (d) the equatorial zonule (or cilioequatorial fibres) which originate from the pars plicata of the ciliary body and insert into the lens capsule at the equator. ⊃ canal of Petit, ciliary body, ciliary processes, Hannover's canal, ora serrata.

zonulolysis enzymic breakdown of the zonula ciliaris of the eye. Previously used prior to intracapsular lens extraction.

zo/o- a prefix that means 'animal', e.g. *zoonosis*.

zoonosis *n* disease in humans transmitted from animals, e.g. anthrax, brucellosis, leptospirosis, rabies—**zoonoses** *pl*.

zoophilia 1. an abnormal and excessive liking for animals. **2.** a psychosexual disorder in which an individual derives sexual gratification from close contact with animals (e.g. fondling/stroking), sexual activity with animals or fantasy involving animals.

zoophobia an excessive and irrational fear of animals, such as mice, rats, snakes, dogs, etc.

zoster *n* herpes zoster. ⊃ herpes zoster, shingles.

Z-plasty in plastic surgery, the use of a Z-shaped incision to relieve scar tissue or contractures.

Y
Z

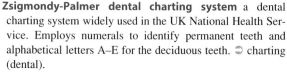

(A) Subcutaneous tissue   (B) Muscle

Z.1 Z-track intramuscular injection technique (reproduced from Downie et al 2003)

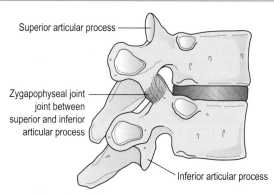

Z.2 Zygapophyseal joint (reproduced from Porter 2005 with permission)

Zsigmondy-Palmer dental charting system a dental charting system widely used in the UK National Health Service. Employs numerals to identify permanent teeth and alphabetical letters A–E for the deciduous teeth. ⊃ charting (dental).

Z-track a technique used during intramuscular injection of substances that can irritate or stain the tissues if tracking and leakage occurs, for example preparations of iron (Figure Z.1).

zwitterions molecules that contain both negatively and positively charged regions, such as amino acids in neutral solutions.

zygapophyseal joint also known as facet joint. The pairs of spinal joints between the superior articular process of the lower vertebra and the inferior articular process of vertebra above (Figure Z.2). These are plane synovial joints and they may be affected by degenerative changes in spondylosis. Their orientation serves to either allow or limit movement of the spine, e.g. in the thoracic spine they permit a great deal of rotation but block rotation in the lumbar spine.

zygoma a synonym for the zygomatic process of the temporal bone. ⊃ zygomatic arch, zygomatic (cheek) bones.

zygomatic arch an arch of bone arising from three bones; the zygomatic process of the temporal bone, the temporal process of the zygomatic bone and the zygomatic process of the maxilla. It passes backwards to rejoin the skull just in front of the external opening to the ear. It serves to protect the eye. The temporal muscle of mastication passes under it for attachment to the coronoid process of the mandible.

zygomatic (cheek) bones also called malar or cheek bones. The two irregular bones of the cheek. They form the prominent part of the cheek and contribute to the orbit. The temporal process of the zygomatic bone articulates with the zygomatic process of the temporal bone and the maxilla to form the zygomatic arch. The masseter muscle of mastication runs from the zygomatic arch to be attached to the outer aspect of the ramus of the mandible.

zygote *n* the fertilized ovum. The diploid cell derived from the fusion after fertilization of the female and male pronuclei, each of which has the haploid, chromosome complement.

zygote intrafallopian tube transfer (ZIFT) a technique used in assisted conception whereby the fertilized conceptus is transferred laparoscopically into the uterine (fallopian) tube.

-zyme a suffix that means 'enzyme, ferment', e.g. *coenzyme*.

zym/o- a prefix that means 'enzyme, ferment', e.g. *zymogen*.

zymogen *n* a proenzyme. An inactive precursor of a proteolytic enzyme, e.g. a clotting factor, or the precursor of proteolytic enzymes produced by the stomach and pancreas, e.g. pepsinogen, trypsinogen. May be activated by another enzyme.

Appendices

Appendix 1

Prefixes and suffixes

Prefixes

Prefix	Meaning	Example
a-	without, not	amenorrhoea
ab-, abs	away from, from, off	abductor
abdo-	abdomen	abdominal
abdomin/o-	abdomen	abdominoplasty
acanth/o-	spiny	acantholysis
acetabul/o-	acetabulum	acetabuloplasty
acro-	extremity	acrocyanosis
ad-	towards	adduction
aden/o-	gland, glandular	adenopathy
aer/o-	air, gas	aerophagia
alb-	white	albino
amb-/ambi-	both, on both sides	ambidexter
amin/o-	containing a NH$_2$ group	amine
amphi/amph-	on both sides, double	amphodiplopia
amyl/o-	starch	amyloid
an-	not, without	anaerobic
andro-	male	androgen
angi/o-	vessel (blood)	angiography
aniso-	unequal	anisocytosis
ant-	against, counteracting	antacid
ante-	before, in front	antemortem
antero-	front	anterograde
anti-	against	anticoagulant
antr/o-	antrum	antroscopy
aorto-	aorta	aortography
ap-/apo	away, derived from	aponeurosis
arachn-	spider	arachnodactyly
arteri/o	artery	arterioplasty
arthr/o-	joint	arthritis
auto-	self	autocrine
bacter/io	bacteria	bacteriology

Prefix	Meaning	Example
bi-	twice, two	biceps
bili-	bile	biliary
bio-	life	biofeedback
blast/o-	immature cell	blastocyst
blenno-	mucus	blennorrhagia.
bleph-	eyelid	blepharoplasty
brachi/o-	arm	brachioradialis
brachy-	short	brachycephaly
brady-	slow	bradypnoea
bronch/i/o-	bronchi	bronchioles
calc/i-	chalk, calcium or heel	calcification
carcin/o-	cancer	carcinoma
cardi/a/o-	heart	cardiogenic
carp/o-	wrist	carpal
cat/a-	down	catabolism
cav-	hollow	cavernous
centi-	hundredth	centigrade
cephal/o-	head	cephalhaematoma
cerebr/i/o-	brain	cerebrovascular
cervic/o-	neck	cervicectomy
cheil/o-	lip	cheiloplasty
cheir/o, chir/o-	hand	chiropractic
chemo-	chemical	chemonucleolysis
chlor/o-	green	chlorolabe
chol/e, chol/o-	bile	cholestasis
cholecyst/o-	gallbladder	cholecystitis
choledoch/o-	common bile duct	choledochostomy
chondr/i, chondr/o-	cartilage	chondrodystrophy
chrom/o, chromat/o-	colour	chromophore
cine-	film, motion	cinematography
circum-	around	circumcorneal

Prefix	Meaning	Example
co-	together	cofactor
col-	together, colon	colitis
coli-	bowel	coliform
colp/o	vagina	colpocentesis
com-	together	combination
con-	together	concomitant
contra-	against	contraindication
costo-	rib	costochondritis
cox-	hip	coxa valga
crani/o-	skull	cranioplasty
cryo-	cold	cryoglobulin
crypt/o-	hidden, concealed	cryptomenorrhoea
cyan/o-	blue	cyanopsia
cyst/i/o-	bladder	cystography
cyt/o-	cell	cytology
dacry/o-	tear	dacryolith
dactyl/o-	finger	dactylitis
de-	away, from, down, off of, reversing	dehydration
deca-	ten	decade
deci-	tenth	decilitre
dent/a, dent/i, dent/o-	tooth	dental
derma, dermat/o, dermo-	skin	dermatome
dextr/o-	to the right	dextral
dia-	through, across, between, apart	diaphragm
di-/dip-	twos, double	dipeptide
dis-	separation, reversal, opposite	disinfection
dors/o, dors/i-	dorsal, back, posterior	dorsum
dys-	difficult, painful, abnormal	dyschezia
ecto-	outside, without, external	ectoderm
electro-	electricity	electrocoagulation
em-	in, into, within	embed
en-	in, into, within	encapsulated
end, endo, ent, ento-	inner, within	endocrine
entero, enter-	intestine	enterocele
ep, epi-	on, above, upon	epicondyle

Prefix	Meaning	Example
erythr/o-	red	erythroblastosis
eu-	well, normal	euhydration
ex, exo-	away from, out, outside, outward, out of	exocytosis
extra, extro-	outside, in addition to, beyond	extrafusal
faci/o-	face	facial
ferro, ferr, ferri-	iron	ferritin
fet/i, fet/o-	fetus	fetoscopy
fibr/o-	fibre, fibrous tissue	fibroadenoma
flav-	yellow	flavonoids
fore-	before, in front of	foregut
galact/a, galact/o-	milk	galactorrhoea
gastr/o-	stomach	gastrectomy
genito-	genitals, reproductive	genitourinary
gero, geronto-	old age	gerodontics
glosso-	tongue	glossodynia
gluco, glyco-	sugar, glucose	glycosuria
gnath/o-	jaw	gnathoplasty
gynae, gyno-	female	gynaecoid
haema, haemat, haemo-	blood	haematemesis
hemi-	half	hemianopsia
hepa-	liver	hepar
hepat/ico, hepato-	liver	hepatic
heter/o-	unlikeness, dissimilarity	heterogametic
hex/a-	six	hexosamine
hist/o-	tissue	histiocytes
hom/eo-	like	homeopathy
homo-	same	homograft
hydro-	water or hydrogen	hydrocele
hygro-	moisture	hygrometer
hyper-	above, excessive	hyperaemia
hypno-	sleep	hypnosis
hypo-	below, deficient	hypocapnia
hyster/o-	uterus	hysterectomy
iatr/o-	physician	iatrogenic
idio-	private, peculiar to the individual	idiosyncrasy

Prefix	Meaning	Example
ileo-	ileum	ileocolitis
ilio-	ilium	iliopectineal
immun/o-	immunity	immunology
in-	not, lack of, in, on, into, within	inappetence
infra-	below	infrapatellar
inter-	between	interarticular
intra-	within	intracellular
intro-	inward	introspection
ischi/o-	ischium	ischiococcygeus
iso-	equal, alike	isograft
jejun/o-	jejunum	jejunectomy
karyo-	nucleus	karyolysis
kerat/o-	horn, skin, cornea	keratomycosis
kin/e, kinesi/o, kin/o-	motion, movement	kinesiology
kypho-	rounded, humped	kypholordosis
lact/o-	milk	lactogenic
lapar/o-	flank, abdomen	laparotomy
laryng/o-	larynx	laryngotracheitis
lepto-	thin, soft	leptophonia
leuco, leuko-	white, white blood cell	leucopenia
lymph/o-	lymph, lymphatic	lymphocele
macro-	large	macroglobulin
mal-	abnormal, poor	malalignment
mamm-	breast	mammaplasty
mast/o-	breast	mastitis
medi-	middle	medial
mega, megalo, mego-	large	megacolon
melano, melan, mel-	pigment, black, dark	melatonin
mening/o, mening/i-	membranes covering brain/spinal cord, the meninges	meningocele
meso-	middle	mesiodens
meta-	change, between, beyond	metacarpus
metro, metra-	uterus	metrostaxis
micro-	small	microcephaly
milli-	a thousandth	millilitre
mio, meio-	smaller, less	meiosis
mono-	one, single	monoamine

Prefix	Meaning	Example
muc/o-	mucus	mucociliary
multi-	many	multigravida
myc, myco, myceto-	fungus	mycotoxins
myelo, myel-	spinal cord, bone marrow	myeloproliferative
my/o-	muscle	myocele
narc/o-	stupor	narcosis
nas/o-	nose	nasogastric
necr/o-	corpse, dead	necrosis
neo-	new	neonate
nephr/o-	kidney	nephron
neur/o-	nerve	neuroblast
noci	pain, injury	nociceptive
noct-	night	nocturnal
normo-	normal	normotension
nucle/o-	nucleus	nucleotoxic
nyct/o, nyctal/o-	night	nyctalopia
occipit/o-	back of the head	occipitobregmatic
oculo-	eye	oculogyric
odont/o, odontia, odontic-	tooth	odontology
oesophag/o-	oesophagus	oesophagitis
olig/o-	few, deficiency, diminution	oligohydramnios
onc/o-	mass, tumour swelling	oncotic
onych/o-	nail	onycholysis
oo-	egg, oocyte, ovum	oocyte
oophor/o-	ovary	oophoropexy
ophthalm/o-	eye	ophthalmoplegia
opisth/o-	backward	opisthotonic
orchi/o, orchido-	testis	orchitis
or/o-	mouth	orogenital
ortho-	straight	orthosis
oss/eo, oss/i	bone	osseous
oste/o-	bone	osteoblast
ot/o-	ear	otoliths
ovari/o-	ovary	ovaritis
ovi, ovo-	egg, oocyte, ovum	oviduct
pachy-	thick	pachyderma
paed-	child	paediatrics

Prefix	Meaning	Example
pan-	all	pancarditis
para-	beside, beyond	paracrine
path/o-	disease	pathogenicity
ped/o-	foot	pedal
pent/a, pent/o-	five	pentosuria
per-	by, through	permeable
peri-	around	perimenopause
perineo-	perineum	perineorrhaphy
pharma, pharmaco	drug	pharmacopoeia
pharyng/o-	pharynx	pharyngotympanic
phleb/o-	vein	phlebotomist
phono-	sound, voice	phonophoresis
phot/o-	light	photoablation
phren/i, phrenic/o, phren/o-	diaphragm, mind	phrenicotomy
physio-	form, nature	physiology
pleur/o-	pleura	pleurodesis
pluri-	many	pluripotent
pneum/o, pneum/a, pneumat/o -	lung	pneumonitis
pod/o-	foot	podalic
polio-	grey (as in grey matter)	polioviruses
poly-	many, much, excessive	polyuria
post-	after, behind	postcoital
pre-	before, in front	pregonal
pro-	before, in front	prodromal
proct/o-	anus	proctitis
prostat/o	prostate gland	prostatectomy
proto-	first	prototype
pseud/o-	false	pseudocyesis
psych/o-	mind	psychopathic
puerper/o-	childbirth	puerperal
pyelo-	pelvis of the kidney	pyelonephritis
py/o-	pus	pyocolpos
pyr/o-	fever	pyrogen
quadr/i-	four	quadriplegia
quint-	five	quintuplets
radic/o, radicul/o-	nerve root	radiculopathy

Prefix	Meaning	Example
radio-	radiation	radioisotope
re-	again, back	reflux
rect/o-	rectum	rectovaginal
ren/i, ren/o-	kidney	renography
retin/o	retina	retinitis
retro-	backward	retrograde
rhin/o-	nose	rhinorrhoea
rhiz/o	nerve root	rhizotomy
rub, rube-	red	rubefacients
sacchar/i, sacchar/o-	sugar	saccharide
sacr/o-	sacrum	sacroanterior
salping/o-	uterine (fallopian) tube	salpingectomy
sapro-	dead, decaying	saprophytic
sarc/o-	flesh	sarcoma
scler/o-	hard	sclerotherapy
scoto-	darkness	scotopic
semi-	half	semiprone
sept/i-	seven	septuagenarian
sept/o-	septum	septal
sero-	serum	seropurulent
socio-	sociology	sociocultural
somatic/o, somat/o	body	somatoform
somn/i	sleep	somnolence
sphygm/o-	pulse	sphygmomanometer
spleno-	spleen	splenocaval
spondyl/o-	vertebra	spondylosis
steat/o-	fat	steatorrhoea
stere/o-	three dimensional, solid	stereognosis
stern/o-	sternum	sternocostal
sub-	below, beneath	subcutaneous
supra, super-	above, excess, superior	suprarenal
sym, syn-	together, union, with	synechia
tabe-	wasting	tabes
tachy-	fast	tachyphasia
tars/o-	foot, edge of eyelid	tarsus
tendin/o, tend/o, teno-	tendon	tenosynovitis
tetra-	four	tetralogy

Prefix	Meaning	Example
therm/o-	heat	thermophiles
thorac/o-	thorax	thoracoscope
thromb/o-	blood clot	thrombogenic
thyr/o, thyroid/o-	thyroid gland	thyroidectomy
tibi/o-	tibia	tibiofibular
tox, toxic/o-	poison	toxin
trache/o-	trachea	tracheal
trans-	across, through	transudation
tri-	three	trigeminal
trich/o-	hair	tricology
troph/o-	nourishment	trophic
tympan/o	eardrum, middle ear	tympanum
ultra-	beyond, excess	ultrafiltration
uni-	one	uniovular
ureter/o-	ureter	ureterolith
urethr/o-	urethra	urethritis
uri, urin/o-	urine	urinalysis
ur/o-	urine, urinary organs	urography
uter/o-	uterus	uteroplacental
vas/o-	vessel, duct	vasopressor
ven/e, ven/i, veno-	vein	venepuncture
ventricul/o	ventricle	ventriculography
vesic/o-	bladder	vesicoureteric
vulv/o	vulva	vulvectomy
xanth/o-	yellow	xanthochromia
xer/o-	dry	xerophthalmia
xiph/i, xiph/o-	ensiform cartilage of sternum	xiphoid process
zo/o-	animal	zoophilia
zym/o-	enzyme, ferment	zymogen

Suffixes

Suffix	Meaning	Example
-able, ible	able to, capable of	transferable
-aemia	blood	anaemia
-aesthesia	sensibility, sense-perception	hyperaesthesia
-al, ale	characterized by, pertaining to	popliteal
-algia	pain	antalgia

Suffix	Meaning	Example
-an, ian	belonging to, pertaining to	amphibian
-ase	catalyst, enzyme	dehydrogenase
-blast	cell (immature)	lymphoblast
-caval	pertaining to venae cavae	portacaval
-cele	tumour, swelling	lymphocele
-centesis	to puncture	thoracentesis
-cide	destructive, killing	insecticide
-clysis	infusion, injection	hypodermoclysis
-coccus	spherical cell	staphylococcus
-cule	little	minuscule
-cyte	cell	monocyte
-derm/a, -dermia, -dermic	skin	pachyderma
-desis	to bind together	pleurodesis
-dynia	pain	proctodynia
-ectasis	dilation, extension	telangiectasis
-ectomy	removal of	orchidectomy
-facient	making	rubefacient
-form	having the form of	fusiform
-fuge	expelling	vermifuge
-genesis	formation, origin	pathogenesis
-genetic	formation, origin	oogenetic
-gen, genic	capable of causing	pathogen
-gogue	increasing flow	cholagogue
-gram	a tracing	electrocardiogram
-graph	instrument for writing or recording	electromyograph
-iasis	condition of, state	myiasis
-iatric	practice of healing	paediatric
-itis	inflammation of	laryngitis
-kinesis, kinetic	motion	hyperkinesis
-lith	calculus, stone	faecalith
-lithiasis	presence of stones	cystolithiasis
-logy	science of, study of	cytology
-lysis	breaking down, separation	hydrolysis
-lytic	disintegration	proteolytic
-malacia	softening	osteomalacia
-megaly	enlargement	splenomegaly
-meter, metry	measure	thermometer
-morph	form	dysmorphic

Suffix	Meaning	Example
-odynia	pain	athrodynia
-ogen	precursor	pepsinogen
-oid	likeness, resemblance	rheumatoid
-ol	alcohol	sterol
-ology	the study of	psychology
-oma	tumour	neuroma
-opia	eye	diplopia
-opsy	looking	cystoscopy
-ose	sugar	glucose
-osis	condition, disease, excess	psychosis
-ostomy	to form an opening or outlet	tracheostomy
-otomy	incision of	osteotomy
-ous	like, having the nature of	insidious
-pathy	disease	nephropathy
-penia	lack of	thrombocytopenia
-pexy	fixation	cryopexy
-phage	ingesting	macrophage
-phagia, phagy	swallowing	dysphagia
-phasia	speech	aphasia
-philia, phily	affinity for, loving	zoophilia
-phobia	fear	photophobia
-phylaxis	protection	chemoprophylaxis
-plasty	reconstructive surgery	arthroplasty
-plegia	paralysis	monoplegia
-pnoea	breathing	dyspnoea
-poiesis	making	thrombopoiesis

Suffix	Meaning	Example
-ptosis	falling	blepharoptosis
-rhythmia	rhythm	dysrhythmia
-rrhage, rrhagia	to burst forth	menorrhagia
-rrhaphy	suturing	herniorrhaphy
-rrhoea	flow, excessive discharge	galactorrhoea
-saccharide	basic carbohydrate molecule	monosaccharide
-scope	instrument for visual examination	cystoscope
-scopy	to examine visually	colposcopy
-somatia, somatic	pertaining to the body	macrosomia
-somy	pertaining to chromosomes	monosomy
-sonic	sound	ultrasonic
-stasis	stagnation, cessation of movement	haemostasis
-sthenia	strength	asthenia
-stomy	to form an opening or outlet	caecostomy
-taxia, taxis, taxy	arrangement, coordination, order	dystaxia
-tome	cutting instrument	dermatome
-tomy	incision of	thoracotomy
-trophy	nourishment	dystrophy
-tropic/tropy	affinity for	neurotropic
-uria	urine	haematuria
-y	condition, process, state	itchy
-zyme	enzyme, ferment	lysozyme

Appendix 2

SI units and the metric system

Acknowledgement

Conversion scales are taken from Goodsell D (1975) Coming to terms with SI metric. *Nursing Mirror* 141: 55–59 and are reproduced by kind permission of the author and *Nursing Mirror*.

Système International (SI) Units

At an international convention in 1960, the General Conference of Weights and Measures agreed to promulgate an International System of Units, frequently described as SI or Système International. This is merely the name for the current version of the metric system, first introduced in France at the end of the 18th century.

In any system of measurement, the magnitude of some physical quantities must be arbitrarily selected and declared to have unit value. These magnitudes form a set of standards and are called *base units*. All other units are *derived units*.

The SI measurement system is used for medical, scientific and technical purposes in most countries and comprises seven base units with several derived units. Each unit has its own symbol and is expressed as a decimal multiple or submultiple of the base unit by use of the appropriate prefix; for example, millimetre is one thousandth of a metre.

Base units

Name of SI Unit	Symbol for SI Unit	Quantity
metre	m	length
kilogram	kg	mass
second	s	time
mole	mol	amount of substance
ampere	A	electric current
kelvin	K	thermodynamic temperature
candela	cd	luminous intensity

Derived units

Derived units are obtained by dividing or multiplying any two or more of the seven base units.

Name of SI unit	Symbol for SI unit	Quantity
joule	J	work, energy, quantity of heat
pascal	Pa	pressure
newton	N	force
watt	W	power
volt	V	electrical potential, potential difference, electromotive force
hertz	Hz	frequency
becquerel	Bq	radioactivity
gray	Gy	adsorbed dose of radiation
sievert	Sv	dose equivalent

Decimal multiples and submultiples

The metric system uses multiples of 10 to express number.

Multiples and submultiples of the base unit are expressed as decimals and the following prefixes are used:

The most widely used prefixes are kilo, milli and micro:

$0.000\ 001\ g = 10^{-6}\ g = 1$ microgram (microgram is used in full for drug prescriptions to avoid dose errors)

Multiples and submultiples of units

Multiplication factor		Prefix	Symbol
1 000 000 000 000	10^{12}	tera	T
1 000 000 000	10^{9}	giga	G
1 000 000	10^{6}	mega	M
1 000	10^{3}	kilo	k
100	10^{2}	hecto	h
10	10^{1}	deca	da
0.1	10^{-1}	deci	d
0.01	10^{-2}	centi	c
0.001	10^{-3}	milli	m
0.000 001	10^{-6}	micro	μ
0.000 000 001	10^{-9}	nano	n
0.000 000 000 001	10^{-12}	pico	p
0.000 000 000 000 001	10^{-15}	femto	f
0.000 000 000 000 000 001	10^{-18}	atto	a

Rules for using units

a. The symbol for a unit is unaltered in the plural and should not be followed by a full stop except at the end of the sentence:

5 cm *not* 5 cm. or 5 cms.

b. The decimal sign between digits is indicated by a full stop positioned near the line. No commas are used to divide large numbers into groups of three, but a half-space (whole space in typing) is left after every third digit. If the numerical value of the number is less than 1 unit, a zero should precede the decimal sign:

0.123 456 *not* .123,456

c. The SI symbol for 'day' (i.e. 24 hours) is 'd', but urine and faecal excretion of substances should preferably be expressed as 'per 24 hours':

g/24 h

d. 'Squared' and 'cubed' are expressed as numerical powers and not by abbreviation:

square centimetre is cm^{2} *not* sq cm.

Commonly used measurements

a. The SI base unit for temperature is the kelvin; however, temperature is expressed as degrees Celsius (°C).

1° Celsius = 1° Centigrade

b. The calorie is replaced by the joule:

1 calorie = 4.2 J

1 kilocalorie (dietetic 'large' Calorie) = 4.2 kilojoules

The energy of food or individual requirements for energy are measured in kilojoules (kJ), but in practice the kilocalorie (kcal) is still in common use.

c. The SI base unit for amount of substance is the mole (mol). The concentration of many substances is expressed in moles per litre (mol/L) or millimoles per litre (mmol/L), which replaces milliequivalents per litre (mEq/L). Some exceptions exist and include: haemoglobin expressed in grams per litre (g/L) or grams per decilitre (g/dL) and plasma proteins expressed in g/L. Enzyme activity is expressed in International Units (IU, U or iu).

d. The SI unit of pressure is the pascal (Pa), and the kilopascal (kPa) replaces millimetres of mercury pressure (mmHg) for blood pressure and blood gases.

1 mmHg = 133.32 Pa

1 kPa = 7.5006 mmHg

However, blood pressure is still widely measured in mmHg pressure and cerebrospinal fluid in millimetres of water (mmH_2O). Central venous pressure may be measured in centimetres of water (cmH_2O) using manual systems with a water manometer, and in either mmHg or cmH_2O using a pressure transducer.

e. Volume is calculated by multiplying length, width and depth. The SI unit for length, the metre (m), is not appropriate, as a cubic metre is not practical for most purposes. The volume of a 10 cm cube; the litre (L), is used instead. The millilitre (mL) is commonly used in clinical practice.

Weights and measures

Linear measure

1 kilometre (km)	= 1000 metres (m)
1 metre (m)	= 100 centimetres (cm) or 1000 millimetres (mm)
1 centimetre (cm)	= 10 millimetres (mm)
1 millimetre (mm)	= 1000 micrometres (µm)
1 micrometre (µm)	= 1000 nanometres (nm)

Conversions

Metric	Imperial
1 metre (m)	= 39.370 inches (in)
1 centimetre (cm)	= 0.3937 inches (in)
30.48 centimetres (cm)	= 1 foot (ft)
2.54 centimetres (cm)	= 1 inch (in)

Volume

1 litre (L)	= 1000 millilitres (mL)
1 millilitre (mL)	= 1000 microlitres (µL)

Conversions

Metric	Imperial
1 litre (L)	= 1.76 pints (pt)
568.25 millilitres (mL)	= 1 pint (pt)
28.4 millilitres (mL)	= 1 fluid ounce (fl oz)

Weight (mass)

1 kilogram (kg)	= 1000 grams (g)
1 gram (g)	= 1000 milligrams (mg)
1 milligram (mg)	= 1000 micrograms (µg)
1 microgram (µg)	= 1000 nanograms (ng)

NB. in order to avoid any confusion with milligram (mg) the word microgram should be written in full on prescriptions.

Conversions

Metric	Imperial
1 kilogram (kg)	= 2.204 pounds (lb)
1 gram (g)	= 0.0353 ounce (oz)
453.59 grams (g)	= 1 pound (lb)
28.34 grams (g)	= 1 ounce (oz)

Temperature

$$°\text{Fahrenheit} = \left(\frac{9}{5} \times x°C\right) + 32$$

$$°\text{Centigrade} = \frac{5}{9} \times (x°F - 32)$$

where x is the temperature to be converted

Conversion scales for certain chemical pathology tests and units of measurement

Chemical pathology blood plasma

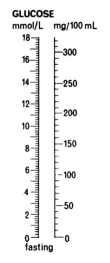

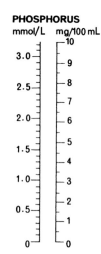

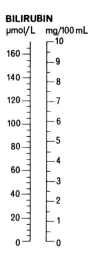

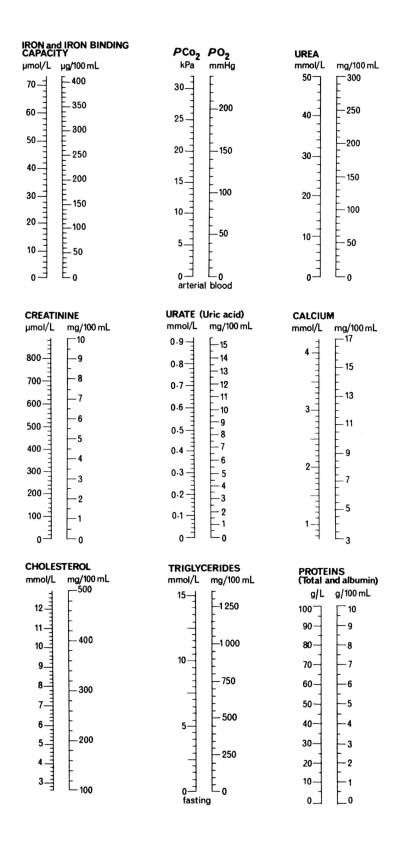

IRON and IRON BINDING CAPACITY

µmol/L	µg/100 mL
70	400
60	350
50	300
40	250
30	200
20	150
10	100
0	50
	0

***P*Co₂** kPa   ***P*o₂** mmHg

arterial blood

UREA

mmol/L	mg/100 mL

CREATININE

µmol/L   mg/100 mL

URATE (Uric acid)

mmol/L   mg/100 mL

CALCIUM

mmol/L   mg/100 mL

CHOLESTEROL

mmol/L   mg/100 mL

TRIGLYCERIDES

mmol/L   mg/100 mL

fasting

PROTEINS
(Total and albumin)

g/L   g/100 mL

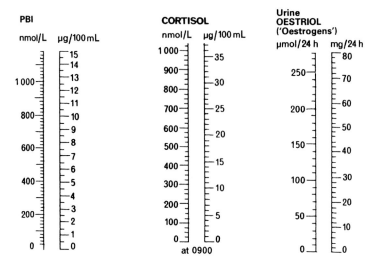

PBI

nmol/L   µg/100 mL

CORTISOL

nmol/L   µg/100 mL

at 0900

Urine OESTRIOL ('Oestrogens')

µmol/24 h   mg/24 h

General measurements

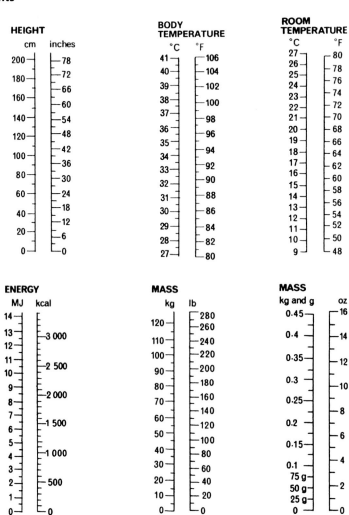

HEIGHT

cm   inches

BODY TEMPERATURE

°C   °F

ROOM TEMPERATURE

°C   °F

ENERGY

MJ   kcal

MASS

kg   lb

MASS

kg and g   oz

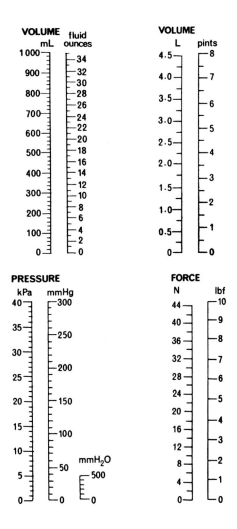

VOLUME
mL — fluid ounces

VOLUME
L — pints

PRESSURE
kPa — mmHg — mmH$_2$O

FORCE
N — lbf

Appendix 3

Normal values

The values below represent an 'average' reference range, in adults, for blood, cerebrospinal fluid, faeces and urine, and should only be used as a guide. Reference ranges vary between laboratories and readers should consult their own laboratory for those used locally.

Blood 861
CSF 862
Faeces 862
Urine 862

Blood—biochemistry (venous serum or plasma unless otherwise stated)

Test	Reference range
Acid phosphatase	0.1–0.6 U/L
Alanine aminotransferase (ALT)	10–40 U/L
Albumin	35–50 g/L
Alkali phosphatase	40–125 U/L
α_1-antitrypsin	1.1–2.1 g/L
Amylase	25–125 U/L
Aspartate aminotransferase (AST)	10–45 U/L
Base excess	−2 to +2
Bicarbonate (arterial blood analysis)	22–28 mmol/L
Bilirubin—total	2–17 µmol/L
Caeruloplasmin	150–600 mg/L
Calcium	2.1–2.6 mmol/L
Chloride	97–106 mmol/L
Cholesterol (total)	Less than 5.0 mmol/L ideal 5.2–6.5 mmol/L mild increase 6.5–7.8 mmol/L moderate increase greater than 7.8 mmol/L severe increase
HDL cholesterol	Greater than 1.0 mmol/L
$PaCO_2$ (arterial blood analysis)	4.6–6.0 kPa
Copper	13–24 µmol/L
C-reactive protein	< 5 mg/L

Test	Reference range
Creatine kinase (total)	
Female	30–135 U/L
Male	55–170 U/L
Creatine kinase MB isoenzyme	< 6% of total creatine kinase
Creatinine	60–120 µmol/L
Ferritin	
Female	7–280 µg/L premenopausal 4–233 µg/L postmenopausal
Male	17–300 µg/L
Gamma-glutamyl transferase (GGT)	5–55 U/L
Glucose (venous blood, fasting)	3.6–5.8 mmol/L
Glycosylated (glycated) haemoglobin (HbA_{1c})	4–6% (from 2011 results will be reported in mmol/mol and percentages)
Hydrogen ion concentration (arterial blood analysis)	35–44 nmol/L
Immunoglobulins	
Ig A	0.8–4 g/L
Ig G	5.5–16 g/L
Ig M	0.4–2.9 g/L
Iron	
Female	10–28 µmol/L
Male	14–32 µmol/L
Iron-binding capacity total (TIBC)	45–80 µmol/L
Lactate (arterial blood)	0.6–1.7 mmol/L
Lactate dehydrogenase (total)	230–460 U/L
Lead	< 1.0 µmol/L
Magnesium	0.75–1.0 mmol/L
Osmolality	275–295 mOsm/kg
Osmolarity	275–295 mOsm/L
Oxygen saturation	More than 97%
PaO_2 (arterial blood analysis)	10.0–13.3 kPa
pH (arterial blood analysis)	7.35–7.45
Phosphate (fasting)	0.8–1.4 mmol/L
Potassium (plasma)	3.3–4.7 mmol/L
Potassium (serum)	3.6–5.0 mmol/L
Protein (total)	60–80 g/L

Test	Reference range
Sodium	135–143 mmol/L
Transferrin	2.0–4.0 g/L
Triglycerides (fasting)	0.5–1.7 mmol/L
Urates	
Female	0.12–0.36 mmol/L
Male	0.12–0.42 mmol/L
Urea	2.5–6.5 mmol/L
Vitamin A	0.5–2.01 µmol/L
Vitamin D	
25-hydroxy	15–100 nmol/L depending on season
1,25-dihydroxy	20–120 nmol/L
Zinc	11–22 µmol/L

Blood—haematology

Activated partial thromboplastin time (APTT)	20–35s
Bleeding time (Ivy)	2–8 min
Erythrocyte sedimentation rate (ESR) (adult)	
Female	0–15 mm/h
Male	0–10 mm/h
NB. Older people may have higher values	
Fibrinogen	1.5–4.0 g/L
Folate (serum)	2.0–13.5 µg/L
Folate (red blood cell)	95–570 µg/L
Haematocrit see PCV	
Haemoglobin	
Female	115–165 g/L (11.5–16.5 g/dL)
Male	130–180 g/L (13–18 g/dL)
Haptoglobins	0.3–2.0 g/L
Mean cell haemoglobin (MCH)	27–32 pg
Mean cell haemoglobin concentration (MCHC)	30–35 g/dL
Mean cell volume (MCV)	78–94 fL
Packed cell volume (PCV) (haematocrit)	
Female	0.37–0.47 (37–47%)
Male	0.40–0.54 (40–54%)
Platelets	150–400 × 10⁹/L
Prothrombin time	11–14s
Red cell count	
Female	3.8–5.3 × 10¹²/L
Male	4.5–6.5 × 10¹²/L
Reticulocytes (adults)	25–85 × 10⁹/L
White blood cells	

Total	4.0–11.0 × 10⁹/L
Differential	
Neutrophils	2.0–7.5 × 10⁹/L
Eosinophils	0.04–0.4 × 10⁹/L
Basophils	0.01–0.10 × 10⁹/L
Lymphocytes	1.5–4.0 × 10⁹/L
Monocytes	0.2–0.8 × 10⁹/L

Cerebrospinal fluid

Pressure (adult)	50–200 mm water
Cells	<5 × 10⁶ all mononuclear
Glucose	2.5–4.0 mmol/L
Protein	150–450 mg/L
IgG index	<0.6

Faeces

Fat content (daily output on normal diet)	less than 7 g/24 h
Fat (as stearic acid)	11–18 mmol/24 h

Urine

Albumin/creatinine ratio (ACR) (used to detect microalbuminuria)	less than 3.5 mg albumin/mmol creatinine
Albumin excretion rate (AER) (used to detect microalbuminuria)	less than 20 µg albumin/min
Calcium (depends on diet)	up to 12 mmol/24 h (normal diet)
Copper	0.2–0.6 µmol/24 h
Cortisol (24 h urine collection)	25–250 nmol/24 h
Creatinine	10–20 mmol/24 h
5-Hydroxyindole-3-acetic acid (5HIAA)	10–60 µmol/24 h
Metadrenaline	0.3–1.7 µmol/24 h
Magnesium	3.3–5.0 mmol/24 h
Normetadrenaline	0.4–3.4 µmol/24 h
Oxalate	0.04–0.49 mmol/24 h
Phosphate	15–50 mmol/24 h
pH	4–8
Potassium (depends on dietary intake)	25–100 mmol/24 h
Protein (total)	<0.3 g/L
Sodium (depends on dietary intake)	100–200 mmol/24 h
Urate	1.2–3.0 mmol/24 h
Urea	170–500 mmol/24 h

Appendix 4

Nutrients

The maintenance of health requires the correct intake of nutrients for the production of energy and the molecules needed for cell growth and repair. These nutrients are the energy-yielding macronutrients—carbohydrate (including non-starch polysaccharide), protein and fat; and the micronutrients—vitamins (water-soluble and fat-soluble) and minerals (including trace elements).

Macronutrients

Nutrient and energy value	RNI (DoH 1991)	Sources	Action/ functions	Deficiency	Excess	Special points
Carbohydrate 1 g yields 16 kJ (3.75 kcal)	A minimum of 47% of total daily energy intake should be provided by carbohydrate this should include no more than 10% as non-milk extrinsic sugars. The RNI for non-starch polysaccharide is 18 g/d	Rice, pasta, noodles, chapatti, bread, breakfast cereals, sugar, yam, plantain and potato	Provides energy for metabolic processes	Weight loss, ketosis	Obesity, hypertrigly-ceridaemia	Diets high in carbohydrate tend to be low in fat
Protein 1 g yields 17 kJ (4 kcal)	Female 45 g/d Male 55 g/d	Meat, fish, eggs, nuts, pulses, dairy products, tofu, and Quorn	A component of all body tissues; energy source in some situations	Retarded growth; weight loss and muscle wasting, poor wound healing; impaired immune system; fat deposition in the liver	Possible link with loss of minerals from bone and age-related deterioration in renal function	Protein content of Western diets usually higher than the RNI
Fat 1 g yields 37 kJ (9 kcal)	Should not exceed 33% of total daily energy intake and of this no more than 10% should be saturated fatty acids	Pastry, cakes, biscuits, chocolate and crisps, cooking oils, ghee, margarine, fried foods, full fat dairy products, meat, oily fish, seeds, nuts	Source of energy, energy storage, absorption of fat-soluble vitamins, synthesis of steroid hormones, integrity of nerve and cell membranes, insulation	Weight loss; deficiency of EFAs can lead to neurological damage	Obesity; increased risk of many conditions including cardiovascular disease and some cancers	The normal development of the nervous system depends on two essential fatty acids—linoleic acid and alpha-linolenic acid

Micronutrients: Vitamins—water-soluble

Vitamin	RNI (DoH 1991)	Sources	Action/ functions	Deficiency	Excess	Special points
Vitamin B group: (i) B_1 Thiamin(e)	0.4 mg/1000 kcal	Fortified breakfast cereals, yeast extract, vegetables, fruit, wholegrain cereals, milk, liver, eggs, pork,	Coenzyme for carbohydrate metabolism	Beri-beri; neuritis; mental confusion; fatigue; poor growth in children. Wernicke–Korsakoff syndrome occurring with alcohol misuse	Headache, insomnia, irritability, contact dermatitis	Requirement related to the amount of carbohydrate intake
(ii) B_2 Riboflavin	Female 1.1 mg/d Male 1.3 mg/d	Milk, milk products, offal, yeast extract, fortified breakfast cereals	Coenzyme for the metabolism of carbohydrate, fat and protein	Fissures at corner of mouth; tongue inflammation; corneal vascularization	Large quantities are not absorbed thus preventing toxicity	Destroyed by sunlight
(iii) B_3 Niacin (nicotinic acid and nicotinamide)	6.6 mg/1000 kcal as nicotinic acid equivalents	Meat, fish, yeast extract, pulses, wholegrains, fortified breakfast cereals	Energy metabolism, as part of coenzymes NAD and NADP involved in oxidation and reduction reactions	Pellagra—dermatitis, diarrhoea and dementia	Liver damage, skin irritation	Also synthesized from the amino acid tryptophan
(iv) B_5 Pantothenic acid	None set	Widespread in food, e.g. liver, eggs, yeast, vegetables, pulses, cereals	Protein, fat, carbohydrate and alcohol metabolism	Vomiting, insomnia	Not reported	
(v) B_6 Pyridoxine	Female 1.2 mg/d Male 1.4 mg/d	Meat, fish, eggs, some vegetables, wholegrains	Amino acid metabolism. Needed for haemoglobin production	Rare; metabolic abnormalities and convulsions	Peripheral nerve damage	Requirement is related to protein intake
(vi) Biotin	None set	Widely distributed in many foods, e.g. offal, egg yolk, legumes, etc. Can be synthesized by intestinal bacteria	Essential in fat metabolism	Rare; dermatitis, hair loss, nausea, fatigue and anorexia. May be seen in patients having long-term total parenteral nutrition and where large quantities of raw egg are eaten	None known	
(vii) B_{12} Cobalamins	15 µg/g of protein	Animal products, meat, eggs, fish, dairy products, yeast extract	Essential for red blood cell formation and nerve myelination. Needed for folate use	Megaloblastic anaemia. Irreversible spinal cord damage	Not reported	Requires the intrinsic factor produced by the stomach for absorption; only found in foods of animal origin; therefore, strict vegetarians and vegans require a dietary supplement

Continued

Micronutrients: Vitamins—water-soluble—Cont'd

Vitamin	RNI (DoH 1991)	Sources	Action/functions	Deficiency	Excess	Special points
(viii) Folates (folic acid)	200 µg/d	Green leaf vegetables, bread, fortified breakfast cereals, yeast extract, liver	Red blood cell production, DNA synthesis	Megaloblastic anaemia; growth retardation	Can mask the megaloblastic anaemia of B_{12} deficiency	Supplement recommended prior to conception and during first 3 months of pregnancy to reduce the incidence of neural tube defects
Vitamin C (ascorbic acid)	40 mg/d	Citrus fruits, kiwi fruit, blackcurrants; green peppers, green leaf vegetables; potato; strawberries; tomatoes. Content decreases with storage	Collagen synthesis, formation of bones, connective tissue, teeth. Iron absorption for red blood cell production. Acts as an antioxidant	Sore mouth and gums; capillary bleeding; scurvy; delayed wound healing, scar breakdown	Diarrhoea; oxalate stones in kidneys	Destroyed by cooking in the presence of air and by plant enzymes released when cutting and grating raw food

Micronutrients: Vitamins—fat-soluble

Vitamin	RNI (DoH 1991)	Sources	Action/functions	Deficiency	Excess	Special points
Vitamin A— retinol	Female 600 µg/d Male 700 µg/d	As retinol in liver, kidney, oily fish, egg yolk, full fat dairy produce. As the provitamin carotenes in green, yellow, orange and red fruit and vegetables, e.g. broccoli, carrots, apricots, mangoes, sweet potatoes and tomatoes	Visual pigments in retina, aids night vision. Normal growth and development of tissues; essential for healthy skin and mucosae. Acts as an antioxidant	Poor growth; rough, dry skin and mucosae; xerophthalmia and eventual blindness; increased risk of infection; poor night vision	High doses are teratogenic	Synthesized in the body from carotenes present in the diet
Vitamin D— cholecalciferol and ergosterol	10 µg/d for the house-bound	Oily fish, egg yolk, butter, fortified margarine; action of ultraviolet rays (sunlight) on the provitamin (7-dehydro-cholesterol) in the skin	Calcium and phosphorus homeostasis	Rickets (children); osteomalacia (adults)	Rare; weight loss and diarrhoea	Produced in the body by action of sunlight on a provitamin in the skin, deficiency develops in those who are not exposed to sun, for example the housebound
Vitamin E— tocopherols and tocotrienes	None set	Wheat germ, vegetable oils, nuts, seeds, egg yolk, cereals, dark green vegetables	An antioxidant. Protects against cell membrane damage	Haemolytic anaemia, can develop in premature infants and malabsorption syndrome	Breast pain, muscle weakness, gastrointestinal disorders	Requirement is increased with increased intake of PUFAs

Micronutrients: Vitamins—fat-soluble—Cont'd

Vitamin	RNI (DoH 1991)	Sources	Action/functions	Deficiency	Excess	Special points
Vitamin K— phylloquinones and menaquinones	None set	Green leafy vegetables, fruit and dairy products	Needed for the production of prothrombin and other coagulation factors	Impaired clotting; liver damage	Not yet observed from naturally occurring vitamin	Synthesized by intestinal bacteria so deficiency unusual; can occur in newborns (haemorrhagic disease of the newborn) and those on anticoagulant therapy

Micronutrients—minerals

Mineral and chemical symbol	RNI (DoH 1991)	Sources	Action/functions	Deficiency	Excess	Special points
Calcium—Ca	700 mg/d	Milk and milk products, green leafy vegetables, soya beans, white bread and hard water	Strengthening the skeleton and teeth; blood coagulation; normal neuromuscular function	Osteomalacia; rickets; tetany. Reduced bone density, osteoporosis	Calcium deposits in soft tissue, hypercalcaemia	Absorption helped by vitamin D and parathyroid hormone
Iodine—I	140 µg/d	Seafood; iodized salt; milk and milk products, meat and eggs	Production of the thyroid hormones: thyroxine and triiodothyronine	Goitre; retarded growth; impaired brain development; congenital abnormalities	Goitre and hyperthyroidism	Some vegetables contain goitrogens that inhibit iodine absorption
Iron—Fe	Female 14.8 mg/d Male 8.7 mg/d	Liver, kidney, red meat, egg yolk, wholegrains, pulses, dark green vegetables, dried fruit, treacle, cocoa, molasses	Component of haemoglobin, myoglobin and many enzymes	Iron deficiency anaemia. Poor growth; impaired intellectual development	Liver damage	Absorption is aided by vitamin C and inhibited by phytates and tannins
Magnesium—Mg	Female 270 mg/d Male 300 mg/d	Cereals, milk, nuts, seeds, and green vegetables	Cofactor for many enzymes essential for carbohydrate and protein metabolism; important role in calcium homeostasis and skeletal development. Neuromuscular function	Unlikely, mainly in cases of chronic malabsorption and chronic renal failure when it will accompany hypocalcaemia	Unlikely from dietary sources	Absorption inhibited by phytate
Potassium—K	3500 mg/d	Fruit, vegetables, meat, wholegrains	Major intracellular electrolyte; influences muscle contraction and nerve excitability. Regulation of acid–base balance	Muscular weakness; depression; confusion; arrhythmias; cardiac arrest	Hyperkalaemia, cardiac arrest	Kidney controls secretion and absorption; deficiency is rare due to poor dietary intake but can occur following prolonged use of diuretics and purgatives

Continued

Micronutrients—minerals—Cont'd

Mineral and chemical symbol	RNI (DoH 1991)	Sources	Action/functions	Deficiency	Excess	Special points
Sodium—Na	1600 mg/d	Table salt, milk, meat, vegetables, sauces, pickles, processed foods and snacks, cheese	Major extracellular electrolyte; important for regulating water balance. Regulation of acid–base balance	Weakness; cramp; faintness	Oedema, hypertension	Lost through fever, sweat and diarrhoea
Zinc—Zn	Female 7.0 mg/d Male 9.5 mg/d	Red meats, eggs, wholegrains	Cofactor needed for many enzymes. Structural role in some proteins; wound healing; functioning of immune system; sexual and physical development	Fatigue; retarded growth and sexual maturity. Acute deficiency may occur during prolonged zinc-free parenteral nutrition; causes diarrhoea, apathy, a moist eczematoid dermatitis especially around the mouth, and loss of hair	Nausea, vomiting, fever, or anaemia with chronic excess	Present in all tissues

Plus other minerals, such as chloride, and trace elements (needed in minute quantities) that include: copper; chromium; fluoride; phosphorus as phosphates; manganese; molybdenum and selenium

Further reading

Geissler C, Powers H 2005 Human Nutrition, 11th edn. Churchill Livingstone, Edinburgh.

Reference

Department of Health (DoH) 1991 Report on Health and Social Subjects 41. Dietary Reference Values for Food Energy and Nutrients for the United Kingdom. London: HMSO.

Appendix 5

Drugs—the law, measurement and drug groups in common use

Drugs and the law

The main Acts governing the use of medicines in the UK are the Medicines Act 1968, the Misuse of Drugs Act 1971, the Medicinal Products: Prescription by Nurses Act 1992 and the Health and Social Care Act 2001.

At the time of writing there are proposals to extend the prescribing of controlled drugs by independent nurse prescribers, and under patient group directions. Readers are advised to check new legislation that may affect practice.

The Medicines Act 1968

Under this Act, medicines are divided into three groups:

- Prescription Only Medicines (POM)—includes most of the potent drugs in common use, from antibiotics to hypnotics. These are drugs that may only be supplied or administered to a patient on the instructions of an appropriate registered practitioner.
- Pharmacy Only Medicines (P)—drugs supplied under the control and supervision of a registered pharmacist without the need for a prescription.
- General Sales List Medicines (GSL)—includes commonly used drugs such as aspirin and paracetamol, available through many retail outlets.

These distinctions of POM, P and GSL medicines do not apply to hospitals where it is accepted practice that medicines are supplied only on prescription.

The Misuse of Drugs Act 1971

This Act imposes controls on those drugs liable to cause dependency and harm when misused, e.g. for recreational purposes. It grades drugs into three classes based on their potential harmfulness:

- Class A—e.g. cocaine, diamorphine, lysergide (LSD), methadone, methylenedioxymethamfetamine (ecstasy), morphine, pethidine and injectable class B drugs. (The 2005 Drugs Act gives the police increased powers to test for class A drugs.)
- Class B—e.g. oral amphetamines, barbiturates, cannabis, cannabis resin, codeine, pentazocine, pholcodine.
- Class C—e.g. androgenic and anabolic steroids, benzfetamine (amphetamine related drug), most benzodiazepines, buprenorphine, chorionic gonadotrophin (human and non-human), diethylpropion, meprobamate, somatropin, zolpidem.

Note. Debate continues in the UK about the desirablity of reclassifying drugs according to the harm they cause in society. For example, downgrading the classification of ecstasy. Readers should be aware that drug classification is subject to continued scrutiny and changes may occur.

The Act categorizes these drugs into five separate schedules according to different levels of control over production, supply, possession, prescribing and record-keeping. The current level of control is defined by the Misuse of Drug Regulations 2001 (see table below). Healthcare practitioners should be familiar with regulations governing Schedule 2 and 3 drugs, which are frequently referred to as 'Controlled Drugs' (CDs); although all five schedules are technically controlled drugs.

Schedule	Examples
1	Drugs that have no medicinal use, e.g. cannabis and hallucinogens such as LSD (lysergide). Possession and supply are only permitted with Home Office authority.
2	Addictive drugs including: amfetamine, cocaine, diamorphine (heroin), morphine, pethidine, secobarbital. Their prescription, safe custody (except secobarbital) must fulfil the full controlled drug requirements, which includes maintaining registers.
3	These include barbiturates (except secobarbital), buprenorphine, phentermine and temazepam. All schedule 3 drugs, except temazepam, are subject to special prescription requirements, but not to safe custody requirements with some exceptions (e.g. buprenorphine). CD registers are not required.
4	These are subject neither to controlled drug prescription rules nor to safe custody requirements. Part I includes benzodiazepines (except temazepam) and zolpidem, in which some controls exist. Part II includes androgenic and anabolic steroids, clenbuterol, chorionic gonadotrophin (hCG), somatropin.
5	These medicines, such as some cough mixtures and kaolin and morphine, contain only small amounts of the CD and so are exempt from most CD regulations except the keeping of invoices for 2 years.

Amendments in 2006 to the Misuse of Drugs Regulations 2001 means that prescriptions involving Controlled Drugs can now be computer-generated, except for the signature. It must include:

- Patient's name and address.
- Dose and dosage form, e.g. tablets, capsules.
- Total quantity to be supplied written in words and figures.
- Prescriber's signature in ink and the date.

In hospital Controlled Drugs must be:

- Stored in a double-locked cupboard attached to the wall and reserved for Controlled Drugs alone, with the key being kept and carried by the Nurse-in-Charge.
- Obtained by a prescription signed by a medical officer. Alternatively, ward stocks of Controlled Drugs in frequent use can be ordered in special Controlled Drugs Order Books. Each order must be signed by the Nurse-in-Charge.
- Recorded in a special book every time a dose is given. The record must state the date, patient's name, time administered and dosage. This record is signed by the nurse giving the drug and another person who has checked the source of the drug as well as the dosage against the prescription.
- Checked regularly to ensure that the contents of the Controlled Drugs cupboard match the record books. Any discrepancies require full investigation, which may involve the police.

As a result of the Shipman Enquiry legislation has been introduced to tighten controls over the management of controlled drugs and to ensure there is an audit trail to monitor their movement from prescriber, through dispenser to patient. For example, people collecting controlled drugs need to provide proof of identity.

Until recently, only registered medical practitioners and dentists could prescribe preparations containing Controlled Drugs, with a special licence being required from the Home Office to prescribe Controlled Drugs for the treatment of addiction. However, the Misuse of Drugs (Amendment) (no. 3) Regulations 2003 allow specialist nurses to prescribe diazepam, lorazepam, midazolam, codeine phosphate, dihydrocodeine, and co-phenotrope for minor ailments and in some specific situations. Furthermore nurses will also be able to prescribe the following drugs under a Patient Group Direction:

- Diamorphine, but only for the treatment of cardiac pain by specialist nurses in accident and emergency and coronary care units in hospitals.
- All drugs listed in Schedule 4 (except anabolic steroids) and Schedule 5 of the 2001 Regulations.

Medicinal Products: Prescription by Nurses Act 1992 and Health and Social Care Act 2001

These two acts contain the primary legislation to allow nurse prescribing and its subsequent extension to 'non-medical prescribing'. Initially nurses and health visitors working in the community who had completed an appropriate educational programme were able to prescribe from a limited formulary. This formulary was expanded in 2002 and nurses in secondary care were enabled to take on a prescribing role. In May

2006 amendments to the legislation enabled nurses, midwives and pharmacists to prescribe, in theory, any drug in the British National Formulary, with the exception of unlicensed drugs and most controlled drugs. These prescribers are referred to as independent prescribers as they take responsibility for the clinical assessment of the patient, establishing a diagnosis and the clinical management required, as well as taking responsibility for prescribing where necessary. However, the Commission on Human Medicines (Formerly Committee on Safety of Medicines and the Medicines Commission) advise that the these Independent Prescribers should **only** prescribe medicines for an identified list of medical conditions (www.bnf.org.uk)

As well as independent prescribers, supplementary or dependent prescribing was introduced in 2003 allowing first level registered nurses, registered midwives and pharmacists, who have undertaken appropriate training, to implement an agreed patient-specific Clinical Management Plan once the patient has been clinically assessed by an independent prescriber (a doctor or dentist). The Clinical Management Plan specifies the range and circumstances within which the supplementary prescriber can vary the dosage, frequency and formulation of the medicines identified and contains relevant warnings about known sensitivities of the patient to particular medicines and includes arrangements for notification of adverse drug reactions. Other healthcare professionals, including optometrists, physiotherapists, podiatrists and radiographers are now also able to become supplementary prescribers.

Although, not considered a form of 'prescribing', Patient Group Directions' allow a variety of health professionals, including nurses, physiotherapists, paramedics and radiographers to supply or administer a named medicine in an identified clinical situation.

Further reading and information sources

British National Formulary and *British National Formulary for Children*—revised twice yearly (March and September) by the British Medical Association and the Royal Pharmaceutical Society of Great Britain. Also available online at www.bnf.org.uk
Department of Heath—www.dh.gov.uk
Medicines and Health Products Regulatory Agency (MHRA) www.mhra.gov.uk
National Prescribing Centre—www.npc.co.uk

Drug measurement

The International System of Units (SI) is used for drug doses and concentrations and for patient data (including weight and body surface area), drug levels in the body and other measurements (see Appendix 2).

Weight

Grams (g) and milligrams (mg) are the units most often encountered in drug dosages. Doses of less than 1 g should be expressed in milligrams, e.g. 250 mg rather than 0.25 g.

Similarly, doses less than 1 mg should be expressed in micrograms, e.g. 200 micrograms, rather than 0.2 mg. Whenever drugs are prescribed in microgram dosages, the units should be written in full, e.g. digoxin 250 micrograms, as the use of the contracted terms μg or mcg may in practice be mistaken for mg and, as this dose is one thousand times greater, disastrous consequences may follow.

Drug dosages are often described in terms of unit dose per kilogram of body weight, i.e. mg/kg, microgram/kg, etc. This method of dosage is frequently used for children and allows dosages to be tailored to the individual patient's size.

Volume

Litres (L rather than 'l' which can be misread as 'one') and millilitres (mL) account for almost all measurements expressed in unit volume for the prescription and administration of drugs.

Concentration

When expressing concentration of dosages of a medicine in liquid form, several methods are available:

- Unit weight per unit volume—describes the unit of weight of a drug contained in unit volume, e.g. 1 mg in 1 mL, 40 mg in 2 mL. For examples pethidine injection 100 mg in 2 mL; chloral hydrate mixture 500 mg in 5 mL.
- Percentage (weight in volume)—describes the weight of a drug expressed in grams (g) which is contained in 100 mL of solution, e.g. calcium gluconate injection 10% which contains 10 g in each 100 mL of solution, or 1 g in each 10 mL, or 100 mg (0.1 g) in each 1 mL.
- Percentage (weight in weight)—describes the weight of a drug expressed in grams (g) which is contained in 100 g of a solid or semi-solid medicament, such as ointments and creams, e.g. fusidic acid ointment 2% which contains 2 g of fusidic acid in each 100 g of ointment.
- Volume containing '1 part'—a few liquids and to a lesser extent gases, particularly those containing drugs in very low concentrations, are often described as containing 1 part per 'x' units of volume. For liquids, 'parts' are equivalent to grams and volume to millilitres, e.g. adrenaline injection 1 in 1000 which contains 1 g in 1000 mL or expressed as a percentage (w/v)—0.1%.
- Molar concentration—only very occasionally are drugs in liquid form expressed in molar concentration. The mole is the molecular weight of a drug expressed in grams and a one molar (1 M) solution contains this weight dissolved in each litre. More often the millimole (mmol) is used to describe a medicinal product, e.g. potassium chloride solution 15 mmol in 10 mL indicates a solution containing the molecular weight of potassium chloride in milligrams × 15 dissolved in 10 mL of solution.

Body height and surface area

Drug doses may be expressed in terms of microgram, milligram or gram per unit of body surface area. This is frequently the case where precise dosages tailored to individual patients'

needs are required. Typical examples may be seen in cytotoxic chemotherapy or in drugs given to children. Body surface area is expressed as square metres or m^2 and drug dosages as units per square metre or units/m^2, e.g. cytarabine injection 100 mg/m^2.

Formulae for calculation of drug doses and drip rates

Oral drugs (solids, liquids)

$$\text{Amount required} = \frac{\text{Strength required} \times \text{Volume of stock strength}}{\text{Stock strength}}$$

Parenteral drugs

(a) Solutions (IM, IV injections)

$$\text{Volume required} = \frac{\text{Strength required} \times \text{Volume of stock strength}}{\text{Stock strength}}$$

(b) Powders
It is essential to follow the manufacturer's directions for dilution, then use the appropriate formula.

(c) IV infusions

$$\text{Rate (drops/min)} = \frac{\text{Volume of solution (mL)} \times \text{Number of drops/mL}}{\text{Time (minutes)}}$$

Macrodrip (20 drops/mL)—clear fluids

$$\text{Rate (drops/min)} = \frac{\text{Volume of solution (mL)} \times 20}{\text{Time (minutes)}}$$

Macrodrip (15 drops/mL)—blood

$$\text{Rate (drops/min)} = \frac{\text{Volume of solution (mL)} \times 15}{\text{Time (minutes)}}$$

(d) Infusion pumps

$$\text{Rate (mL/hr)} = \frac{\text{Volume (mL)}}{\text{Time (hour)}}$$

(e) IV infusions with drugs

$$\text{Rate (mL/hr)} = \frac{\text{Amount of drug required (mg/hr)} \times \text{Volume of solution (mL)}}{\text{Total amount of drug (mg)}}$$

NB After selecting the appropriate formula, ensure that all strengths are in the same units, otherwise convert.

1% solution contains 1 g of solute dissolved in 100 mL of solution.

1:1000 means 1 g in 1000 mL of solution, therefore 1 g in 1000 mL is equivalent to 1 mg in 1 mL.

Other useful formulae

Children's dose (Clarke's Body Weight Rule)

$$\text{Child's dose} = \frac{\text{Adult dose} \times \text{Weight of child (kg)}}{\text{Average adult weight (70 kg)}}$$

NB Young children may require higher doses per kg than adults because of their higher metabolic rates. In obesity calculation by body weight can result in higher than necessary doses; so doses should be calculated from ideal weight, related to age and height.

Children's dose (Clarke's Body Surface Area Rule)

$$\text{Child's dose} = \frac{\text{Adult dose} \times \text{Surface area of child (m}^2\text{)}}{\text{Surface area of adult (1.8 m}^2\text{)}}$$

Acknowledgement

The measurement section was adapted from Henney CR et al 1995 Drugs in Nursing Practice, 5th edn. Churchill Livingstone, Edinburgh, with permission; and the formulae from Havard M 1994 A Nursing Guide to Drugs, 4th edn. Churchill Livingstone, Edinburgh, with permission.

Drug groups in common use

Drug groups and subgroups	Examples	Main indications
Acetylcholinesterase inhibiting drugs	Donepezil, galantamine, rivastigmine	Alzheimer's disease, dementia associated with Parkinson's disease,
Alpha$_1$-adrenoceptor antagonists (alpha blockers)	Doxazosin, prazosin	Benign prostatic enlargement, hypertension
Anabolic steroids	Nandrolone, stanozolol	Aplastic anaemia, pruritus in palliative care
Analgesics		
1. Non-opioids (see also NSAIDs)	1. Aspirin, paracetamol	1. Mild to moderate pain, e.g. simple headache and pyrexia
2. Opioids	2. Diamorphine, morphine, dihydrocodeine, fentanyl, tramadol, etc.	2. Moderate to severe pain, e.g. post-op, palliative care
3. Used for neuropathic pain	3. Amitriptyline, carbamazepine, gabapentine	3. Trigeminal neuralgia, complex regional pain syndrome
Antacids	Aluminium hydroxide, magnesium trisilicate, simeticone, alginate	Dyspepsia, gastro-oesophageal reflux disease (GORD)
Anthelmintics		
1. Benzimidazoles	1. Mebendazole, tiabendazole	1. Intestinal nematodes, e.g. threadworm, roundworm, whipworm, hookworm
2. Filaricides	2. Ivermectin	2. Tissue nematodes, e.g. onchocerciasis. Also cutaneous larva migrans, strongyloidiasis
3. Taenicides	3. Praziquantel	3. Tapeworm. Also schistosomiasis (bilharziasis)
Antiandrogens	1. Cyproterone acetate	1. Male hypersexuality, prostate cancer, acne and hirsutism in women
	2. Dutasteride, finasteride (5α-reductase inhibitors)	2. Benign prostatic enlargement.
Antiarrhythmics		
1. Supraventricular arrhythmias	1. Verapamil, adenosine	1. Supraventricular tachycardia
2. Ventricular arrhythmias	2. Lidocaine (lignocaine)	2. Ventricular tachycardia
3. Both supraventricular and ventricular arrhythmias	3. Amiodarone, disopyramide	3. Atrial fibrillation and flutter, ventricular tachycardia
Antibacterials (antibiotics), antiprotozoals		
1. Aminoglycosides	1. Gentamicin, netilmicin	1. Life-threatening Gram-negative infections, e.g. septicaemia, acute pyelonephritis, etc.
2. Antituberculosis	2. Initial phase—ethambutol, isoniazid, pyrazinamide, rifampicin (in combination)	2. Tuberculosis

Drug groups in common use—Cont'd

Drug groups and subgroups	Examples	Main indications
3. Carbapenems	3. Meropenem	3. Aerobic and anaerobic Gram-positive and Gram-negative bacteria
4. Cephalosporins	4. Cefadroxil, cefuroxime, ceftazidime	4. Meningitis, pneumonia, septicaemia
5. Fluoroquinolones	5. Ciprofloxacin	5. Gram-positive and negative infections, e.g. *Escherichia coli, Pseudomonas, Salmonella, Campylobacter*
6. Glycopeptides	6. Vancomycin, teicoplanin	6. Gram-positive cocci infections, e.g. meticillin-resistant *Staphylococcus aureus* (MRSA), septicaemia, endocarditis
7. Macrolides	7. Erythromycin, clarithromycin	7. Gram-positive infections in penicillin-sensitive patients, *Mycoplasma* pneumonia, Legionnaires' disease
8. 5-Nitroimidazoles	8. Metronidazole	8. Anaerobic infections and protozoal infections with *Trichomonas vaginalis*
9. Oxazolidones	9. Linezolid	9. Gram-positive infections including those caused by meticillin-resistant *Staphylococcus aureus* (MRSA) and vancomycin-resistant enterococci (VRE).
10. Penicillins	10 (a) Broad spectrum, e.g. ampicillin	10 (a) Gram-positive infections, e.g. bronchitis, gonorrhoea, otitis media
	10 (b) Beta-lactamase resistant, e.g. flucloxacillin	10 (b) Staphylococcal cellulitis, pneumonia, etc.
11. Streptogramin	11. Quinupristin and dalfopristin (as a combination)	11. Gram-positive infections that have not responded to other drugs
12. Sulphonamides and trimethoprim	12. Co-trimoxazole	12. Urinary tract infection, *Pneumocystis jirovecii* (formerly *P. carinii*) pneumonia, toxoplasmosis, etc.
13. Tetracyclines	13. Tetracycline, doxycycline	13. Chlamydial infections, rickettsia, Lyme disease
Anticholinesterases	Neostigmine	Myasthenia gravis
Anticoagulants		
1. Coumarins	1. Warfarin	1. Deep vein thrombosis, pulmonary embolus, and patients with mechanical prosthetic heart valves
2. Heparin	2. Standard and low molecular weight heparin	2. Treatment and prophylaxis of deep vein thrombosis and pulmonary embolus
Antidepressants		
1. Monoamine oxidase inhibitors (MAOI)	1. Phenelzine	1. Depressive illness, severe phobias
2. Selective serotonin reuptake inhibitors (SSRI)	2. Citalopram, fluoxetine	2. Depressive illness, obsessive-compulsive disorder and panic disorders
3. Tricyclic antidepressants (TCA)	3. Amitriptyline	3. Depressive illness; neuropathic pain, bedwetting in children
Antidiabetic drugs (oral hypoglycaemics)		
1. Alpha-glucosidases inhibitor	1. Acarbose	1. Type 2 diabetes
2. Biguanides	2. Metformin	2. Type 2 diabetes
3. Glitazones (thiazolidinediones)	3. Pioglitazone, rosiglitazone	3. Type 2 diabetes
4. Prandial glucose regulators	4. Repaglinide	4. Type 2 diabetes
5. Sulphonylureas	5. Glipizide, tolbutamide	5. Type 2 diabetes
6. Dipeptidyl peptidase 4 inhibitors (DPP-4 inhibitors)	6. Sitagliptin	6. Type 2 diabetes
7. Glucagon-like peptide-1 (GLP-1) mimetics	7. Exenatide (by s.c. injection)	7. Type 2 diabetes

Continued

Drug groups in common use—Cont'd

Drug groups and subgroups	Examples	Main indications
Antidiarrhoeals	Codeine phosphate, loperamide (antimotility drugs)	Adjuncts to rehydration in acute diarrhoea
Antiemetics		Nausea and vomiting:
1. Cannabinoids	1. Nabilone	1. Caused by cytotoxic chemotherapy
2. Drugs that act centrally on the chemoreceptor trigger zone	2. Domperidone	2. Caused by cytotoxic chemotherapy
3. D_2-receptor antagonists—phenothiazines	3. Prochlorperazine Metoclopramide acts in a similar way to the phenothiazines but also directly affects the gastrointestinal tract	3. Caused by gastrointestinal disorders, radiation and chemotherapy
4. H_1-receptor antagonists (antihistamines)	4. Cinnarizine, cyclizine	4. Caused by motion sickness, vestibular disorders
5. 5-HT_3-receptor antagonists	5. Dolasetron, ondansetron	5. Caused by chemotherapy, radiation and postoperatively
6. Muscarinic (acetylcholine) receptor antagonists	6. Hyoscine hydrobromide	6. Caused by motion sickness
7. Neurokinin 1 receptor antagonist	7. Aprepitant	7. Used with other drugs to prevent nausea and vomiting associated with cisplatin-based chemotherapy
Antiepileptic (anticonvulsant)	Carbamazapine, gabapentin, phenytoin	Seizure control
Antifibrinolytics and haemostatics	Tranexamic acid, aprotinin	Prevention of bleeding, menorrhagia
Antifungal		
1. Imidazoles	1. Clotrimazole, miconazole	1. Topical candidiasis
2. Polyenes	2 (a) Amphotericin	2 (a) Systemic aspergillosis, candidasis, crytococcosis
	2 (b) Nystatin	2 (b) Topical candidiasis
3. Triazoles	3. Fluconazole	3. Systemic candidiasis, cryptococcal meningitis in patients with AIDS
4. Others	4. Griseofulvin, terbinafine	4. Dermatophytosis, e.g. scalp ringworm
Antihistamines	Chlorphenamine, cetirizine, loratadine	Hay fever; emergency treatment of anaphylactic reactions
Antihypertensives		
1. Angiotensin-converting enzyme inhibitor (ACE inhibitor)	1. Captopril, ramipril	1. Hypertension; also heart failure, left ventricular dysfunction, diabetic nephropathy
2. Angiotensin-II receptor antagonists	2. Candesartan, losartan	2. Hypertension; also in heart failure, diabetic nephropathy
3. Beta-adrenoreceptor antagonists (beta-blockers)	3. Propranolol (non-selective), atenolol (selective for β_1 receptors)	3. Hypertension; also angina, myocardial infarction, arrhythmias, heart failure, hyperthyroidism, anxiety
4. Calcium channel blockers	4. Verapamil, nifedipine, diltiazem	4. Hypertension; also angina, arrhythmias
5. Centrally acting	5. Clonidine, methyldopa	5. Hypertension, migraine
6. Vasodilators	6. Hydralazine	6. Hypertension; also heart failure
Antileprotics	Dapsone, rifampicin, clofazimine	Leprosy
Antimalarials	Chloroquine, mefloquine, primaquine, proguanil, quinine	Malaria—chemoprophylaxis and treatment

Drug groups in common use—Cont'd

Drug groups and subgroups	Examples	Main indications
Antimigraine 5-HT$_1$ agonists	Sumatriptan	Migraine—treatment
Anti-obesity		
1. Lipase inhibitor	1. Orlistat	1. Adjunct in obesity—weight loss
2. Appetite suppressant (centrally acting)	2. Sibutramine	2. Adjunct in obesity—weight loss
Antioestrogens		
1. Negative feedback inhibitor	1. Clomifene	1. Anovulatory infertility
2. Oestrogen-receptor antagonist	2. Tamoxifen	2. Breast cancer; female infertility
3. Aromatase inhibitors	3. Anastrozole, letrozole	3. Metastatic breast cancer
Antiparkinson		
1. Dopaminergics	1 (a) Amantadine	1. Parkinsonism
	1 (b) Catechol-*O*-methyltransferase inhibitors, e.g. entacapone	
	1 (c) Dopamine-receptor agonists, e.g. bromocriptine, pergolide, rotigotine	
	1 (d) Levodopa, e.g. co-beneldopa (levodopa plus benserazide)	
	1 (e) Monoamine-oxidase-B inhibitor, selegiline	
2. Antimuscarinics	2. Orphenadrine	2. Parkinsonism, drug-induced extrapyramidal effects
Antiplatelet drugs	Aspirin, clopidogrel, dipyridamole, tirofiban	Prophylaxis of thrombotic cerebrovascular and cardiovascular disease
Antipsychotics (neuroleptics)		
1. Typical (phenothiazines)	1. Fluphenazine, chlorpromazine	1. Disturbed individuals, e.g. agitated depression. Short-term treatment of severe anxiety. Long-term management of schizophrenia
2. Atypical	2. Clozapine, risperidone	2. as above
Antirheumatics (see Disease modifying antirheumatic drugs [DMARD])		
Antispasmodics	Dicycloverine, mebeverine, peppermint oil	Gastrointestinal smooth muscle spasm, irritable bowel syndrome (IBS)
Antithyroid	Carbimazole	Hyperthyroidism
Antivirals		
1. Nucleoside reverse transcriptase inhibitors	1. Zidovudine	1. HIV infection
2. Protease inhibitors	2. Ritonavir	2. Progressive or advanced HIV infection
3. Non-nucleoside reverse transcriptase inhibitors	3. Efavirenz	3. HIV infection
4. Nucleic acid synthesis inhibitors	4. Aciclovir	4. Herpes simplex, varicella-zoster
Anxiolytics		
Benzodiazepines	Diazepam, temazepam	Short term for anxiety and insomnia, status epilepticus, alcohol withdrawal (acute), etc.
Bisphosphonates	Alendronic acid, disodium etidronate	Osteoporosis, Paget's disease, hypercalcaemia of cancer

Continued

Drug groups in common use—Cont'd

Drug groups and subgroups	Examples	Main indications
Bronchodilators		
1. Beta$_2$-adrenoceptor agonists	1. Salbutamol, salmeterol	1. Asthma, chronic obstructive pulmonary disease (COPD)
2. Muscarinic antagonists	2. Ipratropium, tiotropium	2. Asthma, chronic obstructive pulmonary disease
3. Xanthines	3. Aminophylline, theophylline	3. Asthma, chronic obstructive pulmonary disease
Cardiac glycosides	Digoxin (positive inotropic)	Supraventicular tachycardia
Central nervous system stimulants	Atomoxetine, dexamfetamine methylphenidate, modafinil	Attention deficit hyperactivity disorder (ADHD); narcolepsy; sleepiness due to obstructive sleep apnoea syndrome
Chelating agents	(a) Desferrioxamine	(a) Poisoning with iron salts, treatment for iron overload
	(b) Penicillamine	(b) Copper deposition in Wilson's disease
Contraceptives		
1. Combined contraceptive (an oestrogen and a progestogen in various formulations)	1 (a) Oral—ethinylestradiol + a progestogen, e.g. norethisterone or levonorgestrel	1. Contraception, menstrual problems
	1 (b) Transdermal patch—ethinylestradiol + norelgestromin	
2. Progestogen-only	2 (a) Parenteral—long acting medroxyprogesterone acetate administered by intramuscular injection	2 (a), (b), (c) Contraception
	2 (b) Intrauterine device—levonorgestrel	2 (b) also used for primary menorrhagia
	2 (c) Oral daily (continuous)—desogestrel, levonorgestrel, norethisterone	
3. Emergency contraception—hormonal	3. Levonorgestrel	3. Emergency contraception used within 72 hours of unprotected intercourse
Corticosteroids (see Glucocorticoids and Mineralocorticoids)		
Cromoglicate	Sodium cromoglicate (cromoglycate)	Asthma prophylaxis, food allergy, allergic rhinitis and conjunctivitis
Cytokine inhibitor (see monoclonal antibodies)		
Cytotoxic agents		
1. Alkylating agent	1. Chlorambucil, cyclophosphamide, mephalan	1. Chronic lymphocytic leukaemia, Hodgkin's disease, ovarian cancer etc.
2. Antimetabolite	2. Fluouracil, methotrexate	2. Acute lymphoblastic leukaemia, non-Hodgkin's lymphoma, solid tumours, etc. Methotrexate is used for rheumatoid arthritis and psoriasis. Also unlicensed use for severe inflammatory bowel disease (IBD)
3. Cytotoxic antibiotics including the anthracyclines	3. Bleomycin doxorubicin	3. Acute leukaemia, lymphomas, solid tumours
4. Vinca alkaloids and etoposide	4. Vincristine, etoposide	4. Acute leukaemias, lymphomas, solid tumours (lung, breast, testicular)
5–9. Selection of other anticancer drugs		
5. Monoclonal antibodies (see also separate entry for Monoclonal antibodies)	5. Alemtuzumab, rituximab, trastuzumab	5. Chronic lymphocytic leukaemia, non-Hodgkin's lymphoma, HER2-positive breast cancers

Drug groups in common use—Cont'd

Drug groups and subgroups	Examples	Main indications
6. Platinum compounds	6. Carboplatin, cisplatin	6. Solid tumours (ovarian, lung, testicular, bladder, cervical)
7. Protein kinase inhibitors	7. Dasatinib, erlotinib, etc.	7. Various leukaemias, some metastatic lung cancer
8. Taxanes	8. Docetaxel, paclitaxel	8. Solid tumours (ovarian, breast, lung)
9. Topoisomerase I inhibitors	9. Irinotecan, topotecan	9. Colorectal cancer (metastatic), ovarian cancer (metastatic)
Decongestant	Pseudoephedrine	Nasal congestion
Dementia drugs (see Acetylcholinesterase inhibiting drugs)		
Disease modifying antirheumatic drugs (DMARD)	Gold, penicillamine, chloroquine, sulfasalazine	Suppression of juvenile and rheumatoid arthritis
Diuretics		
1. Aldosterone antagonists	1. Spironolactone	1. Oedema, primary hyperaldosteronism
2. Carbonic anhydrase inhibitors	2. Acetazolamide	2. Glaucoma
3. Loop diuretic	3. Furosemide (frusemide)	3. Oedema, heart failure
4. Osmotic diuretic	4. Mannitol	4. Cerebral oedema, glaucoma
5. Potassium sparing	5. Amiloride, triamterene	5. Oedema, conservation of potassium
6. Thiazide	6. Bendroflumethiazide (bendrofluazide)	6. Heart failure, oedema, hypertension.
Fibrinolytic drugs	Streptokinase, alteplase, reteplase	Deep vein thrombosis, pulmonary embolus, acute myocardial infarction, arterial thromboembolism, etc.
Glucocorticoids (corticosteroids)	Beclometasone, cortisone, dexamethasone, hydrocortisone, prednisolone	Replacement, acute transplant rejection, asthma, dermatitis, inflammatory bowel disease, malignant disease, rheumatoid arthritis
H$_2$-receptor antagonists (see Ulcer healing drugs)		
HMG-CoA reductase inhibitors (see Lipid regulators)		
5-HT$_1$ agonists (see Antimigraine)		
Hypnotics	Zaleplon	Insomnia (short-term only)
Immunosuppressants (see also Glucocorticoids)	Azathioprine, ciclosporin, sirolimus, basiliximab	Organ transplantation, autoimmune and chronic inflammatory diseases
Inotropic sympathomimetics	Dobutamine, dopamine	Cardiogenic shock after cardiac surgery or infarction
Insulin	Short-acting—soluble insulin, insulin analogues (e.g. insulin lispro); Intermediate, long-acting—insulin zinc suspension, protamine zinc suspension, biphasic isophane insulin, analogues (e.g. insulin glargine)	Type I and II diabetes mellitus
Laxatives (aperients)		
1. Bulk-forming laxatives	1. Ispaghula, methylcellulose	1. Constipation
2. Faecal softeners	2. Arachis oil (enema)	2. Constipation
3. Osmotic laxative	3. Lactulose, phosphate and sodium citrate (enema)	3. Constipation
4. Stimulant	4. Senna, bisacodyl (oral and suppositories), glycerol (suppositories), sodium picosulfate (oral)	4. Constipation
5. Bowel cleansing	5. Sodium picosulfate (oral)	5. Prior to examination, barium enema or bowel surgery

Continued

Drug groups in common use—Cont'd

Drug groups and subgroups	Examples	Main indications
Lipid regulators		
1. Anion-exchange resins	1. Colestyramine	1. Hypercholesterolaemia, hyperlipidaemia; also pruritus associated with biliary obstruction and diarrhoea
2. Fibrates	2. Ciprofibrate, gemfibrozil	2. Hyperlipidaemia, prevention of coronary events in patients with coronary heart disease (CHD)
3. Statins (HMG-CoA reductase inhibitors)	3. Pravastatin, simvastin	3. Hypercholesterolaemia, hyperlipidaemia, prevention of coronary events in patients with CHD
Mineralcorticoids	Fludrocortisone	Adrenocortical insufficiency
Miotics	Pilocarpine	Glaucoma
Monoclonal antibodies (2 examples only)	Infliximab (a cytokine inhibitor)	Inflammatory bowel disease, ankylosing spondylitis, rheumatoid arthritis
	Ranibizumab	A vascular endothelial growth factor inhibitor; used in wet age-related macular degeneration.
Mucolytics	Dornase alpha (inhaled)	Cystic fibrosis
Mydriatics	Tropicamide	Pupil dilatation for ophthalmic examination
Myometrial relaxants (tocolytics)	Atosiban, terbutaline sulphate	Uncomplicated premature labour
Neuroleptics (see Antipsychotics)		
Nitrates	Glyceryl trinitrate, isosorbide dinitrate	Angina, left ventricular failure
Non-steroidal anti-inflammatory drugs (NSAIDs)	Diclofenac, ibuprofen, indomethacin, naproxen, rofexcoxib	Pain relief, dental pain, dysmenorrhoea, antipyretic, reduction of inflammation and stiffness in arthritis
Oestrogens	Oestrodiol, oesterone	Hormone replacement therapy (with progesterone for women with an intact uterus)
Opioids (see Analgesics)		
Oxytocics	Oxytocin	Induction of labour, prevention and treatment of postpartum haemorrhage
Potassium channel activator	Nicorandil	Angina
Progestogens	Medroxyprogesterone, progesterone	Dysmenorrhoea, with hormone replacement therapy, infertility, premenstrual syndrome, post-natal depression
Prostaglandins	Gemprost, mifepristone	Induction of labour, termination of pregnancy
Proton pump inhibitors (see Ulcer healing drugs)		
Retinoids	Acitretin, isotretinoin	Severe psoriasis, acne
Selective (o)estrogen receptor modulators (SERMS)	Raloxifene	Prevention and treatment of postmenopausal osteoporosis
Skeletal muscle relaxants	Baclofen, dantrolene, diazepam	Chronic muscle spasm, e.g. multiple sclerosis; malignant hyperthermia
Stimulants (see Central nervous system stimulants)		
Thyroid hormones	Thyroxine (levothyroxine)	Hypothyroidism
Tocolytics (See Myometrial relaxants)		
Tranquillizers (see: Antipsychotics, Anxiolytics)		

Drug groups in common use—Cont'd

Drug groups and subgroups	Examples	Main indications
Ulcer healing drugs		
1. H_2-receptor antagonists	1. Cimetidine, ranitidine	1. Peptic ulceration, gastro-oesophageal reflux disease
2. Proton pump inhibitors	2. Omeprazole, lansoprazole	2. Peptic ulceration, eradication of *Helicobacter pylori* *(with two antibacterials)*, gastro-oesophageal reflux disease, Zollinger–Ellison syndrome
Uricosuric	Probenecid	Prevention of gout
Vasoconstrictor sympathomimetics	Phenylephrine	Acute hypotension

(Readers should be aware that some drugs used as examples for a particular drug group may also have other uses; for example, acetazolamide, a carbonic anhydrase inhibitor, is occasionally used as a second-line antiepileptic drug.)

(Adapted from an appendix revised by Jennifer Kelly for Churchill Livingstone Medical Dictionary 16th edn. 2006)

5

Appendix

Appendix 6

Abbreviations and acronyms—medical terms and related organizations

A	ampere
AA	Alcoholics Anonymous
AAA	abdominal aortic aneurysm
AABR	automated auditory brainstem response
AACG	acute angle-closure glaucoma
AAMI	age-associated memory impairment
AAT	alpha$_1$ (α)-antitrypsin deficiency
ABGs	arterial blood gases
ABPA	allergic bronchopulmonary aspergillosis
ABPI	ankle-brachial pressure index
AC	**1.** alternating current. **2.** approved clinician
ACBT	active cycle of breathing technique
ACD	anaemia of chronic disease
ACE	angiotensin-converting enzyme
ACG	angle-closure glaucoma
ACh	acetylcholine
ACJ	acromioclavicular joint
ACL	anterior cruciate ligament
ACPSM	Association of Chartered Physiotherapists in Sports Medicine
ACTH	adrenocorticotrophic hormone
ADD	attention deficit disorder
ADE	acute demyelinating encephalitis
ADH	antidiuretic hormone
ADHD	attention deficit hyperactivity disorder
ADI	acceptable daily intake
ADLs	activities of daily living
ADP	adenosine diphosphate
ADRs	adverse drug reactions
AE	air entry
AED	automated external defibrillator
AF	atrial fibrillation
AFB	acid-fast bacilli
AfC	Agenda for Change
AFD	anode to film distance

AFI	amniotic fluid index
AFLP	acute fatty liver of pregnancy
AFO	ankle foot orthosis
AFP	alphafetoprotein
AHF/G	antihaemophilic factor/globulin
AGA	appropriate for gestational age
AHI	apnoea hypopnoea index
AHP	allied health professional
AICD	automatic implantable cardioverter defibrillator
AID	artificial insemination using donor semen
AIDS	acquired immune deficiency syndrome
AIH	artificial insemination using husband's (partner's) semen
AIP	acute interstitial pneumonia
AIS	abbreviated injury scale
AJC	acrylic jacket crown
A-K	above knee
ALA	alpha (α)-linolenic acid
ALD	adrenoleucodystrophy
ALG	antilymphocyte globulin
ALL	acute lymphoblastic leukaemia
ALS	**1.** advanced life support **2.** amyotrophic lateral sclerosis
ALT	alanine aminotransferase
AMA	antimitochondrial antibody
amATPase	actomyosin ATPase
AMD	age-related macular degeneration
AMED	Allied and Complementary Medicine Database
aMCI	amnestic mild cognitive impairment
AMF	amplitude modulated frequency
AMHP	approved mental health professional
AMI	acute myocardial infarction
AML	acute myeloblastic/myeloid leukaemia
AMP	adenosine monophosphate
AMS	acute mountain sickness

AN	anorexia nervosa	ATN	acute tubular necrosis
ANA	antinuclear antibody	ATP	adenosine triphosphate
ANCA	antineutrophil cytoplasmic antibody	ATPS	ambient temperature and pressure saturated
ANOVA	analysis of variance	AUG	acute ulcerative gingivitis
ANP	atrial natriuretic peptide	AUNG	acute ulcerative necrotizing gingivitis
ANS	**1.** anterior nasal spine. **2.** autonomic nervous system	A-V	**1.** arteriovenous **2.** atrioventricular
ANT	adverse neural tension	AV ECCO$_2$R	arteriovenous extracorporeal membrane carbon dioxide removal
ANTT®	Aseptic Non Touch Technique	AVM	arteriovenous malformations
ANUG	acute necrotizing ulcerative gingivitis	AVP	arginine vasopressin
AOM	acute otitis media	BACUP	British Association of Cancer United Patients
AP	**1.** anaesthesia practitioner. **2.** anterioposterior	BAL	**1.** British antilewisite **2.** bronchoalveolar lavage
APC	antigen-presenting cell	BAN	**B**ritish **A**pproved **N**ame
APD	**1.** auditory processing disorder. **2.** automated peritoneal dialysis	BAOT/COT	British Association/**C**ollege of **O**ccupational **T**herapists
APEL	accreditation of prior experiential learning	BAS	behavioural activation system
APF	acidulated phosphate fluoride	BASES	**B**ritish **A**ssociation for **S**port and **E**xercise **S**cience
APH	antepartum haemorrhage	BASIC	**B**eginners **A**ll-purpose **S**ymbolic **I**nstruction **C**ode
APKD	adult polycystic kidney disease		
APL	accreditation of prior learning	BBA	born before arrival (at hospital)
Apo-A1	apolipoprotein A1	BBB	**1.** blood–brain barrier **2.** bundle branch block
Apo-B	apolipoprotein B	BBV	blood-borne virus
APTT	activated partial thromboplastin time	BCAA	branched-chain amino acid
AR	antireflection coating	BCC	basal cell carcinoma
ARC	**1.** abnormal retinal correspondence **2.** AIDS related complex	BCG	bacille Calmette–Guérin
		BDA	**1.** British Dental Association **2.** British Dietetic Association
ARDS	acute/adult respiratory distress syndrome		
ARF	**1.** acute renal failure **2.** acute respiratory failure	BDD	body dysmorphic disorder
ARM	**1.** age-related maculopathy **2.** artificial rupture of the membranes	BDHA	British Dental Hygienists' Association
		BED	**b**iological **e**ffective **d**ose
ARMD	age-related macular degeneration	BEI	bioelectrical impedance
AROM	active range of motion	BFI	Baby Friendly Initiative
ART	**a**nti**r**etroviral **t**herapy during pregnancy	BHF	Bolivian haemorrhagic fever
ASCII	**A**merican **S**tandard **C**ode for **I**nformation **I**nterchange	BHL	bilateral hilar lymphadenopathy
		BHN	Brinell hardness scale/number
ASD	atrial septal defect	BID	brought in dead
ASIS	anterior superior iliac spine	BIH	benign intracranial hypertension
ASO	antistreptolysin O	BIO	binocular indirect ophthalmoscope
ASOM	acute suppurative otitis media	BIOS	basic input/output system
AST	aspartate aminotransferase	BIPAP	biphasic positive airways pressure
ASW	approved social worker	BIS	behavioural inhibition system
AT	anaerobic threshold	BLISS	**B**aby **LI**fe **S**upport **S**ystems
ATF	anterior talofibular ligament	BLS	basic life support
ATLS	advanced trauma life support	BM	bowel movement

BMA	British Medical Association
BMD	bone mineral density
BME	benign myalgic encephalomyelitis
BMI	body mass index
BMR	basal metabolic rate
BMT	bone marrow transplant
BMUS	British Medical Ultrasound Society
BN	bulimia nervosa
BNF	British National Formulary
BNR	beam non-uniformity ratio
BOD	biochemical oxygen demand
BOOP	bronchiolitis obliterans organizing pneumonia
BOP	bleeding on probing (index)
BOS	bronchiolitis obliterans syndrome
BP	**1.** blood pressure **2.** British Pharmacopoeia
BPD	**1.** biparietal diameter **2.** bronchopulmonary dysplasia
BPE	**1.** basic periodontal examination **2.** benign prostatic enlargement
BPF	bronchopleural fistula
BPH	benign prostatic hyperplasia
bpm	beats per minute
BPPV	benign paroxysmal positional vertigo
Bq	becquerel
BRAO	branch retinal arterial occlusion
BRM	biological response modifier
BRSC	British Red Cross Society
BRVO	branch retinal vein occlusion
BSA	body surface area
BSE	**1.** bovine spongiform encephalopathy **2.** breast self-examination
BSL	British sign language
BST	bovine somatotrophin
BULL	**B**uccal of **U**pper; **L**ingual of **L**ower (cusps)
BUN	**b**lood **u**rea **n**itrogen
BUT	break-up time (BUT) test
BV	**1.** biological value **2.** bacterial vaginosis
BVP	back vertex power
BW	**1.** birth weight **2.** bite wing radiograph **3.** body weight
Bx	biopsy
BXO	balanitis xerotica obliterans
C	**1.** Celsius (centigrade) **2.** coulomb
CA-125	cancer cell surface antigen 125

CAB	**c**ellulose **a**cetate **b**utyrate
CABG	coronary artery bypass graft
CACG	chronic angle-closure glaucoma
CAD	**1.** **c**omputer-**a**ided **d**rawing **2.** **c**oronary **a**rtery **d**isease
CAH	congenital adrenal hyperplasia
CAL	computer assisted learning
CAM	**1.** **c**ell **a**dhesion **m**olecule **2.** **c**omplementary and **a**lternative **m**edicine
CAMI	Carers Assessment of Managing Index
cAMP	cyclic adenosine monophosphate
CAPD	continuous ambulatory peritoneal dialysis
CAPE	**C**lifton **A**ssessment **P**rocedures for the **E**lderly
C&S	culture and sensitivity
CAT	**c**omputed **a**xial **t**omography
CBA	cost-benefit analysis
CBC	complete blood count
CBF	cerebral blood flow
CBT	cognitive behaviour therapy
CCF	congestive cardiac failure
CCK	cholecystokinin
CCPNS	cell cycle phase non-specific
CCPS	cell cycle phase specific
CCU	coronary care unit
CD	controlled drug
Cd	candela
CDC	Centers for Disease Control and Prevention
CDH	congenital dislocation of the hip
CDROM	compact disk read-only memory
CDRW	compact disk re-writer
CEA	**1.** carcinoembryonic antigen **2.** cost-effectiveness analysis
CEHR	Commission for Equality and Human Rights
CF	cystic fibrosis
CFA	cryptogenic fibrosing alveolitis
CFC	chlorofluorohydrocarbons
CFM	cerebral function monitor
CFS/ME	chronic fatigue syndrome/myalgic encephalomyelitis
CFT	complement fixation test
CFTR	cystic fibrosis transmembrane regulator
CGD	chronic granulomatous disease
CGM	continuous glucose monitoring
CH50	classical haemolytic pathway 50

CHART	continuous hyperfractionated accelerated radiotherapy	COSHH	Control of Substances Hazardous to Health
CHD	1. congenital heart disease 2. coronary heart disease	COT	College of Occupational Therapists
CHF	congestive heart failure	COX-2	cyclo-oxygenase-2
CHI	creatinine height index	CPA	care programme approach
CHM	Commission on Human Medicines	CPAP	continuous positive airways pressure
CHO	carbohydrate	CPD	continuing professional development
CHRE	Council for Healthcare Regulatory Excellence	CPEO	chronic progressive external ophthalmoplegia
ci	curie	CPITN	community periodontal index of treatment needs
CI	1. cardiac index 2. confidence interval	CPK/CP	creatine phosphokinase
CIE	Commission Internationale de l'Eclairage	CPM	continuous passive motion (movement)
CILs	centres of integrated (or independent) living	CPN	Community Psychiatric Nurse
CIN	cervical intraepithelial neoplasia	CPP	cerebral perfusion pressure
CINAHL	Cumulative Index to Nursing and Allied Health Literature	CPR	cardiopulmonary resuscitation
		CPS	characters per second
CIP	continuous inflating pressure	CPT	carnitine palmitoyltransferase
CIS	carcinoma in situ	CPU	central processing unit
CIVD	cold-induced vasodilatation	CQC	Care Quality Commission
CJD	Creutzfeldt–Jakob disease	Cr	creatine
CK	creatine kinase	CRAO	central retinal arterial occlusion
CLAPC	contact lens associated papillary conjunctivitis	CRE	cumulative radiation effect
CLL	chronic lymphocytic leukaemia	CREST	calcinosis, Raynaud's phenomenon, (o)esophageal dysfunction, sclerodactyly and telangiectasis
CLO	columnar-lined oesophagus		
CLPC	contact lens papillary conjunctivitis		
CML	chronic myeloid leukaemia	CRF	chronic renal failure
CMO	1. chief medical officer 2. cystoid macular oedema	CRH	corticotrophin-releasing hormone
		CRL	crown–rump length
CMV	1. controlled mandatory ventilation 2. cytomegalovirus	CrP	creatine phosphate
		CRP	C-reactive protein
CNHC	Complementary and Natural Healthcare Council	CRPS	complex regional pain syndrome
CNMES	chronic neuromuscular electrical stimulation	CRT	cathode ray tube
		CRS	(NHS) care record service
CNO	Chief Nursing Officer	CRVO	central retinal vein occlusion
CNS	1. central nervous system 2. clinical nurse specialist	CS	caesarean section
		CSA	Child Support Agency
CNV	choroidal neovascularization	CSF	1. cerebrospinal fluid 2. colony stimulating factor
CO	cardiac output		
COC	combined oral contraceptive	CSI	Caregiver Strain Index
CoG	centre of gravity	CSII	continuous subcutaneous insulin infusion
CoM	centre of mass	CSM	Committee on Safety of Medicines
COMA	Committee on Medical Aspects of Food Policy	CSOM	chronic suppurative otitis media
COP	1. centre of pressure 2. cryptogenic organizing pneumonia	CSP	Chartered Society of Physiotherapy
		CSR	central serous retinopathy
COPD	chronic obstructive pulmonary disease	CSS	Churg–Strauss syndrome
COR	critical oxygen requirement		

6

Appendix

CSSD	central sterile supplies department
CSSU	central sterile supply unit
CST	contraction stress test
CT	**1.** cerebral tumour **2.** computed tomography **3.** coronary thrombosis **4.** cover test
CTG	cardiotocography
CTZ	chemoreceptor trigger zone.
CUA	cost-utility analysis
CUS	continuous ultrasound
CUT	**C**ity **U**niversity **t**est
CV	curriculum vitae
CVA	cerebrovascular accident
CVD	cardiovascular disease
CVID	common variable immunodeficiency
CVP	central venous pressure
CVS	**1.** cardiovascular system **2.** chorionic villus sampling **3.** computer vision syndrome
CVVH	continuous veno-venous haemofiltration
CVVHD	continuous veno-venous haemodiafiltration (haemodialysis)
CW (probe)	continuous wave probe
CX	circumflex artery
CXR	chest X-ray
DAD	diffuse alveolar damage
DADL	domestic activities of daily living
D and C	dilatation and curettage
D and E	dilatation and evacuation
DAS	disease activity score
DAT	direct antiglobulin test
Db	decibel
DBP	diastolic blood pressure
DC	direct current
DCIS	ductal carcinoma in situ
DCP	dental care professional
DCR	dacryocystorhinostomy
DCSS	diffuse cutaneous systemic sclerosis
DDE	developmental defects of enamel (index)
DDH	developmental dysplasia of the hip
DEF	decayed, extracted, filled
DEL	dose-equivalent limit
DEM	developmental eye movement (test)
DEXA	dual-energy X-ray absorptiometry
DHA	docosahexaenoic acid

DHEA	dehydroepiandrosterone
DHS	dynamic hip screw
DIC	disseminated intravascular coagulation
DICOM	digital imaging and communications in medicine
DIDMOAD	diabetes insipidus, diabetes mellitus, optic atrophy and deafness
DIP	**d**esquamative **i**nterstitial **p**neumonia
DISH	**d**iffuse **i**diopathic **s**keletal **h**yperostosis
DMARD	disease modifying antirheumatic drug
D Max	maximum density
DMD	Duchenne muscular dystrophy
DMF	decayed, missing, filled
DMFS	decayed, missing and filled surfaces
DMS	Director of Medical Services
DNA	deoxyribonucleic acid
DNAR	do not attempt resuscitation
DNase	deoxyribonuclease
DNR	do not resuscitate
DO_2	oxygen delivery
DOA	dead on arrival
DOB	date of birth
DOMS	delayed onset muscle soreness
DOS	disk operating system
DOT	**d**irectly **o**bserved **t**reatment
DPF	Dental Practitioners' Formulary
2,3-DPG	2,3-diphosphoglycerate
DPLD	diffuse parenchymal lung disease
DPT	dental pantomogram
DQE	detected quantum efficiency
DR	**1.** diabetic retinopathy **2.** digital radiography
DRVs	dietary reference values
DRVVT	dilute Russell viper venom time
DSA	digital subtraction angiography
DSH	deliberate self-harm
DSM	Diagnostic and Statistical Manual of Mental Disorder
DTs	delerium tremens
DUB	dysfunctional uterine bleeding
DVD	digital versatile disk
DVI	direct video interface
DVT	deep vein thrombosis
DWSIs	dentists with special interests

e$^-$	electron
E	**1.** energy **2.** exposure
EAR	**e**stimated **a**verage **r**equirement
EAMC	exercise-associated muscle cramp
EB	epidermolysis bullosa
EBA	**1.** epidermolysis bullosa acquista **2.** ethoxybenzoic acid cement
EBM	**1.** evidence-based medicine **2.** expressed breast milk
EBP	evidence-based practice
EBV	Epstein–Barr virus
ECCE	extracapsular cataract extraction
ĒCF	extracellular fluid
ECG	electrocardiogram
ECI	Experience of Caregiving Inventory
ECM	extracellular matrix
ECMO	extracorporeal membrane oxygenator
ECoG	electrocochleography
ECT	electroconvulsive therapy
ECV	external cephalic version
ED	erectile dysfunction
EDB	estimated date of birth
EDD	expected date of delivery
EDRF	endothelium-derived relaxing factor
EDSS	expanded disability status scale
EDTA	ethylene diamine tetra-acetic acid
EDV	end diastolic volume
EEG	electroencephalogram
EFAs	essential fatty acids
EFSA	European Food Safety Authority
EFM	electronic fetal monitor
EGF	epidermal growth factor
EHEC	enterohaemorrhagic Escherichia coli
EIA	exercise induced asthma
EIEC	enteroinvasive Escherichia coli
EIT	electrically initiated torque
ELISA	enzyme-linked immunosorbent assay
EMD	electromechanical dissociation
EMEA	European Medicines Agency
EMF	electromotive force
EMG	electromyogram
EMLA	eutectic mixture of local anaesthetics
EMRSA	epidemic meticillin (methicillin)-resistant Staphylococcus aureus

EMS	early morning stiffness
ENT	ear, nose and throat
EOG	electro-oculogram
EOP	equivalent oxygen pressure
EOT	extraoral traction
EP	evoked potentials
EPA	**1.** eicosapentaenoic acid **2.** electrophysical agent.
EPEC	enteropathic Escherichia coli
EPI	electronic portal imaging
EPO	erythropoietin
EPOC	elevated or excess post-exercise oxygen consumption
EPP	equal pressure point
EPR	electronic patient record
EPROM	erasable programmable read only memory
EPSP	excitatory post synaptic potential
ER	endoplasmic reticulum
ERA	effective radiating area
ERCP	endoscopic retrograde cholangiopancreatography
ERG	electroretinogram
ERPC	evacuation of retained products of conception
ERV	expiratory reserve volume
ESP	**1.** extended scope physiotherapy practitioner **2.** extrasensory perception
ESR	erythrocyte sedimentation rate
ESRD/F	end-stage renal disease/failure
ESWL	extracorporeal shock wave lithotripsy
ESV	end-systolic volume
ET	endotracheal tube
ETCO$_2$	end-tidal carbon dioxide
ETEC	enterotoxigenic Escherichia coli
ETL	echo train length
ETT	exercise tolerance test
EUA	examination under anaesthetic
EW	extended wear (contact lens)
EV	exposure value
F	**1.** farad **2.** field size
f	frequency of radiation
FAD/FADH$_2$	flavin adenine dinucleotide (oxidized and reduced forms respectively)
FAM	Functional Assessment Measure
F(A)ROM	full (active) range of motion
FAS	fetal alcohol syndrome

FAST	**F**ace **A**rm and **S**peech **T**est	FTA-Abs	fluorescent treponemal antibody absorbed test
FB	foreign body	FVC	forced vital capacity
FBC	full blood count	FVP	front vertex power
FBS	**1.** fasting blood sugar **2.** fetal blood sampling	GABA	gamma aminobutyric acid
FDD	**1.** floppy disk drive **2.** focus to diaphragm distance	gamma-GT (γ-GT)	gamma-glutamyltransferase
FDDI	fibre distribution data interface	GAS	**g**eneral **a**daptation **s**yndrome
FDP	**1.** fibrin degradation product **2.** frequency doubling perimetry	GBM	glomerular basement membrane
		GBS	Guillain–Barré syndrome
FEF	forced expiratory flow	GCA	giant cell arteritis
FER	forced expiratory ratio	GCS	Glasgow Coma Scale
FES	functional electrical stimulation	G-CSF	granulocyte colony-stimulating factor
FESS	functional endoscopic sinus surgery	GDC	General Dental Council
FET	forced expiration technique	GDP	general dental practitioner
FEV	forced expiratory volume	GDS	geriatric depression scale
FFA	free fatty acid	GE	gradient echo
FFD	focus to film distance	GFR	glomerular filtration rate
FFM	fat-free body mass	GGT	gamma-glutamyltransferase
FH	**1.** familial hypercholesterolaemia **2.** family history **3.** fetal heart	GH	growth hormone
		GHb	total glycated (glycosylated) haemoglobin
FHS	Family Health Services	GHRH	growth hormone releasing hormone
FI	fatigue index	GHRIH	growth hormone release inhibiting hormone
FID	free induction decay	GI	**1.** gastrointestinal **2.** gingival index **3.** glycaemic index
FIGLU	**f**orm**imino**g**lu**tamic (FIGLU) acid		
FIM	Functional Independence Measure	GIF	graphics interchange format
FiO$_2$	fractional inspired oxygen concentration	GIFT	**g**amete **i**ntra**f**allopian **t**ransfer
FISH	**f**luorescence **in** **s**itu **h**ybridization	GIP	gastric inhibitory peptide
FL	femur length	GLA	gamma (γ)-linolenic acid
FLAIR	**f**luid **a**ttenuation **i**nversion **r**ecovery	GMC	General Medical Council
FM	Fugel-Meyer	GM-CSF	granulocyte-macrophage colony stimulating factor
FMNF	fetal movements not felt		
FMN/FMNH$_2$	flavin mononucleotide (oxidized and reduced form respectively)	GMS	general medical services
		GnRH	gonadotrophin releasing hormone
FMPA	Frankfort mandibular plane angle	GOO	gastric outlet obstruction
FMRI	functional magnetic resonance imaging	GORD	gastro-oesophageal reflux disease
FNA	fine needle aspirate	GP	**1.** general practitioner **2.** gas permeable (contact lens)
FOB	**f**aecal **o**ccult **b**lood		
FOV	field of view	G6P	glucose-6-phosphate
FPA	Family Planning Association	GPC	giant papillary conjunctivitis
FR	functional reach (test)	GPCL	gas permeable contact lens
FRC	functional residual capacity	G6PD	glucose-6-phosphate dehydrogenase
FSA	Food Standards Agency	GPI	general paralysis of the insane
FSD	focus to skin distance	GPL	gas permeable lens
FSH	**1.** facioscapulohumeral muscular dystrophy **2.** follicle stimulating hormone	GSD	glycogen storage diseases
		GSL	general sales list

GTR	guided tissue regeneration
GTT	**1.** gestational trophoblastic tumour **2.** glucose tolerance test.
GTV	gross tumour volume
GU	genitourinary
GUM	genitourinary medicine
GVHD	graft versus host disease
Gy	gray
HAI	hospital acquired infection
HAART	highly active antiretroviral therapy
HACE	high-altitude cerebral (o)edema
HAPE	high-altitude pulmonary (o)edema
HAV	hepatitis A virus
HAVS	hand-arm vibration syndrome
Hb	haemoglobin
HbA	adult haemoglobin
HbA_{1c}	glycated (glycosylated) haemoglobin
HbA_2	adult haemoglobin
HbA_o	non-glycated (non-glycosylated) adult haemoglobin
HbF	fetal haemoglobin
HBIG	hepatitis B immunoglobulin
HBV	hepatitis B virus
HCA	healthcare assistant
HCAI	healthcare-associated infection
hCG (HCG)	human chorionic gonadotrophin
HCV	hepatitis C virus
HDD	hard disk drive
HDL	high-density lipoprotein
HDR	high dose rate
HDU	high dependency unit
HELLP	haemolysis, elevated liver enzymes and low platelets
HEMA	hydroxyethyl methacrylate
HER2	human epidermal growth factor receptor-2
HET	human enhancement technologies
HFEA	Human Fertilisation and Embryology Authority
HFJV	high frequency jet ventilation
HFOV	high frequency oscillation ventilation
HFPPV	high frequency positive pressure ventilation
HGH	human growth hormone
HGP	hard gas permeable (contact lens)
HHNK	hyperglycaemic hyperosmolar non-ketotic (coma)

5-HIAA	5-hydroxyindoleacetic acid
Hib	*Haemophilus influenzae* type B
HIFU	high intensity focused ultrasound
HIS	**H**ospital **I**nformation **S**ystem
HIT	**h**eparin-**i**nduced **t**hrombocytopenia
HIV	human immunodeficiency virus
HK	hexokinase
HLA	human leucocyte antigen
HMB	beta-hydroxy beta-methylbutyrate
HMM	'heavy meromyosin'
HO	heterotophic ossification
HNPCC	hereditary non-polyposis colorectal cancer
HOCM	hypertrophic obstructive cardiomyopathy
HONK	**h**yper**o**smolar **n**on-**k**etotic (coma)
HP	hypersensitivity pneumonitis
HPA	Health Protection Agency
HPC	**1.** Health Professions Council **2.** history of present complaint
HPL	human placental lactogen
HPV	human papilloma virus
HRCT	high-resolution computed tomography
HRmax	maximal heart rate
HRR	heart rate reserve
HRT	hormone replacement therapy
HSC	Health and Safety Commission
HSCT	haemopoietic stem cell transplantation
HSDU	hospital sterilization and disinfection unit
HSE	Health and Safety Executive
HSSU	hospital sterile supply unit
HSV	herpes simplex virus
5-HT	5-hydroxytryptamine
HTLV	human T-cell lymphotropic virus
HUS	haemolytic uraemic syndrome
HV	health visitor
HVPS	high-voltage pulsed stimulation
HVS	**1.** high vaginal swab **2.** hyperviscosity syndrome
HVT	half-value thickness
IABP	intra-aortic balloon pump
IADL	instrumental activities of daily living
IAT	indirect antiglobulin test
IBD	inflammatory bowel disease
IBL	inquiry-based learning
IBS	irritable bowel syndrome

6

Appendix

IBW	ideal body weight
IC	inspiratory capacity
ICCE	intracapsular cataract extraction
ICD-10	International Classification of Diseases
ICE	**i**ce, **c**ompress and **e**levation
ICF	**1.** International Classification of Functioning, Disability and Health **2.** intracellular fluid
ICON	**i**ndex of **c**omplexity of **o**rthodontic **n**eed
ICP	**1.** integrated care pathway **2.** intercuspal position **3.** intracranial pressure.
ICS	inhaled corticosteroids
ICSH	interstitial cell stimulating hormone
ICSI	intracytoplasmic sperm injection (transfer)
ICU	intensive care unit
IDDM	insulin dependent diabetes mellitus
IE	infective endocarditis
IEP	isoelectric point
IFG	impaired fasting glucose/glycaemia
IFN	interferon
IFT	inferential therapy
Ig	immunoglobulin
IGF	insulin-like growth factors
IGT	impaired glucose tolerance
IHD	ischaemic heart disease
IHE	integrated health enterprise
IIMs	idiopathic inflammatory myopathies
IL	interleukin
ILD	interstitial lung disease
IM	**1.** Index Medicus **2.** intramedullary **3.** intramuscular
IMRT	intensity modulated radiotherapy
IMTG	intramuscular triacylglycerol
IMV	intermittent mandatory ventilation
INH	inhalation
INR	international normalized ratio
IOC	International Olympic Committee
IOFB	intraocular foreign body
IOL	intraocular lens
IOP	intraocular pressure
IORT	intraoperative radiotherapy
IOTN	index of orthodontic treatment need
IP_3	inositol triphosphate
IP address	Internet Protocol address
IPD	interpupillary distance

IPE	interprofessional education
IPF	idiopathic pulmonary fibrosis
IPH	intrapartum haemorrhage
IPPB	intermittent positive pressure breathing
IPPV	intermittent positive pressure ventilation
IPSP	inhibitory post synaptic potential
IQ	intelligence quotient
IRR	**1.** infrared radiation/rays **2.** ionizing radiation regulations
IRT	immune-reactive trypsin test
ISC	intermittent self-catheterization
ISD	interventricular septal defect
ISDN	integrated services digital network
ISO	International Standards Organization
ISP	internet service provider
ITM	index of tooth mobility
ITP	idiopathic thrombocytopenic purpura
ITU	intensive therapy unit
IUCD	intrauterine contraceptive device
IUD	**1.** intrauterine (contraceptive) device **2.** intrauterine death (of a fetus)
IUGR	intrauterine growth restriction/retardation
IUI	intrauterine insemination.
IV	intravenous
IVC	inferior vena cava
IVF	in vitro fertilization
IVH	intraventricular haemorrhage
IVI	intravenous infusion
IVIG	intravenous immunoglobulin
IVU/IVP	intravenous urogram/pyelogram
IZOF	individual zone of optimal functioning
J	joule
JCA	juvenile chronic arthritis
JGA	juxtaglomerular apparatus
JND	just noticeable difference
JPEG	joint picture experts group
JVP	jugular venous pressure
KC	keratoconus
KCS	keratoconjunctivitis sicca
KHN	Knoop hardness scale/number
kJ	kilojoule
KP	**1.** keratic precipitates **2.** knowledge of performance
KR	knowledge of results

KUB	kidney, ureter and bladder
LA	left atrium
LABAs	long-acting β₂ agonists
LAD	left anterior descending artery
LAK-cells	lymphokine-activated killer cells
LAN	local area network
LASER	**l**ight **a**mplification by **s**timulated **e**mission of **r**adiation
LASIK	laser insitu keratomileusis or laser assisted intrastromal keratoplasty
LAUP	laser-assisted uvulopalatoplasty
LAVH	laporoscopic-assisted vaginal hysterectomy
LBC	liquid-based cytology
LBM	lean body mass
LBP	low back pain
LBW	low birthweight
LCA	longitudinal chromatic aberration
LCMV	lymphocytic choriomeningitis virus
LCSS	limited cutaneous systemic sclerosis
LD₅₀	lethal dose in 50%
LDH	lactate dehydrogenase
LDL	low-density lipoprotein
LE	lupus erythematosus
LET	**l**inear **e**nergy **t**ransfer
LFA	low-friction arthroplasty
LFTs	liver function tests
LGB	lateral geniculate bodies
LGVCFT	lymphogranuloma venereum complement fixation test
LH	luteinizing hormone
LIP	**l**ymphocytic **i**nterstitial **p**neumonia
LISP	**LIS**t **P**rocessor language
LJP	localized juvenile periodontitis
LMA	laryngeal mask airway
LMN	'light meromyosin'
LMP	last menstrual period
LMPA	low-melting point alloy
LMWH	low-molecular-weight heparin
LOA	left occipitoanterior
LOC	level of consciousness
LOP	**l**eft **o**ccipito**p**osterior
LOS	lower oesophageal sphincter
LP	lumbar puncture

LPL	lipoprotein lipase
LRK	laser refractive keratoplasty
LRNI	lower reference nutrient intake
LRTI	lower respiratory tract infection
LS	**1.** lecithin-sphingomyelin ratio **2.** lichen sclerosis
LSA	**1.** lichen sclerosus et atrophicus **2.** local supervising authority
LSCS	lower segment caesarean section
LSD	lysergic acid diethylamide
LSI	large scale integration
LSP	local service provider
LT	lactate threshold
LTG	low tension glaucoma
LTM	long-term memory
LTOT	long-term oxygen therapy
LUTS	lower urinary tract symptoms
LV	left ventricle
LVA	low vision aids
LVAD	left ventricular assist device
LVF	left ventricular failure
LVRS	lung volume reduction surgery
LWUS	longwave ultrasound
ma	metre angle
MAb	monoclonal antibody
MABP	mean arterial blood pressure
MAC	**1.** mid-arm circumference **2.** *Mycobacterium avium* complex
MAG3	mercaptoacetlytriglycine
MAI	*Mycobacterium avium intracellulare*
MALT	**m**ucosa-**a**ssociated **l**ymphoid **t**issue
MAOI	monoamine oxidase inhibitor
MAP	**m**ean **a**rterial **p**ressure
MAR	**m**inimum **a**ngle of **r**esolution
MAST	**m**iltary **a**nti**s**hock **t**rousers
mATPase	myosin ATPase
Mb	myoglobin
MBC	maximal breathing capacity
MBP	mean (arterial) blood pressure
MCA	**1.** Medicines Control Agency ⊃ MHRA **2.** middle cerebral artery
MCADD	medium chain acyl-CoA dehydrogenase deficiency
MCH	mean cell haemoglobin

MCHC	mean cell haemoglobin concentration		MLNS	mucocutaneous lymph node syndrome
MCID	minimal clinical important difference (of outcome scores)		MLSO	Medical Laboratory Scientific Officer
MCL	medial collateral ligament		MLSS	maximum lactate steady state
MCP	multiple cosmetic phlebectomy		mm	millimetre
MCT	medium chain triglycerides (triacylglycerols)		MMAS	Modified Motor Assessment Scale
MCU	micturating cystourethrogram		mmHg	millimetres of mercury
MCV	mean cell volume		mmol	millimole
MDA	Medical Devices Agency ⊃ MHRA		MMR	measles, mumps and rubella (vaccine)
MDI	metered-dose inhaler		MMSE	Mini Mental State Examination
MDM	mental defence mechanism		MND	motor neuron disease
MDR-TB	multidrug resistant tuberculosis		MO	Medical Officer
MDS	myelodysplastic syndrome		MOA	medium opening activator
MDT	multidisciplinary team		MODEM	**mo**dulator-**dem**odulator
ME	myalgic encephalomyelitis		MODS	multiple organ dysfunction syndrome
MEDLARS	medical literature analysis retrieval system		MODY	maturity onset diabetes of the young
MELAS	mitochondrial encephalopathy lactic acidosis and stroke-like episodes		MOH	Medical Officer of Health
MEN	**m**ultiple **e**ndocrine **n**eoplasia		mol	mole
MEP	**1.** maximum expiratory pressure **2.** motor evoked potential		MOM	multiple of the median
			MPA	microscopic polyangiitis
MERRF	myoclonic epilepsy with ragged red fibres		MPD	monocular pupillary distance
MESA	**m**icrosurgical **e**pididymal **s**perm **a**spiration		MRC	Medical Research Council
MESH/MeSH	**Me**dical **S**ubject **H**eadings		MRI	magnetic resonance imaging
METS	metabolic equivalents		mRNA	messenger ribonucleic acid
MFAC	medium frequency current		MRSA	meticillin (methicillin)-resistant *Staphylococcus aureus*
mg	milligram			
MGD	meibomian gland dysfunction		MS	**1.** multiple sclerosis **2.** musculoskeletal system
MGUS	monoclonal gammopathy of uncertain significance		MSA	multiple system atrophy
MHC	**1.** major histocompatibility complex **2.** myosin heavy chain		MSCC	metastatic spinal cord compression
			MSH	melanocyte stimulating hormones
MHN	Mohs hardness scale/number		MSK	musculoskeletal
MHRA	Medicines and Healthcare products Regulatory Agency		MSP	Munchausen syndrome by proxy
			MSU/MSSU	midstream specimen of urine
MI	myocardial infarction		MSW	Medical Social Worker
MICRR	multiple idiopathic cervical root resorption		MTA	mineral trioxide aggregate
MIME	**m**ultipurpose **i**nternet **m**ail **e**xtensions		MTF	modulation transfer function
MIMS	Monthly Index of Medical Specialties		MUA	manipulation under anaesthetic
MIP	maximum inspiratory pressure		MUAC	mid-upper arm circumference
MIS	minimally invasive surgery		MUFA	monounsaturated fatty acid
mL	millilitre		MVC	maximum voluntary contraction
MLC	**1.** multi-leaf collimation **2.** myosin light chains		MVIT	maximal voluntary isometric torque
			MVT	maximum voluntary ventilation
			MxMnPA	maxillary-mandibular planes angle

N	newton	NMR	nuclear magnetic resonance
NACNE	National Advisory Committee on Nutrition Education	NNT	numbers needed to treat
		NNU	neonatal unit
NAD	**1.** nicotinamide adenine dinucleotide **2.** nothing abnormal detected	NOF	neck of femur
		NPC	near point of convergence
NADP	nicotinamide adenine dinucleotide phosphate	NPDR	non-proliferative diabetic retinopathy
		NPF	Nurse Prescribers' Formulary
NAI	non-accidental injury	NPL	National Physical Laboratory
NAMCW	National Association for Maternal and Child Welfare	NPN	non-protein nitrogen
		NPSA	National Patient Safety Agency
NAWCH	National Association for the Welfare of Children in Hospital	NRDS	neonatal respiratory distress syndrome
		NREM	non-rapid eye movement (sleep)
NBAS	Neonatal Behavioural Assessment Scale	NRPB	National Radiological Protection Board
NBI	no bony injury	NSAIDs	non-steroidal anti-inflammatory drugs
NBM	nil (nothing) by mouth	NSCLC	non-small cell lung carcinoma
NBT	nitroblue tetrazolium reduction test	NSFs	National Service Frameworks
NCT	National Childbirth Trust	NSIP	non-specific interstitial pneumonia
NCVQ	National Council for Vocational Qualifications	NSP	non-starch polysaccharide
NDT	neurodevelopmental therapy	NSU	non-specific urethritis
Nd-Yag laser	neodymium-yag (Nd-Yag) laser	NT	nuchal translucency
NEC	necrotizing enterocolitis	NTD	neural tube defect
NEFA	non-esterified free fatty acid	NUG	necrotizing ulcerative gingivitis
NEQ	noise equivalent quanta	NVQ	National Vocational Qualification
ng	nanogram	NWB	non-weight bearing
NG	nasogastric	OA	osteoarthritis
NGF	nerve growth factor	OAE	otoacoustic emission
NGU	non-gonococcal urethritis	OBLA	onset of blood lactate accumulation
NHL	non-Hodgkin's lymphoma	OBS	organic brain syndrome
NHS	National Health Service	OCD	obsessive compulsive disorder
NHSLA	NHS Litigation Authority	OCR	optical character recognition
NIBUT	non-invasive break-up time (test)	ODA	operating department assistant
NICE	National Institute for Health and Clinical Excellence	ODD	oppositional defiant disorder
		ODP	operating department practitioner
NICU	neonatal intensive care unit	OFD	object-to-film distance
NIDDM	non-insulin dependent diabetes mellitus	OFG	orofacial granulomatosis
NIHL	noise induced hearing loss	OGD	oesophagogastroduodenoscopy
NIPPV	non-invasive intermittent positive pressure ventilation	OHI	oral hygiene index
		OHSS	ovarian hyperstimulation syndrome
NIV	non-invasive ventilation	OID	object-to-image distance
NK	natural killer (cell)	OME	otitis media with effusion
NLH	National Library for Health	OPG®	orthopantomograph
NLP	neurolinguistic programming	ORIF	open reduction internal fixation
nm	nanometre	ORS	oral rehydration solution
NMC	Nursing and Midwifery Council		
NMES	neuromuscular electrical stimulation		

ORT	oral rehydration therapy
OSAS	obstructive sleep apnoea (hypopnoea) syndrome
OSAHS	obstructive sleep apnoea hypopnoea syndrome
OT	occupational therapy/therapist
OTC	over-the-counter (medicines)
OVD	occlusal vertical dimension
Pa	pascal
PA	**1.** pantoscopic angle **2.** pernicious anaemia **3.** posteroanterior
PACG	primary angle-closure glaucoma
$PaCO_2$	partial pressure of carbon dioxide in arterial blood
$PACO_2$	partial pressure of carbon dioxide in alveolar air
PACS	picture archiving communication system
PADL	personal activities of daily living
PAFC	pulmonary artery flotation catheter
PAI	plasminogen activator inhibitor
PAIVMs	passive accessory intervertebral movements
PAL	**1.** physical activity level **2.** progressive addition lens
PALS	**1.** paediatric advanced life support **2.** patient advocacy liaison service
PAM	potential acuity meter
PAN	**p**oly**a**rteritis **n**odosa
PAO	peak acid output
PaO_2	partial pressure of oxygen in arterial blood
PAO_2	partial pressure of oxygen in alveolar air
PAOP	pulmonary artery occlusion pressure
Pap	Papanicolaou smear test
PAPP-A	pregnancy associated plasma protein-A
PAR	**1.** peer assessment review **2.** physical activity ratio
PARNUTS	foods for particular nutritional purposes
PAS	periodic acid–Schiff (reagent)
PATF	professionally applied topical fluoride
PAWP	pulmonary artery wedge pressure
PBD	peak bone density
PBI	papillary bleeding index
PBL	problem-based learning
PBM	peak bone mass
PBMC	peripheral blood mononuclear cells
PCAG	primary closed-angle glaucoma
PCA(S)	patient controlled analgesia (system)
PCEA	patient controlled epidural analgesia

PCI	percutaneous coronary intervention
PCL	posterior cruciate ligament
PCM	protein-calorie malnutrition
PCO_2	partial pressure of carbon dioxide
PCOS	polycystic ovary syndrome
PCP	*pneumocystis* pneumonia
PCr	phosphocreatine
PCR	**1.** plaque control record **2.** polymerase chain reaction
PCT	Primary Care Trust
PCV	packed cell volume
PCWP	pulmonary capillary wedge pressure
PD	interpupillary distance
PDA	patent ductus arteriosus
PDB	Paget's disease of bone
PDGF	platelet-derived growth factor
PDH	pyruvate dehydrogenase
PDI	periodontal disease index
PDP	personal development plan
PDR	proliferative diabetic retinopathy
PDT	photodynamic therapy
PE	pulmonary embolus
PEA	**p**ulseless **e**lectrical **a**ctivity
PEEP	**p**ositive **e**nd **e**xpiratory **p**ressure
PEFR	peak expiratory flow rate
PEG	**p**ercutaneous **e**ndoscopic **g**astrostomy
PEK	punctate epithelial keratitis
PEM	protein-energy malnutrition
PERLA	pupils equal, reacting to light, accommodation
PERRLA	pupils equal, round, react to light, accommodation
PESA	percutaneous epididymal sperm aspiration
PET	**p**ositron **e**mission **t**omography
PFI	private finance initiative
PFJ	patello-femoral joint
PFK	phosphofructokinase
PFM	porcelain fused to metal
PFMC	preformed metal crown
PGD	pre-implantation genetic diagnosis
PGDRS	psychogeriatric dependency rating scale
PGH	pre-implantation genetic halotyping
pH	hydrogen ion concentration
Ph	Philadelphia chromosome

PHC	primary health care
PHPV	persistent hyperplastic primary vitreous
PI	**1.** performance indicator **2.** peridontal (Russell) index
PICC	peripherally inserted central catheter
PICH	primary intracerebral haemorrhage
PICU	Paediatric Intensive Care Unit
PID	**1.** pelvic inflammatory disease **2.** position indicating device **3.** prolapsed inntervertebral disc.
PIH	pregnancy induced hypertension
PJC	porcelain jacket crown
PKB	prone knee bend
PKU	phenylketonuria
PLB	pursed lip breathing
PMA	papillary, marginal and attached gingivae
PMB	postmenopausal bleeding
PMH	past medical history
PMI	point of maximum impulse
PMMA	polymethylmethacrylate
PMR	polymyalgia rheumatica
PMS	premenstrual syndrome
PND	paroxysmal nocturnal dyspnoea
PNF	proprioceptive neuromuscular facilitation
PNH	paroxysmal nocturnal haemoglobinuria
PNI	psychoneuroimmunology
PNS	**1.** peripheral nervous system **2.** posterior nasal spine
PO$_2$	partial pressure of oxygen
POA	pancreatic oncofetal antigen
POAG	primary open-angle glaucoma
POM	prescription only medicine
POMC	pro-opiomelanocortin
POMR	problem-orientated medical record
PONV	postoperative nausea and vomiting
POP	**1.** plaster of Paris **2.** post office protocol **3.** progestogen-only pill
PPE	personal protective equipment
PPH	post partum haemorrhage
PPL	phosphorylase
PPLO	pleuropneumonia-like organism
ppm	parts per million
PPP	pentose phosphate pathway
PPS	pelvic pain syndrome

PPV	positive pressure ventilation
PR	**1.** per rectum **2.** peripheral resistance
PRK	photorefractive keratectomy
PRL	prolactin
PROM	**1.** patient reported outcome measures **2.** programmable read only memory
PROMM	proximal myotonic myopathy
PRP	panretinal photocoagulation
PRR	preventive resin restoration
PRV	polycythaemia rubra vera
PSA	prostate specific antigen
PSR	positive supporting reaction
PSTT	placental site trophoblastic tumour
PSV	pressure supported ventilation
PT	**1.** physiotherapist **2.** prothrombin
PTA	**1.** percutaneous transluminal angioplasty **2.** post-traumatic amnesia
PTC	percutaneous transhepatic cholangiography
PTCA	percutaneous transluminal coronary angioplasty
PTFE	polytetrafluoroethylene
PTH	parathyroid hormone
PTM	pterygo-maxillare
PTSD	post-traumatic stress disorder
PTV	planning target volume
PUBS	**p**ercutaneous **u**mbilical cord **b**lood **s**ampling
PUFA	polyunsaturated fatty acid
PUJ	pelviureteric junction
PUO	pyrexia of unknown origin
PUS	**p**ulsed **u**ltra**s**ound
PUVA	psoralen plus ultraviolet light A
PV	per vagina
PVD	peripheral vascular disease
PVL	Panton-Valentine leukocidin
PVR	pulmonary vascular resistance
PVS	persistent vegetative state
PWB	partial weight bearing
PXF	pseudoexfoliation
PXS	pseudoexfoliation syndrome
QALYs	quality-adjusted life years
QF-PCR	quantitative fluorescence-polymerase chain reaction
QoL	quality of life

RA	1. refractory anaemia 2. rheumatoid arthritis 3. right atrium		RMR	resting metabolic rate
RADAR	Royal Association for Disability and Rehabilitation		RNA	ribonucleic acid
			RNI	reference nutrient intake
RADC	Royal Army Dental Corps		RNIB	Royal National Institute of Blind People
RAEB	refractory anaemia with excess blasts		RNID	Royal National Institute for Deaf People
RAM	random access memory		RO	reality orientation
RAMC	Royal Army Medical Corps		ROA	right occipitoanterior
RAPD	relative afferent pupillary defect		ROM	1. range of motion 2. read only memory 3. resisted range of movement
RARS	refractory anaemia with sideroblasts			
RAS	reticular activating system		ROP	right occipitoposterior
RAST	radioallergosorbent test		ROS	reactive oxygen species
RBC	red blood cell		RP	retinitis pigmentosa
RB-ILD	respiratory bronchiolitis–interstitial lung disease		RPD	removable partial denture
RCA	right coronary artery		RPE	1. rating of perceived exertion 2. retinal pigment epithelium
RCMD	refractory cytopenias with multilineage dysplasia			
			RPP	rapidly progressive periodontitis
RCP	retruded cuspal position		RPR	rapid plasma reagin test
RCT	randomized controlled trial		RQ	respiratory quotient
RD	retinal detachment		rRNA	ribosomal ribonucleic acid
RDA	recommended daily allowance		RSD	reflex sympathetic dystrophy
RDI	recommended daily intake		RSI	repetitive strain injury
RDS	1. random-dot stereogram 2. respiratory distress syndrome		RSV	respiratory syncytial virus
			RTA	1. renal tubular acidosis 2. road traffic accident
REF	renal erythropoietic factor			
REM	rapid eye movement (sleep)		RV	1. residual volume 2. right ventricle
RER or R	respiratory exchange ratio		RVF	right ventricular failure
RES	reticuloendothelial system		S1	first heart sound
RF	rheumatoid factor		S2	second heart sound
RFLP	restriction-fragment length polymorphism		S3	third heart sound
RGP	rigid gas permeable (contact lens)		S4	third heart sound
Rh	Rhesus factor		SA	sinoatrial
RHD	rheumatic heart disease		SACN	Scientific Advisory Committee on Nutrition
RI	retention index		SAD	seasonal affective disorder
RICE	rest, ice, compress, elevation		SADS	sudden adult/arrhythmia death syndrome
RIDDOR	Reporting of Injuries, Diseases and Dangerous Occurrences Regulations		SAH	subarachnoid haemorrhage
			SAID	specific adaptation to imposed demands
RIHSA	radioiodinated human serum albumin		SANDS	Stillbirth and Neonatal Death Society
rINN	Recommended International Non-proprietary Name		StAAA	St Andrew's Ambulance Association
			StJAA	St John Ambulance Association
RIP	raised intracranial pressure		StJAB	St John Ambulance Brigade
RIS	radiology information system		SaO$_2$	arterial oxygen saturation
RK	radial keratotomy		SARA	sexually acquired reactive arthritis
RMO	resident medical officer		SARS	severe acute respiratory syndrome.
			SATA	spatial average temporal average

SATF	self-applied topical fluoride
SATP	spatial average temporal peak
SBLA syndrome	sarcoma, breast, leukaemia and adrenal gland syndrome
SBP	systolic blood pressure
SBS	short bowel syndrome
SC	subcutaneous
SCAT	sheep cell agglutination test
SCBU	special care baby unit
SCC	1. spinal cord compression 2. squamous cell carcinoma
SCID	severe combined immunodeficiency
SCJ	squamocolumnar junction
SCL	soft contact lens
SCT	supervised community treatment
SD	standard deviation
SDA	specific dynamic action
SDH	subdural haematoma
SE	standard error
SEM	scanning electron microscope
SEN	special educational needs
SEP	sensory evoked potentials
SERMs	selective (o)estrogen receptor modulators
SF	synovial fluid
SFA	saturated fatty acid
SFD	1. small for dates 2. source-to-film distance
SFS	Social Functioning Scale
SGA	small for gestational age
SGOT	serum glutamic oxaloacetic transaminase (aspartate aminotransferase)
SGPT	serum glutamic pyruvic transaminase (alanine aminotransferase)
SH	standard (unfractionated) heparin
SHO	Senior House Officer
SI Units	Système International d'Unités
SIADH	syndrome of inappropriate antidiuretic hormone
SIB	self-injurious behaviour
SID	source-to-image distance
SIDS	sudden infant death syndrome
SIJ	sacroiliac joint
SILO	**s**mall **i**n **l**arge **o**ut
SIMA	system for identifying motivated abilities
SIMV	synchronized intermittent mandatory ventilation
SIN	**s**everity, **i**rritability and **n**ature factors
SIR	**s**erial **i**nfra **r**ed
SIRS	**s**ystemic **i**nflammatory **r**esponse **s**yndrome
SL	sublingual
SLAP	**s**uperior **l**abrum **a**nterior-**p**osterior lesion
SLE	systemic lupus erythematosus
SLK	superior limbic keratoconjunctivitis
SLO	scanning laser ophthalmoscope
SLOB	**s**ame **l**ingual:**o**pposite **b**uccal (rule)
SLR	straight leg raise
SLT	speech and language therapist/therapy
SMA	spinal muscular atrophy
SMART (goals)	**s**pecific-**m**easurable-**a**chievable-**r**ealistic-**t**ime orientated
SMBG	self-monitoring blood glucose
SMBR	standardized morbidity ratio
SMR	1. standardized mortality ratio 2. submucous resection
SNB	sentinel node biopsy
SNL	sesorineural hearing loss
SNP	single-nucleotide polymorphism
SOAP	**s**ubjective-**o**bjective-**a**ssessment-**p**lan
SOB	**s**hortness **o**f **b**reath
SOBOE	short of breath on exertion
SOD	**s**ource to **o**bject **d**istance
SOLI	small out large in
SP	spatial peak
SPECT	single-photon emission computed tomography
SPK	superficial punctate keratitis
SPMSQ	Short Portable Mental State Questionnaire
SPOD	sexual problems of the disabled
SPSS	Statistical Package for Social Sciences
SR	sarcoplasmic reticulum
SRBC	sheep red blood cells
SSL	secure socket layer
SSPE	subacute sclerosing panencephalitis
SSRIs	selective serotonin reuptake inhibitors
SSSS	staphylococcal scalded skin syndrome
STD	sexually transmitted disease
STI	sexually transmitted infection

STM	short-term memory		TIBC	total iron binding capacity
STPD	standard temperature and pressure dry		TIFF (TIF)	tagged information file format
SUDI	sudden unexpected death in infancy		TIPSS	transjugular intrahepatic portasystemic stent shunting
SUF(c)E	slipped upper femoral (capital) epiphysis		TIVA	total intravenous anaesthesia
Sv	sievert		TKR	total knee replacement
SV	**1.** single-vision (SV) lens **2.** stroke volume		T_{LAC}	lactate threshold
SVD	spontaneous vaginal delivery		TLC	total lung capacity
SVQs	Scottish Vocational Qualifications		TLS	tumour lysis syndrome
SVR	systemic vascular resistence		TMJ	temporomandibular joint
SVT	supraventricular tachycardia		TMS	transcranial magnetic stimulation
SWAP	**s**hort **w**avelength **a**utomated **p**erimetry		TNF	tumour necrosis factor
T	tesla		TNM	tumour, node (lymph), metastasis
T_3	triiodothyronine		TOP	**t**ermination **o**f **p**regnancy
T_4	thyroxine		TP	temporal peak
$t_{1/2}$	half-life		t-PA, tPA	tissue plasminogen activator
TA	temporal average		TPHA	*Treponema pallidum* haemagglutination assay
TACI	total arterial cerebral infarction		TPN	total parenteral nutrition
T_{AN}	anaerobic threshold		TPR	temperature, pulse, respiration
TAR	**t**otal **a**nkle **r**eplacement		TQM	total quality management
TB	tuberculosis (tubercle bacillus)		TRAM	**t**ransverse **r**ectus **a**bdominis **m**yocutaneous
TBA	traditional birth attendant		TRH	thyrotrophin-releasing hormone
TBI	**1.** total body irradiation **2.** traumatic brain injury		TRIC	trachoma inclusion conjunctivitis
TBSA	total burn surface area		tRNA	transfer ribonucleic acid
TCA	**1.** transverse chromatic aberration **2.** tricyclic antidepressant		TRUS	transrectal ultrasonography
TCR	T-cell receptor		TSE	testicular self-examination
TCRE	transcervical resection of endometrium		TSF	triceps skinfold thickness
TE	echo time		TSH	thyroid-stimulating hormone
TEA	**t**hermic **e**ffect of **a**ctivity		TSS	toxic shock syndrome
TEDs	thromboembolic deterrents		TT	tetanus toxoid
TEF	thermic effect of food		TTTS	twin to twin transfusion syndrome
TEN	**t**oxic **e**pidermal **n**ecrolysis		TUE	therapeutic use exemption
TENS	**t**ranscutaneous **e**lectrical **n**erve **s**timulation		TUR/TURP	transurethral resection of the prostate
TEPP	tetraethyl pyrophosphate		TUVP	transurethral vaporization of the prostate
TFR	total fertility rate		TV	**1.** tidal volume/air **2.** transvaginal **3.** *Trichomonas vaginalis*
TFT	thin film transistor			
TG	**1.** triacylglycerol **2.** triglyceride		T_{vent}	ventilatory threshold
TGC	time gain control		UE_3	unconjugated oestriols
TGF	transforming growth factor		UIP	usual interstitial pneumonia
THC	total haemolytic complement		UNICEF	United Nations International Children's Emergency Fund
THR	total hip replacement			
TI	**1.** inversion time **2.** treatment index		UPPP	uvulopalatopharyngoplasty
TIA	transient ischaemic attack		UPS	underperformance syndrome

URL	uniform resource locator
URTI	upper respiratory tract infection
US, U/S	ultrasound
USB	universal serial bus
USS	ultrasound scan
UTI	urinary tract infection
UUPS	unexplained under performance syndrome
UV	ultraviolet
UVPPP	uvulopalatopharyngoplasty
UVR	ultraviolet radiation
v	volt
VA	visual acuity
VADAS	voice activated domestic appliance system
VAP	ventilator-associated pneumonia
VAS	visual analogue scale
VATS	videoassisted thoracoscopy
VBI	vertebrobasilar insufficiency
VC	vital capacity
VDRL	venereal disease research laboratory (test)
VDT	visual display terminal
VDU	visual display unit
VECP	visual-evoked cortical potential
VEP	visual-evoked potentials
VF	ventricular fibrillation
VFM	value for money
VHF	1. very high frequency 2. viral haemorrhagic fever
VHN	Vickers hardness scale/number
VIN	vulval intraepithelial neoplasia
VIP	vasoactive intestinal peptide
VKC	vernal keratoconjunctivitis
VLBW	very low birth weight
VLDL	very-low-density lipoprotein
VMA	vanillylmandelic acid
VMC	vasomotor centre
VMO	vastus medialis obliquus
VO_2	oxygen consumption
VO_{2max}	maximum oxygen consumption/uptake

V/Q	ventilation perfusion ratio
VRE	vancomycin resistant enterococci
VRSA	vancomycin resistant *Staphylococcus aureus*
VSD	ventricular septal defect
VSO	Voluntary Service Overseas
VT	1. ventilatory threshold 2. ventricular tachycardia
V_T	tidal volume
VTE	venous thromboembolism
VUR	vesicoureteric reflux
VZIG	varicella-zoster (hyperimmune) immunoglobulin
VZV	varicella-zoster virus
W	watt
WADA	World Anti-Doping Agency
WAN	wide area network
WAP	wireless application protocol
WBC	white blood cell
WD	working distance
WFP	World Food Programme
WG	Wegener's granulomatosis
WHO	World Health Organization
WHR	waist-hip ratio
WNV	West Nile virus
WOB	work of breathing
WORM	write once read many
WPW	Wolff–Parkinson–White (syndrome)
WRULD	work-related upper limb disorder
www	World Wide Web
YAG	yttrium aluminium garnet
XCP	extension-cone paralleling technique
XDR-TB	extensively drug-resistant tuberculosis
XLA	X-linked agammaglobulinaemia
XHIM	X-linked hyper-IgM syndrome
Z	1. acoustic impedance 2. atomic number
ZIFT	zygote intrafallopian tube transfer
ZN	Ziehl–Neelsen (stain)
ZOF	zone of optimal functioning

Appendix 7

Useful web sites

Action for Sick Children http://www.actionforsickchildren.org/

Action on Smoking and Health (ASH) http://www.ash.org.uk/

Age Concern England http://www.ace.org.uk/

Alcoholics Anonymous http://www.alcoholics-anonymous. org.uk/

Alzheimer's Society http://www.alzheimers.org.uk/

Arthritis Care http://www.arthritiscare.org.uk/

Asthma UK http://www.asthma.org.uk/

AVERT (HIV/AIDS charity) http://www.avert.org/

BACUP (British Association of Cancer United Patients and their Families and Friends) http://www.cancerbacup.org.uk

Bandolier-Evidence based thinking about healthcare http:// www.jr2.ox.ac.uk/Bandolier/

Breast Cancer Care http://www.breastcancercare.org.uk/

British Allergy Foundation http://www.allergyfoundation.com

British Association/College of Occupational Therapists (BAOT/COT) http://www.cot.org.uk/

British Deaf Association http://www.bda.org.uk/

British Heart Foundation http://www.bhf.org.uk/

British Liver Trust http://www.britishlivertrust.org.uk/

British Medical Association http://www.bma.org.uk

British National Formulary http://www.bnf.org.uk/

British Organ Donor Society http://www.argonet.co.uk/body

British Pregnancy Advisory Service (BPAS) http://www. bpas.org/

British Red Cross Society (BRCS) http://www.redcross.org.uk/

British Society of Hearing Therapists http://www. hearingtherapy.org/

Cancer Research UK http://www.cancerresearchuk.org/

Cardiomyopathy Association http://www.cardiomyopathy.org/

Care Quality Commission http://www.cqc.org.uk

Carers UK http://www.carersonline.org.uk/

Centers for Disease Control and Prevention (US agency) http://www.cdc.gov/

Centre for Reviews and Dissemination (York) http://www. york.ac.uk/inst/crd

Chartered Society of Physiotherapists http://www.csp.org.uk/

Clean, Safe Care. Reducing MRSA and other healthcare associated infections http://www.clean-safe-care.nhs.uk

Cochrane Library http://www.cochrane.co.uk/

Coeliac Society http://www.coeliac.co.uk/

College of Optometrists http://www.college-optometrists.org/

Commission for Equality and Human Rights http://www. cehr.org.uk/

Council for Healthcare Regulatory Excellence http://www. chre.org.uk/

Cruse http://www.crusebereavementcare.org.uk/

Department for Environment, Food and Rural Affairs (defra) http://www.defra.gov.uk/

Department of Health http://www.dh.gov.uk/

Diabetes UK http://www.diabetes.org.uk/

Disabled Living Foundation http://www.dlf.org.uk/

Eating Disorders Association http://www.b-eat.co.uk/

epic2: National Evidence-Based Guidelines for Preventing Healthcare-Associated Infections http://www.epic.tvu. ac.uk

Epilepsy Action http://www.epilepsy.org.uk/

Equal Opportunities Commission http://www.eoc.org.uk

Food Standards Agency www.food.gov.uk

General Medical Council http://www.gmc-uk.org/

Guide Dogs for the Blind Association http://www.gdba.org.uk/

Guillain–Barré Syndrome Society http://www.gbs.org.uk/

Haemophilia Society http://www.haemophilia.org.uk/

Headway—brain injury association http://www.headway.org.uk/

Health & Safety Executive http://www.hse.gov.uk

Health Professions Council http://www.hpc-uk.org/

Health Protection Agency http://www.hpa.org.uk/

Health Protection Scotland http://www.hps.scot.nhs.uk

Healthcare Commission http://www.healthcarecommission. org.uk/

Help the Aged http://www.helptheaged.org.uk/

Ileostomy & Internal Pouch Support Group http://www. ileostomypouch.demon.co.uk/

Infection Protection Society (IPS) incorporating Infection Control Nurses' Association (ICNA) http://www.ips.uk.net

Institute of Complementary Medicine http://www.icmedicine. co.uk/

International Glaucoma Association (IGA) http://www.iga. org.uk

Joint Committee on Vaccination and Immunisation (JCVI) http://www.advisorybodies.doh.gov.uk

King's Fund http://www.kingsfund.org.uk/

Leukaemia Care Society http://www.leukaemiacare.org.uk/

Leukaemia Society http://www.leukaemiasociety.org.uk/

Macmillan Cancer Support http://www.macmillan.org.uk/

Marie Curie Cancer Care http://www.mariecurie.org.uk/

Medicines and Healthcare Products Regulatory Agency http://www.mhra.gov.uk/

Mencap http://www.mencap.org.uk/

Meningitis Research Foundation http://www.meningitis. org.uk/

Migraine Action Association http://www.migraine.org.uk/

MIND—National Association for Mental Health http://www.mind.org.uk/

Multiple Sclerosis Society http://www.mssociety.org.uk/

Muscular Dystrophy Campaign (MDC) http://www.muscular-dystrophy.org/

National Aids Trust http://www.nat.org.uk/

National Childbirth Trust (NCT) http://www.nctpregnancyandbabycare.com/

National Institute for Health and Clinical Excellence (NICE) http://www.nice.org.uk/

National Institute of Medical Herbalists http://www.nimh.org.uk/

National Library for Health http://www.library.nhs.uk/

National Osteoporosis Society http://www.nos.org.uk/

National Patient Safety Agency (NPSA) http://www.npsa.nhs.uk/

National Resource for Infection Control (NRIC) http://www.nric.org.uk

National Society for the Prevention of Cruelty to Children (NSPCC) http://www.nspcc.org.uk/

National Travel Health Network and Centre (NaTHNaC) http://www.nathnac.org/

NHS 24 http://www.nhs24.com/content/

NHS Centre for Reviews and Dissemination (York) http://www.york.ac.uk/inst/crd

NHS Immunisation Information http://www.immunisation.nhs.uk

Nursing and Midwifery Council http://www.nmc-uk.org

Parkinson's Disease Society http://www.parkinsons.org.uk/

Resuscitation Council UK http://www.resus.org.uk/

Royal Association for Disability and Rehabilitation (RADAR) http://www.radar.org.uk/

Royal College of Nursing http://www.rcn.org.uk

Royal National Institute for Deaf People (RNID) http://www.rnid.org.uk/

Royal National Institute of Blind People (RNIB) http://www.rnib.org.uk/

Royal Society for the Prevention of Accidents (RoSPA) http://www.rospa.co.uk/

Royal Society of Medicine http://www.rsm.ac.uk/

Samaritans http://www.samaritans.org.uk/

Scoliosis Association (UK) http://www.sauk.org.uk/

Scottish Executive http://www.scotland.gov.uk/

Scottish Intercollegiate Guidelines Network (SIGN) http://www.sign.ac.uk/

Sickle Cell Society http://www.sicklecellsociety.org/

Society & College of Radiographers http://www.sor.org/

Society of Chiropodists & Podiatrists http://www.scpod.org/

St Andrews Ambulance Association http://www.firstaid.org.uk/

St John Ambulance Association & Brigade http://www.sja.org.uk/

Stillbirth & Neonatal Death Society (SANDS) http://www.uk-sands.org/

Stroke Association http://www.stroke.org.uk/

Terrence Higgins Trust http://www.tht.org.uk/

The Royal College of Anaesthetists http://www.rcoa.ac.uk

The Royal College of General Practitioners http://www.rcgp.org.uk

The Royal College of Obstetricians and Gynaecologists http://www.rcog.org.uk/

The Royal College of Ophthalmologists http://www.rcophth.ac.uk

The Royal College of Paediatrics and Child Health http://www.rcpch.ac.uk

The Royal College of Pathologists http://www.rcpath.org

The Royal College of Physicians http://www.rcplondon.ac.uk

The Royal College of Physicians, Edinburgh http://www.rcpe.ac.uk

The Royal College of Physicians and Surgeons, Glasgow http://www.rcpsglas.ac.uk

The Royal College of Psychiatrists http://www.rcpsych.ac.uk

The Royal College of Radiologists http://www.rcr.ac.uk/enquiries/

The Royal College of Surgeons of Edinburgh http://www.rcsed.ac.uk/

The Royal College of Surgeons of England www.rcseng.ac.uk/

UK National Poisons Information Services http://www.npis.org/

UK Thalassaemia Society http://www.ukts.org/

VSO http://www.vso.org.uk/

World Health Organization http://www.who.org

Appendix 8

Chemical symbols and formulae

Aluminium	Al		Hydrogen bromide	HBr
Aluminium chloride	$AlCl_3$		Hydrogen phosphate	HPO_4
Aluminium hydroxide	$Al(OH)_3$		Hydroquinone	$C_6H_6O_2$
Aluminium oxide	Al_2O_3		Hydroxide	OH
Aluminium sulphate	$Al_2(SO_4)_3$		Iodine	I
Ammonia	NH_3		Iridium	Ir
Ammonium	NH_4		Iron	Fe
Ammonium thiosulphate	$(NH_4)_2S_2O_3$		Lanthanum	La
Barium	Ba		Lanthanum oxybromide	LaOBr
Barium fluorochloride	BaFCl		Lanthanum oxybromide with terbium activator	LaOBr . Tb
Barium fluorochloride with europium activator	BaFCl . Eu		Lead	Pb
Bicarbonate (hydrogen carbonate)	HCO_3		Lithium	Li
Cadmium	Cd		Magnesium	Mg
Caesium	Cs		Magnesium sulphate	$MgSO_4$
Calcium	Ca		Manganese	Mn
Calcium carbonate	$CaCO_3$		Mercury	Hg
Calcium chloride	$CaCl_2$		Molybdenum	Mo
Calcium hydroxide	$Ca(OH)_2$		Nickel	Ni
Calcium sulphate	$(CaSO_4)_2$		Nitrogen	N
Calcium tungstate	$CaWO_4$		Nitrate	NO_3
Carbon	C		Nitric acid	HNO_3
Carbonic acid	H_2CO_3		Oxygen	O
Carbon dioxide	CO_2		Phosphate	PO_4
Chlorine	Cl		Phosphorus	P
Chromium	Cr		Potassium	K
Cobalt	Co		Potassium bromide	KBr
Copper	Cu		Potassium chloride	KCl
Fluorine	F		Potassium nitrate	KNO_3
Gadolinium	Gd		Potassium sulphite	K_2SO_3
Gadolinium oxysulphide	Gd_2O_2S		Radium	Ra
Gadolinium oxysulphide with terbium activator	Gd_2O_2S . Tb		Selenium	Se
Gold	Au		Silicon	Si
Helium	He		Silver	Ag
Hydrochloric acid	HCl		Silver bromide	AgBr
Hydrogen	H		Silver chloride	AgCl

Silver iodide	AgI	Sulphur	S
Silver nitrate	AgNO$_3$	Sulphuric acid	H$_2$SO$_4$
Silver sulphide	Ag$_2$S	Technetium	Tc
Sodium	Na	Terbium	Tb
Sodium bicarbonate	NaHCO$_3$	Thallium	Tl
Sodium chloride	NaCl	Titanium dioxide	TiO$_2$
Sodium hydroxide	NaOH	Vanadium	V
Sodium thiosulphate	Na$_2$S$_2$O$_3$	Water	H$_2$O
Sodium sulphite	Na$_2$SO$_3$	Xenon	Xe
Strontium	Sr	Yttrium	Y
Sulphate	SO$_4$	Zinc	Zn

Appendix 9

Radionuclide applications

Radionuclide	Chemical form	Application
Chromium-51	Sodium chromate solution	Red blood cells Spleen Glomerular filtration rate (GFR)
Cobalt-57	Cyanocobalamin	Pernicious anaemia Vitamin B_{12}
Cobalt-58	Cyanocobalamin	Gastrointestinal malabsorption
Gallium-67	Gallium citrate	Infections Tumour seeking
Indium-111	Indium oxine labelled white blood cells	Infections Abscesses
Iodine-123	Sodium iodide capsules and solutions	Renography Thyroid gland
Iodine-125	o-Iodohippurate Human serum albumin	Plasma volume
Iodine-131	Sodium iodide	Thyroid diagnosis and treatment
Iodine-131 hippuran	o-Iodohippurate	Renography
Iodine-123 MIBG	Meta-iodo-benzylguanidine	Adrenal glands
Krypton-81 m	Gas	Pulmonary ventilation
Phosphorus-32	Sodium phosphate	Treatment of polycythaemia vera
Selenium-75	Seleno-norcholesterol	Adrenal glands
Selenium-75 (seHCAT)	23-seleno-25- homo-taurocholate Selenium-tagged bile salt	Diarrhoea Bile salt absorption
Technetium-99 m	Sodium pertechnetate	Brain Thyroid gland
Technetium-99 m	Exametazine HMPAO	Cerebral blood flow Leucocyte labelling

Radionuclide	Chemical form	Application
Technetium-99 m colloid	Tin colloid	Liver Sites of gastrointestinal bleeds
Technetium-99 m	Succimer (DMSA)	Static renal imaging
Technetium-99 m	Pentetate (DTPA)	Renal imaging, lung ventilation
Technetium-99 m	Etefenin (EHIDA) injection	Biliary function
Technetium-99 m	Albumin aggregated (MAA) Albumin microspheres (HAM)	Perfusion lung scanning
Phosphates labelled with technetium-99 m	HDP hydroxydisophosphate	Bone scanning
Technetium-99 m pertechnetate	Sodium pertechnetate	Testicular torsion Thyroid gland Salivary glands Meckel's diverticulum
Technetium-99 m Pyrophosphates	Phosphonates and phosphates	Acute myocardial infarct Myocardial imaging
Technetium-99 m	Glucoheptonate	Brain Kidneys
Technetium-99 m	Stannous fluoride	Heart blood pool
Technetium cardiolite	Thallous chloride	Myocardial ischaemia
Xenon-133	Gas	Pulmonary ventilation Cerebral blood flow

Basic Life Support (BLS)

Algorithms from the *2005 Resuscitation Guidelines* (Reproduced by permission of the Resuscitation Council UK)

Adult Basic Life Support

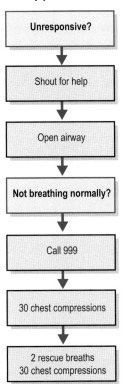

```
Unresponsive?
      ↓
Shout for help
      ↓
Open airway
      ↓
Not breathing normally?
      ↓
Call 999
      ↓
30 chest compressions
      ↓
2 rescue breaths
30 chest compressions
```

AED algorithm

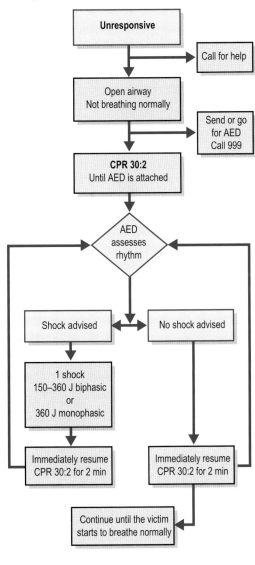

```
Unresponsive
      ↓ → Call for help
Open airway
Not breathing normally
      ↓ → Send or go for AED
            Call 999
CPR 30:2
Until AED is attached
      ↓
AED assesses rhythm
   ↙          ↘
Shock advised    No shock advised
   ↓
1 shock
150–360 J biphasic
or
360 J monophasic
   ↓
Immediately resume    Immediately resume
CPR 30:2 for 2 min    CPR 30:2 for 2 min

Continue until the victim
starts to breathe normally
```

Adult Choking Treatment algorithm

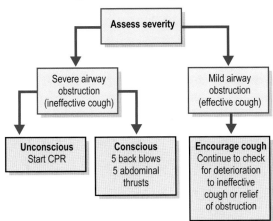

```
Assess severity
   ↙            ↘
Severe airway        Mild airway
obstruction          obstruction
(ineffective cough)  (effective cough)
   ↙        ↘              ↓
Unconscious  Conscious    Encourage cough
Start CPR    5 back blows  Continue to check
             5 abdominal   for deterioration
             thrusts       to ineffective
                           cough or relief
                           of obstruction
```

Paediatric Basic Life Support (Healthcare professionals with a duty to respond)

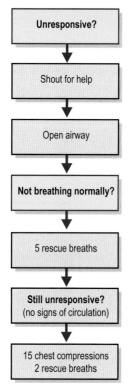

Unresponsive?

↓

Shout for help

↓

Open airway

↓

Not breathing normally?

↓

5 rescue breaths

↓

Still unresponsive?
(no signs of circulation)

↓

15 chest compressions
2 rescue breaths

After 1 minute
call resuscitation team
then continue CPR

Paediatric FBAO treatment

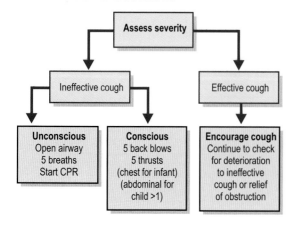

Assess severity

Ineffective cough | Effective cough

Unconscious
Open airway
5 breaths
Start CPR

Conscious
5 back blows
5 thrusts
(chest for infant)
(abdominal for
child >1)

Encourage cough
Continue to check
for deterioration
to ineffective
cough or relief
of obstruction

Newborn life support

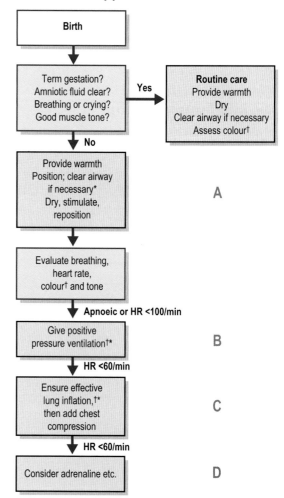

Birth

↓

Term gestation?
Amniotic fluid clear?
Breathing or crying?
Good muscle tone?

— Yes → **Routine care**
Provide warmth
Dry
Clear airway if necessary
Assess colour†

↓ No

Provide warmth
Position; clear airway
if necessary*
Dry, stimulate,
reposition

A

↓

Evaluate breathing,
heart rate,
colour† and tone

↓ Apnoeic or HR <100/min

Give positive
pressure ventilation†*

B

↓ HR <60/min

Ensure effective
lung inflation,†*
then add chest
compression

C

↓ HR <60/min

Consider adrenaline etc.

D

* Tracheal intubation may be considered at several steps
† Consider supplemental oxygen at any stage if cyanosis persists

2005 Resuscitation Guidelines available in full on the Resuscitation Council UK website www.resus.org.uk/

NB Readers should be aware that new Resuscitation Guidelines will be published in the Autumn of 2010.

Chronological development and eruption of the teeth

Primary dentition

Tooth	Commences to calcify (months before birth)	Eruption (months)	Crown calcification complete (months)	Root calcification complete (months)	Resorption commences (years)
A	3–4	5–7	4	18–24	4
B	4–5	7–8	5	18–24	5
C	5	16–20	9	30–36	7
D	5	12–16	6	24–30	6
E	7–9	20–30	12	36	6

Note: 1. A = central or first incisor; B = lateral or second incisor; C = canine; D = first molar; E = second molar.
Note: 2. The lower incisors tend to erupt shortly before the upper incisors.

Permanent dentition

Tooth	Commences to calcify	Eruption (years)	Crown calcification complete (years)	Root calcification complete (years)
1	3–4 months	6–7	4–5	10
2	10–12 months	7–8	4–5	11
3	4–5 months	10–12	6–7	12–13
4	1.5–2 years	9–11	5–6	12–13
5	2–2.5 years	10–11	6–7	12–14
6	Just before birth	5–7	3	10
7	3–4 years	12–13	8	15
8	8 years	When sufficient room. Usually between 18 and 24	12–16	18–25

Note: 1. 1 = central or first incisor; 2 = lateral or second incisor; 3 = canine; 4 = first premolar; 5 = second premolar; 6 = first molar; 7 = second molar; 8 = third molar or wisdom tooth.
Note: 2. The lower incisors and canine tend to erupt 1 year earlier than the upper incisors. They also complete their calcification 1 year earlier.

Appendix **12**

The Nursing & Midwifery Council NMC
The Code
Standards of conduct, performance and ethics for nurses and midwives (2008)

(Reproduced from the Nursing and Midwifery Council with permission)

The people in your care must be able to trust you with their health and wellbeing.

To justify that trust, you must:

- make the care of people your first concern, treating them as individuals and respecting their dignity
- work with others to protect and promote the health and wellbeing of those in your care, their families and carers, and the wider community
- provide a high standard of practice and care at all times
- be open and honest, act with integrity and uphold the reputation of your profession

As a professional, you are personally accountable for actions and omissions in your practice and must always be able to justify your decisions.

You must always act lawfully, whether those laws relate to your professional practice or personal life.

Failure to comply with this Code may bring your fitness to practise into question and endanger your registration.

This Code should be considered together with the Nursing and Midwifery Council's rules, standards, guidance and advice available from www.nmc-uk.org.

Make the care of people your first concern, treating them as individuals and respecting their dignity

Treat people as individuals

- You must treat people as individuals and respect their dignity
- You must not discriminate in any way against those in your care
- You must treat people kindly and considerately
- You must act as an advocate for those in your care, helping them to access relevant health and social care, information and support

Respect people's confidentiality

- You must respect people's right to confidentiality
- You must ensure people are informed about how and why information is shared by those who will be providing their care
- You must disclose information if you believe someone may be at risk of harm, in line with the law of the country in which you are practising

Collaborate with those in your care

- You must listen to the people in your care and respond to their concerns and preferences
- You must support people in caring for themselves to improve and maintain their health
- You must recognize and respect the contribution that people make to their own care and wellbeing
- You must make arrangements to meet people's language and communication needs
- You must share with people, in a way they can understand, the information they want or need to know about their health

Ensure you gain consent

- You must ensure that you gain consent before you begin any treatment or care
- You must respect and support people's rights to accept or decline treatment and care
- You must uphold people's rights to be fully involved in decisions about their care
- You must be aware of the legislation regarding mental capacity, ensuring that people who lack capacity remain at the centre of decision making and are fully safeguarded
- You must be able to demonstrate that you have acted in someone's best interests if you have provided care in an emergency

Maintain clear professional boundaries

- You must refuse any gifts, favours or hospitality that might be interpreted as an attempt to gain preferential treatment
- You must not ask for or accept loans from anyone in your care or anyone close to them
- You must establish and actively maintain clear sexual boundaries at all times with people in your care, their families and carers

Work with others to protect and promote the health and wellbeing of those in your care, their families and carers, and the wider community

Share information with your colleagues

- You must keep your colleagues informed when you are sharing the care of others

- You must work with colleagues to monitor the quality of your work and maintain the safety of those in your care
- You must facilitate students and others to develop their competence

Work effectively as part of a team

- You must work cooperatively within teams and respect the skills, expertise and contributions of your colleagues
- You must be willing to share your skills and experience for the benefit of your colleagues
- You must consult and take advice from colleagues when appropriate
- You must treat your colleagues fairly and without discrimination
- You must make a referral to another practitioner when it is in the best interests of someone in your care

Delegate effectively

- You must establish that anyone you delegate to is able to carry out your instructions
- You must confirm that the outcome of any delegated task meets required standards
- You must make sure that everyone you are responsible for is supervised and supported

Manage risk

- You must act without delay if you believe that you, a colleague or anyone else may be putting someone at risk
- You must inform someone in authority if you experience problems that prevent you working within this Code or other nationally agreed standards
- You must report your concerns in writing if problems in the environment of care are putting people at risk

Provide a high standard of practice and care at all times

Use the best available evidence

- You must deliver care based on the best available evidence or best practice
- You must ensure any advice you give is evidence based if you are suggesting healthcare products or services
- You must ensure that the use of complementary or alternative therapies is safe and in the best interests of those in your care

Keep your skills and knowledge up to date

- You must have the knowledge and skills for safe and effective practice when working without direct supervision
- You must recognize and work within the limits of your competence
- You must keep your knowledge and skills up to date throughout your working life
- You must take part in appropriate learning and practice activities that maintain and develop your competence and performance

Keep clear and accurate records

- You must keep clear and accurate records of the discussions you have, the assessments you make, the treatment and medicines you give and how effective these have been
- You must complete records as soon as possible after an event has occurred
- You must not tamper with original records in any way
- You must ensure any entries you make in someone's paper records are clearly and legibly signed, dated and timed
- You must ensure any entries you make in someone's electronic records are clearly attributable to you
- You must ensure all records are kept confidentially and securely

Be open and honest, act with integrity and uphold the reputation of your profession

Act with integrity

- You must demonstrate a personal and professional commitment to equality and diversity
- You must adhere to the laws of the country in which you are practising
- You must inform the NMC if you have been cautioned, charged or found guilty of a criminal offence
- You must inform any employers you work for if your fitness to practise is impaired or is called into question

Deal with problems

- You must give a constructive and honest response to anyone who complains about the care they have received
- You must not allow someone's complaint to prejudice the care you provide for them
- You must act immediately to put matters right if someone in your care has suffered harm for any reason
- You must explain fully and promptly to the person affected what has happened and the likely effects
- You must cooperate with internal and external investigations

Be impartial

- You must not abuse your privileged position for your own ends
- You must ensure that your professional judgment is not influenced by any commercial considerations

Uphold the reputation of your profession

- You must not use your professional status to promote causes that are not related to health
- You must cooperate with the media only when you can confidently protect the confidential information and dignity of those in your care
- You must uphold the reputation of your profession at all times

Information about indemnity insurance

- The NMC recommends that a registered nurse, midwife or specialist community public health nurse, in advising, treating and caring for patients/clients, has professional indemnity insurance. This is in the interests of clients, patients and registrants in the event of claims of professional negligence.

- Whilst employers have vicarious liability for the negligent acts and/or omissions of their employees, such cover does not normally extend to activities undertaken outside the registrant's employment. Independent practice would not be covered by vicarious liability. It is the individual registrant's responsibility to establish their insurance status and take appropriate action.
- In situations where an employer does not have vicarious liability, the NMC recommends that registrants obtain adequate professional indemnity insurance. If unable to secure professional indemnity insurance, a registrant will need to demonstrate that all their clients/patients are fully informed of this fact and the implications this might have in the event of a claim for professional negligence.

Contact

Nursing & Midwifery Council
23 Portland Place
London W1B 1PZ
020 7333 9333
advice@nmc-uk.org
www.nmc-uk.org

Healthcare professionals have a shared set of values, which find their expression in this Code for nurses and midwives. These values are also reflected in the different codes of each of the UK's healthcare regulators. This Code was approved by the NMC's Council on 6 December 2007 for implementation on 1 May 2008.

Appendix 13

Career development via your curriculum vitae (CV). Personal development and structured networking

Over the past decades, the pattern of work for everyone inside and outside the healthcare sector has changed. Structures have been flattened and management responsibility pushed further down the hierarchy. There are fewer posts that give an opportunity to 'try out' the job. Many 'support posts' and middle management posts have disappeared, with the result that the more senior you become, the fewer posts there are.

Parallel with this, both in the health sector and beyond, there has been real and explicit acknowledgement of the processes and value of lifelong learning. Put simply, the philosophy of lifelong learning accepts and encourages individuals to apply and see as relevant any experience they have had in their life, and shape that into a contribution to further learning. Lifelong learning accepts that skills and knowledge learnt in one context can be transferable to another.

The introduction of formal human resource practices, including equal opportunities legislation, into the NHS does mean that formal job application processes are well established. Gone are the days when a little chat with a senior manager would suffice. Professionals who are already employed in an organization, and who may even be 'acting' into post, still are required to submit formal applications for the post.

Thus, from day one of their working life, practioners need to be developing the skills and tools to 'sell' themselves in the market place, as the exciting concept of portfolio careers gains ground.

Apart from the obvious things, like being able to do the job, and holding the relevant licence to practise, there is a number of 'career skills' to collect in a personal development toolbox. Three of the key skills are; the ability to produce a focused and 'living' curriculum vitae (CV), proactive personal development planning via your Personal Development Plan (PDP) and structured networking. In support of this, many professionals are now keeping a current reflective portfolio that contains evidence of their various experiences. The evidence can be in the form of certificates (such as a Diploma), which state that the individual has achieved given academic outcomes, or evidence can demonstrate skills and knowledge, gained experientially. Both types of evidence have real value in your curriculum vitae to support an application for a new post.

Preparing a curriculum vitae

An up-to-date CV is an important tool for all those working in health care. It serves three purposes:

- It acts as a focal point to assist you to capture your skills, knowledge and achievements;

- It serves as a basis for your PDP and is therefore likely to inform your appraisal process at work;
- It acts as a marketing tool to 'sell' yourself when you are seeking new opportunities, whether that is a particular new job, or just testing the market.

The preparation of this important document follows a number of stages. Most people, however, find that one CV is not enough. That is not to say that a CV represents someone other than yourself—quite the reverse. Your CV gives you the opportunity to add emphasis to your experience and to show the transferability of your knowledge and skills in the workplace. Clearly, a number of circumstances unique to you will inform your CV and CV preparation. If you qualified last week, and went to university straight from school, you will have less material to include in your CV than someone who has been in the profession for many years. The important fact to remember is that the principles and processes involved in crafting a CV are the same. Your CV is not a fixed document; it grows and develops and evolves with your growth, development and evolution, and thus you should get into the habit of updating it regularly.

An effective CV puts the right emphasis upon your experience, and clearly, that emphasis is informed and shaped by the purpose for which the CV is prepared. As a means of illustrating this, it is assumed that individuals might want to have three current CVs. CV1 will be a baseline, a generic collection of information capturing their uniqueness as a professional and as a person.

Subsequent CVs will take the same material as in CV1 and address the emphasis to match the purpose. If an individual were applying for a clinical post, then the emphasis in CV2 would be on clinical experience. There could be two ways of dealing with this. If applying for a job requiring very specialized clinical expertise, for example, clinical nurse specialist in renal nursing, CV2 would need to highlight a detailed clinical focus. If, however, the role/job required a more general focus, then the skills and experience should be differently packaged. There would be less emphasis on the individual's clinical expertise in renal nursing, generalizing his/her clinical experience to a broader perspective, for example to enable him/her to manage a medical unit. The applicant would not be expected to be an expert in all specialities represented in the medical unit, but would draw on overall experience to manage the unit as a whole.

The person would need to make a judgement about the culture and values of the organization. An aggressively business-oriented organization may want to see a different emphasis in a CV than a charitable organization.

All CVs will include the individual's professional and educational qualifications, as well as professional and personal experiences. In the two hypothetical scenarios above (i.e. renal nursing and medical unit), it is more likely that clinical/management experience would be the crucial focus.

However, if the individual was applying for an academic post, in preparing CV3, more detail about the types and levels of academic courses would need to be included, along with details of publications, conference papers, etc. This is not to say that these are not of interest in CV1 and CV2, but it is a matter of emphasis. An emphasis on the number and range of academic courses when applying for a job in a business culture might cause the manager looking at the CV to worry that the individual is more interested in courses than doing the job. It is all a matter of organizational culture and core values.

Conversely, the organizational culture of an academic establishment values as currency the academic processes and achievement the applicant can offer, and these must be given in detail. A word of warning here though—the level of detail must be appropriate—from present times, backwards. A 2-hour in-house course completed 20 years ago is unlikely to have value today.

The one thing that all versions of the CV can have in common is the structure. One structure is offered here, but this is not the only one. Some readers may be surprised that it appears, at first glance, the wrong way round. Most people, on the front page of the CV, include all personal details, name, address, etc. Pause for a moment to think about this. In a job application, the purpose of the CV is to get you an interview (the interview then gets you the job!). When the person short listing for the post is reading the CV, they are looking for a vignette of the person and his/her ability, not their address, etc. Capitalize on this; use the first page for impact and include:

On page 1

- Name, qualifications and current post.
- Roles or experiences that are unique to you outside your post, e.g. advisor to another organization, chair of a professional group.
- Key personal skills, your strengths and attributes. Word these to match the organizational culture in which the job is based, e.g. effective communicator; understands the importance of working within resource; effective change agent; can work within a team, etc. Present these in a bullet pointed list to give impact and to 'catch the eye' of the reader.
- Two or three sentences that capture what you have to offer to the profession/organization. For example 'I can bring to the organization in-depth knowledge of 'x', enthusiasm and ability to get the job done through motivating my staff'.

On page 2

- *Current post . . . .(wef 1st June 2005)*

  Responsibilities and achievements
  Try to write these as outcome statements, rather than just describing a part of your role.
  For example:

  1. Initiated and coordinated a journal club within the unit. As a result the unit has a collection of review notes on relevant topics which act as a resource; or
  2. Led an outreach service to support renal patients in the community. As a result, the number of readmissions to the unit has decreased by 20% over a period of 6 months.

  Finish with...
  My current post gives me ... *one* or *two sentences*

- Previous post ... 1st July 2003–31st May 2005

  Responsibilities and achievements
  You can include a little less detail here. The detail will get less as you move backwards in time.
  Finish with...
  The focus of this post was ...

- Previous post ... 1st August 1999–30th June 2003

  Responsibilities and achievements
  Finish with a sentence highlighting the key issue of this experience.

If your career spans more than 10–15 years, it is usually only necessary to refer to the earliest experience in brief terms, e.g. January 1988–March 1994—various posts at staff nurse grade.

- Career breaks

A great deal of debate has been generated—should career breaks (usually in relation to women) be recorded in the CV? The feminist view may believe that there is no need to explain/apologize for a break. A more pragmatic view is to include a statement something like: 'during the period April 1994 to July 1999 I took a career break'. This ensures that the potential employer can track the person's experience and this is important in ensuring safety for patients and clients. Since recent years have shown examples of unscrupulous individuals gaining employment falsely, more organizations now are demanding a complete work history. Many organizations positively welcome those people with life experience, as this brings an added dimension and balance to the workplace, and fits into the ethos of lifelong learning.

On the final page

This should include the 'nut and bolts' about you. A layout is suggested below:

- Personal details
  - Name/date of birth
  - Address (home), tel/fax, e-mail
  - Business address (optional), tel/fax, e-mail
- Educational and professional qualifications (most recent first)

- Professional body membership
- Publications
- Current studies
- Personal interests and activities include ... *Usually two or three sentences are enough.*
- A person may also include their referees here, with their contact details, having first spoken to them about your intentions.

The first rule of CV writing is to have 'one you prepared earlier'. Often, when you decide to apply for a job, the turn around date for applications is quite tight. You need that time to gather information about the particular organization, so having a CV ready to adjust, rather than having to start from scratch, is a real bonus.

A CV should be prepared on good quality white or cream paper, using a basic, plain typeface and black ink. Resist the temptation to use graphics and colour. Unless they are in the world of the arts/media, this is considered inappropriate and it can cause problems in reproducing the CV. Many organizations now scan CVs to copy them, and colours and graphics do not survive this process well. Organizations are increasingly asking applicants to carry out their application online including the completion of the organization's CV template, or to submit their CVs electronically. However, it is worth remembering that some organizations require a hand written application form and some type of personal statement.

Proactive personal development planning

The value of preparing and maintaining a personal development plan (PDP) has never been more apparent than today. In the healthcare industry, as in others, the picture of career profile, career portfolio and career development has changed dramatically. It is a more complex process than many believe.

Within the spirit of lifelong learning every bit of your work and life experience can contribute to your future career. Activities undertaken during career breaks, or when working abroad or not working in health care, can offer something of value to your future. The structure of the 'portfolio' career has been formalized, and is now valued for its eclecticism, rather than being labelled fragmented and piecemeal.

However, the important thing is to take charge of your career—do not assume that someone else will do it for you. For example, if you see an opportunity at work, once you have done your homework about what it entails and how it might fit into the 'big picture' you have in mind for your own development, put yourself forward and suggest how you might tackle it. In this way, your own personal development is contributing to the well being of the organization and vice versa. Development is about doing things 'on the job', as well as formal study. PDPs should be congruent with the organizational development plan—in that way the optimum outcome emerges from the effort everyone puts into a project.

The timeframe for the PDP is important. Five years is now considered long term, normally 3 years is considered to be medium term and 1 year is a short-term view. This has arisen because of the rapid and continuous pace of change in the world of work. It is too easy to be shell-shocked by this and think that planning is futile because, by the time one has developed a plan, it is irrelevant because the world has changed. This gives a clue to how to prepare a PDP: keep it flexible and responsive. The portfolio of experience you, as a practitioner, are required to produce in order to remain on the live register is an excellent basis for their PDP. Preparing it provides the opportunity to reflect on what you have done, what you enjoyed and what you think you do well. Remember to capture your experiences, and what you have learnt from them, as well as any academic study you have done.

When looking ahead, try not to think in defined roles. For example, it is not helpful to think that in 3–5 years time 'I want to be a *xx*'. The way things are changing, it is unlikely that there will be a post called *xx*, and in any case, different organizations call the same post different things. Be open to opportunities that present themselves. One danger of planning too far ahead is that you overlook exciting things available now. The thing to do is to record the sort of things you would like to be doing in your role in 1, 3, and 5 years' time. For example, you may want to work in a team, or in an autonomous post. You may prefer a big hospital or a remote community. When you have collected this information, you may find it helpful to skim the job advertisements in a number of professional journals. Look at the description of the job rather than the title and match it to your 'wish list'. You may be surprised and begin to look at different roles in different contexts.

Another important activity when working on a PDP is to consider, objectively, your strengths and development needs. Brainstorming these on paper allows you to consider ways to capitalize on strengths and develop those skills and knowledge areas they have identified as priority. Be careful not to fall into the trap of thinking that you must do a course for everything. Some areas of development are best achieved, for example, by shadowing a colleague. For example, if you think you are weak on chairing meetings, ask a colleague whom you feel is good at chairing if you can sit in. Then watch the process of meeting management. Normally people concentrate on the content of the meeting. Making notes on what you felt worked well and why, and try it out for yourself.

A mentor can be a good resource to help you to consider different career opportunities. This is not the same sort of relationship you may have had with your allotted mentor/preceptor on a clinical placement. Clearly it is important that you feel comfortable with your mentor, so take time choosing the right person. The person does not have to be from the same professional background as yourself—in fact sometimes someone outside your professional group can provide a fresh perspective. You may only need to visit this person two or three times a year, so you may choose someone from another area of the country. You may meet your mentor as a result of networking.

Structured networking

Structured networking is an excellent and cost-effective way of developing your career and tapping into a plethora of resources relevant to your area of practice. Most people find that they are networking automatically, but you may find it helpful to consider one or two basic activities as a way to develop your networking skills further. Always keep a note of telephone numbers/e-mail and addresses of people you meet. This may be from conferences, visitors to your place of work, or people with a high professional profile you feel could contribute to your development. Providing you have a focused objective, you will find that the majority of professionals are happy to give time to others and many more senior/experienced people see this as an overt responsibility. If you wish to contact someone who you do not know personally, either write to him/her or telephone his/her personal assistant, explaining who you are and how you feel the person can help you. You must be very focused and succinct. Ask for a 30-minute appointment. Be on time, have your questions ready, ensuring you lead the meeting, and conclude the interview within the allotted time. Be sure to follow up the meeting with a thank-you letter.

Keep contact details of those who have published an interesting journal article. If you feel you would like to ask a question, write to them. Professional groups, such as the relevant specialist forum or group offer a good way of networking with people who have similar professional interests.

The key points to remember are: be proactive, be focused, be reliable and be prepared to give your time to others when approached.

(Adapted from an appendix written by Julie Hyde for Churchill Livingstone Dictionary of Nursing 18th edn. 2002)

Appendix 14

Research, evidence-based practice and web sources

This appendix briefly discusses how research is undertaken; however, dissemination is vital if research is not to simply gather dust in libraries. A short discussion follows of the barriers and bridges to implementing research.

The use of libraries to obtain research-based information is discussed. The need for clinical practice to use research as its base, with reference to literature reviews is outlined. Finally a list of web resources is offered that covers the areas in greater detail.

Research

Research has many definitions, for example: 'a scientific process of inquiry and/or experimentation that involves purposeful, systematic, and rigorous collection of data' (Dempsey and Dempsey 1996).

There are several research paradigms, and the methodology employed will depend on the nature of the enquiry. Broadly there are two types of research: quantitative and qualitative.

Implementation of research

There is an acknowledged theory-practice gap in nursing (and other disciplines). Key aspects (Tierney 1997) are:

- Research education
- Research activity
- Dissemination
- National professional organizations' support
- Funding.

These are inter-related. For if practitioners are to value research they need to understand the process through education. Knowledge of research methods allows the practitioner to understand papers, and thus dissemination will be more effective. Some practitioners will undertake research, requiring institutional support and funding. National professional organizations can take a lead in providing support for research.

Barriers to research implementation are the perception of research as remote, and absence of supporting infrastructure (Wuest 1995). Highest rated barriers in a further study have been understanding of research and acquisition of research skills, lowest rated was a need for research as basis for nursing practice (Lynn and Moore 1997). In nurse education, with a history of teaching rather than research, teachers worry about neglect of teaching excellence (Lorentzon et al 1998).

Funding is an issue, and previously some groups (e.g. nurses) have not been as successful in gaining research funds as other professional groups, in particular medical staff. In one study there were limited regional applications from nurses

for research and development (R&D), and proposals were withdrawn voluntarily, typically after insensitively worded referees' comments, although vigorously pursued nursing proposals rated higher than medical-led proposals (Mead et al 1997). It may be thought that nurses and other health professionals should adopt the strategies employed by doctors, performing quantitative studies (typically randomized controlled trials—RCTs), working in partnership with doctors, and working with other organizations. All these may be useful; however, none should be adopted without good reason.

Projects in one study were more likely to succeed if the method was qualitative and the lead researcher was a nurse (Brooker et al, 1997), and no more likely to succeed if a medical collaborator, a statistician or a health economist was involved, or if there were more than three collaborators, or if they came from more than one university (Brooker et al 1997).

Bridges from the literature have included:

- staff recruitment and retention, funding, contracts, support and publication (Cleverly 1998)
- funding councils, the National Health Service (NHS) (e.g. Department of Health, Training Consortia), professional bodies, medical charities (e.g. Help the Aged), industry and nursing charities (e.g. Foundation of Nursing Studies)
- non-funding bridges have included creating agenda of agreed problems (e.g. inter-professionalism, community health), issues of communication and dissemination and methodological mix (Watson 1998)
- dissemination/communication bridges include practice development practitioners, clinical nurse specialists, link nurses, tutorial series, study days, journals, clinical guidelines, research networks (e.g. Royal College of Nursing), clinical networks (e.g. Wound Care Society) and local groups (Brooks and Anthony 2000).

Local initiatives have been shown to be effective. Bridges implemented in one trust include a research development facilitator, a centre for nursing research and partnership between trust and university (Martin et al, 1998). For example, in Sydney, Australia, a reward system for research productivity (funding designated research groups/faculty support units), the creation of a nursing clinical development unit, and a leadership programme (new clinical chairs) and nursing research seminars were considered successful initiatives in research implementation (Greenwood and Gray 1998).

Research can be effective in stimulating clinical staff, e.g. research is greater in Nursing Development Units than comparators, and networking higher, though the number of audits was the same (Redfern and Murrells 1998). Networking facilitates research, promotes quality, quantity and usefulness of research, and places research into patient care (Leighton-Beck 1997).

Strategies to implement and encourage research include communication with top management, provision of development opportunities, technical research support, building on completed research and use of multidisciplinary teams (Gaynor and Verdin 1973).

Thus nurses and other practitioners can do quality research, and this research does not have to be quantitative. For research to be successful support, education and professional development are needed. Clinical Nurse Specialists have a special role to play as they are opinion leaders, and nurse consultants have a similar or stronger role. Dissemination and networking is helpful, and both traditional and electronic modes should be considered, for example e-mail lists and newsgroups as well as newsletters and conferences.

Having shown that research is needed, and a range of practitioners are capable of conducting or using research, we shall discuss some types of research.

Quantitative research methods

Quantitative research deals with data that may be counted or measured in numerical format. This may be further split into:

- Descriptive studies—where the data are recorded in tables, graphs or measures of central tendency (mean, mode, median) and spread of data (variance, range for example).
- Inferential studies—where hypotheses are proposed, and these are tested with statistical tests. An example would be: there is no significant difference in serum albumin between two groups, those with a pressure ulcer and those with none.

Typical quantitative research designs include:

- Surveys using either interviews or questionnaires to obtain data that can be expressed in numerical terms, e.g. numbers of nurses with a higher degree, age of students enrolling on nursing courses.
- Quasi-experimental studies, for example comparing the pressure ulcer incidence in two hospitals with different treatment regimens.
- Parallel double-blind randomized studies, for example comparing two barrier creams randomly allocated to patients, where neither researcher nor patient knows which cream is allocated to each patient.
- Double blind RCTs, the 'gold standard' where a placebo is compared with an active treatment, where neither researcher nor patient knows whether the patient has received a treatment or placebo (control).

Qualitative research methods

In qualitative studies, the data are richer, often not capable of being expressed in numerical form, and typically using small numbers of subjects, from whom large quantities of data are obtained. Typical qualitative studies might include:

- Historical studies, where primary and secondary sources are examined and analysed to uncover patterns, trends, political and economic outcomes, etc., 'Studying the past facilitates understanding of the present and future.' (Hewitt 1997)
- Focus groups, where a group of subjects are interviewed together.
- Phenomenological studies, which attempt to capture the lived experience of the subjects.
- Interviews and surveys using open-ended questions that do not lend themselves to numerical coding.
- Narrative biography.
- Case studies.

Evidence-based practice

Research should be the basis behind clinical practice: this is evidence-based practice. Practice should be evidence-based as far as is possible. Increasingly clinical guidelines employ a specific defined research base. The Scottish Intercollegiate Guidelines Network (SIGN), Cochrane and NHS Centre for Reviews and Dissemination (York) all use some variant of a numerical classification system that gives most weight to studies with strong evidence. In this scheme a meta-analysis of many RCTs is the best form of evidence, and expert opinion at the other extreme.

Where do you find the research articles on which to base your practice? Typically libraries are the best source, but these may not be local, and can be difficult to access.

Libraries can be accessed via universities and hospitals. However, increasingly these are accessed via the Internet. Many universities use the OPAC system making titles and booking available on the Internet. COPAC (www.copac.ac.uk) is a system where several university libraries are combined, so you may identify the nearest (for example) library that has a book you need.

Bibliographic databases are available at libraries, typically on CD-ROM. However, many of these are available on the Internet, some for free. For example Medline is available via the US National Library of Medicine (among others) for no charge.

Research is cumulative; any study is likely to be a step in a series of work, and itself to add to that body of knowledge. Thus any research report will probably need to refer to earlier work using a review of relevant literature. Ideally a review should be systematic, that is performed according to a specific set of criteria. These include a search strategy, inclusion and exclusion criteria for studies, and methods of evaluation of studies. A systematic review can form the basis for a clinical guideline.

In practice, due to resource constraints, reviews are often narrative rather than systematic. However, some components of a systematic method increase rigour at low cost, for example specification of the search strategy employed.

The use of a systematic approach aids in maintaining validity by ensuring as far as possible that relevant articles are located, and the use of assessment criteria further help by ranking the quality of material.

Summary

Research is needed, but that there is a gap between theory and practice. To ensure practice is research based (evidence-based) appropriate access to library material, often via the Internet, is vital. Dissemination of research does not occur simply by publication, and strategies should be employed by clinical leaders, such as education, use of link nurses and other practitioners, etc.

There is a huge variety of research methods, but these fall mainly into two groups, qualitative and quantitative. The best research is valid research, and the most valid approach (qualitative or quantitative) will depend on the context of the study. All research should build on prior work, and this needs to be referenced in a clear and consistent fashion. Web resources are an excellent way of accessing all types of research, bibliographic databases, and centres with advice on carrying on research, though they should be quality assessed in a similar way as any printed material.

References

Brooker C, Read S, Morrell CJ, Repper J, Jones R, Akehurst R 1997 Coming in from the cold? An analysis of research proposals submitted by the Nursing Section at ScHARR, 1994–1997. Nt Res 423; 2 (6):405–413.

Brooks N, Anthony D 2000 Clinical guidelines in community hospitals. Nurs Stand; 15 (1):35–39.

Cleverly D 1998 Nursing research—taking an active interest. Nurse Educ Today; 18 (4):267–272.

Dempsey P, Dempsey D 1996 Nursing research: text and workbook, 4th edn. Little, Brown and Company: Boston.

Gaynor S, Verdin JA 1973 Conducting unit-based research to improve quality of care. J Nurs Care Qual; 12 (2):63–71.

Greenwood J, Gray G 1998 Developing a nursing research culture in the university and health sectors in Western Sydney, Australia. Nurse Educ Today; 18 (8):642–648.

Hewitt LC 1997 Historical research in nursing: standards for research and evaluation. J NY State Nurses Assoc; 28 (3):16–19.

Leighton-Beck L 1997 Research networking. Networking: putting research at the heart of professional practice. Br J Nurs; 6 (2):120–122.

Lorentzon M, Gass L, Wimpenny P, Gibb S 1998 Protectionism or competition in managing British nursing research? Current debate among nurse and midwifery teachers. J Nurs Manage; 6 (1):29–35.

Lynn MR, Moore K 1997 Research utilization by nurse managers: current practices and future directions. Semin Nurse Managers; 5 (4):217–223.

Martin CR, Bowman GS, Knight S, Thompson DR 1998 Progress with a strategy for developing research in practice. Including commentary by Bartlett H. Nt Res; 3 (1):28–35.

Mead D, Moseley L, Cook R 1997 The performance of nursing in the research stakes: lessons from the field. Nt Res; 2 (5):335–344.

Redfern S, Murrells T 1998 Occasional paper. Research, audit and networking: who's in the lead. Nurs Times; 94 (28):57–60.

Tierney AJ 1997 Organization report. The development of nursing research in Europe. Eur Nurse; 2 (2):73–84.

Watson D 1998 Developing the capacity of nursing and midwifery research: the view from higher education. Nt Res; 3 (2):93–99.

Wuest J 1995 Breaking the barriers to nursing research. Can Nurse; 91 (4):29–33.

Web resources

Agency for Healthcare Research and Quality (US) http://www.ahrq.gov

Centers for Disease Control and Prevention CDC (US) http://www.cdc.gov/

DH Department of Health Research and Development (UK) http://www.dh.gov.uk/en/Researchanddevelopment/index.htm

Medicine http://www.intute.ac.uk/healthandlifesciences/medicine/

National Guideline Clearing House (US) http://www.guideline.gov

National Institute for Health and Clinical Excellence (UK) http://www.nice.org.uk

National Library for Health (UK) http://www.library.nhs.uk/

NHS Centre for Reviews and Dissemination http://www.york.ac.uk/inst/crd/

Nursing, Midwifery and Allied Health http://www.intute.ac.uk/healthandlifesciences/nursing/

Qualitative Research Resources on the Internet http://www.nova.edu/ssss/QR/qualres.html

QualPage: Resources for qualitative research for nurses (papers, conferences, links to other sites, electronic journals, etc.) http://www.qualitativeresearch.uga.edu/QualPage/

Scottish Intercollegiate Guidelines Network (UK) http://www.sign.ac.uk

Social science http://www.intute.ac.uk/socialsciences/

Statistics glossary http://www.stats.gla.ac.uk/steps/glossary/

UK Clinical Research Network (UKCRN) http://www.ukcrn.org.uk/index.html

US National Library of Medicine http://www.nlm.nih.gov/

(Adapted from an appendix written by Dennis Anthony for Churchill Livingstone Dictionary of Nursing 18th edn. 2002)

14

Appendix